Barts and The London
Queen Mary's School of Medicine and Dentistry
WHITECHAPEL LIBRARY, TURNER STREET, LONDON E1
020 7882 7110

WEEK LOAN

the last date belo:

D1423574

ESSENTIALS
OF PSYCHIATRY

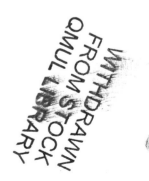

ESSENTIALS OF PSYCHIATRY

Jerald Kay
Professor and Chair
Department of Psychiatry
Wright State University School of Medicine
Dayton, Ohio
USA

Allan Tasman
Professor and Chair
Department of Psychiatry and Behavioral Sciences
University of Louisville School of Medicine
Louisville, Kentucky
USA

John Wiley & Sons, Ltd

Copyright © 2006   John Wiley & Sons Ltd, The Atrium, Southern Gate, Chichester,
West Sussex PO19 8SQ, England
Telephone   (+44) 1243 779777

Email (for orders and customer service enquiries): cs-books@wiley.co.uk
Visit our Home Page on www.wileyeurope.com or www.wiley.com

Other Wiley Editorial Offices

John Wiley & Sons Inc., 111 River Street, Hoboken, NJ 07030, USA

Jossey-Bass, 989 Market Street, San Francisco, CA 94103-1741, USA

Wiley-VCH Verlag GmbH, Boschstr. 12, D-69469 Weinheim, Germany

John Wiley & Sons Australia Ltd, 42 McDougall Street, Milton, Queensland 4064, Australia

John Wiley & Sons (Asia) Pte Ltd, 2 Clementi Loop #02-01, Jin Xing Distripark, Singapore 129809

John Wiley & Sons Canada Ltd, 6045 Freemont Blvd, Mississauga, ONT, L5R 4J3

Wiley also publishes its books in a variety of electronic formats. Some content that appears in print may not be available in electronic books.

Library of Congress Cataloging-in-Publication Data

Kay, Jerald.
Essentials of psychiatry / Jerald Kay, Allan Tasman.
      p. ; cm.
    Includes bibliographical references.
    ISBN-13: 978-0-470-01854-5 (alk. paper)
    ISBN-10: 0-470-01854-2 (alk. paper)
    1. Psychiatry.   I. Tasman, Allan, 1947-. II. Psychiatry. III. Title.
    [DNLM: 1. Psychiatry–methods.   2. Mental Disorders.
    3. Psychotherapy–methods.   WM 100 K225e 2006]

    RC454.K395 2006
    616.89–dc22   2006001884

British Library Cataloguing in Publication Data

A catalogue record for this book is available from the British Library

ISBN-10 0 470 01854 2
ISBN-13 978-0-470-01854-5

Typeset in 9/11pt Times New Roman by Thomson Digital.
Printed and bound in Grafos S.A., Barcelona, Spain.
This book is printed on acid-free paper responsibly manufactured from sustainable forestry in which at least two trees are planted for each one used for paper production.

Dedication

With love and thanks to my family, and especially my father Goodman Tasman, for your inspiration and support.

Allan

To Rena, Jonathan, Rachel, and Sarah with appreciation for all that you have given me.

Jerry

Table of Contents

Preface

Essentials of Psychiatry is a synopsis of the 2400 page *Psychiatry Second Edition* also published by John Wiley and Sons. *Psychiatry* has received exceptional reviews in the leading medical and psychiatric journals within the United States and abroad. *Essentials of Psychiatry* provides a broad overview to clinical psychiatry for beginning psychiatry residents, nonpsychiatric physicians, medical students, and people working in related mental health disciplines such as psychology, social work, psychiatric nursing and counseling. We hope that family members of patients may find this abbreviated text accessible and helpful as well. *Essentials of Psychiatry* differs from the comprehensive two-volume text in that it does not include such an extensive discussion of the neural and social sciences that underlie the practice of psychiatry.

The 112 chapters by more than 270 authors of the *Psychiatry Second Edition* have been condensed by approximately 50% for this new book. All chapters have been updated to include the latest advances in psychopharmacology, psychopathology and psychosocial treatment. Clinical vignettes, as well as DSM-IV™

and ICD 10 related material, have been retained from the original book to preserve an international scope. As indicated in the initial chapters of the *Essentials*, we have also maintained the focus on the centrality of the doctor–patient relationship.

The challenge of condensing a text as large as *Psychiatry Second Edition* was daunting. We are indebted to all of our colleagues who wrote for the original work. We pay homage to these authors at the start of this book. Since the two of us reviewed all 112 chapters, we accept responsibility for any omissions. We are also indebted to those who provided strong support for this effort. At Wiley, this included our editor Deborah Russell and her associate Andrea Baier. In Dr Kay's and Dr Tasman's offices, Edward Depp and Joan Lucas, respectively, were invaluable to the completion of this project.

JERALD KAY, MD

ALLAN TASMAN, MD

Acknowledgements

We would like gratefully to acknowledge the authors of those chapters in *Psychiatry Second Edition* from which material in this book was adapted.

Paul C. Mohl	Listening to the Patient
Laurence J. Kirmayer	The Cultural Context of Clinical Assessment
Cécile Rousseau	The Cultural Context of Clinical Assessment
G. Eric Jarvis	The Cultural Context of Clinical Assessment
Jaswant Guzder	The Cultural Context of Clinical Assessment
Edward K. Silberman	The Psychiatric Interview: Settings and Techniques
Kenneth Certa	The Psychiatric Interview: Settings and Techniques
Stephen M. Sonnenberg	Physician–Patient Relationship
Amy M. Ursano	Physician–Patient Relationship
Robert M. Ursano	Physician–Patient Relationship
Richard S. Epstein	Professional Ethics and Boundaries
Ahmed Okasha	Professional Ethics and Boundaries
Ken Duckworth	Law, Ethics and Psychiatry
Lester Blumberg	Law, Ethics and Psychiatry
David Bienenfeld	Law, Ethics and Psychiatry
Michael Kahn	Law, Ethics and Psychiatry
Marshall Kapp	Law, Ethics and Psychiatry
David A. Mrazek	A Psychiatric Perspective on Human Development
Andrew E. Skodol	Psychopathology Across the Life Cycle
David Shaffer	Psychopathology Across the Life Cycle
Barry Gurland	Psychopathology Across the Life Cycle
Philip S. Wang	Psychiatric Epidemiology
Mauricio Tohen	Psychiatric Epidemiology
Evelyn Bromet	Psychiatric Epidemiology
Jules Angst	Psychiatric Epidemiology
Carol A. Tamminga	Psychiatric Pathophysiology: Schizophrenia
Arvid Carlsson	Psychiatric Pathophysiology: Schizophrenia
Leo Sher	Psychiatric Pathophysiology: Mood Disorders
J. John Mann	Psychiatric Pathophysiology: Mood Disorders
Phil Skolnick	Psychiatric Pathophysiology :Anxiety Disorders
Peter W. Kalivas	Psychiatric Pathophysiology : Addiction
Krista McFarland	Psychiatric Pathophysiology : Addiction
Ronald E. See	Psychiatric Pathophysiology : Addiction
Vahram Haroutunian	Psychiatric Pathophysiology : Dementia
Kenneth L. Davis	Psychiatric Pathophysiology : Dementia
Robert S. Goldman	Cognitive Neuroscience and Neuropsychology
Karen M. Emberger	Cognitive Neuroscience and Neuropsychology
Irma C. Smet	Cognitive Neuroscience and Neuropsychology
Malini Singh	Cognitive Neuroscience and Neuropsychology
Richard S. E. Keefe	Cognitive Neuroscience and Neuropsychology
W. Edward Craighead	Cognitive Psychology: Basic Theory and Clinical Implications
Stephen S. llardi	Cognitive Psychology: Basic Theory and Clinical Implications
Akira Miyake	Cognitive Psychology: Basic Theory and Clinical Implications
Linda W. Craighead	Cognitive Psychology: Basic Theory and Clinical Implications

Michael D. Greenberg	Cognitive Psychology: Basic Theory and Clinical Implications
Genevieve Garratt	Cognitive Psychology: Basic Theory and Clinical Implications
Eugene W. Farber	Social Psychology: Theory, Research, and Mental Health Implications
Nadine J. Kaslow	Social Psychology: Theory, Research, and Mental Health Implications
Andrew C. Furman	Psychoanalytic Theories
Steven T. Levy	Psychoanalytic Theories
Mark E. James	Psychoanalytic Theories
Arnold D. Richards	Psychoanalytic Theories
Lawrence B. Inderbitzen	Psychoanalytic Theories
Beth Seelig	Psychoanalytic Theories
Sybil A. Ginsburg	Psychoanalytic Theories
Henry F. Smith	Psychoanalytic Theories
Robert M. Galatzer-Levy	Psychoanalytic Theories
Ralph E. Roughton	Psychoanalytic Theories
Jonathan E. Dunn	Psychoanalytic Theories
Francine Cournos	Clinical Evaluation and Treatment Planning: A Multimodal Approach
Deborah L. Cabaniss	Clinical Evaluation and Treatment Planning: A Multimodal Approach
Susan C. Vaughan	Behavior and Adaptive Functioning
John M. Oldham	Behavior and Adaptive Functioning
Joan E. Mezzich	The Cultural Framework of Psychiatric Disorders
Roberto Lewis-Fenández	The Cultural Framework of Psychiatric Disorders
Maria Angeles Ruiperez	The Cultural Framework of Psychiatric Disorders
Michael B. First	Psychiatric Classification
Stanley I. Greenspan	Diagnostic Classification in Infancy and Early Childhood
Serena Wieder	Diagnostic Classification in Infancy and Early Childhood
Ludwik S. Szymanski	Childhood Disorders: Mental Retardation
Maija Wilska	Childhood Disorders: Mental Retardation
Larry B. Silver	Childhood Disorders: Learning and Motor Skills Disorders
William M. Klykylo	Childhood Disorders: Communication Disorders
Thomas Owley	Childhood Disorders: The Autism Spectrum Disorders
Bennett L. Leventhal	Childhood Disorders: The Autism Spectrum Disorders
Edwin H. Cook	Childhood Disorders: The Autism Spectrum Disorders
Vanshdeep Sharma	Childhood Disorders: Attention-Deficit and Disruptive Behavior Disorders
Jeffrey H. Newcorn	Childhood Disorders: Attention-Deficit and Disruptive Behavior Disorders
Kurt P. Schulz	Childhood Disorders: Attention-Deficit and Disruptive Behavior Disorders
Jeffey M. Halperin	Childhood Disorders: Attention-Deficit and Disruptive Behavior Disorders
Irene Chatoor	Childhood Disorders: Feeding and Other Disorders of Infancy and Early Childhook
John T. Wlakup	Childhood Disorders: Tic Disorders
Mark A. Riddle	Childhood Disorders: Tic Disorders
Christopher P. Lucas	Childhood Disorders: Elimination Disorders and Childhood Anxiety Disorders
David Shaffer	Childhood Disorders: Elimination Disorders and Childhood Anxiety Disorders
Robert L. Frierson	Delirium and Dementia
David P. Moore	Mental Disorders Due to a General Medical Condition
Thomas R. Kosten	General Approaches to Substance and Polydrug Use Disorders
Thomas F. Barbor	Substance Abuse: Alcohol Use Disorders
Henry R. Kranzler	Substance Abuse: Alcohol Use Disorders
Carlos A. Hernandez-Avila	Substance Abuse: Alcohol Use Disorders
Jane A. Ungemack	Substance Abuse: Alcohol Use Disorders
Eric C. Strain	Substance Abuse: Caffeine Use Disorders
Roland R. Griffiths	Substance Abuse: Caffeine Use Disorders
Amada J. Gruber	Substance Abuse: Cannabis-Related Disorders
Harrison G. Pope, Jr.	Substance Abuse: Cannabis-Related Disorders
Charles Y. Jin	Substance Abuse: Cocaine Use Disorders
Elinore F. McCance-Katz	Substance Abuse: Cocaine Use Disorders
Stephen R. Zukin	Substance Abuse: Phencyclidine Use Disorders
Joyce H. Lowinson	Substance Abuse: Phencyclidine Use Disorders
Ilana Zylberman	Substance Abuse: Phencyclidine Use Disorders
Rif S. El-Mallakh	Substance Abuse: Hallucinogen- and MDMA-Related Disorder
John Halpern	Substance Abuse: Hallucinogen- and MDMA-Related Disorder
Henry David Abraham	Substance Abuse:Hallucinogen- and MDMA-Related Disorders
Charles W. Sharp	Substance Abuse: Inhalant-Related Disorders
Neil Rosenberg	Substance Abuse: Inhalant-Related Disorders

George E. Woody	Substance Abuse: Opioid Use Disorders
Laura F. McNicholas	Substance Abuse: Opioid Use Disorders
Paul J. Fudala	Substance Abuse: Opioid Use Disorders
Douglas Ziedonis	Substance Abuse: Nicotine Dependence
Susan J. Fiester	Substance Abuse: Nicotine Dependence
Donald R. Wesson	Substance Abuse: Sedative, Hypnotic, or Anxiolytic Use Disorders
Walter Ling	Substance Abuse: Sedative, Hypnotic, or Anxiolytic Use Disorders
David E. Smith	Substance Abuse: Sedative, Hypnotic, or Anxiolytic Use Disorders
Jayendra K. Patel	Schizophrenia and Other Psychoses
Debra A. Pinals	Schizophrenia and Other Psychoses
Alan Breier	Schizophrenia and Other Psychoses
Alan M. Gruenber	Mood Disorders: Depression
Reed D. Golstein	Mood Disorders: Depression
Mark S. Bauer	Mood Disorders: Bipolar (Manic–Depressive) Disorders
Teri Pearlstein	Mood Disorders: Premenstrual Dysphoric Disorders
Goron J.G. Asmundson	Anxiety Disorders: Panic Disorder With and Without Agoraphobia
Steven Taylor	Anxiety Disorders: Panic Disorder With and Without Agoraphobia
Marin M. Antony	Anxiety Disorders: Social and Specific Phobias
Randi E. McCabe	Anxiety Disorders: Social and Specific Phobias
Michele T. Pato	Obsessive–Compulsive Disorder
Jane L. Eisen	Obsessive–Compulsive Disorder
Katharine A. Phillips	Obsessive–Compulsive Disorder
Jean C. Beckham	Anxiety Disorders: Traumatic Stress Disorders
Jonathan R.T. Davidson	Anxiety Disorders: Traumatic Stress Disorders
John S. March	Anxiety Disorders: Traumatic Stress Disorders
Jeannine Monnier	Anxiety Disorders: Generalized Anxiety Disorder
R. Bruce Lydiard	Anxiety Disorders: Generalized Anxiety Disorder
Olga Brawman-Mintzer	Anxiety Disorders: Generalized Anxiety Disorder
Sean H. Yutzy	Somatoform Disorders
Anne Fleming	Factitious Disorders
Stuart Eisendrath	Factitious Disorders
David Spiegel	Dissociative Disorders
José R. Maldonado	Dissociative Disorders
Stephen B. Levine	Sexual Disorders
B. Timothy Walsh	Eating Disorders
J. Christian Gillin	Sleep and Sleep–Wake Disorders
Sonia Ancoli-Israel	Sleep and Sleep–Wake Disorders
Milton Erman	Sleep and Sleep–Wake Disorders
Ronald M. Winchel	Impulse Control Disorders
Daphne Simeon	Impulse Control Disorders
Yoram Yovell	Impulse Control Disorders
James J. Strain	Adjustment Disorders
Jeffrey H. Newcorn	Adjustment Disorders
Thomas A. Widiger	Personality Disorders
Stephanie Mullins	Personality Disorders
James L. Levenson	Psychological Factors Affecting Medical Condition
Dilip V. Jeste	Medication-Induced Movement Disorders
Christian R. Dolder	Medication-Induced Movement Disorders
Martha C. Tompson	Relational Problems
David J. Miklowitz	Relational Problems
John F. Clarkiin	Relational Problems
Rena L. Kay	Individual Psychoanalytic Psychotherapy
Walter N. Stone	Group Psychotherapy
Holly A. Swartz	Time-Limited Psychotherapy
John C. Markowitz	Time-Limited Psychotherapy
Edward S. Friedman	Cognitive and Behavioral Therapies
Michael E. Thase	Cognitive and Behavioral Therapies
Jesse H. Wright	Cognitive and Behavioral Therapies
James L. Griffiths	Family Therapy
Lois Slovik	Family Therapy
Eva Ritvo	Couples Therapy
Ira D. Glick	Couples Therapy

José R. Maldonado	Hypnosis
David Spiegel	Hypnosis
Alan S. Bellack	Psychosocial Rehabilitation
Matthew V. Rudorfer	Electroconvulsive Therapy
Michael E. Henry	Electroconvulsive Therapy
Harold A. Sackeim	Electroconvulsive Therapy
Brian Martis	Neurosurgery for Treatment-Refractory Psychiatric Disorders: Obsessive–Compulsive Disorder and Major Depressive Disorder
Rees Cosgrove	Neurosurgery for Treatment-Refractory Psychiatric Disorders: Obsessive–Compulsive Disorder and Major Depressive Disorder
Michael Jenike	Neurosurgery for Treatment-Refractory Psychiatric Disorders: Obsessive–Compulsive Disorder and Major Depressive Disorder
Keh-Ming Lin	Psychopharmacology: Ethnic and Cultural Perspectives
Michael W. Smith	Psychopharmacology: Ethnic and Cultural Perspectives
Margaret T. Lin	Psychopharmacology: Ethnic and Cultural Perspectives
Anri Aoba	Antipsychotic Drugs
W. Wolfgang Fleischhacker	Antipsychotic Drugs
Stephen R. Marder	Antipsychotic Drugs
Seiya Miyamoto	Antipsychotic Drugs
Jeffrey L. Lieberman	Antipsychotic Drugs
Marlene P. Freeman	Mood Stabilizers
Alan J. Gelenberg	Mood Stabilizers
John Misiaszek	Mood Stabilizers
Scott E. Moseman	Mood Stabilizers
Robert J. Boland	Antidepressants
Martin B. Keller	Antidepressants
Rachel E. Maddux	Anxiolytic Drugs
Mark H. Rapaport	Anxiolytic Drugs
Richard I. Shader	Sedative-Hypnotic Agents
Douglas A. Songer	Sedative-Hypnotic Agents
Laurence L. Greenhill	Stimulants
Jeffrey Halperin	Stimulants
John March	Stimulants
Erin Shockey	Stimulants
Lon S. Schneider	Cognitive Enhancers and Treatments for Alzeimer's Disease
Pierre N. Tariot	Cognitive Enhancers and Treatments for Alzeimer's Disease
Karon Dawkins	Therapeutic Management of the Suicidal Patient
Robert N. Golden	Therapeutic Management of the Suicidal Patient
Jan A. Fawcett	Therapeutic Management of the Suicidal Patient
Lesile Citrome	Treatment of Violent Behavior
Jan Volavka	Treatment of Violent Behavior
Richard P. Brown	Complementary and Alternative Treatments in Psychiatry
Patricia L. Gerbarg	Complementary and Alternative Treatments in Psychiatry
Philip R. Muskin	Complementary and Alternative Treatments in Psychiatry
Michelle B. Riba	Combined Therapies: Psychotherapy and Pharmacotherapy
Robyn R. Miller	Combined Therapies: Psychotherapy and Pharmacotherapy
Mehul V. Mankad	Medication Compliance
Marvin S. Swartz	Medication Compliance

Approaches to
the Patient

Listening to the Patient

Listening: The Key Skill in Psychiatry

It was Freud who raised the psychiatric technique of examination – listening – to a level of expertise unexplored in earlier eras. As Binswanger (1963) has said of the period prior to Freudian influence: psychiatric "auscultation" and "percussion" of the patient was performed as if through the patient's shirt with so much of his essence remaining covered or muffled that layers of meaning remained unpeeled away or unexamined.

This metaphor and parallel to the cardiac examination is one worth considering as we first ask if listening will remain as central a part of psychiatric examination as in the past. The explosion of biomedical knowledge has radically altered our evolving view and practice of the doctor–patient relationship. Physicians of an earlier generation were taught that the diagnosis is made at the bedside – that is, the history and physical examination are paramount. Laboratory and imaging (radiological, in those days) examinations were seen as confirmatory exercises. However, as our technologies have blossomed, the bedside and/or consultation room examinations have evolved into the method whereby the physician determines what tests to run, and the tests are often viewed as making the diagnosis. A cardiologist colleague expresses the opinion that, given the growing availability of non-invasive tests – echocardiograms, for example – he is not sure this is a bad thing (Hillis, 2001, personal communication).

So can one imagine a time in the not-too-distant future when the psychiatrist's task will be to identify that the patient is psychotic and then order some benign brain imaging study which will identify the patient's exact disorder?

Perhaps so, but will that obviate the need for the psychiatrist's special kind of listening? Indeed, there are those who claim that psychiatrists should no longer be considered experts in the doctor–patient relationship (where expertise is derived from their unique training in listening skills) but experts in the brain (Nestler, 1999, personal communication). As we come truly to understand the relationship between brain states and subtle cognitive, emotional, and interpersonal states, one could also ask if this is a distinction that really makes a difference. On the other hand, the psychiatrist will always be charged with finding a way to relate effectively to those who cannot effectively relate to themselves or to others. There is something in the treatment of individuals whose illnesses express themselves through disturbances of thinking, feeling, perceiving and behaving that will always demand special expertise in establishing a therapeutic relationship – and that is dependent on special expertise in listening.

Clinical Vignette 1

A 28-year-old white married man suffering from paranoid schizophrenia and obsessive–compulsive disorder did extremely well in the hospital, where his medication had been changed to clozapine with good effects. But he rapidly deteriorated on his return home. It was clear that the ward milieu had been a crucial part of his improvement, so partial hospitalization was recommended. The patient demurred, saying he didn't want to be a "burden". The psychiatrist explored this with the patient and his wife. Beyond the obvious "burdens" of cost and travel arrangements, the psychiatrist detected the patient's striving to be autonomously responsible for handling his illness. By conveying a deep respect for that wish, and then educating the already insightful patient about the realities of "bearing schizophrenia", the psychiatrist was able to help the patient accept the needed level of care.

Traditionally, this kind of listening has been called "listening with the third ear" (Reik, 1954). Other efforts to label this difficult-to-describe process have developed other terms: the interpretive stance, interpersonal sensitivity, the narrative perspective (McHugh and Slavney, 1986). All psychiatrists, regardless of theoretical stance, must learn this skill and struggle with how it is to be defined and taught. The biological or phenomenological psychiatrist listens for subtle expressions of symptomatology; the cognitive–behavioral psychiatrist listens for hidden distortions, irrational assumptions, or global inferences; the psychodynamic psychiatrist listens for hints at unconscious conflicts; the behaviorist listens for covert patterns of anxiety and stimulus associations; the family systems psychiatrist listens for hidden family myths and structures.

This requires sensitivity to the storyteller, which integrates a patient orientation complementing a disease orientation. The listener's intent is to uncover what is wrong and to put a label on it. At the same time, the listener is on a journey to discover who the patient is, employing tools of asking, looking, testing and clarifying. The patient is invited to collaborate as an active informer. Listening work takes time, concentration, imagination, a sense of humor, and an attitude that places the patient as the hero of his or her own life story. Key listening skills are listed in Table 1.1.

The enduring art of psychiatry involves guiding the depressed patient, for example, to tell his or her story of loss in addition to having him or her name, describe, and quantify symptoms

Essentials of Psychiatry   Jerald Kay and Allan Tasman
© 2006 John Wiley & Sons, Ltd.

Table 1.1	Key Listening Skills
Hearing	Connotative meanings of words
	Idiosyncratic uses of language
	Figures of speech that tell a deeper story
	Voice tones and modulation (e.g., hard edge, voice cracking)
	Stream of associations
Seeing	Posture
	Gestures
	Facial expressions (e.g., eyes watering, jaw clenched)
	Other outward expressions of emotion
Comparing	Noting what is omitted
	Dissonances between modes of expression
Intuiting	Attending to one's own internal reactions
Reflecting	Thinking it all through outside the immediate pressure to respond during the interview

of depression. The listener, in hearing the story, experiences the world and the patient from the patient's point of view and helps carry the burden of loss, lightening and transforming the load. In hearing the sufferer, the depression itself is lifted and relieved. The listening is healing as well as diagnostic. If done well, the listener becomes a better disease diagnostician. The best listeners hear both the patient and the disease clearly, and regard every encounter as potentially therapeutic.

The Primary Tools: Words, Analogies, Metaphors, Similes and Symbols

To listen and understand requires that the language used between the speaker and the hearer be shared – that the meanings of words and phrases are commonly held. Common language is the predominant factor in the social organization of humanity (Chomsky, 1972) and is probably the single most important key to the establishment of an active listener/engaged storyteller dyad which the helping alliance represents. Indeed, the Sapir–Whorf hypothesis suggests that what we are able to think is limited/determined by the language with which we are working (Carroll and Whorf, 1956; Sapir, 2000). Patients are storytellers who have the hope of being heard and understood (Edelson, 1993). Their hearers are physicians who expect to listen actively and to be with the patient in a new level of understanding. Because all human beings listen to so many different people every day, we tend to think of listening as an automatic ongoing process, yet this sort of active listening remains one of the central skills in clinical psychiatry. It underpins all other skills in diagnosis, alliance building and communication. In all medical examinations, the patient is telling a story only she or he has experienced. The physician must glean the salient information and then use it in appropriate ways. Inevitably, even when language is common, there are subtle differences in meanings, based upon differences in gender, age, culture, religion, socioeconomic class, race, region of upbringing, nationality and original language, as well as the idiosyncrasies of individual history. These differences are particularly important to keep in mind in the use of analogies,

similes and metaphors. Figures of speech, in which one thing is held representational of another by comparison, are very important windows to the inner world of the patient. Differences in meanings attached to these figures of speech can complicate their use. In psychodynamic assessment and psychotherapeutic treatment, the need to regard these subtleties of language becomes the self-conscious focus of the psychiatrist, yet failure to hear and heed such idiosyncratic distinctions can affect simple medical diagnosis as well.

Clinical Vignette 2

A psychiatric consultant was asked to see a 48-year-old man on a coronary care unit for chest pain deemed "functional" by the cardiologist who had asked the patient if his chest pain was "crushing". The patient said no. A variety of other routine tests were also negative. The psychiatrist asked the patient to describe his pain. He said, "It's like a truck sitting on my chest, squeezing it down". The psychiatrist promptly recommended additional tests which confirmed the diagnosis of myocardial infarction. The cardiologist may have been tempted to label the patient a "bad historian", but the most likely culprit of this potentially fatal misunderstanding lies in the connotative meanings each ascribed to the word "crushing" or to other variances in metaphorical communication.

In psychotherapy, the special meanings of words become the central focus of the treatment.

Clinical Vignette 3

A psychiatrist had been treating a 35-year-old man with a narcissistic personality and dysthymic disorder for 2 years. Given the brutality and deprivation of the patient's childhood, the clinician was persistently puzzled by the patient's remarkable psychological strengths. He possessed capacities for empathy, self-observation, and modulation of intense rage that were unusual, given his background. During a session the patient, in telling a childhood story, began, "When I was a little fella...". It struck the psychiatrist that the patient always said "little fella" when referring to himself as a boy, and that this was fairly distinctive phraseology. Almost all other patients will say, "When I was young/a kid/a girl (boy)/in school", designate an age, etc. On inquiry about this, the patient immediately identified "The Andy Griffith Show" as the source. This revealed a secret identification with the characters of the TV show, and a model that said to a young boy, "There are other ways to be a man than what you see around you". Making this long-standing covert identification fully conscious was transformative for the patient.

How Does One Hear Words in This Way?

The preceding clinical vignettes, once described, sound straightforward and easy. Yet, to listen in this way the clinician must acquire specific yet difficult-to-learn skills and attitudes. It is extremely difficult to put into words the listening processes embodied in these examples and those to follow, yet that is what this chapter must attempt to do.

Students, when observing experienced psychiatrists interviewing patients, often express a sense of wonder such as: "How did she know to ask that?" "Why did the patient open up with him but not with me?" "What made the diagnosis so clear in that interview and not in all the others?" The student may respond with a sense of awe, a feeling of ineptitude and doubt at ever achieving such facility, or even a reaction of disparagement that the process seems so indefinable and inexact. The key is the clinician's ability to listen. Without a refined capacity to hear deeply, the chapters on other aspects of interviewing in this textbook are of little use. But it is neither mystical nor magical nor indefinable (though it is very difficult to articulate); such skills are the product of hard work, much thought, intense supervision, and extensive in-depth exposure to many different kinds of patients.

Psychiatrists, more than any other physicians, must simultaneously listen symptomatically and narratively/experientially. They must also have access to a variety of theoretical perspectives that effectively inform their listening. These include behavioral, interpersonal, cognitive, sociocultural and systems theories. Symptomatic listening is what we think of as traditional medical history taking, in which the focus is on the presence or absence of a particular symptom, the most overt content level of an interview. Narrative–experiential listening is based on the idea that all humans are constantly interpreting their experiences, attributing meaning to them, and weaving a story of their lives with themselves as the central character. This process goes on continuously, both consciously and unconsciously, as a running conversation within each of us. The conversation is between parts of ourselves and between ourselves and what Freud called "internalized objects", important people in our lives whose images, sayings, and attitudes become permanently laid down in our memories. This conversation and commentary on our lives includes personal history, repetitive behaviors, learned assumptions about the world and interpersonal roles. These are, in turn, the products of individual background, cultural norms and values, national identifications, spiritual meanings and family system forces.

Clinical Vignette 4

A 46-year-old man was referred to a psychiatrist from a drug study. The patient had both major depression and dysthymic disorder since a business failure 2 years earlier. His primary symptoms were increased sleep, decreased mood, libido, energy and interests. After no improvement during the "blind" portion of the study, he had continued to show little response once the code was broken, and he was treated with two different active antidepressant medications. He was referred for psychotherapy and further antidepressant trials. The therapy progressed slowly with only episodic improvement. One day, the patient reported that his wife had been teasing him about how, during his afternoon nap, his snoring could be heard over the noise of a vacuum cleaner. The psychiatrist immediately asked additional questions, eventually obtained sleep polysomnography and, after appropriate treatment for sleep apnea, the patient's depression improved dramatically.

It seems that three factors were present that enabled the psychiatrist in the above vignette to listen well and identify an unusual diagnosis that had been missed by at least three other excellent clinicians who had all been using detailed structured interviews that were extremely inclusive in their symptom reviews. First, the psychiatrist had to have readily available in mind all sorts of symptoms and syndromes. Secondly, he had to be in a curious mode. In fact, this clinician had a gnawing sense that something was missing in his understanding of the patient. There is a saying in American medicine designed to focus students on the need to consider common illnesses first, while not totally ignoring rarer diseases: when you hear hoofbeats in the road, don't look first for zebras. We would say that this psychiatrist's mind was open to seeing a "zebra" despite the ongoing assumption that the weekly "hoofbeats" he had been hearing represented the everyday "horse" of clinical depression. Finally, he had to hear the patient's story in multiple, flexible ways, including the possibility that a symptom may be embedded in it, so that a match could be noticed between a detail of the story and a symptom. Eureka! The zebra could then be seen although it had been standing there every week for months.

Looking back at Clinical Vignette 3, we see the same phenomenon of a detail leaping out as a significant piece of missing information that dramatically influences the treatment process. To accomplish this requires a cognitive template (symptoms and syndromes; developmental, systemic and personality theories; awareness of cultural perspectives), a searching curious stance, and flexible processing of the data presented. If one is able to internalize the skills listed in Table 1.1, the listener begins automatically to hear the meanings in the words.

Listening as More Than Hearing

Listening and hearing are often equated in many people's minds. However, listening involves not only hearing and understanding the speaker's words, but attending to inflection, metaphor, imagery, sequence of associations and interesting linguistic selections. It also involves seeing – movement, gestures, facial expressions, subtle changes in these – and constantly comparing what is said with what is seen, looking for dissonances, and comparing what is being said and seen with what was previously communicated and observed. Further, it is essential to be aware of what might have been said but was not, or how things might have been expressed but were not. This is where clues to idiosyncratic meanings and associations are often discovered. Sometimes, the most important meanings are embedded in what is conspicuous by its absence.

It was Darwin (1955) who first observed that there appears to be a biogrammar of primary emotions that all humans share and express in predictable, fixed action patterns. The meaning of a smile or nod of the head is universal across disparate cultures. This insight was lost until the late 1960s when several researchers from different fields (Tiger and Fox, 1971; Tomkins and McCarter, 1964) returned to it and demonstrated empirically the cross-cultural consistency of emotional expression. LeDoux (1996) has been a leader in identifying the neurobiological substrate for these primary emotions. Leslie Brothers (1989), using this work and her own experiments with primates, developed a hypothesis about the biology of empathy based on seeing as well as hearing. Both she and Damasio (1994) have identified the amygdala and the inferior temporal lobe gyrus as the neurobiological substrate for recognition of and empathy for others and their emotional states. Further research has identified that these parts of the brain are, on the one hand, prededicated to recognizing certain gestures, facial expressions, and so on, but require effective maternal–infant interaction in order to do so (Schore, 2001). The "gleam in the mother's eye" of Mahler and colleagues (1975) is literally translated into the reflection of the mother's fovea as she gazes at her infant, stimulating the nondominant orbital frontal cortex which, in turn, completes the key temporal circuits.

All of this is synthesized in the listener as a "sense" or intuition as to what the speaker is saying at multiple levels. The availability of useful cognitive templates and theories enables the listener to articulate what is heard.

Clinical Vignette 5

A 38-year-old Hispanic construction worker presented himself to a small-town emergency department in the Southwest, complaining of pain on walking, actually described in Spanish-accented English as "a little pain". His voice was tight, his face was drawn, and his physical demeanor was burdened and hesitant. His response to the invitation to walk was met by a labored attempt to walk without favor to his painful limb. A physician could have discharged him from the emergency department with a small prescription of ibuprofen. The careful physician in the emergency department responded to the powerful visual message that he was in pain, was beaten down by it, and had suffered long before coming in. This recognition came first to the physician as an intuition that this man was somehow more sick than he made himself sound. A radiograph of the femur revealed a lytic lesion that later proved to be metastatic renal cell carcinoma. To hear the unspoken, one had to be keenly aware of the patient's tone and how he looked, and to keep in mind, too, the cultural taboos forbidding him to give in to pain or to appear to need help.

As has been implied, not only must one affirmatively "hear" all that a patient is communicating, one must overcome a variety of potential blocks to effective listening.

Common Blocks to Effective Listening

Many factors influence the ability to listen. Psychiatrists come to the patient as the product of their own life experiences. Does the listener tune in to what he or she hears in a more attentive way if the listener and the patient share characteristics? What blocks to listening (Table 1.2) are posed by differences in sex, age, religion, socioeconomic class, race, culture, or nationality (Kleinman, 2001; Comas-Diaz and Jacobsen, 1991; Kochman, 1991)? What blind spots may be induced by superficial similarities in different personal meanings attributed to the same cultural symbol? Separate and apart from the differences in the development of empathy when the dyad holds in common certain features, the act of listening is inevitably influenced by similarities and differences between the psychiatrist and the patient.

Would a woman have reported the snoring in Clinical Vignette 4 or would she have been too embarrassed? Would she have reported it more readily to a woman psychiatrist? What about the image in Clinical Vignette 2 of a truck sitting on someone's chest? How gender and culture bound is it? Would "The

Table 1.2   **Blocks to Effective Listening**

Patient–psychiatrist dissimilarities	Race
	Sex
	Culture
	Religion
	Regional dialect
	Individual differences
	Socioeconomic class
Superficial similarities	May lead to incorrect assumptions of shared meanings
Countertransference	Psychiatrist fails to hear or reacts inappropriately to content reminiscent of own unresolved conflicts
External forces	Managed care setting
	Emergency department
	Control-oriented inpatient unit
Attitudes	Need for control
	Psychiatrist having a bad day

Andy Griffith Show", important in Clinical Vignette 3, have had the same impact on a young African-American boy that it did on a Caucasian one? In how many countries is "The Andy Griffith Show" even available, and in which cultures would that model of a family structure seem relevant? Suppose the psychiatrist in that vignette was not a television viewer or had come from another country to the USA long after the show had come and gone? (Roughly 50% of current residents in psychiatry in the USA are foreign born and trained [American Psychiatric Association, 2001].) Consider these additional examples.

Clinical Vignette 6

A female patient came to see her male psychiatrist for their biweekly session. Having just been given new duties on her job, she came in excitedly and began sharing with her therapist how happy she was to have been chosen by her male supervisor to help him with a very important project at their office. The session continued with the theme of the patient's pride in having been recognized for her attributes, talents and hard work. At the next session, she said that she had become embarrassed after the previous session at the thought that she had been "strutting her stuff". The therapist reflected back to her the thought that she sounded like a rooster strutting his stuff, connecting her embarrassment at having revealed that she strove for the recognition and power of men in her company, and that she, in fact, envied the position of her supervisor. The patient objected to the comparison of a rooster, and likened it more to feeling like a woman of the streets strutting her stuff. She stated that she felt like a prostitute being used by her supervisor. The psychiatrist was off the mark by missing the opportunity to point out in the analogous way that the patient's source of embarrassment was in being used, not so much in being envious of the male position.

It is likely that different life experiences based on gender fostered this misunderstanding. How many women easily identify with the stereotyped role of the barnyard rooster? How many men readily identify with the role of a prostitute? These are but two examples of the myriad different meanings our specific gender may incline us towards. Although metaphor is a powerful tool in listening to the patient, cross-cultural barriers pose potential blocks to understanding.

Clinical Vignette 7

A 36-year-old black woman complained to her therapist (of the same language, race, and socioeconomic class) that her husband was a snake, meaning that he was no good, treacherous, a hidden danger. The therapist, understanding this commonly held definition of a snake, reflected back to the patient pertinent, supportive feedback concerning the care and caution the patient was exercising in divorce dealings with the husband.

In contrast, a 36-year-old Chinese woman, fluent in English, living in her adopted country for 15 years and assimilated to Western culture, represented her husband to her Caucasian, native-born psychiatrist as being like a dragon. The therapist, without checking on the meaning of the word "dragon" with her patient, assumed it connoted danger, one of malicious intent and oppression. The patient, however, was using "dragon" as a metaphor for her husband – the fierce, watchful guardian of the family – in keeping with the ancient Chinese folklore in which the dragon is stationed at the gates of the lord's castle to guard and protect it from evil and danger.

Even more subtle regional variations may produce similar problems in listening and understanding.

Clinical Vignette 8

In a family session, a psychiatrist from the South referred to the mother of her patient as "your mama", intending a meaning of warmth and respect. The patient instantly became enraged at the use of such an offensive term toward her mother. Although being treated in Texas, the patient and her family had recently moved from a large city in New Jersey. The use of the term "mama" among working class Italians in that area was looked upon with derision among people of Irish descent, the group to which the patient was ethnically connected. The patient had used the term "mother" to refer to her mother, a term the psychiatrist had heard with a degree of coolness attached. What she knew of her patient's relationship with her mother did not fit in with a word like mother, hence almost out of awareness she switched terms leading to a response of indignation and outrage from the patient.

Psychiatrists discern meaning in that which they hear through filters of their own – cultural backgrounds, life experiences, feelings, the day's events, their own physical sense of themselves, nationality, sex roles, religious meaning systems and intrapsychic conflicts. The filters can serve as blocks or as magnifiers if certain elements of what is being said resonate with something within the psychiatrist. When the filters block, we call it countertransference or insensitivity. When they magnify, we call it empathy or sensitivity. One may observe a theme for a long time repeated with a different tone, embellishment, inflection, or context before the idea of what is meant comes to mind. The "little fella" example in Clinical Vignette 3 illustrates a message that had been communicated in many ways and times in exactly the same language before the psychiatrist "got it". On discovering a significant meaning that had been signaled before in many ways, the psychiatrist often has the experience, "How could I have been so stupid? It's staring me in the face for months!"

Managed care and the manner in which national health systems are administered can alter our attitudes toward the patient and our abilities to be transforming listeners. The requirement for authorization for minimal visits, time on the phone with utilization review nurses attempting to justify continuing therapy, and forms tediously filled out can be blocks to listening to the patient. Limitations on the kinds and length of treatment can lull the psychiatrist into not listening in the same way or as intently. With these time limits and other "third party payer" considerations (i.e., need for a billable diagnostic code from the *Diagnostic and Statistical Manual of Mental Disorders*, Fourth Edition [DSM-IV-TR] or the *International Classification of Diseases*, 10th Revision [ICD-10]), the psychiatrist, as careful listener, must heed the external pressures influencing the approach to the patient. Many health benefits packages will provide coverage in any therapeutic setting only for relief of symptoms, restoration of minimal function, acute problem solving, and shoring up of defenses. In various countries, health care systems have come up with a variety of constraints in their efforts to deal with the costs of care. Unless these pressures are attended to, listening will be accomplished with a different purpose in mind, more closely

Clinical Vignette 9

An army private was brought to the emergency room in Germany by his friends, having threatened to commit suicide while holding a gun to his head. He was desperate, disorganized, impulsive, enraged, pacing and talking almost incoherently. Gradually, primarily through his friends, the story emerged that his first sergeant had recently made a decision for the entire unit that had a particularly adverse effect on the patient. He was a fairly primitive character who relied on his wife for a sense of stability and coherence in his life. The sergeant's decision was to send the entire unit into the field for over a month just at the time the patient's wife was about to arrive, after a long delay, from the USA. After piecing together this story, the psychiatrist said to the patient, "It's not yourself you want to kill, it's your first sergeant!" The patient at first giggled a little, then gradually broke out into a belly laugh that echoed throughout the emergency room. It was clear that, having recognized the true object of his anger, a coherence was restored that enabled him to feel his rage without the impulse to act on it. The psychiatrist then enlisted the friends in a plan to support the patient through the month and to arrange regular phone contact with the wife as she set up their new home in Germany. No medication was necessary. Hospitalization was averted, and a request for humanitarian dispensation, which would have compromised the patient in the eyes of both his peers and superiors, was avoided as well. And, with luck, the young man had an opportunity to grow emotionally as well.

approximating the crisis intervention model of the emergency room or the medical model for either inpatient or outpatient care. In these settings, the thoughtful psychiatrist will arm himself or herself with checklists, inventories, and scales for objectifying the severity of illness and response to treatment: the ear is tuned only to measurable and observable signs of responses to therapy and biologic intervention.

With emphasis on learning here and now symptoms that can bombard the dyad with foreground static and noise, will the patient be lost in the encounter? The same approach to listening occurs in the setting of the emergency department for crisis intervention. Emphasis is on symptom relief, assurance of capacities to keep oneself safe, restoration of minimal function, acute problem solving and shoring up of defenses. Special attention is paid to identifying particular stressors. What can be done quickly to change stressors that threw the patient's world into a state of disequilibrium? The difference in the emergency room is that the careful listener may have 3 to 6 hours, as opposed to three to six sessions for the patient with a health maintenance organization or preferred provider contract, or other limitations on benefits. If one is fortunate and good at being an active listener–bargainer, the seeds of change can be planted in the hope of allowing them time to grow between visits to the emergency department. If one could hope for another change, it would be for a decrease in the chaos in the patient's inner world and outer world.

Crucial Attitudes that Enable Effective Listening

The first step in developing good listening skills involves coming to grips with the importance of inner experience in psychiatric treatment and diagnosis. The *Diagnostic and Statistical Manual of Mental Disorders*, Fourth Edition (American Psychiatric Association, 1994) and *International Classification of Diseases*, 10th Revision (World Health Organization, 1992) have been enormous advances in reliability and accuracy of diagnosis, but their emphasis on seemingly observable phenomena has allowed the willing user to forget the importance of inner experience even in such basic diagnoses as major depressive disorder. Consider the symptom "depressed mood most of the day" or "markedly diminished interest or pleasure" or even "decrease or increase in appetite". These are entirely subjective symptoms. Simply reporting depression is usually not sufficient to convince a psychiatrist that a diagnosis of depression is warranted. In fact, the vast majority of psychiatric patients are so demoralized by their illnesses that they often announce depression as their first complaint. Further, there are a significant number of patients who do not acknowledge depression yet are so diagnosed. The clinician might well comment, "Sitting with him makes me feel very sad".

The psychiatrist must listen to much more than the patient's overt behavior. There are qualities in the communication, including the inner experiences induced in the listener, that should be attended to. The experienced clinician listens to the words, watches the behavior, engages in and notices the ongoing interaction, allows himself/herself to experience his/her own inner reactions to the process, and *never forgets that depression and almost all other psychiatric symptoms are exclusively private experiences*. The behavior and interactions are useful insofar as they assist the psychiatrist in inferring the patient's inner experience.

Therefore, to convince a clinician that a patient is depressed, not only must the patient say she/he is depressed, but the observable behavior must convey it (sad-looking face, sighing, unexpressive intonations, etc.); the interaction with the interviewer must convey depressive qualities (sense of neediness, sadness induced in the interviewer, beseeching qualities expressed, etc.). In the absence of both of these, other diagnoses should be considered, but in the presence of such qualities, depression needs to remain in the differential diagnosis.

Even when we make statements about brain function with regard to a particular patient, we use this kind of listening, generally, by making at least two inferences. We first listen to and observe the patient and then infer some aspect of the patient's private experience. Then, if we possess sufficient scientific knowledge, we make a second inference to a disturbance in neurochemistry, neurophysiology, or neuroanatomy. When psychiatrists prescribe antidepressant medication, they have inferred from words, moved into inner experiences, and come to a conclusion that there is likely a dysregulation of serotonin or norepinephrine in the patient's brain.

As one moves towards treatment from diagnosis, the content of inner experience inferred may change to more varied states of feelings, needs, and conflicts, but the fundamental process of listening remains the same. The psychiatrist listens for the meaning of all behavior, to the ongoing interpersonal relationship the patient attempts to establish, and to inner experiences as well.

Despite all of the technological advances in medicine in general and their growing presence in psychiatry, securing or eliciting a history remains the first and central skill for all physicians. Even in the most basic of medical situations, the patient is trying to communicate a set of private experiences (how does one describe the qualities of pain or discomfort?) that the physician may infer and sort into possible syndromes and diagnoses. In psychiatry, this process is multiplied, as indicated in Figure 1.1. William Styron (1990), a prizewinning novelist, had to go to extraordinary lengths in his eloquent attempt to convey the "searing internal mental pain" that he experienced when suffering from a major depression.

The qualitative aspects of private experience remain, to this day, a major problem in philosophy. It was the basis of Rene Descartes' (1991) philosophical doubting that became the fundamental intellectual underpinning of Western thought for so long. Edmund Husserl (1977) used it as the basis for an entire philosophical system, phenomenology, which was a forerunner of existentialism, which was so influential in both American and European psychiatry in the 1950s and 1960s (May *et al.*, 1958; Binswanger, 1963).

Silvano Arieti (1967) hypothesized that cognitive development produces changes over time in the inner experience of various affects. Does a person with borderline personality disorder experience "anxiety" in the same qualitative and quantitative manner in which a neurotic person does? What is the relationship between sadness and guilt and the empty experiences of depression? This perspective underlies the principle articulated in text after text on interviewing that emphasizes the importance of establishing rapport in the process of history taking. It is incredibly easy for the psychiatrist to attribute to the patient what she/he would have meant and what most people might have meant in using a particular word or phrase. The sense in the narrator that the listener is truly present, connected, and with the patient enormously enhances the accuracy of the story reported.

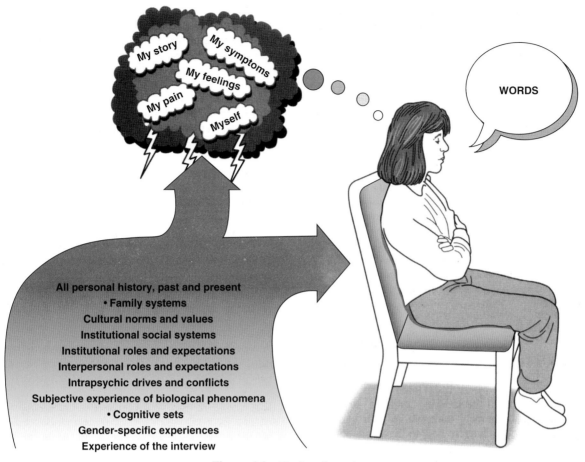

Figure 1.1 *Finding the patient.*

Words that have been used to describe this process of constant attention to and inference of inner experience by the listener include interest, empathy (Rogers, 1951; Kohut, 1991; Truax, 1963), attentiveness and noncontingent positive regard (Truax, 1963). However, these are words that may say less than they seem to. It is the constant curious awareness on the listener's part, that she/he is trying to grasp the private inner experience of the patient, and the storyteller's sense of this stance by the psychiatrist that impels the ever more revealing process of history taking. This quality of listening produces what we call rapport, without which psychiatric histories become spotty, superficial and even suspect. There are no bad historians, only patients who have not yet found the right listener.

In treatment, we even find empirical data to support this perspective. The two most powerful predictors of outcome in any form of psychotherapy are empathy and the therapeutic alliance (Horvath and Luborsky, 1993; Greenson, 1978). This has been shown again and again in study after study for dynamic therapy, cognitive therapy, behavior therapy and even medication management (Elkin *et al.*, 1989). This led some researchers and theorists to propose that the power of psychotherapy can be understood solely as a remoralization phenomenon based on support and empathy (Frank, 1973; Omer and London, 1989). The truth of this can be seen in the remarkable therapeutic success of the "clinical management" cell of the National Institutes of Mental Health Collaborative Study on the Treatment of Major Depression. Although the Clinical Management Cell was not

as effective as the cells that included specific drugs or specific psychotherapeutic interventions, 35% of patients with moderate to severe major depressive disorder improved significantly with carefully structured supportive clinical management alone (Elkin *et al.*, 1989).

Helpful psychiatric listening requires a complicated attitude toward control and power in the interview (see Table 1.3). The psychiatrist invites the patient/storyteller to collaborate as an active informer. He is invited, too, to question and observe himself. This method of history taking remains the principal tool of general clinical medicine. However, as Freud pointed out, these methods of active uncovering are more complex in the psychic

Table 1.3   Attitudes Important to Listening
The centrality of **inner experience**
There are no bad historians
The answer is always inside the patient
Control and power are shared in the interview
It is OK to feel confused and uncertain
Objective truth is never as simple as it seems
Listen to yourself, too
Everything you hear is modified by the patient's filters
Everything you hear is modified by your own filters
There will always be another opportunity to hear more clearly

realm. The use of the patient as a voluntary reporter requires that the investigator keep in mind the unconscious and its power over the patient and listener. Can the patient be a reliable objective witness of himself or his symptoms? Can the listener hold in mind his own set of filters, meanings, and distortions as he hears? The listener translates for himself and his patient the patient's articulation of his experience of himself and his inner world into our definition of symptoms, syndromes, and differential diagnoses which make-up the concept of the medical model.

Objective–descriptive examiners are like detectives closing in on disease. The psychiatric detective enters the inquiry with an attitude of unknowing and suspends prior opinion. The techniques of listening invoke a wondering and a wandering with the patient. Periods of head scratching and exclamations of "I'm confused", or "I don't understand", or "That's awful!" or "Tell me more", allow the listener to follow or to point the way for the dyad. Finally, clear and precise descriptions are held up for scrutiny, with the hope that a diagnostic label or new information about the patient's suffering and emotional pain is revealed.

It is embarking on the history taking journey together – free of judgments, opinions, criticism, or preconceived notions – that underpins rapport. Good listening requires a complex understanding of what objective truth is and how it may be found. The effective psychiatrist must eschew the traditional medical role in interviewing and tolerate a collaborative, at times meandering, direction in which control is at best shared and sometimes wholly with the patient. The psychiatrist constantly asks: What is being said? Why is it being said at this moment? What is the meaning of what is being said? In what context is all this emerging? What does that tell me about the meaning and what does it reflect about the doctor–patient relationship?

Theoretical Perspectives on Listening

Listening is the effort or work of placing the therapist where the patient is ("lives"). Greenson (1978) would call it "going along with"; Rogers (1951) "centering on the client". The ear of the empathic listener is the organ of receptivity – gratifying and, at times, indulging the patient. Greenson would say that it is better to be deceived going along with the patient than to reject him/her prematurely and have the door slammed to the patient's inner world. That is what is meant by the suspension of beliefs for the discovery of the true self. Harry Stack Sullivan, the father of interpersonal psychiatry, would remind us to heed those shrewd, small questions: "What is he up to?" "Where is he taking us?" Every human being has a preferred interpersonal stance, a set of relationships and transactions with which she or he is most comfortable and feels most gratified. The problem is that for most psychiatric patients they do not work well. This is the wisdom that Sullivan (1953) was articulating.

Beyond attitudes that enable or prevent listening there is a role for specific knowledge. It is important to achieve the cognitive structure or theoretical framework and use it with rigor and discipline in the service of patients so that psychiatrists can employ more than global "feelings" or "hunches". In striving to grasp the inner experience of any other human being, one must know what it is to be human; one must have an idea of what is inside any person. This provides a framework for understanding what the patient – who would not be a patient if he fully understood what was inside of him – is struggling to communicate. Personality theory is absolutely crucial to this process.

Whether we acknowledge it or not, every one of us has a theory of human personality (in this day and age of porous boundaries between psychology and biology, we should really speak of a psychobiological theory of human experience) which we apply in various situations, social or clinical. These theories become part of the template alluded to earlier that allow certain words, stories, actions, and cues from the patient to jump out with profound meaning to the psychiatrist. There is no substitute for a thorough knowledge of many theories of human functioning and a well disciplined synthesis and internal set of rules to decide which theories to use in which situations.

Different theoretical positions offer slightly different and often complementary perspectives on listening (Table 1.4). The basic tools of therapeutic power and diagnostic acumen spring from the following:

1. Freud's associative methods (Brill, 1938) and ego psychology (Freud, 1946), in which one listens for the associative trends and conflicts.
2. Melanie Klein's (1975) and Harry Stack Sullivan's (1953) object relations theory. The former discovered the story through inner world exploration and recognized the introjected

Table 1.4	Theoretical Perspectives on Listening	
Theory	Focus of Attention	Listening Stance
Ego psychology	Stream of associations	Neutral, hovering attention
Object relations	Introjects (internalized images of others within the patient)	Neutral, hovering attention
Interpersonal	What relationship is the patient attempting to construct?	Participant observer
Existential	Feelings, affect	Empathic identification with the patient
Self-psychology	Sense of self from others	Empathic mirroring and affirmation
Patient centered	Content control by patient	Noncontingent positive regard, empathy
Cognitive	Hidden assumptions and distortions	Benign expert
Behavioral	Behavioral contingencies	Benign expert
Family systems	Complex forces maneuvering each member	Neutral intruder who forces imbalance in the system

persons of the past who live within the patient's mind, comprising the person's psychic structure; the latter discovered the knowing through the interpersonal experience of the therapeutic dyad (Greenberg and Mitchell, 1983).

3. Binswanger's (1963) understanding of the condition of empathy, in which the listener gives up his or her own position for that of the storyteller.

4. Kohut's (1991) self-psychology, which emphasizes the use of vicarious introspection to reflect (mirror) back to the patient what is being understood. This mirroring engenders in the storyteller a special sense of being "found", that is, of being known, recognized, affirmed, and heard. This feeling of being heard helps to undo the sense of aloneness so common in psychiatric patients.

Each of the great schools of psychotherapy places the psychiatrist in a somewhat different relationship to the patient. This may even be reflected in the physical placement of the therapist in relation to the patient. In a classical psychoanalytic stance, the therapist, traditionally unseen behind the patient, assumes an active, hovering attention. Existential analysts seek to experience the patient's position and place themselves close to and facing the patient. The interpersonal psychiatrist stresses a collaborative dialogue with shared control. One can almost imagine the two side by side as the clinician strives to sense what the storyteller is doing to and with the listener. Interpersonal theory stresses the need for each participant to act within that interpersonal social field.

In the object relations stance, the listener keeps in mind the "other people in the room" with him and the storyteller, that is, the patient's introjects who are constantly part of the internal conversation of the patient and thus influence the dialogue within the therapeutic dyad. In connecting with the patient, the listener is also tuned in to the fact that parts and fragments of him or her are being internalized by the patient. The listener becomes another person in the room of the patient's life experience, within and outside the therapeutic hour. Cognitive and behavioral psychiatrists are kindly experts, listening attentively and subtly for hidden assumptions, distortions, and connections. The family systems psychiatrist sits midway among the pressures and forces emanating from each individual, seeking to affect the system so that all must adapt differently.

Referring again to Clinical Vignette 3, we can see the different theoretical models of the listening process in the discovery of the meaning of "little fella". Freud's model is that the psychiatrist had listened repeatedly to a specific association and inquired of its meaning. Object relations theorists would note that the clinician had discovered a previously unidentified, powerful introject within the therapeutic dyad. The interpersonal psychiatrist would see the shared exploration of this idiosyncratic manner of describing one's youth; the patient had been continually trying to take the therapist to "The Andy Griffith Show". That is, the patient was attempting to induce the clinician to share the experience of imagining and fantasizing about having Andy Griffith as a father.

Existentialists would note how the psychiatrist was changed dramatically by the patient's repeated use of this phrase and then altered even more profoundly by the memory of Andy Griffith, "the consummate good father" in the patient's words. The therapist could never see the patient in quite the same way again, and the patient sensed it immediately. And Kohut would note the mirroring quality of the psychiatrist's interpreting the meaning of this important memory. This would be mirroring at its most powerful, affirming the patient's important differences from his family, helping him to consolidate the memories. The behavioral psychiatrist would note the reciprocal inhibition that had gone on, with Andy Griffith soothing the phobic anxieties in a brutal family.

A cognitive psychiatrist would wonder whether the patient's depression resulted from a hidden assumption that anything less than the idyllic images of television was not good enough. The family systems psychiatrist would help the patient see that he had manipulated the forces at work on him and actually changed the definition of his family.

The ways and tools of listening also change, according to the purpose, the nature of the therapeutic dyad. The ways of listening also change depending upon whether or not the psychiatrist is preoccupied or inattentive. The medical model psychiatrist listens for signs and symptoms. The analyst listens for the truth often clothed in fantasy and metaphor. The existentialist listens for feeling, and the interpersonal theorist listens for the shared experiences engendered by the interaction. Regardless of the theoretical stance and regardless of the mental tension between the medical model's need to know symptoms and signs and the humanistic psychiatrist's listening to know the sufferer, the essence of therapeutic listening is the suspension of judgment before any presentation of the story and the storyteller. The listener is asked to clarify and classify the inner world of the storyteller at the same time he is experiencing it – no small feat!

Using Oneself in Listening

Understanding transference and countertransference is crucial to effective listening. Tomkins, LeDoux, Damasio and Brothers have given us a basic science, biological perspective on this process. However one defines these terms, whatever one's theoretical stance about these issues, Harry Stack Sullivan (1969) had it right when he said that schizophrenics are more human than anything else. To know ourselves is to begin to know our patients more deeply. There are many ways to achieve this. Personal therapy is one. Ongoing life experience is another. Supervision that emphasizes one's emotional reactions to patients is still a third. Once we have started on the road to achieving this understanding by therapy, supervision, or life experience, continued listening to our patients, who teach us about ourselves and others, becomes a lifelong method of growth.

To know oneself is to be aware that there are certain common human needs, wishes, fears, feelings and reactions. Every person must deal in some way with attachment, dependence, authority, autonomy, selfhood, values and ideals, remembered others, work, love, hate and loss. It is unlikely that the psychiatrist can comprehend the patient without his own self-awareness. Thus, Figure 1.1 should really look like Figure 1.2. The most psychotic patient in the world is still struggling with these universal human functions.

In this case, the psychiatrist was able to connect with a patient's inner experience in a manner that had a fairly dramatic impact on the clinical course. That is the goal of listening. The art is hearing the patient's inner experience and then addressing it empathically, enabling the patient to feel heard and affirmed. There are no rules about this, and at any given point in a clinical encounter there are many ways to accomplish it.

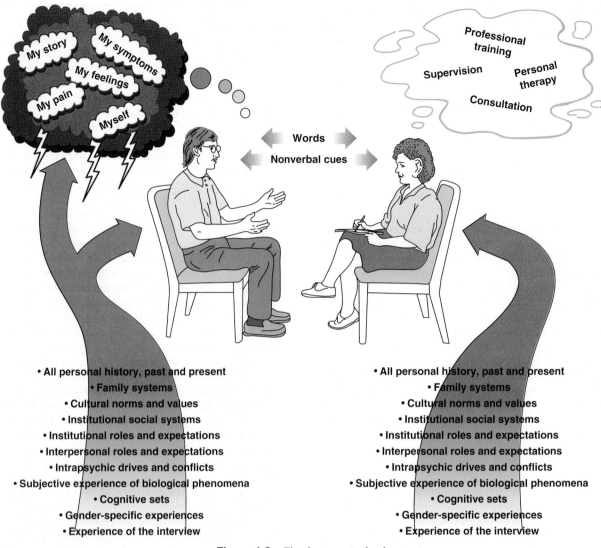

My story
My symptoms
My feelings
My pain
Myself

Professional
training
Supervision
Personal
therapy
Consultation

Words
Nonverbal cues

• All personal history, past and present
• Family systems
• Cultural norms and values
• Institutional social systems
• Institutional roles and expectations
• Interpersonal roles and expectations
• Intrapsychic drives and conflicts
• Subjective experience of biological phenomena
• Cognitive sets
• Gender-specific experiences
• Experience of the interview

• All personal history, past and present
• Family systems
• Cultural norms and values
• Institutional social systems
• Institutional roles and expectations
• Interpersonal roles and expectations
• Intrapsychic drives and conflicts
• Subjective experience of biological phenomena
• Cognitive sets
• Gender-specific experiences
• Experience of the interview

Figure 1.2   *The therapeutic dyad.*

Clinical Vignette 10

A young man with paranoid schizophrenia had been admitted in 1979 to the hospital following a near lethal attack on his father. When asked about this incident, he became frankly delusional, speaking of the Arab-Israeli conflict, the preciousness of Jerusalem, how the Israelis must defend it at all costs. Unspoken was his conviction that he was like the Israelis, with the entire world attacking and threatening him. He believed his father had threatened and attacked him when, in fact, his father had done little more than seek to be closer, more comforting and advising with the patient. The psychiatrist understood the patient to be speaking of that core of selfhood that we all possess, which, when threatened, creates a sense of vulnerability and panic, a disintegrating anxiety unlike any other. The psychiatrist spoke to the patient of Anwar Sadat's visit to Jerusalem and engaged him in a discussion of how that had gone, what the outcome had been, had the threat been lessened or increased? The patient, although still delusional, visibly relaxed and began to speak much more directly about

his own sense of vulnerability and uncertainty over his personal integrity and its ability to withstand any closeness. He still required neuroleptic medication for his illness; however, his violent thoughts and behaviors reduced dramatically. He was able to begin interacting with his father, and his behavior on the ward changed as well.

There are also many ways to respond that are unhelpful and even retraumatizing. The skilled psychiatrist, just as she/he never forgets that it is the patient's inner experience that is to be heard, also never stops struggling to find just the right words, gestures, expressions and inflections that say to a patient, "you have been understood". The most clever diagnostician or insightful interpreter who cannot "connect" with the patient in this manner will miss valuable information. This issue has been addressed by writers who have pointed out how little understood are the concepts of support and empathy (Peteet, 1982).

Being human is also to be a creature of habit and pattern in linguistic, interpersonal, and emotional realms. The skilled psychiatrist listens with this ever in mind. What we see in the interview, what we hear in interactions, may be presumed to be repetitions of many other events. The content may vary, but the form, motive, process and evolution are generally universal for any given individual. This, too, is part of listening. To know what is fundamentally human, to have a well-synthesized rigorous theory, and to hear the person's unique but repetitive ways of experiencing are the essence of listening. These skills "find" the patient in all his/her humanity, but then the psychiatrist must find the right communication that allows the patient to feel "found".

To Be Found: The Psychological Product of Being Heard

Psychiatric patients may be lonely, isolated, demoralized, and desperate, regardless of the specific diagnosis. They have lost themselves and their primary relationships, if they ever had any. Stanley Jackson (1992) makes the point that before anything else can happen, they must be found, and feel found. They can only be found within the context of their own specific histories, cultures, religions, genders, social contexts, and so on. There is nothing more healing than that experience of being found by another. The earliest expression of this need is in infancy and we refer to it as the need for attachment. Referring to middle childhood, Harry Stack Sullivan spoke of the importance of the pal or buddy. Kohut spoke of the lifelong need for **self-objects**. In lay terms, it is often subsumed under the need for love, security, and acceptance. Psychiatric patients have lost or never had this experience. However obnoxious or destructive or desperate their overt behavior, it is the psychiatrist's job to seek and find the patient. That is the purpose of listening.

If we look back to Clinical Vignette 3, wherein the phrase "little fella" bespoke such deep and important unverbalized meaning, the patient's reaction to the memory and recognition by the psychiatrist was dramatic. He had always known he was different in some indefinable ways from his family. That difference had been both a source of pride and pain to him at various developmental stages. However, the recognition of the specific source, its meaning, and its constant presence in his life created a whole new sense of himself. He had been found by his psychiatrist, who echoed the discovery, and he had found an entire piece of himself that he had enacted for years, yet which had been disconnected from any integrated sense of himself.

Sometimes objectifying and defining the disease/disorder enables the person to feel found. One of the most challenging patients to hear and experience is the acting out, self-destructive, demanding person with borderline personality disorder. Even as the prior sentence conveys, psychiatrists often experience the diagnosis as who the patient is rather than what she suffers. The following case conveys how one third year resident was able to hear such a patient, and in his listening to her introduce the idea that the symptoms were not her but her disorder.

Gender can play a significant role in the experience of feeling found. Some individuals feel that it is easier to connect with a person of the same sex; others, with someone of the opposite sex. Clinical Vignette 6 is an excellent example of this. In these days of significant change in and sensitivity to sex roles, a misinterpretation such as that early in treatment could result in a permanent rupture in the alliance. Psychiatrists vary in their sensitivity to the different sexes. Some may do better with those who have chosen more traditional roles; others may be more sensitive to those who have adopted more modern roles.

Clinical Vignette 11

He was working the midnight Friday to 11 AM Saturday shift in a Psychiatric Emergency Room. The patient was a 26-year-old woman brought in by ambulance after overdosing on sertraline following an argument with her boyfriend. She had been partying with him and became enraged at the attention he was paying to the date of a friend who was accompanying them. After being cleared medically, the patient was transferred to psychiatry for crisis intervention. It was about 4 AM when she arrived. She was crying and screaming for the psychiatric staff to release her. In the emergency department she had grabbed a suture scissors attached to the uniform of the charge nurse. The report was given to the psychiatric resident that she had been a "management problem" in the medicine ER.

The psychiatrist sat wearily and listened to the patient tell her story with tears, shouts, and expletives sputtered through clenched teeth. She stated that she did not remember ever being happy, that she frequently had thoughts of suicide, and that she had overdosed twice before, following a divorce from her first husband at the age of 19 and then 8 months prior to this episode when she had been fired from a job for arguing with her supervisor. Her parents had kept her 6-year-old and 7-year-old sons since her divorce. She was currently working as a file clerk and living with her boyfriend of 2 months. She stated that she felt like there was a cold ice cube stuck in her chest as she watched her boyfriend flirting with the other woman. She acknowledged that she felt empty and utterly alone even in the crowded bar. She created an unpleasant scene and they continued to argue until they got home. Then he had laughed at her and left, stating that he would come back when she had cooled down.

The resident sat quietly and listened. He looked dreary. The night had been a busy one. She looked at him and complained, "Don't let me and my problems bore you!" He looked at her and said, "Quite the contrary. I've been thinking as you speak that I know what disorder you suffer from". With that statement, he pulled out the DSM-IV and read with her the description of the symptoms and signs of borderline personality disorder. She had been in therapy off and on since she was 16 years old. No one had ever shared with her the name of the diagnosis but instead had responded to her as if the disorder was the definition of who she was. In his listening, he was able to hear her symptoms as a disorder and not the person. And in his ability to separate the two, he was able to allow her to distance herself from the symptoms, too, and see herself in a new light with her first inkling of her own personhood.

We now know that just as there is a neurobiological basis for empathy and countertransference, there is a similar biological basis for the power of listening to heal, to lift psychological burdens, to remoralize and to provide emotional regulation to patients who feel out of control in their rage, despair, terror, or other feelings (Table 1.5). Attachment and social support are psychobiological processes that provide the necessary physiological regulation to human beings. This has been shown by the work of Hofer (1996), Cobb (1976), Meaney (2001), Nemeroff (Heim and Nemeroff, 2001), and many others. Additional work of Paul

Table 1.5	The Basic Sciences of Listening

Neurobiology of primary affects
Universality of certain affective expressions
Neurobiology of empathy
Biological need for interpersonal regulation
Psychobiology of attachment
Biological impact of social support
Environmental impact on central nervous system structure
    and function

Ekman (1992) supports the notion of the patient's capacity to perceive empathy through the powerful nonverbal, universally understood communication of facial expressions. His research in basic human emotions sets forth the idea of their understanding across cultures and ages. It further supports the provocative idea that facial expressions of the listener may generate autonomic and central nervous system changes not only within the listener but within the one being heard, and vice versa. Indeed, the evidence is growing that new experiences in clinical interactions create learning and new memories, which are associated with changes in both brain structure and function (Kandel, 1999; Gabbard, 2000; Mohl, 1987; Liggan and Kay, 1999). When we listen in this way, we are intervening not only in a psychological manner to connect, heal, and share burdens but also in a neurobiological fashion to regulate, modulate and restore functioning. When patients feel found, they are responding to this psychobiological process.

Listening to Oneself to Listen Better

To hold in mind what has been said and heard after a session and between sessions is the most powerful and active tool of listening. It is a crucial step often overlooked by students and those new at listening. It is necessary to hear our patients in our thoughts during the in-between times in order to pull together repetitive patterns of thinking, behaving, and feeling, giving us the closest idea of how patients experience themselves and their world. In addition, many of our traumatized patients have not had the experience of being held inmind, of being remembered, and their needs being thought of by significant others. These key experiences of childhood affirm the young person's psychological being. It is important to distinguish this kind of "re-listening" to the patient – an important part of the psychiatrist's ongoing processing and reprocessing of what has been heard and experienced – from what some may leap to call countertransference. One way of identifying this distinction would be to differentiate listening to oneself as one reviews in one's mind the patient's story versus

---

Clinical Vignette 12

A second year resident, rotating through an inpatient unit which serves the psychiatric needs of very severely ill psychotic patients with multiple admissions, dual diagnoses, homelessness, criminal records, significant histories of medical noncompliance, and, in some, unremitting psychosis, was particularly struggling with a 33-year-old white woman admitted for the 11th time

---

since age 19. The patient invariably stopped medications shortly after discharge, never kept follow-up appointments, and ended up on the streets psychotic and high on crack cocaine. She would then be involuntarily committed for restabilization. And so the cycle would repeat itself. The resident would see the patient on daily rounds. The patient's litany was the same day after day: "I'm not sick. I don't need to be here. I don't need medicines". And regularly she refused doses.

The resident spoke often of her patient to other residents in her class and often found herself ruminating about the patient's abject lostness. She began her regular supervision hours either frustrated or feeling hopeless that anything would change with this patient because the patient flatly refused to acknowledge her disorder. The patient's level of denial was of psychotic proportions. Shortly after a particularly difficult encounter with the patient concerning her refusal to take an evening dose of haloperidol, the resident came to supervision with the report that she had awakened terrorized by dreaming the night before that she had been diagnosed with schizophrenia. She had been intensely affected by overwhelming pain, confusion and despair as she heard the diagnosis in her dream. "IT CAN'T BE!" she screamed, waking herself with a shaking start. "I'M NOT SICK! I DON'T NEED TO BE HERE! I DON'T NEED MEDICINE!" The words of her patient echoed in her mind as her own echoed in her ears. She had taken the patient's story and words home with her and kept them in mind at an unconscious level to be brought up in her dream, the ultimate identification with the patient. How more intensely can one be empathic with her patient than to dream as if she is experiencing the same horrifying reality? The patient and resident continued to struggle, but after the dream the resident was able to approach the patient and her story from a position of understanding the patient's need to maintain a lack of awareness or absence of insight. To acknowledge the presence of the disorder was more than the patient's already fragmented ego could bear. And now the resident "heard" it.

becoming preoccupied and stuck with one's thoughts and feelings about a particular aspect of a patient.

As the verbal interaction with the patient occurs, psychiatrists may find themselves expressing thoughts and feeling in ways that may be quite different from their usual repertoire. The following case is an example.

Clinical Vignette 13

A 45-year-old divorced white woman, being followed for bipolar disorder and borderline personality traits and stable for several years on lithium, was in weekly psychotherapy. During the prior weekend she had moved into another apartment closer to her work. On the day of the move, she overslept and woke up with a start. The admonition to herself as she awoke was, "You lazy bitch! You can never manage on your own". She had earlier, as a child, experienced a mother who was needy, engulfing, punishing, hostile, critical and dependent upon the patient. Her therapist, having some knowledge of the patient and her background, said, "Your mother is still with you. It was she in your head continuing to bombard you with derogatory statements". The same patient was often 10 or 15 minutes late for sessions, and her therapist found herself irritated at the patient's habitual tardiness. To her own surprise and enlightenment, the therapist also found herself thinking, "What a chaotic woman! She'll never manage to be here on time". She, too, had heard the voice of her patient's mother. In the next session she wondered with her patient if she found herself wishing to place her therapist in the position of her mother, wanting at once to be engulfed and punished.

Clinical Vignette 14

A psychiatrist was treating a 40-year-old man who was in the process of recognizing his own primary homosexual orientation. In the course of treatment he became enraged, suicidal, and homicidal. After one session, the psychiatrist, while driving home, experienced the fantasy that when he got home he would find his patient already there, having taken the psychiatrist's family hostage. The psychiatrist became increasingly terrified, even outright paranoid that this fantasy might actually come to pass. The patient was a computer expert who had indeed discovered the unlisted phone number and address of his therapist. But the psychiatrist realized that this fantasy was far out of keeping with his own usual way of feeling and the patient's way of behaving and viewing him. On arriving home to discover his family quite safe, the psychiatrist called the patient and scheduled him as his first for appointment the following morning. When the patient arrived, the psychiatrist said, "You know, I think I'm only now beginning to appreciate just how terrified and desperate all of this makes you". The patient slumped down into his chair, heaved a sigh, and said, "Thank God!"

This sort of listening to oneself in order to understand the patient requires a good working knowledge of projective identification (Ogden, 1979). Projective identification, first defined by Melanie Klein, describes a defense mechanism in which the patient, in an effort to master intolerably terrifying emotions, unconsciously seeks to engender them in the therapist and to identify with the psychiatrist's ability to tolerate and handle the feelings.

Listening in Special Clinical Situations

Children

Listening to younger children often involves inviting them to play and then engaging them in describing what is happening in the play action. The psychiatrist pays careful attention to the child's feelings. These feelings are usually attributed to a doll, puppet, or other humanized toy. So if a child describes a stuffed animal as being scared, the psychiatrist may say, "I wonder if you, too, are scared when…" or "That sounds like you when…". The following case is an example.

Clinical Vignette 15

A 4-year-old boy was brought in for psychiatric evaluation. He and his father had come upon a very serious automobile accident. One person had been thrown from the car and was lying clearly visible on the pavement with arms and legs positioned in grotesque angles, gaping head wound, obviously dead. The child's father was an off duty police officer who stopped to assist in the extraction of two other people trapped in the car. The father kept a careful eye on the youngster who was left in the car. The child observed the scene for about 30 minutes until others arrived on the scene and his dad was able to leave. That night and for days to come, the child preoccupied himself with his toy cars which he repetitiously rammed into each other. He was awakened by nightmares three times in the ensuing weeks. During his evaluation in the play therapy room he engaged in ramming toy cars together. In addition, he tossed dolls about and arranged their limbs haphazardly. As he was encouraged to put some words to his action, he spoke of being frightened of the dead body and of being afraid to be by himself. He was afraid of the possibility of being hurt himself. He came in for three more play sessions which went much the same way. His preoccupation with ramming cars at home diminished and disappeared as did the nightmares. The content of his play was used to help him put words and labels on his scare.

Geriatric Patients

Working with the elderly poses its own special challenges. These challenges include not only the unique developmental issues they face but also the difficulty in verbalizing a lifetime of experience and feelings and, commonly, a disparity in age and life experience between the clinician and the patient.

Clinical Vignette 16

A psychiatrist was asked to examine an 87-year-old white man whom the family believed to be depressed. They stated that he was becoming increasingly detached and disinterested in the goings-on around him. When seen, he was cooperative and compliant, but he stated that he didn't believe he needed to be evaluated. The patient had faced multiple losses over the past few years. After retiring at the age of 65, he had developed the habit of meeting male friends at a coffee shop each morning at 7 am. Now, all but he and one other were dead, and the other was in a nursing home with the cognitive deficits of primary dementia of the Alzheimer's type, preventing his friend from recognizing him when visiting. The patient's wife had died 15 years before after many years of marriage. He had missed her terribly at first but then after a year or so he got on with his life. Several years later, he suffered a retinal detachment that impaired his vision to the point that he was no longer able to drive himself to get about as he once had. What he missed most was the independence of going places when it suited him, rather than relying on his son or grandson to accommodate him within their busy schedules. He had taken to watching televised church services rather than trouble his son to drive him to church. His mind

Clinical Vignette 16 *continued*

remained sharp, he said, but his body was wearing out, and all the people with whom he had shared a common history had died. His answers were "fine" and "all right" when questions of quality of sleep and mood were asked – despite the fact that he had experienced significant nocturia. When questioned about his ability to experience joy, he retorted, "Would you be?" His youngest sister had died the year prior to the evaluation. She was 76 years old and had been on home oxygen for the last 18 months of her life for end-stage chronic obstructive pulmonary disease. He had been particularly close to her because she had been only 3 years old when their mother had died. He had been her caretaker all her life.

Although he denied feelings of guilt, he said that it "wasn't right" that he had outlived the youngest member of his family. His family said that he had taken her death especially hard and was tearful and angry. The focus of his anger during the final stages of her illness was at the young doctors whom he perceived as having given up on her. After her death, it fell to him to dispose of her accumulated possessions as she had no children and her husband had preceded her in death many years before. At first he said that he couldn't face the task. Finally, some 2 months later, he was able to close her estate. During that period of time, he had significant sleep disturbance, reduced energy and his family often experienced him as crotchety and complaining. They and the patient attributed it to mourning her loss. However, recently he was emotionally detached, not very interested in life around him, and they found it particularly alarming that he had said to his son that he was "ready to die". What did all this mean? Was he depressed? Was he physically ill, creating the sense of apathy and disinterest? Was he grieving? He was not suicidal. He did not suffer negative thoughts about his own personhood. He was not having thoughts that he had let anyone down. Together, he and the psychiatrist decided that he was indeed grieving. This time, he was grieving for his own decline and imminent death. He, in fact, was in the final acceptance phase of that process. In a family meeting, in the discussions about the feelings of each member of the family, it became apparent that he was facing the end of life, which evoked many emotions in those who loved him.

It is challenging to elicit the elements of a story especially when they span generations. The elderly are often stoic. In the face of losses that mark the closing years of life, denial often becomes a healthy tool allowing one to accept and cope with declining abilities and the loss of loved ones. The psychiatrist must appreciate that grief and depression can often be similar in some respects.

Chronically Mentally III

Listening to the chronically mentally ill can be especially challenging, too. The unique choice of words characteristic of many who have a thought disorder requires that the physician search for the meanings of certain words and phrases that may be peculiar and truly eccentric. Clinical Vignettes 1, 10 and 12 are examples of this important challenge for the psychiatric listener.

Clinical Vignette 17

A young man with schizotypal personality disorder and obsessive–compulsive disorder presented for months using adjectives describing himself as "broken and fragmented". Only after listening carefully, not aided by the expected or normal affect of a depressed person, was the psychiatrist able to discern that his patient was clinically depressed but did not have the usual words to say it or was unable to discuss it.

Clinical Vignette 18

A 32-year-old black woman who had multiple hospitalizations for schizophrenia and lived with her mother was seen in the community psychiatric center for routine medication follow-up. Her psychiatrist found her to have an increase in the frequency of auditory hallucinations, especially ones of a derogatory nature. The voices were tormenting her with the ideas that she was not good, that she should die, that she was worthless and unloved. Her psychiatrist heard her say that she had wrecked her mother's car 2 weeks previously. The streets had been wet and the tires worn. She had slid into the rear of a car that had come to an abrupt stop ahead of her on a freeway. Although her mother had not been critical or judgmental, the patient felt overwhelming guilt as she watched her mother struggle to arrange transportation for herself each day to and from work.

Chronically psychiatrically disabled patients may have a unique way of presenting their inner world experiences. Sometimes the link to the outer world is not so apparent. The psychiatrist is regularly challenged with making sense of the meanings of the content and changes in intensity or frequency of the psychotic symptoms.

Physically III Patients

In consultations with a colleague in a medical or surgical specialty one is evaluating a patient who has a chronic or acute physical illness. The psychiatrist must listen to the story of the patient but also keep in mind the story as reflected in the hospital records and medical and nursing staff. Then the psychiatrist serves as the liaison not only between psychiatry and other medical colleagues, but also between the patient and his caregivers.

Clinical Vignette 19

A 35-year-old woman was hospitalized for complications of a pancreas/kidney transplant that was completed 20 months previously. Prior to surgery she had been on dialysis for over a year awaiting a tissue match for transplantation. That year she had been forced to take a leave of absence from her job as a social worker with a local child and adolescent community center. At the time of this hospitalization, she had been back at work for only 8 months when she developed a urinary tract infection that did not respond to several antibiotics. Her renal function was deteriorating and her doctors found her to be paranoid, hostile and labile. Her physicians dreaded going into her room each morning and began distancing themselves from her.

Psychiatric consultation was sought following a particularly difficult interaction between the patient and her charge nurse, the leader of the transplant team and the infectious disease expert. She was hostile, blaming, agitated, circumstantial, refused further medications and pulled out her intravenous lines. The consultation requested assistance in hospital management.

When interviewed, the patient was lying quietly in bed but visibly stiffened when the psychiatrist introduced herself. She very quickly exhibited the symptoms described in the consultation. This patient had struggled with juvenile onset diabetes since the age of nine. Despite the fact that she consistently complied with diet and insulin, control of blood sugars had always been difficult. As complication after complication occurred, she often developed the belief that her physicians thought that she was a "bad" patient. And now, the hope that her life would normalize to the point that she could carry on with her career was dashed. She felt misunderstood and alone in her struggle with long-term, chronic illness. The psychiatrist resonated with the story emotionally and listened for ways to address symptoms from a biological standpoint as well. The patient felt reassured that someone was there to appreciate the tragic turn that her life had taken.

Growing and Maturing as a Listener

Transference/countertransference influence not only relationships in traditional psychotherapy but also interactions between all physicians and patients and is always present as a filter or reverberator to that which is heard. However, even the most experienced of listeners are not always aware of the ways in which their patients' stories are impacted by countertransference. Patients come, too, with tendencies and predispositions to experience the listener, the other person in the therapeutic dyad, in familiar but distorted fashion. The patient may idealize and adapt to interpretations. She/he may be hostile and distrustful, identifying the psychiatrist in an unconscious way with one who has been rejecting in the past. Listening to the "flow of consciousness", the psychiatrist discerns a thread of continuity and purposefulness in the patient's communications. As the psychiatrist becomes more and more familiar with his patient, he will discover the connections between threads and the meaning will become apparent. This awareness may come as a sign and symptom, fantasy, feeling, or fact.

There is an increasing recognition that to be a healing listener one must be able to bear the burden of hearing what is told. Like the patient, we fear what might be said. A patient's story may be one of rage in response to early childhood attachment ruptures or abuse, of sadness as losses are remembered, or of terror in response to disorganization during the experience of perceptual abnormalities accompanying psychotic breaks. The patient's stories invariably invoke anger, shame, guilt, abject helplessness, or sexual feelings within the listener. These feelings, unless attended to, appreciated and understood will block the listening that is essential for healing to take place.

Every insight is colored by what the listener has known. It is impossible to know that which is not experienced. The psychiatrist comes with his own experiences and the experiences he has had with others. To listen in the manner we are describing here is another way of truly experiencing the world. The experiences include the imaginings of how it must be to be 87 years old as a patient when one is a 35-year-old doctor just finishing residency; to be female when one is male; to be a child again; to grow up African-American in a small white suburb of a large city; to be an immigrant in a new country; to be Middle Eastern when one is Western European, and so on. One comes to know by listening with imagination, allowing the words of the patient to resonate with one's own experiences or with what one has come to know through hearing with imagination the stories of other patients or listening to the thoughts or insights of supervisors.

The best psychiatrists continue all their professional lives to learn how to listen better. This may be thought of not only as a matter of mastering countertransference but of self-education. One must learn to recognize when there are impasses in the treatment and to seek education, from a colleague or, perhaps, even from the patient. Consider these two examples.

Clinical Vignette 20

A Jewish resident was treating an 8-year-old Catholic boy who came in one day and mentioned offhandedly that he was about to go to his first confession. The psychiatric resident made no particular note of the issue and kept on listening to the boy's play and its themes. He noted that guilt, which had been an ongoing theme, was prominent again. When he presented the session in supervision the supervisor wondered about the connection. It emerged that there was a large gulf between the therapist and the boy. Jewish concepts of sin and atonement are different from Christian ones, and the rituals surrounding them have rather different intentions and ideas of resolution. The resident had missed the opportunity to explore the young boy's first introduction, within his religious context, to the belief in a forgiving God, a potentially important step in helping the child to resolve his ongoing struggles with guilt over his own greedy impulses.

Clinical Vignette 21

A psychiatrist began treating a Nigerian native who was suffering from post traumatic stress disorder (PTSD) after being assaulted at work. After several sessions, the psychiatrist felt a sense of being at a loss in terms of what the patient was expecting out of their work and how the therapist was being seen by the patient. He then took several sessions to inquire of the patient about his tribe, its structure, family roles, definitions of healing, ideas of illness and wellness, etc. After this exploration, the psychiatrist adopted a different stance with the patient, heard the patient's communications very differently, and the therapy proceeded much more smoothly and comfortably to a successful conclusion.

How can the psychiatrist's demeanor convey to the patient that he is safe to tell his story, that the listener is one who can be trusted to be with him, to worry with him, and serve as a helper? Much is written about the demeanor of the psychiatrist. The air, deportment, manner, or bearing is one of quiet anticipation – to receive that which the patient has come to tell and share in the telling. Signals of anticipation and curiosity may be conveyed by such statements as "I've thought about what you said last time," "How do you feel about…?" "What if…?"

Efforts of clarification often serve as bridges between sessions and communicate that the listener is committed to a fuller understanding of the patient. Patients have the need to experience the psychiatrist as empathic. Empathy describes the feeling one has in hearing a story which causes one to conjure up or imagine how it would have been to have actually have had an experience oneself. How does one integrate all this so that it is automatic but not deadened by automaticity? How does the psychiatrist continue to hear the "same old thing" with freshness and renewal? How does one encourage the patient with consistency, clarity, and assurance in the face of uncertainty and occasional confusion? Not by assurance that everything will be all right when things might probably not be. Not by attempting to talk the patient into seeing things the clinician's way but rather by the psychiatrist's having the capacity to hear things his patient's way, from the patient's perspective.

Psychiatry is one of those rare disciplines where the experience of listening over and over again allows the listener to grow in their capacities to hear and to heal. Hopefully, we get better and better as the years advance, become smoother, and develop a style which blends with our personality and training. We are renewed by the shared experiences with our patients.

To hear stories of the human condition reminds the psychiatrist that he, too, is human. There is time to make discoveries in the patient's stories from previous times, and maybe in previous patients. Patients will always endeavor to tell their stories. The psychiatrist continues to grow by being the perpetual student, always with the ear for the lesson, the remarkable life stories of his patients.

References

American Psychiatric Association (1994) *Diagnostic and Statistical Manual of Mental* Disorders, 4th edn. APA, Washington DC.

American Psychiatric Association (2001) *Annual Survey of Residents.* APA, Washington DC.

Arieti S (1967) *The Intrapsychic Self Feelings, Cognitions, and Creativity in Mental Health* and Mental Illness. Basic Books, New York.

Binswanger L (1963) *Being in the World.* Basic Books, New York.

Brill AA (ed) (1938) *The Basic Writings of Sigmund Freud.* Random House Modern Library, New York.

Brothers L (1989) A biological perspective on empathy. *Am J Psychiatr* 146, 10–19.

Carroll J and Whorf B (1956) *Language, Thought and Reality.* MIT Press, Boston, MA.

Chomsky N (1972) *Language and Mind.* Harcourt Brace Jovanovich, New York.

Cobb S (1976) Social support as a moderator of life stress. *Psychosom Med* 38(5), 300–314.

Comas-Diaz L and Jacobsen S (1991) Ethnocultural transference and Countertransference in the therapeutic dyad. *Am J Orthopsychiatr* 61, 392–402.

Damasio AR (1994) *Descartes' Error: Emotion, Reason and the Human Brain.* Avon Books, New York.

Darwin C (1955) *The Expression of Emotion in Man and Animals.* Philosophical Library, New York.

Descartes R (1991) *The Philosophical Writings of Descartes.* Cambridge University Press, Cambridge, UK.

Edelson M (1993) telling and enacting stories in psychoanalysis and psychotherapy. *Psychoanal Stud Child* 48, 293–325.

Ekman P (1992) Facial expressions of emotion: an old controversy and new findings. *Transact Roy Soc Lond Biol* 335, 63–69.

Elkin I, Shea MT, Watkins JT *et al.* (1989) National Institute of Mental Health Treatment of Depression Collaborative Research Program: General effectiveness of treatments. *Arch Gen Psychiatr* 46(11), 971–982.

Frank JD (1973) *Persuasion and Healing: A Comparative Study of Psychotherapy.* Schocken Books, New York.

Freud A (1946) *The Ego and the Mechanisms of Defense.* International Universities Press, New York.

Gabbard GO (2000) A neurobiologically informed perspective on psychotherapy. *Br J Psychiatr* 177, 117–122.

Greenberg JR and Mitchell SA (1983) *Object Relations in Psychoanalytic Theory.* Harvard University Press, Cambridge, MA.

Greenson RR (1978) *Explorations in Psychoanalysis.* International Universities Press, New York.

Heim C and Nemeroff CB (2001) The role of childhood trauma in the neurobiology of mood and anxiety disorders: Preclinical and clinical studies. *Biol Psychiatr* 49(12), 1023–1039.

Hofer MA (1996) On the nature and consequences of early loss. *Psychosom Med* 58(6), 570–581.

Horvath AO and Luborsky L (1993) The role of the therapeutic alliance in psychotherapy. *J Consult Clin Psychol* 61(4), 561–573.

Husserl E (1977) *Cartesian Meditations: An Introduction to Phenomenology.* Martinus Nijhoff Publishers, Dordrecht, Netherlands.

Jackson S (1992) The listening healer in the history of psychological healing. *Am J Psychiatr* 149(12), 1623–1632.

Kandel ER (1999) Biology and the future of psychoanalysis: A new intellectual framework for psychiatry revisited. *Am J Psychiatr* 156(4), 505–524.

Klein M (1975) *Envy and Gratitude.* Dell, New York, pp. 1946–1973.

Kleinman A (2001) Cross-cultural psychiatry: A psychiatric perspective on global change. *Harv Rev Psychiatr* 9(1), 46–47.

Kochman T (1991) *Black and White: Styles in Conflict.* University of Chicago Press, Chicago, IL.

Kohut H (1991) *The Search for the Self: Selected Writings of Heinz Kohut.* International Universities Press, Madison, CT, pp. 1978–1981.

LeDoux J (1996) *The Emotional Brain: The Mysterious Underpinnings of Emotional Life.* Simon & Shuster, New York.

Liggan DY and Kay J (1999) Some neurobiological aspects of psychotherapy. A review. *J Psychother Pract Res* 8(2), 103–114.

Mahler M, Pine F and Bergman A (1975) *The Psychological Birth of the Human Infant.* Basic Books, New York.

May R, Angel E and Ellenberger HF (eds) (1958) *Existence: A New Dimension in Psychiatry and Psychology.* Basic Books, New York.

McHugh PR and Slavney PR (1986) *Perspectives of Psychiatry.* Johns Hopkins University Press, Baltimore, MD.

Meaney MJ (2001) Maternal care, gene expression, and the transmission of individual differences in stress reactivity across generations. *Annu Rev Neurosci* 24, 1161–1192.

Mohn PC (1987) Should psychotherapy be considered a biological treatment? *Psychosomatics* 28(6), 321–326.

Ogden TH (1979) On projective identification. *Int J Psychoanal* 60(Pt 3), 357–373.

Omer H and London P (1989) Signal and noise in psychotherapy: The role and control of nonspecific factors. *Br J Psychiatr* 155, 239–245.

Peteet JR (1982) A closer look at the concept of support: Some application to the care of patients with cancer. *Gen Hosp Psychiatr* 4(1), 19–23.

Reik T (1954) *Listening with the Third Ear. Inner Experience of a Psychoanalyst.* Farrar, Straus, New York.

Rogers CR (1951) *Client Centered Therapy: Its Current Practice, Implications and Theory.* Houghton Mifflin, Boston, MA.

Sapir E (2000) *Language, An Introduction to the Study of Speech.* Bartleby.com, New York.

Schore AN (2001) The effects of a secure attachment relationship. Right brain development, affect regulation, and infant mental health. *Inf Ment Health* J 22, 7–66.

Sullivan HS (1953) *Conceptions of Modern Psychiatry.* WW Norton, New York.

Sullivan HS (1969) *Schizophrenia as a Human Process.* WW Norton, New York.

Styron W (1990) *Darkness Visible.* Random House Books, New York.

Tiger L and Fox R (1971) *The Imperial Animal.* Holt, Rinehart & Winston, New York.

Tomkins SS and McCarter R (1964) What and where are the primary affects? Some evidence for a theory. *Percept Motor Skills* 18, 119–158.

Truax CB (1963) The empirical emphasis in psychotherapy: A symposium. Effective ingredients in psychotherapy: An approach to unraveling the patient–therapist interaction. *J Counsel Psychol* 10(3), 256–263.

World Health Organization (1992) *International Classification of Diseases*, 10th Rev. WHO, Geneva.

The Cultural Context of Clinical Assessment

Introduction: The Cultural Matrix of Psychiatry

Although it has long been recognized that the mode of expressing psychological distress and behavioral disturbances varies with cultural beliefs and practices, a growing body of evidence shows that the effects of culture are more far-reaching. Research has clearly demonstrated that the causes, course and outcome of major psychiatric disorders are influenced by cultural factors (Kleinman, 1988; Kirmayer, 2001; Leff, 2001; Lopez and Guarnaccia, 2000). Wide variations in the prevalence of many psychiatric disorders across geographic regions and ethnocultural groups have been documented with current standardized epidemiological survey methods (Canino et al., 1997; Kirmayer and Groleau, 2001). In addition, social and cultural factors are major determinants of the use of health care services and alternative sources of help (Rogler and Cortes, 1993).

For all of these reasons, careful assessment of the cultural context of psychiatric problems must form a central part of any clinical evaluation (GAP, 2002). Beyond this, culturally based attitudes and assumptions govern the perspectives that both patient and clinician bring to the clinical encounter. Lack of awareness of important differences can undermine the development of a therapeutic alliance and the negotiation and delivery of effective treatment.

The changing demography of North America and around the world has made the recognition and response to cultural diversity increasingly important in psychiatric practice (GAP, 2002). The overarching ideology took for granted that newcomers would gradually become just like all others through a process of cultural assimilation (Portes and Rumbaut, 1996; Susser and Patterson, 2001). However, sociological research has shown a high degree of retention of ethnic culture with the persistence of religious practices, family life-cycle rituals and ethnic enclaves in many cities. Added to this is the recognition of the importance of maintaining and renewing ethnocultural identity to combat the legacy of racial discrimination. This has led to rethinking the notion of assimilation to take into account other modes of acculturation including the development of multiple cultural identities. More recent waves of global migration from south to north and east to west have brought together new mixes of peoples with greater differences in their cultural assumptions, with corresponding challenges for intercultural clinical work.

These changes, along with larger forces of globalization, have encouraged a fresh look at culture in every area of psychiatry. In clinical practice, "cultural competence" has become the rubric under which to advance a broad range of skills and perspectives pertinent to working with a culturally diverse clinical population (GAP, 2002). In the sections that follow, we will summarize some of the concepts and approaches that can inform culturally competent clinical practice.

What Is Culture?

There is a famous saying to the effect that we do not know who discovered water but it was not the fish. So it is with culture: we are immersed in our own cultural worlds from birth, and consequently our culture is largely implicit and unexamined. Just as we are unconscious of many of our own motivations and patterns of thought and behavior until they are reflected back to us by others, so too are we unconscious of our cultural background knowledge and assumptions. Bringing the cultural unconscious to light may be more difficult than facing the individual unconscious because institutions and others around us may reinforce our assumptions and resist any attempt to question them. Our explicit appreciation of culture usually comes from intercultural encounters, which make us suddenly aware of culture through difference. More formally, anthropological research comparing different cultures allows us to see the tacit assumptions of our own worldviews. There is no substitute for this sort of systematic reflection on cultural difference, which should extend to the critical analysis of the construction of psychiatric knowledge (Lock and Gordon, 1988; Young, 1995).

Older views of culture were based on ethnographic studies of relatively isolated small-scale societies. Many accounts tended to assume that cultures were finely balanced systems and that, as a result, everything was for a purpose and had an adaptive function for the group (if not always for the individual). The outsider was thus cautioned not to pass judgment on cultural differences or to see pathology where there was simply difference. This is still wise advice. However, it is clear that cultures are not homeostatic systems in a steady state or equilibrium but are constantly shifting and evolving systems. They may be riven by conflict and create maladaptive circumstances not only for disadvantaged individuals but for specific groups or even the society as a whole. Thus, while refraining from prejudging specific cultural values or practices, the clinician must nevertheless consider that every culture encompasses practices that may help or hinder patients, and aggravate or ameliorate any given type of psychopathology. Each society tends to cultivate blind spots around the specific forms of social suffering that it produces (Kleinman et al., 1997). Openness, respect and capacity for collective self-criticism are thus key elements of any transcultural clinical encounter.

Essentials of Psychiatry   Jerald Kay and Allan Tasman
© 2006 John Wiley & Sons, Ltd.

At the same time, anthropologists have come to recognize the high level of individual variability within even small cultural groups and the active ways in which individuals and groups make use of a variety of forms of knowledge to fashion an identity and a viable way of living. In urban settings where many cultures meet, individuals have a wide range of options available and can position themselves both within and against any given ethnocultural identity or way of living. This has led anthropologists to rethink the notion of culture or even to suggest that it has outlived its usefulness.

Indeed, the modern world includes forms of electronic communication and rapid transportation that have begun to weave the whole globe together in new ways. This results in the intermixing of cultural worlds and the creation of new ethnocultural groups and individuals with multiple or hybrid identities. Many people now see themselves as transnational, with networks of affiliation and support that span great distances. The mental health implications of these new forms of identity and community have been little explored and will be an increasingly important issue for psychiatry in the years to come (Bibeau, 1997; Kirmayer and Minas, 2000).

As this brief discussion makes clear, the notion of culture covers a broad territory. It is useful precisely because of this breadth, but to apply it to clinical practice we need to make some further specifications and distinctions. In the North American context, it is useful to distinguish notions of race, ethnicity and social class from culture.

Race is a term used to mark off groups within and between societies. Racial distinctions generally reflect a few superficial physical characteristics and hence have little correlation with clinically relevant genetic variation. The boundaries of any racial group are socially defined and have no biological reality (Graves, 2001). Race is usually ascribed by others and cannot readily be changed or discarded unless larger social criteria change. Race is significant as a social category that is employed in racist and discriminatory practices. Racism is clinically important because of its effects on mental and physical health and the challenge it presents to both individual and collective self-esteem.

Ethnicity refers to the collective identity of a group based on common heritage, which may include language, religion, geographic origin and specific cultural practices. Ethnic identity is often constructed *vis-à-vis* others and a dominant society. Hence, it is sometimes assumed that "foreigners" or minorities have ethnicity while the dominant group (e.g., Americans of British or northern European extraction) does not. This obscures the fact that everyone may become aware of an ethnic identity in the right context (in China, an American clearly has a distinct ethnicity). Ethnicity may be chosen or ascribed by others. For example, the US census defined five ethnoracial blocs: White, African-American, Hispanic, Asian-American and Pacific Islander, and American Indian and Alaska Native. These are heterogeneous categories variously based on race, language, geographic origin and ethnicity. Although the categories are fictive, they have acquired practical and political reality because they have been used to present epidemiological findings and define health service needs (Hollinger, 1995). Nevertheless, the clinician must recognize that to meet the patient on a common ground requires a much more fine-grained notion of ethnocultural identity than afforded by these crude categories.

Finally, social class reflects the fact that most societies are economically stratified and individuals' opportunities, mobility, lifestyle and response to illness are heavily constrained by their economic position. Issues of poverty, unemployment, powerlessness and marginalization may overshadow cultural factors as causes of illness and influences on identity and help-seeking behavior. Violence is a particularly striking example in North American society of the overlap of exclusion, poverty, discrimination and intergenerational transmission of trauma.

The notion of culture is sometimes extended to speak of various subcultures or the cultures of professions. In this sense, we can speak of the cultures of biomedicine and of psychiatry. Each of these systems of knowledge includes a wide range of behavioral norms and institutional practices that may be familiar to clinicians but novel and confusing to patients. However, familiar cultural notions of self and personhood underwrite these technical domains, which therefore serve to reinforce larger cultural ideologies (Lock and Gordon, 1988). This becomes clear when we consider alternative systems of medicine such as traditional Chinese medicine or Indian Ayurveda, which are based on different notions of the person (ethnopsychology), the body (ethnophysiology), different roles for patient and healer, and, indeed, different epistemologies (Leslie and Young, 1992). Even the understanding and practice of biomedicine may differ across countries, so the clinician should not assume that familiar terms always refer to the same practice.

Culture and Gender

Gender refers to the ways in which cultures differentiate and define roles based on biological sex or reproductive functions. Because of this link with physical aspects of sex, there is a tendency to view gender differences as biological givens. However, while some distinctions may be closely related to the physiological differences between males and females, most are assigned to the sexes on the basis of specific cultural beliefs and social organization (Comas-Diaz and Greene, 1994).

Men and women do have some fundamentally different experiences of their bodies, of their social worlds and of their life course. It has been suggested that women are more in touch with their bodies because of the experiences of menstruation, childbearing, childbirth, breast-feeding and menopause. These differences may be as substantial as any between disparate cultures. At the same time, there is much evidence that these bodily grounded experiences vary substantially across cultures. For example, the anthropologist Margaret Lock (1993) has shown that Japanese women report fewer bodily symptoms of menopause and do not think of the end of menstruation as a distinctive "change of life" in the same terms as many women in North America.

There are also important gender differences in styles of emotional expression, symptom experience, and help-seeking. In epidemiological surveys in the USA, women tend to report more somatic symptoms as well as more emotional distress and they are more likely to seek help for psychological or interpersonal problems. However, the gender difference in symptom reporting varies significantly cross-nationally (Piccinelli and Simon, 1997).

In North America, important differences have been documented in male and female styles of conversation that are relevant to the clinical context (Tannen, 1994). In general, women tend to give more frequent acknowledgments that they are listening to a speaker. They may give signs of assent simply to indicate they are following the conversation. Men tend to be more taciturn and, if they signal assent, it usually means they actually agree with the speaker. These differences in communication style may lead to systematic misunderstandings between men and women that are further aggravated by cultural differences in gender roles and etiquette.

Clinical Vignette 1

When an ultra-orthodox Jewish family arrives for their consultation, the female psychiatrist, who is dressed in a short skirt, welcomes them offering her hand to the father in greeting. He is confused and offended, avoiding eye contact and reluctant to proceed with the session. The female doctor's style of dress and friendly handshake were viewed as disrespectful or as indicating her lack of familiarity with norms of conduct with observant orthodox families.

In many societies, gender is associated with marked differences in power and social status. For example, in patriarchal societies, men have specific power and privileges that give them a measure of control over the lives of women. This is often coupled with responsibilities for maintaining family honor and well-being. In recent years, North American society has espoused social and political equality in gender roles. From this egalitarian point of view, patriarchal families may seem oppressive to women. However, women may accept and participate in cultural definitions of their roles that appear restrictive by North American cultural norms but that make family life meaningful. Any judgment as to whether a given family's relationships are oppressive or pathological must not only take into account social norms and practices but also explore the meaning of issues and events for the individuals involved.

Clinical Vignette 2

A 29-year-old East Indian woman, in the US for 6 months, presents with symptoms of depression and PTSD. Throughout the initial evaluation, the patient looks away from the male psychiatrist, never making eye contact. The interviewer is concerned that he may have offended the woman in some way. The female interpreter explains that the patient is showing respect by not looking directly at a male in authority.

Differences in cultural definitions of gender roles may become sources of conflict after migration. Culturally prescribed patterns of marriage and child bearing may be central to the social status, identity and self-esteem of men and women even when they are not given the same importance in the dominant culture.

Clinical Vignette 3

A 28-year-old woman from South Asia has an arranged marriage with an older man from the same religious community, who has lived all of his life in the USA. The couple has been unable to conceive for 5 years and is in the midst of extensive infertility treatments. The husband complains that she is paranoid and does not want to work or go out of the house. The woman tearfully relates that she feels depressed and ashamed because of her predicament and fears that her marriage will end if she cannot bear children.

Table 2.1   DSM-IV Outline for the Cultural Formulation

- identity of the individual
- explanations of the illness
- psychosocial environment and levels of functioning
- relationship between the individual and the clinician
- overall assessment with implications for diagnosis and care

Reprinted with permission from the Diagnostic and Statistical Manual of Mental Disorders, Fourth Ed, Text revision. Copyright 2000, American Psychiatric Association.

The Cultural Formulation

In an effort to address the cultural dimensions of clinical assessment, DSM-IV-TR introduced an outline for a cultural formulation (Table 2.1). This outline covers major areas that a clinician should explore in a comprehensive evaluation. These are integrated in a formulation that helps to account for symptomatology, diagnosis, prognosis and appropriate treatment (Lewis-Fernandez, 1996; see also Chapter 21). The formulation may go well beyond the DSM-IV-TR categories to consider many sorts of problems and predicaments relevant to the patient's well-being.

The cultural formulation is merely intended as a checklist or reminder to encourage the clinician to perform the needed exploration and integration of a broad range of relevant social and cultural information. Clearly, cultural considerations may apply to every aspect of the clinical assessment and interview and must not be used only as an afterthought to the standard psychiatric interview.

Ethnocultural Identity

The first dimension of the cultural formulation involves ethnocultural identity. This includes the individual's ethnic or cultural reference groups and the position of these groups *vis-à-vis* the larger society. Certain groups have a specific ethnocultural identity ascribed to them by others; this may have an impact on individuals' everyday experience and narratives of identity whether or not they are explicitly aware of it.

In a world of mass migration and intermingling of peoples over generations, identity is very often hybrid, multiple and fluid (Bibeau, 1997). For immigrant and ethnic minorities it is important to understand the degree of involvement with both the culture of origin and the host culture. Ethnic identity may be situational and shift with social context. The ethnocultural and religious groups with which the patient most identifies may depend on who asks the question and in what context. For example, whether someone self-identifies as Canadian, West Indian or Trinidadian may depend on the perceived identity of the interviewer and the setting where the interview takes place.

Language is central to identity for many people and has a profound effect on clinical encounters. Individuals who speak multiple languages, learned at different stages in their life, may have different memories, affect and interpersonal schemas associated with the use of each language. Languages may be associated with developmentally important relationships and tied to specific areas of conflict or mastery. Personal and political allegiances within the family and community may be expressed through choice of language.

Language is the medium through which experience is articulated; hence, the assessment of higher cognitive functions, complex emotions and experiential symptoms of pathology all depend on the clinician's access to the patient's language. Patients who are hobbled in a second language may be misjudged as less intelligent or competent than they are in fact; wishing to avoid such bias, clinicians may be overly generous in their assessment and miss significant problems or pathology.

Even where patients have a moderate level of facility in the clinician's preferred language, they may not express themselves fully in a second language so that important details are not conveyed. The use of a second language not only affects doctor–patient communication, it also influences individuals' ability to reflect about themselves. When patients are forced to formulate their problems in a language in which they are not proficient, they may be less creative and effective as problem solvers. When patients are able to use their own best language, their accounts of experience become much richer, more complex and nuanced; their thinking is subtler; they can express a wider range of affect and engage in playful therapeutic exchanges.

Multilingual people sometimes report that they feel and think differently when using a second language. In part, this is due to the cognitive effort of having to find words in a language in which one is not totally fluent. Since each language favors certain modes of expression and ways of thinking, bilingual speakers may report that they feel like a different person in their other language. It follows that aspects of the history and experience of a patient can be less accessible in a clinical evaluation if patients are not able to express themselves in the appropriate language. Of course, use of a second language may also afford the patient some distance from intense emotions and painful memories, and so assist in coping and affect regulation. Careful attention to spontaneous or strategic shifts in use of language in a multilingual assessment can provide the clinician with important information about areas of conflict and strengths. Often this requires the use of a trained interpreter, as discussed later in this chapter.

Religion is another key marker of identity. For many individuals and communities, it may structure the moral world more strongly than ethnic or national identity. The term "spirituality" has gained currency to acknowledge the fact that many individuals maintain deeply held personal beliefs about God, the meaning of life and what happens after death, without being formally affiliated with one religion or another. Religious affiliation is also a frequent source of discrimination.

Despite the ubiquity of religious and spiritual experience, it is frequently neglected during routine psychiatric evaluation. A thorough cultural formulation requires consideration of the patient's religion and spirituality. Areas to cover include religious identity, the role of religion in the family of origin, current religious practices (attendance at services, public and private rituals), motivation for religious behavior (i.e., religious orientation), and specific beliefs of individuals and of their family and community.

Illness Explanations and Help-seeking

The second major dimension of the cultural formulation concerns cultural explanations of symptoms and illness. Cultures provide systems of diagnosis and treatment of illness and affliction that may influence patients' experience of illness and help-seeking behavior. People label and interpret their distress based on these systems of knowledge, which they share with others around them. Much

Table 2.2	Explanatory Model Interview

1. What do you call your problem?
2. What causes your problem?
3. Why do you think it started when it did?
4. How does it work?
5. What is going on in your body?
6. What kind of treatment do you think would be best for this problem?
7. How has this problem affected your life?
8. What frightens or concerns you most about this problem or treatment?

Source: Kleinman A, Eisenberg L and Good B (1978) Culture, illness, and care: Clinical lessons from anthropologic and cross-cultural research. *Ann Intern Med* 88, 251–258. Reproduced by permission of American College of Physicians.

research in medical anthropology has developed the idea of explanatory models, which may include accounts of causality, mechanism or process, course, appropriate treatment, expected outcome and consequences. Not all of this knowledge is related directly to personal experience – much of it resides in cultural knowledge and practices carried by others. Hence, understanding the cultural meanings of symptoms and behavior may require interviews with other people in the patient's family, entourage, or community.

Table 2.2 provides questions for eliciting patients' explanatory models. These questions should be modified based on the patient's responses. For example, the origins of problems may be located not in the body but in the workings of the mind, the family, the community, the realms of ancestors or spirits, or in mythological accounts that explain the social and moral order.

In many cases, particularly with acute illness, patients may not have well-developed explanatory models. Instead, they reason by analogy on the basis of past experiences of their own or other prominent prototypes encountered in family, friends, or mass media. Once an explanatory model is evoked in conversation, however, patients may give formulaic accounts that accord with that cultural model or script. Therefore, to obtain more complete information about the cognitive and social factors that are actually influencing the patients' illness experience and behavior, it is useful to begin with an open-ended interview that simply aims to reconstruct the events surrounding symptoms and the illness experience. This will reveal idiosyncratic temporal patterns of contiguity and association that may not fit any explicit cultural model. Following this, the clinician can ask about prototypes (Have you ever had anything like this before? Has anyone you know ever had anything like this before?) This will uncover salient models of illness that may shape illness experience and be used to reason analogically about the current episode. Finally, it is important to inquire into explicit cultural models using the sorts of questions devised for the explanatory model interview.

The ethnomedical systems described in anthropological texts often are idealized and complex portraits pieced together by working with cultural experts. In clinical practice, patients usually have only partial or fragmentary knowledge of the traditional explanations and treatment for their problem. Depending on the knowledge and attitudes of family and kin, and on the availability of practitioners of traditional medical systems, patients may be influenced by larger cultural systems to which they themselves do not fully subscribe.

Clinical Vignette 4

A family from Nigeria consults for developmental delay in their 4-year-old son. Problems had become evident when they attempted to integrate the child into a preschool program. The child presents a classical profile of pervasive developmental disorder. The parents comment that their family doctor raised the possibility of autism but that they did not consider that what he described applied to their son. They explain that the migration process, when the child was two, had hindered his acquisition of speech and social activities. After a few sessions it becomes apparent that the child's difficulties had already been recognized in Nigeria but were attributed by both the maternal and the paternal lineage to sorcery on the other side of the family because they were in conflict.

In everyday life, people use culturally prescribed idioms to discuss their problems. These cultural idioms of distress cut across specific diagnostic categories. They may be used to talk about ordinary problems as well as to shape the expression of distress associated with major psychiatric disorders. For example, many cultures have notions of "nerves" (in Spanish, *nervios*), which signal emotional distress that may range from mild upset with life events to disabling anxiety or psychosis. Appendix I of DSM-IV-TR provides a list of some common idioms of distress. The same appendix also lists some well-described culture bound syndromes, culturally distinctive clusters of symptoms that may be of pathological significance. Many culture-specific terms, however, do not refer to syndromes or idioms of distress but are actually symptoms or illness attributions that reference folk models of causality. For example, **susto**, a term used in Central and South America, attributes a wide range of bodily symptoms and diseases (including infectious diseases and congenital malformations) to the damaging effects of sudden fright.

Many cultural idioms of distress use bodily metaphors for experience. In seeking medical help, patients usually try to present the sort of problems they believe the clinician is competent to treat. Consequently, in biomedical settings patients tend to emphasize physical symptoms. This pattern of clinical presentation combined with the wide currency of somatic idioms of distress has led to a characterization of many ethnocultural groups as prone to somatize their distress (Kirmayer, 2001). The social stigma commonly associated with psychiatric symptoms and disorders, as well as with substance abuse, antisocial behavior and various other behaviors also may prevent patients from acknowledging such problems and events. However, with clear communication and a respectful stance, the clinician may be able to build sufficient trust over time for patients to disclose shameful or potentially stigmatizing information.

Similarly, people commonly use multiple remedies or consult various healers for their symptoms, and may be reluctant to disclose treatments they think the clinician will not understand or accept. They may also omit mention of preparations they view as "natural" or as foods and hence not included under the rubric of medications or drugs. Commonly used remedies like ginseng, St John's Wort and *Gingko biloba* have significant effects on pharmacokinetics and drug metabolism (see Chapter 76) and are, therefore, important for their potential impact on physiology as well as their role in patients' belief systems and sense of control over their illness. A nonjudgmental inquiry by the clinician will enable patients more freely to discuss their use of traditional and alternative treatments.

Psychosocial Environment and Levels of Functioning

Cultural factors have a dual influence on the psychosocial environment: they determine life circumstances and, at the same time, provide interpretations of their meaning and significance for the individual. This dual effect of culture means that the clinician must explore both events and their personal and cultural meanings to understand the impact of the social environment.

There are wide cultural variations in the composition and functioning of families including the variety of people living together in a household (not always identical to the family or kin); who is considered close or distant kin; hierarchy, power structure and economic arrangements; age and gender roles; organization of household activities and routines; styles of expression of emotion and distress; body practices (arrangements and procedures for sleeping, eating, washing, dressing, recreation and use of physical remedies for ailments); conflict management strategies; and the relationship of family to larger social networks and communities.

Social support must be assessed with attention to cultural configurations of the family and community. Extended multigenerational families, tightly knit religious and ethnocultural communities, and transnational networks all may provide specific forms of instrumental and emotional support. Often these supports are inextricably intertwined with interpersonal obligations and demands that may constitute burdens for the individual. This complex relationship of burden and support may have crucial implications for clinical interventions.

Clinical Vignette 5

A woman from South Asia appears to have a severe depression with vegetative symptoms and persistent suicidal ideation. She does not respond to trials of several antidepressant medications. On reassessment with a clinician who speaks her language, she reveals that her husband has an unpaid debt of honor to her daughter's husband's family, and she is suffering from the ongoing feud, which has barred her from seeing her daughter and grandchildren. When this is addressed in a series of family therapy sessions, her "depression" lifts dramatically.

Similarly, levels of functioning and disability must be assessed against culturally determined notions of social roles and values. It is important to recognize that the clinician's priority may not be the most important issue for patients or their families.

In addition to these general cultural considerations, certain social situations present specific stressors with which the clinician must become familiar. All immigrants and refugees have arrived in the host country after a migration experience. For some, migration is a personal choice taken in the hope of bettering personal and family prospects; for others the experience is borne of extreme difficulty and is only taken under threat of harm or death. Many new arrivals face bleak job prospects, are isolated from family and cultural institutions, and have an uphill battle as they adapt to a new language and unfamiliar social rules and obligations. Furthermore, the path that some immigrants take prior to arriving at their final destination is often lengthy, circuitous and costly, in addition to being dangerous. It is crucial, therefore, to take into account the migration experience when evaluating immigrants and refugees. Questions must be carefully phrased and asked in a judicious manner, as not all patients will be ready to discuss their reasons for leaving their homeland. Important points to cover include the premigration lifestyle of the patient, the context of migration, the experience of migration, the postmigration experience, and the "aftermath" of migration, or the long-term adjustment and acculturation to the host society (Beiser, 1999).

The stresses experienced by refugees may include the confusion and disorientation of unplanned flight and exile; loss of social status, wealth, security and community; and worry about the safety of family left behind and still in peril. Refugee claimants or asylum seekers usually face a stressful period of uncertainty while waiting to have their status determined. The refugee review process itself may be traumatic because it often occurs in an adversarial atmosphere that questions the veracity of the refugee's story even as it foregrounds traumatic memory (Silove *et al.*, 2000). Individuals who have endured war-related trauma, torture, or other forms of organized violence have special needs to insure the safety of the clinical setting and relationship (Silove, 1999).

Clinical Vignette 6

A 35-year-old professional from Peru visited the emergency room because of high fever caused by pneumonia. While waiting to be seen, he suddenly became agitated and fled the hospital, breaking through the parking lot barrier. After his arrest the judge ordered a psychiatric assessment. The patient explained that on seeing the medical instruments in the ER he was reminded of his torture in Peru and felt convinced that he was back there and that his life was in danger. The combined effects of fever and reminders of the trauma had triggered a dissociative episode.

The growing number of undocumented people around the world also presents ethical and pragmatic challenges to the medical profession. These illegal immigrants and families may have particular mental health needs, which are largely unrecognized because there is almost no funded research or services to address them.

Clinician–Patient Relationship

The roles of healer, helper and physician differ across cultural contexts, and patients may have correspondingly different expectations of their relationship with clinicians, including the duration, level of disclosure, formality and emphasis on technical competence. These expectations often need to be explored, with opportunities for patients and clinicians to negotiate or explain limits to the roles they are able and willing to adopt. Once these differing perspectives are made explicit, a culturally appropriate and professionally acceptable relationship and working alliance can be negotiated.

Clinicians must become aware of their own ethnocultural background and identity and reflect on how it is perceived by patients from their own and different backgrounds. The terms

"cultural transference" and "cultural countertransference" have been used to acknowledge that both patient and clinician may have fantasies and responses to the other that are based on earlier relationships with others from that culture or on culturally rooted associations to the other, rather than to strictly personal characteristics (Adams, 1996; Comas-Diaz and Jacobsen, 1991).

Clinical Vignette 7

Sent by her 8-year-old son's school, a university-educated woman from Somalia consults for his conduct problems which are not responding to stimulant medication prescribed by a pediatrician for attention deficit hyperactivity disorder. She is obviously reticent about the assessment process. The white clinician explicitly addresses the difficulty of being a black, veiled woman in North America because of the strong prejudices against both Islam and Africa. The woman visibly relaxes and begins to explain that she feels that she is being treated as though she is intellectually handicapped or as a child by the school. They use a loud voice and simplistic formulations when they speak to her, and she finds this very humiliating. Later in the interview, after further strengthening of the alliance with the clinician, she discloses the war trauma to which the boy was exposed.

Overall Assessment

The aim of the cultural assessment is to integrate all of the pertinent elements of the cultural context of the patient's identity, illness and social context in a formulation that can guide diagnosis and treatment (Hays, 2001; Tseng and Streltzer, 1997). Factors associated with one aspect of the formulation may have an impact that cuts across many dimensions of illness experience and behavior. The salient aspects of culture vary across cases and may reflect issues in the dominant society as much as any intrinsic characteristics of the patient's ethnocultural group.

For example, cultural notions of race and racism may profoundly affect every aspect of the cultural formulation (Pinderhughes, 1989; Patel *et al.*, 2000; GAP, 2002). Racial categories may impose a disvalued identity on the patient; this may be resisted by reconstructing identity in a fashion that imbues one's background with dignity and "cultural capital" (Comas-Diaz and Greene, 1994; Kareem and Littlewood, 1992). Race may figure in explanations of the nature of illness. For example, some Native peoples have come to view alcoholism, diabetes and other conditions as "white man's illnesses", which they suffer in large numbers precisely because of the history of colonization and racist practices. High blood pressure among African-Americans has been linked to the stresses of racial prejudice and related economic and educational disparities (Dressler *et al.*, 1998). Institutionalized racism may have a powerful impact on the level of stress and social support for individuals, families and communities, which may fracture or unite around this issue. The legacy of racism may define the clinician–patient relationship, where it may influence the transference and undermine rapport.

Cultural Competence

Recent years have seen the development of professional standards for training and quality assurance in cultural competence (Lopez, 1997; Sue, 1998). This term stands for a range of

Table 2.3 Strategies to Elicit Cultural Information

- Present an open, friendly face of the institution (have the diversity of the community represented within the diversity of the institution, with attention to not simply reproducing the class structure of the society in the institutional hierarchy).
- Make explicit the clinician's position and identity, explain goals and methods, use self-disclosure appropriately.
- Ask for clarification of unfamiliar terms or key terms that may be mistakenly assumed to be familiar.
- Ask for detailed description of practices related to health, illness and coping.
- Have the patient compare situation with previous events or experiences of others from similar background.
- Interview other family members and patient's entourage to obtain normative framework and identify consensus and conflicting perspectives.
- Consult knowledgeable clinicians, culture-brokers, interpreters, anthropologists and ethnographic literature.

approaches aimed at improving the delivery of appropriate services to a culturally diverse population. Cultural competence may involve both culture-specific and generic strategies to address a range of practical issues in intercultural work (Okpaku, 1998). This includes the clinician's ability to elicit cultural information during the clinical encounter (Table 2.3), to understand how different cultural worlds of patients and their families influence the course of the illness, and to develop a treatment plan that empowers the patient by acknowledging cultural knowledge and resources while allowing appropriate psychiatric intervention.

Clinical Vignette 8

A 16-year-old girl from Haiti presents with disorganized schizophrenia, which began around age 14 years. Her family has not been compliant with treatment and this had led to several hospitalizations of the patient in a dehydrated state. During the third hospitalization, the clinical team decide to explore the family's interpretation of the illness. A grand-aunt insists on sending the girl to Haiti for a traditional diagnosis. The traditional healer indicates that the problem is due to an ancestor's spirit in the mother's family and that for this reason it will be a prolonged illness. This explanation helps to restore cohesion in the extended family by rallying people around the patient, and her family receives much support. The traditional interpretation and treatment has broken the family sense of shame and isolation and promoted an alliance with the medical team and the acceptance of antipsychotic medication.

Specific cultural competence has to do with knowledge and skills pertaining to a single cultural group, which may include history, language, etiquette, styles of child-rearing, emotional expression and interpersonal interaction as well as cultural explanations of illness and specific modalities of healing. Often, it is assumed that specific cultural competence is assured when there is an ethnic match between clinician and patient (e.g., a

Hispanic clinician treating a client from the same background). However, ethnic matching without explicit training in models of culture and intercultural interaction may not be sufficient to ensure that clinicians become aware of their tacit cultural knowledge or biases and apply their cultural skills in a clinically effective manner.

Ethnic matching can occur at the level of the individual, the technique, the institution, or any combination of these levels (Weinfeld, 1999). At the level of the individual, it may be easier to establish rapport when clinician and patient share a common background. However, there is a risk that some issues may be left unexplored because they are taken for granted, or are taboo and awkward to approach. There is also difficulty when the patient's expectations of a fellow community member are not met because the clinician applies the rules and limits dictated by professional training. This may include expectations of receiving special treatment, of being cured quickly, of becoming friends, or intervening inappropriately on behalf of other family or community members.

In many cases, however, ethnic matching is only crude or approximate. For example, the term **Hispanic** covers a broad territory with many cultural, educational and social class differences that transcend language. Indeed, there is enormous intracultural variation and no one person carries comprehensive knowledge of his or her own cultural background, so there is always the need to explore local meanings with patients.

In the course of professional training, clinicians may distance themselves from their own culture of origin and become reluctant or unable to use (or understand the impact of) their tacit cultural knowledge in their clinical work. Clinicians from ethnic minority backgrounds may resent being pigeon-holed and expected to work predominately with a specific ethnocultural group. Patients may have complex reactions to meeting a clinician from the same background. These issues require attention and sensitive exploration just as much as the feelings evoked by meeting someone from a different background.

At the level of technique, the clinician familiar with a specific ethnocultural group learns to modify his or her approach to take advantage of culturally supported coping strategies. For example, religious practices, family and community supports, and appeals to specific cultural values may all provide useful strategies for symptom management and improved functioning. Traditional diagnostic and treatment methods may be used in concert with conventional psychiatric treatments. The clinician may use his or her own person differently in recognition of cultural notions of healing relationships, adopting a more authoritative stance, making selective use self-disclosure, or participating in symbolic social exchanges with patients and their extended families to establish trust and credibility.

At the level of institutions, ethnic match is represented in the organization of the clinical service, which should reflect the composition of the communities it serves (Kareem and Littlewood, 1992). This is not merely a matter of hiring practices but also involves creating structures that allow a measure of community feedback and control of the service institution. When people feel a sense of ownership in an institution, they will evince a higher level of trust and utilization. It is important, therefore, for clinicians to understand how the institutional setting in which they are working is seen by specific ethnocultural communities.

Increasingly, clinicians work in settings where there is great cultural diversity that precludes reaching a high level of specific competence for any one group. Changes in migration patterns and new waves of immigrants and refugees lead to corresponding changes in patient populations. For all of these reasons, it is crucial to supplement specific cultural competence with more generic competence that is based on a broad theoretical understanding of culture and ethnicity. Generic cultural competence abstracts general principles from specific examples of cultural differences. The core of generic competence resides in clinicians' understanding of their own cultural background and assumptions, some of which are related to ethnicity and religion and many of which derive from professional training and the context of practice. Appreciating the wide range of cultural variation in gender roles, family structures, developmental trajectories, explanations of health and illness, and responses to adversity allows the clinician to ask appropriate questions about areas that would otherwise be taken for granted. The culturally competent clinician has a keen sense of what he or she does not know and a solid respect for difference. While empathy and respectful interest allow the clinician gradually to come to know another's world, the clinician must tolerate the ambiguity and uncertainty that comes with not knowing. In the end, patients are the experts on their own experiential worlds and cultural context must be reconstructed simultaneously from the inside out (through the patient's experience) and from the outside in (through an appreciation of the social matrix in which the patient is embedded).

The wide range of specific and generic skills needed for competent intercultural work means that most clinicians will find it helpful to work in multidisciplinary teams that contain cultural diversity that reflects the patient population. A variety of models for such teamwork have been developed (Kareem and Littlewood, 1992; Kirmayer *et al.*, 2003).

Working with Interpreters and Culture-brokers

A key skill which has not been addressed in many training programs concerns how to work with interpreters (Table 2.4). In the absence of familiarity with this technique and quality assurance standards insisting on appropriate use of interpreters, many clinicians simply try to avoid the situation, relying on patients' sometimes limited command of the clinician's language. This is unfortunate and may lead to errors in diagnosis and management as well as the failure to engage and help many patients.

There are several models of working with interpreters (Westermeyer, 1989). Medical interpreters have adopted a code of ethics and model of working that owes much to forensic and political interpreting. Their goal is to provide accurate, complete and literal translation of the statements of patient and physician. This model tends to portray the interpreter as providing a transparent window or conduit of communication between clinician and patient. In this approach, the clinician addresses the patient directly as though the interpreter is not present. The interpreter may speak in the first person for the patient and for the clinician alternately. The model assumes that it is possible to achieve complete and accurate translation of message in both directions and treats the interpersonal triad of doctor–interpreter–patient as if it was a dyad. To do so assumes that the interpreter does not have an independent relationship with patient or clinician. Of course, this is certainly not the case in any clinical encounter that goes on for a time or involves repeated meetings. Indeed, at the level of transference it is never the case because the mere presence of another person immediately evokes distinctive thoughts, feelings

Table 2.4	Guidelines for Working with Interpreters and Culture-Brokers
Before the Interview	

* Explain the goals of the interview to the interpreter
* Clarify the roles of interpreter and clinician, and the conduct of the interview
* Discuss the interpreter's social position in country of origin and local community as it may influence the relationship with the patient
* Explain the need for literal translation in the Mental Status Examination (e.g., to ascertain thought disorder, emotional range and appropriateness, and suicidality)
* Ask for feedback when something is hard to translate
* Discuss etiquette and cultural expectations

After the Interview

* Debrief the interpreter to address any of their own emotional reactions and concerns
* Discuss the process of the interview, any significant communication that was not translated, including paralanguage
* Assess the patient's degree of openness or disclosure
* Consider translation difficulties, misunderstandings
* Plan future interviews
* Work with same interpreter/culture-broker for the same case whenever possible

and fantasies. Then too, the presence of the interpreter inevitably changes a dyad into a triadic social system with its own complex interpersonal dynamics. These dynamics are complicated by the ethnocultural background of the interpreter and his or her own cultural assumptions.

The very idea of literal translation is also problematic. Across languages, words and phrases with similar denotation often have different sets of connotations. Every translation, therefore, is an interpretation that emphasizes some potential meanings while muting or eliding others. Interpreters tend to smoothe out fragmentary, incomplete, or incoherent statements and so may mask thought disorder or other idiosyncrasies of speech with diagnostic relevance. The clinician needs to understand the choice of alternatives made by the interpreter in order to appreciate the connotations of the patient's words and to convey his or her own nuanced meanings. These requirements place much higher demands on interpreting in mental health setting than in other medical or legal settings.

A slightly different model views the interpreter as a "go-between". In this approach, the interpreter takes turns interacting with clinician and patient to clarify what is being said and to find a means of conveying it. This model acknowledges the interpreter as an active intermediary and allows the interpreter some autonomy. The sequential dyadic interaction puts greater time and distance between clinician and patient. This demands that the interpreter have a high degree of clinical knowledge and interpersonal skill, which is possible when the interpreter has been trained as a clinician. Taking this autonomy further, the interpreter may be viewed as a cotherapist. In this approach, the interpreter with clinical skills develops his or her own working alliance with the patient. The interpreter may respond independently to the patient and initiate interventions. This sometimes happens because of language barriers, when patients may contact the interpreter to ask for help with practical issues.

Given the complexities of interpreting, we prefer to view the interpreter as a culture-broker who works to provide both the patient and the clinician with the cultural context needed to understand each other's meanings. To do this, the interpreter must understand something of the perspectives, cultural background and social positions of both patient and clinician and appreciate the goals of the clinical task. Based on this knowledge, the culture-broker can enhance patient and clinician understanding of each other and can help negotiate compromises when there are widely divergent understandings of a problem and its solutions.

Despite increasing recognition of the importance of adequate interpretation, many clinicians or institutions use lay interpreters who are directly available at no cost, usually family members (even children) or other workers within the institution. Except in emergency situations, this practice should be avoided because it exerts a strong censorship on what may be disclosed in the encounter and because it may damage relationships that are very important to the patient by transgressing certain social and familial taboos.

Both interpreters and culture brokers need training to perform competently, and clinicians need training, in turn, to work with these allied professionals. The clinician must take a systemic approach, understanding the other people in the room as part of an interactional system. Clinicians must also understand the interpreter's position in the larger community. Some of this training can go on when clinicians have an opportunity to work repeatedly with the same interpreters, who thus become part of a treatment team.

Clinical Vignette 9

A 42-year-old man from the Congo is referred for psychiatric consultation because of concern that he is depressed following chemotherapy for leukemia. The patient lies in bed staring out the window and complaining of poor appetite, headache and fatigue. At first he says little to the Euro-Canadian interviewer. After a few minutes of stilted conversation, the culture-broker, a psychologist from central Africa, stands at the foot of the bed and delivers a lecture full of exhortations to the patient. He explains that the doctor has come to help, urges the patient to cooperate with the doctor and insists that he must try to get better. After this intervention, the patient speaks more openly, clarifying that his fatigue and poor appetite are not due to depression or the lingering effects of chemotherapy but stem from the absence of appropriate African foods in his diet and the fear that he will die an improper death, far from home. His symptoms improve markedly once suitable food is arranged by contacting supportive members of his cultural community.

Conclusion: The Limits of Culture

The cultural formulation and the basic strategies of cultural competence represent useful initial approaches to exploring clinically relevant dimensions of patients' cultural backgrounds. However, to apply these tools successfully, the clinician must avoid some biases implicit in psychiatric assessment and in the concept of culture itself.

Psychiatric diagnosis tends to be individual-centered, locating problems inside the individual, in their psychology, or neurophysiology. Cultural psychiatry, in agreement with family theory and therapy, recognizes that many problems are systemic and reside in interpersonal interactions or social contexts.

In the cultural formulation, culture tends to appear as something distinctive of patients who come from ethnocultural minorities, migrants, or indigenous peoples. The clinician too has a culture that is distinctive from the patients' point of view. Indeed, culture also constitutes the larger social matrix in which the clinical encounter is embedded. The cultural critique of psychiatric theory and practice are important correctives to this view of culture as something only possessed by the "other".

Talk of culture tends to reify and essentialize it as a fixed set of traits or characteristics shared by all members of a group. However, there is enormous diversity and individual variation within any cultural group, and many divergent perspectives. The integrated whole of culture then appears to be a fiction or idealization. Contemporary anthropologists have argued for entirely dispensing with the notion of culture or else viewing it as an abstraction for a shifting set of perspectives, discourses and resources used by individuals and groups to construct and position socially viable selves. This perspective recognizes that cultures are flexible frameworks that provide both opportunities and constraints but do not wholly determine the trajectories of individual lives.

With these caveats in mind, the clinician can apply the cultural formulation by approaching each case as unique, with a focus on the social and cultural context of the behavior and experience of the identified patient and his or her family. Cultural competence involves using one's knowledge of culture, language and etiquette as modes of inquiry rather than as *a priori* answers to the dilemmas of a specific case. With the help of cultural experts, the clinician can appreciate the range of variation in a cultural group and its significance for individuals and the community. In this way, it is possible to recognize when culture is a camouflage for problems at other levels and when it is constitutive of problems itself. In assessment the aim is to formulate cultural dynamics as part of a comprehensive process model of pathology. This can then be used to design interventions to address the most flexible or accessible level of the individual, family, or social system. Whenever possible, clinical interventions should mobilize and work with the family and ethnocultural community, who will have their own strategies and resources for problem solving and coping with adversity.

Cultural competence is based on respect for and interest in difference. It requires that clinicians become familiar with and comfortable talking about cultural differences rather than attempting to "treat everyone the same" in a misguided sense of "colorblindness" or "neutrality"; lack of recognition of important differences results in ethnocentrism, seeing the world strictly from one's own cultural point of view. Instead, the clinician must learn to de-center, to encounter the other on a more equal footing that allows some questioning of cultural assumptions relevant to psychiatric practice.

Mainstream care cannot respond adequately to the needs of a diverse population unless it gives explicit attention to cultural issues. The ethnocultural diversity of mental health professionals represents an invaluable resource. Training programs must recognize this and make it safe for clinicians to explore their own ethnocultural background and assumptions as a path to more sensitive and responsive work with others.

References

Adams MV (1996) *The Multicultural Imagination: "Race", Color, and the Unconscious*. Routledge, London.

American Psychiatric Association (1994) *Diagnostic and Statistical Manual of Mental Disorders*, 4th edn. APA, Washington DC, pp. 843–849.

Beiser M (1999) *Strangers at the Gate: The "Boat People's" First Ten Years in Canada*. University of Toronto Press, Toronto.

Bibeau G (1997) Cultural psychiatry in a creolizing world: Questions for a new research agenda. *Transcult Psychiatr* 34(1), 9–41.

Canino G, Lewis-Fernandez R and Bravo M (1997) Methodological challenges in cross-cultural mental health research. *Transcult Psychiatr* 34(2), 163–184.

Comas-Diaz L and Greene B (eds) (1994) *Women of Color: Integrating Ethnic and Gender Identities in Psychotherapy*. Guilford Press, New York.

Comas-Diaz L and Jacobsen FM (1991) Ethnocultural transference and countertransference in the therapeutic dyad. *Am J Orthopsychiatr* 61(3), 392–402.

Dressler WW, Bindon JR and Neggers YH (1998) John Henryism, gender, and arterial blood pressure in an African-American community. *Psychosom Med* 60, 620–624.

GAP (Group for the Advancement of Psychiatry) (2002) *Cultural Assessment in Clinical Psychiatry*. American Psychiatric Press, Washington DC.

Graves JL Jr. (2001) *The Emperor's New Clothes: Biological Theories of Race at the Millennium*. Rutgers University Press, New Brunswick, NJ.

Hays PA (2001) *Addressing Cultural Complexities in Practice: A Framework for Clinicians and Counsellors*. American Psychological Association, Washington DC.

Hollinger DA (1995) *Postethnic America: Beyond Multiculturalism*. Basic Books, New York.

Kareem J and Littlewood R (eds) (1992) *Intercultural Therapy: Themes, Interpretations and Practice*. Blackwell Scientific, Oxford, UK.

Kirmayer LJ (2001) Cultural variations in the clinical presentation of depression and anxiety: Implications for diagnosis and treatment. *J Clin Psychiatr* 62(Suppl 13), 22–28.

Kirmayer LJ and Groleau D (2001) Affective disorders in cultural context. *Psychiatr Clin N Am* 24(3), 465–478.

Kirmayer LJ and Minas H (2000) The future of cultural psychiatry: An international perspective. *Can J Psychiatr* 45(5), 438–446.

Kirmayer LJ, Rousseau C and Santhanam R (2003) Models of diagnosis and treatment planning in multicultural mental health, in *Immigration, Health and Ethnicity* Rummens A, Beiser M, and Noh S (eds). University of Toronto Press, Toronto.

Kleinman A (1988) *Rethinking Psychiatry*. Free Press, New York.

Kleinman A, Eisenberg L and Good B (1978) Culture, illness, and care: Clinical lessons from anthropologic and cross-cultural research. *Ann Int Med* 88, 251–258.

Kleinman A, Das V and Lock M (eds) (1997) *Social Suffering*. University of California Press, Berkeley, CA.

Leff J (2001) *The Unbalanced Mind*. Columbia University Press, New York.

Leslie C and Young A (eds) (1992) *Pathways to Asian Medical Knowledge*. University of California Press, Berkeley, CA.

Lewis-Fernandez R (1996) Cultural-formulation of psychiatric diagnosis. *Cult Med Psychiatr* 20, 133–144.

Lock M (1993) *Encounters with Aging: Mythologies of Menopause in Japan and North America*. University of California Press, Berkeley, CA.

Lock M and Gordon D (eds) (1988) *Biomedicine Examined*. Kluwer Academic, Dordrecht, Netherlands.

Lopez SR (1997) Cultural competence in psychotherapy: A guide for clinicians and their supervisors, in *Handbook of Psychotherapy Supervision* (eds Watkins CE). John Wiley, New York.

Lopez S and Guarnaccia PJ (2000) Cultural psychopathology: Uncovering the social world of mental illness. *Annu Rev Psychol* 51, 571–598.

Okpaku S (1998) *Clinical Methods in Transcultural Psychiatry*. American Psychiatric Press, Washington DC.

Patel N, Bennet E, Dennis M *et al.* (eds) (2000) *Clinical Psychology, "Race" and Culture: A Training Manual*. British Psychological Society, Leicester, UK.

Piccinelli M and Simon G (1997) Gender and cross-cultural differences in somatic symptoms associated with emotional distress. An international study in primary care. *Psychol Med* 27, 433–444.

Pinderhughes E (1989) Understanding Race, Ethnicity, and Power: The Key to Clinical Efficacy. Free Press, New York.

Portes A and Rumbaut RG (1996) *Immigrant America: A Portrait*, 2nd edn. University of California Press, Berkeley, CA.

Rogler LH and Cortes DE (1993) Help-seeking pathways: A unifying concept in mental health care. *Am J Psychiatr* 150(4), 554–561.

Silove D (1999) The psychosocial effects of torture, mass human rights violations, and refugee trauma. *J Nerv Ment Dis* 187(4), 200–207.

Silove D, Steel Z and Watters C (2000) Policies of deterrence and the mental health of asylum seekers. *J Am Med Assoc* 284(5), 604–611.

Sue S (1998) In search of cultural competence in psychotherapy and counseling. *Am Psychol* 53(4), 440–448.

Susser I and Patterson TC (eds) (2001) *Cultural Diversity in the United States*. Blackwell, Malden, MA.

Tannen D (1994) *Gender and Discourse*, 2nd edn. Oxford University Press, New York.

Tseng W-S and Streltzer J (1997) *Culture and Psychopathology: A Guide to Clinical Assessment*. Brunner/Mazel, New York.

Weinfeld M (1999) The challenges of ethnic match: Minority origin professionals in health and social services, in *Ethnicity, Politics, and Public Policy: Case Studies in Canadian Diversity* (eds Troper H and Weinfeld M). University of Toronto Press, Toronto, pp. 117–141.

Westermeyer J (1989) *Psychiatric Care of Migrants: A Clinical Guide*. American Psychiatric Press, Washington DC.

Young A (1995) *The Harmony of Illusions: Inventing Posttraumatic Stress Disorder*. Princeton University Press, Princeton, NJ.

3

The Psychiatric Interview: Settings and Techniques

The interview is the principal means of assessment in clinical psychiatry. Despite major advances in neuroimaging and neurochemistry, there are no laboratory procedures as informative as observing, listening to, and interacting with the patient, and none as yet are more than supplementary to the information gathered by the psychiatric interview. This chapter deals with the interview as a means of assessing the patient and developing an initial treatment plan in clinical situations.

Psychiatric interviews are analogous to the history and physical in a general medical assessment, and they share the major features of other types of medical interviews (Mackinnon and Yudofsky, 1986); they systematically survey subjective and objective aspects of illness, and generate a differential diagnosis and plan for further evaluation and treatment. They differ from other medical interviews in the wide range of biological and psychosocial data which they must take into account, and in their attention to the emotional reactions of the patient and the process of interaction between the patient and interviewer. The nature of the interaction is informative diagnostically and is a means of building rapport and eliciting the patient's cooperation, which is especially important in psychiatry (Reiser and Schroder, 1980). The style and content of a psychiatric interview are necessarily shaped by the interviewer's theory of psychopathology (Lazare, 1973). Thus, a biological theory of illness leads to an emphasis on signs, symptoms and course of illness; a psychodynamic theory dictates a focus on motivations, attitudes, feelings and personal interactions; a behavioral viewpoint looks at antecedents and consequences of symptoms or maladaptive behaviors. In past times, when these and other theories competed for theoretical primacy, an interviewer might have viewed exploration from a particular single perspective as adequate. However, modern psychiatry views these perspectives as complementary rather than mutually exclusive, and recognizes the contributions of biological, intrapsychic, social and environmental factors to human behavior and its disorders (Leigh and Reiser, 1992b). The interviewer, therefore, faces the task of understanding each of these dimensions, adequately surveying them in the interview, and making informed judgments about their relative importance and treatment implications (Shea, 1990).

The written psychiatric database, the mental organization which the interviewer maintains during the interview, and the structure of the interview itself may differ considerably from one another. The written psychiatric database is an orderly exposition of information gathered in the interview, presented in a relatively fixed format. The mental organization of the interviewer consists of questions and tentative hypotheses. It evolves flexibly over the course of the interview, and is determined by the goals of the interview and emerging information which indicates needed areas of focus (Lazare, 1976).

The third structure is that of the interview itself. While guided by general principles of interviewing, this structure is the most flexible of the three, being determined not only by the purpose of the interview and the type of problem which the patient presents, but also by the patient's mode of communication and style of interaction with the interviewer. Thus, the interviewer must hold his/her own structure in mind while responding flexibly to the patient.

Goals of the Psychiatric Interview

The interviewer may be thought of as seeking the answers to several basic questions about the patient and the presenting problems. These questions provide the mental framework of the interview (although not its explicit form). They begin with triaging of patients into broad categories of type and severity and progress to inquiry about details in each salient area. Table 3.1 lists the questions which the interview addresses and the implications of each for understanding and treating the patient. The answers to the questions in Table 3.1 are presented here in greater detail.

Does the Patient Have a Psychiatric Disorder?

This is the most basic question which the psychiatrist is called upon to answer, and determines whether or not there is any need for further psychiatric assessment or treatment.

How Severe Is the Illness?

The answer to this question determines the necessary level of treatment, ranging from hospitalization with close observation to infrequent outpatient visits. The main determinants of severity are dangerousness to self and others and impairment in ability to care for oneself and function in social and occupational roles.

What Is the Diagnosis?

In psychiatry, as in the rest of medicine, descriptive information about signs, symptoms and course over time is used to assign a diagnosis to the presenting problem. Not all psychiatric diagnoses have well-established validity, but most convey knowl-

Essentials of Psychiatry   Jerald Kay and Allan Tasman
© 2006 John Wiley & Sons, Ltd.

Table 3.1	Issues to be Addressed in a Psychiatric Assessment
Question	**Implications**
Does the patient have a psychiatric disorder?	Need for treatment
How severe is the disorder?	Need for hospitalization Need for structure or assistance in daily life Ability to function in major life roles
Are there abnormalities of brain function?	Degree of dysfunction of major mental processes such as perception, cognition, communication, regulation of mood and affect Responsivity of symptoms to environmental and motivation features Responsivity of symptoms to biological treatment
What is the diagnosis?	Description of the illness Prognosis and treatment response
What is the patient's baseline level of functioning?	Determination of onset of illness State vs. trait pathology Goals for treatment Capacity for treatment
What environmental issues contribute to the disorder?	Prediction of conditions which may trigger future episodes of illness Need for focus on precipitating stressors Prevention of future episodes through amelioration of environmental stressors and/or increased environmental/social support
What biological factors contribute to the disorder?	Need for biological therapy Place of biological factors in explanation of illness presented to the patient Focus on biological factors as part of ongoing therapy
What psychological factors contribute to the disorder?	Responsivity of the symptoms to motivational, interpersonal, reinforcement factors Need to deal with psychological or interpersonal issues in therapy
What is the patient's motivation and capacity for treatment?	Decision to treat Choice of treatment

edge of prognosis, comorbidity, treatment response, occurrence in family members, or associated biological or psychological findings (Tischler, 1987). Even in the case of poorly understood entities, our present system of diagnosis using specific criteria maximizes uniformity in the description and naming of psychiatric disorders.

One important implication of diagnoses is whether there may be reduced plasticity of brain functioning due to anatomical or physiological abnormalities. Symptoms, deficits and behaviors which stem from such abnormalities vary less in response to environmental and motivational factors than those behaviors which arise in the context of normal brain function. For example, mood swings in a patient with bipolar disorder, a condition for which there is strong evidence of a biological–genetic etiology, typically recur at regular time intervals, often independently of the patient's life situation. By contrast, mood swings in a patient with narcissistic personality disorder are much more likely to be triggered by interactions with other people. Furthermore, when brain function is impaired, biological treatments are more likely to be necessary, and verbal, interpersonal, or environmental interventions are less likely to be sufficient. Thus, the likelihood of altered brain function has major implications for understanding and treating the patient's problems.

Although the question of brain abnormalities is basic to psychiatric triaging, we do not yet have a clearcut biological etiology for any disorder outside of those historically classified as "organic". Standard laboratory studies (such as brain imaging or electroencephalography) are not generally diagnostic of psychopathology; however, there is research-based evidence of altered brain function in many psychiatric disorders. Table 3.2 presents an overview of the current state of knowledge of brain abnormalities in psychiatric disorders, along with known responses to biological and psychosocial treatments.

What Is the Patient's Baseline Level of Functioning?

Determining what the patient has been like in his/her best or most usual state is a vital part of the assessment. This information allows the interviewer to gauge when the patient became ill, and how he/she is different when ill versus well. Environmental, biological and psychological factors that contribute to low baseline levels of functioning may also predispose a patient to the development of psychiatric disorders. Thus, information about baseline functioning provides clues about the patient's areas of vulnerability to future illness as well as his/her capacity to benefit from treatment. It is also an important guide to realistic goals and expectations for such treatment. Table 3.3 lists major components of functioning with examples of elements of each.

Table 3.2 Brain Dysfunction in Psychiatric Disorders

Disorder	Evidence for Brain Dysfunction	Response to Biological Treatments	Response to Psychosocial Treatments
Delirium, dementia, amnestic and cognitive disorders (Popkin 1994; Lipowski 1984; Lishman 1978; Leigh and Reiser, 1992a)	Well established	Reversible causes respond to appropriate treatment, neuroleptics, anxiolytics, antidepressants, lithium and anticonvulsants. Beta-blockers may be helpful	Environmental support and supportive psychotherapy may be helpful
Schizophrenia (Carpenter and Buchanan, 1994; Kotrla and Weinberger, 1995; Davis, 1975; Bellack and Mueser, 1993; Sensky *et al.*, 2000)	Strong evidence	Most respond to antipsychotics; antidepressants, mood stabilizers, and anxiolytics may be helpful adjunctively	Environmental support, supportive psychotherapy, cognitive–behavioral therapy, family therapy, and skills training are helpful
Delusional disorder (Maber 1992; Manschreck, 1996)	Little evidence – few studies	Poor to fair response to psychotics	Poor response to psychotherapy
Schizoaffective disorder (Kendler, 1991; Winokur *et al.*, 1996; Keck *et al.*, 1996)	Evidence for relationship to schizophrenia and mood disorders	Most respond to combinations of antipsychotics, antidepressants, mood stabilizers, carbamazepine, ECT	Not well established. Similar range of treatments as for schizophrenia may be helpful
Brief psychotic disorder (Susser *et al.*, 1995; Jorgensen *et al.*, 1996)	Little evidence – few studies	Not well established	Environmental support and supportive psychotherapy helpful
Bipolar disorder (Goodwin and Jaminson, 1990, Janowsky *et al.*, 1974; Tsuang and Faraone, 1990)	Strong evidence	Most respond to lithium, antidepressants, anticonvulsants, neuroleptics, or ECT	Supportive and educative psychotherapy and family therapy helpful
Major depressive disorder (Siever and Davis, 1985; Thase and Howland, 1995; Elkin *et al.*, 1989)	Evidence suggestive – considerable heterogeneity	Often responds to antidepressants or ECT	Less severe cases respond to cognitive, interpersonal and psychodynamic psychotherapy
Panic disorder (Barlow, 1988; Barlow *et al.*, 2000; Goddard and Charney, 1997; Milrod *et al.*, 2000)	Evidence suggestive	Most respond to anxiolytics or antidepressants	Variable. Cognitive – behavioral therapy more effective than psychodynamic
Generalized anxiety disorder (Blazer *et al.*, 1991)	Little evidence	Variable. Anxiolytics may be helpful	Variable. Psychodynamic, or cognitive–behavioral psychotherapies are often helpful
Simple phobia (Fyer *et al.*, 1990; Marks, 1987)	Little evidence	Medications not usually helpful	Most respond to behavioral therapy
Post traumatic stress disorder (Heim *et al.*, 2000; Marks *et al.*, 1998; Katz *et al.*, 1996)	Evidence suggestive	Variable. Antidepressants and mood stabilizers may be helpful	Psychotherapy with exploratory, supportive, and behavioral features usually helpful
Obsessive–compulsive disorder (Baxter *et al.*, 1992; Insel, 1992; Abramowitz, 1997)	Evidence suggestive	Most respond to selective serotonin reuptake inhibitors	Rituals but not obsessive thoughts respond to behavioral therapy
Somatization disorder (Cloninger *et al.*, 1986; Min and Lee, 1997)	Preliminary evidence	Poor. Medication for comorbid depression or anxiety may help	Poor. Supportive psychotherapy may help

Continues

Table 3.2   Brain Dysfunction in Psychiatric Disorders *Continued*

Disorder	Evidence for Brain Dysfunction	Response to Biological Treatments	Response to Psychosocial Treatments
Conversion disorder (Lazare, 1981; Ford and Foulks, 1985)	None known	Amytal interview may help; otherwise not indicated	Most respond to psychotherapy with exploratory, expressive and behavioral features. May remit spontaneously
Hypochondriasis (Kellner, 1987; Ford, 1995)	None known	No direct response. Medications may help for treatment of comorbid depression and anxiety	Variable. Supportive–educative psychotherapy may be helpful
Dissociative disorders (Brenner and Marmer, 1998; Kluft and Fine, 1993)	None known	No direct response. Medications may help for treatment of comorbid depression and anxiety	Variable. Many respond to expressive–exploratory psychotherapy
Alcoholism (Prescott and Kendler, 1999; Merlett, 1998)	Strong evidence in subgroups	No well-demonstrated direct effects. Opiate antagonists may be helpful	Group and individual psychotherapies most common treatment modalities. Response variable, relapse high
Psychoactive substance use disorders (Banmohl and Jaffe, 1995; Nesse and Berridge, 1997)	Little evidence – some subgroups	No well-demonstrated direct effects	Group and individual psychotherapies most common treatment modalities. Response variable, relapse high
Sexual disorder (LoPiccolo, 1985; Marshall and Barbaree, 1990)	May be due to metabolic disorders; otherwise little evidence	Medications for underlying medical conditions may be necessary. Antiandrogens or serotonergic antidepressants may be helpful for paraphilias	Sexual dysfunctions often respond to behavior therapy. Couples therapy or exploratory therapy may also be helpful
Eating disorders (Johnson and Connors, 1987; Halmi, 1992)	Evidence suggestive	Antidepressants may help ameliorate symptoms	Expressive exploration, family and behavioral therapy often helpful
Adjustment disorders (Andreasen and Hoevk, 1982; Greenberg *et al.*, 1995)	None known	Medications may alleviate symptoms of anxiety or depression	Supportive psychotherapy often helpful
Personality disorders: Cluster A (Kendler *et al.*, 1984; Siever *et al.*, 1991)	Evidence for relationship of schizotypal personality to schizophrenia; otherwise none known	Schizotypal patients may improve on antipsychotic medication; otherwise not indicated	Poor. Supportive psychotherapy may help
Personality disorders: Cluster B (Coccaro and Kavoussi, 1997; Tarnepolsky and Berlowitz, 1987; Bateman and Fonagy, 2001; Zuckerman, 1996	Evidence suggestive for antisocial and borderline personalities; otherwise none known	Antidepressants, antipsychotics, mood stabilizers may help for borderline personality; otherwise not indicated	Poor in antisocial personality. Variable in borderline, narcissistic and histrionic personalities
Personality disorders: Cluster C (Cloninger *et al.*, 1993; Cloninger, 1987; Millon, 1996)	None known	No direct response. Medications may help with comorbid anxiety, depression	Most common treatment for these disorders. Response variable

Table 3.3	Assessment of Baseline Functioning
Component	**Examples**
Level of symptoms	Depression
	Anxiety Obsessions and compulsions
	Delusion
	Hallucinations
Interpersonal relations	Sexual relationships and marriage
	Quality and longevity of friendships
	Capacity for intimacy and commitment
Work adjustment	Employment history
	Level of responsibility
	Functioning in nonpaid roles, e.g., homemaker, parent
	Satisfaction with work life
Leisure activities	Hobbies and interests
	Group and social activities
	Travel
	Ability to take pleasure in nonwork activities
Ego functions	Talents, skills, intelligence
	Ability to cope; reality testing
	Control over affects and behaviors
	Ability to formulate and carry through plans
	Stable sense of self and others
	Capacity for self-observation

What Environmental Factors Contribute to the Disorder?

Environmental contributions to the presenting problem are factors external to the patient. They may be acute events which precipitate illness, or longstanding factors which increase general vulnerability. Loss, change and traumatic events are very common acute precipitants (Paykel, 1978). Longstanding environmental stressors may predispose the patient to the development of illness and may also worsen the outlook for recovery.

It is important to identify adverse environmental influences which can be modified, and to help the patient or family make necessary changes. For example, a patient with recurrent paranoid psychosis needed yearly hospitalization as long as she worked in an office with many other people. However, she no longer suffered severe relapses when she was helped to find work which she could do in her own home. However, even irreversible precipitants, such as death of a loved one, must be identified and dealt with in the treatment plan.

What Biological Factors Contribute to the Disorder?

Biological factors may contribute to psychiatric disorders directly by their effects on the central nervous system and indirectly through the effects of pain, disability, or social stigma. Thus, biological factors must be assessed through both the psychiatric history and diagnosis, and the general medical history.

Biological factors affecting the central nervous system may be genetic, prenatal, perinatal, or postnatal. There is strong evidence of genetic contributions to schizophrenia, bipolar disorder and alcoholism, among others (Carpenter and Buchanan, 1994; Jorgensen *et al.*, 1996; Kluft and Fine, 1993); conditions such as maternal substance abuse or intrauterine infections may affect fetal brain development; birth complications may cause cerebral hypoxia with resultant brain damage. In postnatal life, the entire range of diseases which affect the brain may alter mental function and behavior, as may exposure to toxins at work, in the environment, and through substance abuse. In addition, medical conditions which do not directly affect brain functioning may have profound effects on the patient's state of mind and behavior.

Biological factors may both predispose to and precipitate episodes of illness. Thus, a patient with a genetic vulnerability to schizophrenic illness may have an episode of acute psychosis precipitated by heavy cocaine use. Similarly, a patient with borderline low intellectual capacity due to hypoxia at birth may have marginal ability to care for herself. An accident resulting in a fractured arm might overwhelm this person's coping capacity and precipitate a severe adjustment disorder.

What Psychological Factors Contribute to the Disorder?

Psychological factors are mental traits which the patient brings to life situations. While they interact with social and environmental factors, they are intrinsic to the individual, and not readily changed by outside influences.

Psychological factors predisposing to illness include both general and focal deficits in coping adaptability. General deficits encompass the entire range of ego functioning, including poor reality testing, rigid or maladaptive psychological defense mechanisms, low ability to tolerate and contain affects, impulsivity, poorly formed or unstable sense of self, low self-esteem and hostile, distant, or dependent relationships with others (Valliant, 1977). Patients with such deficits generally meet diagnostic criteria for one or more personality disorders and are at increased risk for episodes of acute psychiatric illness. An example of general deficits in psychological functioning is illustrated by the following case.

Clinical Vignette 1

A 30-year-old married woman suffers from chronic low mood and lack of enjoyment of life. She is highly dependent on her husband for practical and emotional support, although she frequently flies into rages at him, feeling that he is cold and uncaring. She has had a series of secretarial jobs which she begins enthusiastically, but soon comes to feel that her employers are highly critical and belittling, whereupon she resigns. Her friendships are limited to people with whom she can have very special, exclusive relationships. She deals poorly with change or loss, which frequently trigger episodes of acute dysfunction. When a friend is not sufficiently available to her, she feels betrayed and worthless, her mood plummets, she becomes lethargic, has eating binges, and is unable to work or pursue her usual routine for up to weeks at a time.

Focal psychological issues may also contribute to mental disorders. These issues, which typically involve conflicts between opposing motivations, may affect the patient in certain specific areas of function or life situations, leaving other broad areas of function intact (Nemiah, 1961a). Such conflicts are most likely to cause maladaptive behaviors or symptoms when the patient is not clearly aware of them.

Clinical Vignette 2

A patient functions well in a responsible job and has had a long-standing, stable marriage. However, he is driven by the need to be liked and accepted by all who know him, and has a deep-seated, but not conscious, belief that he must continually fulfil the wishes of others in order to accomplish this. At the same time, he has a chronic feeling of powerlessness and an unarticulated wish to be able to say no. At times of increased demands by family members or coworkers, he develops flu-like symptoms and stays home from work "recuperating", relieved of responsibility for fulfilling the expectations of others.

The meaning of an event in the context of the patient's life course is another focal issue which may contribute to illness.

Clinical Vignette 3

A young woman became acutely depressed upon receiving her acceptance to medical school. She was the oldest of four children and had been expected to assume a major caretaking role with her younger siblings. Her mother, a busy physician, wished for her daughter to have a similar career. To the patient, entering medical school meant accepting a lifelong role as a caretaker and forever relinquishing her own wishes to be taken care of.

What Is the Patient's Motivation and Capacity for Treatment?

Whatever the physician's view of the presenting problem, the patient's wishes and capacities are a major determinant of treatment choice (Lazare *et al.*, 1975). Some patients seek relief of symptoms; some wish to change their behavior or the nature of their relationships; some want to understand themselves better. Patients may wish to talk or to receive medication or instructions.

The patient's capacity for treatment must also be considered in the treatment plan. For example, a patient with schizophrenia may agree to medication but be too disorganized to take it reliably without help. Suitability for exploratory psychotherapy depends upon such factors as the ability to observe oneself, tolerate unpleasant affects, and establish and maintain a working relationship with the treater (Strupp and Binder, 1984). Such factors must be evaluated in the interview.

The Psychiatric Database

The body of information to be gathered from the interview may be termed the psychiatric database (Tables 3.2 to 3.4). It is a variable set of data: either very specific or general, mainly limited to the present state or focused on early life, dominated by neurological questions or inquiry into relationships. To avoid setting the impossible task of learning everything about every patient, one must consider certain factors which modify the required database.

Whose questions are to be answered – the patient's concern about himself, a family or friend's concern about him, another physician's diagnostic dilemma, a civil authority's need to safeguard the public, or a research protocol requirement? Who will have access to the data gathered and under what circumstances? What is the setting of the interview? Priorities in an emergency room differ from those in an office setting (Meyers and Stein, 2000). Is the interview to be the first session of a psychotherapy regimen, or is it a one time only evaluation? What is the nature of the pathology? For example, negative responses regarding the presence of major psychotic symptoms, coupled with a history of good occupational function, will generally preclude a detailed inventory of psychotic features. A missed orientation or memory question will require careful cognitive testing. Patients with personality disorder symptoms warrant careful attention to the history of significant relationships (Nurnberg *et al.*, 1991), work history and the feelings evoked in the interviewer during the evaluation process. The database should be expanded in areas of diagnostic concern to support or rule out particular syndromes. The amount and nature of the data obtained is also, of necessity limited, by the patient's ability to communicate and his cooperativeness.

Database Components

Identifying Data

This information establishes the patient's identity, especially for the purpose of obtaining past history from other contacts, when necessary, as well as to fix his/her position in society. The patient's name should be recorded, along with any nickname or alternative names he/she may have been known by in the past. This

Table 3.4	Core Database		
	Identifying Data	Chief Complaint	History of Present Illness
	Name	**Reason for consultation**	**Major symptoms**
	Age/date of birth Next of kin		**Time course**
			Stressors
			Change in functioning
			Current medical problems and treatment
	Past Psychiatric History	Past Medical History	Family History
	Any previous psychiatric treatmen	Ever hospitalized	Psychiatric illness
		Surgery	
		Medications	
	History of suicide attempts		
	Functioning problems secondary to psychiatric symptoms		
	Alcohol/drug abuse		
	Personal History	Mental Status	
	Educational level	Appearance	
	Ever married/committed relationship	Attitude	
		Affect	
		Behavior	
	Work history	Speech	
	Means of support	Thought process	
	Living situation	Thought content	
		Perception	
		Cognition	
		Insight	
		Judgment	

is important for women who might have been treated previously under a maiden name, or a patient who has had legal entanglements and so has adopted aliases.

Date of birth, or at least age, and race are other essential parts of every person's database. A number of different classifications for race exist, as well as different terms and controversies (Porter, 1993). In the USA and Canada, the categories of white, black (or African-American), Asian, Native American, and others are generally accepted. The additional modifier of ethnicity, especially Hispanic/nonHispanic, is becoming more widely used. If a patient is a member of a particular subculture based on ethnicity, country of origin, or religious affiliation, it may be noted here.

A traditional part of the identifying data is a reference to the patient's civil status: single, married, separated, divorced, or widowed. The evolution of relationship patterns over the last two decades, with less frequent formalization of relationships, has made classification more difficult (Ishii-Kuntz and Tallman, 1991), especially in the case of homosexual patients, whose relationships are not legally recognized in most jurisdictions.

The patient's social security number (or other national ID number) can be a very useful bit of data when seeking information from other institutions.

In most cases, it is assumed that the informant (supplier of the history) is the patient. If other sources are used, and espe-

cially if the patient is not the primary informant, this should be noted at the beginning of the database.

Chief Complaint

The chief complaint is the patient's responses to the question, "What brings you to see me/to the hospital today?" or some variant. It is usually quoted verbatim, placed within quotation marks, and should be no more than one or two sentences.

Even if the patient is very disorganized or hostile, quoting his response can give an immediate sense of where the patient is as the interview begins. If the patient responds with an expletive, or a totally irrelevant remark, the reader of the database is immediately informed about how the rest of the information may be distorted. In such cases, or if the patient gives no response, a brief statement of how the patient came to be evaluated should be made and enclosed in parentheses.

History of the Present Illness

Minimum Essential Database

The present illness history should begin with a brief description of the major symptoms which brought the patient to psychiatric attention. The most troubling symptoms should be detailed initially; later a more thorough review will be stated. As a minimum, the approximate time since the patient was last at his baseline level of functioning, and in what way he is different from that now, should be described, and any known stressors, the sequence of symptom development, and the beneficial or deleterious effects of interventions included.

How far back in a patient's history to go, especially when he has chronic psychiatric illness, is sometimes problematic. In patients who have required repeated hospitalization, a summary of events since last discharge (if within 6 months) or last stable baseline is indicated. It is rare that more than 6 months of history be included in the history of the present illness, and detailed history is more commonly given on the past month.

Expanded Database
A more expanded description of the history of the present illness would include events in a patient's life at the onset of symptoms, as well as exactly how the symptoms have affected the patient's occupational functioning and important relationships. Any concurrent medical illness symptoms, medication usage (and particularly changes), alterations in the sleep–wake cycle, appetite disturbances and eating patterns should be noted; significant negative findings should also be remarked upon.

Past Psychiatric History

Minimum Essential Database
Most of the major psychiatric illnesses are chronic in nature. For this reason, often patients have had previous episodes of illness with or without treatment. New onset of symptoms, without any previous psychiatric history, becomes increasingly important with advancing age in terms of diagnostic categories to be considered. At a minimum, the presence or absence of past psychiatric symptomatology should be recorded, along with psychiatric interventions taken and the result of such interventions. An explicit statement about past suicide and homicide attempts should be included.

Expanded Database
A more detailed history would include names and places of psychiatric treatment, dosages of medications used, and time course of response. The type of psychotherapy, the patient's feelings about former therapists, his compliance with treatment as well as circumstances of termination are also important. Note what the patient has learned about the biological and psychological factors predisposing him/her to illness, and whether there were precipitating events.

Past Medical History

Minimum Essential Database
In any clinical assessment, it is important to know how a patient's general health status has been. In particular, any current medical illness and treatment should be noted (Slaby and Andrew, 1987), along with any major past illness requiring hospitalization. Previous endocrine or neurological illness are of particular pertinence (Flomenbaum and Altman, 1985).

Expanded Database
An expanded database could well include significant childhood illnesses, how these were handled by the patient and his fam-

ily, and therefore the degree to which the patient was able to develop a sense of comfort and security about his physical well-being. Illnesses later in life should be assessed for the degree of regression produced. The amount of time a patient has had to take off work, how well he/she was able to follow a regimen of medical care, his/her relationship with the family physician or treating specialist can all be useful in predicting future response to treatment. A careful past medical history can also at times bring to light a suicide attempt, substance abuse, or dangerously careless behavior, which might not be obtained any other way.

Family History

Minimum Essential Database
Given the evidence for familial, genetic factors in so many psychiatric conditions, noting the presence of mental illness in biological relatives of the patient is a necessary part of any database (Hammen *et al.*, 1987). It is important to specify during questioning the degree of family to be considered – usually to the second degree: aunts, uncles, cousins and grandparents, as well as parents, siblings and children.

Expanded Database
A history of familial medical illness is a useful part of an expanded database. A genogram (pedigree), including known family members with dates and causes of death and other known chronic illnesses is helpful. Questioning about causes of death will also occasionally bring out hidden psychiatric illness, for example, sudden, unexpected deaths which were likely suicides or illness secondary to substance abuse.

Personal History

Minimum Essential Database
Recording the story of a person's life can be a daunting undertaking and is often where a database can expand dramatically. As a minimum, this part of the history should include where a patient was born and raised, and in what circumstances – intact family, number of siblings and degree of material comfort. Note how far the patient went in school, how he/she did there, and what his/her occupational functioning has been. If he/she is not working, why not? Has the patient ever been involved in criminal activity, and with what consequences? Has the patient ever married or been involved in a committed relationship? Are there any children? What is his/her current source of support? Does he/she live alone or with someone? Has he/she ever used alcohol or other drugs to excess, and is there current use? Has he/she ever been physically or sexually abused or been the victim of some other trauma?

Expanded Database
An expanded database can include a great deal of material beginning even prior to the patient's conception. What follows is an outline of the kind of data which may be gathered, along with an organizational framework.

Family of Origin

Were parents married or in committed relationships?

Personality and significant events in life of mother, father, or other significant caregiver.

Siblings: how many? their ages, significant life events, personality, relationship to patient.

Who else shared the household with the family?

Prenatal and Perinatal

Was the pregnancy planned? Quality of prenatal care; mother's and father's response to pregnancy.

Illness, medication or substance abuse, smoking, trauma during pregnancy; labor – induced or spontaneous?

Weeks gestation, difficulty of delivery, vaginal or Caesarean section.

Presence of jaundice at birth, birth weight, Apgar score.

Baby went home with mother or stayed on in hospital.

Early Childhood

Developmental milestones: smiling, sitting, standing, walking, talking, type of feeding – food allergies or intolerance.

Consistency of caregiving: interruptions by illness, birth of siblings.

Reaction to weaning, toilet-training, maternal separation.

Earliest memories: problematic behavior (tantrums, bedwetting, hair-pulling or nail-biting).

Temperament (shy, overactive, outgoing, fussy).

Sleep problems: insomnia, nightmares, enuresis, parasomnias.

Later Childhood

Early school experiences: evidence of separation anxiety.

Behavioral problems at home or school: firesetting, bedwetting, aggressive toward others, cruelty to animals, nightmares.

Developmental milestones: learning to read, write.

Relationships with other children and family: any loss or trauma.

Reaction to illness.

Adolescence

School performance: ever in special classes?

Athletic abilities and participation in sports.

Evidence of gender identity concerns: overly "feminine" or "masculine" in appearance/behavior, or perception by peers.

Ever run away? Able to be left alone and assume responsibility.

Age onset of puberty (menarche or nocturnal emissions), reaction to puberty.

Identity

Sexual preference and gender identity, religious affiliation (same as parents?).

Career goals: ethnic identification.

Sexual History

Early sexual teaching: earliest sexual experiences, experience of being sexually abused, attitudes toward sexual behavior.

Dating history, precautions taken to prevent sexually transmitted diseases and/or pregnancy.

Episodes of impotence and reaction.

Masturbating patterns and fantasies.

Preoccupation with particular sexual practices, current sexual functioning, length of significant relationships, ages of partners.

Adulthood

Age at which left home, level of educational attainments.

Employment history, relationships with supervisors and peers at work, reasons for job change.

History of significant relationships including duration, typical roles in relationships, patterns of conflict: marital history, legal entanglements and criminal history, both covert and detected, ever victim or perpetrator of violence.

Major medical illness as adult.

Participation in community affairs.

Financial status: own or rent home, stability of living situation.

Ever on disability or public assistance?

Current family structure, reaction to losses of missing members (parents, siblings), if applicable.

Substance abuse history.

Mental Status Examination

It can be helpful to conceptualize the recording of the Mental Status Examination as a progression. One begins with a snapshot: what can be gained from a cursory visual exam, without any movement or interaction – appearance and affect. Next, motion is added: behavior. Then comes sound: the patient's speech, though initially only as sound. The ideas being expressed come next: the thought process and content, perception, cognition, insight, and judgment. Table 3.5 gives a summary of areas to be commented on, along with common terms.

At every level of the Mental Status Examination, preference should be given for explicit description over jargon. Stating that a patient is delusional is less helpful than describing him as believing that his neighbors are pumping poisonous gases into his bedroom while he sleeps.

Conduct of the Interview: Factors Which Affect the Interview

A skillful interview will not necessarily yield all the relevant information but will make the most of the opportunities in a clinical situation, given the limitations which both the patient and interviewer bring. Factors which influence the development of an alliance and the amount which can be learned in the interview include the following:

The Patient's Physical or Emotional Distress

Patients who are in acute distress either from physical discomfort or from emotional factors such as severe depression or anxiety will be limited in their motivation and ability to interact with the interviewer. The interviewer may be able to enhance communication by addressing the patient's discomfort in a supportive manner. However, he/she must also recognize times when the patient's discomfort necessitates a more limited interview.

The Cognitive Capacities of the Patient

Patients who are demented, retarded, disorganized, thought-disordered, amnesic, aphasic, or otherwise impaired in intellectual or cognitive capacity have biologically based deficits which limit the amount of information they can convey.

Table 3.5　Mental Status Examination

Appearance

Level of consciousness (alert, hypervigilant, somnolent, stuporous)
Dress (casual, appropriate for weather, eccentric, careless, disheveled)
Grooming (style of hair, degree of makeup, shaven/unshaven, clean, malodorous)
Idiosyncracies – tattoos (professional or amateur), prominent scars, religious emblems

Attitude

Cooperative, hostile, evasive, threatening, obsequious

Affect

Range (restricted, expansive, blunted, flat)
Appropriateness to items discussed
Stability (labile, shallow)
Quality (silly, anxious)

Mood

Response to question: "How are you feeling/How's your mood been?"

Behavior

Psychomotor agitation or retardation

Speech

Rate (rapid, slowed, pressured, hard to interrupt)
Volume (loud, soft, monotone, highly inflected or dramatic)
Quality (neologisms, fluent, idiosyncratic)

Thought Process

Goal directed, disorganized, loose associations, tangential, circumstantial, flight of ideas

Thought Content

Major preoccupations, ideas of reference, delusions (grandiose, paranoid, bizarre, state exactly what it is the patient appears to believe)
Thought broadcasting, insertion, or withdrawal
Suicidal or homicidal ideation. Plan and intent to carry out ideas

Perception

Illusions and hallucinations – type (auditory, visual, olfactory, tactile, gustatory), evidence (patient spontaneous report, answer to interviewer question, observation of patient attending or responding to nonexistent external stimuli).
Patient's beliefs about hallucinatory phenomenon (do they seem to originate from the outside or inside, how many voices, what gender, talking to patient or to other voices, are they keeping up constant commentary on the patient.)

Cognition

Orientation: time, place, person, situation
Memory: number of remembered objects, digit span, presidents backward, recent events
Concentration: serial 7s, *world* spelled backwards
Abstraction: proverb interpretation – what would someone mean by "The grass is always greener on the other side of the fence", ("Get off my back".)
Similarities: (How are these things alike – apple–orange, table–chair, eye–ear, praise–punishment?)
Computation: number of digits successfully added or subtracted, ability to calculate change
(How many quarters are in $1.50? If you bought a loaf of bread for 89 cents and gave the cashier a dollar, what change would you get back?)

Insight

Knows something is wrong, that he/she is ill, that illness is psychiatric; understands ways in which illness disrupts function

Judgment

Response to standard questions (If you found a sealed, addressed, stamped letter, what would you do? If you smelled smoke in a crowded theater?)
Evidence from behavior prior to and during interview (Was the patient caring for himself/herself properly, handling business affairs well? Does the behavior during the interview match his/her stated goals, e.g., if he/she wishes to be thought to be in control, is he/she keeping the voice down and movement in check?)

The Emotionally Based Biases of the Patient

Patients bring to the interview a wide variety of preconceptions, expectations and tendencies toward distortion, which influence how they view and relate to the interviewer. Such biases are commonly referred to as **transference** because they frequently can be understood as arising from interactions with important figures in childhood, such as parents, which then color perceptions of others during adult life (Nemiah, 1961b). Transferential biases may be positive or negative. Thus, even before the start of the interview, one patient may be primed to view the doctor as a wise and kindly healer, while another will be predisposed to see him/her as an exploitative charlatan. Clearly, such biases affect the amount of openness and trust which the patient brings to the interview and the quality of information he/she provides.

The Emotionally Based Biases of the Interviewer

The interviewer, like the patient, may have feelings stirred up by the interaction. The interviewer's emotional reactions to the patient can be an invaluable asset in assessment if he/she can be conscious of them and reflect on their causes. For example, an interviewer finds himself becoming increasingly annoyed at a highly polite patient. On reflection, he realizes that the politeness serves to rebuff his attempts to establish a warmer, more spontaneous relationship and is a manifestation of the patient's underlying hostile attitude.

When the interviewer is unable to monitor and examine his/her emotional reactions, they are more likely to impede rather than enhance understanding of the patient. This is most likely to happen when emotional reactions are driven more by the interviewer's own biases than by the patient's behavior. Such reactions are referred to as the interviewer's **countertransference** (Mackinnon and Michels, 1971). In the example cited in the previous paragraph, the interviewer might inaccurately perceive a polite patient as rigid and hostile due to unconscious biases (countertransference) based on his relationship with his own rigidly polite parent. The entire range of countertransferential interviewer attitudes toward the patient, from aversion to infatuation, might similarly bias judgment.

Situational Factors

Patients' attitudes toward the interview will be strongly influenced by the situation in which the consultation arises. Some patients decide for themselves that they need treatment, while others come reluctantly, under pressure from others. Patients who are being evaluated for disability or in connection with a lawsuit may feel a need to prove that they are ill, while those being evaluated for civil commitment or at the insistence of family members may need to prove that they are well. Similarly, a patient's past history of relationships with psychiatrists or with health professionals in general is likely to color his/her attitude toward the interviewer.

The interviewer may also be affected by situational factors. For example, pressure of time in a busy emergency service may influence the interviewer to omit important areas of inquiry and reach premature closure; the experience of a recent patient suicide may bias the interviewer toward overestimation of risk in someone with suicidal thoughts. As with countertransference reactions, it is important for the interviewer to minimize distortions due to situational factors by being as aware of them as possible.

Racial, Ethnic and Cultural Factors

The degree of racial, ethnic, cultural, and socioeconomic similarity between the patient and interviewer can influence the course and outcome of the interview in many ways. (see also Chapters 2 and 21.) It may affect the level of rapport between patient and interviewer, the way both view the demands of the situation, the way they interpret each other's verbal and nonverbal communications, and the meaning the interviewer assigns to the patient's statements and behaviors (Gaw, 1993). Not only racial or cultural prejudice but also well-intentioned ignorance can interfere with communication and accurate assessment.

Some cultures, for example, place a higher value on politeness and respect for authority than does western culture. A patient from such a background might be reluctant to correct or disagree with the interviewer's statements even when they are erroneous. The interviewer might not suspect that he/she was hearing distorted information, or conversely, might see the patient as pathologically inhibited or unemotional. Many nonwestern cultures place a higher value on family solidarity than on individuality. Pressing a patient from such a culture to report angry feelings toward family members might raise his/her anxiety, decrease rapport with the interviewer and produce defensive distortions in the material.

General Features of Psychiatric Interviews

Setting

The ideal interview setting is one which provides a pleasant atmosphere and is reasonably comfortable, private and free from outside distractions. Such a setting not only provides the physical necessities for an interview but conveys to the patient that he/she will be well cared for and safe. Providing such a setting may pose special problems in certain interviewing situations. For example, it may be necessary to interview highly agitated patients in the presence of security personnel; interviewers on medical–surgical units must pay special attention to the patient's comfort and privacy.

Verbal Communication

Verbal communication may be straightforward imparting of information: "Every year around November, I begin to lose interest in everything and my energy gets very low". However, patients may convey information indirectly through metaphor, or use words for noninformational purposes such as to express or contain emotions or to create an impact on the interviewer.

In metaphorical language, one idea is represented by another with which it shares some features. For example, when asked how she gets along with her daughter-in-law, a woman replies, "I can never visit their house because she always likes to keep the thermostat down. It's never as warm as I need". Such a reply suggests that the woman may not feel "warmly" accepted and welcomed by her son's wife. Metaphor may also use the body to represent ideas or feelings. A man who proved to meet the diagnostic criteria for major depressive disorder described his mood as "OK" but complained that his life was being ruined by constant aching in his chest for which the doctors could find no cause. In this instance, the pain of depression was experienced and described metaphorically as a somatic symptom.

Language may be used to express emotions directly ("I'm afraid of you and I don't want to talk to you"), but more often is used indirectly by influencing the process of the interview (Bernstein and Bernstein, 1985). Patients may shift topics, make off-hand remarks or jokes, ask questions, and compliment or belittle the interviewer as a way of expressing feelings. The process of the interview frequently expresses the patient's feelings about his/her immediate situation or interaction with the interviewer (Malan, 1979). For example, a woman being evaluated for depression and anxiety suddenly said, "I was just wondering doctor, do you have any children?" The further course of the interview revealed that she was terrified of being committed to a hospital and abandoned. The question was an attempt to establish whether the interviewer was a good parent and therefore safe as a caretaker for her.

Language may also be used in the service of psychological defense mechanisms to contain rather than express emotions (Freud, 1946). For example, a young man with generalized anxiety was asked whether he was sexually active. He replied by talking at length about how all the women he knew at college were either unappealing or attached to other men. Further discussion revealed that he developed severe symptoms of anxiety whenever he was with a woman to whom he felt sexually attracted. His initial reply represented an automatic, verbal mechanism (in this case, a rationalization) for keeping the anxiety out of awareness.

Another form of process communication is the use of language to make an impact on the interviewer (Casement, 1985). A statement such as "If you can't help me I'm going to kill myself", might convey suicidal intent, but may also serve to stir up feelings of concern and involvement in the interviewer. Similarly, the patient who says, "Dr X really understood me, but he was much older and more experienced than you are", may be feeling vulnerable and ashamed, and unconsciously trying to induce similar feelings in the interviewer. When language is used in this way, the interviewer's subjective reaction may be the best clue to the underlying feelings and motivations of the patient.

Nonverbal Communication

Emotions and attitudes are communicated nonverbally through facial expressions, gestures, body position, movements of the hands, arms, legs, and feet, interpersonal distance, dress and grooming, and speech prosody (Knapp, 1978). Some nonverbal communications such as gestures are almost always conscious and deliberate, while others often occur automatically outside one's awareness. The latter type are particularly important to observe during an interview because they may convey messages entirely separate from or even contradictory to what is being said.

Facial expression, body position, tone of voice, and speech emphasis are universal in the way they convey meaning (Ekman *et al.*, 1972). The interviewer will automatically decode these signals but may ignore the message due to coun-

tertransference or social pressure from the patient. For example, a patient may say, "I feel very comfortable with you, doctor", but sit stiffly upright and maintain a rigidly fixed smile, conveying a strong nonverbal message of tension and mistrust. The nonverbal message may be missed if, for example, the interviewer has a strong need to be liked by the patient. Another patient denies angry feelings while sitting with a tightly clenched fist. The interviewer may unconsciously collude with the patient's need to avoid his anger by ignoring the body language.

As with any medical examination, observation of nonverbal behavior may provide important diagnostic information. For example, a leaden body posture may indicate depression, movements of the foot may arise from anxiety or tardive dyskinesia, and sudden turning of the head and eyes may suggest hallucinations.

Nonverbal communication proceeds in both directions, and the nonverbal messages of the interviewer are likely to have a considerable effect on the patient. Thus, the interviewer who sits back in his chair and looks down at his notes communicates less interest and involvement than one who sits upright and makes eye contact. Similarly, an interviewer who gives a weak handshake and sits behind a desk or far across the room from the patient will communicate a sense of distance which may interfere with establishing rapport. It is important that the interviewer be aware of his/her own nonverbal messages and adapt them to the needs of the patient.

Listening and Observation

The complexity of communication in the psychiatric interview is mirrored by the complexity of listening (Luborsky, 1984). The interviewer must remain open to literal and metaphorical messages from the patient, to the impact the patient is trying to make, and to the degree to which nonverbal communication complements or contradicts what is being said. Doing this optimally requires that the interviewer also be able to listen to his/her own mental processes throughout the interview, including both thoughts and emotional reactions. Listening of this kind depends upon having a certain level of comfort, confidence and space to reflect, and may be very difficult when the patient is hostile, agitated, demanding, or putting pressure on the interviewer in any other way. With such patients, it may take many interviews to do enough good listening to gain an adequate understanding of the case.

Another important issue in listening is maintaining a proper balance between forming judgments and remaining open to new information and new hypotheses. On the one hand, one approaches the interview with knowledge of diagnostic classifications, psychological mechanisms, behavioral patterns, social forces and other factors which shape one's understanding of the patient. The interviewer hears the material with an ear to fitting the information into these preformed patterns and categories. On the other hand, the interviewer must remain open to hearing and seeing things which extend or modify his/her judgments about the patient. At times the interviewer may listen narrowly to confirm a hypothesis, while at others he/she may listen more openly, with relatively little preconception. Thus, listening must be structured enough to generate a formulation but open enough to avoid premature judgments.

Attitude and Behavior of the Interviewer

The optimal attitude of the interviewer is one of interest, concern and intention to help the patient. While the interviewer must be tactful and thoughtful about what he/she says, this should not preclude behaving with natural warmth and spontaneity. Indeed, these qualities may be needed to support patients through a stressful interview process. Similarly, the interviewer must try to use natural, commonly understood language and avoid jargon or technical terms. The interviewer must communicate his/her intention to keep the patient as safe as possible, whatever the circumstances. Thus, while one must at times set limits on the behavior of an agitated, threatening, or abusive patient, one should never be attacking or rejecting.

Empathy is an important quality in psychiatric interviewing. While sympathy is an expression of agreement or support for another, empathy entails putting oneself in another's place and experiencing his/her state of mind. Empathy comprises both one's experiencing of another person's mental state and the expression of that understanding to the other person (Barrett-Lennard, 1981). For example, in listening to a man talk about the death of his wife, the interviewer may allow himself to resonate empathetically with the patient's feelings of loneliness and desolation. Based on this resonance, he might respond, "After a loss like that, it feels as if the world is completely empty".

As a mode of listening, empathy is an important way of understanding the patient; as a mode of response, it is important in building rapport and alliance. Patients who feel great emotional distance from the interviewer may make empathic understanding difficult or impossible. Thus, the interviewer's inability to empathize may itself be a clue to the patient's state of mind.

Structure of the Interview

The overall structure of the psychiatric interview is generally one of reconnaissance and detailed inquiry (Sullivan, 1970). In reconnaissance phases, the interviewer inquires about broad areas of symptomatology, functioning, or life course: "Have you ever had long periods when you felt very low in mood?" "How have you been getting along at work?" "Tell me what you did between high school and when you got married". In responding to such questions, patients give the interviewer leads which then must be pursued with more detailed questioning. Leads may include references to symptoms, difficulty in functioning, interpersonal problems, ideas, states of feeling, or stressful life events. Each such lead raises questions about the nature of the underlying problem, and the interviewer must attempt to gather enough detailed information to answer these questions. Reliance on yes or no "gate questions" to rule out areas of pathology has been shown to increase the risk of missing important information. This risk may be minimized by asking about important areas in several ways (Barber et al., 2001).

In general, the initial reconnaissance consists of asking how the patient comes to treatment at this particular time. This is done by asking an open-ended question such as "What brings you to see me today?" or "How did you come to be in the hospital right now?" A well-organized and cooperative patient may spontaneously provide most of the needed information, with little intervention from the interviewer. However, the patient may reveal deficits in thought process, memory, or ability to communicate, which dictate more structured and narrowly focused questioning.

The patient's emotional state and attitude may also impede a smooth flow of information. For example, if the patient shows evidence of anxiety, hostility, suspiciousness, or indifference, the interviewer must first build a working alliance before trying to collect information. This usually requires acknowledging the emotions which the patient presents, helping the patient to express his/her feelings and related thoughts, and discussing these concerns in an accepting and empathic manner (Strean, 1985). As new areas of content open up, the interviewer must continue to attend to the patient's reactions, both verbal and nonverbal, and to identify and address resistance to open communication.

Setting an appropriate level of structure is an important aspect of psychiatric interviewing. Psychiatric patients may spontaneously report a low number of symptoms, and initial diagnostic impressions may be misleading (Herran et al., 2001). Over the past two decades, a variety of structured interview formats have been developed for psychiatric assessment (Wiens, 1990; Spitzer et al., 1978). In these interviews, the organization, content areas, and, to varying degrees, wording of the questions are standardized; vague, overly complex, leading or biased, and judgmental questions are eliminated, as is variability in the attention given to different areas of content. The major benefits of such interviews are that they ensure complete coverage of the specified areas and greatly increase the reliability of information gathered and diagnostic judgments. In addition, formats which completely specify the wording of questions can be administered by less highly trained interviewers or even as patient self-reports.

The disadvantages of highly structured interviews are that they diminish the ability to respond flexibly to the patient and preclude exploration of any areas not specified in the format (Groth-Marnat, 1990). They are therefore used to best advantage for interviews with focused goals. For example, such interviews may aim to survey certain DSM IV Axis I disorders, to assess the type and degree of substance abuse, or to delineate the psychological and behavioral consequences of a traumatic event. They are less useful in a general psychiatric assessment where the scope and focus of the interview cannot be preordained.

In the usual clinical situation, while the interviewer may have a standardized general plan of approach, he/she must adapt the degree of structure to the individual patient. Open-ended, nondirective questions derive from the psychoanalytic tradition. They are most useful for eliciting and following emotionally salient themes in the patient's lifestory and interpersonal history. Focused, highly structured questioning derives from the medical/descriptive tradition and is most useful for delineating the scope and evolution of pathological signs and symptoms. In general, one uses the least amount of structure needed to maintain a good flow of communication and cover the necessary topic areas.

Phases of the Interview

The typical interview comprises an opening, middle and closing phase. In the opening phase, the interviewer and patient are introduced, and the purposes and procedures of the interview are set. It is generally useful for the interviewer to begin by summarizing what he/she already knows about the patient and proceeding to the patient's own account of the situation. For example, the interviewer may say, "Dr Smith has told me that you have had several episodes of depression in the past, and now you may be going into another one", or "I understand that you were brought in by the police because you were threatening people on the street. What do you think is happening with you?" or "When we spoke on the phone you said you thought your marriage was in trouble. What has been going wrong?" Such an approach orients the patient and sets a collaborative tone.

The opening phase may also include clarification of what the patient hopes to gain from the consultation. Patients may sometimes state this explicitly, but often do not, and the interviewer should not assume that his/her goals are the same as the patient's (Lazare *et al.*, 1975). A question such as "How were you hoping I could help you with the problem you have told me about?" invites the patient to formulate and express his/her request and avoids situations in which the patient and interviewer work at cross-purposes. The interviewer must also be explicit about his/her own goals and the extent to which they fit with the patient's expectations. This is especially important when the interests of a third party, such as an employer, a family member, or a court of law is involved.

The middle phase of the interview consists of assessing the major issues in the case and filling in enough detail to answer the salient questions and construct a working formulation. Most of the work of determining the relative importance of biological, psychological, environmental and sociocultural contributions to the problem is done during this phase. The patient's attitudes and transferential perceptions are also monitored during this phase so that the interviewer can recognize and address barriers to communication and collaboration.

When appropriate, formal aspects of the Mental Status Examination are performed during the middle phase of the interview. While most of the mental status evaluation is accomplished simply by observing the patient, certain components such as cognitive testing and review of psychotic symptoms may not fit smoothly into the rest of the interview. These are generally best covered toward the end of the interview, after the issues of greatest importance to the patient have been discussed and rapport has been established. A brief explanation that the interviewer has a few standard questions he/she needs to cover before the end of the interview serves as a bridge and minimizes the awkwardness of asking questions which may seem incongruous or pejorative.

In general, note-taking during an assessment interview is helpful to the interviewer and not disruptive of rapport with the patient. Notes should be limited to brief recording of factual material such as dates, durations, symptom lists, important events and past treatments, which might be difficult to keep in memory accurately. The interviewer must take care not to become so involved in taking notes as to lose touch with the patient. It is especially important to maintain a posture of attentive listening when the patient is talking about emotionally intense or meaningful issues. When done with interpersonal sensitivity, note-taking during an assessment interview may actually enhance rapport by communicating that what the patient says is important and worth remembering. This is to be distinguished from note-taking during psychotherapy sessions, which is more likely to diminish the treater's ability to listen and respond flexibly.

In the third or closing phase of the interview, the interviewer shares his/her conclusions with the patient, makes treatment recommendations and elicits reactions. In situations where the assessment runs longer than one session, the interviewer may sum up what has been covered in the interview and what needs to be done in subsequent sessions. Communications of this kind serve several purposes. They allow the patient to correct or add to the salient facts as understood by the interviewer. They contribute to the patient's feeling of having gained something from the interview. They are also the first step in initiating the treatment process because they present a provisional understanding of the problem and a plan for dealing with it. All treatment plans must be negotiated with the patient, including discussion of mutual goals, expected benefits, liabilities, limitations and alternatives, if any. In many cases, such negotiations extend beyond the initial interview and may constitute the first phase of treatment.

Dimensions of Interviewing Techniques

Although many systems have been suggested for classifying interview techniques (Elliott *et al.*, 1987), it is convenient to think about four major dimensions of interviewing style: degree of directiveness, degree of emotional support, degree of fact versus feeling orientation and degree of feedback to the patient. The interviewer must seek a balance among these dimensions to best cover the needed topics, build rapport, and arrive at a plan of treatment.

Directiveness

Directiveness in the interview ensures that the necessary areas of information are covered and supplies whatever cognitive support the patient needs in discussing them. Table 3.6 lists interventions which are low, moderate and high in directiveness.

Low-directive interventions request information in the broadest, most open-ended way and do not go beyond the material supplied by the patient. Moderately directive interventions are narrower in focus and may extend beyond what the patient himself/herself has said. For example, confrontation makes the patient aware of paradoxes or inconsistencies in the material and requests him/her to resolve them; interpretation requests the patient to consider explanations or connections that had not previously occurred to him/her. Highly directive interventions aim to focus and restrict the patient's content or behavior. Such interventions include yes–no or symptom-checklist type questions and requests for the patient to modify behaviors that impede the progress of the interview.

Supportiveness

Patients vary considerably in the degree of emotional and cognitive support they need in the interview. Table 3.7 lists examples of emotionally supportive interventions. Each such intervention supports the patient's sense of security and self-esteem. While some patients may come to the interview feeling safe and confident, others have considerable anxiety about being criticized, ridiculed, rejected, taken advantage of, or attacked (literally so in the case of some psychotic patients).

Overt manifestations of insecurity range widely, from fearful demeanor and tremulousness to requests for reassurance to haughty contemptuousness. The interview's task is to identify such anxiety when it arises and respond in a manner

Table 3.6   Degrees of Directiveness in the Interviewer

Directiveness	Intervention	Examples
Low	Open-ended questions	"What brings you to the hospital?" "Tell me about your current situation in life."
Low	Repetition	*Patient:* "Last night I suddenly started to feel so terrible I was afraid I was going to die." *Interviewer:* "You were afraid you were going to die."
Low	Restatement	*P:* "Nobody is on my side anymore – even my family is out to get me." *I:* "So it seems as if everyone has turned against you."
Low	Summarization	"To review what we have been discussing, over the last month you've been very low in mood, you felt overwhelmed even by small chores, and you no longer want to see any of your friends."
Low	Clarification	"You told me that it "upsets" you to have to say no. It seems that when you say no to your boss your feeling is fear, but when you say no to your children you feel guilty."
Low	Nonverbal Acknowledgment	"Uh-huh"; nodding of head
Low	Attentive listening	In talking about the recent death of his wife, the patient became tearful and hesitant in speech. The interviewer remains silent, but attentive, allowing the patient time to express himself
Moderate	Broad-focus questions	"What do you notice about yourself lately that is different from usual?" "What is it about your job that you find stressful?"
Moderate	Use of examples	"Sometimes illness seems to be triggered by something that happens, like a change in finances or living situation, or losing someone who's close to you. Has anything like that been happening to you?"
Moderate	Confrontation	"You told me you got a "terrible" evaluation at work, but in 9 of 10 categories your rating was actually excellent." "You don't feel the medicine does you Any good, but whenever you've stopped It you've had to go back into the hospital. How do you account for that?"
Moderate	Interpretation	"Part of the tension between you and your wife is that you forget things she tells you. Perhaps this is what you do when you are angry at her."
High	Narrow-focus questions	"Do you have trouble getting to sleep or staying asleep? "How much alcohol do you drink in a week?"
High	Question repetition	*I:* "How has your daily routine changed in the last month?" *P:* "I used to like to read, but now I don't anymore. My husband thinks I would feel better if I pushed myself to keep busy, but I tell him that this dizziness makes it impossible for me to do anything. I don't know what to think anymore." *I:* "How else has your routine changed lately?"
High	Redirection	*P:* "I've always thought that my father's personality caused a lot of my troubles in life." *I:* "I'd like to hear more of your thoughts about that, but first I need to get a clearer picture of what's been happening with you lately. When did you decide to make the appointment with me?"
High	Change of topics	"You mentioned before that your brother had similar problems to yours. Can you tell me how many brothers and sisters you have, and if they've had any emotional problems?" "We've been talking about your marriage, but now I'd like to know something about your work."
High	Limit-setting	"I'm going to have to interrupt you because there are a few more things we need to cover in the time left." "I know you feel restless, but I have to ask you to try to stay in your chair and concentrate on what we're talking about."

Table 3.7   Supportive Interventions

Intervention	Examples
Encouragement	*Patient:* "I'm not sure I'm making any sense today doctor." *Interviewer:* "You're doing very well at describing the troubles you've been having."
Approval	"You did the right thing by coming in for an appointment." "You've been doing your best to keep going under very difficult circumstances."
Reassurance	"What you are telling me about may seem very strange to you, but many people have had similar experiences." "You feel like you will be sick forever, but with treatment you have a very good chance of feeling better soon."
Acknowledgment of affect	"You look very sad when you talk about your brother." "I have the impression that my question made you angry."
Empathic statements	"When your boyfriend doesn't call you, you feel completely helpless and unloved." "It seems unfair for you to get sick so many times while others remain well."
Nonverbal communication	Smiling, firm handshake, attentive body posture, gentle touch on shoulder.
Avoidance of affect-laden material	Interviewer elects to defer discussion or probing of topics that arouse intense feelings of anxiety, shame, or anger.

that conveys empathic understanding, acceptance and positive regard.

Obstructive interventions are one which (usually unintentionally) impede the flow of information and diminish rapport. Table 3.8 lists common examples of such interventions. Compound or vague questions are often confusing to the patient and may produce ambiguous or unclear answers. Biased or judgmental questions suggest what answer the interviewer wants to hear or that he/she does not approve of what the patient is saying. "Why" questions often sound critical or invite rationalizations. "How" questions better serve the purposes of the interview ("How did you come to change jobs?" rather than "Why did you change jobs?"). Other interventions are obstructive because they disregard the patient's feeling state or what he/she is trying to say. Paradoxically, this may include premature reassurance or advice. When given before the interviewer has explored and understood the issue, this has the effect of cutting off feelings and coming to a premature closure.

Fact Versus Feeling Orientation

Interviews differ in the degree to which they focus on factual–objective versus feeling–meaning oriented material. Tables 3.9 and 3.10 provide examples of interventions of both types. The interviewer must determine what the salient issues are in a given case and develop the focus accordingly. For example, at one extreme, the principal task in assessing a cyclically occurring mood disorder might be to delineate precisely the symptoms, time course and treatment response of the illness. At the other end of the spectrum might be a patient with a circumscribed difficulty in living, such as the inability to achieve an intimate, lasting love relationship. In such a case, the interviewer may focus not only on the facts of the patient's interactions with others but also on the feelings, fantasies and thoughts associated with such relationships.

Feedback

Interviews differ in how much the interviewer conveys to the patient of his/her own thoughts, feelings, conclusions and recommendations. Table 3.11 presents common types of feedback from the interviewer. Judicious statements about the interviewer's ongoing thoughts and feelings can be used to pose questions or make clarifications or interpretations while enhancing rapport and trust. Communication of factual information, formulations of the problem and treatment recommendations are the foundations of joint treatment planning with the patient. Responding to questions and giving advice may serve an educational purpose as well as enhancing the alliance. When responding to requests for advice or information, the interviewer must first take care to be sure of what is being asked, and for what reason.

There is little systematic data on the superiority of one clinical interviewing style over another, but what there are suggest that many styles can be used effectively. Rutter and his colleagues have investigated this question in a series of naturalistic and experimental studies of interviews of parents in a child psychiatry clinic (Rutter *et al.*, 1981; Cox *et al.*, 1981, 1988). The major findings of these studies are:

1. Active, structured techniques are no better than nondirective styles in eliciting positive findings (i.e., areas of pathology). However, active techniques are better in eliciting more detailed and thorough information in areas where pathology is found and are also better at delineating areas without pathology.
2. An active, fact-gathering style does not prevent the interviewer from effectively eliciting emotional reactions from informants.
3. Use of open questions, direct requests for feelings, interpretations of feelings, and expressions of sympathy are associated with greater expression of emotions by informants.

Table 3.8   Obstructive Interventions

Intervention	Examples
Suggestive or biased questions	"You haven't been feeling suicidal, have you?" "You've had six jobs in the last 2 yr I guess none of them held your interest."
Judgmental questions or statements	"How long have you been behaving so selfishly?" "What you've told me is typical of delusional thinking."
"Why" questions	"Why can't you sit still?" "Why do you keep choosing men who can't make a commitment to you?"
Ignoring the patient's leads	*Patient:* "I'm afraid I'm going to fall apart". *Interviewer:* "Have you had any odd experiences, such as hearing voices?" *P:* "No, but I just feel as though I can't cope and I wanted to talk to someone about it." *I:* "Has your sleep pattern or appetite changed?" *P:* "Well, I don't sleep as well as I used to, but it's getting through the days that's the hardest." *I:* Have you had any suicidal thought?", etc.
Crowding the patient with questions	*P:* "I just can't get it out of my mind that this cancer of mine is a punishment of some kind because I…" *I:* "Have you been in a low mood or been tearful?"
Compound questions	"Have you ever heard voices or thought that other people were out to harm you?"
Vague questions	"Do you feel socially self-conscious a lot?" "How much trouble do you have with your memory?"
Minimization or dismissal	*P:* "I don't seem to be able to enjoy my life as much as I think I should". *I:* "You're doing well at your job and have a nice family – you're probably just feeling some minor stress".
Premature advice or reassurance	*P:* "I've been having terrible headaches and I forget a lot of things. There's nothing wrong with my brain, is there?" *I:* "Headaches and forgetfulness are very common and are probably due to some minor cause in your case." *P:* "I've started to have thoughts that I married the wrong man and I should leave my husband." *I:* "Maybe the two of you ought to take some time away together."
Nonverbal questions	Sitting at a distance, yawning, looking at watch, fidgeting, frowning, rolling of eyes.

Table 3.9   Fact-oriented Interventions in the Psychiatric Interview

Intervention	Examples
Questions about symptoms	"Do the voices seem to come from within your own head or from outside?" "When did you first begin to check your door lock many times before going out?"
Questions about behavior	"What do you do when you fly into a rage – do you yell, hit the furniture, or hit people?" "Since you've had your pain, how is your daily routine different than it used to be?"
Questions about events	"What was the next thing you did after you took the overdose of medication?" "What led up to your decision to move out of your parents' home?"
Request for biographical data	"Who lived with you when you were growing up?" "How many times have you been in a psychiatric hospital?" "Tell me about your close relationships with women."
Requests for medical data	"What medicines do you take?" "What conditions do you see a doctor for?"

Table 3.10	**Feeling-oriented Interventions in the Psychiatric Interview**
Intervention	Examples
Questions about feelings in specific situations	"Some people might have been angry in the situation you told me about. Did you feel that way?" "How did you feel when your doctor told you that you had a heart attack?" "I've noticed your voice got much quieter when you answered my last question. What were you feeling just then?"
Questions or comments about emotional themes or patterns Questions or comments about the personal meaning of events	"Growing up, you never felt like you measured up to your mother's expectations. Do you feel that same way in your marriage?" "You are concerned about becoming enraged at your daughter. When she disregards your wishes, what do you feel that means about you as a parent?"

Table 3.11	**Feedback in the Psychiatric Interview**
Intervention	Examples
Sharing of ongoing thoughts	"As you were talking I began to wonder if you had ever lost anyone very close to you". "As I hear your story it occurs to me that you've been an outsider every place you've lived in."
Sharing of subjective reactions	"What you are saying makes me feel quite sad." "You've told me how you left treatment with your last psychiatrist, but I still feel a bit confused about what happened." "I notice I'm feeling somewhat tense right now and I wonder if you might be feeling it too."
Imparting of information	"About 75% of people with your condition respond well to medication." "The tendency to develop the kind of symptoms you have described runs in families, and probably is inherited."
Proposing a formulation	"I think the immediate cause of your depression and insomnia is your heavy drinking." "When you are under stress you tend not to think clearly and to develop unrealistic fears. It seems as though your present stress comes from the way you and your family are getting along at home."
Making treatment recommendations	"In order for you to keep safe and begin treatment I think it would be best to go into the hospital for a while." "Medication should help you get out of your depression much faster. When you are feeling better, it would be a good idea for us to try to understand how you got so isolated from your friends and family."
Advice	"It might be better not to decide about changing jobs until you're feeling back to your regular self."
Response to questions	*Patient:* "What type of psychiatrist are you, doctor?" *Interviewer:* "I'm a general psychiatrist who uses medication and psychotherapy. I also have a special interest in anxiety disorder." *P:* "Have you ever seen another patient like me?" *I:* "I can answer your question better if you tell me what there is about you that I might have never seen before." *P:* "Do you think I'm a terrible person?" *I:* "I don't think you are terrible, but I wonder what you think about yourself that you would ask me that."

4. Less activity on the interviewer's part is associated with more informant talkativeness and spontaneous emotional expression. Less directive techniques also tend to produce more emotional responses at times when they are not specifically requested. Conversely, more active styles of asking about feelings may be more effective for informants who are low in spontaneous emotional expression.

5. In summary, techniques which actively elicit both facts and emotions are likely to produce the richest, most detailed database. When skillfully used, these do not impair the doctor–patient relationship.

References

Abramowitz JS (1997) Effectiveness of psychological and pharmacological treatments for obsessive–compulsive disorder: A quantitative review. *J Consult Clin Psychol* 65, 44–52.

Andreasen N and Hoevk PR (1982) The predictive value of adjustment disorders. A follow-up study. *Am Psychiatr* 134, 584–590.

Banmohl J and Jaffe JH (1995) History of alcohol and drug abuse treatment in the United States, in *Encyclopedia of Drugs and Alcohol*, Vol. 3. (ed Jaffe JM). Macmillan, New York.

Barber M, Marzuk P, Leon A *et al.* (2001) Gate questions in psychiatric interviewing. The case of suicide assessment. *Psychiatr Res* 35, 67–69.

Barlow DH (1988) *Anxiety and its Disorders—The Nature and Treatment of Anxiety and Panic*. Guilford Press, New York.

Barlow DM, Gorman JM, Shear MK *et al.* (2000) Cognitive–behavioral therapy, imipramine, or their combination for panic disorder: A randomized controlled trial. *JAMA* 283, 2629–2536.

Barrett-Lennard GT (1981) The empathy cycle. Refinement of a nuclear concept. *J Couns Psychol* 28, 91–100.

Bateman A and Fonagy P (2001) Treatment of borderline personality disorder with psychoanalytically oriented partial hospitalization: An 18-month follow-up. *Am J Psychiatr* 158, 36–42.

Baxter LR (1992) Neuroimaging studies of obsessive–compulsive disorder. *Psychiatr Clin N Am* 15(1), 841–884.

Bellack AS and Mueser KT (1993) Psychosocial treatment of schizophrenia. *Schizophr Bull* 19, 317–336.

Bernstein L and Bernstein R (1985) An overview of interviewing techniques, in *Interviewing, A Guide for Health Professionals*. Appleton-Century-Crofts, New York, pp. 21–33.

Blazer DC, Hughes D and George LK (1991) Generalized anxiety disorder, in *Psychiatric Disorders in America. The Epidemiologic Catchment Area Study* (ed Robins LN). Free Press, New York, pp. 180–203.

Brenner JD and Marmer CR (1998) *Trauma, Memory and Dissociation*. American Psychiatric Press, Washington DC.

Carpenter W and Buchanan RW (1994) Schizophrenia. *New Engl J Med* 330, 681–690.

Casement P (1985) Forms of interactive communication, in *On Learning for the Patient* (ed Casement P). Guilford Press, New York, pp. 72–101.

Cloninger CR (1987) A systematic model for clinical description and classification of personality variants. *Arch Gen Psychiatr* 44, 573–588.

Cloninger R, Martin RL, Guze SB *et al.* (1986) A prospective follow-up and family study of somatization in men and women. *Am J Psychiatr* 143, 873–878.

Cloninger CR, Surakic DM and Przybeck TR (1993) A psychobiological model of temperament and character. *Arch Gen Psychiatr* 50, 975–990.

Coccaro ER and Kavoussi RJ (1997) Fluoxetine and impulsive-aggressive behavior in personality-disordered subjects. *Arch Gen Psychiatr* 45, 1081–1088.

Cox A, Holbrook D and Rutter M (1981) Psychiatric interviewing techniques VI. Experimental study. Eliciting feelings. *Br J Psychiatr* 139, 144–152.

Cox A, Rutter M and Holbrook D (1988) Psychiatric interviewing techniques. A second experimental study: Eliciting feelings. *Br J Psychiatr* 152, 64–72.

Davis JM (1975) Overview: Maintenance therapy in psychiatry. I. Schizophrenia. *Am J Psychiatr* 132, 1237–1245.

Ekman, Friesen W and Ellsworth P (1972) *Emotion in the Human Face*. Pergamon Press, New York.

Elkin I, Shea T, Watkins J *et al.* (1989) National Institute of Mental Health Treatment of Depression Collaborative Research Program. General effectiveness of treatments. *Arch Gen Psychiatr* 46, 971–982.

Elliott R, Stiles W, Mahrer A *et al.* (1987) Primary therapist response modes. Comparison of six rating systems. *J Consult Clin Psychol* 55, 218–223.

Flomenbaum N and Altman M (1985) Medical aspects of emergency psychiatry. *New Dir Ment Health Serv* 28, 55–66.

Ford CV (1995) Dimensions of somatization and hypochondriasis. *Neurol Clin* 13, 241–253.

Ford CV and Foulks DG (1985) Conversion disorders. An overview. *Psychosomatics* 26, 371–374.

Freud A (1946) *The Ego and the Mechanisms of Defense*. International Universities Press, New York.

Fyer AJ, Munnuzza S, Gallops MS *et al.* (1990) Familial transmission of simple phobias and fears: A preliminary report. *Arch Gen Psychiatr* 47, 252–256.

Gaw A (ed) (1993) *Culture, Ethnicity, and Mental Illness*. American Psychiatric Press, Washington DC.

Goddard AW and Charney DS (1997) Toward an integrated neurolobiology of panic disorder. *J Clin Psychiatr* 58(Suppl), 4–11.

Goodwin FK and Jamison KR (1990) *Manic–Depressive Illness*. Oxford University Press, New York.

Greenberg WM, Rosenfeld D and Ortege E (1995) Adjustment disorder: An admission diagnosis. *Am J Psychiatr* 152, 459–461.

Marnat G, (1990) The assessment interview, in *Handbook of Psychological Assessment*, 2nd edn. (ed Groth-Marnat G). John Wiley, New York, pp. 57–79.

Halmi K (ed) (1992) *The Psychobiology and Treatment of Anorexia Nervosa and Bulimia Nervosa*. American Psychiatric Press, Washington DC.

Hammen CL, Gordon D, Burge D *et al.* (1987) Maternal affective disorders, illness and stresses. *Am J Psychiatr* 144, 736–741.

Heim C, Ehlert U and Helhammer DH (2000) The potential role of hypocortisolism in pathophysiology of stress related bodily disorders. *Psychoneuroendocrinology* 25, 1–35.

Herran A, Sierra-Biddle D, deSantiago A *et al.* (2001) Diagnostic accuracy in the first 5 minutes of a psychiatric interview. *Psychother Psychosom* 70, 141–144.

Insel TR (1992) Toward a neuroanatomy of obsessive–compulsive disorder. *Arch Gen Psychiatr* 49, 739–744.

Ishii-Kuntz M and Tallman M (1991) The subjective well-being of parents. *J Fam Issues* 12, 58–68.

Janowsky DS, El-Yousef MK and Davis JM (1974) Playing the name game. Interpersonal maneuvers of manic patients. *Am J Psychiatr* 131, 250–255.

Johnson C and Connors ME (1987) *The Etiology and Treatment of Bulimia Nervosa*. Basic Books, New York.

Jorgensen P, Bennedson B, Christensen J *et al.* (1996) Acute and transient psychotic disorder. Comorbidity with personality disorder. *Acta Psychiatr Scand* 94(6), 460–464.

Katz L, Fleisher W, Kjernisted K *et al.* (1996) A review of the psychobiology and pharmacotherapy of posttraumatic stress disorder. *Can J Psychiatr* 41, 233–238.

Keck PE, McElroy SL and Strakowski SM (1996) New developments in the pharmacological treatments of schizoaffective disorder. *J Clin Psychiatr* 57, 41–48.

Kellner R (1987) Hypochondriasis and somatization. *JAMA* 258, 2718–2722.

Kendler KS (1991) Mood-incongruent psychotic affective illness. A historical empirical review. *Arch Gen Psychiatr* 48, 362–369.

Kendler KS, Masterson CL, Ungaro R *et al.* (1984) A family history study of schizophrenia-related personality disorders. *Am J Psychiatr* 143, 424–427.

Kluft RP and Fine CG (1993) *Clinical Perspectives on Multiple Personality Disorder.* Psychiatric Press, Washington DC.

Knapp ML (1978) *Nonverbal Communication in Human Interaction.* Holt, Rinehart & Winston, New York.

Kotrla KJ and Weinberger DR (1995) Brain imaging in schizophrenia. *Annu Rev Med* 46, 113–122.

Lazare A (1973) Hidden conceptual models in psychiatry. *New Engl J Med* 288, 345–351.

Lazare A (1976) The psychiatric examination in the walk-in clinic. Hypothesis generation and hypothesis testing. *Arch Gen Psychiatr* 33, 96–102.

Lazare A (1981) Current concepts in psychiatry. Conversion symptoms. *New Engl J Med* 305, 745–748.

Lazare A, Eisenthal S and Wasserman L (1975) The customer approach to patienthood. Attending to patients requests in a walk-in clinic. *Arch Gen Psychiatr* 32, 553–558.

Leigh H and Reiser M (1992a) Confusion, delerium, and dementia. Organic brain syndromes and the elderly patient, in *The Patient: Biological, Psychological, and Social Dimensions of Medical Practice*, 3rd edn. Plenum Press, New York.

Leigh M and Reiser M (1992b) Approach to a patient: The patient evaluation grid, in *The Patient. Biological, Psychological, and Social Dimensions of Medical Practice*, 3rd edn. Plenum Press, New York.

Lipowski ZJ (1984) Organic mental disorders – an American perspective. *Br J Psychiatr* 144, 542–546.

Lishman WA (1978) *Organic Psychiatry.* Blackwell Scientific, Oxford, UK.

LoPiccolo J (1985) Diagnosis and treatment of male sexual dysfunction. *J Sex Marital Ther* 2, 215–232.

Luborsky L (1984) Expressive techniques. Listening and understanding, in *Principles of Psychoanalytic Psychotherapy* (ed Luborsky L). Basic Books, New York, pp. 90–93.

Maber BA (1992) Delusions. Contemporary etiological hypotheses. *Psychiatr Ann* 22, 260–264.

Mackinnon R and Michels R (1971) *The Psychiatric Interview in Clinical Practice.* WB Saunders, Philadelphia, pp. 28–33.

Mackinnon RA and Yudofsky SC (1986) The psychiatric interview, in *The Psychiatric Interview in Clinical Practice* (eds Mackinnon RA and Yudofsky SC). Lippincott, Philadelphia.

Malan DH (1979) Unconscious communication, in *Individual Psychotherapy and the Science of Psychodynamics* (ed Malan DH). Butterworth, London, pp. 16–23.

Manschreck TC (1996) Delusional disorder. The recognition and management of paranoia. *J Clin Psychiatr* 57(Suppl), 32–38.

Marks I, Lovell K, Noshirvani H *et al.* (1998) Treatment of post-traumatic stress disorder by exposure and/or cognitive restructuring: A controlled study. *Arch Gen Psychiatr* 55, 317–325.

Marks IM (1987) *Fears, Phobias and Rituals: Panic, Anxiety and Their Disorders.* Oxford University Press, New York.

Marshall WL and Barbaree HE (1990) An integrated theory of the etiology of sexual offending, in *Handbook of Sexual Assault. Issues, Theories, and Treatment of the Offender* (eds Marshall WL, Laws DN, and Barbaree HE). Plenum Press, New York, pp. 257–275.

Merlett GA (1998) Addictive behaviors, etiology and treatment. *Annu Rev Psychol* 39, 223–252.

Meyers J and Stein S (2000) The psychiatric interview in the emergency department. *Emerg Med Clin N Am* 18, 173–183.

Millon T (1996) *Disorders of Personality: DSM-IV and Beyond.* John Wiley, New York.

Milrod B, Busch F, Leon AC *et al.* (2000) Open trial of psychodynamic therapy for panic disorder: A pilot study. *Am J Psychiatr* 157, 1878–1880.

Min SK and Lee BO (1997) Laterality in somatization. *Psychosom Med* 59, 236–240.

Nemiah J (1961a) Psychological conflict, in *Foundations of Psychopathology* (ed Nemiah H). Oxford University Press, New York, pp. 35–55.

Nemiah J (1961b) The doctor and his patient, in *Foundations of Psychopathology* (ed Nemiah H). Oxford University Press, New York, pp. 289–304.

Nesse RM and Berridge KC (1997) Psychoactive drug use in evolutionary perspective. *Science* 278, 63–66.

Nurnberg HG, Raskin M, Levine PE *et al.* (1991) Hierarchy of DSM-III R. Criteria efficiency for the diagnosis of borderline personality disorder. *J Pers Disord* 5, 211–244.

Paykel ES (1978) Contribution of life events to causation of psychiatric illness. *Psychol Med* 8, 245–253.

Popkin MK (1994) Syndromes of brain dysfunction presenting with cognitive impairment or behavioral disturbance. Delirium, dementia, and mental disorders due to a general medical condition, in *The Medical Basis of Psychiatry*, 2nd edn. (eds Winokur G and Clayton PJ). WB Saunders, Philadelphia, pp. 17–37.

Porter TL (1993) The use of race in case presentation (letter). *Am J Psychiatr* 150, 1129.

Prescott CA and Kendler KS (1999) Genetic and environmental contributions to alcohol abuse and dependence in a population-based sample of male twins. *Am J Psychiatr* 156, 34–40.

Reiser D and Schroder A (1980) The interview process, in *Patient Interviewing. The Human Dimension.* Williams & Wilkins, Baltimore, MD, pp. 111–136.

Rutter M, Cox A, Egert S *et al.* (1981) Psychiatric interviewing techniques IV. Experimental study. Four contrasting styles. *Br J Psychiatr* 138, 456–465.

Sensky T, Turkington D, Kingdon D *et al.* (2000) A randomized controlled trail of cognitive–behavioral therapy for persistent symptoms in schizophrenia resistant to medication. *Arch Gen Psychiatr* 57, 165–272.

Shea S (1990) Contemporary psychiatric interviewing. Integration of DSM III R, psychodynamic concerns, and mental status, in *Handbook of Psychological Assessment*, 2nd edn. (eds Goldstein G and Hersen M). Pergamon Press, New York, pp. 283–307.

Siever LJ and Davis KL (1985) Overview: Toward a dysregulation hypothesis of depression. *Am J Psychiatr* 142, 1017–1033.

Siever LJ, Bernstein DP and Silverman JM (1991) Schizotypal, paranoid, and schizoid personality disorders: A review of their current status. *J Pers Disord* 5, 178–193.

Slaby A and Andrew E (1987) The emergency treatment of the depressed patient with physical illness. *Int J Psychiatr Med* 17, 71–83.

Spitzer RL, Endicott JO and Robins E (1978) Research diagnostic criteria. Rationale and reliability. *Arch Gen Psychiatr* 35, 773–782.

Strean H (1985) *Resolving Resistances in Psychotherapy.* John Wiley, New York.

Strupp H and Binder J (1984) Assessment, in *Psychotherapy in a New Key* (eds Strupp H and Binder J). Basic Books, New York.

Sullivan HS (1970) *The Psychiatric Interview.* WW Norton, New York.

Susser E, Fennig S, Jandorf L *et al.* (1995) Epidemiology, diagnosis and course of brief psychoses. *Am J Psychiatr* 152, 1745–1748.

Tarnepolsky A and Berlowitz M (1987) Borderline personality – a review of recent research. *Br J Psychiatr* 151, 724–734.

Thase M and Howland RH (1995) Biological processes in depression. An updated review and integration, in *Handbook of Depression* (eds Beckham E and Leber W). Guilford Press, New York.

Tischler GL (ed) (1987) *Diagnosis and Classification in Psychiatry. A Critical Appraisal of DSM III.* Cambridge University Press, Cambridge, UK.

Tsuang M and Faraone S (1990) *The Genetics of Mood Disorders*. Johns Hopkins University Press, Baltimore, MA.

Valliant GE (1977) *Adaptation to Life*. Little Brown, Boston.

Wiens A (1990) Structured clinical interview for adults, in *Handbook of Psychological Assessment*, 2nd edn. (eds Goldstein G and Hersen M). Pergamon Press, New York, pp. 324–341.

Winokur G, Monahan P, Coryell W *et al.* (1996) Schizophrenia and affective disorder – distinct entities or a continuum? An analysis based on a 6-year follow-up. *Compr Psychiatr* 37, 77–87.

Zuckerman M (1996) The psychobiological model for impulsive unsocialized sensation seeking. A comparative approach. Neuropsychobiology 34, 125–129.

Physician–Patient Relationship

For centuries, healers had little understanding of disease and lacked the technologies we now know are necessary for the treatment and cure of many diseases. Physicians had few medications, and surgery was only a last resort. In fact, the most important tool for healing was the relationship between the physician and the patient. Interpersonal relationships have a powerful influence on both morbidity and mortality (House *et al.*, 1988). Social connectedness enhances health in both direct and indirect ways: directly regulating many biological functions, decreasing anxiety, providing opportunities for new information, and fostering alternative behaviors (Hofer, 1984). We know little about the basic mechanisms by which interpersonal relationships, and the physician–patient relationship in particular, operate (Ursano and Fullerton 1991). However, clinical wisdom holds that both the reality-based elements of the physician–patient relationship – in modern times referred to as the working alliance or the therapeutic alliance (Zetzel, 1956; Greenson, 1965) – and the fantasy-based elements of that relationship affect the patient's pain, suffering and recovery from illness.

Physicians learned through trial and error to interact with their patients in ways that relieved pain and promoted health (Frank, 1971). Often the physician's only interventions were reassuring patients, providing knowledge about the patient's disease, accepting the patient's feelings of distress as normal, and maximizing the patient's hope for the future. Although these interventions, based on wisdom and intuition, are no longer the only tools available to the physician, they continue to be an important part of the physician's and particularly the psychiatrist's therapeutic armamentarium.

Such nonspecific aspects of cure are often thought to be mystical or mysterious. In fact, in biological studies they are recognized as the placebo effect. Oddly, these effects of interpersonal relationships are both one of the prized and one of the most denigrated aspects of all of medicine. Yet, as clinicians, we all strive to alleviate our patients' pain and suffering and return them to health as soon as possible with whatever tools may help. Many well-designed studies show that 20 to 30% of subjects respond to the placebo condition. Recent studies show that analgesic placebo has similar neural mechanisms to opioid analgesia (Petrovic *et al.*, 2002). The problem with placebos is not whether they work but that we do not understand how they work and, therefore, we do not have control over their effects. As a physician, one strives to maximize one's interpersonal healing effects and, in this way as well as with other healing tools, increase the chances of our patients' relief from pain and of recovery.

The physician–patient relationship includes specific roles and motivations. These form the core ingredients of the healing process. In its most generic form the physician–patient relationship is defined by the coming together of an expert and a help seeker to identify, understand and solve the problems of the help seeker. The help seeker (in modern terms, the patient) is motivated by the desire and hope for assistance and relief from pain (Sullivan, 1954). A physician is required to have a genuine interest in people and a desire to help (Lidz, 1983). Simply stated, "the secret of the care of the patient is in caring for the patient" (Peabody, 1927). Caring about and paying attention to a patient's suffering can yield remarkable therapeutic dividends. More than one attending physician has been reminded of this when a patient deferred making a treatment decision until he or she was able to consult with "my doctor", who turned out to be the medical student.

In today's technology-driven medicine, the importance and complexity of the physician–patient interaction are often overlooked. The amount of information the medical student or resident must learn frequently takes precedence over learning the fine points of helping the patient relax sufficiently to provide a thorough history or to allow the physician to palpate a painful abdomen. Talking with patients and understanding the intricacies of the physician–patient relationship may be given little formal attention in the medical school curriculum. Even so, medical students, residents and staff physicians recognize, often with awe, the skill of the senior physician who uncovers the lost piece of history, motivates the patient who had given up hope, or is able to talk to the distressed family without increasing their sense of hopelessness or fear.

The relationship between the physician and the patient is essential to the healing of many patients, perhaps particularly so for many psychiatric patients. The physician who can skillfully recognize the patient's half-hidden comment that he or she has not been taking the prescribed medication, perhaps hidden because of feelings of shame, anger, or denial, is better able to ensure long-term compliance with medication as well as to motivate the patient to stay in treatment. Regardless of the type of treatment – medication, biofeedback, hospitalization, psychotherapy, or the rearrangement of the demands and responsibilities in the patient's life – the relationship with the physician is critical to therapeutic outcome.

Modern medicine emphasizes a specific role for the physician in the relationship with the patient. In many Western countries, the patient comes for help with a specific problem, the doctor's office staff secures permission from a third party payer for the doctor to conduct a particular treatment, a prescribed intervention, which will take a specified amount of time. Decades ago, when the doctor was neighbor, advisor and friend to the patient and routinely invited to important family events in

Essentials of Psychiatry   Jerald Kay and Allan Tasman
© 2006 John Wiley & Sons, Ltd.

the patient's life such as weddings of children, and when doctors routinely cared for more than one generation of the same family, the physician typically assumed that he or she would be a source of strength and assistance to the patient throughout the cycle of life. This meant more than curing a specific disease or relieving a specific pain.

While today's patients may not consciously expect that the physician's influence and healing powers will take many forms in a complex interpersonal relationship, human nature is still the same, and patients still want from their doctors many nonspecific forms of emotional support which can promote a sense of well-being and better health. Though modern doctors may feel a great deal of time pressure to see many patients each day and to focus narrowly their healing efforts, the physician must also be sensitive to the many needs of patients, who believe that the physician is possessed of wisdom and understanding. Sensitivity to such desires and needs will promote effective medical care in all specialties, with all patients. A view that such patients are unusually needy and demanding will not serve the cause of effective medical care.

Finally, in today's mobile and geographically evermore united world, the importance of recognizing the needs of patients from parts of the world other than that of the physician's is a challenge to the practitioner. The physician must be open to the limitations of his or her knowledge of the expectations, beliefs and likely behavior of patients from different cultures, nations, religions, and ethnic and socioeconomic backgrounds. The physician must recognize this challenge and one hopes, embrace it with enthusiasm. It can make the practice of medicine a more exciting experience.

Clinical Vignette 1

A 20-year-old female patient suffered a painful athletic injury. She was unsure exactly how her injury had occurred, but she did recall falling on her shoulder on the tennis court while running after a sharply hit ball. She went to the physician fearing that she had damaged her collarbone. When she was informed that there was no fracture, that her pain was due to a bruised muscle and would go away with ice, heat and aspirin, she immediately felt better. Not only was she relieved but also her perception and experience of the pain actually changed: "It doesn't seem to hurt as much now".

Clinical Vignette 2

Somewhat different was the situation of a 30-year-old male patient who developed chronic pain after an athletic injury. The patient had to convince himself to visit the physician. He felt he was being a "baby" to complain. One week after the injury, he went to his family physician who perfunctorily prescribed a strong painkiller and offered a follow-up appointment a month later. He left feeling that he had been a nuisance. The following week was a particularly bad one for the patient; the pain was severe. But the patient stopped taking the prescribed medication, did not keep the follow-up appointment, and never returned for help. This patient continued to experience pain, unnecessarily, for years. In large part, this was because the physician offered no hope; therefore follow-up care, including physical therapy and alternative medications, could not be provided

The physician–patient relationship is also a source of information for the physician. The way the patient relates to the physician can help the physician understand the problems the patient is experiencing in her or his interpersonal relationships. The nature of the physician–patient relationship can also provide information about relationships in the patient's childhood family, in which interpersonal patterns are first learned. With this information, the physician can better understand the patient's experience, promote cooperation between the patient and those who care for her or him, and teach the patient new behavioral strategies in an empathic manner, understanding the patient's subjective perspective, that is, feelings, thoughts and behaviors.

Clinical Vignette 3

A 45-year-old single man was hospitalized for treatment of a bleeding ulcer. The patient had no past history of ulcers. Despite reassurance, he continued to feel hopeless. A psychiatric consultant was called to evaluate the patient. She found him to be needy, but could not understand why he was so pessimistic. The psychiatrist recognized the importance to this patient of showing interest in him, showing concern for his condition, and spending time with him. The patient's response was noteworthy; he clearly enjoyed the psychiatrist's company but seemed unusually sad when their times together ended. The psychiatrist asked the patient if this was a correct perception and, if so, why it was the case. The patient responded that the psychiatrist reminded him of his mother. Further inquiry revealed that the patient's mother had died several years ago of colon cancer. The psychiatrist inquired about the symptoms the mother had during her terminal illness. The symptoms were similar to the patient's symptoms: bleeding in the digestive tract and gastrointestinal pain.

The psychiatrist then understood the complex process through which the patient was feeling inordinately pessimistic. Transference was evident in his experience of each departure as an unconscious reminder of the loss of his mother. The patient's identification with his mother (as part of managing her death) was also the source of his unspoken expectation that he, too, was dying of colon cancer. It was the pattern of the relationship between the psychiatrist and the patient, the sadness shown whenever the psychiatrist left, that provided the information necessary to help the patient. Increasing the patient's understanding of his medical condition, specifically how it was different from his mother's, relieved his emotional pain, and he began on the road to recovery.

These clinical vignettes illustrate that the physician–patient relationship is composed of both the reality-based component (the working alliance or therapeutic alliance) and the fantasy-based component (the transference) derived from the patient's patterns of interpersonal behavior learned in childhood. Either or both of these may maximize or limit the patient's sense of reassurance, available information, feelings of comfort and sense of hope (Meissner, 1996). In this way, the nonspecific curative aspects of the physician–patient relationship may be enhanced or diminished.

Formation of the Physician–Patient Relationship

Assessment and Evaluation

The physician–patient relationship develops during the assessment and evaluation of the patient. The patient observes the thoroughness and sensitivity with which the physician collects information, performs the physical examination, and explains needed tests. At each step, the physician's clarification of the treatment goals and interventions either builds up the patient's expectation of help and feelings of safety or creates increasing disease for the patient. In many aspects and, in particular, in the physician's compassion and patience, he/she is like a good teacher, establishing the context in which learning and growth may occur and anxiety decrease (Banner and Cannon, 1997). Alertness to the patient's fears and misunderstandings of the evaluation process can minimize unnecessary disruptions of the relationship and provide information on the patient's previous experiences with medical care and important authority figures. These past experiences form the patient's present expectations of either help or disappointment (Smith and Thompson, 1993) (Table 4.1).

Rapport

Early in the relationship between a psychiatrist and a patient, the patient requests help with his or her pain, uncertainty, or discomfort. The psychiatrist initiates the "contract" of the relationship by acknowledging the patient's pain and offering help. In this action, the psychiatrist has recognized the patient's ill-health and acknowledged the need for and possibility of removing the disease or illness. In this first stage of the development of rapport, the way of relating between the physician and the patient, the physician–patient relationship has begun to organize the interactions. Through the physician's and the patient's shared recognition of the patient's pain, the basis for rapport – a comfortable pattern of working together – is established.

The psychiatrist's ability to empathize, to understand in feeling terms every patient's subjective experience, is important to the development of rapport. Empathy is particularly important in complex interpersonal behavioral problems in which the environment (family, friends, caretakers) may wish to expel the patient, and the patient has therefore lost hope. Suicidal patients, adolescents involved in intense family conflicts and patients in conflict with their medical caregivers can often be convinced to cooperate with the evaluation only when the psychiatrist has shown accurate empathy early in the first meeting with the patient. When the physician acknowledges the patient's pain, the patient feels less alone and inevitably more hopeful (Marziali and Alexander, 1991). This rapport establishes a set of principles of

and expectations for the physician–patient interaction. On this basic building block more elaborate goals and responsibilities of the patient can be developed.

Clinical Vignette 4

A young man sought treatment for ill-defined reasons: he was dissatisfied with his work, his social life and his relationship with his parents. He was unable to say how he thought the psychiatrist could help him, but he knew he was experiencing emotional pain: he felt sadness, anxiety, inhibition and loss of a lust for living. He wanted help. The psychiatrist noted the patient's tentative style and heard him describe his ambivalence toward his controlling and directing father. With this in mind, the psychiatrist articulated the patient's wish for help and recognized with him his confusion about what was troubling him. She suggested that through discussion they might define together what he was looking for and how she might help him. This description of the evaluation process as a joint process of discovery established a rapport based on shared work that removed the patient's fears of control and allowed him to feel heard, supported, and involved in the process of regaining his health.

The Therapeutic or Working Alliance

For a patient to trust and work closely with a physician it is essential that there be a reality-based relationship outside the conflicted ones for which the patient is seeking help (Rawn, 1991; Friedman, 1969). With more disturbed patients considerable skill is required of the physician to reach this reality-based part of the patient and decrease the patient's fears and expectations of attack or humiliation. Even for healthy patients, the physician must bridge the gap between the patient and the physician that is always present because of their different backgrounds and perceptions of the world. This gap is an expectable result of differences between the physician's and the patient's culture, gender, ethnic background, socioeconomic class, religion, age, or role in the physician–patient relationship. The experienced physician makes communication across the gap seem effortless, using a different "language" for each patient. The student often sees this as an art rather than as a skill to be learned.

The therapeutic alliance is extremely important in times of crisis such as suicidality, hospitalization and aggressive behavior. But it is also the basis of agreement about appointments, fees and treatment requirements. In psychiatric patients, this core component of the physician–patient relationship can be disturbed and requires careful tending. Frequently, the psychiatrist may feel that he or she is "threading a needle" to reach and maintain the therapeutic alliance while not activating the more disturbed elements of the patient's patterns of interpersonal relating.

The therapeutic or working alliance must endure in spite of what may, at times, be intense, irrational, delusional, characterologic, or transference-based feelings of love and hate. The working alliance must outweigh or counterbalance the distorted components of the relationship. It must provide a stable base for the patient and the physician when the patient's feelings or behaviors may impair reflection and cooperation. The working alliance embodies the mutual responsibilities both physician and patient have accepted to restore the patient's health. Likewise, the working alliance must be strong enough to ensure that the

Table 4.1 Mechanisms for the Formation of the Physician–Patient Relationship

Assessment and evaluation process
Development of physician–patient rapport
Therapeutic or working alliance
Transference
Countertransference
Defense mechanisms
Patient's mental status

treatment goes forward even when both members of the dyad may doubt that it can. The alliance requires a basic trust by the patient that the physician is working in his or her best interests, despite how the patient may feel at a given moment. Patients must be taught to be partners in the healing process and to recognize that the physician is a committed partner in that process as well. The development of common goals fosters the physician and patient seeing themselves as having reciprocal responsibilities: the physician to work in a physician-like fashion to promote healing; the patient to participate actively in formulating and supporting the treatment plan, "trying on" more adaptive behaviors in the chosen mode of treatment, and taking responsibility for his or her actions to the extent possible (Ursano and Silberman, 1988).

Important to the reality-based relationship with the patient is the physician's ability to recognize and acknowledge the limitations of her or his knowledge and to work collaboratively with other physicians. When this happens, patients are most often appreciative, not critical, and experience a strengthening of the alliance because of the physician's commitment to finding an answer. When a patient loses confidence in the physician, it is often because of unacknowledged shortcomings in the physician's skills. The patient may lose motivation to maintain the alliance and seek help elsewhere. Alternatively, the patient may seek no help.

Transference and Countertransference

Transference is the tendency we all have to see someone in the present as being like an important figure from our past (Freud, 1958). This process occurs outside our conscious awareness; it is probably a basic means used by the brain to make sense of current experience by seeing the past in the present and limiting the input of new information. Transference is more common in settings that provoke anxiety and provide few cues to how to behave – conditions typical of a hospital. Transference influences the patient's behavior and can distort the physician–patient relationship, for good or ill (Adler, 1980).

Although transference is a distortion of the present reality, it is usually built around a kernel of reality that can make it difficult for the inexperienced clinician to recognize rather than react to the transference. The transference can be the elaboration of an accurate observation into the "total" explanation or the major evidence of some expected harm or loss. Often the physician may recognize transference by the pressure she or he feels to respond in a particular manner to the patient, for example, always to stay longer or not abruptly leave the patient (Sandler *et al*., 1973).

Transference is ubiquitous. It is a part of day-to-day experience, although its operation is outside conscious awareness. Recognizing transference in the physician–patient relationship can aid the physician in understanding the patient's deeply held expectations of help, shame, injury, or abandonment that derive from childhood experiences.

Transference reactions, of course, are not confined to the patient; the physician also superimposes the past on the present. This is called countertransference, the physician's transference to the patient (Table 4.2). Countertransference usually takes one of two forms: concordant countertransference, in which one empathizes with the patient's position; or complementary countertransference, in which one empathizes with an important figure from the patient's past (Racker, 1968). For example, concordant countertransference would be evident if a patient were describing

Table 4.2	Types of Countertransference

Concordant countertransference
  The physician experiences and empathizes with **the patient's** emotional experience and perception of reality
Complementary countertransference
  The physician experiences and empathizes with the emotional experience and perception of reality of **an important person from the patient's life**

an argument with his or her boss, and the psychiatrist, perhaps after a disagreement with the psychiatrist's own supervisor and without having collected detailed information from the patient, felt, "Oh yeah, what a terrible boss". Similarly, complementary countertransference would be evident if the same psychiatrist felt, "This person (the patient) does not work very hard, no wonder the boss is dissatisfied," and felt angry with the patient as well. Paying close attention to our personal reactions while refraining from immediate action can inform us in an experiential manner about subtle aspects of the patient's behavior that we may overlook or not appreciate. In the preceding example, the psychiatrist with the concordant countertransference might be identifying with the patient's subtle need to fight with authority. The psychiatrist with the complementary countertransference might have identified with the patient's boss, seeing only the patient's more passive wishes.

Countertransference occurs in all "sizes and shapes", more or less mixed with the physician's past but often greatly influencing the physician–patient relationship. The wish to save or rescue a patient is commonly experienced and indicates a need to look for countertransference responses. When a patient is seriously ill, such as with cancer, we may increasingly want to treat the patient more aggressively, with procedures that may hold little hope, create substantial pain, and perhaps even be against the patient's wishes. The physician's feelings of loss of a valued person (in the present and as a reminder of the past) or feelings of failure (loss of the physician's own power and ability) can often fuel such reactions. More subtle factors, such as the effects of being overworked, can result in unrecognized feelings of deprivation leading to unspoken wishes for a patient to quit treatment. When these feelings appear in subtle countertransference reactions, such as being late to appointments, becoming tired in an hour, or being unable to recall previous material, they can have powerful effects on the patient's wish to continue treatment.

Major developmental events in physicians' lives can also influence their perceptions of their patients. When a psychiatrist is expecting the birth of a child, she or he may be overly sensitive to or ignore the concerns of a patient worried about a significant illness in the patient's child. Similarly, a physician with a dying parent or spouse may be unable to empathize with a patient's concerns about loss of a job, feeling that it is trivial.

Defense Mechanisms

All people, including patients, employ mechanisms of defense to protect themselves from the painful awareness of feelings and memories that can provoke overwhelming anxiety. Defense mechanisms are specific cognitive processes: ways of thinking that the mind employs to avoid painful feelings (Freud, 1966). They are often characteristic of a person and form a style of

Clinical Vignette 5

A psychiatrist was called to evaluate an agitated older adult resident of a nursing home. After she had interviewed the energetic, sad and anxious patient, the psychiatrist found herself unexpectedly sad, confused and unsure about what to do. This was not a new case for the psychiatrist, who had treated many similar cases. In considering her response, her thoughts turned to her grandmother with whom she had lived when she was 8 years old, and who had been displaced from her residence and moved to a nursing home in another city by well-meaning children who wanted her near them. After the move, her grandmother had become depressed and disoriented and died 3 months later. The psychiatrist recalled feeling confused at the time of her grandmother's death, wondering why she had died when she had just moved to an attractive new home. Recalling her confusion, the psychiatrist could think more clearly about her present patient and wondered if the patient might be depressed. She talked further with the nurses and found symptoms of depression in addition to the nighttime agitation. This new information altered her decision on the type of medication to begin with and the need for psychotherapy in addition to medication.

cognition (Shapiro, 1965). Common defense mechanisms include projection, repression, displacement, intellectualization, humor, suppression and altruism (Table 4.3).

Defense mechanisms may be more or less mature depending on the degree of distortion of reality and interpersonal disruption to which they lead. This patterning of feelings, thoughts and behaviors by defense mechanisms is involuntary and arises in response to perceptions of psychic danger (Vaillant, 1992). The patient's characteristic defense mechanisms, the cognitive processes used to lower anxiety and unpleasant feelings, can greatly affect the physician–patient relationship. Defense mechanisms operate all the time; however, in times of high anxiety, such as in a hospital or during a life crisis, patients may become much less flexible in the defenses they use and may revert to using less mature defenses.

Table 4.3 Common Defense Mechanisms

Healthier Defenses	More Primitive Defenses
Sublimation	Splitting
Humor	Projection
Repression	Projective identification
Displacement	Omnipotence
Intellectualization	Devaluing
Reaction formation	Primitive idealization
Reversal	Denial
Identification with the aggressor	Conversion
Asceticism	Avoidance
Altruism	
Isolation of affect	

Clinical Vignettes 6 and 7 are examples of defense mechanisms (conversion and avoidance or repression) affecting the treatment relationship. In Vignette 6, the conversion reaction that resulted in the paralysis expressed both the patient's anger and his conflict over what to do. In Vignette 7, the physician knew that the

Clinical Vignette 6

A 36-year-old army first sergeant was hospitalized for the evaluation of acute paralysis of his right hand. When the results of a neurological work-up revealed no evidence of organic pathology, psychiatric consultation was obtained. The patient denied any past psychiatric history or significant alcohol or other substance abuse. He described a healthy family support system but then hesitated, saying, "You know, Doc, there's one thing I just haven't been able to talk about with anyone." He proceeded to speak of the extreme pressure he was feeling on the job, where he had found out that his boss (the company commander) was behaving unethically. The patient stated, "I feel like I'm between a rock and a hard place – if I report it, I'm being disloyal to my boss, but if I don't, I'm betraying my soldiers and the army". After further elaborating his feelings of anger and disgust toward his boss, the patient asked to terminate the interview but agreed to talk with the psychiatrist again in the morning.

Returning the next morning, the psychiatrist was greeted by the patient, who was brushing his teeth, using his right hand. "Hey, Doc, I'm good to go!" The patient then described what happened the evening before. "I was telling my wife about how I've got to get out of here and get back to work, because, after all, I'm the commander's right-hand man. And you know what, Doc? My hand started to work! Get me out of here, I'm not crazy after all!" The patient then reviewed the process, aided by the psychiatrist, and was able to further his understanding of the link between his conflicted rage toward his boss and how it was expressed symbolically as an involuntary physical paralysis of his right hand. He resolved: "I'm gonna do the right thing. I got to live with myself", and planned to report the commander's misconduct on return to work. He was discharged from the hospital later that day, having regained full use of his hand.

Clinical Vignette 7

A 20-year-old man came for consultation because of uncertainty about his career. He soon revealed that he felt profoundly sad, hopeless, helpless and even suicidal. He had a family history of depression. The physician and patient agreed to employ antidepressant medication aggressively. Yet over a period of several weeks the patient did not improve. When the physician asked why that might be happening, the patient revealed that he had frequently forgotten to take the prescribed medication and had forgotten to tell the physician that this was the case during two meetings. The physician explored the reasons for this, and together the physician and the patient learned that the patient felt ashamed of having been diagnosed as depressed and of having been considered to require medication. He felt he was not his own master and had experienced this as a severe blow to his self-esteem. Taking the medication was a reminder of this "flaw". Hearing himself say this and feeling the physician's empathic support, the patient recognized the irrationality of his behavior and felt relieved. In addition, the physician now understood better the intensity of the patient's feelings and changed the prescription to once-a-day dosage at bedtime to decrease the patient's sense of shame and increase compliance with the treatment.

forgetting was neither intentional nor conscious but was directed at denying the need for treatment. In these cases, recognizing the defenses was important to knowing how to relate to the patient (Clinical Vignette 6) and avoid a countertransference reaction of anger at the patient for lack of compliance (Clinical Vignette 7).

Mental Status of the Patient

The patient's mental status is a major determinant of the formation and nature of the relationship with the physician. A young, healthy patient with an acute disorder has different needs and expectations than a somewhat older person who comes for help with a condition that has been present for a number of years. Both differ from the older adult who comes to the physician expecting that the future will be filled with physical and emotional losses.

It can be seen when comparing these two clinical vignettes that the mental status of the patient helps define the nature of

A 25-year-old recent law school graduate came to a psychiatrist following a romantic disappointment. He reported that he was very sad because his girlfriend had chosen to move to a different city, which he believed foretold the end of their relationship. He added that he had been having trouble sleeping for several weeks, and was worried because his exhaustion was causing problems in his ability to perform his work. When the physician took a careful history, he learned that this young man had led a successful life, and that his social and sexual development had been quite unremarkable. He had had good friends and close friendships, and several girlfriends in his life. He said he would miss his girlfriend, but that he never intended to marry her. The doctor indicated to her patient that sometimes, after such a disappointment, it was quite common for there to be a period of anxiety and that his sadness was a good sign, showing that he had a good capacity to attach and mourn the loss of a close friend. The psychiatrist also suggested that the patient may be more angry with the girlfriend than he had recognized, with which the patient agreed. The doctor prescribed a mild sleep medication, suggesting it may not even be required, and scheduled a follow-up appointment in a month. When the patient returned, he reported that he had used only two of the sleeping pills and had thrown the rest away. He did not want to schedule another appointment; he expressed gratitude to the psychiatrist and they parted company.

A 70-year-old widowed lawyer was vigorous, active, financially comfortable, with many friends and professional associates. She explained to the psychiatrist that the last year had, however, been very difficult for her. Six months before, her husband of 45 years had died after a 2-year struggle with congestive heart failure. She now found herself seriously depressed, despite her active life. She was thinking actively about giving up her law practice, though she was very involved in several ongoing cases, which she had previously found interesting and which held the promise of significant financial reward. She went on to say that she had no appetite. She was chronically sleep deprived and was losing interest in her friends, children and grandchildren. When taking a careful history, the psychiatrist also learned that this patient had suffered from a serious depression 35 years earlier, when she lost a pregnancy, and that this depression lasted for a year. It eventually resolved after she took a tricyclic antidepressant and engaged in brief, insight-oriented psychotherapy. In that therapy, her relationship with her own depressed mother had been discussed. With all this information, the psychiatrist suggested she and her patient meet weekly and that the treatment include a pharmacological intervention to help with the patient's current depression. This treatment ended successfully 1 year later.

the physician–patient relationship, though in both cases the treatment relationship was of relatively brief duration and ended successfully.

The patient's mental status in this case was the focus of and major factor in the structure of a long psychotherapy that greatly assisted the rehabilitation of interpersonal skills and the

A 40-year-old man came to a psychiatrist with a long history of emotional difficulties. He had been a healthy and happy college student when he developed a skin abscess, which caused a septicemia and a brain infection. After this, his entire life changed. Although college was quite challenging, he was able to finish it, but had difficulty concentrating, his judgment was poor, his impulse control impaired. He had difficulty remembering words, and he realized that his previously adequate social skills had been lost. Where once he had been charming and known for his sense of humor, now he was dull and in many ways boring. Yet there was more to him than that, and he longed for an opportunity to speak with an understanding listener in the hope that through such a relationship he might be able to make constructive changes in his life. He knew what had been lost, he wanted to understand his limitations better, and he wanted to be able to function well enough to keep a job. A more remote goal was to have a long-term relationship with a woman. His consulting psychiatrist knew that were she to take on this patient it would be for the long haul. Fortunately, there were no financial barriers to treatment, and the pair worked together on a weekly basis for many years. In the course of that treatment, the patient came to understand the social situations that made him anxious and the way his emotional states of mind influenced changes in his cognitive function. He developed the ability to work and love more effectively; he met a woman who was kind and loving. The psychiatrist was invited to his wedding. She attended the religious service but quietly left the reception after congratulating her patient and his wife. By that time, years into the physician–patient relationship, the patient saw his physician as a wise observer, an advisor and a trusted friend. To the physician, her patient was a happy reminder of how much a person can strive to improve his life, and a rich source of learning about the interaction of emotion, cognitive function and behavior.

understanding of his cognitive limitations and newly changed cognition. The ability to work with an empathic listener while confronting limitations and feelings of shame and embarrassment is a special opportunity of the well-formed doctor–patient relationship.

Special Issues in the Physician–Patient Relationship

Phase of Treatment

The treatment phase – early, middle, or late (Table 4.4) – affects the structure of the physician–patient relationship in terms of both the issues to be addressed and the task to be accomplished by the physician and the patient. The early stage of treatment involves developing a rapport, forming shared initial goals, and initiating the working alliance. Education of the patient is important to the success of the physician–patient relationship in this stage, so that the patient learns what he or she can expect. In the middle stage of treatment, the physician and patient continuously refine their shared goals, and various interventions are tried. While this takes place, transference and countertransference are likely to emerge. How these are recognized and managed is critical to whether the relationship continues and is therapeutic.

In the later phase of treatment, the assessment of the outcome and plans for the future are the primary focus. The physician and the patient discuss the end of their relationship in a process known as termination. Successes and disappointments associated with the treatment are reviewed. The physician must be willing to acknowledge the patient's disappointments, as well as recognize her or his own disappointments in the treatment. The therapeutic alliance is strengthened in this stage when the physician accepts expressions of the patient's disappointments, encourages such expressions when they are not forthcoming,

---

Table 4.4 Key Features of Treatment Phases

Early: developing rapport, forming shared initial goals, initiating the working alliance

Middle: refining shared goal, using a variety of trial interventions

Late: assessing outcome, resolving presenting problems, planning for future

---

Table 4.5 Factors Affecting the Physician–Patient Relationship

Phases of treatment: early, middle, late
Treatment setting
Transition between inpatient and outpatient treatment
Managed care
Health and illness of the physician

---

and prepares the patient for the future. Such preparations include orienting the patient as to when he or she might seek further treatment (Ursano and Silberman, 2002). Solidifying the physician–patient relationship at the end of the treatment can be critical to the patient's self-esteem and willingness to return if symptoms reappear (Table 4.5).

As a part of the termination process the physician and the patient must review what has been learned, discuss what changes have taken place in the patient and the patient's life, and acknowledge together the sadness and joy of their leave-taking. The termination involves a mourning process even when treatment has been brief or unpleasant. Of course, when the physician–patient relationship has been rewarding, and both physician and patient are satisfied with what they have accomplished, mourning is more intense and often characterized by a bittersweet sadness.

Treatment Settings

The physician–patient relationship takes place in a variety of treatment settings. These include the private office, community clinic, emergency room, inpatient psychiatric ward and general hospital ward. Psychiatrists treating patients in a private office may find that the relative privacy of this setting enhances the early establishment of trust related to confidentiality. In addition, the psychiatrist's personality is more evident in the private office where personal factors influencing choice of decor, room arrangement and location play a role. However, in contrast to the hospital or community setting, the private office generally lacks other evidence of the physician's competence and humanness. In hospital and community settings, when a colleague greets the physician and the patient in the hall, or the physician receives a call for a consultation by a colleague or for a meeting, it indicates to the patient that the physician is qualified, skilled and humane.

On the other hand, therapeutic work conducted in the community clinic, emergency room and general hospital ward often requires the psychiatrist and patient to adapt rapidly to meeting one another, assessing the problem, establishing treatment goals, and ensuring the appropriate interventions and follow-up. The importance of protecting the patient's needs for time, predictability and structure can run counter to the demands of a busy service and unexpected clinical and administrative requirements. The psychiatrist must stay alert to the patient's perspective but not all interruptions can be avoided. The patient can be informed and accommodated as much as possible, and any feelings of hurt, disappointment, or anger can be listened for by the physician and responded to empathically. At times, patients, particularly those with borderline personality disorder, may require transfer to another psychiatrist whose schedule can accommodate the patient's exquisite needs for stability.

The boundaries of confidentiality are necessarily extended in hospital and community settings to include consultation with other physicians, nursing staff and often family members (Wise and Rundell, 2002). Particular attention must always be given to the patient's need for and right to respect and privacy. Regardless of the setting, patients receiving medication must be fully informed about the potential risks and benefits of and alternatives to the recommended pharmacological treatment (Kessler, 1991). Patients must be educated about the risks and benefits of receiving prescribed treatment and of not receiving treatment. This is an important component of maintaining the physician–patient relationship. Patients who are informed about and involved in decisions about medication respect the physician's role and interest in their welfare. Psychiatrists must also pay particular attention to the meaning a patient attaches to any prescribed medication, particularly when the time comes to alter or discontinue its use (Ursano *et al.*, 1991).

The change from inpatient to outpatient therapy involves the resumption of a greater degree of autonomy by the patient in the physician–patient dyad. The physician must actively encourage this separation and its hope for the future. This transition is delicate for any therapeutic pair.

Managed Care

Managed care, broadly defined as any care of patients that is not determined solely by the provider, currently focuses on the economic aspects of delivering medical care, with little attention thus far to its potential effects on the physician–patient relationship (Goodman et al., 1992). Discontinuity of care and the creation of unrealistic expectations on the part of patients have been raised as likely deleterious effects on that relationship (Emanuel and Brett, 1993). Other issues that can affect the physician–patient relationship include the erosion of confidentiality, shrinkage of the types of reimbursable services, and diminished autonomy of the patient and the physician in medical decision-making. Additionally, many managed care systems dictate a split treatment model, with the psychiatrist prescribing psychopharmacologic treatment and a separate clinician providing psychotherapy. In such a system, there are complicated challenges faced both by clinicians and patients. With neither party in complete control of decisions, the physician–patient relationship can become increasingly adversarial and subservient to external issues such as cost, quality of life, political expediency and social efficiency (Siegler, 1993).

The Physician–Patient Relationship in Specific Populations of Patients

Cross-cultural and Ethnic Issues

Addressing cross-cultural issues such as race, ethnicity, religion and gender is vital to the establishment and maintenance of an effective physician–patient relationship (see Chapter 2 and 21). Failure to clarify cultural assumptions, whether stemming from differences or similarities in background, may impede the establishment of a trusting therapeutic alliance, making effective treatment unlikely (Cheng and Lo, 1991).

Children, Adolescents and Families

Establishing an effective physician–patient relationship with children, adolescents and families is one of the most challenging and rewarding tasks in the practice of psychiatry. Rather than being treated as "little adults", children and adolescents must be approached with an appreciation for their age-appropriate developmental tasks and needs. When physicians treat this population, they must establish a trusting relationship with both the patient and the parents. Preadolescent children face the psychosocial developmental tasks of establishing trust, autonomy, initiative and achievement. By understanding the facets of normal childhood development, physicians may help parents understand the nature of their child's disturbance and work within the family system to establish effective mechanisms for coping and recovery (Angold, 2000; Erikson, 1950).

Adolescent patients, facing the task of establishing an individual identity, pose particular challenges to the physician–patient relationship. Adolescents are particularly sensitive to any signals from the physician that their powers of decision, their intelligence, or their perceptions are being ignored. The critical time for engagement with the adolescent is often in the first session, sometimes even in the first few minutes (Katz, 1990). Defiance, detachment and aggression may be anticipated and defused with a steady therapeutic presence grounded in consistent boundaries and open acknowledgment of the adolescent patient's distress (Colson *et al.*, 1991).

In working with families, physicians in general and psychiatrists in particular must clearly address questions and concerns regarding all aspects of treatment and convey respectful compassion for all members. The therapeutic alliance, or "joining" with the family and patient, requires developing enough of a family consensus that treatment is worth the struggle involved. Taking sides and engaging with individual and family power struggles can be particularly destructive to the physician–patient relationship in families. Rather, it is the physician's ability to relate to the family as a multifaceted organism, massively interconnected, transcending the sum of its parts, that often allows treatment to progress and, in the best scenarios, allows for growth and understanding to occur (Fleck, 1985; Ziegler, 1999).

Terminally Ill Patients

Terminally ill patients share concerns related to the end of the life-cycle. Elderly patients at all levels of health face the developmental task of integrating the various threads of their life into a figurative tapestry that reflects their lifelong feelings, thoughts, values, goals, beliefs, experiences and relationships, and places them into a meaningful perspective. Patients newly diagnosed with a terminal illness such as metastatic cancer or acquired immunodeficiency syndrome may be particularly overwhelmed and initially unable to deal with the demands of their illness, especially if the patient is a younger adult or child. Psychiatrists may enhance the terminally ill patient's ability to cope by addressing issues related to medical treatment, pharmacotherapy, psychotherapy, involvement of significant others, legal matters and institutional care (Lederberg and Holland, 2000). Patients struggling with spiritual or religious concerns may benefit from a religious consultation, a resource that is frequently unused.

Countertransference feelings ranging from fear to helplessness to rage to despair can assist the therapist greatly in maintaining the physician–patient relationship and ensuring appropriate care. Physicians working with patients with acquired immunodeficiency syndrome must frequently confront their own feelings and attitudes toward homosexuality (McKusick, 1988). Issues commonly encountered with disabled patients include inaccurate assumptions about their ability to function fully in all areas of human activity, including sex and vocation. Terminally ill patients may evoke reactions of unwarranted pessimism, thwarting the physician's ability to help the patient maximize hope for the quality of whatever time may remain. Patients and their family members often look to their physician for guidance.

Conclusion

The physician–patient relationship is essential to the healing process and is the foundation on which an effective treatment plan may be negotiated, integrating the best of what medical technology and human caring can provide. The centrality of this relationship is particularly true for psychiatric physicians and their patients. In the psychiatrist–patient relationship, empathy, compassion and hope frequently serve as the major means of alleviating pain and enhancing active participation in all treatment interventions: biological, psychological and social.

The development of the physician–patient relationship depends on skilled assessment, the development of rapport through empathy, a strong therapeutic alliance and the effective understanding of transference, countertransference and defense mechanisms. Current research findings support the purposeful use of common therapy factors, of which the therapeutic alliance is the most powerful, to enhance clinical outcome.

The development of the physician–patient relationship is influenced by numerous factors, including the phase of treatment, the treatment setting, transitions between inpatient and outpatient care, managed care and changes in the physician's health. The astute physician is attuned to the needs and characteristics of specific populations of patients, adopting the therapeutic approach that most effectively bridges the gap between physician and patient and leads to a healing relationship.

References

Adler G (1980) Transference, real relationship and alliance. *Int J Psychoanal* 61, 547–558.

Angold A (2000) Assessment in child and adolescent psychiatry, in *New Oxford Textbook of Psychiatry* (eds Gelder MG, Lopez-Ibor JJ, and Andreasen N). Oxford University Press, Oxford, pp. 1700–1705.

Banner JM and Cannon H (1997) *The Elements of Teaching.* Yale University Press, New Haven, pp. 81–106.

Cheng LY and Lo HT (1991) On the advantages of cross-cultural psychotherapy: The minority therapist/mainstream patient dyad. *Psychiatry* 54, 386–396.

Colson DB, Cornsweet C, Murphy T *et al.* (1991) Perceived treatment difficulty and therapeutic alliance on an adolescent psychiatric hospital unit. *Am J Orthopsychiatr* 61, 221–229.

Emanuel EJ and Brett AS (1993) Managed competition and the patient–physician relationship. *New Engl J Med* 329, 879–882.

Erikson EH (1950) *Childhood and Society.* WW Norton, New York.

Fleck S (1985) The family and psychiatry, in *Comprehensive Textbook of Psychiatry*, Vol. 4 (eds Kaplan HI and Saddock BJ). Williams & Wilkins, Baltimore, pp. 273–294.

Frank JD (1971) Therapeutic factors in psychotherapy. *Am J Psychother* 25, 350–361.

Freud A (1966) *The Ego and the Mechanisms of Defense*, Rev. ed. International Universities Press, New York.

Freud S (1958) The dynamics of transference, in *The Standard Edition of the Complete Psychological Works of Sigmund Freud*, Vol. 12 (trans-ed Strachey J). Hogarth Press, London, pp. 97–108. (Originally published in 1912).

Friedman L (1969) The therapeutic alliance. *Int J Psychoanal* 50, 139–153.

Goodman M, Brown J and Dietz P (1992) *Managing Managed Care: A Mental Health Practitioner's Survival Guide.* American Psychiatric Press, Washington DC.

Greenson R (1965) The working alliance and the transference neurosis. *Psychoanal Q* 34, 155–181.

Hofer MA (1984) Relationships as regulators: A psychobiologic perspective on bereavement. *Psychosom Med* 46, 183–197.

House JS, Landis KR and Umberson D (1988) Social relationships and health. *Science* 241, 540–545.

Katz P (1990) The first few minutes: The engagement of the difficult adolescent. *Adolesc Psychiatr* 17, 69–81.

Kessler DA (1991) Communicating with patients about their medications. *New Engl J Med* 325, 1650–1652.

Lederberg MS and Holland JC (2000) Psycholoncology. In Comprehensive Textbook of Psychiatry, Saddock BJ and Saddock VA (eds). Williams & Wilkins, *Baltimore*, pp. 1850–1875.

Lidz T (1983) *The Person*, Rev. ed. Basic Books, New York.

Marziali E and Alexander L (1991) The power of the therapeutic relationship. *Am J Orthopsychiatr* 61, 383–391.

McKusick L (1988) The impact of AIDS on practitioner and client. Notes for the therapeutic relationship. *Am Psychol* 43, 935–940.

Meissner W (1996) *The Therapeutic Alliance.* Yale University Press, New Haven, pp. 62–106.

Peabody FW (1927) The care of the patient. *J Am Med Assoc* 88, 877–882.

Petrovic P, Kalso E, Petersson KM *et al.* (2002) Placebo and opioid analgesia – imaging a shared neuronal network. *Science* 295, 1737–1740.

Racker H (1968) *Transference and Countertransference.* International Universities Press, New York.

Rawn M (1991) The working alliance: Current concepts and controversies. *Psychoanal Rev* 78, 379–389.

Sandler J, Dare C and Holder A (1973) *The Patient and the Analyst: The Basis of the Psychoanalytic Process.* International Universities Press, New York.

Shapiro D (1965) *Neurotic Styles.* Basic Books, New York.

Siegler M (1993) Falling off the pedestal: What is happening to the traditional doctor–patient relationship? *Mayo Clin Proc* 68, 461–467.

Smith TC and Thompson TL (1993) The inherent, powerful therapeutic value of a good physician–patient relationship. *Psychosomatics* 34, 166–170.

Sullivan HS (1954) *The Psychiatric Interview.* WW Norton, New York.

Ursano RJ and Fullerton CS (1991) Psychotherapy: Medical intervention and the concept of normality. In The Diversity of Normal Behavior: Further Contributions to Normatology, Offer D and Sabshin M (eds). Basic Books, New York, pp. 39–59.

Ursano RJ and Silberman EK (1988) Individual psychotherapies in *The American Psychiatric Press Textbook of Psychiatry* (eds Talbott JA, Hales RE and Yudofsky SC). American Psychiatric Press, Washington DC, pp. 876–884.

Ursano RJ and Silberman EK (2002) Psychoanalysis, psychoanalytic psychotherapy and supportive psychotherapy, in *American Psychiatric Press Textbook of Psychiatry* (eds Hales RE, Yudofsky SC and Talbot JA). American Psychiatric Press, Washington DC.

Ursano RJ, Sonnenberg SM and Lazar SG (1991) *Concise Guide to Psychodynamic Psychotherapy.* American Psychiatric Press, Washington DC.

Vaillant G (1992) *Ego Mechanisms of Defense.* American Psychiatric Press, Washington DC, pp. 237–248.

Wise MG and Rundell JR (eds) (2002) *Textbook of Consultation Liaison Psychiatry: Psychiatry in the Medically Ill.* American Psychiatric Publishing, Washington DC.

Zetzel ER (1956) Current concepts of transference. *Int J Psychoanal* 37, 369–376.

Ziegler RG (1999) *Sharing Care: The Integration of Family Approaches with Child Treatment.* Brunner/Mazel, New York, pp. 7–58.

5 Professional Ethics and Boundaries

Introduction

In the last several decades, advances in psychiatry have made it possible to treat mental disorders that were previously unamenable to successful intervention. There has been a dark side to this progress, however, because futuristic anticipation of subduing disease and forcing nature to surrender her secrets has led many practitioners to outrun their headlights. Like technical sorcerers of science fiction confusing promise with reality, we are in danger of being lulled into an intellectual arrogance that can cause us to forget what it means to be professionals. One manifestation of this process has been the defensive reliance by clinicians on reductionistic explanations for complex and multidetermined disorders, combined with a neglect of the important role of trust and empathy as a curative factor in treating mental disorders.

A bewildering potpourri of treatment options and methods for financing healthcare present psychiatrists with other sources of confusion. Patients' health and safety often depend upon our ability to make rapid clinical decisions regarding diagnosis and to utilize an optimal psychotherapeutic or psychopharmacologic approach. The psychiatrist's dilemma is similarly compounded by conflicts between the cost-determined restrictions of managed care and the sacred promise to advocate primarily for patients' welfare.

Building a cooperative and trusting relationship with patients has always been an essential factor enabling clinicians to foster the healing process. In ancient times, when there were few specific remedies available, physicians relied on a highly integrative view of the sick person. For example, ancient Egyptian medicine did not make a special distinction between soma and psyche in considering physical and mental disorders, and therefore attached no special stigma to the mentally ill (Okasha and Okasha, 2000). Similarly, the Rabbinic sage and physician Maimonides (1135–1204 AD) (1944), relying on scriptural and clinical wisdom, taught that both physical and mental illness resulted from imbalances in somatic and mental processes, and that physical health and mental health are interdependent (Gorman, 2001).

In most instances, modern technology augments but cannot substitute for a trusting doctor–patient relationship. Patients seeking medical care must suspend ordinary social distance and critical judgment if they are to allow physicians to enter their physical and psychological space. While neither the law nor medical ethics relieve patients from taking an active responsibility for treatment outcome (American Medical Association, 1993), society places a greater burden upon the healer – a mandate to act with the special care and vigilance expected of a fiduciary (Frank and Frank, 1991; Simon, 1987) or of a Common Carrier (Epstein, 1994, pp. 59–61) as a precondition for granting licenses to practice.

As we review in this chapter, the ability to sustain a professional attitude and to practice within a set of coherent boundaries forms the foundation of proper psychiatric treatment, regardless of theoretic orientation or treatment modality. An understanding of psychiatric ethics plays a vital role in the psychiatrist's ability to keep proper boundaries because these values provide a stable beacon in the cognitively perplexing fog that so often pervades the treatment situation.

Ethical Behavior and its Relationship to the Professional Attitude

The term **professional** derives from medieval times, when scholastics were expected to "profess" their belief in a doctrine (Dyer, 1988, p. 17). In modern times, a professional is expected to be a learned person who has acquired special knowledge of a subject that is of vital importance for the welfare of the community. Having expertise is not enough, however. A professional is also obliged to adhere to certain societal responsibilities that are founded upon a code of ethical behavior and an attitude of service to those in need. A professional commitment to ethical behavior and service must take precedence over monetary compensation (Dyer, 1988, p. 16). All physicians, including psychiatrists, are bound by such a covenant – a sacred vow to place patient well-being before other considerations (Webb, 1986). In Western medical tradition, this obligation primarily derives from the teachings of Hippocrates in the 5th century BC. Hippocrates' Oath is the predominant pledge recited at the graduation exercises at American medical schools (Dickstein *et al.*, 1991), and contains three of the six core principles of modern medical ethics: **beneficence**, **nonmalfeasance**, and **confidentiality**:

> I will follow that system of regimen which according to my ability and judgment, I consider for the benefit of my patients, and abstain from whatever is deleterious and mischievous .... With purity and holiness I will pass my life and practice my Art .... Into whatever houses I enter, I will go into them for the benefit of the sick, and will abstain from every voluntary act of mischief and corruption; and, further, from the seduction of females or males, of freemen and slaves. Whatever, in connection with my professional practice or not, in connection with it, I see or hear, in the life of men, which ought not to be spoken of abroad, I will not divulge, as reckoning that all such should be kept secret (Hippocrates, 1929).

Essentials of Psychiatry   Jerald Kay and Allan Tasman
© 2006 John Wiley & Sons, Ltd.

Table 5.1   Six Basic Principles of Medical Ethics

Principle	Description
Beneficence Nonmalfeasance	Applying one's abilities solely for the patient's well-being Avoiding harm to a patient
Autonomy	Respect for a patient's independence
Justice	Avoiding prejudicial bias based on idiosyncrasies of the patient's background, behavior, or station in life
Confidentiality	Respect for the patient's privacy
Veracity	Truthfulness with oneself and one's patients

Reprinted with permission from Epstein RS (1994) *Keeping Boundaries. Maintaining Safety and Integrity in the Psychotherapeutic Process.* Copyright, American Psychiatric Press, Washington DC.

The other three general principles of medical ethics include autonomy, justice and veracity (see Table 5.1 for a description and summary of all six ethical principles; Epstein 1994, p. 20). The American Psychiatric Association (APA) (1973) adopted the American Medical Association's (AMA) *Principles of Medical Ethics*, publishing it along with special annotations applicable for psychiatric practice. The APA has produced six revisions of these annotations. The seven sections of the AMA principles are summarized in Table 5.2. Table 5.3 summarizes some of the salient ethical annotations for psychiatrists (American Psychiatric Association, 1993).

The World Psychiatric Association (World Psychiatric Association [WPA] 1999–2002; World Psychiatric Association Ethical Statements, 2000) developed and approved ethical guidelines, starting with the Declaration of Hawaii in 1977, galvanized by concerns about the abuse of psychiatry. A long process of investigation within the domain of professional ethics provided the foundation for the Declaration of Madrid that was endorsed by the General Assembly of the WPA in 1996. In its final form, the Declaration of Madrid included seven general guidelines that focused on the aims of psychiatry. They are summarized as follows:

1. Psychiatry's concern should be to provide the best treatment and rehabilitation for persons with mental disorders, consistent with scientific knowledge, ethical principles, and with the least possible restriction on the freedom of the patient.
2. Psychiatrists have a duty to keep abreast of scientific developments. Psychiatrists trained in research should seek to advance the frontiers of knowledge.
3. The psychiatrist–patient relationship must be based on mutual trust and respect, and should allow the patient to make free and informed decisions. The psychiatrist has a duty to accept the patient as a partner in the therapy and to empower the patient with necessary information for rational treatment decisions.
4. Psychiatrists should consult with families of incapacitated patients to safeguard the human dignity and the legal rights of the patient. Treatment should not be given against the patient's will, unless withholding treatment would endanger the life of the patient or others. Treatment must always be in the best interest of the patient.

Table 5.2   Summary of the Principles of Ethics of the American Medical Association

Section	Statement of Principle
Preamble	The medical profession's ethical standards are designed primarily for the well-being of patients. As professionals, physicians are required to acknowledge a responsibility to patients, to society, to self and to their colleagues.
Section I	Dedication to competent, compassionate care. Respect for human dignity.
Section II	Obligation to deal honestly with patients and colleagues and to expose physicians who are incompetent or fraudulent.
Section III	Respect for the law. Obligation to seek changes in laws harmful to patient's care.
Section IV	Respect for the rights of patients and colleagues. Within legal constraints, preservation of confidentiality.
Section V	Commitment to continued education, sharing of relevant knowledge, and obtaining necessary consultation.
Section VI	Except in emergency, freedom to decide whom to treat, with whom to associate, and the setting in which one serves.
Section VII	Acknowledge the responsibility to contribute to improving the community.

Reprinted with permission from American Psychiatric Association (1993) *Principles of Medical Ethics with Annotations Especially Applicable to Psychiatry.* Copyright, American Psychiatric Association, Washington DC.

Table 5.3   Summary of Selected Ethical Principles for Psychiatrists

Principle	Annotations
Competent care	The psychiatrist must scrutinize the effect of his/her conduct on the boundaries of the treatment relationship.
Honest dealing	Sex with a current or former patient is unethical. Information given by patients should not be exploited. Contractual arrangements should be explicit. Fee splitting is unethical.
Confidentiality, respecting colleagues	Restraint in release of information to third parties. Adequate disguise of case presentations. Disclosure of lack of confidentiality in nontreatment situations. Sex with students or supervisees may be unethical.

Reprinted with permission from American Psychiatric Association (1993) *Principles of Medical Ethics with Annotations Especially Applicable to Psychiatry.* Copyright, American Psychiatric Association, Washington DC.

5. Psychiatrists performing assessments, especially when retained by a third party, have a duty to inform the person being examined about the purpose of the intervention, the use of the findings, and the possible repercussions of the assessment.
6. Unless there is a threat of serious harm to the patient or other persons, psychiatrists should keep all patient information in confidence, and use such information only for the purpose of helping the patient. Psychiatrists are prohibited from making use of such information for personal, financial, or academic benefits.
7. It is unethical to conduct research that is not in accordance with the canons of science. Research activities should be approved by an appropriate and ethically constituted oversight committee. Because of the vulnerability of psychiatric patients, extra caution and strict ethical standards should be employed to safeguard patients' autonomy, patients' mental and physical integrity, and the selection of population groups.

An appendix in the Declaration of Madrid includes additional guidelines on specific ethical issues in psychiatry, including the following (World Psychiatric Association, 1999–2000; World Psychiatric Association Ethical Statements, 2000):

WPA Guidelines on Euthanasia
The physician's role, first and foremost, is to promote health, reduce suffering, and protect life. The psychiatrist, whose patients may include those who are severely incapacitated or incompetent to reach an informal decision, should be particularly careful about actions that could lead to the death of individuals who cannot protect themselves because of disability, and should be vigilant to the possibility that a patient's views could be distorted by mental illness such as depression. In such situations, the psychiatrist's role is to treat the illness.

WPA Guidelines on Torture
A psychiatrist should not take part in any process of mental or physical torture even when authorities attempt to force their involvement in such acts. Furthermore, a psychiatrist should not participate under any circumstances in legally authorized executions, nor participate in assessments of competency to be executed.

WPA Guidelines on Sex Selection
It is unethical for a psychiatrist to participate in decisions to terminate pregnancy for the purpose of sex selection.

WPA Guidelines on Organ Transplantation
Psychiatrists should seek to protect their patients and help them exercise self-determination to the fullest extent possible. The role of the psychiatrist is to clarify the issues surrounding organ donations and to deal with the religious, cultural, social and family factors to ensure that informed and proper decisions be made by all concerned.

WPA Guidelines on Genetic Research and Counseling in Psychiatric Patients
Psychiatrists participating in genetic research should be mindful that the ramifications of genetic information are not limited to the individual subject or patient but can lead to far-reaching repercussions and consequences that can have a negative and disruptive effect on the larger family or community. Psychiatrists are ethically obligated to observe proper practice, avoid the risks associated with premature disclosure, misinterpretations, or misuse of genetic information, and should never advise a pregnant woman with mental disorders to get an abortion based on the medical or genetic basis of her mental illness. They should not refer patients to genetic testing unless there are satisfactory levels of quality assurance and adequate genetic counseling available to the patient.

Further guidelines on the relationship between psychiatrists and the media, ethnic discrimination, ethnic cleansing, and genetic research and counseling were endorsed by the WPA General Assembly in 1999.

WPA Guidelines on Ethnic Discrimination and Ethnic Cleansing
The Madrid Declaration defines ethnic discrimination as basically racist, as it fails to accept diversity and humanity's common heritage. In its most malignant form, ethnic cleansing is a crime against humanity. In this regard, psychiatrists should not discriminate nor help to discriminate against patients on ethnic grounds, nor be involved in any activity that promotes ethnic cleansing.

WPA Guidelines on Psychiatrists Addressing the Media
It is important that psychiatrists use the media in an affirmative way for a variety of goals that promote good mental health care, such as advocating for the destigmatization of mental disorder and mental patients. In all their interactions with the media, psychiatrists are obliged to advocate for the mentally ill and to maintain the dignity of the profession. Psychiatrists should be mindful of the effect of their statements on the public perception of the profession and patients, and abstain from making statements or undertaking public activities that may be demeaning to either. Patients' confidentiality should be maintained, and the sensationalization of mental illness should be avoided. Regarding the disclosure of research findings, psychiatrists should be cautious to report only results that are generally accepted by experts, and to convey the presentation of such results in a way that serves patients' welfare and dignity.

The Coherent Treatment Frame and the Role of Therapeutic Boundaries in Effective Psychiatric Treatment
The "frame" of a social interaction was defined by Goffman (1974) as consisting of the spoken and unspoken expectations defining meaning and involvement in a given situation. For example, patients seek out psychiatrists based on a tacit assumption that the doctor is a reliable and experienced clinician who has the ability to assist them in finding relief for distress. However, many patients tend to frame their treatment in pathological ways. For example, some will attempt to pressure the psychiatrist into the role of a magical wizard who will confer unconditional love and pleasure. Whatever method the patient employs to frame the relationship, any abrupt disappointment or rupture of these unspoken expectations often results in intense and disruptive feelings of mortification and betrayal. A sudden breach of a social frame can lead to the dissolution of one's sense of meaning and connection, and is often accompanied by intense feelings of shame. By examining verbal and behavioral responses following violations of the treatment frame, Langs (1984–1985) was able to document that

Principle	Method Applied
Inspiring trust	The therapist establishes an emotionally arousing, trusting, and confidential relationship.
Coherent structure	A structured setting is formed that is associated with the healing process.
Rationale explained	A reasoned treatment method is offered that plausibly explains the patient's problems.
Cooperative engagement	Therapist and patient actively work together in the program. Both believe that it will work.

Table 5.4 Factors Common to All Successful Psychotherapy

Source: Frank JD and Frank JB (1991) *Persuasion and Healing. A Comparative Study of Psychotherapy*, 3rd edn. Johns Hopkins University Press, Baltimore.

patients usually perceive the offending therapist as an unreliable and mentally unstable person – someone seeking perverse pleasure at another person's expense.

The psychiatrist's task is to provide a coherent therapeutic frame within which to contain the patient's illness. The psychiatrist's frame makes it secure to proceed with the specific therapeutic modality, just as the surgical suite provides a safe environment for operative techniques. The treatment frame enables the patient to maintain a feeling of trust and connectedness while learning to deal with the unrealistic nature of his/her expectations. The frame comprises various boundary factors that include acting in a reliable way, showing respect for the patient's autonomy by explaining the potential risks and benefits of the treatment method, maintaining confidentiality, avoiding exploitation of the patient's sexual feelings, and resisting the patient's manipulative efforts by explaining the maladaptive nature of such behavior (Epstein, 1994; Simon, 1992).

Frank and Frank (1991) conducted an extensive review of the literature concerning psychotherapy outcome. They determined that there were four basic factors common to all successful psychotherapies (see Table 5.4), and that treatment efficacy relied upon the ability of the therapist to form a structured, mutually trusting, confidential and emotionally arousing relationship. Their findings sustain the argument that maintaining a coherent treatment frame is an essential part of all psychiatric treatment, regardless of the therapeutic paradigm being employed. These issues are important whether the patient is being treated solely with psychotropic medication management, cognitive–behavioral therapy, or psychoanalysis.

Boundary Violations

Psychiatric treatment cannot be conducted without doctor and patient entering into each other's space, just as it is impossible to perform a bloodless laparotomy. Gutheil and Gabbard (1993) termed such incursions occurring during the therapeutic process **boundary crossings**. They defined boundary violations as boundary crossings that cause injury to the patient. However, it is not always easy to be sure of the consequences of such a

"crossing", since harmful effects may be delayed or concealed. Many patients are unable to articulate their sense of injury because the psychiatrist's aberrant behavior may appear so similar to exploitation they have experienced in previous pathological relationships. For example, patients who were sexually abused in childhood are more likely to acquiesce to an amorous advance by a psychiatrist and to avoid complaining about feeling used, because they fear the threat of the psychiatrist's rejection and retaliation. Certain nonsexual boundary crossings such as conflicts of interest might seem harmless on the surface but can interfere with patients' ability to feel safe in their psychiatrist's care and will diminish their chances for optimal recovery. In this context, a boundary violation can be defined as any infringement that interferes with the primary goal of providing care or causes harm to the patient, the therapist, or the therapy itself (Epstein, 1994, p. 2).

Prior to the 1970s, open discussion on the topic of psychiatrist–patient sex was virtually taboo and considered "too hot to handle" as a subject for publication in scientific journals (Dahlberg, 1970). Professional societies demonstrated an inconsistent and ambiguous attitude of "amused tolerance" (Pope and Bouhoutsos, 1986, p. 161) towards mental health practitioners engaging in sexual behavior with their patients.

The public has become increasingly interested in the subject of psychiatric boundary violations in the past 25 years, particularly those involving sexual exploitation. State licensing boards, professional ethics committees and civil juries are much more likely to mete out strong sanctions against violators than ever before. These attitudinal changes have taken place in spite of the fact that popular movies continue to romanticize the idea of psychiatrist–patient sexuality, and almost always seem oblivious to the horrendous feelings of shame, betrayal and devastation that patients experience when these things happen to them in real life.

The public's intolerance of sexual involvement between psychiatrists and patients has resulted in part from the increasing empowerment of the victims of incest, rape and spousal abuse, and a better understanding of the psychological sequelae that follow mental trauma such as post traumatic stress disorder (PTSD). In addition, psychiatric patients have become more willing to expose unethical or exploitative behavior on the part of clinicians, particularly when it involves sexual activity. This trend has been augmented by the fact that courts and professional licensing bodies are now more inclined to render sanctions for injuries that are solely psychological in nature.

Quantitative estimates of the frequency of sexual boundary violations among mental health professionals derive from survey studies conducted over the last 20 years (Pope and Bouhoutsos, 1986; Kardener et al., 1973; Perry, 1976; Holroyd and Brodsky, 1977; Gartrell et al., 1986; Borys and Pope, 1989; Schoener, 1990). A review of these studies shows that from 5.5 to 13.7% of male mental health clinicians admitted to engaging in sexual activity with patients. Epstein (1994, pp. 207–208) calculated a crude weighted average from Schoener's (1990) comprehensive review of survey studies reporting frequency of sexual violations by clinicians' gender. From ten studies involving a total of 5 816 respondents (excluding a large survey of nurses), an average of 7.4% of male and 2.3% of female clinicians admitted to engaging in sexual behavior with patients. These data suggest that male clinicians are about three times more likely to admit they have become sexually involved with patients. Although more recent studies suggest that sexual exploitation by mental health practitioners might be occurring less frequently, increasing media reports of severe sanctions taken against offending therapists have probably diminished the validity of self-report questionnaires.

Studies of nonsexual violations suggest that many mental health clinicians still have serious problems maintaining professional boundaries with patients (Borys and Pope, 1989; Epstein *et al.*, 1992). Epstein and colleagues (1992) queried 532 psychiatrists practicing in the USA about their behavior with patients within a prior 2-year period, using the Exploitation Index (EI) developed by Epstein and Simon (1990). They found that 19% of respondents reported engaging in a personal relationship with patients after treatment was terminated, 17% told patients personal details of their life in order to impress them, and 17% joined in activities with patients to deceive a third party such as an insurance company (see Table 5.5, reviewing the frequency of nonsexual boundary violations among respondents in this study). Xiangyi and Tiebang (2001) surveyed mental health clinicians in China using a Chinese translation of the EI. They found a rate of endorsement of boundary violations that was similar to the findings in the US study, although there were distinct variations in the pattern of certain responses that the authors attributed to cultural differences between the two populations.

Simon (1989) emphasized that when clinicians engage in nonsexual infringements of the treatment relationship, it is often a prelude to subsequent sexual behavior. Sexual involvement with patients often starts with excessive personal disclosure, accepting and giving gifts, requesting favors, and meeting patients outside of the office setting. Like a seduction, the behavior escalates over time until it culminates in sexual contact (Simon, 1989).

Regardless of the specific type of infringement involved, there are common elements to all boundary violations. Peterson (1992) argued that such activity emanated from a disturbed and disconnected relationship. She suggested four basic behavioral themes in this regard, including efforts on the part of the clinician to reverse roles with the patient, to intimidate the patient to maintain secrecy, to place the patient in a double bind, and to indulge professional privilege. Indulgence of privilege is often accompanied by a sense of entitlement on the clinician's part, such that he/she regards the patient as a wholly owned subsidiary.

Epstein (1994, pp. 89–110) outlined the progression of boundary violations as they originate from dysregulation in the clinician's personal ego boundaries. Circumstances impairing the clinician's ability to cope with patients and their problems may include deficient knowledge, general stress, mental disorder, or a treatment-induced regression. These factors may lead the clinician to employ maladaptive intrapsychic or behavioral coping mechanisms that manifest in the form of therapeutic boundary violations. Other general factors common to all boundary violations include a slippage of the original purpose of the treatment (Epstein, 1994, pp. 97–98), pseudoeclecticism (Epstein and Janowsky, 1969), a narcissistic sense of specialness (Epstein, 1994, pp. 107–110; Epstein and Simon, 1990), and efforts to deprofessionalize the relationship by fostering an atmosphere of "pseudoequality" between clinician and patient (Peterson, 1992).

The double-binding messages that exploitive clinicians employ often represent a way for them to project their own disavowed feelings of shame and inadequacy onto vulnerable patients. For example, a therapist may deceive a patient suffering from low self-esteem and sexual dysfunction by encouraging her to have sex with him. He may rationalize:

> You have told me that you feel unattractive and inadequate as a woman. Since therapy is supposed to help you with your problems, I will help show you how attractive and effective you are as a woman by having sex with you.

Psychotherapy and erotic behavior can both be construed as subcategories of the superordinate class of "activities that help people feel better" (Epstein, 1994, p. 102). In the example cited above, the exploitive therapist blurs the logical boundaries between the two subcategories and fails to inform the patient that sexual behavior with him is likely to be harmful to her. Blurring of logical categories is an essential aspect of double-binding messages. Patients who are subjected to such reasoning are often in a dependent and cognitively regressed state and are unable to understand the logical absurdity of the double bind. They fear that if they refuse to comply with the therapist's suggestions, they will be rejected for failing to cooperate with the therapist.

It is important to place the burgeoning literature on boundary violations in its social context. An aroused public has been exposed to recurring reports of psychiatrists and other mental health professionals, who have been disciplined or sued for behavior such as sexual involvement with patients and spouses of patients; using information learned in patients' psychotherapy sessions to gain inside data on financial investments; and accepting large bequests from elderly patients. Each new scandal serves to erode society's trust in the integrity of psychiatry as a profession and makes it more difficult for the mentally ill to obtain needed treatment. Compounding this problem is the fact that some of these well-publicized reports of boundary violations involved highly trained psychiatrists who were leaders in their field and who served as important role models for students in professional training.

As has occurred many times before in history, societal changes tend to overshoot the mark, leading some observers to caution against an hysterical "witch hunt" against suspected offenders. Slovenko (1991) cautioned that the current climate has become ripe for an increasing number of false accusations to be made against innocent clinicians. Gutheil (1992) has documented such cases and provided guidelines for proper forensic psychiatric evaluation following allegations of sexual misconduct.

Table 5.5	Summary of Survey Results of Nonsexual Boundary Violations Among 532 Psychiatrists	
Behavior		**Percentage**
Using touch (exclusive of handshake)		45
Treating relatives or friends		32
Personal relationships post termination		19
Personal disclosure		17
Colluding with patient against third party		17
Influencing patient for political causes		10
Using patient communication for financial gain		7

Reprinted with permission from Epstein RS, Simon RI, and Kay GG (1992) Assessing boundary violations in psychotherapy: Survey results with the exploitation index. *Bull Menn Clin* 56, 150–166. Copyright, Guildford Publications, Inc.

Components of the Coherent Psychiatric Frame

The purpose of the therapeutic frame is to protect the patient's safety and to promote recovery. It is the therapist's responsibility to structure the frame through word and deed. Langs (1984–1985) stressed that a healthy and secure therapeutic environment is predicated on reducing variability and uncertainty in the treatment setting as much as possible. Table 5.6 summarizes the major boundary factors comprising the coherent treatment frame. Careful attention to these boundary issues can assist treating psychiatrists to communicate defining messages that strengthen the differentiation of role and identity between patient and practitioner.

The diversity of opinion regarding optimal methods of treatment for specific psychiatric disorders makes it very difficult to devise a set of specific guidelines that are appropriate for psychiatrists adhering to a wide spectrum of theoretical orientations. Dyer (1988, pp. 45–57) emphasized how problematic it is to define a comprehensive ethical system, whether it is based on a set of specific rules (deontological ethics), on a list of values and goals (teleological ethics), or from consideration of the emotional and practical consequences of a given course of action (consequentialist ethics). A parallel dilemma exists when it comes to defining psychiatric boundaries. For this reason, guidelines for psychiatrists should enhance patient safety, foster adherence to established clinical principles, and help to avoid specific consequences that are detrimental to either patient or practitioner. Such an approach is consistent with an intensifying interest in reducing preventable medical error. In his seminal work on human error, Reason (1990, p. 69) outlined three major types of performance as a way to address the sources of preventable human error. These categories include rule-based performance, skill-based performance and knowledge-based performance. As an example, Reason described how the use of inadvisable rules leads to rare but preventable collisions at sea, citing studies reporting how experienced maritime pilots expose themselves and others to unnecessary and potentially serious risk by allowing their own vessel to navigate too closely to adjacent ships even when there is plenty of sea room to avoid such proximity:

> The confidences these and other experienced operators have in their ability to get themselves out of trouble can maintain inadvisable rule behavior. This is particularly so when a high value is attached to recovery skills and where the deliberate courting of a moderate degree of risk is seen as a necessary way of keeping these skills sharp.

With regard to rule-based procedures for reducing error in psychiatric practice, each boundary issue can be examined from the point of view of clearly **indicated** procedures, **relatively risky** procedures and **contraindicated** procedures (Epstein, 1994, pp. 113–117). In the ensuing discussion of components of the psychiatric frame, lists of these various types of procedures are adapted from Epstein's earlier work on boundaries (Epstein, 1994, pp. 119–236).

Riskier procedures that fall into the "gray zone" are not necessarily unethical or unsound. However, psychiatrists engaging in such activities should be aware of the circumstances under which they increase or reduce the chance for injury either to the patient or themselves. For example, under most conditions, it is probably unwise to attempt psychiatric treatment of one's next-door neighbor. Nevertheless, practitioners living in remote areas or working in confined ethnic communities might, as a matter of

Boundary Issue	Function and Purpose	Implicit Message to Patient
Stability	Consistency as to time, place, location, parties involved and treatment method	"The doctor is reliable. This treatment can contain my irrationality."
Avoiding dual relationships	Utmost fidelity to the primary purpose of helping the patient	"The doctor focuses his/her attention on my problem, and is not sidetracked."
Neutrality and promoting patient autonomy	Avoiding abuse of power and promoting the patient's independence	"The doctor values my ideas and encourages me to exercise choices."
Noncollusive compensation	Scrupulous and forthright terms of remuneration for the clinician	"Aside from the payment, I don't have to gratify the doctor."
Confidentiality	To protect the patient's privilege of keeping his/her communications secret	"My thoughts and feelings belong to me, not to the doctor."
Anonymity	Avoids seductiveness and role reversal	"This is a place to bring my issues, not a forum for the doctor's personal problems."
Abstinence	Encourages verbalization rather than action in dealing with feelings and conflicts	"There is a big difference between wishes and reality."
Preserving the clinician's safety and self-respect	Discourages the patient's destructive behavior, sets a good role model for establishing healthy self-esteem.	"It is possible to have a close relationship without someone getting hurt."

Table 5.6 Major Boundary Issues Contributing to the Formation of a Coherent Treatment Frame

practicality, be forced to treat such a patient for whom no reasonable alternative exists. The hazard of no treatment may outweigh other factors in the situation. However, the fact that psychiatrists sometimes must treat patients under risky circumstances does not mean they should disregard the increased hazard they are assuming or forget about optimal treatment standards, just as the exigencies of battlefield surgery do not obviate the need to strive for aseptic technique.

Psychiatrists should safeguard against any semblance of inappropriate behavior even if the activity can be justified as seemingly harmless. For example, seeking social activities with patients outside of the treatment setting can be interpreted by patients or their family members as seductive. Gutheil and Gabbard (1993) have emphasized that the very appearance of undue familiarity with a patient may, in and of itself, hamper successful defense against false allegations of professional wrongdoing.

Stability

Configuring a stable and consistent treatment setting is analogous to the "holding environment" provided by parents in early childhood (Winnicott, 1960). Patients with psychiatric illnesses will find it very difficult to entrust their lives to a psychiatrist whom they perceive to be unreliable. Indicated measures regarding stability include formulating an agreement with the patient for a treatment regimen that will take place according to a specific method and schedule, encouraging truthful disclosure and cooperation; establishing a commitment to beginning and ending sessions on time, discouraging interruptions during treatment sessions; offering advance notice as to when the psychiatrist will be absent, providing for coverage by another practitioner when the psychiatrist is off duty, maintaining coherent therapeutic demeanor; and maintaining relative consistency as to who participates in the treatment situation.

It is generally unwise for a psychiatrist to disparage a patient's complaints about issues like the doctor's tardiness in starting sessions or to become defensive when explaining the meaning of the patient's distress about such complaints. Many psychiatrists experience patients' demands for consistency as a form of control and imprisonment. Out of anger, they may react to these patients as if their wishes for reliability and concern were infantile and irrational:

> Your complaints about my lateness are a reflection of your need to control me.

The psychiatrist's tardiness might in fact be creating tremendous anxiety because it reminds the patients of parents who never took their feelings into account.

Avoiding Dual Relationships

Psychiatrists should avoid treatment situations that place them in a conflict between therapeutic responsibility to patients and third parties. Examples of dual relationships in psychiatric practice include clinicians treating their own relatives and friends, the same therapist employing concurrent family and individual therapy paradigms with a given patient, and clinicians testifying as forensic witnesses for current psychotherapy patients. Although it is a very common practice (Epstein *et al.*, 1992), accepting psychotherapy patients referred by one's current or former patients embraces certain risks that must be considered (Pope and Vetter, 1992). For example, a current patient might refer an attractive friend for therapy as a way of either seducing the therapist or sabotaging the treatment (Langs, 1973).

Role conflicts are quite widespread (Pope and Vetter, 1992) and interfere with the practitioner's single-mindedness of purpose as a healer. Chodoff (1993, pp. 457–459) placed special emphasis on this issue by arguing that advocating for the needs of the mentally ill was one of psychiatry's primary societal responsibilities. By eroding public trust, dual relationships interfere with the ability of psychiatrists to carry out their vital functions in the community.

The burgeoning expansion of prepaid care in the USA in the last two decades has provoked concern about a new source of role conflict for psychiatrists. Managed care has been espoused as an important modality to reduce unnecessary treatment by encouraging preventive care and promoting cost-consciousness among physicians (Fries *et al.*, 1993). Stephen Appelbaum (1992) argued that psychotherapists practicing under the old fee-for-service model were more inclined to provide unnecessarily prolonged treatment than those working under an organizational system that prevented direct monetary involvement between patient and practitioner.

On the other hand, increasing coverage of the population of the USA under a system of managed care has generated serious concerns regarding potential conflicts of interest (McKenzie, 1990). This disquietude is particularly noticeable in the field of psychiatry. Many managed care organizations (MCOs) have severely restricted the number of psychiatrists within a given community allowed to serve on their treatment panels. Patients' access to their regular treating practitioner have been further limited, even when the doctor is allowed to enroll on the panel. For example, under the rules of some MCOs, a psychiatrist might be prevented from maintaining continuity of care for outpatients needing hospitalization. During their hospital stay, such patients must be attended by a preselected group of psychiatrists who conduct all hospital treatment for the plan.

Although there is little scientific data to support the contention that restricted managed care panels are necessary for lowering costs, it is important that both patients and clinicians be informed about the hazard such a system of care entails. Since participation on a panel is often contingent on cost-efficiency profiles, psychiatrists who derive a significant portion of their income from a given MCO are discouraged from advocating for patients needing more expensive care. In addition, some MCOs refuse to pay for integrated treatment for mentally ill patients by psychiatrists enrolled in their panel. Instead, these MCOs insist on a split treatment model in which the patient obtains psychotherapy from a social worker or psychologist and is allowed only brief medication management visits with a psychiatrist. Psychiatrists attempting to do medication management under this model often have little contact with the psychotherapist, are very restricted in the frequency and duration of visits with the patient, and are thereby limited in making overall clinical decisions that might become necessary. Such a situation creates an ethical bind for the psychiatrist in which the medical responsibility is not accompanied by a commensurate degree of authority to direct the treatment process.

In the face of reports of physicians claiming they were terminated from managed care contracts because they protested treatment denials, fear of retaliation for patient advocacy has mounted (McCormick, 1994). Judge Marvin Atlas (1993) has suggested that psychiatrists who fail to give informed consent regarding the risks to the patient of their role conflicts would be exposing themselves to civil damages in the event of an adverse outcome. Although the extent of the legal duty to disclose risk factors under managed care is unresolved, Paul Appelbaum (1993) proposed that mental health clinicians inform beginning patients that payment for treatment under managed care might be stopped before the patient feels ready to terminate.

Limitations as to who may serve on a managed care panel and what functions the clinician may perform are other factors that have strong potential for creating disruption in the continuity of care. For example, Westermeyer (1991) described seven case histories in which psychiatric patients treated under managed care committed suicide or suffered serious clinical deterioration. Clinically uninformed managed care practices appeared to serve as critical aggravating factors for each of these patients. In the cases of two individuals who killed themselves, the employer had switched contracts to different managed care companies and the patients were forced to transfer to new clinicians. These disruptions appeared to play an important role in the patients' suicides.

Although more research is required to evaluate the full ramifications of managed care on psychiatric populations, recent studies suggest that some groups face adverse outcomes under this system. For example, Rogers and colleagues (1993) found that, on average, patients with depression who were treated by psychiatrists under prepaid treatment plans acquired new limitations in their physical or day-to-day functioning over a 2-year period, whereas those treated in the traditional fee-for-service setting did not.

Autonomy and Neutrality

Freud (1912, 1913) recommended that psychoanalysts adhere to a position of neutrality with their patients by refraining from the temptation to take sides in the patient's internal conflicts or life problems. This advice has relevance for all psychiatric treatment, insofar as it espouses the idea that practitioners should maintain profound respect for their patients' autonomy and individuality. This is a fundamental therapeutic stance that fosters independence, growth and self-esteem. It reinforces the idea that the clinician believes the patient to be the owner of his/her body, life and problems. The patient receives the following message:

> The doctor tries to help by assisting me to learn about myself, not by trying to take control of me.

Patient autonomy has not always been accorded its current importance in the hierarchy of priorities in medical practice in the USA. According to Blackhall and colleagues (1995), in 1961, 90% of physicians in the USA did not inform their patients of a diagnosis of cancer. By 1979, 97% of American physicians made it their policy to inform patients with cancer of their diagnosis (Blackhall *et al.* 1995). This change appears to be the result of physicians assuming less of a paternalistic attitude and becoming more enlightened and respectful of patients' right to participate in medical decisions. In some parts of the world, similar changes have occurred in clinical practice with mentally ill patients.

Cultural, ethnic and probably sociodemographic factors strongly shape attitudes regarding patient autonomy and informed consent. In some cultures, a higher value may be placed on the harmonious functioning in the interlocking pattern of family relationships than on the autonomy of individual family members. For example, according to Okasha (2000), patients reared in some cultures may not wish to continue treatment with a physician who is not sensitive to the importance of involving the family directly in communications about the patient's illness. The psychiatrist should diligently explore the role that cultural and family relationships play in the patient's healthy mental functioning and be guided primarily by the patient's communications about their degree of comfort or conflict with these family relationships. Psychiatrists should be considerate and respectful of cultural differences between themselves and their patients and be particularly cautious about interpreting those differences as a pathological process.

Mindful of cultural issues, indicated ways of encouraging autonomy include encouraging informed consent by outlining the potential benefits, risks and alternatives for a proposed treatment approach; explaining the rationale for the treatment; and fostering the patient's participation in the treatment process. Paradoxically, acutely suicidal patients often require the psychiatrist to assume temporary responsibility for their safety. In most cases this serves to augment the patient's sense of autonomy through a coherent modeling process (Bratter, 1975), because true independence is impossible without self-governance.

Clinical actions that may interfere with the patient's autonomy include advice regarding nonurgent, major life decisions, attempting to exert undue influence on issues unrelated to the patient's health, reluctance to allow patients to terminate treatment, seeking gratification by exerting power over patients, and using power over patients as a form of retaliation.

Coherent and Noncollusive Compensation

Although there are rewards to be obtained from working in an interesting and creative profession, this is best applied to one's collective professional endeavors. With a specific patient, monetary compensation is the only gratification psychiatrists should realistically expect (Epstein and Simon, 1990). When compensation is direct, there should be a set fee, and the patient should be responsible for the scheduled appointment time. When compensation is indirect or salaried, the psychiatrist must avoid colluding either with the patient against the party paying for the treatment or with the third party against the patient (see the previous section on avoiding dual relationships). Whatever method is being used for paying for mental health treatment, a coherent and noncollusive arrangement imparts the message to the patient:

> The doctor has needs of his/her own, but they are limited to a salary or fee. Aside from financial obligations, I don't have to please, gratify, or nurture my doctor.

The practice of charging for missed appointments under the traditional fee-for-service paradigm is often misunderstood by patients because their experience with physicians in other branches of medicine has usually been that they were charged on a fee-for-procedure, rather than fee-for-time, basis. Charging for missed appointments is justifiable from an ethical standpoint as long as the rationale is clearly explained to the patient at the beginning of treatment and the patient agrees to it. In addition, no attempt should be made to hide the fact of billing for missed appointments from third-party payers. Some states have an absolute prohibition against billing for missed appointments under entitlement programs such as Medicaid and Medicare (Epstein, 1994, p. 169). Within certain guidelines, it is permissible to bill the patient (but not Medicare) for missed appointments under the Medicare program (Epstein, 1994, pp. 169–170). Readers are cautioned that regulations regarding Medicaid and Medicare are subject to periodic legislative revisions and may vary according to jurisdiction.

Generally risky compensation arrangements include working for a treatment organization one perceives to be financially exploitive, accepting inexpensive gifts from patients especially when such gifts are not part of a culturally expected mode of behavior, bartering goods or services in return for treatment, referring patients for treatments or procedures in which one has a proprietary financial interest, and neglecting the patient's failure to adhere to the original agreement regarding payment of fees. Certain practices are absolutely contraindicated and likely to be destructive, including fraudulent billing, accepting expensive gifts, fee splitting, colluding with the patient or third party, and use of financial insider information.

Confidentiality

It is essential that psychiatrists treat their patients' communications as privileged. This means that patients alone retain the right to reveal information about themselves. The advent of managed care has raised even greater concern about the privacy of patients' personal communications with their psychiatrists because of the potential for an increasing number of persons connected with the MCO to have access to material from patients' files. Psychiatrists should caution their patient about the potential limitations to confidentiality and be prepared to explore the consequences of these exceptions. For example, if a patient is raising his/her mental health as an issue in litigation, some or all communications to a psychiatrist could be legally discoverable. Coherent boundaries with regard to confidentiality send the message to the patient:

> My thoughts and feelings belong to me. The doctor does not treat them as if they belong to him/her.

Indicated means of preserving confidentiality include obtaining proper authorization from patients before releasing information, explaining the need for confidentiality with parents of children and adolescents, and involving all participants in family and group psychotherapy in agreements about confidentiality. Problematic activities that may endanger confidentiality include stray communications with concerned relatives of patients in individual psychotherapy, where there is no prior expectation on the patient's part about discussions with relatives; discussion of privileged information with the psychiatrist's own family members; releasing information about deceased patients; and failure to properly disguise case presentations.

Anonymity

Many psychiatrists associate the principle of relative anonymity with Freud's advice to psychoanalysts (Freud, 1912):

> The doctor should be opaque to his patients and, like a mirror, should show them nothing but what is shown to him.

Freud argued that it was dangerous for psychoanalysts to expose their own mental problems or intimate life details in a spurious attempt to place themselves on an "equal footing" with patients (Freud, 1912, pp. 117–118). The merit of this recommendation extends beyond its origin in psychoanalytic technique to a fundamental boundary issue applicable to all forms of psychiatric treatment. It serves as a reminder to both patient and clinician of the professional purpose of the relationship. Avoiding unnecessary personal disclosure to patients protects both patient and practitioner from a reversal of roles – one of the critical themes recurring in boundary violations in general (Peterson, 1992). Many patients experience excessive self-disclosure by the psychiatrist as seductive and it has been frequently observed to be a precursor to subsequent sexual involvement (Schoener and Gonsiorek, 1990, p. 403). By maintaining a policy of relative anonymity, the patient receives the following message about the treatment:

> This is a place where I can bring my issues. The doctor doesn't burden me with his/her stuff.

Certain forms of self-disclosure are indicated in the course of work with psychiatric patients, including appraising patients of the clinician's qualifications and treatment methods as part of informed consent, discussing reality factors about the psychiatrist's health status or intentions regarding retirement that will impact on the patient's treatment decisions, and using "reality checks" to help patients contain disturbed and frightening fantasies.

Abstinence

Abstinence means that psychiatrists should discourage direct forms of pleasure such as touching or sexuality in the course of their interactions with patients. In the therapeutic relationship, the patient's ability to consent to sexual activity with the psychiatrist is vitiated by the knowledge the latter possesses over the patient and by the power differential that vests the psychiatrist with special authority.

For patients, actual gratification from the psychiatrist is best confined to realistic goals for recovery and emotional growth. Psychiatrists should limit themselves to the pleasure of getting paid for a job well done and for the opportunity to participate in an interesting and creative profession. Although steadfast application of this boundary can be quite frustrating for both doctor and patient, it pays excellent dividends in the long run by encouraging autonomy and a more mature way of dealing with impulses. The rule of abstinence as a therapeutic boundary has an analogous function to the incest taboo as a social organizer. In all known human cultures, the incest taboo has survival value because, during childhood development, it serves to strengthen the sense of individuality and personal boundaries so necessary for growth, independence and social responsibility (Parker, 1976).

From a practical standpoint, psychiatrists can strengthen their patients' boundaries in this regard by resisting behaviors such as physical touching, accepting gifts, socialization outside treatment and sexual involvement. The patient receives the following messages from a clinician who is able properly to adhere to this principle:

> The doctor is more interested in my health than his/her own gratification and doesn't try to take possession of me. I am learning that I can have wishes that needn't result in action.

There are occasions when psychiatrists are obligated to employ physical procedures such as taking blood pressures, checking for extrapyramidal symptoms, restraining dangerous patients, or administering electroconvulsive therapy. Indeed, clinical touching of patients is considered an integral part of the physician–patient relationship because of its important role in physical examination and therapeutic procedures. Even though psychiatrists are physicians, they are obligated to use much more restraint in this regard than is expected of colleagues in other branches of medicine. It is probably too invasive for the same physician, on a protracted basis, simultaneously to intrude both into the patient's psychological and physical spaces.

Other risky forms of gratification include embracing or kissing patients, eating and drinking with patients, socializing with patients outside of the therapy setting, and failure to understand and resolve recurrent or obsessive sexual fantasies about a patient. Engaging in sexual behavior with current or former patients is contraindicated because it is almost invariably destructive, even though the damage may not be immediately manifest.

The APA (American Psychiatric Association, 1993) took a principled and unequivocal stand regarding sexual activity between psychiatrists and their current or former patients:

> Additionally, the inherent inequality in the doctor–patient relationship may lead to exploitation of the patient. Sexual activity with a current or former patient is unethical.

The APA's position is in agreement with the principles espoused in the Hippocratic Oath, which clearly mandates that a physician approach a patient "for the benefit of the sick, and… abstain from every voluntary act of mischief and corruption; and, further, from the seduction of females or males, of freemen and slaves".

Despite the ancient basis of this proscription and convincing evidence in our times of the damaging effects of sexual relationships between therapists and former patients (Epstein, 1994, pp. 218–220; Luepker, 1990; Brown *et al.*, 1992), some authors have raised legal and theoretical challenges to the permanent prohibition contained in the APA guidelines (Appelbaum and Jorgenson, 1991). While refraining from calling for a repeal of APA's ethical proscription against sex with former patients, Malmquist and Notman (2001) argued that legal misapplications of imprecise and unproven concepts of transference and countertransference have exposed therapists who enter post termination sexual liaisons with their patients to inappropriate legal liability.

Research examining the causation and prevention of human error have provided neurocognitive evidence supporting the ancient wisdom of Hippocrates' injunction. Skilled performance is subject to potentially calamitous error when experts fail to follow empirically derived safety guidelines or lack an adequate knowledge base upon which to initiate critical interventions (Reason, 1990, pp. 76, 84, 86, 146–147). Skillful performance in conducting medical procedures are acquired from overlearned behavior that enables an expert to undertake complex cognitive and behavioral operations in a smooth and rapid fashion. Performance skills in which success depends on overlearned and automatic processes rely primarily on the procedural memory system (Cabeza and Nyberg, 2000). The Hippocratic mandate of approaching the patient solely for their benefit and to avoid mischief is a prime example of an overlearned, automatically embedded, error protection message acquired through years of medical training. Anything that interferes with such an intensively elaborated internal safeguard endangers patients' well-being.

Whether they realize it or not, psychiatrists who justify the permissibility of post termination sexual relationships are sabotaging their own overlearned commitment to act primarily in their patient's best interest and are exposing their patient to a biased and error prone treatment. This self-permissive attitude would make a psychiatrist more prone to engage in seductive grooming of a patient during the treatment process in anticipation of termination. In addition, biased by this attitude, a psychiatrist is likely to avoid making any communication to the patient that would discourage a subsequent romantic post termination liaison (Epstein, 2002). While a psychiatrist might consciously deny that this attitude is a violation of the Hippocratic dictum, in actual cases where psychiatrists have engaged in post termination sex with patients, their pretermination subliminal thinking ran like this:

> I'm treating this patient only for her/(his) benefit. Like Hippocrates, I will abstain from every voluntary act of mischief and corruption and, further, from seduction. However, after I cure this very attractive patient, I will keep his/(her) phone number, and after a respectable period of time, it will be a different matter, and we will see what will happen.

Note that this reasoning represents a form of dissociative thinking based on a primitive wish for inappropriate gratification with a patient that magically disavows the connection between post treatment behavior and pretreatment reality. All psychiatric treatment is based on the assumption that a psychiatrist's interventions by means of positive attitudes, words, deeds and medical interventions will have a lasting beneficial effect on the patient after the treatment has ended. There is no realistic escape from the fact that the reverse is also true, namely, that inappropriate attitudes, words, deeds and interventions are likely to have a lasting harmful effect on the patient after the treatment has ended.

Self-respect and Self-protection

It is essential that psychiatrists protect themselves from being exploited by patients. This principle is necessary to protect clinicians and patients alike. Many patients seeking treatment have endured abusive relationships in which being victimized became the price for maintaining human connectedness. For such patients, efforts to exploit the psychiatrist may be an action-question that inquires:

> Must one of us be injured in order for us to have a close relationship?

By setting a proper role model for self-respect and self-caretaking, the psychiatrist imparts the following message to the patient:

> Relationships need not be structured on the basis that one or both parties must be exploited. If I as the doctor allow you to hurt me, I am setting a poor role model.

Psychiatrists should attempt to discuss the meaning of any exploitive behavior on the patient's part as soon as possible. With unstable or impulsive patients who are prone to acting out, confrontation should be timed to maximize safety. For example, it would be more prudent to interpret the manipulative aspects of a patient's suicidal behavior after the patient is admitted to a hospital. If a patient makes a sudden physical overture such as attempting a sexually provocative embrace, it must be dealt with the same urgency as a physical assault. The psychiatrist should inform the patient that such behavior is inconsistent with coherent treatment (Epstein, 1994; Shor and Sanville, 1974, pp. 228–231; 58). It is generally risky to allow repeated exceptions such as last-minute prolongation of sessions, repeated lateness in paying fees, excessive intrusion into the psychiatrist's personal space in the form of regular and frequent late night phone calls, or taking items from the office.

Certain psychiatrists find themselves avoiding confrontation with an exploitive patient out of fear of the latter's narcissistic rage. This is an indication of an escalating situation that may lead to further boundary violations either by the patient or the psychiatrist. A useful explanation of this behavior is provided in Gabbard's (1994) description of a subgroup of clinicians who become sexually involved with patients as part of a self-defeating pattern of behavior he termed "masochistic surrender". These practitioners are unable to defend against being tormented by certain highly demanding patients. They succumb to the patient's importunings, sometimes while in a dissociated state, even though they may know their behavior is wrong. Gabbard (1994) argued that the aberrant behavior of these clinicians is rooted in an impaired ability to cope with their own aggressive feelings, resulting in their feeling that it would be sadistic to set limits on the patient.

Table 5.7   Indicators of Potential Boundary Violations with Suggested Remedial Responses

Indicator	Suggested Remedial Response for Clinician
Clinician is frequently tardy starting sessions	Avoid criticizing patient for complaining about lateness. Reexamine reasons for tardiness in light of patients' need for a stable treatment frame.
Clinician changes the treatment paradigm in "midstream", i.e., switching from individual therapy with Mr A to couples therapy with Mr A and his wife.	Avoid dual relationships that may interfere with primary loyalty to the first patient. If dual relationships cannot be avoided, explain risks to patient(s) according to principle of informed consent.
Clinician frequently advises patients on matters not related to treatment process.	Consider if this is a general pattern of need for control in one's nonclinical relationships. If so, consider ways to help patient to make his/her own decisions.
Clinician often relates to patient as if he/she were a personal friend.	Listen for signs that the patient feels burdened. Acknowledge pattern of role reversal and importance of clinician's fiduciary obligations to patient.
Clinician accepts gifts from patient.	Try to explore patient's motive for the gift. Consider refusing the gift by explaining that it might interfere with the effectiveness of treatment. Be prepared to work with patient's shame in this regard.
Clinician feels overly resentful about having to keep boundaries because they feel too constraining and spoil the "fun" and creativity of being a therapist.	Remember that therapy is hard work that is often burdensome and frustrating, and that boundaries are necessary for the patient's safety.
Clinician seeks contact with patient outside therapy setting.	Avoid contact, and explain the reason to patients. In settings where social contact is likely, discuss problems and options with the patient in advance.
Clinician is unable to confront patients who are late paying fees, remove items from the office, repeatedly try to prolong sessions, or torment therapist with insatiable demands.	Listen to the content of patient's communications and dreams regarding people injuring one another. Explore fear of one's own anger, the patient's anger, or of setting limits.
Clinician often tries to impress patients with personal information about himself/herself.	Refrain from further disclosure and examine one's possible motives. Consider how such activity might relate to sexual feelings to patient or need to control patient.
Clinician becomes sexually preoccupied with patient, for example, feels a pleasurable sense of excitement or longing when thinking of patient or anticipating his/her visit.	Consider that one's sexual feelings may portend the reenactment of an actual or symbolic incestuous scenario from the patient's past. Remember that incestuous behavior or its symbolic equivalent infantilizes the victim. Obtain supervision and/or personal psychotherapy if sexual preoccupations continue unabated.

Summary

The ethical and boundary issues discussed in this chapter were designed to stimulate a better understanding of an extremely thorny topic rather than to provide an exhaustive compendium. Table 5.7 summarizes selected indicators of potential boundary violations, along with remedial responses clinicians might employ to deal with these situations. A burgeoning literature regarding the psychological characteristics of clinicians who have problems with maintaining proper boundaries (Epstein, 1994; Gutheil and Gabbard, 1993; Epstein and Simon, 1990; Schoener and Gonsiorek, 1990; Gabbard, 1994; Twemlow and Gabbard, 1989; Gabbard, 1991; Geis et al., 1985) provides useful guidance in this regard.

The difficulties psychiatrists may encounter in keeping boundaries derive from many sources. In the past, professional training programs have not addressed this issue systematically. Recent proposals to bolster the study of ethics and boundaries in medical school and residency programs (Roman and Kay, 1997; Kay and Roman, 1999) will help to remediate this problem. It behoves psychiatrists to determine whether they have suffered deficiencies in training or adverse role modeling during the course of their professional development and whether their own emotional problems significantly interfere with maintaining coherent professional boundaries.

References

American Medical Association (1993) *Report Number 52. Patient Responsibilities*. Council on Ethical and Judicial Affairs, Code of Medical Ethics Reports IV, 190–191.

American Psychiatric Association (1973) Principles of Medical Ethics with annotations especially applicable to psychiatry. *Am J Psychiatr* 130, 1057–1064.

American Psychiatric Association (1993) *Principles of Medical Ethics with Annotations Especially Applicable to Psychiatry.* American Psychiatric Association, Washington DC.

Appelbaum PS (1993) Legal liability and managed care. *Am Psychol* 48, 251–257.

Appelbaum PS and Jorgenson L (1991) Psychotherapist–patient sexual contact after termination of treatment: An analysis and a proposal. *Am J Psychiatr* 148, 1466–1473.

Appelbaum SA (1992) Evils in the private practice of psychotherapy. *Bull Menn Clin* 56, 141–149.

Atlas M (1993) *Forum on Health Care Reform*, American Psychiatric Association Assembly meetings, November 5. Washington DC.

Blackhall L, Murphy S, Frank G *et al.* (1995) Ethnicity and attitudes towards patient autonomy. *JAMA* 274, 10.

Borys DS and Pope KS (1989) Dual relationships between therapist and client: A national study of psychologists, psychiatrists, and social workers. *Profess Psychol Res Pract* 20, 283–293.

Bratter TE (1975) Responsible therapeutic eros: The psychotherapist who cares enough to define and enforce behavior limits with potentially suicidal adolescents. *Couns Psychol* 5, 97–104.

Brown LS, Borys DS, Brodsky AM *et al.* (1992) Psychotherapist–patient sexual contact after termination of treatment. *Am J Psychiatr* 149, 979–980.

Cabeza R and Nyberg L (2000) Imaging Cognition II. An empirical review of 275 PET and fMRI studies. *J Cogn Neurosci* 12, 1–47.

Chodoff P (1993) Responsibility of the psychiatrist to his society, in *Psychiatric Ethics*, 2nd edn. (eds Bloch S and Chodoff P). Oxford University Press, New York.

Dahlberg CC (1970) Sexual contact between patient and therapist. *Contemp Psychoanal* 6, 107–124.

Dickstein E, Erlen J and Erlen JA (1991) Ethical principles contained in currently professed medical oaths. *Acad Med* 66, 622–624.

Dyer AR (1988) *Ethics and Psychiatry. Toward Professional Definition.* American Psychiatric Press, Washington DC.

Epstein RS (1994) *Keeping Boundaries. Maintaining Safety and Integrity in the Psychotherapeutic Process.* American Psychiatric Press, Washington DC.

Epstein RS (2002) Post-termination boundary issues (Letter). *Am J Psychiatr* 159, 877–878.

Epstein RS and Janowsky DS (1969) Research on the psychiatric ward. The effects on conflicting priorities. *Arch Gen Psychiatr* 21, 455–463.

Epstein RS and Simon RI (1990) The Exploitation Index: An early warning indicator of boundary violations in psychotherapy. *Bull Menn Clin* 54, 450–465.

Epstein RS, Simon RI and Kay GG (1992) Assessing boundary violations in psychotherapy: Survey results with the exploitation index. *Bull Menn Clin* 56, 150–166.

Frank JD and Frank JB (1991) *Persuasion and Healing. A Comparative Study of Psychotherapy*, 3rd edn. Johns Hopkins University Press, Baltimore.

Freud S (1912) Recommendations to physicians practicing psychoanalysis in *The Standard Edition of the Complete Psychological Works of Sigmund Freud*, Vol. 12, (trans-ed Strachey J). Hogarth Press, London, pp. 118–119. (Volume published in 1958).

Freud S (1913) On beginning the treatment. Further recommendations on the technique of psychoanalysis, in *The Standard Edition of the Complete Psychological Works of Sigmund Freud*, Vol. 12. (trans-ed Strachey J). Hogarth Press, London, p. 140. (Volume published in 1958).

Fries JF, Koop CE, Beadle CE *et al.* (1993) Reducing health care costs by reducing the need and demand for medical services. *New Engl J Med* 329, 321–325.

Gabbard GO (1991) Psychodynamics of sexual boundary violations. *Psychiatr Ann* 21, 651–655.

Gabbard GO (1994) Psychotherapists who transgress sexual boundaries with patients. *Bull Menn Clin* 58, 124–134.

Gartrell N, Herman J, Olarte S *et al.* (1986) Psychiatrist–patient sexual contact: Results of a national survey: I—Prevalence. *Am J Psychiatr* 143, 1126–1131.

Geis G, Pontell HN, Keenan C *et al.* (1985) Peculating psychologists: Fraud and abuse against Medicaid. *Profess Psychol Res Pract* 16, 823–832.

Goffman E (1974) *Frame Analysis. An essay on the organization of experience.* Harvard University Press, Cambridge.

Gorman JM (2001) Images in Psychiatry. Maimonides, 1135–1204 (AD). *Am J Psychiatr* 158, 376.

Gutheil TG (1992) Approaches to forensic assessment of false claims of sexual misconduct by therapists. *Bull Am Acad Psychiatr Law* 20, 289–296.

Gutheil TG and Gabbard GO (1993) The concept of boundaries in clinical practice: Theoretical and risk-management dimensions. *Am J Psychiatr* 150, 188–196.

Hippocrates (1929) *The Genuine Works of Hippocrates.* Adams F (trans). William Wood, New York.

Holroyd JC and Brodsky AM (1977) Psychologists' attitudes and practices regarding erotic and nonerotic physical contact with patients. *Am Psychol* 32, 843–849.

Kardener SH, Fuller M and Mensh IN (1973) A survey of physicians' attitudes and practices regarding erotic and nonerotic contact with patients. *Am J Psychiatr* 130, 1077–1081.

Kay J and Roman B (1999) The prevention of sexual misconduct at the medical school, residency, and practitioner levels, in *Current Dilemmas in the Approach to the Sexual Misconduct of Physicians.* (eds Bloom JD and Nadelson CC). American Psychiatric Press, Washington DC, pp. 153–177.

Langs R (1973) *The Technique of Psychoanalytic Psychotherapy*, Vol. 1, Aronson, New York, pp. 60–62.

Langs R (1984–1985) Making interpretations and securing the frame: Sources of danger for psychotherapists. *Int J Psychoanal Psychother* 10, 3–23.

Luepker E (1990) Clinical assessment of clients who have been sexually exploited by their therapists and development of differential treatment plans, in *Psychotherapist's Sexual Involvement with Clients: Intervention and Prevention.* (eds Schoener GR, Milgrom JH, Gonsiorek JC *et al.*). Walk-In Counseling Center, Minneapolis, pp. 172–174.

Maimonides M (1944) *Mishneh Torah Hilchot Deot.* (ed Birnbaum P). Hebrew Book Publishing, New York, p. 12.

Malmquist CP and Notman MT (2001) Psychiatrist–patient boundary issues following treatment termination. *Am J Psychiatr* 158, 1010–1018.

McCormick B (1994) What price patient advocacy? *Am Med News* 28 (Mar), 1 and 6.

McKenzie NF (1990) The new ethical demand in the crisis of primary care medicine, in *The Crisis in Health Care. Ethical Issues.* (ed McKenzie NF). Meridian, New York, pp. 113–126.

Okasha A (2000) The impact of Arab culture on psychiatric ethics, in *Ethics, Culture and Psychiatry. International Perspectives.* (eds Okasha A, Arboleda-Florez J and Sartorius N). American Psychiatric Press, Washington DC, pp. 15–28.

Okasha A and Okasha T (2000) Notes on mental disorders in Pharoanic Egypt. *Hist Psychiatr* 11, 413–424.

Parker S (1976) The precultural basis of the incest taboo: Toward a biosocial theory. *Am Anthropol* 78, 285–305.

Perry JA (1976) Physicians' erotic and nonerotic physical involvement with patients. *Am J Psychiatr* 133, 838–840.

Peterson MR (1992) *At Personal Risk. Boundary Violations in Professional–client Relationships.* WW Norton, New York.

Pope KS and Bouhoutsos JC (1986) *Sexual Intimacy between Therapists and Patients.* Praeger, New York.

Pope KS and Vetter VA (1992) Ethical dilemmas encountered by members of the American Psychological Association. A national survey. *Am Psychol* 47, 397–411.

Reason J (1990) *Human Error*. Cambridge University Press, Cambridge, UK.

Rogers WH, Wells KB, Meredith LS *et al.* (1993) Outcomes for adult outpatients with depression under prepaid or fee-for-service financing. *Arch Gen Psychiatr* 50, 517–525.

Roman B and Kay J (1997) Residency education on the prevention of physician–patient sexual misconduct. *Acad Psychiatr* 21, 26–34.

Schoener GR (1990) A look at the literature, in *Psychotherapists' Sexual Involvement with Clients: Intervention and Prevention* (eds Schoener GR, Milgrom JH, Gonsiorek JC *et al.*). Walk-In Counseling Center, Minneapolis, pp. 11–50.

Schoener GR and Gonsiorek JC (1990) Assessment and development of rehabilitation plans for the therapist, in *Psychotherapist's Sexual Involvement with Clients: Intervention and Prevention* (eds Schoener GR, Milgrom JH, Gonsiorek JC *et al.*). Walk-In Counseling Center, Minneapolis, pp. 401–420.

Shor J and Sanville J (1974) Erotic provocations and alliances in psychotherapeutic practice: Some clinical cues for preventing and repairing therapist–patient collusions. *Clin Soc Work J* 2, 83–95.

Simon RI (1987) The psychiatrist as a fiduciary. Avoiding the double agent role. *Psychiatr Ann* 17, 622–626.

Simon RI (1989) Sexual exploitation of patients. How it begins before it happens. *Psychiatr Ann* 19, 104–112.

Simon RI (1992) Treatment boundary violations: Clinical, ethical and legal considerations. *Bull Am Acad Psychiatr Law* 20, 269–286.

Slovenko R (1991) Undue familiarity or undue damages? *Psychiatr Ann* 21, 598–610.

Twemlow SW and Gabbard GO (1989) The lovesick therapist in *Sexual Exploitation in Professional Relationships* (ed Gabbard GO). American Psychiatric Press, Washington DC, pp. 71–87.

Webb WL (1986) The doctor–patient covenant and the threat of exploitation. *Am J Psychiatr* 143, 1149–1150.

Westermeyer J (1991) Problems with managed psychiatric care without a psychiatrist-manager. *Hosp Comm Psychiatr* 42, 1221–1224.

Winnicott DW (1960) Ego distortion in terms of true and false self, in *The Maturational Processes and the Facilitating Environment*. Studies in the Theory of Emotional Development. Collected papers, published 1965. International Universities Press, New York.

World Psychiatric Association Ethical Statements (2000) In Ethics, Culture and Psychiatry. International Perspectives (appendix), (eds Okasha A, Arboleda-Florez J, and Sartorius N). American Psychiatric Press, Washington DC, pp. 211–214.

World Psychiatric Association Informational Folder (1999–2002) World Psychiatric Association, New York.

Xiangyi C and Tiebang L (2001) The survey of therapeutic relationship in psychotherapy. *Chin J Psychiatr* 34, 117–120.

6 Law, Ethics and Psychiatry

Introduction

Psychiatrists' efforts to be helpful to their patients are driven by the desire to act in the "right" or ethical way. They also work within the context of the legal system which will often impact the way in which they provide care. While psychiatrists do not need to become experts in the practice of law or in the study of ethics, they should have an appreciation of how clinical work intersects with the law and the ethical foundations upon which their own decisions are made.

This chapter will begin by surveying the principles underlying the legal system, highlighting some of the landmark cases that impact our work as psychiatrists, and illustrating common clinical sources of interest and relevance to clinical practice. The chapter will conclude by reviewing the sources of psychiatric ethics, outlining the consensus principles of psychiatric ethics, and illustrating some important clinical areas which generate issues of ethical concern.

Overview of Legal Principles

The development of legal principles is the result of the interplay of legislatures that enact laws, executive branches that enforce them and courts that interpret them. The first level of courts are trial courts, where cases are tried and decided. Appeals courts generally hear arguments by parties who feel that lower courts have made errors of law which require reversal of the lower court decision. The federal and most state court systems have two levels of appeals courts (an Appeals Court and a Supreme Court, although terminology varies among jurisdictions). The highest court in the land is the US Supreme Court, which is the final arbiter of questions of Federal and Constitutional Law.

Cases decided in state courts set the law only for the state in which the case is decided. Although state decisions may ultimately influence one another, no state is required to abide by the precedent of a different state's courts. For instance, the Tarasoff case discussed below set standards in California for a mental health professional's duty to protect a third party from the danger posed by a client. Although that case only applied to practice in California, it has had a great influence on legal and clinical practice in other states. Similarly, federal Appeals Courts set precedent only for the Circuits in which they sit. Only when the US Supreme Court has ruled on a matter of law are all other state and federal courts required to follow the precedent.

Each state also has a constitution that may be more protective of individuals' rights or more limiting of the states' power than the federal constitution. State courts can make decisions interpreting their own constitutions or the federal constitution. While federal

Appeals Courts and ultimately the US Supreme Court can overrule a state court's interpretation of the federal constitution, the state supreme court has the final word on the state's constitution, so long as the state constitution does not violate the federal constitution. (For instance, a state constitution may provide greater protection against police searches than the federal constitution, but not less.)

The specific legal rights and principles with which we will concern ourselves are found in the amendments to the US Constitution. Of particular interest to psychiatry are the following constitutional amendments: the First Amendment, which embodies the right to freedom of speech and religion; the Third and Fourth Amendments, which have been interpreted as implying a right to privacy; the Fifth Amendment, which grants the right to remain silent in a criminal case; the Sixth Amendment, which discusses the rights of defendants to fair and speedy trials; the Eighth Amendment, which proscribes cruel and unusual punishment; and the Fourteenth Amendment, which embodies the "due process" and "equal protection of the law" clauses (Table 6.1).

Rights and Responsibilities

Right to Treatment

Although the US Supreme Court has expounded no national, constitutionally based right to treatment, there has been a substantial amount of activity in this area since Birnbaum published "The Right to Treatment" in 1960. At the time the article was published, it was common for psychiatric patients to spend decades in hospitals, at times involuntarily, while receiving little treatment or only custodial care. The article attempted to upgrade the quality of care in hospitals by creating a hospitalization-treatment quid pro quo. Birnbaum (1965) later criticized state hospital conditions, declaring that "Personally, I should like to state that as a doctor I often find it repugnant to use the term 'patient' to describe persons in certain mental hospitals". He instead argued that "inmate" was a better term if no treatment were given. Birnbaum's landmark articles generated interest in this key area of mental health policy.

Birnbaum's quid pro quo rationale was endorsed in *Rouse v. Cameron* (1966) decided by Judge Bazelon of the District of Columbia Circuit Court. Rouse was found not guilty by reason of insanity on a misdemeanor charge and was thereafter civilly committed to St Elizabeth's Hospital. He petitioned for his release based on the argument that he was not receiving treatment. Judge Bazelon ruled that hospitals must make real efforts to improve patients' conditions and that lack of resources was not an adequate defense. In his decision he wrote, "The hospital need not show that the treatment will cure or improve him but only that there is a bona fide effort to do so".

Essentials of Psychiatry   Jerald Kay and Allan Tasman
© 2006 John Wiley & Sons, Ltd.

Table 6.1   US Constitutional Amendments Relevant to the Practice of Psychiatry

First Amendment

Congress shall make no law respecting an establishment of religion, or prohibiting the free exercise thereof; or abridging the freedom of speech, or of the press; or the right of the people to peaceable assemble, and to petition the Government for a redress of Grievances.

Fourth Amendment

The right of the people to be secure in their persons, houses, papers and effects. Against unreasonable searches and seizures, shall not be violated, and no Warrants shall issue, but upon probable cause, supported by Oath or affirmation, and particularly describing the place to be searched, and the persons or things to be seized.

Fifth Amendment

No person shall be held to answer for a capital, or otherwise infamous crime, unless on a presentment or indictment of a Grand Jury. Except in cases arising in the land or naval forces, or in the Militia, when in actual service in time of War or public danger; nor shall any person be subject for the same offence to be twice put in jeopardy of life or limb; nor shall be compelled in any criminal case to be a witness against himself, nor be deprived of life, liberty, or property, without due process of law; nor shall private property be taken for public use, without just compensation.

Sixth Amendment

In all criminal prosecutions, the accused shall enjoy the right to a speedy and public trial, by an impartial jury of the State and district wherein the crime shall have been committed, which district shall have been previously ascertained by law, and to be informed of the nature and cause of the accusation; to be confronted with the witnesses against him: to have compulsory process for obtaining witnesses in his favor, and to have the Assistance of Counsel for his defense.

Eighth Amendment

Excessive bail shall not be required, nor excessive fines imposed, nor cruel and unusual punishments inflicted.

Fourteenth Amendment

Section 1. All persons born or naturalized in the United States, and subject to the jurisdiction thereof, are citizens of the United States and of the State wherein they reside. No State shall make or enforce any law which shall abridge the privileges or immunities of citizens of the United States, or shall any state deprive any person of life, liberty, or property, without due process of law; nor deny to any person within its jurisdiction the equal protection of the laws.

The case of *Wyatt v. Stickney* (1972), a class action suit against an Alabama hospital with poor conditions for patients, led to definitions of humane environment, which have been incorporated into a patient's bill of rights in many states. Chief Judge Johnson wrote for the US District Court, "[Involuntarily committed patients] unquestionably have a constitutional right to receive such individual treatment as will give each of them a realistic opportunity to be cured or to improve his or her mental condition". Although this case was not heard by the US Supreme Court, it did have far-reaching social consequences for institutions in that it prompted scrutiny of the services they provide.

It was not until 1982, in the case of *Youngberg v. Romeo* (1982), that the Court held that a person who is involuntarily confined has a right to "minimally adequate training". Romeo was a profoundly retarded man who suffered injuries "on at least 63 occasions … by his own violence and by the reactions of other residents to him" while he was an inpatient at Pennhurst State Hospital in Pennsylvania. His mother sued, arguing that Romeo's Eighth and Fourteenth Amendment rights were being violated. The US Supreme Court agreed that Romeo had "constitutionally protected liberty interests under the Due Process Clause of the Fourteenth Amendment to reasonably safe conditions of confinement, freedom from unreasonable bodily restraints, and such minimally adequate training as reasonably may be required by these interests". "Minimally adequate training" required the exercise of professional judgment, which was held to be presumptively valid and to which "courts must show deference".

Most of the right to treatment cases attacked institutional standards of care, and were based on efforts to expand the scope of constitutional rights of inpatients. As will be seen below, current litigation seeking to establish rights to treatment in the community focuses largely on the statutory rights afforded by such anti-discrimination statutes as the Americans with Disabilities Act (ADA).

Right to Refuse Treatment

Patients with little or no insight into the nature of their psychiatric illness often refuse treatment. A compelling set of ethical and legal questions arises when a person's stated choice (not to receive treatment) appears to conflict with medical prediction that the person's insight and mental status would probably improve with treatment. In the past, a general assumption that mentally ill patients were, by definition, incompetent, led society to grant psychiatrists a great deal of autonomy in selecting and administering treatments to patients. With the consumer activism of the 1960s and 1970s and the accompanying development of patients' rights, however, psychiatrists and legal authorities have come to see that involuntarily committed patients are not always globally incompetent, and efforts to support patients' rights to refuse treatment have increased.

Although the US Supreme Court has not declared a federal right to refuse treatment, federal Appeals Courts and most state courts have found such rights in the federal or state constitutions, citing the due process clause of the Fourteenth

Amendment, within the right to privacy, bodily integrity, or personal security.

Appelbaum (1988) has described two broad models of treatment refusal. The "rights-driven" model seeks to maximize patient autonomy. It is based on the principle that competent adults have the right to reject treatment, even if the rejection of such treatment may result in harm or even death. States that adopt this model focus on the patient's competence to make the decision and often have considerable judicial procedures protecting patients. The laws of these states typically remove decision-making power from the psychiatrist and vest it in a guardian or the court. In these states the guardian or court decides what the patient would want if he or she were competent (the "substituted judgment" standard). The substituted judgment doctrine requires a challenging decision: it means that the judicial decision-maker must decide, based not on his or her own values and interests, or even on what may objectively be in the patient's best interests, but instead on what the patient would decide if he or she were competent.

The "treatment-driven" model tends to view treatment as an essential element of commitment to a hospital. States with this model tend to give psychiatrists more autonomy in making decisions for patients. Procedural review is done primarily by psychiatrists and is usually focused on whether the treatment is appropriate to the patients' conditions. A series of cases emanating from Massachusetts is emblematic of the rights-driven model. In the matter of *Guardianship of Richard Roe III* (1981), the court noted on involuntary psychiatric medication for psychiatric outpatients, stating, "If an incompetent individual refuses antipsychotic drugs, those charged with his protection must seek judicial determination of substituted judgment".

A later Massachusetts case, *Rogers v. Commissioner of Mental Health* (1983), applied this rationale to involuntary inpatients. Incompetent patients at Boston State Hospital were being given antipsychotic medication without the opportunity to give informed consent. The Rogers case upholds the right of committed mentally ill patients to make treatment decisions unless they have been adjudicated incompetent by a court. The Rogers court also affirmed the holding that treatment with antipsychotic medication constituted extraordinary treatment, and that authority to administer such medication to an incompetent individual required the exercise of the individual's substituted judgment. The court outlined six factors that a judge must assess when determining whether a patient should be permitted to refuse treatment: 1) the patient's previously expressed preference; 2) the patient's religious convictions; 3) the impact on family of the patient's preference; 4) probable side effects; 5) prognosis with treatment; and 6) prognosis without treatment. Several cases illustrate the treatment-driven model. *Rennie v. Klein* (1983), decided in the Third Circuit of the US Court of Appeals, held that New Jersey's procedures for reviewing the administration of antipsychotics to an unwilling patient were consistent with due process: the "decision to administer such drugs against a patient's will must be based on accepted professional judgment". Rather than have the courts superimpose procedural safeguards, treatment-driven model cases defer to medical judgment. The Rennie decision relied on the US Supreme Court's deference to professional judgment in *Youngberg v. Romeo* (1982).

Liberty and Civil Commitment

Although it is generally agreed that patients have a right to be treated in the least restrictive setting, there are times when a person's mental illness is such that he or she must be hospitalized involuntarily. Each state has different provisions for short-term emergency commitment. Many states have removed this process from the judicial setting; some states, however, require a probable cause hearing before even an emergency commitment. The purpose of such a hearing is to determine whether there is probable cause to believe that the person meets the legal criteria for involuntary hospitalization. If the patient is hospitalized after such a hearing, it is generally for a short period of time for evaluation; if it is determined that the patient needs longer involuntary hospitalization, then the statutory procedures for long-term commitment must be followed.

In the case of *O'Connor v. Donaldson* (1975), the US Supreme Court set a minimum below which states cannot set their standards for civil commitment. The Court wrote: "The state cannot constitutionally confine without more, a nondangerous, mentally ill person who is capable of surviving safely by himself or with the help of family or friends". While the Court did not state what it meant by "more", most states now require a finding of dangerousness in addition to mental illness.

In *Addington v. Texas* (1979), the US Supreme Court recognized the substantial liberty interest involved in a commitment, and set the minimum standard of proof for commitment cases as "clear and convincing". The court ruled: "The individual's liberty interest in the outcome of a civil commitment proceeding is of such weight and gravity, compared with the state's interests in providing care to its citizens who are unable, because of emotional disorders, to care for themselves...that due process requires the State to justify commitment by proof more substantial than mere preponderance of the evidence.... The reasonable-doubt standard is inappropriate in civil commitment proceedings because, given the uncertainty of psychiatric diagnosis, it may impose a burden the state cannot meet and thereby erect an unreasonable barrier to needed medical treatment". (A few states do interpret their own constitutions to require proof beyond a reasonable doubt.)

The standards for long-term commitment vary from state to state, but they all rely on two broad principles of state power. One is the *parens patriae* power; the other, the police power. *Parens patriae*, translated from Latin as "father of the country", historically referred to the sovereign's power to make decisions for the subjects. A more contemporary translation is "state as parent", which refers to the government's interest in, and responsibility to act for, individuals who are unable to care for themselves. *Parens patriae* is used as a rationale for commitment when a person is unable to care for herself or himself as a result of a mental illness or when he or she poses a danger to self. The police power stems from the state's interest in maintaining public safety. The commitment criterion of "dangerousness to others" is derived from the police power. Over time, the trend in legislation and in court action has been more toward the dangerousness standard and less toward disability. Under all current statutes, a finding of mental illness is a prerequisite to commitment Table 6.2.

The notion of dangerousness to others or to self is a problematical one for psychiatrists, given that prediction of harm is an inexact science. Complicating the picture is the fact that states also require different levels of proof that people are dangerous to themselves. Some states require imminent harm, while others are more tolerant of general predictions of future dangerousness based on a patient's pattern of treatment noncompliance and decompensation.

Finally, many states require a finding that hospitalization is the least restrictive method to prevent the harm the patient

Table 6.2	Principles Underlying Involuntary Commitment
Parens Patriae	• State as parent: acts for those who cannot • "*Unable to care for self*" and "*danger to self*" criteria
Police Power	• State as protector: acts to preserve public safety • "*Danger to others*" criterion

faces. In *Lake v. Cameron* (1966), the District of Columbia Court of Appeals held that a 60-year-old demented homeless woman could not be involuntarily hospitalized if there were other alternatives. This case is most famous for the concept of "least restrictive alternative", as it focused on the place of confinement as well as the fact of confinement.

The issues underlying the threshold for commitment are fundamentally social, not psychiatric. They entail a balancing of rights and liberty interests with needs for treatment and safety. This balance has historically shifted with changes in the political and social climate, and continues to be a source of debate in both the legal and mental health fields.

In 1985, the APA developed a Model Law for Commitment, which generated considerable debate in the profession: "[I]t was conceived in response to the ... 'libertarian model,' which many mental health professionals and growing numbers of families believed was unworkable, unrealistic and inhumane" (Stone, 1985). Stone added that "the liberty of psychotic persons to sleep in the streets of America is hardly a cherished freedom" and advocated for greater discretion for psychiatric commitment as well as greater resources for treatment once the patient is hospitalized.

Outpatient Commitment

Progress in the treatment of severe and chronic mental illness often depends upon the patient's compliance with medication and other treatment regimens in the community. This has been a source of challenge and frustration for psychiatrists who treat such patients. In recent years there has been a growth of interest in the possibility that outpatient commitment may offer a way to ensure that those who most need treatment will in fact receive it. In principle, an outpatient commitment law allows the same sort of treatment options as already exist with inpatient commitment: a patient may be deprived of liberty and, if found to be incompetent to make medication decisions, may be made to take medication against his will. While inpatient commitment is justified when a patient represents a danger or cannot care for himself, how does one justify coercing a patient who may be stable, relatively symptom-free and functioning in the community?

Here the legal debate splits into two camps. Those in favor of outpatient commitment make several arguments: 1) the treatments are safe and effective; 2) untreated mental illness may increase the likelihood of violence, homelessness, incarceration and suicide; and, more controversially, 3) patients with severe mental illness frequently lack awareness of their condition, and are therefore not really free when ill (Torrey and Zdanowicz, 2001). Those opposing outpatient commitment counter that: 1) better funded and staffed outpatient programs would provide the kind of outreach which would make coercion unnecessary; 2) the prospect of coercion may actually drive certain patients away

from help; 3) public safety would not be enhanced by outpatient commitment; and 4) even the most ill patient is, in the eyes of the law, still competent to refuse treatment (Allen and Smith, 2001).

At least 41 states permit some form of outpatient commitment, yet the first two randomized trials examining its use (Steadman *et al.*, 2001; Swartz *et al.*, 2001) provided equivocal evidence of efficacy (Appelbaum, 2001). The actual mechanics of apprehending a nondangerous person, taking him/her to some facility, and injecting him/her involuntarily with medication, all because he/she had not followed through on a treatment plan, has proven difficult both to implement and to tolerate in a society which still places great value on maintaining its citizens' liberty interests. The debate will continue as psychiatrists try to reduce the aggregate suffering imposed on individuals and society by the effects of untreated mental illness.

Confidentiality and Privilege

The principles of confidentiality and privilege have a long and still evolving historical connection with the practice of medicine and the role of the physician. The Hippocratic Oath states, "And about whatever I may see or hear in treatment, or even without treatment, in the life of human beings – things that should not ever be blurted out outside – I will remain silent, holding such things to be unutterable [sacred, not to be divulged]" (Von Staden, 1996). The elegant simplicity of this statement of principle is now pitted against conflicting legal demands and societal values. The *Tarasoff* case (discussed below) and its progeny, the increasing use of subpoenas for psychiatric records, the complexity of interfacing with managed care, and confidentiality guidelines related to human immunodeficiency virus infection (HIV) are just some of the issues that complicate the psychiatrists' oath of confidentiality.

Confidentiality

In the APA's *Principles of Medical Ethics with Annotations Especially Applicable to Psychiatry* (1993), Section 4, Annotation 1 reads, "Confidentiality is essential to psychiatric treatment. This is based in part on the special nature of psychiatric therapy as well as on the traditional ethical relationship between physician and patient". The constitutional right of privacy has been discussed elsewhere in this chapter. Confidentiality is defined as the clinician's obligation to keep information learned in that relationship unavailable to third parties (Appelbaum and Gutheil, 2000; Gutheil, 1994, pp. 1–13).

Appelbaum and Gutheil (2000) looked at practice in psychiatric facilities, and devised the concept of a "circle of confidentiality" (Figure 6.1). Within the circle, information about the patient is shared without the patient's consent. For instance, for a hospitalized patient, the resident psychiatrist, the psychiatrist's supervisor, the staff and essential consultants are considered to be within the circle of confidentiality. The patient's family, the patient's attorney, the patient's outside psychiatrist, the patient's previous psychiatrist and the police are outside the circle. As Appelbaum and Gutheil note, although the patient is inside the circle, the patient may speak to anyone outside the circle without restriction.

The duty of confidentiality is sometimes understood in terms of the treatment contract between the patient and psychiatrist. There is agreement between the legal system and the psychiatric profession that confidentiality is not an absolute value. There are several major exceptions to the obligation of

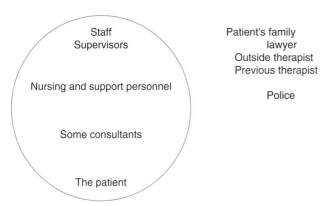

Staff
Supervisors

Patient's family
lawyer
Outside therapist
Previous therapist

Nursing and support personnel

Police

Some consultants

The patient

Figure 6.1 *The circle of confidentiality. Reprinted with permission from Appelbaum PS and Gutheil TG (2000) Clinical Handbook of Psychiatry and the Law, Baltimore Psychiatric press. Washington DC, pp. 1–29. Copyright, Lippincott, Williams & Wilkins.*

confidentiality, the most common of which is when the patient consents to information being released. Psychiatrists and their patients should be aware of the implications of releasing information to insurance companies, family members, employers and so forth and should work collaboratively in making these decisions (Table 6.3).

As a rule, the psychiatrist should get the patient's consent in writing and, optimally, the patient should read any information that leaves the office before it is released.

The second exception is based on the duty to protect, wherein the value of safety is given priority over the value of confidentiality. This is discussed later in the chapter.

The third set of exceptions includes reporting statutes, which mandate physician reporting of certain conditions. All states have such laws in one form or another, and generally include incidents of infectious diseases, child abuse and elder abuse. If they are following any of these statutes in good faith, psychiatrists run little risk of liability. See the discussion of child abuse reporting, below.

The fourth set of exceptions includes emergencies. For instance, when a psychiatrist is evaluating a patient in an emergency department and the patient is grossly psychotic and unwilling to participate in the interview, the psychiatrist is presented with the dilemma of whether to contact family members or prior treaters without the expressed written consent of the patient. This involves a risk–benefit assessment that the evaluating psychiatrist must make. Psychiatrists must be aware of their states' standards concerning emergency breach of confidentiality; one state may require an identifiable harm to be prevented, while another may permit breach when it is necessary in the clinician's judgment to gather the relevant information to make a proper diagnosis or disposition for the patient.

Table 6.3 Major Exceptions to Confidentiality
• Patient consents to release of information
• Duty to protect
• Emergencies
• Mandatory reporting statutes
• Court-ordered evaluations
• Patient initiates litigation

Medical insurance has brought its own challenges to the issue of confidentiality. Insurance companies may ask mental health providers to sign a contract agreeing to release information to the insurer. Patients may ultimately have to decide which they value more: their privacy or the benefits obtained through the managed health company. Mental health providers who are negotiating contracts with insurers should be mindful of any obligation to provide confidential information without the patient's consent.

Appelbaum and Gutheil (1991) state that psychiatrists in the position of having to breach confidentiality should observe certain basic principles. First, they should alert patients, whenever possible, of their intention to breach confidentiality before doing so. Secondly, psychiatrists should use a hierarchy of confidentiality. Psychiatrists do not need to jump to breach confidentiality in all situations where it is necessary to communicate confidential information. They often have time to discuss issues with a patient, to consider alternatives and thus avoid such confrontations. Finally, Appelbaum and Gutheil state that psychiatrists should bear in mind that the alliance is based on the "healthy side" of the patient against the patient's illness. They suggested that when the patient is experiencing impulses to harm another person, the psychiatrist and the patient should attempt to make the call to warn the person together. The healthy side of the patient is thus supported actively by the psychiatrist, as opposed to having the psychiatrist "blow the whistle" on a patient who has become dangerous. These recommendations emphasize the importance of the therapeutic alliance and remind us that confidentiality is an important aspect of that alliance.

Psychiatrist–Patient Privilege

Privilege is defined as the patient's right to prevent testimony by a psychiatrist in a court setting (Gutheil, 1994; Appelbaum and Gutheil, 1991). It rests on two primary justifications: 1) it protects the patient's interests in the privacy of treatment matters; and 2) it may encourage patients to speak openly with their psychiatrists. The scope of privilege is generally limited to the patient's communications with the psychiatrist. Observations of the patient's demeanor, or his or her conduct or even words in a public setting may not be covered within the privilege.

Privilege is a right belonging to the patient and may be waived by the patient. Although the privilege does not belong to the psychiatrist, he or she may have a duty to assert it in legal proceedings, unless and until one of the exceptions to privilege applies. In the absence of a release or waiver of privilege by the patient, psychiatrists should consult with legal counsel if they are called to testify about their communications with a patient.

Exceptions to the doctrine of privilege vary from state to state and include situations when a patient has introduced his or her mental state into litigation to which the patient is a party. In some states, privilege does not apply in competence to stand trial, or criminal responsibility evaluations. There are often exceptions in cases of child custody, involuntary commitment proceedings, will contests, or malpractice claims filed by the patient against a psychiatrist. Finally, state law may vary on the scope of the exception once it is invoked.

Informed Consent

Psychiatrists, like all other medical practitioners, face a dilemma: patients come to them for answers and treatment, and they expect the psychiatrist to have those answers; however, treatment of mental illness is an uncertain process, and is not without risks. In order to give informed consent to treatment, patients must be given sufficient information concerning the risks and benefits of the proposed treatment; where outcomes are uncertain, they must also be informed of that uncertainty. The doctrine of informed consent has evolved considerably in the past several decades. The need to obtain a patient's consent for treatment is grounded in the legal theory of battery, which is defined as an intentional touching of a person without that person's consent. Provision of medical treatment is considered an intentional touching; if it is provided without the patient's consent (and without other exceptions, such as provision of emergency medical care), then it is a battery. Only after obtaining consent from a competent person may the physician treat the patient without risking liability for the tort of battery. As medical treatment has become more complex, and as concern for patients' rights has grown, the notion of informed consent has evolved to require provision of ever more information to assist patients in making informed medical decisions.

Courts began setting modern standards for informed consent in the 1960s. The Kansas Supreme Court held that the quantum of information that a physician was required to provide was that which a "reasonable medical practitioner" would divulge (*Natanson v. Kline*, 1960). In 1972, the US Court of Appeals for the District of Columbia decided the landmark case of *Canterbury v. Spence*, in which the court ruled that the physician had the duty to "advise patient of need for or desirability of any alternative treatment". Although the majority of states determine the sufficiency of disclosure by the standard of that which the reasonable practitioner would deem significant, some states take a more patient centered approach in which the quantum of information is that which "would be regarded as significant by a reasonable person in the patient's position" (*Truman v. Thomas*, 1980).

In general, then, the psychiatrist is obligated to disclose likely material risks of treatment, but not all possible risk, that is, the likelihood and severity of injurious side effects or death. Also, the psychiatrist should explain the need for treatment, and risks and the benefits of receiving or refusing the treatment. Finally, there should be a discussion of possible alternative treatments.

Obtaining informed consent for psychopharmacological treatment of children presents a particular challenge, since many psychoactive medications have not received FDA approval for use with children. Psychiatrists should be as clear as possible when explaining the state of knowledge regarding use of particular medications with children, so that the parent's or guardian's consent is as fully informed as possible.

Exceptions to Informed Consent

There are four primary exceptions to the general rule that the patient receiving treatment must give informed consent (Table 6.4). The first is a medical emergency. Consent is presumed when a person is suffering from an emergent situation that requires treatment, but is unable to give consent. Thus, for example, when a di-

abetic patient is in a coma and consent cannot be obtained before giving the patient insulin, the treating physician may rely on presumed consent for treatment as a defense to a claim of battery. In psychiatry, the definition of an emergency has been somewhat more ambiguous. Because there is no national standard of what constitutes a psychiatric emergency, clinicians should know the definitions (if any) in their state. They should consider how emergent the situation is, document their assessment, and note that it was not possible to gain the patient's informed consent at the time. Intervention in a psychiatric emergency, especially administration of medication, is often not considered treatment in the same sense as emergency treatment of a traditional medical condition. It is for this reason that many states regulate administration of emergency psychiatric medications as restraint, rather than as treatment.

Incompetence is the second exception to the need to obtain informed consent from a patient. An incompetent person, by definition, is incapable of giving informed consent; it can be granted only by that person's guardian, or other entity charged under state law with the authority to give consent. (It is thus not truly an exception to the need for informed consent, but a situation in which the consent is obtained from a surrogate.) Even incompetent patients should be engaged in the making of treatment decisions, to the extent of their ability, and gaining their assent to treatment is important, even if they do not have the legal capacity to render informed consent. All states have procedures by which a person can be declared incompetent; such a declaration usually requires a judicial finding, though some states have administrative proceedings for resolving treatment issues that do not require judicial intervention.

The third exception to informed consent arises from the concept of therapeutic privilege. Psychiatrists use privilege when they withhold information in the belief that giving a patient all of the information necessary to make a decision would harm the patient. Invocation of therapeutic privilege, rare in medicine, is even rarer in psychiatry, in which sharing information is central to the work of the psychiatrist. Psychiatrists should use this exception to the informed consent doctrine exceedingly sparingly, with extreme caution, and with great thought; here, the psychiatrist is taking a maximally paternalistic posture in presuming what is not useful for a patient to know. The psychiatrist assumes a grave risk of liability if the patient suffers harm, and subsequently proves that a reasonable patient would have wanted to have the withheld information in order to make an informed choice about treatment.

Waiver is the fourth exception in the informed consent doctrine. Competent patients may request that their physicians not give them information, effectively waiving their right to know. This circumstance has become increasingly unusual over time as physicians are less likely to withhold this information and patients less likely to request such a waiver.

Consent to the Treatment of Minors

Minors are considered to be incompetent for almost all purposes, including the right to make medical decisions. Each state has its own definition of the age that minors must attain to consent to different treatments, and the age requirements may vary with the type of treatment. For instance, a state may have a lower age of consent for treatment of sexually transmitted diseases or mental illness than for traditional medical treatment. Psychiatrists must become familiar with the law of the state or states in which they practice.

Table 6.4   Exceptions to Informed Consent
• Emergencies
• Therapeutic privilege
• Incompetence
• Waiver

Psychiatrists who work in schools must obtain the consent of parents before initiating ongoing treatment. An emergency evaluation of a student – performed without such consent – is permissible for the most part under the doctrine of emergencies and must be documented as such (see earlier discussion). Psychiatrists who work in school settings also have to work with parents who are separated or divorced. Psychiatrists are obligated to determine which parent has legal custody and to obtain the consent of that parent for the treatment of the child; documented proof of custody must be obtained. Most states have laws by which minors may become emancipated, and therefore are deemed competent to make their own decisions. The conditions of emancipation typically include marriage, becoming a parent, entry into the armed services, and sometimes a demonstrated ability of a minor to manage his or her own financial affairs and to live on his or her own.

Medicolegal Aspects of Clinical Practice

Malpractice and Risk Management

A lawsuit in which a plaintiff sues a defendant for damages resulting from some act of negligence is called a tort (which is characterized as a civil, as opposed to a criminal, wrong). A malpractice suit is a type of negligence case; it shares with all negligence cases four broad elements – the "four Ds" – which must be proved if the plaintiff is to be awarded damages (Table 6.5).

The first element involves duty. A psychiatrist in private practice has no duty to treat or care for a patient unless he or she has made an agreement to do so. Once the psychiatrist agrees to treat the patient, however, the psychiatrist is legally and ethically obligated to treat the patient until treatment is properly terminated.

Once the psychiatrist–patient relationship is established, the psychiatrist is obligated to provide treatment at the standard of care. Since the duty comes into being when the relationship is established, psychiatrists need to be mindful of whether they are in fact entering into a psychiatrist–patient relationship. Commonly, psychiatrists in private practice see patients for a one-time consultation and then decide whether they wish to provide treatment. The psychiatrist should make it clear at the time of the initial contact that the first appointment is an opportunity for the psychiatrist and patient to see if their relationship is going to be a useful one. If this is not clearly spelled out and agreed to, it might be argued that the psychiatrist assumed a duty to provide care at the initial consultation. The second element of malpractice is negligence (or dereliction of duty). The test of negligence is whether the psychiatrist's actions deviated from the standard of care practiced by other professionals of the same level of training.

The third element that needs to be demonstrated is harm or damage. Once the plaintiff has proven that the psychiatrist has a duty to the patient and has performed in a derelict manner, there must be proof that the patient has suffered harm. Even a grossly

Table 6.5	The Four Ds of Malpractice
• Dereliction of	
• Duty	
• Directly causing	
• Damage	

negligent act that results in no harm will not result in a finding of liability for malpractice.

The fourth factor is direct or proximate cause. The damage that the patient has suffered must directly result from the dereliction of duty by the psychiatrist. Without this connection, a claim of malpractice will not be successful.

Third Party Payers and the Psychiatrist

The increasing role that insurers play in determining the type of treatment patients receive has increased the complexity of the psychiatric–legal interface. A major public policy issue in this area is whether, and to what extent, insurance companies may be held responsible when a denial of coverage results in harm to a patient. Health care providers are faced with difficult legal and ethical decisions when their professional judgment calls for provision of a particular service in the face of an insurance company denial. The law in this area is evolving; whereas early cases seemed to cloak managed care payers with a great deal of protection, later cases and some statutory changes are increasing their exposure.

The 1987 case, *Wickline v. the State of California*, illustrates the relationship between the treating physician and the third party payer in a relatively early stage of the development of this area of law. The message of the case is that a denial of coverage does not obviate a physician's duty to render treatment to the appropriate standard of care. Where coverage is denied, physicians are nonetheless obligated to exercise their medical judgment, and, where necessary, to challenge the denial through whatever mechanisms are available.

Three years later, the same California court made it clear that insurance companies may indeed share liability with physicians when the denial of benefits results in harm to the patient. In the case of *Wilson v. Blue Cross of California* (1990), the patient, Wilson, was admitted to a hospital in Los Angeles, suffering from depression, substance dependence and anorexia. His treating physician determined that he required 3 or 4 weeks of inpatient care, but on his 10th day in the hospital his insurance company stated that it would not pay for any further hospital care. When the family made it clear that they could not afford to pay for the hospitalization, the patient was discharged; 20 days later he committed suicide. Although the treating physician did not appeal the denial of coverage, he later testified that he was reasonably sure that Wilson would not have committed suicide had he been permitted to remain in the hospital. The court ruled that the insurance company's denial of coverage might have been a proximate cause of Wilson's suicide, and it permitted the case to go to trial where the plaintiff would have had to prove the elements of negligence to a jury. The intersection of the demands of confidentiality with those of managed care presents a second major area of complexity. At the beginning of therapy, the psychiatrist should outline the scope of utilization review and should obtain the consent of the patient before releasing any information to the reviewing companies. Once a patient gives consent for a psychiatrist to speak to a utilization review committee, the psychiatrist should give only the minimal amount of information necessary to facilitate the utilization review decision. Patients should also be made aware of the possibility that payment for recommended services may be denied by the insurance company. The treatment agreement between the patient and psychiatrist should make clear the patient's financial responsibilities in the event of such a denial. However, a psychiatrist may face liability for failure to provide, or arrange for, necessary care in the community, just as in the hospital setting, even when coverage is denied.

Finally, there is a potential for conflict and liability when health care providers sign contracts with managed care companies. Whether the contract is based on a capitated scale or fee for service, providers often have a financial incentive to limit the care they provide (just as they have a financial incentive to inflate costs under traditional indemnity arrangements). In addition, some managed care companies are making an effort to transfer their financial liability for treatment denials to their psychiatrists by having them sign "hold harmless" or "indemnification" agreements. Psychiatrists must be aware that such arrangements may have an impact on their relationships with their patients, and must guard against the possibility that their clinical judgment may be influenced thereby.

Liability for Supervising Other Professionals

Psychiatrists work in a variety of settings and interact in many different ways with other mental health professionals. One aspect of this interaction is the liability potential that psychiatrists undertake in each of these relationships. The APA publication entitled "Guidelines for psychiatrists in consultative, supervisory, or collaborative relationships with nonmedical therapists" (1980) outlines the typical consultative relationships and their corresponding degree of responsibility. Broadly, the degree of liability correlates with the extent of authority to make (as opposed to recommend) treatment decisions (Table 6.6).

Supervisory relationships are relationships in which the psychiatrist is hierarchically and legally responsible for the overall care of the patient, and will be held responsible for the treatment provided by those he or she supervises. The American Psychiatric Association (1980) guidelines state that:

> In a supervisory relationship the psychiatrist retains direct responsibility for patient care and gives professional direction and active guidance to the therapist. In this relationship the nonmedical therapist may be an employee of an organized health care setting or of the psychiatrist. The psychiatrist remains ethically and medically responsible for the patient's care as long as the treatment continues under his or her supervision. The patient should be fully informed of the existence and nature of, and any changes in, the supervisory relationship.

Consultative relationships are different in terms of the level of responsibility and liability undertaken. Consultative advice is given on a "take it or leave it" basis. Consultants are outside the decision-making chain of command; they do not make

Table 6.6	**Psychiatrists' Relationships with Nonmedical Therapists**
Supervisory	• Psychiatrist has treatment responsibility • Psychiatrist may hire or fire • Psychiatrist has final authority
Collaborative	• Responsibility shared between parties • Delineation of responsibilities required
Consultative	• Consultee may take advice or not • Consultant is not responsible for supervision • Consultant has no hire or fire authority

treatment decisions, and do not have hiring and firing authority. As such, they generally are not held liable for treatment decisions (though psychiatrists practicing as consultants should be aware of any unusual legal provisions in the state in which they practice). The American Psychiatric Association (1980) guidelines state that in this type of relationship the psychiatrist does not assume responsibility for the patient's care. The psychiatrist evaluates the information provided by the therapist and offers a medical opinion which the therapist may or may not accept. Consultation is not a one-way process and psychiatrists do and should seek appropriate consultation from members of other disciplines in order to provide more comprehensive services to patients.

Risk Management Techniques

There is consensus among risk management experts that various strategies can reduce medico–legal liability. The clinical strategies of obtaining consultation on difficult cases, documenting the rationale behind critical decisions, and using informed consent to build rapport are valuable risk management techniques. In documentation, "thinking for the record" is advocated by Gutheil. The psychiatrist thus demonstrates the use of judgment and ongoing risk benefit assessments. Institutional strategies include regular quality assurance monitoring, training in documentation, a system for working with patients and families on adverse effects, and providing access to expert consultation.

In psychiatry, several areas deserve special mention. Suicide and attempted suicide represent one of the most common and expensive sources of lawsuits in psychiatry (Slawson, 1989). Psychiatrists should assess the level of suicidality and the ability of patients to monitor and report their suicidality (Gutheil *et al.*, 1986) and plan an appropriate strategy based on that assessment. In lawsuits involving suicide, the patients are more commonly portrayed as the victims, rather than agents in their own deaths. The psychiatrist who both fosters and documents active collaboration with the patient demonstrates good risk management practice as well as clinical skill. Prescribing medications also raises psychiatrists' liability risk. Solid documentation of history, examinations, laboratory tests, indications for a medication and risk assessment are essential to reduce liability. Consultation with a colleague should be sought for difficult cases.

Duty to Warn, Duty to Protect

> When a psychotherapist determines (or, pursuant to the standards of the profession, should determine) that his/her patient represents a serious danger of violence to another, he/she incurs an obligation to use reasonable care to protect the intended victim against such danger. The discharge of such duty, depending on the nature of the case, may call for the therapist to warn the intended victim or others likely to appraise the victim of the danger, to notify the police, or to take whatever other steps are reasonably necessary under the circumstances.

This is the so-called Tarasoff principle, established by California Judge Tobrinen in 1976 in the case of *Tarasoff v. Regents* (1976). It has generated controversy, spawned lawsuits, and initiated a fundamental reexamination of the psychiatrist's role *vis-à-vis* members of the public.

The *Tarasoff* case involved the tragic death of a University of California student, Tatiana Tarasoff, who was murdered by a fellow student, Prosenjit Poddar. Poddar was an outpatient at the campus mental health clinic. He stated to his psychologist that he intended to kill Tarasoff. The therapist completed paperwork to have Poddar committed for 72-hour emergency psychiatric detention. The local police detained Poddar, but released him when he stated that he would "stay away from that girl". Two months later he successfully carried out his threat to kill Tarasoff.

This case, as well as subsequent cases and legislation in other states, created new clinical and ethical dilemmas for psychiatrists, as they now must balance confidentiality with the safety of third parties in outpatient settings as well. At what point is the inherently trusting nature of the psychiatrist–patient relationship impaired by the legally driven obligation to report threats of harm? When should a psychiatrist report a patient's vague statement wishing to harm a third party? How should the patient's violent history be weighed in the assessment of whether to violate confidentiality? Does the circle of responsibility include only named third parties, or does it extend to groups of reasonably identifiable potential victims? Is a warning sufficient? Although these questions are ultimately matters of clinical judgment, psychiatrists need to know whether their states have established specific guidelines for settling them.

Criminal Law and Psychiatry

The psychiatrist's role in the courtroom is substantially different from that in the clinical setting (Rappeport, 1982). In criminal cases, psychiatrists are commonly called on to evaluate defendants' competence to stand trial or (less commonly) criminal responsibility. In perhaps the most challenging of situations, psychiatrists are faced with the ethically challenging task of evaluating defendants' competence to understand the death penalty.

The Psychiatrist as Expert Witness

Psychiatrists may work in forensic settings as agents of the court, providing impartial evaluations for the judge, or may function as experts for the defense or prosecution. As opposed to fact witnesses, who can testify only as to facts that they have observed, expert witnesses may review records, conduct tests, perform evaluations or other research, and provide opinions (such as diagnoses) in court. Expert witnesses, by definition, are familiar with a body of professional knowledge that is not well known to the layperson (Table 6.7).

When asked to serve as an expert witness, the psychiatrist should have a clear understanding of the legal question or standard being addressed. The expert witness should inform the client that patient–psychiatrist confidentiality is not to be expected and that the information being elicited will be presented to the court to help the judge or jury make a decision. In general, attorneys attempt to establish the credibility of their experts by presenting their qualifications to the court, either by testimony, or by admitting the expert's resumé. Psychiatrists who offer themselves as expert witnesses should be prepared to have their credentials challenged by the attorney for the opposing side. Good expert witnesses take these challenges in stride. They respond to questions calmly, without becoming defensive or arrogant. Good expert testimony is given in understandable, jargon-free language, with short, concise answers. Expert testimony is a challenging and difficult professional task.

Competence to Stand Trial Evaluations

In order for a criminal case to proceed, the defendant must be competent to stand trial. This is a constitutional standard that has its roots in old English law. Although specific standards of competence are determined on a state-by-state basis, the federal standard has provided the basis for each state's law. The test is "whether [the defendant] has sufficient present ability to consult with his lawyer with a reasonable degree of rational understanding and whether he has a rational as well as a factual understanding of the proceedings against him" (*Dusky v. United States*, 1960)." The legal standard is not an exacting one. Only a small proportion of criminal defendants are referred for competency evaluations.

Although there is no universally accepted clinical standard for assessing competence, the McGarry (McGarry *et al.*, 1973) criteria have been empirically validated and are the most commonly used sources of evaluation. This standard encourages the psychiatrist to assess 13 different areas of functioning, including the patient's behavior, ability to relate to an attorney, ability to plan a legal strategy, and motivation and capacity to testify, in addition to the patient's understanding of the charges, possible consequences, and likely outcomes.

Psychiatrists must remember that when they are conducting evaluations on behalf of the court, they are agents of the court; the usual rules of the psychiatrist–patient relationship (including confidentiality and privilege) are thereby waived. Those being examined must be informed of these different ground rules, in accordance with the requirements of the particular state. Since the defendant's understanding of his or her waiver of confidentiality is often an issue, the evaluator should carefully document the defendant's response to the information, using direct quotes, when possible. States have different requirements in cases where the patient appears incompetent to give informed consent for a "stand trial" evaluation. The psychiatrist needs to be aware of these requirements, and to be prepared to proceed accordingly (some states permit the evaluation to proceed; others might require further hearings). The fate of defendants found incompetent to stand trial was addressed in *Jackson v. Indiana* (1972). Jackson was mentally retarded, deaf and mute; he was charged with two counts of petty larceny. The psychiatrist who evaluated Jackson concluded that he was almost completely unable to communicate; in addition to his lack of hearing, his mental deficiency left him unable to understand the nature of the charges against him or to participate in his defense. Based on this evidence, the trial court found that Jackson "lacked comprehension sufficient to make his defense" and ordered him committed to the Indiana Department of Mental Health until that department could certify to the court that he was "sane".

Since it was clear that Jackson would never become "sane", (that is, competent to stand trial), his commitment essentially amounted to imposition of a life sentence, without his ever being convicted of a crime. The court held that this outcome violated Jackson's Fourteenth Amendment right to due process and that a defendant cannot be committed indefinitely just because he is incompetent to stand trial. His commitment must be for a purpose permitted under state law (and the Constitution).

Table 6.7	**The Psychiatrist as Expert Witness**
Fact Witness	Expert Witness
• No specialized knowledge • No special fee • Does not offer opinion	• Has special knowledge base • May offer opinions • Receives compensation

Thus, if the defendant may reasonably be restored to competence with treatment, he may be committed for that purpose. If it is unlikely that the defendant will be restored to competence (as in Jackson's case), then his commitment must meet other legitimate state purposes, such as prevention of harm under civil commitment standards. If the defendant does not meet the criteria for such a commitment, he must be released.

Insanity Defense

There is an important distinction between a finding of incompetence to stand trial and a finding of not guilty by reason of insanity (NGRI). The former means that defendants do not have a chance to defend themselves until competence is restored. The latter is a not guilty finding, based on the defendant's inability to have formed the state of mind requisite for a criminal conviction. It is not a matter of restoration or recovery from mental illness; once a defendant is found NGRI, the criminal case is permanently resolved. Criminal responsibility and competency evaluations are often requested together, but they are separate and distinct.

In order to be convicted, a defendant must be shown both to be guilty of committing an illegal act (*actus reus*) and to have had the intention of committing the crime (*mens rea*). Criminal responsibility evaluations focus on the *mens rea* component of criminal acts. The psychiatrist involved in an insanity defense is presented with a more challenging assignment than that of the competence to stand trial evaluation. Assessing a patient's mental state retrospectively is a task fraught with difficulties. The defendant may forget, lie, or "fill in" details of the events. For this reason, this evaluation typically involves more collateral investigation, such as reviewing the prosecutor's file including police, witness, victim and perhaps even autopsy reports, in addition to standard history such as past psychiatric records. The clinical interview should include the confidentiality warning, a detailed present-day mental status examination, and direct queries into the defendant's recollected mental state and in-depth recall of the crime. This detective work, together with careful questioning, as well as psychological or neurological assessment when indicated, is necessary to enable the psychiatrist to present as clear a picture as possible of the defendant's state of mind at the moment of the crime.

The first appellate decision in English law involving the insanity defense was *M'Naghten*'s case. In 1843, Daniel M'Naghten shot and killed Edward Drummond, who was secretary to the prime minister. Apparently, M'Naghten was under the delusion that he was being persecuted by the prime minister as well as other people throughout all of England. After this case, the standard for criminal responsibility became known as the M'Naghten rule: "To establish a defense on the grounds of insanity it must be conclusively proved that, at the time of committing the act, the party accused was laboring under such a defect of reason, from the disease of the mind, as to not know the nature and quality of the act he was doing; or if he did know it that he did not know what he was doing was wrong". This standard allows either a cognitive test (did he know what he was doing?) or a moral test (did he know it was wrong?). It addresses itself to the specific criminal act, as opposed to assessing the defendant from the perspective of a broad-reaching sense of right and wrong.

The American Law Institute standard provides: "A person is not responsible for criminal conduct if at the time of such conduct as a result of a mental disease or defect he lacks substantial capacity either to appreciate the wrongfulness of his conduct or

to conform his conduct to the requirements of the law" (Model Penal Code, 1955). This test incorporates the cognitive component of the M'Naghten rule but, by use of the terms "mental disease or defect", allows for the possibility that conditions other than psychotic illnesses (such as impulse disorders) may result in a lack of criminal responsibility. Contrary to public perception, a successful insanity defense does not usually result in freedom. In fact, when a defendant is found not guilty by reason of insanity, he or she may face years of confinement in a hospital setting. As Elliot and colleagues (1993) note:

> Acquittals by reason of insanity are unlike acquittals in criminal law. The criminal defendant who wins an outright acquittal is free of state control and may simply walk away from the court house after the trial. But the defendant found [NGRI] typically remains confined….

The hurdles to commitment are typically much lower and the barriers to release much higher. Especially when charged with misdemeanors, insanity acquittees generally remain hospitalized far longer than ordinary civil acquittees and may remain confined for periods greater than the maximum sentence that would have been possible on conviction of the criminal charges.

Civil Litigation

Tort Liability

The tort system is designed to compensate individuals or groups who are injured by the acts of other individuals or entities, including corporations and sometimes government agencies. As in malpractice cases (which are a category of tort), the four Ds (**dereliction** of a **duty**, **directly** causing **damage**) are the standard by which tort liability is assessed. Unlike most criminal cases, where the conduct of the victim is not relevant to the defendant's guilt, the injured party's (or plaintiff's) conduct is often a factor in determining the legal result. Thus, in a motor vehicle case, if the plaintiff was also operating his or her vehicle negligently, and thus contributed to the accident, the defendant's liability will be reduced in proportion to the plaintiff's comparative negligence. Where a party's mental state is at issue, or where there are claims for emotional damages, psychiatrists may be called upon to conduct evaluations and testify.

Psychiatrists performing an evaluation for psychic harm must evaluate the person's mental state before and after the act. For instance, if a person had a preexisting history of affective disorder and had recurrent episodes after an injury, that would be noteworthy for a psychic harm report. The question would be whether the traumatic event exacerbated the preexisting condition. Not unlike criminal responsibility evaluations, these assessments may rely heavily on collateral documentation of the event and interviews with other witnesses. Emotional injury evaluations often focus heavily on functional deficits that the plaintiff may be exhibiting, since damages are related to loss of function; it is not sufficient to simply meet diagnostic criteria for mental illness. As in all such evaluations, especially where the subject is aware of the consequences of the process, malingering should always be considered.

Disability

Psychiatrists may perform disability evaluations for both workers' compensation and Social Security disability claims. Workers' compensation is an alternative system of compensation that does not involve the complexity of the tort system. Workers' compensation, which is paid when a disabling injury occurs in the course of employment, is an exclusive remedy based on the worker's prior salary and the degree and duration of disability. In general, there are no awards for pain and suffering as there are in tort cases. In this system, evaluations focus on functional limitations and require assessment of credibility, as well as corroboration of the person's prior mental state and its connection to the work environment.

Since workers' compensation systems are created by legislatures, it is important to know the statutory definitions of the conditions under evaluation; this is particularly true for mental disability. The typical categories of mental disability are as follows: 1) physical trauma causing mental injury; 2) mental injury causing physical effects; and 3) mental stress causing mental injury.

Social Security Disability Insurance was established in 1956 for people who had contributed to the fund while working. Supplemental Security Income was developed in 1972 to establish federal matching payment for state benefit programs for the disabled, regardless of work history. The Social Security disability programs use definitions of mental disorders that resemble, but are not identical with, those of the *Diagnostic and Statistical Manual of Mental Disorders*, Fourth Edition (DSM-IV) (American Psychiatric Association, 1994). The evaluating clinician must determine whether a qualifying condition exists, and assess the degree of disability it produces, as measured against standards of the American Medical Association's guidelines (Linda *et al.*, 2001).

Competence, Capacity and Guardianship

Competence is best understood as a legal term referring to an individual's capacity to make informed decisions. Adult individuals are presumed to be legally competent, unless and until there is a court finding of incompetence. A finding of incompetence means that a physical or mental illness has caused a defect in cognition or judgment, regarding the specific area in question, such that the individual lacks the capacity to make informed decisions. When a court determines that an individual is incompetent, a guardian may be appointed to make decisions for that person.

Competence is often used as a general term, but it should be defined specifically. With the advent of modern psychopharmacology, competence in severely mentally ill patients is often related to medication compliance. Even floridly psychotic patients may become competent after they are stabilized on medications. Since the legal decision-making for incompetent patients often involves determining what the individual would want if he or she were competent to choose, it is important that the psychiatrist assess the person's capacity when he/she is doing clinically well, in addition to when he/she is doing poorly.

Assessing a patient's capacity to give consent is based on several general principles (Appelbaum and Grisso, 1988). The patient must be able to 1) communicate choices, 2) understand the relevant information, 3) appreciate the situation and its consequences, and 4) manipulate the information rationally (Table 6.8).

There is general agreement that the standard for judging competence also varies with the presented task. For instance the standard for competence to consent to take an experimental drug is higher than for taking an aspirin. The greater the risk in the

Table 6.8	Assessment of Capacity

- Ability to communicate choices
- Understand relevant information
- Appreciate the situation and its consequences
- Rationally manipulate information

intervention, the more the psychiatrist needs to be clear about the four elements noted in the preceding paragraph.

Several other competencies require attention in civil matters. For example, testamentary capacity (the capacity to make a will) may be challenged by disgruntled and disinherited parties. For this reason, some people obtain an evaluation of their capacity to make a will before their death. Testamentary capacity requires that individuals understand 1) the nature of a will, 2) the extent of their assets, 3) the identity of their natural heirs, and 4) that they should not be under undue influence. Decision-making can be based on either the "best interests" standard or the "substituted judgment" model. The best interests model is a paternalistic approach that assumes that decision-makers know what is in the patient's best interests, and that they will act accordingly. It is a value laden paradigm that requires guardians to be aware of their own value systems, and to be on guard against the risk that their values may conflict with those that might apply to the patient. Perhaps more onerous, but more individualized, is the substituted judgment model, discussed briefly above in the section on informed consent. Here, the guardian attempts to act in the manner the person would want under the circumstances. This is a difficult task. When an individual has never considered a possibility, such as being in a coma, it cannot be known with certainty what the individual's wishes would be. While it might be generally agreed that individualized decision-making is a preferable model, it is easy to see why the relative comfort of the best interest approach makes this model the one that is most widely applied.

Special Issues

Child Abuse Reporting

Kempe and colleagues in a 1962 paper, "The Battered Child Syndrome", began an awareness of child abuse and neglect that continues to grow. Before this seminal paper, many psychiatrists considered children's allegations of sexual and physical abuse to be fantasy that was to be interpreted and not acted on. Child abuse is now recognized to be widespread, and for the individual child, a potentially devastating reality.

All states place an affirmative duty on the professional to report suspicions of abuse. Even though many adult psychiatrists receive relatively little training in child psychiatry and in child development, all psychiatrists are mandated reporters of suspicions of child abuse and neglect. Psychiatrists who treat patients with alcoholism, serious mental illness, and a history of abuse are working with populations who have increased risk of child abuse. While pediatricians file the majority of child abuse reports, psychiatrists may be called to consult in cases requiring additional clinical judgment.

Neglect is a most difficult form of abuse to identify. Although the laws are written to encourage reporting in the "gray" cases, clinicians must still exercise a level of clinical judgment. One person's view of neglect may be another person's view of bad parenting. Clearly, a child who is malnourished is being neglected. A child who is left alone for a significant period may have been neglected, but this depends on the age and developmental stage of the child. Clinicians must also guard against cultural or racial bias. Hampton and Newberger (1985) studied child abuse reporting and noted that physicians are more likely to file child abuse reports involving people who are of a different race or class than themselves. Psychiatrists also worry about the damage a report will do to the alliance between the psychiatrist and the patient. Clinical experience demonstrates that, in most cases, an explanation of the practitioner's legal obligation to file a report maximizes the potential to maintain the clinical alliance. That reassurance aside, psychiatrists must be aware that the legal obligation to report supersedes the value of the alliance.

A child abuse report is usually made to the state's child welfare agency, sometimes called the "Department of Social Services" or "Children and Family Services". Most commonly, the call is screened in or out over the phone and, if screened in, then the agency begins an investigation into the allegations. If the report is substantiated the child may be taken out of the home, and the parents may eventually lose custody. Less draconian measures often include mandatory treatment of psychiatric or substance abuse disorders for both parents and children. These are painful clinical realities, but psychiatrists should not hesitate to file a child abuse report when, in their judgment, they have reason to believe a child is suffering from either abuse or neglect.

Elder or Disabled Abuse Reporting

Over 40 states have also enacted statutes mandating reporting of abuse or neglect of elderly or disabled individuals. These statutes often mirror the state's child abuse reporting laws, though they may contain broader exceptions to mandated reporting in certain circumstances. The remaining states provide legal immunity for professionals who voluntarily report abuse or neglect of the aged or disabled.

Child Custody Evaluations

Divorce has an impact on all children, but where the parents are unable to agree, especially around custody, children face more stress. Psychiatrists have responded to this burgeoning need by developing expertise in the clinical issues that surround custody decisions. A number of psychiatrists offer consultation and mediation services to divorcing couples who wish to resolve custody issues between themselves. However, when custody disputes become adversarial, formal child custody assessments are often ordered by the court. These assessments present unique clinical, legal and ethical challenges. The APA has written recommendations for conducting child custody evaluations (Child Custody Consultation, 1982).

Psychiatrists performing a child custody evaluation should have training in child work or at least have a child psychiatrist with whom to confer. As with forensic evaluations, the parents (and where appropriate, the child) should be informed that the usual rules of confidentiality and privilege will not apply.

In conducting custody evaluations, it is important to know the legal standard which the court will apply. The standard adopted in many states provides that judges making custody decisions shall "consider all relevant factors including 1) the wishes of the child's parents as to his custody, 2) the wishes of the child as to his custodian, 3) the interaction and interrelationship of the child with his parent or parents, his siblings, and any other

persons who may significantly affect the child's best interest, 4) the child's adjustment to his home, school, and community, and 5) the mental and physical health of all individuals involved. The court shall not consider conduct of a proposed custodian that does not affect his relationship to the child'' (Child Custody Consultation, 1982). The judge is required to balance these factors against the legal standard, which in most states is a "best interests of the child'' standard. The psychiatrist should thus conduct the evaluation in such a way as to provide information that will assist the judge in weighing the relevant factors.

The Americans with Disabilities Act and the Olmstead Case

In 1990, Congress enacted the Americans with Disabilities Act (ADA), with the goal of eliminating discrimination against individuals with disabilities. The Act is divided into four major sections, which prohibit discrimination in employment (Title I), public services provided by government entities (Title II), public accommodations provided by private entities (Title III) and telecommunications (Title IV).

Although discrimination in employment has been the focus of most ADA enforcement activity, advocates for the mentally ill have been litigating under Title II of the ADA, arguing that institutionalization of individuals with mental disabilities who could be appropriately treated in a less restrictive setting constitutes illegal discrimination by the state. The issue came to a head in the case of *Olmstead v. L.C.*, decided by the US Supreme Court in 1999.

Title II of the ADA states that "no qualified individual with a disability'' shall be discriminated against by a public entity (such as a state) in the provision of services, programs, or activities. In order to enable such individuals to participate on a par with nondisabled individuals, public entities are required to make "reasonable accommodations'' in the operation of services, programs, or activities. The federal Court of Appeals noted that when "treating professionals find that a community-based placement is appropriate [for an individual with a disability], the ADA imposes a duty to provide treatment in a community setting – the most integrated setting appropriate to that [individual's] needs''. The US Supreme Court agreed, ruling that "unjustified isolation is properly regarded as discrimination based on disability''.

For psychiatrists who practice in state institutions, the case is significant for the importance placed on clinical judgment about whether the patient can be adequately treated in a community setting. It is this judgment that triggers the right to community placement under the ADA, according to the Supreme Court. Clinicians making these determinations are confronted with a myriad of sometimes conflicting pressures. Is the patient really ready for the community? What kinds of accommodations might be needed in the standard community programs in order to enable the patient to function? Are these accommodations reasonable? What is the role of the clinician in advocating for individual patients versus maximizing scarce resources to benefit the greatest number of patients?

Psychiatric Ethics

Ethics, from the Greek word *ethikos*, meaning customary, or nature, is the study of standards of conduct and moral judgment. These two definitions summarize the core features of ethics. The term customary speaks to the social component of ethics, while nature emphasizes that the actor's own character is an important component. Ethics also refers to the system or code of morals of a particular person, religion, group, or profession (*Webster's*, 1980). In recent years, professional ethics have evolved from widely understood principles of etiquette and consideration for dealing with other members of the profession, to sets of rules that govern the relationship between a professional and a client or patient (Kelly, 1998). These modern principles are built upon the most ancient ideal of medical ethics: first do no harm.

Certain basic assumptions form the framework of psychiatric ethics. Society and the medical profession expect the physician to do the following:

- Deliver competent, compassionate, and respectful care.
- Deal honestly with patients and colleagues.
- Act within the bounds of the law.
- Respect the rights and autonomy of the patient.
- Be responsible to the community and society.

Sources of Psychiatric Ethics

Law

Ethics and law are closely related, but they are not synonymous (Ellis, 1991). Courts and legislatures attempt to embody ethical principles in their creation and interpretation of law. But not every ethically supportable course of conduct is, or should be, codified in the form of mandatory or prohibitory legal provisions backed up by the government's authority to punish, and not every legal mandate is consistent with medical ethics.

Religion

It is beyond the scope of this chapter to deal comprehensively with the ethical codes established by the world's various religions. Suffice it to say that many ethical decisions that confront psychiatrists have their roots in religion. Indeed, almost to the end of the 19th century, the treatment of mental disorders was conducted, to a great extent, under the auspices of religious institutions or at least in concert with the prevailing religious ideas of the time. Today's issues include treatment refusal, abortion and end of life decisions, among many others. Psychiatrists must be sensitive to the impact that their own and their patients' religious beliefs have on their understanding of human behavior.

Professional Associations

One of the hallmark characteristics of a learned profession is its development and adoption of a unique code of ethics to guide its practitioners. The APA has adopted such a code since 1989. Although "psychiatrists are assumed to have the same goals as all physicians", these principles have been revised "with annotations especially applicable to psychiatry". The rationale was that "there are special ethical problems in psychiatric practice that differ in coloring and degree from ethical problems in other branches of medical practice" (Table 6.9).

Potential Consequences of Diagnostic Labels

Diagnoses of mental disorders carry implications that are different from diagnoses of purely somatic illnesses, in part because of the societal stigma attached to mental illness. This stigma has ancient roots. Humankind attaches great power to the mind but finds it deeply mysterious. One of the worst fears is the loss of

control of meaningful communication, decision-making ability and intellectual capacity (Trad, 1991). Even accepting the medical model that grants validity to the diagnosis of mental disorders, the psychiatrist still faces ethical tensions in making such diagnoses.

Because confidentiality is not absolute, a patient's diagnosis is available to many parties, with practical consequences. Opportunities to obtain employment or insurance may be constrained by the documented presence of a psychiatric illness. Conversely, such a diagnosis may make tangible assistance and subsidies available based on the psychiatrist's assessment of the patient's disability. The clinician performing an evaluation is obliged to pay attention to any internal prejudices about patients' entitlements and to perform the assessment as fairly as possible. Another realm of prejudice that can enter the diagnostic arena relates to cultural perceptions of behavior. Although there is abundant statistical validity to the diagnostic schema of the DSM-IV, its validity is based on the norms of the majority culture. Patients who are members of cultural minority groups may express distress in ways that are inappropriately labeled as diagnosable psychopathology (Siantz, 1993).

Ethics and Patient–Therapist Boundaries

There are abundant clinical reasons for maintaining clear and predictable boundaries in the patient's relationship to the psychiatrist. Among other justifications, a clear therapeutic framework makes the psychotherapeutic environment one in which the patient can feel safe to disclose sensitive information without fear of punishment, and in which the care received is not dependent on the patient's meeting the needs or earning the approval of the caregiver.

Maintaining the principles of respect, honesty and autonomy of patients, all major organizations of medical and mental health professionals specifically condemn sexual contact between physicians or therapists and their patients, regardless of the form or intensity of the psychiatric treatment being provided. The ethical background for this blanket prohibition stems from the nature of the therapeutic relationship. Although many of the features of the psychiatrist–patient relationship are the same as those that exist with any other physician, there are some specific facets of the psychiatric alliance that lend the issue particular distinction.

The patient enters the relationship in pain and is therefore vulnerable. Not infrequently, issues of unresolved feelings about sexuality, intimacy and dependence may be part of the problem brought to the psychiatrist. The psychiatrist is seen by society, and usually by the patient, as possessing education, authority and experience. Therefore, there is an imbalance of power in the relationship from the beginning. Because the patient has brought his or her problem to the trusted psychiatrist with the expectation of assistance, courts and society have maintained that the therapeutic alliance constitutes a fiduciary relationship, wherein the psychiatrist is obliged to act scrupulously in the patient's best interests, eschewing any personal advantage (Carr and Robinson, 1990; Strasburger *et al.*, 1992).

This absolute prohibition, however, has not yielded absolute abstinence. Numerous surveys conducted from the mid-1970s through the late 1980s found that 7 to 10% of male therapists and 2 to 3% of female therapists admitted to erotic contact with patients (Strasburger *et al.*, 1992). Rarely does sexual contact with patients occur in isolation. Rather, it usually represents the last in a series of steps eroding the professional and clinical boundaries of therapy. The earlier steps may include extending

Table 6.9	Ethical Principles for Psychiatric Practice

Principles of Medical Ethics: American Medical Association	Annotations Especially Applicable to Psychiatry: American Psychiatric Association
"A physician shall be dedicated to providing competent medical service with compassion and respect for human dignity."	1. The psychiatrist shall be vigilant about the boundaries of the doctor–patient relationship. 2. A psychiatrist should not be party to any discriminatory policy. 3. It is ethical for a physician to cooperate with peer review. 4. A psychiatrist should not be a participant in a legally authorized execution.
"A physician shall deal honestly with patients and colleagues, and strive to expose those physicians deficient in character or competence, or who engage in fraud or deception."	1. Sexual activity with a current or former patient is unethical. 2. The psychiatrist should not exploit information furnished by the patient, and should not influence a patient in any way not directly relevant to the treatment goals. 3. A psychiatrist should not practice outside his/her area of professional competence. 4. When patient welfare is jeopardized by the mental illness of a psychiatrist, it is encouraged for other psychiatrists to intercede. 5. The treatment contract should be explicitly established. 6. It is ethical to charge for missed appointments within the terms of the treatment contract. 7. Fee-splitting arrangements for administration or supervision are not acceptable.
"A physician shall respect the law and also recognize a responsibility to seek changes in those requirements which are contrary to the best interests of the patient."	1. The right to protest social injustices, which may violate certain laws, may not be professionally unethical. 2. Where not prohibited by local laws, a qualified psychiatrist may practice acupuncture.
"A physician shall respect the rights of patients, of colleagues, and of other health professionals, and shall safeguard confidences within the constraints of the law."	1. Psychiatric records must be protected with extreme care. Where information must be released, the welfare of the patient must be a continuing consideration. 2. A psychiatrist may release confidential information only with the authorization of the patient or under proper legal compulsion. 3. Material used in teaching and writing must be adequately disguised. 4. The same responsibility to confidentiality holds for consultations in which the patient was not present and the consultee was not a physician. 5. The psychiatrist may disclose only that information which is relevant to a given situation. 6. When performing nonconfidential examinations, the psychiatrist must reveal the nonconfidential nature of the interview at the outset. 7. The psychiatrist must execute careful judgment in providing or withholding information to the parents of a minor patient. 8. Psychiatrists may reveal confidential information to protect the safety of the patient or the community. 9. When ordered by a court to reveal information, the psychiatrist may ethically dissent within the framework of the law. 10. With informed consent, a patient may be presented to a scientific gathering, with the audience's understanding of the confidentiality of the material. 11. It is ethical to present a patient to the public or news media only with fully informed, written consent.

Continues

Table 6.9	Ethical Principles for Psychiatric Practice *Continued*
Principles of Medical Ethics: American Medical Association	Annotations Especially Applicable to Psychiatry: American Psychiatric Association
	12. When involved in funded research, the psychiatrist will reveal to patients the source of funding and the nonconfidentiality of data. 13. It is unethical to evaluate a person charged with a crime prior to availability of legal counsel, except if the sole purpose is for medical treatment. 14. Sexual involvement between a teacher or supervisor and a trainee may be abusive of power and unethical.
"A physician shall continue to study, apply and advance scientific knowledge, make relevant information available to patients, colleagues, and the public, obtain consultation, and use the talents of other health professionals when indicated."	1. Psychiatrists are responsible for their own continuing education. 2. The psychiatrist should work respectfully with nonphysician therapists and consultants, and with nonpsychiatric physicians. He/she should not refer to anyone whose training, skill or ethics are in doubt. 3. When supervising or collaborating with another mental health worker, the psychiatrist should expend adequate time to assure that proper care is given. 4. The physician should not delegate to any nonmedical person any matter requiring professional medical judgment. 5. The psychiatrist should agree to the request of a patient for consultation from another clinician.
"A physician shall, in the provision of appropriate patient care, except in emergencies, be free to choose whom to serve, with whom to associate, and the environment in which to provide medical services."	1. Preservation of optimal conditions for the development of a sound working relationship should take highest precedence. Professional courtesy may lead to poor psychiatric care. 2. A psychiatrist may refuse to provide psychiatric treatment to a person who cannot be diagnosed as having a mental illness amenable to psychiatric treatment.
"A physician shall recognize a responsibility to participate in activities contributing to an improved community."	1. Psychiatrists are encouraged to serve society by advising and consulting with government agencies. In so doing, the psychiatrist should clarify whether he/she speaks as an individual or a representative of an organization. Personal opinions should not be cloaked with the authority of the profession. 2. Psychiatrists may share with the public their expertise in psychosocial issues that may affect mental health and illness. 3. It is unethical for a psychiatrist to offer a public professional opinion regarding someone he/she has not personally examined, or without proper authorization. 4. The psychiatrist may permit his/her certification to be used for involuntary treatment of a person only following a personal examination.

Adapted with permission from *The Principles of Medical Ethics With Annotations Especially Applicable to Psychiatry.* Copyright 1993, American Psychiatric Association, Washington DC.

sessions beyond the usual time, scheduling a patient for an hour when no one else is in the office or clinic, meeting the patient for meals or elsewhere outside the treatment setting, and accepting invitations that place the therapist and patient in intimate social situations. Such compromises erode the structure that is necessary for therapy to be a healing process and pave the way for a destructive relationship. After the termination of therapy. Most maintain, that the fiduciary obligation does not end; that transference, despite the most intense and successful analysis, never disappears; that the therapist always maintains the power of confidences divulged in the treatment; and that a therapist who begins

any therapy without having first excluded the possibility of any future sexual contact with the patient may be seen as lying in wait for the opportunity to exploit (Murphy, 1992). The consensus of practitioners and ethicists remains that, "Once a patient, always a patient".

Ethics of Psychiatric Research

The conduct of psychiatric research often presents a paradox with troubling ethical ramifications. In many circumstances, particularly in clinical investigations, worthwhile research that is primarily intended to benefit individuals with mental illnesses as a group demands that the human subjects taking part in the protocols themselves be drawn from the ranks of the mentally ill community. The central dilemma, of course, is that the very psychiatric illness that makes an individual a desirable, even necessary, subject for a particular research project may compromise that individual's own capacity to give voluntary, informed and competent consent to research participation. No subjects may be involved in research unless legally effective informed consent has been obtained and it is clear that undue influence and coercion are eliminated. The best research asks a specific and relevant question that will advance the field of knowledge, has a hypothesis, and has an investigator who has thoughtfully considered the risks of the study for subjects and the process for obtaining informed consent. The investigator presents the study to an Institutional Review Boards (IRB) which is comprised of institutionally-appointed assessors of risk and informed consent. IRBs have membership from the consumer community, the scientific community and others. IRBs are free to reject research, to amend the informed consent procedure, and to demand additional protections for the subjects. Although IRBs are a legally mandated check, which can also provide resources on the ethics of research, the responsibility for conducting ethical research lies with the investigator.

Ethics and Suicide

Much has been written about the ethics of suicide (Heyd and Bloch, 1991), and a number of philosophers, as well as physicians, have argued that suicide may be rational under some circumstances. Although US society no longer criminalizes attempted suicide, neither does it condone it. Thus, the strong current weight of ethical opinion, based on a commitment to the sanctity of life, is that usually psychiatrists ought to intervene to prevent or disrupt suicide attempts by patients. Further, according to this view, the psychiatrist's duty to intervene may justify a breach of the ordinary obligation of confidentiality (see earlier discussion) and initiation of involuntary commitment and forced treatment proceedings because of the patient's danger to self. Yet the obligation to respect the patient's autonomy requires the psychiatrist to ask whether the intent to commit suicide in a particular case is sick and justifying – even mandating – intervention or whether it is a rational decision with which the physician has no ethical justification to interfere.

In a related vein, much debate has emerged in the past few years surrounding the ethical permissibility of physician-assisted suicide (Quill, 1991). Advocates for permissibility cite unbearable pain as a justification and submit that a regimen of procedural safeguards could adequately ensure against abuse (Quill, 1993). Among these safeguards would be the presence of a terminal or disabling condition from which there is no reasonable likelihood of recovery, the existence of an ongoing physician–patient relationship, a patient capable of making decisions, and repeated and unequivocal requests by the patient for the physician's assistance in hastening death.

Ethical Dimensions of Health System Changes

The US health care system, including its mental health components, exists in a tremendous state of turbulence and flux at the beginning of the 21st century. The continuing quest for simultaneous achievement of the three goals of quality, accessibility and affordability continues to frustrate health policymakers in both public and private sectors. This quest has resulted in dramatic changes in the structure of our health care delivery system, with the growing replacement of fee-for-service professionals and institutions by large managed care networks. These structural and operational changes are radically altering the financial incentives that influence provider behavior by rewarding cost containment, rather than generous provision of services.

The proper ethical stance of the psychiatrist in a changing health system is not clear, but the psychiatrist ought to be clear whether he/she is acting as a doctor or citizen. Doctors ethically and zealously advocate for getting whatever they feel is in the best interests for their patients. This may be done without regard for the bigger picture of resource allocation. For the doctor, the patient comes first.

As citizens, however, psychiatrists also have a responsibility. Society makes determinations of how big the pool of resources will be, what illnesses are covered under insurance, and how much a clinician will be paid. Psychiatrists have a unique perspective and expertise on the consequences of these decisions, and in their citizen and public policy role will do well to participate in the difficult and ethically challenging work of creating and influencing policy decisions affecting their patients, profession and society.

Conclusion

Psychiatrists can anticipate further developments in the clinical/legal interface, and that ethical challenges will be a core element of the work. This chapter has attempted to outline the most relevant legal and ethical issues and principles facing psychiatrists today. Many of these principles, such as society's value of individual liberty, are stable, and will endure throughout the entire careers of today's students. Others are in flux, such as the balance between confidentiality and public safety. Still others have yet to be identified and are unforeseen. As psychiatrists try to implement the ancient ethical principle, "first do no harm", in today's complex legal, social and financial environment, continued education and reflection in all these areas will be required of all of us.

References

Addington v. Texas, 441 US 418, 99 S C1 1804 (1979).

Allen M and Smith VF (2001) Opening Pandora's box: The practical and legal dangers of involuntary outpatient commitment. *Psychiatr Serv* 52(3) (Mar), 342–346.

American Psychiatric Association (1980) Guidelines for psychiatrists in consultative, supervisory, or collaborative relationships with non-medical therapists. *Am J Psychiatr* 1489–1491.

American Psychiatric Association (1993) *The Principles of Medical Ethics with Annotations Especially Applicable to Psychiatry*. APA, Washington DC.

American Psychiatric Association (1994) *Diagnostic and Statistical Manual of Mental Disorders, 4th edn*. APA, Washington DC.

Americans with Disabilities Act (1990) Congressional Findings, 42 USC 12101(a).

Appelbaum PS and Gutheil TG (2000) Clinical Handbook of Psychiatry and the Law. Williams & Wilkins, Baltimore (for a detailed discussion of the concept of confidentiality, see pp. 1–13).

Appelbaum PS (1988) The right to refuse treatment with antipsychotic medications: Retrospect and prospect. *Am J Psychiatr* 145, 413–419.

Appelbaum PS (2001) Thinking carefully about outpatient commitment. *Psychiatr Serv* 52(3) (Mar), 347–350.

Appelbaum PS and Grisso T (1988) Assessing patients' capacities to consent to treatment. *New Engl J Med* 319, 1635–1638.

Appelbaum PS and Gutheil TG (2000) *Clinical Handbook of Psychiatry and the Law.* Williams & Wilkins, Baltimore (for a detailed discussion of the concept of confidentiality, see pp. 1–13).

Birnbaum M (1960) The right to treatment. *Am Bar Assoc J* 46, 499.

Birnbaum M (1965) Some comments on "the right to treatment". *Arch Gen Psychiatr* 13, 34–45.

Canterbury v. Spence (1972) 150 US App DC 263, 464 F2d 772.

Carr M and Robinson GE (1990) Fatal attraction: The ethical and clinical dilemma of patient–therapist sex. *Can J Psychiatr* 35, 122–127.

Child Custody Consultation (1982) American Psychiatric Press, Washington DC.

Dusky v. United States (1960) 362 US 402, 80 S Ct 788.

Elliott RL, Nelson E, Fitch WL *et al.* (1993) Informed decision-making in persons acquitted not guilty by reason of insanity. *Bull Am Acad Psychiatr Law* 21, 309–320.

Ellis T (1991) The nature of morality. In Ethical Issues in Mental Health Care, Barker PJ and Baldwin S (eds). Chapman & Hall, London, pp. 13–26.

Guardianship of Richard Roe III (1981) 383 Mass 415, 421 NE2d 40.

Gutheil TG, Bursztajn H and Brodsky A (1984) supra, note 33.

Gutheil TG, Bursztajn H and Brodsky A (1986) The multidimensional assessment of dangerousness: Competence assessment in patient care and liability prevention. *Bull Am Acad Psychiatr Law* 14, 123–129.

Gutheil TG (1994) Personal communication, for a detailed discussion of the concept of privilege, see pp. 14–17 of Appelbaum and Gutheil, see footnote 31.

Hampton RL and Newberger EH (1985) Child abuse incidence and reporting by hospitals: Significance of severity, class, and race. *Am J Publ Health* 75, 56–60.

Heyd D and Bloch S (1991) The ethics of suicide, in *Psychiatric Ethics*, 2nd edn. (eds Bloch S and Chodoff P). Oxford Medical Publications, New York, pp. 243–264.

Jackson v. Indiana (1972) 406 US 715, 92 S Ct 1845.

Kelly Kevin V (1998) *Psychiatric Times*, Vol. 15(6).

Kempe CH, Silverman FN, Steele BF *et al.* (1962) The battered child syndrome. *JAMA* 181, 17–24.

Lake v. Cameron (1966) 124 US App DC 264, 364 F2d 657.

Linda Cocchiarella and Gunnar BJ Andersson (eds) (2001) *Guides to the Evaluation of Permanent Impairment*, 5th edn. American Medical Association, Chicago.

M'Naghten's Case (1843) 8 Eng Rep 718, 8 Eng Rep 722.

Massachusetts General Laws, Chapter 111, section 70F.

McGarry AL, Curran WJ *et al.* (1973) *Competency to Stand Trial and Mental Illness.* National Institute of Mental Health, Rockville, MD.

Model Penal Code (1955) American Law Institute, Philadelphia, 401.1(1).

Murphy GE (1992) Psychotherapist–patient sexual contact after termination of therapy. *Am J Psychiatr* 149, 985–986.

Natanson v. Kline (1960) 186 Kan 393, 350 P2d 1093.

O'Connor v. Donaldson, 422 US 563, 95 S Ct 2486 (1975).

Olmstead v. L.C. (1999) 527 US 581.

Quill T (1991) Death and dignity: A case of individualized decision-making. *New Engl J Med* 324, 691–694.

Quill T (1993) *Death and Dignity: Making Choices and Taking Charge.* WW Norton, New York.

Rappeport JR (1982) Differences between forensic and general psychiatry. *Am J Psychiatr* 139, 331–334.

Rennie v. Klein, 720 F2d 266 (3d Circ 1983).

Rogers v. Commissioner (1983) 390 Mass 489, 458 NE2d 308 (1983).

*Rouse v. Cameron,** 125 US App DC 366, 373 F2d 451 (1966).

Sapir PE (1992) Patient–therapist sexual contact after termination of treatment. *Am J Psychiatr* 149, 984.

Siantz ML (1993) The stigma of mental illness on children of color. *J Child Adolesc Psychiatr Merit Health Nurs* 6, 10–17.

Slawson P (1989) Psychiatric malpractice: Ten years loss experience. *Med Law* 8, 415–527.

Slobogin C (1985) The guilty but mentally ill verdict: An idea whose time should not have come. *George Wash Law Rev* 53, 494–527.

Special section on APA's Model Commitment Law (1985) *Hosp Comm Psychiatr* 36, 966–989.

Steadman HJ *et al.* (2001) Assessing the New York City Involuntary Outpatient Commitment Pilot Program. *Psychiatr Serv* 52 (Mar) 3, 330–336.

Stone AA (1985) A response to comments on APA's Model Commitment Law. *Hosp Comm Psychiatr* 36, 984–989.

Strasburger LH, Jorgenson L and Sutherland P (1992) The prevention of psychotherapist sexual misconduct: Avoiding the slippery slope. *Am J Psychother* 46, 544–555.

Swartz MS *et al.* (2001) A randomized controlled trial of outpatient commitment in North Carolina. *Psychiatr Serv* 52 (Mar)(3), 325–329.

Tarasoff v. Regents (1976) 17 Ca 3d 425, 551 P2d 334, 131 Cal Rptr 14.

Torrey EF and Zdanowicz M (2001) Outpatient commitment: What, why, and for whom? *Psychiatr Serv* 52(3), (Mar) 337–341.

Trad PV (1991) The ultimate stigma of mental illness. *Am J Psychother* 45, 463–466.

Truman v. Thomas (1980) 27 Cal3d 285, 611 P2d 902.

Von Staden H. (trans) (1996) "In a pure and holy way": Personal and professional conduct in the hippocratic oath. *J His Med Allied Sci* 51, 406–408.

Webster's New World Dictionary (1980) 2nd College Edition.

Wickline v. State (1987) 192 Cal App3d 1630, 239 Cal Rptr 810.

Wilson v. Blue Cross (1990) 222 Cal App3d 660, 271 Cal Rptr 876.

Wyatt v. Stickney, 344 F Supp 387 (MD Ala 1972).

Youngberg v. Romeo, 457 US 307, 102 S Ct 2452 (1982).

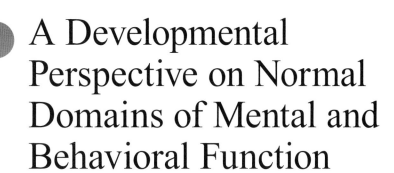

A Developmental Perspective on Normal Domains of Mental and Behavioral Function

A Psychiatric Perspective on Human Development

The miracle of human development has always fascinated physicians. Psychiatrists and pediatricians have formally studied developmental processes and used the knowledge gained from these investigations to create more effective strategies for care of patients. With the evolution of the specialty of geriatrics, interest in the developmental changes that occur after having achieved full maturation has further expanded the scope of investigations. With better understanding of the changes that predictably occur in the last half of life, it has become possible to link more effectively early precursors of illnesses to the later expression of developmental delays and deviations.

There are two classical approaches to the study of human development: the stage model and the longitudinal lines of development model. Each has distinct advantages and disadvantages. The more traditional approach is to examine each stage of development. Consequently, the unfolding of the many new capabilities of the infant is reviewed chronologically so the child as a whole can be better understood. Thinking about development as a series of stages is a particularly useful approach for clinicians. In this regard, it is traditional to address the development of 1) infants, 2) preschool children, 3) school-age children, 4) adolescents, and 5) adults. Sometimes it is helpful to distinguish phases within these groups. For example, it is common to describe adolescence as being comprised of early, middle, and late phases as illustrated in Table 7.1.

An alternative strategy used to teach development is to choose a particular aspect of human development and track it

Table 7.1	**Phases of Adolescence**	
Phase	Age (Years)	Characteristic
Early	11–13	Growth spurt, development of secondary sex characteristics, beginning of social separation from parents and family, greater affinity with peers
Middle	14–16	Consolidation of sense of self, increased sexual experimentation, decreased sense of threat from adults
Late	17–19	Concerns about entering adult life – work, independence, intimacy

from birth until death. This is a helpful strategy for understanding the process of development and is useful for researchers who are searching for the antecedents of characteristics that occur during later developmental periods. However, accurately charting these lines of development has proved to be difficult. Clearly, it is not feasible for a single investigator to study the extensive changes that occur over the lifespan. In the rare longitudinal studies that span at least 10 years, it is usually necessary for a series of principal investigators to work sequentially in order to achieve continuity. Consequently, most investigators become specialists in narrow age ranges of the developmental process and must work collaboratively with colleagues to link together the transitions from infancy to childhood or adolescence to the adult years.

Theories and Models of Development

Theories of Development

Theories are important to the study of development for a number of reasons. They organize and prioritize large amounts of data regarding infant development, indicating which are the most salient and why. Often, they also explain the importance of the early years for subsequent development, indicating how developmental issues are related to broader issues of the lifespan. Generally, they move beyond mere descriptions of behavior and attempt to explain why individuals are motivated to behave in certain ways at certain times. Finally, they may generate meaningful and testable hypotheses for empirical research.

On the other hand, theories have inherent liabilities. A selective focus on one theory may obscure others of equal or greater value. Theories also inevitably lead to oversimplification of complex processes and events. They may create biases that affect how we interpret observations and how we make inferences from these observations. The history of psychology is filled with examples of adherence to a particular point of view, making it impossible to see disconfirming information. All of these factors warrant caution about the uncritical use of theories to understand development. A useful theory is one which is developmental, integrative, contextualist, constructionist and perspectivist in nature, discounting its own absolute claim to truth and integrating as many relevant approaches as possible. An integrative developmental theory accounts for the dynamic interactions of biology (including neuroanatomy, genetics, neurotransmitters, etc.), relationships (including parental, sibling, peer and wider social

Essentials of Psychiatry   Jerald Kay and Allan Tasman
© 2006 John Wiley & Sons, Ltd.

Table 7.2   Some Developmental Theories and the First 3 Years of Life

Theorist	Type and Focus of Theory	Stages or Phases
Sigmund Freud (1940)	Psychoanalytic drive theory (psychosexual stages)	Oral (birth–18 mo) Anal (18–36 mo)

Jean Piaget (1952)	Cognitive	Sensory–motor intelligence (first 2 yr)
		    Modification of reflexes (birth–1 mo)
		    Primary circular reactions (1–4 mo)
		    Secondary circular reactions (4–10 mo)
		    Coordination of secondary schemas (10–12 mo)
		    Tertiary circular reactions (12–18 mo)
		    Representational thinking (18–24 mo)
		Preoperational intelligence (2–6 yr)

Erik Erikson (1951)	Psychoanalytic theory (psychosocial stages)	Trust vs. mistrust (birth–18 mo) Autonomy vs. shame or doubt (18–36 mo)

Margaret Mahler (1975)	Psychoanalytic theory (separation and individuation)	Autistic phase (birth–2 mo)
		Symbiosis (2–4 or 5 mo)
		Differentiation (4 or 5–8 or 9 mo)
		Practising
		    Early practising (8 or 9–12 mo)
		    Practising proper (12–18 mo)
		Rapprochement (18–24 mo)
		On the way to object constancy (24–36 mo)

John Bowlby (1969, 1973, 1980)	Attachment theory	Phase of limited discrimination (birth–2 mo) Phase of limited preference (2–7 mo) Phase of focused attachment and secure base (7–24 mo) Phase of goal-corrected partnership (24–36 mo)
Daniel Stern (1985)	Psychoanalytic theory (sense of self-development)	Sense of emergent self (birth–2 mo) Sence of core self (2–3 mo) Sense of subjective self (7–9 mo) Sense of verbal self (18–20 mo)

groups), culture (including cultural norms for individual and collective development), and technology (including medication, informatics, etc.) (Wilber, 2000).

Table 7.2 presents a brief summary of some of the major theories of development as they pertain to the first 3 years of life. Although others could have been selected, those presented have been most influential with regard to clinical practice and research on early development. As noted in Table 7.2, the theories vary with regard to their particular focus of development, although most use stages to describe periods of discontinuity.

In this chapter, an overview of five prominent lines of human development is presented so that the reader can quickly obtain a sense of the timetable of normal development. These are 1) biological development, 2) cognitive social development, 3) emotional development, 4) social development, and 5) moral development.

In addition, a longitudinal review of periods of development that are associated with an increased risk for specific psychiatric disturbances is provided.

There has been a scientific preoccupation with defining the relative contributions of genetic endowment and environmental experience on the course of human development. While early behavioralists took the extreme view that children can be shaped almost exclusively by their environments, today evidence supports the view that genes and experience interact continuously over time in a transactional manner that leads to the unique development of an individual. The study of environmental contributions has steadily improved through the application of more careful methods of assessment and an appreciation of the value of examining the many components of the early experience of children.

However, the most explosive advances in the understanding of human development have been made as specific gene sequences have been identified and linked to physical and behavioral outcomes. In the past decade, the pace of new gene discovery has increased exponentially as a consequence of the success of the Human Genome Project. It is now estimated that human beings have approximately 38 000 to 40 000 genes. Determining the precise number has been elusive as it has been necessary gradually to understand that human genes are more complex than the genes of simpler organisms. Specifically, many human genes produce multiple proteins. We are now learning about the degrees of genomic variability that exist between individuals, as well as beginning to understand how genes interact with each other and how they are regulated by the environment. A key focus of new research is the discovery of how the passage of time and the gradual maturation of the individual affect the expression of genes that have remained silent but potentially ominous from the beginning of fetal development. Future studies of cohorts of infants who are at known genetic risk for a trait or illness may well identify environmental factors associated with both the expression and the suppression of gene expression.

The concept of studying development longitudinally has its origin in the studies of lives and was well established by Plutarch and popularized by Shakespeare. In many ways, biographers strive to examine the origins of adult traits through consideration of the early experiences of their particular subject. This tradition was adopted by psychoanalysts who searched for the origins of psychopathology through the exposition of a "genetic formulation". The choice of the word "genetic" to modify a conceptual formulation based on the experience of the individual is somewhat ironic. The term has largely been abandoned, as these formulations had little to do with the function of individual genes. Nonetheless, this focus on the influence of early experience on development may well have been a foreshadowing of the importance of intense early experience on gene expression. In all likelihood, the genetic formulations of the future will focus on how experience regulates gene expression at the molecular level.

The concept of parallel yet interacting lines of development was popularized by Anna Freud (1946) who created a classical monograph that articulated nine lines of development that were well described through adolescence. Although some of these conceptual lines have been abandoned, the overarching principle of a line of development has proven to have heuristic value. Table 7.3 lists four relevant developmental lines.

Other psychoanalysts have built on her model to create parallel lines extending into adulthood. Erikson (1963) further elaborated the evolution of domains of function in the creation of his epigenetic stage model, as presented in Figure 7.1. His paradigm continues to have a strong influence on psychiatric theory,

as is well illustrated by Vaillant's work who has extended the Eriksonian model by proposing two additional phases of the adult life-cycle, career-consolidation vs. self-absorption and keeper of the meaning vs. rigidity. The former acknowledges the importance of achieving a stable career identity in addition to the achievement of identity within one's family of origin. The latter describes further Erikson's concept of generativity beyond assuming sustained responsibility for building the community and for the growth, well-being and leadership of others. "Keeper of the meaning" and its virtue, wisdom, involve a nonpartisan and less personal approach to others and is to be distinguished from the tasks of a generative coach, partisan parent, or mentor from the tasks of a Supreme Court judge or chair of a historical society.

Although lines of development are attractive conceptually, they are a deceptively simplistic representation of the complex evolution of personality. The concept of "decalage" was put forward by Piaget (1952) to refer to a disengagement in the normal evolution of the parallel development of specific cognitive abilities. However, decalage is equally salient in the conceptualization of major distortions in emotional or social development. In this chapter, five broad lines of development are reviewed as they evolve over the course of the lifespan, and developmental timelines for each line are included.

Biological Development

Genetic Considerations
The genes that an individual possesses contain all of the information required to define the individual. Some genes have strong pen-

Table 7.3	Kohlberg's Stages of Moral Development	
Preconventional: Emphasis on avoiding punishments and getting rewards	Stage 1 Might makes right (punishment and obedience orientation)	Children at this stage are egocentric and experience difficulty with perspective taking when considering moral dilemmas. Motives and intentions are ignored when judging the goodness or badness of a behavior.
	Stage 2 Look out for number one (instrument and relativist orientation)	Recognition that others have different points of view occurs at this stage, but this understanding is still somewhat limited. Action is viewed as right if it satisfies one's needs. The reason to be nice to people is so they will be nice to you.
Conventional: Emphasis on social rules and conformity to social norms	Stage 3 "Good girl" and "nice boy"	Approval is more important than any specific reward. The individual has newly acquired abilities for mutual perspective taking. In this stage, a person can anticipate what another person is feeling and knows that other people also have this ability.
	Stage 4 Law and order	The individual can now take into consideration societal laws when deciding a course of action. A behavior is considered right if it involves obeying rules established by authority.
Postconventional: Emphasis on moral principles and values	Stage 5 Social contract, legalistic	Rules are regarded as more flexible, with the aim of furthering human values. They are not absolute. This stage emphasizes fair procedures for interpreting and changing the law when the law is destructive or unethical. Ethics are considered when evaluating laws.
	Stage 6 Universal ethical principles	At this stage, there is the recognition that some principles and values (i.e., "life is sacred") transcend laws, and that some moral obligations are valid for humanity.

Source: Kohlberg L (1964) Development of moral character and moral ideology. In Review of Child Development Research, Hoffman ML and Hoffman LW (eds). Russell Sage Foundation, New York, pp. 383–432.

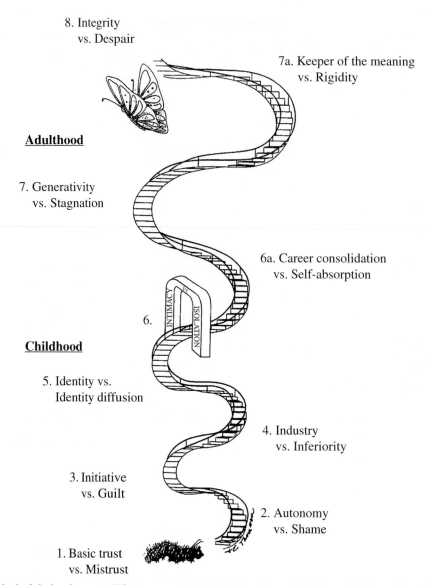

8. Integrity
vs. Despair

7a. Keeper of the meaning
vs. Rigidity

Adulthood

7. Generativity
vs. Stagnation

6a. Career consolidation
vs. Self-absorption

6.

Childhood

5. Identity vs.
Identity diffusion

4. Industry
vs. Inferiority

3. Initiative
vs. Guilt

2. Autonomy
vs. Shame

1. Basic trust
vs. Mistrust

Figure 7.1   *A model of adult development. (This is essentially Erik Erikson's model of the adult life-cycle with the addition of stages 6a and 7a.) Reprinted with permission from Valient GE (1993). The Wisdom of the Ego. Harvard University Press.*

etrance and express themselves in virtually all environments. This is the traditional view of the influence of genes, which if taken literally leads to the erroneous conclusion that any genetic influence is immutable. It is now clear that many genes have only partial penetrance and that there are both physical and emotional–environmental factors associated with the expression of these genes.

In considering the biological development of an individual, it is apparent that single genes that control such critical functions as physical growth have a high degree of penetrance in a wide range of environments. For example, while malnutrition, maltreatment and medications can retard growth, genes have a powerful impact on adult height. This is demonstrated by the observation that monozygotic twins are nearly identical in adult height. Interestingly, the same is not true of weight, which suggests that a wider range of environmental factors lead to adult variation in weight. In monozygotic twin pairs, adult weight can vary by more than 20%, although the majority of twins are actually much closer in size.

A timeline of biological development over the course of the lifespan is presented in Figure 7.2.

Neurological Considerations

Brain growth is one of the most basic indicators of neurological development. The brain is already at approximately one-third of its adult size at birth, and it grows rapidly, reaching 60% by approximately 1 year and 90% by 5 years of age. The final 10% of growth occurs during the next 10 years with attainment of full weight by 16 years of age. The processes of myelinization, synapse proliferation and synaptic pruning occur in the course of the lifespan, but they are particularly active in the first years of life when the functional structure of the brain is becoming defined. Maximum synaptic density is reached at different development time points in different brain regions. Maximum density in the auditory cortex is achieved by 3 months, whereas maximum density in the middle frontal gyrus is not reached until 15 months of age (Huttenlocher and Dabholkar, 1997). After this point, the density of dendritic spines generally decreases as glucose metabolism becomes fully developed. The establishment of biological rhythms occurs in early infancy and sleep becomes more organized and of shorter nocturnal duration. A stable pattern of temperament cannot be documented in the first months of life, but it gradually

Biological Development

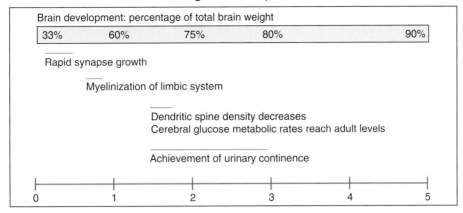

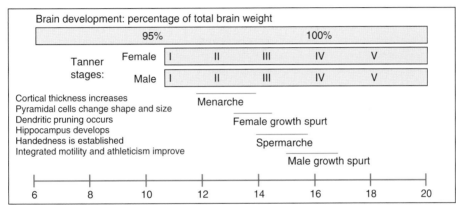

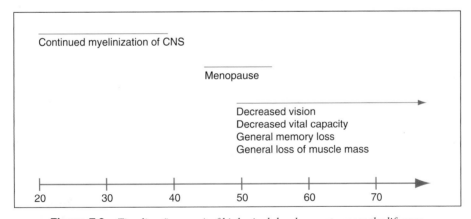

Figure 7.2 *Timeline (in years) of biological development across the lifespan.*

becomes established during the second year. All of the major theories of temperament endorse the idea that temperament is rooted in biological differences (Goldsmith *et al.*, 1987). The most influential view has been that of Thomas and colleagues (1968). In the New York Longitudinal Study which viewed temperament as a child's behavioral style, the "how" of behavior as opposed to its content or motivation. This work addressed dimensions such as activity level, intensity of emotional expression, adaptability to changes in routine and the tendency to approach or avoid novel situations. This work elucidated distinct temperament clusters, the easy, slow to warm-up and difficult child. The difficult child was characterized as having a negative mood, irregular biological rhythms, slower adaptability, intensity of reactions and a negative response to novelty. Difficult children often express early behaviors that are correlated with later school problems, social difficulties and psychiatric disorders. Behavioral inhibition is

a trait that has been reliably identified after 18 months and has been associated with the Hypothalamic-Pituitary-Adrenal (HPA) axis activation and right frontal asymmetry (Fox *et al.*, 2001), the latter being predictative of social wariness at 4 years for boys more so than girls (Henderson *et al.*, 2001). During the preschool period, individual neurons and neural networks are preferentially preserved if they receive stimulation. Motor skills emerge as a reflection of the underlying neuronal development of the central nervous system.

By the age of 7 years, considerable sensory integration has occurred. Handedness has been clearly established, and brain plasticity has decreased. By 10 years of age, limitations in the ability to learn to speak an unaccented second language reflect further changes in the development of the motor linguistic pathways. In the years of adolescence, full brain weight is achieved, but myelinization continues well into the fourth decade. As well, the dorsolateral

Table 7.4   Patterns of Attachment

Characteristics	Secure Pattern	Avoidant Pattern	Resistant Pattern	Disorganized Pattern
Distress	Open display of distress and need for comfort	Inhibited display of distress	Exaggerated display of distress	Odd or contradictory display of distress
Soothing	Effective soothing; positive greeting	No soothing; avoidance instead of greeting	Ineffective soothing; no positive greeting because of distress	Ineffective soothing; usually no positive greeting; often odd or ambivalent greeting
Anger	Little angry behavior	Displaced anger	Angry, resistant behaviors	No predictable pattern
Stress	Low cortisol secretion	High cortisol secretion	No cortisol data	No cortisol data
Strategy for obtaining comfort	Coherent strategy of seeking comfort directly when needed	Coherent strategy of minimizing distress by displaced attention	Coherent strategy of exaggerating distress to mobilize caregiver	Incoherent strategy or significant lapse in organization of strategy
Parental characteristics	Sensitive, emotionally available caregiving; balanced perspective on childhood relationship experiences	Emotionally restricted caregiving; dismissing of painful relationship experiences and their effects	Inconsistent caregiving; unintegrated emotional response to relationship experiences	No data on caregiving; unresolved losses or traumatic childhood experiences

prefrontal cortex (DLPFC) has a protracted developmental course, given that its functional specificity is not fully determined until puberty. By the end of the fifth decade, there is often evidence of the beginning of decline in specific neuronal functions, with vision and memory being particularly vulnerable. However, integrative capacities may reach a peak during the later decades.

Endocrinological Considerations

While interesting changes in hormonal development occur in the first years of life, dramatic changes in both physical and emotional functions are triggered by the hormonal shifts associated with puberty that characterize the adolescent years. In girls, estradiol and progesterone production results in the onset of breast development, followed by the onset of pubic hair growth and vaginal elongation. Axillary hair subsequently develops during stage 3 of pubic hair development. Although there is wide variability in different cultural environments, menarche is usually attained 2 years after the onset of breast development and has been reported to occur at an average of 12.8 years of age in population studies (Zacharias et al., 1976), the range is between 10–16 years. Menarche appears to be affected by nutrition, genetic endowment, general health status and environmental factors such altitude and light. In boys, puberty begins when rising levels of pituitary hormone result in enlargement of the testes and subsequent increases in circulating testosterone. Spermatogenesis occurs after testicular enlargement at approximately 14 years of age. Pubic hair development is triggered by adrenal androgens and occurs in five stages during the course of about 2.5 years. Facial hair tends to develop between 14 and 15 years of age.

Growth hormone and gonadal hormones are both necessary to initiate the adolescent growth spurt. This occurs earlier in girls, usually during Tanner's breast stages 2 and 3, whereas in boys it does not occur until stage 4 of genital development. Both an acceleration of bone growth and a maturation of the skeletal structure as reflected by increased bone density and closing of epiphyses occur during this process.

Sexual function peaks early in the adult years in men but there is only a gradual decline in sexual function as measured by frequency of orgasm from 20 to 70 years. Women have consistent sexual functioning throughout the childbearing years and frequently become more orgasmic in their 30s. However, decreases in estrogen levels associated with menopause usually occur between 45 and 54 years of age. Men have no comparable menopausal change in hormonal levels.

Cognitive Development

The study of cognitive development provides a perspective on the evolution of the capacity to think. Increased cognitive abilities are an integral component required for the onset of language. Changes in thinking ultimately shape the course of emotional, social and moral development. Recent investigations of the relation of brain development to cognitive development have attempted to attribute specific developmental changes in central nervous system function with the achievement of new cognitive abilities (Casey et al., 2000; Anderson, 2001).

However, the acquisition of mental abilities has been charted as an independent sequence of mental accomplishments. Piaget established the field of cognitive development, and his stage theory of the evolution of cognitive processes has dominated this field (Piaget and Inhelder, 1969). Although specific aspects of his four primary stages have been modified by subsequent empirical experiments as well as by the development of a greater appreciation of the role of emotions and context in the utilization of cognitive abilities, his careful observations and brilliant deductions have provided the framework on which much of our knowledge of cognitive development has been built. In contrast, Vygotsky (1978) provided a model of early cognitive development that placed greater importance on the influence of culture and language-mediated guidance by adults.

Piaget introduced the concept of "schemas" which he defined as units of cognition. He further described processes that result in schema modification, which begin in infancy as a child assimilates new information and accommodates to novel stimuli. A particularly important Piagetian concept has been that of a decalage within cognitive development, which refers to an unevenness in cognitive development. For example, a child may demonstrate cognitive abilities at the concrete operational stage of development with regard to conservation of volume and at the same time retain preoperational forms of thinking such as persistent egocentrism. Such an unevenness can also be seen across lines of development. The concept of interlineal decalages is described more fully in the last section of this chapter.

Even newborns have the ability to learn through making associations between different states or experiences. There is evidence that cognitive "prewiring" exists, which allows for the perceptual capacities of infants that are necessary to seek stimulation and interaction with adult caregivers. A key capacity required for these early cognitions is recognition of the invariant features of perceptual stimuli coupled with the ability to translate these invariant features across sensory modalities. Interestingly, infants can differentiate the human voice from other sounds innately without "learning" the complex characteristics of the structure and pitch of speech.

By 2 to 3 weeks of age, cross-modal fluency is demonstrated by the ability of infants to imitate facial expression. This requires the recognition of a visual schema of a facial expression to be linked with a proprioceptive tactile schema of producing a facial expression. By 3 months of age, infants can be classically conditioned, and their interest in stimuli led Piaget to suggest this was a period dominated by attempts to make "interesting spectacles last" (Piaget and Inhelder, 1969).

By 6 months of age, associations between "means" and "ends" have been demonstrated. This is followed by object permanence, which evolves during the second half of the first year. During the second year, infants can infer cause after observing an effect as well as anticipate effects after producing a causal action. A corollary of this new ability is that they are now able correctly to sequence past events.

By the third year of life, children enter the preoperational stage. This form of thinking is more similar to adult cognition, but it incorporates magical explanations and is marked by a tendency to focus on one perceptual attribute at a time (centration). Idiosyncratic cosmological theories are common and are usually dominated by transductive reasoning, which attributes causality based exclusively on temporal or spatial juxtaposition. Throughout the preschool period, attention span and memory are limited while pretend play and fanciful thinking are common. Animism is frequently used and refers to endowing inanimate objects with the qualities of living things. Not surprisingly, children having imaginary friends and talking pets characterize this cognitive period. The preoperational stage is also the time during which explosive language development occurs. This development appears to be made possible by a genetically determined capacity for language. However, language development is clearly enhanced by experiential support and parental communication that is sensitive to the child's ability to process new words and grammatical structure.

By age 6 or 7 years, children begin to use operational thinking. The child who has attained concrete operational thought has the ability to conserve both volume and quantity as well as being able to appreciate the reversibility of events and ideas. A shift from an egocentric perspective results in a new capacity to appreciate the perspective of others. These new cognitive skills demonstrate an ability to engage in logical dialogue and to develop an appreciation of more complex causal sequences. These new cognitive abilities are clearly required for a child to benefit from the grade school curriculum.

Adolescence results in the development of a new processing capacity that involves the manipulation of ideas and concepts.

Furthermore, the informational fund of knowledge is dramatically expanded and serves as a referent for verification of new data that are assimilated. A final major transition is possible with the development of the ability to reflect on cognition as a process. This is referred to as the development of a metacognitive capacity. Achievement of this capacity allows adolescents to understand and empathize with the divergent perspectives of others to a greater degree than was previously possible. This capacity is necessary for recursive thinking which involves an awareness that others can think about the domain of the adolescent's own thought. These cognitive skills represent the transition into the final stage of cognitive ability, which is referred to as the use of formal operations. One capacity characteristic of this stage is the ability to understand complex combinatorial systems that require a well-developed sense of reversibilities that include inversion, reciprocity and symmetry. New levels of problem solving are achieved that include the ability to recognize a core problem or core isomorph within a more complex new problem. The adult with formal operational ability can recognize a previously successful solution and use this knowledge to develop a parallel innovative solution to the complex problem. It is important to appreciate that many adults remain at the stage of concrete operations and never develop these more advanced capacities.

A timeline of cognitive development during the course of the lifespan is presented in Figure 7.3.

Emotional Development

The emotional state of the newborn is largely assessed by facial expression and accompanying vocalizations. However, the communicative capacity of young infants has become increasingly well appreciated. In the first weeks of life, contentment and distress have been reliably monitored (Lewis, 1994). These primary emotions further differentiate during the first months of life. It is clear from work beginning in the late 1960s and 1970s that the infant is not a passive recipient of external influences, a tabla rasa or blank slate. Freud's idea about a stimulus barrier, which was postulated to protect a young infant from overstimulation, and Mahler *et al.*, (1975) notion that the first 2 months can be conceptualized as a relatively autistic phase of development are no longer supported. By 7 to 9 months, a transition occurs that is based on the earliest attainment of intersubjectivity. At this point, infants begin to understand that their own inner experiences and feelings can be appreciated by other individuals (Trevarthen, 1979; Emde, 1984). This leads to the possibility of developing affect attunement as parents match their own behavior with the behavior of their infant, while experiencing shared internal feeling states. An infant pouting to elicit a parental response evidences the instrumental use of emotions. Social referencing is usually evident by 12 months of age, when infants turn to examine their mothers' facial expressions at times when they are confronted with potentially fearful situations or objects (Klinnert, 1984).

In the second year of life, the rapprochement crisis occurs, as infants become aware of their separateness from their primary attachment figure and the limitations of their control on her behavior. After the infant has attained self-cognition, new, more complex emotions of embarrassment and envy emerge that further evolve to feelings of shame, pride and then guilt by the end of the second year. Object constancy, or the ability to reduce anxiety in response to the separation from the primary caretaker, reflects the association of an emotional state with the memory of the sense of internal security provided by the attachment figure.

Cognitive Development

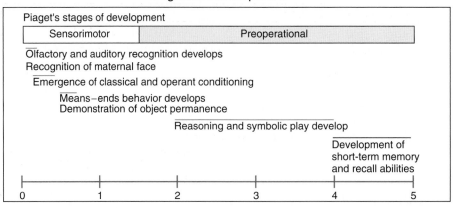

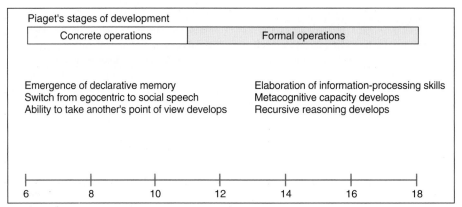

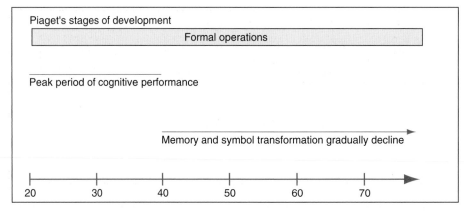

Figure 7.3   *Timeline (in years) of cognitive development across the lifespan.*

The role of implicit memory through the experience of synchrony, reciprocity and affect attunement between parent and infant in numerous modalities is substantial in early emotional development and has been related to sense of self and emotional regulation. Affect attunement beween mother and infant involves an emotional interchange in which the mother matches her behavior to the infant's behavior. This matching is not merely imitative but involves some aspect of the internal feeling state that is shared. An attuned mother exaggerates her responses which allow the infant to begin to recognize his own emotional response as being separate from that of his mother's. Affective attunement appears to be an essential ingredient of empathy, intimacy, mirroring and other clinical phenomena. Fonagy's (2001) concept of mentalization is predicated on the mother's ability to promote both relatedness and separateness in the infant through

her marked affective responses. Mentalization is the capacity of the infant to ascertain the mental states of the self and of others. It describes a process of the infant's recognition that someone else has a different mind from his own. It is acquired through repeated experiences in judging facial expression, tone of voice and other nonverbal communications. These experiences are encoded in implicit (nondeclarative) memory and in parallel with explicit (declarative) memory which has a temporal dimension. This is a critical accomplishment in that it establishes the basis for secure attachment. Conversely, the failure to mirror the child's affective state often results in disorganized attachment through problematic internalization and therefore less than optimal identity formation and individuation. These infants are at extreme risk for attentional, behavioral and emotional disturbance in early childhood often with enduring consequences in

Emotional Development

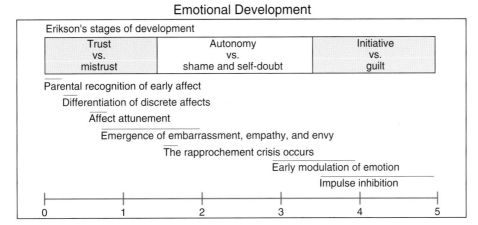

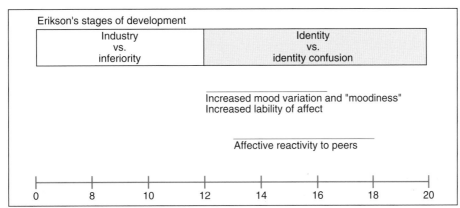

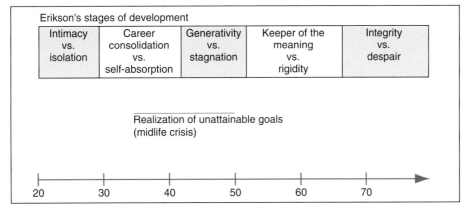

Figure 7.4 *Timeline (in years) of emotional development across the lifespan.*

development at later stages of childhood, adolescence, and even adulthood.

During the preschool years, children begin to learn the nature of the relationship between emotions and behaviors. They begin to understand the culturally defined rules associated with affect expression and consequently begin to mask their emotions. This is also the period when the Oedipus impulses are most evident and children must deal with both their conscious attraction to the parent of the opposite sex and their fear of potential retaliation from the same-sex parent.

As children move into the school years, they experience the full range of adult emotions, although there is at least a qualitative sense that during the prepubertal period there is less intense expression of affect. Although sadness is easily recognized from the second year of life, prolonged periods of depressed affect are rare during this period. However, temperamental styles tend to emerge and, specifically, behavioral inhibition can become more clearly appreciated within the context of increasing social and educational demands (Kagan *et al.*, 1989).

In adolescence, emotions are more intensely displayed. Capacities for abstraction permit adolescents to consider factors outside their own immediate emotional experience and they are, therefore, more emotionally interactive than at any previous period of development. Emotions in adolescence exert an increasingly important role in guiding behavior and become a sustaining motivation for behaviors and mediate relationships with peers and family. During this period, there is an emergence of a greater incidence of affective disorder and anxiety. Similarly, there is a dramatic increase in suicidal behavior that is in part associated with cognitive ability. At this point, there is a greater reflection

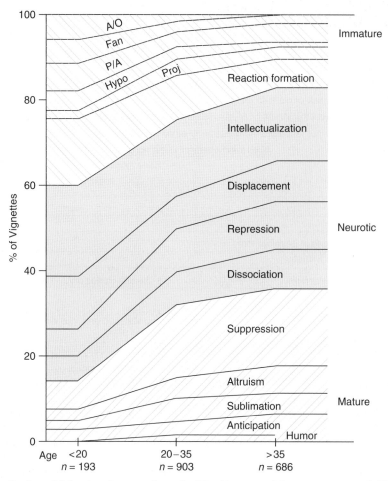

Figure 7.5   *Shifts in distribution of defensive vignettes shown by 95 subjects at adolescence, young adulthood, and middle age (A/O indicates acting out; Fan, fantasy; P/A, passive aggression; Hypo, hypochondriasis; Proj, projection). (Source: Vaillant GE [1976] Natural history of male psychological health. Arch Gen Psychiatr 33, 535–545. Copyright 1976 American Medical Association.)*

on aspects of existential crisis, which can be experienced from more complex vantage points.

A perspective on the evolution of defense mechanisms as regulators of affect suggests that a hierarchy of more sophisticated and effective defensive strategies emerge throughout adolescence and adulthood (Vaillant, 1993). Figure 7.5 illustrates the evolution of defense mechanisms during adulthood. A timeline of emotional development during the course of the lifespan is presented in Figure 7.5.

Social Development

It has become widely appreciated that infants are socially interactive from the first days of life. The strong tie that parents feel for their infants has been referred to as the parent–infant bond. Between 7 and 9 months of age, infants develop separation protest and a negative reaction to the approach of a stranger. During the second half of the first year, the attachment of the infant to his or her parents evolves. The primary role of the attachment figure is the provision of a secure base from which the infant can begin to explore a wider social environment (Ainsworth *et al.*, 1978). It is within the context of the attachment relationship that the first Eriksonian state of "basic trust" is achieved.

Attachment is the affectional connection that a baby develops with its primary caregiver, most often the mothering per-

son, which becomes increasingly discriminating and enduring. It is the availability and responsiveness of the mother or other caretaker that is ultimately the most influential in determining the strength and safety of the attachment system. The infant's attachment behavior is an attempt to bring stability, predictability and consistency to his or her world through drawing the mother closer. There is an extensive literature on and theories about what occurs in the mental life of infants and children during the attachment process. At the risk of over-simplifying, the most intriguing and clinically useful of these theories focuses on the process of internalization. Internalization is the mechanism for building psychological structure. More specifically, it is an attempt to describe how the child achieves an increasingly stable and sophisticated view of himself and the world around him. The acquisition of internal representations of the infant and those who care for him are the building blocks of identity formation and individuation. The former includes the capacity for relatedness and cohesiveness of self and the latter refers to the establishment of autonomy or separateness. Table 7.4 summarizes patterns of attachment. There is an extensive literature on attachment patterns and subsequent development of psychopathology (Kay, 2005).

By 18 months, play begins to be more directed toward peers, but this does not become the predominant form of play until the third year. Along with the striving toward autonomy that characterizes Erikson's second stage, there emerge more negative

Table 7.4	Newborn States of Arousal
States of Arousal	**Characteristics**
Quiet sleep	Regular respirations, limited movements
Active sleep	Rapid eye movements, irregular respirations, large muscle paralysis. Most common state in newborn period
Drowsy	Transitional state between sleep states and waking states
Quiet alert	Sustained gaze, limited movements, maximal alertness. Limited in first few weeks
Active alert	Active movements, mild distress occasionally
Crying	Unable to attent to other stimuli

affective interactions within the context of the attachment relationship. This phenomenon is widely recognized within the popular culture as the arrival of the "terrible twos". However, the quality of the attachment relationship earlier in life has been shown to predict better preschool social adaptation and a stronger sense of self-worth. Included in it is the observation that patterns of social dominance become established during the third year of life and that insecurely attached preschoolers exhibit more conflict and aggression in the establishment of their social status. These early social strivings are compatible with Erikson's third stage, which has as its central developmental objective the achievement of initiative within the context of potential failure and guilt.

Gender differences emerge by 2 years of age. Boys are more aggressive and tend to play with toys that can be manipulated. Girls prefer doll play and artwork. However, boys and girls also engage in both types of play. By the end of the third year, gender preference in play has emerged, and the preference is to play with children of the same sex. This preference remains throughout childhood. Associative play, which refers to play that involves other children and the sharing of toys but does not include the adopting of roles or working toward a common goal, becomes more prominent during the preschool years. Cooperative play also emerges along with a strong tendency to include elements of pretend play into the cooperative sequences. The cultural context begins to shape the nature of social interaction even at these earliest stages of development.

During the school years, the role of peers in shaping social behavior becomes predominant. Small groups form, and the concept of clubs becomes important. Shared activities, including the collection of baseball cards or doll clothes, are a common

Table 7.5	Ideal Task Accomplishment to Attain Adolescence

- Disengagement from parents along with ability to make decisions about onw's life
- Value system respecting self and others
- Solid employment, possibly beginning a vocation
- Fixed sexual identity
- Long-term sexual relationship

and important characteristic of this period. Sharing secrets and making shared rules also serve as organizing social parameters. Social humor develops, and appearance and clothing become an important social signaling system. It is a time of practicing and developing athletic, artistic and social skills that are associated with Erikson's fourth stage of achievement of industry within the context of a sense of potential interpersonal inferiority.

In adolescence and throughout the adult years, social and sexual relationships play a complex and powerful role in shaping experience. With the onset of strong sexual impulses and increasing academic and social demands in adolescence, the role of peer influences in shaping both prosocial and deviant behavior becomes powerful. Adolescence is the period during which Erikson described the central objective to be the establishment of an individual identity, and there has been wide acceptance of this sense of self-occurring within the context of the social and cultural experience. Table 7.5 describes the tasks of adolescence.

The roles of adulthood are complex and focused on the most basic issues of marriage, parenting, working and dealing with death. The key to understanding the sequential nature of adult development lies in the appreciation of both the relative complexity and the inner threat of the tasks and commitments that must be mastered. The twin anxieties of young adulthood involve the abilities to commit to one person and one job without sacrificing autonomy. Prospective studies suggest that by midlife a major developmental task for women is to achieve traits of independence, rationality and self-direction. Similarly it becomes equally enriching for men in midlife to achieve warmth, emotional expressiveness and relatedness (Vallant, 1977; Gutttman, 1977). Individuals who achieve generativity almost always have evolved to stages of identity formation, achievement of intimacy and career consolidation. It is important to note that within the various Eriksonian stages, a selfless generativity reflects a clear capacity to care for and guide the next generation. The final stage of adult development, achieving integrity, may be compared to putting a garden to bed for the winter. Reflection on one's life facilitates coming to terms with it and accepting the past.

A timeline of social development during the course of the lifespan is presented in Figure 7.6.

Moral Development

The newborn infant lives in an interactive world but one that is free of moral directives or structure. However, by the second year of life, the emergence of "moral emotions" such as empathy, pride, embarrassment, shame and guilt demonstrates that the beginning of a code of moral behavior, in the most primitive sense, is being established. Moral emotions evoke a sense of shared experience with important others that is central to the process of moral internalization. By 36 months, most children demonstrate the internalization of parental standards even when their parents are not available to provide cues or reinforcement. The importance of emotions in the early evolution of moral behavior during the preschool years represents a distinct departure from the more traditional perspective that moral development does not occur until the establishment of concrete operation.

During the school years, the importance of rules and adhering to them becomes well defined. The moral code tends to be one of absolutes with strong consequences for transgressors. Extreme examples of children turning their parents into authorities because of political resistance provide a sobering perspective on the strength of the convictions of some children. However, for most boys and girls during this period, interpersonal relationships with

Social Development

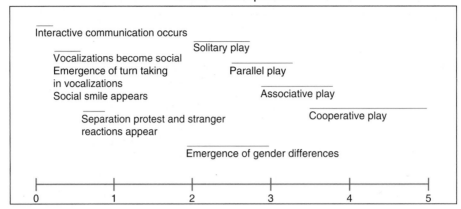

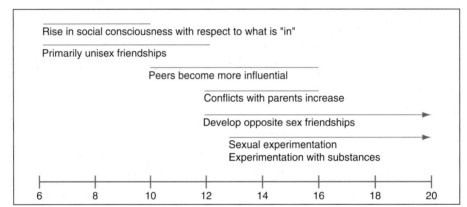

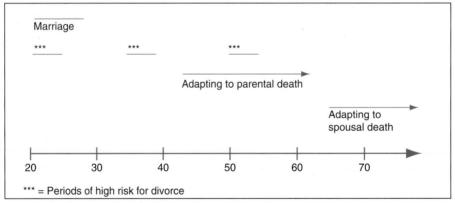

Figure 7.6   *Timeline (in years) of social development across the lifespan.*

peers or siblings are a consideration in the determination of "cho-sen outcomes" when situational paradigms designed to clarify moral priorities are presented (Smetana *et al.*, 1991). There appears to be some gender difference in the quality of mercy demonstrated during the school years. Girls are more concerned with aspects of human interaction and boys preferentially seek blind justice.

The later evolution of moral principles is a complex pro-cess. With the development of abstract reasoning, adolescents progress through Kohlberg's (1964) stages of conventional mo-rality, which entail meeting the expectations of others (stage 3) and subsequently accepting the maintenance of societal norms and rules as an appropriate standard (stage 4). These stages do not progress in a strictly sequential manner. Stages 5 and 6, which ultimately lead to the conviction that moral principles of justice should supersede those of human-made laws, have not been eas-

ily codified either, given the influence of complex emotions on behavior and the well-documented moral inconsistencies that oc-cur over the course of adult development (Gibbs, 1979).

A timeline of moral development during the course of the lifespan is presented in Figure 7.7.

Developmental Psychopathology

Risk and Protective Factors

The risk and protective factor model is a paradigm that facilitates the understanding of developmental deviations. It can be applied at any stage of development. Risk factors have been divided into three large categories: those at the level of the individual, the family and the community.

Moral Development

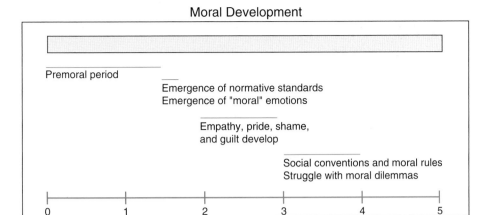

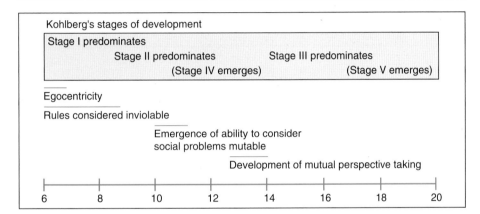

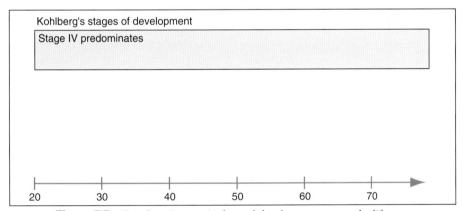

Figure 7.7 *Timeline (in years) of moral development across the lifespan.*

The first category of risk factors is defined at the level of the individual. Both physical and emotional considerations are relevant. Examples include atypical genetic polymorphisms, deficits in perception and high levels of generalized anxiety. Variable possibilities for adaptation exist, but for a trait or condition to be considered a risk factor there must be a demonstrated increase in the probability of subsequent emotional or behavioral disorder associated with the factor.

The second category of risk factors is conceptualized at the level of the family. One of the classic examples of a familial risk factor is a parent with a serious mental illness. It is difficult to define the mechanism by which this risk is transmitted. Each parent provides exactly one-half of the genome of the child. However, parents are also in a powerful position to shape the early environment of their children. The full range of family risk factors is quite broad, and extends beyond the influence of single individuals within the

family to include the impact of family dynamics which influence the development of the child. For example, a scapegoated child in a family environment that tolerates overt child maltreatment is at particularly high risk for the development of psychopathology.

The third category of risk factors is defined at the level of the community. Discrimination based on ethnic or racial status falls into this group of risk factors, as does social disadvantage. Although there is little controversy regarding the negative consequences of discrimination and poverty, the quantification of this risk has been problematic. Community risk factors rarely occur in the absence of individual and familial risk factors, making it difficult fully to understand their specific influence. Table 7.6 elucidates some important developmental risk factors.

One strategy that has been used to determine the overall risk for developmental psychopathology is to add up the specific factors

Table 7.6   Development Risk Factors

Risk Factors	Biological Effect	Psychological Effect	Social Effect
Poverty	Malnutrition	Attachment problems	Family dysfunction, environmental threat
Child maltreatment	Trauma effects, failure to thrive	Disturbed affective responsiveness, poor social interaction, attachment problems	Antisocial behavior and conduct disorder
Maternal substance abuse	Impaired prenatal central nervous system development	Inconsistent and unpredictable parenting, attachment problems	Family dysfunction
Premature birth and serious illness in infancy	Delayed or disrupted central nervous system development, increased development disorders	Increased parental stress	Environmental destabilization

that a child must deal with, creating an adversity index. This has been accomplished for young children (Sameroff, 1986) as well as applied to risk factors occurring later in development (Rutter, 1985a, 1985b). Most individuals can cope with a small number of risk factors, particularly if protective factors are also present. However, under the weight of multiple risk factors, most individuals begin to show signs of disturbance. Sophisticated research designs have been developed to estimate relative contributions (Topolski *et al.*, 1997). Curiously, the quantitative effects of protective factors have been less extensively studied, although investigations into the life course of resilient individuals provide some understanding of these factors (Mrazek and Mrazek, 1987).

Resilient children represent one of the most fascinating opportunities to understand the mechanisms by which risk and protective factors interact. The study of the children of mothers with schizophrenia or bipolar disorder has been an area of investigation that is of particular interest to psychiatrists. Perhaps this is because these children have been perceived to have had both a high risk for the inheritance of genes that confer poor adaptive skills and the misfortune of having a parent with impaired capacities for sensitive responses to their early developmental needs. What is striking is that some of these children turn out to be productive and happy adults despite what appear to be overwhelming odds.

In adulthood, resilience depends on the ability to find, use and internalize social supports. Throughout the life span, maturity of ego defense is an important characteristic of resilience (Vaillant, 1993). The use of mature defenses has been associated with health – whether health was defined as the presence of successful objective life adjustment, the absence of psychopathology, or the achievement of subjective self-satisfaction. The number of risk and protective factors appears to be more significant than the specificity of stressors.

A timeline of the development of psychopathology during the course of the lifespan is presented in Figure 7.8.

High-Risk Periods for Psychopathology

Psychiatrists who treat children and adolescents are particularly aware of the precursors and onset of psychiatric illnesses. Two examples of age-specific vulnerabilities will be discussed, but Figure 7.8 gives an overview of the periods of most probable onset for many of the major psychiatric disor-

ders. The first example is autism, which is unusual in both its invariant early onset and its striking presentation. The second is suicide, which is particularly interesting because of episodic periods of particularly high risk during the developmental course.

Autism is a disease of early onset that has been shown to have a strong genetic basis. Nevertheless, the role of the environment in affecting the onset of autism is still striking, as demonstrated by the quite dramatic variability in the symptom presentations and ultimate adaptations of monozygotic twins. Autistic children appear normal at birth. During their first months of life, they begin to develop severe deficits in their capacity to form relationships and communicate with others. Once fully expressed, autism has a devastating impact on the subsequent development of afflicted children. What is perhaps most striking is the inevitability of early expression as there are no examples of onset later in childhood or adolescence.

Suicide provides a sharp contrast to autism. Suicide is highly associated with mental disorder in general and affective disorder in particular. It has also been shown to be moderately heritable. Whereas the onset of suicidal thoughts does occur in rare cases in the preschool period, the capacity to commit suicide increases with age. After puberty the rate of suicide increases nearly tenfold. The underlying explanation for this dramatic increase is complex and involves consideration of risk factors at the level of the individual, family and community. However, the ultimate life course pattern is striking, as there is a second dramatic increase in suicidality in the later years of life. The explanation for this second increase usually focuses on the increase in medical problems of the elderly, but the multiple emotional losses of these years also provide a vulnerable context for depression and despair.

Interlineal Decalage

Piaget and Inhelder defined uneven developmental progress of specific cognitive abilities as a decalage (1969). Psychiatrists must often help patients deal with a decalage across lines of development. Although this chapter is largely devoted to the explanation of normal development, there has been a systematic effort to illustrate how deviations in development may lead to the onset of developmental psychopathology. Normality can be defined as a multilineal progression of development without a decalage, or unevenness of progress, across any of the primary domains of

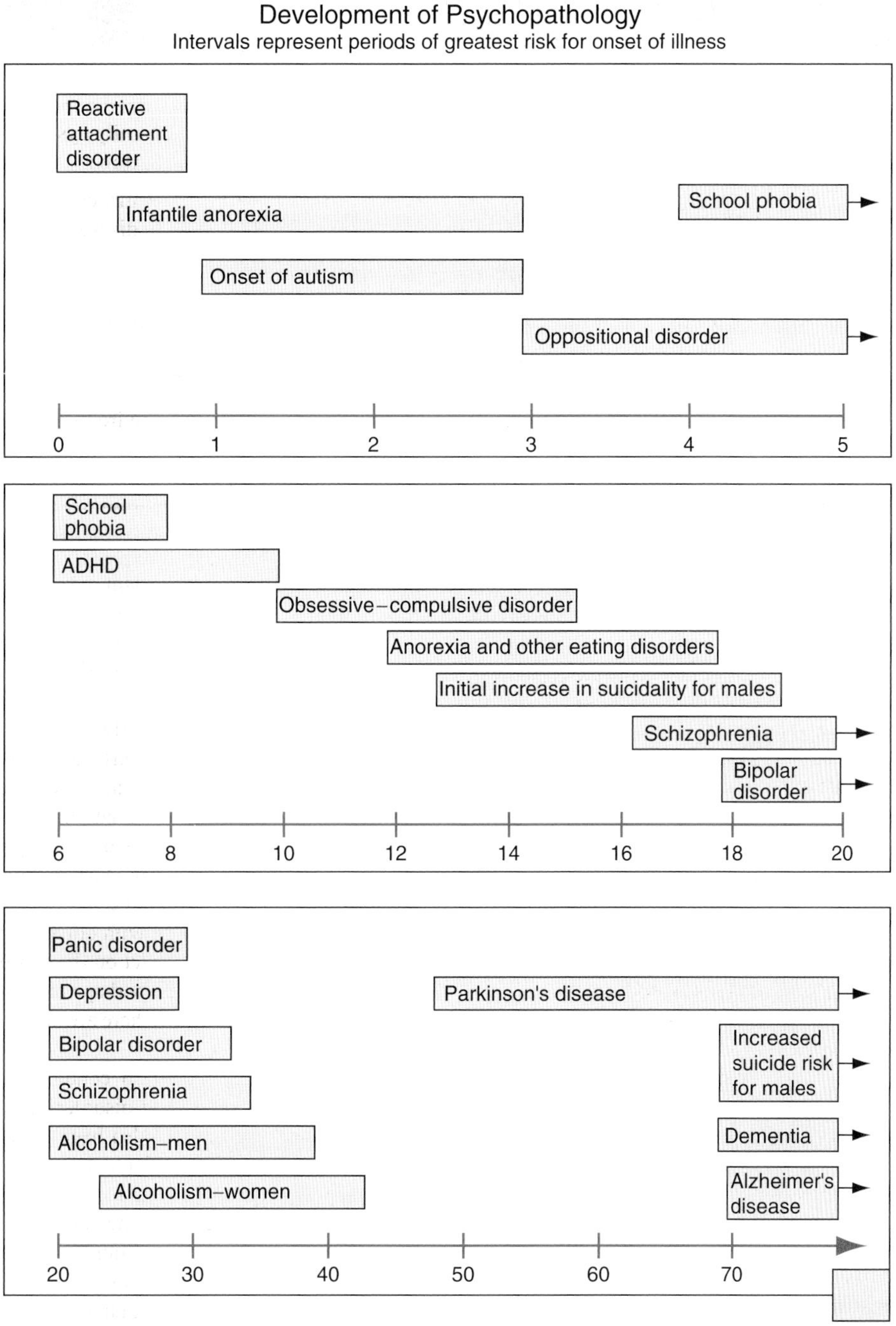

Development of Psychopathology
Intervals represent periods of greatest risk for onset of illness

Reactive attachment disorder

Infantile anorexia

Onset of autism

School phobia

Oppositional disorder

0   1   2   3   4   5

School phobia

ADHD

Obsessive–compulsive disorder

Anorexia and other eating disorders

Initial increase in suicidality for males

Schizophrenia

Bipolar disorder

6   8   10   12   14   16   18   20

Panic disorder

Depression

Parkinson's disease

Bipolar disorder

Increased suicide risk for males

Schizophrenia

Alcoholism–men

Dementia

Alcoholism–women

Alzheimer's disease

20   30   40   50   60   70

Figure 7.8 *Timeline (in years) showing the development of psychopathology across the lifespan.*

function. Normal children learn to think, to make friends, to deal with intense affects, and to honor the customs of their society. Problems occur when development is uneven. The patterns of these interlineal decalages are varied and their complexity is in large part one of the persistent areas of fascination for psychiatrists. To illustrate this process, two straightforward decalages are discussed. Finally, a more complex example of a severe arrest in development is presented.

Cognitive delays can result in a decalage in which a teenager has the mental capacity of a second-grader while having the sexual urges and emotional swings of a normal adolescent in high school. The cognitive ability of such a teenager may not be perceived as abnormal in the context of a protected classroom. However, within the general population, he will be clearly labeled as

deviant and will be at high risk for experiences that will place him in jeopardy for negative social and academic outcomes. Beyond dealing with the obvious limitations in achievement, there are also emotional risks to be considered if intellectual limitations cannot be placed within a context that protects such an adolescent from ridicule and humiliation.

Emotional delays provide a similar potential for a variety of decalages. A child who is cognitively normal or even precocious may remain emotionally immature. The decalage can be widened if intensive academic effort and subsequent successes become the predominant strategy that the child develops for dealing with social awkwardness or peer rejection. Temper tantrums that were expected in the early years become less easily tolerated in the child "genius" who repeatedly demands to have family and social events orchestrated on her or his terms. In more severe cases, frustration and despair may interfere with adaptation in the same way that they do in the child who is cognitively delayed.

If a domain of function becomes arrested, the decalage becomes more severe. In these cases, overt psychopathology often results. A clear example is the development of conduct disorder and, subsequently, antisocial personality disorder. In these individuals, physical, cognitive and social developments appear to be progressing well, but a specific deficit in the development of moral judgment occurs. In some cases, the deficit is best described as the persistence of an immature sense of right and wrong, but in other adolescents there is a deviant development of amorality that is abnormal at any stage of development. Given the resistance of adults with antisocial personality disorder to current treatments, there is a strong case for focusing on the origins of this developmental decalage with the expectation that earlier intervention may be more effective than later efforts to treat.

The Psychiatrist as a Developmentalist

All psychiatrists inevitably become students of development. The life histories of their patients demand developmental formulations to achieve a sense of understanding of the origins of the presenting symptoms and disturbing behaviors that bring the patients to psychiatric treatment. Perhaps one of the most poignant examples is Huntington's chorea. The gene that causes this disease has been identified, and it is possible to know accurately whether an infant is destined to struggle with the symptoms of this crippling disability many decades in the future. Yet it is the life experiences of this individual that shape many of the coping strategies that determine the ultimate outcomes of these future struggles. Anticipating the challenges of later life and understanding the origins of the strengths and weaknesses of each patient are at the core of the therapeutic process, whether it involves influencing the balance of the central neurotransmitters or identifying and supporting available community resources.

References

Ainsworth MDS, Blehar MD, Waters E *et al.* (1978) *Patterns of Attachment: A psychological study of the strange situation.* Lawrence Erlbaum, Hillsdale, NJ.

Anderson V (2001) Assessing executive functions in children: Biological, psychological, and developmental considerations. *Pediatr Rehabil* 4, 119–136.

Casey BJ, Giedd JN and Thomas KM (2000) Structural and functional brain development and its relation to cognitive development. *Biol Psychiatr* 54, 241–257.

Emde RN (1984) The affective self: Continuities and transformations from infancy, in *Frontiers of Infant Psychiatry II* (eds Call J, Galenson E, and Tyson RL). Basic Books, New York, pp. 38–54.

Erikson E (1963) *Childhood and Society*, 2nd edn., revised and expanded. W W Norton, New York.

Fonagy P (2001) *Attachment Theory and Psychoanalysis.* Other Press, New York.

Fox NA, Henderson HA, Rubin KH *et al.* (2001) Continuity and discontinuity of behavioral inhibition and exuberance: Psychophysiological and behavioral influences across the first four years of life. *Chil Dev* 72(1) (Jan–Feb), 1–21.

Freud A (1946) *The Ego and the Mechanisms of Defence.* International Universities Press, New York.

Gibbs JC (1979) Kohlberg's moral stage theory: A Piagetian revision. *Hum Dev* 22, 89–112.

Goldsmith HH, BUss AH, Plomin R *et al.* (1987) Roundtable: What is temperament? Four approaches. *Child Dev* 58, 505–529.

Guttman D (1977) The cross-cultural perspective: Notes toward a comparative psychology of aging, in *Handbook of the Psychology of Aging* (eds Birren JE and Schaie KW). Van Nostrand Reinhold, New York, pp. 302–326.

Henderson HA, Fox NA and Rubin KH (2001) Temperamental contributions to social behavior: The moderating roles of frontal EEG asymmetry and gender. *JAACAP* 40 (Jan), 1.

Huttenlocher PR and Dabholkar AS (1997) Regional differences in synaptogenesis in human cerebral cortex. *J Comp Neurol* 387, 167–178.

Kagan J, Reznick JS and Gibbons J (1989) Inhibited and uninhibited types of children. *Child Dev* 60, 838–845.

Kay J (2005) Attachment and its disorders, in *Clinical Child Psychiatry* (eds Klykylo W and Kay J). John Wiley and Sons, Chichester, England.

Klinnert MD (1984) The regulation of infant behavior by maternal facial expression. *Inf Behav Dev* 7, 447–465.

Kohlberg L (1964) Development of moral character and moral ideology, in *Review of Child Development Research* (eds Hoffman ML and Hoffman LW). Russell Sage Foundation, New York, pp. 383–432.

Lewis M (1994) The emergence of human emotions, in *Handbook of Emotions* (eds Lewis M and Haviland J). Guilford Press, New York, pp. 223–226.

Mahler M, Pine F and Bergman A (1975) *The Psychological Birth of the Human Infant.* Basic Books, New York.

Mrazek PJ and Mrazek DA (1987) Resilience in child maltreatment victims: A conceptual exploration. *Child Abuse Neglect* 11, 357–366.

Piaget J (1952) *The Origins of Intelligence in Children.* International Universities Press, New York.

Piaget J and Inhelder B (1969) *The Psychology of the Child.* Basic Books, New York.

Rutter M (1985a) Resilience in the face of adversity: Protective factors and resistance to psychiatric disorder. *Br J Psychiatr* 147, 598–611.

Rutter M (1985b) Family and school influences on behavioral development. *J Child Psychol Psychiatr* 26, 349–368.

Sameroff AJ (1986) Environmental context of child development. *J Pediatr* 109, 192–200.

Smetana JG, Killen M, and Turiel E (1991) Children's reasoning about interpersonal and moral conflicts. *Child Dev* 52, 629–644.

Thomas A, Chess S and Birch HG (1968) *Temperament and Behavior Disorders in Children.* New York University Press, New York.

Topolski T, Hewitt J, Leaves L *et al.* (1997) Genetic and environmental influences on child reports of manifest anxiety and symptoms of separation anxiety and overanxious disorders: A community-based twin study. *Behav Genet* 27, 15–28.

Trevarthen C (1979) Communication and cooperation in early infancy: A description of primary intersubjectivity, in *Before Speech: The Beginning of Interpersonal Communication* (ed Bullowa MM). Cambridge University Press, New York, pp. 321–347.

Vaillant GE (1977) *Adaptation to Life.* Little, Brown & Co, Boston.

Vaillant GE (1993) *The Wisdom of the Ego.* Harvard University Press, Cambridge, MA.

Vygotsky LS (1978) *Mind in Society: The Development of Higher Psychology Processes.* Harvard University Press, Cambridge, MA.

Wilber K (2000) *Integral Psychology.* Shambala Publications, Boston.

Zacharias L, Rand WM and Wurtman RJ (1976) A prospective study of sexual development and growth in American girls: The statistics of menarche. *Obstet Gynecol Surv* 31, 325–337.

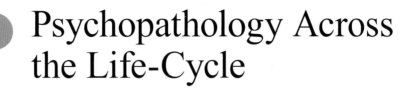

CHAPTER

8

Psychopathology Across the Life-Cycle

Psychopathology is the study of the nature and causes of mental disorders. Because definitive etiologies for most mental disorders have not been identified, psychopathology for the most part is focused on the myriad manifestations of psychiatric illness. An elusive concept itself, mental disorder has been defined in the *Diagnostic and Statistical Manual of Mental Disorders*, Fourth Edition, Text Revision (DSM-IV-TR) (American Psychiatric Association, 2000, p. xxxi) as "a clinically significant behavioral or psychological syndrome or pattern that occurs in an individual and that is associated with present distress (e.g., a painful symptom) or disability (i.e., impairment in one or more important areas of functioning) or with a significantly increased risk of suffering death, pain, disability, or an important loss of freedom".

The manifestations of psychiatric illness can be grouped into five broad domains of human functioning: 1) consciousness, orientation, memory, and intellect; 2) speech, thinking, perception, and self-experience; 3) emotions; 4) physical functioning; and 5) behavior and adaptive functioning. These five areas encompass the processes by which humans know about themselves and the world around them; how they think, reason, learn, and express themselves; how they feel and express these feelings; how they perceive their bodies and experience their sensations and essential functions; and how they act and react to both internal and external stimuli.

In this chapter, we discuss the ways in which psychiatric illness presents across the life-cycle and in which the manifestations of disorder may vary according to the patient's developmental life stage (e.g., infancy, childhood, adolescence, adulthood and late life). We also discuss variation by gender, because psychiatric disturbance often takes different forms in men and in women. Fundamental to our discussion is the notion that different life stages (and genders) are associated with differential incidence and prevalence rates of particular mental disorders as a result of the developmental tasks of the epoch and corresponding stressors (Rutter, 1989a). Thus, developmental considerations may help to explain both the origins of individual disorders and their course (Rutter *et al.*, 1994). In addition, age appears to have a pathoplastic effect on the manifestations of psychiatric illness such that the same disorder may have different manifestations at different ages.

Continuity, Persistence and Progression Across the Life-Cycle

Epidemiological research suggests that considerable stability or continuity of mental disorders can be observed from childhood into adolescence, at least for broad diagnostic groupings.

In particular, behavior disorders in childhood are associated with increased risk of behavior disorders in adolescence, especially for boys, and childhood emotional disorders are associated with increased risk of adolescent emotional disorders, especially for girls (Costello and Angold, 1995). The more severe the disorder, the more likely it is to persist (Cohen *et al.*, 1993a). In addition, epidemiological surveys of adults indicate that the age at onset of disorders for many patients was during adolescence, further reinforcing the notion of persistence or progression of disorders from childhood across the life-cycle (Burke *et al.*, 1990).

Stress-diathesis Model of Psychopathology

Theories of the causes of mental disorders are many and are the subjects of other chapters. For simplicity, we take the position that etiology in psychopathology is multifactorial. Most mental disorders are likely to be caused by both a predisposition or vulnerability at the level of brain biochemistry and experience with acute life events or chronic stressful life circumstances. Such a model helps to explain why a person with a strong family history of depression, for example, may be asymptomatic for long periods but may experience depression after a loss.

Pathoplastic Effects of Age

Age appears to influence psychopathology in three ways (Table 8.1). A few mental disorders appear almost to be age-specific and not to occur outside a certain age range. Feeding disorder of infancy or early childhood (failure to thrive) is a disturbance restricted to the first several years of life because of a child's total dependence on caregivers for food during this time. Dementia of the Alzheimer's type is much more common after the age of 65 years; few cases develop before age 50 years.

More commonly, disorders that may occur at virtually any age have an usual onset at certain stages in life. Mental retardation, learning disorders, disruptive behavior disorders and elimination disorders, among others, usually have their onset and are first diagnosed during childhood. The median age at onset for

Table 8.1	Pathoplastic Effects of Age
Age specificity of disorders	
Usual age at onset	
Age effects on symptom expression	

Essentials of Psychiatry   Jerald Kay and Allan Tasman
© 2006 John Wiley & Sons, Ltd.

the first psychotic episode of schizophrenia is in the early to mid-twenties for men and in the late twenties for women (American Psychiatric Association, 2000).

Most mental disorders can occur at various times in life's stages. Some of these are expressed differently depending on age. For example, although the core symptoms of major depression are the same regardless of a person's age, in children somatic symptoms, irritable mood and social withdrawal may be especially common. In depressed elderly persons, cognitive symptoms such as memory loss, disorientation and distractibility may predominate.

Problems of Childhood

Individual Differences

Children differ from each other in ways that affect their psychological functioning from birth. They differ in intelligence, in temperament and in genetic endowment for both risk for and resilience against mental disorder.

Intelligence is the ability to reason, plan, think abstractly, solve problems, understand and learn. Average intelligence is associated with a score of 100 (IQ) on a standardized intelligence test. About 67% of children have IQs between 85 and 115 and about 95% between 70 and 130. Estimates of the heritability of IQ range from 0.4 to 0.8 (Plomin, 1990) indicate that heredity plays a larger role than environment. Higher intelligence is correlated with successful adaptation in life, and substantially reduced intelligence is associated with developmental and behavioral problems and functional impairment (see the discussion of mental retardation).

Types of Problems

Psychopathology in childhood falls into four major groups of problems (Table 8.2). Many of the disorders of childhood appear to be severe forms of problems that are more or less continuously distributed, common and "normal" occurrences. Thus, clinical depression may appear to be a severe form of sadness and disappointment, conduct disorder a severe form of aggressiveness, and anorexia nervosa a severe form of adolescent dieting and dissatisfaction with body shape (Rutter and Sandberg, 1985).

Estimates are that 5 to 15% of 9- to 10-year-old children suffer from an emotional or behavior disorder of sufficient severity to cause impairment in everyday functioning (Cox, 1994). The co-occurrence of several disorders (i.e., comorbidity) is common in childhood (Caron and Rutter, 1991). As can be seen in Table 8.3, comorbidity both within and between disorder types can be observed.

Developmental Problems

Childhood is a time of growth, physical and social maturation, and the acquisition of skills necessary to deal independently and

Table 8.2	Psychopathology in Childhood
Developmental problems	
Emotional problems	
Behavioral problems	
Problems in physical functioning	

Table 8.3	Common Patterns of Comorbidity in Childhood
Disorder Type or Specific Disorder	Comorbid Disorders
Intellectual (mental retardation)	Attention-deficit/hyperactivity disorder Pervasive developmental disorders Stereotyped movement disorder Mood disorders Disorders due to general medical condition
Learning disorders	Other learning disorders Conduct disorder Oppositional defiant disorder Attention-deficit/hyperactivity disorder Major depressive disorder Dysthymic disorder Communication disorders Medical conditions (e.g., lead poisoning, fetal alcohol syndrome)
Motor skills disorders (developmental coordination disorder)	Communication disorders
Communication disorders	Other communication disorders Learning disorders Motor skills disorders Enuresis Attention-deficit/hyperactivity disorder
Pervasive developmental disorders	Mental retardation Pica Communication disorders General medical conditions
Anxiety disorders	Other anxiety disorders Major depressive disorder Behavioral disorders
Depressive disorders	Anxiety disorders
Behavioral disorders	Other behavioral disorders Learning disorders Communication disorders Mood disorders Anxiety disorders Substance use disorders Somatoform disorders Tourette's disorder Mental retardation
Feeding disorders	Mental retardation
Elimination disorders	Other elimination disorders Parasomnias Oppositional defiant disorder Conduct disorder

Continues

Table 8.3	Common Patterns of Comorbidity in Childhood *Continued*
Disorder Type or Specific Disorder	Comorbid Disorders
Tourette's disorder	Obsessive–compulsive disorder Attention-deficit/hyperactivity disorder Learning disorders

successfully with the environment. Children who are greatly delayed in their development or who never acquire the requisite skills or maturity associated with their developmental stage have developmental problems. Developmental disorders fall into five main types: intellectual, learning, motor skills, communication and pervasive developmental disorders.

The most severe developmental problems are evident in infancy. For example, the infant with autism may manifest limited eye contact, facial responsiveness and smiling, and may be difficult to hug or may appear to dislike physical contact. Restricted social relationships emerge, however, after the third or fourth year of life. For children with other pervasive developmental disorders, infancy may be normal, with the onset of the abnormal behavior occurring months or even years after birth. In milder forms, such as Asperger's syndrome (Tantum, 1988), in which communication skills are spared, a pervasive developmental disorder may not be recognized until preschool or the actual beginning of school. The course after diagnosis is variable, depending on the subtype.

Emotional Problems
The emotional problems of children involve anxiety and depression. Although these problems have counterparts in adults, children frequently experience and express their disturbances of feelings or emotions differently from adults. Because of their more limited vocabulary and understanding of emotional life, children may not express their emotional distress verbally as well as some adults do. Thus, even in the emotional disorders of childhood, disturbances in behavior and in physical functioning are apt to be prominent in the clinical presentation. Children are not unlike so-called alexithymic adults, whose expression of emotions is indirect and nonverbal.

Some children may be excessive worriers in general. They may worry about school performance, athletic prowess, appearance and popularity, parental expectations, potential catastrophic events, and so on. Children who worry excessively are said to have generalized anxiety disorder. Moody periods are common in children, but children may also exhibit prolonged and persistent disturbances of mood, usually depression.

The manifestations of mania in younger children may involve irritability, emotional lability, or admixtures of dysphoria and hypomania, as well as more typical symptoms of hyperactivity, grandiosity, pressure of speech and distractibility (Carlson, 1990; Strober *et al.*, 1989). As many as one-third of children with major depressive episodes may show bipolar disorder by adolescence (Geller *et al.*, 1994). Early-onset bipolar disorders may have a poorer prognosis than later onset disorders. Childhood major depressive disorder also appears to

increase the risk for the development of personality disorders in young adulthood (Kasen *et al.*, 2001).

Behavior Problems
Behavior problems in children fall into the general groupings of oppositional behavior, hyperactivity, excessive aggressiveness and conduct disturbance. An appropriate degree of control over behavior is a necessary development for a child to function in a family, in school, and with peers.

Disturbances in Physical Functioning
A number of developmental tasks of childhood involve primarily physical functions. These include developing proper eating and sleeping habits (Wolke, 1994), bowel (Hersov, 1994) and bladder (Shaffer, 1994) control and sexual identity (Paikoff and Brooks-Gunn, 1994). Disturbances may occur in these functions during childhood.

Table 8.4 summarizes the estimated prevalence and sex distribution of DSM-IV-TR mental disorders seen in children.

Problems of Adolescence
Adolescence is the period of life between puberty and age 19 years. For the great majority of children, the physiological events of puberty signify the end of childhood. Achievement of financial independence from the family of origin through work and formation of love relationships outside the family usually signify the end of adolescence and the beginning of adulthood. In the modern world, these goals may not be attained until the early or middle twenties or later. There are many important developmental phases in adolescence. Although moody, confused and rebellious "adolescent turmoil" is no longer considered the norm for young people, some emotional troubles are fairly common. These may turn out to be symptomatic of nothing more than the stresses and strains of normal development, or they may be the early signs of significant psychological disturbance.

Types of Problems
Common problems of adolescence are listed in Table 8.5. Rarely, schizophrenia may have a late adolescent onset. As might be expected, comorbidity is common among disorders of adolescence. Table 8.6 summarizes these patterns.

Problems in Self-image and Physical Functioning
Disturbances in body image and eating behavior have peak ages at onset during adolescence and early adulthood. Persistence of disturbed eating behaviors into early adulthood is often accompanied by the development of personality disorders in many cases. Bulimia nervosa has been shown to be associated with borderline personality disorder in contrast with anorexia nervosa, which was found to be associated with avoidant personality disorder (Skodol *et al.*, 1993).

Although adolescents tend to sleep late, excessive daytime sleepiness may become a problem during adolescence. Excessive sleepiness may indicate the onset of narcolepsy, a rare disorder characterized by sleep attacks, accompanied by cataplexy (sudden, bilateral loss of muscle tone), and/or hypnopompic or hypnogogic hallucinations or sleep paralysis (Regestein, 1994).

Table 8.4   Prevalence and Sex Distribution of Mental Disorders of Childhood

Type of Problem	Specific Disorder	Estimated Prevalence*	Predominant Sex
Developmental	Mental retardation	Rare	Male
Intellectual	Reading disorder	Less common	Male
Learning	Developmental coordination disorder	Common	Male
Motor skills			
Communication	Expressive language disorder	Less common	Male
	Mixed receptive–expressive language disorder	Less common	Male
	Phonological disorder		
	Stuttering	Less common	Male
		Rare	Male
Pervasive	Autistic disorder	Very rare	Male
	Rett's disorder	Very rare	Female (only)
	Childhood disintegrative disorder	Very rare	Male
	Asperger's disorder	Very rare	Male
Emotional Anxiety	Separation anxiety disorder	Less common	Female
	Specific phobia	Less common	Female
	Social phobia	Rare	Female
	Generalized anxiety disorder	Less common	Female
	Obsessive–compulsive disorder	Rare	Equal
	Posttraumatic stress disorder	NK	Female
	Selective mutism	Very rare	Female
Mood	Major depressive disorder	Rare	Equal
Behavioral	Oppositional defiant disorder	Common	Male
	Attention-deficit/hyperactivity disorder	Less common	Male
	Conduct disorder, childhood onset	Common	Male
Physical functioning	Rumination disorder	NK	Male
Eating	Feeding disorder	NK	Equal
	Pica	NK	NK
Sleep	Nightmare disorder	NK	Female
	Sleep terror disorder	NK	Male
	Sleepwalking disorder	Less common	Equal
Elimination	Encopresis	Rare	Male
	Enuresis	Common	Male
Sexual	Gender identity disorder	Less common	Male
Tic	Tourette's disorder	Very rare	Male

*Prevalence estimates are as follows: common, .5%; less common, 2–5%; rare, 1–2%; very rare, ,1%; NK, not known.

A preoccupation with an imagined or exaggerated defect in appearance may develop in adolescence. Unlike the normal concerns of adolescents with their physical appearances, excessively time-consuming concerns that cause great distress or interfere with functioning suggest body dysmorphic disorder.

Table 8.7 summarizes the estimated prevalence and sex distribution of DSM-IV mental disorders commonly seen in adolescents.

Problems of Early Adulthood

The period between the ages of 20 and 30 years is commonly referred to as early adulthood.

Early Adult Development

Developmental tasks of early adulthood include achieving emotional and financial independence from parents and forming intimate relationships with people outside the family of origin. Stage-specific stressors include leaving home, education and

Table 8.5   Psychopathology in Adolescence

Identity problems
Emotional problems
Behavioral problems
Problems in self-image and physical functioning

Table 8.6	Common Patterns of Comorbidity in Adolescence
Disorder Type or Specific Disorder	Comorbid Disorders
Mood disorders	Anxiety disorders
	Substance use disorders
	Eating disorders
Anxiety disorders	Other anxiety disorders
	Mood disorders
Substance use disorders	Substance-induced disorders
	Other substance use disorders
Conduct disorder	Conduct disorder
	Substance use disorders
	Mood disorders
Pathological gambling	Mood disorders
	Substance use disorders
	Anxiety disorders
Trichotillomania	Substance use disorders
	Mood disorders
	Anxiety disorders
Eating disorders	Major depressive disorder
Anorexia nervosa	Obsessive–compulsive disorder
	Substance use disorders
	Avoidant personality disorder
	General medical conditions
Bulimia nervosa	Major depressive disorder
	Dysthymic disorder
	Anxiety disorders
	Substance use disorders
	Borderline personality disorder
Narcolepsy	Mood disorders
	Substance-related disorders
	Generalized anxiety disorder
	Sleepwalking disorder
	Enuresis
Body dysmorphic disorder	Mood disorders
	Anxiety disorders
	Personality disorders

Table 8.7	Prevalence and Sex Distribution of Mental Disorders of Adolescence		
Type of Problem	Specific Disorder	Estimated Prevalence*	Predominant Sex
Emotional Mood	Major depressive disorder	Common	Female
	Bipolar disorder	NK	Equal
Anxiety	Panic disorder	Very rare	Female
	Social phobia	Rare	Female
	Obsessive–compulsive disorder	Rare	Male
Behavioral Substance related	Alcohol intoxication	Very common	Male
	Substance abuse	Common	Male
Disruptive	Conduct disorder	Very common	Male
Impulse control	Pathological gambling	Very rare	Male
	Trichotillomania	Rare	Female
Self-image and physical functioning			
Eating	Anorexia nervosa	Very rare	Female
	Bulimia nervosa	Less common	Female
Sleep	Narcolepsy	Very rare	Equal
	Body dysmorphic disorder	NK	Equal
Somatoform			

*Prevalence estimates are as follows: very common, .0%; common, 5–10%; less common, 2–5%; rare, 1–2%; very rare, ,1%; NK, not known.

The relationships between comorbid "disorders" are complex. Whether they indeed represent independent entities with distinctive etiologies, pathogenetic mechanisms and outcomes, or merely reflect different ways in which fundamental psychopathological disturbances are manifest over time, between sexes, or across aspects of psychological functioning remains to be determined. In some cases, one disorder is clearly antecedent to another. Examples include disorders of childhood, such as separation anxiety disorder or conduct disorder, that evolve into adult versions – in these cases, panic disorder with agoraphobia or antisocial personality disorder, respectively. Sometimes, as in the case of attention-deficit/hyperactivity disorder, residual symptoms persist and form the basis for developing problems such as substance abuse or personality dysfunction. At other times, a second disorder may develop as a consequence of a primary disorder – in reaction to it or as a complication. Examples include

career choice, in some cases service in the armed forces, finding and maintaining employment, courtship and marriage, and sexual relations, among others.

Types of Problems

Problems of young adulthood fall mostly into the categories listed in Table 8.8. By the end of early adulthood, people have passed through the ages of greatest risk for first onset of the majority of recognized mental disorders. Comorbidity between disorders becomes the rule rather than the exception. In a population survey in the USA, 14% of those evaluated had three or more lifetime disorders and accounted for more than 50% of the mental disorders found, both on a lifetime basis and in the year before the assessment (Kessler *et al.*, 1994).

Table 8.8	Psychopathology in Early Adulthood
Emotional problems	
Problems of behavior and adaptive functioning	
Problems in physical functioning	
Problems in reality testing	

major depressive disorder developing after a person has been incapacitated by panic disorder with agoraphobia, or sedative, anxiolytic, or alcohol abuse developing because the person attempted to self-medicate for the condition. Alternatively, disorders appear more or less contemporaneously and reflect an underlying diathesis or vulnerability. Thus, patients present with several disorders, all suggestive of a problem of generalized impulsivity, such as bulimia nervosa, a substance use disorder and an impulse control disorder (e.g., kleptomania). Personality disorders often develop in the context of underlying traits affecting specific capacities such as impulse control or interpersonal relatedness, as dysfunction becomes widespread.

Table 8.9 summarizes patterns of comorbid mental disorders in early adulthood.

Emotional Problems

Although disturbances in mood can occur at any age, the peak ages of onset of mood disorders are probably in the twenties. Mood disturbances may be acute and episodic or insidious and chronic. They may be relatively mild or severe and may be accompanied by psychotic features or suicidal behavior. The most common mood disorders are major depressive disorder, dysthymic disorder, bipolar disorder and cyclothymic disorder.

Although several anxiety disorders have their onset most often in childhood or adolescence, as previously described, others have increased risk for onset in early adult life. In particular, many cases of acrophobia (fear of heights) and situational phobias, such as of elevators, flying, or closed places, develop in early adulthood (American Psychiatric Association, 2000). There is a rise in the rate of panic disorder in women in early and middle adult life (Regier *et al.*, 1988). Obsessive–compulsive disorder has a later age at onset in women than in men, during the twenties rather than the teens. Acute stress disorder and PTSD can occur at any age but are prevalent in young adults.

Disorders such as panic disorder, other specific phobias, social phobia and generalized anxiety disorder, which are more likely to begin in childhood or adolescence, may persist or recur during early adult life.

The severity, duration and proximity of a person's exposure to a traumatic event influence the risk of developing either an acute stress disorder or PTSD (March, 1993). Acute stress reactions which do not resolve (Classen *et al.*, 1998), peritraumatic dissociation (Shalev *et al.*, 1996) or emotional numbing in response to the stressor (Epstein *et al.*, 1998) predict later PTSD. Social support, family history, childhood experiences, personality variables and preexisting mental disorders also affect risk. Men and women appear equally vulnerable. Dissociative disturbances may occur in the absence of reexperiencing or avoidance symptoms, often in response to severe stress (Spiegel and Cardena, 1991).

Milder, time-limited reactions to stressors of any severity may also occur. These are common occurrences that might follow the breakup of a romantic relationship or the loss of a job. The symptoms may be of depression, anxiety, or disturbance of conduct. They cause temporarily decreased performance at school or work or impairment in social relationships. Provided that the consequences of the stressor are resolved (i.e., the person resumes dating or obtains a new job), the course of the symptoms and impairment should be less than 6 months.

Behavior and Adaptive Functioning

Problems with various types of impulsive behaviors and problems with adaptive functioning in general seem particularly prone to

Table 8.9   Common Patterns of Comorbidity in Early Adulthood

Disorder Type	Comorbid Disorders
Mood disorders	Other mood disorders Anxiety disorders Eating disorders Substance-related disorders Personality disorders
Anxiety disorders	Other anxiety disorders Mood disorders Substance-related disorders Eating disorders Somatization disorder Personality disorders
Dissociative disorders	Mood disorders Post traumatic stress disorder Substance-related disorders Somatoform disorders Personality disorders
Substance use disorders	Other substance-related disorders Mood disorders Anxiety disorders Personality disorders Schizophrenia and other psychotic disorders Eating and sleep disorders Impulse control disorders
Impulse-control disorders	Mood disorders Anxiety disorders Substance-related disorders Eating disorders Personality disorders
Personality disorders	Other personality disorders Psychotic disorders Mood disorders Anxiety disorders Eating disorders Substance-related disorders Impulse control disorders Somatoform disorders
Sexual disorders Sexual dysfunctions	Other sexual dysfunctions Mood disorders Anxiety disorders
Paraphilias	Substance-related disorders Sexual dysfunction Personality disorders
Somatoform disorders	Mood disorders Anxiety discorders Substance-related disorders Dissociative disorders Personality disorders
Factitious disorders	Substance-related discorders Personality disorders

Source: Data from American Psychiatric Association (2000) *Diagnostic and Statistical Manual of Mental Disorders*, 4th edn., Text Rev. APA, Washington DC.

become manifest in early adulthood. These problems may develop, in part, secondary to the increased stresses of movement away from the protective environments of school and family that characterize the period.

Of major significance in the twenties is the stabilization of patterns of perceiving, relating to, and thinking about the environment and oneself that we call personality. Also, however, in the twenties, the potential for the development of inflexible and maladaptive traits that cause distress or interfere with effective social and occupational functioning may arise. Thus, personality disorders may become evident.

Disturbances in Physical Functioning

Certain disturbances in physical functioning are likely to become manifest in early adult life. These include disturbances in sexual functioning, sleep disturbances and some physical complaints that cannot be fully explained on the basis of a known general medical condition.

Certain disturbances characterized by physical complaints without known medical etiology have a high incidence rate in early adulthood. Specifically, conversion reactions, hypochondriasis and somatization disorder can be first diagnosed in this age group.

Problems in Reality Testing

Problems in reality testing are reflected in abnormalities of speech, thinking, perception and self-experience. They are suggestive of psychotic disorders such as schizophrenia. Although schizophrenia and its counterpart disorder of briefer duration, schizophreniform disorder, may have an onset in late adolescence (or in later adulthood), the most common age at onset is in early adult life.

Patients who have illness episodes that are characterized by major episodes of mood disturbance, either depressed or manic, accompanied by schizophrenia-like psychotic symptoms and whose delusions and hallucinations are also present when mood symptoms are not, are said to have schizoaffective disorder.

The vast majority of disorders with typical onset in early adult life persist or recur in middle adult life. Some of these disorders may also have their initial onset after age 30 years. Table 8.10 summarizes the estimated prevalence and sex distribution of mental disorders of early adulthood.

Problems of Middle Adult Life

Middle Adult Development

Middle adult life may be applied to ages 30 to 65 years, which are characterized developmentally by consolidation and generativity in career and family life. Although potentially the most productive years of life, they are also fraught with obstacles and frustrations in the achievement of personal goals. Common stressors include marriage and divorce, parenting, career setbacks, recognition of unattainable goals and death of parents. Any of these may serve as the focus of a midlife crisis.

Types of Problems

Psychosocial stressors may precipitate episodes of already existing disorders of virtually any type or initiate disorders *de novo*. Relatively few disorders have a typical onset between 30 and 65 years (Table 8.11). They include particular anxiety, psychotic, sleep and substance-related disorders, and disorders associated with general medical conditions.

General Medical Conditions

Because medical conditions have increased incidence during adult life, psychopathological conditions resulting from the direct physiological effects of general medical conditions are on the rise. General medical conditions (and their treatments) can cause delirium, dementia, amnestic disorder, psychotic disorder, mood

Table 8.10   Prevalence and Sex Distribution of Mental Disorders in Early Adulthood and Middle Adult Life

Type of Problem	Specific Disorder	Estimated Prevalence*	Predominant Sex†
Emotional			
Mood	Major depressive disorder	Very common	Female
	Dysthymic disorder	Very common	Female
	Bipolar I disorder	Rare	Equal
	Bipolar II disorder	Very rare	Female
	Cyclothymic disorder	Very rare	Equal
Anxiety	Specific phobia	Very common	Female
	Social phobia	Very common	Female
	Panic disorder‡	Less common	Female
	Obsessive–compulsive disorder	Less common	Equal
	Acute stress disorder	NK	NK
	Post traumatic stress disorder	Less common or common	NK
	Generalized anxiety disorder	Less common	Female
Dissociative	Dissociative amnesia	NK	NK
	Dissociative fugue	Very rare	NK
	Depersonalization disorder	NK	NK
	Dissociative identity disorder	NK	Female
Adjustment	Adjustment disorder	Very common	Equal

Continues

Table 8.10 Prevalence and Sex Distribution of Mental Disorders in Early Adulthood and Middle Adult Life *Continued*

Type of Problem	Specific Disorder	Estimated Prevalence*	Predominant Sex†
Behavior, adaptive functioning Substance use	Alcohol dependence	Very common	Male
	Amphetamine dependence	Less common	Male
	Cannabis dependence	Less common	Male
	Cocaine abuse	Very rare	Equal
	Hallucinogen abuse	Very rare	Male
	Inhalant abuse	NK	Male
	Nicotine dependence	Very common	Male
	Opioid dependence	Very rare	Male
	Sedative dependence	Rare	Female
Substance-induced Impulse control	Alcohol-induced persisting amnestic disorder§	NK	Male
		Rare	Male
	Intermittent explosive disorder	Rare	Female
	Kleptomania	Rare	Male
	Pyromania	Less common	Male
	Pathological gambling		
Personality	Paranoid personality disorder	Rare	Male
	Schizoid personality disorder	NK	Male
	Schizotypal personality disorder	Less common	Male
	Antisocial personality disorder	Less common	Male
	Borderline personality disorder	Less common	Female
	Histrionic personality disorder	Less common	Female
	Narcissistic personality disorder	Very rare	Male
	Avoidant personality disorder	Very rare	Equal
	Dependent personality disorder	NK	Female
	Obsessive–compulsive personality disorder	Rare	Male
Physical functioning Sexual dysfunction	Premature ejaculation	NK	Male (only)
	Vaginismus	NK	Female (only)
Paraphilias	All	NK	Male
Sleep	Primary insomnia	NK	Female
	Primary hypersomnia	NK	NK
	Breathing-related sleep disorder§	Common	Male
Somatoform	Conversion disorder	Very rare	Female
	Hypochondriasis	NK	Equal
	Somatization disorder	Rare	Female
	Pain disorder§	Very common	Female
Factitious	Factitious disorder	NK	Male
Reality testing	Schizophrenia	Very rare	Equal
	Schizophreniform disorder	Very rare	Female
	Schizoaffective disorder	Very rare	Female
	Delusional disorder§	Very rare	Equal

*Prevalence estimates are as follows: very common, .10%; common, 5–10%; less common, 2–5%; rare, 1–2%; very rare, ,1%; NK, not known.
†NK, Not known.
‡Second peak in incidence in middle adult life.
§Peak in age at onset in middle adult life

Table 8.11 Disorders with Onset in Middle Adult Life

Panic disorder
Delusional disorder
Breathing-related sleep disorder
Substance-induced disorders
Disorders due to general medical conditions
Pain disorder

disorder, anxiety disorder, catatonic disorder, sexual dysfunction, sleep disorder and personality disorder.

Medical conditions can also act as psychosocial stressors (Popkin *et al.*, 1987), in which case the prognosis also depends on the management of the stress and the treatment of the mental disorder.

The estimated prevalence and sex distribution of the few mental disorders with a peak in age at onset in middle adult life are included in Table 8.10.

Table 8.12 Psychopathology in Late Life
Memory impairment
Emotional problems
Substance abuse
Problems in physical functioning
Problems in reality testing

Problems of Late Life

Late Life Development

The developmental demands of late life are many. Coping with physical illness, disability, or a diminished capacity for physical activity; adapting to retirement or reduced productivity at work; and dealing with grief after the loss of friends or a spouse are all frequent and challenging tasks. Maintaining emotional equilibrium by finding a new balance between desirable and undesirable events and circumstances (Baltes, 1987) is a major undertaking.

Types of Problems

Risk for mood disturbances in late life remains high. Other emotional problems, substance abuse and problems in physical functioning and in reality testing may occur. However peak age of risk is mainly for memory, or other impairment associated with the dementias (Gurland, 1996), or delirium (Table 8.12).

Table 8.13 summarizes the estimated prevalence and sex ratio of selected mental disorders of late life.

Conclusion

Psychopathology occurs throughout the life-cycle, from infancy to death. Certain forms of psychopathology are limited to specific stages in life, but most can occur at any stage. Particular disorders have a peak age at onset during specific intervals of the life-cycle. Some seem related to the developmental themes of the stage in which they tend to develop. The manifestations of psychopathology may change in expression in relationship to age. Men and women differ in their susceptibilities to certain disorders, the age at which they are at greatest risk, certain symptom patterns, and, in some cases, in their prognoses.

Given the wide range of psychopathology encountered in the life-cycle, clinicians must cast a wide net in collecting diagnostically relevant information. They must exert good clinical judgment in interpreting the information collected, including a judicious weighing of the evidence supporting diagnostic criteria. They must view patients through the filter of their cultural context. And they must apply accepted diagnostic algorithms to reach the most accurate diagnosis for each patient's problem. The remaining chapters in this section are meant to assist in these endeavors.

References

American Psychiatric Association (2000) *Diagnostic and Statistical Manual of Mental Disorders*, 4th edn. Text Rev. APA, Washington DC.

Baltes PB (1987) Theoretical propositions of life-span developmental psychology: On the dynamics between growth and decline. *Dev Psychol* 23, 611–626.

Burke KC, Burke JD Jr., Regier DA *et al.* (1990) Age at onset of selected mental disorders in five community populations. *Arch Gen Psychiatr* 47, 511–518.

Carlson GA (1990) Child and adolescent mania – diagnostic considerations. *J Child Psychol Psychiatr* 31, 331–341.

Caron C and Rutter M (1991) Comorbidity in child psychopathology: Concepts, issues, and research strategies. *J Child Psychol Psychiatr* 32, 1064–1080.

Classen C, Koopman C, Hales R, et al. (1998) Acute stress disorder as a predictor of posttraumatic stress symptoms. *Am J Psychiatr* 155, 620–624.

Cohen P, Cohen J, Kasen S *et al.* (1993a) An epidemiological study of disorders in late childhood and adolescence. I. Age- and gender-specific prevalence. *J Child Psychol Psychiatr* 34, 851–867.

Table 8.13 Prevalence and Sex Distribution of Mental Disorders in Late Life			
Type of Problem	Specific Disorder	EstimatedPrevalence*	Predominant Sex
Memory impairment	Dementia of Alzheimer's type	Less common	Female
	Vascular dementia	Rare	Male
Emotional			
Mood	Major depressive disorder	Rare	Female
	Other depressive disorders	Less common	Female
	Minor depression	Very common	Female
Anxiety	Specific phobia	Common	Female
	Panic disorder	Very rare	Female
	Generalized anxiety disorder	Rare	Female
	Obsessive–compulsive disorder	Very rare	Equal
Substance use	Alcohol abuse or dependence	Rare	Male
Physical functioning	All sleep disorders	Very common	NK
Sleep	Pain disorder	Very common	NK
Somatoform			
Reality testing	All nonaffective psychotic disorders	Very rare	Equal

*Prevalence estimates are as follows: very common, >10%; common, 5–10%; less common, 2–5%; rare, 1–2%; very rare, <1%; NK, not known.

Costello EJ and Angold A (1995) Developmental epidemiology, in *Developmental Psychopathology*, Vol. 1, *Theory and Methods* (eds Cicchetti D and Cohen DJ). John Wiley, New York, pp. 23–56.

Cox AD (1994) Diagnostic appraisal. In Child and Adolescent Psychiatry: Modern Approaches, 3rd ed., Rutter M, Taylor E, and Hersov L (eds). Blackwell Scientific, Oxford, UK, pp. 22–33.

Epstein RS, Fullerton CS and Ursano RJ (1998) Posttraumatic stress disorder following an air disaster: A prospective study. *Am J Psychiatr* 155, 934–938.

Geller B, Fox L and Clark K (1994) Rate and predictors of prepubertal bipolarity during follow-up of 6- to 12-year-old depressed children. *J Am Acad Child Adolesc Psychiatr* 33, 461–468.

Gurland B (1996) Epidemiology of psychiatric disorders, in *Comprehensive Review of Geriatric Psychiatry*, 2nd edn. (eds Sadavoy J, Lazarus LW, Jarvik LF *et al.*). American Psychiatric Press, Washington DC, pp. 3–41.

Hersov L (1994) Faecal soiling, in *Child and Adolescent Psychiatry: Modern Approaches*, 3rd edn. (eds Rutter M, Taylor E and Hersov L). Blackwell Scientific, Oxford, UK, pp. 520–528.

Kasen S, Cohen P, Skodol AE *et al.* (2001) Childhood depression and adult personality disorder: Alternative pathways of continuity. *Arch Gen Psychiatr* 58, 231–236.

Kessler RC, McGonagle KA, Zhao S *et al.* (1994) Lifetime and 12-month prevalence of DSM-III-R psychiatric disorders in the United States: Results from the National Comorbidity Survey. *Arch Gen Psychiatr* 51, 8–19.

March JS (1993) What constitutes a stressor? The "criterion A" issue, in *Posttraumatic Stress Disorder: DSM-IV and Beyond* (eds Davidson JRT and Foa EB). American Psychiatric Press, Washington DC, pp. 37–54.

Paikoff RL and Brooks-Gunn J (1994) Psychosexual development across the lifespan, in *Development Through Life: A Handbook for Clinicians* (eds Rutter M and Hay DF). Blackwell Scientific, Oxford, UK, pp. 558–582.

Popkin MK, Callies AL, and Colon EA (1987) A framework for the study of medical depression. *Psychosomatics* 28, 27–33.

Regestein QR (1994) Primary hypersomnia, in *DSM-IV Sourcebook*, Vol. 1 (eds Widiger TA, Frances AJ, Pincus HA *et al.*). American Psychiatric Association, Washington DC, pp. 619–626.

Regier DA, Boyd JH, Burke JD Jr. *et al.* (1988) One-month prevalence of mental disorders in the United States, based on five Epidemiologic Catchment Area sites. *Arch Gen Psychiatr* 45, 977–986.

Rutter M (1989a) Pathways from childhood to adult life. *J Child Psychol Psychiatr* 30, 23–51.

Rutter M and Sandberg S (1985) Epidemiology of child psychiatric disorder: Methodological issues and some substantive findings. *Child Psychiatr Hum Dev* 15, 209–233.

Rutter M, Taylor E and Hersov L (eds) (1994) *Child and Adolescent Psychiatry: Modern Approaches*, 3rd edn. Blackwell Scientific, Oxford, UK.

Shaffer D (1994) Enuresis, in *Child and Adolescent Psychiatry: Modern Approaches*, 3rd edn. (eds Rutter M, Taylor E and Hersov L). Blackwell Scientific, Oxford, UK, pp. 505–519.

Shalev AY, Peri T, Canetti L *et al.* (1996) Predictors of PTSD in injured trauma survivors: A prospective study. *Am J Psychiatr* 153, 219–225.

Skodol AE, Oldham JM, Hyler SE *et al.* (1993) Comorbidity of DSM-III-R eating disorders and personality disorders. *Int J Eat Disord* 14, 403–416.

Spiegel D and Cardena E (1991) Disintegrated experience: The dissociative disorders revisited. *J Abnorm Psychol* 100, 366–378.

Strober M, Hanna G and McCracken J (1989) Bipolar disorder, in *Handbook of Child Psychiatric Diagnosis* (eds Last CG and Hersen M). John Wiley, New York, pp. 299–316.

Tantum D (1988) Asperger's syndrome. *J Child Psychol Psychiatr* 29, 245–253.

Wolke D (1994) Sleeping and feeding across the lifespan, in *Development Through Life: A Handbook for Clinicians* (eds Rutter M and Hay DF). Blackwell Scientific, Oxford, UK, pp. 517–557.

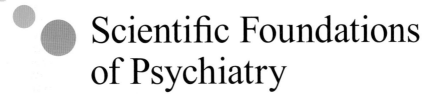

Scientific Foundations
of Psychiatry

9 Psychiatric Epidemiology

Overview

At its most basic level, the discipline of psychiatric epidemiology is the study of the patterns of mental disorders, including how frequently disorders occur, how they are distributed in populations, and what are associated risk factors. Psychiatric epidemiology also defines the time course of mental disorders including their onset, duration and recurrence. Recently, the field has greatly expanded and now includes detailed examinations of the natural history of psychiatric disorders, genetic epidemiology, the relationships between physical and mental disorders, and studies of the use and outcomes of mental health treatments. This expansion has required significant advances and developments in psychiatric epidemiologic methods (Tsuang and Tohen, 2002).

Important characteristics that distinguish psychiatric epidemiological research from other clinical investigations are the inclusion of representative samples and the application of systematic methods for determining diagnosis or outcome. The specific type of sample and choice of mental health measure depend on the goal of the study. Three types of samples are generally used in epidemiology. For studies aimed at establishing prevalence and incidence rates, the population-based survey is the optimal method. Complex sampling procedures have been developed to ensure random selection for both single-stage and two-stage studies. For studies of rare disorders, identified patients are usually ascertained from registries or a representative set of psychiatric treatment facilities. However, because only a minority of individuals with diagnosable disorders are ever treated for psychiatric problems within the mental health care system (Regier et al., 1993; Kessler et al., 1994; Wang et al., 2000), these sources may omit true case patients who do not present for treatment.

The development of structured diagnostic interview schedules tailored to clear operationalized diagnostic criteria was the crucial element underlying the recent progress in psychiatric epidemiology. As a result of the development of structured diagnostic interview schedules, the need to establish the prevalence of specific disorders was finally realized, at least within the limits of our current ability to operationalize mental disorders and within the constraints inherent in interview data (Fennig and Bromet, 1992). Estimates suggest that approximately 12% of children (Institute of Medicine, 1989) and 15% of adults (Regier et al., 1988) currently meet criteria for one or more mental disorders. More precise estimates will be possible as more sensitive diagnostic tools become available.

The Scope of Inquiry in Psychiatric Epidemiology

"Epidemiology" is derived from the Greek words *epidemos*, meaning "among the people", and is defined as the study of "the patterns of disease occurrence in human populations and of the factors that influence these patterns" (MacMahon and Pugh, 1970). Because the ultimate goal of epidemiological research is to understand the cause of disease and prevent its occurrence, epidemiology is the backbone of public health.

Important advances have been made in psychiatric epidemiology, largely since World War II. To make such advances, investigators have had to overcome formidable problems that are unique to the study of psychiatric disorders. Foremost among their achievements has been the development of the ability to define mental disorders reliably and efficiently. This accomplishment has in turn allowed investigators to conduct descriptive analyses that have yielded much-needed estimates of the incidence, prevalence, age at onset, and frequency of recurrence of mental disorders.

The ability to accurately categorize cases and noncases has also been essential for allowing psychiatric epidemiologists to progress from simple descriptive work establishing rates to analytical research aimed at identifying risk factors, as well as biological and psychosocial variables that modify the effects of these risk factors. Examples of promising areas in which there has been significant research activity recently include investigations of the genetic bases for psychiatric disorders (Risch and Merikangas, 1990) and the modification of risk by environmental exposures, especially in the prenatal period (Neugebauer et al., 1999).

Whereas traditional epidemiology has largely been concerned with the occurrence and causes of disease, clinical epidemiology has emerged as a closely related discipline which seeks to identify the occurrence and determinants of clinical outcomes from illnesses (Weiss, 1985; Sackett et al., 1985). Clinical epidemiologic studies employ the same principles and methods of population-based epidemiology, but are usually conducted among clinical samples. Recent clinical epidemiologic investigations such as the NIMH Collaborative Program on the Psychobiology of Depression (CPPD) and the Harvard–Brown Anxiety Research Program have provided important information on prognostic factors associated with the natural history of psychiatric disorders (Judd et al., 1998; Rogers et al., 1999). Other examples include two countywide longitudinal studies of first-admission psychosis (Beiser et al., 1989; Bromet et al., 1992), which included patients from all facilities in the respective geographical regions, or a follow-up study of first-episode psychotic patients admitted to the McLean Hospital in Belmont, Massachusetts (Tohen et al., 1992). Psychopharmacoepidemiology has been an especially fast growing component of clinical epidemiologic inquiry (Wang et al., 2002b), in part because psychotropic medications are now widely used in both general medical and psychiatric populations. Many psychopharmacoepidemiologic studies have consisted of

Essentials of Psychiatry   Jerald Kay and Allan Tasman

descriptions of the patterns and predictors of psychiatric medication use (Olfson *et al.*, 2002; Wang *et al.*, 2000) as well as investigations of unanticipated hazards from psychiatric medications (Wang *et al.*, 2001a, 2001b, 2001c, 2002a, 2002c).

Clinical epidemiologic research has also begun to evaluate the economic costs associated with mental disorders, both the direct costs for provision of mental health services as well as the indirect costs to society, secondary to the disability caused disorders. The WHO Global Burden of Disease (GBD) study (Murray and Lopez, 1996) identified mental disorders as among the most costly diseases in the world. For example, major depression was the single most burdensome disease in the world among individuals under 45 years of age. Another closely related area of inquiry is that of mental health services research. This discipline investigates the patterns of utilization of mental health services, unmet needs for treatment, barriers to help seeking, the appropriateness and quality of treatments, and premature dropout from treatment (Kessler *et al.*, 2001; Wang *et al.*, 2000, 2002; Edlund *et al.*, 2002).

The accumulation of information on risk factors for mental disorders, their outcomes, and treatment has in turn led to another important line of inquiry in psychiatric epidemiology, namely, interventional research. In addition to efficacy trials of psychiatric treatments conducted under rigorously controlled conditions (Tohen *et al.*, 2000, 2002), recent experimental studies have also begun to include effectiveness trials of "real-world" treatment strategies (Katon *et al.*, 1995, 1996; Simon *et al.*, 2000; Wells *et al.*, 2000). Finally, the proliferation of effective but costly interventions, coupled with growing constraints on health care budgets, have also made it imperative to study not only the effectiveness of interventions but also their cost-effectiveness and cost-benefits. For this reason, economic analyses now frequently accompany efficacy and effectiveness trials of interventions (Schoenbaum *et al.*, 2001).

Epidemiological Methods

Conducting investigations across this broad scope of inquiry has required the development of rigorous psychiatric epidemiologic methods. The following section contains a brief description of some of the basic elements of this methodology.

Measures of Disease Frequency

Epidemiological studies examine the incidence and prevalence rates of disorders in populations at risk and the factors associated with onset and recurrence. A rate is determined by the number of cases (the numerator) divided by the population at risk (the denominator).

Incidence

Incidence rates refer to new cases that arise in a healthy population during a fixed time. The most commonly applied incidence rate in psychiatric epidemiology is the cumulative incidence rate, also known as the "incidence proportion" (Selvin, 1991), that is, the proportion of a population at risk that has a disease during a specified time. The range is from 0 to 1. The numerator includes new cases of the illness, and the denominator is composed of individuals at risk of becoming diseased for the first time. In cumulative incidence, the duration of the observation needs to be defined (e.g., new cases in 1 month, 1 year, or 5 years).

Cumulative incidence is appropriate when a study has a fixed cohort design (i.e., when all of the members of the cohort are observed for the same time). However, when attrition occurs, the cumulative incidence rate is a less desirable measure. Individuals lost to follow-up who would have become case patients are excluded from the numerator, whereas the denominator, which is the total population, remains unchanged. Moreover, those who become lost to follow-up are often a biased subgroup of the original study population (Eaton *et al.*, 1992). Therefore, cumulative incidence should be considered most reliable when there is a small loss to follow-up during the specified time. When loss to follow-up occurs or when the occurrence of a health outcome is measured in a dynamic cohort (i.e., when members of the cohort come in and out) different statistical adjustments must be employed (Selvin, 1991).

$$\text{Cumulative incidence} = \frac{\text{number of new cases}}{\text{total population at risk}}$$

In epidemiology, incidence rate refers to the number of new cases occurring in a specified time period divided by the sum of time periods of the observation for all individuals in the population at risk, or person-time (Rothman and Greenland, 1998). In effect, this statistic measures the instantaneous force of morbidity or disease occurrence (Rothman and Greenland, 1998). Miettinen (1985) also referred to it as incidence density. The denominator person-time is the observational experience during which a particular outcome may occur. The range of an incidence rate is 0 to infinity. The incidence rate is measured in units of the reciprocal of time (time^{-1}). The units of incidence rates are time^{-1}. Because the units and the numerical value of an incidence rate are difficult to interpret, incidence rates are usually compared with each other to obtain incidence rate ratios.

$$\text{Incidence rate} = \frac{\text{number of new cases}}{\text{person-years}}$$

Prevalence

Prevalence rates measure the proportion of individuals who have the disease at a specified point or period in time. Incidence refers only to new-onset cases, whereas prevalence includes all new, recurrent, or chronic cases in the numerator and the entire population, including those with a history of the disorder, in the denominator. The point prevalence rate is the proportion of a population affected by a disease at a given point in time. Period prevalence refers to the proportion of a population affected by a disease during a specified time period, such as 6 months, 1 year, or lifetime. Prevalence rates are influenced by the duration of a disease. For nonchronic disorders, such as major depression, the point prevalence is usually lower than the period prevalence. For chronic conditions, such as schizophrenia, the point prevalence and period prevalence are expected to be similar.

$$\text{Prevalence rate} = \frac{\text{number of cases}}{\text{total population at risk}}$$

In general, prevalence data are less useful than incidence data for etiological research. Prevalence is determined not just by factors that cause a disease but also by factors secondary to the disease itself. On the other hand, prevalence measures are useful in public health or service utilization situations. For instance, the geographical location and planning of specific services of a community mental health center are usually based on findings from prevalence studies.

Measures of Association

Incidence rates can be used to calculate two types of effects. One is the attributable risk, or the absolute effect. The attributable risk is the difference between two incidence rates. This is most commonly used in comparing rates of exposed with nonexposed populations. The second type of effect is the relative risk, which is the ratio of the incidence rates of the exposed and unexposed groups. In case–control studies, it is not possible to estimate incidence rates. Relative risks, however, can be calculated with an odds ratio, which is the ratio of the odds of exposure of the case patients to that of the control subjects.

Instruments to Identify Cases

The calculations defined in the preceding assume a fundamental requirement of epidemiological research, the ability to define a case. Historically, defining "caseness" in psychiatric epidemiologic studies has been difficult. The development of structured diagnostic interview schedules tailored to clear operationalized diagnostic criteria has been the crucial element underlying the recent progress in psychiatric epidemiology.

The feasibility and benefits of structured, or semistructured, interview schedules that could systematically elicit criteria for objectively defined disorders further became evident after the appearance and widespread use of instruments such as the Schedule for Affective Disorders and Schizophrenia (SADS) (Endicott and Spitzer, 1978), the companion interview for the Research Diagnostic Criteria (Spitzer et al., 1978). The SADS and the Research Diagnostic Criteria were originally developed for use by psychiatrists in the multisite collaborative study of the psychobiology of depression sponsored by the NIMH (Katz et al., 1979). Other standardized psychiatric interviews that have been commonly used are the present state examination (Wing et al., 1974) and its successor, the schedule for clinical assessment in neuropsychiatry (Wing et al., 1990); the structured clinical interview for DSM-III-R (Spitzer et al., 1992); and the diagnostic interview for genetic studies developed by the NIMH-sponsored centers for genetic linkage research (Nurnberger et al., 1994). Puig-Antich and colleagues have also developed an instrument for use with children, the Kiddie-SADS, that has been modified for epidemiological studies (Orvaschel, 1985).

The first widely used of a new family of instruments is the Diagnostic Interview Schedule (Robins et al., 1981). The Diagnostic Interview Schedule was originally designed for the five-site epidemiological catchment area (ECA) study of DSM-III disorders (Regier et al., 1984). The ECA methodology and findings are described in more detail later. Subsequent versions of the Diagnostic Interview Schedule incorporated revised DSM-III (DSM-III-R) as well as *Diagnostic and Statistical Manual of Mental Disorders*, Fourth Edition (DSM-IV) criteria. In the field of children's mental health, fully structured diagnostic interview schedules have also been designed, such as the Diagnostic Interview Schedule for children (Costello et al. 1988; Jensen et al., 1995).

Another fully structured instrument is the composite international diagnostic interview (CIDI), developed in collaboration with the World Health Organization (WHO 1990) and NIMH (Wittchen et al., 1991). The CIDI was designed to be used with both DSM and ICD diagnostic criteria and to be available in multiple languages.

Psychometric Properties of Instruments

Because classification in psychiatric epidemiology is based on self-report or interviewer-based rating scales and questionnaires, several features of an instrument must be tested and quantified. An instrument's sensitivity (proportion of those with true-positive results identified as such by the study instrument) and specificity (proportion of those with true-negative results identified as such by the study instrument) are one set of measures. For an instrument to be useful in epidemiology, it should have high sensitivity and at least moderately high specificity.

To identify cases accurately, an instrument used for case identification must be reliable and valid. Reliability refers to the reproducibility of a measure (i.e., the consistency of measurement regardless of the rater, the situation, or the time of administration). Interrater agreement is usually calculated with statistical methods, such as the kappa statistic, that control for chance agreement. Test–retest reliability, or temporal stability, is calculated with product-moment or intraclass correlation coefficients. Validity refers to whether a construct is measured accurately. This concept is more difficult to establish in psychiatry because there is no "gold standard" or biological marker for the disorders under study.

Risk Factor Identification

Risk factors are characteristics whose presence increases the chances for development of a disease. A true risk factor must exist before a disease develops. For example, being male and having a family history of alcoholism are risk factors for the development of alcoholism (Merikangas, 1990). When a variable cannot be definitively proved to predate the onset of a disorder, it is best conceptualized as a correlate. For example, socioenvironmental factors, such as adverse life events and chronic strain, that are statistically associated with the development of depressive disorders should usually be regarded as correlates because it is usually not possible to disentangle the causal sequence of these relationships.

Types of Epidemiological Studies

In general, epidemiological studies are designed to find associations between exposures and health outcomes. A main concern in epidemiological studies is the selection of study groups on the basis of either disease status or exposure status. Epidemiological studies (Table 9.1) can be classified as 1) experimental, 2) quasi-experimental, and 3) nonexperimental or observational.

Experimental Studies

The main distinction of experimental studies is that the investigator assigns the status of exposure or nonexposure to each subject.

Table 9.1 Types of Study Designs
Experimental
Quasi-experimental
Nonexperimental (observational)
Longitudinal
Case–control studies
Cohort studies
Prospective
Retrospective
Cross-sectional

The assignment to the exposure group becomes part of the study protocol. Once subjects are assigned to exposed or nonexposed groups, they are observed for a time, and observations about changes in morbidity are recorded. The most common experimental design is the clinical trial, in which clinical populations are exposed to a specific treatment protocol to measure an outcome, usually resolution of symptoms. To ensure the integrity of a clinical trial, three main elements are necessary (Miettinen, 1985): 1) "randomization", to ensure comparability of the populations; 2) "placebo", to ensure comparability of the effects; and 3) "blinding", to ensure comparability of information.

In randomization, subjects are randomly assigned to different exposure groups to attempt to ensure that subjects in each group have similar clinical and demographic characteristics. Randomization should theoretically achieve a balance of unknown factors in the different groups.

To control comparability of extraneous effects of a specified treatment, experimental studies use placebo-controlled groups. A placebo controls for factors that may affect the outcome of the study independently of the exposure status. For example, if subjects in an open trial are aware of what medication they receive, this knowledge could bias their response to the treatment. Similarly, subjects who are aware of being in an untreated control group could respond over time in a biased fashion. Thus, one goal in assigning patients at random to treatment or placebo-control groups is to minimize observation bias. In a single-blind study, only the patient is unaware of the actual treatment. In a double-blind study, the investigator and the subject of investigation are unaware of treatment assignment. In a triple-blind study, the data analyst is also not informed of the meaning of the group assignment code.

Quasi-experimental Studies

Natural experiments that permit comparisons of two populations, one that receives an exposure and the other that does not, are referred to as quasi-experimental studies. To be considered quasi-experimental, baseline data must have been collected before the exposure event. Without that requirement, the study is simply a retrospective observational study.

Nonexperimental Studies

Nonexperimental studies are divided into cross-sectional and longitudinal designs.

Cross-sectional Designs

Cross-sectional designs are typically employed in surveys aimed at providing data on the distribution of disorders in the population. Differences in rates by basic demographic data are also usually derived. In epidemiology, cross-sectional designs are usually best employed when causal hypotheses are not being tested. For example, when a community wants to investigate the distribution of an illness to decide on the need for psychiatric services, a cross-sectional survey is highly appropriate.

Longitudinal Designs

Longitudinal designs are divided into case–control and cohort studies and are characterized by a time interval between cause and effect. In cross-sectional studies, there is no interval between exposure and illness, which are measured at the same point in time.

Case–Control Studies.   In case–control studies, subjects are defined in terms of having (case patients) or not having (control patients) the disease of interest. The groups are compared in terms of history of exposure. In general, two types of control groups are used: hospital control groups and population control groups. The selection of the control group is a key point in terms of validity. Control subjects should be selected independently of exposure status. Case and control patients may be matched on different characteristics, the key issue being that control patients should represent those individuals who, if they had the disease, would be selected as case patients (Miettinen, 1985).

Case–control studies can assess whether a risk factor is more prevalent in case than in control patients but may not be able to establish the rate of disease after exposure to that risk factor. For the purpose of estimating the true rate of disease associated with an exposure, the prospective cohort study design is the preferable methodology.

Cohort Studies.   In cohort studies, subjects are identified in terms of exposure or nonexposure status and are observed for a specified time to determine the presence or absence of a health outcome. Cohort studies are divided into prospective and retrospective. In prospective cohort studies, the exposure or nonexposure status is defined when the study is initiated. The subjects of investigation are followed up into the future to determine disease or nondisease status. In retrospective studies, the status of exposed or nonexposed is defined in the present. In prospective cohort studies, exposures of the present are evaluated; in retrospective cohort studies, exposures of the past are being evaluated. Cohort groups share the common exposure status and are observed to ascertain the presence or absence of a disease or outcome.

For comparison groups, a cohort study can use an internal subset of the population under study, by comparing exposed with unexposed members of the cohort, or an external comparison. A comparison cohort can be selected from a similarly defined population.

The major strength of the cohort design is the possibility of estimating a temporal relationship between exposure and disease. With a cohort study, it is possible to study rare exposures and to evaluate multiple outcomes from a single exposure. The limitation of cohort studies is primarily one of feasibility because most such studies are expensive and involve study populations who are difficult to recruit and maintain for follow-up.

Threats to Validity in Epidemiological Studies

An essential feature of epidemiological studies is a comparison of two groups in terms of presence or absence of exposure or presence or absence of disease. For the measurements to be comparable, the investigator should ensure absence of bias. Biases can be divided into three general types: 1) selection bias; 2) information or observation bias; and 3) confounding bias.

Selection Bias

Selection bias can arise when the sampling procedure is influenced *a priori* by the disease or the exposure.

Another example, referred to as self-selection bias, occurs when subjects who have been exposed to an event are more likely to participate in a study if they have the disease or prodromal stages of the disease under study. A similar type of selection bias can occur when subjects are solicited from newspaper or other similar advertisements.

Information (Observation) Bias

In case–control studies, information bias occurs when the details about prior exposure are obtained in a noncomparable manner or are subject to poor recall. To minimize such bias, exposure data should be collected without knowledge of disease status. This procedure is known as blindness. However, because of selective recall, when the sole source of information is the affected individual, this type of bias sometimes presents insurmountable problems.

Confounding Bias

Confounding bias results when a third factor that is a cause of the disease under study is also associated with the exposure. A confounding factor is a cause of the disease under study independent of its association with the exposure.

Examples of Psychiatric Epidemiologic Studies

Dohrenwend and Dohrenwend (1982) have divided the growth of psychiatric epidemiological research into three periods, or generations. This section describes the key studies and prevalence rates from the most recent of these periods.

Third-generation Studies

The methodology for the third-generation epidemiological studies reflected the view in American psychiatry in the early 1970s that mental illness could be delineated into discrete, operational categories. These changes in nosology were exemplified in the 1970s with the development of the Feighner criteria at Washington University in St Louis (Robins and Guze, 1970; Feighner et al., 1972) and culminated in the creation of DSM-III a decade later. By operationalizing diagnoses with specific criteria, it was possible to create structured diagnostic assessments to elicit the symptoms needed for these categories. Preliminary evidence about the utility of using diagnostic procedures in community samples was obtained in a third-wave follow-up of the New Haven Study noted before. In this study, Weissman and colleagues (1978) successfully administered the SADS-L in a community population. This and other studies (Bromet et al., 1982) demonstrated that structured diagnostic instruments designed for clinical investigations could produce meaningful findings when administered in population-based studies.

The third-generation studies, thus, are characterized primarily by the use of structured diagnostic assessment procedures. In the next sections, we describe two of the largest third-generation studies, the NIMH-sponsored ECA project (Regier et al., 1984, 1985, Robins et al., 1991) and the NCS (Kessler et al., 1994).

The Epidemiological Catchment Area Study

In response to the 1978 President's Commission on Mental Health Report, NIMH sponsored the Epidemiological Catchment Area (ECA) project to determine the prevalence of mental disorders in specific sites and the proportion receiving mental health services (Regier et al., 1984). Parallel to the planning of the ECA study, the APA published the DSM-III (American Psychiatric Association, 1980), which had clearly defined operational criteria that facilitated case definition. Thus, the concept of a case as a discrete entity that had been achieved in the late 1970s permitted the categorical determination of psychiatric caseness as opposed to the dimensional assessment of symptom impairment. As a prelude to the ECA, the NIMH cosponsored the development of the Diagnostic Interview Schedule (reviewed above).

The basic design involved face-to-face baseline interviews with random samples of adults selected from the catchment areas, 6-month telephone follow-up interviews to obtain interim information on medical and psychiatric service use, and 1-year face-to-face interviews with the original sample. The initial response rate ranged from 68% (Los Angeles) to 79% (St Louis and Durham) (Leaf et al., 1991). Overall, 12% of the original respondents were lost to or refused to participate in the follow-up interview. Eaton and collaborators (1992) reported that failure to be tracked was associated with being male, young, unmarried and Hispanic; refusal to participate was associated with being older, married and uneducated.

Prevalence

Overall, 32.2% of the adults included in the five sites met criteria for one or more of the assessed mental disorders during their lifetime (Table 9.2. Phobias and alcohol abuse and dependence were the most common mental disorders (Regier et al., 1985). The lifetime prevalence for phobia was 12.5%, and the 1-month prevalence was 6.2%. The rates for drug abuse and dependence were 5.9% for lifetime and 1.3% for 1-month prevalence.

The ECA study investigators did extensive analyses of the variation in prevalence rates by demographic characteristics.

Table 9.2	Lifetime Prevalence Rate of Specific Diagnostic Interview Schedule (DIS)/DSM-III Disorders*

Disorder	Estimated Prevalence Rate (% Population)
Any DIS disorder covered	32.2
Any DIS disorder except cognitive impairment, personality disorder, and substance abuse	19.6
Substance use disorders	16.4
Alcohol abuse and dependence	13.3
Drug abuse and dependence	5.9
Schizophrenia and schizophreniform disorders	1.5
Affective disorders	8.3
Manic episode	0.8
Major depressive episode	5.8
Dysthymia	3.3
Anxiety disorders	14.6
Generalized anxiety disorder	8.5
Phobia	12.5
Panic	1.6
Obsessive–compulsive disorder	2.5
Somatization disorder	0.1
Personality disorder	
Antisocial personality	2.5
Cognitive impairment (severe)	1.3

*Based on five ECA sites standardized to the 1980 US census.
Source: Regier DA, Boyd JH, Burke JD Jr. *et al.* (1988) One-month prevalence of mental disorders in the United States. Based on five Epidemiologic Catchment Area sites. *Arch Gen Psychiatr* 45, 977–986. Copyright 1988 American Medical Association.

Table 9.3	Epidemiological Catchment Area Study: Lifetime Prevalence Rate of Any Psychiatric Disorder	
	N	Lifetime Prevalence (%)
Total	19 640	
Sex		
Men	8419	36
Women	11 221	30
Age (yr)		
<30	4872	37
30–44	4650	39
45–64	4194	27
65+	5912	21
Ethnicity		
White	13 091	32
Black	4697	38
Hispanic	1606	33
Education		
Not completed high school	8818	36
High school or more	10 565	30
Occupational status of men (30–64 yr)		
Total	3452	35
Unemployed	774	48
Unskilled	599	40
Skilled or higher	2061	30
Rural/urban		
Urban	4694	34
Rural	2107	32
Marital history		
Married and never divorced or separated	9216	24
Single and never cohabited for 1 yr	3424	33
Ever divorced or separated	5906	44
Unmarried and cohabited	986	52

For lifetime diagnosis, 36% of men at some point suffered from an addictive or mental disorder, compared with 30% of women (Table 9.3).

The pooled 1-month prevalence rates for the five sites (see Table 9.4) was 15.4% for all ages for any DSM-III disorder. The age group 25 to 44 years had the highest overall rate of 17.3%. Although this age pattern was also true for women, men aged 18 to 24 years had the highest overall rate. This occurred because of the peak in rates of drug abuse and dependence in men in this age group. Anxiety disorders were most prevalent at 11.7% in women 25 to 44 years old, compared with only 4.7% for men in the same group. The overall prevalence for all affective disorders was 5.1%; the age group with the highest prevalence was women 25 to 44 years old.

Incidence

Incidence rates were calculated based on the 12-month follow-up assessments of healthy individuals found during the initial assessments (Regier *et al.*, 1993).

During the 1-year follow-up period, 6% of the total population had one or more new disorders (Regier *et al.*, 1993). Also, 5.7% of those with a history of a mental disorder suffered a relapse or a new condition in the 1-year period for a total of 12.3% of new cases in 1 year.

Use of Mental Health Services

Although 28.1% of the sample had diagnosable mental or addictive disorders, only 14.7% (23 million) received care, indicating that a disproportionate number of individuals suffering from mental and addictive disorders did not receive treatment. Conversely, although 22% of respondents who had recently used a medical care facility met criteria for a DSM-III disorder, 17% of nonusers had a diagnosable illness (Regier *et al.*, 1993; Eaton *et al.*, 1992; Narrow *et al.*, 1993, Kessler *et al.*, 1987). The disorders making the greatest contribution were alcohol abuse and dependence in men and major depression in women. The ECA study found that 0.9% received inpatient treatment in a specialty mental and addictive disorders facility during a 1-year period. Among individuals with any DSM-III disorder who received mental health services, 28.5% sought treatment from either a mental health clinician or medical physician (see Table 9.5).

Comorbidity of Mental and Substance Use Disorders

The ECA study provided valuable data about the prevalence of comorbidity of alcohol and substance use disorders with mental disorders (Regier *et al.*, 1985, 1990). Before the ECA study, most of the information about comorbidity came from populations in treatment settings. Since the early 1950s, it has repeatedly been found that patients in clinical settings typically present themselves for treatment because they have more than one disorder, a phenomenon first described by Berkson (1946). Thus, clinical populations provide a biased (and inflated) view of comorbidity.

The ECA study defined comorbidity as the occurrence of more than one disorder and did not require that the disorders overlap temporally. Up to 29% of individuals with a mental disorder suffer from a comorbid substance use disorder. Similarly, individuals with alcohol use disorder have twice the risk of having a comorbid mental disorder and more than five times the risk of having a comorbid drug use disorder. Among individuals with alcohol use disorders, the most common comorbid mental disorder was anxiety disorder, with a prevalence of 19.4%. For individuals with drug use disorder, 22% suffered from a mental disorder.

In summary, findings from the ECA confirmed the widespread and impairing nature of mental disorders reported in the second-generation community studies described above. The methodologic rigor with which the ECA was conducted was instrumental at dispelling the disbelief and criticism of methodology that frequently accompanied second-generation studies. The rates in the five ECA sites confirmed the high prevalence of untreated mental disorder. ECA results, such as the finding that individuals with mental disorders were relatively more likely to use general medical services compared with those without disorders, raised provocative questions for a new generation of psychiatric epidemiologists.

The National Comorbidity Survey

Because the ECA study was conducted in five specific sites, each selected because it contained unique population characteristics,

Table 9.4   One-Month Prevalence Rate (%) of Specific Diagnostic Interview Schedule (DIS)–DSM-III Disorders*

	Any DIS Disorder	Any DIS Disorder Except Cognitive Impairment, Substance Use, and Antisocial Personality	Drug Abuse and Dependence	Schizophrenia	Schizophreniform Disorders	Anxiety Disorders	Phobia	Panic	Obsessive–Compulsive Disorder	Affective Disorders	Manic Episode	Manic–Depressive Episode	Dysthymia
Both Sexes													
All ages	15.4	11.2	1.3	0.6	0.1	7.3	6.2	0.5	1.3	5.1	0.4	2.2	3.3
18–24	16.9	11.0	3.5	0.7	0.1	7.7	6.4	0.4	1.8	4.4	0.6	2.2	2.2
25–44	17.3	13.0	1.5	0.9	0.1	8.3	6.9	0.7	1.6	6.4	0.6	3.0	4.0
45–64	13.3	10.7	0.1	0.4	0.0	6.6	6.0	0.6	0.9	5.2	0.2	2.0	3.8
65+	12.3	7.4	0.0	0.1	0.0	5.5	4.8	0.1	0.8	2.5	0.0	0.7	1.8
Men													
All ages	14.0	7.6	1.8	0.6	0.1	4.7	3.8	0.3	1.1	3.5	0.3	1.6	2.2
18–24	16.5	8.4	4.8	0.7	0.2	4.9	3.6	0.4	1.7	3.4	0.4	1.5	2.2
25–44	15.4	8.2	2.3	0.8	0.1	4.7	3.5	0.3	1.2	4.5	0.5	2.2	2.8
45–64	11.9	7.5	0.1	0.6	0.1	5.1	4.8	0.5	0.6	3.1	0.2	1.2	2.0
65+	10.5	4.5	0.0	0.1	0.0	3.6	2.9	0.0	0.7	1.4	0.0	0.4	1.0
Women													
All ages	16.6	14.5	0.7	0.6	0.1	9.7	8.4	0.7	1.5	6.6	0.4	2.9	4.2
18–24	17.3	13.5	2.4	0.7	0.0	10.4	9.1	0.4	1.8	5.3	0.8	2.9	2.2
25–44	19.2	17.7	0.8	1.1	0.2	11.7	10.2	1.1	1.9	8.2	0.6	3.9	5.1
45–64	14.6	13.7	0.0	0.3	0.0	8.0	7.0	0.7	1.2	7.2	0.2	2.6	5.4
65+	13.6	9.4	0.0	0.1	0.0	6.8	6.1	0.2	0.9	3.3	0.0	0.9	2.3

*Based on five ECA sites.

Reprinted with permission from Regier DA, Boyd JH, Burke JD Jr. *et al.* (1988) One-month prevalence of mental disorders in the United States. Based on five Epidemiologic Catchment Area sites. *Arch Gen Psychiatr* 45, 977–986. Copyright 1988 American Medical Association.

the findings could not be readily extrapolated to the USA as a whole. Therefore, the NCS was designed to estimate the prevalence and comorbidity of psychiatric and substance use disorders in the mainland USA. The NCS was designed by Kessler and colleagues (1994) as the first population-based study administered to a nationally representative sample in the USA using a structured diagnostic interview. It built upon a history of conducting (second-generation) national studies of the prevalence of psychiatric symptoms in the USA at the University of Michigan. The NCS also built on the knowledge and experience of the ECA study. Among its many advantages, it uniformly included a set of demographic and psychosocial risk factors.

Table 9.5	Epidemiological Catchment Area Study: Mental Health Visits in Service Sector in 1 Year	
Diagnosis	Proportion with Mental Health Visits (%)
Any Diagnostic Interview Schedule/DSM-III disorder	28.5
Any Diagnostic Interview Schedule/DSM-III disorder except substance abuse	31.9
Any mental disorder with comorbid substance use	37.4
Substance use disorder	23.6
Alcohol abuse and dependence	22.0
Drug abuse and dependence	29.8
Schizophrenia and schizophreniform disorders	64.3
Affective disorders	45.7
Manic episode	60.9
Major depressive episode	53.9
Dysthymia	42.1
Anxiety disorders	32.7
Phobia	31.1
Panic	58.8
Obsessive–compulsive disorder	45.1
Somatization disorder	69.7
Antisocial personality	31.1
Severe cognitive impairment	17.0

Prevalence

Table 9.6 presents the NCS 1-year and lifetime prevalence rates of the various psychiatric disorders. Lifetime prevalence rates are the proportion of individuals who ever experienced a disorder, and 1-year prevalence represents the proportion of individuals who experienced a disorder in the year before the interview. The lifetime prevalence for any DSM-III-R disorder was 48.7%, and the 12-month prevalence was 27.7%. When grouped by diagnostic category, the lifetime prevalence rates were 24.9% for anxiety disorders, 26.6% for substance abuse and dependence, and 19.3% for affective disorders. As expected, anxiety and affective disorders were more common in women, and substance abuse was more common in men.

Comorbidity

An important focus of the NCS was the assessment of comorbidity. Interestingly, whereas 21% of the sample experienced only one disorder, 14% met criteria for three or more lifetime disorders. Furthermore, among individuals with a lifetime disorder, 53.9% had three or more lifetime disorders. Among individuals with a disorder occurring in the past 12 months, 58.9% experienced three or more disorders. The level of comorbidity was most dramatic for individuals with a severe disorder in the past 12 months, defined as active mania, nonaffective psychosis, or active disorder of other types that either resulted in hospitalization or created severe role impairment. In that subset of respondents, 89.5% had three or more disorders.

Risk Factors and Correlates

The NCS also yielded important data on demographic correlates and potential risk factors for mental disorders. Several earlier patterns of association observed for gender and other characteristics were confirmed.

Use of Mental Health Services

The NCS also examined the patterns of use of health services by the respondents. Only 40% of individuals with a mental disorder ever received professional care, and only 25% received their care in the mental health specialty sector. On the other hand, 60% of individuals with three or more comorbid disorders received professional help, 40% in the mental health specialty sector. Furthermore, one third of persons with three or more comorbid disorders received professional help in the past year compared with only 20% of those with one disorder. These findings indicate that the use of health services is concentrated in the segment of the population with a high degree of comorbidity.

Subsequent analyses of service utilization in the NCS have shed light on the magnitude and potential determinants of important subcomponents of the problem of unmet needs for mental health treatment. For example, while only a minority with active major depression received any care in the prior year, an even smaller percentage (7%) received treatment that could be considered minimally adequate (Katz et al., 1998). Even among the extremely vulnerable and impaired population that met criteria for active serious mental illness (SMI), only 40% received any treatment in the prior year (Kessler et al., 2001) and only 15% received care that could be considered minimally adequate (Wang et al., 2002). Among NCS respondents with mental disorders who received treatment in the prior year, 19% dropped out prematurely (Edlund et al., 2002).

The Ongoing NCS Research Program

The NCS will continue to yield important new findings in the future, though a new series of landmark studies are currently in the field (Kessler and Walters, 2002). In one ongoing component of this research, the National Comorbidity Survey-2 (NCS-2), the baseline NCS respondents were reinterviewed a decade later. When linked with the prospectively-collected data that respondents had provided in the baseline NCS, the NCS-2 will be an important source of information on the patterns and predictors of the course of mental disorders. The NCS-2 will also provide investigators with the ability to study the effects of primary disorders on the development and course of secondary disorders. An additional survey with a new national sample of 10 000 respondents, the national comorbidity survey-replication (NCS-R), is also being conducted together with the NCS-2. The NCS-R data will provide much needed data on temporal changes that may have occurred in the past decade. The tremendous utility of such analyses is perhaps best illustrated in mental health services research, where the last decade has seen dramatic changes in treatments and service delivery systems, yet the impact of these changes on unmet needs for treatment remains largely unknown. A survey is also being conducted among 10 000 adolescents, the NCS-A, and will yield much needed information on the occurrence and correlates of mental disorders in this population. Finally, as part of the WHO WMH (Womens Health and Gender) 2000 initiative, the NCS-R is being administered as parallel community epidemiological survey in over 20 developing as well developed countries throughout the world. The cross-national comparisons made possible by these surveys will provide a unique look at the occurrence, burdens and patterns of treatment for mental disorders around the globe.

Table 9.6 National Comorbidity Survey: Lifetime and 12-Month Prevalence Rates (%)

Disorders	Male		Female		Total	
	Lifetime Rate	12-Month Rate	Lifetime Rate	12-Month Rate	Lifetime Rate	12-Month Rate
Affective disorders						
Major depressive episode	12.7	7.7	21.3	12.9	17.1	10.3
Manic episode	1.6	1.4	1.7	1.3	1.6	1.3
Dysthymia	4.8	2.1	8.0	3.0	6.4	2.5
Anxiety disorders						
Panic disorder	2.0	1.3	5.0	3.2	3.5	2.3
Agoraphobia without panic disorder	3.5	1.7	7.0	3.8	5.3	2.8
Social phobia	11.1	6.6	15.5	9.1	13.3	7.9
Simple phobia	6.7	4.4	15.7	13.2	11.3	8.8
Generalized anxiety disorder	3.6	2.0	6.6	4.3	5.1	3.1
Substance use disorders						
Alcohol abuse without dependence	12.5	3.4	6.4	1.6	9.4	2.5
Alcohol dependence	20.1	10.7	8.2	3.7	14.1	7.2
Drug abuse without dependence	5.4	1.3	3.5	0.3	4.4	0.8
Drug dependence	9.2	3.8	5.9	1.9	7.5	2.8
Any substance abuse and dependence	35.4	16.1	17.9	6.6	26.6	11.3
Nonaffective psychosis*	0.6	0.5	0.8	0.6	0.7	0.5
Any National Comorbidity Survey disorder	48.7	27.7	47.3	31.2	48.0	29.5

*Schizophrenia, schizophreniform disorder, schizoaffective disorder, delusional disorder and atypical psychosis.

References

Beiser M, Iacono WG and Erickson D (1989) Temporal stability in the major mental disorders, in *The Validity of Psychiatric Diagnosis* (eds Robins LN and Barrett JE). Raven Press, New York, pp. 77–98.

Berkson J (1946) Limitations of the application of fourfold table analysis to hospital data. *Biometrics* 2, 47–53.

Bromet EJ, Schwartz JE, Fennig S *et al.* (1992) The epidemiology of psychosis: The Suffolk County Mental Health Project. *Schizophr Bull* 18, 243–255.

Costello E, Costello A, Edelbrock C *et al.* (1988) Psychiatric disorders in pediatric primary care. *Arch Gen Psychiatr* 45, 1107–1116.

Dohrenwend BP and Dohrenwend BS (1982) Perspectives on the past and future of psychiatric epidemiology: The 1981 Rema Lapouse lecture. *Am J Pub Health* 72, 1271–1279.

Eaton WW, Anthony JC, Tepper S *et al.* (1992a) Psychopathology and attrition in the Epidemiologic Catchment Area Study. *Am J Epidemiol* 135, 1051–1059.

Eaton WW, Kramer M, Anthony JC *et al.* (1992) The incidence of specific DIS/DSM-III mental disorders: Data from the NIMH Epidemiologic Catchment Area Program. *Acta Psychiatr Scand* 79, 163–178.

Edlund M, Wang PS, Berglund P *et al.* (2002) Patterns and predictors of dropping out of treatment for mental disorders: An examination of the United States and Ontario. *Am J Psychiatr* 159, 845–851.

Endicott J and Spitzer RL (1978) A diagnostic interview: The Schedule for Affective Disorders and Schizophrenia. *Arch Gen Psychiatr* 35, 837–844.

Feighner JP, Robins E, Guze SB *et al.* (1972) Diagnostic criteria for use in psychiatric research. *Arch Gen Psychiatr* 26, 57–63.

Fennig S and Bromet E (1992) Issues of memory in the Diagnostic Interview Schedule. *J Nerv Ment Dis* 180, 223–224.

Institute of Medicine (1989) Research on Children and Adolescents with Mental, Behavioral, and Developmental Disorders: Mobilizing a National Initiative. National Academy Press, Washington DC.

Jensen P, Roper M, Fisher P *et al.* (1995) Test–retest reliability of the Diagnostic Interview Schedule for Children (DISC 2.1). *Arch Gen Psychiatr* 52, 61–71.

Judd LL, Akiskal HS, Maser JD *et al.* (1998) A prospective 12-year study of subsyndromal and syndromal depressive symptomatology in unipolar depressive disorders. *Arch Gen Psychiatr* 55, 694–701.

Katon WJ, VonKorff M, Lin E *et al.* (1995) Collaborative management to achieve treatment guidelines: Impact on depression in primary. *JAMA* 273, 1026–1031.

Katon WJ, Robinson P, VonKorff M *et al.* (1996) A multifaceted intervention to improve treatment of depression in primary care. *Arch Gen Psychiatr* 53, 924–932.

Katz MM, Secunda SK, Hirschfeld RMA *et al.* (1979) NIMH clinical research branch collaborative program on the psychobiology of depression. *Arch Gen Psychiatr* 36, 765–771.

Katz SJ, Kessler RC, Lin E *et al.* (1998) Medication management of depression in the United States and Ontario. *J Gen Intern Med* 13, 77–85.

Kessler LG, Burns BJ, Shapiro S *et al.* (1987) Psychiatric diagnoses of medical service users: Evidence from the Epidemiologic Catchment Area Program. *Am J Pub Health* 77, 18–24.

Kessler RC and Walters E (2002) The National Comorbidity Survey. In *Textbook in Psychiatric Epidemiology*, 2nd edn., (eds Tsuang MT and Tohen M). John Wiley, New York.

Kessler RC, McGonagle KA, Zhao S *et al.* (1994) Lifetime and 12-month prevalence of DSM-III-R psychiatric disorders in the United States: Results from the National Comorbidity Survey. *Arch Gen Psychiatr* 51, 8–19.

Kessler RC, Berglund PA, Bruce ML *et al.* (2001) The prevalence and correlates of untreated serious mental illness. *Health Serv Res* 36, 987–1007.

Leaf PJ, Myers JK and McEvoy LT (1991) Procedures used in the Epidemiologic Catchment Area study, in *Psychiatric Disorders in*

America (eds Robins LN and Regier DA). Free Press, New York, pp. 11–32.

MacMahon B and Pugh TF (1970) *Epidemiology: Principles and Methods*. Little, Brown Co, Boston.

Merikangas KR (1990) The genetic epidemiology of alcoholism. *Psychol Med* 20, 11–22.

Miettinen OS (1985) *Theoretical Epidemiology*. John Wiley, New York.

Murray CJL and Lopez AD (1996) *The Global Burden of Disease*: A comprehensive assessment of mortality and disability from diseases, injuries, and risk factors in 1990 and projected to 2020. Harvard University Press, Cambridge.

Narrow WE, Regier DA, Rae DS *et al.* (1993) Use of services: Findings from the National Institute of Mental Health Epidemiologic Catchment Area Program. *Arch Gen Psychiatr* 50, 95–107.

Neugebauer R, Hoek HW and Susser E (1999) Prenatal exposure to wartime famine and development of antisocial personality disorder in early adulthood. *JAMA* 282, 455–462.

Nurnberger JI, Blehar MC, Kaufman CA *et al.* (1994) Diagnostic Interview for Genetic Studies. Rationale, unique features and training. *Arch Gen Psychiatr* 51, 849–859.

Olfson M, Marcus SC, Druss B *et al.* (2002) National trends in the outpatient treatment of depression. *JAMA* 287, 203–209.

Orvaschel H (1985) Psychiatric interviews suitable for use in research with children and adolescents. *Psychopharmacol Bull* 21, 737–745.

Regier DA, Myers JK, Kramer M *et al.* (1984) The NIMH Epidemiologic Catchment Area (ECA) Program: Historical context, major objectives, and study population characteristics. *Arch Gen Psychiatr* 41, 934–941.

Regier DA, Boyd JH and Burke JD (1985) One-month prevalence of mental disorders in the United States based on five Epidemiologic Catchment Area sites. *Arch Gen Psychiatr* 45, 977–986.

Regier DA, Boyd JH Burke JD Jr. *et al.* (1988) One-month prevalence of mental disorders in the United States. Based on five Epidemiologic Catchment Area sites. *Arch Gen Psychiatr* 45, 977–986.

Regier DA, Farmer ME, Rae DS *et al.* (1990) Comorbidity of mental health disorders with alcohol and other drug abuse. *JAMA* 264, 2511–2518.

Regier DA, Narrow WE, Rae DS *et al.* (1993) The de facto US mental and addictive disorders service system: Epidemiologic Catchment Area prospective 1-year prevalence rates of disorders and services. *Arch Gen Psychiatr* 50, 85–94.

Risch N and Merikangas KR (1996) The future of genetic studies of complex human disease. Science 273, 1516–1517.

Robins E and Guze SB (1970) Establishment of diagnostic validity in psychiatric illness: Its applications to schizophrenia. *Am J Psychiatr* 126, 983–988.

Robins LN, Helzer JE, Croughan JL *et al.* (1981) National Institute of Mental Health Diagnostic Interview Schedule: Its history, characteristics, and validity. *Arch Gen Psychiatr* 38, 381–389.

Robins LN, Locke BZ, and Regier DA (1991) An overview of psychiatric disorders in America. In Psychiatric Disorders in America: The Epidemiologic Catchment Area Study, Robins LN and Regier DA (eds). Free Press, New York, pp. 328–366.

Rogers MP, Warshaw MG, Goisman RM *et al.* (1999) Comparing primary and secondary generalized anxiety disorder in a long-term naturalistic study of anxiety disorders. *Depress Anx* 10, 1–7.

Rothman KJ and Greenland S (1998) Matching, in *Modern Epidemiology*, 2nd edn., (eds Rothman KM and Greenland S). Lippincott-Raven, Philadelphia, PA.

Sackett DL, Haynes RB and Tugwell P (1985) *Clinical Epidemiology*. Little, Brown Co, Boston.

Schoenbaum M, Unutzer J, Sherbourne C *et al.* (2001) Cost-effectiveness of practice-initiated quality improvement for depression: Results of a randomized controlled trial. *JAMA* 286, 1325–1330.

Selvin S (1991) *Statistical Analysis of Epidemiologic Data*. Oxford University Press, New York.

Simon GE, VonKorff M and Rutter C (2000) Randomised trial of monitoring, feedback, and management of care by telephone to improve treatment of depression in primary care. *BMJ* 320, 550–554.

Spitzer RL, Endicott J, and Robins E (1978) Research diagnostic criteria: Rationale and reliability. *Arch Gen Psychiatr* 35, 773–782.

Spitzer RL, Williams JBW, Gibbon M *et al.* (1992) The Structured Clinical Interview for DSM-III-R (SCID). I: History, rationale, and description. *Arch Gen Psychiatr* 49, 624–629.

Tohen M, Chengappa KNR, Suppes T *et al.* (2002) Efficacy of olanzapine in combination with valproate or lithium in the treatment of mania in patients partially nonresponsive to valproate or lithium monotherapy. *Arch Gen Psychiatr* 59, 62–69.

Tohen M, Jacobs TG, Grundy SL *et al.* (2000) Efficacy of olanzapine in acute bipolar mania. *Arch Gen Psychiatr* 57, 841–849.

Tohen M, Stoll AL, Strakowski SM *et al.* (1992) The McLean First-Episode Psychosis Project: Six-month recovery and recurrence outcome. *Schizophr Bull* 18, 273–282.

Tsuang MT and Tohen M (eds) (2002) *Textbook in Psychiatric Epidemiology*, 2nd edn. John Wiley, New York.

Wang PS, Berglund PA and Kessler RC (2000) Recent care of common mental disorders in the US: Prevalence and conformance with evidence-based recommendations. *J Gen Intern Med* 15, 284–292.

Wang PS, Bohn RL, Glynn RJ *et al.* (2001a) Zolpidem use and hip fractures in the elderly. *J Am Geriatr Soc* 49, 1685–1690.

Wang PS, Bohn RL, Glynn RJ *et al.* (2001b) Hazardous benzodiazepine regimens in the elderly: Effects of half-life, dosage, and duration on risk of hip fracture. *Am J Psychiatr* 158, 892–898.

Wang PS, Demler O and Kessler RC (2002) The adequacy of treatment for serious mental illness in the United States. *Am J Pub Health* 92, 99–104.

Wang PS, Gilman SE, Guardino M *et al.* (2000) Initiation and adherence to treatment for mental disorders: Examination of patient advocate group members in eleven countries. *Med Care* 38, 926–936.

Wang PS, Glynn RJ, Ganz DA, Schneeweiss S, Levin R and Avorn J (2002a) Clozapine use and the risk of diabetes mellitus. *J Clin Psychopharmacol* 22, 236–243.

Wang PS, Walker AM and Avorn J (2002b) The pharmacoepidemiology of psychiatric medications, in *Textbook in Psychiatric Epidemiology*, 2nd edn., (eds Tsuang MT and Tohen M). John Wiley, New York.

Wang PS, Walker AM, Tsuang MT, Orav EJ, Glynn RJ, Levin RL and Avorn J (2002c) Dopamine antagonists and the development of breast cancer. *Arch Gen Psychiatr* 59, 1147–1154.

Wang PS, Walker AM, Tsuang MT *et al.* (2001c) Antidepressant use and the risk of breast cancer. *J Clin Epidemiol* 54, 728–734.

Weiss NS (1985) *Clinical Epidemiology*. Oxford University Press, New York.

Weissman MM, Myers JK and Harding PS (1978) Psychiatric disorders in a US urban community: 1975–1976. *Am J Psychiatr* 135, 459–461.

Wells KB, Sherbourne C, Schoenbaum M *et al.* (2000) Impact of disseminating quality improvement programs for depression in managed primary care: A randomized controlled trial. *JAMA* 283, 212–220.

Wing JK, Cooper JE and Sartorius N (1974) *Measure and Classification of Psychiatric Symptoms: An Instructional Manual for the PSE and CATEGO Programs*. Cambridge University Press, Cambridge, UK.

Wing JK, Babor T, Brugha T *et al.* (1990) SCAN: Schedule for Clinical Assessment in Neuropsychiatry. *Arch Gen Psychiatr* 47, 589–593.

Wittchen H-U, Robins LN, Cottler LB *et al.* (1991) Cross-cultural feasibility, reliability and sources of variance in the Composite International Diagnostic Interview (CIDI). *Br J Psychiatr* 159, 645–653.

World Health Organization (1990) Composite International Diagnostic Interview (CIDI), Version 1.0. World Health Organization, Geneva.

10 Psychiatric Pathophysiology: Schizophrenia

Pursuing the Pathophysiology of Schizophrenia

For decades there existed only indirect techniques to study the living human brain. Now, with the advent of *in vivo* brain imaging, the structure, chemistry and function of the living human brain in health and disease and in multiple behavioral and pharmacologic states can be directly assessed. With the characterization of the human genome, we can begin to link disease characteristics with abnormal regional protein alterations to begin to draw together disease characteristics with tissue targets of illness. This will provide critical direct information about brain behavior in schizophrenia to enable productive and integrative data collection.

The observation that persons with schizophrenia perform poorly on tasks that require frontal neocortical function has long suggested that the frontal cortex is involved in the mechanisms of schizophrenia (Bleuler, 1978). Several laboratories have developed this idea further, showing that frontal function is abnormal in schizophrenia (Ingvar and Franzen, 1974; Weinberger *et al.*, 1986), proposing that the disturbed frontal function can influence dopamine dynamics in the striatum (Meyer-Lindenberg *et al.*, 2002), and that symptomatic (Andreasen, 1991), cellular (Lewis, 2000), neurochemical (Akbarian *et al.*, 1993), dendritic (Selemon *et al.*, 1995), and expression differences (Middleton *et al.*, 2002) exist in this area in persons with the illness. Other brain regions have also been the focus of considerable productive study in schizophrenia, including the hippocampus (Benes *et al.*, 1991; Gao *et al.*, 2000; Heckers *et al.*, 1998), thalamus (Andreasen *et al.*, 1994; Pakkenberg, 1990), and the cerebellum (Andreasen *et al.*, 1994). Within these brain areas, evidence exists for neurochemical abnormalities in dopaminergic transmission (Laruelle *et al.*, 1996), in excitatory synaptic function (Gao *et al.*, 2000; Olney and Farber, 1995; Tsai *et al.*, 1995), and in GABA-mediated inhibition (Benes *et al.*, 1996). Multiple formulations of pathophysiology in schizophrenia have been articulated, each based on a body of knowledge and an orientation to the illness.

Clinical Pharmacology in Schizophrenia

Pharmacologic data collected from living persons with schizophrenia has implicated two neurotransmitter systems in the pathophysiology of the illness. These include both the midbrain dopamine system and the cortical NMDA-sensitive glutamate system. For dopamine-mediated neurotransmission, comprehensive evidence exists that blockade of dopamine-mediated neurotransmission in the central nervous system reduces the psychosis of schizophrenia (Davis, 1969; Seeman, 1995), thus suggesting the involvement of dopamine dynamics in psychosis pathways. Because other strategies to diminish dopaminergic transmission, e.g., partial dopamine agonist action (Tamminga 2002), and dopamine synthesis blockade (Walinder *et al.*, 1976), are also antipsychotic, the hypothesis has broad pharmacological support. Indeed, a treatment based on the action of a low intrinsic-activity partial dopamine agonist is now on the market, namely aripiprazole. Moreover, the recent data that schizophrenia is associated with increased dopamine release (Laruelle *et al.*, 1996) are consistent with the hypothesis that a hyperactive dopamine system may be a pivotal part of the pathophysiology in schizophrenia.

A putative role for glutamatergic transmission at the NMDA receptor in schizophrenia is based on more recent pharmacologic observations. The action of NMDA-sensitive glutamate antagonists (specifically, the noncompetitive antagonist ketamine) in causing psychotomimetic symptoms in normal persons (Krystal *et al.*, 1994; Lahti *et al.*, 2001; Malhotra *et al.*, 1996) and in worsening psychosis in schizophrenia (Lahti *et al.*, 1995) implicates this system in mediating psychosis. These data suggest that reduced glutamatergic transmission at the NMDA receptor in the brain could be associated with psychosis in schizophrenia, especially given the supportive tissue histology (Harrison, 1999) and neurochemistry (Gao *et al.*, 2000). Most studies suggest that it is in the limbic cortex, including the anterior cingulate, hippocampus and ventral striatum, where this change is most critical.

Preclinical Studies Relevant to the Pathophysiology of Schizophrenia

Several classes of drugs capable of inducing psychosis in humans act as behavioral stimulants in animals, for example, rodents. In general, such behavior differs from the activity pattern caused by exposing normal animals to a new environment in that it is more primitive in its stereotyping and has lost the rich exploratory repertoire. Tentatively, such abnormal behavior can be looked upon as a model of psychosis with both positive and negative symptom elements and a cognitive deficit component. Examples of psychotomimetic drugs inducing such abnormal behavior are the dopamine-receptor agonists acting directly or indirectly and the glutamatergic antagonists acting on the NMDA-sensitive glutamate receptor.

Essentials of Psychiatry   Jerald Kay and Allan Tasman
© 2006 John Wiley & Sons, Ltd.

Multiple observations regarding these systems suggest that glutamatergic pathways, presumably emanating from the cerebral cortex, exert a strong inhibitory and stabilizing effect on an array of subcortical, potentially psychosis-inducing mechanisms, involving both monoaminergic and cholinergic pathways. The mechanism underlying this stabilizing glutamatergic function appears to be complex. In part it seems to be located postsynaptically to the (limbic) striatum, where corticostriatal pathways control both direct and indirect striatopallidothalamic pathways, as detailed in Figure 10.1. These pathways appear to regulate the sensory input to the cerebral cortex as well as the arousal. The direct and indirect pathways are mutually antagonistic, the former being activating and the latter inhibitory on the thalamocortical glutamatergic projections. Both the direct and the indirect pathways are also controlled by dopaminergic projections, whereby the former are activating (via D_1 receptors) and the latter inhibitory (via D_2 receptors). In addition, glutamatergic and glutamatergic/GABAergic pathways seem to control the monoaminergic neurons themselves by means of an accelerator and a brake mechanism, respectively (Carlsson et al., 2001). These observations support glutamatergic involvement in schizophrenia and emphasize the interaction of glutamate with other, largely subcortical transmitter systems and open up possibilities for a multifactorial dysregulation in complex neurocircuits where,

besides glutamate, GABAergic, monoaminergic and cholinergic systems participate in the psychotogenic process (Carlsson and Carlsson, 1990).

Several drugs in different states of development will probably shed additional light on the multifactorial aspects of psychotogenesis, for example, agonists acting at the glycine site of the NMDA receptor, glycine-reuptake inhibitors, ampakines, drugs acting on the metabotropic glutamate receptors, partial dopamine receptor agonists and dopaminergic stabilizers lacking intrinsic activity on dopamine receptors (Carlsson et al., 2001).

Systems Pathology in Schizophrenia: The Limbic Cortex

In looking for sites of pathophysiology in the cerebral cortex, several lines of evidence point to abnormal limbic function. Decades of postmortem research in schizophrenia have reported structural, histologic, and neurochemical changes in limbic cortex (Jakob and Beckmann, 1989). Abnormalities in hippocampal size (Bogerts et al., 1985), axial orientation (Scheibel and Kovelman, 1981), neuronal and nonneuronal number (Benes et al., 1991, 1998; Heckers et al., 1991; Jeste and Lohr, 1989), and changes in neurochemical markers of transmission and development (Akbarian et al., 1993; Gao et al., 2000; Tsai et al.,

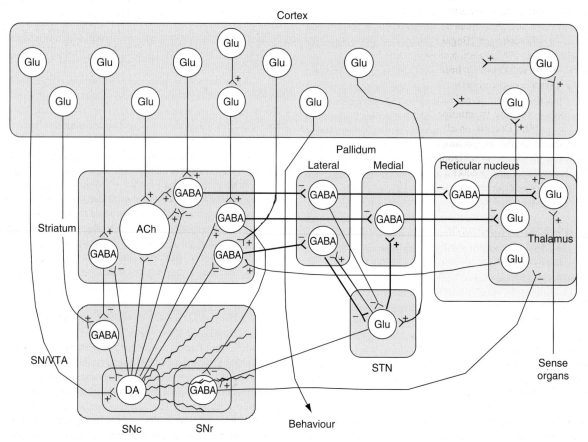

Figure 10.1   *Neurocircuitries of the basal ganglia. Detail of the striatopallidothalamic pathways. Among these, the top and bottom pathways drawn with thick lines contain three GABAergic neurons and are referred to as "indirect", i.e., inhibitory pathways. The pathway in between contains two GABAergic neurons and is referred to as "direct", i.e., excitatory. Explanation: SNc, = substantia nigra, pars compacta; SNr, = substantia nigra, pars reticulata; VTA, = ventral tegmental area; STN, = subthalamic nucleus; Glu, = glutamate; ACh, = acetylcholine; and DA, = dopamine. Reproduced with permission from Carlsson and Carlsson A (1990) Interactions between glutamtic and manoaminergic systems within the Basal Ganglia: Implications for schizophrenia and Parkinsons disease. Trends Neurosci 13, 272–276.*

1995) have all been reported in postmortem schizophrenia tissue, although not always reliably replicated (Altshuler *et al.*, 1987; Jakob and Beckmann, 1989). Curiously, often more pronounced or significant changes are reported in the left compared with the right hemisphere (Zaidel *et al.*, 1997).

Postmortem Limbic Cortex Abnormalities in Schizophrenia: Structural Changes

Much focused work in the human limbic cortex in schizophrenia began after Scheibel and Kovelman (1981) described an alteration in pyramidal cell apical dendrite orientation in the hippocampus, in its anterior and middle section, particularly at the subicular-CA_1 border. In a later extension of this work, they correlated symptom severity with the extent of the dendritic disorientation (Kovelman and Scheibel, 1984). However, other studies have not uniformly replicated these findings (Altshuler *et al.*, 1987; Christison *et al.*, 1989; Vogel *et al.*, 1997), but the original findings are still often referenced as evidence for neuroanatomical abnormalities in the hippocampus. Weinberger (1996) highlights several studies describing cytoarchitectural abnormalities in the entorhinal cortex (including the specific loss of NADPH-diaphorase neurons Nicotinamide Adenosine Dinucleotide Phosphate) as providing the best evidence for neuropathological findings (Akbarian *et al.*, 1993; Arnold *et al.*, 1991; Jakob and Beckmann, 1986). Other studies have reported significant reductions in the volumes or cross-sectional areas of the entorhinal cortex or hippocampus in schizophrenia (Bogerts *et al.*, 1985; Brown *et al.*, 1986; Colter *et al.*, 1987; Falkai and Bogerts, 1986; Falkai *et al.*, 1988), but these results have not been uniformly replicated (Benes *et al.*, 1991; Heckers *et al.*, 1991).

Hippocampal size is reduced bilaterally, albeit mildly, in the illness especially in anterior areas (Becker *et al.*, 1996; Bilder *et al.*, 1995; Bogerts *et al.*, 1990; Suddath *et al.*, 1989. Shape analyses of the hippocampus have suggested regional abnormalities of volume in schizophrenia. Importantly, regional shape abnormalities are predominantly localized to the head, implicating only a delimited area within hippocampus as abnormal (Csernansky *et al.*, 1998).

Neurochemical Changes

Changes in $GABA_A$ receptor density, in GABA release and in glutamate-related transmitters and their enzymes in hippocampus have been reported in the illness (Simpson *et al.*, 1992; Tsai *et al.*, 1995). While there appears to be no change in the density of hippocampal NMDA glutamate receptors (Ishimaru *et al.*, 1992; Kerwin *et al.*, 1990; Kornhuber *et al.*, 1989), kainate binding, particularly in CA_2 has been found reduced in several studies (Kerwin *et al.*, 1988, 1990; Simpson *et al.*, 1992) but not consistently (Deakin *et al.*, 1989). Reduced levels of non-NMDA receptor binding (Kerwin *et al.*, 1990) and lower concentrations of non-NMDA receptor mRNA (Harrison *et al.*, 1991), have both been reported in CA_3. The previous finding of an alteration in the NR_1 subunit and an increase in NR_{2B} in postmortem tissue from schizophrenia (Gao *et al.*, 2000) suggests a reduction in excitatory glutamate transmission at hippocampal NMDA receptors in this illness.

In addition, considerable evidence of compromised cognitive function, especially short-term memory and attention, exists in schizophrenia (Green, 1996; Gruzelier *et al.*, 1988; Venables, 1992). These dysfunctions may represent the behavioral correlates of hippocampal pathology.

In Vivo

Functional Limbic Cortex Change in Schizophrenia

Functional studies of human brain in schizophrenia have directly demonstrated an alteration in neuronal activity in the limbic cortex in the illness (Fletcher, 1998; Haznedar *et al.*, 1997; Heckers *et al.*, 1998; Medoff *et al.*, 2001; Nordahl *et al.*, 1996; Tamminga *et al.*, 1992). Anterior cingulate cortex consistently shows alterations in schizophrenia when persons are imaged medication-free and matched for performance. Moreover, connectivity analyses suggest that the anterior cingulate rCBF is not tightly coupled to hippocampal activity during tasks of learning and memory, as it is in normal persons. Although the entire body of these data have not yet suggested the pivotal limbic pathology, they do implicate abnormal function of these structures in the illness. Moreover, as suggested in the preclinical studies, such pathology could destabilize the function of subcortical brain areas in psychosis.

An analysis of connectivity in auditory discrimination experiments directly suggests that a systems failure occurs within limbic cortex in schizophrenia. A malfunction within the limbic cortex and the subsequent disruption of related neocortical areas and secondary dysregulation of subcortical structures may underlie the manifestations of schizophrenia. This working hypothesis suggests that it may be the resultant "misbehavior" of the limbic system itself that generates positive and cognitive symptoms in schizophrenia, possibly through its connections with neocortical and subcortical structures. These speculations raise the possibility that the primary origin of the circuit dysfunction could be varied, but inevitably result in a characteristic "psychosis" circuit abnormality (Figure 10.2).

Functional Effects of D_2 Dopamine Receptor Blockade

The clinical evidence of a systems basis of psychosis, along with the preclinical data suggesting multiple and complex neurotransmitter interactions within these symptoms, builds a plausible "psychosis circuit" for schizophrenia and potentially for its treatment. The effective functioning of the human brain to facilitate cognitive, motor and affective performance, is dependent not only on the proper functioning of individual regional neuronal groups dedicated to specific tasks, but also to interacting brain systems which function to connect neural systems to perform a particular mental task and systematically to direct information flow in the brain. Because schizophrenia is not characterized primarily by a neural or behavioral deficit, but rather by productive symptoms and by a "confusion" of neural activity with resulting mental malfunction, a system hypothesis of schizophrenia pathology is plausible. The idea that psychosis is the consequence of dysfunction somewhere within the limbic cortex, seen during cognitive work and even during routine mental function is supported by a great deal of research. This putative dysfunction is prominently manifest in the anterior components of the limbic system. Hence this change primarily influences the frontal regions of the neocortex, leaving the posterior hippocampus and the posterior neocortex relatively unaffected. Exactly where the primary limbic pathology is located within these anterior areas is a matter of speculation, but it could be multiple sites with a single resultant systems dysfunction.

Importantly, this idea allows for the real possibility that other drug actions can be exerted at other sites within the relevant

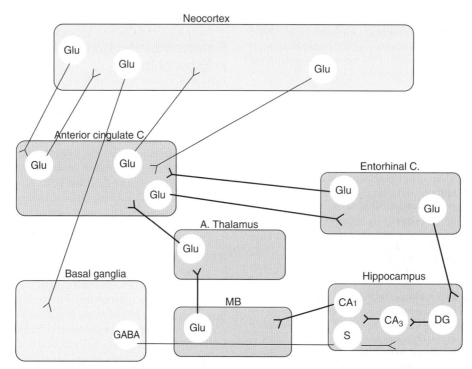

Figure 10.2   *Neurocircuitries of the limbic system. This illustration of limbic connectivity provides a depiction, albeit simplistic, of the flow of information within limbic regions. Information transfer is bidirectional in all instances except in the hippocampal trisynaptic pathway where transmission is unidirectional (forward only). At many junctures, the limbic cortex influences subcortical structures, particularly those in the ventral basal ganglia, and in the neocortex, particularly the frontal cortex.*

circuits. The 5HT$_{2A}$ antagonist activity of the second generation drugs may well be exerted, either partially or wholly, in frontal cortex. Moreover, the glutamate-enhancing activity of the second generation drugs at the NMDA receptor, whether tied to this serotonin action or independent from it, may well be a cortical action. This formulation increases the complexity but also the therapeutic potential of psychosis treatment (Carlsson and Carlsson, 1990).

References

Akbarian S, Bunney WE Jr., Potkin SG *et al.* (1993) Altered distribution of nicotinamide-adenine dinucleotide phosphate-diaphorase cells in frontal lobe of schizophrenics implies disturbances of cortical development. *Arch Gen Psychiatr* 50(3), 169–177.

Altshuler LL, Conrad A, Kovelman JA *et al.* (1987) Hippocampal pyramidal cell orientation in schizophrenia. A controlled neurohistologic study of the Yakovlev collection. *Arch Gen Psychiatr* 44(12), 1094–1098.

Andreasen NC (1991) Schizophrenia: The characteristic symptoms (review). *Schizophr Bull* 17(1), 27–49.

Andreasen NC, Arndt S, Swayze VW *et al.* (1994) Thalamic abnormalities in schizophrenia visualized through magnetic resonance image averaging. *Science* 266(5183), 294–298.

Arnold SE, Hyman BT, Van Hoesen GW *et al.* (1991) Some cytoarchitectural abnormalities of the entorhinal cortex in schizophrenia. *Arch Gen Psychiatr* 48(7), 625–632.

Becker T, Elmer K, Schneider F *et al.* (1996) Confirmation of reduced temporal limbic structure volume on magnetic resonance imaging in male patients with schizophrenia. *Psychiatr Res* 67, 135–143.

Benes FM, Kwok EW, Vincent SL *et al.* (1998) A reduction of nonpyramidal cells in sector CA$_2$ of schizophrenics and manic depressives. *Soc Biol Psychiatry* 44, 88–97.

Benes FM, Sorensen I and Bird ED (1991) Reduced neuronal size in posterior hippocampus of schizophrenic patients. *Schizophr Bull* 17, 597–608.

Benes FM, Vincent SL, Marie A *et al.* (1996) Up-regulation of GABA$_A$ receptor binding on neurons of the prefrontal cortex in schizophrenic subjects. *Neuroscience* 75(4), 1021–1031.

Bilder RM, Bogerts B, Ashtari M *et al.* (1995) Anterior hippocampal volume reductions predict frontal lobe dysfunction in first episode schizophrenia. *Schizophr Res* 17, 47–58.

Bleuler M (1978) *The Schizophrenic Disorders: Long-term Patient and Family Studies.* Yale University Press, New Haven, CT.

Bogerts B, Meertz E and Schonfeldt-Bausch R (1985) Basal ganglia and limbic system pathology in schizophrenia. A morphometric study of brain volume and shrinkage. *Arch Gen Psychiatr* 42(8), 784–791.

Bogerts B, Falkai P, Haupts M *et al.* (1990) Post-mortem volume measurements of limbic system and basal ganglia structures in chronic schizophrenics. Initial results from a new brain collection. *Schizophr Res* 3(5–6), 295–301.

Brown R, Colter N, Corsellis J *et al.* (1986) Postmortem evidence of structural brain changes in schizophrenia, differences in brain weight, temporal horn area and parahippocampal gyrus compared with affective disorder. *Arch Gen Psychiatr* 43, 36–42.

Carlsson M and Carlsson A (1990) Interactions between glutamatergic and monoaminergic systems within the basal ganglia – implications for schizophrenia and Parkinson's disease. *Trends Neurosci* 13, 272–276.

Carlsson A, Waters N, Holm-Waters S *et al.* (2001) Interactions between monoamines, glutamate, and GABA in schizophrenia: New evidence. *Annu Rev Pharmacol Toxicol* 41, 237–260.

Christison GW, Casanova MF, Weinberger DR *et al.* (1989) A quantitative investigation of hippocampal pyramidal cell size, shape, and variability of orientation in schizophrenia. *Arch Gen Psychiatr* 46, 1027–1032.

Colter N, Battal S, Crow TJ *et al.* (1987) White matter reduction in the parahippocampal gyrus of patients with schizophrenia (letter). *Arch Gen Psychiatr* 44(11), 1023.

Csernansky JG, Joshi S, Wang L *et al.* (1998) Hippocampal morphometry in schizophrenia by high dimensional brain mapping. *Proc Nat Acad Sci USA* 95, 11406–11411.

Davis JM (1969) Review of antipsychotic drug literature, in *Diagnosis and Drug Treatment of Psychiatric Disorders* (eds Klein DF and Davis JM). Williams & Wilkins, Baltimore, pp. 52–138.

Deakin JF, Slater P, Simpson MD *et al.* (1989) Frontal cortical and left temporal glutamatergic dysfunction in schizophrenia. *J Neurochem* 52, 1781–1786.

Falkai P and Bogerts B (1986) Cell loss in the hippocampus of schizophrenics. *Eur Arch Psychiatr Neurol Sci* 236(3), 154–161.

Falkai P, Bogerts B and Rozumek M (1988) Limbic pathology in schizophrenia: The entorhinal region – a morphometric study. *Biol Psychiatr* 24(5), 515–521.

Fletcher P (1998) The missing link: A failure of fronto-hippocampal integration in schizophrenia. *News Views* 1(4), 266–267.

Gao XM, Sakai K, Roberts RC *et al.* (2000) Ionotropic glutamate receptors and expression of N-methyl-D-aspartate receptor subunits in subregions of human hippocampus: Effects of schizophrenia. *Am J Psychiatr* 157(7), 1141–1149.

Green MF (1996) What are the functional consequences of neurocognitive deficits in schizophrenia? *Am J Psychiatr* 153, 321–330.

Gruzelier J, Seymour K, Wilson L *et al.* (1988) Impairments on neuropsychologic tests of temporohippocampal and frontohippocampal functions and word fluency in remitting schizophrenia and affective disorders. *Arch Gen Psychiatr* 45(7), 623–629.

Harrison PJ (1999) The neuropathology of schizophrenia. A critical review of the data and their interpretation. *Brain* 122 (Pt 4), 593–624.

Harrison PJ, McLaughlin D and Kerwin RW (1991) Decreased hippocampal expression of a glutamate receptor gene in schizophrenia. *Lancet* 337(8739), 450–452.

Haznedar MM, Buchsbaum MS, Luu C *et al.* (1997) Decreased anterior cingulate gyrus metabolic rate in schizophrenia. *Am J Psychiatr* 154, 682–684.

Heckers S, Heinsen H, Geiger B *et al.* (1991) Hippocampal neuron number in schizophrenia. *Arch Gen Psychiatr* 48, 1002–1008.

Heckers S, Rauch SL, Goff D *et al.* (1998) Impaired recruitment of the hippocampus during conscious recollection in schizophrenia. *Nature* 1(4), 318–323.

Ingvar DH and Franzen G (1974) Abnormalities of cerebral blood flow distribution in patients with chronic schizophrenia. *Acta Psychiatr Scand* 50(4), 425–462.

Ishimaru M, Kurumaji A and Toru M (1992) NMD$_A$-associated glycine binding site increases in schizophrenic brains (letter). *Biol Psychiatr* 32, 379–381.

Jakob H and Beckmann H (1989) Gross and histological criteria for developmental disorders in brains of schizophrenics (review). *J Roy Soc Med* 82(8), 466–469.

Jeste DV and Lohr JB (1989) Hippocampal pathologic findings in schizophrenia. A morphometric study. *Arch Gen Psychiatr* 46(11), 1019–1024.

Kerwin RW, Patel S, Meldrum B *et al.* (1988) Asymmetrical loss of glutamate receptor subtype in left hippocampus in schizophrenia. *Lancet* i, 583–584.

Kerwin R, Patel S and Meldrum B (1990) Quantitative autoradiographic analysis of glutamate binding sites in the hippocampal formation in normal and schizophrenic brain postmortem. *Neuroscience* 39, 25–32.

Kornhuber J, Mack-Burkhardt F, Riederer P *et al.* (1989) [3H] MK-801 binding items in postmortem brain regions of schizophrenic patients. *J Neur Transm* 77, 231–236.

Kovelman JA and Scheibel AB (1984) A neurohistological correlate of schizophrenia. *Biol Psychiatr* 19(12), 1601–1621.

Krystal JH, Karper LP, Seibyl JP *et al.* (1994) Subanesthetic effects of the noncompetitive NMDA antagonist, ketamine, in humans: Psychotomimetic, perceptual, cognitive, and neuroendocrine responses. *Arch Gen Psychiatr* 51, 199–214.

Lahti AC, Holcomb HH, Medoff DR *et al.* (1995) Ketamine activates psychosis and alters limbic blood flow in schizophrenia. *Neuro Report* 6(6), 869–872.

Lahti AC, Weiler MA, Tamara Michaelidis BA *et al.* (2001) Effects of ketamine in normal and schizophrenic volunteers. *Neuropsychopharmacology* 25(4), 455–467.

Laruelle M, Abi-Dargham A, van Dyck CH *et al.* (1996) Single photon emission computerized tomography imaging of amphetamine-induced dopamine release in drug-free schizophrenic subjects. *Proc Nat Acad Sci USA* 93(17), 235–240.

Lewis DA (2000) GABAergic local circuit neurons and prefrontal cortical dysfunction in schizophrenia. *Brain Res Rev* 31(2–3), 270–276.

Malhotra AK, Pinals DA, Weingartner H *et al.* (1996) NMDA receptor function and human cognition: The effects of ketamine in healthy volunteers. *Neuropsychopharmacology* 14(5), 301–307.

Medoff DR, Holcomb HH, Lahti AC *et al.* (2001) Probing the human hippocampus using rCBF: Contrasts in schizophrenia. *Hippocampus* 11, 543–550.

Meyer-Lindenberg A, Miletich RS, Kohn PD *et al.* (2002) Reduced prefrontal activity predicts exaggerated striatal dopaminergic function in schizophrenia. *Nat Neurosci* 5(3), 267–271.

Middleton FA, Mirnics K, Pierri JN *et al.*, (2002) Gene expression profiling reveals alterations of specific metabolic pathways in schizophrenia. *J Neurosci* 22(7), 2718–2729.

Nordahl TE, Kusubov N, Carter C *et al.*, (1996) Temporal lobe metabolic differences in medication-free outpatients with schizophrenia via the PET-600. *Neuropsychopharmacology* 15(6), 541–554.

Olney JW and Farber NB (1995) Glutamate receptor dysfunction and schizophrenia. *Arch Gen Psychiatr* 52(12), 998–1007.

Pakkenberg B (1990) Pronounced reduction of total neuron number in mediodorsal thalamic nucleus and nucleus accumbens in schizophrenics. *Arch Gen Psychiatr* 47(11), 1023–1028.

Scheibel AB and Kovelman JA (1981) Disorientation of the hippocampal pyramidal cell and its processes in schizophrenic patients (letter). *Biol Psychiatr* 16, 101–102.

Seeman P (1995) Dopamine receptors and psychosis. *In Sci Med* 5, 28–37.

Selemon LD, Rajkowska G and Goldman-Rakic PS (1995) Abnormally high neuronal density in the schizophrenic cortex. A morphometric analysis of prefrontal area 9 and occipital area 17. *Arch Gen Psychiatr* 52(10), 805–818.

Simpson MD, Slater P, Royston MC *et al.* (1992) Regionally selective deficits in uptake sites for glutamate and gamma-aminobutyric acid in the basal ganglia in schizophrenia. *Psychiatr Res* 42(3), 273–282.

Suddath RL, Casanova MF, Goldberg TE *et al.* (1989) Temporal lobe pathology in schizophrenia: A quantitative magnetic resonance imaging study. *Am J Psychiatr* 146(4), 464–472.

Tamminga CA (2002) Partial dopamine agonists in the treatment of psychosis. *J Neural Transm* 109(3), 411–420.

Tamminga CA, Thaker GK, Buchanan R *et al.* (1992) Limbic system abnormalities identified in schizophrenia using positron emission tomography with fluorodeoxyglucose and neocortical alterations with deficit syndrome. *Arch Gen Psychiatr* 49(7), 522–530.

Tsai G, Passani LA, Slusher BS *et al.* (1995) Abnormal excitatory neurotransmitter metabolism in schizophrenic brains. *Arch Gen Psychiatr* 52(10), 829–836.

Venables PH (1992) Hippocampal function and schizophrenia. Experimental psychological evidence. *Ann NY Acad Sci* 658, 111–127.

Vogel MW, Jin W, Roberts RC *et al.* (1997) Variations in hippocampal pyramidal neuron orientation in schizophrenia. *Soc Neurosci Abstr* 23, 2199.

Walinder J, Skott A, Carlsson A *et al.* (1976) Potentiation by metyrosine of thioridazine effects in chronic schizophrenics. A long-term trial using double-blind crossover technique. *Arch Gen Psychiatr* 33(4), 501–505.

Weinberger DR (1996) On the plausibility of "The Neurodevelopmental Hypothesis" of schizophrenia. *Neuropsychopharmacology* 14, 1S–11S.

Weinberger DR, Berman KF and Zec RF (1986) Physiologic dysfunction of dorsolateral prefrontal cortex in schizophrenia. I. Regional cerebral blood flow evidence. *Arch Gen Psychiatr* 43(2), 114–124.

Zaidel DW, Esiri MM and Harrison PJ (1997) The hippocampus in schizophrenia: Lateralized increase in neuronal density and altered cytoarchitectural asymmetry. *Psychol Med* 27, 703–713.

11 Psychiatric Pathophysiology: Mood Disorders

Genetic Factors

The familial nature of mood disorders has long been observed. It has been established that bipolar I disorder is more heritable than the other mood disorders, that an early age of onset is associated with greater heritability, and that heritable risk decreases in proportion to the amount of genetic material shared by members of a pedigree (Kelsoe, 2000). Genetic factors can interact with environmental factors to influence the vulnerability to mood disorders in different ways. For example, Kendler (1998) explored two such mechanisms: "genetic control of sensitivity to environment", and "genetic control of exposure to the environment". "Genetic control of sensitivity to the environment" suggests that genes, in part, render individuals relatively vulnerable or relatively invulnerable to the pathogenic effects of environmental stress. The depressogenic effect of stressful life events is substantially greater in those at high versus low genetic risk to the mood disorders. "Genetic control of exposure to the environment" suggests that genetic factors influence the probability that individuals will select themselves into high versus low risk environments. The genetic risk factors for major depression in part express themselves by influencing the probability that individuals will experience stressful life events, particularly of an interpersonal nature.

Molecular Genetic Research

Molecular biology studies have reported, replicated, or failed to replicate various associations between several specific genes or gene markers and mood disorders (Sevy *et al.*, 1995; Reus and Freimer, 1997; Sherman *et al.*, 1997; Kendler, 1998; Dubovsky and Buzan, 1999; Kelsoe, 2000; Berrettini, 2000; Craddock and Jones, 2001; Johansson *et al.*, 2001).

Why have no genetic associations been consistently replicated? Reasons include: 1) complexity of the phenotype; 2) the likelihood that multiple genes and gene combinations contribute to the phenotypes; 3) gene–environment effects; 4) the complexity of the environment; and 5) the low power of sample sizes studied to date (Dubovsky and Buzan, 1999; Kelsoe, 2000; Mann *et al.*, 2001). A major problem of studies in psychiatric genetics is that psychiatric diagnoses are not known to be biologically homogeneous entities. Syndromal psychiatric diagnostic categories such as depression or anxiety disorders potentially include etiologically, pathologically and prognostically heterogeneous disorders (Charlton, 1997; Sher, 2000a). However, behavioral geneticists remain cautiously optimistic and hope that genetic studies promise a new era of understanding and treatment of mood disorders. There is confidence in the existence of genetic factors in mood disorders without having as yet succeeded in identifying the responsible genes.

Monoamine Alterations

Serotonergic System

Serotonin has been implicated in the pathophysiology of depression and bipolar disorder (for reviews, see Mann, 1999; Oquendo and Mann, 2000; Shiah and Yatham, 2000; Mann *et al.*, 2001; Nemeroff *et al.*, 1997; Meltzer and Lowy, 1987; Coppen, 1969; Mace and Taylor, 2000; Kandel, 2000; Charney *et al.*, 1981) (Table 11.1 and Figure 11.1). This hypothesis proposed that the vulnerability to either depression or mania was related to low serotonergic activity, attributable to either less serotonin release or fewer serotonin receptors or impaired serotonin receptor-mediated signal transduction. Prange *et al.*, (1974) formulated a permissive hypothesis of serotonin function in bipolar disorder. They suggested that a deficit in central serotonergic neurotransmission permits the expression of bipolar disorder, and that both the manic and depressive phases of bipolar disorder are characterized by low central serotonergic neurotransmission. Over the last 30 years, a variety of studies of the serotonergic system have reinforced its role in major depression and identified additional associations with suicidal behavior, impulsivity, aggression, eating disorders, obsessive–compulsive disorder, anxiety disorders, personality disorders, seasonal changes in mood and behavior, and alcohol abuse and dependence. The serotonergic system also plays a role in the regulation of a variety of basic biological functions including sleep, appetite, circadian rhythm and cognitive function.

Medications that target the serotonin transporter site and selectively inhibit reuptake of serotonin (e.g., fluoxetine, sertraline, paroxetine, fluvoxamine, citalopram) have all been shown to be effective antidepressants (Nemeroff *et al.*, 1997; Sampson, 2001;

Table 11.1	Studies of the Serotonergic System in Major Depression
CSF 5-HIAA levels	$\downarrow$?
Postsynaptic 5-HT$_{2A}$ receptors in brain and platelets	$\uparrow$
Serotonin transporter binding in brain and platelets	$\downarrow$
Platelet serotonin uptake	$\downarrow$
Prolactin response to fenfluramine, clomipramine, and l-tryptophan	$\downarrow$

$\uparrow$ higher; $\downarrow$ lower

Essentials of Psychiatry   Jerald Kay and Allan Tasman
© 2006 John Wiley & Sons, Ltd.

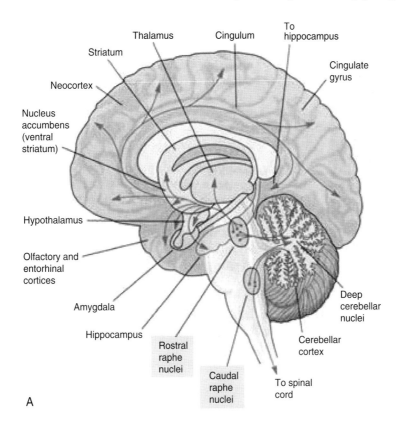

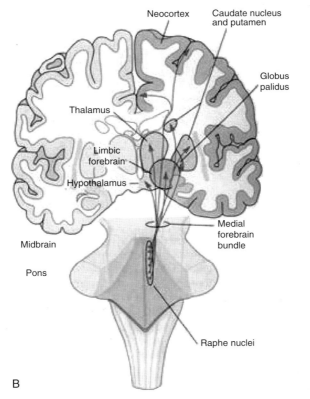

Figure 11.1   *The major serotonergic pathways. (A) A lateral view of the brain shows the course of the major serotonergic pathways. Although the raphe nuclei form a continuous collection of cell groups throughout the brain stem, they are graphically shown here as two groups, one rostral and one caudal. (B) A coronal view of the brain demonstrates some of the major targets of the serotonergic neurons. Reproduced with permission from Principles of Neural Science 4th Ed. Kandel ER (2000) Disorders of Mood: depression, Mania and Anxiety Disorders. Copyright McGraw Hill Education.*

Mace and Taylor, 2000). Some antidepressant drugs specifically act at one of the many serotonin receptor subtypes. For example, suggested antidepressive/anxiolytic medications buspirone and gepirone are 5-HT$_{1A}$ receptor agonists, and fewer 5-HT$_{1A}$ receptors are implicated in the pathophysiological mechanism of depression and anxiety (Yocca, 1990; Apter and Allen, 1999).

Considered together, studies of serotonin function in major depression suggest both hypofunction and likely compensatory changes that would increase serotonergic activity (Brown et al., 1994; Leonard, 1994; Dubovsky and Buzan, 1999). Findings such as 1) lower serotonin and 5-HIAA levels in postmortem brain stem and lower CSF 5-HIAA; 2) relapse of depression with diet acute depletion of tryptophan; 3) fewer serotonin transporter sites in prefrontal cortex; 4) fewer postsynaptic 5-HT$_{1A}$ receptors; and 5) the antidepressant properties of medications that enhance serotonergic transmission suggest that underactivity of the serotonin system is part of the pathogenesis of depression. Conversely, more 5-HT$_{2A}$ receptor binding in the frontal cortex of depressed individuals who committed suicide, fewer brainstem 5-HT$_{1A}$ autoreceptors and fewer serotonin transporters in the raphe nuclei would tend to increase serotonergic transmission in major depression. There is evidence for the contribution of serotonin in mania and in the mechanism of action of mood stabilizers (Shiah and Yatham, 2000); however, the data on the role of the serotonergic system in mania are fewer and not consistent. Alterations in functioning of other neurotransmitters in mania such as norepinephrine, dopamine, acetylcholine and GABA, and their interaction with serotonin may also contribute. Future studies of serotonergic activity in mood disorders will need further to differentiate primary pathogenesis from compensatory changes.

Noradrenergic System

There are multiple lines of evidence that the noradreneric system is disordered in depression (Berman et al., 1996; Charney, 1998; Heninger et al., 1996; Leonard, 1997; Owens, 1997; Kandel, 2000; Potter et al., 1993; Schatzberg and Schildkraut, 1995; Nemeroff et al., 1997; Ressler and Nemeroff, 1999) (Table 11.2 and Figure 11.2).

A large body of metabolite data are consistent with the hypothesis that there are abnormalities in the noradrenergic system in depression. The conflicting findings, however, are not consistent with simple increased or decreased noradrenergic activity.

Dopaminergic System

Some studies have found that CSF levels of the dopamine metabolite homovanillic acid (HVA) are lower in patients with major depression than in controls and that lower CSF HVA levels are found in more severely depressed patients (see Kapur and Mann, 1992; Brown et al., 1994, for a summary) (Table 11.3). However, other studies failed to replicate these findings or found higher CSF HVA in patients with depression (Jimerson, 1987; Vestergaard et al., 1978).

Table 11.2	Studies of the Noradrenergic System in Major Depression	
CSF and urinary MHPG	↑↓	
Plasma norepinephrine and epinephrine levels	↑ in mania than in depression	
α$_2$-adrenergic binding in platelets	↑	
Growth hormone response to clonidine and platelet α$_2$-adrenergic responses	↓	

↑ higher; ↓ lower

Gamma-aminobutyric Acid

Gamma-aminobutyric acid (GABA) is the major inhibitory neurotransmitter in almost all areas of the CNS and regulates many CNS functions (Nemeroff et al., 1997). A decrease in GABAergic activity may play a role in depression by regulating receptor responses to catecholamines (Enna et al., 1986; Nemeroff et al., 1997). Pathophysiological contributions of GABA and therapeutic effects of GABAergic medications in mood disorders may be mediated via effects on other neurotransmitter systems (Dubovsky and Buzan, 1999; Nemeroff et al., 1997).

Other Neurotransmitters

Cholinergic neurons containing acetylcholine project diffusely throughout the cortex (Thase, 2000). The involvement of cholinergic system in the pathogenesis of depression is supported by the following findings: cholinergic input reduces REM latency (decreased REM latency is seen in depression); some antidepressants have anticholinergic properties; lecithin, an acetylcholine precursor, reduces mania in some cases and can induce depression; and cholinergic rebound following abrupt withdrawal of anticholinergic medications can cause a relapse of depression (Dubovsky and Buzan, 1999; Dilsaver and Coffman, 1989; Janowsky and Risch, 1984; Keshavan, 1985).

There are emerging data that drugs that antagonize NMDA receptors have antidepressant effects (Przegalinski et al., 1997; Papp and Moryl, 1994; Trullas and Skolnick, 1990).

It is important to note that all neurotransmitters and receptors interact with and influence each other (Brown et al., 1994; Leonard, 1994; Dubovsky and Buzan, 1999). Most cerebral functions are the result of the converging action of many different neurotransmitters. It is not likely that the pathophysiology of mood disorders is due to a single neurotransmitter (Brown et al., 1994). More probably, mood disorders are disorders of the overall interaction of multiple transmitter systems. Alternatively, different components of depression may be related to different neurotransmitter dysfunction.

The binding of a neurotransmitter to a postsynaptic receptor triggers a cascade of chemical processes that include the second messenger systems (Thase, 2000; Dubovsky and Buzan, 1999; Thase and Howland, 1995). The bidirectional actions of second messengers allow unitary changes in second messenger function to produce diverse changes in transmitter synthesis and release, and in receptor activity, leading to complex neurotransmitter and receptor effects. There is evidence that mood-stabilizing drugs (e.g., lithium) act upon G proteins or other second messengers (Jesberger and Richardson, 1985; Kofman and Belmaker, 1993; Wang et al., 2001; Chen et al., 2001).

Neuropeptides and Hormones

Cortical–Hypothalamic–Pituitary–Adrenal Axis

The cortical–hypothalamic–pituitary–adrenal axis has been intensely studied in patients with major depression (Carroll et al., 1968; Sachar et al., 1970; Stokes and Sikes, 1987; Brown et al., 1994; Nemeroff et al., 1997; Thase, 2000). The cortical–hypothalamic–pituitary–adrenal axis hyperactivity in depressed patients can be explained by hypersecretion of CRF and secondary pituitary and adrenal gland hypertrophy, although impaired negative feedback at various CNS sites including hippocampus and the pituitary are also likely to contribute. Downregulation of hippocampal mineralocorticoid receptors and expression is reported in depressed suicides (Lopez et al., 1998). Hyperactivity of the cortical–hypothalamic–pituitary–adrenal axis also occurs in patients with bipolar disorder (Kiriike et al., 1988; Stokes and Sikes, 1987). This increased cortical–hypothalamic–pituitary–adrenal axis activity has

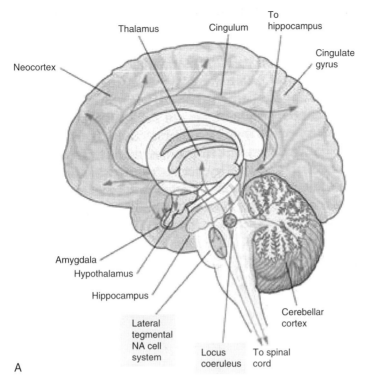

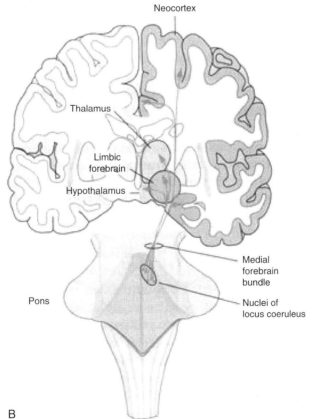

Figure 11.2 *The major noradrenergic pathways.* (A) *A lateral view of the brain shows the course of the major noradrenergic pathways. The major noradrenergic pathways emanate from the locus coeruleus and from the lateral brain stem tegmentum.* (B) *A coronal view of the brain demonstrates some of the major targets of the noradrenergic neurons. (Source: Kandel ER [2000] Disorders of mood: depression, mania, and anxiety disorders, in Principles of Neural Science, 4th ed., [eds Kandel ER, Schwartz JH, and Jessell TM]. McGraw-Hill, New York.)*

Table 11.3	Studies of the Dopaminergic System in Major Depression
CSF HVA levels	↓ (psychomotor retardation)
Plasma dopamine and HVA levels	↑ in psychotic depression
Plasma HVA and dopamine levels in response to the administration of glucocorticoids	↑ in controls, may contribute to the development of psychotic depression
Platelet MAO activity	↑ in unipolar ↓ in bipolar
Serum dopamine β-hydroxylase activity	↓

↑ higher; ↓ lower

been observed in mixed mood states (Evans and Nemeroff, 1983; Krishnan *et al.*, 1983; Swann *et al.*, 1992), mania (Godwin, 1984), and in depression in rapid-cycling patients (Kennedy *et al.*, 1989). Effect of treatment and recovery from depression are associated with partial reversal of HPA overactivity and may be required for recovery (Garlow *et al.*, 1999; Christensen and Kessing, 2001).

Hypothalamic–Pituitary–Thyroid Axis
About 5 to 10% of people evaluated for depression have previously undetected or subclinical thyroid dysfunction (Thase, 2000). Jackson (1998) suggests that some patients with depression, although generally viewed as chemically euthyroid, have alterations in their thyroid function including slight elevation of the serum thyroxine (T4), blunted thyrotropin (TSH) response to thyrotropin-releasing hormone (TRH) stimulation, and loss of the nocturnal TSH rise. One possible explanation for the blunting of the TSH response to TRH challenge is a downregulation of TRH receptors in the pituitary, in response to the increased levels of TRH secreted into the hypophyseal–portal circulation (Garlow *et al.*, 1999). Elevated CSF concentrations of TRH in depressed patients were reported by Kirkegaard *et al.* (1979) and Banki *et al.* (1988), but not by Roy *et al.* (1994). It has been proposed that brain thyroid hormones may play a role in the mechanisms of seasonal affective disorder and light therapy (Sher, 2000b, 2001).

Hypothalamic–Growth Hormone Axis
Mood disorders are associated with alterations in the activity of the growth hormone axis (Toivola *et al.*, 1972; Schilkrut *et al.*, 1975; Mendlewicz *et al.*, 1985; Nemeroff *et al.*, 1997; Garlow *et al.*, 1999; Thase, 2000). The most consistent finding in depression is a blunted growth hormone response to clonidine, an alpha-2 receptor agonist (Toivola *et al.*, 1972; Thase, 2000).

Brain Growth Factor
Multiple neurochemical factors, including thyroid hormones, somatostatin, growth hormone and brain-derived neurotrophic factor (BDNF) may affect brain growth and development (Krawiec *et al.*, 1969; Leroux *et al.*, 1995; Oppenheimer and Schwartz, 1997; Duman *et al.*, 2000). BDNF, a major neurotrophic factor in the brain, is critical for the survival and guidance of neurons during development, but is also required for the survival and function of neurons in the adult brain (McAllister *et al.*, 1999; Duman *et al.*, 2000).

Recent studies demonstrate that antidepressant treatment upregulates the cyclic adenosine monophosphate (cAMP)-response element-binding protein (CREB) cascade and expression of BDNF (Duman *et al.*, 1999). Upregulation of CREB and BDNF raises the possibility that antidepressant treatment could oppose the cell death pathway. These findings suggest that regulation of the cell death pathways could also contribute to the actions of agents used for the treatment of bipolar disorder.

Substance P
Substance P, an undecapeptide, is abundant both in the periphery and in the CNS, where it is usually colocalized with one of the classical neurotransmitters, most commonly serotonin (Baby *et al.*, 1999; Argyropoulos and Nutt, 2000; Stout *et al.*, 2001). A role for substance P is proposed in the regulation of pain, asthma, psoriasis, inflammatory bowel disease and, in the CNS, emesis, migraine, schizophrenia, depression and anxiety. Drug development has focused most intensively on the substance P-preferring receptor, neurokinin-1. Although originally studied as potential analgesic compounds, recent evidence suggests that neurokinin-1 receptor antagonists may possess antidepressant and anxiolytic properties. If confirmed by further controlled clinical studies, this will represent a mechanism of action distinct from all existing antidepressant agents. The existing preclinical and clinical literature is suggestive of, but not conclusive, concerning a role of substance P and neurokinin-1 receptors in the pathophysiology of depression and/or anxiety disorders.

Neuroimaging Studies
Neuroimaging technology provides opportunities for elucidating the anatomic correlates of mood disorders (Thase and Howland, 1995; Kegeles and Mann, 1997; Soares and Mann, 1997a, 1997b; Dougherty and Rauch, 1997; Drevets *et al.*, 1999, 2000, 2001). Neuroimaging studies of major depression have identified structural and functional abnormalities in multiple areas of the orbital and medial prefrontal cortex, the amygdala, and related parts of the striatum and thalamus (Thase and Howland, 1995; Soares and Mann, 1997a, b; Dougherty and Rauch, 1997; Drevets *et al.*, 1999; Dubovsky and Buzan, 1999, Drevets, 2000, 2001).

The most consistently indentified functional neuroimaging finding has been prefrontal lobe dysfunction, as indicated by reduced blood flow and glucose metabolism (Soares and Mann, 1997b; Drevets, 2000, 2001). There is evidence of abnormalities in basal ganglia, temporal lobe and related limbic structures. Unipolar depression is associated with dysfunction primarily in the prefrontal cortex and basal ganglia, while bipolar depression may be associated with dysfunction in the temporal lobe, in addition to these other areas. Some of these functional abnormalities appear mood-state-dependent and are located in regions where cerebral blood flow increases during normal and some pathologic emotional states. These neurophysiologic differences between depressives and control subjects may thus implicate areas where physiologic activity changes to mediate or respond to the emotional, behavioral and cognitive manifestations of major depressive episodes. Other abnormalities persist following symptom remission, and are found in orbital and medial prefrontal cortex areas where postmortem studies demonstrate reductions in cortex volume and histopathologic changes in primary mood disorders (Mann and Arango, 1999). These areas appear to modulate emotional behavior and stress responses, based upon evidence from brain mapping, lesion analysis and electrophysiologic studies of humans and experimental animals. Dysfunction involving these regions is thus hypothesized to play a role in the pathogenesis of depressive symptoms. Taken together, these findings implicate interconnected neural circuits in which pathologic patterns of neurotransmission may result in the emotional, motivational, cognitive and behavioral manifestations of primary and secondary affective disorders.

The development of selective ligands for neuroreceptor imaging is providing rapidly expanding capabilities for noninvasive quantitation of *in vivo* receptor binding and neurotransmitter function. PET and SPECT studies provided important information regarding the role of serotonergic receptors in the pathogenesis of mood disorders. Such studies will permit more complete characterization of the neurotransmitter abnormalities suggested by studies of body fluids, postmortem tissue and neuroendocrine function. This area is becoming one of the most important applications for PET and SPECT technologies.

References

Apter JT and Allen LA (1999) Buspirone: Future directions. *J Clin Psychopharmacol* 19, 86–93.

Argyropoulos SV and Nutt DJ (2000) Substance P antagonists: Novel agents in the treatment of depression. *Exp Opin Invest Drugs* 9, 1871–1875.

Banki CM, Bissette G, Arato M et al. (1988) Elevation of immunoreactive CSF TRH in depressed patients. *Am J Psychiatr* 145, 1526–1531.

Baby S, Nguyen M, Tran D, et al. (1999) Substance P antagonists: The next breakthrough in treating depression? *J Clin Pharmacol Therap* 24, 461–469.

Berman R, Krystal J and Charney D (1996) Mechanism of action of antidepressants: Monoamine hypotheses and beyond, in *Biology of Schizophrenia and Affective Disease* (ed Watson S). American Psychiatric Press, Washington DC, pp. 295–368.

Berrettini W (2000) The search for susceptibility genes in bipolar disorder, in *Genetic influences on Neural and Behavioral Functions* (eds Pfaff DW, Berrettini WH, Joh TH et al.). CRC Press, Boca Raton, pp. 31–45.

Brown SL, Steinberg RL and van Praag HM (1994) The pathogenesis of depression: reconsideration of neurotransmitter data, in *Handbook of Depression and Anxiety* (eds den Boer JA and Sitsen JMA). Marcel Dekker, New York, pp. 317–347.

Carroll BJ, Martin FI, and Davies B (1968) Pituitary–adrenal function in depression. *Lancet* i, 1373–1374.

Charleton BG (1997) Natural kinds, natural history and the clinician-researcher. *QJM-Monthly J Assoc Phys* 90, 707–709.

Charney D (1998) Monoamine dysfunction and the pathophysiology and treatment of depression. *J Clin Psychiatr* 59(Suppl 14), 11–14.

Charney DS, Menkes DB and Heninger GR (1981) Receptor sensitivity and the mechanism of action of antidepressant treatment. Implications for the etiology and therapy of depression. *Arch Gen Psychiatr* 38, 1160–1180.

Chen G, Huang LD, Zeng WZ et al. (2001) Mood stabilizers regulate cytoprotective and mRNA-binding proteins in the brain: long-term effects on cell survival and transcript stability. *Int J Neuropsychopharmacol* 4, 47–64.

Christensen MV and Kessing LV (2001) The hypothalamo–pituitary–adrenal axis in major affective disorder: A review. *Nord J Psychiatr* 55, 359–363.

Coppen AJ (1969) Biochemical aspects of depression. *Int Psychiatr Clin* 6, 53–81.

Craddock N and Jones I (2001) Molecular genetics of bipolar disorder. *Br J Psychiatr* 41(Suppl), 128–133.

Dilsaver SC and Coffman JA (1989) Cholinergic hypothesis of depression: A reappraisal. *J Clin Psychopharmacol* 9, 173–179.

Dougherty D and Rauch SL (1997) Neuroimaging and neurobiological models of depression. *Harv Rev Psychiatr* 5, 138–159.

Drevets WC (2000) Neuroimaging studies of mood disorders. *Biol Psychiatr* 48, 813–829.

Drevets WC (2001) Neuroimaging and neuropathological studies of depression: implications for the cognitive-emotional features of mood disorders. *Curr Opin Neurobiol* 11, 240–249.

Drevets WC, Frank E, Price JC, et al. (1999) PET imaging of serotonin 1A receptor binding in depression. *Biol Psychiatr* 46, 1375–1385.

Dubovsky SL and Buzan R (1999) Mood disorders, in *The American Psychiatric Press Textbook of Psychiatry* (eds Hales RE, Yudofsky SC and Talbott JA). American Psychiatric Press, Washington DC, pp. 479–565.

Duman RS, Malberg J and Thome J (1999) Neural plasticity to stress and antidepressant treatment. *Biol Psychiatr* 46, 1181–1191.

Duman RS, Malberg J, Nakagawa S, et al. (2000) Neuronal plasticity and survival in mood disorders. *Biol Psychiatr* 48, 732–739.

Enna SJ, Karbon EW and Duman RS (1986) GABA-B agonist and imipramine-induced modifications in rat brain beta-adrenergic receptor binding and function, in *GABA and Mood Disorders: Experimental and Clinical Research* (eds Bartholine G, Lloyd KG, and Morselli PL). Raven Press, New York, pp. 23–49.

Evans DL and Nemeroff CB (1983) Use of the dexamethasone suppression test using DSM-III criteria on an inpatient psychiatric unit. *Biol Psychiatr* 18, 505–511.

Garlow SJ, Musselman DL and Nemeroff CB (1999) The neurochemistry of mood disorders: Clinical studies, in *Neurobiology of Mental Illness* (eds Charney DS, Nestler EJ, and Bunney BS). Oxford University Press, New York, pp. 348–364.

Godwin CD (1984) The dexamethasone suppression test in acute mania. *J Affect Disord* 7, 281–286.

Heninger G, Delgado P and Charney D (1996) The revised monoamine theory of depression: A modulatory role for monoamines, based on new findings from monoamine depletion experiments in humans. *Pharmacopsychiatry* 29, 2–11.

Jackson IM (1998) The thyroid axis and depression. *Thyroid* 8, 951–956.

Janowsky DS and Risch SC (1984) Adrenergic–cholinergic balance and affective disorders: a review of clinical and therapeutic implications. *Psychiatr Hosp* 15, 163–171.

Jesberger JA and Richardson JS (1985) Neurochemical aspects of depression: the past and the future? *Int J Neurosci* 27, 19–47.

Jimerson DC (1987) Role of dopamine mechanisms in affective disorders, in *Psychopharmacology: The Third Generation of Progress* (ed Mettzer HY. Raven Press, New York, pp. 505–511.

Johansson C, Jansson M, Linner L et al. (2001) Genetics of affective disorders. *Eur Neuropsychopharmacol* 11, 385–394.

Kandel ER (2000) Disorders of mood: depression, mania, and anxiety disorders, in *Principles of Neural Science*, 4th edn (eds Kandel ER, Schwartz JH, and Jessell TM). McGraw-Hill, New York, pp. 1209–1226.

Kapur S and Mann JJ (1992) Role of the dopaminergic system in depression. *Biol Psychiatr* 32, 1–17.

Kelsoe JR (2000) Mood disorders: Genetics, in *Kaplan and Sadock's Comprehensive Textbook of Psychiatry*, Vol. 2 (eds Sadock BJ and Sadock VA). Lippincott Williams & Wilkins, Philadelphia, pp. 1308–1318.

Kendler KS (1998) Major depression and the environment: a psychiatric genetic perspective. *Pharmacopsychiatry* 31, 5–9.

Kennedy SH, Tighe S, McVey G et al. (1989) Melatonin and cortisol "switches" during mania, depression, and euthymia in a drug-free bipolar patient. *J Nerv Ment Dis* 177, 300–303.

Keshavan MS (1985) Bezhexol withdrawal and cholinergic mechanisms in depression. *Br J Psychiatr* 147, 560–564.

Kegeles LS and Mann JJ (1997) In vivo imaging of neurotransmitter systems using radiolabeled receptor ligands. *Neuropsychopharmacology* 17, 293–307.

Kiriike N, Izumiya Y, Nishiwaki S et al. (1988) TRH test and DST in schizoaffective mania, mania, and schizophrenia. *Biol Psychiatr* 24, 415–422.

Kirkegaard C, Faber J, Hummer L et al. (1979) Increased levels of TRH in cerebrospinal fluid from patients with endogenous depression. *Psychoneuroendocrinol* 4, 227–235.

Kofman O and Belmaker RH (1993) Ziskind-Somerfeld Research Award 1993. Biochemical, behavioral, and clinical studies of the role of inositol in lithium treatment and depression. *Biol Psychiatr* 34, 839–852.

Krawiec L, Garcia Argiz CA, Gomez CJ, et al. (1969) Hormonal regulation of brain development. 3. Effects of triiodothyronine and growth hormone on the biochemical changes in the cerebral cortex and cerebellum of neonatally thyroidectomized rats. *Brain Res* 15, 209–218.

Krishnan RR, Maltbie AA and Davidson JR (1983) Abnormal cortisol suppression in bipolar patients with simultaneous manic and depressive symptoms. *Am J Psychiatr* 140, 203–220.

Leonard BE (1994) Effects of antidepressants on specific neurotransmitters: are such effects relevant to the therapeutic action? In *Handbook of Depression and Anxiety* (eds den Boer JA and Sitsen JMA). Marcel Dekker, New York, pp. 379–404.

Leonard BE (1997) The role of noradrenaline in depression: A review. *J Psychopharmacol* 11(Suppl 4), S39–S47.

Leroux P, Bodenant C, Bologna E, et al. (1995) Transient expression of somatostatin receptors in the brain during development. *Ciba Found Symp* 190, 127–137.

Lopez JF, Chalmers DT, Little KY et al. (1998) Regulation of serotonin1A, glucocorticoid, and mineralocorticoid receptor in rat and human hippocampus: implications for the neurobiology of depression. *Biol Psychiatr* 43, 547–573.

Mace S and Taylor D (2000) Selective serotonin reuptake inhibitors: a review of efficacy and tolerability. *Exp Opin Pharmacother* 1, 917–933.

Mann JJ (1999) Role of serotonergic system in the pathogenesis of major depression and suicidal behavior. *Neuropsychopharmacology* 21, 99S–105S.

Mann JJ, Brent DA and Arango V (2001) The neurobiology and genetics of suicide and attempted suicide: A focus on the serotonergic system. *Neuropsychopharmacology* 24, 467–477.

Mann JJ and Arango V (1999) Abnormalities of brain structure and function in mood disorders. In Neurobiology of Mental Illness, Charney DS, Nestler EJ, and Bunney BS (eds). Oxford University Press, Oxford, New York, pp. 385–393.

McAllister AK, Katz LC, and Lo DC (1999). Neurotrophins and synaptic plasticity. *Annu Rev Neurosci* 22, 295–318.

Meltzer HY and Lowy MT (1987). The serotonin hypothesis of depression, in *Psychopharmacology: The Third Generation of Progress* (ed Meltzer HY). Raven Press, New York, pp. 513–526.

Mendlewicz J, Linkowski P, Kerkhofs M, et al. (1985) Diurnal hypersecretion of growth hormone in depression. *J Clin Endocrinol Metabol* 60, 505–512.

Nemeroff CB, Musselman DL, Nathan KI et al. (1997) Pathophysiological basis of psychiatric disorders: Focus on mood disorders and schizophrenia, in *Psychiatry* (eds Tasman A, Kay J, and Lieberman JA). WB Saunders, Philadelphia, PA, pp. 258–311.

Oppenheimer JH and Schwartz HL (1997) Molecular basis of thyroid hormone-dependent brain development. *Endocrinol Rev* 18, 462–475.

Oquendo MA and Mann JJ (2000) Serotonergic dysfunction in mood disorders, in *Bipolar Disorders: Basic Mechanisms and Therapeutic Implications* (eds Soares JC and Gershon S). Marcel Dekker, New York, pp. 121–142.

Owens MJ (1997) Molecular and cellular mechanisms of antidepressant drugs. *Depress Anx* 4, 153–159.

Papp M and Moryl E (1994) Antidepressant activity of noncompetitive and competitive NMDA receptor antagonists in a chronic mild stress model of depression. *Eur J Pharmacol* 263, 1–7.

Potter W, Grossman G and Rudorfer M (1993) Noradrenergic function in depressive disorders, in *Biology of Depressive Disorders, Part A: A Systems Perspective* (eds Mann J and Kupfer D). Plenum Press, New York, pp. 1–27.

Prange AJ Jr., Wilson IC, Lynn CW, et al. (1974). L-tryptophan in mania. Contribution to a permissive hypothesis of affective disorders. *Arch Gen Psychiatr* 30, 56–62.

Przegalinski E, Tatarczynska E, Deren-Wesolek A et al. (1997) Antidepressant-like effects of a partial agonist at strychnine-insensitive glycine receptors and a competitive NMDA receptor antagonist. *Neuropharmacology* 36, 31–37.

Ressler KJ and Nemeroff CB (1999) Role of norepinephrine in the pathophysiology and treatment of mood disorders. *Biol Psychiatr* 46, 1219–1233.

Reus VI and Freimer NB (1997) Understanding the genetic basis of mood disorders: where do we stand? *Am J Hum Gen* 60, 1283–1288.

Roy A, Wolkowitz OM and Bissette G (1994) Differences in CSF concentrations of thyrotropin-releasing hormone in depressed patients and normal subjects: negative findings. *Am J Psychiatr* 151, 600–602.

Sachar EJ, Hellman L, Fukushima DK, et al. (1970) Cortisol production in depressive illness. A clinical and biochemical clarification. *Arch Gen Psychiatr* 23, 289–298.

Sampson SM (2001) Treating depression with selective serotonin reuptake inhibitors: a practical approach. *Mayo Clin Proc* 76, 739–744.

Schatzberg A and Schildkraut J (1995) Recent studies on norepinephrine systems in mood disorders, in *Psychopharmacology: The Fourth Generation of Progress* (eds Bloom F and Kupfer D). Raven Press, New York, pp. 911–920.

Schilkrut R, Chandra O, Osswald M, et al. (1975) Growth hormone release during sleep and with thermal stimulation in depressed patients. *Neuropsychobiology* 1, 70–79.

Sevy S, Mendlewicz J and Mendelbaum K (1995) Genetic research in bipolar illness, in *Handbook of Depression*, 2nd edn., (eds Beckham EE and Leber WR). Guilford Press, New York, pp. 203–212.

Sher L (2000a) Psychiatric diagnoses and inconsistent results of association studies in behavioral genetics. *Med Hypoth* 54, 207–209.

Sher L (2000b) The role of brain thyroid hormones in the mechanisms of seasonal changes in mood and behavior. *Med Hypoth* 55, 56–59.

Sher L (2001) Possible role of brain thyroid hormones in the effects of bright light on mood and behavior. *Med Hypoth* 57, 602–605.

Sherman SL, DeFries JC, Gottesman II et al. (1997) Recent developments in human behavioral genetics: past accomplishments and future directions. *Am J Hum Genet* 60, 1265–1275.

Shiah IS and Yatham LN (2000) Serotonin in mania and in the mechanism of action of mood stabilizers: A review of clinical studies. *Bipol Disord* 2, 77–92.

Soares JC and Mann JJ (1997a) The anatomy of mood disorders: Review of structural neuroimaging studies. *Biol Psychiatr* 41, 86–106.

Soares JC and Mann JJ (1997b) The functional neuroanatomy of mood disorders. *J. Psychiatr Res* 31, 393–432.

Stokes PE and Sikes CR (1987) Hypothalamic–pituitary–adrenal axis in affective disorders, in *Psychopharmacology: The Third Generation of Progress* (ed Meltzer HY). Raven Press, New York, pp. 589–607.

Stout SC, Owens MJ, and Nemeroff CB (2001) Neurokinin(1) receptor antagonists as potential antidepressants. *Ann Rev of Pharmacol Toxicol* 41, 877–906.

Swann AC, Stokes PE, Casper R et al. (1992) Hypothalamic–pituitary–adrenocortical function in mixed and pure mania. *Acta Psychiatr Scand* 85, 270–274.

Thase ME (2000) Mood disorders: neurobiology, in *Kaplan & Sadock's Comprehensive Textbook of Psychiatry*, Vol. 2, 7th edn., (eds Sadock BJ and Sadock VA). Lippincott Williams & Wilkins, Philadelphia, pp. 1318–1328.

Thase ME and Holland RH (1995) Biological processes in depression: An updated review and integration, in *Handbook of Depression* (eds Beckham EE and Leber WR). Guilford Press, New York, pp. 213–279.

Toivola PT, Gale CC, Goodner CJ, et al. (1972) Central-adrenergic regulation of growth hormone and insulin. *Hormones* 3, 192–213.

Trullas R and Skolnick P (1990) Functional antagonists at the NMDA receptor complex exhibit antidepressant actions. *Eur J Pharmacol* 185, 1–10.

Vestergaard P, Sorensen T, Hoppe E et al. (1978) Biogenic amine metabolites in cerebrospinal fluid of patients with affective disorders. *Acta Psychiatr Scand* 58, 88–96.

Wang JF, Bown CD, Chen B et al. (2001) Identification of mood stabilizer-regulated genes by differential-display PCR. *Int J Neuropsychopharmacol* 4, 65–74.

Yocca FD (1990) Neurochemistry and neurophysiology of buspirone and gepirone: interactions at presynaptic and postsynaptic 5-HT1A receptors. *J Clin Psychopharmacol* 10(Suppl 3), 6S–12S.

Psychiatric Pathophysiology: Anxiety Disorders

One thing is certain, that the problem of anxiety is a nodal point, linking up all kinds of important questions: a riddle, of which the solution must cast a flood of light upon our whole mental life.

Freud 1917

Introduction

In the 50 years since DSM-I, the rubric of "anxiety disorder" has evolved and expanded to encompass generalized anxiety disorder (GAD), panic disorder (PD), phobias, obsessive–compulsive disorder (OCD) and post traumatic stress disorder (PTSD) (Rickels and Rynn, 2001). Given the complex circuitry required to integrate behaviors characteristic of the anxiety disorders (Lang et al., 1998; Coplan and Lydiard, 1998; Davis 1998), it seems implausible that a single gene product or transmitter system will ultimately be identified as the sole mediator of any anxiety disorder.

Most contemporary neurobiological theories of anxiety disorders are grounded on the molecular mechanisms of drugs used to treat these disorders. Despite the ever-increasing use of genetically engineered mice (which has certainly added to our knowledge base), this "reverse engineering" approach remains the standard in biological psychiatry, in part because of the difficulties inherent in validating animal models of psychiatric disorders. Further, when a drug is shown to be effective, variants of the drug (differing in potency and/or efficacy) often facilitate hypothesis testing in both animals and humans. This chapter describes preclinical studies linking four major transmitter systems (GABA, glutamate, serotonin and norepinephrine) to anxiety disorders. This selection was based on the mechanism of action of drugs currently approved to treat one or more of the anxiety disorders.

Gamma-aminobutyric Acid (GABA)

GABA is the principal inhibitory transmitter in the vertebrate central nervous system, with about one-third of all synapses using GABA as a transmitter. Fifteen years after their introduction into clinical practice, benzodiazepines were shown to augment the actions of GABA (Haefely and Polc, 1986). A compelling body of evidence indicates that augmentation of GABAergic transmission mediates the principal pharmacological actions of the benzodiazepines. The efficacy of benzodiazepines in the treatment of anxiety disorders (including GAD, PD and social phobia) has been well documented by double-blind, placebo-controlled studies (Ballenger, 1999; Blanco et al., 2002).

From a cellular perspective, benzodiazepines act as allosteric modulators, increasing the apparent affinity of GABA at $GABA_A$ receptors (Figure 12.1). By binding to a specific subset of amino acids on the N-terminal of the $GABA_A$ receptor alpha and gamma subunits (Wong et al., 1992; Tretter et al., 1997), benzodiazepines (and structurally unrelated compounds that bind to overlapping sequences on these subunits) effect this increase in the apparent affinity of GABA to its recognition site (Haefely and Polc, 1986).

Despite the evidence that benzodiazepines and other strategies directed at augmenting GABAergic transmission are effective in the treatment of anxiety disorders, this evidence does not directly implicate $GABA_A$ receptors in their pathophysiology. Nonetheless, convergent pharmacological and physiological evidence are consistent with the hypothesis that GABAergic pathways are intimately involved in the behavioral, somatic and endocrine manifestations of anxiety.

There are two principal lines of pharmacological evidence implicating GABAergic pathways in anxiety. The first involves the demonstration that so-called benzodiazepine receptor *inverse agonists* produce a constellation of actions (behavioral, somatic and endocrine) reminiscent of anxiety in rodents and primates, including man. Recall that the principal cellular action of benzodiazepines is to increase the apparent affinity of GABA at $GABA_A$ receptors, manifested as a left shift of the GABA concentration effect curve (Figure 12.2).

The second line of pharmacological evidence linking $GABA_A$ receptor dysfunction to anxiety disorders stems from reports that flumazenil is panicogenic in PD patients but not in control subjects (Nutt et al., 1990; Woods et al., 1991). It can be hypothesized that flumazenil acts as a GABA negative (inverse agonist) compound in some subsets of PD patients with an **atypical** $GABA_A$ receptor composition in circumscribed areas of the central nervous system (CNS). While there is no direct evidence to support this hypothesis, positron emission tomography (PET) studies have demonstrated a global reduction in the binding of ^{11}C flumazenil throughout the brain in patients with PD compared with controls.

Findings from multiple lines of research indicate that $GABA_A$ receptors may have evolutionary significance as a **bio-warning** system and perhaps as a means of compensating for perturbations in the environment. If stress-induced activation of $GABA_A$ receptors (manifested in these studies as increases

Essentials of Psychiatry   Jerald Kay and Allan Tasman
© 2006 John Wiley & Sons, Ltd.

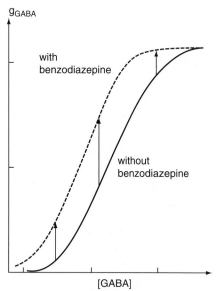

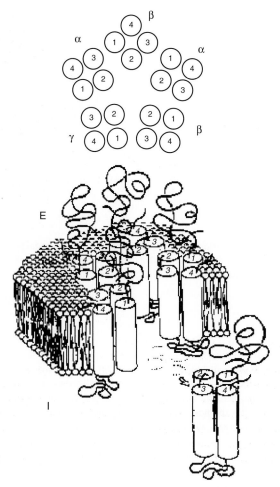

Figure 12.1 *Benzodiazepines augment GABAergic transmission. Ordinate: Magnitude of GABA-induced (chloride) currents (g_{GABA}); abcissa: concentration of GABA applied. In systems expressing $GABA_A$ receptors (ranging from spinal neurons to cells transfected with mRNAs encoding $GABA_A$ receptor subunits), application of GABA increases chloride conductance, generally producing membrane hyperpolarization. While unable either to gate (like GABA and GABAmimetics) or directly open (like anesthetic concentrations of barbiturates) these GABA-gated chloride channels, benzodiazepines increase the apparent affinity of GABA, producing the illustrated left shift in its concentration-effect curve. An increase in the apparent affinity of endogenous GABA produced by benzodiazepines (and related compounds) is thought to mediate the principal pharmacological actions of these compounds, including their antianxiety actions. Reproduced with permission from Physiology of GABA enhancement by benzodiazepines and barbiturates. In Benzodiazepine/GABA Receptors and Chloride Channels, Haefley W and Polc P [1986] Olsen R and Venter C [eds]. Alan R. Liss, New York. With permission from John Wiley, New York.*

Figure 12.2 *Model of the $GABA_A$ receptor. $GABA_A$ receptors are hetero-oligomers, with the great majority of native receptors containing α, β, and γ subunits. The stoichiometry of a recombinant receptor containing an $α_1$, $β_{2 or 3}$, and $γ_2$ subunit (this subunit combination represents the majority of $GABA_A$ receptors in mammalian brain) (De Blas AL [1996] Brain $GABA_A$ receptors studied with subunit-specific antibodies. J Mol Neurobiol 12, 55–71) is 2α, 2β, and 1γ, arranged as illustrated in the top panel (Klausberger T, Sarto I, Ehya N et al. [2001] Alternate use of distinct intersubunit contacts controls $GABA_A$ receptor assembly and stoichiometry. J Neurosci 21, 9124–9133). Binding sites for benzodiazepines (and related compounds) are formed by the amino-terminal domains (located in the extracellular space, E) of the α and γ subunits. Each subunit possesses four transmembrane spanning domains (illustrated as cylinders 1–4), with the second transmembrane spanning domain forming the lumen of the GABA-gated chloride channel. Symbols: E, extracellular space; I, intracellular space. (Source: Modified from Olsen R and Towin A [1990] Molecular biology of $GABA_A$ receptors Faseb J 4, 1469–1480; Klausberger T, Sarto I, Ehya N et al. [2001] Alternate use of distinct intersubunit contacts controls $GABA_A$ receptor assembly and stoichiometry. J Neurosci 21, 9124–9133.)*

in TBPS binding) is an attempt to compensate for environmental perturbations, then benzodiazepines (and low doses of barbiturates which increase the frequency of channel opening) (Study and Barker, 1981) may be viewed as pharmacological mimicry of the organism's initial attempts to cope with the disruption of its environment.

Glutamate

Glutamate is the principal excitatory transmitter in the mammalian CNS. A discussion of the role of glutamatergic transmission is included in this overview based on an extensive preclinical literature linking modulation of both ionotropic (*N*-methyl-D-aspartate) and metabotropic (mGluR2) glutamate receptor subtypes (Figure 12.3) to anxiety (Skolnick, 2000). Further, a recent, albeit preliminary, clinical study

(Levine *et al.*, 2001) appears to validate preclinical findings indicating that glutamate receptors are a valid target for the

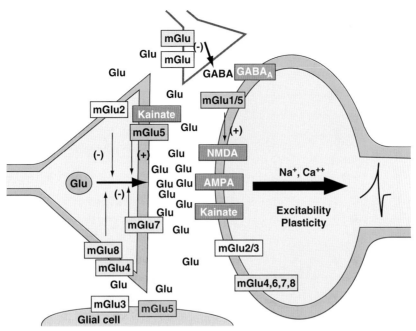

Figure 12.3   *Glutamate receptors: cellular localization and function. The majority of ionotropic glutamate (AMPA, kainate and NMDA) receptors are postsynaptic. These glutamate receptors mediate fast excitatory transmission through associated ligand-gated cation (sodium and calcium permeant). Among ionotropic glutamate receptors, the NMDA subfamily has been most closely linked to anxiety disorders (see text for details). Metabotropic glutamate receptors are distributed across the synapse region (including neighboring glia) and appear to serve modulatory roles via coupling to phospholipase C or adenylate cyclase. Among metabotropic glutamate receptors, group II (mGluR2 and mGluR3) have been most closely linked to anxiety disorders (see text for details). (Schoepp DD [2001] Unveiling the functions of presynaptic metabotropic glutamate receptors in the central nervous system. J Pharmacol Exp Ther 299, 12–20. Reproduced by permission of American Society for Pharmacology and Experimental Therapeutics).*

development of novel anxiolytics. Like serotonin receptors, the glutamate receptor superfamily includes both ionotropic and G-protein coupled receptors (GPCR). The structural and molecular details of both receptor classes have been reviewed in detail (Schoepp, 2001; Conn and Pin, 1997; Palfreyman *et al.*, 1994; Cotman *et al.*, 1995). A brief overview of two glutamate receptor subtypes is provided as a background to place preclinical and clinical findings in context.

NMDA Receptors
NMDA receptors are broadly and unevenly distributed across the mammalian CNS.

In addition to reports that NMDA antagonists are anxiolytic, there is a body of preclinical literature indicating that NMDA receptor activation is **anxiogenic**. These studies are reminiscent of, and in some sense parallel, studies with benzodiazepine receptor inverse agonists.

Linking NMDA Receptors to Biogenic Amine-based Anxiolytics
In preclinical studies, chronic treatment with biogenicamine–based antidepressants used in the treatment of anxiety disorders blunts NMDA receptor function (Skolnick, 1999). In view of the anxiolytic-like actions of NMDA antagonists in

preclinical tests, the body of evidence indicates that NMDA receptors may represent a downstream target for biogenic amine-based antidepressants. While this hypothesis has been used to explain the **therapeutic lag** associated with biogenic amine-based antidepressants (Skolnick, 1999), it may also contribute to the delay in onset of these serotonin and norepinephrine modulators used to treat anxiety disorders (Figure 12.4).

Group II Metabotropic Glutamate Receptors
Metabotropic glutamate receptors are classified as "family 3" G-protein coupled receptors (GPCRs). Group II metabotropic receptors (that include mGluR2 and mGluR3 receptors) are negatively coupled to adenylate cyclase, and the mGluR2 receptor subclass is found both pre- and extrasynaptically. Several lines of evidence indicate that glutamate activates these mGluR2 receptors, resulting in a rapid inhibition of glutamate release, creating a negative feedback loop (Schoepp, 2001; Scanzfani *et al.*, 1997). Since activation of Group II metabotropic receptors appears to require an elevated glutamate concentration, an agonist at these receptors would effectively dampen glutamatergic transmission (including activation of NMDA receptors) without remarkably affecting synaptic glutamate under resting conditions.

Based on these data and reports that telencephalic glutamate concentrations are rapidly elevated during stress

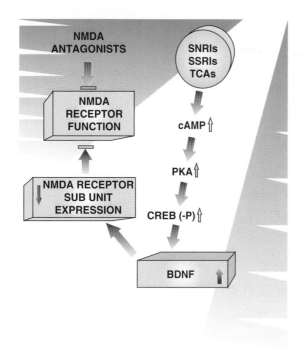

Figure 12.4 *Linking NMDA receptors to biogenic amine-based anxiolytics: By increasing the synaptic availability of biogenic amines, MAOIs, TCAs, and SSRIs can activate adenylate cyclase through G_s-coupled receptors. Increases in intracellular cyclic AMP increase protein kinase A activity, which may then phosphorylate a cyclic AMP response element binding protein (CREB), increasing the transcription of BDNF. Exposure to BDNF can diminish NMDA receptor function (see text and Skolnick [1999] for details). In view of preclinical studies linking NMDA receptors to anxiety disorders, downregulation of NMDA may represent a downstream target for biogenic amine-based agents. While this hypothesis has been used to explain the therapeutic lag associated with biogenic amine-based antidepressants, it may also contribute to the delay in onset of these serotonin and norepinephrine modulators used to treat anxiety disorders. Reprinted from European Journal of Pharmacology 375, Skolnick, Antidepressants for the new millennium. Copyright 1999, with permission from Elsevier.*

(Moghaddam, 1993), it may be hypothesized that activation of Group II metabotropic receptors and the subsequent reduction in glutamate release will result in an anxiolytic action. An emerging body of preclinical data (Skolnick, 2000) as well as a recent clinical report (Levine *et al.*, 2001) support this hypothesis.

Serotonin

An association between serotonergic transmission and anxiety disorders was established more than 30 years ago with reports (Graeff and Schoenfeld, 1970; Geller and Blum, 1970) that inhibitors of serotonin synthesis (such as *p*-chlorophenylalanine) reduced the ability of punishment (e.g., footshock) to suppress operant responding. Many studies have confirmed and embellished the basic findings that destruction of serotonergic pathways and/

or a reduction in the synthesis of this biogenic amine results in an animal behaving as if it had been administered an anxiolytic. There is a complementary body of evidence that serotonin receptor activation exacerbates anxiety. For example, challenge doses of meta-chlorphenylpiperazine (a serotonin agonist) were anxiogenic in PD patients (Charney *et al.*, 1987b), individuals with OCD (Zohar *et al.*, 1987) and in patients with GAD (Nutt, 2001). The observation that anxiety can initially be exacerbated in GAD patients receiving SSRIs (Nutt, 2001) provides perhaps the most compelling evidence that acute elevation of synaptic serotonin is anxiogenic.

Norepinephrine

Like serotonergic neurons, noradrenergic neurons are anatomically restricted, with the majority (>70%) found in the nucleus locus coeruleus. Noradrenergic neurons also possess an extensively ramified system of efferent projections, diffusely innervating brain regions (e.g., cortex, amygdala, hippocampus, hypothalamus) associated with anxiety disorders. From a historical perspective, the evidence linking norepinephrine (and by implication, the recognition sites subserving this transmitter) to anxiety disorders clearly predates (Blaschko, 1972) the other transmitters described in this chapter. The ability of stress to impact brain norepinephrine levels has been known for almost 40 years (e.g., Barchas and Freedman, 1963; Maynert and Levi, 1964). A wide range of stressors have been reported to increase norepinephrine turnover in the CNS (Stone, 1975; Tilson *et al.*, 1975). This activation of noradrenergic neurons by stress can be attenuated by benzodiazepines (Taylor and Laverty, 1973; Ida *et al.*, 1985).

The locus coeruleus sends projections to many forebrain areas associated with fear and anxiety via the dorsal noradrenergic bundle. Redmond and his colleagues (Redmond and Huang, 1979) provided perhaps the most compelling preclinical data linking noradrenergic pathways to anxiety disorders. Thus, it was demonstrated that electrical stimulation of the locus coeruleus in monkeys produced fear-like behaviors, and that "symptom" severity appeared dependent on the strength of the applied stimulus. Bilateral ablation of the locus coeruleus blunted the behavioral responses of animals to threatening environmental stimuli (Redmond and Huang, 1979). Pharmacological studies in humans have also implicated noradrenergic pathways in some of the anxiety disorders.

A variety of clinical and preclinical findings indicate that physiological or pharmacological activation of noradrenergic pathways mimics or exacerbates anxiety. At face value, these findings are at odds with the reported efficacy of TCAs and MAOIs in anxiety disorders (Hoehn-Saric, 2000; Buller and Jorga, 2000). In a broad sense, this body of evidence parallels the apparent contradictory findings that increasing serotonergic transmission is associated with anxiety, yet drugs whose primary neurochemical action (e.g., SSRIs) results in increased synaptic concentrations of serotonin are useful in the treatment of anxiety disorders.

Future studies on potential targets downstream of the monoaminergic synapse (e.g., Rossby and Sulser, 1997) (Figure 12.5) may result in a better understanding of the antianxiety actions of these compounds and the neurochemical substrates of anxiety.

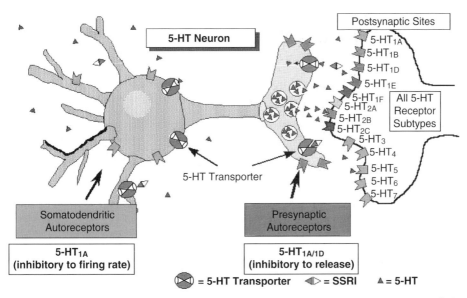

Figure 12.5 *Serotonin receptor heterogeneity. The cell bodies of serotonin-containing neurons are primarily located in or near the brain stem raphe nuclei. These neurons possess long, extraordinarily arborized axons. Serotonin signaling is largely effected through G-protein–coupled receptors, although one ionotropic (5-HT$_3$) receptor has been identified. The G-protein–coupled serotonin receptors include representatives of the Gs family (e.g., 5-HT$_6$ receptors) positively coupled to adenylate cyclase, the Gi family (e.g., 5-HT$_{1A}$ receptors) inhibiting adenylate cyclase, and receptors coupled to phopholipase C activation (e.g., 5-HT_{2C} receptors). Drugs that increase synaptic serotonin concentrations (e.g., SSRIs, TCAs) are effective in treating anxiety disorders. However, the functional and anatomical diversity of serotonergic pathways may contribute to both a delay in onset and a body of evidence that acute activation of serotonergic transmission is anxiogenic. (Reprinted with the permission of Dr David Nelson, Lilly Research Laboratories.)*

References

Ballenger JC (1999) Current treatments of the anxiety disorders in adults. *Biol Psychiatr* 46, 1579–1594.

Barchas JD and Freedman D (1963) Response to physiological stress. *Biochem Pharmacol* 12, 1232–1235.

Blanco C, Antia SX and Liebowitz MR (2002) Pharmacotherapy of social anxiety disorder. *Biol Psychiatr* 51, 109–120.

Blaschko H (1972) Catecholamines (1922–1971), in *Catecholamines, Handbook of Experiment Pharmacology*, Vol. 33 (eds Blaschko H and Muscholl E). Springer-Verlag, Berlin, pp. 1–15.

Buller R and Jorga KM (2000) Monoamine oxidase inhibitors (including the newer reversible compounds), in *Anxiolytics* (eds Briley M and Nutt D). Birkhauser Verlag, Basel, pp. 41–53.

Charney DS, Woods SW, Goodman WK *et al.* (1987b) Serotonin function in anxiety: II. Effects of the serotonin agonist mCPP in panic disorder patients and healthy subjects. *Psychopharmacology* 92, 14–24.

Conn PJ and Pin JP (1997) Pharmacology and functions of metabotropic glutamate receptors. *Annu Rev Pharmacol Toxicol* 37, 205–237.

Coplan JD and Lydiard RB (1998) Brain circuits in panic disorder. *Biol Psychiatr* 44, 1264–1276.

Cotman CW, Kahle JS, Miller SE *et al.* (1995) Excitatory amino acid neurotransmission, in *Psychopharmacology: The Fourth Generation of Progress* (eds Bloom FE and Kupfer DJ). Raven Press, New York, pp. 75–85.

Davis M (1998) Are different parts of the extended amygdala involved in fear versus anxiety? *Biol Psychiatr* 44, 1239–1247.

Geller I and Blum K (1970) The effect of 5-HTP on para-chlorophenylalanine (*p*-CPA) attenuation of conflict behavior. *Eur J Pharmacol* 9, 319–324.

Graeff FG and Schoenfeld RI (1970) Tryptaminergic mechanisms in punished and nonpunished behavior. *J Pharmacol Exp Ther* 173, 277–283.

Haefely W and Polc P (1986) Physiology of GABA enhancement by benzodiazepines and barbiturates, in *Benzodiazepine/GABA Receptors and Chloride Channels* (eds Olsen R and Venter C). Alan R. Liss, New York, pp. 97–133.

Hoehn-Saric R (2000) Tricyclic antidepressants, in *Anxiolytics* (eds Briley M and Nutt D). Birkhauser Verlag, Basel, pp. 27–39.

Ida Y, Tanaka M, Tsuda A *et al.* (1985) Attenuating effect of diazepam on stress-induced increases in noradrenaline turnover in specific brain regions of rats: Antagonism by Ro 25-1788. *Life Sci* 37, 2491–2498.

Lang PJ, Bradley MM and Cuthbert BN (1998) Emotion, motivation and anxiety: Brain mechanisms and psychophysiology. *Biol Psychiatr* 44, 1248–1263.

Levine LR, Gaydos B, Sheehan D *et al.* (2001) The mGlu2/3 receptor agonist, LY354740, reduces panic anxiety induced by a CO2 challenge in patients diagnosed with panic disorder. *Abs Am College Neuropsychopharmacol Ann Meet 40* (Abstract #58), p. 134.

Maynert EW and Levi R (1964) Stress induced release of brain norepinephrine and its inhibition by drugs. *J Pharmacol Exp Ther* 143, 90–95.

Moghaddam B (1993) Stress preferentially increases extraneuronal levels of excitatory amino acids in the prefrontal cortex: Comparison to the hippocampus and basal ganglia. *J Neurochem* 60, 1650–1657.

Nutt DJ (2001) Neurobiological mechanisms in generalized anxiety disorder. *J Clin Psychiatr* 62(Suppl 11), 22–27.

Nutt DJ, Glue P, Lawson CW *et al.* (1990) Flumazenil provocation of pain attacks: Evidence for altered benzodiazepine receptor sensitivity in panic disorder. *Arch Gen Psychiatr* 47, 917–925.

Palfreyman MG, Reynolds IJ and Skolnick P (eds) (1994) *Pharmacology and Toxicology: Basic and Clinical Aspects: Direct and Allosteric Control of Glutamate Receptors*. CRC Press, Boca Raton.

Redmond DE and Huang YH (1979) New evidence for a locus coeruleus-norepinephrine connection with anxiety. *Life Sci* 25, 2149–2162.

Rickels K and Rynn MA (2001) What is generalized anxiety disorder? *J Clin Psychiatr* 62(Suppl 11), 4–12.

Rossby SP and Sulser F (1997) Antidepressants: Beyond the synapse, in *Antidepressants: New Pharmacological Strategies* (eds Skolnick P). Humana Press, Totowa, pp. 195–212.

Scanzfani M, Salin PA, Vogt KE *et al.* (1997) Use-dependent increases in glutamate concentrations activate presynaptic metabotropic glutamate receptors. *Nature* 385, 630–634.

Schoepp DD (2001) Unveiling the functions of presynaptic metabotropic glutamate receptors in the central nervous system. *J Pharmacol Exp Ther* 299, 12–20.

Skolnick P (1999) Antidepressants for the new millennium. *Eur J Pharmacol* 375, 31–41.

Skolnick P (2000) Glutamate receptor ligands, in *Anxiolytics* (eds Briley M and Nutt D). Birkhauser Verlag, Basel, pp. 139–150.

Stone EA (1975) Stress and catecholamines, in *Catecholamines and Behavior*, Vol. 2, (ed Friedhoff AJ). Plenum Press, New York, pp. 31–72.

Study R and Barker J (1981) Diazepam and (−) pentobarbital: Fluctuation analysis reveals different mechanisms for potentiation of gamma-aminobutyric acid response in cultured central neurons. *Proc Natl Acad Sci USA* 78, 7180–7184.

Taylor KM and Laverty R (1973) The interaction of chlordiazepoxide, diazepam and nitrazepam with catecholamine and histamine in regions of the rat brain, in *The Benzodiazepines* (eds Garattini S, Mussini E, and Randall LO). Raven Press, New York, pp. 191–202.

Tilson HA, Rech RH and Sparber SB (1975) Release of 14C-norepinephrine into the lateral cerebroventricle of rats by exposure to a conditioned aversive stimulus. *Pharmacol Biochem Behav* 3, 385–392.

Tretter V, Ehya N, Fuchs K *et al.* (1997) Stoichiometry and assembly of a recombinant GABAA receptor subtype. *J Neurosci* 17, 2728–2737.

Wong G, Sei Y and Skolnick P (1992) Stable expression of type 1 γ-aminobutyric acid$_A$/benzodiazepine receptors in a transfected cell line. *Mol Pharmacol* 42, 996–1003.

Woods SW, Charney DS, Silver JM *et al.* (1991) Behavioral, biochemical, and cardiovascular responses to the benzodiazepine receptor antagonist flumazenil in panic disorder. *Psychiatr Res* 36, 115–127.

Zohar J, Mueller EA, Insel TR *et al.* (1987) Serotonergic responsivity in obsessive–compulsive disorder. Comparison of patients and healthy controls. *Arch Gen Psychiatr* 44, 946–951.

13 Psychiatric Pathophysiology: Addiction

Addiction is a complex maladaptive behavior produced by repeated exposure to rewarding stimuli (O'Brien, 2001). There are two primary features common to both natural and pharmacological stimuli that elicit addiction. First, the rewarding stimulus associated with the addiction is a compelling motivator of behavior at the expense of behaviors leading to the acquisition of other rewarding stimuli. Thus, individuals come to orient increasing amounts of their daily activity around the acquisition of the rewarding stimulus to which they are addicted. Secondly, there is a persistence of craving for the addictive stimulus, combined with an inability to regulate the behaviors associated with obtaining that stimulus. Thus, years after the last exposure to an addictive stimulus, re-exposure or environmental cues associated with that stimulus will elicit behavior aimed at obtaining the reward.

During the course of repeated exposure to strong motivationally relevant stimuli, specific brain nuclei and circuits become engaged that mediate the addicted behavioral response. It is generally thought that different rewarding stimuli involve different brain circuits, but also that there are regions of overlap forming a common substrate for all addictive stimuli. Studies using animal models of reward and addiction have focused on subcortical brain circuits known to be involved in drug reward, such as the dopamine projection from the ventral mesencephalon to the nucleus accumbens (Koob and LeMoal, 2001; Everitt and Wolf, 2002). Accordingly, molecular and electrophysiological studies of the cellular plasticity mediating the emergence of addictive behaviors have focused on the nucleus accumbens and ventral mesencephalon. However, over the last decade studies have emerged from both the animal literature and neuroimaging of drug addicts indicating that the expression of addicted behaviors such as sensitization and craving involves regions of the cortex and allocortex (Pierce and Kalivas, 1997; Volkow and Fowler, 2000; Grant et al., 1996; Childress et al., 1999). In this regard, two regions have come to be most closely associated with craving, the amygdala and frontal cortex (including the anterior cingulate and ventral orbitofrontal cortex). Prior to describing circuitry underlying the state of addiction, we will briefly examine the neurobiology associated with the development of the addicted state.

The Development of Addiction

The acute administration of all addictive drugs, with the possible exception of the benzodiazepines, stimulates dopamine transmission in the projection from the ventral mesencephalon to the nucleus accumbens. This projection is generally referred to as the mesolimbic dopamine system; Figure 13.1

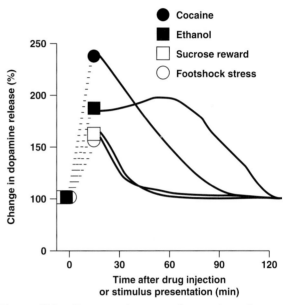

Figure 13.1 *Changes in dopamine release in the nucleus accumbens of rats treated acutely with various classes of addictive drugs, or exposed to positive (sucrose) or negative (footshock) environmental stimuli. The changes in dopamine levels were determined with microdialysis and the data are an idealized portrayal derived from the majority of extant literature. For specific examples of experimental measurements the reader is referred to the following references (Nisell M, Nomikos GG and Svensson TH [1994] Systemic nicotine-induced dopamine release in the rat nucleus accumbens is regulated by nicotinic receptors in the ventral tegmental area. Synapse 16, 36–44; Kalivas PW and Duffy P [1993] Time course of extracellular dopamine and behavioral sensitization to cocaine. I. Dopamine axon terminals. J Neurosci 13, 266–275; Yim HJ, Schallert T, Randall PK et al. [1998] Comparison of local and systemic ethanol effects on extracellular dopamine concentration in rat nucleus accumbens by microdialysis. Alcohol Clin Exp Res 22[2], 367–374; Salamone J, Cousins M, McCullough L et al. [1994] Nucleus accumbens dopamine release increases during instrumental lever pressing for food but not free food consumption. Pharmacol Biochem Behav 49, 25–31; Deutch AY and Roth RH [1990] The determinants of stress-induced activation of the prefrontal cortical dopamine system. Prog Brain Res 85, 357–393). Note that the effect of addictive substances on extracellular dopamine levels is of greater intensity and duration than the effect of motivationally relevant environmental stimuli.*

Essentials of Psychiatry Jerald Kay and Allan Tasman
© 2006 John Wiley & Sons, Ltd.

illustrates the capacity of two drugs of abuse – cocaine and ethanol – to increase dopamine transmission in the nucleus accumbens. The pharmacological site of action by which different classes of drugs of abuse activate dopamine transmission varies and includes three general cellular mechanisms that encompass all drugs of abuse: 1) Receptors for the drug are on dopamine cell bodies and dendrites, and through these receptors drug administration directly stimulates dopamine neurons. Nicotine and marijuana are examples of drugs working in part through this mechanism (Cheer *et al.*, 2000; Nisell *et al.*, 1994). 2) Receptors are located primarily on GABAergic inhibitory afferents to the dopamine cells, and drug binding to these receptors reduces GABA release, thereby disinhibiting dopamine neuronal activity. Opioids and ethanol produce reward in part by this mechanism (Bunney *et al.*, 2001; Cameron *et al.*, 1997). 3) Finally, drugs can bind to presynaptic receptors to increase the presynaptic release of dopamine without directly altering the activity of dopamine neurons. The primary mechanism in this category is exemplified by amphetamine-like psychostimulants which bind to the dopamine transporter and increase dopamine release by blocking reuptake and/or promoting the release of dopamine by reverse transport (Seiden *et al.*, 1993).

Figure 13.1 also illustrates that mesolimbic dopamine is released by environmental stimuli that are motivationally relevant to the organism, regardless of the valence of the stimulus. For example, either positive motivational stimuli such as sex and food, or negative stressful stimuli will increase dopamine release. However, as indicated in Figure 13.1, regardless of the intensity of the natural stimulus, the extent of dopamine release is far less than that produced by drugs. This is especially true for the duration of dopamine release induced by a typical dose of addictive drugs that will endure for many minutes to hours, while a natural stimulus is thought to elevate dopamine for a period of only a few minutes, even if the stimulus itself is present for a greater length of time.

Unlike physiological stimuli, the increase in dopamine transmission does not diminish following repeated drug administration (although this varies with drug class, and some tolerance can be demonstrated to all drugs during a binge of drug taking). Thus, repeated drug use is associated with repeated increase in dopamine, thereby providing a repeated stimulus for cellular adaptation. Due to both the relative lack of tolerance to drug-induced dopamine release as well as to the fact that the quantity of release is well in excess of what is seen physiologically with naturally rewarding stimuli (see Figure 13.1), it is thought that dopamine-dependent neuroplastic changes induced by repeated drug use are beyond the physiological range of normal cellular adaptation. This pathological event precipitates a sequence of cellular changes that ultimately produce neuroadaptations that are widespread in cortical and limbic circuitry, and these adaptations constitute the underlying pathophysiology of addiction. Although the addiction-associated neuroadaptations are impacted by drug class, dose and withdrawal period, it is thought that excessive, nonphysiological release of dopamine is a critical initiator of the pathology.

Identifying the specific changes in gene expression and cellular function that are associated with the development of addiction is an area of active research, and the interested reader is referred to recent reviews of this literature (Nestler, 2001; Kalivas, 2002).

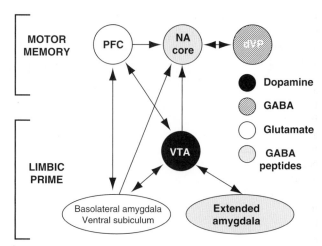

Figure 13.2   *Motive circuit thought to be involved in addiction. A role for these nuclei and interconnections between nuclei in addiction has been revealed using neuroimaging techniques in addicts and/or reinstatement animal models of drug-seeking behavior. (dVP-dorsal ventral pallidum, NAcore-core of the nucleus accumbens, PFC-prefrontal cortex, and VTA-ventral tegmental area.)*

Brain Circuitry and Addiction

Figure 13.2 will be used as a guide for this portion of the chapter and outlines the nuclei and the interconnections between these nuclei, which will be discussed. This circuit has been previously characterized as the motive circuit and contains brain nuclei that are considered critical substrates for drug reward and the development of addiction (as outlined above), such as the dopamine neurons in the ventral tegmental area and projections to the nucleus accumbens. In addition, the circuit contains prefrontal cortical and allocortical brain regions now known to be critical for the expression of behaviors commonly associated with addiction, such as drug craving.

Human Neuroimaging and Animal Models Reveal Addiction Circuitry

The majority of our recent understanding of how the motive circuit (in Figure 13.2) is involved in addiction is derived from neuroimaging studies in human addicts and animal studies employing the reinstatement model of drug craving. The neuroimaging studies typically involve functional imaging of brain activity in addicts that are exposed to evocative stimuli, such as an injection of a low dose of drug or stimuli (e.g., the drug paraphernalia) that the addict associates with drug taking (Volkow and Fowler, 2000).

The Motive Circuit as a Substrate of Addiction

The circuit illustrated in Figure 13.2 consists of interconnected nuclei that have been shown to be involved in the processing of drug reinforcement and in initiating behaviors to obtain such reinforcement. Neuroimaging studies have clearly identified cortical circuits that are activated by drug-associated stimuli in addicts. This includes areas of the prefrontal cortex, such as the anterior cingulate and the ventral orbital cortex, as well as some allocortical regions including the amygdala (Pierce and

Kalivas, 1997; Volkow and Fowler, 2000; Grant *et al.*, 1996; Childress *et al.*, 1999; Porrino and Lyons, 2000). In addition, some neuroimaging studies have revealed involvement of the ventral striatum (including the nucleus accumbens), especially in response to a small challenge dose of drug (Porrino and Lyons, 2000; Breiter *et al.*, 1997). In addition, the animal literature has identified two other brain regions to be critical in models of primed relapse. One area is the ventral tegmental area that, as outlined above, contains dopamine cells projecting to the cortex and nucleus accumbens. The other region that has been associated with stress-induced relapse is the bed nucleus of the stria terminalis, and probably the accompanying nuclei of the extended amygdala. Finally, recent evidence has emerged indicating a possible role for the ventral subiculum, where electrical stimulation was found to induce reinstatement of drug seeking for cocaine (Vorel *et al.*, 2001).

There is a growing realization that stimulus-evoked drug-seeking behavior is comprised of two circuits, a motor memory circuit and a limbic priming circuit (see Figure 13.2). The motor memory circuit consists of the motor nuclei in the motive circuit including the dorsal prefrontal and ventral orbital cortex, core of the nucleus accumbens and dorsolateral ventral pallidum. The limbic priming circuit activates the motor memory circuit in response to various stimuli. The stimuli activate the motor memory circuit via limbic circuitry, and the limbic nuclei involved are somewhat distinct depending upon stimulus modality. The ventral tegmental area is integral to all stimulus modalties, and the extended amygdala and basolateral amygdala contribute differentially depending on whether the stimulus is a stressor or a drug-associated cue, respectively (Figure 13.3).

Motor Memory Circuit

This portion of the circuit may be integral to all forms of drug-taking behavior. Priming stimuli access this circuit primarily via the prefrontal cortex and evoke behaviors organized to obtain drug reward. Thus, the motor memory circuit functions akin to a procedural memory circuit and, when accessed by a priming stimulus, provides a programmed sequence of learned behaviors to obtain drug.

The regions of the prefrontal cortex most clearly shown in neuroimaging studies to be activated by drug-associated environmental or pharmacological cues are the anterior cingulate and ventral orbital cortices (Volkow and Fowler, 2000; Childress *et al.*, 1999). Both of these cortical areas make substantial glutamatergic projections to the nucleus accumbens (Groenewegen *et al.*, 1996).

Although the role of the accumbens to pallidum projection in primed reinstatement is only just emerging, this projection has long been known to mediate motor activity initiated by motivationally relevant stimuli (Mogenson *et al.*, 1980, 1993; Burns *et al.*, 1994). From this literature it is clear that both dopamine and glutamate transmission in the nucleus accumbens are necessary conditions for normal motor stimulation to occur (Burns *et al.*, 1994; Robbins and Everitt, 1996; Vanderschuren and Kalivas, 2000). The data show an association between glutamate, but not dopamine transmission in the nucleus accumbens and drug-seeking behavior. However, in contrast to the nucleus accumbens, dopamine transmission in the dorsal prefrontal cortex or basolateral amygdala has been shown to be critical to the execution of cocaine- or cue-primed reinstatement, respectively (See *et al.*, 2001; McFarland and Kalivas, 2001).

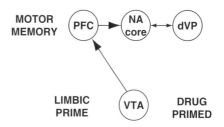

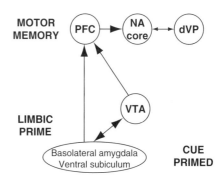

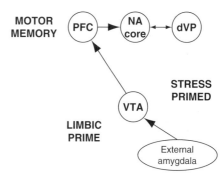

Figure 13.3 *Hypothesized circuits involved in the priming of craving and drug-seeking behavior by stress, learned associations, or an acute drug administration. While the motor memory circuit is postulated to be involved, regardless of the modality of the priming stimulus, the priming circuitry differs between the three classes of stimuli.*

Limbic Priming Circuit

Drug-primed Reinstatement

Acute administration of a drug that was previously self-administered is known to elicit craving and drug-seeking behaviors in experimental animals and human addicts (O'Brien 2001; Markou *et al.*, 1993). The role of dopamine at inducing priming is well established since both systemic and intra-cortical administration of dopamine blockers have been shown to inhibit drug-primed reinstatement. However, activation of dopamine neurons is apparently not a prerequisite, although having an intact dopamine system is permissive. Figure 13.3 illustrates the circuit critical for cocaine-primed reinstatement. It is proposed that this is a minimal circuit and that other drugs of abuse may involve additional brain nuclei that activate dopamine cells. For example, disinhibition of GABAergic input to dopamine cells in the ventral tegmental area by a microinjection of morphine is known to elicit reinstatement in animals trained to self-administer heroin (Stewart, 1984).

Cue-primed Reinstatement

When animals or humans experience drug effects in the presence of an environmental stimulus (cue), a learned association develops such that presentation of that cue will elicit craving and behavior organized to obtain drug reward. Cue-primed reinstatement of drug-seeking behavior is clearly dependent upon the functional integrity of the basolateral amygdala (Meil and See, 1997; Grimm and See, 2000). This region of the amygdala has also been shown to be critical for many forms of stimulus-reinforcer associations (Everitt et al., 1999). Moreover, it was recently shown that in a manner analogous to the role of the prefrontal cortex in drug-primed reinstatement, blockade of D_1 dopamine receptors in the basolateral amygdala prevents cue-primed reinstatement (See et al., 2001). This effect implies that presentation of the cue activates the projection from the ventral tegmental area to the basolateral amygdala, and is consistent with a well-developed electrophysiological literature showing that dopamine neurons in the ventral tegmental area increase burst firing following presentation of a cue that predicts a reward (Schultz, 1998).

Stress-primed Reinstatement

Addicts often report that environmental stress can precipitate craving and drug-taking behavior (O'Brien, 2001; Lyvers, 2000). The regions of the brain most clearly associated with stress-primed reinstatement are associated with extended amygdala (Shaham et al., 2000; Heimer et al., 1993).

Integration of Findings

Present knowledge suggests the possibility of a final common pathway for addiction, and possibly similar brain circuits between drugs and stimuli that provoke craving and relapse. The extant data support a common role of the motor memory circuit shown in Figure 13.3 that consists of the series projection from the prefrontal cortex to nucleus accumbens to ventral pallidum. Moreover, there is abundant evidence for enduring neuroadaptations in gene expression and neuronal function in the nucleus accumbens and prefrontal cortex following a bout of drug taking (Nestler, 2001; Kalivas, 2002). While the finding from multiple lines of research are promising in pointing towards a common site of intervention in addiction, it is important to note that such a generalization based primarily on work with psychostimulants is premature and requires substantially more research using other classes of drugs to validate. Similarly, the proposal for a final common motor memory pathway mediating craving and relapse induced by different modalities of stimuli is based on only a modest number of neuroimaging studies in addicts and experimental models of relapse. Nonetheless, sufficient supportive data has accrued to at least speculate on the prepotent involvement of the motor memory pathway in addiction, especially the glutamatergic projection from regions of the prefrontal cortex including the anterior cingulate and ventral orbital cortex to the core of the nucleus accumbens. Likewise, dopamine projections to prefrontal cortex and allocortical areas such as the basolateral amygdala are also critical.

These emerging hints and hypotheses pose directions for novel pharmacological therapeutic strategies for ameliorating craving and relapse associated with addiction. Notably, pharmacological regulation of glutamate transmission in the cortical projection to the nucleus accumbens would seem to be a potential target. Given that enhanced release of glutamate appears to be associated with cue-, drug-, and perhaps, stress-primed relapse, diminishing that release would be one possible mechanism for pharmacotherapeutic intervention.

References

Breiter HC, Gollub RL, Weisskoff RM et al. (1997) Acute effects of cocaine on human brain activity and emotion. Neuron 19, 591–611.

Bunney E, Appel S and Brodie M (2001) Electrophysiological effects of cocaethylene, cocaine, and ethanol on dopaminergic neurons of the ventral tegmental area. J Pharmacol Exp Ther 297(2), 696–710.

Burns LH, Everitt BJ, Kelley AE et al. (1994) Glutamate-dopamine interactions in the ventral striatum: Role in locomotor activity and responding with conditioned reinforcement. Psychopharmacology 115, 516–528.

Cameron DL, Wessendorf MW and Williams JT (1997) A subset of ventral tegmental area neurons is inhibited by dopamine, 5-hydroxytryptamine and opioids. Neuroscience 77, 155–166.

Cheer J, Kendall D and Marsden C (2000) Cannabinoid receptors and reward in the rat: A conditioned place preference study. Psychopharmacology 151(1), 25–30.

Childress AR, Mozley PD, McElgin W et al. (1999) Limbic activation during cue-induced cocaine craving. Am J Psychiatr 156, 11–18.

Deutch AY and Roth RH (1990) The determinants of stress-induced activation of the prefrontal cortical dopamine system. Prog Brain Res 85, 357–393.

Everitt BJ and Wolf MG (2002) Psychomotor stimulant addiction: A neural systems perspective. J Neuroscience 22, 3312–3320.

Everitt BJ, Parkinson JA, Olmstead MC, et al. (1999) Associative processes in addiction and reward. The role of amygdala-ventral striatal subsystems. Ann NY Acad Sci 877, 412–438.

Grant S, London ED, Newlin DB et al. (1996) Activation of memory circuits during cue-elicited cocaine craving. Proc Natl Acad Sci (USA) 93, 12040–12045.

Grimm J and See R (2000) Dissociation of primary and secondary reward-relevant limbic nuclei in an animal model of relapse. Neuropsychopharmacology 22, 473–479.

Groenewegen HJ, Wright CI and Beijer VJ (1996) The nucleus accumbens: Gateway for limbic structures to reach the motor system? Prog Brain Res 107, 485–551.

Heimer L, Alheid GF, and Zahm DS (1993) Basal forebrain organization: An anatomical framework for motor aspects of drive and motivation. In Limbic motor circuits and neuropsychiatry, Kalivas PW and Barnes CD (eds). CRC Press, Boca Raton, FL, pp. 1–32

Kalivas PW (2002) The development and expression of behavioral sensitization: Temporal profile of changes in gene expression, in Molecular Biology of Drug Addiction (ed Moldanado R). Humana Press, Totowa, NJ.

Koob GF and LeMoal M (2001) Drug addiction, dysregulation of reward and allostasis. Neuropsychopharmacology 24, 97–129.

Lyvers M (2000) "Loss of control" in alcoholism and drug addiction: A neuroscientific interpretation. Exp Clin Psychopharmacol 8(2), 225–249.

Markou A, Weiss F, Gold LH, et al. (1993) Animal models of drug craving. Psychopharmacology 112, 163–182.

McFarland K and Kalivas PW (2001) The circuitry mediating cocaineinduced reinstatement of drug-seeking behavior. J Neurosci 21(21), 8655–8663.

Meil WM and See RE (1997) Lesions of the basolateral amygdala abolish the ability of drug associated cues to reinstate responding during withdrawal from self-administered cocaine. Behav Brain Res 87, 139–148.

Mogenson GJ, Jones DJ, and Yim CY (1980) From motivation to action: Functional interface between the limbic system and the motor system. Prog Neurobiol 14, 69–97.

Mogenson GJ, Jone DJ, and Yim CY (1980) From motivation to action: Functionl interface between the limbic system and the motor system. Prog Neurobiol 14, 69–97

Nestler E (2001) Molecular basis of long-term plasticity underlying addiction. *Nat Rev* 2, 119–128.

Nisell M, Nomikos GG and Svensson TH (1994) Systemic nicotine-induced dopamine release in the rat nucleus accumbens is regulated by nicotinic receptors in the ventral tegmental area. *Synapse* 16, 36–44.

O'Brien C (2001) Drug addiction and drug abuse. In The Pharmacological Basis of Therapeutics, Hardman J, Limbird L, and Gilman AG (eds). McGraw-Hill, New York, pp. 621–642.

Pierce RC and Kalivas PW (1997) A circuitry model of the expression of behavioral sensitization to amphetamine-like psychostimulants. *Brain Res Rev* 25, 192–216.

Porrino LJ and Lyons D (2000) Orbital and medial prefrontal cortex and psychostimulant abuse: Studies in animal models. *Cereb Cortex* 10(3), 326–333.

Robbins T and Everitt B (1996) Neurobehavioural mechanisms of reward and motivation. *Curr Opin Neurobiol* 6, 228–236.

Salamone J, Cousins M, McCullough L *et al.* (1994) Nucleus accumbens dopamine release increases during instrumental lever pressing for food but not free food consumption. *Pharmacol Biochem Behav* 49, 25–31.

Schultz W (1998) Predictive reward signal of dopamine neurons. *Am J Physiol* 80, 1–27.

Seiden LS, Sabol KE and Ricuarte GA (1993) Amphetamine: Effects on catecholamine systems and behavior. *Annu Rev Pharmacol Toxicol* 33, 639–677.

Shaham Y, Erb S, and Stewart J (2000) Stress-induced drug seeking to heroin and cocaine in rats: A review. Brain Res Rev 33, 13–33.

Stewart J (1984) Reinstatement of heroin and cocaine self-administration behavior in the rat by intracerebral application of morphine in the ventral tegmental area. *Pharmacol Biochem Behav* 20, 917–923.

Vanderschuren LJ and Kalivas PW (2000) Alterations in dopaminergic and glutamatergic transmission in the induction and expression of behavioral sensitization: A critical review of preclinical studies. *Psychopharmacology (Berl)* 151(2–3), 99–120.

Volkow ND and Fowler JS (2000) Addiction, a disease of compulsion and drive: Involvement of the orbitofrontal cortex. *Cereb Cortex* 10(3), 318–325.

Vorel SR, Liu X, Hayes R *et al.* (2001) Relapse to cocaine-seeking after hippocampal theta burst stimulation. *Science* 292, 1175–1178.

Yim HJ, Schallert T, Randall PK *et al.* (1998) Comparison of local and systemic ethanol effects on extracellular dopamine concentration in rat nucleus accumbens by microdialysis. *Alcohol Clin Exp Res* 22(2), 367–374.

Psychiatric Pathophysiology: Dementia

Neuropathological Causes of Dementia in the Elderly

The most common neuropathological findings in demented elderly individuals are lesions associated with Alzheimer's disease (AD) and with cerebrovascular disease. Diseases such as Parkinson's disease, diffuse Lewy body disease, Pick's disease, and a constellation of heterogeneous diseases collectively identified as frontotemporal dementia and characterized by pronounced frontotemporal atrophy are also identified, albeit, less frequently (Green *et al.*, 2000; Xuereb *et al.*, 2000; Hachinski and Munoz, 2000; Perl, 2000; Dickson, 2001; Mckhan *et al.*, 2001). Often, AD and cerebrovascular disease, or AD and Parkinson's disease-like lesions (Perl *et al.*, 1998), are comorbid, making it difficult to ascribe dementia to either disease entity alone and blurring the distinctions between them (Xuereb *et al.*, 2000; Hachinski and Munoz, 2000; Perl *et al.*, 1998; Aguero-Torres and Winbald, 2000; Snowdon *et al.*, 1997; Hardy and Gwinn-Hardy, 1999).

Neuropathology of Alzheimer's Disease

In his original work, Alzheimer described the plaques and tangles that have not only withstood modern scrutiny of the original index case (Graeber and Mehraein, 1999) but have become the diagnostic hallmarks of the disease known as Alzheimer's disease. Neurofibrillary tangles (NFT) and senile/neuritic plaques (NP) are the principal lesions of Alzheimer's disease (Rogers and Morrison, 1985; Tomlinson *et al.*, 1970) and form the basis for the neuropathological diagnosis of AD (Mirra *et al.*, 1991; Khachaturian, 1985; NIA-Reagan, 1997). In addition to NPs and NFTs, there is generally macroscopic evidence of cerebral cortical atrophy, reduced brain weight, and enlargement of the ventricles; however, because of the considerable overlap between AD and normal control subjects and the frequency of similar changes in other degenerative diseases (e.g., Pick's disease), these macroscopic findings are not diagnostically informative (Perl, 2000; Dickson, 2001; Adams and Duchen, 1992).

Neuritic plaques are extracellular spheroid elements (10–120 μm in diameter) with complex structures that include amyloid fibrils and dystrophic neurites (Figure 14.1) that are frequently surrounded by microglia and reactive astrocytes. The core of the plaque is composed of amyloid beta-peptide (Aβ) surrounded by abnormal neuronal processes and fragments (Glenner and Wong, 1984; Selkoe, 1991, 1994, 2000). Aβ is derived from the sequential proteolytic cleavage of a larger protein known as amyloid precursor protein (APP). APP is highly conserved in evolution being expressed in all mammals studied and in most organs. An above-normal accumulation of NPs with Aβ cores in the cerebral cortex, hippocampal formation and subcortical structures has constituted the principal diagnostic measure of AD (Mirra, 1991; Khachaturian, 1985).

The precise mechanism(s) by which Aβ causes cell damage and neuronal degeneration are not presently understood. It should be kept in mind, however, that although it is broadly accepted that Aβ plays an important role in AD, its role as the primary etiological agent in the disease process is not universally accepted with certainty (Davies, 2000). Furthermore, how, if at all, NPs and NFTs interact and influence each other is far from being understood.

Neurofibrillary tangles constitute the second hallmark of AD. Although the most commonly used formal neuropathological diagnostic criteria for AD rely almost exclusively on the density of neocortical NPs (Mirra *et al.*, 1991; Khachaturian, 1985), a number of studies have argued that the development of NFTs, especially in the entorhinal cortex, represents the earliest neuropathological change in AD (Jellinger *et al.*, 1991; Braak and Braak, 1996b; Braak *et al.*, 1996; Hyman, 1997; Bouras *et al.*, 1993).

NFTs are intracellular coarse fibrillary structures that can surround the neuronal nucleus and extend into the neuronal processes. Although NFTs are observed in neurons that are otherwise apparently "healthy", it is generally, but not universally assumed that NFT formation leads to eventual neuronal death (Davies, 2000). NFTs are composed of pairs of approximately 10 nm filaments entwined into helices with a signature periodicity of approximately 160 nm.

Although neurons bearing NFTs in the hippocampus and the entorhinal cortex are observed in many if not most elderly individuals, the "spread" of NFTs to the neocortex (Braak stage III and above) is almost always associated with some level of dementia.

Despite considerable advances in understanding the neurobiology and genetics of Aβ and NFTs (see later), linkage between these two apparently diverse lesions has not been clearly established. It may be tempting to argue that AD is the result of the coincidence of two relatively independent neurobiological abnormalities. It is well established that a single mutation in the APP or an APP-related gene can cause AD. Thus, there are considerable gaps in our knowledge of the mechanisms by which the full spectrum of AD neuropathology is expressed and a more complete understanding of the etiology of AD must await further research.

Neurochemical Deficits in Alzheimer's Disease

The neuropathology of AD is accompanied with significant neurochemical pathology and dysfunction. A central tenet of

Figure 14.1   *Typical appearance of a neuritic plaque in the neocortex of an Alzheimer's disease patient. Section stained using a modified Bielschowsky silver impregnation method. (Image courtesy: Dr Dushyant Purohit, The Mount Sinai School of Medicine, New York.)*

Alzheimer's disease, established 20 years ago and repeatedly replicated, is the loss of cortical cholinergic markers, specifically the reduction of the activities of the enzymes choline acetyltransferase (ChAT) and acetylcholinesterase (AChE), in postmortem tissue from Alzheimer's patients (Perry *et al.*, 1977; Davies and Maloney, 1976; Bowen *et al.*, 1982). This abnormality has been shown to correlate with neuropathological markers and with the severity of dementia (Perry *et al.*, 1978; Bierer *et al.*, 1995a). Other neurochemical abnormalities that exist in the AD brain include loss of corticotropin releasing factor (CRF) (De Souza *et al.*, 1986; Nermeroff *et al.*, 1991) and somatostatin immunoreactivity (Davies and Terry, 1981; Davies *et al.*, 1980), and decreases in noradrenergic (Adolfsson *et al.*, 1979; Gottfries *et al.*, 1989; Chan-Palay and Asan, 1989; Teicher *et al.*, 1988), serotonergic (Cross *et al.*, 1986a, 1986b; Gottfries, 1990), GABAergic (Ellison *et al.*, 1986; Sasaki *et al.*, 1986; Simpson *et al.*, 1988; Chu *et al.*, 1987a, 1987b; Hardy *et al.*, 1987) and glutamatergic (Ellison *et al.*, 1986; Kowall and Beal, 1991; Chalmers *et al.*, 1990) markers in some patients. Table 14.1 summarizes some of the principal neuropathologic and neurochemical findings in AD.

Synapses and Synaptic Proteins in Alzheimer's Disease

Given the neuronal degeneration and the reductions in neuronal size and arborization in AD, it is only reasonable that the numbers of synapses and their integrity should be compromised in AD. Synaptic neurotransmission, like all forms of exocytosis, requires an array of proteins. These proteins have varying ion

Table 14.1   Most Frequently Observed Neuropathological and Neurochemical Features of Alzheimer's Disease Pathology

Neuropathology	Neurochemistry
• Neuritic plaques in hippocampus, entorhinal cortex, cerebral cortex, and some subcortical nuclei.	• Profound cholinergic deficits including reduced activity of acetylcholine synthesizing (choline acetyltransferase) and degrading (acetylcholinesterase) enzymes.
• Neurofibrillary tangles in hippocampus, entorhinal cortex, cerebral cortex and some subcortical nuclei	• Reduced levels and immunoreactivity of neuropeptides, somatostatin and corticotrophin releasing factor/hormone.
• Neuronal loss in hippocampus, entorhinal cortex, cerebral cortex and some subcortical nuclei including the forebrain cholinergic nuclei, nucleus basalis of Meynert, medial septum and diagonal band of Broca.	• Reduced levels of norepinephrine and serotonin and reduced numbers of neurons in their respective nuclei (locus coeruleus and Raphe, respectively) observed in some, but not all cases.

and guanine nucleotide sensitivities, and possess intricate functional and biochemical kinships. Synaptic proteins on vesicles within the synapse and on synaptic membranes interact to enable neurotransmitter-bearing vesicles to dock with synaptic membranes and become ready for neurotransmitter release. Although losses of synaptic proteins are not unexpected in a degenerative disease, the fact that the loss of synaptic marker proteins significantly and profoundly correlate with the severity of dementia (Terry *et al.*, 1991; Masliah *et al.*, 1989; Lassmann *et al.*, 1993; Heinonen *et al.*, 1995; Tiraboschi *et al.*, 2000) suggest that the loss of synapses may play a pivotal role in the expression of the symptoms of AD.

Inflammatory Processes in Alzheimer's Disease

The identification or recognition of neurobiological indices of inflammation in the AD brain was initially controversial because of the belief that the brain was immunologically privileged (Rogers and Shen, 2000). More than a decade of research and hundreds of studies have now confirmed the presence of inflammatory responses in the AD brain (Akiyama *et al.*, 2000) and have raised the possibility of the potential benefit of anti-inflammatory therapeutic avenues (Akiyama *et al.*, 2000; Aisen, 2000; Anthony *et al.*, 2000). It is generally acknowledged that inflammation of the brain or its neurons is unlikely to be the primary etiological factor in AD, but that it is initiated by AD-specific pathogenic processes such as deposition of NPs and/or NFTs. However, as in many other diseases, once initiated, inflammatory responses may contribute to the progression of the disease and its malignancy (Rogers and Shen, 2000).

Genetic Factors in Alzheimer's Disease

Much has been learned regarding the contribution of genetic factors to AD over the past two decades (George-Hyslop, 2000a, 2000b). However, the impact of these genetic contributors to dementia severity is not yet well understood. Significant evidence has accumulated for genetic traits that confer susceptibility to AD. Four genes, beta-amyloid precursor protein (β-APP) (Selkoe, 1997, 2000b; George-Hyslop *et al.*, 1987; Robakis *et al.*, 1987; Goate *et al.*, 1991), presenilin-1 (PS1) (Selkoe, 1997, 2000b; Robakis *et al.*, 1987; Sherrington *et al.*, 1995), presenilin-2 (PS2) (Selkoe, 1997, 2000b; Robakis *et al.*, 1987; Rogaev *et al.*, 1995), and apolipoprotein E (APOE) (Selkoe, 1997, 2000b; Robakis *et al.*, 1987; Saunders *et al.*, 1993; Poirier, 2000) are of particular note. The fact that the three most prominent AD-associated mutations all affect APP processing, albeit by different mechanisms, increase Aβ production, strongly suggests that Aβ is a prominent pathogenetic agent in AD and strongly supports the amyloid hypothesis of AD (George-Hyslop, 2000a, 2000b), especially since emerging data suggest that even the epsilon-4 allele of APOE may influence Aβ processing.

Although a thorough understanding of the development of different neuropathological features of AD and their relationship to the progression of dementia must await the development of sensitive *in vivo* markers of neuropathology, the existing evidence supports the hypothesis that NPs and NFTs are "dose-dependently" associated with the earliest manifestations of AD-type dementia and that inflammatory responses and neurochemical deficits such as the cholinergic deficit become evident as dementia severity becomes more pronounced.

Dementia in Schizophrenia and its Neuropathological and Neurochemical Sequelae

Chronic schizophrenia, with its onset in early adulthood can in geriatric years become a disorder that is commonly associated with dementia (Davidson and Haroutunian, 1995; Harvey *et al.*, 1992, 1996; Davidson *et al.*, 1995). The findings of continuing deterioration of the symptoms of schizophrenia, the cognitive performance of schizophrenics, especially the apparent dementia that has been documented in elderly schizophrenics (Davidson and Haroutunian, 1995; Harvey *et al.*, 1997, 1999a, 1999b;), and progressive enlargement of the ventricles, especially in poor-outcome schizophrenics (Davis *et al.*, 1998) has raised the possibility of a neurodegenerative component to the disease process or to its dementia.

The age-related emergence of cognitive impairment in schizophrenia fueled hypotheses linking dementia in elderly schizophrenics to AD and positing that the dementia of late-life schizophrenia was a consequence of comorbid AD (Davidson and Haroutunian, 1995; Arnold *et al.*, 1994). However, several large postmortem studies failed to support this hypothesis. Thus, although there is clear evidence for dementia in at least a subpopulation of elderly schizophrenics, the neuropathological and neurobiological substrates of this dementia have remained elusive and, as of yet, undetermined.

References

Adams JH and Duchen LW (1992) *Greenfield's Neuropathology*, 5th edn. Oxford University Press, New York, pp. 1317–1341.

Adolfsson R, Gottfries CG, Roos BE *et al.* (1979) Changes in the brain catecholamines in patients with dementia of Alzheimer-type. *Br J Psychiatr* 135, 216–223.

Aisen PS (2000) Anti-inflammatory therapy for Alzheimer's disease. *Neurobiol Aging* 21, 447–448.

Akiyama H, Barger S, Barnum S, *et al.* (2000) Inflammation and Alzheimer's disease. *Neurobiol Aging* 21, 383–421.

Anthony JC, Breitner JC, Zandi PP, *et al.* (2000) Reduced prevalence of AD in users of NSAIDs and H2 receptor antagonists: The Cache County study. Neurology 54, 2066–2071.

Arnold SE (2001) Contributions of neuropathology to understanding schizophrenia in late life. Harv Rev Psychiatr 9, 69–76.

Arnold SE, Franz BR, and Trojanowski JQ (1994) Elderly patients with schizophrenia exhibit infrequent neurodegenerative lesions. Neurobiol Aging 15, 299–303.

Bierer L, Haroutunian V, Gabriel S, *et al.* (1995a) Neurochemical correlates of dementia severity in Alzheimer's disease: Relative importance of the cholinergic deficits. *J Neurochem* 64, 749–760.

Bouras C, Hof PR, and Morrison JH (1993) Neurofibrillary tangle densities in the hippocampal formation in a nondemented population define subgroups of patients with differential early pathologic changes. *Neurosci Lett* 153, 131–135.

Bowen DM, Benton JS, Spillane JA, *et al.* (1982) Choline acetyltransferase activity and histopathology of frontal neocortex from biopsies of demented patients. *J Neurol Sci* 57, 191–202.

Braak H and Braak E (1996) Development of Alzheimer-related neurofibrillary changes in the neocortex inversely recapitulates cortical myelogenesis. *Acta Neuropathol (Berl)* 92, 197–201.

Braak E, Braak H, and Mandelkow EM (1994) A sequence of cytoskeleton changes related to the formation of neurofibrillary tangles and neuropil threads. *Acta Neuropathol (Berl)* 87, 554–567.

Braak H and Braak E (1996a) Development of Alzheimer-related neurofibrillary changes in the neocortex inversely recapitulates cortical myelogenesis. *Acta Neuropathol (Berl)* 92, 197–201.

Braak H and Braak E (1996b) Evolution of the neuropathology of Alzheimer's disease. *Acta Neurol Scan* 165(Suppl), 3–12.

Braak H, Braak E, Bohl J, *et al.* (1996) Age, neurofibrillary changes, A beta-amyloid and the onset of Alzheimer's disease. Neurosci Lett 210, 87–90.

Chalmers DT, Dewar D, Graham DI, *et al.* (1990) Differential alterations of cortical glutamatergic binding sites in senile dementia of the Alzheimer type. Proc Natl Acad Sci USA 87, 1352–1356.

Chalmers DT, Dewar D, Graham DI *et al.* (1990) Differential alterations of cortical glutamatergic binding sites in senile dementia of the Alzheimer type. *Proc Natl Acad Sci USA* 87, 1352–1356.

Chan-Palay V and Asan E (1989) Alterations in catecholamine neurons of the locus coeruleus in senile dementia of the Alzheimer-type and in Parkinson's disease with and without dementia and depression. *J Comp Neurol* 287, 373–392.

Chu DC, Penney JB Jr. and Young AB (1987a) Quantitative autoradiography of hippocampal GABAB and GABAA receptor changes in Alzheimer's disease. *Neurosci Lett* 82, 246–252.

Chu DC, Penney JB Jr. and Young AB (1987b) Cortical GABAB and GABAA receptors in Alzheimer's disease: A quantitative autoradiographic study. *Neurology* 37, 1454–1459.

Cross AJ, Crow TJ, and Peters TJ (1986a) Cortical neurochemistry in Alzheimer-type dementia. *Prog Brain Res* 70, 153–169.

Cross AJ, Crow TJ, Ferrier IN *et al.* (1986b) The selectivity of the reduction of serotonin S2 receptors in Alzheimer-type dementia. *Neurobiol Aging* 7, 3–7.

Davidson M and Haroutunian V (1995) Cognitive impairment in geriatric schizophrenic patients: Clinical and postmortem characterization, in Psychopharmacology: The Fourth Generation of Progress, Bloom FE and Kupfer DJ (eds). Raven Press, New York.

Davies P (2000) A very incomplete comprehensive theory of Alzheimer's disease. Ann NY Acad Sci 924, 8–16.

Davies P and Maloney AJF (1976) Selective loss of central cholinergic neurons in Alzheimer's disease. Lancet 2, 1403.

Davidson M, Harvey P, Powchik P *et al.* (1995) Severity of symptoms in chronically institutionalized geriatric schizophrenic patients. *Am J Psychiatr* 152, 197–206.

Davies P and Terry RD (1981) Cortical somatostatin-like immunoreactivity in cases of Alzheimer's disease and senile dementia of Alzheimer's type. *Neurobiol Aging* 2, 9–14.

Davies P, Katzman R and Terry RD (1980) Reduced somatostatin-like-immunoreactivity in cerebral cortex from cases of Alzheimer's disease Alzheimer's senile dementia. *Nature (Lond)* 288, 279–280.

Davis KL, Buchsbaum MS, Shihabuddin L *et al.* (1998) Ventricular enlargement in poor-outcome schizophrenia. *Biol Psychiatr* 43, 783–793.

De Souza EB, Whitehouse PJ, Kuhar MJ *et al.* (1986) Reciprocal changes in corticotropin-releasing factor (CRF-like) immunoreactivity and CRF receptors in cerebral cortex of Alzheimer's disease. *Nature* 319, 593–595.

Dickson DW (2001) Neuropathology of Alzheimer's disease and other dementias. *Clin Geriatr Med* 17(2) (May), 209–228.

Ellison DW, Beal MF, Mazurek MF *et al.* (1986) A postmortem study of amino acid neurotransmitters in Alzheimer's disease. *Ann Neurol* 20, 616–621.

George-Hyslop PH, Tanzi RE, and Polinsky RJ (1987) The genetic defect causing familial Alzheimer's disease maps on chromosome 21. Science 235, 885–890.

George-Hyslop PH (2000a) Genetic factors in the genesis of Alzheimer's disease. *Ann NY Acad Sci* 924, 1–7.

George-Hyslop PH (2000b) Molecular genetics of Alzheimer's disease. Biol Psychiatr 47, 183–199.

Glenner GG and Wong CW (1984) Alzheimer's disease and Down's syndrome: Sharing of a unique cerebrovascular amyloid fibrile protein. *Biochem Biophys Res Comm* 120, 1131–1135.

Goate A, Chartier-Harlin M-C, Mullan M *et al.* (1991) Segregation of a missense mutation in the amyloid precursor protein gene with familial Alzheimer's disease. *Nature* 349, 704–706.

Gottfries CG (1990) Disturbance of the 5-hydroxytryptamine metabolism in brains from patients with Alzheimer's dementia. *J Neural Trans* 30(Suppl), 33–43.

Gottfries CG, Adolfsson R, Aquilonius SM *et al.* (1989) Biochemical changes in dementia disorders of the Alzheimer-type (AD/SDAT). *Neurobiol Aging* 4, 261–271.

Hardy J, Cowburn R, Barton A *et al.* (1987) A disorder of cortical GABAergic innervation in Alzheimer's disease. *Neurosci Lett* 73, 192–196.

Harvey PD, Davidson M, Powchik P, *et al.* (1992) Assessment of dementia in elderly schizophrenics with structured rating scales. *Schizophr Res* 7, 85–90.

Harvey P, Lombardi J, Leibman M *et al.* (1997) Age-related differences in formal thought disorder in chronic schizophrenic patients: A cross-sectional study across 9 decades. *Am J Psychiatr* 154, 205–210.

Harvey PD, Parrella M, White L *et al.* (1999b) Convergence of cognitive and adaptive decline in late-life schizophrenia. *Schizophr Res* 35, 77–84.

Harvey PD, Silverman JM, Mohs RC *et al.* (1999a) Cognitive decline in late-life schizophrenia: A longitudinal study of geriatric chronically hospitalized patients. *Biol Psychiatr* 45, 32–40.

Heinonen O, Soininen H, Sorvari H *et al.* (1995) Loss of synaptophysin-like immunoreactivity in the hippocampal formation is an early phenomenon in Alzheimer's disease. *Neuroscience* 64, 375–384.

Hyman BT (1997) The neuropathological diagnosis of Alzheimer's disease: Clinical-pathological studies. *Neurobiol Aging* 18, S27–S32.

Jellinger K, Braak H, Braak E, et al. (1991) Alzheimer lesions in the entorhinal region and isocortex in Parkinson's and Alzheimer's diseases. Ann NY Acad Sci 640, 203–209.

Kowall NW and Beal MF (1991) Glutamate-, glutaminase-, and taurine-immunoreactive neurons develop neurofibrillary tangles in Alzheimer's disease. *Ann Neurol* 29, 162–167.

Lassmann H, Fischer P and Jellinger K (1993) Synaptic pathology of Alzheimer's disease. *Ann NY Acad Sci* 695, 59–64.

Masliah E, Terry RD, DeTeresa RM *et al.* (1989) Immunohistochemical quantification of the synapse-related protein synaptophysin in Alzheimer disease. *Neurosci Lett* 103, 234–239.

Mirra SS, Heyman A, McKeel D, *et al.* (1991) The Consortium to Establish a Registry for Alzheimer's Disease (CERAD). Part II. Standardization of the neuropathologic assessment of Alzheimer's disease. Neurology 41, 479–486.

Nermeroff CB, Bissette G, Slotkin TA *et al.* (1991) Recent advances in the neurochemical pathology of Alzheimer's disease. Studies of neuropeptides, cholinergic function and Alzheimer's disease-associated protein. *Ann NY Acad Sci* 640, 193–196.

Perl DP, (2000) Neuropathology of Alzheimer's disease and related disorders. Neurol Clin 18(4) (Nov), 847–864.

Perry EK, Perry RH, Blessed G, *et al.* (1977) Necropsy evidence of central cholinergic deficits in senile dementia. Lancet 1, 189.

Perry EK, Tomlinson BE, Blessed G *et al.* (1978) Correlation of cholinergic abnormalities with senile plaques and mental test scores in senile dementia. *Br Med J* 2, 1457–1459.

Poirier J (2000) Apolipoprotein E and Alzheimer's disease: A role in amyloid catabolism. *Ann NY Acad Sci* 924, 81–90.

Robakis N, Ramakrishna N, Wolfe G *et al.* (1987) Molecular cloning and characterization of a cDNA encoding the cerebrovascular and the neuritic plaque amyloid peptides. *Proc Natl Acad Sci USA* 84, 4190–4194.

Rogaev EI, Sherrington R, Rogaeva EA *et al.* (1995) Familial Alzheimer's disease in kindreds with missense mutations in a gene on chromosome 1 related to the Alzheimer's disease type 3 gene. *Nature* 376, 775–778.

Rogers J and Morrison JH (1985) Quantitative morphology and regional and laminar distribution of senile plaques in Alzheimer's disease. *J Neurosci* 5, 2801–2808.

Rogers J and Shen Y (2000) A perspective on inflammation in Alzheimer's disease. *Ann NY Acad Sci* 924, 132–135.

Sasaki H, Muramoto O, Kanazawa I *et al.* (1986) Regional distribution of amino acid transmitters in postmortem brains of presenile and senile dementia of Alzheimer type. *Ann Neurol* 19, 263–269.

Saunders A, Strittmatter W, Scdhmechel D *et al.* (1993) Association of apolipoprotein E allele epsilon-4 with late-onset familial and sporadic Alzheimer's disease. *Neurology* 43, 1467–1472.

Selkoe DJ (1991) The molecular pathology of Alzheimer's disease. *Neuron* 6, 487–498.

Selkoe DJ (1994) Normal and abnormal biology of the B-amyloid precursor protein. *Annu Rev Neurosci* 17, 489–517.

Selkoe DJ (1997) Alzheimer's disease: Genotypes, phenotype, and treatment. *Science* 275, 630–631.

Selkoe DJ (2000) The genetics and molecular pathology of Alzheimer's disease: Roles of amyloid and the presenilins. *Neurol Clin* 18, 903–922.

Sherrington R, Rogaev EI, Liang Y *et al.* (1995) Cloning of a gene bearing missense mutations in early-onset familial Alzheimer's disease. *Nature* 375, 754–760.

Simpson MD, Cross AJ, Slater P *et al.* (1988) Loss of cortical GABA uptake sites in Alzheimer's disease. *J Neural Transm* 71, 219–226.

Snowdon DA, Greiner LH, Mortimer JA, *et al.* (1997) Brain infarction and the clinical expression of Alzheimer disease. The Nun Study. JAMA 277, 813–817.

Teicher MH, Barber NI, Baldessarini RJ *et al.* (1988) Amphetamine accelerates and attenuates ultradian activity rhythms in preweaning rats. *Pharmacol Biochem Behav* 29, 517–523.

Terry RD, Masliah E, Salmon DP, *et al.* (1991) Physical basis of cognitive alterations in Alzheimer's disease: Synapse loss is the major correlate of cognitive impairment. *Ann Neurol* 30, 572–580.

Tiraboschi P, Hansen LA, Alford M, *et al.* (2000) The decline in synapses and cholinergic activity is asynchronous in Alzheimer's disease. *Neurology* 55, 1278–1283.

Tomlinson BE, Blessed G and Roth M (1970) Observations on the brains of demented old people. *J Neurol Sci* 11, 205–242.

Xuereb JH, Brayne C, Dufouil C, *et al.* (2000) Neuropathological findings in the very old. Results from the first 101 brains of a population-based longitudinal study of dementing disorders. *Ann NY Acad Sci* 903, 490–496.

Cognitive Neuroscience and Neuropsychology

What Is Cognitive Neuroscience?

In the past two decades, much has been learned about cognitive phenomena from the constituent disciplines of cognitive neuroscience: neuropsychology, neurology, psychiatry, neuroimaging, neurobiology, computer science and cognitive psychology. The emergence of cognitive behavior from the underlying neuroanatomical substrate represents a fascinating, if elusive, process of scientific discovery. Although cognitive neuroscience is represented by a collection of disciplines, its goal is to provide a framework or process for integration in the study of cognitive phenomena. That is, the experimental information gained from these disciplines allows coordinated knowledge of brain systems to proceed both reductionistically (from macrocognitive to cellular levels) and laterally (from cognitive theories to neuropsychological theories).

The proper domain of cognitive neuroscience is vast. Motor functioning, attention, language, memory, executive control, vision, emotion, sensory functions and consciousness are only subsets of this domain. In this chapter, we selectively focus on a few critical areas of cognitive neuroscience – namely, memory, executive functions and language – and discuss these areas in depth. We highlight the structural and functional organization of these systems and discuss the relevant research from the cognitive neurosciences that address these areas. The reader is referred to a number of more comprehensive sources, where appropriate, for greater detail and discussion.

Beginning in 1901, Korbinian Brodmann undertook a series of landmark studies on the cytoarchitectonics of the mammalian cortex. It had been known before Brodmann that there were six layers of the human isocortex based on cell type and size. Brodmann extended this work on cytoarchitectonics to the subdivision of areas of cortex with similar cellular and laminar structure; he subdivided the human cerebral cortex into 47 areas. The result is a cytoarchitectonic map of the human cerebral cortex. Its development is critical to the interpretation and replication of findings in cortical localization. This system is the predominant one utilized today, especially with the use of single-cell recordings in animals and functional neuroimaging studies in humans. In a number of places we refer to Brodmann's areas with respect to localization of particular cognitive functions. Brodmann's map is depicted in Figure 15.1.

Current Theoretical Conceptualization of Brain Organization

Current thinking in the cognitive neurosciences strikes a balance between local and holistic organization of functions. The current emphasis is on "connectivity", as both a theoretical heuristic and a set of models of neural behavior. The localizationist perspective of Wernicke introduced the rudimentary idea that interconnected brain regions could work in a serial fashion to perform a set of operations such as language. The Russian neuropsychologist Alexander Luria, who influenced much contemporary thinking in cognitive neuroscience, was himself influenced by the idea of connectivity.

By borrowing from the then emerging field of machine intelligence, the model of the brain as a digital computer operating in a serial processing framework was introduced. In this model, brain functions were seen as the constellation of interconnected neural networks, each operating in serial fashion, to produce macrocognitive processes from series of local microcognitive operations. Although the early artificial intelligence and information-processing traditions of cognitive psychology offered elegant models, they were limited by their underlying assumptions. First, the cognitive models that postulated the premise of connectivity between local networks did not explicitly link the cognitive realm with the underlying anatomical substrate, lending these theories a lack of neural reality. For example, this yielded models of attention that "worked" from a cognitive perspective but did not suggest an underlying neural mechanism.

Connectionist theories of the brain within the cognitive sciences have begun to offer models with greater neural and computational realism. In the computer realm, the development of massively parallel computing has suggested that extremely complex functions can be performed simultaneously, not in a serial fashion. The obvious extrapolation to neural science is to think of brain functions as having a parallel architecture, which would perform several operations simultaneously. In contrast to serial processing, parallel processing allows the relatively slow individual neurons to accomplish tasks in rapid real time. The other current concept applied to neural processing is that of distributed processing. Distributed processing refers to the coordination of functions that are distributed within and across brain regions. A particular function is therefore emergent from neural processing that is both parallel and distributed. This concept of neural function represents a compromise between local and holistic perspectives. The model of the brain in terms of parallel distributed processing (PDP) is both a heuristic framework from which to view neural organization and a formal set of models within cognitive science. The formal elements of PDP involve the relationship of neural science and computer science and have been applied to the development of models of language, vision, motor learning and memory. As a heuristic framework, the notion that

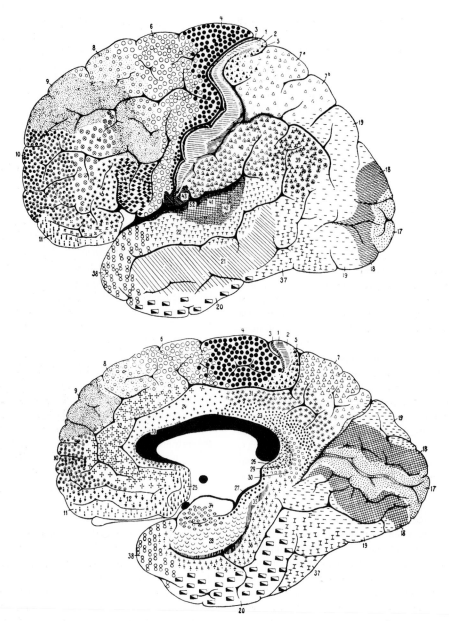

Figure 15.1 *Brodmann's cytoarchitectural map of the human cerebral cortex, lateral view; each symbol represents a distinct area of the cerebral cortex, numbered as shown. (Source: Brodmann K [1909] Vegleichende Lokalisation lehre der Grosshirnrinde ihren Prinzipien dargestelt auf Grund des Zellenbaues. JA Barth, Leipzig.)*

higher cortical functions are best described as parallel and distributed is quite influential to most current thinking in the cognitive neurosciences.

Memory

Memory functioning – broadly defined as the storage and recall of past experience – is of major interest and importance in cognitive neuroscience. The intensity of research in the area of memory has been especially great in the past decade, when the fields of cognitive psychology and neuropsychology converged to offer unified models of memory functioning on the basis of experimentation in normal and brain-damaged humans, as well as lesion studies in animals. Functional neuroimaging has also begun to yield valuable insights into the patterns of neuroanatomical connectivity involved in aspects of memory. Because this field is relatively

massive, the reader is referred to comprehensive sources for further details (Christianson, 1992; Squire and Butters, 1992).

Historically, the debate between the localizationist and holistic views of neural processing has been nowhere sharper than in the search for regionally specific entities involved in memory. The search for the "engram" or memory trace led Lashley (1950) to conclude that memories are distributed throughout the brain, not localized within a discrete or unitary structure. The debate has been given a more sophisticated focus with the realization that although there is regional specificity in aspects of memory, the complexity of the processes requires multiple brain regions, probably operating in a parallel fashion.

The initial contributions to the present knowledge of memory were from two methodologies. These are the lesion analytical method and cognitive studies of normal individuals. The lesion analytical method has contributed the most to an understanding of both the cognitive and neuroanatomical aspects of memory functioning.

In the last 10 years, functional neuroimaging techniques (particularly positron emission tomography [PET] and functional magnetic resonance imaging [fMRI]) have become increasingly popular and provide an alternative method of studying human cognition. These techniques have the dual potential to validate existing models of memory and to suggest newer theories based on patterns of anatomical connectivity observed during the performance of memory tasks. Furthermore, unlike the lesion analytical method, they afford the ability to observe cognitive processes in healthy human brains. Neither PET nor fMRI directly measures neural activity; rather, they rely on changes in regional cerebral blood flow (rCBF) that result from the metabolic demands of neural activity. As neural activity occurs, the demand for oxygen causes an increase in the relative concentration of deoxyhemoglobin in the surrounding region.

There are several things to keep in mind when considering findings from neuroimaging studies. First, it is important to remember that PET and fMRI are based on relative blood flow. Therefore, the baseline task subtracted from the events of interest must be tightly controlled to ensure that the finding is as specific as possible. Furthermore, although functional neuroimaging can suggest brain regions functionally involved in performing a cognitive operation, blood flow studies cannot suggest what is unique about that brain region. Also, when distributed brain regions are simultaneously activated, the technique itself does not immediately reveal the functional connectivity between those regions. Unlike the electrophysiological studies of working memory, imaging cannot suggest whether a brain region is in a sense storing information or transmitting information or is in some other way involved in the performance of an operation.

Cellular Basis of Memory

On the basis of lesion analytical studies, the hippocampus and related structures have been implicated as a site for the consolidation of memory. The question naturally arises out of the properties of the neurons in this area that might permit the association of information. Neuroanatomically (Figure 15.2), the hippocampal formation consists of the fields of Ammon's horn (regions CA_1, CA_2, CA_3), the dentate gyrus and the subiculum. Afferent pathways from the entorhinal cortex project to the hippocampus via the perforant pathway and synapse on the granular cells in the dentate gyrus. The entorhinal cortex itself receives cortical inputs from polysensory associational regions in the frontal, temporal and parietal lobes. Within the hippocampal formation, the granule cells in region CA_3 also project to the CA_1 region through the fimbria fornix, which also projects to the subiculum. The subiculum is the major efferent pathway, projecting to a number of cortical regions but also projecting back to the entorhinal cortex, completing the loop.

For learning and memory to occur, there must be plastic changes such that the structure and functional characteristics of nerve cells and their interconnections are altered. Much of the research into the processes of synaptic plasticity underlying learning and memory has been conducted in invertebrates (Kandel *et al.*, 1983; Kandel, 1991) through examination of reflexive learning processes (habituation, sensitization and classical conditioning).

Regarding the mammalian brain, Bliss and Lomo (1973) were the first to demonstrate that repeated stimulation of the

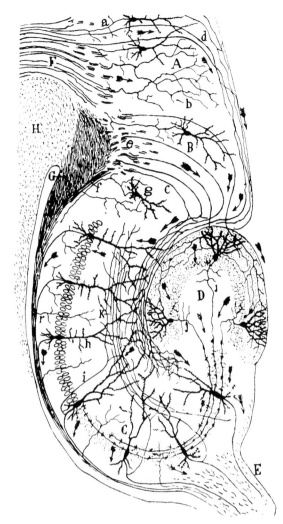

Figure 15.2 *Some of the structure and connections of the hippocampus (Ammon's horn) as drawn by Ramon y Cajal. A, Entorhinal cortex; B, subiculum; C, hippocampus; D, dentate gyrus; E, fimbria of fornix; F, fibers of the cingulum entering the entorhinal cortex (A); K, Schaffer collaterals; a, axons entering the cingulum; b, fibers of the cingulum terminating in the entorhinal cortex; g, pyramidal cell of the subiculum; h, pyramidal cells of the hippocampus; i, ascending collaterals from the hippocampal pyramidal cells; j, granule cell axons; r, collaterals from axons in the alveus. (Source: Ramon y Cajal S [1911] Histologie du Système Nerveux de l'Homme et des Vertébrés. Maloine, Paris.)*

afferent pathways to the dentate granule cells of the hippocampus of the rabbit produced an excitatory potential in the postsynaptic hippocampal neurons lasting for hours. Recording in intact animals has shown potentials that lasted for days and weeks. They termed this increased facilitation as a result of repeated stimulation long-term potentiation (LTP).

With respect to area CA_1 of the hippocampus, studies have shown that LTP occurs only when a number of input pathways have been stimulated. This is known as the criterion of cooperativity. When distinct weak and strong excitatory inputs impinge on a pyramidal nerve cell, the weak input becomes potentiated through association with a strong input. This is known as the criterion of associativity. Finally, the criterion of specificity refers to

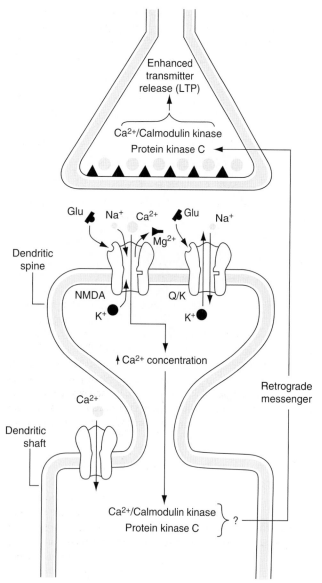

Figure 15.3 *The events surrounding the induction of LTP are portrayed. As a result of the tetanic stimulation of the postsynaptic membrane, depolarization relieves the magnesium (Mg²⁺) blockade of the NMDA channel allowing sodium (Na⁺), potassium (K⁺) and calcium (Ca²⁺) to flow through the NMDA channel. The increase of calcium in the dendritic spine then triggers calcium-dependent kinases, which induce LTP. The maintenance of transmitter release is thought to occur by release of a retrograde messenger that acts on the presynaptic terminal. The voltage-dependent calcium channels in the dendritic shaft remain closed. (Source: Adapted from Kandel ER [1991] Cellular mechanisms of learning and the biological basis of individuality, in Principles of Neural Science, 3rd edn. [eds Kandel E, Schwartz JH, and Jessell TM]. Appleton & Lange, Norwalk, CT, pp. 1009–1031. Copyright, the McGraw-Hill Companies, Inc.)*

the fact that strong repeated stimulation in one synaptic pathway is specific only to that stimulated pathway. Unstimulated synapses on the same cell do not demonstrate LTP.

The events surrounding LTP are schematically described here (Figure 15.3); the reader is referred to a detailed explanation of the cellular and molecular aspects of LTP (Kandel, 1991;

Shepherd, 1994). Studies of the CA₁ region of the hippocampus reveal that LTP is mediated by the neurotransmitter glutamate.

LTP has been stressed as a cellular mechanism of informational connectivity in the hippocampus. Brief mention should also be made of long-term depression (LTD). LTD is the opposite of LTP and refers to "use-dependent long-lasting decreases in synaptic strength" (Linden and Connor, 1995). LTD may have a number of advantages and work in parallel with LTP with respect to memory functioning. LTD may help reset synapses that have been potentiated by LTP, to prevent saturation. It may serve as a cellular mechanism of forgetting (Tsumoto, 1993) and, finally, may also form an active inhibitory system to attenuate signals from adjacent potentiated synapses. The specific role of LTD in the coordination of memory is still unclear. For a detailed description of the potential cellular and molecular mechanisms involved in LTD, the reader is referred to other sources (Linden and Connor, 1995; Linden, 1994). The phenomena of LTP and LTD provide an example in which neural cytoarchitecture and the underlying cellular and molecular levels may actually conform to the principles of association and connectivity. Computational models have been developed to further our understanding of the manner in which learning and memory emerge from the properties of synaptic plasticity embodied in the circuitry of the hippocampus (Churchland and Sejnowski, 1992; Traub and Miles, 1991). The attraction of computational models is that they may clarify the link between aspects of LTP and LTD within local networks of associated neurons at the cellular level and the events at the behavioral level.

Major Subdivisions of Memory Systems

Current research on the cognitive neuroscience of memory has considered memory from the perspective of multiple systems rather than a unitary system. Figure 15.4 illustrates the subdivisions between memory systems. A number of systems have been proposed, and the distinction between these systems is not impermeable. The most basic distinction between memory systems is that of explicit versus implicit memory. Explicit memory is also referred to as declarative memory and implicit memory is also known as nondeclarative memory. What is considered explicit about this type of memory is that it requires conscious awareness of past experience (Cohen and Squire, 1980). There are two major components of explicit memory: episodic memory and semantic memory. Episodic or autobiographical memory is the

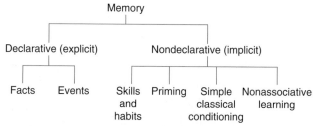

Figure 15.4 *Subdivision of major memory systems. Declarative (explicit) memory requires conscious awareness of past experience; nondeclarative (implicit) memory refers to the effects of previous experience on current behavior without conscious recollection. Reprinted with permission from Squire LR and Zola-Morgan S [1991] The medial temporal lobe memory system. Science 253, 1380–1386. Copyright 1991, American Association for the Advancement of Science.*

ability to remember personal events over time. This refers to the individual's ability to remember not only that something occurred but also the context in which it occurred. Semantic memory, in contrast, refers to knowledge without context. Another type of explicit memory system that involves the short-term registering of information is termed working memory, which will be discussed in the executive functions section of this chapter. Memory systems research in the past several years has also focused on implicit memory. Implicit memory does not involve conscious awareness. It refers to the effects of previous experience on current behavior without conscious recollection.

On the basis of cases of medial temporal lobe damage in humans, it has been concluded that the medial temporal lobe, including the hippocampus, and adjacent anatomical structures enable the formation of explicit memories. In humans, it has been shown that a lesion confined solely to the hippocampus (field CA_1 of the hippocampus) can produce a mild amnestic syndrome (Zola-Morgan *et al.*, 1986). It would then appear that the parahippocampal and perirhinal cortical regions are also necessarily involved in explicit memory. According to Zola-Morgan and Squire (1993), the medial temporal lobe system essentially coordinates the organization of information that originated in other brain regions. The medial temporal lobe system may thereby act as a temporary site to store information that is cortically distributed until the information is permanently coded.

Diencephalon and Explicit Memory

Neuropsychological studies of patients with Wernicke–Korsakoff disease have yielded insight into the contribution of the diencephalon (dorsal and anterior thalamic nuclei and the mamillary bodies of the hypothalamus) to memory. Wernicke–Korsakoff disease is usually associated with a thiamine deficiency and is typically seen in individuals with alcoholism, nutritional deficiencies, infections and brain tumors (Markowitsch and Pritzel, 1985). The memory deficit is characterized by impairment of explicit memory as seen by dense anterograde amnesia and variable retrograde amnesia. These patients are also frequently apathetic and indifferent and have diminished initiative.

The effects of damage caused by alcoholic and nonalcoholic lesions to the anterior and medial thalamic nuclei as well as to the mamillary bodies are diverse. The diencephalic region is connected with the hippocampal region; the mamillary bodies are connected to the hippocampus via the fornix and to the anterior thalamus via the mamillothalamic tract. The mediodorsal thalamic component of the system is also interconnected with the frontal lobes. Patients with Korsakoff's disease typically manifest frontal lobe damage, which is seen in the phenomenon of confabulation. Aside from this frontal component, which is often seen in alcoholism and may represent an independent lesion, the diencephalic amnesia is largely similar to the kinds of memory deficits observed with damage to the medial temporal lobe system. This suggests that, at least at a functional level, anatomical damage in this subcortical system produces an impairment in the consolidation of information.

Basal Forebrain and Memory

Another neuroanatomical region that plays a direct role in explicit memory is the basal forebrain. The basal forebrain region is located where the diencephalon meets the cerebral hemispheres and includes a number of brain structures such as the septal area, diagonal band of Broca, nucleus accumbens septi, olfactory tubercle, and substantia innominata. Figure 15.5 illustrates the rostral cholinergic projections in the rat brain. The contribution of this brain region to memory has been a relatively recent discovery. The cholinergic system plays a role in memory (although its full role is not clear at this time), and is implicated in normal and pathological aging, but is only one locus in the network of brain regions involved in memory.

Affective Valence and Neuromodulatory Systems

Memory functioning requires a system for establishing valence between memorable events. That is, some events are more memorable than others. Affect and its associated chemical neuromodulators probably serve a valence capacity by facilitating the storage of emotionally charged experiences. The underlying

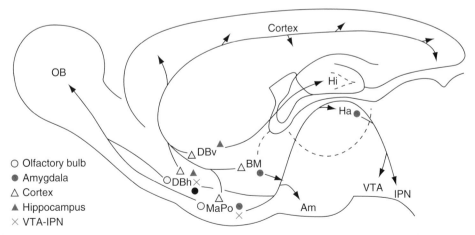

Figure 15.5   *Sagittal view of some projections of the rostral cholinergic column in the rat. The symbols ([Page No. 371]) refer to the origin within the rostral cholinergic column of afferents to the olfactory bulb, amygdala, and so on. Am, Amygdala; BM, nucleus basalis; DBh, horizontal limb of diagonal band; DBv, vertical limb of diagonal band; Ha, habenula; Hi, hippocampus; IPN, interpeduncular nucleus; MaPo, magnocellular preoptic area; OB, olfactory bulb; VTA, ventral tegmental area. Reprinted with permission from Fibiger HC and Vincent SR [1987] the Anatomy of the central cholinergic neurons. In Psychopharmacology: The third Generation of Progress, Meltzer (Ed). Copyright, Lipincott Williams and Wilkins (1987).*

assumption here is that emotionally tinged experiences activate neurobiological pathways that facilitate their storage. In evolutionary terms, it is highly adaptive to remember experiences that are learned under arousing conditions. Neuroimaging studies have provided evidence for the role of the amygdala in forming declarative memories. A number of neuromodulators play a role in affective responding and also influence memory storage. Chief among them is the noradrenergic system. The central noradrenergic system involves the locus coeruleus in the midbrain reticular formation, the amygdala and the stria terminalis (a major afferent and efferent pathway to the amygdala). A number of findings have converged to suggest that central norepinephrine (NE) receptors in the amygdala are involved in the postlearning consolidation of information (Liang *et al.*, 1986).

Overall, the role of the noradrenergic and other systems, such as GABA and opioid peptides, in memory may lie in the release of adrenal epinephrine after stressful or emotional stimuli. Activation of NE in the locus coeruleus–amygdala system, which ultimately has extensive connectivity with a number of brain regions, then serves to consolidate the storage of these memories. On a cellular level this may occur by the production of LTP, because noradrenergic compounds have been found to enhance LTP (Gold *et al.*, 1984).

Frontal Lobe Contribution to Explicit Memory

It is probable that interactive processing between the medial temporal lobe system and the frontal lobes is necessary for explicit memory. The frontal lobe provides an executive input to the medial temporal lobe system, imbuing memory with "intelligence" (Moscovitch, 1992). The frontal lobes, through their extensive reciprocal connectivity with the hippocampal formation, probably provide input to ordering and placing experience in a spatial–temporal context. The frontal lobes in a sense add goal orientation to memory.

Implicit Memory

As defined earlier, implicit memory refers to the influence of past experience on current behavior that is not conscious or intentional. In other words, retention of linguistic, visual, or motor information can occur in the absence of explicit retrieval of that information. An example of the manner in which explicit memory and implicit memory can be dissociated is given by the results of a fragment stem completion task (Tulving *et al.*, 1982), which illustrates the priming effect. Priming refers to the increased facilitation of identifying a stimulus that occurs as a result of having had prior exposure to that stimulus (Schacter *et al.*, 1993), even though the individual may have no conscious recollection of the exposure. On the basis of numerous studies with brain-damaged and normal individuals, it is probable that the perceptual representation subsystems for priming are a visual word form system representing the orthographical features of words, a system that represents structural relations among parts of objects, and an auditory word form system that mediates phonological or acoustic information. The likely brain regions associated with each of these subsystems are the extrastriate cortex, inferior temporal region and perisylvian cortex.

Although the priming effect is the most extensively studied aspect of implicit memory, it is important to note that the learning of motor skills and habits and the phenomenon of classical conditioning fall under the rubric of implicit memory. These processes may be considered as part of implicit memory because behavior changes and learning occur without conscious. This behavioral dissociation between priming and skill learning suggests that the latter may be mediated by the corticostriatal loop that mediates motor programming, namely the basal ganglia, thalamus, and motor, premotor and sensorimotor cortex (Heindel *et al.*, 1991).

Executive Functioning and the Frontal Lobes

Most researchers now agree that the study of frontal lobes represents an important aspect of attempts to understand of humans' higher mental functions, such as planning, decision-making, reasoning and judgment, which are often referred to as executive processes.

The frontal lobes of the human brain comprise all the tissue anterior to the central sulcus. Four major subdivisions of the frontal lobes have been suggested: 1) the motor area; 2) the premotor area; 3) the prefrontal area, and 4) the basomedial portion of the lobes (Walsh, 1994).

Two prefrontal areas, namely, the orbitomedial prefrontal cortex and the dorsolateral prefrontal cortex, have been targeted in much of the research concerning executive processes. The functional role of the frontal system in providing executive control to behavior is probably related to the extensive reciprocal anatomical connectivity between the frontal lobes and other brain regions involved in information processing. Numerous afferent and efferent connections of the frontal lobe have been demonstrated. The extracortical and transcortical connections of the frontal lobes are exceedingly complex, especially where the prefrontal cortex is involved (Kolb and Wishaw, 1990). In general, brain connectivity encompasses three major types: cortical–cortical, thalamic–cortical, and subcortical–cortical (Figure 15.6). For a detailed review of brain connectivity, the reader is referred to the works of Pandya and Yeterian (1984) and Goldman-Rakic (1988).

Cortical–cortical connections of the frontal lobes take on a number of distinct forms (Kolb and Wishaw, 1990). First, as previously mentioned, connections within the frontal lobes themselves involve projections from tertiary cortex in the prefrontal areas to the premotor cortex and to the motor cortex. Secondly, there are reciprocal connections between the prefrontal cortex (Brodmann's areas 8, 9 and 46) and the temporal, auditory and visual association regions, as well as the medial temporal lobes. Thirdly, there is another set of reciprocal connections connecting the prefrontal areas and the anterior and medial temporal regions. Fourthly, there are connections between prefrontal areas and the limbic system, including a reciprocal connection between the amygdala and the frontal lobe.

Thalamic–cortical connections include projections to the prefrontal lobe from the pulvinar, anterior nuclei and dorsomedial nucleus of the thalamus. In addition, via the dorsomedial nucleus, information from limbic areas and the hypothalamus is relayed to the frontal lobes for processing of emotions and internal states.

Subcortical–cortical connections include projections from the frontal cortex to various subcortical structures including the caudate nucleus, superior colliculus and hypothalamus. Particular attention has been paid to the interconnectivity of the frontal lobe and basal ganglia via the corticostriate projection system. Lesions in either area are associated with similar cognitive impairments, such as decreased cognitive flexibility or set switching (Eslinger and Grattan, 1993).

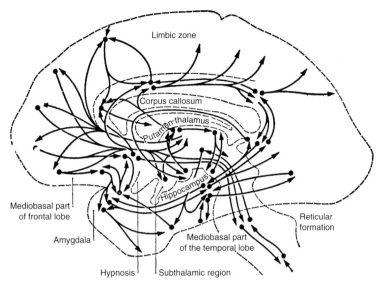

Figure 15.6 *Illustration of some of the patterns of frontal lobe connectivity. (Source: Luria AR [1973b] The Working Brain: An Introduction to Neuropsychology. Penguin Books, London, p. 85.)*

Examination of the connectivity of the frontal lobes has revealed that the pattern of connectivity is best viewed from within the context of a parallel and distributed anatomical network (Figure 15.7).

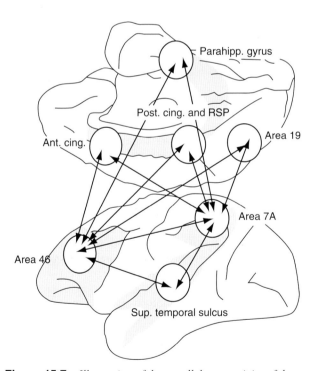

Figure 15.7 *Illustration of the parallel connectivity of the frontal and parietal regions. Area 46 and area 7A project to more than a dozen common targets; five of these areas are illustrated. (Source: Goldman-Rakic PS [1988] Changing concepts of cortical connectivity: Parallel distributed cortical networks, in Neurobiology of Neocortex [eds Rakic P and Singer W], p. 187. Copyright 1988 John Wiley. Reprinted by permission of John Wiley.)*

Working Memory

We have previously discussed in general terms the frontal contribution to memory at the level of encoding and retrieving. However, memory researchers believe that the frontal lobes modulate the use of memory in executive functions such as planning and decision-making. This kind of memory is referred to as "working memory" (Miller *et al.*, 1960). In their recent comprehensive review of working memory models, Miyake and Shah (1999) proposed that working memory "is those mechanisms or processes that are involved in the service of complex cognition, including novel as well as familiar, skilled tasks". This definition differentiates working memory from short-term memory because it suggests that working memory goes beyond simply keeping information "in mind"; rather, working memory brings or keeps information online in a goal-directed fashion. Baddeley and Hitch (1974) were the first to provide a human cognitive model for the concept of working memory, and the neuroanatomical localization of this to the frontal lobes has been largely advanced by the extensive work of Goldman-Rakic and colleagues (Goldman-Rakic, 1987, 1988; Baddeley and Hitch, 1974).

Figure 15.8 illustrates the major components of the Baddeley and Hitch model of working memory. This model (Baddeley and Hitch, 1974) provides for a dynamic system of temporary and limited storage. It is composed of a central executive and two "slave" systems, a visual–spatial sketchpad, and a phonological loop.

The central executive aspect of the working memory system appears to exert control over the flow of activity between the slave systems and provides the input to long-term memory. However, this is also the least well-understood component of working memory. The interaction of slave systems with the central executive probably reflects the interplay between the frontal lobe mechanisms of executive control of input received from parietal, temporal and occipital systems of perception and association. Although the detailed role of the central executive remains unclear, evidence from the animal and human experimental literature suggests that the prefrontal cortex is specialized with respect to working memory.

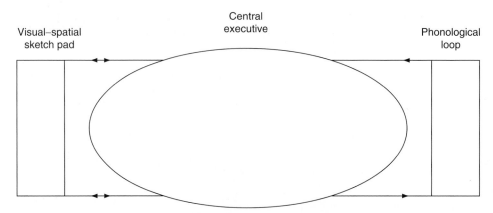

Figure 15.8 *A simplified representation of the Baddeley and Hitch (1974) working memory model. Reprinted with permission from Working memory. In The Cognitive Neurosciences, Gazzaniga MS, Bizzi E, Black IB, et al. [eds]. Baddeley A [1995] Copyright Elsevier Baddeley AD and Hitch G [1974] Working memory. In The Psychology of Learning and Motivation, Vol. 8, Bower GA [ed]. Academic Press, New York, pp. 47–89.*

Anatomical Evidence of Working Memory

The prefrontal cortex may be a kind of multipurpose working memory center, with each area concerned with a different domain. The prefrontal cortex would then function as the coordinating element in a parallel distributed cortical–cortical network.

Theories of Frontal Lobe Functioning

Some of the influential theories of the role of the prefrontal cortex and behavior are shown in Table 15.1. All theories impute to the frontal lobes a functional role as an executive control system for other cognitive and motor processes. The theories differ with respect to the specific mechanisms involved and the extent to which cognitive and neuroanatomical parameters are delineated.

Assessment of Frontal Lobe Functioning

Neuropsychological Assessment

There is an extensive literature concerning the evaluation of frontal lobe functioning with various neuropsychological assessment

Table 15.1	**Theories of Frontal Lobe Functioning**	
Basis	Author	Description
Psychological assessment	Miller *et al.* (1960)	Postulated test-operate-test-exit feedback loops by which the frontal lobe organizes and coordinates behaviors transferred from the posterior brain.
Psychological assessment	Teuber (1964)	Postulated that anticipatory discharges travel from the frontal lobe to the posterior brain influencing motor system and sensory functions.
Psychological or anatomical	Luria (1973a)	Postulated three brain units, each unit having different neuroanatomical representation. Unit 3 is located in frontal lobes and exerts regulatory functions over the behavior of the other two units in the posterior brain through interactive and sequential processing.
Psychological or information processing	Norman and Shallice (1986)	Postulated that the frontal lobes primarily function as an SAS over cognitive units and schemas during nonroutine behavior.
Anatomical or animal studies	Fuster (1989)	Postulated that frontal lobes generally function in the temporal integration of behavior through three subordinate functions: anticipation, provisional memory and control of interference.
Neuroanatomical or animal studies	Goldman-Rakic (1987)	Postulated that prefrontal cortex maintains a representational memory of symbolic, mnemonic, and sensory information from nonprefrontal areas. These memory units exert inhibitory and excitatory influences on behavior through PDP.
Neuroanatomical or computational neuroscience	Mesulam (1990)	Postulated that the frontal lobes, through interconnectivity with other brain areas, exert executive control over neural networks subserving different information processing capacities via PDP.

techniques. The majority of these studies are based on assessment of individuals with known frontal lobe damage or animals with experimentally induced lesions. Dubois and colleagues (1994) suggested that the skills needed for the elaboration, control and execution of goal-directed behaviors form the basis of studies involving the prefrontal cortex. These abilities would necessarily include planning, mental flexibility, impulse control, working memory and evaluation of one's behavior, that is, executive processes.

Evaluation of executive processes is fraught with numerous obstacles. First, there are few assessment procedures that allow enough flexibility in response or ability to consider alternative ways of thinking, which are central elements of executive processing. Consider the paradox of having to structure an examination technique that assesses the ability of subjects to make structure for themselves (Lezak, 1995). Secondly, executive functioning is the final stage of a processing sequence, relying heavily on information provided by other brain areas. It follows that successful execution of the frontal lobe functions depends, in great part, on the integrity of the remainder of the brain. Effective executive processing is an unlikely occurrence if the information needed from nonfrontal lobe regions is missing or inaccurate. Thirdly, frontal lobe functioning encompasses a number of abilities, making a complete assessment of such processes an arduous, if not impossible, task at best. Fourthly, many of the neuropsychological instruments used in the assessment of executive processes are weakly constructed and insensitive to obscure changes in the

presence of compensatory strategies that occur after frontal lobe damage. Despite these obstacles, the quest better to understand the cognitive processes that belie the functioning of the frontal lobes, as well as the desire to prognosticate level of adaptive functioning in patients with known impairment, has maintained the strong interest in employing neuropsychological assessment techniques. Many of these neuropsychological tasks have also been used in the context of functional neuroimaging to better delineate cognitive and neuroanatomical correlates. Table 15.2 details several of the assessment procedures used to evaluate the integrity of the frontal lobes in performing cognitive operations.

Behavioral–Neuroanatomical Correlates

Disrupted neurobehavioral functioning in a number of psychiatric and neurological disorders has revealed several interesting aspects of the role of the frontal lobes in behavior. Studies involving dementias of the frontal lobe type, particularly Pick's disease, have provided some information concerning the role of the frontal lobes. Pick's disease is quite distinguishable from the better known Alzheimer's type in that in the former basic memory functions are relatively spared early in the disease course. The initial presentation of Pick's disease largely involves the presence of striking changes in personality and social appropriateness. Memory dysfunction, if apparent, is secondary to motivational or attentional factors rather than faulty learning. Patients with Pick's disease consistently perform poorly on a wide variety of tests sensitive to frontal lobe dysfunction.

Many of the studies involving the association of affective disorders and frontal lobe functioning have emerged from the literature on stroke. Starkstein and associates (1987) have found that the left frontal opercular region is the area most frequently damaged in patients suffering from poststroke depression. Similarly, using computed tomography, Robinson and Szetela (1981) have demonstrated that the closer the lesion is to the frontal pole, the more severe the ensuing depression. After reviewing the relationship between frontal lobe impairment and affective dysfunction in poststroke depression, Baxter and colleagues (1989) concluded that left prefrontal hypometabolism was the most consistent and severe finding in major depression, bipolar depression and obsessive–compulsive disorders.

A surge in the study of schizophrenia has provided a wealth of knowledge concerning the functioning of the prefrontal cortex. It is generally agreed that cognitive abnormalities associated with schizophrenia often involve difficulties in executive processing. Some of the earliest and best known studies involving neuroimaging techniques in the assessment of cognitive abilities in this population were carried out by Weinberger and colleagues. Many other studies employing rCBF (Buchsbaum *et al.*, 1984; Weinberger *et al.*, 1988; Sagawa *et al.*, 1990) and functional brain imaging (Buchsbaum *et al.*, 1990) have found evidence to support the "hypofrontality" hypothesis in schizophrenia. However, not all studies have found frontal hypometabolism in patients with schizophrenia (Gur *et al.*, 1985; Berman *et al.*, 1988). The heterogeneous nature of schizophrenia probably accounts for these contradictory findings. A number of researchers including Volkow and colleagues (1987) and Andreasen and associates (1992) have found that hypofrontality was most related to patients with a predominance of negative symptoms.

Table 15.2	Tests Commonly Used to Assess Executive Functions
Function	**Test**
Abstract thinking	Comprehension subtest of Wechsler Adult Intelligence Scale–Revised, Gorham's Proverbs Test
Concept formation, social judgment	Similarities subtest of Wechsler Adult Intelligence Scale–Revised
Concept formation and cognitive flexibility including establishing, maintaining and shifting cognitive set	Wisconsin Card Sorting Test Halstead Categories Test
Cognitive flexibility and psychomotor speed	Trail Making Test, part B
Cognitive set maintenance and impulse control	Stroop Color–Word Test
Planning and impulse control	Porteus Maze Test
Visual–spatial working memory and problem solving	Tower of London
Cognitive productivity	Controlled Oral Word Association Test (verbal fluency) Ruff Figure Fluency Test (design fluency)

Attention

In view of what is known about the role of the prefrontal cortex, it is readily apparent that the primary role of this brain region involves the integration and modulation of cognitive functioning. Given the onerous task of managing vast amounts of incoming and outgoing information, it stands to reason that attentional abilities are of great importance to frontal lobe functioning.

The area of attention as it relates to the frontal lobes has provided a rich field of study. Like many of the other general areas of cognition (e.g., memory, language), attention represents a vast and complex phenomenon. This is, in part, due to the many facets of attention itself. Underlying all cognitive activity, there must be some tonic form of activation that provides the background in which all other cortical activity occurs. Luria (1973a) referred to this capacity as his first functional brain area and noted that the reticular activating system in the brain stem provided the core structure subserving brain activation. In general, this is referred to as alertness or wakefulness. However, one's ability to pay attention to specific stimuli is thought to be subserved by higher cortical areas, including the prefrontal cortex. The psychological process of attention can broadly be defined in terms of divided, focused and sustained abilities. Divided attention occurs when multiple stimuli are attended to simultaneously. We can often find ourselves participating in divided attention tasks at parties when we tune into two different conversations at one time. Focused attention refers to the ability to inhibit irrelevant stimuli in the service of attending to a particular stimulus. Often this type of attention requires one to inhibit automatic responses that conflict with the task at hand. Sustained attention requires the ability to maintain attention over time.

As suggested earlier, Mesulam (1990) has proposed a neurocognitive network of attention involving a number of neural circuits participating in PDP. According to this model, interactive, multifocal neural pathways that are both localized and distributed give rise to multiple possibilities and flexibility with respect to attentional behavior. Much of this model is based on neglect behavior, which can be separated into perceptual, motor and limbic components. In general, the perceptual component refers to the diminished awareness that a sensory event has occurred within the neglected field, the motor component refers to the diminution or absence of exploratory behaviors, and the limbic component refers to a devaluation or amotivation of the neglected hemispace. According to Mesulam, neglect behavior in both humans and monkeys consistently follows lesions to one of three areas: the dorsolateral parietal cortex, the dorsolateral premotor–prefrontal cortex and the cingulate gyrus. These three areas provide local networks that provide the basis for a large-scale neural model of attention. Each local network or component participates in mapping the environment in slightly different ways. For example, in the case of visual hemineglect, Mesulam suggested that the posterior parietal cortex provides sensory (visual) awareness, the prefrontal area provides a map of exploratory movements (i.e., eye movements), and the cingulate gyrus provides a map for assigning value to the spatial coordinates. Within these areas, specific cytoarchitectonic structures interact through extensive reciprocal and monosynaptic connections. In the area of the dorsolateral prefrontal cortex, the frontal eye fields (Brodmann's area 8) play a critical role in directed attention. Although lesions in other brain regions, such as subcortical structures, are known to cause neglect, these areas have been found to connect to at least two of the three central components.

Language

Language as a species-specific ability in humans is intrinsic to the development of knowledge and understanding. It endows us with a capacity unique to the human species to structure and organize experiences through the manipulation of categorical and abstract concepts. With increasing internalization of language comes the capacity for disengagement from the environment so that concepts exist independently of their immediate context, as internal representations. Through this capacity to organize and form internal representations of experiences, a stable construction of reality is made possible (Bunowski and Bellugi, 1970; Guidano and Liotti, 1983).

Language is thus an integral part of mentation. Language is also central to modes of communication. Both of these aspects of language have been subjects of study for many disciplines, including philosophy, psycholinguistics, psychology and cognitive sciences. Furthermore, the disconnection of language from other cognitive processes and the disruptions in its communicative functions have been subjects of investigation in the fields of neurology, neurosurgery, neurophysiology and neuropsychology. Multidisciplinary efforts have led to a burgeoning body of research on language in normal and brain-damaged individuals, and the converging findings have greatly advanced our understanding of language as a complex human ability.

Regardless of the discipline within which the study of language is attempted, its essential features are common. Language is governed by a set of rules that link its various components. The basic units of a sound-based language (e.g., as opposed to a sign-based language) are classified in terms of phonemes, morphemes, lexicon, syntax, semantics, prosody and discourse. Phonemes are the smallest units of sound; morphemes are the smallest meaningful word units that when combined form words; syntax refers to the relational features by which words are combined, that is, grammar; lexicon refers to the words or vocabulary of a language; semantics refers to the meaning of words and sentences; prosody means the inflection and rhythm of utterances; and discourse involves the combination of sentences within any given context and constitutes narratives (Damasio and Damasio, 1992).

Important Issues in Language Research

From a historical standpoint, one of the earliest questions about language has pertained to the concept of cerebral dominance and differential lateralization. A second area of investigation that has gained considerable interest because of cross-disciplinary research efforts is concerned with structural and functional localization of language. Researchers are concerned with whether specific regions of the brain are specialized for specific linguistic functions, including speaking, comprehending, reading and writing. Furthermore, with the growing influence of cognitive neuroscience, researchers are investigating whether specific language operations are localized in different levels of processing (e.g., phonological, orthographical, lexical, syntactic) and studying specific neural substrates associated with these processing networks. They are also interested in studying the patterns of connectivity between these neural networks. A third area that continues to generate great interest relates to neurodevelopmental aspects of language. Some of the questions in this area deal with the acquisition and development of language, as well as with the organization of the brain for language abilities in children.

The centrality of these issues to an understanding of language is reflected in the emergence of different models for language, which are described in greater detail in later sections. Briefly, these models can be broadly classified into traditional and current models when placed in a historical context. The traditional models were essentially localizationist (Wernicke, Broca, early contributions of Geschwind); the current models are more "hybrid" (Mesulam, 1990) in that they reflect a conceptualization of language processing as being both localized and distributed.

Because a great deal of what is understood about language and continues to intrigue investigators has emerged from studies of deficits and their neuroanatomical correlates in the various language disorders, especially aphasia, a description of these is important and is provided next. For more detailed reviews of language disorders, the reader is referred to other sources (Benson and Geschwind, 1985; Heilman and Valenstein, 1993).

Acquired Language Disorders: The Example of Aphasia

The longstanding finding of different patterns of language impairment linked with specific neuroanatomical sites has led to several classification schemes for organizing clinical and research data on aphasia. Classifications based on syndromes or clusters of symptoms have been most favored. The major aphasia subtypes that are now widely accepted are presented in Table 15.3. The subtypes of aphasia have been further subdivided in terms of their neuroanatomical loci into perisylvian (Broca's, Wernicke's, conduction and global) and extrasylvian (transcortical-motor, transcortical-sensory, mixed, anomic and subcortical) aphasias (Benson and Geschwind, 1985). The impairment and preservation of the ability to repeat appear to coincide with this dichotomy. Figure 15.9 depicts some of the regions of the left cerebral cortex that are involved in language functioning.

Table 15.3 Clinical Features Associated with Subtypes of Aphasia

Type of Aphasia	Speech or Verbal Output	Repetition	Comprehension	Naming	Other Features*	Regions Involved
Broca's	Nonfluent	Impaired	Largely preserved	Often impaired	Right hemiparesis; may be depressed	Left posterior inferior frontal
Wernicke's	Fluent; paraphasic	Impaired	Impaired	Impaired	May be agitated; ambiguous; paranoid	Left posterior superior temporal
Conduction	Fluent; paraphasic	Impaired	Impaired	Often impaired	†Right hemisensory defect †Right arm and facial weakness	Left supramarginal gyrus or left auditory cortex
Global	Nonfluent	Impaired	Impaired	Impaired	Right hemiparesis; right hemisensory defect	Left frontal parietal temporal
Transcortical motor	Nonfluent	Intact or largely preserved	Impaired	Impaired	‡Right hemiparesis	Left frontal, anterior or superior to Broca's area
Transcortical sensory	Fluent; paraphasic	Intact or largely preserved	Impaired	Impaired	†Right hemiparesis	Left temporoparietal areas surrounding Wernicke's area
Anomic	Fluent	Intact or largely preserved	Largely preserved	Impaired	No definite motor signs	Left temporoparietal or frontal
Subcortical*	Fluent or articulatory disturbances may be present	Intact or may be impaired	Impaired	Intact or impaired	†Right hemiparesis	Caudate; thalamus

*Variable symptoms depending on subcortical area affected;
†sometimes present;
‡often present.

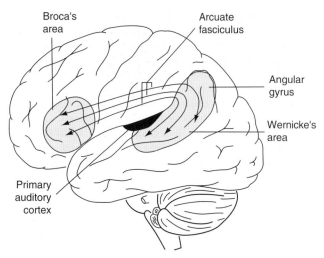

Figure 15.9 *Left cerebral hemisphere showing areas of particular relevance to language processing. Reprinted from Burt AM [1993] Textbook of Neuroanatomy. WB Saunders, Philadelphia, p. 469. Copyright 1993, with permission from Elsevier.*

Computed tomographic studies have linked aphasia with left-sided lesions in areas lying outside the cerebral cortex. This finding suggests that language is also subserved by subcortical areas. Subcortical aphasia is characterized by mutism in the early stage of the disorder, followed by articulatory disturbances and paraphasic output. Paraphasia appears to resolve when the patient has to repeat sentences. Comprehension is commonly impaired, and other language disturbances may also be involved. One distinguishing feature of this type of aphasia is the transient nature of the severe language defects seen in the early stages (Benson and Geschwind, 1985). The neuropathology in subcortical aphasia has been found to vary in terms of localization. Most commonly, subcortical aphasia is associated with lesions in the thalamus, caudate, and putamen (Naeser *et al.*, 1982).

Some inconsistent findings have raised questions about the role of subcortical damage in aphasia. For example, it has been noted that aphasia can resolve even in the presence of persisting subcortical abnormalities. Conversely, in some cases, aphasia does not follow damage to subcortical areas. In some instances, evidence from functional neuroimaging studies has been used to understand such discrepancies. PET studies reveal that structural damage in an area might result in hypometabolism in distant, intact areas. Metter and coworkers (1987) found that aphasia was associated with the presence of cortical hypometabolism after structural lesions in subcortical areas. Thus, there is some suggestion that changes in cortical hypometabolism accompanying subcortical lesions might be a factor associated with the presence or absence of aphasia rather than the lesion in the subcortical region.

Concepts of Neuroanatomical Dominance and Localization in Language

Dominance

As previously noted, Broca's discovery of the connection between aphasia and damage to the left hemisphere was the precursor of all contemporary investigations of the structural and functional organization of the brain. Broca pointed out the significance of the left inferior frontal area, and Wernicke predicted the importance of the left temporoparietal region. In the past

two decades, functional mapping studies of language disorders have clearly established dominance of the left hemisphere for language functions through the use of radiological techniques. Studies of the relationship between handedness and dominance for language have suggested that in about 98 to 99% of right-handed individuals the left side is dominant for language. About 1 to 2% of right-handed individuals show right side dominance (Gling *et al.*, 1969). This reversed pattern of dominance (i.e., right side dominance) is therefore considered to be exceptional and has been reported in a few studies (Fischer *et al.*, 1991).

Localization

Although the issue of neuroanatomical dominance for language abilities in right-handed adults has been more or less settled for many years, the debate over localization has evolved into new directions. One classical approach to localization has been syndromic, with attempts made to find structural substrates for each of the subtypes of aphasia. This method involves lesion-syndrome correlations (Cappa and Vignolo, 1983).

An approach to localization that has yielded an extensive literature on neuroanatomical correlates of language focuses on specific linguistic functions and processes. This approach uses data from lesion-deficit correlational studies and functional neuroimaging techniques have further made it possible to identify brain regions that are activated during the performance of language tasks even in normal individuals. In the past few years, investigations into the neural correlates of specific functions, such as naming, comprehension and reading, have led to the well-established conclusion that these functions are not unitary. Rather, they are complex language processes that involve various components of language, including phonology, lexicon, syntax and semantics. Thus, the new direction in localization research involves attempts to find the loci for specific language operations within the various component processes and, in turn, to map these components onto brain regions.

Evidence from various sources has clearly established that linguistic functions are multifaceted in terms of both neural mechanisms and components of processing. As a result, impairment of a function does not involve global loss; instead, there are selective patterns of dissociation even between aspects of a specific linguistic function. This finding has given rise to the view that the various aspects of a function have corresponding neural mechanisms that are localized in different regions of the brain. The different regions are interconnected in ways that are thought of as forming neural networks. A breakdown in their connections results in selective patterns of dissociation. Because these networks can involve distant regions of the brain, the earlier ideas of localization of a function in terms of dichotomous subdivisions such as anterior versus posterior and sensory versus motor regions are now considered untenable. In addition, the patterns of dissociation suggest differential breakdown of the interconnections between levels of processing. Some of the patterns of dissociation observed in functions such as word finding and comprehension are presented to elucidate the involvement of different regions.

Model of Language

In the past two decades, neurolinguistic research has been greatly influenced by the application of cognitive theories and computational models to the study of language processes. Combined with functional neuroimaging techniques, these methodologies have enabled the analyses of much smaller units of language processing. The evidence has led to the development of the current information-processing or PDP model for language that has supplemented the traditional Wernicke–Geschwind model as well as earlier cognitive models of language.

The traditional Wernicke–Geschwind model was more anatomically based and reflected a view of language functioning in terms of interconnections and disconnections between hierarchically arranged regions of the brain. According to this view, language was processed through a serial flow of information in the interconnecting pathways and cortical regions. For example, in a simple repetition task, the information flows through the following pathways: auditory input received by the auditory apparatus passes through the medial geniculate nucleus, primary auditory cortex (Brodmann's area 41), and higher order auditory cortex (area 42) to the angular gyrus (area 39) and Wernicke's area (area 22). Thereupon, the arcuate fasciculus transfers the information to Broca's area, where syntactic processing and articulatory programming for production take place.

The application of cognitive theories to neuropsychological processes led to the development of information-processing models for language (as for other mental activities). However, the earlier models also tended to posit that information traversed across regions and across levels of processing (phonological, syntactic, semantic) in a serial fashion.

Within the framework of the current PDP model, linguistic operations are considered to be performed in more complex ways. One feature that characterizes this model is that any given task is thought to involve many operations that are localized within the various components of language (e.g., orthographical, semantic, phonetic, syntactic). These components, in turn, are subserved by different regions in the brain; that is, they are distributed (Paulesu *et al.*, 1993). Investigations in this area therefore entail two stages: first, an attempt is made to locate the operations within the components or levels of processing; secondly, attempts are made to map these components onto specific brain areas. A second feature of this model is that it posits a view that the various linguistic operations that constitute performance are carried out interactively through various routes in a parallel, concurrent and simultaneous fashion. At least, in normal or near-normal performance this is the case. In defective language processing, the flow of information through the expected routes is disturbed. As suggested earlier, the concept of parallel processing emerged from a realization that the notion of a serial transfer of information did not account for the rapidity with which mental processes are carried out.

Given the complexity of linguistic phenomena and the technical and methodological limitations involved in applying a heuristic computational model to the empirical analyses of language processes, this field of inquiry is still in its infancy.

Neurodevelopmental Aspects of Language

Any description of the relationship between the brain and language would be incomplete without considering some neurodevelopmental aspects of language. As a comprehensive discussion of this subject is beyond the scope of this section, the focus here is on presenting central theoretical issues. Some of these issues help shed light on the ways in which the brain is organized for language in children. For discussions of language disorders in children, the reader is referred to Yule and Rutter (1987).

Language Acquisition

One central issue addresses the notion of the innateness of language. Interest in this concept was stimulated by the pioneering work of Chomsky (1988), who espoused the view of an innate human capacity to know the universal rules of grammar. Chomsky drew attention to the fact that despite differences in the languages of the world, all human languages have the same universal features. Consequently, learning a language is something that "happens" to a child (Goldberg, 1989).

The fact that there are universal regularities in the acquisition of language supports the notion of an innate capacity. Thus, according to Lenneberg (1967, 1969), an infant's language capabilities are linked with physical maturation and there is therefore a correlation between language development and motor development. Thus, by about 15 months of age, when the motor milestone of self-propulsive gait is attained, an infant has a vocabulary of three to 50 words; by 18 to 24 months, when a child begins to run (with falls), many two-word utterances are observed (Lenneberg, 1969; Brown, 1973). By about 3 to 4 years of age, a child acquires the capability for many fully grammatical utterances (Stromswold, 1995).

In the literature dealing with the issue of language acquisition, much consideration has been given to the relative influences of genetic and environmental factors. Individual differences in performance raise questions about the relative contributions of these factors in language acquisition. On the one hand, it has been thought that if language is indeed an innate capacity with associated neural mechanisms, then language functions and malfunctions must also have a genetic basis.

Evidence for a genetic basis has come from many sources, especially from research in the area of developmental language disorders. Based on a review of relevant studies, Stromswold (1995) reported the finding of a higher incidence of language impairment in families of children with developmental disorders than in families of children without such impairment.

With respect to the view of language as an innate capacity, it is generally believed that language can be acquired without explicit instruction. For example, Stromswold (1995) reported that even children who are unable to speak and therefore cannot be corrected are capable of acquiring normal receptive language. In addition to the evidence that supports genetic contributions to language functions and dysfunctions, there is indirect support for the role of environmental exposure from studies of individuals raised in severely deprived environments. Studies of "wild" children raised in conditions of extreme linguistic, social and emotional deprivation essentially suggested an innate hypothesis for language acquisition but also suggested that the environment can have some modifying influences.

Brain Organization and Language Development

It is thought that if language is indeed an innate capacity, there must be a neural basis for this capacity that is present from birth. In this regard, there has been some debate about the concepts of equipotentiality and differential lateralization at birth.

Equipotentiality of the brain for language means that both sides are capable of performing linguistic functions. Equipotentiality also suggests plasticity of the brain and a capacity for reorganization even after injury so that language functions can be transferred from one hemisphere to the other. Indeed, lesion data for childhood aphasia and earlier reports of hemispherectomy studies have suggested functional recovery with respect to language until puberty, as evidenced by ipsilateral and contralateral transfer of linguistic functions. Thus, it has been reported that if there is damage to the left side in infancy but the right side remains intact, the child can still develop normal language (Curtiss, 1989; Dennis and Whitaker, 1976).

In early childhood, after the onset of language but before age 4 years, damage to the language areas results in transient aphasia. After puberty, by about age 14 years, the prognosis begins to worsen, and similar lesions in adulthood can cause irreversible deficits (Lenneberg, 1967, 1969). Some authors, such as Lenneberg (1967), have taken these findings about the capacity for transfer of function in young children to mean that the brain is symmetrically organized to begin with and only gradually becomes asymmetrically specialized, resulting in a diminished capacity for recovery with age. However, there is now increasing evidence that the brain is asymmetrical with respect to linguistic ability from birth.

If the brain is lateralized for linguistic functions from birth, a question arises about the evidence for greater recoverability of language when damage occurs early enough in life. One interpretation of this recoverability is that there is greater neuroplasticity in the young brain, as evident from the capacity of surviving neurons to make new synaptic connections even after injury.

Lenneberg's view of the critical period for language development (from birth to the early teens) was that both hemispheres are involved in language functions at first, but by puberty the left becomes more specialized. A later view relates the concept of critical period to the notion of neural plasticity. In any case, it is thought that the critical period is correlated with innate mechanisms, and that language development is most susceptible to the limiting effects of both biological and environmental factors if these extend beyond this critical period.

Conclusion

The focus of this chapter has been the cognitive neuroscience of memory, language and executive functions. As stated earlier, the term cognitive neuroscience does not refer to a single discipline; it connotes the integration of work from several fields examining brain–behavior relationships as they subserve specific mental processes. The exciting research that has emanated from *in vivo* functional imaging, especially with respect to memory, holds promise for further understanding of the manner in which the brain is specialized to process and store information.

Within the realm of theory, we have also stressed the growing consensus that neural processing and the emergence of cognition occur in a parallel and distributed fashion. Although this idea may be heuristically tenable, the specific mechanisms allowing simultaneity in information processing are difficult to model, from both cognitive and neuroanatomical perspectives. Work in computational neuroscience, aided by functional imaging and electrophysiological techniques, should permit the development of increasingly realistic and integrated models of cognition and brain. Rather than localizing whole functions to discrete areas of damage (as was the earlier tradition), the current emphasis continues to be on the contribution of a discrete area to a particular functional network. This approach characterizes present research on language, in which the role of regional specificity is understood within the context of a distributed functional and neuroanatomical system. The frontal lobes and executive control of behavior have proved to be an area that is rich in theory, but delineating the specific role of the frontal lobes in behavior and underlying neuronatomical mechanisms has proved somewhat elusive. Advances in characterizing frontal circuitry and the specialized role of the prefrontal cortex in such functions as representational memory have elucidated the complex contribution of this region to the regulation of behavior.

References

Andreasen NC, Rezai K, Alliger R *et al.* (1992) Hypofrontality in neuroleptic naive patients and in patients with chronic schizophrenia. *Arch Gen Psychiatr* 49, 943–958.

Baddeley A (1995) Working memory, in *The Cognitive Neurosciences* (eds Gazzaniga MS, Bizzi E, Black IB *et al.*). The MIT Press, Cambridge, MA, p. 760.

Baddeley AD and Hitch G (1974) Working memory, in *The Psychology of Learning and Motivation*, Vol. 8, (ed Bower GA). Academic Press, New York, pp. 47–89.

Baxter LR, Schwartz JM, Phelps ME *et al.* (1989) Reduction of prefrontal cortex glucose metabolism common to three types of depression. *Arch Gen Psychiatr* 46, 243–250.

Benson DF and Geschwind N (1985) Aphasia and related disorders: A clinical approach. In Principles of Behavioral Neurology, 3rd ed., Mesulam MM (ed). FA Davis, Philadelphia, pp. 193–238.

Berman KF, Illowsky BP and Weinberger DR (1988) Physiological dysfunction of dorsolateral prefrontal cortex in schizophrenia. IV. Further evidence for regional and behavioral specificity. *Arch Gen Psychiatr* 45, 616–622.

Bliss TVP and Lomo T (1973) Long-lasting potentiation of synaptic transmission in the dentate area of the anaesthetized rabbit following stimulation of the perforant path. *J Physiol (Lond)* 232, 331–356.

Brown R (1973) *A First Language: The Early Stages*. Harvard University Press, Cambridge, MA.

Buchsbaum MS, Cappelletti J, Ball R *et al.* (1984) Positron emission tomographic image measurement in schizophrenia and affective disorders. *Ann Neurol* 15(Suppl), 157–165.

Buchsbaum MS, Nuechterlein KH, Haier RJ *et al.* (1990) Glucose metabolic rate in normals and schizophrenics during the Continuous Performance Test assessed by positron emission tomography. *Br J Psychiatr* 156, 216–227.

Bunowski J and Bellugi U (1970) Language, name, and concept. *Science* 168, 669–673.

Burt AM (1993) *Textbook of Neuroanatomy*. WB Saunders, Philadelphia, p. 469.

Cappa SF and Vignolo LA (1983) CT scan studies of aphasia. *Hum Neurobiol* 2, 129–134.

Chomsky N (1988) *Language and Problems of Knowledge*. The MIT Press, Cambridge, MA.

Churchland PS and Sejnowski TJ (1992) The Computational Brain. The MIT Press, Cambridge, MA.

Christianson SA (ed) (1992) *The Handbook of Emotion and Memory: Research and Theory*. Lawrence Erlbaum, Hillsdale, NJ.

Cohen NJ and Squire LR (1980) Preserved learning and retention of pattern-analyzing skill in amnesia: Dissociation of knowing how and knowing that. *Science* 210(4466), 207–210.

Curtiss S (1989) The independence and task-specificity of language. In Interaction in Human Development, Bornstein A and Bruner J (eds). Lawrence Erlbaum, Hillsdale, NJ, pp. 105–137.

Damasio AR and Damasio H (1992) Brain and language. *Sci Am* 267(3), 89–95.

Dennis M and Whitaker HA (1976) Language acquisition following hemi-decortication: Linguistic superiority of the left over the right hemisphere. *Brain Lang* 3, 404–433.

Dubois B, Verin M, Teixeira-Ferreira C *et al.* (1994) How to study frontal lobe functions in humans, in *Motor and Cognitive Functions of the Prefrontal Cortex* (eds Thierry AM, Glowinski J, Goldman-Rakic PS *et al.*). Springer-Verlag, New York, pp. 1–16.

Eslinger PJ and Grattan LM (1993) Frontal lobe and frontal-striatal substrates for different forms of human cognitive flexibility. *Neuropsychologia* 31, 17–28.

Fibiger HC and Vincent SR (1987) Anatomy of central cholinergic neurons, in *Psychopharmacology: The Third Generation of Progress* (ed Meltzer HY). Raven Press, New York, p. 213.

Fischer RS, Alexander MP, Gabriel C *et al.* (1991) Reversed lateralization of cognitive functions in right handers: Exceptions to classical aphasiology. *Brain* 744, 245–261.

Fuster JM (1989) The Prefrontal Cortex: Anatomy, Physiology, and Neuropsychology of the Frontal Lobe. Raven Press, New York.

Gling I, Gloning K, Haub G et al. (1969) Comparison of verbal behavior in right-handed and non-right-handed patients with anatomically verified lesion of one hemisphere. Cortex 5, 43–52.

Gold PE, Delanoy RL and Merrin J (1984) Modulation of long-term potentiation by peripherally administered amphetamine and epinephrine. Brain Res 305, 103–107.

Goldberg E (1989) Gradiential approach to neocortical functional organization. J Clin Exp Neuropsychol 11, 489–517.

Goldman-Rakic PS (1987) Circuitry of the prefrontal cortex and the regulation of behavior by representational knowledge. In Handbook of Physiology, Section 1, The Nervous System, Vol. 5, Higher Functions of the Brain, Plum F (ed). American Physiological Society, Bethesda, MD, pp. 373–417.

Goldman-Rakic PS (1988) Changing concepts of cortical connectivity: Parallel distributed cortical networks. In Neurobiology of Neocortex, Rakic P and Singer W (eds). John Wiley, New York, pp. 177–202.

Guidano VF and Liotti G (1983) Cognitive Processes and Emotional Disorders. Guilford Press, New York.

Gur RE, Gur RC, Skolnick BE et al. (1985) Brain function in psychiatric disorders. III. Regional cerebral blood flow in unmedicated schizophrenics. Arch Gen Psychiatr 42, 329–334.

Heilman KM and Valenstein E (1993) Clinical Neuropsychology, 3rd edn. Oxford University Press, New York.

Heindel WC, Salmon DP and Butters N (1991) The biasing of weight judgements in Alzheimer's and Huntington's disease: A priming or programming phenomenon? J Clin Exp Neuropsychol 13, 189–203.

Kandel ER (1991) Cellular mechanisms of learning and the biological basis of individuality, in Principles of Neural Science, 3rd edn., (eds Kandel E, Schwartz JH, and Jessell TM). Appleton & Lange, Norwalk, CT, pp. 1009–1031.

Kandel ER, Abrams T, Bernier L et al. (1983) Classical conditioning and sensitization share aspects of the same molecular cascade in Aplysia. Quant Biol 48, 821–830.

Kolb B and Wishaw IQ (1990) Fundamentals of Human Neuropsychology, 3rd edn. WH Freeman, New York.

Lashley KS (1950) In search of the engram. Symp Soc Exp Biol 4, 454–482.

Lenneberg EH (1967) Biological Foundations of Language. John Wiley, New York.

Lenneberg EH (1969) On explaining language. Science 164, 635–643.

Liang KC, Juler R and McGaugh JL (1986) Modulating effects of post-training epinephrine on memory: Involvement of the amygdala noradrenergic system. Brain Res 368, 125–133.

Linden DJ (1994) Long-term synaptic depression in the mammalian brain. Neuron 12, 457–472.

Linden DJ and Connor JA (1995) Long-term synaptic depression. Annu Rev Neurosci 18, 319–357.

Lezak MD (1995) Neuropsychological Assessment, 3rd ed. Oxford University Press, New York.

Luria AR (1973a) The Working Brain. Basic Books, New York.

Luria AR (1973b) The Working Brain: An Introduction to Neuropsychology. Penguin Books, London, p. 85.

Markowitsch HJ and Pritzel M (1985) The neuropathology of amnesia. Prog Neurobiol 25, 189–287.

Mesulam MM (1990) Large scale neurocognitive networks and distributed processing for attention, language, and memory. Ann Neurol 28, 587–613.

Metter EJ, Kempler D, Jackson C, et al. (1987) Cerebellar glucose metabolism in chronic aphasia. Neurology 37, 1599–1606.

Miller GA, Gallanter EH and Pribram KH (1960) Plans and the Structure of Behavior. Holt, Reinhart & Winston, New York.

Miyake A and Shah P (1999) Models of Working Memory: Mechanisms of Active Maintenance and Executive Control. Cambridge University Press, New York.

Moscovitch M (1992) A neuropsychological model of memory and consciousness, in Neuropsychology of Memory, 2nd edn., (eds Squire LR and Butters N). Guilford Press, New York, pp. 5–22.

Naeser MA, Alexander MP, Helm-Estabrooks N et al. (1982) Aphasia with predominantly subcortical lesion sites: Description of three capsular/putaminal aphasia syndromes. Arch Neurol 39, 2–14.

Norman DA and Shallice T (1986) Attention to action: Willed and automatic control of behavior, in Consciousness and Self-regulation: Advances in Research and Theory (eds Davidson RJ, Schwartz GE, and Shapiro D). Plenum Press, New York, pp. 1–18.

Pandya DN and Yeterian EH (1984) Architecture and connections of cortical association areas, in Cerebral Cortex, Vol. 4 (eds Peters A and Jones EG). Plenum Press, New York, pp. 3–61.

Paulesu E, Frith CD, and Frackowiak RSJ (1993) The neural correlates of the verbal component of working memory. Nature 362, 342–345.

Ramon y Cajal S (1911) Histologie du Système Nerveux de l' Homme et des Vertbrs. Maloine, Paris.

Robinson RG and Szetela B (1981) Mood change following left hemispheric injury. Ann Neurol 9, 447–453.

Sagawa K, Kawakatsu S, Shibuya I et al. (1990) Correlation of regional cerebral blood flow with performance on neuropsychological tests in schizophrenic patients. Schizophr Res 3, 241–246.

Schacter DL, Chiu P, and Ochsner KN (1993) Implicit memory: A selective review. Annu Rev Neurosci 16, 159–182.

Shepherd GM (1994) Neurobiology, 3rd edn. Oxford University Press, New York.

Squire LR and Butters N (eds) (1992) Neuropsychology of Memory. Guilford Press, New York.

Squire LR and Zola-Morgan S (1991) The medial temporal lobe memory system. Science 253, 1380–1386.

Starkstein SE, Robinson RG, and Price TR (1987) Comparison of cortical and subcortical lesions in the production of post-stroke mood disorders. Brain 110, 1045–1059.

Stromswold K (1995) The cognitive and neural bases of language acquisition. In Cognitive Neuroscience, Gazzaniga M (ed). The MIT Press, Cambridge, MA, pp. 855–870.

Teuber HL (1964) The riddle of frontal lobe function in man. In The Frontal Granular Cortex and Behavior, Warren JM and Akert K (eds). McGraw-Hill, New York, pp. 410–444.

Traub RD and Miles R (1991) Neuronal Networks of the Hippocampus. Cambridge University Press, Cambridge, UK.

Tsumoto T (1993) Long-term depression in cerebral cortex: A possible substrate of "forgetting" that should not be forgotten. Neurosci Res 16, 263–270.

Tulving E, Schacter DL, and Stark H (1982) Priming effects in word-fragment completion are independent of recognition memory. J Exp Psychol Learn Mem Cogn 8, 336–342.

Volkow ND, Wolf AP, VanGelder P et al. (1987) Phenomenological correlates of metabolic activity in 18 patients with chronic schizophrenia. Am J Psychiatr 144, 151–158.

Walsh KW (1994) Neuropsychology: A Clinical Approach. Churchill Livingstone, New York.

Weinberger DR, Berman KF, and Illowsky BP (1988) Physiological dysfunction of the dorsolateral prefrontal cortex in schizophrenia. Arch Gen Psychiatr 454, 609–615.

Yule W and Rutter M (1987) Language Development and Disorders. MacKeith Press, Oxford, UK.

Zola-Morgan S, Squire LR, and Amaral DG (1986) Human amnesia and the medial temporal region: Enduring memory impairment following a bilateral lesion limited to field CA$_1$ of the hippocampus. J Neurosci 6, 2950–2967.

Zola-Morgan S and Squire LR (1993) Neuroanatomy of memory. Annu Rev Neurosci 16, 547–563.

16 Cognitive Psychology: Basic Theory and Clinical Implications

A number of factors, including the development of complex learning theories, discussions regarding language development, use of computers as a metaphor for human information processing and practical applications needed during World War II, all contributed to the cognitive revolution in psychological research during the 1950s and 1960s. Cognitive psychology is now one of the major areas of psychological inquiry alongside experimental, developmental, social and personality, and clinical psychologies.

The major synthesis of cognitive psychology with clinical practice has been forged by cognitive–behavior therapists. There are, however, other major applications and implications of cognitive psychology regarding attention, memory and higher order cognitive processes such as problem solving, schema construction and modification, and automatic processing.

The purposeful allocation of one's finite mental resources is a process known as attention (Ashcraft, 1994). Attentional processes have profound implications regarding adaptive functioning, inasmuch as it falls to the attentional system to identify and select the most salient pieces of information in need of processing at each moment. Inefficient or erratic allocation of attention may engender maladaptive behavioral responses. Furthermore, it has been noted that a subset of cognitive processes appears to occur in the absence of attentional focus; such processes are often referred to as automatic (Posner and Snyder, 1975). Dysregulations of the attentional system appear to play a central role in several clinical disorders, such as Generalized Anxiety Disorder (GAD), Major Depressive Disorder (MDD), Attention-Deficit/Hyperactivity Disorder (ADHD) and Borderline Personality Disorder (BPD). Consequently, efficacious cognitive–behavioral interventions for these disorders have accorded considerable attention to the development of strategies designed to facilitate more efficient and adaptive functioning of the attentional system.

Human memory is the central, essential ingredient in an information-processing system. Human cognition supports operations more diverse by far than those of a computer, ranging from complex mathematical and spatial reasoning, to artistic and literary endeavors, to athletic prowess and interpersonal awareness. During the past century, empirical research has led to an increasingly refined understanding of the interlocking mechanisms of human memory. This understanding has now been applied to the domain of clinical assessment and psychopathology. Researchers have documented the role of memory deficits and biases in several mental disorders, including (but not limited to) depression and PTSD. The results of these investigations have suggested that memory, just as it plays an essential role

in adaptive human functioning, may also play a central role in maladaptive, pathological functioning. The cognitive perspectives on psychopathology place an emphasis on the role of schematic memory bias in its contribution to various forms of psychiatric disorder, and corresponding psychotherapy techniques have been developed to address bias in memory (Beck, 1976; Beck et al., 1979).

Problem solving is the complex mental process of using previously learned information to identify solutions to new problems. Although specific empirical links between basic research and clinical practice have been sparse, the conceptual connections have provided several clinical procedures that are identifiable within self-control, cognitive–behavioral and interpersonal psychotherapies.

Cognitive psychologists studying memory developed the concept of schema, which can be understood as templates used to make sense of and draw conclusions about new sensory affective, of cognitive information. The schema construct was formulated to explain how memory is organized and why it produces the inaccuracies and incompleteness often observed in human recall. The incorporation and abstraction of new experiences into relevant schemata serve to influence the interpretation of future experience and thereby the encoding and recollection of new memories. Schemata, therefore, affect all levels of human cognitive processing and may well be the most significant regarding a theoretical model contribution to date in cognitive psychology. The development and modification of schemata are central to Beck and others' models of cognitive–behavioral conceptualizations of psychopathology and therapeutic change.

Finally, material is frequently processed automatically while conscious processing occurs on a parallel cognitive track. This raises intriguing questions regarding the similarities and differences in various conceptualizations of the unconscious. Answers to questions raised about automatic processes may well be the most significant future contributions cognitive psychology and neuroscience integration can offer clinical practice.

Piaget's work in the mid-20th century helped delineate the subsequent areas of inquiry about human psychological functioning and adaptation, and to some extent it has influenced the mainstream of cognitive psychology; however, his greatest legacy is clearly his seminal contributions to the study of human development and developmental psychology, of which cognitive development is only a portion. The focus of Piaget's theory was also considered cognitive when set in apposition to Freud's focus on emotion in his theory of psychosexual development. This chapter focuses on major areas of cognitive psychology: attention, memory and several of the most important "higher order"

Essentials of Psychiatry Jerald Kay and Allan Tasman
© 2006 John Wiley & Sons, Ltd.

cognitive processes. Neisser (1967) provided a seminal summary of cognitive psychology reviewing in detail information-processing approaches, findings from related models, and empirical data regarding internal mental processes of human functioning.

Although the information-processing paradigm is still dominant in cognitive psychology, two new paradigms became influential during the last 10 to 15 years of the last century. The more established one is called **connectionism** (or parallel distributed processing, see Chapter 16) (McClelland *et al.*, 1986). This approach addresses an inherent limitation of the traditional computer metaphor of the mind – the fact that the brain's information processing operations differ dramatically from those of serial symbol-processing computers, inasmuch as the former occur within a distributed architecture of parallel interconnected elemental (neural) arrays. In other words, the connectionist approach attempts to gain insights into human information processing by attending closely to the manner in which the brain's own neurons process information. Accordingly, this approach uses neural network computational modeling techniques (simulations) as useful theoretical tools in the specification of the actual neural mechanisms and processes that underlie human cognition.

An even newer cognitive paradigm is the so-called ecological approach, although it is not yet as well established or as conceptually coherent as are the information-processing and connectionist paradigms. The ecological approach emphasizes that cognition does not occur in isolation from larger environmental (e.g., cultural) contexts, and argues that it is essential to study cognition in the natural context in which it occurs.

In the following sections, we review the general findings regarding attention, memory and higher order cognitive processes and give examples of their application to various areas of psychopathology and treatment interventions. Figure 16.1 provides an overall schematic of the interactions of the cognitive processes that are discussed.

Attention

The purposeful allocation of one's finite mental resources is a process known as **attention** (Ashcraft, 1994). Attentional processes have profound implications regarding adaptive functioning, inasmuch as it falls to the attentional system to identify and select the most salient pieces of information in need of processing at each moment. Inefficient or erratic allocation of attention may engender maladaptive behavioral responses. Furthermore,

it has been noted that a subset of cognitive processes appears to occur in the absence of attentional focus; such processes are often referred to as automatic (Posner and Snyder, 1975). Some automatic processes may also be etiologically involved in certain forms of psychopathology to the extent that automatic thoughts, which occur without the benefit of attentional inspection, turn out to be aberrant or distorted (Beck, 1976). Dysregulations of the attentional system appear to play a central role in several clinical disorders.

The following sections examine various ways in which the functioning, or malfunctioning, of attentional processes may be involved in four relatively common psychiatric disorders: anxiety disorders (AD), major depressive disorder (MDD), attention-deficit/hyperactivity disorder (ADHD) and borderline personality disorder (BPD).

Anxiety Disorders

An individual in an anxious state gives heightened attention to threat-related cues (MacLeod *et al.*, 1986; Matthews and MacLeod, 1985; Brosschot *et al.*, 1999; Bradley *et al.*, 2000; Fox *et al.*, 2001; Lundh and Oest, 2001; Bradley *et al.*, 1999; Mogg *et al.*, 2000), as such cues are usually particularly salient to the feelings of anxiety; this selectivity process may in turn filter out and discard information not congruent with the anxious mood state. Such a mood-congruent attentional bias helps orient the individual to the source of danger, which may in turn help ensure that the individual formulates an appropriate response to the threatening situation. To the extent that there is a reasonable goodness of fit between the level of anxious arousal and the level of genuine threat posed to the individual by the environment, the mood-congruence attentional bias serves an adaptive function. When the level of anxiety is consistently incommensurate with the environmental context, however, a state of pathological anxiety ensues.

Barlow's (1988) anxious apprehension model suggests that pathological anxiety, such as that observed in GAD, may arise from a chronic misapprehension or overestimation of the level of threat posed by a wide array of situations, many of them benign. It is further proposed that, once the anxious arousal of a patient with GAD is triggered by the misapprehension of threat, there is a narrowing of external attention to the perceived danger, concurrent with a ruminative internal self-focus on negative expectancies regarding the situation's

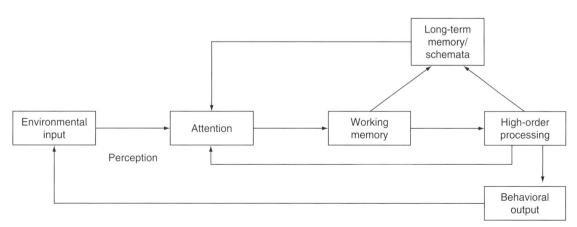

Figure 16.1 *Human cognition.*

outcome. Two deleterious consequences of such an attentional bias predictably ensue: 1) the patient disregards or discounts information that could serve to correct the original misapprehension of threat and 2) the patient's attentional resources are so thoroughly consumed by the focus on negative expectancies that few resources are available for constructive problem solving and adaptive responding.

A somewhat related cognitive model of pathological anxiety has been proposed by Beck and Emery (1985) in the schema theory of anxiety. Central to this theory is the mechanism of cognitive appraisal, with anxiety as the feeling state resulting from the appraisal of threatening stimuli. The appraisal process, in turn, is believed to be influenced by cognitive structures known as schemata, which consist of stored information abstracted from previous experience (Dombeck and Ingram, 1993; Dibartolo *et al.*, 1997). Schema-guided appraisal is held to take place automatically.

Schema theory views pathological anxiety as the result of faulty schemata that lead to habitual, and largely automatic, overappraisal of danger; pathological appraisal often takes place automatically without benefit of the scrutiny that accompanies attentional focus. Accordingly, Beck's therapeutic approach to ameliorating pathological anxiety involves helping the patient allocate more attentional resources to the appraisal process, as a corrective to faulty schematic processing. Applications from cognitive psychology to the treatment of anxiety disorders are presented in Table 16.1.

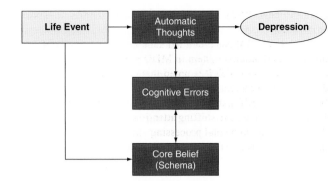

Figure 16.2 *Beck's model of depression.*

Major Depressive Disorder (MDD)

It has been consistently observed that individuals suffering from major depression are prone to a negativistic bias in cognitive processing. Within Beck's influential cognitive model of depression (Figure 16.2) (Beck, 1976; Beck *et al.*, 1979), these depressotypic negative thoughts are held to be centrally involved in the onset and maintenance of the depressive episode (Figure 16.2). In addition, Beck's model proposes that many depressive thoughts occur automatically, in the absence of attentional awareness. In a manner similar to that observed with anxiety disorders, it appears that the attention of depressed patients is selectively focused on environmental cues congruent with the depressed state (Engel

Table 16.1   Prominent Clinical Exemplars of Cognitive Psychology

DSM Syndrome	Relevant Cognitive Psychological Finding	Clinical Application*
Major depressive disorder	Mood-congruent bias in recall and encoding of memory	CBT: Patient is trained to examine noncongruent memories (positive or neutral) to compensate for schematic distortion.
	Occurrence of negativistic automatic thoughts regarding self, world and future	CBT: Patient is directed to challenge automatic thoughts and to generate rational alternatives and is subsequently taught to challenge underlying negative beliefs.
	Deficits in problem solving	IPT: Patient is instructed in the use of problem-solving techniques, primarily in the interpersonal domain.
Generalized anxiety disorder	Heightened attention to environmental threat cues	CBT: Patient is directed to use relaxation techniques as means of ameliorating the anxiety state, thereby attenuating attentional bias.
	Overestimation of environmental threat	CBT: Patient is trained to undertake rational evaluation of all relevant environmental stimuli.
	Schematic bias in retrieval of threat-related memories	CBT: Threat-related schemata are modified via integration of successful coping experiences.
DSM Syndrome	Relevant Cognitive Psychological Finding	Clinical Application*
Borderline personality disorder	Poor regulation of emotion secondary to lack of attentional control	DBT: Patient is trained in the use of numerous attentional control techniques (e.g., core mindfulness; see Linehan, 1989).
	Deficits in problem solving secondary to attentional dyscontrol	DBT: Patient is directed to shift attention from rumination over difficulties to discovery of more adaptive responses to problem. Also, patient receives direct training in social problem-solving skills.

*CBT, Cognitive–behavioral therapy; IPT, Interpersonal psychotherapy; DBT, Dialectical behavioral therapy.

and DeRubeis, 1993), such as cues related to themes of failure or rejection.

Rehm (1974) has identified another prominent dysregulation of the attentional system in MDD in the self-control model of depression, in which it is noted that depressed patients often devote excessive attentional focus to ruminative appraisal of self. By extension, self-management therapy for depression (Rehm, 1984) assists patients in shifting attentional focus away from self, thereby freeing up mental processing resources for the formulation of more effective behavioral responses.

Attention-deficit/Hyperactivity Disorder

In general, it appears that the attentional system of children with ADHD frequently functions inefficiently, so that relevant stimuli often go unidentified, irrelevant stimuli (distractors) are accorded disproportionate attention, and even on occasions when attention is paid to appropriate environmental information, such attention is often broken off prematurely; that is, the children frequently respond to environmental stimuli before consideration of all relevant data (Douglas, 1980).

These attentional difficulties seem to be strongly related to problems with behavioral inhibition (Barkley, 1999), a finding that still obtains even when global intelligence, reading achievement and comorbid psychopathology are taken into account (Chhabildas *et al.*, 2001; Nigg *et al.*, 1998; Nigg 1999; Seidman *et al.*, 1997). Within this perspective, treatments need to include components which address the fundamental problems regarding behavioral inhibition.

Various stimulant medications, most notably methylphenidate, have been shown to be efficacious in the acute treatment of ADHD. As noted by Kendall and MacDonald (1993), there are limitations to stimulant therapy that highlight the need for also developing effective psychosocial interventions for ADHD: 1) some children with ADHD do not respond to stimulant medication; 2) medication appears to be limited in its effect on some higher order cognitive processes, such as problem solving; 3) medication may not ameliorate longstanding deficits in social skills; 4) some children experience difficulties complying with medication regimens; and 5) gains made during medication therapy are often not maintained after termination of treatment. Cognitive–behavioral treatment interventions for ADHD, therefore, would appear to constitute a potentially valuable supplement and/or alternative to medication.

Borderline Personality Disorder

Inability to regulate emotional states has been identified as one of the hallmarks of BPD (Grotstein, 1987; Linehan, 1993a; Herpertz *et al.*, 2001). The significance of this finding for the present discussion lies in the fact that there exists a strong reciprocal relationship between emotion regulation and attentional focus: an increase in emotional arousal narrows attention to a focus on emotion-relevant stimuli. Conversely, the ability to shift attention away from affect-inducing stimuli may be central to the process of emotion modulation. Therefore, it has been hypothesized that the characteristic difficulties with emotion regulation of the patient with BPD may be directly linked to a relative lack of attentional control (Linehan, 1993a; Coolidge *et al.*, 2000).

Linehan's (1989, 1993a) dialectical behavior therapy (DBT) has been shown in a series of clinical trials to be effective in ameliorating many of the more serious symptoms of BPD, including parasuicidal behavior and impulsive angry outbursts (Linehan *et al.*, 1991, 1993; Shearin and Linehan, 1994; Koons *et al.*, 2001). Significantly, the DBT protocol includes numerous interventions that seek to address the dysregulations in attention characteristic of patients with BPD.

A central goal of DBT is the cultivation of core mindfulness, a frame of mind described by Linehan as "[being] in control of attentional processes – that is, what one pays attention to and how long one pays attention to it" (Linehan, 1993b, p. 65). The patient with BPD is taught to recognize the connection between attentional fixation on distressing stimuli and a commensurate escalation in affective arousal, especially problematical negative affective states such as rage and depression. Thus, in DBT there is explicit recognition that enhanced attentional control is a primary treatment goal.

Memory

The second major area of study in cognitive psychology involves the investigation of memory. In the most generic sense, memory refers to the components of an information-processing system that support the encoding, storage and retrieval of information over time. Memory is the central, essential ingredient in the human information-processing system. Human cognition supports operations more diverse by far than those of a computer, ranging from complex mathematical and spatial reasoning, to artistic and literary endeavors, to athletic prowess and interpersonal awareness. Memory is the substrate of these many skills and the foundation for human consciousness. To the extent that we are each more than the sum of our biological components, it is in large part the texture of our own unique memories that makes us so.

Over the course of the past century, the empirical efforts have led to an increasingly refined understanding of the interlocking mechanisms that constitute human memory. This understanding has begun to be applied to the domain of clinical assessment and psychopathology. Researchers have documented the role of memory deficits and biases in several mental disorders. The results of these investigations have suggested that memory, just as it plays an essential role in adaptive human functioning, may also play a central role in maladaptive, pathological functioning. The cognitive perspectives on psychopathology place an emphasis on the role of schematic memory bias in its contribution to various forms of psychiatric disorders, and corresponding psychotherapeutic techniques have been developed to address bias in memory (Beck, 1976; Beck *et al.*, 1979).

For the purposes of this discussion, it is necessary to point out that the study of memory has become a useful adjunct to the cognitive perspectives on psychopathology. The central theme of these perspectives is an emphasis on maladaptive thinking in the genesis and maintenance of psychiatric disorders. Once granted the premise that dysfunctional thoughts and/or cognitive biases may play a pivotal role in the dynamics of psychopathology (Beck, 1976, 1983; Beck *et al.*, 1979), it follows that memory may serve as a cognitive mediator in many forms of mental disorders; an extensive empirical literature has developed through efforts to test this premise.

The following sections of this chapter present a brief discussion of memory-related research for two particular psychiatric disorders, MDD and post traumatic stress disorder (PTSD). Because researchers have substantially documented the memory deficits associated with these disorders, a review of the findings may prove useful for clinical and diagnostic purposes.

Clinical Depression, Memory and Schemata Bias

Depression (clinical and subclinical) has been linked to impaired performance in a variety of memory experiments, and additional research has suggested that the effect may partly reflect deficits in the recognition or employment of informational structure in stimulus materials. It remains to be demonstrated conclusively whether similar impairments obtain for implicit memory processes (in which the subject is unaware of any conscious recollection). There is a different line of research, however, that bears more directly on depression and automatic (or unconscious) memory processes. According to the theory of depression of Beck and colleagues (Beck, 1976; 1983; Beck *et al.*, 1979), the depressed individual is prone to make negativistic inferences and generalizations and prone to consequent biases in recall and recognition memory (e.g., through selective abstraction, overgeneralization, magnification, minimization). These memory biases have been more broadly described as mood-congruent recall, referring to distortions in memory based on current mood state. Mood-congruent recall is an implicit, automatic memory process (to the extent that mood state may exert a systematic effect on the content of memory retrieval, without conscious awareness or intention on the part of the individual).

For clinical purposes, two generic findings from cognitive research on depression are important to remember. First, depression is associated with general impairment for explicit memory tasks (recognition and recall). Secondly, depression is also associated with a mood-congruent memory bias. Taken individually, either of these symptoms may interfere with adaptive coping, because accurate memory is necessary for adaptive and intelligent behavioral responses. In combination, the two memory difficulties can have a substantial impact on an individual's perceptions of the self, the world and the future (Beck's cognitive triad [Beck, 1976; Beck *et al.*, 1979]), serving both to impair behavior and to maintain depressive affect. In consequence, memory disturbance in depression can be an important focus for clinical intervention (Beck *et al.*, 1979), and it should ideally be considered in the formulation of a comprehensive treatment package.

Posttraumatic Stress Disorder, Repression and Memory Impairment

Survivors of PTSD suffer from a persistent and aversive tendency to reexperience the traumatic event, as manifested by symptoms of intrusion, dissociation and hyperarousal. These symptoms can include recurrently intrusive images or dreams, hallucinatory flashbacks, intense psychological distress (caused by symbolic reexposure), blunted affect, social withdrawal, hopelessness, amnesia, avoidant behavior, irritability, insomnia, hypervigilance and impaired concentration. When experienced in combination, these symptoms may often result in a highly debilitating syndrome that operates to the exclusion of adaptive coping behavior.

PSSD by definition involves a pathological response to memories that are so traumatic as to be at once unforgettable (hence the intrusive symptoms) and intolerable to remember (hence the dissociation). The resulting heterostasis is posited to lead to emotional and physical dysregulation and presents a challenge to fundamental beliefs regarding security, efficacy and prospect for future well-being (Herman, 1992).

It is currently unclear whether PTSD memory deficits derive from some (unidentified) neuropsychological sequelae of extreme stress exposure or are simply concomitant to prolonged symptoms of hypervigilance, emotional distress, or comorbid depression. It is clear that PTSD is associated with significant proactive interference in memory, such that survivors are impaired in their ability to encode and to retrieve new information.

The second type of memory deficit in PTSD involves symptoms of amnesia for, and intrusion of, memories for the initial traumatic event. These symptoms represent a functional deficit in memory, such that the survivor is alternately confronted with emotionally disturbing recollections and unable to access the traumatic memory.

In addition to deficits in memory, individuals with PTSD complain about the intrusion of memories for the traumatic event. In a pattern similar to that observed in MDD, individuals with PTSD appear to demonstrate both overgeneral autobiographical recall and a negativistic memory bias.

Questions about the accuracy (or inaccuracy) of repressed memory are difficult to address. Although the prevalence of amnesic and dissociative symptoms in PTSD has been validated by studies of trauma survivors (Herbst, 1992; Zimering *et al.*, 1993), these studies do not address the validity of more controversial cases that reportedly involve complete (and asymptomatic) repression over long periods. Empirical efforts to document long-term traumatic repression continue to meet with significant methodological and conceptual criticisms (Williams, 1994; Loftus *et al.*, 1994).

The practicing psychiatrist must recognize the possibility of suggestibility and bias in retrieval of traumatic memories (Loftus, 1993; Berliner and Loftus, 1992; Gutheil, 1993), while maintaining a stance of openness and compassion in helping trauma survivors to clarify and to reintegrate their memories of traumatic events (Alloy *et al.*, 1990). In sum, PTSD is a disorder of unbearable and inescapable recollection, and both research and therapy will continue to focus on the elucidation of memory for trauma.

Higher Order Cognitive Processing

Problem Solving

Newell and Simon (1972) exemplified the modern approach to the study of problem solving. Their methodology involved the extensive analysis of verbal protocols, that is, subjects' verbalizations as they attempted to solve (often lengthy) mental problems. Their in-depth analyses of human mental processes ultimately led Newell and Simon to their most important conceptual contribution – the idea that human thought could be conceived of as internal symbol manipulation, or the processing of information. Their analogy to algorithmic information processing in computers proved useful; data input was similar to perception, data representation was similar to memory and data manipulation was similar to problem solving.

Goldfried and Davison (1994, p. 186) concluded that "much of what we view clinically as 'abnormal behavior'...may be more usefully construed as ineffective behavior with its negative consequences, such as anxiety, depression, and the creation of secondary problems". Deficits in problem solving have been documented as nonspecific deficits associated with many psychiatric disorders (e.g., schizophrenia). Problem-solving techniques are considered standard cognitive–behavioral interventions with applications to such diverse problems as depression, suicidal behavior, anxiety, marital problems and adolescent social problems (D'Zurilla, 1986; Nezu *et al.*, 1989; Nezu and D'Zurilla, 1980; Robin, 1981). Applications with children have focused on reducing aggressive behavior (Camp and Bash, 1985), reducing impulsive behavior (Kendall and Braswell, 1985), and teaching social competence in prevention programs (Kirschenbaum and Ordman, 1984).

In the current practice of problem-solving therapies, there is general agreement on the five steps central to most problem-solving applications. These steps may be traced to observations derived from empirical work on problem solving in cognitive psychology, although actual explicit empirical links have never been established. These five steps, first enumerated by D'Zurilla and Goldfried (1971), are: 1) developing a general orientation or set to recognize problems, 2) defining the specifics of the problem and what needs to be accomplished, 3) generating alternative courses of action, 4) deciding among the alternatives by evaluating their consequences, and 5) verifying the results of the decision process and determining whether the alternative selected is achieving the desired outcome. If the outcome is not satisfactory, the process is repeated. These basic steps of clinical problem solving, at times combined with components of Spivak and Shure's (1974) program (e.g., taking the perspective of other persons), have formed the core of the empirically validated problem-solving therapies that are usually identified as a type of cognitive–behavioral therapy.

Schema Theory and Reasoning

Beck and colleagues (1979) suggested that new information about particular experiences or situations is processed through the medium of an established, organized, cognitive structure based on abstractions from relevant prior experience. This organized, cognitive structure is called a **schema**, and it has become one of the primary elements in the cognitive perspective on depression (as well as the cognitive perspective on other forms of psychiatric disorders). Cognitive schemata are believed to exert their influence at many different levels of information processing. Schemata are hypothesized to direct the selectivity of attention, as well as the interpretation of ambiguous information, and the integration of new experiences into an existing cognitive matrix. For this reason, schema theory can be used as an overarching, explanatory framework for much of the clinical psychopathology research on attentional mechanisms, memory biases and reasoning processes.

The application of schema theory to the study of psychiatric disorders represents one of the important elements in the cognitive perspective on psychopathology. Although Beck is most widely known for his theories about depression, he has also written about the cognitive bases for other emotional disorders including anxiety and anger (Beck, 1976), as well as the cognitive bases for personality disorders (Beck and Freeman, 1990). In all of these theories, the central credo involves the influence of schematic bias in the interpretation of new information and the encoding of new memory. Thus (for example) in depression, the overgeneralized operation of negativistic schemata is hypothesized to lead to faulty and depressogenic inferences about events and experiences in an individual's life (Beck *et al.*, 1979). Another example of the role of schemata in psychopathology is observed among personality disorders, wherein an individual is hypothesized to suffer from a self-perpetuating and treatment-resistant "early maladaptive schema", which essentially involves a dysfunctional set of assumptions and interpretations regarding oneself in relation to other people and/or the environment (Young, 1990). Cognitive theory can be extended, by analogy, to many of the other forms of psychiatric disorders.

Automatic Versus Conscious Processing

As noted previously, mental processes exist that appear to occur in the absence of attentional focus and thus outside conscious awareness; these processes are frequently described as being automatic (Logan and Klapp, 1991; Posner and Snyder, 1975; Shiffrin and Schneider, 1977). It was further noted that complex mental processes, such as driving to work, initially require considerable attentional focus but may eventually become automatic as a result of overlearning (Craighead *et al.*, 1994). Automatic cognitive processes often facilitate adaptive functioning, inasmuch as they permit the individual to engage in numerous cognitive operations concurrently (i.e., parallel processing). However, it has also been suggested that some automatic thoughts, such as appraisals, may turn out to be aberrant or distorted (Beck and Emery, 1985), and because such thoughts are not subjected to the scrutiny that accompanies conscious attentional focus, aberrant automatic thoughts are unlikely, under most circumstances, to be corrected. We know that schema-based inferences fill in the gaps in memory of prior events so that humans reconstruct that which they cannot completely recall. Thus, what is recalled is integrated in memory with that which is reconstructed and the relevant schema is thereby modified, many times in a self-defeating or negativistic manner by patients. Although this is an efficient mechanism that facilitates functioning in our complex world, it can lead to schematic errors of which the individual may not have full awareness – she or he only is aware of the outcome and not the process. One of the fundamental goals of cognitive–behavioral therapy is the development of the understanding of both the content and functioning of such automatic processes.

This model of automatic cognitive processes has been implicated in the etiology and maintenance of numerous forms of psychopathology, most prominently GAD (Wolpe, 1958; Barlow, 1988) and MDD (Beck, 1976; Beck *et al.*, 1979). For example, the patient with GAD is hypothesized to engage in automatic overestimation of potential threat in a variety of environmental contexts, many of them benign (Beck and Emery, 1985). This automatic misappraisal is believed to be influenced, in large measure, by the operation of faulty schemata, cognitive structures that represent the preprocessed distillation of various threat-related experiences stored in long-term memory. Likewise, depressed patients have been observed to engage frequently in a variety of negativistic automatic thoughts, presumably influenced by the operation of schemata concerning themes of rejection and failure.

References

Alloy LB, Albright JS, Abramson LY *et al.* (1990) Depressive realism and nondepressive optimistic illusions: The role of self, in *Contemporary Psychological Approaches to Depression*, (ed Ingram RE). Plenum Press, New York.

Ashcraft MH (1994) *Human Memory and Cognition*, 2nd edn. Harper-Collins College Publishers, New York.

Barkley RA (1999) Theories of attention-deficit/hyperactivity disorder, in *Handbook of Disruptive Behavior Disorders* (eds Quay H and Hogan A). Kluwer Academic/Plenum Publishing, New York, pp. 295–316.

Barlow DH (1988) *Anxiety and Its Disorders: The Nature and Treatment of Anxiety and Panic*. Guilford Press, New York.

Beck AT (1976) *Cognitive Therapy and the Emotional Disorders*. International Universities Press, New York.

Beck AT (1983) Cognitive therapy of depression: New perspectives, in *Treatment of Depression: Old Controversies, New Approaches*. (eds Clayton PJ, Barren JE). Raven Press, New York, pp. 265–290.

Beck AT and Emery G (1985) *Anxiety Disorders and Phobias: A Cognitive Perspective*. Basic Books, New York.

Beck AT and Freeman AM (1990) *Cognitive Therapy of Personality Disorder*. Guilford Press, New York.

Beck AT, Rush Aj, Shaw BE *et al.* (1979) *Cognitive Therapy of Depression: A Treatment Manual*. Guilford Press, New York.

Berliner L and Loftus E (1992) Sexual abuse accusations: Desperately seeking reconciliation. *J Interpers Violence* 7, 570–578.

Bradley B, Mogg K, White J *et al.* (1999) Attentional bias for emotional faces in generalized anxiety disorder. *Br J Clin Psychol* 38, 267–278.

Bradley B, Mogg K and Millar N (2000) Covert and overt orienting of attention to emotional faces in anxiety. *Cogn Emotion* 14, 789–808.

Brosschot J, deRuiter C and Kindt M (1999) Processing bias in anxious subjects and repressors, measured by emotional Stroop interference and attentional allocation. *Pers Individ Differ* 26, 777–793.

Camp BW and Bash MAS (1985) *Think Aloud: Increasing Social and Cognitive Skills – A Problem Solving Program for Children*. Research Press, Champaign, IL.

Chhabildas NA, Pennington BF and Willcutt EG (2001) A comparison of the cognitive deficits in the DSM-IV subtypes of ADHD. *J Abnorm Child Psychol* 29, 529–540.

Coolidge FL, Segal DL, Stewart SE *et al.* (2000) Neuropsychological dysfunction in children with borderline personality disorder features: A preliminary investigation. *J Res Pers* 34, 554–561.

Craighead LW, Craighead WE, Kazdin AE *et al.* (1994) *Cognitive and Behavioral Interventions: An Empirical Approach to Mental Health Problems*. Allyn & Bacon, Needham, MA.

Dibartolo P, Brown TA and Barlow DH (1997) Effects of anxiety on attentional allocation and task performance: An information processing analysis. *Behav Res Ther* 35, 1101–1111.

Dombeck MI and Ingram RE (1993) Cognitive conceptions of anxiety, in *Psychopathology and Cognition*, (eds Dobson KS and Kendall PC). Academic Press, San Diego, CA, pp. 54–81.

Douglas VI (1980) Treatment and training approaches to hyperactivity: Establishing internal or external control, in *Hyperactive Children: The Social Ecology of Identification and Treatment* (eds Whalen C and Henker B). Academic Press, New York.

D'Zurilla T (1986) *Problem-Solving Therapy: A Social Competence Approach to Clinical Intervention*. Springer-Verlag, New York.

D'Zurilla TJ and Goldfried MR (1971) Problem solving and behavior modification. *J Abnorm Psychol* 78, 107–126.

Engel RA and DeRubeis RJ (1993) The role of cognition in depression, in *Psychopathology and Cognition* (eds Dobson KS and Kendall PC). Academic Press, San Diego, CA, pp. 83–119.

Fox E, Russo R, Bowles R *et al.* (2001) Do threatening stimuli draw or hold visual attention in subclinical anxiety? *J Exp Psychol* 130, 681–700.

Goldfried MR and Davison GC (1994) *Clinical Behavior Therapy*. John Wiley, New York.

Grotstein JS (1987) The borderline as a disorder of self-regulation, in *The Borderline Patient: Emerging Concepts in Diagnosis, Psychodynamics, and Treatment* (eds Grotstein JS, Solomon MF, and Lang JA). The Analytic Press, Hillsdale, NJ, pp. 347–384.

Gutheil TG (1993) True or false memories of sexual abuse? A forensic psychiatry view. *Psychiatr Ann* 23, 527–531.

Herbst PR (1992) From helpless victim to empowered survivor: Oral history as a treatment for shattered survivors of torture. *Women Ther* 13, 141–154.

Herman JL (1992) *Trauma and Recovery*. Basic Books, New York.

Herpertz SC, Dietrich TM, Wenning B *et al.* (2001) Evidence of abnormal amygdale functioning in borderline personality disorder: A functional MRI study. *Biol Psychiatr* 50, 292–298.

Kendall PC and Braswell L (1985) *Cognitive–Behavioral Therapy for Impulsive Children*, 2nd edn. Guilford Press, New York.

Kendall PC and MacDonald JP (1993) Cognition in the psychopathology of youth and implications for treatment, in *Psychopathology and Cognition*, (eds Dobson KS and Kendafl PC). Academic Press, San Diego, CA, pp. 387–427.

Kirschenbaum DS and Ordman AM (1984) Prevention interventions for children: Cognitive–behavioral perspectives, in *Cognitive–Behavior Therapy with Children* (eds Meyers AW and Craighead WE). Plenum Press, New York, pp. 377–409.

Koons CR, Robins CJ, Tweed JL *et al.* (2001) Efficacy of dialectical behavior therapy in women veterans with borderline personality disorder. *Behav Ther* 32, 371–390.

Linehan MM (1989) Cognitive and behavior therapy for borderline personality disorder, in *American Psychiatric Press Review of Psychiatry*, Vol. 8, (eds Tasman A, Hales RE, and Frances AJ). American Psychiatric Press, Washington, DC, pp. 84–102.

Linehan MM, Armstrong HE, Suarez A, et al. (1991) Cognitive–behavioral treatment of chronically parasuicidal borderline patients. *Arch Gen Psychiatr* 48, 1060–1064.

Linehan MM (1993a) *Cognitive–Behavioral Treatment of Borderline Personality Disorder*. Guilford Press, New York.

Linehan MM (1993b) *Skills Training Manual for Treating Borderline Personality Disorder*. Guilford Press, New York.

Linehan MM, Heard HL and Armstrong HE (1993) Naturalistic follow-up of a behavioral treatment for chronically parasuicidal borderline patients. *Arch Gen Psychiatr* 50, 971–974.

Loftus EF (1993) The reality of repressed memories. *Am Psychol* 48, 518–537.

Loftus EF, Garry M and Feldman J (1994) Forgetting sexual trauma: What does it mean when 38% forget? *J Consult Clin Psychol* 62, 1177–1181.

Logan GD and Klapp ST (1991) Automatizing alphabet arithmetic: 1. Is extended practice necessary to produce automaticity. *J Exp Psychol Learn Mem Cogn* 17, 179–195.

Lundh G and Oest G (2001) Attentional bias, self-consciousness and perfectionism in social phobia before and after cognitive–behaviour therapy. *Scand J Behav Ther* 30, 4–16.

MacLeod C, Matthews AM and Tata P (1986) Attentional bias in emotional disorders. *J Abnorm Psychol* 95, 15–20.

Matthews AM and MacLeod C (1985) Selective processing of threat cues in anxiety states. *Behav Res Ther* 23, 563–569.

McClelland JL, Rumulhart DE and Hinton GE (1986) The appeal of parallel distributed processing, in *Parallel Distributed Processing* (eds Rumulhart DE, McClelland JL, and PDP Research Group). Vol. 1. MIT Press, Cambridge, MA, pp. 3–44.

Mogg K, Bradley BP, Dixon C *et al.* (2000) Trait anxiety, defensiveness and selective processing of threat: An investigation using two measures of attentional bias. *Pers Individ Diff* 28, 1063–1077.

Neisser U (1967) *Cognitive Psychology*. Appleton-Century-Crofts, New York.

Newell A and Simon HA (1972) *Human Problem Solving*. Prentice-Hall, Englewood Cliffs, NJ.

Nezu A and D'Zurilla T (1980) Social problem-solving and negative affective conditions, in *Anxiety and Depression: Distinctive and Overlapping Features* (eds Kendall PC and Watson D). Academic Press, New York, pp. 285–315.

Nezu AM, Nezu CM and Perri MG (1989) *Problem Solving Therapy for Depression*. John Wiley, New York.

Nigg JT (1999) The ADHD response inhibition deficit as measured by the Stop Task: Replication with DSM-IV combined types, extension, and qualification. *J Abnorm Child Psychol* 27, 391–400.

Nigg JT, Hinshaw SP, Carte E *et al.* (1998) Neuropsychological correlates of childhood attention-deficit/hyperactivity disorder: Explainable by comorbid disruptive behavior or reading problems? *J Abnorm Psychol* 107, 468–480.

Posner MI and Snyder CRR (1975) Facilitation and inhibition in the processing of signals, in *Attention and Performance* V (eds Rabbitt PMA and Domic S). Academic Press, New York.

Rehm LP (1974) A self-control model of depression. *Behav Ther* 8, 787–804.

Rehm LP (1984) Self-management therapy for depression. *Adv Behav Res Ther* 6, 83–98.

Robin AL (1981) A controlled evaluation of problem-solving communication training with parent adolescent conflict. *Behav Ther* 12,
593–609.

Seidman LJ, Biederman J, Faraone SV *et al.* (1997) Toward defining a neuropsychology of attention-deficit hyperactivity disorder:
Performance of children and adolescents from a large clinically referred sample. *J Consult Clin Psychol* 65, 150–160.

Shearin EN and Linehan MM (1994) Dialectical behavior therapy for
borderline personality disorder: Theoretical and empirical foundations. *Acta Psychiatr Scand* 89(Suppl), 61–68.

Shiffrin RM and Schneider W (1977) Controlled and automatic human
information processing. II. Perceptual learning, automatic attending,
and a general theory. *Psychol Rev* 84, 127–190.

Spivak G and Shure MB (1974) *Social Adjustment of Young Children: A
Cognitive Approach to Solving Real-life Problems.* Jossey-Bass, San
Francisco.

Williams LM (1994) Recall of childhood trauma: A prospective study
of women's memories of childhood abuse. *J Consult Clin Psychol* 62,
1167–1176.

Wolpe J (1958) *Psychotherapy by Reciprocal Inhibition.* Stanford
University Press, Stanford, CA.

Young JE (1990) *Cognitive Therapy for Personality Disorders: A Schema-
Focused Approach.* Professional Resource Exchange, Sarasota, FL.

Zimering R, Cadell JM, Fairbank JA *et al.* (1993) Posttraumatic stress
disorder in Vietnam veterans: An experimental validation of the
DSM-III diagnostic criteria. *J Traumatic Stress* 6, 327–342.

CHAPTER

17

Social Psychology

Social psychology, defined broadly as the study of social influences on psychological functioning, is highly relevant to a biopsychosocial perspective in that it focuses on understanding the person–environment relationship. Environmental factors are presumed to influence psychological functioning. Individuals are defined as active interpreters of the environmental contexts in which they live such that individual construals of events influence psychological life and behavior.

The chapter begins with a discussion of how social factors influence the psychological processes of the individual, including self-functioning and social cognition processes. This is followed by a review of interpersonal processes. Next, attention is turned to the functioning of social groups, including the family. Finally, the influence of culture is considered.

The Self

Theory and Research Findings

Historical Precedents
Current social psychological efforts to understand the self in the context of the person–environment relationship, particularly the social world of the individual, are not without significant historical precedence. For example, James (1890/1981) posited that one component of the self was a social self determined in part by relationships with significant others. James maintained that because one's social roles and impact on others are varied, each individual has multiple social selves (e.g., self at work, self with family) with varying degrees of integration and internal consistency. Cooley's (1902) concept of the looking-glass self referred to the idea that the self emerges from one's interpretations of the reactions of important others in the social environment. Similarly, Mead's (1934) symbolic interactionism approach posited that self-knowledge derives from a process of taking the role of the other in social interaction. According to this view, the individual internalizes norms and expectations of the social group (the generalized other) in the course of social interaction. This internalization of the generalized other provides the basis for self-reflection, including the capacity to evaluate one's gestures and deeds, and anticipate others' responses to one's behavior. Social psychological inquiries into the self in the middle decades of the 20th century were sparse, but over the past 20 years interest in self-functioning has dramatically increased, in part spurred by social cognition research (Taylor, 1998). While a comprehensive review of this now voluminous literature is beyond the scope of this discussion, a sampling of representative, contemporary social psychological perspectives on self is presented here.

Social Psychological Models of Self
Consistent with trends toward systematic examination and articulation of the person–environment relationship in personality functioning as a whole (Baumeister, 1999; Curtis, 1991; Mitchell, 2000), social psychological models presume that self-functioning is influenced both by intrapersonal and situational context factors (Baumeister, 1998; Tesser *et al.*, 2000). From this perspective, self-functioning may be understood in terms of personal traits and dispositions (individual self), interpersonal roles and relationship patterns (relational self), and larger group identifications (collective self) (Sedikides and Brewer, 2001).

Investigations of the self have produced myriad conceptualizations of self-functioning. To organize the diverse strands of theory and research on self, Baumeister (1998) has proposed three dimensions central to the construction of self, including reflexive consciousness, interpersonal being and executive function. Reflexive consciousness refers to the human capacity to reflect on personal thoughts, feelings and behavior, and is the mechanism that makes possible the construction of self-conceptions and self-knowledge. Interpersonal being connotes the relational component of self that develops within ongoing interpersonal transactions and serves the vital psychological function of negotiating the relational world. Executive function refers to the capacity for agency, decision-making and initiative in living, and is the basis for active engagement with the environment. Social psychological models of self-functioning typically presuppose and/or focus on one or more of these dimensions of self.

To illustrate current social psychological thinking with regard to self-functioning, a few examples of recent social psychological theories of self are outlined briefly in the table: the self-verification theory, self-evaluation maintenance, self-discrepancy theory and self-determination theory (Table 17.1). Each of these models represents a significant contribution to the social psychological perspective on self, and although not clinically derived, has significant relevance to the clinical situation.

Self-presentation, Impression Management and Personal Identity
Along with specific theoretical models of self, social psychology has examined the impact of self-presentation and impression management on self-functioning. Specifically, people are invested in presenting themselves in certain ways (performing) in social situations and endeavor to control the impressions that others have of them in those situations (Goffman, 1959; Leary, 1995). These modes of self-presentation have some degree of influence on

Essentials of Psychiatry   Jerald Kay and Allan Tasman
© 2006 John Wiley & Sons, Ltd.

Table 17.1	Theories of Self: Representative Examples
Model	**Basic Tenets**
Self-verification theory	Individuals use their social relationships to validate core aspects of their self-concepts.
Self-evaluation maintenance	Regulation of self-regard is influenced by the performance of others in one's social environment.
Self-discrepancy theory	Persons seek a state of affairs in which their self-concept (qualities that oneself/others presume that one possesses) is perceived to be congruent with how they and others believe they should or ought to be.
Self-determination theory	Behavior is directed by a core self-organization consisting primarily of intrinsic motivation, innate needs, and integrative psychological functions.

self-definition and personal identity (Tice and Baumeister, 2001). Successful impression management requires an awareness of social expectations regarding behavior in a specific situation, a desire to act within social expectations, and a capacity to present oneself in such a way that the desired impression is conveyed. One's behavior in social interactions also is guided by the impressions one forms of others. Generally speaking, it is adaptive to be cognizant of others' views of oneself and to portray oneself in particular ways because these interpersonal strategies can enhance one's capacity to comprehend, regulate and anticipate social interaction patterns (Schlenker and Pontari, 2000). In deciding how to present themselves in a social interchange, people stress the commonalities between themselves and what is expected of them and present a personally and socially desirable public image to assure social compatibility, solidarity with others and social approval.

Self in Health and Illness

Issues of physical health and illness influence both one's self-definition and the quality and nature of one's interpersonal world. In turn, one's self-definition influences how one responds to health-related concerns. Self-efficacy (Bandura, 1997), which connotes beliefs regarding one's capacity to perform a required action, is an especially important variable in predicting individual responses to health-related concerns (Salovey et al., 1998). To heighten the extent to which individuals can exercise control over their own health behaviors and associated environmental stresses, individuals may be taught self-management and self-control techniques. Learning the array of cognitive and behavioral coping strategies that increase people's ability to manage their illness and associated affective responses also enhances self-efficacy and overall capacity for effective self-regulation.

Mental Health Implications

Mental health professionals increasingly have appreciated the need to understand self-functioning in a relational context. This shift in focus has been influenced by attachment theory (Bowlby, 1982), interpersonal psychiatry (Sullivan, 1953), psychoanalytic object relations theory (Greenberg and Mitchell, 1983), feminism (Jordan, 1997) and family systems theory (Gurman and Kniskern, 1981, 1991). For example, Sullivan's (1953) clinical theory included a characterization of the self-system as composed of the good-me bad-me and not-me personifications, with the self-system defined interpersonally on the basis of perceived responses of significant others beginning early in life. Within the psychoanalytic tradition, adherents to object relations theory (Fairbairn, 1954; Guntrip, 1969; Winnicott, 1965), self-psychology (Kohut, 1977), and relational psychoanalysis (Mitchell, 2000) have underscored the importance of the interpersonal contributions to self-development and functioning. Each of these approaches emphasizes that the nature and quality of the relationship between the therapist and patient is centrally relevant to helping the patient make changes in self-functioning.

Models of Self and Clinical Intervention

Based on a synthesis of theoretical models and empirical research findings, Deaux (1992) has developed a social psychological model of relationships between self and mental health that revolves around self-definition and the impact of challenges to self-definition on mental health functioning. In the model, self-definition is conceptualized as consisting of 1) specific domains of functioning (e.g., social and personal identities, life tasks) rather than as a global entity; 2) goals and aspirations as motivational elements; and 3) active interpretations of experience and personal meaning constructions. Demographic and sociocultural variables, social structure and socialization processes are viewed as distal influences on self-definition. Although the self-definition is presumed to be relatively stable, it is subject to challenge by internal factors (e.g., perceived discrepancies between the self-definition and internally defined expectations for oneself, negative social comparisons) and/or external factors (e.g., illness, change of employment status, changes in significant relationships). Challenge triggers a self-evaluation process to deal with information that is inconsistent with one's predominant self-definition. Self-evaluation results in regulation and reconstruction activities focused internally on the self (e.g., self-esteem maintenance, self-affirmation, self-esteem protection, activities associated with alterations in self-definition) and/or externally on the external world (e.g., self-verification, self-monitoring, behavioral disconfirmation activities associated with presentation of the reformulated self-definition in the social world). Negative outcomes of the self-evaluation process are presumed in the model to be associated with adverse mental health outcomes.

Drawing from myriad theories and concepts from within social psychology, Deaux's (1992) model acknowledges the centrality of self-regulation processes in the maintenance of overall mental health as individuals respond to challenges to existing self-definitions. Self-regulation processes are a core element of the social psychological theories of self summarized herein, including self-verification theory (Swann, 1983, 1997), self-evaluation maintenance (Tesser, 1991; Beach and Tesser, 1995), self-discrepancy theory (Higgins, 1987; Moretti and Higgins, 1999) and self-determination theory (Deci and Ryan, 2000; Ryan and Deci, 2000). Each of these models provides insights for the clinical understanding and treatment of mental health problems as they relate to challenges to self-definition and the self-evaluation processes that ensue in response to such challenges. Examples of the clinical relevance and utility of these models for clinical work now will be considered.

Self-presentation and Impression Management in Clinical Perspective

While the maintenance of a specific social image through impression management can yield psychological benefit, certain patterns of self-presentation can also have a negative psychological impact. For example, preoccupation with presenting oneself as competent in a particular pursuit when realistic appraisal suggests otherwise can give rise to pursuit of goals for which one is not suited, generating impractical expectations for self and precipitating associated frustration and disappointment. Extreme efforts to present oneself in a particular light can lead to maladaptive states of mind, response patterns and relationships (Shepperd and Kwavnick, 1999).

Impression management also has implications for the self-relevant social emotions of guilt and shame. Both guilt and shame are responses to perceived transgressions on the part of the self, but differ in that guilt involves condemnation of a particular behavior and is accompanied by remorse or regret, whereas shame involves condemnation of one's self and is accompanied by feelings of being exposed as objectionable and bad (Tangney and Salovey, 1999). Both guilt and shame are emotional experiences tied to one's perceived failure to maintain a positive self-presentation, and each propels specific patterns of impression management. For instance, guilt tends to spark interpersonal efforts to make reparation for one's behavior, whereas shame may prompt social avoidance associated with a wish to hide the self from view (Tangney and Salovey, 1999). Although guilt and shame are expectable emotional dimensions of everyday psychological life, their problematic manifestations can adversely affect both self-regulation and interpersonal relationships, and therefore must be considered in clinical evaluation and treatment of psychological dysfunction.

Social Cognition

Social cognition – the ways social events are interpreted, analyzed and mentally represented – provides an information-processing framework for understanding how construals of self and others affect social discourse and psychological life (Fiske and Taylor, 1991). Social cognition concepts have influenced traditional areas of social psychological theory and research, including attribution processes, person perception, and attitude formation and change. Over time, the information processing emphasis of social cognition has been integrated with concepts of motivation and emotion to create a fuller view of the individual in relation to the social world (Taylor, 1998).

Attribution Processes

Attribution processes refer to causal explanations generated by an individual to account for why a particular event or set of outcomes has occurred. People use attributions to make sense of their own behavior and that of others, and, therefore, attribution processes influence individual actions, affective experiences and

Table 17.2	Attribution Theories: Representative Examples
Model	Basic Tenets
Heider's model	Individuals attribute the causes of events to dispositional or situational factors.
Jones and Davis' model	Individuals make inferences about the dispositions of an actor based on observations of the noncommon effects of the actor's behavior.
Kelley's model	Individuals attribute the causes of behavior to the actor, the entity, or the circumstances. Consensus, consistency and distinctiveness information are used to formulate an attribution to one of these three sources.
	Causal schemas also influence attributions when one or more of these types of information is not available.
Achievement model	Affective responses in achievement situations are influenced by the extent to which success or failure is attributed to internal/external causes, stable/variable causes and controllable/uncontrollable causes.
Depression model	Risk of depression increases as a result of attribution of negative events to internal, stable and global causes.

interpersonal behavior (Weiner and Graham, 1999). Attribution theory (Table 17.2) and research has been a mainstay of social psychology and has led to important clinical mental health applications (Bell-Dolan and Anderson, 1999; Forsterling, 2001; Graham and Folkes, 1990).

Attribution Biases

Based on the proliferation of research stimulated in the 1970s by social psychological models of causal attribution, three major types of attribution biases in everyday social interactions were illuminated: the fundamental attribution error (Ross, 1977), the actor–observer bias (Jones and Nisbett, 1971) and the self-serving (hedonic) attribution bias (Bradley, 1978) (Table 17.3).

The fundamental attribution error – a bias toward attributing behavior to dispositional factors in the actor while underestimating the influence of situational variables – typically occurs in the context of understanding the behavior of others.

Table 17.3	Major Attributional Biases
Bias	**Description**
Fundamental attribution error	A bias toward attributing behavior to dispositional factors and underestimating situational influences on the behavior in question
Actor–observer bias	A bias toward attributing one's own acts to situational factors while attributing others' behavior to dispositional factors
Self-serving (hedonic) bias	A propensity to attribute one's own successes to dispositional factors while attributing failures to situational factors

The actor–observer bias refers to instances in which individuals attribute their own acts to situational factors and minimize the role of dispositional qualities, attributing the others' behavior to dispositional factors. Actor–observer differences may be a function of greater self-knowledge than knowledge of others, or related to differing perspectives between actors and observers that lead to different causal interpretations. The self-serving (hedonic) attribution bias involves a propensity to attribute one's successes to dispositional factors and one's failures to situational causes. Specifically, the self-serving bias reflects a wish to present oneself in the best possible light. People tend to extend this attribution bias to important others in their interpersonal sphere (e.g., spouse). Multiple explanations have been offered in the literature regarding the causal underpinnings of these attribution biases (Forsterling, 2001).

Attributions in Health and Illness

Given that attribution processes tend to be activated by negative, unanticipated, or ambiguous events, it is logical to assume that attribution theory would have a useful role in conceptualizing how people come to understand the causes of their illness as well as processes of stress and coping with illness (Amirkhan, 1990; Salovey et al., 1998). Empirical evidence supports this view, as exemplified in a recent meta-analytic study that suggested that attributions influence illness-related coping and adjustment (Roesch and Weiner, 2001). Attributions influence one's self-definitions in relation to the illness, as well as one's perceptions of control over illness-related contingencies and outcomes. However, associations between specific attributions and illness should not be interpreted to mean that certain attribution patterns cause illness, but rather that they may be among a complex set of factors affecting responses to illness.

It is clear that causal attributions are important in facilitating health promotion and positive health practices (Rodin and Salovey, 1989; Salovey et al., 1998). To the extent possible, treatment interventions with medically ill persons should incorporate a focus upon enhancing the individual perceptions of control over health and treatment regimens with the aim of increasing adherence to medical regimens and improving adjustment to medical procedures and conditions. Existing research also underscores the importance of considering locus, stability and controllability dimensions of the attribution process in understanding illness-related attribution processes and their role in predicting patient perceptions of medical treatment (Amirkhan, 1990).

Mental Health Implications: Attribution Processes

Theoretical models and research have significant implications for mental health treatment (Bell-Dolan and Anderson, 1999; Forsterling, 2001; Weiner and Graham, 1999). Presumably, attribution models can be instructive for designing interventions that target causal inferences associated with problematic emotion states (e.g., guilt), moods (e.g., depression) and behavioral constellations (e.g., social avoidance) (Bell-Dolan and Anderson, 1999). The application of attribution models to depression is illustrative of this point.

Hopelessness Theory of Depression

The use of attribution concepts, including the notion of attributional style, in understanding learned helplessness and depression led to the formulation that the presence of a pessimistic attributional style increased the risk that an individual would experience helplessness, hopelessness and depression (Abramson et al., 1978). This attribution dimension was later incorporated as a key component of the hopelessness theory of depression (Abramson et al., 1989; Gotlib and Abramson, 1999). This model predicts that an individual is at risk for hopelessness depression to the extent that negative events are attributed to internal, stable and global causes, and that these causes are perceived as both likely to prompt other negative consequences and to be reflective of deficiencies or shortcomings of self. The model also posits that a given individual's causal attributions are a function of both situational factors and individual differences in attributional style. Further, cognitive vulnerability to hopelessness depression is conceptualized as a function of individual differences in attributional style as well as the propensity to infer negative consequences and negative self-evaluation in response to adverse events (Gotlib and Abramson, 1999).

Person Perception and Implicit Personality Theories

Person perception, also referred to as social perception, pertains to the ways in which people formulate impressions of others (Leyens and Fiske, 1994). Person perception can be conceptualized broadly as involving three sequential processes: 1) the identification of meaningful acts by observation of overt actions based on the actor's intentions or traits; 2) the formation of attributions about the acts; and 3) the integration of attribution inferences into a unified impression of an individual (Gilbert, 1998). Social psychologists have long suggested that people formulate implicit personality theories that consist of general beliefs about human characteristics and patterns of covariation among personality traits (Schneider, 1973). These knowledge systems facilitate rapid formation of inferences about the enduring personality qualities of other people in everyday life by using assumptions about interrelationships among dispositional qualities to draw conclusions about observed behavior. More recently, schema concepts in social cognition have been investigated in order to specify cognitive processes through which individuals organize and represent coherent and meaningful impressions of others (Leyens and Fiske, 1994).

Although person perception variables per se have not been explicitly discussed in the context of health issues, one particularly useful application of this literature is in understanding relationships between patients and their health care providers. The doctor–patient relationship is influenced in part by the affective and cognitive evaluations that each make regarding the other. These person perception variables affect interaction styles between physicians and their patients which, in turn, may influence the nature and quality of medical care. Patients' perceptions of their physicians as paternalistic, interested in mutuality in decision-making regarding care, or expecting them (the patient) to have primary responsibility for decision-making will contribute to differential doctor–patient interaction dynamics (Shelton, 1998). Similarly, the degree to which the physician's impression of the patient is that of a passive novice, informed partner, or the consumer in charge of care will affect doctor–patient interactions.

Person perception has clinical relevance for the cognitive interpretation of interpersonal situations. Many of the cognitive distortions (e.g., overgeneralization, magnification and minimization) observed in depressed persons (Beck *et al.*, 1979), anxious individuals (Beck *et al.*, 1985), and people with personality disorders (Beck and Freeman, 1990) influence person perception in a maladaptive fashion. Thus, while person perception research has demonstrated a normative tendency to make rapid evaluations of others and interpersonal situations based on limited information, this process is apt to become problematic when cognitive distortions are operative. For example, the depressed person with low self-esteem and a pessimistic attributional style who, based on a few experiences of being criticized, perceives others as judgmental in virtually every interpersonal interaction is overgeneralizing based upon limited data (i.e., "others are always critical of me"). This is likely to interfere with the development of trusting relationships.

Implicit personality theories and schemas in social cognition are clinically applicable to understanding chronically maladaptive person perception processes. This may have particular relevance for the clinical understanding of personality disorders. For example, the patient with paranoid personality disorder may hold a pervasive view of others as potentially attacking, blaming and controlling (Benjamin, 1996). The patient with borderline personality disorder may perceive others as simultaneously rejecting, abandoning and needing dependent others (Benjamin, 1996). The patient with obsessive–compulsive personality disorder may believe that others expect perfection regardless of the individual's own wants and needs (Benjamin, 1996). To address these maladaptive implicit personality theories, schemas and associated interaction patterns, effective psychotherapy helps patients identify dysfunctional person perceptions, develop an affective and cognitive awareness of the etiology of these beliefs and the functions they serve, and form more adaptive schemas of self in relation to others (Benjamin, 1996). Additionally, therapists' awareness of problematic schemas and implicit personality theories early in treatment can assist in assessment and identification of interpersonal patterns that are likely to be enacted in the therapeutic relationship.

Attitudes

Attitudes refer to evaluations made by people along a continuum from positive to negative about specific entities called attitude objects (e.g., ideas, concrete things, life events, social groups, classes of behavior, persons) (Eagly and Chaiken, 1998). Individual attitudes consist of three elements: cognitive (beliefs about attitude objects), affective (emotions elicited by attitude objects) and behavioral (action intentions or overt behavior directed toward attitude objects). Additionally, individual attitudes may be associatively or logically linked to form broader inter-attitudinal structures consisting of two or more attitudes (Eagly and Chaiken, 1998). Attitudes provide a framework for rapid appraisal and evaluative interpretation of one's world, thereby allowing one to formulate responses to the complexities and ambiguities of daily living in an economical fashion, often without the need for deliberate, conscious processing (Cooper and Aronson, 1992). Fundamentally, attitudes serve an important adaptive function by virtue of their evaluative properties involving distinctions of good stimuli presumed to enhance well-being from bad stimuli that could endanger well-being (Eagly and Chaiken, 1998).

Attitude Theories

Attitude theory and research has a rich history as one of the great areas of inquiry within social psychology (Eagly and Chaiken, 1998; Petty and Wegener, 1998). However, this voluminous and intricate literature can be encapsulated only briefly here. Theoretical frameworks developed in the 1950s, 1960s and 1970s that laid the foundation for later social psychological inquiries into attitudes (Table 17.4).

Learning and reinforcement theories of attitude formation and change, founded on principles of behaviorism, were derived

Table 17.4	Attitude Theories: Representative Examples
Model	Basic Tenets
Learning and reinforcement theories	Environmental contingencies, including conditioning and association processes, determine the formation, maintenance and alteration of attitudes.
Social judgment theory	Attitudes are most likely to be influenced by information that is similar to one's own attitudinal set, may be influenced by information about which one's attitudes are not clearly defined, and are least likely to be influenced by information that is inconsistent with one's attitudinal set.
Consistency theories	Attitude formation and change are organized by a need to impose structure and order on one's understanding of the environment.
Functional theories	Individuals form and maintain attitudes that are consistent with their needs and motives.

from basic experimental psychology. Two major examples are conditioning (Staats and Staats, 1958) and associationist (stimulus–response) (Hovland *et al.*, 1953) perspectives. These approaches emphasize the influence of stimulus pairing and stimulus–response patterns in attitude formation (Eagly and Chaiken, 1998).

Social judgment theory emphasizes the interplay of cognitive and affective attitudinal components and posits that perceptions and judgments mediate attitude change (Sherif *et al.*, 1965). According to this approach, attitudes are most likely to be influenced by information that is similar to one's existing attitudinal set (i.e., latitude of acceptance), may be influenced by information about which one's attitudinal set is not clearly defined and affectively neutral (i.e., latitude of noncommitment), and least likely to be influenced by information that is inconsistent with one's attitudinal set (i.e., latitude of rejection).

Consistency theories posit that attitude formation and change are organized by a need to impose structure and order on one's understanding of the environment. Cognitive dissonance theory (Festinger, 1957) posited that discrepancies between simultaneously held attitudinal cognitions (dissonance) produced psychological tension, requiring attitudinal changes to reestablish consistency (consonance). The degree to which this dissonance causes psychological tension is a function of the personal importance of the cognitions and the number of dissonant cognitions relative to consonant cognitions.

An alternative approach that proposed to account for research findings regarding dissonance was self-perception theory (Bem, 1972). According to this perspective, individuals infer their attitudes through observing their own behavioral responses and the conditions under which they occur. From this view, attitudes are formed on the basis of self-attributions (Cooper and Aronson, 1992).

The final group of attitude theories – functional theories – hold that individuals form and maintain attitudes consistent with their needs and motives (Katz, 1960; Kelman, 1961; Smith *et al.*, 1956). For example, particular attitudes may be adopted for adjustment, instrumental, or utilitarian purposes, as they maximize rewards and minimize punishments. Attitudes also may serve a value expression function. Ego-defensive or externalizing functions of attitudes allow for maintenance of desired views of self and the world, while protecting the individual from acknowledgement of unpleasant realities. Attitudes serving a knowledge function assist people in formulating meaning about events in their world. Functional models suggest a complex interplay among different attitudinal beliefs, necessitating different change strategies based upon the function of the attitude being targeted for change (Eagly and Chaiken, 1998).

Interest in enhancing precision in the prediction of behavioral responses from attitudinal beliefs prompted efforts to develop models of the attitude–behavior relationship (Table 17.5). Two broad types of models include those focusing on attitudes toward targets of behavior and those focusing on attitudes toward behavior (Eagly and Chaiken, 1998).

Attitudes in Health and Illness

People's attitudes affect whether or not they practice adaptive or maladaptive health behaviors. Accordingly, it has been suggested that information aimed at promoting behaviors that reduce health risk should focus on attitudinal and normative beliefs influencing the behavior in question. The goal of such

Table 17.5	Models of Attitude–Behavior Relationships: Representative Examples	
Model	**Basic Tenets**
Reasoned action model	The strength of intentions to act is determined by one's attitudes toward the behavior and perceptions of the social desirability of the behavior.
Cognitive dissonance model	Individuals alter attitudes in a manner consistent with their behavior to reduce dissonance.
Self-perception model	Individuals infer their attitudes through observation of their own behaviors and the conditions under which they occur.

interventions is to bolster intentions to engage in or abstain from the target behavior.

Although not an attitude theory per se, the health belief model (Rosenstock *et al.*, 1988; Strecher *et al.*, 1997) is a well-known social psychological model explicitly formulated to understand health-related behavior practices. The health belief model posits that individuals are motivated to respond to perceived threats of illness, with threat defined in terms of perceptions regarding seriousness of and personal susceptibility to an illness. Behavioral responses to health-related threats are influenced by expectations regarding the ability to minimize such a threat, including perceived benefits and problems associated with a given response pattern. Sociocultural and demographic factors as well as personal and environmental cues regarding appropriate courses of action also are considered in the model. The model predicts that people are likely to take steps to minimize the risk of contracting a medical problem if the following conditions occur: 1) they view themselves as vulnerable to a particular health condition; 2) they deem the condition to be personally consequential; 3) they believe that a specific course of action would minimize vulnerability to the condition and that limitations associated with such actions are outweighed by the potential benefits to be accrued; and 4) they perceive themselves as capable of performing these actions (i.e., self-efficacy). Researchers have examined the utility of the health belief model in informing prevention and intervention approaches for medically ill individuals and those at risk for specific illnesses (Salovey *et al.*, 1998).

Attitudes can have an important impact on psychological outlook and functioning. Whereas individuals who evidence positive mental health possess flexible attitudes that are adaptive to the context, persons with psychological difficulties evidence rigidly held maladaptive attitudes that impair their capacity to cope effectively with life's challenges. This suggests that helping patients identify and modify maladaptive attitudes about self and others can be an important component of psychotherapeutic intervention (Cooper and Aronson, 1992).

Interpersonal Processes

Recent multidisciplinary trends in theory and research on interpersonal phenomena have converged in scientific efforts to elucidate relationship dynamics, including their antecedents and consequences (Reis *et al.*, 2000). Underlying these efforts is the assumption that, since human behavior takes place within a relational context, a comprehensive scientific understanding of human behavior requires careful study of interpersonal relationships (Reis *et al.*, 2000). Although there have been differences of opinion regarding how to define the term relationship, there is loose agreement that a relationship involves an interaction between relational partners that affects the subsequent behavior of each partner in the interaction (Berscheid and Reis, 1998).

The study of interpersonal relationships spans a multitude of behavioral domains relevant to social psychology. Although recognition of the limits of the traditional individualistic focus of social psychological theory and research recently has prompted calls for a more systemic conceptual approach to research on interpersonal relationships, the vast majority of work to date has examined relationships between individual variables and relationship experiences (Reis *et al.*, 2000). It is important to emphasize that the nature and qualities of human social interaction are not attributable solely to evolutionary and biological influences and processes and are not directly parallel to animal behavior (Hinde, 1987). Further, while an evolutionary perspective can provide useful insights, adoption of such a viewpoint does not imply strict genetic determinism or unmodifiability of evolved behavioral patterns (Buss and Kenrick, 1998).

Attachment

Bowlby (1982) regarded attachment between infants and caregivers as an innate relational pattern that evolved in order to ensure the survival of the infant. Attachment phenomena are common in birds and mammals, with extended dependency periods in which offspring are fed, cleaned, sheltered and protected by the parent. In many species, attachment is enhanced by imprinting (Lorenz, 1970), a learned attachment that forms at the earliest phases of development. Imprinting is most likely to occur during specific, critical periods of development. If imprinting is not achieved during those times, it is difficult to attain. Attachment facilitates survival of the offspring, and investment in parental care for offspring is theorized to involve a cost–benefit trade off; the increased likelihood that offspring will survive is weighed against potential costs of parental care.

Attachment theory has as its cornerstone a system of reciprocal interactions that facilitate psychological safety and security (i.e., attachment behavioral system) (Bowlby, 1973, 1980, 1982). According to Bowlby's theory of attachment, as a consequence of evolutionary processes, children possess emotional and behavioral systems that organize and direct them to seek proximity and to bond with their primary caretakers when they feel distressed or threatened. The nature and quality of parental response in such instances influences the child's development. Children's internal working models of the attachment figure and the self in relation to this figure (i.e., self- and object-representations and schemas of interaction patterns between self and attachment figures) influence their attachment style and the quality of their interpersonal relationships (Bretherton and Munholland, 1999).

The bulk of attachment research has been conducted with young children and their primary caretakers. This research reveals four attachment bonds types (i.e., secure, avoidant, anxious/ambivalent, disorganized/disoriented) most noted when

Table 17.6	Types of Childhood Attachment Bonds and Behavioral Correlates
Attachment Bond	Behavioral Hallmarks
Secure	Social, freely explore the environment, respond with resilience to stress
Avoidant	Anxious with primary caretaker, angry or attention-seeking with others
Anxious/Ambivalent	Fearful, affectively unstable, excessive clinging behavior
Disorganized/Disoriented	Disorganized and contradictory behaviors, particularly upon reunion with primary caretaker

infants and their primary caretaker are reunited following a brief, experimentally controlled separation (Ainsworth *et al.*, 1978; Hesse and Main, 2000; Main, 2000) (Table 17.6).

Securely attached children are social, able to explore their environment freely, and resilient when faced with stressful situations. In contrast, avoidant children tend to be anxious with their primary caretaker(s) and angry or attention-seeking with others. Anxious/ambivalent children typically are fearful of the environment, affectively unstable, and cling inordinately to others. Finally, disorganized/disoriented children often exhibit signs of disorganization and contradictory behaviors, particularly upon reunion with their primary caretaker. Longitudinal research shows that attachment behavior patterns are stable over time, predictive of school behavior and peer interactions, and consistent with the quality of parenting received and parental attachment style (Bowlby, 1988; Sroufe, 2002; Sroufe *et al.*, 1990).

Adult Attachment

Recently, clinicians and researchers have begun to turn their attention to attachment patterns in adults (Sperling and Berman, 1994; West and Sheldon-Keller, 1994). Similar to infant attachment patterns, adult attachment is presumed to be rooted in evolutionarily significant biological adaptation processes (Hazan and Diamond, 2000) and is characterized by a strong interest in the other, a desire to remain physically close to and spend time with the other, reliance on ongoing access to the other, dependence upon the other for support in the face of physical or emotional threats, and feelings of discomfort and distress upon separation (Feeney, 1999; Shaver and Hazan, 1993; West and Sheldon-Keller, 1994). However, unlike attachment patterns in children, the primary adult attachment objects typically are peers, adult patterns of relating are more reciprocal, and attachment figures often also are sexual partners (Feeney *et al.*, 2000). Adult attachment is influenced significantly by working models of the attachment object and self that have their origins in childhood attachment experiences with primary caretakers (Bartholomew and Horowitz, 1991). Work in adult attachment theory addresses the establishment and maintenance of primary emotional partnerships in adult life, the effects of early and current attachment experiences on the development of psychopathology, and the use of attachment theory to guide therapeutic interventions.

Among the most compelling questions in research on close relationships are those that pertain to relationship satisfaction and stability. Work in this area has been influenced (see Table 17.7) heavily by the social exchange tradition, which assumes that the exchange of rewards and costs is a key influence on relationships (Berscheid and Reis, 1998). Specifically, social exchange theory suggests that people are motivated to maximize rewards and minimize costs, with the favorability of relational outcomes being defined by the relative balance of rewards and costs for each relationship participant. Within the social exchange framework, interdependence theory (Thibaut and Kelley, 1959; Rusbult and Van Lange, 1996) has been especially useful in making predictions about relationship satisfaction and stability. This model posits that people evaluate relationship satisfaction according to expectancy standards for relationship outcomes (comparison level), and that relationship satisfaction is a function of the extent to which outcomes meet or exceed these expectancy standards. The model also posits an additional evaluative standard employed by individuals to determine whether or not to stay in a given relationship (comparison level for alternatives). This standard is relevant to predicting relationship stability, as it represents the minimal acceptable relationship outcome level for remaining in a given relationship when outcomes associated with available alternative relationships are taken into consideration. According to the model, therefore, relationship stability is related to the combined influence of relationship attractiveness and the availability of desirable alternatives external to the relationship. Relationship stability is likely to be compromised to the extent that relationship attractiveness is lower than the appeal of available relationship alternatives. In general, relationship stability is influenced by degree of commitment to the relationship, availability in the social environment of viable relationship alternatives, perceived approval for the relationship by the social networks of the respective partners, and partner perceptions of the relative equity/inequity in gains as a result of being in the relationship (Berscheid and Reis, 1998).

Sexual behavior is an important channel of expression in certain types of interpersonal relationships (e.g., romantic relationships) and its patterns of expression may symbolize underlying relational dynamics (Mason, 1991). While some social psychological perspectives have explored sexuality as it relates to romantic love, much of the extant theory and research related to sexuality has focused on mate selection (Berscheid and Reis, 1998). Evolutionary psychology, in particular, has examined mate selection in detail (Buss and Kenrick, 1998).

In humans, sexual behavior serves more than the purely biological functions of procreation and physiological release, as it is also an important means of expressing love, closeness and the need for human contact. Sexual behavior is manifested in diverse ways determined by a complex interplay among one's relationships, life situations and the broad sociocultural context. Although normative sexual behavior has received systematic empirical study, beginning with the survey research of Kinsey and colleagues (1948, 1953) and continuing to the present day (Janus and Janus, 1994), much of the emphasis of psychological research has been on sexual dysfunction and its treatment (Kaplan, 1974; Masters and Johnson, 1970).

Considerable evidence has accrued that social integration in general, and social support in particular, are related both to enhanced health and lowered risk of mortality (Berscheid and Reis, 1998; Stroebe and Stroebe, 1996). Both main effect models and

Table 17.7	Attraction Theories: Representative Examples
Model	Basic Tenets
Cognitive-consistency theories	Attraction is influenced by the need for internally consistent beliefs.
Reinforcement theories	Attraction is influenced by patterns of reinforcement and punishment.
Exchange theories	Attraction is influenced by mutuality of rewards.
Developmental theories	Attraction occurs according to a sequence of deepening involvement from casual contact to increased degrees of intimacy.

stress-buffering models have been employed to explain observed relationships between social support and health factors (Stroebe and Stroebe, 1996). Main effect models assume that a specific factor, such as social influence, may directly affect health and well-being via its impact on health beliefs, attitudes and behavior. By contrast, stress-buffering models presume that social support confers health benefits only to the extent that an individual is experiencing stress. According to this perspective, social support may provide health benefits indirectly by serving as a resource to help the individual cope with health-related stress.

Several factors influence the likelihood of social-support provision. Among these are social-exchange processes and social norms surrounding provision of help for individuals in ill-health, as well as causal attributions made about the recipient of social support (Stroebe and Stroebe, 1996). For example, social psychological research suggests that a curvilinear relationship exists between degree of distress and likelihood of an individual receiving social support, with moderate distress eliciting the greatest degree of supportive actions by others. Further, individuals perceived by others as responsible for their plight may be less likely to receive social support than those whose ill-health is perceived by others as caused by uncontrollable circumstances. Additionally, social support may be withheld if individuals are perceived as not trying hard enough to manage their illness or are not showing sufficient improvement in response to social support provision. These patterns may have unfortunate implications for individuals with disease syndromes that cause high stress levels, are highly stigmatized, and/or are chronic or progressive, as they may find themselves socially isolated at times of high need for social contact.

As has already been mentioned, there is a vast scientific literature in support of the idea that relationships contribute both to physical and mental well-being (Berscheid and Reis, 1998; Reis *et al.*, 2000; Stroebe and Stroebe, 1996). This empirical base complements the widespread clinical regard for the treatment relationship as a primary tool of influence and therapeutic change (Mitchell, 2000). As such, social psychological theory and research on relationships can contribute substantively to current thinking about how to structure the clinician–patient relationship to maximize mental health treatment benefit (Derlega *et al.*, 1991).

The Treatment Relationship

Derlega and colleagues (1991) have delineated specific mental health applications of social psychological research on interpersonal relationships. For instance, they suggest that principles from social exchange theory can be applied to clinical formulation of the patient–therapist relationship dynamics, including the influence of rewards and costs on decisions to initiate a therapy relationship, levels of satisfaction with and commitment to the relationship, and the overall quality of an ongoing therapeutic relationship. They also point out that application of findings from interpersonal attraction research can enhance clinical understanding of the goodness of fit and working alliance between a therapist and patient. For example, patient attraction to the therapist may be influenced by the extent to which the therapist is perceived as similar on domains that the patient considers highly significant (e.g., gender, cultural background, beliefs and values, personality style). The therapist's experience of rapport with the patient may be similarly influenced. The attraction between therapist and patient is likely strengthened by the extent to which time is shared, as increased experience allows for greater mutual understanding, which in turn enhances the experience of interpersonal attraction and compatibility. Different types of therapeutic alliances tend differentially to influence the course and nature of the treatment. Finally, Derlega and colleagues (1991) point out that social psychological models of relationship development, such as social penetration theory, can provide some insight into the understanding of how therapeutic relationships unfold and deepen.

The benefits of social support for psychological well-being have been clearly established in the research literature (Stroebe and Stroebe, 1996). It follows, therefore, that an important objective of therapy is to assist patients in building adequate social support. Further, it is useful also to conceptualize the therapeutic relationship itself as a source of social support for the patient. Among the therapist activities that can be regarded as aspects of social support are the communication of positive feelings toward the patient, attending to patient feelings and beliefs, encouraging patient expression and providing help with solving problems and completing tasks (Derlega *et al.*, 1991).

Attachment theory and the associated empirical findings have useful clinical implications for assessing and treating dysfunctional parent–child, peer, dyadic romantic and family relationships, and for understanding therapist–patient relationships (Doane and Diamond, 1994; Sperling and Berman, 1994). Attachment theory also provides a meaningful framework for conceptualizing various psychiatric disorders in individuals and families (Doane and Diamond, 1994; Sperling and Berman, 1994). In an attachment theory based approach to psychotherapy, the therapist provides new and more adaptive models of relating such that individuals may move from insecure and/or anxious attachments to the development and maintenance of secure attachments (West and Sheldon-Keller, 1994). This process is facilitated by the therapist's provision of a secure base, examination of relationships and expectations of significant people in the patient's life, exploration of the therapist–patient relationship, reflection on links between parental expectations and the patient's working models of relationships, and development of an understanding of the appropriateness of these working models for guiding current and future relationships (Bowlby, 1988).

The Egoism–Altruism Debate

Historically, the Western perspective has been that human beings tend to be motivated by self-interest (egoism). It is therefore not surprising that investigators concerned with prosocial behavior have debated the veracity of the concept of altruistically motivated prosocial acts in which others are benefited with no apparent short-term or long-term benefits for the helper. A model proposed by Batson (1987, 1998) is intended to account for altruism without invoking self-serving motives by establishing empathy as a key factor that drives altruistic behavior. According to this empathy–altruism hypothesis, empathy provides a vehicle for adopting the perspective of the other in need that then motivates the helper to act with the goal of benefiting the other. Because empathic emotion is distinguished from that of a distress response, it is argued that helpful acts resulting from empathic determinants are carried out with the intention of enhancing the welfare of the other rather than the self. Three types of self-serving motives have been proposed to challenge the empathy–altruism hypothesis, including the prospect of self and social rewards for providing help, avoidance of self or social punishment for failing to help, and reduction of aversive arousal associated with feelings of empathy. In reviewing existing research, Batson (1998) concluded that none of these self-serving motives could adequately account for the relationship between empathy and helping behavior, and that, on balance, empirical findings generally support the empathy–altruism hypothesis that there are instances of altruism that can be distinguished from helping behavior involving self-serving motives. Batson (1998) further proposed a general model involving four categories of prosocial motivation, each of which is linked to specific values. These include egoism (valuing self-enhancement), altruism (valuing other-enhancement at the level of the individual), collectivism (valuing other-enhancement at the level of the social group), and principlism (valuing maintaining faithfulness to specific moral ideals). Although ideally these four categories of prosocial motivation operate in cooperative and complementary ways, they also may at times come into conflict. In investigations of helping behavior, factors that influence whether or not an individual will engage in helping others, focus on characteristics of the helper, the person who is in need of help, and the situation (Batson 1998) (Table 17.8).

The high value placed on aiding those in ill-health is ubiquitous in human life, exemplified at the cultural level by health care professions and health care institutions entrusted to care for those in need of medical intervention. Although multiple factors

Table 17.8   Factors Influencing Helping Behavior

Mood of the helper
Empathy for the needs of the one in need of help
View of the one in need of help as similar to oneself
Perception of the one in need of help as attractive and likeable
Attribution processes
Diffusion of responsibility
Ambiguity regarding whether or not the situation is one in which help is needed
Concerns that one might do more harm than good
Evaluation apprehension

contribute to the existence of health care institutions and personal decisions to work in health-related fields, prosocial motivations are key among them. At the level of the individual, the family and peer group, caring and empathy may propel the desire to help those who are ill by providing emotional and instrumental support. As myriad empirical investigations have shown, these prosocial acts of social support provide beneficial health effects for individuals who receive them (Stroebe and Stroebe, 1996).

Empathy engenders a sense of interest in and care for others (Batson, 1998). The capacity for empathy is an important part of healthy social relationships in that it enhances understanding of others and thereby facilitates social connection and the supportive dimensions of relationships. As such, clinical assessment should incorporate an evaluation of empathy skills, especially in instances where clinical difficulties stem from maladaptive relational patterns. Consideration of the balance of empathic versus self-serving interpersonal stances of the patient can be useful, not only in individual psychotherapy but also in work with couples seeking help in resolving conflictual relationship patterns.

The clinical relevance of empathy extends to the clinical practitioner. Therapist empathy is crucial to the understanding of the patient and to the maintenance of the therapist's concern for and desire to enhance patient well-being. It is, therefore, hard to imagine the practice of psychotherapy without empathic investment of the therapist (Watson, 2002). Although a powerful tool of therapeutic change, accurate empathy requires that the therapist bear witness to considerable emotional pain in the process of helping the patient. In some instances, the therapist may be overwhelmed by the clinical issues of a given patient, and in response may retreat from an empathic stance by distancing from, avoiding, or becoming numb to the experience of the patient. It has been suggested that this empathic retreat is a factor in the phenomenon of clinician burnout (Batson, 1998). As such, empathic availability is an important variable for therapists to attend to in their day-to-day work with patients.

Aggressive Behavior

Multiple definitions of aggression have been proposed by social scientists (Baron and Richardson, 1994). This reflects both the diverging views regarding the nature and determinants of aggressive behavior and the social norms that provide a context for evaluating whether or not an aggressive behavior is socially sanctioned. For this discussion, aggressive action is defined as any verbal or physical behavior or set of behaviors emitted with the intention to harm or damage someone or something. Biological, affective, social cognitive, social learning, personality and sociocultural influences on aggressive behavior are reviewed here in the table (Table 17.9).

Aggressive behavior has implications both for overall public health and individual health. For instance, aggression as it relates to interpersonal violence has obvious public health implications. One clear example of this is family violence, which threatens the physical health and lives of those toward whom this behavior is directed. At the individual level, anger and hostility, which play some role in aggression (though are distinct from aggressive behavior), have been associated with specific health effects. The most well-known example is research showing increased risk of subsequent coronary heart disease in individuals with high levels of anger and hostility (Salovey *et al.*, 1998; Contrada *et al.*, 1999). Hypothesized mechanisms for these health effects include psychophysiological processes (e.g., blood

Table 17.9	Factors that Influence Aggression
Factor	Behavioral Correlates
Biological	Instinctual processes and/or specific physiological systems influence aggressive behavior.
Affective	Aggression is a response to frustration or general negative affect states.
Social cognitive	Aggression is influenced by social cognition processes (e.g., attributions, attitudes).
Social learning	Aggression is influenced by one's history of reinforcement and modeling of aggressive behavior.
Personality	Aggression is influenced by dispositional factors in the actor.
Sociocultural	Aggression is influenced by social norms, laws, and customs.

pressure, stress hormone secretion, heart rate), health-compromising lifestyle patterns (e.g., poor self-care, cigarette smoking, limited exercise), and reactions to illness (e.g., compromises in adherence to medical treatment).

Multiple clinical techniques have been developed for helping individuals effectively modulate and manage aggression. These include exploring interpersonal patterns in which aggression arises, teaching cognitive restructuring techniques to address attribution processes (e.g., hostile attribution bias) that make aggressive behavior more likely to occur, employing family therapy approaches (e.g., functional family therapy; Alexander *et al.*, 1990) and parent management training, and utilizing cognitive–behavioral therapy techniques (e.g., problem-solving skills training, social skills training and aggression-related reinforcement contingencies). These techniques may be used individually or in combination, depending upon the clinical indications derived from a multidimensional assessment of factors contributing to aggressive behavior. Where indicated, addressing the role of psychoactive substance use in aggressive behavior is also important, given research suggesting that use of substances such as alcohol can be an antecedent to aggression (Baron and Richardson, 1994).

Behavior in Groups

An individual's social world is comprised largely of group affiliations (Levine and Moreland, 1998). A group is a social unit in which members interact and are interdependent, such that there is mutual influence among the members. Groups vary across such dimensions as size, duration, purpose, tasks, goals, and patterns and rules of communication. Involvement in familial, work, social and/or activity groups provides several potential benefits, including the satisfaction of survival, psychological, informational and identity needs. In some instances, however, the group dynamics and organization may compromise or hinder the gratification of these needs. As such, groups can both positively and adversely influence psychological adjustment (Forsyth and Elliott, 1999; Levine and Moreland, 1992).

Research on groups has revealed specific structural dimensions (Levine and Moreland, 1998). One such dimension is the status system, which reflects the power status of each group member relative to the other members. Additionally, groups are characterized by group norms, consisting of rules and expectations for behavior and interaction in the group. Individual group members typically adopt specific roles in the group *vis-à-vis* other group members and the group as a whole. Further, groups vary in their degree of cohesion, which refers to the extent to which group members experience a sense of connectedness to the group. Each of these structural dimensions affect the group culture, which can be broadly conceptualized as the group's shared knowledge systems and customs.

The study of group influence on behavior has elucidated several dynamics of group influence (Table 17.10).

Group Decision-making

An important function of many groups is that of decision-making (Levine and Moreland, 1998). It has been suggested that groups often are more effective than individuals in making decisions or solving problems, particularly when the collective and cooperative efforts of the individuals in the group are needed to accomplish the various components of the task at hand. In general, however, research suggests that the nature of a given task makes a difference in whether a group shows greater decision-making effectiveness than an individual. Successful group performance is aided

Table 17.10	Group Influence Factors
Factor	Description
Social facilitation	The presence of others enhances performance on simple or familiar tasks.
Social inhibition	The presence of others inhibits performance on complex or novel tasks.
Social loafing	The presence of others leads to lowered work effort when individual efforts are perceived to be anonymous and not subject to social evaluation.
Identity functions	Social identity may in part be defined by group affiliations.
Conformity	Uniformity of group opinion and/or behavior resulting from group pressure.
Minority influence	The influence of a minority faction in a group on the majority viewpoints.

Table 17.11	Problematic Group Decision-Making Processes
Group polarization	The tendency for groups to arrive at more extreme positions (i.e., more risky or conservative decisions) than would individual group members alone
Groupthink	A phenomenon in which cohesive groups make faulty decisions because intragroup dissent is discouraged.

by a cooperative, rather than competitive, group atmosphere in which members work together to attain goals that benefit the group as a whole. Group conflict may arise when there is disagreement about decisions, tasks, roles and objectives of a group, prompting the emergence of specific group processes to address group differences (e.g., negotiation, coalition formation) (Levine and Moreland, 1998). Groups are susceptible to specific social processes that may exert a potentially deleterious influence on the process of making thoughtful and productive decisions (Table 17.11).

The Familial Group

The family is one of the most powerful and important group structures in our society (for a review of family theory, see Kaslow *et al.*, 1999), and there are many similarities between the functioning of familial and nonfamilial groups (McGrath, 1984). Further, one's roles and functions in social groups are influenced by one's roles and functions in one's family of origin (i.e., parents, grandparents, extended family, siblings) and family of creation (i.e., partner, children, grandchildren).

General systems theory (von Bertalanffy, 1968), which provides the theoretical underpinnings of family systems theory, is also applicable to nonfamilial groups. According to systems theory, a system is a group of interacting elements. Family systems attempt to find a balance between change and homeostasis to facilitate adaptation of the family and its individual members across the life-cycle. Family systems exchange information via feedback loops, circular response patterns in which there is a return flow of information within the system. Interactions reflect circular causality, in which single events are viewed as both cause and effect. Families may be characterized in terms of their structure (i.e., organization) and function. The key structural property is wholeness (i.e., the whole is greater than the sum of its parts). Family units consist of interdependent subsystems that carry out distinctive functions to maintain themselves and sustain the system as a whole. Boundaries separate these subsystems and protect their integrity, while allowing interaction between subsystems. To maintain their structure, family systems have rules that enable them to function productively. Within each unit, individuals play a number of roles, exhibiting a predictable set of behaviors that may be influenced by family of origin, gender and generation within the nuclear family. All family behavior (e.g., roles, communication patterns, symptoms) is presumed to serve a systemic function.

Collaboration among medical providers is central to effective patient care. As medical providers routinely make important decisions in the context of work groups, it is important for health providers to be cognizant of the dynamics of group behavior. Where decisions are being made about such matters as delicate health procedures that have life and death ramifications, efforts should be made to foster a group environment that minimizes the likelihood of faulty group decision-making stemming from group polarization or groupthink phenomena. This process will increase the chances that an integrated biopsychosocial strategy will be adopted and maintained.

Cognizance of group process also is important in family medicine, where major patient-care decisions often are best managed by involving patients, their families and health care providers in a collaborative process (McDaniel *et al.*, 1992). Given the systemic phenomena that typify family functioning as described above, the family context within which illness progression unfolds is a key component in developing and implementing effective treatment strategies as well as maximizing treatment adherence. Further, families can provide significant social support resources for patients living with illness-related challenges.

Groups can serve an important social support function for individuals with severe illnesses. One example is the peer-led support group. Such groups include members who share common concerns, and tend to be characterized by group autonomy, self-governance, freedom of expression, equal distributions of power and mutual helping, including problem-solving and support (Forsyth and Elliott, 1999). Clinician-led group psychotherapy also has been shown to benefit patients with diseases such as cancer, both in terms of emotional adjustment and health effects (Spiegel and Kimerling, 2001; Spira, 1997).

Given the profound influence of group involvement on one's sense of self and interpersonal relationships, it is reasonable to assume that membership in family groups, groups at work or school, or community-based groups are associated with the quality of one's mental health functioning (Forsyth and Elliott, 1999; Levine and Moreland, 1992). Group involvement often is sought as a means of gaining help in managing personal and social problems. In clinical mental health practice settings, various forms of both group therapy (Yalom, 1995) and family therapy (Gurman and Kniskern, 1981, 1991) have been employed routinely to treat psychiatric disorders.

Psychotherapy groups are organized for the specific purpose of dealing with intrapsychic, behavioral and interpersonal difficulties encountered in daily living. For illustrative purposes, a brief review of the interpersonal or transactional approach to group psychotherapy will be presented, as social psychological principles can be applied easily to understanding the nature and efficacy of this commonly used approach. Yalom (1995), who has contributed substantively to the understanding and implementation of psychotherapy groups, posits that groups provide an interpersonal context within which the members manifest their maladaptive interpersonal patterns, receive feedback about these patterns, and gain opportunities to learn new and more authentic modes of relating to others. In this regard, groups function as social microcosms reflecting each participant's social universe. According to Yalom, there are a number of therapeutic factors that facilitate change in group therapy. These include the instillation of hope, universality, imparting of information, altruism, corrective recapitulation of the primary family group, development of socializing techniques, imitative behavior, interpersonal learning, group cohesiveness, catharsis and existential factors. Forsyth (1991) has evaluated these change factors from a social psychological perspective, suggesting that social comparison,

social learning, self-insight, social influence and social provisions processes are all relevant to the understanding of change processes in therapeutic groups.

Many social psychological concepts regarding small group behavior may have particular applicability to group psychotherapy. For example, it is essential for the therapist to facilitate establishment of group norms that maximize the likelihood that the therapeutic factors associated with change will exert full influence. Such norms may pertain to group procedure (e.g., attendance, participation and communication rules, length, frequency and duration of sessions), communication of support and empathy, values (e.g., self-disclosure, honesty, acceptance) and goals (e.g., improved psychological adjustment, enhanced relationship satisfaction). Additionally, group cohesiveness is a key component to a successful therapeutic group in that group cohesion is associated with acceptance and support among group members, along with the formation of authentic intragroup relationships. Further, high levels of group cohesion are associated with more stable group functioning (Yalom, 1995).

The therapist's awareness of some potential pitfalls of group decision-making processes also is essential (i.e., group polarization, groupthink). For instance, the group polarization phenomenon (e.g., risky shift) may be addressed effectively by the presence of a cotherapy team rather than a single therapist, as the two therapists may assist group members in arriving at more moderate positions (Yalom, 1995). Careful attention to minimizing the conditions under which groupthink may occur also is important in order to sidestep potentially catastrophic group decisions. In this regard, it is crucial that group leaders monitor their own inclinations to dominate group processes and suppress intragroup dissent.

Culture and Social Psychology

Social psychologists increasingly have appreciated the influence of culture on psychological functioning (Fiske *et al.*, 1998; Kim and Berry, 1993; Moghaddam *et al.*, 1993; Matsumoto, 2001). Consistent with this trend, Fiske and colleagues (1998) have proposed a mutual constitution of psychological and cultural life. Specifically, these investigators suggest that culture influences psychological functioning which in turn can change cultural expressions. They further argue that although the human tendency to form cultures sprang from evolutionary processes, culture, in turn, has exerted an influence on the subsequent course of evolution.

Myriad definitions of culture have been proposed by social scientists across a range of disciplines. Culture can be defined as a collective organization of behaviors, ideas, attitudes, values, beliefs and customs shared by a group of people, and socially transmitted across generations through language and/or other modes of communication. As this definition suggests, cultural processes are of core importance to individual psychological functioning, as they influence the cognitive, affective and behavioral aspects of a range of personal and social activities. Factors that influence the manner in which cultural patterns are manifested in interpersonal relationships include gender, ethnicity, race, socioeconomic status, educational background, neighborhood and geographic region of residence, country of origin, transmigration patterns, religious and political affiliations, and stage in the life-cycle.

Social psychological researchers have emphasized the importance of distinguishing culture-specific from universal

Table 17.12	Social Psychological Factors Influenced by Culture
Internal Processes	**Interpersonal Processes**
Self	Relationships
Person perception	Aggression
Social cognition	Group behavior

psychological findings (Triandis, 1997). This is illustrated by the conceptual distinction between **emics** (findings that differ across cultures and suggest culture-specific psychological principles) and **etics** (findings that apply across cultures and suggest universal psychological principles) (Matsumoto, 1994). Given cultural influences on psychological phenomena, a cross-cultural approach is presumed to be essential for the articulation of universal principles (Moghaddam *et al.*, 1993). Theorists and researchers who take a cultural perspective have argued persuasively that many findings from social psychological research in the USA reflect specific cultural dynamics and are not necessarily universally applicable (Moghaddam *et al.*, 1993; Triandis, 1997). Culture influences the understanding of self, social cognition, relationships and group behavior (Table 17.12).

Culture affects definitions and causal explanations of health and illness, as well as the nature and quality of help-seeking behavior (Kazarian and Evans, 2001; MacLachlan, 1997). Given that one's ethnomedical system influences one's involvement in the health care system as either patient or health professional, it is essential to inquire about the patient's "explanatory models" of health and illness and to be cognizant of the match between the doctor's and patient's world view *vis-à-vis* illness and its treatment (Kleinman, 1988). Further, it behoves health providers and patients to acknowledge that medicine as practiced in hospitals forms a subculture consisting of specific values, beliefs, and practices (i.e., the culture of medicine). In this regard, interactions between patients and health care providers can be viewed as cross-cultural communications, with all participants working to comprehend one another's world views.

Recent work emphasizing the understanding of psychological functioning from a cultural perspective has led mental health practitioners to recognize culture as central to the conceptualization, assessment, and treatment of clinically significant emotional and behavioral problems (Gopaul-McNicol and Armour-Thomas, 2002; Kleinman, 1988; Tseng 2001; Tseng and Streltzer, 2001). A cultural perspective has important implications for defining and conceptualizing normal and abnormal behavior, with some arguing that dichotomizing behavior as either normal or abnormal reflects historically Western scientific cultural constructions (Foulks, 1991). A cultural perspective is also important for developing and implementing culturally sensitive interventions. There is considerable evidence to suggest that culture influences many of the psychological and social variables typically associated with psychological development, including child-rearing practices and customs, constellation and structure of family life, communication and emotional expression, social support networks, frequency and quality of life stress, the ways in which difficulties are defined and managed, and values regarding help-seeking behavior for emotional distress (Foulks, 1991). As cultural differences across these domains vary, manifestations of psychological and personality dysfunction also will differ (Foulks, 1991). This particularly is applicable to disorders that are thought to derive more from social and environmental influences than from biological factors.

Implicit in Western models of psychiatric nosology are a number of culture-bound assumptions regarding mental health and psychiatric disorder. Examples of North American culture-bound biases articulated by Lewis-Fernandez and Kleinman (1994) include: 1) an emphasis on individuality and autonomy (egocentric view of self) as opposed to a more interdependent emphasis (sociocentric view of self); 2) a view that psychopathological conditions have either an organic or a psychological etiology but not both simultaneously (mind–body dualism versus a more integrated somatopsychological view); and 3) an assumption that cultural effects on psychological functioning are epiphenomena underneath which can be found a universally knowable biological reality. The tendency to organize one's understanding of behavior according to these biases must be monitored carefully in work with patients. Further, clinicians and researchers need to contextualize behavior and experience, and use relevant cultural norms to understand behavioral difficulties and their adaptive value (Lewis-Fernandez and Kleinman, 1994).

The importance of cultural considerations in psychiatric diagnosis has increasingly been recognized (Mezzich *et al.*, 1996). Cross-cultural social scientists have investigated psychiatric epidemiology in different cultures, with particular attention to schizophrenia spectrum disorders and mood disorders. This work primarily has been conducted using an etic approach. Although there is considerable evidence that supports the universality of schizophrenia, cross-cultural differences in symptom expression and course have been reported (Kulhara and Chakrabarti, 2001). An additional area of work that approaches diagnostic classification from an emic perspective is that of culture-bound syndromes or folk diagnostic categories, defined as "… certain recurrent, locality-specific patterns of aberrant behavior and experience that appear to fall outside conventional Western psychiatric diagnostic categories" (Simons and Hugnes, 1993, p. 75). These disorders reflect symptom patterns that are linked to the cultural context within which they are embedded. Examples of culture-bound syndromes in Western societies include anorexia nervosa and the type A behavior pattern (Simons and Hugnes, 1993).

In addition to influencing assessment and diagnosis, cultural variables should be taken into account in psychotherapeutic endeavors. In this regard, cultural considerations are important in understanding the conditions under which mental health treatment may be sought, the type of approaches that would be most effective, the clinical stance of the therapist within the treatment setting, and the nature of the therapeutic relationship. Effective psychotherapy requires sensitivity to differences that may affect the therapist's and the patient's perspective on the problem, treatment method, and therapeutic process and objectives. Thus, it is important for therapists to be cognizant of the patient's culturally defined values and belief systems, definitions of normality and psychopathology, problem-solving styles, communication patterns, interpersonal customs and family role behaviors. This cultural perspective is essential when working with adults (Tseng and Streltzer, 2001), children (Canino and Spurlock, 1994; Vargas and Koss-Chioino, 1992) and families (McGoldrick *et al.*, 1996).

Conclusion

Several basic assumptions, articulated cogently by Leary and Maddux (1987), guide the work of mental health professionals whose clinical activities incorporate a social psychological perspective. First, emotional and behavioral dysfunction is understood within the interpersonal and sociocultural context within which it is embedded. Secondly, the social milieu and its associated norms and values contribute to definitions of normality and abnormality. Thirdly, clinical conceptualization, diagnosis and assessment involve the clinician's attribution and attitudinal processes, and those person perception operations that contribute to impression formation and maintenance. Fourthly, psychotherapeutic interventions with individuals, couples, families, or groups are conceptualized as quintessentially social relationships that have as major objectives the enhancement of both individual identity and healthy interpersonal relatedness, which are inextricably interwoven processes.

In a discussion of the place of social psychology in the "Decade of the Brain" (the 1990s), Cacioppo and Berntson (1992) proposed a multilevel analysis for understanding psychological phenomena, integrating various biopsychosocial variables and the interactions among them. In this regard, they maintained that "the level of organization of psychological phenomena can vary from the molecular, to the cellular, to the tissue, to the organ, to the system, to the organism, to the physical environment, to the sociocultural context" (Cacioppo and Berntson, 1992, p. 1020). This so-called social neuroscience approach assumes that the integration of neural and social standpoints on social psychological phenomena can lead to a more comprehensive set of psychological principles based on multiple levels of analysis (Cacioppo *et al.*, 1996; Ito and Cacioppo, 2001). The focus of this chapter has been to highlight the social, interpersonal and sociocultural tiers of this multilevel approach to understanding psychological functioning.

References

Abramson LY, Seligman MEP and Teasdale JT (1978) Learned helplessness in humans: Critique and reformulation. *J Abnorm Psychol* 87, 49–74.

Abramson LY, Metalsky GI and Alloy LB (1989) Hopelessness depression: A theory-based subtype of depression. *Psychol Rev* 96, 358–372.

Ainsworth MDS, Blehar MC, Waters E *et al.* (1978) *Patterns of Attachment: A Psychological Study of the Strange Situation.* Lawrence Erlbaum, Hillsdale, NJ.

Alexander J, Waldon HB, Newberry AM *et al.* (1990) The functional family therapy model, in *Family Therapy for Adolescent Drug Abuse* (eds Friedman AS and Granick S). Lexington Books, Lexington, MA, pp. 183–199.

Amirkhan JH (1990) Applying attribution theory to the study of stress and coping, in *Attribution Theory: Applications to Achievement, Mental Health, and Interpersonal Conflict* (eds Graham S and Folkes VS). Lawrence Erlbaum, Hillsdale, NJ, pp. 79–102.

Bandura A (1997) *Self-Efficacy: The Exercise of Control.* WH Freeman, New York.

Baron RA and Richardson DR (1994) *Human Aggression*, 2nd edn. Plenum Press, New York.

Bartholomew K and Horowitz L (1991) Attachment styles among young adults: A test of a four category model. *J Pers Soc Psychol* 61, 226–244.

Batson CD (1987) Prosocial motivation: Is it ever truly altruistic? In *Advances in Experimental Social Psychology*, Vol. 20 (ed, Berkowitz L). Academic Press, New York, pp. 65–122.

Batson CD (1998) Altruism and prosocial behavior, in *The Handbook of Social Psychology*, Vol. 2, 4th edn. (eds Gilbert DT, Fiske ST, and Lindzey G). McGraw-Hill, New York, pp. 282–316.

Baumeister RF (1998) The self. In The Handbook of Social Psychology, Vol. 1, 4th ed., Gilbert DT, Fiske ST, and Lindzey G (eds). McGrawHill, New York, pp. 680–740.

Baumeister RF (1999) On the interface between personality and social psychology, in *Handbook of Personality: Theory and Research*, 2nd edn. (eds Pervin LA and John OP). Guilford Press, New York, pp. 367–377.

Beach SRH and Tesser A (1995) Self-esteem and the extended self-evaluation maintenance model, in *Efficacy, Agency, and Self-Esteem* (ed Kernis MH). Plenum Press, New York, pp. 145–170.

Beck AT and Freeman A (eds) (1990) *Cognitive Therapy of Personality Disorders.* Guilford Press, New York.

Beck AT, Rush J, Shaw B *et al.* (1979) *Cognitive Therapy of Depression.* Guilford Press, New York.

Beck AT, Emery G, and Greenburg RL (1985) *Anxiety Disorders and Phobias: A Cognitive Perspective.* Basic Books, New York.

Bell-Dolan D and Anderson CA (1999) Attributional processes: An integration of social and clinical psychology, in *The Social Psychology of Emotional and Behavioral Problems: Interfaces of Social and Clinical Psychology* (eds Kowalski RM and Leary MR). American Psychological Association, Washington DC, pp. 37–67.

Bem DJ (1972) Self-perception theory, in *Advances in Experimental Social Psychology*, Vol. 6 (ed Berkowitz L). Academic Press, New York, pp. 1–62.

Benjamin LS (1996) *Interpersonal Diagnosis and Treatment of Personality Disorders*, 2nd edn. Guilford Press, New York.

Berscheid E and Reis HT (1998) Attraction and close relationships, in *The Handbook of Social Psychology*, Vol. 2, 4th edn. (eds Gilbert DT, Fiske ST, and Lindzey G). McGraw-Hill, New York, pp. 193–281.

Bowlby J (1973) *Attachment and Loss, Vol. 2. Separation: Anxiety and Anger.* Basic Books, New York.

Bowlby J (1980) *Attachment and Loss, Vol. 3. Loss: Sadness and Depression.* Basic Books, New York.

Bowlby J (1982) *Attachment and Loss, Vol. 1. Attachment, 2nd edn.* Basic Books, New York.

Bowlby J (1988) *A Secure Base.* Basic Books, New York.

Bradley GW (1978) Self-serving biases in the attribution process: A reexamination of the fact or fiction question. *J Pers Soc Psychol* 13, 420–432.

Bretherton I and Munholland KA (1999) Internal working models in attachment relationships: A construct revisited, in *Handbook of Attachment: Theory, Research, and Clinical Applications* (eds Cassidy J and Shaver PR). Guilford Press, New York, pp. 89–111.

Buss DM and Kenrick DT (1998) Evolutionary social psychology, in *The Handbook of Social Psychology*, Vol. 2, 4th edn. (eds Gilbert DT, Fiske ST, and Lindzey G). McGraw-Hill, New York, pp. 982–1026.

Cacioppo JT and Berntson GG (1992) Social psychological contributions to the Decade of the Brain: Doctrine of multilevel analysis. *Am Psychol* 47, 1019–1028.

Cacioppo JT, Berntson GG and Crites SL Jr. (1996) Social neuroscience: Principles of psychophysiological arousal and response, in *Social Psychology: Handbook of Basic Principles* (eds Higgins ET and Kruglanski AW). Guilford Press, New York, pp. 72–101.

Canino IA and Spurlock J (1994) *Culturally Diverse Children and Adolescents: Assessment, Diagnosis, and Treatment.* Guilford Press, New York.

Contrada RJ, Cather C and O'Leary A (1999) Personality and health: Dispositions and processes in disease susceptibility and adaptation to illness, in *Handbook of Personality: Theory and Research*, 2nd edn. (eds Pervin LA and John OP). Guilford Press, New York, pp. 576–604.

Cooley CF (1902) *Human Nature and the Social Order.* Scribner, New York.

Cooper J and Aronson JM (1992) Attitudes and consistency theories: Implications for mental health, in *The Social Psychology of Mental Health: Basic Mechanisms and Applications* (eds Ruble DN, Constanzo PR, and Oliveri ME). Guilford Press, New York, pp. 279–300.

Curtis RC (ed) (1991) *The Relational Self: Theoretical Convergences in Psychoanalysis and Social Psychology.* Guilford Press, New York.

Deaux K (1992) Focusing on the self: Challenges to self-definition and their consequences for mental health, in *The Social Psychology of Mental Health: Basic Mechanisms and Applications* (eds Ruble

DN, Constanzo PR, and Oliveri ME). Guilford Press, New York, pp. 301–327.

Deci EL and Ryan RM (2000) The "what" and "why" of goal pursuits: Human needs and the self-determination of behavior. *Psychol Inq* 11, 227–268.

Derlega VJ, Hendrick SS, Windstead BA *et al.* (1991) *Psychotherapy as a Personal Relationship*. Guilford Press, New York.

Doane JA and Diamond D (1994) *Affect and Attachment in the Family: A Family-Based Treatment of Major Psychiatric Disorder*. Basic Books, New York.

Eagly AH and Chaiken S (1998) Attitude structure and function, in *The Handbook of Social Psychology*, Vol. 1, 4th edn. (eds Gilbert DT, Fiske ST, and Lindzey G). McGraw-Hill, New York, pp. 269–322.

Fairbairn WRD (1954) *Psychoanalytic Studies of Personality*. Tavistock, London.

Feeney JA (1999) Adult romantic attachment and couple relationships, in *Handbook of Attachment: Theory, Research, and Clinical Applications* (eds Cassidy J and Shaver PR). Guilford Press, New York, pp. 355–377.

Feeney JA, Noller P and Roberts N (2000) Attachment and close relationships, in *Close Relationships: A Sourcebook* (eds Hendrick C and Hendrick SS). Sage Publications, Thousand Oaks, CA, pp. 185–201.

Festinger LA (1957) *A Theory of Cognitive Dissonance*. Row, Peterson, Evanston, IL.

Fiske AP, Kitayama S, Markus HR *et al.* (1998) The cultural matrix of social psychology, in *The Handbook of Social Psychology*, Vol. 2, 4th edn. (eds Gilbert DT, Fiske ST and Lindzey G). McGraw-Hill, New York, pp. 915–981.

Fiske ST and Taylor SE (1991) *Social Cognition*, 2nd edn. McGraw-Hill, New York.

Forsterling F (2001) *Attribution: An Introduction to Theories, Research and Applications*. Psychology Press/Taylor & Francis, Philadelphia.

Forsyth DR (1991) Change in therapeutic groups, in *Handbook of Social and Clinical Psychology: The Health Perspective* (eds Snyder CR and Forsyth DR). Pergamon Press, New York, pp. 664–680.

Forsyth DR and Elliot TR (1999) Group dynamics and psychological well-being: The impact of groups on adjustment and dysfunction, in *The Social Psychology of Emotional and Behavioral Problems: Interfaces of Social and Clinical Psychology* (eds Kowalski RM and Leary MR). American Psychological Association, Washington DC, pp. 339–361.

Foulks EF (1991) Transcultural psychiatry and normal behavior, in *The Diversity of Normal Behavior: Further Contributions to Normatology* (eds Offer D and Sabshin M). Basic Books, New York, pp. 207–238.

Gilbert DT (1998) Ordinary personology, in *The Handbook of Social Psychology*, Vol. 2, 4th edn. (eds Gilbert DT, Fiske ST and Lindzey G). McGraw-Hill, New York, pp. 89–150.

Goffman E (1959) *The Presentation of Self in Everyday Life*. Doubleday Anchor, Garden City, NY.

Gopaul-McNicol SA and Armour-Thomas E (2002) *Assessment and Culture: Psychological Tests with Minority Populations*. Academic Press, San Diego, CA.

Gotlib IH and Abramson LY (1999) Attributional theories of emotion, in *Handbook of Cognition and Emotion* (eds Dalgleish T and Power MJ). John Wiley, New York, pp. 613–636.

Graham S and Folkes VS (1990) *Attribution Theory: Applications to Achievement, Mental Health, and Interpersonal Conflict*. Lawrence Erlbaum, Hillsdale, NJ.

Greenberg JR and Mitchell SA (1983) *Object Relations in Psychoanalytic Theory*. Harvard University Press, Cambridge, MA.

Guntrip H (1969) *Schizoid Phenomena, Object Relations and the Self*. International Universities Press, New York.

Gurman AS and Kniskern DP (eds) (1981) *Handbook of Family Therapy*, Vol. 1. Brunner/Mazel, New York.

Gurman AS and Kniskern DP (eds) (1991) *Handbook of Family Therapy*, Vol. 2. Brunner/Mazel, New York.

Hazan C and Diamond LM (2000) The place of attachment in human mating. *Rev Gen Psychol* 4, 186–204.

Hesse E and Main M (2000) Disorganized infant, child, and adult attachment: Collapse in behavioral and attentional strategies. *J Am Psychoanal Assoc* 48, 1097–1127.

Higgins ET (1987) Self-discrepancy: A theory relating self and affect. *Psychol Rev* 94, 319–340.

Hinde RA (1987) *Individuals, Relationships and Culture: Links Between Ethology and the Social Sciences*. Cambridge University, New York.

Hovland C, Janis I and Kelley HH (1953) *Communication and Persuasion: Psychological Studies of Opinion Change*. Yale University Press, New Haven, CT.

Ito TA and Cacioppo JT (2001) Affect and attitudes: A social neuroscience approach, in *Handbook of Affect and Social Cognition* (ed Forgas JP). Lawrence Erlbaum, Mahwah, NJ, pp. 50–74.

James W (1981) *The Principles of Psychology*. Harvard University Press, Cambridge, MA. (Originally published in 1890).

Janus SS and Janus CL (1994) *The Janus Report on Sexual Behavior*. John Wiley, New York.

Jones EE and Nisbett RE (1971) The actor and the observer: Divergent perceptions of the cases of behavior, in *Attribution: Perceiving the Cause of Behavior* (eds Jones EE, Kanouse DE, Kelley HH *et al.*). General Learning Press, Morristown, NJ, pp. 79–94.

Jordan JV (ed) (1997) *Women's Growth in Diversity: More Writings from the Stone Center*. Guilford Press, New York.

Kaplan HS (1974) *The New Sex Therapy: Active Treatment of Sexual Dysfunction*. Brunner/Mazel, New York.

Kaslow NJ, Kaslow FW and Farber EW (1999) Theories and techniques of marital and family therapy, in *Handbook of Marriage and the Family* (eds Sussman MB, Steinmetz SK, and Peterson GW). Kluwer Academic/Plenum Publishers, New York, pp. 767–792.

Katz D (1960) The functional approach to the study of attitudes. *Pub Opin Q* 24, 163–204.

Kazarian SS and Evans DR (eds) (2001) *Handbook of Cultural Health Psychology*. Academic Press, San Diego, CA.

Kelman HC (1961) Processes of opinion change. *Pub Opin Q* 25, 57–78.

Kim U and Berry JW (eds) (1993) *Indigenous Psychologies: Research and Experience in Cultural Context*. Sage Publications, Newbury Park, CA.

Kinsey AC, Pomerory WB, Martin CE, et al. (1953) Sexual Behavior in the Human Female. WB Saunders, Philadelphia.

Kinsey AC, Pomerory WB, and Martin CE (1948) *Sexual Behavior in the Human Male*. WB Saunders, Philadelphia.

Kleinman A (1988) *Rethinking Psychiatry: From Cultural Category to Personal Experience*. Free Press, New York.

Kohut H (1977) *The Restoration of the Self*. International Universities Press, New York.

Kulhara P and Chakrabarti S (2001) Culture and schizophrenia and other psychotic disorders. *Psychiatr Clin N Am* 24, 449–464.

Leary MR (1995) *Self-Presentation: Impression Management and Interpersonal Behavior*. Westview Press, Boulder, CO.

Leary MR and Maddux JE (1987) Progress toward a viable interface between social and clinical-counseling psychology. *Am Psychol* 42, 904–911.

Levine JM and Moreland RL (1992) Small groups and mental health, in *The Social Psychology of Mental Health: Basic Mechanisms and Applications* (eds Ruble DH, Costanzo PR and Oliveri ME). Guilford Press, New York, pp. 126–165.

Levine JM and Moreland RL (1998) Small Groups, in *The Handbook of Social Psychology*, Vol. 2, 4th edn. (eds Gilbert DT, Fiske ST and Lindzey G). McGraw-Hill, New York, pp. 415–469.

Lewis-Fernandez R and Kleinman A (1994) Culture, personality, and psychopathology. *J Abnorm Psychol* 103, 67–71.

Leyens JP and Fiske ST (1994) Impression formation: From recitals to symphonie fantastique, in *Social Cognition: Impact on Social Psychology* (eds Devine PG, Hamilton DL and Ostrom TM). Academic Press, New York, pp. 39–75.

Lorenz KZ (1970) *Studies on Animal and Human Behavior.* Harvard University Press, Cambridge. MA.

MacLachlan M (1997) *Culture and Health.* John Wiley, New York.

Main M (2000) The organized categories of infant, child and adult attachment: Flexible vs. inflexible attention under attachment-related stress. *J Am Psychoanal Assoc* 48, 1055–1096.

Mason MJ (1991) Family therapy as the emerging context for sex therapy, in *Handbook of Family Therapy*, Vol. 2 (eds Gurman AS and Kniskern DP). Brunner/Mazel, New York, pp. 479–507.

Masters WH and Johnson VE (1970) *Human Sexual Inadequacy.* Little Brown, Boston, MA.

Matsumoto D (1994) *People: Psychology from a Cultural Perspective.* Brooks/Cole, Pacific Grove, CA.

Matsumoto D (ed) (2001) *The Handbook of Culture and Psychology.* Oxford University Press, London.

McDaniel SH, Hepworth J and Doherty WJ (1992) *Medical Family Therapy: A Biopsychosocial Approach to Families with Health Problems.* Basic Books, New York.

McGoldrick M, Giordano J and Pearce JK (eds) (1996) *Ethnicity and Family Therapy*, 2nd edn. Guilford Press, New York.

McGrath JE (1984) *Groups: Interaction and Performance.* Prentice-Hall, Englewood Cliffs, NJ.

Mead GH (1934) *Mind, Self and Society.* University of Chicago Press, Chicago.

Mezzich JE, Kleinman A, Fabrega H Jr., et al. (eds) (1996) Culture and Psychiatric Diagnosis: A DSM-IV Perspective. American Psychiatric Press, Washington DC.

Mitchell SA (2000) *Relationality: From Attachment to Intersubjectivity.* Analytic Press, Hillsdale, NJ.

Moghaddam FM, Taylor DM and Wright SC (1993) *Social Psychology in Cross-Cultural Perspective.* WH Freeman, New York.

Moretti MM and Higgins ET (1999) Own versus other standpoints in self-regulation: Developmental antecedents and functional consequences. *Rev Gen Psychol* 3, 188–223.

Petty RE and Wegener DT (1998) Attitude change: Multiple roles for persuasion variables, in *The Handbook of Social Psychology*, Vol. 1, 4th edn. (eds Gilbert DT, Fiske ST and Lindzey G). McGraw-Hill, New York, pp. 323–390.

Reis HT, Collins WA and Berscheid E (2000) The relationship context of human behavior and development. *Psychol Bull* 126, 844–872.

Rodin J and Salovey P (1989) Health psychology. *Annu Rev Psychol* 10, 533–579.

Roesch SC and Weiner B (2001) A meta-analytic review of coping with illness: Do causal attributions matter? *J Psychosom Res* 50, 205–219.

Rosenstock IM, Strecher VJ and Becker MH (1988) Social learning theory and the health belief model. *Health Educ Q* 15, 175–183.

Ross L (1977) The intuitive psychologist and his shortcomings: Distortions in the attribution process, in *Advances in Experimental Social Psychology*, Vol. 10, (ed Berkowitz L). Academic Press, New York, pp. 173–220.

Rusbult CE and Van Lange PAM (1996) Interdependence processes, in *Social Psychology: Handbook of Basic Principles* (eds Higgins ET and Kruglanski AW). Guilford Press, New York, pp. 564–596.

Ryan RM and Deci EL (2000) Self-determination theory and the facilitation of intrinsic motivation, social development, and well-being. *Am Psychol* 55, 68–78.

Salovey P, Rothman AJ and Rodin J (1998) Health behavior, in *The Handbook of Social Psychology*, Vol. 2, 4th edn. (eds Gilbert DT, Fiske ST and Lindzey G). McGraw-Hill, New York, pp. 633–683.

Schlenker BR and Pontari BA (2000) The strategic control of information: Impression management and self-presentation in daily life, in *Psychological Perspectives on Self and Identity* (eds Tesser A, Felson RB and Suls JM). American Psychological Association, Washington DC, pp. 199–232.

Schneider DJ (1973) Implicit personality theory: A review. *Psychol Bull* 79, 294–309.

Sedikides C and Brewer MB (2001) Individual self, relational self, and collective self: Partners, opponents, or strangers? In *Individual Self, Relational Self, Collective Self* (eds Sedikides C and Brewer MB). Psychology Press, Philadelphia, pp. 1–4.

Shaver PR and Hazan C (1993) Adult romantic attachment: Theory and evidence, in *Advances in Personal Relationships*, Vol. 4 (eds Perlman D and Jones W). Jessica Kingsley, London, 29–70.

Shelton S (1998) The doctor–patient relationship, in *Human Behavior: An Introduction for Medical Students*, 2nd edn. (ed Stoudemire A). Lippincott-Raven, Philadelphia, pp. 3–35.

Shepperd JA and Kwavnick KD (1999) Maladaptive image maintenance. In The Social Psychology of Emotional and Behavioral Problems: Interfaces of Social and Clinical Psychology, Kowalski RM and Leary MR (eds). American Psychological Association, Washington DC, pp. 249–277.

Sherif CW, Sherif M and Nebergall RE (1965) *Attitude and Attitude Change: The Social Judgment–Involvement Approach.* WB Saunders, Philadelphia.

Simons RC and Hugnes CC (1993) Culture-bound syndromes, in *Culture, Ethnicity, and Mental Illness* (ed Gaw AC). American Psychiatric Press, Washington DC, pp. 75–99.

Smith MB, Bruner JS and White RW (1956) *Opinions and Personality.* John Wiley, New York.

Sperling MB and Berman WH (eds) (1994) *Attachment in Adults: Clinical and Developmental Perspectives.* Guilford Press, New York.

Spiegel D and Kimerling R (2001) Group psychotherapy for women with breast cancer: Relationships among social support, emotional expression, and survival, in *Emotion, Social Relationships, and Health* (eds Ryff CD and Singer BH). Oxford University Press, New York, pp. 97–123.

Spira JL (ed) (1997) *Group Therapy for Medically Ill Patients.* Guilford Press, New York.

Sroufe LA (2002) From infant attachment to promotion of adolescent autonomy: Prospective, longitudinal data on the role of parents in development, in *Parenting and the Child's World: Influences on Academic, Intellectual, and Social-Emotional Development. Monographs in Parenting* (eds Borkowski JG and Ramey SL). Lawrence Erlbaum, Mahwah, NJ, pp. 187–202.

Sroufe LA, Egeland B and Kreutzer T (1990) The fate of early experience following developmental change: Longitudinal approaches to individual adaptation in childhood. *Child Dev* 61, 1363–1373.

Staats AW and Staats CK (1958) Attitudes established by classical conditioning. *J Abnorm Soc Psychol* 57, 37–40.

Strecher VJ, Campion VL and Rosenstock IM (1997) The health belief model and health behavior, in *Handbook of Health Behavior Research I: Personal and Social Determinants* (ed Gochman DS). Plenum Press, New York, pp. 71–91.

Stroebe W and Stroebe M (1996) The social psychology of social support, in *Social Psychology: Handbook of Basic Principles* (eds Higgins ET and Kruglanski AW). Guilford Press, New York, pp. 597–621.

Sullivan HS (1953) *The Interpersonal Theory of Psychiatry.* WW Norton, New York.

Swann WB Jr (1983) Self-verification: Bringing social reality into harmony with self, in *Psychological Perspectives on the Self*, Vol. 2 (eds Suls J and Greenwald AG). Lawrence Erlbaum, Hillsdale, NJ, pp. 33–66.

Swann WB Jr. (1997) The trouble with change: Self-verification and allegiance to the self. *Psychol Sci* 8, 177–180.

Tangney JP and Salovey P (1999) Problematic social emotions: Shame, guilt, jealousy, and envy, in *The Social Psychology of Emotional and Behavioral Problems: Interfaces of Social and Clinical Psychology* (eds Kowalski RM and Leary MR). American Psychological Association, Washington DC, pp. 167–195.

Taylor SE (1998) The social being in social psychology, in *The Handbook of Social Psychology*, Vol. 1, 4th edn. (eds Gilbert DT, Fiske ST, and Lindzey G). McGraw-Hill, New York, pp. 58–95.

Tesser A (1991) Social versus clinical approaches to self psychology: The self-evaluation maintenance model and Kohutian object relations theory, in *The Relational Self: Theoretical Convergences in Psychoanalysis and Social Psychology* (ed Curtis RC). Guilford Press, New York, 257–281.

Tesser A, Felson RB and Suls JM (eds) (2000) *Psychological Perspectives on Self and Identity.* American Psychological Association, Washington DC.

Thibaut JW and Kelley HH (1959) *The Social Psychology of Groups.* John Wiley, New York.

Tice DM and Baumeister RF (2001) The primacy of the interpersonal self, in *Individual Self, Relational Self, Collective Self* (eds Sedikides C and Brewer MB). Psychology Press, Philadelphia, pp. 71–88.

Triandis HC (1997) A cross-cultural perspective on social psychology, in *The Message of Social Psychology: Perspectives on Mind in Society* (eds McGarty C and Haslam SA). Blackwell, Cambridge, MA, pp. 342–354.

Tseng WS (2001) *Handbook of Cultural Psychiatry.* Academic Press, San Diego, CA.

Tseng WS and Streltzer J (eds) (2001) *Culture and Psychotherapy: A Guide to Clinical Practice.* American Psychiatric Press, Washington DC.

Vargas LA and Koss-Chioino JD (eds) (1992) *Working with Culture: Psychotherapeutic Interventions with Ethnic Minority Children and Adolescents.* Jossey-Bass, San Francisco, CA.

von Bertalanffy L (1968) *General Systems Theory: Foundations, Development, and Applications*, Rev. edn. George Braziller, New York.

Watson JC (2002) Re-visioning empathy, in *Humanistic Psychotherapies: Handbook of Research and Practice* (eds Cain DJ and Seeman J). American Psychological Association, Washington DC, pp. 445–471.

Weiner B and Graham G (1999) Attribution in personality psychology, in *Handbook of Personality: Theory and Research*, 2nd edn. (eds Pervin LA and John OP). Guilford Press, New York, pp. 605–628.

West ML and Sheldon-Keller AE (1994) *Patterns of Relating: An Adult Attachment Perspective.* Guilford Press, New York.

Winnicott DW (1965) *The Maturational Processes and the Facilitating Environment: Studies in the Theory of Emotional Development.* International Universities Press, New York.

Yalom ID (1995) *The Theory and Practice of Group Psychotherapy*, 4th edn. Basic Books, New York.

CHAPTER

18 Psychoanalytic Theories

Psychoanalysis is a clinical therapy originally developed by Sigmund Freud (1856–1939) for the treatment of neuroses. The term refers as well to a theory of psychopathology underlying the therapeutic practice; a general theory of the mind based on the understanding arising from the clinical procedure and other sources, and a mode of research into mental life that is inherent in, and inextricably intertwined with, the therapeutic process. Although the contemporary practice of psychoanalysis derives historically from Freud's original contributions, it has evolved like any other discipline. Beginning with Freud and the inception of psychoanalysis, the section traces the important trends in the maturation of analytic theory and its current state of development.

Development and Major Concepts

Freud's Contributions

Dreams

Freud's study (1900, 1901) of dreams during his self-analysis and in his work with patients resulted in an elaborate understanding of the workings of the mind. The analysis of dreams continues to hold a prominent position in psychoanalytic practice. Dreams give expression to unconscious wishes in disguised form and generally represent their fulfillment or gratification. Analysis of dreams can provide conscious access to unconscious drives, wishes, fantasies and associated repressed infantile memories, providing what Freud called the "royal road to the unconscious".

The dream that is remembered on awakening is referred to as the **manifest dream**. Its component elements include sensory stimuli occurring during sleep, the **day residue** and the **latent dream content**. The day residue consists of experiences of events of the preceding day or days, often associated in the mind with unconscious wishes. The latent dream content is the set of unconscious infantile urges, wishes, and fantasies that seek gratification during the dreaming state of blocked motor discharge and regression.

Freud hypothesized a **dream censor** whose function is to keep the unconscious latent content from conscious awareness, thereby preventing the emergence of anxiety and awakening from sleep. The surreal and fantastic quality of the remembered manifest dream is a reflection of the influence of **dream work** and **primary process** unconscious mentation (Table 18.1): depiction of immediate gratifications, absence of the rules of logic of conscious thought, merging of past and present, absence of negatives, loss of distinction between opposites and representation of a whole by a part. The activity of the dream work involves a set of mental mechanisms designed to disguise and distort the latent content in keeping with the function of the dream censor.

Table 18.1 Primary Process Thinking
Does not follow rules of logic
Spatial and temporal relationships are not preserved
Thoughts and actions are equivalent
"Dream language"

In psychoanalytic treatment, the analysis of dreams attempts to take this process backward, starting with the patient's narration of the dream and then observing the patient's associations to the manifest elements, with the goal of obtaining insight into the dreamer's unconscious wishes, memories and infantile fantasies, and processes of defense.

Childhood Sexuality

In his analyses of adult patients and observations of children, Freud (1905) became convinced of the influence of early sexual fantasies on the formation of neurotic symptoms and of the universality of sexual wishes throughout life including early childhood. The term **sexuality** is used in this context to refer not exclusively to adult genital sexuality but to a variety of body stimulations that are pleasurable and sensually gratifying. He postulated a developmental sequence of body zones that become primary foci of erotic sensations and mental organization (Table 18.2): oral, anal (including perianal and urethral) and genital (phallic). During development, there is a more or less orderly progression from one zone to the next, with pleasure being derived from sucking, biting, tasting, touching, looking, smelling, filling, emptying, penetrating and being penetrated. In the neuroses, the repressed component instincts become an unconscious source of symptom formation.

Fixation (Table 18.3) at a particular phase of development may occur if there is insufficient mastery of issues pertinent to that phase. Fixations result in continued manifestations of phase specific issues in a person's behavior, influencing later personality adjustment (e.g., the anal organization of the obsessional character). **Regression** (Table 18.3), a return to a less mature level

Table 18.2 Freud's Stages of Psychosexual Development
Oral: birth to 18 mo
Anal: 18 mo to 3 yr
Genital: 3 to 6 yr
Latency: 6 yr to puberty
Adolescence: puberty

Essentials of Psychiatry   Jerald Kay and Allan Tasman

Table 18.3	Responses to Developmental Stress
Regression	
Use of behavioral and emotional solutions from a developmental phase earlier than the present conflict	
Fixation	
Overreliance on behavioral and emotional solutions from the phase in which the conflict occurs	

of mental organization, may occur in the context of stressors or conflict that overtaxes the adaptive capacities of an individual.

The first of the phases described by Freud is the **oral phase** (Table 18.4), which encompasses approximately the first 18 months of life. During this phase, the mouth, lips and tongue are the primary sources of sensual gratification. The activities of sucking, swallowing, mouthing and biting, as well as the experience of being held during feeding, form a cognitive template for the organization of fantasy and relatedness to others. The infant at this stage is dependent on mother for nurturance, protection and sustenance. A favorable outcome of this stage is the establishment of a capacity to feel trust and safety in a dependent

Table 18.4	Characteristics of Developmental Phases
Oral	
Urgency of needs	
Extreme dependency	
No consideration of others	
Low frustration tolerance	
Separation anxiety	
Anal	
Need for control and autonomy	
Orderliness, obstinacy, punctuality	
Beginning dyadic relationships	
Conflict over autonomy and compliance	
Guilt	
Genital	
Oedipus complex	
Emergence of genital sexuality	
Concerns about self-image	
Shift from dyadic to triadic relationships	
Latency	
Waning of Oedipus complex	
Decreased emphasis on sexual gratification	
Focus on same-sex relationships	
Emphasis on development of autonomous ego functions	
Adolescence	
Recapitulates early phases	
Separation from family	
Important bonds with peers	
Revival of sexual interest	
Identity formation	

relationship, a sureness that needs will be recognized and gratified, and a minimum of conflict about aggressive wishes occurring during moments of frustration. Excessive neglect or deprivation during this period may result in adult feelings of interpersonal insecurity, mistrust, envy, depression, excessive dependency, anticipation of rejection by others and proneness to moments of diffuse rage.

The **anal phase** (see Table 18.4) emerges with the development of increasing neuromuscular control of the anal and urethral sphincters and takes place from about 18 months to 3 years. Fantasy organizes around anal pleasure and anal functions such as withholding, expelling and controlling. Because of the child's increased motor skills, language development and emerging autonomy, she or he is expected to take more of an active part in self-care activities, including using the toilet. Related to toileting, power struggles may ensue around the child's soiling or withholding. Anger is felt toward those in control of this educative process, but the child also wishes to please them. The child in the anal phase experiences considerable ambivalence around expelling versus retaining (giving versus keeping), obedience and submission versus defiance and protest, and cleanliness and orderliness versus messiness. Fixation at this stage results in a personality organized around anal erotism and its associated conflicts, characterized by wishes to dominate and control people or life situations, rigidity, defiance and anger toward authority, neatness, orderliness, messiness, parsimony, frugality and obstinacy.

The **phallic** or **phallic–oedipal** or **genital phase** (see Table 18.4) occurs from the ages of 3 to about 5 or 6 years. At the onset of this period, sensual pleasure has become most highly focused around the genitals, and masturbatory sensations more closely resemble the usual sense of the word **sexual**. The child at this time has become even more autonomous and has more sophisticated motor and language skills, conceptual capabilities and elaborate fantasies. The child is better able to recognize feelings of love, hate, jealousy and fear; has a more distinct recognition of the anatomical difference between the sexes; and appreciates that the parents have an intimate sexual relationship from which the child is excluded. Thinking about relatedness to others shifts from the largely dyadic (mother–child) quality of the prephallic phases to an appreciation of relational triangles.

Freud recognized in his patients' associations that there were regularly occurring incestuous fantasies and wishes toward the parent of the opposite sex that were involved in the formation of neurotic difficulties. He termed this phenomenon the **Oedipus complex**, in reference to the story of Oedipus, who unknowingly killed his father and married his mother. In the midst of the Oedipus complex, the child wishes to possess exclusively the parent of the opposite sex and to eliminate the parent of the same sex. The jealousy and murderous rage felt toward the same-sex parent are accompanied by fears of retaliation and physical harm. Because these fantasies are associatively linked to pleasurable genital sensations, the child has specific unconscious fears of being castrated, which Freud referred to as the **castration complex**. The oedipal phase proceeds differently in boys and girls.

Successful passage through the phallic phase includes resolution of the Oedipus complex and repression of oedipal fantasies. The child internalizes the parental prohibitions and moral values and demonstrates a greater capacity to channel instinctual energies into constructive activities. Excessive conflict or traumatization during this phase may lead to a personality organized around oedipal fantasies and conflicts or a proneness defensively to regress to anal or oral organization.

During the **latency phase** (see Table 18.4), from age 6 years to puberty, play and learning take a prominent position in the child's behavioral repertoire as cognitive process matures further. Although Freud believed that the sexual urges become relatively quiescent during this phase, observation indicates that they are expressed in derivative form in the child's play. At puberty and through adolescence, genital urges once again predominate, but there is now a consolidation of sexual identity and a movement toward adult sexuality (Figure 18.1).

Libido Theory

Freud's continued consideration of the sources and nature of the sexual drives led to his dynamic model of the mind referred to as

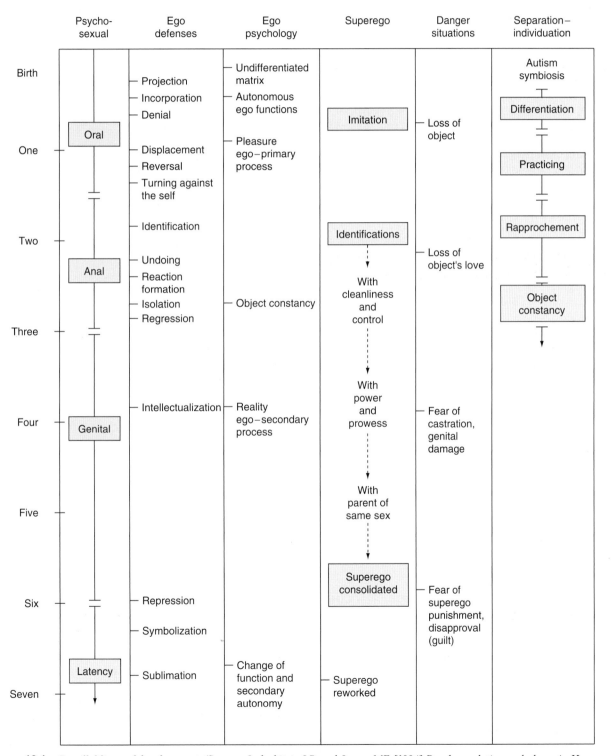

Figure 18.1 *Parallel lines of development. (Source: Inderbitzin LB and James ME [1994] Psychoanalytic psychology, in Human Behavior: An Introduction for Medical Students, 2nd edn. [ed. Stoudemire A]. JB Lippincott, Philadelphia, p. 131.)*

Table 18.5	Libido (Drive) Theory
Assumes that biological "needs" (drives) fuel behavior	
The aim of behavior is to gratify the drive	
Drives are either sexual or aggressive in nature	

libido theory (Table 18.5). This theory attempted to explain the observation that behavior and mental activity are not only triggered by external stimuli (as in the reflex arc) but also generated by primary internal processes. Freud defined instinct as "a concept on the frontier between the mental and the somatic, as the psychical representative of the stimuli originating within the organism and reaching the mind, as a measure of the demand made upon the mind for work in consequences of its connection with the body". Regardless of the specifics of their origins, derivatives of the instincts are experienced mentally as compelling urges and a source of motivation.

Although Freud had given up the idea that sexual traumatization was always the cause of psychoneurotic symptoms, he maintained the view that the sexual instinct played an etiological role in the neuroses and that sexual stimulation exerted a predominant force on mental activity throughout life. Freud termed this force **libido**. The discharge of libido is experienced as pleasure; the welling up of libido without discharge is felt as tension or unpleasure. According to the **pleasure principle**, the individual seeks pleasure (through the discharge of libidinal tension) and avoids unpleasure. The primary process quality of unconscious mentation follows the pleasure principle as it maintains its focus on the gratification of wishes. As the mind develops, conscious mentation becomes more governed by the **reality principle** (Freud, 1911) involving a shift from fantasy to perception of and action on reality. The secondary process form of conscious thought follows the reality principle. Under the influence of the reality principle, gratification of wishes may be delayed with the aim of eventually achieving greater and/or safer pleasure.

The sexual instinct has four defining components: **source**, **pressure** (or **impetus**), **aim**, and **object**. **Source** refers to the biological substrate of the instinct. **Pressure** is the amount of force or "demand for work" of the instinct. The **aim** is the action designed to accomplish release of tension and satisfaction. An **object** is the target of desire, the person or thing through which gratification is accomplished. Although the libido theory has been criticized because it was based on 19th century German scientism, it has served as a useful metaphor to understand pleasure, attachments, and the dynamic processes of mental activity.

From the Topographical to the Structural Model

According to the topographical theory, three regions or systems of the mind exist as defined by their relationship to conscious thought: the conscious, preconscious and unconscious. The **conscious** mind registers sensations from the outside world and from internal processes, and is the agency of ordinary wakeful thought. Conscious mentation follows the reality principle and uses secondary process logic. The **preconscious** includes mental contents that can gain access into consciousness by the focusing of attention. The **unconscious** is defined from three basic angles: descriptively, it consists of all mental processes and contents operating outside conscious awareness; dynamically, these processes and contents are kept actively repressed or censored by the expenditure of mental energy to prevent the anxiety or repugnance that would accompany their conscious recognition; and as a mental system, it is a part of the mind that operates in accordance with the pleasure principle using primary process logic.

Over time, Freud encountered clinical phenomena that were not adequately accounted for by the topographical model. Freud revised his theory of mental systems to include the structural model, but the useful conception of the dynamic unconscious and the particular qualities of conscious, preconscious and unconscious mentation have been retained.

Theory of Narcissism

In all mental functioning, it is possible to observe the balance between libido deployed toward objects and libido directed toward the self. For example, when a person is in love, much libido is attached to the loved object, even to the extent that the person feels himself or herself diminished (from decreased ego libido). During physical illness or hypochondriacal states, libido is pulled toward the ego so the person appears preoccupied with the body and uninterested in the world. According to the pleasure principle, the mind seeks to discharge libido, and if it is dammed up, symptoms will result. In neurotic persons, excess object libido has accumulated and, undischarged, produces anxiety. In psychotic persons, ego libido has been prevented from being discharged outward, so it is discharged inward, resulting in hypochondriacal anxiety and megalomania.

Internal judgmental processes and self-regard are also addressed by the theory of narcissism. In normal adults, most evidence of the operation of ego libido has been repressed. A new target of self-love has been constructed, the **ego ideal**, a forerunner of the superego concept, consisting of ideas and wishes for how one would like to be. Similarly, love objects may become the subject of idealization. Freud theorized a separate psychic agency, which he called the superego (see below), that attends to ensuring narcissistic satisfaction and measuring self-reflection, censoring and repression. Living up to the ideal, loving oneself and being loved, reflects attempts to restore a state comparable to the primary narcissism of infancy.

Melancholia

In *Mourning and Melancholia* Freud (1917), developed a theory to explain processes of guilt, internal self-punishment and depression. To do this, he contrasted states of grief or mourning with the condition of melancholia, now called depression. Both have in common the experience of pain and sadness, and both are brought on by the experience of loss, but the person in mourning maintains her or his positive self-regard, whereas the person with melancholia feels dejected, loses interest in the world, shows a diminished capacity to love, inhibits all activities and exhibits low self-regard in the form of self-reproaches. In mourning, libido is gradually withdrawn from the object attachment; in melancholia, the ego feels depleted or comes under attack as though "one part of the ego sets itself over against the other, judges it critically, and as it were, takes it as its object". This critical agency (again a theoretical forerunner of the superego) comes to operate independently of the ego.

The self-accusations of the person with melancholia seem to fit best with criticism that might be leveled against the lost object. In the case of suicidal impulses, the melancholic person

Table 18.6	Structural Theory

Id

First to develop
Completely unconscious
Contains all drives
Ruled by pleasure principle
No awareness of reality

Ego

Second structure to develop
Operates on reality principle
Mediates conflict among id, ego, and superego
Provides reality testing
Monitors quality of interpersonal relations
Provides synthesis and coordination
Carries out primary autonomous functions
Defends against anxiety

Superego

Third structure to develop
Self-criticism based on moral values
Self-punishment
Self-praise based on ego ideal
Most functions are unconscious

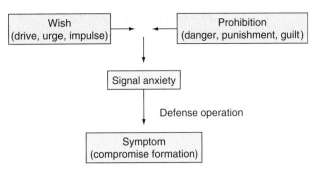

Figure 18.2 *Freud's theory of symptom formation.*

id generates the motivational push for gratification of sexual and aggressive wishes.

The **ego** grows out of the id early in human development. Its functions include perception, interpretation of perceptions, voluntary movement, modulation of affects and impulses, cognition, memory, judgment and adaptation to reality. Subject to conflicting forces from the id, the superego and reality, the ego synthesizes mental compromises that provide gratification of instinctual wishes in accord with reality considerations and the moral demands of the superego.

The **superego**, which develops as an outgrowth of both the ego and id, consists of the moral standards, values and prohibitions that have been internalized throughout childhood and adolescence. It is the source of internal punishment, which is felt as guilt, and of internal reward. Early in development, the superego has a harsh and archaic quality. During maturation under optimal conditions, it becomes less harsh and comes to include loving components as well. In the structural model, the ego ideal (discussed earlier) is considered a component of the superego, accounting for feelings of shame and pride.

Anxiety and Symptom Formation

With the elaboration of the structural theory, Freud progressively viewed the nature of anxiety and the origin of symptoms (Figure 18.2) differently. According to his original theory, anxiety resulted from the accumulation of undischarged sexual tensions caused by inadequate sexual activity in the actual neuroses or by inhibitions due to repression in the psychoneuroses. Later, it became clear that anxiety was more closely related to fear occurring in response to perceived dangers, either external or internal. This led to a focus on the ego, one of whose functions is to anticipate and negotiate danger situations. A dangerous or traumatic situation is one in which excessive stimulation threatens to overwhelm the ego's capacity for delay and compromise.

The ego has as one of its tasks the continual formation of **compromises** among id wishes, the prohibitions and moral standards of the superego, and the dictates of reality. If these

seems to be directing at himself or herself the sadism and murderous wishes felt toward the disappointing or lost other. Freud theorized that in the context of the loss of an ambivalently held object, the ego incorporates, or forms a narcissistic identification with, the object. Hostility originally felt toward the object is now directed at the self, giving rise to feelings of torment, suffering and self-debasement. A predisposition to melancholia may thus result from forming narcissistic object attachments and identifications.

Dual-instinct Theory

Freud had originally considered two types of instincts, the sexual and the ego (self-preservative) instincts, and considered sadism to represent a fusion of the two, with hostility occurring in the context of frustrated libidinal strivings. However, this theory did not adequately address psychological situations in which destructive tendencies seem to be operating independently of libidinal or self-preservative drives.

Freud concluded that there must be a separate instinct of aggression, whose aim is destructiveness. The aggressive drive is at work in impulses to harm, in the desire for control and power, in sadistic or masochistic behaviors, in guilt and depression, and in the persecutory fears of paranoid individuals.

Structural Model

On the basis of the preceding considerations, Freud revised his theory of the mind into what is now known as the structural or tripartite model (Table 18.6). He conceived of three mental agencies operating in the psyche: the id, the ego and the superego. The **id** is the biological source of instinctual drives, operating unconsciously and following the pleasure principle. The activity of the

Table 18.7	Typical Situations of Danger

Fear of instincts (traumatic overstimulation)
Fear of object loss
Fear of loss of love
Fear of castration (body injury)
Fear of guilt (moral anxiety)

Table 18.8	Characteristic Defenses of Paranoid–Schizoid Position

Projection
Introjection
Projective identification
Splitting
Idealization
Omnipotence
Denial

compromises are successful, anxiety will operate predominantly on a signal level and behavior will be both sufficiently gratifying and acceptable in reality. A **symptom neurosis** occurs if these compromises are felt as uncomfortable, painful, or maladaptive.

Post-freudian Ego Psychology

Ego, Defense and Adaptation

Anna Freud laid out a categorization of defense mechanisms (1936) (Table 18.8). In discussing the preliminary stages of defense that are first used by the ego to avoid pain from the external world, she succeeded in integrating two main themes in the development of the ego concept: defense and relations with external reality. Anna Freud advocated a shift of the analyst's attention to the ego as the proper field for observation, in order to gain a picture of its functioning in relation to the other two psychic structures, **id** and **superego**. This more detailed methodical attention to the mind's surface, which includes manifestations of unconscious ego activities, provides a much clearer view of the actual workings of the mind. Her recommendation that the analyst listen from a point equidistant from id, ego and superego emphasized the importance of observing neutrally the influence of all three psychic agencies. The ego wards off not only derivatives of instinctual drives but also **affects** that are intimately connected with the drives. She advocated that priority be given to the interpretation of the defenses against affects, as well as defenses against instinctual drives.

Other Psychoanalytic Perspectives

Object Relations Theory

There is no unitary theory of object relations; rather, it is a variety of theories that differ from each other in important ways and are often contradictory. For some theorists, object relations refers primarily to interpersonal relations; others emphasize that the concept refers not to external interpersonal relationships but to specific intrapsychic structures. The concept of an inner world inhabited by mental representations of the self and of objects is central to all object relations theories. This inner world is constructed by the individual through the more or less successful integration of the internalized representations of real significant external figures with whom the subject has interacted.

Melanie Klein

Klein's (Klein, 1937, 1946) theoretical formulations grew out of her observations of the psychotic children she treated. Although some of her controversial ideas have never gained acceptance in mainstream American psychoanalytic thought, her formulations

about the importance of aggression and envy, particularly in more primitively organized patients, as well as her understanding of primitive defensive operations have been central in the thinking of later object relations theorists.

Klein believed that fantasy exists from the beginning of life and is by definition the mental expression of the instincts. She conceptualized the neonate as having an active inner world of fantasy based on its innate libidinal and aggressive drives and their aims. The death instinct is central to Klein's theories. It finds its expression in earliest infancy in aggression against the object and the self.

Klein modified Freud's theories of psychological development drastically. As mentioned, she focused predominantly on infancy, describing two psychological "positions" during the first year of life (which was for Freud the oral stage of development). These are the paranoid–schizoid position (Table 18.8) during the first 6 months of life and the depressive position during the second 6 months. The paranoid–schizoid position is characterized by the defenses of projection, introjection, projective identification, splitting, idealization, omnipotence and denial (Klein, 1946).

These defenses are termed primitive defenses because they have their origin in early development, in contrast to the higher-level defenses that evolve later. **Projection** is the defensive externalization of a threatening internal impulse, ideal, or feeling. Because this is the predominant defense of earliest infancy, the young infant believes that the dangerous impulse, idea, or feeling, which actually originated from within as a manifestation of its own intense drives, is coming from an external source. Therefore, the feared threat is perceived as external rather than internal. This results in anxiety about being attacked from without, termed paranoid anxiety.

Introjection takes place when an external object is taken inside (in fantasy) and becomes part of the internal rather than

Table 18.9	Erikson's Stages of Development	
Psychosexual Stage	Psychosocial Crisis	Basic Strength
Oral–sensory (infancy)	Basic trust vs. basic mistrust	Hope
Anal–muscular (early childhood)	autonomy vs. shame and doubt	Will
Genital–locomotor (play age)	Initiative vs. shame and guilt	Purpose
Latency (school age)	Industry vs. inferiority	Competence
Puberty (adolescence)	Identity vs. identity confusion	Fidelity
Genitality (young adulthood)	Intimacy vs. isolation	Love
Procreativity (adulthood)	Generativity vs. stagnation	Care
Generalization of sensual modes (old age)	Integrity vs. despair	Wisdom

Source: Modified from Erikson EH (1982) *The Life Cycle Completed*. WW Norton, New York, pp. 32–33. Copyright 1985, WW Norton.

the external world. The paranoid position is characterized by projection and introjection taking place in cycles.

Projective identification, as conceptualized by Klein, is a complicated primitive defense that involves the projection of an internal object (usually a bad one) into an external object, followed by identification with the external object that is now experienced by the infant as having been contaminated by the bad object.

Splitting is the intrapsychic separation of the object into different partial objects. Typically, an unrealistically all-good (idealized) object and an equally unrealistically all-bad object are constructed. In the course of normal development, in the presence of adequate parenting that provides the consistent availability of predominantly benign external objects, the cycle of projection and introjection gradually results in the introjection of more benign aspects of the external object (parent or other caretaker), and the bad internal object is gradually detoxified.

Donald W. Winnicott

Donald W. Winnicott was both a practicing pediatrician and a psychoanalyst for most of his professional life. He worked with many categories of patients – including regressed adults, disturbed and delinquent adolescents, and problem children – and treated mother–infant-toddler pairs. Working with such a diverse population of patients, he experienced the deficiencies of both the libido and the structural theories. The libido theory focuses on drives and anergic concepts; the structural theory concentrates on oedipal development and, in Freud's formulation, places the "narcissistic neuroses" (i.e., the psychoses) in a separate group without a framework for treatment. Although he found the existing theories to be problematic, Winnicott attempted to fit his ideas within them. He handled his disagreements with Freud's ideas by reinterpreting them to meet his need to deal with highly disturbed early relationships. For example, he reworked the Oedipus complex to emphasize Klein's conflict between love and hate, rather than Freud's conflict between instinctual desires and fear of castration. (Winnicott acknowledged his debt to Klein, particularly with reference to the depressive position; Winnicott, 1954–55). Another way in which Winnicott reinterpreted Freudian theory was to focus on the central function of an early maternal "holding environment". This primacy of early bonding contradicted Freud's concept of "primary narcissism", which held that the infant is at first not oriented toward others and that relationships become important only later, secondary to drive frustration.

Every individual, according to Winnicott (1960), develops **true** and **false selves**. Insofar as the mother is empathically attuned to her child, without intruding on the child, there is a core feeling of wholeness and goodness from which the true self develops. With appropriate "mirroring", the child learns to play, to be creative and to be alone with comfort. Those developmental achievements create the **fundamental organizer**, the true self (at times also called the **ego** by Winnicott). However, insofar as there is a mismatch in the relationship, the child's development is stunted, and the child develops a false self. In healthy people, the false self is relatively minimal. It is represented by politeness and social manners; however, in extreme states of illness, it may be the main self-representation. A lifelong feeling of unreality and futility results, with a severely unempathic mother, in Winnicott's view. One positive function of the false self is that it protects the nascent true self from a damaging environment.

Winnicott's (1951) **transitional object** is a concrete, real external object (unlike the intrapsychic objects that we have been discussing). It is the infant's first "not me" possession and is imbued psychologically with attributes of both mother and infant. The transitional object evolves out of activities occurring in the "space" between infant and mother. These activities generally have close links to the mouth or the mother's body. For example, the child may at first put a fist or thumb in the mouth or stroke the corner of a blanket. The blanket gradually becomes special and essential to the child (the familiar security blanket). A stuffed toy such as teddy bear or even a hard toy may become a transitional object. This process is based on the facilitating, appropriate response of the mother. The blanket may become smelly, yet it must not be washed; and the teddy bear may become tattered, yet it must accompany the toddler everywhere. The evolution of the transitional object is the precursor of the child's ability to play. As an intermediary object, the transitional object also serves as a precursor of the ability to be alone. There is wide variation as to when the transitional object develops, but it usually evolves from about 4 to 12 months.

John Bowlby

Bowlby began his study of the attachment of children to their caregivers in the late 1940s. The observations clearly confirmed that early separation produced extreme distress in children and that there were significant long-term adverse effects on the children as a result of even relatively brief separations. These initial observations, combined with the fact that there was at the time no adequate theoretical framework for understanding the profound effects of separation, led Bowlby to research and formulate theories about attachment, separation reactions, related anxiety, depression and psychopathological processes originating in disturbances in attachment.

Bowlby's major thesis was that the child's tie (attachment) to the object, for which he preferred the term **attachment-figure**, is primary and instinctive (in the sense of instincts shared by humans and animals rather than in Freud's sense of instinctual drives). This attachment is **not** secondary to the gratification of any drive. It is independent of the need for food and warmth and of any other striving. He strongly opposed the theoretical position that there is **ever** an early objectless state.

Bowlby went on to extend his observations of attachment behaviors and responses to separation across various cultures, citing anthropological observations. "No form of behavior is accompanied by stronger feeling than is attachment behavior. The figures towards whom it is directed are loved and their advent is greeted with joy. So long as a child is in the unchallenged presence of a principal attachment-figure, or within easy reach, he feels secure. A threat of loss creates anxiety, and actual loss sorrow: both, moreover, are likely to arouse anger" (Bowlby, 1969, p. 209). For Bowlby, the unpleasurable affects of anxiety, grief and anger were **secondary** to the thwarting of attachment.

Margaret Mahler

According to Mahler (1975) the newborn does not differentiate internal from external stimuli; there is only tension and satiation. By the second month, the infant begins the "normal symbiotic phase", in which there is a relationship characterized by an "omnipotent fusion", a "delusion of a common boundary" with "the need-satisfying object". From the infant's perspective, mother and child are a "dual unity". If the symbiotic period progresses normally, the infant begins to develop "memory islands" and a "core sense of self", which are preparatory for the "hatching" that will occur at about 5 months. In her description of this period, Mahler used the concepts of libido theory but also referred to both Rene Spitz's observations of the first months of life* and to Winnicott's concept of the holding environment.

What follows these earliest months, the period from about 5 months to beyond 3 years, is termed "the psychological birth of the human infant" by Mahler. During this time, the stages of the separation–individuation process occur. Mahler formulated a series of subphases of this process. In summary, the subphases are:

1. Differentiation: 4 to 8 or 9 months. During these months, there is the "first tentative" pushing away from "completely passive lap-babyhood". The 5- to 6-month-old infant gradually begins to creep. During this time, transitional objects develop (a term coined by Winnicott and discussed earlier in this section). The infant soon begins differentiating, with more or less anxiety, the faces of strangers from primary caretakers.
2. Practicing
   a. Early: 7 months to about 1 year. This subphase overlaps with differentiation. Infants begin to crawl and stand. They become upset if they end up too far away, frequently paddling back to mother for "emotional refueling".
   b. Practicing subphase proper: about 12 to 18 months. This subphase begins with walking and ushers in a "love affair with the world". The children are frequently elated, curious and adventurous. They are delightful to observe but must be carefully watched because they are likely to dash blithely into precarious situations. They tend to be impervious to minor falls and other mishaps.
3. Rapprochement: gradually, from about 15 to 22 months or more, the carefree behavior gives way to anxiety about separation and fear of "object loss". The toddler is learning that "the world is **not** his oyster" (Mahler *et al.*, 1975, p. 78). The child alternates between demanding, negativistic, challenging behavior and seeking love and approval by "wooing" behavior.
4. "The child on the way to object constancy": 24 months to 3 years and beyond.

The optimal unfolding of phases depends on the emotional availability of the mothering person. If it is disrupted in the earliest months, the result can be the development of an infantile psychosis either because of lack of maternal availability or empathy or because, for constitutional reasons, the infant is unable to respond to the mothering. Regardless of whether the cause is environmental or constitutional, if the symbiotic mother–infant relationship fails to provide safe "anchoring" or discourages hatching, the separation–individuation process cannot proceed normally. Later phases may also be disrupted, for example, by overprotective mothering, which inhibits independence, or because of precocious motor development, which may lead the infant to separate physically from the mother before psychological readiness for that degree of separation. In addition, Mahler believed that the success or failure of the rapprochement subphase lays the foundation for subsequent relatively stable mental health or borderline pathology.

Otto Kernberg

Kernberg's major contributions have stemmed from his work on the psychoanalysis and psychotherapeutic treatment of patients with severe character disorders, particularly those with borderline personality organization (Kernberg, 1968), as well as patients with narcissistic character.

The primitive defenses of splitting and projective identification, first described by Klein, are central to the diagnosis of borderline personality disorder as conceived by Kernberg (1979). His depiction of the landscape of the mind also owes some of its salient features to Jacobson, who first suggested that internal representations of self and object with an associated affect are the nuclei of the early development of the psyche. Kernberg's depiction of the inner world of borderline and psychotic patients is, however, uniquely his own. Splitting breaks up the internal representation of objects and of the self into part object representations, each with an associated affect. The central feature of projective identification, a primitive defense according to Kernberg, is that it always involves the projection of an internal object relation with its associated affect. When projection is effective, the subject eliminates the unacceptable impulse or idea from any connection with the self. In contrast, in projective identification, the connection to the unacceptable contents is preserved along with the tie between the part self and the part object. The connection cannot be totally eliminated.

Kernberg envisioned the inner world of the borderline or psychotic patient as being populated by numerous unintegrated part self–part object dyads that are each linked by a predominant affect. These internal nuclei are kept separate by the defense of splitting. The borderline individual projects these pathological inner contents onto any significant other with whom he or she interacts. Which of these self-object–affect structures is active can shift from moment to moment; this results in the chaotic and shifting pattern of relationships that is the essence of what is observed clinically in patients with borderline psychopathological disorders (who can be described as being stably unstable).

Erik H. Erikson

Erikson divided the entire life-cycle into eight stages, thus extending into adulthood Freud's notion of infantile psychosexual stages while at the same time broadening Anna Freud's concept of the developmental lines of childhood. As shown in Table 18.10, Erikson (1982) linked each **psychosexual** stage to a particular body zone or zones. In each stage, the individual negotiates a phase-specific **psychosocial** developmental task toward the achievement of specific strengths. In this model, each individual evolves a mode of interpersonal and intrapsychic functioning with emergent social capacities uniquely adapted to a particular social milieu. The crises of each stage are normative, not pathological ones, and the developmental tasks are never fully resolved in each stage but continue to be worked out throughout the life span.

Far from being a simple linear model, Erikson used his hierarchical schema to explore increasingly complex interactions between earlier and later stages over time and between internal and external factors that influence development. Erikson integrated so many separate components of the individual's development and provided tools for their investigation in research models.

Erikson's work has had a lasting impact on our understanding of adolescence and the concept of identity. Each of the developmental stages has a psychosocial crisis. For the adolescent it is an identity crisis. Whereas the term identity crisis has come into popular use to denote troubled teenagers with pathological antisocial behavior, Erikson's original intention, as with

Table 18.10	Erikson's Stages of Development	
Psychosexual Stage	Psychosocial Crisis	Basic Strength
Oral–sensory (infancy)	Basic trust vs. basic mistrust	Hope
Anal–muscular (early childhood)	Autonomy vs. shame and doubt	Will
Genital–locomotor (play age)	Initiative vs. shame and guilt	Purpose
Latency (school age)	Industry vs. inferiority	Competence
Puberty (adolescence)	Identity vs. identity confusion	Fidelity
Genitality (young adulthood)	Intimacy vs. isolation	Love
Procreativity (adulthood)	Generativity vs. stagnation	Care
Generalization of sensual modes (old age)	Integrity vs. despair	Wisdom

Source:Modified Erikson EH (1982) The Life Cycle Completed. WW Norton, New York, pp. 32-33). Copyright 1985 WW Norton.

the crises of each of the other developmental stages, was to designate a normative phase-specific internal conflict.

It is the concept of individual development within a social matrix and the interaction between the two to which Erikson gave his stamp. He had a complex view of this interaction, describing how at each stage of development the specific caretaker within the social matrix responds to the individual's stage and needs in accordance with the caretaker's own phase-specific capacities and needs. Thus, the developing individual and his or her caretaker mutually influence each other in a manner specific to each dyad. The paradigm of this mutual interplay can be used to describe the interaction between parents and children, children and their teachers, psychotherapists and patients, societies and their members, or any one individual and another throughout the life-cycle.

Erikson concluded that every society responds to each developmental phase with institutions specific to that culture and so determines for each individual growing up in that culture the manner and extent of resolution of every developmental phase. Through this process, a given community preserves its own ecological balance.

Heinz Kohut: Self-psychology

Conceptual Background

Freud and his followers tried to understand psychological life in terms of biology. Their ideal was scientific objectivity. They believed the analyst's human tendency to identify with the subjects of study impeded objectivity. In contrast, Kohut viewed empathic comprehension as the fundamental mode of psychoanalytic investigation. It is the knowledge of the other's experience, what it is like to be in that person's shoes. Empathy is the understanding of another's complex psychological experience as whole. Using this empathic method, Kohut attempted to create an "experience-near" psychology, explaining psychological events in terms of meanings and motives comprehensible from ordinary experience. He contrasted this to Freudian metapsychology with its postulated experience-distant forces, energies and structures.

The concept of **bipolar self** (Figure 18.3) refers to Kohut's metaphorical description of the self as having two poles, one of ideals and ambitions, the other a sense of the grandiose self. The former involves the sense of being vigorous and coherent because one is associated with what is good and powerful, for example, that an adult might have when working in accord with professional ideals. The grandiose pole of the self consists in the sense of being personally valuable and appreciated, as a child may feel by virtue of the glowing enthusiasm of parents.

Kohut's singular contribution was the idea of the **self-object**. Clinical observations led him to believe, like of object relations theorists, that the self could survive and prosper only in the context of experience with others. These experiences

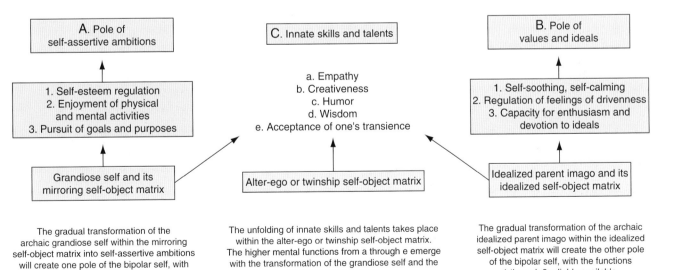

Figure 18.3 *Structure and functions of the supraordinate bipolar self (normal development). (Source: Ornstein P and Kay J [1990] Developments of psychoanalytic self-psychology: A historical-conceptual overview. Annu Rev Psychiatr 9, 303–322.)*

Kohut called self-objects, that is, objects (in the psychoanalytic sense of intrapsychic representation of other people) that are necessary for the well-being of the self. Kohut was speaking of intrapsychic experiences, not interpersonal relations. Intrapsychic experience may be contingent on interpersonal events. For example, the sense that one is appreciatively responded to usually requires some sort of active response from another person, but how that person's actions are experienced depends on many factors besides the actions themselves.

Kohut (1971) described two main types of self-object. **Idealized self-objects** embody what is admirable, strong and vigorous. The self feels alive and coherent by virtue of proximity to the idealized self-object. The youngster who feels like "a chip off the old block", the student who is enlivened in the presence of a brilliant teacher, and the religious person who feels safe in God's presence have idealized self-object experiences. **Mirroring self-objects** contribute to the sense through their support of the grandiose pole of the self. Kohut described three major types of mirroring self-object:

- In **merger**, the self is maintained through the sense that the person and self-object form a unity that is powerful and alive in a way the person could not be by himself or herself. The sense of merger can be found in the feeling that "we" do something. Outside the analytical situation, it is commonly seen in athletic, professional, and military activities.
- **Alter ego (or twinship) self-object** induces a sense of personal coherence by virtue of having a partner who is like oneself.

- The **mirroring self-object proper** supports the sense of personal value and coherence through its accurate, valuing appreciation of the person. The person who feels valuable and whole when a parent's or friend's eyes light up as she or he comes into a room or who feels similarly in response to authentic praise of accomplishment is experiencing such a mirroring self-object.

Self-objects remain essential throughout life. Contrary to psychoanalytic theories that characterize maturity in terms of autonomy, self-psychology views mature people as ordinarily dependent on others for appreciation, comradeship, meaning and solace. The nature of the people and institutions that embody self-objects changes with maturation. They become more numerous and more complex, often serving many psychological functions beyond their self-object function. It refers to the total experience of people and institutions that sustain and support the development of the self.

Disorders of the Self

The study of self-psychology began with the realization that many symptoms of psychological distress could be understood as arising from disorders of the self. These include symptoms involving direct experiences of an endangered, enfeebled, or fragmented self, and symptoms arising from unsatisfactory attempts to protect an endangered self. In practice, these symptoms may appear in the same patient, but for expository purposes, separating them is useful. Sometimes the symptoms of self-pathology are acute (Figure 18.4), but more often they are chronic states

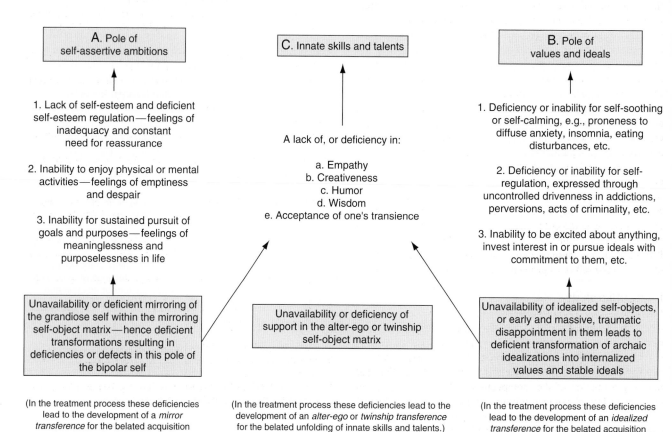

Figure 18.4   *Structure and functions of the supraordinate bipolar self (deficient or derailed development). (Source: Ornstein P and Kay J [1990] Developments of psychoanalytic self-psychology: A historical-conceptual overview. Annu Rev Psychiatr 9, 303–322.)*

whose intensity varies as the self is felt to be more or less in danger.

Symptoms that directly express the enfeeblement or fragmentation of the self include certain depressive states, traumatic states, hypochondriasis, some forms of rage, called narcissistic rage, and direct experiences of profound disorganization.

A common response to feeling the self-endangered is rage (Kohut, 1972). Narcissistic rage is a major public health problem. The most common cause of violence and homicide is the rage engendered when people feel "disrespected". Spousal murders most commonly result when an already demoralized person is confronted by apparently trivial inconsiderate behavior and responds with murderous rage. Communal chronic narcissistic rage may be a major factor in world history when maintaining group dignity or seeking compensation for past inequities may lead to hatred and destructiveness lasting for centuries. Narcissistic rage varies from the momentary fury to lifelong states. Like many activities in the service of the self, narcissistic rage is often rationalized. Perpetrators often describe violence as necessary to achieve a goal but closer examination usually shows that violence does little to effect its supposed aim. Physical child abuse, often a manifestation of narcissistic rage resulting from a sense of inadequacy in caring for children, is commonly rationalized as "educating" the youngster. Narcissistic rage often joins other psychological action designed to invigorate the self.

States involving the direct experience of fragmentation, in which patients cannot organize experience or recognize their coherent wishes, are overwhelmingly distressing. Any solution to this state, including the psychotic reorganization of experience, feels better. Indeed, such states are most commonly seen briefly with the onset of overt psychosis. Patients commonly describe this state as "going crazy" and may attempt desperately to hang on to some organizing principle. These states are psychiatric emergencies because many patients report that death is preferable to the continuation of the intense anxiety they experience. Many other symptoms are understandable as attempts to repair an impaired or endangered self. These include relations with others designed to achieve urgently needed self-object experiences and activities designed to soothe or stimulate the self.

When self-object functions become unavailable to such an extent that the person cannot provide for himself or herself these functions based upon personal abilities and memories already available, a psychological emergency ensues. In this circumstance, the person uses less broadly adaptive means to try to compensate for the missing but needed psychological functions. Pathological functioning is manifested either in direct expression of a distressed self or as problematic compensatory activities.

Intersubjectivity

Intersubjectivity in psychoanalysis refers to the dynamic interplay between the analyst's and the patient's subjective experiences in the clinical situation. To some extent, all schools of psychoanalysis agree on the significance of intersubjectivity in psychoanalytic work. Intersubjectivity embodies the notion that the very formation of the therapeutic process is derived from an inextricably intertwined mixture of the clinical participants' subjective reactions to one another. Knowledge of the patient's psychology is considered contextual and idiosyncratic to the particular clinical interaction. This interaction nexus is considered the primary force of the psychoanalytic treatment process.

The intersubjective position is that mental phenomena cannot be sufficiently understood if approached as an entity that exists within the patient's mind, conceptually isolated from the social matrix from which it emerges. Intersubjectivists see the analyst and the patient together constructing the clinical data from the interaction of both members' particular psychic qualities and subjective realities. The analyst's perceptions of the patient's psychology are always shaped by the analyst's subjectivity. Conversely, the patient's psychology is not conceptualized as something discoverable by the external, unbiased observer (Hoffman, 1991; Ogden 1992a, 1992b, 1994; Spezzano, 1993).

References

Bowlby J (1969) *Attachment and Loss*. Basic Books, New York.
Erikson EH (1982) *The Life Cycle Completed*. WW Norton, New York.
Freud A (1936) *The Ego and the Mechanisms of Defense*. International Universities Press, New York.
Freud S (1900) *The Interpretation of Dreams*. Standard Edition, 4 and 5. Hogarth Press, London.
Freud S (1901) *On Dreams*. Standard Edition, 5. Hogarth Press, London.
Freud S (1905) *Three Essays on the Theory of Sexuality*. Standard Edition, 7. Hogarth Press, London.
Freud S (1911) *Formulations on the Two Principles of Mental Functioning*. Standard Edition, 12. Hogarth Press, London.
Freud S (1917) *Mourning and Melancholia*. Standard Edition, 14. Hogarth Press, London.
Hoffman IZ (1991) Toward a social-constructivist view of the psychoanalytic situation. *Psychoanal Dial* 1, 74–105.
Kernberg OF (1968) The treatment of patients with borderline personality organization. *Int J Psychoanalysis* 49:600-619.
Kernberg OF (1979) Some implications of object relations theory for psychoanalytic technique, *J Am Psychoanalytic Ass* 27 (Suppl.): 207–239.
Klein M (1937) Love, guilt, and reparation, in *Love, Guilt and Reparation, 1921–1945*. Free Press, New York, pp. 306–343.
Klein M (1946) Notes on some schizoid mechanisms, in *Envy and Gratitude, 1946–1963*. Dell Books, New York, pp. 43–47.
Kohut H (1971) *The Analysis of the Self*. International Universities Press, New York.
Kohut H (1972) Thoughts on narcissism and narcissistic rage. *Psychoanal Study Child* 27, 360–400.
Mahler MS, Pine F, and Bergman A (1975) *The Psychological Birth of the Human Infant*. Symbiosis and Individuation. Basic Books, New York.
Ogden TH (1992a) The dialectically constituted/decentered subject of psychoanalysis. I. The Freudian subject. *Int J Psychoanal* 73, 517–526.
Ogden TH (1992b) The dialectically constituted/decentered subject of psychoanalysis. II. The contributions of Klein and Winnicott. *Int J Psychoanal* 73, 613–626.
Ogden TH (1994) The analytic third: Working with intersubjective clinical facts. *Int J Psychoanal* 75, 3–19.
Spezzano C (1993) *Affects in Psychoanalysis: A Clinical Synthesis*. Analytic Press, Hillsdale, NJ.
Winnicott, DW (1951) *Transitional Objects and Transitional Phenomena: A Study of the First Not-Me Possession*.
Winnicott, DW (1954–55) *Through Paediatrics to Psycho-Analysis*, Basic Books 1975.
Winnicott, DW (1960) *Ego Distortion in Terms of True and False Self, Maturation Processes*, 1965 Hogarth Press, London.

Glossary of Psychoanalytic Terms

Abreaction The discharge of affect associated with a traumatic memory. Abreaction may be brought about by hypnosis or free association.

Adaptive point of view   A metapsychological framework that considers how the developing mind is influenced by environmental realities. In this model, the ego is thought of as the "organ" of adaptation.

Aggressive drive   One of the primary instinctual drives, aggression includes the urge to harm or destroy, the urge to dominate or prevail over others, and strivings toward mastery. The aggressive drive is a major source of intrapsychic conflict.

Anal   Stage of psychosocial development from about 18 months to 3 years during which pleasures and conflicts center on defecation and urination and their symbolic derivatives. In addition, with increased cognitive and motor development, issues of mastery, autonomy, obedience and defiance are observed.

Cathexis   The attachment of mental energy to a thought or memory, resulting in an increased emotional or motivational intensity associated with the thought or memory.

Character (personality) disorder   Habitually and generally inflexible patterns of behavior that are ego-syntonic, that is, cause little subjective discomfort and are experienced as appropriate, reasonable, and justified. Such behavior may actually cause problems in adaptive functioning and interpersonal relationships.

Compromise formation   An activity of the ego that attempts to solve conflicts between opposing forces operating in the mind, in particular the gratification of instinctual wishes that are prohibited by the superego or by reality. Compromises may take many forms including character traits, neurotic symptoms, dreams and fantasies, adaptive behavior and transference.

Conscious   The portion of mental activity and content that is directly available to immediate perception (as opposed to unconscious or preconscious). Conscious mentation obeys rational, secondary process logic.

Countertransference   Attitudes and feelings of the psychiatrist toward the patient. As narrowly defined, countertransference comes about as a result of activation of wishes, fantasies, or conflicts from the psychiatrist's life. More broadly defined, countertransference also includes reactions to the patient's projections or role enactments. Countertransference responses have the potential to have a negative impact on the therapeutic approach to the patient and also to provide data about unconscious processes occurring in patient and psychiatrist.

Defense mechanism   Specific unconscious operations used by the ego to protect against the fantasied danger associated with conscious awareness or unconscious wishes. Examples include repression, displacement, reaction formation, projection, isolation and undoing.

Depressive position   In Kleinian theory, a constellation of internal object relations, defenses and anxieties in which others are viewed ambivalently as containing both goodness and badness (as opposed to the split objects of the paranoid–schizoid position) and in which fear and guilt are felt around the fantasy that one's aggressive impulses may destroy the needed and loved object.

Developmental point of view   Metapsychological perspective that emphasizes the progressive unfolding of stages of development and focuses on the contribution of childhood experience to the psychology of the adult.

Dynamic motivational point of view   Metapsychological perspective that considers the actions of mental forces (wishes or needs inherent in the nature of humans), which may be in opposition to one another, resulting in conflict and compromise.

Dynamic unconscious   The content and processes of the system unconscious, which are kept outside conscious awareness by repression.

Ego   In structural model, the mental agency that is positioned between the physiologically based instinctual urges and the outer world. Its functions include mediating between the pressures of the id, superego and reality and the variety of processes of perception, cognition, memory, motor behavior and learning.

Ego ideal   The portion of superego functions that includes goals, ideals, and standard of thought and behavior. It is involved in the experience of self-esteem, pride and shame.

Empathy   A mode of knowing or perceiving the emotional or psychological state of another, in which the quality of experience of one person is momentarily shared by another.

Envy   A primitive emotion of desire, of wanting what the other has, combined with a hostile wish to destroy or spoil the source of that which is desired.

Fixation   The persistence of modes of gratifying impulses, reacting defensively to perceived danger, and relating to objects that belong to earlier stages of psychosexual development. Points of fixation can be returned to in the process of regression.

Free association   The basic activity in psychoanalytic treatment in which the patient reports everything that comes to mind without the usual selectiveness used in conventional discourse.

Id   In the structural model, the collection of unconscious drives and drive derivatives that continually push for gratification.

Insight   The conscious recognition and comprehension of previously unconscious mental content and conflicts, as occurs during psychoanalytic treatment. Insight is typically accompanied by adaptive behavioral changes.

Instinctual drives   Innate motivational forces originating within the organism that seek discharge or gratification. In Freud's theory, drives are characterized by their source, aim and object. The two basic instincts are the sexual and the aggressive.

Internalization   A process by which aspects and functions of need-gratifying relationships are taken into the self and represented in its psychic structure. Types of internalization include incorporation, introjection and identification.

Interpretation   The principle type of therapeutic intervention in psychoanalytic treatment that brings to the patient's attention observations about his or her mental processes and their underlying motives, conflicts, compromises, wishes, needs and patterns of object relations. The expected outcome of interpretation is insight, psychic structural change and symptomatic improvement.

Latency   Stage of psychosexual development between the approximate ages of 5 and 12 years in which the sexual drives and conflicts are less apparent and the major activities of the child are learning and other socially approved channels of gratification.

Libido   Term originally used to refer to sexual desire but later used by Freud to describe the metapsychological concept of mental "energy" that could be deployed toward and attached to various mental representations or psychic structures.

Metapsychology   An abstract conceptual framework used to organize, systematize, and orient clinical observations.

Narcissism   In its original use, narcissism refers to self-love, but the term was elaborated theoretically by Freud to refer to the libidinal cathexis of the self (or ego). In modern theory, aspects of character organization, self-experience, affect regulation and object relations are discussed along the dimension of normal versus pathological narcissism.

Neurosis   A set of psychiatric syndromes characterized by abnormalities of emotions, attitudes, behavior and thought and that have in common (in psychoanalytic theory) their origins in unconscious psychic conflict. Classic neuroses include hysteria, obsessions, phobias and certain types of neurosis are ego-dystonic and are recognized by the patient as abnormal and alien to the self.

Object As defined by Freud, a person or thing through which instinctual needs can be gratified. The inner mental schemas or constructions that conceptualize other persons are referred to as object representations. The theory of object relations examines the relationship of the self to internal objects and the interpersonal enactments of those mental phenomena.

Object constancy A developmental achievement in which mental representations of love objects are experienced as constant and stable, despite their availability or unavailability.

Oral The stage of psychosexual development occurring in the first 18 months of life, during which the oral and perioral areas provide the major source of sensual pleasure. Because the infant is extremely dependent during this stage, optimal development requires considerable parental attunement to the needs of the infant; if this is provided satisfactorily, the infant should acquire a sense of trust and a sense that the world is safe and that the infant's needs will be met.

Paranoid–schizoid position In Kleinian theory, the earliest and most primitive mental organization, in which there is a predominance of the defenses of projective identification, splitting, primitive denial and idealization. During moments of frustration in this stage, there is the experience of diffuse rage and persecutory anxiety.

Phallic–oedipal Stage of psychosexual development for approximately 3 to 6 years of age, during which the genitals become the major source of sensual pleasure. During this stage, the child develops an intense desire to possess exclusively the parent of the opposite sex and to eliminate the other parent who is perceived as a rival. The jealous conflict of this triangular relationship, with accompanying fantasies of retaliation by castration, leads eventually to identification with the parents and the development of the superego.

Pleasure–unpleasure principle The tendency of the mental apparatus to seek pleasure and avoid principle unpleasure. According to Freud's libido theory, pleasure is attained through drive discharge, and unpleasure represents the build-up of undischarged mental energy.

Preconscious In the topographical theory, mental content and processes that are not conscious but can be readily accessed by the direction of attention.

Primary process Type of mentation associated with the unconscious, characterized by irrationality and a predominant emphasis on wish fulfillment and drive discharge. Primary process logic involves many of the mechanisms and qualities seen in dreams including symbolization, displacement, condensation, absence of negatives and timelessness.

Psychic determinism A central idea of psychoanalysis, which asserts that all psychological events are influenced and shaped by past experiences that nothing in mental life occurs solely by chance.

Psychosexual development The sequence of development of the instinctual drives as theorized by Freud, in which the expression of drives centers on and is organized around specific erotogenic zones (oral, anal, genital) that shift in emphasis as the infant grows and develops.

Regression A shift in the organization of mental functioning to a more developmentally immature level, often occurring defensively in the context of anxiety associated with higher-level functioning but also seen in sleep and dreaming, love and sex, esthetic and religious experiences, and psychoanalytic treatment.

Repetition compulsion A controversial concept that descriptively refers to the tendency to repeat certain distressing or painful experiences during the course of life; also referred to as the neurosis of destiny.

Resistance The opposition to free association and other aspects of participation in psychoanalytic treatment, activated to prevent the emergence of unconscious wishes and their associated anxieties.

Secondary process Rational, logical, linear, controlled thought that characterizes conscious mentation and follows the rules of Aristotelian logic.

Self The total person including the body and the psychic organization; the center of subjectivity; the nuclear core of the personality.

Self-object In self-psychology as developed by Kohut, objects who provide an interpersonal function that optimally contributes to the maintenance of cohesive self-experience (e.g., mirroring or idealizability).

Separation–individuation Developmental process elaborated by Mahler in which the infant progressively emerges from the symbiotic unity with mother and forms a sense of individual selfhood and a sense of differentiation from love objects. The subphases of this process include "hatching" (differentiation), practicing, rapprochement, and "on the way to object constancy".

Structural model Also known as the tripartite model, Freud's later model of the mind that divides the mind into three structures: id, ego and superego.

Superego Mental structure that includes the functions of moral standards, ideals, prohibitions and conscience, and generates the affects of guilt and shame.

Therapeutic alliance The rational, conscious relationship between patient and psychiatrist based on the mutual agreement to work together cooperatively for the patient's benefit.

Topographical model Freud's first systematic model of the mind classifying three regions of mental functioning: conscious, preconscious and unconscious.

Transference The unconscious displacement of feelings, attitudes, and expectations from important persons of childhood onto the person of the analyst or the analytic relationship.

Unconscious Set of mental processes and content that operates outside conscious awareness. Unconscious mentation tends to be irrational; obeys primary process logic; and may be revealed through dreams, parapraxes, and free associations.

Source: Abstracted from Moore and Fine (1990).

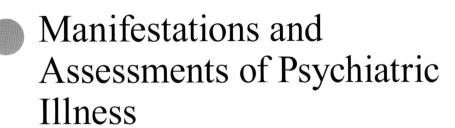

Manifestations and Assessments of Psychiatric Illness

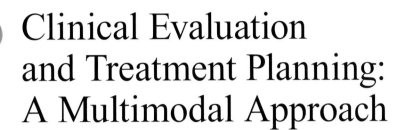

19 Clinical Evaluation and Treatment Planning: A Multimodal Approach

Every psychiatric evaluation must be specific to the context in which it occurs. The evaluation of a patient in the psychiatric emergency room is different from the evaluation of a graduate student applying for psychoanalysis, a member of a couple who seeks consultation for marital distress, or an indicted prisoner who is being evaluated for competence to stand trial. In each case, the evaluation and treatment plan are tailored to the situation.

In this chapter, we present an outline of a comprehensive approach to psychiatric evaluation. The complete psychiatric evaluation consists of the psychiatric interview; physical examination, including neurological assessment; laboratory testing; and, as appropriate, neuropsychological testing, structured interviews and brain imaging. The results of the evaluation are then used to assess risk, reach tentative and, if possible, definitive diagnoses, and complete initial and comprehensive treatment plans. Clearly, the length, detail and order of the evaluation need to be modified when it is conducted in different settings. The clinician needs to assess the goals of the interview, the patient's tolerance for questioning, and the time available. Table 19.1 shows the variation of the psychiatric evaluation with the type of setting.

| | Table 19.1 Psychiatric Evaluation and Treatment Planning | | |
Setting	Psychiatric Interview and Mental Status Examination (MSE)	Physical or Neurological Examination, Laboratory Assessments, Brain Imaging	Treatment Planning
Emergency room	Most often lengthy and extensive, except as limited by patient's ability or willingness to communicate.	Physical examination is often performed; other tests and examinations are ordered as indicated.	Primary focus is on disposition.
Psychiatric inpatient unit	Extensive, but complete information may be obtained in a series of interviews over time.	Physical and neurological examinations and laboratory tests are always performed. Other tests and examinations are ordered as indicated.	Comprehensive and formal plans are developed.
Consultation liaison service	Depth of interview is highly variable depending on reasons for referral and patient's medical condition. An attempt is made to obtain a complete MSE.	Most medical information is obtained from the chart. Psychiatric consultant may request further assessment.	Recommendations focus on reasons for referral and are made to the primary treatment team.
Outpatient office or clinic	Urgency of situation is assessed. In nonurgent situations, the initial interview usually focuses on the chief complaint and MSE.	Medical information is obtained as needed, usually by referral to a general practitioner or specialist.	Planning may be formal or informal, depending on applicable regulatory and reimbursement requirements.
Third-party interviews (e.g., for court, disability determinations)	Interview addresses the reason for referral and may be narrowly focused but contains a complete MSE.	Assessments are ordered according to the purpose of the interview.	Not usually relevant except for recommendations pertaining to the purpose of the interview.

Table 19.2	**Psychiatric Interview**
Greeting	
Identifying information	
Chief complaint	
History of present illness	
Past psychiatric history	
Personal history	
Family history	
Medical history	
Substance use history	
Mental status examination	

Psychiatric Interview

Despite the advent of brain imaging tests, standardized diagnostic criteria and structured rating scales, the psychiatric interview (Table 19.2) remains the cornerstone of clinical evaluation in psychiatry. Whether it is conducted in a busy psychiatric emergency room, an inpatient ward, or an outpatient office, the psychiatric interview is essential for establishing rapport with the patient, initiating the therapeutic alliance, eliciting the psychiatric history and performing the Mental Status Examination. When conducted skillfully, the interview may appear to be a relaxed and casual conversation, but it is actually an extremely precise diagnostic tool composed of specific elements: the identifying information, the chief complaint, the history of present illness, the past psychiatric history, the personal history, the family history, the medical history, the substance use history and the Mental Status Examination (MSE). The essential features of the psychiatric interview are highlighted here.

Before beginning, the psychiatrist should introduce himself or herself, explain the purpose of the interview, and try to make the patient as comfortable as possible. The interview gives the most accurate information when the psychiatrist and patient speak in a language in which they are both fluent. When this is not possible, a translator should be used, preferably one with mental health training or experience. Even then, some of the subtleties of the patient's communications are lost.

Identifying Information

Most interviewers find it helpful to begin with a few questions designed to identify the patient in a general way. Asking the patient's name, age, address, marital status and occupation provides a quick general picture and begins the interview with emotionally neutral material. If the interviewer chooses to begin in this way, it is important to complete this section rapidly and then give the patient a chance to respond to open-ended questions. This allows the interviewer to gain a more accurate sense of the patient's spontaneous speech patterns, thought processes and thought content. If the patient becomes too disorganized in response to this change, the psychiatrist can revert to more focused questions to structure and organize the interview. If it is possible, within the context of the interview, other pieces of identifying information, such as the patient's ethnic group and religious affiliation, should be obtained.

Chief Complaint

At the start, the interviewer wants to ascertain exactly why the patient is seeking psychiatric help at this time. The interviewer may begin with a fairly general question, such as "What brings you

to treatment at this time?" The patient may have a long history of psychiatric illness, but the chief complaint refers only to the acute problem that necessitates the current intervention. The interviewer should try to help the patient distinguish the chief complaint from any chronic problems, as in the following example:

> *Interviewer: Can you tell me what brings you to see a psychiatrist at this time?*
>
> *Patient: Well, I have had schizophrenia for 25 years.*
>
> *Interviewer: I see. But my guess is that something happened recently that has prompted you to come in today, rather than several months ago.*
>
> *Patient: Oh, yes. Yesterday my wife kicked me out of the house. I'm homeless.*

Here the patient's chief complaint is homelessness; the schizophrenia is part of his psychiatric history. Although a psychotic patient may offer a chief complaint that seems incoherent or unrealistic, it is important to collect the chief complaint in the patient's words and later look to other sources of information for additional history. Similarly, in response to the question, "What brings you to seek psychotherapy at this time?" a patient may begin to answer by detailing his or her childhood, but the interviewer should help the patient to focus on current issues that precipitated the consultation. Some patients may not be able to cite a chief complaint: "My wife sent me" or "There's no problem. I don't know why the police picked me up". Even these answers give the interviewer information about the patient's current situation, which can be elaborated on by asking the patient for more details.

When the interview is being conducted for a third party – for example to determine whether a patient is eligible for disability – the chief complaint is replaced by the purpose of the interview. The psychiatrist should review such purpose with the patient and discuss the limits of confidentiality.

History of Present Illness

Having obtained the chief complaint, the interviewer should clarify the nature of the present illness. By definition, the present illness begins with the onset of signs and symptoms that characterize the current episode of illness. For example, the present illness of a manic patient with chronic bipolar disorder who was asymptomatic for the past 3 years would begin with the onset of the current episode of mania. The interviewer should determine the duration of the present illness, as well as precipitating factors such as psychosocial stressors, substance use, discontinuing medication and medical illnesses. The patient should be allowed to tell the story, and the clinician should follow-up with specific diagnostic questions. For example, a patient who tells a story of 6 months of sadness after the death of a relative should then be asked about vegetative symptoms of depression, suicidal ideation and guilty rumination.

Past Psychiatric History

The interviewer should ask for information regarding any previous episodes of psychiatric illness or treatment, including hospitalization, medications, outpatient therapy, substance use treatment, self-help groups and consultation with culture-specific healers such as shamans. The duration and effectiveness of treatment should be ascertained, as well as the patient's general experience of her or his psychiatric treatment to date.

Table 19.3	Personal History

Prenatal History

Wanted vs. unwanted pregnancy
History of maternal malnutrition or maternal drug use (including prescription drugs)
Circumstances of birth (vaginal delivery vs. cesarean section)
History of birth trauma
Birth order

Early Childhood (0–3 yr)

Temperament
Major milestones, including speech and motor development
History of toilet training
Early feeding history, including breast-feeding
Early behavioral problems, (e.g., nightmares and night terrors, enuresis and encopresis, aggressive behavior)
Early relationships with parents and siblings
History of significant early illnesses or hospitalizations
History of early separations from caregivers

Middle Childhood – Latency (3–11 yr)

Early school history, including any evidence of cognitive impairment
Relationships with siblings and peers
Early personality development
History of behavioral problems (e.g., separation anxiety, school phobia, aggressive behavior)

Adolescence (12–18 yr)

Psychosexual development, including experience of puberty and menarche, masturbatory history and early sexual behavior
Later school history
Later personality development
History of behavioral or emotional problems (e.g., substance abuse, eating disorders)

Adulthood

Marital history or history of relationships with significant others
History of child-rearing
Sexual history
Occupational and educational history
Religious history
Current living situation

Personal History

No interview is complete without some understanding of the patient's background and life circumstances (Table 19.3). Within the constraints of the interviewer's time and the patient's tolerance for further questioning, the clinician should inquire about the patient's upbringing, educational and vocational history, interpersonal relations and current social situation. It is important to inquire about the patient's sexual history and to ask about risk factors for human immunodeficiency virus (HIV) infection, such as a history of multiple partners, unprotected vaginal and anal intercourse, and intravenous drug use. This information is relevant not only for the assessment and diagnosis of the present illness but also for treatment planning.

Family History

The interviewer should ask the patient specifically about any relatives with a history of psychiatric illness or treatment, suicide, or substance use. This information may be of diagnostic importance. For example, a patient who presents with a first episode of acute psychosis may have any one of a number of disorders, but a family history of affective disorders may lead the interviewer to suspect a diagnosis of bipolar disorder or major depression with psychotic features rather than schizophrenia. This information is also important for treatment planning, particularly if the patient's primary caregivers are also psychiatrically ill or also abuse substances.

Medical History

A careful review of a patient's medical history is an important part of the psychiatric interview because medical conditions can dramatically affect psychiatric status. Many medical disorders such as endocrinological conditions (thyroid disease, pheochromocytomas, pituitary adenomas), neurological disorders (Parkinson's disease, central nervous system neoplasms, Wilson's disease, stroke syndromes, head trauma) and infectious diseases (HIV infection, meningitis, sepsis) can have manifestations that include psychiatric symptoms (see Chapter 33). When such a disorder is suspected, rigorous inquiry is essential. A review of all of the patient's medications, including over-the-counter preparations and alternative remedies, is important because many of these substances can produce or exacerbate psychiatric symptoms. For example, propranolol taken for hypertension may produce symptoms of depression, and scopolamine taken for motion sickness may induce delirium. Finally, the toll of chronic, debilitating medical conditions or the acute onset of a catastrophic physical illness may be accompanied by secondary psychiatric symptoms that can be fully understood only in the context of the patient's medical condition.

Substance Use History

The interviewer should inquire about which substances are used, under what circumstances, and the quantity, variety, and duration of use (Table 19.4). A question such as "Do you drink alcohol?" is likely to be answered with a quick "No". A better question, such as "How much alcohol do you drink?" communicates to the patient that the clinician is not making a value judgment and is more likely to elicit an accurate answer. The interviewer must be sure to ask about past and current drug injection, including the sharing of injection equipment, to assess for HIV risk factors (Table 19.5).

Mental Status Examination

The MSE is a structured way to assess a patient's mental state at a given time. Unlike the parts of the interview that focus on the history, the MSE provides a descriptive snapshot of the patient at the interview. Much of the information needed for the evaluation of appearance, behavior and speech is gathered without specific questioning during the course of the interview. However, the interviewer generally wants to ask specific questions to assess the patient's mood, thought process and content and cognitive functioning. Bearing in mind the outline of the MSE (Table 19.6) ensures that the interview is comprehensive. The components of the MSE are described in the following paragraphs.

Table 19.4   Substance Use History
Survey of drugs that have been used include: Alcohol
Opioids (heroin, methadone, analgesics)
Stimulants (cocaine, crack, amphetamines, ecstasy)
Depressants (benzodiazepines, barbiturates)
Hallucinogens (cannabis, lysergic acid diethylamide [LSD], mescaline)
Phencyclidine
Nicotine
Caffeine
Over-the-counter preparations
Pattern of usage
Age of first use
Period of heaviest use
Pattern or frequency of current use
Route of administration (injected, intranasal, inhaled, oral)
Periods of sobriety
Symptoms of tolerance or dependence.
Medical history, including HIV status and other substance use-related disorders. Note ongoing substance use despite knowledge that it could worsen medical conditions.
History of treatment for substance use.
Legal history. Note relationship to drug use.

Table 19.5   Human Immunodeficiency Virus Risk Factors
Parenteral
Use of shared needles or drug works in the course of drug injection or amateur tattooing
Receipt of blood, blood products, or organ transplant in the USA between 1978 and 1985
Maternal–fetal transmission (pediatric cases)
Occupational exposure among health care workers and laboratory technicians through needle-stick injuries and other significant exposures (uncommon)
Unsafe Sexual Activity
Most common for men: unprotected anal intercourse with other men; unprotected vaginal or anal intercourse with women who are known to be HIV-positive, engage in prostitution, or are injection drug users or sexual partners of injection drug users; multiple heterosexual partners
Most common for women: unprotected anal or vaginal intercourse with men who are known to be HIV-positive, are injection drug users, are the sexual partners of injection drug users, are bisexual, or were treated for hemophilia or coagulation disorder when blood products were contaminated; multiple heterosexual partners
Cofactors
Compromise of the skin or mucous membranes, especially through the presence of sexually transmitted diseases, which increases the likelihood of transmission on exposure to HIV-infected body fluids
Use of noninjection drugs, especially alcohol and crack cocaine, through association with high-risk sexual activity
Environmental Context
Risk behavior while living or traveling in geographic areas with high rates of HIV infection, through increased likelihood of exposure to HIV-infected body fluids

Appearance

The interviewer should note the patient's general appearance, including grooming, level of hygiene and attire.

Behavior

This includes patient's level of cooperativeness with the interview, motor excitement or retardation, abnormal movements (e.g., tardive dyskinesia, tremors), and maintenance of eye contact with the interviewer.

Speech

The psychiatrist should carefully assess the patient's speech for rate, fluency, clarity and softness or loudness. The interviewer may want to question the patient directly about his or her speech. For example, the psychiatrist can gain valuable diagnostic information by asking a patient with pressured speech if she or he is able to modulate the rate of the speech or by asking whether a dysarthric patient is aware of not speaking clearly. A bipolar patient who is in the midst of a manic episode is not able to slow down her or his speech; a fast-talking anxious person is able to do so. Similarly,

Table 19.6	Mental Status Examination

I. Appearance
II. Behavior (includes attitude toward the interviewer)
III. Speech
IV. Mood and affect V. Thought
    A. Thought process
    B. Thought content
VI. Perception
    A. Hallucinations
        1. Auditory
        2. Visual
        3. Other (somatic, gustatory, tactile)
    B. Illusions VII. Cognition
    A. Level of awareness
    B. Level of alertness
    C. Orientation
        1. Person
        2. Place
        3. Time
    D. Memory
        1. Immediate
        2. Short term
        3. Long term
    E. Attention (digit span)
    F. Calculations
    G. Fund of knowledge
    H. Abstractions
        1. Similarities
        2. Proverbs
    I. Insight
    J. Judgment

a patient whose dysarthria is secondary to ill-fitting dentures is aware of this problem whereas an intoxicated person is not. It is helpful to clarify whether patients with a speech abnormality feel that this is their normal speech pattern or a new problem.

Mood and Affect

The interviewer should be aware of the patient's mood and affect. This may be evident from the way in which the patient answers other questions and tells the history, but specific questions are often indicated. The patient's mood is a pervasive affective state, and it is often helpful simply to ask, "What has your mood been like lately?" or "How would you describe your mood?" In contrast, affect is the way in which one modulates and conveys one's feeling state from moment to moment. The clinician judges the congruity between the material the patient is presenting and the accompanying affect, that is, sadness when discussing the death of a loved one or happiness when describing a child's accomplishments. This reveals whether the affect is labile (shifts too rapidly) and whether it is appropriate to the content of the material (see Chapter 17).

Thought

The clinician should assess the patient's thought process and content. Thought process is the form of the patient's thoughts – are they organized and goal directed or are they tangential, circumstantial, or loosely associated? (See Chapter 45 for definitions and examples.) If the patient's thought processes are difficult to

understand, the clinician can indicate his or her difficulty in following what is being said and then assess the patient's response to this intervention. Some patients – such as patients with stroke who have nonfluent aphasias – may appear to have disorganized speech but are aware that they are not making sense, whereas those with fluent aphasias, psychosis and delirium are not necessarily aware of their impairment. The psychiatrist should ask specifically about the patient's thought content, including delusions (grandiose, persecutory, somatic), hallucinations (auditory, visual, tactile and olfactory), obsessions, phobias, and suicidal and homicidal ideation. Although these questions should be asked with tact and empathy, they should always be asked. Patients are generally relieved that the interviewer has broached the subject of suicide, and simply asking the question does not give patients ideas they have not had before.

Cognition

Every psychiatric interview should include some assessment of the patient's cognitive functioning (see also Chapter 8). This includes the patient's level of awareness, alertness and orientation (to person, place and time). If there is a question about the patient's memory, formal memory testing may be done to assess short-term, intermediate and long-term memory. A patient who can answer questions for 30 minutes is clearly attentive, but any doubts about the patient's attentiveness should prompt a formal assessment, for example, asking the patient to recite a series of digits forward and backward. Before assessing the patient's calculations and fund of knowledge, it is important to ascertain the patient's level of education. Formal assessment of the patient's ability to abstract may be unnecessary for a patient who has used abstract constructions throughout the interview, but the interviewer may want to ask formally for interpretations of similes and proverbs. It is often helpful to begin with simple constructions, for example, asking the patient the meaning of such phrases as "He has a warm heart" or "Save your money for a rainy day". Patients whose native language is not English may have difficulty in this area that does not reflect a lack of ability to abstract.

The interviewer should gain a full understanding of the patient's insight into the illness by asking why, in the patient's opinion, he/she is currently in need of psychiatric care and what has caused problems. Finally, the interviewer should learn about the patient's judgment. This is best assessed in terms of the circumstances of the patient's life, for example, asking a mother how she would deal with a situation in which she had to leave her children to go to the store or asking a chronically ill person what he does when he sees that he is running out of medicine.

The interviewer may want to use the Mini-Mental State Examination (Mini-MSE) to quantify the degree of cognitive impairment of a patient with obvious cognitive abnormalities. This can be useful as an initial diagnostic tool, as well as a means of assessing changes in cognitive function over time. The Mini-MSE is outlined in Figure 19.1.

Physical Examination

The physical examination is an important part of the comprehensive psychiatric evaluation for several reasons. First, many patients who present with psychiatric symptoms may have underlying medical problems that are causing or exacerbating the presenting symptoms. For example, an agitated, delirious patient may be septic or a patient being treated for an autoimmune disorder who develops new onset paranoia may have a steroid-induced

Maximum Score	Score	ORIENTATION
5	( )	What is the (year) (season) (date) (day) (month)?
5	( )	Where are we: (state) (county) (town) (hospital) (floor)?
		REGISTRATION
3	( )	Name 3 objects: 1 second to say each. Then ask the patient all 3 after you have said them. Give 1 point for each correct answer. Then repeat them untill he learns all 3. Count trials and record. Trials
		ATTENTION AND CALCULATION
5	( )	Serial 7's. 1 point for each correct. Stop after 5 answers. Alternatively spell "world" backwards.
		RECALL
3	( )	Ask for the 3 objects repeated above. Give 1 point for each correct.
		LANGUAGE
9	( )	Name a pencil, and a watch (2 points) Repeat the following "No ifs, ands or buts." (1 point) Follow a 3-stage command: "Take a paper in your right hand, fold it in half, and put it on the floor" (3 points) Ready and obey the following: CLOSE YOUR EYES (1 point) Write a sentence (1 point) Copy design (1 point)
_____		Total score ASSESS level of consciousness along a continuum _____

Alert	Drowsy	Stupor	Coma

Figure 19.1   *Mini-Mental State Examination. (Source: Folstein MF, Folstein SE and McHugh PR [1975] "Mini-mental state". A practical method for grading the cognitive state of patients for the clinician. J Psychiatr Res 12, 189–198. Reprinted with permission from Elsevier Science, Pergamon Imprint, Oxford, England.)*

psychosis. Secondly, the patient's physical capacity to tolerate certain psychiatric medications, such as tricyclic antidepressants or lithium, must be assessed. Finally, many patients who present to a psychiatrist have had inadequate medical care and should be routinely examined to assess their general level of physical health. This is especially true for patients with chronic mental illness or substance abuse. In some settings, such as emergency rooms and inpatient wards, the psychiatrist may want to perform the physical examination; in others, it may be more appropriate to refer the patient to a general practitioner for this purpose. Genital, rectal and breast examinations can usually be included even for anxious and paranoid patients, but when they must be postponed, care should be taken to complete them at a later time. A same-sex chaperone is necessary for the security of both the patient and the examiner.

Certain aspects of the information obtained in the psychiatric interview should alert the psychiatrist to the need for a physical examination. Any indication (Table 19.7) from the history that the psychiatric symptoms followed physical trauma, infection, medical illness, or drug ingestion should prompt a full physical examination. Similarly, the acute onset of psychiatric symptoms in a previously psychiatrically healthy individual, as well as symptoms arising at an unusual age, should raise questions about potential medical causes (Table 19.8).

New-onset psychosis or mania in a previously healthy 65-year-old is representative of a case requiring pursuit of a medical condition as the cause because these disorders do not commonly present at this age. Any gross physical abnormalities, such as gait disturbances, skin lesions, eye movement abnormalities, lacerations, flushed skin, or drooling, should raise the interviewer's

Table 19.7   Indications for Physical Examination

History of medical illness
Current symptoms of medical illness, particularly fever, neurological symptoms, or cardiovascular abnormalities
Evidence while taking history of altered mental status or cognitive impairment
History or physical evidence of trauma, particularly head trauma
Rapid onset of symptoms
New onset of psychosis, depression, mania, panic attacks
New onset of visual, tactile, or olfactory hallucinations
New onset psychiatric symptoms after age 40
Family history of physical illness that could cause psychiatric illness

Table 19.8	Physical Illnesses That May Present with Psychiatric Symptoms

Neurological	Metabolic
Amyotrophic lateral sclerosis	Acute intermittent porphyria
Epilepsy – particularly partial complex seizures (e.g., temporal lobe epilepsy)	Electrolyte imbalance
	Hepatic encephalopathy
Huntington's disease	Hepatolenticular degeneration (Wilson's disease)
Multi-infarct dementia	Hypoxemia
Normal-pressure hydrocephalus	Uremic encephalopathy
Parkinson's disease	**Nutritional**
Pick's disease	
Stroke syndromes (cerebrovascular disease)	Vitamin B_{12} deficiency
Rheumatological (Autoimmune)	Central pontine myelinolysis
	Folate deficiency (megaloblastic anemia)
Systemic lupus erythematosus	General malnutrition
Temporal arteritis	Nicotinic acid deficiency (pellagra)
Infectious	Thiamine deficiency (Wernicke-Korsakoff syndrome)
	Infectious
Acquired immunodeficiency syndrome	**Traumatic, Particularly Head Trauma Toxic**
Brain abscess	
Encephalitis	
General infection (e.g., urinary tract)	Environmental toxins
Meningitis	Intoxication with alcohol or other drugs
Syphilis, particularly neurosyphilis	**Neoplastic**
Tuberculosis	
Viral hepatitis	Carcinoma (general)
Endocrine	Central nervous system tumors (primary or metastatic)
	Endocrine tumors
Adrenal hyperplasia (Cushing's syndrome)	Pancreatic carcinoma
Diabetes mellitus	
Hypo- or hyperparathyroidism	
Hypo- or hyperthyroidism	
Hypothalamic dysfunction	
Panhypopituitarism	
Pheochromocytoma	

suspicion that there might be an underlying medical condition. Urinary or fecal incontinence is also highly suggestive of a medical etiology. Stigmata of drug or alcohol use or abuse, such as dilated or pinpoint pupils, track marks, evidence of skin popping, or frank evidence of intoxication (e.g., alcohol on the breath) should also signal the need for a more thorough physical examination. Abnormalities of speech, such as impaired fluency or dysarthria, may indicate the presence of an underlying medical disturbance. Many mood problems may be caused by physical disorders, and even apparently healthy patients with dysthymia may have hypothyroidism that can be treated medically. Finally, any cognitive disturbances, such as disorientation, fluctuating level of alertness, inattentiveness, or memory problems are, until proved otherwise, evidence of a physical problem that is causing psychiatric symptoms. In such situations, careful attention should be paid to the patient's vital signs, neurological examination (See section on Neurological Examination), and any indications of infection. In a hospital setting, a physical examination, including a careful assessment of the patient's vital signs (including orthostatic measurements), cardiovascular status and pulmonary status precedes the prescription of most psychiatric medications. Psychiatrists should pay particular attention to a patient's cardiovascular

status (e.g., electrocardiographic abnormalities, orthostatic hypotension, decreased cardiac ejection fraction) before beginning tricyclic antidepressants, which may induce cardiac conduction disturbances and thus must be used with caution for patients with such cardiac abnormalities as arrhythmias or other conduction abnormalities. Patients taking medications such as low-potency neuroleptics, monoamine oxidase inhibitors and tricyclic antidepressants should be assessed for orthostatic hypotension, especially if they are elderly. If beta-blockers such as propranolol are being considered, patients should be evaluated for the presence of asthma, which may be exacerbated by these drugs.

Physical examination may also be warranted during treatment with medication if physical symptoms arise. For example, fever and a change of mental status during a course of neuroleptics require a full physical and neurological examination to rule out neuroleptic malignant syndrome. Urinary retention induced by medications with anticholinergic side effects requires an abdominal examination to assess bladder fullness. Anticholinergic-induced constipation may warrant abdominal or rectal examination to assess for impaction. When patients are seen in office-based practices, the psychiatrist most often obtains a careful medical history and may complete simple procedures such as blood pressure checks but may refer the patient to another physician for a complete physical examination.

Neurological Examination

With every patient, the psychiatrist should consider a thorough neurological examination, especially for hospitalized patients. Patients who have a history of neurological disturbances, such as strokes, seizure disorders, central nervous system neoplasms, dementias and movement disorders, should be carefully evaluated, perhaps by a neurologist. The neurological examination should be particularly designed to rule out any lateralizing neurological signs which would point toward the presence of a focal lesion. Unilateral weakness or abnormalities in pupil size or eye movements might suggest a focal neoplasm, infection (such as toxoplasmosis), intracranial bleeding, or a stroke, which may explain such psychiatric symptoms as confusion, sudden onset of speech difficulties, psychosis, or even depression. Stiffness and cogwheel rigidity are classical signs of Parkinson's disease, a disorder which may be associated with such psychiatric symptoms as depression, psychosis and dementia.

Patients with acquired immunodeficiency syndrome should also be carefully evaluated neurologically because many neurological manifestations of advanced HIV-related illness (including HIV-associated dementia and CNS opportunistic infections) and the medicines administered to treat these illnesses may produce psychiatric symptoms, including depression, delirium, mania and psychosis. Gait should be carefully examined in psychiatric patients because certain neurological conditions in which gait disturbances are prominent, such as normal-pressure hydrocephalus, tertiary syphilis (tabes dorsalis) and combined system disease (caused by vitamin B_{12} deficiency) may produce a variety of psychiatric symptoms.

Psychological and Neuropsychological Testing

Psychological and neuropsychological tests are standard instruments used to measure specific aspects of mental functioning. They are usually administered by psychologists or other professionals who have been trained in their use and interpretation. In most cases, several tests, often referred to as a **battery**, are performed together. These test results must then be interpreted in the context of the broad clinical picture of the patient.

Because of the time and expense involved, testing is usually reserved for situations in which there is some uncertainty about a patient's diagnosis, cognitive capacity, or psychological functioning. There are, however, times when psychological testing is essential, for example, IQ testing to establish the severity of mental retardation. In addition, giving simple tests of cognitive functioning, such as asking the patient to copy Bender Gestalt diagrams (Figure 19.2), can be helpful as one aspect of assessing central nervous system impairment caused by a medical condition. Psychological and neuropsychological testing can be particularly useful in the assessment of children with academic or behavioral difficulties in school. Table 19.9 lists some of the most commonly used tests.

Neuropsychological Examination Compared with Other Examinations

Neuropsychological testing provides information regarding diagnosis; cognitive, perceptual and motor capacities or deficits;

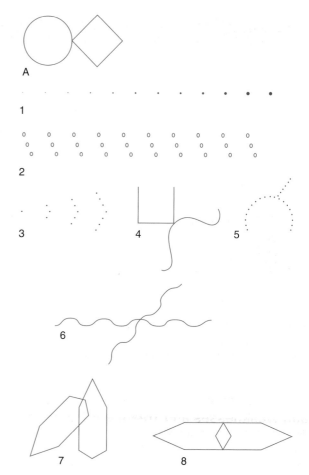

Figure 19.2   *Bender Gestalt diagram.*

and treatment recommendations (Table 19.10). Experienced clinicians use test data to determine the presence or absence of brain dysfunction, to localize the damage, and to establish the etiology (Milberg *et al.*, 1996). Moreover, a comprehensive functional assessment can lead to neurologically meaningful subgroups of disorders (as in different types of developmental disorders, verbal and nonverbal) that may have relevance to treatment, such as in the application of different strategies of cognitive rehabilitation or school placement (Weinstein and Seidman, 1994).

All neuropsychological approaches assess some aspects of intelligence, reasoning and abstraction, attention (sustained and selective), "executive" and self-control functions (set shifting, planning and organizational capacity), learning and memory (e.g., working memory, declarative), language, perceptual (i.e., auditory and visual) and constructional tasks, and sensory and motor functions. Comprehensive test batteries can be quite lengthy, because the human brain–behavior relationship is quite complex. Test data are interpreted in the context of many factors including the age, sex, education, and handedness of the patient.

Types of Referral Questions for Neuropsychological Evaluation

The neuropsychological examination has three general aims: 1) identification of neuropsychological dysfunction leading to inferences regarding the presence, type and etiology of brain dysfunction; 2) comprehensive assessment of cognitive, perceptual, and

Table 19.9   Common Psychological and Neuropsychological Tests

Name of Test	General Purpose
Bender Gestalt Test	Subject's reproduction of geometric designs used to screen for neuropsychiatric impairment
Halstead-Reitan Battery	Complex battery of tests that give a detailed picture of neuropsychiatric functioning
Minnesota Multiphasic Personality Inventory*	Multiple true–false questions designed to assess psychopathology and personality
Rorschach Test	Ten inkblot designs; subject's associations used to assess thinking disturbances and psychological conflicts and defenses
Thematic Apperception Test	Emotionally suggestive pictures portraying one or more people; used to elicit stories that reveal psychological development and motivation
Wechsler Adult Intelligence Scale – Revised	Eleven subscales; used to assess verbal and performance IQ in adults
Wechsler Intelligence Scale for Children – Revised	Twelve subscales; used to assess verbal and performance IQ in children 6 to 16 yr old

motor strengths and weaknesses as a guide for treatment; 3) assessment of the level of performance over a broad range, for both initial evaluation and measurement of change over time.

Characterization of Adaptive Strengths and Weaknesses and Treatment Planning

Probably the greatest contribution of the neuropsychological examination compared with that of neurological or other neurodiagnostic evaluation is in providing a broad description of the patient's capacities and deficits and the impact of these resources and limitations on the patient's adaptation to the world. This

Table 19.10   Typical Goals of Neuropsychological Testing

Reliably, validly, and as completely as possible, measure the behavioral correlates of brain functions.

Differential diagnosis – identify the characteristic profile associated with a neurobehavioral syndrome.

Establish possible localization, lateralization and etiology of a brain lesion.

Determine whether neuropsychological deficits are present (i.e., cognitive, perceptual, or motor) regardless of diagnosis.

Describe neuropsychological strengths, weaknesses, and strategy of problem solving.

Assess the patient's feelings about his or her syndrome.

Provide treatment recommendations (i.e., to patient, family, school).

Indications for Clinical EEG Assessment of Psychiatric Patients

1. Rule out possible organic brain disorders
2. History of head trauma or suspicion of epilepsy
3. Differentiating pseudodementia secondary to depression and true dementia
4. First presentation of psychosis
5. Pre- and post-electroconvulsive therapy
6. Evaluating sleep disorders

profile is essential for treatment planning, which may include rehabilitation efforts generally and psychotherapy specifically (Weinstein *et al.*, 1991).

Assessment of Change of State

Many patients have fluctuating mental states, such as in schizophrenia and affective disorder, medical illness (e.g., renal disease, diabetes), or abuse of drugs or alcohol, or as a result of somatic therapies (medication or electroconvulsive therapy). Repeated testing is often desirable to clarify the patient's cognitive capacities. The effects of a treatment such as electroconvulsive therapy on cognitive function (e.g., verbal memory functions) can persist for months (Squire and Shimamura, 1996). Monitoring cognitive status by repeated testing allows an objective measure of subjective complaints and of recovery of function. Baseline testing early in the course of an illness such as schizophrenia or brain tumor can be compared with later evaluations to clarify the course of the disorder or to assess the impact of various interventions.

Neuropsychological evaluations differ not only in length but also in conceptual focus and in selection of the particular instruments that compose a battery of tests. In general, three batteries are used commonly throughout the USA: the Halstead–Reitan Battery (Reitan and Wolfson, 1993), the Luria–Nebraska Battery (Golden *et al.*, 1980), and a flexible, hypothesis-testing approach typified by the Boston process neuropsychological approach (Goodglass and Kaplan, 1979; Holmes-Bernstein and Waber, 1990; Kaplan, 1990; Milberg *et al.*, 1996). The decision to use one or the other of these approaches depends to some extent on the training of the practitioner, the nature of the referral questions, and a number of other factors discussed in more detail elsewhere (Seidman and Toomey, 1999).

Limitations of Reliability and Validity

Despite the obvious role of quantification in neuropsychological testing, interpretation of test data ultimately depends on the knowledge base, training and skill of the clinician. Neuropsychological test scores are an indirect measure of the status of the brain, as contrasted with direct measures of structure by magnetic resonance imaging (MRI) or function by positron emission tomography (PET), functional MRI, or EEG. In a psychiatric setting, where problems of motivation, effort, cooperation and stage of the illness are ubiquitous, analysis of neuropsychological data must go beyond the level of performance deficits because many studies have shown performance to be especially affected by functional (emotional) factors. Process analyses oriented to focal syndromes and focused on the relative efficiency of the two sides of the body and hemispace may enhance predictive validity.

The patient's clinical state may change, and repeated testing when the patient's clinical status is optimal often clarifies the nature of the diagnosis. Selective deficits found in the context of otherwise good performance when patients are tested in their best state can be considered most valid. Neuropsychologists must also take into account the effect of medication on neuropsychological function and distinguish medication effects from the patient's adaptive ability. Different medications are likely to produce different effects. For example, Trimble and Thompson (1986) have demonstrated that, for epileptic patients and normal subjects, anticonvulsants have negative effects on most measures of neuropsychological testing. On the other hand, Cassens and colleagues (1990) have demonstrated that (traditional) antipsychotic medications have negligible or mildly positive effects on most measures of neuropsychological testing in chronic schizophrenia, with the exception of a negative effect on motor performance. Spohn and Strauss (1989) have indicated that typical antipsychotic medications tend to improve attentional performance, such as on versions of the CPT.

Structured Clinical Instruments and Rating Scales

Structured instruments and rating scales have been developed primarily for research purposes. They allow investigators to compare findings in different studies by ensuring that similar data and criteria have been used to establish diagnoses and to measure the presence and severity of psychiatric symptoms and their response to treatment. Many types of mental health professionals and, in some cases, nonclinicians can be trained to administer these rating scales.

Although most practicing clinicians do not commonly use structured instruments to assess or follow-up patients, a small number of rating scales have come to be used routinely in clinical practice. For example, the Abnormal Involuntary Movement Scale (Figure 19.3) is often used to monitor patients receiving antipsychotic medication for the presence of tardive dyskinesia, and the Global Assessment of Functioning Scale (Figure 19.4), which is a slight modification of the Global Assessment Scale, is now used in Axis V in the *Diagnostic and Statistical Manual of Mental Disorders*, Fourth Edition (DSM-IV-TR).

Table 19.11 shows some of the most commonly cited structured instruments and rating scales. Hundreds of other specialized scales are also in use to assess such diverse areas as personality disorder, aggressive behavior, sexual practices, stressful life events and quality of life.

Table 19.12 gives an example of how these different rating scales approach the assessment of two symptoms: guilt, a purely subjective state of mind, and suicide risk, an inclination that is assessed using both subjective and behavioral components.

Laboratory Assessments

A variety of laboratory tests can aid in the clinical evaluation of the psychiatric patient (Table 19.13). (Councilon Scientific Affairs, 1987; Gold and Dackis, 1986).

Serological Evaluations

Blood tests are particularly helpful in ruling out medical causes of psychiatric symptoms.

Toxicology

When the clinician suspects that the ingestion of a substance has caused the presenting symptoms, a urine toxicology screen and blood alcohol level determination (Table 19.14) are indicated. (It is important to remember that an alcohol level of zero may indicate that the symptoms are due to a withdrawal syndrome and thus does not rule out alcohol as an inciting factor.) If the patient is known to be taking certain psychiatric medications, such as lithium, tricyclic antidepressants and anticonvulsants, levels of these medications should be tested as toxic levels may cause a variety of psychiatric symptoms.

Complete Blood Count

The complete blood count is part of the general laboratory evaluation of a new patient. It is used to screen for multiple problems, most commonly infections and anemia. In cases in which alcoholism is suspected or the mean corpuscular volume indicates a macrocytic anemia, vitamin B_{12} and folate levels should be tested. Vitamin B_{12} deficiency may lead to combined system disease, which can present with psychiatric symptoms such as irritability and forgetfulness in the early stages and dementia or frank psychosis in the later stages. The complete blood count is routinely used to monitor white blood cell counts in patients taking clozapine. Additional emergency complete blood counts may be necessary if such a patient develops fever, malaise, or other symptoms of infection. Certain mood stabilizers, such as carbamazepine and divalproex sodium, can induce a variety of blood dyscrasias.

Blood Glucose

The blood glucose test is an inexpensive, essential test in the evaluation of patients with a new onset of central nervous system dysfunction, psychosis, affective disorders and anxiety disorders. Hypoglycemia may produce lethargy and vegetative symptoms that may mimic those of depression, and hyperglycemia may produce anxiety and delirium. This test is clearly indicated for known diabetics who present with the first onset of psychiatric symptoms. The atypical antipsychotic olanzapine can elevate blood sugar.

Kidney Function Tests

The blood urea nitrogen and creatinine levels are important measures of kidney function. Kidney function tests are used to screen for kidney failure and hypovolemic states (in which blood urea nitrogen and creatinine levels increase). It is essential to perform these tests before beginning therapy with lithium, which is cleared by the kidneys.

Liver Function Tests

These tests, which check for levels of various enzymes in the liver, are indicated when there is some suspicion that liver

INSTRUCTIONS: Complete Examination Procedure before making ratings.
MOVEMENT RATINGS: Rate highest severity observed. Rate movements that occur upon activation one *less* than those observed spontaneously.

Code: 0 = None
1 = Minimal, may be extreme normal
2 = Mild
3 = Moderate
4 = Severe

		(Circle One)				
FACIAL AND ORAL MOVEMENTS:	1. Muscles of facial expression e.g., movements of forehead, eyebrows, periorbital area, cheeks; include frowning, blinking, smiling, grimacing	0	1	2	3	4
	2. Lips and perioral area e.g., puckering, pouting, smacking	0	1	2	3	4
	3. Jaw e.g., biting, clenching, chewing, mouth opening, lateral mavement	0	1	2	3	4
	4. Tongue Rate only increase in movement both in and out of mouth, NOT inability to sustain movement	0	1	2	3	4
EXTREMITY MOVEMENTS:	5. Upper *(arms, wrists, hands, fingers)* include choreic movements, (i.e., rapid, objectively purposeless, irregular, spontaneous), athetoid movements (i.e., slow, irregular, complex, serpentine). Do NOT include tremor (i.e., repetitive, regular, rhythmic)	0	1	2	3	4
	6. Lower *(legs, knees, ankles, toes)* e.g., lateral knee movement, foot tapping, heel dropping, foot squirming, inversion and eversion of foot	0	1	2	3	4
TRUNK MOVEMENTS:	7. Neck, shoulders, hips e.g., rocking, twisting, squirming, pelvic gyrations	0	1	2	3	4

GLOBAL JUDGMENTS:	8. Severity of abnormal movements	None, normal	0
		Minimal	1
		Mild	2
		Moderate	3
		Severe	4
	9. Incapacitation due to abnormal movements	None, normal	0
		Minimal	1
		Mild	2
		Moderate	3
		Severe	4
	10. Patient's awarness of abnormal movements Rate only patient's report	No awarness	0
		Aware, no distress	1
		Aware, mild distress	2
		Aware, moderate distress	3
		Aware, severe distress	4

Figure 19.3 *Abnormal Involuntary Movement Scale. (Source: Guy W [1976] ECDEU Assessment Manual for Psychopharmacology, Rev. National Institute of Mental Health, Rockville, MD. p. 534.)*

disease is present. They help the clinician to screen for hepatitis, alcoholism and biliary tract disease. They include creatine kinase, which is often elevated in neuroleptic malignant syndrome as well as in other conditions in which muscle rigidity is prominent. Monitoring of liver function tests is essential with some psychotropic medications such as divalproex sodium and nefazodone.

Thyroid Function Tests

Both hypothyroidism and hyperthyroidism can mimic the symptoms of psychiatric disorders. Hyperthyroidism may mimic anxiety disorders, psychosis, or mania, and hypothyroidism may mimic dysthymia and depression. Thyroid function tests are therefore indicated in cases of new onset of a major mental illness. In addition, thyroid function should always be tested when initiating lithium therapy because lithium may cause hypothyroidism.

Syphilis Screening

These tests should be done for any patient with new-onset psychosis. They have become particularly important with the increasing incidence of syphilitic infection associated with the HIV epidemic. Positive serologic results in the presence of unexplained psychiatric symptoms necessitate a lumbar puncture to test for neurosyphilis.

Consider psychological, social, and occupational functioning on a hypothetical continuum of mental health-illness. Do not include impairment in functioning due to physical (or environmental) limitations.

Code	(**Note:** Use intermediate codes when appropriate, e.g., 45, 68, 72.)
100 91	**Superior functioning in a wide range of activities, life's problems never seem to get out of hand, is sought out by others because of his or her many positive qualities. No symptoms.**
90 81	Absent or minimal symptoms (e.g., mild anxiety before an exam), **good functioning in all areas, interested and involved in a wide range of activities, socially effective, generally satisfied with life, no more than everyday problems or concerns** (e.g., an occasional argument with family members).
80 71	**If symptoms are present, they are transient and expectable reactions to psychosocial stressors** (e.g, difficulty concentrating after family argument); **no more than slight impairment in social, occupational, or school functioning** (e.g., temporarily falling behind in schoolwork).
70 61	**Some mild symptoms** (e.g., depressed mood and mild insomnia) **OR some difficulty in social, occupational, or school functioning** (e.g., occasional truancy, or theft within the household), **but generally functioning pretty well, has some meaningful interpersonal relationships.**
60 51	**Moderate symptoms** (e.g., flat affect and circumstantial speech, occasional panic attacks) **OR moderate difficulty in social, occupational, or school functioning** (e.g., few friends, conflicts with peers or co-workers).
50 41	**Serious symptoms** (e.g., suicidal ideation, severe obsessional rituals, frequent shoplifting) **OR any serious impairment in social, occupational, or school functioning** (e.g., no friends, unable to keep a job).
40 31	Some impairment in reality testing or communication (e.g., speech is at times illogical, obscure, or irrelevant) **OR major impairment in several areas, such as work or school, family relations, judgment, thinking, or mood** (e.g., depressed man avoids friends, neglects family, and is unable to work; child frequently beats up younger children, is defiant at home, and is failing at school).
30 21	**Behavior is considerably influenced by delusions or hallucinations OR serious impairment in communication or judgment** (e.g., sometimes incoherent, acts grossly inappropriately, suicidal preoccupation) **OR inability to function in almost all areas** (e.g., stays in bed all day; no job, home, or friends).
20 11	**Some danger of hurting self or others** (e.g., suicide attempts without clear expectation of death; frequently violent; manic excitement) **OR occasionally fails to maintain minimal personal hygiene** (e.g., smears feces) **OR gross impairment in communication** (e.g., largely incoherent or mute).
10 1	**Persistent danger of severely hurting self or others** (e.g., recurrent violence) **OR persistent inability to maintain minimal personal hygiene OR serious suicidal act with clear expectation of death.**
0	Inadequate information.

Figure 19.4   *Global Assessment of Functioning Scale. (Source: American Psychiatric Association [2000] Diagnostic and Statistical Manual of Mental Disorders, 4th edn, Text Rev. APA, Washington DC, p. 32.)*

Table 19.11   Common Structured Instruments and Psychiatric Rating Scales

Name of Scale	General Purpose
Abormal Involuntary Movement Scale	Brief structured assessment of abnormal movements; used to rate presence and severity of tardive dyskinesia
Beck Depression Inventory*	Twenty-item rating scale for depression; focuses on mood and cognition
Brief Psychiatric Rating Scale	Eighteen-item scale that rates current severity of psychopathology
Diagnostic Interview Schedule	Diagnostic instrument developed for use by nonclinicians to conduct community surveys
Global Assessment of Functioning Scale	Overall psychosocial functioning rated on a scale from 0 to 100; used as Axis V of DSM-IV
Hamilton Depression Rating Scale	A 17- to 21-item scale that rates the severity of depressive symptoms; strong focus on somatic problems
Nurses' Observation Scale for Inpatient Evaluation	Eighty items used to rate the behavior of hospitalized patients by staff
Overt Aggression Scale	Rates aggression in four categories: verbal, physical against self, physical against objects, physical against other people
Personality Disorder Examination	Items that rate six areas of personality functioning, which are analyzed by computer with a series of algorithms to generate personality disorder diagnoses

Table 19.11   Common Structured Instruments and Psychiatric Rating Scales *Continued*

Name of Scale	General Purpose
Present State Examination	Continually updated semistructured diagnostic interview used in international research and tied to the manual on the International Classification of Diseases (most recently ICD-10)
Schedule for Affective Disorders and Schizophrenia	Semistructured questions, similar to the Structured Clinic Interview for DSM-IV but more detailed, for establishing diagnoses of affective disorders and schizophrenia
Structured Clinical Interview for DSM-IV-TR	Semistructured questions used to establish DSM-IV-TR Axis I and Axis II diagnoses
Symptom Checklist* (SCL-90)	Ninety-item self-report instrument used to assess psychopathology

*These instruments are self-administered.

Table 19.12   Comparison of Rating Scales for Assessing Guilt and Suicide Risk

Rating Scale	Guilt	Suicide Risk
Beck Depression Inventory. Patient picks best answer.	3 = I feel as though I am very bad or worthless. 2 = I feel quite guilty. 1 = I feel bad or unworthy a good part of the time. 0 = I don't feel particularly guilty.	3 = I would kill myself if I had the chance. 2 = I have definite plans about committing suicide. 1 = I feel I would be better off dead. 0 = I don't have any thoughts of harming myself.
Symptom Checklist. Patient rates on 5-point scale from not at all to extremely.	How much were you bothered by: Blaming yourself for things? The idea that you should be punished for your sins? Feelings of guilt?	How much were you bothered by: Thoughts of ending your life? Thoughts of death or dying?
Structured Clinical Interview for DSM-IV. Semistructured interview. Rater selects:	*Interviewer asks:* "How did you feel about yourself? (worthless?)" If no, "What about feeling guilty about things you had done or not done? (nearly every day?)"	*Interviewer asks:* Were things so bad that you were thinking a lot about death or that you would be better off dead? What about thinking of hurting yourself?
1 = Absent or false 2 = Subthreshold 3 = Threshold or true	*Interviewer rates:* Feelings of worthlessness or excessive or inappropriate guilt (which may be delusional) nearly every day (not merely self-reproach or guilt about being sick).	*Interviewer rates:* Recurrent thoughts of death (not just fear of dying), recurrent suicidal ideation without a specific plan, or a suicide attempt or specific plan for committing suicide.
Schedule for Affective Disorders and Schizophrenia. Semistructured interview. Rater selects answers on 6-point scale from not at all to extreme.	*Interviewer asks:* Do you blame yourself for anything you have done or not done? What about feeling guilty? Do you feel you have done anything wrong? (Do you deserve punishment?) Do you feel you have brought this on yourself? *Interviewer rates:* Feelings of self-reproach or excessive or inappropriate guilt for things done or not done, including delusions of guilt. *Further questions:* Assess delusions of guilt or sin.	*Interviewer asks:* When people get upset or depressed or feel hopeless, they may think about dying or even killing themselves. Have you? (Have you thought how you would do it? Have you told anybody about suicidal thoughts? Have you actually done anything?) *Interviewer rates:* Suicidal tendencies, including preoccupation with thoughts of death or suicide. *Further questions:* Assess gestures, attempts, risk-rescue factors, medical lethality.

Continues

Table 19.12 Comparison of Rating Scales for Assessing Guilt and Suicide Risk *Continued*

Rating Scale	Guilt	Suicide Risk
Hamilton Depression Rating Scale. Rater selects best answer.	0 = Feelings of guilt are absent. 1 = Self-reproach, feelings of having let people down. 2 = Ideas of guilt or rumination over past errors or sinful deeds. 3 = Present illness is a punishment; delusions of guilt. 4 = Hears accusatory or denunciatory voices and/or experiences threatening visual hallucinations.	0 = Thoughts of suicide absent. 1 = Feels life is not worth living. 2 = Wishes he or she were dead or any thoughts of possible death to self. 3 = Suicide ideas or gesture. 4 = Attempts at suicide (any serious attempt rates 4).
Brief Psychiatric Rating Scale. Rater selects answer on 7-point scale where 1 = Not present, 7 = Extremely severe	Overconcern or remorse for past behavior. Rate on the basis of patient's subjective experiences of guilt as evidenced by verbal report with appropriate affect; do not infer guilt feelings from depression, anxiety, or neurotic defenses.	

Table 19.13 Common Laboratory Tests for Evaluation of Psychiatric Patients

Serologic
Toxicology screen (blood)
Complete blood count
Blood glucose
Kidney function tests
Liver function tests
Thyroid function tests
Syphilis serology
HIV antibody test
Pregnancy test
Blood cultures
Vitamin B_{12} and folate levels

Urine
Toxicology screen (urine)
Dipstick for protein and glucose
Pregnancy test

Lumbar Puncture
Electrocardiogram
Chest Radiograph

Blood Cultures

Blood cultures are indicated in the evaluation of medically ill patients who develop fever and psychiatric symptoms such as confusion, disorientation and agitation because this delirium may be secondary to sepsis.

HIV Testing

Psychiatric patients who present with known risk factors for HIV infection, including injection drug use and unsafe sexual practices (see Table 19.5), should be approached for consent to HIV testing, especially in geographic areas with high numbers of reported cases of acquired immunodeficiency syndrome. This also applies to patients who present with multiple sexually transmitted diseases or tuberculosis. HIV should always be suspected in cases of unexplained central nervous system dysfunction and when psychiatric illness is accompanied by suggestive medical findings such as thrush or swollen lymph nodes. HIV testing requires consent of the patient and should be preceded and followed by counseling.

Pregnancy Testing

The serologic test for the presence of human chorionic gonadotropin b-subunit may assist in ruling out pregnancy before the initiation of therapy with lithium, benzodiazepines, or other medications associated with fetal malformations. It is advisable

Table 19.14 Toxicology Screens

Drug	Amount per mL	Approximate Duration of Detectability (d)*
Alcohol	300 μg	1
Amphetamines	500 ng	2
Barbiturates	1000 ng	1–3
Benzodiazepines	300 ng	3
Cocaine	150 ng	2–3
Opiates	300 ng	2
Phencyclidine	25 ng	8
Tetrahydrocannabinolcarboxylic acid	<15 ng	3–20

*May vary widely depending on amount ingested, compound, physical state of subject, and other factors.

Table 19.15	Indications for Lumbar Puncture (Cerebrospinal Fluid Evaluation) in Psychiatric Patients

Rapid onset of new psychiatric symptoms, including dementia, delirium, psychosis

New-onset psychiatric symptoms with fever

New-onset neurological symptoms (e.g., seizures, paralysis)

Suspected neuroleptic malignant syndrome (e.g., while taking antipsychotics, patient develops fever, tremor, dystonia, autonomic instability, mental status changes)

New-onset psychiatric symptoms with a known history of HIV infection or neoplasm (if space-occupying lesion is suspected, brain imaging should precede lumbar puncture)

to perform pregnancy testing for all women of childbearing age before initiating therapy with any psychotropic medication.

Urine Testing

Urine testing is indicated in two situations. Urine tests for pregnancy are often indicated in the emergency room setting in which an immediate result is required before the initiation of drug therapy. Urinalysis may be indicated for geriatric patients with new onset of central nervous system dysfunction or psychosis because urinary tract infections may manifest themselves in this manner in the elderly.

Cerebrospinal Fluid Evaluation

Lumbar puncture may be indicated to test for infections, including meningitis, neurosyphilis, toxoplasmosis and cerebrospinal fluid tuberculosis. It is indicated in the evaluation of patients with symptoms such as confusion, disorientation, decreased alertness, or dementia when accompanied by fever (Table 19.15). It is also an important part of the evaluation of patients who have new-onset seizures or who are suspected of having neuroleptic malignant syndrome because these symptoms may be caused by central nervous system infections. In cases in which increased cerebrospinal fluid pressure is suspected, lumbar puncture should be preceded by computed tomographic (CT) scanning to evaluate for mass lesions.

Electrocardiogram

Because it is important to screen for conduction disturbances and cardiac arrhythmias before beginning therapy with tricyclic antidepressants, an electrocardiogram should precede the initiation of therapy. An electrocardiogram is also indicated before beginning certain other psychotropic medications that may produce electrocardiographic changes (Tables 19.16 and 19.17). An

Table 19.16	Indications for Electrocardiography

Assessment of cardiac functioning before beginning

    Tricyclic antidepressants

    Lithium

    Thioridazine

    Ziprasidone

    β-blockers

    Electroconvulsive therapy

    Drug overdoses (need varies with substance or substances ingested)

Table 19.17	Common Electrocardiographic Abnormalities Seen with Psychotropic Medication	
Medication	Abnormality
Tricyclic antidepressants	Increased PR, QRS, or QT intervals
Lithium	T wave flattening or inversion Sinoatrial block Sick sinus syndrome
Antipsychotics	Increased QTc interval
Thioridazine	Increased QTc interval
Ziprasidone	Increased QTc interval
Clozapine	Sinus tachycardia

electrocardiographic tracing of a patient who took an overdose of tricyclic antidepressants is shown in Figure 19.5.

Electroencephalography

A history of brain injury or head trauma is an indication for an electroencephalogram (EEG) in the work-up of mental status changes or psychiatric symptoms. The patient with new-onset psychosis should also have an EEG because partial complex seizures may produce psychosis. Symptoms suggesting temporal lobe epilepsy (Figure 19.6), such as hyperreligiosity, hyposexuality and hypergraphia, also indicate that an EEG should be obtained, including nasopharyngeal leads, to best evaluate electrical activity in the temporal lobes. EEGs may be useful in the assessment of insomnia and other sleep disturbances.

Abrupt onset of psychiatric symptoms such as psychosis, mania, or personality change, or the presence of visual, olfactory and tactile hallucinations suggest central nervous system dysfunction, which may warrant evaluation by electroencephalography.

Neurophysiologic Assessment

A variety of techniques are now available that can provide more direct assessments of brain function in psychiatric patients. These include not only neuroimaging techniques (PET scans and functional MRI), but also electrophysiologic measures, such as the EEG and evoked or event-related potentials (ERPs). Electrophysiologic measures have the advantage of being economical and noninvasive, and allow continuous monitoring of brain electrical activity with a temporal resolution that surpasses that of neuroimaging measures. The EEG has traditionally been used in psychiatry to screen for brain disorders. In a conventional clinical EEG, a highly trained reader uses visual inspection of brain waves recorded from scalp electrodes. The presence of epileptiform discharges, spikes, or generalized slowing of brain electrical activity is associated with known central nervous system pathology. In patients who have a history of head trauma or where epilepsy is suspected, a clinical EEG should be done to rule out organic brain disorders (see Table 19.10). When evaluating for epilepsy, several EEGs may be necessary for accurate results because epileptiform activity is not consistently present (Boutros, 1992). The EEG can also play an important role in the diagnosis of dementia, delirium and other cognitive disorders. Generalized EEG slowing in Alzheimer's dementia is correlated with the degree of cognitive impairment and with decreased

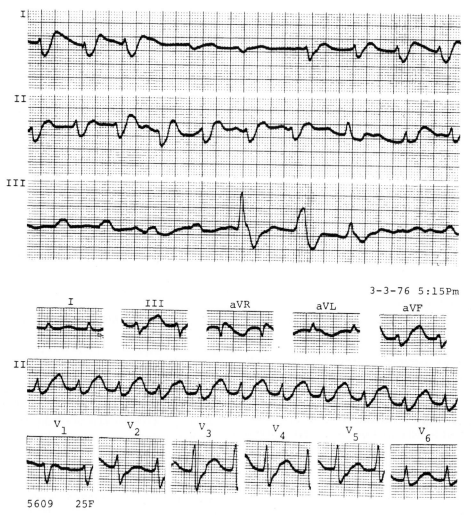

3-3-76 5:15Pm

5609   25F

Figure 19.5 *Tricyclic antidepressant overdose. The patient was a 25-year-old woman who took 500 mg of imipramine (Tofranil) 4 hours before the 5 pm tracing was recorded. The three standard limb leads show wide QRS complexes of varying morphology. The exact rhythm cannot be determined. She had severe hypotension at this time. Fifteen minutes later, the tracing shows probable supraventricular rhythm with intraventricular conduction defect. (Source: Chou TC [1991] Electrocardiography in Clinical Practice, 3rd edn. WB Saunders, Philadelphia, p. 481.)*

regional cerebral blood flow (Hughes and John, 1999). In elderly psychiatric patients, a clinical EEG is of value for distinguishing dementia and pseudodementia associated with depression. This is of importance for treatment selection because EEG abnormality in elderly patients is negatively associated with clinical response to antidepressants (Boutros, 1992).

Patients who experience their first psychotic episode are also candidates for a clinical EEG because brain lesions and seizure disorders, such as temporal lobe epilepsy, can cause psychotic symptoms that are clinically indistinguishable from functional psychoses. EEG recordings before, during and after electroconvulsive therapy (ECT) for depression also have clinical relevance (Hughes, 1996; Small, 1999). Patients with pretreatment EEG abnormalities may respond less well to ECT (Drake and Shy, 1989), and changes in EEG after ECT generally accompany clinical improvement (Sackeim *et al.*, 1996). Reviews of clinical EEG findings in childhood and adult psychiatric disorders show that 30 to 60% of referrals have abnormal EEGs (Hughes, 1996; Small, 1999), which underscores the importance of clinical EEG

evaluations in psychiatry. One of the limitations of routine clinical EEG is that it is dependent on the trained eye of the reader and is therefore subject to human error and may miss subtle abnormalities in the EEG tracing. Brain potentials evoked by auditory or visual stimuli (e.g., clicks or tones) have been used in both clinical and research contexts in psychiatry. Brain stem evoked potentials (BSEPs) refer to seven positive potentials evoked during the first 12 milliseconds after hearing a click. BSEPs have proven useful for assessment of hearing in infants and uncooperative patients, and in the assessment of brainstem lesions and multiple sclerosis (Celesia and Brigell, 1999). A later event-related P3 or P300 potential, typically recorded during an "oddball" target detection task with either auditory or visual stimuli, refers to a positive potential that peaks 300 to 500 milliseconds after onset of an infrequent target stimulus. The strongest case for the clinical utility of the P3 potential is in aging and dementia (Polich, 1999). Longer P3 latency distinguishes patients with dementia from those with pseudodementia secondary to depression, and patients with Alzheimer's disease from healthy subjects

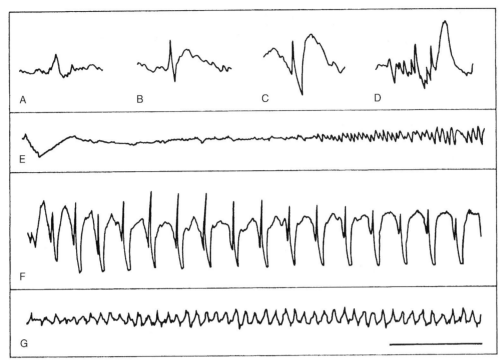

Figure 19.6   *Examples illustrate waveforms of typical interictal EEG transients and ictal EEG discharges. (A) Interictal sharp wave. (B) and (C) Interictal spike-and-wave complexes. (D) Interictal polyspike-and-wave complex. (E) Recruiting rhythm typical of generalized convulsion onsets. (F) Repetitive spike-and-wave discharges typical of absence seizures. (G) Rhythmic pattern seen with temporal lobe seizures. Line at the bottom right of the figure represents 1 second. (Source: Wyngaarden JB, Smith LH, and Bennett JC [1992] Cecil Textbook of Medicine, 19th edn. WB Saunders, Philadelphia, PA. p. 2208.)*

(Ford *et al.*, 1997; Frodl *et al.*, 2002; Polich and Herbst, 2000). Although P3 provides a useful index of cognitive efficiency, it has little value for the differential diagnosis of psychiatric disorders such as schizophrenia because it lacks specificity.

Brain Imaging

Several methods of brain imaging are available to assist in diagnostic assessment. Table 19.17 lists some indications for brain imaging.

Computed tomographic (CT) scans and magnetic resonance imaging (MRI) can be used to assess brain structure and are useful in detecting such abnormalities as mass lesions (central nervous system neoplasms, certain infections and hemorrhage), calcifications, atrophy, or areas of infarction. Mass lesions should be suspected in situations in which focal or lateralizing abnormalities such as focal weakness, unilateral disturbances in reflexes and increased pupillary size are found during the neurological examination. Other situations that call for brain imaging include the work-up of a patient with dementia to look for brain atrophy or lacunar infarctions; the evaluation of new-onset psychosis, acute onset of aphasia or memory loss and neglect syndromes; the evaluation of normal-pressure hydrocephalus (a syndrome characterized by a wide-based gait, dementia and urinary incontinence); and demyelinating conditions.

Whereas CT and MRI provide visualization of brain structure, positron emission tomography (PET), single photon emission computed tomography (SPECT) and regional cerebral blood flow allow investigators to study brain functioning by assessing which areas of the brain are stimulated during various types of mental activity.

Structural Imaging Modalities

Computed Tomography

Advantages and Limitations

1. CT offers excellent spatial resolution (<1 mm) and is effective at distinguishing tissues with markedly different X-ray attenuation properties (e.g., bone versus soft tissue versus fluid versus gas).
2. CT is useful for the detection of acute bleeding (less than 24 to 72 h old) but less helpful in subacute bleeding (more than 72 h old) and in severely anemic patients (hemoglobin below 10 g/dL) (Osborn, 1994). In addition, CT is an excellent modality for imaging bone. CT is the imaging modality of choice for acute trauma or when an acute bleed or ischemia is suspected.
3. CT is not helpful in visualizing subtle white-matter lesions due to CT's poor ability to distinguish between the X-ray attenuation properties of different soft tissue densities.
4. CT uses ionizing radiation and thus is strongly contraindicated in pregnancy. Women of childbearing potential should undergo a pregnancy screen prior to having a CT scan.
5. Patient anxiety is usually less during a CT scan than during an MRI scan because the scanning environment is more open, there is less noise associated with the procedure, and scanning time is relatively brief (~10 minutes for the brain).
6. CT is best for patients with metallic implants (e.g., foreign bodies, some aneurysm clips, pacemakers, etc.) as MRI is contraindicated in this patient population.

Magnetic Resonance Imaging

Advantages and Limitations

1. MRI provides excellent spatial resolution and superior soft-tissue contrast in comparison to CT (i.e., more useful for the visualization of white matter and white matter lesions). Also, while CT images are always axial images, MRI data can be resliced in any plane.
2. MRI is superior for surveying the posterior fossa and brain stem.
3. Fresh blood from an acute bleed (less than 48 to 72 hours) is not easily distinguished from gray matter. However, diffusion-weighted MRI may soon change this. Subacute bleeding (greater than 48 to 72 hours) or chronic hematomas are easily identified with MRI.
4. MRI does not use ionizing radiation, and so it is preferable to CT in pregnancy, but still is relatively contraindicated.
5. MRI is contraindicated in patients with metallic implants for the following reasons:

   - Metal can cause artifacts in MR images.
   - Metal can shift position or absorb heat within the magnetic field, causing burn injuries.
   - Mechanical devices such as pacemakers can malfunction within the magnetic field.

6. As many as 10% of patients undergoing MRI scanning experience significant anxiety during the imaging session. This is likely due to a number of factors. MRI scanners are much deeper (often several feet deep) than CT scanners; patients generally perceive the MRI scanner as more tunnel-like and may experience claustrophobia. Pretreatment of potentially anxious patients with benzodiazepines or other sedatives/hypnotics before undergoing MRI may be helpful in these situations. Also, the noise associated with the procedure is much louder than with CT. Lastly, the scanning time required for MRI is longer than that required for CT (20–40 minutes versus ~10 minutes for a study of the brain).

CT versus MRI

1. CT is the modality of choice for patients with acute bleeds or acute trauma, though diffusion-weighted MRI may soon become the modality of choice for assessing suspected acute brain ischemic events.
2. MRI is superior to CT for the differentiation of white from gray matter and the identification of white matter lesions.
3. MRI is superior to CT for the detection of posterior fossa and brain stem pathology.
4. CT is recommended if MRI is contraindicated (i.e., paramagnetic protheses; inability to tolerate scanner time, noise, or confinement).
5. MRI is recommended if radiation exposure is contraindicated (i.e., young children or women of childbearing potential).

Indications for Use of Structural Imaging Modalities in Psychiatric Populations

General Guidelines for Structural Neuroimaging
On the basis of existing data, we have suggested criteria for appropriate structural brain imaging:

1. Patients with acute changes in mental status (including changes in affect, behavior, or personality) plus at least one of three additional criteria:

   - Age greater than 50 years;
   - Abnormal neurological exam (especially focal abnormalities);
   - History of significant head trauma (i.e., with extended loss of consciousness, neurological sequelae, or temporally related to mental status change in question).

2. New onset psychosis.
3. New onset delirium or dementia of unknown cause.
4. Possibly for treatment refractory patients.
5. Possibly prior to an initial course of electroconvulsive therapy (may be helpful in identifying lesions that may lead to an adverse outcome such as aneurysms, tumors, arteriovenous malformations, hydrocephalus and basal ganglia infarction).

We estimate that adherence to the criteria listed above should yield positive findings in 10 to 45% of cases. However, only 1 to 5% will produce findings that lead to specific medical intervention. Lastly, if structural neuroimaging is indicated, one should use MRI unless the problem is an acute trauma or an acute bleed is suspected.

Functional Imaging Modalities

Positron Emission Tomography

Advantages and Limitations

1. PET is the gold standard of functional neuroimaging modalities.
2. Only PET can measure cerebral glucose metabolism.
3. A larger number of radioligands, especially those used for neuroreceptor characterization, are available for PET.
4. PET offers excellent spatial resolution (~4 mm).
5. PET is very expensive and requires relatively rapid access to a cyclotron, which produces the positron-emitting radionuclides. Most PET centers have a cyclotron on the premises. However, because of the high cost of obtaining and maintaining a functional cyclotron, some centers do not have a cyclotron on the premises. ^{18}F has a longer half-life (110 minutes) than other radionuclides such as ^{11}C (20 minutes), ^{13}N (10 minutes) and ^{15}O (2 minutes), so ^{18}FDG may be prepared using a cyclotron at one site and then transported to other sites as long as they are within hours (generally ~1–3 half-lives) of the site of synthesis.

Single Photon Emission Computed Tomography

Advantages and Limitations

1. SPECT is more affordable than PET and does not require a cyclotron for production of nuclides.
2. Currently, SPECT provides inferior spatial resolution (~6–8 mm) compared with PET.
3. Typically, SPECT spatial resolution worsens as one attempts to image deeper brain structures, although this is becoming less of an issue with the introduction of newer generation SPECT cameras.

PET versus SPECT

1. PET provides superior spatial resolution, especially for deeper brain structures.
2. PET offers a broader array of radioligands for use in receptor studies and is the only modality that allows for the measurement of metabolism.
3. SPECT is less expensive than PET and is more widely available.

Indications for Use of Functional Imaging Modalities in Psychiatric Populations

Although functional neuroimaging modalities include PET, SPECT and functional MRI (to be discussed later), in clinical situations only PET and SPECT are generally used at this time. These modalities are now commonly used as aids for diagnosis and monitoring treatment in cardiology and oncology (including brain tumors). Also, the use of ligands for neuroreceptor characterization is being increasingly used for the diagnosis and assessment of basal ganglia diseases such as Parkinson's disease. Still, most applications of functional neuroimaging in psychiatry occur in the field of research. However, a clinical role for functional neuroimaging in dementia and seizures is evolving and showing promise.

Dementia

As characteristic functional neuroimaging profiles emerge for various forms of dementia, the role of PET and SPECT in the evaluation of dementia is expanding. For example, Alzheimer's disease is associated with characteristic hypoperfusion in bilateral temporoparietal regions. Some studies have indicated that functional neuroimaging can offer better than 90% sensitivity and specificity in distinguishing Alzheimer's disease from other kinds of dementia (Silverman *et al.*, 2001; Bonte *et al.*, 2001). Since the introduction of cholinesterase inhibitors for treatment of dementia, early diagnosis of Alzheimer's disease may have greater import than in the past. Some PET studies of healthy older subjects with normal cognitive function who are homozygous for the apolipoprotein E epsilon 4 allele (a gene associated with the development of Alzheimer's disease) reveal that these subjects have temporo-parietal hypoperfusion before the onset of disease (Small *et al.*, 1995; Reiman *et al.*, 1996). Initiation of treatment, with cholinesterase inhibitors or other drugs being developed, in these individuals prior to the onset of symptoms of dementia may prove to be of great value.

Seizures

Some seizures, especially complex partial seizures, are not always detected by electroencephalogram (EEG). EEG measures cortical surface electrical activity but is less efficacious if the seizure focus is deeper in the brain. PET and SPECT images typically demonstrate ictal hypermetabolism and interictal hypometabolism (Krausz *et al.*, 1996, Theodore and Gaillard 2000). This allows for the detection of seizure foci during the predominant interictal period. To evaluate a possible seizure disorder, functional neuroimaging is usually performed in conjunction with EEG. PET is also useful for more precise localization of seizure foci in a patient with a known seizure disorder, if neurosurgical intervention is indicated.

FMRI

Expanding upon the basic principles underlying standard structural MRI used in clinical situations, functional magnetic resonance imaging (fMRI) allows investigators to assess brain function. Using either a standard or, preferably, a high-speed MR scanner with specific image-acquisition parameters, indices of cerebral blood flow and blood volume can be measured. While structural MRI studies rely on excitation and relaxation of hydrogen atoms in water, fMRI takes advantage of the paramagnetic properties of hemoglobin to measure blood flow and volume.

fMRI has distinct advantages when compared with PET and SPECT, and these include:

1. fMRI does not expose subjects to radiation and its relative safety has been documented.
2. The spatial resolution of fMRI is at least equal to if not superior to that of PET.
3. The temporal resolution of fMRI is vastly superior to that of PET or SPECT. While the temporal resolution of an ^{15}O PET study is 1 to 2 min, multiple time points can be assessed per second with fMRI.

The major disadvantage of fMRI when compared with PET or SPECT is that no satisfactory techniques for receptor neuroimaging have yet been developed for fMRI.

While fMRI currently has little utility, it may be useful in clinical situations in the future. One area of research that shows particular promise is the use of intravenous paramagnetic contrast agents with fMRI. This method, termed tracer kinetic technique, produces maps of cerebral blood volume (CBV) (Belliveau *et al.*, 1991). These CBV maps are relatively well matched to PET images of FDG uptake (Gonzalez *et al.*, 1995) and HM-PAO SPECT images of cerebral blood flow (Johnson *et al.*, 1995). Because these fMRI CBV maps can be obtained after only 1 to 2 min of imaging without exposure to radiation, this technique may be used instead of PET or SPECT for evaluation of dementia or seizures in the future.

Special Assessment Techniques

In certain situations, special assessment techniques may be indicated in the psychiatric evaluation of patients who are unable or unwilling to cooperate. These situations include the assessment of patients who are mute, have amnesia, or intentionally provide false information. In general, special techniques are employed only after all conventional ways to obtain the necessary information have been exhausted, including the use of other informants where available and appropriate.

Hypnosis can aid in the recovery of repressed memories. For example, a patient who presents with a conversion symptom may be able to recall the forgotten traumatic events that precipitated it. The usefulness of hypnosis is limited by the patient's susceptibility to the procedure and by concern that the interviewer's suggestions can produce false memories. (See also Chapter 72.)

Another approach available for similar purposes is to use a sedative during the interview to produce disinhibition and allow the patient to speak more freely or access otherwise unavailable memories. Intravenous amobarbital sodium is the best known of the medications used for this purpose. Caution must be exercised to avoid oversedation, to monitor for side effects of the medication, and to ensure that the interviewer does not inappropriately influence the patient's answers.

The assessment of a patient who is suspected of intentionally providing false information or malingering can become uncomfortable and problematic because it may require techniques that seem at odds with the establishment of the therapeutic alliance. A careful assessment of the patient's motives, confronting the patient with inconsistencies, physical assessment of implausible somatic complaints, and the use of other informants, prior medical records and other documents can all help establish the validity of what the patient is saying. When the case involves the commission of a crime, an assessment of the patient's capacity to understand his or her actions may be important for the disposition plan.

However, because psychiatric evaluation depends on what the patient tells the interviewer and there are few objective means of clarification, it is best for the interviewer not to be overly concerned about the possibility of being intentionally misled. Establishing the truthfulness of the patient's story usually takes place over an extended period.

Treatment Planning

The psychiatric evaluation is the basis for developing the case formulation, initial treatment plan, initial disposition and comprehensive treatment plan.

Case Formulation

The case formulation is the summary statement of the immediate problem, the context in which the problem has arisen, the tentative diagnosis and the assessment of risk. The latter two areas are described next in more detail.

Assessment of Risk

The assessment of risk is the most crucial component of the formulation because the safety of the patient, the clinician and others is the foremost concern in any psychiatric evaluation. Four areas are important: suicide risk, assault risk, life-threatening medical conditions and external threat.

Suicide Risk

The risk of suicide is the most common life-threatening situation mental health professionals encounter. Its assessment is based on both an understanding of its epidemiology, which alerts the clinician to potential danger, and the individualized assessment of the patient. Suicide is the eighth leading cause of death in the USA. In the past century, the rate of suicide has averaged 12.5 per 100 000 people. Studies of adults and adolescents who commit suicide reveal that more than 90% of them suffered from at least one psychiatric disorder and as many as 80% of them consulted a physician in the months preceding the event. An astute risk assessment therefore provides an opportunity for prevention.

For those who complete suicide, the most common diagnoses are affective disorder (45–70%) and alcoholism (25%). In certain psychiatric disorders, there is a significant lifetime risk for suicide, as listed in Table 19.18. Panic disorder is associated with an elevated rate of suicidal ideation and suicide attempts but estimates of rates of completed suicide are not well established.

Suicide rates increase with age, although rates among young adults have been steadily rising. Women attempt suicide more often than men, but men are three to four times more likely than women to complete suicide. Whites have higher rates of suicide than other groups.

A patient may fit the diagnostic and demographic profile for suicide risk, but even more essential is the individualized

Table 19.18	Indications for Brain Imaging

History of head trauma
Focal neurological findings on physical examination
New-onset psychosis
New-onset psychiatric symptoms after age 40 (including affective disorder and personality change)
Rapid onset of psychiatric symptoms
History of neurological symptoms (including seizures)
Evidence of cognitive impairment
Abnormal electroencephalogram
Abnormal lumbar puncture

assessment developed by integrating information from all parts of the psychiatric evaluation. This includes material from the present illness (e.g., symptoms of depression, paranoid ideation about being harmed), past psychiatric history (e.g., prior attempts at suicide or other violent behavior), personal history (e.g., recent loss), family history (e.g., suicide or violence in close relatives), medical history (e.g., presence of a terminal illness) and the MSE (e.g., helplessness, suicidal ideation).

The most consistent predictor of future suicidal behavior is a prior history of such behavior, which is especially worrisome when previous suicide attempts have involved serious intent or lethal means. Among the factors cited as having an association with risk of suicide are current use of drugs and alcohol; recent loss, such as of a spouse or job; social isolation; conduct disorders and antisocial behavior, especially in young men; the presence of depression, especially when it is accompanied by hopelessness, helplessness, delusions, or agitation; certain psychotic symptoms, such as command hallucinations and frightening paranoid delusions; fantasies of reunion by death; and severe medical illness, especially when it is associated with loss of functioning, intractable pain, or central nervous system dysfunction. Table 19.19 lists risk factors for suicide. It should be noted that assisted suicide is now more openly discussed among people with terminal illnesses and has gained some measure of acceptability. Nonetheless, the vast majority of people who are bereaved or suffer from a serious medical illness do not end their lives by suicide. Adequate end-of-life care should forestall requests for assisted suicide. Although suicidal intent may be lacking, patients who are delirious and confused as a result of a medical illness are also at risk of self-injury.

It is essential to be clear about whether the patient has passive thoughts about suicide or actual intent. Is there a plan? If so, how detailed is it, how lethal, and what are the chances of rescue? The possession of firearms is particularly worrisome, because nearly two-thirds of documented suicides among men and more than a third among women have involved this method.

Table 19.19	Estimated Lifetime Rates of Completed Suicide by Diagnosis

Major affective disorders: 10–15%
Alcoholism: 10–15% (comorbid depression usually present)
Schizophrenia: 10% (often during a post-psychotic depressive state)
Borderline and antisocial personality disorders: 5–10%

Factors that may protect against suicide include convictions in opposition to suicide; strong attachments to others, including spouse and children; and evidence of good impulse control.

In addition to the assessment of risk factors, it is important to decide whether the possibility of suicide is of immediate concern or represents a long-term ongoing risk.

Risk of Assault

Unlike those who commit suicide, most people who commit violent acts have not been diagnosed with a mental illness, and data clarifying the relationship between mental illness and violence are limited. The most common psychiatric diagnoses associated with violence are substance-related disorders. Conduct disorder and antisocial personality disorder, by definition, involve aggressive, violent and/or unlawful behavior.

In the absence of comorbid substance-related disorders, most people with such major mental illnesses as affective disorders and schizophrenia are not violent. But data from the National Institute of Mental Health Epidemiological Catchment Area Study suggest that these diagnoses are associated with a higher rate of violence than that found among individuals who have no diagnosable mental illness. The MacArthur Violence Risk Assessment Study found this was only true for psychiatric patients with substance abuse (Steadman *et al.*, 1998).

Table 19.20 lists risk factors for violence. As with suicide, the best predictor of future assault is a history of past assault.

Information from the psychiatric evaluation that helps in this assessment includes the present illness (e.g., preoccupation with vengeance, especially when accompanied by a plan of action), psychiatric history (e.g., childhood conduct disorder), family history (e.g., exposure as a child to violent parental behavior), personal history (e.g., arrest record), and the MSE (e.g., homicidal ideation, severe agitation). Other predictors of violence include possession of weapons and current illegal activities. There is considerable overlap between risk factors for suicide and those for violence.

Life-threatening Medical Conditions

It is essential to consider life-threatening medical illness as a potential cause of psychiatric disturbance. Clues to this etiology can be found in the present illness (e.g., physical complaints), family history (e.g., causes of death in close family members), medical history (e.g., previous medical conditions and treatments), physical examination (e.g., abnormalities identified) and MSE (e.g., confusion, fluctuation in levels of consciousness). Laboratory assessment, brain imaging and structured tests for neuropsychiatric impairment may also be essential.

Probably the most common life-threatening medical situations that the psychiatrist evaluates are acute central nervous system changes caused by medical conditions and accompanied by mental status alterations. These include increased intracranial pressure or other cerebral abnormalities, severe

Table 19.20	Risk Factors for Suicide
Category	Risk Factors for Suicide
Demographic	White Male Older age Divorced, never married, or widowed Unemployed
Historical	Previous suicide attempts, especially with serious intent, lethal means, or disappointment about survival Family history of suicide Victim of physical or sexual abuse
Psychiatric	Diagnosis: affective disorder, alcoholism, panic disorder, psychotic disorders, conduct disorder, severe personality disorder (especially antisocial and borderline) Symptoms: suicidal or homicidal ideation; depression, especially with hopelessness, helplessness, anhedonia, delusions, agitation; mixed mania and depression; psychotic symptoms, including command hallucinations and persecutory delusions Current use of alcohol or illicit drugs Recent psychiatric hospitalization
Environmental	Recent loss such as that of a spouse or job Social isolation Access to guns or other lethal weapons Social acceptance of suicide
Medical	Severe medical illness, especially with loss of functioning or intractable pain Delirium or confusion caused by central nervous system dysfunction
Behavioral	Antisocial acts Poor impulse control, risk taking, and aggressiveness Preparing for death (e.g., making a will, giving away possessions, stockpiling lethal medication) Well-developed, detailed suicide plan Statements of intent to inflict harm on self or others

metabolic alterations, toxic states and alcohol withdrawal. Patients may be at risk of death if these states are not quickly identified.

External Threat

Some patients who present for psychiatric evaluation are at risk as a result of life-threatening external situations. Such patients can include battered women, abused children and victims of catastrophes who lack proper food or shelter. Information about these conditions is usually obtained from the present illness, the personal history the medical history and physical examination.

Differential Diagnosis

The differential diagnosis is best approached by organizing the information obtained in the psychiatric evaluation into five domains of mental functioning according to the disturbances revealed by the evaluation (see Table 19.21 and the subsequent chapters in this section for more detail). After organizing the information into these five domains, the psychiatrist looks for the psychopathological syndromes and potential diagnoses that best account for the disturbances described. A complete diagnostic evaluation includes assessments on each of the five axes of DSM-IV-TR (Table 19.22).

Disturbances of consciousness, orientation and memory are most typically associated with delirium related to a general medical condition or a substance use disorder. Memory impairment and other cognitive disturbances are the hallmarks of dementia. Results of the history, physical examination, laboratory testing and brain imaging often help in defining the specific etiology. It is important to elicit risk factors for HIV infection and, when they are present, to encourage voluntary HIV antibody testing. Neuropsychological testing is particularly useful in the diagnosis of subcortical dementia, such as that caused by Huntington's disease and HIV infection. Dissociative disorders and severe psychotic states may also present with disturbances in this domain without evidence of any medical etiology. Cognitive impairment caused by mental retardation is established by intelligence testing.

Disturbances of speech, thinking, perception and self-experience are common in psychotic states that can be seen in patients with such diagnoses as schizophrenia and mania, as well as in central nervous system dysfunction caused by substance use or a medical condition. Disturbances in self-experience are also common in dissociative disorders and certain anxiety, somatoform and eating disorders. Cluster A personality disorders may be associated with milder forms of disturbances in this domain (American Psychiatric Association, 2000).

Disturbances of emotion are most typical of affective and anxiety disorders. These disturbances may also be caused by substance use disorders and general medical conditions. Mood and affect disturbances accompany many personality disorders and may be especially pronounced in borderline personality disorder.

Physical signs and symptoms and any associated abnormalities revealed by diagnostic medical tests and past medical history are used to establish the presence of general medical conditions, which are coded on Axis III. When a medical disorder is causally related to a psychiatric disorder, a statement of this relationship should appear on Axis I. Physical signs and symptoms

Table 19.21 **Risk Factors for Violence**	
Category	Risk Factors
Demographic	Young Male Limited education Unemployed
Historical	Previous history of violence to self or others, especially with high degree of lethality History of animal torture Past antisocial or criminal behavior Violence within family of origin Victim of physical or sexual abuse
Psychiatric	Diagnosis: substance-related disorders, antisocial personality disorder; conduct disorder; intermittent explosive disorder; pathological alcohol intoxication; psychoses (e.g., paranoid, toxic) Symptoms: physical agitation; intent to kill or take revenge; identification of specific victim(s); psychotic symptoms, especially command hallucinations to commit violence and persecutory delusions Current use of alcohol or other drugs
Environmental	Access to guns or other lethal weapons Living under circumstances of violence Membership in violent group
Medical	Delirium or confusion caused by central nervous system dysfunction Disinhibition caused by traumatic brain injuries and other central nervous system dysfunctions Toxic states related to metabolic disorders (e.g., hyperthyroidism)
Behavioral	Antisocial acts Agitation, anger Poor impulse control; risk taking or reckless behavior Statements of intent to inflict harm

Table 19.22   Categorizing Features of Mental Disturbance

Area of Mental Functioning	Examples of Relevant Evidence of Disturbance
Consciousness, orientation, and memory	Abnormalities on interview or MSE, especially impairments in awareness; alertness; orientation to person, place, time; immediate, short-term or long-term memory; attention; calculations; fund of knowledge; abstractions Past history of foregoing Positive substance use history Risk factors for HIV; positive HIV antibody result Focal neurological findings on physical examination Laboratory and brain imaging abnormalities Impairments on neuropsychological testing
Speech, thinking, perception, and self-experience	Abnormalities on interview or MSE, especially disturbances of speech, thinking, reality testing, and presence of hallucinations, delusions Past history of foregoing
Emotions	Abnormalities on interview or MSE, especially labile, depressed, expansive, elevated, irritable mood, and inappropriate affect, anger, or anxiety Past history of foregoing Positive scores for mood disturbance on structured interviews
Physical signs and symptoms; physiological disturbances	Physical or neurological findings indicative of medical or mental disorder Laboratory abnormalities Past medical illnesses Positive substance use history
Behavior and adaptive functioning	Personality dysfunction Impaired social or occupational functioning Impaired activities of daily living Impulsive, compulsive, or avoidant behaviors History of behavioral or functional disturbances Personal history (highest levels of achievement)

may also suggest diagnoses of mood or anxiety disorders or states of substance intoxication or withdrawal. Physical symptoms for which no medical etiology can be demonstrated after thorough assessment suggest somatoform or factitious disorders or malingering, although the possibility of an as-yet-undiagnosed medical condition should still be kept in mind.

Information about behavior and adaptive functioning is useful for diagnosing personality disorders, documenting psychosocial and environmental problems on Axis IV, and assessing global functioning on Axis V. This information is also useful for diagnosing most psychiatric disorders, which typically include criteria related to abnormal behaviors and functional impairment.

When all information has been gathered and organized, it may be possible to reach definitive diagnoses, but sometimes this must await further evaluation and the development of the comprehensive treatment plan.

Initial Treatment Plan

The initial treatment plan follows the case formulation, which has already established the nature of the current problem and a tentative diagnosis. The plan distinguishes between what must be accomplished now and what is postponed for the future. Treatment planning works best when it follows the biopsychosocial model.

Biological Intervention

This includes an immediate response to any life-threatening medical conditions and a plan for the treatment of other less acute physical disorders, including those that may contribute to an altered mental status. Prescription of psychotropic medications in accordance with the tentative diagnosis is the most common biological intervention.

Psychosocial Intervention

This includes immediate plans to prevent violent or suicidal behavior and address adverse external circumstances. An overall strategy must be developed that is both realistic and responsive to the patient's situation. Developing this strategy requires an awareness of the social support systems available to the patient; the financial resources of the patient; the availability of services in the area; the need to contact other agencies, such as child welfare or the police; and the need to ensure child care for dependent children.

Initial Disposition

The primary task of the initial disposition is to select the most appropriate level of care after completion of the psychiatric evaluation. Disposition is primarily focused on immediate goals. After referral, the patient and the treatment team develop longer term goals.

Hospitalization

The first decision in any disposition plan is whether hospitalization is required to ensure safety. There are times when a patient presents with such severe risk of harm to self or others that hospitalization seems essential. In other cases, the patient could be managed outside the hospital, depending on the availability of other supports. This might include a family who can stay with the patient or a crisis team in the community able to treat the patient at home. The more comprehensive the system of services, the easier it is to avoid hospitalization. Because hospitalization is associated with extreme disruption of usual life activities and in and of itself can have many adverse consequences, plans to avoid hospitalization are usually appropriate as long as they do not compromise safety.

Day Programs, Crisis Residences and Supervised Housing

These interventions provide ongoing supervision but at a lower level than that available within the hospital. They are most often used to treat patients with alcohol and substance use disorders or severe mental illness. Crisis housing can be useful when a patient cannot safely return home, when caregivers need respite, and when the patient is homeless. Other forms of supervised housing usually have a waiting period and may not be immediately available.

There are many different types of and names for day-long programming, including partial hospitalization, day treatment, psychiatric rehabilitation and psychosocial clubs. Depending on the nature of the program, it may provide stabilization, daily medication, training in social and vocational skills, and treatment of alcohol and substance use problems. Long-term day programs should generally be avoided if a patient is functioning successfully in a daytime role, such as in a job or as a homemaker. In these instances, referral to a day program may promote a lower level of functioning than the patient is capable of.

Outpatient Medication and Psychotherapy

The most common referral after psychiatric evaluation is to psychotherapy and/or medication management. In office-based settings, the psychiatrist decides whether she or he has the time and expertise to treat the patient and makes referrals to other practitioners as appropriate. Hospital staff usually have a broad overview of community resources and refer accordingly. There are high rates of dropout when patients are sent from one setting to another. These can be reduced by providing introductions to the treatment setting and/or conducting follow-up to ensure that the referral has been successful.

Comprehensive Treatment Planning

The psychiatric evaluation usually continues beyond the initial disposition. The providers assuming responsibility for the patient, who may be inpatient staff, outpatient staff, or private practitioners, complete the evaluation and take responsibility for developing the comprehensive treatment plan. This plan covers the entire array of concerns that affect the course of the patient's psychiatric problems. In hospital settings, the initial treatment plan is usually completed within 24 to 72 hours after admission, followed by comprehensive treatment plan after more extensive evaluation.

The comprehensive treatment plan usually includes more definitive diagnoses and a well-formulated management plan with central goals and objectives. For severely ill or hospitalized patients, every area is usually covered (Table 19.23 and 19.24). It is best for the patient and, as appropriate, the family, to have input into the plan. The comprehensive treatment plan guides and coordinates the direction of all treatment for an extended time, usually

Table 19.23	DSM-IV-TR Multiaxial System
Axis I	Clinical disorders Other conditions that may be a focus of clinical attention
Axis II	Personality disorders Mental retardation
Axis III	General medical conditions
Axis IV	Psychosocial and environmental problems
Axis V	Global assessment of functioning

months, and is periodically reviewed and updated. For more focal psychiatric problems (e.g., phobias, sexual dysfunctions) and more limited interventions (e.g., brief interpersonal, cognitive, and behavioral therapies in office-based practices), the comprehensive treatment plan may focus on only several of the possible areas.

Conclusion

The psychiatric evaluation is a method of collecting present and past psychological, biological, social and environmental data for the purpose of establishing a comprehensive picture of the patient's strengths and problems, including the psychiatric diagnoses, and developing treatment plans. It is the essential beginning of every course of psychiatric treatment and, when carried out successfully, integrates a multimodal approach to understanding mental illness and providing clinical care.

Table 19.24	Areas Covered by Comprehensive Treatment Plan

Mental health
    Diagnoses on five axes
    Psychiatric management, including medications
Physical health
    Medical diagnoses
    Medical management, including medications
Personal strengths and assets
Rehabilitation needs
    Educational
    Occupational
    Social
    Activities of daily living skills
    Use of leisure time
Living arrangements
Social supports and family involvement
Finances
    Personal finances
    Insurance coverage
    Eligibility for social service benefits
Legal or forensic issues
Central goals and objectives
Listing of treatment team members
Evidence of participation by patient and, as appropriate, family members and others
Criteria for discharge from treatment

References

American Psychiatric Association (2000) *Diagnostic and Statistical Manual of Mental Disorders*, 4th edn, Text Rev. APA, Washington DC.

Belliveau JW, Kennedy D, McKinstry RC *et al.* (1991) Functional mapping of the human visual cortex by magnetic resonance imaging. *Science* 254, 716–719.

Boutros NN (1992) A review of indications for routine EEG in clinical psychiatry. *Hosp Comm Psychiatr* 43, 716–719.

Bonte FJ, Weiner MF, Bigio EH, et al. (2001) SPECT imaging in dementias. *J Nucl Med* 42, 1131–1132.

Cassens G, Inglis AK, Appelbaum PS *et al.* (1990) Neuroleptics: Effects on neuropsychological function in chronic schizophrenic patients. *Schizophr Bull* 16, 477–499.

Celesia GG and Brigell MG (1999) Auditory evoked potentials, in *Electroencephalography: Basic Principles, Clinical Applications, and Related Fields*, 4th edn. (eds Niedermeyer E and Lopes Da Silva F). Lippincott, Williams & Wilkins, Baltimore, MD, pp. 994–1013.

Chou TC (1991) *Electrocardiography in Clinical Practice*, 3rd edn. WB Saunders, Philadelphia, PA, p. 481.

Council on Scientific Affairs (1987) Scientific issues in drug testing. *JAMA* 257, 3110–3114.

Drake ME and Shy KE (1989) Predictive value of electroencephalography for electroconvulsive therapy. *Clin Electroencephalogr* 20, 55–57.

Ford JM, Roth WT, Isaacks BG *et al.* (1997) Automatic and effortful processing in aging and dementia: Event-related brain potentials. *Neurobiol Aging* 18, 169–180.

Frodl T, Hampel H, Juckel G *et al.* (2002) Value of event related P300 subcomponents in the clinical diagnosis of mild cognitive impairment and Alzheimer's Disease. *Psychophysiology* 39, 175–181.

Gold MS and Dackis CA (1986) Role of the laboratory in the evaluation of suspected drug abuse. *J Clin Psychiatr* 47(Suppl), 17–23.

Gonzalez RG, Fischman AJ, Guimaraes AR *et al.* (1995) Functional MR in the evaluation of dementia: Correlation of abnormal dynamic cerebral blood volume measurements with changes in cerebral metabolism on positron emission tomography with fluorodeoxyglucose. *Am J Neuroradiol* 16, 1763–1770.

Golden CJ, Hammeke T and Purisch A (1980) *Manual for The Luria-Nebraska Neuropsychological Battery*. Western Psychological Services, Los Angeles, CA.

Goodglass H and Kaplan E (1979) Assessment of cognitive deficit in the brain-injured patient, in *Handbook of Behavioral Neurobiology*, Vol. 2, *Neuropsychology*, (ed Gazzaniga M). Plenum Press, New York.

Holmes-Bernstein J and Waber DP (1990) Developmental neuropsychological assessment: The systemic approach, in *Neuromethods: Neuropsychology* (eds Boulton AA, Baker GB, and Hiscock M). Humana Press, Clifton, NJ, pp. 311–371.

Hughes JR (1996) A review of the usefulness of the standard EEG in psychiatry. Clin Electroencephalogr 27, 35–39.

Hughes JR and John ER (1999) Conventional and quantitative electroencephalography in psychiatry. *J Neuropsychiatr Clin Neurosci* 11, 190–207.

Johnson KA, Renshaw PF, Becker JA *et al.* (1995) Comparison of functional MRI and SPECT in Alzheimer's disease. *Neurology* 45(Suppl), S874.

Kaplan E (1990) The process approach to neuropsychological assessment of psychiatric patients. *J Neuropsychiatr Clin Neurosci* 2, 72–87.

Krausz Y, Bonne O, Marciano R *et al.* (1996) Brain SPECT imaging of neuropsychiatric disorders. *Eur J Radiol* 21, 183–187.

Milberg WP, Hebben N and Kaplan E (1996) The Boston process neuropsychological approach to neuropsychological assessment, in *Neuropsychological Assessment of Neuropsychiatric Disorders*, 2nd edn. (eds Grant I and Adams KM). Oxford University Press, New York, pp. 58–80.

Osborn AG (1994) *Diagnostic Neuroradiology*. Mosby Year Book, St. Louis.

Polich J (1999) P300 in clinical applications, in *Electroencephalography: Basic Principles, Clinical Applications and Related Fields*, 4th edn. (eds Niedermeyer E and Lopes da Silva F). Lippincott, Williams & Wilkins, Baltimore, MD, pp. 1073–1091.

Polich J and Herbst KL (2000) P300 as a clinical assay: Rationale, evaluation, and findings. *Int J Psychophysiol* 38, 3–19.

Reiman EM, Caselli RJ, Yun LS *et al.* (1996) Preclinical evidence of Alzheimer's disease in persons homozygous for the epsilon 4 allele for apolipoprotein E. *New Engl J Med* 334, 752–758.

Reitan RR and Wolfson D (1993) *The Halstead–Reitan Neuropsychological Test Battery: Theory and Clinical Interpretation*, 2nd edn. Neuropsychology Press, Tucson, AZ.

Sackeim HA, Luber B, Katzman GP *et al.* (1996) The effects of electroconvulsive therapy on quantitative electroencephalograms. *Arch Gen Psychiatr* 53, 814–824.

Seidman LJ and Toomey R (1999) The clinical use of psychological and neuropsychological tests, in *The New Harvard Guide to Psychiatry* (ed Nicholi A). Harvard University Press, Cambridge, MA, pp. 40–64.

Silverman DH, Small GW, Chang CY, et al. (2001) Positron emission tomography in evaluation of dementia: Regional brain metabolism and long-term outcome. *J Am Med Assoc* 286, 2120–2127.

Small GW, Mazziotta JC, Collins MT *et al.* (1995) Apolipoprotein E type 4 allele and cerebral glucose metabolism in relatives at risk for familial Alzheimer's disease. *J Am Med Assoc* 273, 942–947.

Small JG (1999) Psychiatric disorders and EEG, in *Electroencephalography: Basic Principles, Clinical Applications, and Related Fields*, 4th edn. (eds Niedermeyer E and Lopes Da Silva F). Lippincott, Williams & Wilkins, Baltimore, MD, pp. 603–620.

Spohn HE and Strauss ME (1989) The relation of neuroleptic and anticholinergic medication to cognitive functions in schizophrenia. *J Abnorm Psychol* 98, 367–380.

Squire LR and Shimamura A (1996) The neuropsychology of memory dysfunction and its assessment, in *Neuropsychological Assessment of Neuropsychiatric Disorders* (eds Grant I and Adams KM). Oxford University Press, New York, pp. 268–299.

Steadman HJ, Gounis K, Dennis D *et al.* (1998) Violence by people discharged from acute psychiatric inpatient facilities and by others in the same neighborhoods. *Arch Gen Psychiatr* 55, 393–401.

Theodore WH and Gaillard WD (2000) Positron emission tomography in neocortical epilepsies. *Adv Neurol* 84, 435–446.

Trimble MR and Thompson PJ (1986) Neuropsychological aspects of epilepsy, in *Neuropsychological Aspects of Neuropsychiatric Disorders*. Oxford University Press, New York, pp. 321–346.

Weinstein CS and Seidman LJ (1994) The role of neuropsychological assessment in adult psychiatry, in *The Psychotherapist's Guide to Neuropsychiatry: Diagnostic and Treatment Issues* (eds Ellison J, Weinstein CS, and Hodel-Malinofsky T). American Psychiatric Press, Washington DC, pp. 53–106.

Weinstein CS, Seidman LJ, Feldman J *et al.* (1991) Neurocognitive disorders in psychiatry: A case example of diagnostic and treatment dilemmas. *Psychiatry* 54, 65–75.

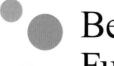

CHAPTER

20

Behavior and Adaptive Functioning

To function adaptively means to behave in such a way that one's attitudes and actions are well matched to the demands and constraints of the external environment and that one's sense of internal discomfort or distress is minimized. Therefore, by definition, the ability to adapt depends both on the individual's behavioral repertoire and on the external environment. A person's capacity for adaptive functioning is so crucial that it has been studied in situations ranging from adaptation to long-term missions in outer space (Eksuzian, 1999) to the self-management of life-threatening illnesses such as chronic heart failure (Buetow *et al.*, 2001). This chapter focuses on the ingredients that shape personality and the ways in which personality in turn affects behavior. In addition, the domains in which individuals are typically expected to function are reviewed, with particular attention to the ways in which various personality styles affect functioning in each domain. Patterns of behavior that are frequently pathological in nature, such as impulsive, compulsive and avoidant behaviors, are examined. Finally, approaches to the assessment of behavior and adaptive functioning in the psychiatric interview are reviewed.

Clinical Vignette 1

Mr C, a young schizophrenic man, attempted to avoid hospitalization by beginning to shave more regularly and cutting his fingernails. However, he remained unwilling and unable to have his hair cut, attempting to disguise its length by wearing it up under a baseball cap when going outside.

Clinical Vignette 2

Ms D, a middle-aged woman, came to the emergency department claiming that she had run out of Valium and that her prescribing physician was out of town. Her story was convincing and the resident physician was about to give her a prescription when he noted on close examination that she had a dirty hem on both her pants and her jacket sleeves, which seemed inconsistent with her presentation of herself as an executive secretary. After pressing her for more details of her story and consulting with another emergency department, he determined that the patient was actually a homeless woman who got prescriptions from hospitals and then sold them on the street.

Personality Style

An individual's personality style has a great influence on his or her behavior and adaptive functioning. Personality is shaped from a blend of inborn temperament, genetic strengths and vulnerabilities, and the impact of positive and negative life experiences. Psychiatry is moving toward an improved understanding of human behavior that focuses on the ways that these factors interact with one another.

There is evidence of striking variation among neonates in their capacity to tolerate frustration, which reflects their inborn temperaments (Thomas *et al.*, 1963). Such individual differences in temperament form the biological substrate that interacts with early development. Temperament affects the degree to which different infants are susceptible to distress as well as their variations in attachment style (Rothbart and Ahadi, 1994).

Genetic factors of various types also play a role in development, particularly when they interact with environmental factors. In general, genetic factors account for between 30 and 60% of the variance in adult personality traits (Carey and DiLalla, 1994).

Life experiences also have an impact on an individual and affect her or his behavior for better or worse. Considering whether particular experiences are the result of fate in contrast to whether they are partially brought about by the person's own actions can be important in thinking about their impact and meaning.

While psychiatrists have long suspected links between early life experiences, especially traumatic ones, and adult psychopathology, these connections are just now being clearly, empirically demonstrated. For example, in one recent study, childhood verbal abuse conferred an increased likelihood of borderline, narcissistic, paranoid, schizoid and schizotypal personality disorder during adolescence which was independent of other facts like temperament, physical and sexual abuse, use of corporal punishment, parental psychopathology and cooccuring psychiatric disorders (Johnson *et al.*, 2001). Further, as the relationships between genetic propensities expressed as temperament or personality factors and environmental influences have been explicated, some fascinating interactions have emerged. For example, one recent study suggested that high levels of the personality trait of sensation seeking, which appears to be genetically mediated, might result in a high incidence of adverse life events that would in turn help to precipitate depression (Farmer *et al.*, 2001) Further, exploration of patterns of disease and personality factors is beginning to shape genetic investigations by serving as guides for genetic linkage studies (Nigg and Goldsmith, 1998). For instance, in one study, twins and siblings who were highly

Essentials of Psychiatry   Jerald Kay and Allan Tasman
© 2006 John Wiley & Sons, Ltd.

concordant and discordant for neuroticism, a personality factor, were examined for evidence of anxiety and depression. Tissue samples were collected to look for areas of genetic overlap and thus to identify potential foci on chromosomes that warranted further exploration (Kirk *et al.*, 2000).

Personality styles have been described in a variety of ways with use of different models of normal personality variation. These models are either categorical or dimensional in nature. In a categorical model, a person is described as meeting or not meeting the criteria for various diagnostic categories. In a dimensional model of personality, a person is evaluated in terms of the blend of various traits or factors he or she possesses, measured on a continuum. In general, as a person moves toward the extreme end of a given continuum in the dimensional model, she or he becomes more likely to meet the criteria for a categorical diagnosis. Some dimensional models set a threshold beyond which a given characteristic is likely to be a problem or pathological.

The categorical model is a more common approach to diagnosis within clinical psychiatry and within medicine in general. It now seems clear that useful information is gained from both categorical and dimensional approaches to examining personality. Thus, although personality disorders as outlined in the *Diagnostic and Statistical Manual of Mental Disorders*, Fourth Edition (DSM-IV-TR) (American Psychiatric Association, 1994) are currently cast in categorical terms, Oldham and Skodol (2000), among others, have suggested that elements of both categorical and dimensional systems be included when revisions are made in DSM-V. Others have proposed a prototype-matching approach to diagnosing personality disorders in which models of various personality styles are constructed and psychiatrists make diagnosis by matching their patient to the best available prototype (Westen and Shedler, 2000).

Oldham and Morris (1995) translated each of the personality disorders of the DSM-IV-TR system into a less pathological collection of categories that describe normal personality styles. In their system, a cross between a categorical and a dimensional model, conscientiousness is the positive personality trait that in excess becomes obsessive–compulsive personality disorder. Table 20.1 summarizes the personality style–personality disorder continuum described by Oldham and Morris.

A continuum model such as this one acknowledges that whereas too much of a good thing may constitute a disorder, everyone's personality consists of traits that can be adaptive or maladaptive. The quantity rather than the quality of a given trait

is often what makes it a problem or adaptive. Similarly, flexibility and variability are important determinants of a person's adaptive capacity.

Examples of dimensional models of personality include the five-factor model (Widiger *et al.*, 1994), Cloninger's seven-factor model (Cloninger, 1987; Cloninger *et al.*, 1993), and the biogenic spectrum model of Siever and Davis (1991). The five-factor model of personality was first suggested by McDougall (1932) and was elaborated and updated by Digman (1990) and McCrae and Costa (1987) among others. In the five-factor model, personality traits are described in terms of a taxonomy of five dimensions. These include neuroticism, extraversion, openness to experience, agreeableness and conscientiousness. Table 20.2 summarizes the factors of the five-factor model and their relationship to DSM-IV-TR categories.

A second dimensional model of personality is Cloninger's seven-factor model of temperament and character (Cloninger, 1987; Cloninger *et al.*, 1993) (Table 20.3). In this model, a patient's behavior is evaluated on seven separate dimensions. Four of the seven dimensions are related to temperament and have been shown to be independently heritable, manifested early in life, and involved in early perceptual memory and habit formation.

Table 20.1	Oldham and Morris' Personality Style–Personality Disorder Continuum
Style	DSM-IV Disorder
Vigilant	Paranoid
Solitary	Schizoid
Idiosyncratic	Schizotypal
Adventurous	Antisocial
Mercurial	Borderline
Dramatic	Histrionic
Self-confident	Narcissistic
Sensitive	Avoidant
Devoted	Dependent
Conscientious	Obsessive–compulsive

Table 20.2	The Five-Factor Model	
Factor	Traits	DSM-IV Example
Neuroticism	Anxiety Hostility Depression Self-consciousness Impulsiveness Vulnerability	High in borderline Low in schizoid
Extraversion	Warmth Gregariousness Assertiveness Activity Excitement seeking Positive emotions	High in histrionic Low in avoidant
Openness	Fantasy Esthetics Feelings Actions Ideas Values	High in schizotypal Low in paranoid
Agreeableness	Trust Straightforwardness Altruism Compliance Modesty Tendermindedness	High in dependent Low in narcissistic
Conscientiousness	Competence Order Dutifulness Achievement striving Self-discipline Deliberation	High in obsessive–compulsive Low in antisocial

Table 20.3   Cloninger's Seven-Factor Model of Temperament and Character

Temperament Factor	Behavioral Effect
Harm avoidance	Behavioral inhibition
Reward dependence	Motivation for behavior
Novelty seeking	Initiation of exploration
Persistence	Maintenance of behavior
Character Factor	Self-Concept Effect
Self-directedness	Sense of self as autonomous
Cooperativeness	Sense of self as part of community
Self-transcendence	Sense of self in the universe

These four dimensions include novelty seeking, harm avoidance, reward dependence and persistence. Figure 20.1 is a schematic representation of Cloninger's model.

Cloninger also describes three dimensions of character, namely, self-directedness, cooperativeness, and self-transcendence. The blend of these three characteristics that an individual possesses helps to determine self-concept, such as whether the individual identifies himself or herself as an autonomous individual, as an integral part of humanity, and as a part of the universe as a whole. Those with low degrees of self-directedness and low degrees of cooperativeness are more likely to have personality disorders (Svrakic *et al.*, 1993).

A third dimensional model of personality is the biogenic spectrum model of Siever and Davis (1991). This model proposes that certain personality styles and disorders are associated with and are characterological variants of various Axis I disorders. Thus, personality disorders are not extreme variants of normal but are characterological variants of Axis I disorders. The biogenic spectrum model may be useful in guiding treatment, such as using anxiolytics to treat avoidant personality disorder because it is considered to be on a spectrum with Axis I anxiety disorders. There is growing evidence that the biogenic spectrum model is useful for at least some Axis I/Axis II disorders. One example is the link between schizophrenia and schizotypal personality disorder in which those with the Axis II disorder demonstrate a better capacity for buffering in certain frontal brain regions as shown by functional imaging as compared with those with the full-blown Axis I disorder (Kirrane and Siever, 2000). Table 20.4 presents details of the biogenic model.

Domains of Functioning

Each person's unique personality style is reflected in the various domains in which the person functions. DSM-IV's Axis V, the

Table 20.4   The Biogenic Model and DSM-IV-TR

Axis I Disorder	Example of Axis II Variant
Mood	Borderline
Anxiety	Avoidant
Impulse control	Antisocial
Psychotic	Schizoid

Global Assessment of Functioning, provides a 100-point scale with which to rate a person's overall level of adaptation. It provides a useful global rating of adaptive function that assesses the degree of symptoms and the capacity to function in social and occupational spheres (American Psychiatric Association, 1994). These domains are somewhat overlapping. Oldham and Morris' model of normal personality derived from the DSM categories provides a framework for thinking about how different personality styles predispose people to emphasize or minimize the importance they assign each domain and to function more or less effectively in each area (Oldham and Morris, 1995).

Social and Interpersonal Functioning

Interpersonal styles greatly affect social functioning, which in turn has a large impact on both work- and leisure-time functioning. Distinctive individual personality styles affect a person's perception of the importance of relationships with others as well as the quality and depth of the bonds they can form. Those with solitary traits are unlikely to crave and seek close relationships, whereas those with a devoted style become uneasy and feel incomplete if they are not with others. Vigilant people are cautious of the attentions of others, whereas dramatic types thrive on the admiration of their peers. Those who are mercurial often run "hot" and "cold" in their relationships with others, sometimes expressing their feelings in ways that offend others; sensitive types are easily affected by the perspectives and behavior of others but tend to keep their feelings to themselves.

The Social Adjustment Scale (Weissman *et al.*, 1974, 2001) provides a quantitative way to investigate several types of interpersonal functioning (Table 20.5) including a person's relationships with family of origin, spouse or partner, children, work colleagues, and friends and acquaintances. Inherent in these assessments of functioning is an assumption that to be successful, relationships should be interpersonally relatively free of friction and arguments, reciprocal and supportive. In addition, each person's experience of the relationship should be comfortable and relatively conflict free.

Benjamin's Structural Analysis of Social Behavior (Figure 20.2) provides another means of assessing recurrent patterns in a person's interactions with others (Benjamin, 1986b). It has three dimensions: 1) the focus of the interaction; 2) the tone of the interaction (loving versus hating); and 3) whether the interaction is characterized by interdependence or independence. The focus in the Structural Analysis of Social Behavior can be on another person, on oneself in relation to another person, or on inward, internal aspects of the self. The Structural Analysis of Social Behavior is widely used in research settings to describe and quantify a person's mode of interpersonal functioning in various relationships.

Occupational Functioning

Assessing adaptive occupational functioning requires examining the ways in which an individual completes tasks, takes and gives orders, delegates responsibilities and cooperates with others. Job situations also require an ability to balance demands, obey regulations and make decisions. Clearly, success in these tasks in part depends on one's capacity for interpersonal functioning.

Weissman's Social Adjustment Scale (Weissman *et al.*, 2001) provides a means of evaluating a person's occupational functioning. The scale focuses on both externally observable

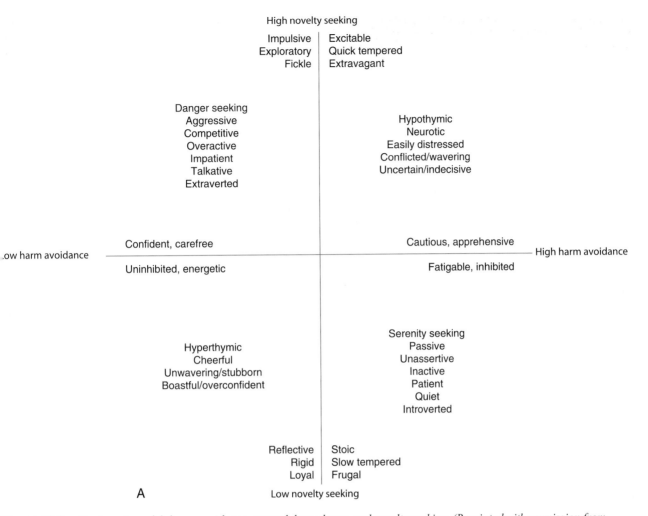

High novelty seeking

Impulsive	Excitable
Exploratory	Quick tempered
Fickle	Extravagant

Danger seeking
Aggressive
Competitive
Overactive
Impatient
Talkative
Extraverted

Hypothymic
Neurotic
Easily distressed
Conflicted/wavering
Uncertain/indecisive

Low harm avoidance ——— Confident, carefree   Cautious, apprehensive ——— High harm avoidance

Uninhibited, energetic   Fatigable, inhibited

Hyperthymic
Cheerful
Unwavering/stubborn
Boastful/overconfident

Serenity seeking
Passive
Unassertive
Inactive
Patient
Quiet
Introverted

Reflective	Stoic
Rigid	Slow tempered
Loyal	Frugal

A   Low novelty seeking

Figure 20.1 *Cloninger's model: harm avoidance, reward dependence, and novelty seeking. (Reprinted with permission from Cloninger CR [1987] A systematic method for clinical description and classification of personality variants: A proposal.* Arch Gen Psychiatr *44, 573–588. Copyright 1987, American Medical Association.)*

behaviors, such as number of days lost in a month and the degree of impairment of performance at work, as well as internal states, such as feeling inadequate, angry and distressed at work. In addition, whether a person is distressed, disinterested and bored by work is also assessed. These questions begin to suggest what adaptive occupational functioning comprises, namely, that it consists of being engaged and feeling satisfied about and competent at work. In addition, the Social Adjustment Scale assesses whether these positive internal states are reflected in work performance and relationships with superiors and subordinates.

Leisure
The capacity to enjoy leisure depends in part on other external demands and responsibilities as well as financial and other resources. Leisure is more than time left over from work and family. The gusto with which leisure activities are pursued and the types of activities that are chosen are affected by a person's characteristic style. In contrast to the work domain, those with a leisurely style are likely to enjoy their free time and to have myriad hobbies and interests; those with conscientious styles may approach leisure as another job, by working hard at trying to have fun. Those with aggressive styles may choose competitive leisure pursuits, such as

sports, in which they can pit their prowess against others; solitary types may prefer solo leisure pursuits that do not involve others.

The Social Adjustment Scale may be used to evaluate how well developed and specific a patient's interests are as well as the frequency with which such activities are pursued. It can be helpful in assessing whether a person's leisure-time contacts with others are diminished. The Social Adjustment Scale quantifies aspects of leisure, such as how many social events one has attended in the last month. The experience of loneliness or boredom during free time as well as the person's ability to compensate for these painful states yields a measure of leisure-time adaptation.

Assessing Behavior and Adaptive Functioning in the Clinical Interview
Finding out about a patient's personality style, level of adaptive functioning and usual patterns of behavior is one of the major tasks of the psychiatric interview. A psychiatrist gains important information from what a patient and those people close to the patient say about her or his behavior. However, a psychiatrist also gains invaluable information by closely observing the person during the interview itself. Whether the psychiatrist is quickly sizing up an agitated patient during a psychiatric emergency or carefully

Table 20.5 The Social Adjustment Scale	
Domain*	**Assessment Questions**
Work	Time lost?
Outside home	Impaired performance?
At home	Feelings of inadequacy?
At school	Friction with coworkers?
	Distress about work?
	Disinterest in work?
Social	Impaired leisure activities?
	Diminished contacts with others?
	Diminished social interactions?
	Reticence to have social contacts?
	Friction within social contacts?
	Hypersensitivity?
	Social discomfort?
	Loneliness?
	Boredom?
	Diminished dating?
	Disinterest in dating?
Interpersonal	Friction?
Extended family	Reticence?
Spouse or partner	Withdrawn?
Parental functioning	Dependency?
Family unit	Rebellion?
	Worry?
	Guilt?
	Resentment?
	Submissiveness?
	Domineering behavior?
	Lack of affection?
	Sexual interest, frequency, problems with partner?
	Lack of involvement?
	Impaired communication?

*Each domain is scored on a 5-point scale ranging from 1 (not a problem) to 5 (an extreme problem). In addition, a global score in each domain is assigned by use of this same scale.

noticing how a patient shifts in the chair during a psychotherapy session, the ability to observe a patient's behavior is one of a psychiatrist's most important tools. A patient's appearance, attitude and motor behaviors during an interaction with the psychiatrist provide important clues to personality, capacity for interpersonal interactions and potentially problematic behavior patterns.

Appearance

Observing a patient's appearance includes making a judgment about the overall physical impression of the person reflected by grooming, clothing, poise and posture. The ability to appear well-kempt is impaired in many psychiatric disorders, ranging from the psychotic patient who appears disheveled after being up for several nights to the depressed patient dressed in dark, somber tones and slumped in the chair. Clothing often reveals aspects

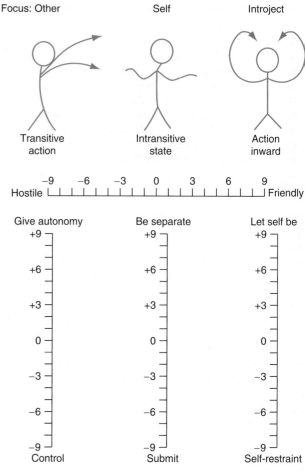

Figure 20.2   *The three dimensions of the Structural Analysis of Social Behavior model. Therapy content and process expressed in interactional terms can be coded in terms of the three dimensions: focus, love versus hate, and interdependence. Viewing all relationships in terms of these dimensions makes parallels among early and current relationships more apparent. (Source: Benjamin LS [1986a] Adding social and intrapsychic description to Axis I of DSM-III, in* Contemporary Directions in Psychopathology: Toward the DSM-IV *[eds Million T and Klerman GL].* Guilford Press, New York, p. 608.)

of personality; patients with extroverted, histrionic, or dramatic personalities often wear brightly colored, unusual clothes and are often garishly made up. Problems with appearance can suggest the possibility of other functional impairments as well. The motivation and degree of volitional control over appearance must usually be inferred. At times, appearance may provide an important clue of an inconsistency in a patient's verbal presentation and suggest a serious behavior problem.

Clinical Vignette 3

Ms G, a 21-year-old woman with borderline personality disorder, carved the word "monster" on her arm. Of this act she said, "I was feeling so tense and angry, like there was a tornado inside of me. As I focused on the small red lines I made with the razor, I began to feel better. The physical pain let me center my attention on my body, and my angry feelings seemed to fade away".

Clinical Vignette 4

Mr H, a 23-year-old college senior, sought help for his paraphilia, namely, exhibitionism. He would resist the urge to exhibit his genitals to a woman for weeks but would eventually feel that the desire was irresistible. As he noted the look of shock or surprise on the woman's face when he exhibited his penis, he would often ejaculate. However, after this, he would feel ashamed, remorseful, afraid that the woman would recognize him on the street, and convinced that she would notify the police and he would be arrested.

Attitude and Cooperation

The interviewer can also detect a patient's attitude and willingness to cooperate during an examination. Attitude and cooperation are related but not identical concepts; a paranoid patient may have a suspicious attitude but may cooperate by answering the interviewer's questions nonetheless. Often, however, a person's attitude and ability to cooperate are both affected by psychiatric illness. Patients may be friendly or hostile, seductive, defensive, or apathetic. During the psychiatric interview, they may seem attentive or disinterested and be frank or evasive and guarded. Again, each of these attitudes and the degree of cooperation a patient exhibits can depend on the underlying psychiatric state or can reflect a conscious manipulation on the part of the patient for the sake of achieving a desired goal. Attitude and degree of cooperativeness with an interviewer yield data about a patient's capacity to establish rapport and relate to others, thereby suggesting the person's general level of interpersonal functioning.

Motor Behavior

The astute examiner can also observe motor behaviors that provide clues to a patient's internal state. First, the overall level of activity should be noted. Behavioral activity is often quantitatively increased in patients with mania or anxiety disorders, whereas it may be decreased in those with depression or intoxication. In addition, impulsivity can sometimes be revealed by motor behaviors, as when a person pounds on a wall or hurls an object. Motor behavior can also provide clues to personality; the dramatic patient often gesticulates freely during conversation, whereas the obsessive patient often conveys a sense of constricted facial movements and gestures. The types of behaviors associated with overactivity may include restlessness, pacing, handwringing, or other forms of agitation. In contrast, psychomotor retardation is a slowing of the usual body movements. A depressed patient with psychomotor slowing may be observed sitting perfectly still, staring into space. Similarly, patients with underlying neurological disorders such as Parkinson's disease or those who are taking medicines that produce parkinsonism may exhibit motor slowing in the form of lack of facial expressiveness and loss of the body movements and gestures that often accompany speech.

Another clinically relevant way of approaching the task of assessing a patient's behavior was suggested by Halleck (1994). He suggested that in addition to focusing on appearance, attitude and cooperation in the clinical evaluation, the interviewer can assess 1) the patient's physical and emotional attractiveness; 2) his or her means of seeking control and whether control is a central issue; and 3) the degree to which the patient is dependent, passive, aggressive, attention seeking, private, or exploitative in his or her behaviors. Although patients with different styles have different motives for and various ways of expressing these types of behaviors, examining their behavior in each of these categories is likely to provide a productive additional approach to evaluating behavior and adaptive functioning.

Problematic Patterns of Behavior

Problematic patterns of behavior, such as impulsivity, compulsivity and avoidance, cut across diagnostic groups; looking for these patterns can be a fruitful way of characterizing aspects of maladaptive functioning. Each of these three patterns can arise from a wide array of psychiatric problems. For example, intoxicated people are often disinhibited and impulsive, acting in ways that they would not act if they were sober. However, a manic patient may also be impulsive, often spending money freely or engaging in sexual activity without considering the consequences of these actions. Labeling each of these patterns of behavior impulsive is an important first step in reaching a diagnosis. In addition, finding one type of impulsive behavior should prompt the psychiatrist to look for others and to predict that the patient may act impulsively in the future.

Impulsive Behaviors

Clinical Vignette 5

Ms I, a 50-year-old financially comfortable housewife, came for treatment after being arrested for shoplifting (kleptomania). She was puzzled by her urges, stating, "I feel compelled to steal things even though I don't need them and could easily buy them. Half the time I throw them away afterward". Although she felt that she could resist these urges if a security guard was in plain view, she recognized that the threat of being arrested did not deter her at the moment of the theft.

Clinical Vignette 6

Mr J, a 43-year-old married executive, engaged in cross-dressing (transvestic fetishism). He frequently masturbated to orgasm while wearing his wife's lingerie, paying little attention to whether his wife would suspect him when she discovered the soiled undergarments.

Impulsive behaviors are actions that arise without much delay between the formation of an idea or desire and its gratification in action. Not all impulsive behavior is pathological; in a muted and well-modulated form, impulsivity is closer to spontaneity. Certain personality styles, such as dramatic characters, are more likely to be spontaneous or impulsive than others. In contrast, a person with a conscientious style might decide to think about the purchase for a few days, then return to buy the necklace only to find it gone.

However, in its more extreme forms, impulsivity is often pathological. A number of behaviors that seem dissimilar may have impulsivity as the common and uniting thread. Another advantage of thinking about impulsivity as a distinct pattern of

Table 20.6	Impulsive, Compulsive and Avoidant Patterns of Behavior
Pattern	**Examples**
Impulsive	Self-mutilation
	Suicide
	Substance abuse
	Pathological gambling
	Binging and purging
	Hair pulling
	Kleptomania
	Pyromania
	Paraphilias
Compulsive	Handwashing, checking
	Sexual compulsions
	Food restriction
Avoidant	Agoraphobia
	Simple phobias (e.g., acrophobia)
	Social phobia

problem behavior is that impulsivity in one sphere is often accompanied by impulsive behaviors in other arenas.

Behaviors that are frequently impulsive in nature include self-mutilation and suicide, substance abuse, pathological gambling, binging and purging eating behaviors, and hair pulling. In addition, urges to steal (kleptomania), to set fires (pyromania), or to engage in sexually perverse or unusual behaviors (paraphilias) also result in impulsive behaviors (Table 20.6).

Different types of impulsive behaviors are often experienced in similar ways by patients. One hallmark of impulsive acts is that they are often preceded by a growing internal sense of tension and discomfort that is reduced by the impulsive act itself. Whether the act is hair pulling (trichotillomania) that results in baldness, or pathological gambling that has severe financial consequences, the person is likely to feel that she or he can no longer tolerate the internal tension and that giving in to the impulse will provide relief to an uncomfortable internal state.

Clinical Vignette 7

Mr K, a 35-year-old construction worker, experienced irresistible urges to set fires (pyromania). He often did so in a hasty and unpremeditated fashion at construction sites where he worked. Because his actions were poorly planned and executed, he was at risk of being seen setting the fires. Firefighters rapidly concluded that the fires were the result of arson. In addition, Mr K tended to feel compelled to stay and watch the consequences of his actions, enjoying the sight of the fire itself as well as the various equipment used to extinguish it. This meant he was remaining at the scene of his crime for an extended time.

A second characteristic of impulsive acts is that they are often frankly pleasurable at the moment of action even if the person is extremely remorseful afterward.

Clinical Vignette 8

Ms N is a 34-year-old woman with obsessive–compulsive disorder who has recurrent, intrusive thoughts about having been contaminated with germs by objects she has touched. These thoughts are pervasive and extremely anxiety producing. She attempts to neutralize them by compulsively cleaning her house and washing her hands. When treated by use of a technique called flooding in which she was not permitted to wash her hands despite her obsessional thought, she became overwhelmingly anxious and panicky.

A third hallmark of impulsive behaviors is that patients are often relatively impervious to the consequences of their actions at the time and tend to underestimate their chances of being caught.

Clinical Vignette 9

Mr O is a 38-year-old man who is distressed by the compulsion to masturbate that he feels nearly every morning on awakening with an erection. He describes the activity in detached terms, stating, "I think it's a waste of time. I don't enjoy it. I'm often making a mental list of things I have to do at work or even watching morning television programs while I'm masturbating. But I feel nervous for the rest of the day if I don't do it".

Patients with impulsive patterns of behavior also tend to underestimate the chances of being caught by a spouse or friend. In addition, the impulsive nature of the action itself may increase the odds of apprehension and punishment.

Clinical Vignette 10

Mr R is a 26-year-old man who had his first panic attack while attending church. Because he was sitting in the middle of a pew, he was forced to climb over several people to flee during the attack. He felt this was both scary and embarrassing. Since this initial attack, he has avoided sitting anywhere other than in the back row at the end of the pew while attending services. He feels relatively comfortable sitting in this location because he can escape quickly if another attack occurs. He is not bothered by sitting in the middle of a row at the movies or in a theater.

Clinical Vignette 11

Mr S is a 38-year-old man who began having panic attacks in his early twenties. After one unexpected attack while he was on the subway, he began to ride the bus instead. Before long, he had another panic attack on the bus, and began walking to work. Walking took about 1 hour, but he persisted until he had a panic attack in the street. After this attack, Mr S avoided leaving his house unless accompanied by another person, often his brother who lives nearby. His agoraphobia forced him to quit work and apply for disability compensation.

Another feature common to impulsive behaviors is that they often involve a binge, an episode of engaging in a behavior that seems out of control and cannot be terminated by the patient. Often, the binge ends only when an external constraint forces the patient to abandon the action. An eating binge and the relapse of an alcoholic person are often similarly described: "Once I started eating (drinking) I couldn't stop. I just kept on stuffing myself (ordering drinks) until I was too exhausted and sick (drunk and broke) to continue".

It is noteworthy that impulsively binging on a substance such as alcohol sets the stage for further impulsive behaviors secondary to intoxication.

Compulsive Behaviors

Clinical Vignette 12

Ms T, a 24-year-old student, recognized that she was mildly afraid of heights. However, she wished to climb the Mayan temple at Chichén Itzáa during her vacation in Mexico. As she started the steep climb to the top, she began to feel anxious and to anticipate arriving at the top and being unable to descend from the monument. Pausing to try to calm down, she turned to look at the ground and began to feel overwhelmingly anxious and afraid of falling. She decided to descend at once but found that her legs felt shaky and weak, making the climb especially frightening. On making it down from the stairs, she vowed never to climb such a monument again.

Clinical Vignette 13

Mr. M is a 48-year-old executive who suffers from obsessive–compulsive disorder. Despite treatment with a variety of medications including fluoxetine and clomipramine, he has been unable to rid himself of the idea that he has accidentally hit someone while driving to work. Any bump in the road that he notices sets off this obsessive worry, and he feels compelled to circle back to the scene to double-check that he is not guilty of a hit-and-run accident. Sometimes he is not reassured by this initial check and continues to circle the area until "something clicks" and he feels certain that he has not hit anyone. This behavior makes Mr. M as much as 2 hours late for work.

In its muted form, compulsivity can be seen as carefulness or attention to detail. It is easy to see how such attention to detail is helpful in a variety of settings in daily life. Many jobs depend on thoroughness and a willingness to keep working until the books are balanced to the last penny. However, compulsive behaviors become a problem when they begin to consume much more time than necessary and when they are a response to nonsensical thoughts (obsessions).

At first glance, compulsive patterns seem to be the opposite of impulsive patterns of behavior. In compulsive behaviors, a person repetitively behaves in a stereotyped way. Yet repeated impulsive behaviors can become difficult to distinguish from compulsive ones. Is a young female patient who repeatedly gives in to the urge to pull her hair out impulsive or compulsive or both?

In fact, there is evidence that impulsive and compulsive behaviors tend to cooccur in the same individual. In one study, impulsive aggression was found to be common in patients with obsessive–compulsive disorder (Stein and Hollander, 1993). The authors theorized that obsessive–compulsive disorder and impulsivity may both arise from a similar problem in the self-regulation of behavior due to a neuroanatomical lesion in the serotoninergic system. They found that treating the obsessive–compulsive disorder with serotonin reuptake inhibitors also decreased these patients' impulsive aggression.

The compulsions of obsessive–compulsive disorder, food-restricting behaviors such as those found in anorexia nervosa, and compulsive sexual behavior are common types of compulsivity (see Table 20.6). Like impulsive behaviors, compulsions share common features and are experienced in similar ways by patients. However, the driving force behind compulsive behaviors is not the gratification of impulses, but rather the prevention or reduction of anxiety and distress.

Clinical Vignette 14

Ms. N is a 34-year-old woman with obsessive–compulsive disorder who has recurrent, intrusive thoughts about having been contaminated with germs by objects she has touched. These thoughts are pervasive and extremely anxiety producing. She attempts to neutralize them by compulsively cleaning her house and washing her hands. When treated by use of a technique called flooding in which she was not permitted to wash her hands despite her obsessional thought, she became overwhelmingly anxious and panicky.

The concept that compulsive behavior is an attempt to reduce anxiety is easy to understand when the behavior is a response to an obsessive thought. However, even when the compulsive behavior is sexual in nature, it is driven by the need for anxiety reduction rather than by sexual desire (Coleman, 1992).

Clinical Vignette 15

Mr. O is a 38-year-old man who is distressed by the compulsion to masturbate that he feels nearly every morning on awakening with an erection. He describes the activity in detached terms, stating, "I think it's a waste of time. I don't enjoy it. I'm often making a mental list of things I have to do at work or even watching morning television programs while I'm masturbating. But I feel nervous for the rest of the day if I don't do it."

Avoidant Behaviors

Clinical Vignette 16

Mr. P is a 55-year-old man who was robbed at gunpoint 1 year ago after visiting an automated teller machine to withdraw money. Since the robbery, he has felt somewhat afraid when using the automated teller machine in the daytime, although this fear has diminished over time. He has avoided needing to use the automated teller machine at night by carefully planning his finances since the robbery.

Clinical Vignette 17

Ms. Q is a 40-year-old woman who works in a university library. She has gradually become more accustomed to dealing with patrons at the reference desk but continues to prefer the solitary task of looking for books that are misshelved. Despite her boss's encouragement, she has decided not to apply for a higher level job that would involve teaching groups of new employees about the library computer system. She realizes that she is passing up a good career opportunity, but she also recognizes that the public speaking and writing on the board that this new position would entail are terrifying to her. She worries that she will stammer and blush and make a fool of herself in front of the group. Even now, she feels uncomfortable on her lunch break because she is reluctant to join other employees in the cafeteria.

As with impulsivity and compulsivity, avoidance in its modulated form can be positive; learning from past negative experiences and avoiding prior mistakes are important capacities.

Avoidant behaviors usually arise from a patient's history of being fearful or concerned that he or she will become fearful in a given situation. Because of the past history or the perceived threat, the anxiety-provoking situation is avoided. Avoiding the situation means avoiding the fear and anxiety the situation threatens to produce.

Clinical Vignette 18

Mr. R is a 26-year-old man who had his first panic attack while attending church. Because he was sitting in the middle of a pew, he was forced to climb over several people to flee during the attack. He felt this was both scary and embarrassing. Since this initial attack, he has avoided sitting anywhere other than in the back row at the end of the pew while attending services. He feels relatively comfortable sitting in this location because he can escape quickly if another attack occurs. He is not bothered by sitting in the middle of a row at the movies or in a theater.

One study showed that fear and avoidance ratings were highly correlated both at baseline level and after behavior therapy for agoraphobia (Cox *et al.*, 1993). In another study, panic disorder patients with agoraphobia were differentiated from panic disorder patients without agoraphobia by increased rates of anxiety-relevant cognitions in the agoraphobic group (Ganellen *et al.*, 1986).

Another feature common to avoidant behaviors is that they become self-reinforcing and tend to worsen in severity over time if left untreated.

Clinical Vignette 19

Mr. S is a 38-year-old man who began having panic attacks in his early twenties. After one unexpected attack while he was on the subway, he began to ride the bus instead. Before long, he had another panic attack on the bus, and

began walking to work. Walking took about 1 hour, but he persisted until he had a panic attack in the street. After this attack, Mr. S avoided leaving his house unless accompanied by another person, often his brother who lives nearby. His agoraphobia forced him to quit work and apply for disability compensation.

Clinical Vignette 20

Ms. T, a 24-year-old student, recognized that she was mildly afraid of heights. However, she wished to climb the Mayan temple at Chichén Itzáa during her vacation in Mexico. As she started the steep climb to the top, she began to feel anxious and to anticipate arriving at the top and being unable to descend from the monument. Pausing to try to calm down, she turned to look at the ground and began to feel overwhelmingly anxious and afraid of falling. She decided to descend at once but found that her legs felt shaky and weak, making the climb especially frightening. On making it down from the stairs, she vowed never to climb such a monument again.

A further common feature of avoidant behaviors is their tendency to heighten anticipatory anxiety and precipitate the very reactions that a person fears.

Conclusion

In evaluating the adaptiveness of a person's behavior, an understanding of the strengths and weaknesses of various character styles and the constraints and demands of the external environment is essential. Behavior is the final common pathway for the expression of genetics, temperament, personality traits and psychiatric symptoms. Behavior is an observable entity in a field where many important aspects of a patient's internal life must be inferred by the psychiatrist. Although some behaviors are clearly more adaptive than others, emphasizing the strengths of a person's capacities is important. Even pathological behaviors often represent a person's best attempt at adaptation; a paranoid patient who installs extra locks on the door may be doing the best she or he can in the face of illness to survive, to cope and to adapt to the environment the patient perceives around her or him.

References

American Psychiatric Association (1994) *Diagnostic and Statistical Manual of Mental Disorders*, 4th edn. APA, Washington DC.

Benjamin LS (1986b) Operational definition and measurement of dynamics shown in the stream of free associations. *Psychiatry* 49, 104–129.

Buetow S, Goodyear-Smith F and Coster G (2001) Coping strategies in the self-management of chronic heart failure. *Fam Pract* 18, 117–122.

Carey G and DiLalla DL (1994) Personality and psychopathology: Genetic perspectives. *J Abnorm Psychol* 103, 32–43.

Cloninger CR (1987) A systematic method for clinical description and classification of personality variants: A proposal. *Arch Gen Psychiatr* 44, 573–588.

Cloninger CR, Svrakic DM and Przybeck TR (1993) A psychobiological model of temperament and character. *Arch Gen Psychiatr* 50, 975–990.

Coleman E (1992) Is your patient suffering from compulsive sexual behavior? *Psychiatr Ann* 22, 320–325.

Cox BJ, Swinson RP and Fergus KD (1993) Changes in fear versus avoidance ratings with behavioral treatments for agoraphobia. *Behav Ther* 24, 619–624.

Digman JM (1990) Personality structure: Emergence of the five-factor model. *Annu Rev Psychol* 50, 116–123.

Eksuzian DJ (1999) Psychological and behavioral health issues of long-duration space missions. *Life Supp Biosph Sci* 6, 35–38.

Farmer A, Redman K, Harris T *et al.* (2001) Sensation-seeking, life events, and depression. The Cardiff Depression study. *Br J Psychiatr* 178, 549–552.

Ganellen RJ, Matuzas W, Uhlenhuth EH *et al.* (1986) Panic disorder, agoraphobia, and anxiety-related cognitive style. *J Affect Disord* 11, 219–225.

Halleck SL (1994) *Evaluation of the Psychiatric Patient: A Primer.* Plenum Press, New York.

Johnson JG, Cohen P, Smailes EM *et al.* (2001) Childhood verbal abuse and risk for personality disorders during adolescence and early adulthood. *Compr Psychiatr* 42, 16–23.

Kirk KM, Birley AJ, Statham DJ *et al.* (2000) Anxiety and depression in twin and sib pairs extremely discordant and concordant for neuroticism: Prodromus to a linkage study. *Twin Res* 3, 299–309.

Kirrane RM and Siever LJ (2000) New perspectives on schizotypal personality disorder. *Curr Psychiatr Rep* 2, 62–66.

McCrae RR and Costa PT Jr (1987) Validation of the five-factor model across instruments and observers. *J Pers Soc Psychol* 52, 81–90.

McDougall W (1932) Of the words character and personality. *Charact Pers* 1, 3–16

Nigg JT and Goldsmith HH (1998) Developmental psychopathology, personality, and temperament: Reflections on recent behavioral genetics research. *Hum Biol* 70, 387–412.

Oldham JM and Morris LB (1995) *The New Personality Self-Portrait: Why You Think, Work, Love and Act the Way You Do.* Bantam Books, New York.

Oldham JM and Skodol AE (2000) Charting the future of Axis II. *J Pers Dis* 14, 17–29.

Rothbart MK and Ahadi SA (1994) Temperament and the development of personality. *J Abnorm Psychol* 103, 55–66.

Siever LJ and Davis KL (1991) A psychobiological perspective on the personality disorders. *Am J Psychiatr* 148, 1647–1658.

Stein DJ and Hollander E (1993) Impulsive aggression and obsessive–compulsive disorder. *Psychiatr Ann* 23, 389–395.

Svrakic DM, Whitehead C, Przybeck TR *et al.* (1993) Differential diagnosis of personality disorders by the seven-factor model of temperament and character. *Arch Gen Psychiatr* 50, 991–999.

Thomas A, Chess S, Birch H *et al.* (1963) *Behavioral Individuality in Early Childhood.* University Press, New York.

Weissman MM, Klerman GL, Paykel ES *et al.* (1974) Treatment effects on the social adjustment of depressed patients. *Arch Gen Psychiatr* 30, 771–778.

Weissman MM, Olfson M, Gameroff MJ *et al.* (2001) A comparison of three scales for assessing social functioning in primary care. *Am J Psychiatr* 158, 460–466.

Westen D and Shedler J (2000) A prototype matching approach to diagnosing personality disorders: Toward DSM-V. *J Pers Dis* 14, 109–126.

Widiger TA, Trull TJ, Clarkin JF *et al.* (1994) A description of the DSM-III-R and DSM-IV personality disorders with the five-factor model of personality, in *Personality Disorders and the Five-Factor Model of Personality* (eds Costa PT and Widiger TA). American Psychological Association, Washington DC, pp. 19–40.

Cultural Aspects of Psychiatric Disorders

Introduction

From the outset, psychopathological research has usually assumed that mental disorders exist as "objective" states and can be evaluated with universal and standardized criteria, forgetting, in part, the impact of social, economic, cultural, and political factors in the explanation of psychopathological disorders. This oversight is all the more critical when comparing culturally distinct groups. However, in the last 30 years this oversight has been mitigated by significant contributions in cross-cultural research, whose objective has been to understand the cultural component of psychopathology.

This research, which has increased dramatically since the 1970s and 1980s, was consolidated via the creation of a group working on cross-cultural studies for the preparation of the *Diagnostic and Statistical Manual of Mental Disorders*, Fourth Edition (DSM-IV-TR) (American Psychiatric Association, 1994; Mezzich *et al.*, 1993). The Manual contains three kinds of information relating to cultural factors: 1) in the clinical presentation of disorders, a discussion of cultural variants of each disorder, called symptoms dependent on culture and gender; 2) guidelines for a "cultural formulation" of the clinical presentation to help clinicians perform a culturally sensitive diagnosis; and 3) a description of "culture-bound" syndromes, including the name of the disorder, the cultures in which it has been diagnosed, and a brief description of the psychopathology associated with each clinical presentation (the last two sections are included in Appendix I of the DSM-IV-TR). The ICD-10 has also been revised and updated to account for cultural factors, as evidenced by the emergence of new diagnostic systems such as the *Chinese Classification of Mental Disorders* and the *Latin American Guide for Psychiatric Diagnosis* (Berganza *et al.*, 2001; Mezzich *et al.*, 2001). While both of these culturally sensitive diagnostic manuals recognize the value of local cultural requirements to enhance the validity of psychiatric diagnosis, they also illustrate the complementary need to integrate such systems of diagnosis into a global and reliable diagnostic language (Lee, 1993; Berganza *et al.*, 2001).

The existence of a rich modern tradition of cross-cultural research and debate led directly to the increased attention to cultural factors in DSM-IV-TR. In turn, the publication of the manual stimulated continued research on the influence of cultural factors on the etiology, symptomatology, course and treatment outcome of psychopathological disorders. In this chapter, we will focus on cultural considerations pertinent to the use of diagnostic criteria in ethnically and culturally diverse populations. We will also comment briefly on related culture-bound syndromes.

Specific Cultural Considerations

Cognitive Disorders

Less attention has been paid to cultural variants of the cognitive disorders than to other psychopathological forms, probably because of the widespread assumption that this group of disorders is influenced exclusively by biological factors. Nevertheless, these disorders show several kinds of social, cultural and ethnic influences. Given the etiologically based subtyping of the cognitive disorders, these influences are exerted, first, by effects on the nature and rates of the diseases that are the causative agents of these disorders (Lin and Fábrega, 1997).

Socioeconomic factors influence the prevalence rates of diseases affecting the brain. Low industrialization of a country or the poverty of a particular social group tends to increase the rates of infectious diseases, nutritional disorders, toxic exposures (e.g., lead), head injuries, endocrinological abnormalities and seizure disorders among others (Cruickshank and Beevers, 1989). This, in turn, may result in differences in the rates of the subtypes of dementia, of delirium, and of other specific cognitive syndromes (Spector, 1979; Westermeyer and Canino, 1997).

Cultural factors, such as prohibitions against substance use and variations in sexual mores, also affect the rates of alcohol- and drug-related syndromes as well as of acquired immunodeficiency syndrome (AIDS) related organic mental disorders (Agarwal and Goedde, 1990; Kaslow and Francis, 1989). Ethnic determinants are also important. Hypertension and strokes have been suggested to be more prevalent among the African-Americans and some Asian groups; this may result in different rates of multi-infarct dementia (de la Monte *et al.*, 1989). In addition, research on Alzheimer's dementia is currently evaluating reports of lower rates among the Chinese and the Chinese-Americans as well as the African-Americans (de la Monte *et al.*, 1989; Zhang *et al.*, 1990). The detection and assessment of the cognitive disorders are also influenced by social and cultural factors. Social groups that tolerate and even expect substantial decreases in decision-making and self-care among older persons may not be regarded as pathological milder degrees of disorientation among the elderly (Ikels, 1991). Educational level and cultural differences appear to exert separate but intermingled effects on the inappropriately high identification of cognitive impairment with the Mini-Mental State Examination (MMSE) among several ethnic groups, including the Hispanic, Taiwanese, Chinese, Southeast Asian (Williams, 1987), and Afro-Caribbean populations (Richards *et al.*, 2000). Based on a review of the literature and consultations with members of the aboriginal community,

Essentials of Psychiatry   Jerald Kay and Allan Tasman
© 2006 John Wiley & Sons, Ltd.

Cattarinich and colleagues (2001) note that differing degrees of acculturation within and between aboriginal groups create problems for cognitive evaluations. On the basis of these and other findings, some researchers have begun to question the adequacy of the MMSE and other cognitive assessment instruments, and as a consequence some practitioners have begun modifying their methods.

Substance Use Disorders

Sociocultural factors exert considerable influence over some aspects of substance use disorders and not others. The prevalence rates of alcohol and drug abuse and dependence vary significantly across cultures. Lifetime rates for alcoholism, for example, range from 23% among the American Indians to 0.45% among the population of Shanghai (Helzer and Canino, 1992). Specific local factors that affect degree of risk for substance-related disorders include patterns of use, attitudes toward substance consumption, accessibility of the drug, physiological reactions to the same drug, and family norms and patterns (Westermeyer and Canino, 1997) (Table 21.1). Recent studies of teenagers find that different ethnic groups in the US experience different rates of substance abuse (Turner and Gill, 2002). Of even greater concern is the epidemiological finding that rates of alcohol and other substance abuse are higher among the US-born Mexican-Americans than among Mexico-born migrants, and increase with length of stay in the USA, indicating either a pathogenic impact of the US residence, a loss of protective social factors with migration, or both. These findings suggest that interventions should be tailored to the needs of different minority and immigrant populations, particularly as substance abuse has been related to other psychological disorders (Vega et al., 1998; Lee, 2001; Griffin et al., 2000). In part, these differences may be influenced by the way the local culture influences the definition of pathological substance use through differences in the perception of the impairment caused by high consumption and frequent intoxication (Osterberg, 1986). Particular cultural views toward drinking in children, the value of moderation, the tolerance for intoxication, and the association of drinking with family activities and special social occasions appear to influence the degree of risk for alcoholism (Valliant, 1986). The availability of a substance also increases its rates of abuse and dependence (Helzer and Canino, 1992). Sociocultural factors such as religious proscriptions may exert their influence in this fashion. Heath (2001) has remarked on the long tradition of drug inhalation, from tobacco to hallucinogens, in tropical South America, which contradicts the perception in North America of drug inhalation as a novel, and therefore aberrant, trend (Kirmayer and Groleau, 2001).

Several aspects of substance use disorders appear to be less affected by cultural factors. Such aspects include the comorbidity patterns, the nature of dependence syndromes, the age at onset, and the results of laboratory tests and physical examinations (Westermeyer, 1989). For example, alcoholism is associated in many societies with abuse of other substances, mania and antisocial personality as well as with depression and anxiety (Anthony and Helzer, 1991). Alcoholism and drug abuse are reliably more common among men, although the sex ratio can vary from 2:1 to 4:1 (Helzer and Canino, 1992; Robins et al., 1981). Drug abuse is also more prevalent among urban populations, the less educated, and the young (Anthony and Helzer, 1991). The physical symptoms as well as the temporal relationship between onset of use and dependence are substance-specific and also fairly similar across cultures (Berger and Westermeyer, 1977).

Schizophrenia and Related Psychotic Disorders

The cross-cultural presentation and course of schizophrenia are among the best-studied aspects of cultural psychiatry. Research has revealed both cross-cultural similarities and differences, both of which are important for elucidating the biological and environmental bases of the disease. A "spectrum" of schizophrenic syndromes – consisting of a combination of certain positive and negative psychotic symptoms – has been found nearly everywhere, although the specific content of hallucinations and delusions as well as the prevalence of visual and other nonauditory hallucinations varies (Krassoievitch et al., 1982; Ndetei and Vadher, 1984). Significant cross-cultural variation has been found, however, in several features of the syndrome. Its distribution is not uniform, ranging from 1 in a 1000 in the nonWestern societies to more than 1% in the West; its highest prevalence is displayed in economically and technologically advanced, urbanized and bureaucratized societies (Kleinman, 1988; Warner, 1985). Its phenomenology varies with cultural setting, with much higher rates of catatonia in India and of hebephrenia in Japan than in the West. Most important, the course and outcome of schizophrenia are markedly better in nonindustrialized countries, even when cultural differences in outcome assessment and in acuteness of presentation are taken into account (Sartorius et al., 1986; Lin and Kleinman, 1988; Kulhara and Chakrabarti, 2001). Variations in outcome are thought to be related in part to different attitudes toward persons with the disorder, a set of culturally patterned interactions studied under the rubric of expressed emotion (Jenkins and Karno, 1992) (Table 21.2). Other cross-cultural variations with regard to schizophrenia include higher misdiagnosis among patients from devalued and ethnic minority groups (Good, 1992/93), differences in cultural and gender-related conceptions

---

Table 21.1 Sociocultural Factors Related to Substance Use Disorders

- Attitudes toward substance consumption
- Accessibility of drugs
- Local patterns of drug use
- Ethnic-specific physiological reactions to various drugs
- Immigrant status (protective in some cases)
- Religious proscriptions
- Male gender
- Urban life
- Lower education

Table 21.2 Sociocultural Factors Associated with Better Outcome in Persons Experiencing Schizophrenia

- Residence in nonindustrialized society
- Social attitudes toward persons experiencing the disorder
- Culturally patterned interactions
- Well-knit support systems

regarding the expression of emotion that complicate the assessment of flat affect (Karno and Jenkins, 1997), and culturally syntonic experiences that may be mistaken for schizophrenic symptoms. The latter include the accepted appearance of hallucinations among the bereaved Native Americans (Hultkrantz, 1979) or reports of perceptual alterations among the distressed Puerto Ricans (Guarnaccia *et al.*, 1992).

Cross-cultural differences have also been detected in emotional processing among the German, American and Indian subjects with schizophrenia. Face discrimination performance was most impaired in the Indian subgroup (Habel *et al.*, 2000). Another study comparing the German natives and the Turkish immigrants with schizophrenia also found cross-cultural differences, this time in higher indices of hostile excitement and depression among the immigrant group (Haasen *et al.*, 2001).

Mood Disorders

Contemporary cross-cultural research on mood disorders has focused on unipolar depression syndromes, revealing extensive cultural patterning as well as significant similarities. For example, the World Health Organization Collaborative Study on Depression found a core depressive syndrome in the five countries studied, but it also revealed substantial cross-cultural differences in symptom presentation, affect conceptualization, level of severity, and influence of acculturation, despite a methodology that tended to accentuate similarities at the expense of local differences (Marsella *et al.*, 1985).

Culture and other social factors, such as class and gender, influence the interpretation of and exposure to stressors that predispose to depression (Brown and Harris, 1978). The specific characteristics of the dysphoria of depressive illness also vary cross-culturally. For example, among the Hopi in North America, feelings of guilt, shame and sinfulness are separate experiences displaying distinct relationships to subtypes of depression (Manson *et al.*, 1985). Whereas reports of irritability, rage and "nervousness" are prominent descriptors of depressive affect among the Puerto Ricans and other Latinos (Lewis-Fernández, 2002). The frequent combination of depression and anxiety noted around the world, particularly in primary care settings, has fueled the DSM-IV-TR proposal for a mixed anxiety–depression disorder (Katon and Roy-Byrne, 1991).

In addition, most cross-cultural studies have found a significantly higher rate of somatic complaints associated with depression (and anxiety) among the nonWestern groups than in the Western settings, including the presence of unique symptoms (e.g., "heat or water in the head" and "crawling sensation of worms and ants" in the Nigerian cultures) (Marsella *et al.*, 1985; Ebigbo, 1982). Emotional complaints are often present as well but may not be considered the source of distress or impairment. The mix of emotional and somatic symptoms has also been found to vary by sex in some studies (Clark *et al.*, 1981; Guarnaccia *et al.*, 1989). For example, a study comparing the Puerto Ricans, Mexican-Americans and Cuban-Americans on the Center for Epidemiologic Studies Depression Scale of depressive symptoms found that the women in all three groups tended to endorse depressive and somatic scale items together as a single factor. This happened significantly more often amongst women than men (Guarnaccia *et al.*, 1989).

Finally, the threshold at which dysphoria becomes disorder is affected by cultural factors. The two-week duration criterion for major depression, an important proxy for pathological intensity, may vary among some nonWestern groups. Manson and colleagues (1985) found that the Hopi identify five distinct indigenous syndromes related to depression, only one of which shares significant parameters with Western depressive disorder. This folk syndrome, however, differed from major depression in its average duration of 1 week, not 2, although still causing comparable morbidity. On the basis of this, duration criterion for major depressive disorder when it is used with the Hopi patients should be shortened (Manson *et al.*, 1985). Conversely, in a study of the Bambui community in Brazil, researchers were surprised to find depressive episodes averaging 1 month, higher than that observed in similar studies in many other societies (Vorcaro *et al.*, 2001).

The substantial overlap of depression with anxiety, somatoform and dissociative disorders implies a higher probability of under-recognition or misidentification of affective disorders in many ethnocultural groups (Kirmayer and Groleau, 2001). These findings raise serious issues about the universality of the prototypical representation of depression in the North American psychiatry and the operational criteria of the depressive disorders, and tend to support the phenomenological expansion of the depression categories (Manson and Good, in press; Kirmayer and Groleau, 2001).

Anxiety Disorders

The effect of culture on anxiety is similar to that on depression, especially since cross-cultural studies have shown a marked tendency for anxiety and depression to overlap (American Psychiatric Association, 1994). Cultural factors affect the precipitants, symptom presentations, pathological thresholds and specific syndrome criteria of the anxiety disorders (Good and Kleinman, 1985). For example, the cross-cultural validity of criterion A for the *Diagnostic and Statistical Manual of Mental Disorders*, Third Edition, Revised (DSM-III-R) generalized anxiety disorder (GAD) has been challenged because it restricts the diagnosis of chronic pathological anxiety to a disturbance stemming from undue worry in the absence of actual stressors or excessive worry after minor stress. This leaves out the much larger group of patients in developing societies and devalued minorities in the West who experience chronic pathological anxiety as a result of recurrent stress (Lewis-Fernández and Kleinman, 1995).

Cultural and ethnic elements have been invoked to explain local differences in anxiety disorder prevalence that persist after controlling for other social factors. For example, the higher rate of simple phobia social phobia and agoraphobia among the African-Americans, as compared with whites (Neal and Turner, 1991), has been attributed to the stress resulting from racial discrimination (Brown *et al.*, 1990). In fact, the cross-cultural epidemiological literature reveals a complex pattern of similarities and differences with regard to the anxiety disorders, and opinions differ as to the role of culture in this process (Guarnaccia and Kirmayer, in press). For example, it is presently unclear why the Mexicans born in Mexico, when compared with those born in the USA, show a markedly lower rate of anxiety and other disorders. Suggested explanations include selective migrations, different thresholds for perceiving and reporting a disorder stemming from distinct cultural interpretations of what constitutes a "hard life" and acceptable suffering, and a combination of both explanations (Shrout *et al.*, 1992).

Multiple cross-cultural studies point to the coappearance of anxiety, depression, somatoform complaints and dissociative symptoms among the nonWestern groups. A markedly somatic idiom predominates, often in the form of culturally specific symptoms (Ebigbo, 1982). These often coalesce distinctively as culture-bound syndromes characterized also by specific etiological factors, demographics, patterns of impairment and help-seeking choices (Hughes *et al.*, in press). It is far from clear that this represents the comorbidity of the Western disorders rather than a different organization of pathological experience (Maser and Dinges, 1992). Examples include *ataque de nervios* among the Latinos, *koro* in the Asian communities and *taijin kyofusho* among the Japanese (Guarnaccia and Kirmayer, in press). Each of these disorders exhibits significant differences that prevent simple one-to-one correlations with the established Western categories (Weiss, 1996).

Somatoform Disorders

In a survey of international use of DSM-III and DSM-III-R, somatoform disorders were among the more problematic diagnoses (Maser *et al.*, 1991), probably because of their cross-cultural limitations (Kirmayer and Weiss, 1997). First, many nosologies around the world do not distinguish between mood, anxiety, somatoform disorders and dissociative disorders, because sufferers report single syndromes that run across boundaries of the diagnostic categories (Lewis-Fernández, 1992). This is similar to the situation with depression, where a single description of the disorder has led to under-recognition and misidentification of depressive syndromes in many ethnocultural groups (Kirmayer and Groleau, 2001). Demarcating somatoform conditions in these settings may create artificial distinctions that confound accurate diagnosis. Examples include neurasthenia in China and other Asian settings, and *nervios* in Latin America (Lin, 1989; Angel and Guarnaccia, 1989).

Secondly, the idioms of distress of many societies rely on somatic complaints for the expression of nonpathological, personal and social predicaments. Interpretations of these communication mechanisms as a somatoform disorder may result in overpathologization (Kirmayer and Robbins, 1991). In addition, the use of somatic idioms varies according to intracultural factors, such as gender and class, which in turn may determine who receives a somatoform diagnosis. For example, conversion symptoms appear to be more common in the rural and less educated sector of nonWestern societies, and particularly in family or social structures that allow few opportunities for protest (Kirmayer and Weiss, 1997; Nichter, 1981).

Thirdly, the symptom lists of DSM-III-R and DSM-IV-TR do not canvas the rich variety of somatic symptoms reported in other parts of the world, such as the complaints of worms and ants in the head described earlier (Ebigbo, 1982). Examples of other common somatic symptoms include chronic fatigue; heat in the feet, chest, or head; painful "gas" that moves from the abdomen around the flank to the back; "brainache"; and feeling presences when alone or among others.

Fourthly, in most of the world, the degree to which symptoms are medically unexplained is difficult to ascertain owing to the marked limitation of diagnostic tests and medical personnel. Moreover, the high prevalence of endemic disease in the underdeveloped countries, often with protean and inchoate manifestations, may also confound the assessment of the somatoform disorders. This may result in overdiagnosis if organic causes are not identified, or underdiagnosis if organic explanations are uncritically accepted for systemic illness (Kirmayer and Weiss, 1997).

Dissociative Disorders

Syndromes characterized by pathological dissociation are common worldwide, but the current concepts of dissociative disorders do not appear to account for their phenomenological variety (Lewis-Fernández, 1992; González *et al.*, 1997). For example, a study performed in an outpatient psychiatric clinic in India found that more than 90% of dissociative disorder cases did not fulfill criteria for the specified categories, ironically receiving instead a DSM-III diagnosis of atypical dissociative disorder. Distressing trance states and possession trance episodes constituted most of these cases (Saxena and Prasad, 1989). These instances of misdiagnosis again call to question the usefulness of some of the standard diagnostic categories of North American psychiatry (Kirmayer and Groleau, 2001). Many indigenous illness syndromes around the world display salient features of pathological dissociation. Some of these syndromes are characterized by involuntary possession trance – dissociative alterations in identity attributed to the invasion by external spirits or agents – distinguished from dissociative identity disorder by their episodic and remitting course, the nature and number of their alternative identities and their gradual response to treatment. These syndromes have been identified in India, western Africa, China, Malaysia, Brazil and the Caribbean, among many other settings (Lewis-Fernández, 1994; Ward, 1989; Spiegel and Cardeña, 1991).

Other dissociative syndromes are characterized by alterations of consciousness and memory, during which the person runs around in an agitated state (Arctic *pibloktoq*); attacks others indiscriminately (Malayo-Indonesian *amok*); undergoes convulsive movements, screaming fits and aggressive acts toward self or others (Caribbean *ataque de nervios*); or lies as if dead, suffering from specific perceptual alterations; hears and understands what is happening but cannot see or move ("falling out" among the African-Americans in southern USA, Bahamian "blacking out", and Haitian *indisposition*) (González *et al.*, 1997; Cardeña *et al.*, 2002, Weidman, 1979). In a recent study, Lewis-Fernández and colleagues (1997) confirmed the association between *ataque de nervios* and dissociation. Among the female Puerto Rican psychiatric outpatients, *ataque* frequency was directly related to self- and clinician-ratings of dissociative symptoms and disorders. Of note, patients with and without *ataque* did not differ on measures of childhood trauma, which was uniformly high among subjects (Lewis-Fernández *et al.*, 1997). The proposed dissociative trance disorder category in DSM-IV-TR would provide a Western nosological niche for these disorders, although not without the risk of overpathologizing some culturally accepted instances of these behaviors (Lewis-Fernández, 1992).

In fact, extensive cross-cultural research reveals that most dissociative experiences around the world are completely normal, usually forming part of religious and ritual events (Lewis-Fernández, 1994). The Western emphasis on pathological experiences of dissociation that result from overwhelming trauma probably stems from the relative absence of normal dissociation among the dominant Western groups and from the acknowledgment by mental health professionals of the sequelae of physical and sexual abuse (Ross, 1991; Martínez-Taboas, 1991). Depersonalization, considered one of the most common psychiatric symptoms in the West (Steinberg, 1991), is a greatly desired goal for Hindu yogis, revealing the substantial cultural patterning of dissociative experience (Castillo, 1991).

Sexual Disorders

Research on cross-cultural influences on sexual disorders is limited, owing to the lack of uniform descriptive methodology and to the fact that the major ethnic minorities in the USA do not seek medical treatment for this class of complaints (Davis and Herdt, 1997). Some cross-cultural studies have concluded that the paraphilias as currently characterized in the DSM-IV-TR are determined by specific features of the Western society, such as demographical size and complexity (whereby individuals may escape social sanction through anonymity), the nonavailability of partners, and the primacy of masturbatory activities as sexual outlets (Rooth, 1973; Gebhard, 1971). Despite a few small clinical studies that found similar rates of sexual dysfunctions among African-American populations (Fisher, 1980; Finkle and Finkle, 1978), most cross-cultural research suggests that sexual response is influenced by cultural and ethnic considerations. Racist stereotypes, machismo, anxiety about infertility, and the tendency toward somatization of mood disorders as impotence have been cited as etiological factors of sexual dysfunction in African-American and Latino populations (Wyatt, 1982; Espín, 1984). In addition, the ethnographical literature shows that standards for sexual competence differ across the cultural spectrum and that many societies display a more flexible approach to issues of sexual orientation than is assumed by the diagnostic categories (Davis and Whitten, 1987; Herdt, 1990).

This cross-cultural diversity complicates the assessment of the sexual disorders. At present, it is unclear whether certain culture-bound syndromes involving sexual organs, such as *koro* among the Asians (characterized by the fear of genital retraction) or *dhat* in India (involving obsession or anxiety about semen loss), should be categorized among the sexual or the somatoform disorders (Davis and Herdt, 1997).

Eating Disorders

Research has disclosed a significant cultural effect on the patterning and distribution of the eating disorders. An important determinant appears to be the Western premium on thinness as an esthetic and moral value (Ritenbaugh, 1982; Nichter and Nichter, 1991; Banks, 1992). Cases of eating disorder have been found in many nonWestern societies and several ethnic minorities in the USA, but their presenting features often differ somewhat from the DSM-IV-TR criteria for anorexia nervosa and bulimia nervosa (Shisslak *et al.*, 1989).

Groups at high risk include those experiencing rapid acculturation to the Western society, such as immigrants or those living in areas undergoing accelerated industrialization (Ritenbaugh *et al.*, 1997). For example, one study found a 12% prevalence of DSM-III eating disorders among the Egyptian female college students in London and no evidence of these conditions among a similar sample in Cairo (Nasser, 1986). Although it is as yet unclear exactly how acculturation predisposes the nonCaucasians to eating disorders, as a rule these conditions are more prevalent among the Caucasians than persons of other ethnic backgrounds (Wildes *et al.*, 2001). Bulimia nervosa appears more common than anorexia nervosa among the US minorities and is often associated with higher than average weight, female sex and sometimes older age, for example, among the American Indian groups (Rosen *et al.*, 1988). Anorexia nervosa has been found among lower socioeconomic class samples in several cultures but often characterized by atypical features, such as the absence of distorted body image or of the fear of gaining weight (Suematsu

et al., 1985; Lee *et al.*, 1989). Cross-cultural studies have proposed more flexible diagnostic criteria for anorexia nervosa so that abdominal fullness, epigastric pain, or distaste for food may be accepted instead of intense fear of weight gain to account for the severe restriction of food intake or other weight-losing behavior (Lee, 1991).

Adjustment Disorders

The effect of culture on the adjustment disorders is pervasive. Culturally based interpretations are essential to the appraisal of the repertoire of behavioral and emotional responses that pattern both normal and disordered reactions to stress (Jenkins and Kinzie 1997). Whereas some experiences are uniformly stressful (e.g. natural disaster), others may make sense only within particular cultural contexts (e.g., facing deadlines, witchcraft accusations (Fábrega and Mezzich, 1987). In addition, the judgment of what constitutes a maladaptive response to a stressor must be made in relation to what exceeds cultural norms (Kleinman, 1988). Diagnosis of an adjustment disorder may be a particular problem among refugee populations. These groups have undergone distressing experiences, but their intensively challenged coping styles may be unknown to caregivers in the host country (Beiser, 1996).

Personality Disorders

The current configuration of the personality disorders has received substantial cross-cultural challenge. Even the basic concept of personality as a set of individual internal traits is considered inseparable from the Western cultural assumptions of individuality by many authors (Lewis-Fernández and Kleinman 1993). Difficulties in the reliable assessment of these disorders within the Western cultures may be due to the degree to which these conditions are determined by social and contextual factors. These factors include adaptational strategies toward adverse communal environments (including the relative value of aggression or avoidance), family-based customs and traditions, occupational and educational options and cultural methods of child-rearing (Alarcón and Foulks, 1997). It is striking, for example, that the antisocial personality disorder is nearly absent among the Hutterites, an ethnoreligious enclave living for more than a century in the USA and Canada (Favazza, 1985). Intracultural diversity may be more important in this respect than cross-cultural difference. For example, in his studies of affective and personality disturbances among the Inuit and the Yoruba, Leighton (1981) was unable to disentangle cultural influences from "the much more powerful effects" of gender, age and class.

Epidemiological assessment of DSM-III antisocial personality disorder has been performed as part of the Epidemiological Catchment Area study using a clearly operationalized survey instrument, the Diagnostic Interview Schedule (Robins *et al.*, 1984). This yielded similar prevalence rates in the USA and Puerto Rico (Canino *et al.*, 1987). However, low reliability rates for the diagnosis of personality disorders across standardized instruments raise serious doubts about the validity of this aspect of the Epidemiological Catchment Area study data (Perry, 1992). One World Health Organization study was able to identify cases of most of the *International Classification of Diseases* personality disorders in 15 urban clinic samples in Africa, Asia, North America and Europe (Paris, 1991), but the cross-cultural validity of the definitions of these categories had been criticized earlier by Shepherd and Sartorius (1974).

The Case of Culture-bound Syndromes and Idioms of Distress

Investigation of so-called culture-bound syndromes was geared for decades toward incorporation of these "exotic" categories into the Western nosologies (Simons and Hughes 1985). The term "culture-bound" (Table 21.3) was used to describe a certain number of psychiatric disorders whose phenomenologies made them distinct from the Western categories and that theoretically could be singled out as unique to a particular cultural setting (Hughes *et al.*, 1997). The clear implication was that the Western categories were not culture-bound but rather universal, and that proper characterization would disclose a translation key for specific nonWestern syndromes. However, these conditions have been studied more critically to understand instead the culture-bound nature of the Western classification schemes themselves and to enable the appropriate treatment of patients whose understandings and presentation of illness conform to these indigenous categories (Good, 1994; Good and Delvecchio Good, 1982).

Contemporary cultural psychiatry recognizes that all classification schemes are inherently cultural and subjects Western nosologies to the same kind of social analysis that it continues to apply to the indigenous nosologies (Lewis-Fernández and Kleinman, 1995). In this modern sense, "cultural-bound syndrome" is an inherited and controversial term that is used in practice to describe psychiatric categories, whether they are part of the Western or nonWestern nosologies, on whose emergence, manifestation, or course culture is thought to exert a particularly strong influence (Hahn, 1985; Guarnaccia, 1993). The term continues to refer to relatively consistent illness categories with characteristic courses ("syndromes") and specific labels, some of which are discussed in this chapter (e.g., *amok, taijin kyofusho,* anorexia nervosa). The organizing principle that unifies a syndrome conceptually can be 1) a collection of symptoms, which can follow diverse classificatory schemes (descriptive); 2) a cause, including an immediate precipitating context (etiological); or 3) a response to treatment (Good and Delvecchio Good, 1982).

"Idiom of distress" is a newer term, which was coined to refer to a more general level of analysis (Nichter, 1981). Rather than denoting specific syndromes, the term refers to the more general illness "languages" of social groups, the culturally preferred ways of expressing distress, such as by somatic complaints, psychologizing explanations, possession or witchcraft terminology, oppositional or violent behavior illnesses due to "nerves", or attributions of inexplicable misfortune. In this sense, a given idiom of distress, such as somatization, can be expressed as multiple culture-bound syndromes such as *ataques de nervios,* neurasthenia, "brain fag", and so on. DSM-IV-TR presented a substantial list of culture-bound syndromes and idioms of distress in one of its appendices.

Contemporary use of this terminology allows us to understand certain difficulties in the integration of the Western and nonWestern categories of psychiatric illness (Lewis-Fernández, 1992; Wig, 1983). First, the Western nosologies are based at present nearly exclusive on descriptive parameters. Wary of "theoretical" causes, our current diagnostic system privileges a formal definition of psychopathological processes. Most indigenous nosologies, on the other hand, distinguish illness from normality at least as much on the basis of contextual characteristics as on descriptive ones. These include assessments regarding appropriateness of the symptom in the particular setting at the specific time in question, the relative sufficiency of precipitating stressors, and the nature and quality of the human relationships of the sufferer. These discrepancies between the organizing principles of the Western and nonWestern nosologies prevent an easy consolidation of psychopathological criteria across cultures.

Secondly, nosologies also differ in the configurations of their phenomenologies (Kleinman, 1988; Weiss, 1996; Good and Delvecchio Good, 1982). The symptoms of many culture-bound syndromes, such as *amok* in Malaysia, or *ataque de nervios* in Puerto Rico, are composed of a variety of behavioral and experiential elements that are considered by the Western nosologists to belong to separate diagnostic categories. The characteristic presentations of these conditions exhibit diverse combinations of dissociative, psychotic, anxiety, depressive, characterological and somatic symptoms (Lewis-Fernández, 1992). Significant phenomenological variation occurs among individual cases, which are nevertheless unifying under a single nosological label.

These differences in definitions of illness and phenomenological organization between the Western and nonWestern categories ensure that the two nosologies are overlapping as global systems. From the psychiatric perspective, a cohort of individuals identified by a cohort indigenous label will prove to be diagnostically heterogeneous or even nonpathological. The obverse is that almost homogeneous psychiatric cohorts will appear locally verse. A nomographical, one-to-one relationship between the Western and nonWestern nosologies appears thus unattainable (Weiss, 1996). What is achievable is the systematic characterization of individual cases of persons suffering from culture-bound syndromes in terms of the Western categories of psychiatric illness, retaining at the same time an account of their distinct definitions of illness, idioms of distress, unique symptoms and other associated factors in the form of a cultural formulation

Table 21.3	Culture-bound Syndromes and Idioms of Distress Listed in DSM-IV

- *amok*
- *ataques de nervios*
- bilis and colera
- *boufée delirante*
- brain fag
- *dhat*
- falling out or blacking out
- ghost sickness
- *hwa-byung*
- *koro*
- *latah*
- *locura*
- *mal de ojo*
- *nervios*
- *pibloktoq*
- *qi-gong* psychotic reaction
- rootwork
- *sangue dormido*
- *shenjing shuairuo*
- *shen-k'uei; shenkui*
- *shin-byung*
- spell
- *susto*
- *taijin kyofusho*
- zar

Table 21.4   Components of the DSM-IV Outline for a Cultural Formulation

- Cultural identity of the individual
- Cultural explanations of the individual's illness
- Cultural factors related to psychosocial environment and levels of functioning
- Cultural elements of the relationship between the individual and the clinician
- Overall cultural assessment for diagnosis and care

(Mezzich and Good, 1997) (Table 21.4). This iterative process of translation will result eventually in a comprehensive cultural psychiatry that integrates diverse local and professional classifications of psychiatric illness with the goal of more effective communication and care of patients.

In spite of the importance of including culture-bound syndromes in the DSM-IV-TR, Guarnaccia and Rogler (1999) warn that important methodological issues remain unaddressed, since DSM-IV-TR does not include a system of norms to delimit the range of psychiatric disorders that relate to particular culture-bound syndromes, nor include these cultural conditions within the established disorder categories.

Conclusion

The importance of culture in the understanding of psychopathology is revealed by the literature summarized in this chapter. However, future studies must evolve to include psychological and psychiatric measures that are relevant and appropriate for distinct cultural groups, since many cross-cultural studies utilize the Western concepts to explain the modes of expression of psychopathological manifestations (Kirmayer and Groleau, 2001), ways of seeking aid, use of mental health services, or treatment outcome, without taking into account their close relationship with cultural factors (Aneshensel and Phelan, 1999). At the same time, new possibilities are emerging for the application of cultural information to diagnostic systems and the diagnostic process. This chapter has focused on some of the most conspicuous contributions aimed at enhancing the cultural suitability of DSM-IV-TR, and thus on the use of diagnostic categories and criteria in multicultural settings. Other contributions, such as the glossary of culture-bound syndromes and idioms of distress and the guidelines for a cultural formulation, have been referred to succinctly. Cultural developments are also being worked into the family of classifications of the *International Classification of Diseases and Related Health Problems*, 10th Revision (Mezzich, 1995). All these efforts promise to increase the applicability and usefulness of the new diagnostic systems for our multicultural world. Further, they may encourage psychiatrists and the field as a whole to stay focused on the person of the patient and his or her context to augment the validity of diagnosis and the effectiveness of clinical care.

References

Agarwal DP and Goedde HW (1990) *Alcohol Metabolism, Alcohol Intolerance, and Alcoholism*. Springer-Verlag, Berlin.

Alarcón RD and Foulks EF (1997) Cultural factors and personality disorders: A review of the literature, in *Sourcebook for DSM-IV* (eds Widiger T, Frances AJ, Pincus HA *et al.*). American Psychiatric Press, Washington DC, pp. 975–982.

American Psychiatric Association (1994) *Diagnostic and Statistical Manual of Mental Disorders*, 4th edn. APA, Washington DC.

Aneshensel C and Phelan J (1999) The sociology of mental health: Surveying the field. In Handbook of the Sociology of Mental Health, Aneshensel C and Phelan J (eds). Kluwer Academic/Plenum Publishers, New York, pp. 3–17.

Angel R and Guarnaccia PJ (1989) Mind, body, and culture: Somatization among Hispanics. *Soc Sci Med* 28, 1229–1238.

Anthony JC and Helzer JE (1991) Syndromes of drug abuse and dependence in America, in *Psychiatric Disorders in America* (eds Robins L and Regier D). Free Press, New York, pp. 116–154.

Banks CG (1992) "Culture" in culture-bound syndromes: The case of anorexia nervosa. *Soc Sci Med* 34, 867–884.

Beiser M (1996) Adjustment disorder in DSM-IV: Cultural considerations, in *Culture and Psychiatric Diagnosis* (eds Mezzich JE, Kleinman A, Fábrega H *et al.*). American Psychiatric Press, Washington DC.

Berganza CE, Mezzich JE, Otero-Ojeda AA *et al.* (2001) The Latin American Guide for Psychiatric Diagnosis. A cultural overview. *Psychiatr Clin N Am* 24(3) (Sept), 433–446.

Berger LJ and Westermeyer J (1977) World traveler addicts in Asia: II. Comparison with "stay at home" addicts. *Am J Drug Abuse* 4, 495–503.

Brown DR, Eaton WW and Sussman L (1990) Racial differences in prevalence of phobic disorders. *J Nerv Ment Dis* 178, 434–441.

Brown GW and Harris T (1978) *Social Origins of Depression: A Study of Psychiatric Disorder in Women*. Free Press, New York.

Canino GJ, Rubio-Stipec M, Shrout P *et al.* (1987) Sex differences in depression in Puerto Rico. *Psychol Women Q* 11, 443–459.

Cardeña E, Lewis-Fernández R, Bear D *et al.* (2002) Dissociative disorders, in *Sourcebook for DSM-IV* (eds Widiger T, Frances AJ, Pincus HA *et al.*). American Psychiatric Press, Washington DC.

Castillo RJ (1991) Culture, Trance, and Mental Illness: Divided Consciousness in South Asia. Doctoral Dissertation in Anthropology, Harvard University.

Cattarinich X, Gibson N and Cave AJ (2001) Assessing mental capacity in Canadian Aboriginal seniors. *Soc Sci Med* 53(11) (Dec), 1469–1479.

Clark VA, Aneshensel CS, Frerichs RR *et al.* (1981) Analysis of effects of sex and age in response to items on the CES-D scale. *Psychiatr Res* 5, 171–181.

Cruickshank JK and Beevers DG (1989) *Ethnic Factors in Health and Disease*. Wright, London.

Davis DL and Herdt G (1997) Cultural issues and the sexual disorders of the DSM-IV, in *Sourcebook for DSM-IV* (eds Widiger T, Frances AJ, Pincus HA *et al.*). American Psychiatric Press, Washington DC.

Davis DL and 1Whitten RG (1987) The cross-cultural study of human sexuality. *Annu Rev Anthropol* 16, 69–98.

de la Monte SM, Hutchins GM and Moore GW (1989) Racial differences in the etiology of dementia and frequency of Alzheimer's lesions in the brain. *J Nat Med Assoc* 81, 644–652.

Ebigbo PO (1982) Development of a culture specific (Nigeria) screening scale of somatic complaints. *Cult Med Psychiatr* 6, 29–44.

Espín OM (1984) Cultural and historical influences on sexuality in Hispanic/Latin women, in *Pleasure and Anger: Exploring Female Sexuality* (ed Boston VC). Routledge & Kegan Paul, New York, pp. 149–164.

Fábrega H and Mezzich JE (1987) Adjustment disorder and psychiatric practice: Cultural and historical aspects. *Psychiatry* 50, 31–49.

Favazza AR (1985) Anthropology and psychiatry, in *Comprehensive Textbook of Psychiatry*, 4th edn. (eds Kaplan HI and Sadock JD). Williams & Wilkins, Baltimore, pp. 247–265.

Finkle A and Finkle C (1978) Sexual impotency. *Urology* 23, 25–30.

Fisher S (1980) Personality correlates of sexual behavior in Black women. *Arch Sex Behav* 9, 27–35.

Gebhard PH (1971) Human sexual behavior, in *Human Sexual Behavior* (eds Marshall DS and Suggs RC). Basic Books, New York, pp. 206–217.

González C, Lewis-Fernández R, Griffith EEH *et al.* (1997) The impact of culture on dissociation: On enhancing the cultural suitability of DSM-IV, in *Sourcebook for DSM-IV* (eds Widiger T, Frances AJ, and Pincus HA *et al.*). American Psychiatric Press, Washington DC, pp. 943–950.

Good BJ (1992/93) Culture, diagnosis, and comorbidity. *Cult Med Psychiatr* 16, 427–447.

Good BJ (1994) *Medicine, Rationality, and Experience: An Anthropological Perspective*. Cambridge University Press, Cambridge, UK.

Good BJ and Delvecchio Good MJ (1982) Toward a meaning-centered analysis of popular illness categories: "Fright-illness" and "heart distress" in Iran, in *Cultural Conceptions of Mental Health and Therapy* (eds Marsella AJ and White GM). Reidel, Dordrecht, pp. 141–166.

Good BJ and Kleinman A (1985) Culture and anxiety: Cross-cultural evidence for the patterning of anxiety disorders, in *Anxiety and the Anxiety Disorders* (eds Tuma A and Maser J). Erlbaum, Hillsdale, NJ.

Griffin KW, Scheier LM, Botvin GJ *et al.* (2000) Ethnic and gender differences in psychosocial risk, protection, and adolescent alcohol use. *Prev Sci* 1(4) (Dec), 199–212.

Guarnaccia PJ (1993) Ataques de nervios in Puerto Rico: Culture-bound syndrome or popular illness? *Med Anthropol* 15, 157–170.

Guarnaccia PJ and Kirmayer LJ (in press) Literature review on culture and the anxiety disorders (DSM-IV), in *Sourcebook for DSM-IV* (eds Widiger T, Frances AJ, Pincus HA *et al.*). American Psychiatric Press, Washington DC.

Guarnaccia PJN and Rogler LH (1999) Research on culture-bound syndromes: new directions. *Am J Psychiatr* 156(9) (Sept), 1322–1327.

Guarnaccia PJ, Angel R and Worobey JL (1989) The factor structure of the CES-D in the Hispanic Health and Nutrition Examination Survey: The influences of ethnicity, gender, and language. *Soc Sci Med* 29, 85–94.

Guarnaccia PJ, Guevara-Ramos LM, Gonzáles G *et al.* (1992) Cross-cultural aspects of psychotic symptoms in Puerto Rico. *Res Comm Ment Health* 7, 99–110.

Haasen C, Yagdiran O, Mass R *et al.* (2001) Schizophrenic disorders among Turkish migrants in Germany. A controlled clinical study. *Psychopathology* 34(4) (July–Aug), 203–208.

Habel U, Gur RC, Mandal MK *et al.* (2000) Emotional processing in schizophrenia across cultures: Standardized measures of discrimination and experience. *Schizophr Res* 42(1) (Mar 16), 57–66.

Hahn RA (1985) Culture-bound syndromes unbound. *Soc Sci Med* 21, 165–171.

Heath DB (2001) Culture and substance abuse. *Psychiatr Clin N Am* 24(3) (Sept), 479–496.

Helzer JE and Canino GJ (eds) (1992) *Alcoholism – North America, Europe, and Asia: A coordinated analysis of population data from ten regions*. Oxford University Press, Oxford, London.

Herdt G (1990) Developmental continuity as a dimension of sexual orientation across cultures, in *Homosexuality and Heterosexuality* (eds McWhirter D, Reinisch J, and Sanders P). Oxford, New York, pp. 208–238.

Hughes CC, Simons RC and Wintrob RM (1997) The "culture-bound syndromes" and DSM-IV, in *Sourcebook for DSM-IV* (eds Widiger T, Frances AJ, Pincus HA *et al.*). American Psychiatric Press, Washington DC, pp. 991–1000.

Hultkrantz A (1979) *The Religions of the American Indians*. University of California Press, Berkeley.

Ikels C (1991) Aging and disability in China: Cultural issues in measurement and interpretation. *Soc Sci Med* 32, 649–665.

Jenkins JH and Karno M (1992) The meaning of expressed emotion: Theoretical issues raised by cross-cultural research. *Am J Psychiatr* 149, 9–21.

Jenkins JH and Kinzie JD (1997) Culture and the diagnosis of adjustment disorders, in *Sourcebook for DSM-IV* (eds Widiger T, Frances AJ, Pincus HA *et al.*). American Psychiatric Press, Washington DC, pp. 969–974.

Karno M and Jenkins JH (1997) Cultural considerations in the diagnosis of schizophrenia and related disorders and psychotic disorders not otherwise classified, in *Sourcebook for DSM-IV* (eds Widiger T, Frances AJ, Pincus HA *et al.*). American Psychiatric Press, Washington DC, pp. 901–908.

Kaslow RA and Francis DP (1989) *The Epidemiology of AIDS*. Oxford University Press, New York.

Katon W and Roy-Byrne PP (1991) Mixed anxiety and depression. *J Abnorm Psychol* 100, 337–345.

Kirmayer LJ and Groleau D (2001) Affective disorders in cultural context. *Psychiatr Clin N Am* 24(3) (Sept), 465–478.

Kirmayer LJ and Robbins JM (1991) Introduction: Concepts of somatization, in *Current Concepts in Somatization: Research and Clinical Perspectives* (eds Kirmayer LJ and Robbins JM). American Psychiatric Press, Washington DC, pp. 1–19.

Kirmayer LJ and Weiss M (1997) On cultural considerations for somatoform disorders in DSM-IV, in *Sourcebook for DSM-IV* (eds Widiger T, Frances AJ, Pincus HA *et al.*). American Psychiatric Press, Washington DC, pp. 933–942.

Kleinman A (1988) *Rethinking Psychiatry*. Free Press, New York.

Krassoievitch M, Pérez-Rincón H and Suárez P (1982) Correlation entre les hallucinations visuelles et auditives dans une population de schizophrenes Mexicains. *Confront Psychiatr* 15, 149–162.

Kulhara P and Chakrabarti S (2001) Culture and schizophrenia and other psychotic disorders. *Psychiatr Clin N Am* 24(3) (Sept), 449–464.

Lee S (1991) Anorexia nervosa in Hong Kong: A Chinese perspective. *Psychol Med* 23(2), 437–451.

Lee S (1993) Side effects of chronic lithium therapy in Hong Kong Chiwesli: An enthropsychiatric perspective. *Cult Med Psychiatr* 17(3), 301–320.

Lee S (2001) From diversity to unity: The classification of mental disorders in 21st-century China. *Psychiatr Clin N Am* 24(3) (Sept), 421–431.

Lee S, Chiu HFK and Chen C (1989) Anorexia nervosa in Hong Kong: Why not more in Chinese? *Br J Psychiatr* 154, 683–688.

Leighton A (1981) Culture and psychiatry. *Can J Psychiatr* 26, 522–529.

Lewis-Fernández R (1992) The proposed DSM-IV trance and possession disorder category: Potential benefits and risks. *Transcult Psychiatr Res Rev* 29, 301–317.

Lewis-Fernández R (1994) Culture and dissociation: A comparison of ataque de nervios among Puerto Ricans and "Possession Syndrome" in India, in *Dissociation: Culture, Mind, and Body* (ed Spiegel D). American Psychiatric Press, Washington DC, pp. 123–167.

Lewis-Fernández R (2002) Puerto Rico, los nervios, y la nueva psiquiatría transcultural. Revista de psiquiatría de Puerto Rico.

Lewis-Fernández R and Kleinman A (1993) Culture, personality, and psychopathology. *J Abnorm Psychol* 103, 67–71.

Lewis-Fernández R and Kleinman A (1995) Cultural psychiatry: Theoretical, clinical and research issues. *Psychiatr Clin N Am* 18(3), 433–448.

Lewis-Fernández R, Garrido P, Bennasar MC *et al.* (1997) The relationship between dissociation, childhood trauma, and ataque de nervios among Puerto Rican psychiatric outpatients. *Am J Psychiatr* 159(9), 1603–1605.

Lin K-M and Fábrega H (1997) Cultural considerations on cognitive impairment in DSM-IV, in *Sourcebook for DSM-IV* (eds Widiger T, Frances AJ, Pincus HA *et al.*). American Psychiatric Press, Washington DC, pp. 885–892.

Lin K-M and Kleinman A (1988) Psychopathology and clinical course of schizophrenia: A cross-cultural perspective. *Schizophr Bull* 14, 555–567.

Lin T-Y (1989) Neurasthenia revisited: Its place in modern psychiatry. *Cult Med Psychiatr* 13, 105–130.

Manson SM and Good BJ (in press) Cultural considerations in the diagnosis of DSM-IV mood disorders, in *Sourcebook for DSM-IV* (eds

Widiger T, Frances AJ, Pincus HA *et al.*). American Psychiatric Press, Washington DC.

Manson SM, Shore JH and Bloom JD (1985) The depressive experience in American Indian communities: A challenge for psychiatric theory and diagnosis, in *Culture and Depression: Studies in the Anthropology and Cross-Cultural Psychiatry of Affect and Disorder* (eds Kleinman A and Good BJ). University of California Press, Berkeley, pp. 331–368.

Marsella AJ, Sartorius N, Jablensky A *et al.* (1985) Cross-cultural studies of depressive disorders: An overview, in *Culture and Depression: Studies in the Anthropology and Cross-Cultural Psychiatry of Affect and Disorder* (eds Kleinman A and Good BJ). University of California Press, Berkeley, pp. 299–324.

Martínez-Taboas A (1991) Multiple personality disorder as seen from a social constructionist viewpoint. *Dissociation* 4, 129–133.

Maser JD and Dinges N (1992) Comorbidity: Meaning and uses in cross-cultural clinical research. *Cult Med Psychiatr* 16, 409–425.

Maser JD, Kaelber C and Weise RE (1991) International use and attitudes toward DSM-III and DSM-III-R: Growing consensus in psychiatric classification. *J Abnorm Psychol* 100, 271–279.

Mezzich JE (1995) International perspectives on psychiatric diagnosis, in *Comprehensive Textbook of Psychiatry*, 6th edn. (eds Kaplan HI and Sadock BJ). Williams & Wilkins, Baltimore, pp. 692–703.

Mezzich JE and Good BJ (1997) On culturally enhancing the DSM-IV multiaxial formulation, in *Sourcebook for DSM-IV (eds*, Widiger T, Frances AJ, Pincus HA *et al.*). American Psychiatric Press, Washington DC, pp. 983–990.

Mezzich JE, Kleinman A, Fábrega H *et al.* (eds) (1993) Revised cultural proposals for DSM-IV. Working document submitted to the DSM-IV Task Force by the NIMH-sponsored Group on Culture and Diagnosis.

Mezzich JE, Berganza CE and Ruiperez MA (2001) Culture in DSM-IV, ICD-10, and evolving diagnostic systems. *Psychiatr Clin N Am* 24(3) (Sept), 407–419.

Mezzich JE, Kleinman A, Fábrega H *et al.* (eds) (in press) *Culture and Psychiatric Diagnosis*. American Psychiatric Press, Washington DC.

Nasser M (1986) Comparative study of the prevalence of abnormal eating attitudes among Arab female students of both London and Cairo Universities. *Psychol Med* 16, 621–625.

Ndetei DM and Vadher A (1984) A comparative cross-cultural study of the frequencies of hallucination in schizophrenia. *Acta Psychiatr Scand* 70, 545–549.

Neal AM and Turner SM (1991) Anxiety disorders research with African-Americans: Current status. *Psychol Bull* 109, 400–410.

Nichter M (1981) Idioms of distress: Alternatives in the expression of psychosocial distress: A case study from South India. *Cult Med Psychiatr* 5, 379–408.

Nichter M and Nichter M (1991) Hype and weight. *Med Anthropol* 13, 249–284.

Osterberg E (1986) Alcohol-related problems in cross-national perspectives: Results of the ISACE study, in *Alcohol and Culture: Comparative Perspectives from Europe and America*, Annals of the New York Academy of Sciences, Vol. 472 (ed Babor T), pp. 10–20.

Paris J (1991) Personality disorders, parasuicide, and culture. *Transcult Psychiatr Res Rev* 28, 25–39.

Perry JC (1992) Problems and considerations in the valid assessment of personality disorders. *Am J Psychiatr* 149, 1645–1653.

Richards M, Brayne C, Dening T *et al.* (2000) Cognitive function in UK community-dwelling African Caribbean and white elders: A pilot study. *Int J Geriatr Psychiatr* 15(7) (July), 621–630.

Ritenbaugh C (1982) Obesity as a culture-bound syndrome. *Cult Med Psychiatr* 6, 347–361.

Ritenbaugh C, Shisslak CL, Teufel N *et al.* (1997) Eating disorders: A cross-cultural review in regard to DSM-IV, in *Sourcebook for DSM-IV* (eds Widiger T, Frances AJ, Pincus HA *et al.*). American Psychiatric Press, Washington DC, pp. 959–968.

Robins LN, Helzer JE, Croughan J *et al.* (1981) National Institute of Mental Health Diagnostic Interview Schedule. *Arch Gen Psychiatr* 38, 381–389.

Robins LN, Helzer JE, Weissman MM *et al.* (1984) Lifetime prevalence of specific psychiatric disorders in three sites. *Arch Gen Psychiatr* 41, 949–958.

Rooth G (1973) Exhibitionism. *Arch Sex Behav* 2, 351–363.

Rosen LW, Shafer CL, Dummer GM *et al.* (1988) Prevalence of pathogenic weight-control behavior among Native American women and girls. *Int J Eat Disord* 7, 807–811.

Ross CA (1991) The dissociated executive self and the cultural dissociation barrier. *Dissociation* 4, 55–61.

Sartorius N, Jablensky A, Korten A *et al.* (1986) Early manifestations and first-contact incidence of schizophrenia in different cultures. *Psychol Med* 16, 909–928.

Saxena S and Prasad KVSR (1989) DSM-III subclassification of dissociative disorders applied to psychiatric outpatients in India. *Am J Psychiatr* 145, 261–262.

Shepherd M and Sartorius N (1974) Personality disorder and the international classification of diseases. *Psychol Med* 4, 141–146.

Shisslak CM, Crago M and Yates A (1989) Typical patterns in atypical anorexia nervosa. *Psychosomatics* 30, 307–311.

Shrout PE, Canino GJ, Bird H *et al.* (1992) Mental health status among Puerto Ricans, Mexican Americans, and nonHispanic Whites. *Am J Comm Psychol* 20, 729–752.

Simons RC and Hughes CC (eds) (1985) *The Culture-Bound Syndromes: Folk Illnesses of Psychiatric and Anthropological Interest.* Reidel, Dordrecht.

Spector RE (1979) *Cultural Diversity in Health and Illness*. Appleton-Century-Crofts, New York.

Spiegel D and Cardeña E (1991) Disintegrated experience: The dissociative disorders revisited. *J Abnorm Psychol* 100, 366–378.

Steinberg M (1991) The spectrum of depersonalization: Assessment and treatment, in *American Psychiatric Press Review of Psychiatry*, Vol. 10 (eds Tasman A and Goldfinger SM). American Psychiatric Press, Washington DC, pp. 223–247.

Suematsu H, Ishikawa H, Kuboki T *et al.* (1985) Statistical studies on anorexia nervosa in Japan: Detailed clinical data on 1,011 patients. *Psychother Psychosom* 43, 96–103.

Turner RJ and Gill AG (2002) Psychiatric and substance use disorders in South Florida: Racial/ethnic and gender contrasts in a young adult cohort. *Arch Gen Psychiatr* 59(1) (Jan), 43–50.

Valliant G (1986) Cultural factors in the etiology of alcoholism: A prospective study, in *Alcohol and Culture: Comparative Perspectives from Europe and America*, Vol. 472 (ed Babor T). Annals of the New York Academy of Sciences, New York, pp. 142–148.

Vega WA, Kolody B, Aguilar-Gaxiola S *et al.* (1998) Lifetime prevalence of DSM-III-R psychiatric disorders among urban and rural Mexican in California. *Arch Gen Psychiatr* 55, 771–778.

Vorcaro CM, Lima-Costa MF, Barreto SM *et al.* (2001) Unexpected high prevalence of 1-month depression in a small Brazilian community: The Bambui Study. *Acta Psychiatr Scand* 104(4) (Oct), 257–263.

Ward CA (ed) (1989) *Altered States of Consciousness and Mental Health: A Cross-Cultural Perspective.* Sage, Newbury Park.

Warner R (1985) *Recovery from Schizophrenia: Psychiatry and Political Economy.* Routledge & Kegan Paul, New York.

Weidman HH (1979) Falling-out: A diagnostic and treatment problem viewed from a transcultural perspective. *Soc Sci Med* 13B, 95–112.

Weiss MG (1996) Culture and the diagnosis of somatoform and dissociative disorders, in *Culture and Psychiatric Diagnosis* (eds Mezzich JE, Kleinman A, Fábrega H *et al.*). American Psychiatric Press, Washington DC.

Westermeyer J (1989) *Mental Health for Refugees and Other Migrants: Social and Preventive Approach.* CC Thomas, Illinois.

Westermeyer J and Canino GJ (1997) Culture and substance related disorders, in *Sourcebook for DSM-IV* (eds Widiger T, Frances AJ,

Pincus HA *et al.*). American Psychiatric Press, Washington DC, pp. 893–900.

Wig NN (1983) DSM-III: A perspective from the Third World, in *International Perspectives on DSM-III* (eds Spitzer RL, Williams JB, and Skodol AE). American Psychiatric Press, Washington DC.

Wildes JE, Emery RE and Simons AD (2001) The roles of ethnicity and culture in the development of eating disturbance and body dissatisfaction: A meta-analytic review. *Clin Psychol Rev* 21(4) (June), 521–551.

Williams CL (1987) Issues surrounding psychological testing of minority patients. *Hosp Comm Psychiatr* 38, 184–189.

Wyatt GE (1982) Identifying stereotypes of Afro-American sexuality and their impact on sexual behavior, in *The Afro-American Family* (eds Bass BA, Wyatt GE, and Powell G). Grune & Straton, New York, pp. 333–346.

Zhang M, Katzman R, Salmon D *et al.* (1990) The prevalence of dementia and Alzheimer's disease in Shanghai, China: Impact of age, gender, and education. *Ann Neurol* 27, 428–437.

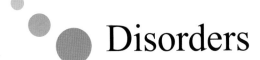

22 Psychiatric Classification

Introduction

There is a natural human predilection to categorize and classify for simplifying and organizing the wide range of observable phenomena and experiences that one is confronted with, thus facilitating both their understanding and their predictability. The current system for the diagnosis of mental disorders, the *Diagnostic and Statistical Manual of Mental Disorders*, Fourth Edition (DSM-IV) (American Psychiatric Association, 1994), is just the latest example from the long and colorful history of psychiatric classification. Although there was a more recent text revision, DSM-IV-TR (American Psychiatric Association, 2000), we will refer to DSM-IV as the "current" version since DSM-IV-TR primarily differs with respect to the textual descriptions of the disorders. The classification, diagnostic terms and virtually all of the diagnostic criteria are identical (First and Pincus, 2002).

Goals of a Classification System

Perhaps the most important goal of a psychiatric classification is to allow mental health practitioners and researchers to communicate more effectively with each other by establishing a convenient shorthand for describing the mental disorders that they see (First, 1992). For example, saying to a colleague that a patient has major depressive disorder can convey a great deal of information in only a few words. First of all, it indicates that depressed mood or loss of interest is a central aspect of the presenting problem and that the depression is not the kind of "normal" mood fluctuation that lasts for only a few days but rather that it persists every day for an extended period of time, for at least 2 weeks. Furthermore, one can expect to find a number of additional symptoms occurring at the same time, like suicidal ideation and changes in appetite, sleep, energy and psychomotor activity. Finally, information is also communicated about what is not to be found in this patient – specifically, that the depression is not caused by the direct physiological effects of alcohol, other drugs, medications, or a general medical condition; that substance use and general medical conditions have been ruled out as etiological factors; and that there is no history of schizophrenia or manic or hypomanic episodes.

DSM-IV also facilitates the identification and management of mental disorders in both clinical and research settings. Most of the DSM-IV diagnostic labels provide considerable and important predictive power. For example, making a diagnosis of bipolar disorder suggests the choice of treatment options (e.g., mood stabilizers), that a certain course may be likely (e.g., recurrent and episodic), and that there is an increased prevalence of this disorder in family members. By defining more or less homogeneous groups of individuals for study, DSM-IV can also further efforts to understand the etiology of mental disorders. The classifications of the manual have been a reflection of, and a major contribution to, the development of an empirical science of psychiatry. DSM-IV also plays an important role in education. In its organization of disorders into major classes, the system offers a structure for teaching phenomenology and differential diagnosis. DSM-IV is also useful in psychoeducation by showing patients that their pattern of symptoms is not mysterious and unique but rather has been identified and studied in others.

Approaches to Classification

Etiological Versus Descriptive

Historically, there have been two fundamental approaches to formulating systems of psychiatric classification: etiological and descriptive. Etiology-based classification systems organize categories around pathogenetic processes so that disorders corresponding to a particular category share the same underlying cause. Because the etiological basis for most psychiatric conditions remains elusive, etiological classification systems tend to be based instead on a particular conceptualization of the process of mental disorders. Although such classifications may be heuristically useful to proponents of the particular conceptualization that forms the basis of the system, they are often considerably less useful for proponents of different etiological principles, which greatly limits their utility. For this reason, a descriptive approach to classification has proved to be of greater utility given our current understanding. The descriptive approach aims to eschew particular etiological theories and instead relies on clinical descriptions of presenting symptoms. This approach, advanced by the work of the 19th century psychiatrist Emil Kraepelin, formed the basis for the system of classification of the *Diagnostic and Statistical Manual of Mental Disorders*, Third Edition (DSM-III) introduced in 1980. As a result, DSM-III and its successors, the *Diagnostic and Statistical Manual of Mental Disorders*, Third Edition, Revised (DSM-III-R) and DSM-IV, have proved to be useful in a variety of different settings and by psychiatrists of widely different backgrounds and conceptual orientations.

Syndrome Versus Symptom

Given that the manual lacks a specific etiological conceptualization, what is its organizing principle? The fundamental element is the syndrome, that is, a group or pattern of symptoms that appear together temporally in many individuals. It is assumed that these symptoms cluster together because they are associated in some clinically meaningful way, which perhaps may reflect a common etiological process, course, or treatment response.

Essentials of Psychiatry   Jerald Kay and Allan Tasman
© 2006 John Wiley & Sons, Ltd.

Table 22.1	Example of DSM-IV Multiaxial Evaluation*
Axis I	296.23 Major depressive disorder, single episode, severe but without psychotic features, with postpartum onset 307.51 Bulimia nervosa
Axis II	301.6 Dependent personality disorder Frequent use of denial
Axis III	Rheumatoid arthritis
Axis IV	Partner relational problem
Axis V	GAF = 35 (current)

*GAF, Global Assessment of Functioning Scale score.

Although it was hoped that the syndromes identified in the DSM represented relatively homogeneous subpopulations of patients, over the past 20 years since the publication of these definitions in DSM-III, the goal of discovering common etiologies for each of the DSM-defined syndromes has remained elusive. Epidemiologic and clinical studies have shown extremely high rates of comorbidities among the disorders, undermining the hypothesis that the syndromes represent distinct etiologies. Furthermore, epidemiologic studies have shown a high degree of short-term diagnostic instability for many disorders. With regard to treatment, lack of specificity in treatment response is the rule rather than the exception. The efficacy of many psychotropic medications cuts across the DSM-defined categories. For example, the selective serotonin reuptake inhibitors (SSRIs) have been demonstrated to be efficacious in a wide variety of disorders from many different sections of the DSM, including major depressive disorder, panic disorder, obsessive–compulsive disorder, dysthymic disorder, bulimia nervosa, social anxiety disorder, post traumatic stress disorder generalized anxiety disorder, hypochondriasis, body dysmorphic disorder and borderline personality disorder. Results of twin studies have also contradicted the DSM assumption that separate syndromes have a different underlying genetic basis. For example, twin studies have shown that generalized anxiety disorder and major depressive disorder may share the same genetic risk factors (Kendler, 1996), and evidence from molecular genetics research (Berrettini, 2000) indicates that three of the putative susceptibility loci associated with DSM-defined bipolar disorder also contribute to the risk of DSM-defined schizophrenia.

Given these clear limitations in the syndromal approach, it is important that users of the DSM resist the temptation to reify the DSM diagnostic categories as if they were actual diseases. They are best viewed as clinically useful constructs that are helpful in facilitating communication and record keeping and in selecting treatment. As more information about the causes of mental disorders become evident over the next decades, it is more than likely that the syndromal approach will be replaced by a classification system that is more reflective of the underlying etiology and pathophysiology.

Categorical Versus Dimensional

The diagnoses included in DSM-IV are defined categorically, that is, diagnostic criteria are provided that indicate whether an individual's clinical presentation either meets or does not meet the diagnostic criteria for a particular disorder. This method of classification is similar to what is used in other fields in medicine, namely that a patient either has or does not have a particular diagnosis, like pneumonia, colon cancer, multiple sclerosis, and so on. This tendency to define illness in terms of categories is undoubtedly due to the fact that it is reflective of basic human thought processes, embodied by the use of nouns in everyday speech to indicate categories of "things" (e.g., chairs, tables, dogs, cats).

In principle, however, variation in the symptomatology can be represented by a set of dimensions rather than by multiple categories. An example of this in medicine is blood pressure, which is measured along a continuum from low to high. (It only becomes categorical when we apply the label "hypertension" to indicate that a patient has a significant elevated level of blood pressure that puts him or her at risk for developing serious illness.) While a categorical approach to classification has important heuristic appeal, it may not represent the true state of things. Implicit in the categorical approach is an assumption that mental disorders are discrete entities, separated from one another and from normality, either by recognizably distinct combinations of symptoms or by demonstrably distinct etiologies. While this has been shown to be the case for a small number of conditions (e.g., Down syndrome, fragile X syndrome, phenylketonuria, Alzheimer's disease, Huntington's disease and Creutzfeldt–Jakob disease), there is little evidence supporting the applicability of this model for most other psychiatric symptoms. Indeed, in the last 20 years, the categorical approach has been increasingly questioned as evidence has accumulated that the so-called categorical disorders like major depressive disorder and anxiety disorders, and schizophrenia and bipolar disorder seem to merge imperceptibly both into one another and into normality (Kendler and Gardner, 1998) with no demonstrable natural boundaries.

Dimensional approaches do have some clear advantages. First of all, the commonly observed phenomena of excessive comorbidity (i.e., an individual receiving multiple, simultaneous DSM diagnoses) is arguably a direct result of having a categorical system with more than 250 categories. A dimensional approach, which would characterize an individual's psychopathology by indicating the extent of his or her psychiatric symptomatology across a number of dimensions, virtually eliminates apparent comorbidity. For example, consider an individual who presents with depression, anxiety and social avoidance. Using the DSM-IV categorical system, criteria might be met for three diagnoses (i.e., major depressive disorder, social phobia and generalized anxiety disorder), thus warranting a diagnosis of all three disorders on Axis I. A dimensional approach may simply indicate that the person has "high scores" on the depression, anxiety and social avoidance dimensions. Another advantage of the dimensional approach is that it avoids setting particular thresholds for distinguishing between pathology and normality. Rather than categorically saying that an individual has major depressive disorder, a dimensional approach might say that the person is high on the depression dimension.

There are a number of practical problems that potentially limit the utility of adopting a dimensional approach. First of all, clinicians are accustomed to thinking in terms of diagnostic categories, and the existing knowledge base about the presentation, etiology, epidemiology, course, prognosis and treatment is based on these categories. Furthermore, decisions about the management of individual patients (e.g., whether to treat and with what type of treatment) are also much easier to make if the patient is thought of as having a particular disorder (with its associated prognostic and treatment implications) rather than as a profile of scores across a series of dimensions. It should be noted that, at least for personality disorders, current dissatisfaction with the categorical approach has led to proposals for research that might allow for the adoption of a dimensional approach to classifying personality functioning in DSM-V (First *et al.*, 2002).

DSM-IV OVERVIEW

The remainder of this chapter provides an overview of the DSM-IV multiaxial system, as well as a presentation of some of the organizational principles of the various diagnostic groupings included in the DSM-IV classification. The succeeding chapters are organized according to the presentation of disorders in the DSM-IV classification and provide detailed information regarding the diagnosis, etiology and pathophysiology, epidemiology, course and treatment of these DSM-IV disorders.

DSM-IV Multiaxial System

The multiaxial system was first introduced by DSM-III in order to encourage the clinician to focus his or her attention during the evaluation process on issues above and beyond the psychiatric diagnosis. Use of the multiaxial system requires that information be noted on each of the five different axes, each axis devoted to a different aspect of the evaluation process. Axes I, II and III are the diagnostic axes that divide up the diagnostic pie into three separate domains. Axis I is for "clinical syndromes and disordersg", an admittedly confusing name since Axis II and Axis III are also diagnostic axes. The most accurate name for Axis I is "diagnoses not coded on Axis II and Axis III", since Axis II and Axis III were carved out of Axis I specifically to draw attention to certain disorders that clinicians were more likely to overlook.

That said, Axis II is designated for coding personality disorders and mental retardation. There have been many recent criticisms of the coding of personality disorders on Axis II. Critics correctly point out that there is no firm conceptual basis for this division. Although disorders on Axis II tend to be lifelong and pervasive, a number of disorders on Axis I (e.g., schizophrenia, autistic disorder, dysthymic disorder) fit this description as well. Others have made the incorrect assumption that categories on Axis II are unresponsive to medication treatment, which is at odds with more recent evidence that medications are often helpful in the treatment of personality disorders. The fact is that the Axis I/Axis II division was made strictly pragmatic. It was introduced in DSM-III as a way of drawing attention to a set of disorders that were thought not to be given adequate attention by mental health professionals. First introduced in DSM-III, Axis II was designed to draw attention to certain disorders that were thought to be overshadowed in the face of the more florid Axis I presentations.. Certainly the placement of personality disorders on a separate axis has increased both their clinical visibility and their importance as a subject for research studies. Whether the Axis I/Axis II division has finally outlived its usefulness remains a topic of heated debate, and will be revisited during the DSM-V deliberations.

Check:

— Problems with primary support group (childhood, adult, parent–child). Specify: _____

— Problems related to the social environment. Specify: _____

— Educational problems. Specify: _____

— Occupational problems. Specify: _____

— Housing problems. Specify: _____

— Economic problems. Specify: _____

— Problems with access to health care services. Specify: _____

— Problems related to interaction with the legal system/crime. Specify: _____

— Other psychosocial problems. Specify: _____

Figure 22.1 *DSM-IV-TR Axis IV: Psychosocial and Environmental Checklist. (Source: Modified from American Psychiatric Association [2000] Diagnostic and Statistical Manual of Mental Disorders, 4th edn., Text Rev. APA, Washington DC, p. 36.)*

Axis III, like Axis II, is intended to encourage clinicians to pay special attention to conditions that they tend to overlook; in this case, clinically relevant general medical conditions. The concept of "clinically relevant" is intended to be broad. For example, it would be appropriate to list hypertension on Axis III even if its only relationship to an Axis I disorder is its impact on the options for the choice of antidepressant medication.

Psychosocial stressors are well known to play an important role in the etiology, maintenance and management of a number of mental disorders. Axis IV provides the psychiatrist with the opportunity to list clinically relevant psychosocial and environmental problems (e.g., homelessness, poverty, divorce). To facilitate a comprehensive evaluation of such problems, DSM-IV includes a psychosocial and environmental checklist that allows the psychiatrist to indicate which types of problems are present and relevant (Figure 22.1).

Mental disorders differentially impact on individual's level of functioning. For example, one patient with schizophrenia may function quite well-being able to live in the community, marry and have a family, and maintain a steady job whereas another patient with schizophrenia may function quite poorly, requiring chronic institutionalization. Since both of these patients have symptoms that meet the diagnostic criteria for schizophrenia, their important differences in functioning are not captured by the clinical diagnosis alone. Some of the differences in functioning may be due to different symptom profiles or symptom severities. Other differences may be related to resilience factors or different levels of psychosocial support. Whatever the reason, the DSM-IV multiaxial system provides the clinician with the ability to indicate the patient's overall level of functioning in addition to the diagnosis on Axis V, using the Global Assessment of Functioning (GAF) Scale (Figure 22.2). This GAF Scale has been criticized because

Consider psychological, social, and occupational functioning on a hypothetical continuum of mental health-illness. Do not include impairment in functioning due to physical (or environmental) limitations.

Code	(Note: Use intermediate codes when appropriate, e.g., 45,68,72.)
100 | 91	Superior functioning in a wide range of activities, life's problems never seem to get out of hand, is sought out by others because of many positive qualities. No symptoms.
90 | 81	Absent or minimal symptoms (e.g., mild anxiety before an examination), good functioning in all areas, interested and involved in a wide range of activities, socially effective, generally satisfied with life, no more than everyday problems or concerns (e.g., an occasional argument with family members).
80 | 71	If symptoms are present, they are transient and expectable reactions to psychosocial stressors (e.g., difficulty concentrating after family argument); no more than slight impairment in social, occupational, or school functioning (e.g., temporarily falling behind in school work).
70 | 61	Some mild symptoms (e.g., depressed mood and mild insomnia) OR some difficulty in social, occupational, or school functioning (e.g., occasional truancy, or theft within the household), but generally functioning pretty well, has some meaningful interpersonal relationships.
60 | 51	Moderate symptoms (e.g., flat affect and circumstantial speech, occasional panic attacks) OR moderate difficulty in social, occupational, or school functioning (e.g., few friends, conflicts with peers or coworkers).
50 | 41	Serious symptoms (e.g., suicidal ideation, severe obsessional rituals, frequent shoplifting) OR any serious impairment in social, occupational, or school functioning (e.g., no friends, unable to keep a job).
40 | 31	Some impairment in reality testing or communication (e.g., speech is at times illogical, obscure, or irrelevant) OR major impairment in several areas, such as work or school, family relations, judgment, thinking, or mood (e.g., depressed man avoids friends, neglects family, and is unable to work; child frequently beats up younger chlidren, is defiant at home, and is failing at school).
30 | 21	Behavior is considerably influenced by delusions or hallucinations OR serious impairment in communication or judgment (e.g., sometimes incoherent, acts grossly inappropriately, suicidal preoccupation) OR inability to function in almost all areas (e.g., stays in bed all day; no job, home or friends).
20 | 11	Some danger of hurting self or others (e.g., suicide attempts without clear expectation of death, frequently violent, manic excitement) OR occasionally fails to maintain minimal personal hygiene (e.g., smears feces) OR gross impairment in communication (e.g., largely incoherent or mute).
10 | 1	Persistent danger of severely hurting self or others (e.g., recurrent violence) OR persistent inability to maintain minimal personal hygiene OR serious suicidal act with clear expectation of death.
0	Inadequate information

Figure 22.2 *DSM-IV-TR Axis V: Global Assessment of Functioning Scale. (Source: American Psychiatric Association [2000] Diagnostic and Statistical Manual of Mental Disorders, 4th ed., Text Rev. APA, Washington DC, p. 34.)*

it is not actually a "pure" measure of an individual's ability to function, since it incorporates symptom severity into the scale, for example, level 41 to 50 is for serious symptoms (e.g., suicidal ideation, severe obsessional rituals, frequent shoplifting) or any serious impairment in social, occupational, or school functioning (e.g., no friends, unable to keep a job). For this reason, the DSM-IV includes a scale (the Social and Occupational Functioning Scale [SOFAS]) that relies exclusively on functioning in its appendix of Criteria Sets and Axes Provided for Further Study (American Psychiatric Association, 2000, pp. 817–818).

DSM-IV-TR Classification and Diagnostic Codes

The "DSM-IV-TR Classification of Mental Disorders" refers to the comprehensive listing of the official diagnostic codes, categories, subtypes and specifiers (see below). It is divided into various "diagnostic classes" which group disorders together based on common presenting symptoms (e.g., mood disorders, anxiety disorders), typical age-at-onset (e.g., disorders usually first diagnosed in infancy, childhood and adolescence), and etiology (e.g., substance-related disorders, mental disorders due to a general medical condition).

DSM-IV-TR CLASSIFICATION

NOS = Not Otherwise Specified.

An x appearing in a diagnostic code indicates that a specific code number is required.

An ellipsis (…) is used in the names of certain disorders to indicate that the name of a specific mental disorder or general medical condition should be inserted when recording the name (e.g., 293.0 Delirium Due to Hypothyroidism).

If criteria are currently met, one of the following severity specifiers may be noted after the diagnosis:

> Mild
> Moderate
> Severe

If criteria are no longer met, one of the following specifiers may be noted:

> In Partial Remission
> In Full Remission
> Prior History

Disorders Usually First Diagnosed in Infancy, Childhood, or Adolescence

MENTAL RETARDATION

Note:	*These are coded on Axis II.*
317	Mild Mental Retardation
318.0	Moderate Mental Retardation
318.1	Severe Mental Retardation
318.2	Profound Mental Retardation
319	Mental Retardation, Severity Unspecified

LEARNING DISORDERS

315.00	Reading Disorder
315.1	Mathematics Disorder
315.2	Disorder of Written Expression
315.9	Learning Disorder NOS

MOTOR SKILLS DISORDER

315.4	Developmental Coordination Disorder

COMMUNICATION DISORDERS

315.31	Expressive Language Disorder
315.32	Mixed Receptive–Expressive Language Disorder
315.39	Phonological Disorder
307.0	Stuttering
307.9	Communication Disorder NOS

PERVASIVE DEVELOPMENTAL DISORDERS

299.00	Autistic Disorder
299.80	Rett's Disorder
299.10	Childhood Disintegrative Disorder
299.80	Asperger's Disorder
299.80	Pervasive Developmental Disorder NOS

ATTENTION-DEFICIT AND DISRUPTIVE BEHAVIOR DISORDERS

314.xx	Attention-Deficit/Hyperactivity Disorder
.01	Combined Type
.00	Predominantly Inattentive Type
.01	Predominantly Hyperactive-Impulsive Type
314.9	Attention-Deficit/HyperactivityDisorder NOS
312.xx	Conduct Disorder
.81	Childhood-onset Type
.82	Adolescent-onset Type
.89	Unspecified Onset
313.81	Oppositional Defiant Disorder
312.9	Disruptive Behavior Disorder NOS

FEEDING AND EATING DISORDERS OF INFANCY OR EARLY CHILDHOOD

307.52	Pica
307.53	Rumination Disorder
307.59	Feeding Disorder of Infancy or Early Childhood

TIC DISORDERS

307.23	Tourette's Disorder
307.22	Chronic Motor or Vocal Tic Disorder
307.21	Transient Tic Disorder
	Specify if: Single Episode/Recurrent
307.20	Tic Disorder NOS

ELIMINATION DISORDERS

—.—	Encopresis
787.6	With Constipation and Overflow Incontinence
307.7	Without Constipation and Overflow Incontinence
307.6	Enuresis (Not Due to a General Medical Condition)
	Specify type: Nocturnal Only/Diurnal Only/Nocturnal and Diurnal

OTHER DISORDERS OF INFANCY, CHILDHOOD, OR ADOLESCENCE

309.21	Separation Anxiety Disorder
	Specify if: Early Onset
313.23	Selective Mutism
313.89	Reactive Attachment Disorder of Infancy or Early Childhood
	Specify type: Inhibited Type/Disinhibited Type
307.3	Stereotypic Movement Disorder
	Specify if: With Self-Injurious Behavior
313.9	Disorder of Infancy, Childhood, or Adolescence NOS

Delirium, Dementia and Amnestic and Other Cognitive Disorders

DELIRIUM

293.0	Delirium Due to … [*Indicate the General Medical Condition*]
—.—	Substance Intoxication Delirium (*refer to Substance-Related Disorders for substance-specific codes*)
—.—	Substance Withdrawal Delirium (*refer to Substance-Related Disorders for substance-specific codes*)
—.—	Delirium Due to Multiple Etiologies (*code each of the specific etiologies*)
780.09	Delirium NOS

DEMENTIA

294.xx	Dementia of the Alzheimer's Type, With Early Onset (*also code 331.0 Alzheimer's disease on Axis III*)

.10	Without Behavioral Disturbance
.11	With Behavioral Disturbance
294.xx	Dementia of the Alzheimer's Type, With Late Onset (*also code 331.0 Alzheimer's disease on Axis III*)
.10	Without Behavioral Disturbance
.11	With Behavioral Disturbance
290.xx	Vascular Dementia
.40	Uncomplicated
.41	With Delirium
.42	With Delusions
.43	With Depressed Mood
	Specify if: With Behavioral Disturbance

Code presence or absence of a behavioral disturbance in the fifth digit for Dementia Due to a General Medical Condition:

294.10 =	Without Behavioral Disturbance
294.11 =	With Behavioral Disturbance
294.1x	Dementia Due to HIV Disease (*also code 042 HIV on Axis III*)
294.1x	Dementia Due to Head Trauma (*also code 854.00 head injury on Axis III*)
294.1x	Dementia Due to Parkinson's Disease (*also code 332.0 Parkinson's disease on Axis III*)
294.1x	Dementia Due to Huntington's Disease (*also code 333.4 Huntington's disease on Axis III*)
294.1x	Dementia Due to Pick's Disease (*also code 331.1 Pick's disease on Axis III*)
294.1x	Dementia Due to Creutzfeldt–Jakob Disease (*also code 046.1 Creutzfeldt–Jakob disease on Axis III*)
294.1x	Dementia Due to … [*Indicate the General Medical Condition not listed above*] (*also code the general medical condition on Axis III*)
—.—	Substance-Induced Persisting Dementia (*refer to Substance-Related Disorders for substance-specific codes*)
—.—	Dementia Due to Multiple Etiologies (*code each of the specific etiologies*)
294.8	Dementia NOS

AMNESTIC DISORDERS

294.0	Amnestic Disorder Due to … [*Indicate the General Medical Condition*]
	Specify if: Transient/Chronic
—.—	Substance-Induced Persisting Amnestic Disorder (*refer to Substance-Related Disorders for substance-specific codes*)
294.8	Amnestic Disorder NOS

OTHER COGNITIVE DISORDERS

| 294.9 | Cognitive Disorder NOS |

Mental Disorders Due to a General Medical Condition Not Elsewhere Classified

293.89	Catatonic Disorder Due to … [*Indicate the General Medical Condition*]
310.1	Personality Change Due to … [*Indicate the General Medical Condition*]
	Specify type: Labile Type/Disinhibited Type/Aggressive Type/Apathetic Type/Paranoid Type/Other Type/Combined Type/Unspecified Type

| 293.9 | Mental Disorder NOS Due to … [*Indicate the General Medical Condition*] |

Substance-related Disorders

The following specifiers apply to Substance Dependence as noted:

[a]*With Physiological Dependence/Without Physiological Dependence*

[b]*Early Full Remission/Early Partial Remission* SustainedFullRemission/SustainedPartialRemission

[c]*In a Controlled Environment*[d]*On Agonist Therapy/*

The following specifiers apply to Substance-Induced Disorders as noted:

[I]With Onset During Intoxication

[W]With Onset During Withdrawal

ALCOHOL-RELATED DISORDERS

Alcohol Use Disorders
| 303.90 | Alcohol Dependence[a,b,c] |
| 305.00 | Alcohol Abuse |

Alcohol-Induced Disorders
303.00	Alcohol Intoxication
291.81	Alcohol Withdrawal
	Specify if: With Perceptual Disturbances
291.0	Alcohol Intoxication Delirium
291.0	Alcohol Withdrawal Delirium
291.2	Alcohol-Induced Persisting Dementia
291.1	Alcohol-Induced Persisting Amnestic Disorder
291.x	Alcohol-Induced Psychotic Disorder
.5	With Delusions[I,W]
.3	With Hallucinations[I,W]
291.89	Alcohol-Induced Mood Disorder[I,W]
291.89	Alcohol-Induced Anxiety Disorder[I,W]
291.89	Alcohol-Induced Sexual Dysfunction[I]
291.89	Alcohol-Induced Sleep Disorder[I,W]
291.9	Alcohol-Related Disorder NOS

AMPHETAMINE (OR AMPHETAMINE-LIKE)-RELATED DISORDERS

Amphetamine Use Disorders
| 304.40 | Amphetamine Dependence[a,b,c] |
| 305.70 | Amphetamine Abuse |

Amphetamine-Induced Disorders
292.89	Amphetamine Intoxication
	Specify if: With Perceptual Disturbances
292.0	Amphetamine Withdrawal
292.81	Amphetamine Intoxication Delirium
292.xx	Amphetamine-Induced Psychotic Disorder
.11	With Delusions[I]
.12	With Hallucinations[I]
292.84	Amphetamine-induced Mood Disorder[I,W]
292.89	Amphetamine-induced Anxiety Disorder[I]
292.89	Amphetamine-induced Sexual Dysfunction[I]
292.89	Amphetamine-induced Sleep Disorder[I,W]
292.9	Amphetamine-related Disorder NOS

CAFFEINE-RELATED DISORDERS

Caffeine-induced Disorders
305.90   Caffeine intoxication
292.89   Caffeine-induced Anxiety Disorder[I]
292.89   Caffeine-induced Sleep Disorder[I]
292.9   Caffeine-related Disorder NOS

CANNABIS-RELATED DISORDERS

Cannabis Use Disorders
304.30   Cannabis Dependence[a,b,c]
305.20   Cannabis Abuse

Cannabis-induced Disorders
292.89   Cannabis Intoxication
            Specify if: With Perceptual Disturbances
292.81   Cannabis Intoxication Delirium
292.xx   Cannabis-induced Psychotic Disorder
    .11   With Delusions[I]
    .12   With Hallucinations[I]
292.89   Cannabis-induced Anxiety Disorder[I]
292.9   Cannabis-related Disorder NOS

COCAINE-RELATED DISORDERS

Cocaine Use Disorders
304.20   Cocaine Dependence[a,b,c]
305.60   Cocaine Abuse

Cocaine-induced Disorders
292.89   Cocaine Intoxication
            Specify if: With Perceptual Disturbances
292.0   Cocaine Withdrawal
292.81   Cocaine Intoxication Delirium
292.xx   Cocaine-induced Psychotic Disorder
    .11   With Delusions[I]
    .12   With Hallucinations[I]
292.84   Cocaine-induced Mood Disorder[I,W]
292.89   Cocaine-induced Anxiety Disorder[I,W]
292.89   Cocaine-induced Sexual Dysfunction[I]
292.89   Cocaine-induced Sleep Disorder[I,W]
292.9   Cocaine-Related Disorder NOS

HALLUCINOGEN-RELATED DISORDERS

Hallucinogen Use Disorders
304.50   Hallucinogen Dependence[b,c]
305.30   Hallucinogen Abuse

Hallucinogen-induced Disorders
292.89   Hallucinogen Intoxication
292.89   Hallucinogen Persisting Perception Disorder
            (Flashbacks)
292.81   Hallucinogen Intoxication Delirium
292.xx   Hallucinogen-induced Psychotic Disorder
    .11   With Delusions[I]
    .12   With Hallucinations[I]
292.84   Hallucinogen-induced Mood Disorder[I]
292.89   Hallucinogen-induced Anxiety Disorder[I]
292.9   Hallucinogen-related Disorder NOS

INHALANT-RELATED DISORDERS

Inhalant Use Disorders
304.60   Inhalant Dependence[b,c]
305.90   Inhalant Abuse

Inhalant-induced Disorders
292.89   Inhalant Intoxication
292.81   Inhalant Intoxication Delirium
292.82   Inhalant-induced Persisting Dementia
292.xx   Inhalant-induced Psychotic Disorder
    .11   With Delusions[I]
    .12   With Hallucinations[I]
292.84   Inhalant-induced Mood Disorder[I]
292.89   Inhalant-induced Anxiety Disorder[I]
292.9   Inhalant-related Disorder NOS

NICOTINE-RELATED DISORDERS

Nicotine Use Disorder
305.1   Nicotine Dependence[a,b]

Nicotine-induced Disorder
292.0   Nicotine Withdrawal
292.9   Nicotine-related Disorder NOS

OPIOID-RELATED DISORDERS

Opioid Use Disorders
304.00   Opioid Dependence[a,b,c,d]
305.50   Opioid Abuse

Opioid-induced Disorders
292.89   Opioid Intoxication
            Specify if: With Perceptual Disturbances
292.0   Opioid Withdrawal
292.81   Opioid Intoxication Delirium
292.xx   Opioid-induced Psychotic Disorder
    .11   With Delusions[I]
    .12   With Hallucinations[I]
292.84   Opioid-induced Mood Disorder[I]
292.89   Opioid-induced Sexual Dysfunction[I]
292.89   Opioid-induced Sleep Disorder[I,W]
292.9   Opioid-related Disorder NOS

PHENCYCLIDINE (OR PHENCYCLIDINE-LIKE) RELATED DISORDERS

Phencyclidine Use Disorders
304.60   Phencyclidine Dependence[b,c]
305.90   Phencyclidine Abuse

Phencyclidine-induced Disorders
292.89   Phencyclidine Intoxication
            Specify if: With Perceptual Disturbances
292.81   Phencyclidine Intoxication Delirium
292.xx   Phencyclidine-induced Psychotic Disorder
    .11   With Delusions[I]
    .12   With Hallucinations[I]
292.84   Phencyclidine-induced Mood Disorder[I]
292.89   Phencyclidine-induced Anxiety Disorder[I]
292.9   Phencyclidine-related Disorder NOS

SEDATIVE-, HYPNOTIC-, OR ANXIOLYTIC-RELATED DISORDERS

Sedative, Hypnotic, or Anxiolytic Use Disorders
304.10   Sedative, Hypnotic, or Anxiolytic Dependence[a,b,c]
305.40   Sedative, Hypnotic, or Anxiolytic Abuse

Sedative-, Hypnotic-, or Anxiolytic-induced Disorders
292.89   Sedative, Hypnotic, or Anxiolytic Intoxication
292.0   Sedative, Hypnotic, or Anxiolytic Withdrawal
          Specify if: With Perceptual Disturbances
292.81   Sedative, Hypnotic, or Anxiolytic Intoxication Delirium
292.81   Sedative, Hypnotic, or Anxiolytic Withdrawal Delirium
292.82   Sedative-, Hypnotic-, or Anxiolytic-induced Persisting Dementia
292.83   Sedative-, Hypnotic-, or Anxiolytic-induced Persisting Amnestic Disorder
292.xx   Sedative-, Hypnotic-, or Anxiolytic-induced Psychotic Disorder
    .11   With Delusions[I,W]
    .12   With Hallucinations[I,W]
292.84   Sedative-, Hypnotic-, or Anxiolytic-induced Mood Disorder[I,W]
292.89   Sedative-, Hypnotic-, or Anxiolytic-induced Anxiety Disorder[W]
292.89   Sedative-, Hypnotic-, or Anxiolytic-induced Sexual Dysfunction[I]
292.89   Sedative-, Hypnotic-, or Anxiolytic-induced Sleep Disorder[I,W]
292.9   Sedative-, Hypnotic-, or Anxiolytic-related Disorder NOS

POLYSUBSTANCE-RELATED DISORDER
304.80   Polysubstance Dependence[a,b,c,d]

OTHER (OR UNKNOWN) SUBSTANCE-RELATED DISORDERS

Other (or Unknown) Substance Use Disorders
304.90   Other (or Unknown) Substance Dependence[a,b,c,d]
305.90   Other (or Unknown) Substance Abuse

Other (or Unknown) Substance-induced Disorders
292.89   Other (or Unknown) Substance Intoxication
          Specify if: With Perceptual Disturbances
292.0   Other (or Unknown) Substance Withdrawal
          Specify if: With Perceptual Disturbances
292.81   Other (or Unknown) Substance-induced Delirium
292.82   Other (or Unknown) Substance-induced Persisting Dementia
292.83   Other (or Unknown) Substance-induced Persisting Amnestic Disorder
292.xx   Other (or Unknown) Substance-induced Psychotic Disorder
    .11   With Delusions[I,W]
    .12   With Hallucinations[I,W]
292.84   Other (or Unknown) Substance-Induced MoodDisorder[I,W]
292.89   Other (or Unknown) Substance-induced Anxiety Disorder[I,W]

292.89   Other (or Unknown) Substance-induced Sexual Dysfunction[I]
292.89   Other (or Unknown) Substance-induced Sleep Disorder[I,W]
292.9   Other (or Unknown) Substance-related Disorder NOS

Schizophrenia and Other Psychotic Disorders
295.xx   Schizophrenia

The following Classification of Longitudinal Course applies to all subtypes of Schizophrenia.

  Episodic With Interepisode Residual Symptoms (*specify if*: With Prominent Negative Symptoms)/Episodic With No Interepisode Residual Symptoms/Continuous (*specify if*: With Prominent Negative Symptoms)
  Single Episode In Partial Remission (*specify if*: With Prominent Negative Symptoms)/Single Episode In Full Remission
  Other or Unspecified Pattern

    .30   Paranoid Type
    .10   Disorganized Type
    .20   Catatonic Type
    .90   Undifferentiated Type
    .60   Residual Type
295.40   Schizophreniform Disorder
          Specify if: *Without Good Prognostic Features/With Good Prognostic Features*
295.70   Schizoaffective Disorder
          Specify type: Bipolar Type/Depressive Type
297.1   Delusional Disorder
          Specify type: Erotomanic Type/Grandiose Type/ Jealous Type/Persecutory Type/Somatic Type/ Mixed Type/Unspecified Type
298.8   Brief Psychotic Disorder
          Specify if: With Marked Stressor(s)/Without Marked Stressor(s)/With Postpartum Onset
297.3   Shared Psychotic Disorder
293.xx   Psychotic Disorder Due to…[*Indicate the General Medical Condition*]
    .81   With Delusions
    .82   With Hallucinations
—.—   Substance-Induced Psychotic Disorder (*refer to Substance-Related Disorders for substance-specific codes*)
          Specify if: With Onset During Intoxication/With Onset During Withdrawal
298.9   Psychotic Disorder NOS

Mood Disorders
Code current state of Major Depressive Disorder or Bipolar I Disorder in fifth digit:
1 =   Mild
2 =   Moderate
3 =   Severe Without Psychotic Features
4 =   Severe With Psychotic Features
          Specify: Mood-congruent Psychotic Features/Mood-Incongruent Psychotic Features
5 =   In Partial Remission
6 =   In Full Remission
0 =   Unspecified

The following specifiers apply (for current or most recent episode) to Mood Disorders as noted:

[a]Severity/Psychotic/Remission Specifiers
[b]Chronic
[c]With Catatonic Features
[d]With Melancholic Features
[e]With Atypical Features
[f]With Postpartum Onset

The following specifiers apply to Mood Disorders as noted:

[g]With or Without Full Interepisode Recovery
[h]With Seasonal Pattern
[i]With Rapid Cycling

DEPRESSIVE DISORDERS

296.xx	Major Depressive Disorder
.2x	Single Episode[a,b,c,d,e,f]
.3x	Recurrent[a,b,c,d,e,f,g,h]
300.4	Dysthymic Disorder
	Specify if: Early Onset/Late Onset
	Specify: With Atypical Features
311	Depressive Disorder NOS

BIPOLAR DISORDERS

296.xx	Bipolar I Disorder
.0x	Single Manic Episode[a,c,f]
	Specify if: Mixed
.40	Most Recent Episode Hypomanic[g,h,i]
.4x	Most Recent Episode Manic[a,c,f,g,h,i]
.6x	Most Recent Episode Mixed[a,c,f,g,h,i]
.5x	Most Recent Episode Depressed[a,b,c,d,e,f,g,h,i]
.7	Most Recent Episode Unspecified[g,h,i]
296.89	Bipolar II Disorder[a,b,c,d,e,f,g,h,i]
	Specify (current or most recent episode): Hypomanic/Depressed
301.13	Cyclothymic Disorder
296.80	Bipolar Disorder NOS
293.83	Mood Disorder Due to… [*Indicate the General Medical Condition*]
	Specify type: With Depressive Features/With Major Depressive-Like Episode/With Manic Features/With Mixed Features
—.—	Substance-Induced Mood Disorder (*refer to Substance-Related Disorders for substance-specific codes*)
	Specify type: With Depressive Features/With Manic Features/With Mixed Features
	Specify if: With Onset During Intoxication/With Onset During Withdrawal
296.90	Mood Disorder NOS

Anxiety Disorders

300.01	Panic Disorder Without Agoraphobia
300.21	Panic Disorder With Agoraphobia
300.22	Agoraphobia Without History of Panic Disorder
300.29	Specific Phobia
	Specify type: Animal Type/Natural Environment Type/Blood-injection-injury Type/Situational Type/Other Type
300.23	Social Phobia
	Specify if: Generalized
300.3	Obsessive–Compulsive Disorder
	Specify if: With Poor Insight

309.81	Post traumatic Stress Disorder
	Specify if: Acute/Chronic
	Specify if: With Delayed Onset
308.3	Acute Stress Disorder
300.02	Generalized Anxiety Disorder
293.89	Anxiety Disorder Due to… [*Indicate the General Medical Condition*]
	Specify if: With Generalized Anxiety/With Panic Attacks/With Obsessive–Compulsive Symptoms
—.—	Substance-induced Anxiety Disorder (*refer to Substance-related Disorders for substance-specific codes*)
	Specify if: With Generalized Anxiety/With Panic Attacks/With Obsessive–Compulsive Symptoms/With Phobic Symptoms
	Specify if: With Onset During Intoxication/With Onset During Withdrawal
300.00	Anxiety Disorder NOS

Somatoform Disorders

300.81	Somatization Disorder
300.82	Undifferentiated Somatoform Disorder
300.11	Conversion Disorder
	Specify type: With Motor Symptom or Deficit/With Sensory Symptom or Deficit/With Seizures or Convulsions/With Mixed Presentation
307.xx	Pain Disorder
.80	Associated With Psychological Factors
.89	Associated With Both Psychological Factors and a General Medical Condition
	Specify if: Acute/Chronic
300.7	Hypochondriasis
	Specify if: With Poor Insight
300.7	Body Dysmorphic Disorder
300.82	Somatoform Disorder NOS

Factitious Disorders

300.xx	Factitious Disorder
.16	With Predominantly Psychological Signs and Symptoms
.19	With Predominantly Physical Signs and Symptoms
.19	With Combined Psychological and Physical Signs and Symptoms
300.19	Factitious Disorder NOS

Dissociative Disorders

300.12	Dissociative Amnesia
300.13	Dissociative Fugue
300.14	Dissociative Identity Disorder
300.6	Depersonalization Disorder
300.15	Dissociative Disorder NOS

Sexual and Gender Identity Disorders

SEXUAL DYSFUNCTIONS

The following specifiers apply to all primary Sexual Dysfunctions:

Lifelong Type/Acquired Type
Generalized Type/Situational Type

Due to Psychological Factors/Due to
Combined Factors

Sexual Desire Disorders

302.71	Hypoactive Sexual Desire Disorder
302.79	Sexual Aversion Disorder

Sexual Arousal Disorders

302.72	Female Sexual Arousal Disorder
302.72	Male Erectile Disorder

Orgasmic Disorders

302.73	Female Orgasmic Disorder
302.74	Male Orgasmic Disorder
302.75	Premature Ejaculation

Sexual Pain Disorders

302.76	Dyspareunia (Not Due to a General Medical Condition)
306.51	Vaginismus (Not Due to a General Medical Condition)

Sexual Dysfunction Due to a General Medical Condition

625.8	Female Hypoactive Sexual Desire Disorder Due to…[*Indicate the General Medical Condition*]
608.89	Male Hypoactive Sexual Desire Disorder Due to…[*Indicate the General Medical Condition*]
607.84	Male Erectile Disorder Due to…[*Indicate the General Medical Condition*]
625.0	Female Dyspareunia Due to…[*Indicate the General Medical Condition*]
608.89	Male Dyspareunia Due to…[*Indicate the General Medical Condition*]
625.8	Other Female Sexual Dysfunction Due to…[*Indicate the General Medical Condition*]
608.89	Other Male Sexual Dysfunction Due to…[*Indicate the General Medical Condition*]
—.—	Substance-induced Sexual Dysfunction (*refer to Substance-related Disorders for substance-specific codes*) *Specify if*: With Impaired Desire/With Impaired Arousal/With Impaired Orgasm/With Sexual Pain *Specify if*: With Onset During Intoxication
302.70	Sexual Dysfunction NOS

PARAPHILIAS

302.4	Exhibitionism
302.81	Fetishism
302.89	Frotteurism
302.2	Pedophilia *Specify if*: Sexually Attracted to Males/Sexually Attracted to Females/Sexually Attracted to Both *Specify if*: Limited to Incest *Specify type*: Exclusive Type/Nonexclusive Type
302.83	Sexual Masochism
302.84	Sexual Sadism
302.3	Transvestic Fetishism *Specify if*: With Gender Dysphoria

302.82	Voyeurism
302.9	Paraphilia NOS

GENDER IDENTITY DISORDERS

302.xx	Gender Identity Disorder
.6	in Children
.85	in Adolescents or Adults *Specify if*: Sexually Attracted to Males/Sexually Attracted to Females/Sexually Attracted to Both/SexuallyAttracted to Neither
302.6	Gender Identity Disorder NOS
302.9	Sexual Disorder NOS

Eating Disorders

307.1	Anorexia Nervosa *Specify type*: Restricting Type; Binge-Eating/Purging Type
307.51	Bulimia Nervosa *Specify type*: Purging Type/Nonpurging Type
307.50	Eating Disorder NOS

Sleep Disorders

PRIMARY SLEEP DISORDERS

Dyssomnias

307.42	Primary Insomnia
307.44	Primary Hypersomnia *Specify if*: Recurrent
347	Narcolepsy
780.59	Breathing-Related Sleep Disorder
307.45	Circadian Rhythm Sleep Disorder *Specify type*: Delayed Sleep PhaseType/Jet Lag Type/Shift Work Type/Unspecified Type
307.47	Dyssomnia NOS

Parasomnias

307.47	Nightmare Disorder
307.46	Sleep Terror Disorder
307.46	Sleepwalking Disorder
307.47	Parasomnia NOS

SLEEP DISORDERS RELATED TO ANOTHER MENTAL DISORDER

307.42	Insomnia Related to…[*Indicate the Axis I or Axis II Disorder*]
307.44	Hypersomnia Related to…[*Indicate the Axis I or Axis II Disorder*]

OTHER SLEEP DISORDERS

780.xx	Sleep Disorder Due to…[*Indicate the General Medical Condition*]
.52	Insomnia Type
.54	Hypersomnia Type
.59	Parasomnia Type
.59	Mixed Type
—.—	Substance-induced Sleep Disorder (*refer to Substance-related Disorders for substance-specific codes*)

Specify type: Insomnia Type/Hypersomnia Type/
Parasomnia Type/Mixed Type
Specify if: With Onset During Intoxication/With
Onset During Withdrawal

Impulse Control Disorders Not Elsewhere Classified

312.34	Intermittent Explosive Disorder
312.32	Kleptomania
312.33	Pyromania
312.31	Pathological Gambling
312.39	Trichotillomania
312.30	Impulse control Disorder NOS

Adjustment Disorders

309.xx	Adjustment Disorder
.0	With Depressed Mood
.24	With Anxiety
.28	With Mixed Anxiety and Depressed Mood
.3	With Disturbance of Conduct
.4	With Mixed Disturbance of Emotions and Conduct
.9	Unspecified

Specify if: Acute/Chronic

Personality Disorders

Note: *These are coded on Axis II*

301.0	Paranoid Personality Disorder
301.20	Schizoid Personality Disorder
301.22	Schizotypal Personality Disorder
301.7	Antisocial Personality Disorder
301.83	Borderline Personality Disorder
301.50	Histrionic Personality Disorder
301.81	Narcissistic Personality Disorder
301.82	Avoidant Personality Disorder
301.6	Dependent Personality Disorder
301.4	Obsessive–Compulsive Personality Disorder
301.9	Personality Disorder NOS

Other Conditions That May Be a Focus of Clinical Attention

PSYCHOLOGICAL FACTORS AFFECTING MEDICAL CONDITION

316   … [*Specified Psychological Factor*]
Affecting… [*Indicate the General Medical Condition*]
Choose name based on nature of factors:
Mental Disorder Affecting Medical Condition
Psychological Symptoms Affecting Medical Condition
Personality Traits or Coping Style Affecting Medical Condition
Maladaptive Health Behaviors Affecting Medical Condition
Stress-Related Physiological Response Affecting Medical Condition
Other or Unspecified Psychological Factors Affecting Medical Condition

MEDICATION-INDUCED MOVEMENT DISORDERS

332.1	Neuroleptic-induced Parkinsonism
333.92	Neuroleptic alignant Syndrome
333.7	Neuroleptic-induced Acute Dystonia
333.99	Neuroleptic-induced Acute Akathisia
333.82	Neuroleptic-induced Tardive Dyskinesia
333.1	Medication-induced Postural Tremor
333.90	Medication-induced Movement Disorder NOS

OTHER MEDICATION-INDUCED DISORDER

995.2	Adverse Effects of Medication NOS

RELATIONAL PROBLEMS

V61.9	Relational Problem Related to a Mental Disorder or General Medical Condition
V61.20	Parent–Child Relational Problem
V61.10	Partner Relational Problem
V61.8	Sibling Relational Problem
V62.81	Relational Problem NOS

PROBLEMS RELATED TO ABUSE OR NEGLECT

V61.21	Physical Abuse of Child (*code 995.54 if focus of attention is on victim*)
V61.21	Sexual Abuse of Child (*code 995.53 if focus of attention is on victim*)
V61.21	Neglect of Child (*code 995.52 if focus of attention is on victim*)
—.—	Physical Abuse of Adult
V61.12	(if by partner)
V62.83	(if by person other than partner) (*code 995.83 if focus of attention is on victim*)
—.—	Sexual Abuse of Adult
V61.12	(if by partner)
V62.83	(if by person other than partner) (*code 995.83 if focus of attention is on victim*)

ADDITIONAL CONDITIONS THAT MAY BE A FOCUS OF CLINICAL ATTENTION

V15.81	Noncompliance With Treatment
V65.2	Malingering
V71.01	Adult Antisocial Behavior
V71.02	Child or Adolescent Antisocial Behavior
V62.89	Borderline Intellectual Functioning

Note: *This is coded on Axis II*

780.9	Age-Related Cognitive Decline
V62.82	Bereavement
V62.3	Academic Problem
V62.2	Occupational Problem
313.82	Identity Problem
V62.89	Religious or Spiritual Problem
V62.4	Acculturation Problem
V62.89	Phase of Life Problem

ADDITIONAL CODES

300.9	Unspecified Mental Disorder (nonpsychotic)
V71.09	No Diagnosis or Condition on Axis I
799.9	Diagnosis or Condition Deferred on Axis I
V71.09	No Diagnosis on Axis II
799.9	Diagnosis Deferred on Axis II

Multiaxial System

Axis I   Clinical Disorders
           Other Conditions That May Be a Focus of Clinical
           Attention
Axis II   Personality Disorders
           Mental Retardation
Axis III   General Medical Conditions
Axis IV   Psychosocial and Environmental Problems
Axis V   Global Assessment of Functioning

The diagnostic codes listed in the DSM-IV are derived from the *International Classification of Diseases*, Ninth Revision, Clinical Modification (ICD-9-CM), the official coding system for reporting morbidity and mortality in the USA. That is the reason why the codes go from 290.00 to 319.00; they are actually derived from the mental disorders section of a much larger coding system for all medical disorders that extends from 001 to 999. Clinicians working in the USA are required to use ICD-9-CM in order to receive reimbursement from both government agencies (e.g., Medicare and Medicaid) and private insurers.

Disorders Usually First Diagnosed in Infancy, Childhood, or Adolescence

The classification begins with disorders usually first diagnosed in infancy, childhood, or adolescence. The provision for a separate section for so-called childhood disorders is only for convenience. Although most individuals with these disorders present for clinical attention during childhood or adolescence, it is not uncommon for some of these conditions to be diagnosed for the first time in adulthood (e.g., attention-deficit/hyperactivity disorder). Moreover, many disorders included in other sections of the DSM-IV have an onset during childhood (e.g., major depressive disorder). Thus, a clinician evaluating a child or adolescent should not only focus on those disorders listed in this section but also consider disorders from throughout the DSM-IV. Similarly, when evaluating an adult, the clinician should also consider the disorders in this section since many of them persist into adulthood (e.g., stuttering, learning disorders, tic disorders).

The first set of disorders included in this diagnostic class (mental retardation, learning and motor skills disorders, and communication disorders). While they are not, strictly speaking, regarded as mental disorders, they are included in the DSM-IV-TR to facilitate differential diagnosis and to increase recognition of these conditions among mental health professionals. Autism and other pervasive developmental disorders are characterized by gross qualitative impairment in social relatedness, in language, and in repertoire of interests and activities. Disorders covered include autistic disorder, Asperger's disorder, Rett's disorder and childhood disintegrative disorder. Attention-deficit/hyperactivity disorder and other disruptive behavior disorders are grouped together because they are all characterized (at least in their childhood presentations) by disruptive behavior. The chapter on feeding disorders includes both the DSM-IV-TR categories of pica, rumination disorder and feeding disorder of infancy and early childhood (also known as "failure to thrive"), as well as several disorders that have been identified by researchers but are not currently included in the DSM-IV-TR (i.e., feeding disorder of state regulation, feeding

disorder of reciprocity, infantile anorexia, sensory food aversions and post traumatic feeding disorder). Tic disorders and elimination and other disorders of infancy and early childhood conclude the childhood disorders.

Delirium, Dementia, Amnestic Disorder and Other Cognitive Disorders

In the previous DSM-III-R, delirium, dementia, amnestic disorder and other cognitive disorders were included in a section called "organic mental disorders", which contained disorders that were due to either a general medical condition or substance use. In DSM-IV-TR, the term **organic** was eliminated because of the implication that disorders not included in that section (e.g., schizophrenia, bipolar disorder) did not have an organic component (Spitzer *et al.*, 1992). In fact, virtually all mental disorders have both psychological and biological components, and to designate some disorders as organic and the remaining disorders as nonorganic reflected a reductionistic mind–body dualism that is at odds with our understanding of the multifactorial nature of the etiological underpinnings of disorders.

DSM-IV-TR replaced each unitary organic mental disorder (e.g., organic mood disorder) with its two component parts: mood disorder due to a general medical condition and substance-induced mood disorder. Because of their central roles in the differential diagnosis of cognitive impairment, delirium, dementia and amnestic disorder are contained within the same diagnostic class in DSM-IV-TR.

Whereas both delirium and dementia are characterized by multiple cognitive impairments, delirium is distinguished by the presence of clouding of consciousness, which is manifested by an inability appropriately to maintain or shift attention. DSM-IV-TR includes three types of delirium: delirium due to a general medical condition, substance-induced delirium and delirium due to multiple etiologies.

Dementia is characterized by clinically significant cognitive impairment in memory that is accompanied by impairment in one or more other areas of cognitive functioning (e.g., language, executive functioning). DSM-IV-TR includes several types of dementia based on etiology, including dementia of the Alzheimer's type, vascular dementia, a variety of dementia due to general medical and neurological conditions (e.g., human immunodeficiency virus infection, Parkinson's disease), substance-induced persisting dementia and dementia due to multiple etiologies.

In contrast to dementia, amnestic disorder is characterized by clinically significant memory impairment occurring in the absence of other significant impairments in cognitive functioning. DSM-IV-TR includes amnestic disorder due to a general medical condition and substance-induced persisting amnestic disease.

Mental Disorders Due to a General Medical Condition Not Elsewhere Classified

This diagnostic class includes all of the specific mental disorders due to a general medical condition.. In DSM-IV-TR, most of the mental disorders due to a general medical condition have been distributed throughout the various diagnostic classes alongside their "nonorganic" counterparts in the classification. For example, mood disorder due to a general medical condition and substance-induced mood disorder are included in the mood disorders section of DSM-IV-TR. Two specific types of mental disorder due to a general medical condition (i.e., catatonic disorder due to a general medical condition and personality change due to a general medical condition) are physically included in this diagnostic class.

Substance-related Disorders

The term **substance** in DSM-IV has a broader meaning than merely a drug of abuse. It also includes medication side effects and the consequences of toxin exposure. Two types of substance-related disorders are included in DSM-IV-TR: substance use disorders (dependence and abuse), which describe the maladaptive nature of the pattern of substance use; and substance-induced disorders, which cover psychopathological processes caused by the direct effects of substances on the central nervous system. Criteria sets for substance dependence, substance abuse, substance intoxication and substance withdrawal that apply across all drug classes are included before the substance-specific sections of DSM-IV.

Schizophrenia and Other Psychotic Disorders

The title of this diagnostic class is potentially misleading for two reasons: 1) there are other disorders that have psychotic features that are not included in this diagnostic class (e.g., mood disorders with psychotic features, delirium) and 2) it may incorrectly imply that the other psychotic disorders included in this section are related in some way to schizophrenia (which is only true for schizophreniform disorder and possibly schizoaffective disorder). Instead, what ties together all of the disorders in this diagnostic class is the presence of prominent psychotic symptoms. Included here are schizophrenia, schizophreniform disorder, schizoaffective disorder, delusional disorder, shared psychotic disorder and brief psychotic disorder..

It should be noted that the definition of the term **psychosis** has been used in different ways historically and is not even used consistently across the various categories in the DSM-IV-TR. The most restrictive definition of psychosis (used in substance-induced psychotic disorder) requires a break in reality testing such that the person has delusions or hallucinations with no insight into the fact that the delusions or hallucinations are caused by taking drugs.

Mood Disorders

This diagnostic class includes disorders in which the predominant disturbance is in the individual's mood. Although the term **mood** is broadly defined to include depression, euphoria, anger and anxiety, the DSM-IV-TR generally restricts mood disturbances to depressed, elevated, or irritable mood.

The mood disorders section begins with the criteria for mood episodes (major depressive episode, manic episode, hypomanic episode, mixed episode), which are the building blocks for the episodic mood disorders. The codable mood disorders come next and are divided into the depressive disorders (i.e., major depressive disorder and dysthymic disorder, and the bipolar disorders (i.e., bipolar I disorder, bipolar II disorder and cyclothymic disorder). Finally, the many specifiers that provide important treatment-relevant information close this section. Several so-called "subthreshold mood disorders" (i.e., they are characterized by depression but fall short of meeting the diagnostic criteria for either major depressive disorder or dysthymic

disorder) are included in DSM-IV-TR appendix B, for Criteria Sets and Axes Provided for Further Study. These include minor depressive disorder, brief recurrent depressive disorder, mixed anxiety depressive disorder, postpsychotic depressive disorder of schizophrenia and premenstrual dysphoric disorder.

Anxiety Disorders

The common element joining these disparate categories together is the fact that the anxiety is a prominent part of their clinical presentation. This grouping has been criticized because of evidence suggesting that at least some of the disorders are likely to be etiologically distinct from the others. Most particularly, obsessive–compulsive disorder and post traumatic stress disorder seem to share little in common with the other anxiety disorders. In fact, separate diagnostic classes for stress-related disorders (that would also include adjustment disorders and perhaps dissociative disorders) and for obsessive–compulsive spectrum disorders (which might also include trichotillomania, tic disorders, hypochondriasis, body dysmorphic disorder and other disorders characterized by compulsive behavior) have been proposed.

Somatoform Disorders

This diagnostic class includes disorders in which the defining feature is a physical complaint or bodily concern that is not better accounted for by a general medical condition or another mental disorder. These disorders can be divided into three groups based on the focus of the individual's concerns: 1) focus on the physical symptoms themselves (somatization disorder, undifferentiated somatoform disorder, pain disorder and conversion disorder); 2) focus on the belief that one has a serious physical illness (hypochondriasis); and 3) focus on the belief that one has a defect in physical appearance (body dysmorphic disorder).

Factitious Disorders

This diagnostic class contains only one disorder: factitious disorder, which describes presentations in which the individual intentionally produces or feigns physical or psychological symptoms in order to fulfill a psychological need to assume the sick role. Factitious disorder should always be distinguished from malingering, in which the individual similarly pretends to have physical or psychological symptoms. The difference is that in malingering, the person's motivation is to achieve some external gain (e.g., disability benefits, lessening of criminal responsibility, shelter for the night). For this reason, unlike factitious disorder, malingering is not considered a mental disorder.

Dissociative Disorders

The common element to this group of disorders is the symptom of dissociation, which is defined as a disruption in the usually integrated functions of consciousness, memory, identity and perception. Four specific disorders are included: dissociative amnesia, dissociative fugue, dissociative identity disorder and depersonalization disorder.

Sexual and Gender Identity Disorders

This diagnostic class contains three relatively disparate types of disorders, linked together only by virtue of their involvement in human sexuality. Sexual dysfunctions refer to disturbances in sexual desire or functioning, paraphilias refer to unusual sexual preferences that interfere with functioning (or in the case of preferences that involve harm to others like pedophilia, merely acting on those preferences), and gender identity disorder refers to a serious conflict between one's internal identity of maleness and femaleness (gender identity) and one's anatomical sexual characteristics.

Eating Disorders

Although the name of this diagnostic class focuses on the fact that the disorders in this section are characterized by abnormal eating behavior (refusal to maintain adequate body weight in the case of anorexia nervosa and discrete episodes of uncontrolled eating of excessively large amounts of food in the case of bulimia nervosa), of near equal importance is the individual's pathological overemphasis on body image. A third category, which is being actively researched but has not been officially added to the DSM-IV-TR, is binge-eating disorder (included in the appendix of Criteria Sets and Axes Provided for Further Study). Like bulimia nervosa, individuals with binge-eating disorder have frequent episodes of binge-eating. However, unlike bulimia nervosa, these individuals do not do anything significant to counteract the effects of their binge-eating (i.e., they do not purge, use laxatives or diet pills, or excessively exercise).

Sleep Disorders

Sleep disorders are grouped into four sections on the basis of presumed etiology (primary, related to another mental disorder, due to a general medical condition, and substance-induced). Two types of primary sleep disorders are included in DSM-IV-TR: dyssomnias (problems in regulation of amount and quality of sleep) and parasomnias (events that occur during sleep). The dyssomnias include primary insomnia, primary hypersomnia, circadian rhythm sleep disorder, narcolepsy and breathing-related sleep disorder, whereas the parasomnias include nightmare disorder, sleep terror disorder and sleepwalking disorder.

Impulse Control Disorders Not Elsewhere Classified

As is suggested by the title of this diagnostic grouping, no one diagnostic class in DSM-IV comprehensively includes all of the impulse control disorders. A number of disorders characterized by impulse control problems are classified elsewhere (e.g., conduct disorder, attention-deficit/hyperactivity disorder, oppositional-defiant disorder, delirium, dementia, substance-related disorders, schizophrenia and other psychotic disorders, mood disorders, antisocial and borderline personality disorders). What ties together the disorders in this class is that they present with clinically significant impulsive behavior and that they are not better accounted for by one of the mental disorders included in other parts of DSM-IV-TR. Five such disorders are included here: intermittent explosive disorder, pathological gambling, pyromania, kleptomania and trichotillomania.

Adjustment Disorders

All DSM-IV categories (except NOS categories) take priority over adjustment disorder. This category is intended to apply to maladaptive reactions to psychosocial stressors that do not meet the criteria for any specific DSM-IV-TR disorder.

Personality Disorders

This diagnostic class is for personality patterns that significantly deviate from the expectations of the person's culture, are pervasive and lead to significant impairment or distress. Ten specific personality disorders are included in DSM-IV: paranoid personality disorder (pervasive distrust and suspiciousness of others), schizoid personality disorder (detachment from social relationships and a restricted expression of emotions), schizotypal personality disorder (acute discomfort with close relationships, perceptual distortions and eccentricities of behavior), antisocial personality disorder (disregard for the rights of others), borderline personality disorder (instability of personal relationships, instability of self-image and marked impulsivity), histrionic personality disorder (extensive emotionality and attention seeking), narcissistic personality disorder (grandiosity, need for admiration and lack of empathy), avoidant personality disorder (social inhibition, feelings of inadequacy and hypersensitivity to negative evaluation), dependent personality disorder (excessive need to be taken care of), and obsessive–compulsive personality disorder (preoccupation with orderliness, perfectionism, and mental and personal control at the expense of flexibility, openness and efficiency).

Other Conditions That May Be a Focus of Clinical Attention

This section of DSM-IV is for problems that are not mental disorders but that may be a focus of attention for treatment by a mental health professional. *Psychological factors affecting medical condition* is intended to allow the psychiatrist to note the presence of psychological factors (e.g., Axis I or II disorder) that adversely affect the course of a general medical condition, including factors that interfere with treatment and factors that constitute health risks to the individual. Six specific *medication-induced movement disorders* are also included because of their importance in treatment and differential diagnosis; five are related to neuroleptic administration and one (medication-induced postural tremor) is most often associated with the use of lithium carbonate. Although these are best considered medical conditions, by DSM-IV-TR convention they are coded on Axis I.

Relational problems include parent–child, partner and sibling relational problems. Relational problem related to a mental disorder or general medical condition applies to situations in which one member of the relational unit has a mental disorder or a general medical condition. In such situations, the relational dynamics can negatively affect the individual's condition or vice versa (or both). *Problems related to abuse or neglect* (physical abuse, sexual abuse and child neglect).

References

American Psychiatric Association (1952) *Diagnostic and Statistical Manual of Mental Disorders*. APA, Washington DC.

American Psychiatric Association (1968) *Diagnostic and Statistical Manual of Mental Disorders*, 2nd edn. APA, Washington DC.

American Psychiatric Association (1980) *Diagnostic and Statistical Manual of Mental Disorders*, 3rd edn. APA, Washington DC.

American Psychiatric Association (1987) *Diagnostic and Statistical Manual of Mental Disorders*, 3rd edn., Rev. APA, Washington DC.

American Psychiatric Association (1994) *Diagnostic and Statistical Manual of Mental Disorders*, 4th edn. APA, Washington DC.

American Psychiatric Association (1996) *Diagnostic and Statistical Manual of Mental Disorders*, 4th edn. Coding Update. APA, Washington DC.

American Psychiatric Association (2000) *Diagnostic and Statistical Manual of Mental Disorders*, 4th edn., Text Rev. APA, Washington DC.

Berrettini WH (2000) Are schizophrenic and bipolar disorders related? A review of family and molecular studies. *Biol Psychiatr* 48(6) (Sept 15), 531–538.

First MB and Pincus HA (2002) The DSM-IV Text Rev. Rationale and potential impact on clinical practice. *Psychiatr Serv* 53(3) (Mar), 288–292.

First MB, Frances A and Widiger TA (1992) DSM-IV and behavioral assessment. *Behav Assess* 14, 297–306.

First MB, Bell CC, Cuthbert B *et al.* (2002) Personality disorders and relational disorders: A research agenda for addressing crucial gaps in DSM, in *A Research agenda for DSM-V* (eds Kupfer DJ, First MB, and Regier DA). American Psychiatric Publishing, Washington DC, pp. 123–200.

Kendler KS (1996) Major depression and generalised anxiety disorder: Same genes, (partly) different environments—revisited. *Br J Psychiatr* 168(Suppl 30), 68–75.

Kendler KS and Gardner CO (1998) Boundaries of major depression: An evaluation of DSM-IV criteria. *Am J Psychiatr* 155, 172–177.

Kraepelin E (1883) *Compendium der Psychiatrie: Zum Gebrauche Adur Studirende und Aerzte.* Verlag von Ambr, Abel, Leipzig.

Spitzer RL, First MB, Williams JBW *et al.* (1992) Now is the time to retire the term "organic mental disorders." *Am J Psychiatr* 149, 240–244.

23 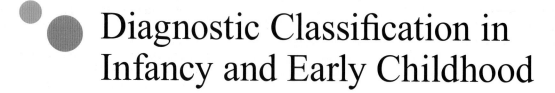 Diagnostic Classification in Infancy and Early Childhood

Knowledge about the mental health and development of infants has grown exponentially in the past two decades. Through systematic observation, research and clinical intervention a more sophisticated understanding has emerged of the factors that contribute to adaptive and maladaptive patterns of development and of the meaning of individual differences in infancy. This knowledge has led to an increasing awareness of the importance of prevention and early treatment in creating or restoring favorable conditions for the young child's development and mental health. Timely assessment and accurate diagnosis can provide the foundation for effective intervention before early deviations become consolidated into maladaptive patterns of functioning.

As a result of this growing knowledge base, a new diagnostic framework was formulated through an 8-year effort of ZERO TO THREE: National Center for Infants, Toddlers, and Families. This framework is presented in detail in *Diagnostic Classification of Mental Health and Developmental Disorders of Infancy and Early Childhood* (DC:0–3) (1994). It seeks to address the need for a systematic, developmentally based approach to the classification of mental health and developmental difficulties in the first 3 years of life. It is designed to complement existing medical and developmental frameworks for understanding mental health and developmental problems in the earliest years.

DC:0–3 categorizes emotional and behavioral patterns that represent significant deviations from normative development in the earliest years of life. Some of the categories presented represent new formulations of mental health and developmental difficulties. Other categories describe the earliest manifestations of mental health problems that have been identified among older children and adults but have not been fully described in infants and young children. In infancy and early childhood, these problems may have different characteristics, and prognosis may be more optimistic if effective early intervention can occur. This chapter summarizes the principles of assessment and diagnosis as well as the new diagnostic classifications for the first 3 years of life.

Discussions of diagnostic categories can be most helpful if they identify challenges to be overcome in the context of an understanding of adaptive coping and development. Understanding both adaptive capacities and challenges is part of the essential foundation for planning and implementing effective interventions. A detailed discussion of the principles of assessment, diagnosis and intervention, along with case studies, is presented in *Infancy and Early Childhood* (Greenspan, 1992).

Reflecting our current state of knowledge, the diagnostic categories presented in this chapter are descriptive, that is, they record presenting patterns of symptoms and behaviors. Some of the categories (e.g., those involving trauma) imply potential etiological factors; some (e.g., regulatory disorders) imply pathophysiological processes. However, at the moment, all that can be stated is that associations have been observed between some of these symptoms and processes (e.g., between a traumatic event and a group of symptoms, or between a sensory or motor pattern and a group of symptoms). Only further research will establish possible pathophysiological or etiological links among these observed phenomena.

As an evolving framework, this conceptualization is not intended to include all possible conditions or disorders. It is an initial guide for mental health professionals and researchers to facilitate clinical diagnosis and planning as well as communication and further research. It is not intended to have legal or nonclinical applications.

Principles of Assessment

Many different assumptions and theories contribute to our approach to diagnosis and treatment. These assumptions come from both clinical practice and research. Developmental, psychodynamic, family systems, relationship and attachment theory inform our work, as do observations of the way infants organize their experience, infant–caregiver interaction patterns, temperament, regulatory patterns and individual differences in many domains of development.

This chapter describes a new diagnostic classification for the first 4 years of life. It is meant to complement the *Diagnostic and Statistical Manual of Mental Disorders*, Fourth Edition (DSM-IV-TR). *Diagnostic Classification of Mental Health and Developmental Disorders of Infancy and Early Childhood*, published in 1994 by ZERO TO THREE/National Center for Clinical Infant Programs (now ZERO TO THREE: National Center for Infants, Toddlers, and Families, Washington DC), describes types of behaviors and problems not addressed in other schemas as well as the earliest manifestations of problems and behaviors that have heretofore been ascribed to older children. Because of the new system's comprehensive clinical and developmental approach, the authors have decided to include this overview, adapted from DC:0-3 with permission from ZERO TO THREE: National Center for Infants, Toddlers, and Families, here. More information about DC:0-3 is available from ZERO TO THREE: National Center for Infants, Toddlers, and Families, 734 15th Street, NW, 10th Floor, Washington DC 20005, Tel: 1-800-899-4301.

Essentials of Psychiatry   Jerald Kay and Allan Tasman
© 2006 John Wiley & Sons, Ltd.

We have formulated a model to characterize the different factors that must be taken into account and understood in an infant's, toddler's, or preschooler's functioning within the context of his family, community and world. We call this model the Developmental, Individual Difference, Relationship-based (DIR) model.

The DIR Model

The DIR model attempts to facilitate understanding of children and their family by identifying, systematizing and integrating the essential functional developmental capacities. These include the child's 1) functional–emotional developmental level; 2) the child's individual differences in sensory reactivity, processing and motor planning; and 3) the child's relationships and interactions with caregivers, family members and others.

Functional Developmental Capacities

Functional–Emotional Developmental Level

The child's functional–emotional developmental level examines how children integrate all their capacities (motor, cognitive, language, spatial, sensory) to carry out emotionally meaningful goals. The support for these functional–emotional developmental levels is reviewed elsewhere (Greenspan, 1979, 1989, 1992, 1997). These capacities include the ability to:

1. Attend to multisensory affective experience and, at the same time, organize a calm, regulated state (e.g., looking at, listening to, and following movement of a caregiver).
2. Engage with and evidence affective preference and pleasure for a caregiver or caregivers (e.g., joyful smiles and affection with a stable caregiver).
3. Initiate and respond to two-way presymbolic gestural communication (e.g., back-and-forth use of smiles and sounds).
4. Organize chains of two-way social problem-solving communications (opening and closing many circles of communication in a row), maintain communication across space, integrate affective polarities, and synthesize an emerging prepresentational organization of self and other (e.g., taking dad by the hand to reach a toy on the shelf).
5. Create and functionally use ideas as a basis for creative or imaginative thinking, giving meaning to symbols (e.g., pretend play, using words to meet needs, "Juice!").
6. Build bridges between ideas as a basis for logic, reality testing, thinking and judgment (e.g., engage in debates, opinion-oriented conversations and/or elaborate, planned pretend dramas).

Individual Differences in Sensory, Modulation, Processing and Motor Planning

These biologically-based individual differences are the result of genetic, prenatal perinatal and maturational variations and/or deficits and can be characterized in at least four ways:

1. Sensory modulation, including hypo- and hyperreactivity in each sensory modality, including touch, sound, smell, vision and movement in space;
2. Sensory processing in each sensory modality, including auditory processing and language and visual–spatial processing. Processing includes the capacity to register, decode, and comprehend sequences and abstract patterns);

3. Sensory–affective processing in each modality (e.g., the ability to process and react to affect, including the capacity to connect "intent" or affect to motor planning and sequencing, language and symbols). This processing capacity may be especially relevant for ASD (Greenspan and Wieder, 1997, 1998).
4. Motor planning and sequencing, including the capacity to sequence actions, behaviors and symbols, including symbols in the form of thoughts, words, visual images and spatial concepts.

Relationships and Interactions

Relationship and affective interaction patterns include developmentally appropriate, or inappropriate, interactive relationships with caregiver, parent and family patterns. Interaction patterns between the child and caregivers and family members bring the child's biology into the larger developmental progression and can contribute to the negotiation of the child's functional developmental capacities. Developmentally appropriate interactions mobilize the child's intentions and affects and enable the child to broaden his/her range of experience at each level of development and move from one functional developmental level to the next. In contrast, interactions that do not deal with the child's functional developmental level or individual differences can undermine progress. For example, a caregiver who is aloof may not be able to engage an infant who is underreactive and self-absorbed.

The DIR model examines the developmental capacities of the children in the context of their unique biologically-based processing profile and their family relationships and interactive patterns. As a functional approach, it uses the complex interactions between biology and experience to understand behavior. Implementation of an appropriate assessment of all the relevant functional areas requires a number of sessions with the child and family. These sessions must begin with discussions and observations.

The assessment process which is described in detail elsewhere (ZERO TO THREE, 1994; Greenspan and Wieder, 1997) includes: 1) two or more clinical observations, of 45 minutes each, of child–caregiver and/or clinician–child interactions; 2) developmental history and review of current functioning; 3) review of family and caregiver functioning; 4) review of current programs and patterns of interaction; 5) consultation with speech pathologists, occupational and physical therapists, educators and mental health colleagues, including the use of structured tests on an as-needed, rather than routine basis; and 6) biomedical evaluation.

The Functional Developmental Profile

The assessment then leads to an individualized functional profile which captures each child's unique developmental features and serves as a basis for creating individually-tailored intervention programs (i.e., tailoring the program to the child rather than fitting the child to a general program). The profile describes the child's functional developmental capacities and contributing biological processing differences and environmental interactive patterns, including the different interaction patterns available to the child at home, at school, with peers, and in other settings. The profile should include all areas of challenge, not simply the ones that are more obviously associated with symptoms of one or another syndrome or disease. For example, the preschooler's lack of ability to symbolize a broad range of emotional interests and themes in either pretend play or talk is just as important, if not more important, than that same preschooler's tendency to be perseverative or self-stimulatory. In fact, clinically we have often seen that as the child's range of symbolic expression broadens, perseverative and self-stimulatory tendencies decrease.

The functional approach to creating a profile enables the clinician to consider each functional challenge separately, explore different explanations for it, and resist the temptation to assume that difficulties are necessarily tied together as part of a syndrome (unless all alternative explanations have been ruled out). For example, hand flapping is often related to motor problems and is seen when children with a variety of motor problems become excited or overloaded. Many conditions, including cerebral palsy, autism, hypotonia and dyspraxia involve motor problems and, at times, hand flapping. Yet this symptom is often assumed to be uniquely a part of the autistic spectrum. Similarly, sensory over- or under-reactivity is present in many disorders and developmental variations. Yet it is also often assumed to be a unique part of autism. The functional approach does not detract from understanding existing syndromes. In fact, over time, it may clarify what symptoms are unique to particular syndromes, lead to new classifications, and further tease out biological and functional patterns.

Constructing the child's profile of functional capacities through appropriate clinical assessments enables the clinician to tailor the intervention program to the child's and family's unique features, rather than have the child fit the program, based on some broad, but nonspecific, diagnostic criteria.

As the DIR model suggests, any intervention or treatment program should be based on as complex an understanding of the child's and family's circumstances as is possible to achieve. It is the responsibility of any psychiatrist who is charged with doing a full diagnostic work-up and planning an appropriate intervention program to take into account **all** the relevant areas of a child's functioning, using state-of-the-art knowledge in each area. These areas include the following:

- Presenting symptoms and behaviors
- Developmental history: past and current affective, language, cognitive, motor, sensory, family and interactive functioning
- Family functioning and cultural and community patterns
- Parents as individuals
- Caregiver–infant (child) relationship and interactive patterns
- The infant's constitutional–maturational characteristics
- Affective, language, cognitive, motor and sensory patterns
- The family's psychosocial and medical history, the history of the pregnancy and delivery, and current environmental conditions and stressors

The process of gaining an understanding of how each area of functioning is developing for an infant or toddler usually requires a number of sessions. A few questions to the parents or caregiver about each area may be appropriate for screening but not for a full evaluation. A full evaluation usually requires a minimum of three to five sessions of 45 minutes or more each. A complete evaluation will usually involve taking the history; direct observation of functioning (i.e., of family and parental dynamics; caregiver–infant relationship and interaction patterns; the infant's constitutional–maturational characteristics; and language, cognitive and affective patterns); and hands-on interaction assessment of the infant, including assessment of sensory reactivity and processing, motor tone and planning, language, cognition and affective expression. Standardized developmental assessments, if needed, should always build on the clinical process described. They may be indicated when they are the most effective way to answer specific questions and when the child is sufficiently interactive and can respond to the requirements of the test.

The result of such a comprehensive evaluation should lead to preliminary notions about the following:

1. The nature of the infant's or child's difficulties as well as her or his strengths; the level of the child's overall adaptive capacity; and functioning in the major areas of development, including social–emotional relationships and cognitive, language, sensory and motor abilities in comparison to age-expected developmental patterns.
2. The relative contribution of the different areas assessed (e.g., family relationships, interactive patterns, constitutional–maturational patterns, stress) to the child's difficulties and competencies.
3. A comprehensive treatment or preventive intervention plan to deal with 1 and 2.

Overview of the Classification System

DC:0–3 proposes a provisional multiaxial classification system. We refer to the classification system as provisional because it is assumed that categories may change as more knowledge accumulates. The diagnostic framework consists of the following:

Axis I   Primary diagnosis
Axis II   Relationship disorder classification
Axis III   Physical, neurological, developmental, and mental health disorders or conditions (described in other classification systems)
Axis IV   Psychosocial stressors
Axis V   Functional–emotional developmental level

The axes in this system are not intended to be entirely symmetrical with such other systems as DSM-IV and the *International Statistical Classification of Diseases and Related Health Problems*, 10th Revision (ICD-10) because this system, in dealing with infants and young children, focuses on developmental issues. Dynamic processes, such as relationship and developmentally based conceptualizations of adaptive patterns (i.e., functional–emotional developmental level), are therefore of central importance.

Use of the system will provide the psychiatrist with a "diagnostic profile" of an infant or toddler. Such a diagnostic profile focuses the psychiatrist's attention on the various factors that are contributing to the infant's difficulties as well as on areas in which intervention may be needed.

Axis I: Primary Diagnoses

The following are the Axis I primary diagnoses that have thus far been suggested:

---

100. Traumatic Stress Disorder

A continuum of symptoms related to a single event, a series of connected traumatic events, or chronic enduring stress.

1. Reexperiencing of the trauma, as evidenced by
   a. post traumatic play
   b. recurrent recollections of the traumatic event outside play
   c. repeated nightmares

d. distress at reminders of the trauma

e. flashbacks or dissociation

2. Numbing of responsiveness or interference with developmental momentum

   a. increased social withdrawal

   b. restricted range of affect

   c. temporary loss of previously acquired developmental skills

   d. a decrease in play

3. Symptoms of increased arousal

   a. night terrors

   b. difficulty going to sleep

   c. repeated night waking

   d. significant attentional difficulties

   e. hypervigilance

   f. exaggerated startle response

4. Symptoms not present before

   a. aggression toward peers, adults, or animals

   b. separation anxiety

   c. fear of toileting alone

   d. fear of the dark

   e. other new fears

   f. self-defeating behavior or masochistic provocativeness

   g. sexual and aggressive behaviors

   h. other nonverbal reactions (e.g., somatic symptoms, motor reenactment, skin stigmas, pain, or posturing)

200. Disorders of Affect

Focuses on the infant's experience and on symptoms that are a general feature of the child's functioning rather than specific to a situation or relationship.

201. Anxiety Disorders of Infancy and Early Childhood

Levels of anxiety or fear, beyond expectable reactions to normal developmental challenges.

1. Multiple or specific fears

2. Excessive separation or stranger anxiety

3. Excessive anxiety or panic without clear precipitant

4. Excessive inhibition or constriction of behavior

5. Lack of development of basic ego functions

6. Agitation, uncontrollable crying or screaming, sleeping and eating disturbances, recklessness, and other behaviors

Criterion: Should persist for at least 2 weeks and interfere with appropriate functioning.

202. Mood Disorder: Prolonged Bereavement–Grief Reaction

1. Possible crying, calling and searching for the absent parent, refusing comfort

2. Emotional withdrawal, with lethargy, sad facial expression, and lack of interest in age-appropriate activities

3. Eating and sleeping possibly disrupted

4. Regression in developmental milestones

5. Constricted affective range

6. Detachment

7. Sensitivity to any reminder of the caregiver

203. Mood Disorder: Depression of Infancy and Early Childhood

Pattern of depressed or irritable mood with diminished interest or pleasure in developmentally appropriate activities, diminished capacity to protest, excessive whining, and diminished social interactions and initiative. Disturbances in sleep or eating.

Criterion: At least 2 weeks.

204. Mixed Disorder of Emotional Expressiveness

Ongoing difficulty expressing developmentally appropriate emotions.

1. The absence or near-absence of one or more specific types of affects

2. Constricted range of emotional expression

3. Disturbed intensity

4. Reversal of affect or inappropriate affect

205. Childhood Gender Identity Disorder

Becomes manifest during the sensitive period of gender identity development (between approximately 2 and 4 years).

1. A strong and persistent cross-sex identification

   a. repeatedly states desire to be, or insistence that he or she is, the opposite sex

   b. in boys, preference for cross-dressing or simulating female attire; in girls, insistence on wearing stereotypical masculine clothing

   c. strong and persistent preferences for cross-sex roles in fantasy play or persistent fantasies of being the opposite sex

   d. intense desire to participate in the games and pastimes of the opposite sex

   e. strong preference for playmates of the opposite sex

4. Persistent discomfort with one's assigned sex or sense of inappropriateness in that role

5. Absence of nonpsychiatric medical condition

206. Reactive Attachment Deprivation–Maltreatment Disorder of Infancy

1. Persistent parental neglect or abuse, of a physical or psychological nature, undermines the child's basic sense of security and attachment.

2. Frequent changes in, or the inconsistent availability of, the primary caregiver.

3. Other environmental compromises that prevent stable attachments.

300. Adjustment Disorder

Mild, transient situational disturbances related to a clear environmental event and lasting no longer than 4 months.

400. Regulatory Disorders

Difficulties in regulating physiological, sensory, attentional, motor, or affective processes and in organizing a calm, alert, or affectively positive state. Observe at least one sensory, sensory–motor, or processing difficulty from the following list, in addition to behavioral symptoms.

1. Overreactivity or underreactivity to loud or high- or low-pitched noises

2. Overreactivity or underreactivity to bright lights or new and striking visual images

3. Tactile defensiveness or oral hypersensitivity

4. Oral–motor difficulties or incoordination influenced by poor muscle tone and oral-tactile hypersensitivity

5. Underreactivity to touch or pain

6. Gravitational insecurity
7. Underreactivity or overreactivity to odors
8. Underreactivity or overreactivity to temperature
9. Poor muscle tone and muscle stability
10. Qualitative deficits in motor planning skills
11. Qualitative deficits in ability to modulate motor activity
12. Qualitative deficits in fine motor skills
13. Qualitative deficits in auditory–verbal processing
14. Qualitative deficits in articulation capacities
15. Qualitative deficits in visual–spatial processing capacities
16. Qualitative deficits in capacity to attend and focus

401. Type I: Hypersensitive

- Fearful and cautious
  - Behavioral patterns: excessive cautiousness, inhibition, or fearfulness
  - Motor and sensory patterns: overreactivity to touch, loud noises, or bright lights
- Negative and defiant
  - Behavioral patterns: negativistic, stubborn, controlling and defiant; difficulty in making transitions; prefers repetition to change
  - Motor and sensory patterns: overreactivity to touch and sound; intact visual–spatial capacities; compromised auditory processing capacity; good muscle tone and motor planning ability; shows some delay in fine motor coordination

402. Type II: Underreactive

- Withdrawn and difficult to engage
  - Behavioral patterns: seeming disinterest in relationships; limited exploratory activity or flexibility in play; appears apathetic, easily exhausted and withdrawn
  - Motor and sensory patterns: underreactivity to sounds and movement in space; either overreactive or underreactive to touch; intact visual–spatial processing capacities, but auditory–verbal processing difficulties; poor motor quality and motor planning
- Self-absorbed
  - Behavioral patterns: creative and imaginative, with a tendency to tune into her or his own sensations, thoughts, and emotions
  - Motor and sensory patterns: decreased auditory–verbal processing capacities

403. Type III: Motorically Disorganized, Impulsive

Mixed sensory reactivity and motor processing difficulties. Some appear more aggressive, fearless and destructive; others appear more impulsive and fearful.
- Behavioral patterns: high activity, seeking contact and stimulation through deep pressure; appears to lack caution
- Motor and sensory patterns: sensory underreactivity and motor discharge

404. Type IV: Other

500. Sleep Behavior Disorder

Only presenting problem; younger than 3 years of age; no accompanying sensory reactivity or sensory processing difficulties. Difficulty in initiating or maintaining sleep; may also have problems in calming themselves and dealing with transitions from one stage of arousal to another.

600. Eating Behavior Disorder

Shows difficulties in establishing regular feeding patterns with adequate or appropriate food intake. Absence of general regulatory difficulties or interpersonal precipitants (e.g., separation, negativism, trauma).

700. Disorders of Relating and Communicating

1. DSM-IV conceptualization pervasive developmental disorder, or
2. Multisystem developmental disorder

Multisystem Developmental Disorder

1. Significant impairment in, but not complete lack of, the ability to form and maintain an emotional and social relationship with primary caregiver
2. Significant impairment in forming, maintaining, or developing communication
3. Significant dysfunction in auditory processing
4. Significant dysfunction in the processing of other sensations and in motor planning

701. Pattern A

These children are aimless and unrelated most of the time, with severe difficulty in motor planning, so that even simple intentional gestures are difficult.

702. Pattern B

These children are intermittently related and capable, some of the time, of simple intentional gestures.

703. Pattern C

These children evidence a more consistent sense of relatedness, even when they are avoidant or rigid.

Axis II: Relationship Disorder Classification

The diagnostic system also includes an Axis II for relationships classification. Three aspects of a relationship are considered: 1) behavioral quality of the interaction, 2) affective tone, and 3) psychological involvement. The types of relationship problems are as follows:

901. Overinvolved Relationship

Physical or psychological overinvolvement.
1. Parent interferes with infant's goals and desires
2. Overcontrols
3. Makes developmentally inappropriate demands
4. Infant appears diffuse, unfocused and undifferentiated
5. Displays submissive, overly compliant behaviors
6. May lack motor skills or language expressiveness

902. Underinvolved Relationship

Sporadic or infrequent genuine involvement.
1. Parent insensitive or unresponsive
2. Lack of consistency between expressed attitudes about infant and quality of actual interactions
3. Ignores, rejects, or fails to comfort
4. Does not reflect infant's internal feeling states
5. Does not adequately protect
6. Interactions underregulated
7. Parent and infant appear to be disengaged
8. Infant appears physically or psychologically uncared for
9. Delayed or precocious in motor and language skills

903. Anxious–Tense Relationship

Tense, constricted with little sense of relaxed enjoyment or mutuality.
1. Parent is overprotective and oversensitive
2. Awkward or tense handling
3. Some verbally and emotionally negative interactions
4. Poor temperamental fit between parent and child
5. Infant compliant or anxious

904. Angry–Hostile Relationship

Harsh and abrupt, often lacking in emotional reciprocity.
1. Parent insensitive to infant's cues
2. Handling is abrupt
3. Infant frightened, anxious, inhibited, impulsive, or diffusely aggressive
4. Defiant or resistant behavior
5. Demanding or aggressive behaviors
6. Fearful, vigilant and avoidant behaviors
7. Tendency toward concrete behavior

905. Mixed Relationship

Combination of the features described above.

906. Abusive Relationships

1. Verbally abusive relationship.
   a. Intended to severely belittle, blame, attack, overcontrol and reject the infant or toddler
   b. Reactions vary from constriction and vigilance to severe acting-out behaviors
2. Physically abusive relationship.
   a. Physically harms by slapping, spanking, hitting, pinching, biting, kicking, physical restraint, isolation
   b. Denies food, medical care, or opportunity to rest
   c. May include verbal and emotional abuse or sexual abuse
3. Sexually abusive relationship.
   a. Parent engages in sexually seductive and overstimulating behavior – coercing or forcing child to touch parent sexually, accept sexual touching, or observe others' sexual behaviors
   b. Young child may evidence sexually driven behaviors such as exhibiting himself or herself or trying to look at or touch other children
   c. May include verbal and emotional abuse or physical abuse

Axis III: Medical and Developmental Diagnoses

On Axis III, one indicates any coexisting physical (including medical and neurological), mental health, or developmental disorders. DSM-IV, ICD-9 or ICD-10 for the primary care setting classifications are used. Occupational therapy, physical therapy, special education and other designations are specified.

Axis IV: Psychosocial Stressors

On Axis IV, one identifies (1) the source of stress (e.g., abduction, adoption, loss of parent, natural disaster, parent's illness), (2) severity (mild to catastrophic), (3) duration (acute to enduring), and (4) overall impact (none, mild, moderate, severe).

Overall Impact of Stress	
Mild effects	Causes recognizable strain, tension, or anxiety but does not interfere with infant's overall adaptation
Moderate effects	Derails child in areas of adaptation but not in core areas of relatedness and communication
Severe effects	Significant derailment in areas of adaptation

Axis V: Functional–Emotional Developmental Level

Axis V profiles the child's functional and emotional developmental level. It involves the following:

A. Essential processes or capacities
   1. Mutual attention: ability of dyad to attend to one another
   2. Mutual engagement: joint emotional involvement
   3. Interactive intentionality and reciprocity: ability for cause-and-effect interaction; infant signals and responds purposefully
   4. Representational–affective communication: language and play communicate emotional themes
   5. Representational elaboration: pretend play and symbolic communication that go beyond basic needs and deal with more complex intentions, wishes, or feelings
   6. Representational differentiation I: pretend play and symbolic communication in which ideas are logically related; knows what is real and unreal
   7. Representational differentiation II: complex pretend play; three or more ideas are logically connected and informed by concepts of causality, time and space
B. Functional–Emotional Developmental Level Summary, which documents the child's achievement
   1. Has fully reached expected levels
   2. At expected level but with constrictions – not full range of affect; not at this level under stress; only with certain caregivers or with exceptional support
   3. Not at expected level but has achieved all prior levels
   4. Not at current expected level but some prior levels
   5. Has not mastered any prior levels

Conclusion

We have briefly reviewed the principles of assessment and diagnosis and outlined the new diagnostic classification system for infants, young children and their families. The field of clinical work with infants and young children is a relatively new one. It has strong empirical support in the numerous studies of both normal and disturbed development and the rapidly expanding experience with a variety of clinical cases. As more experience is accumulated, the classification of challenges and difficulties will be refined and additional clinical strategies developed.

References

Greenspan SI (1979) Intelligence and adaptation: An integration of psychoanalytic and Piagetian developmental psychology. *Psychological Issues* (Monograph No. 47–48). International Universities Press, New York.

Greenspan SI (1989) *The Development of the Ego: Implications for personality theory, psychopathology, and the psychotherapeutic process.* International Universities Press, New York.

Greenspan SI (1992) *Infancy and Early Childhood: The Practice of Clinical Assessment and Intervention with Emotional and Developmental Challenges.* International Universities Press, Madison, CT.

Greenspan SI (1997) *The Growth of the Mind and the Endangered origins of Intelligence.* Addison Wesley Longman, Reading, MA.

Greenspan SI and Wieder S (1997) Developmental patterns and outcomes in infants and children with disorders in relating and communicating: A chart review of 200 cases of children with autistic spectrum diagnoses. *J Dev Learn Dis* 1, 87–141.

Greenspan SI and Wieder S (1998) *The Child with Special Needs: Encouraging Intellectual and Emotional Growth.* Perseus Books, Reading, MA.

ZERO TO THREE Diagnostic Classification Task Force, Greenspan SI (chair), Weider S (cochair and clinical director) (1994) *Diagnostic Classification of Mental Health and Developmental Disorders of Infancy and Early Childhood.* ZERO TO THREE/National Center for Clinical Infant Programs, Arlington, VA.

Childhood Disorders: Mental Retardation

Concept of Mental Retardation

Following are the basic concepts of mental retardation and the psychiatric approaches to it, on which this chapter is based:

1. Mental retardation is not a single, specific disorder. The term refers to a behavioral syndrome, describing the level of a person's functioning in defined domains. It does not have a single cause, mechanism, course, or prognosis and does not necessarily last a lifetime.
2. Mental retardation is not a unitary concept. Persons diagnosed as having mental retardation do not constitute a homogeneous group but represent a wide spectrum of abilities, clinical presentations and behavioral patterns.
3. Persons with mental retardation do not have unique personalities or behavioral patterns that are specific to mental retardation, although certain patterns may be frequently seen in certain mental retardation-associated syndromes.
4. Maladaptive behaviors should not automatically be seen as part of the retardation or an expression of "organicity". As in all individuals, these behaviors may be related to life experiences; they can also be a symptom of mental illness comorbid with the mental retardation.
5. Mental disorders seen in persons with mental retardation are the same as those in the general population.

Some common misconceptions about mental retardation are that it is a specific and lifelong disorder with unique personality pattern, and that comorbid mental disorders existing with mental retardation are different from those encountered in other individuals. Although mental retardation is listed as a mental disorder in the *Diagnostic and Statistical Manual of Mental Disorders*, Fourth Edition, Text Revision (DSM-IV-TR) (American Psychiatric Association, 2000), it is not a unique nosological entity. Instead, diagnosis of mental retardation refers to the level of a person's intellectual and adaptive functioning below a cutoff point that is not even natural but is arbitrarily chosen in relation to the average level of functioning of the population at large. Its chief function is administrative, defining a group of persons who are in need of support and educational services. Thus, mental retardation does not have a single cause, mechanism, course, or prognosis. It has to be differentiated from the diagnosis (if known) of the underlying medical condition.

Epidemiology of Mental Retardation

Prevalence

The results of epidemiological studies of mental retardation depend on two major factors: the definition of mental retardation that is used and how the results are ascertained. There have been various models for estimating the prevalence of mental retardation. A model based on IQ score alone used the expected statistical distribution of intelligence levels. The past definition based only on an IQ that was one standard deviation or greater below the mean implied that almost 15% of the population could be classified as having mental retardation. With the introduction of the diagnostic criterion of impairment in adaptive behavior and an IQ cutoff at two standard deviations below the mean (approximately 70), the prevalence of mental retardation was commonly thought to be 3% of the population. More recent population-based studies, using multiple methods of ascertainment and a current definition of mental retardation, suggest that the prevalence might be closer to 1%. In the study of McLaren and Bryson (1987), the prevalence of mild mental retardation was 0.37 to 0.59%, whereas the prevalence of moderate, severe and profound retardation was 0.3 to 0.4%. When age is considered, the highest prevalence is in the school-age group, when the child cannot meet the expectations of academic learning. United States Department of Education indicated the prevalence of mental retardation among school-age children (6–17 years of age) to be 1.14%, with variations reported by different states (Massey and McDermott, 1995). Conversely, some persons who are diagnosed with mild mental retardation when of school age lose that diagnosis in adulthood when their good adaptive skills are more relevant than their academic achievement.

Etiology and Pathophysiology of Mental Retardation

General Considerations

Intellectual abilities depend to a great degree on the integrity of the CNS. A variety of biomedical causes can disrupt this integrity and start the process leading to mental retardation. It should be kept in mind, however, that the term mental retardation describes the overall level of functioning, encompassing current intellectual and adaptive skills. These, in turn, are shaped by other factors besides CNS integrity, such as the patient's general state of health and associated disabilities, environmental factors (such as nurturing, learning opportunities, supports) and psychological factors (such as the person's self-image, psychopathological characteristics, motivation). Thus, a biomedical cause, whether genetic or acquired, may be a primary cause that will start the process of developmental delay but will not necessarily be the only factor responsible for the functional outcome, which will depend on the synergistic or cumulative effects of all factors involved. It is important to know as much as possible about the "primary" cause for a number of reasons:

Treatment possibilities can include early institution of diet in phenylketonuria (PKU) and thyroid hormone supplementation in congenital hypothyroidism. Primary prevention of the recurrence of the same condition using, for example, parental education to prevent fetal alcohol syndrome and enable genetic counseling for the family. Early recognition and treatment of complications known to be associated with the particular mental retardation syndrome, such as hypothyroidism in Down syndrome. Research on causation and prevention Assessment of epidemiology, which is important in public policy (planning for services) as well as in prevention Understanding of prognosis in association with a particular disorder Support for the family and other caregivers by dispelling misconceptions and anxieties related to uncertainty about the cause

- Treatment possibilities, which can include early institution of diet in phenylketonuria (PKU) and thyroid hormone supplementation in congenital hypothyroidism.

- Prevention, such as primary prevention of the recurrence of the same condition using, for example, parental education to prevent fetal alcohol syndrome and enabling genetic counseling for the family.
- Early recognition and treatment of complications known to be associated with the particular mental retardation syndrome, such as hypothyroidism in Down syndrome.
- Research on causation and prevention.
- Assessment of epidemiology, which is important in public policy (planning for services) as well as in prevention.
- Understanding of prognosis in association with a particular disorder.
- Support for the family and other caregivers by dispelling misconceptions and anxieties related to uncertainty about the cause.

Approaches to Classification of the Causation of Mental Retardation

The prevalence of diagnosable (using current techniques) biomedical causes of mental retardation varies with the degree of the disability. When the retardation is severe, a prenatal cause can be identified in 59 to 73% of patients, but in mild mental retardation such a cause can be identified in only 23 to 43% of patients.

Table 24.1 illustrates the most commonly employed classification system of the etiology of mental retardation. It reflects

Table 24.1   Etiological Classification of Mental Retardation Based on the Timing and Type of the Central Nervous System Insult*†

Division and Group	Percent	Examples
Prenatal: Genetic Disorders	32	
Chromosomal aberrations		Trisomy 21, trisomy 13m cri du chat syndromes
Malformations due to microdeletions		Angelman's and Prader–Willi syndromes, William's syndrome, Rubinstein–Taybi syndrome
Monogenic mutations		Tuberous sclerosis, metabolic disorders, fragile X syndrome
Multifactorial mental retardation		"Familial" mental retardation
Malformations, Cause Unknown	8	
Malformations of the CNS		Holoprosencephaly, lissencephaly, neural tube defects
Multiple malformation syndromes		de Lange's syndrome, Sotos' syndrome
Prenatal: Disorders due to External Causes	12	
Maternal infections		Rubella and HIV, cytomegalovirus and *Toxoplasma* infections
Toxins		Fetal alcohol syndrome, fetal hydantoin syndrome
Toxemia, placental insufficiency		IUGR, prematurity
Other		Radiation, trauma
Perinatal Causes	11	
Infections		Meningitis, herpes
Delivery problems		Asphyxia, trauma
Other		Hypoglycemia, hyperbilirubinemia
Postnatal Causes	8	
Infections		Meningitis, encephalitis
Toxins		Lead poisoning
Other CNS disorders		Cerebrovascular accidents, tumors, traumas
Psychosocial problems		
Unknown Causes	25	

*These data are based on the Finnish National Board of Social Welfare registry of persons, with mental retardation, who were receiving special services in the 1980s. There were about 19 000 persons in that registry. In about 4%, no etiological information was recorded (unpublished data).
†CNS, central nervous system; HIV, human immunodeficiency virus; IUGR, intrauterine growth retardation.

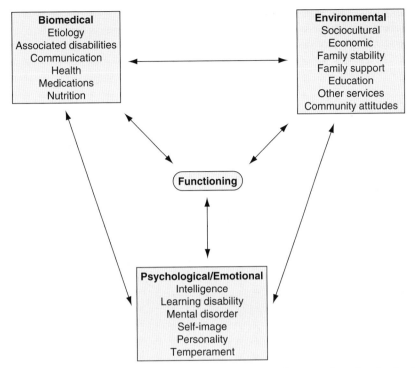

Figure 24.1 *Schematic representation of transactional relationship of various factors influencing the development of adaptive and maladaptive behaviors in persons with mental retardation.*

both the timing and the type of the causative process which will affect the development and function of the CNS (Wilska and Kaski, 1999). The goal of the etiological assessment is to elucidate the earliest developmental cause as well as other coexisting causative factors because their effects are usually interactive and cumulative (McLaren and Bryson, 1987)

Phenomenology and Variations in Presentation

The clinical presentation of persons with mental retardation is influenced by multiple factors, which can be grossly divided into biological (such as syndromes underlying the retardation), psychological (the level of the person's intellectual and adaptive functioning), and environmental (such as cultural expectations and services received). Their mutual relationship is illustrated in Figure 24.1.

The more severe the mental retardation, the earlier the child will come to medical attention because the developmental delay will be obvious earlier, and associated physical impairments will be more prevalent. Conversely, children with mild mental retardation may not be diagnosed until they reach school age, when they fail in academic learning. If the sociocultural environment does not value and stress early academic learning and early education is not available, mild mental retardation might go undetected, especially if the person has relatively good adaptive skills. A false-positive diagnosis of mental retardation can also occur, especially if psychological tests are not sensitive to cultural background, and there is a language barrier between the child and the tester.

The importance of the earliest diagnosis possible cannot be overstated because the prognosis will be much better if the intervention which results from the diagnostic knowledge is begun as early as possible.

Assessment of Mental Retardation

American Association on Mental Retardation's Classification of Mental Retardation

The American Association on Mental Retardation has published in 2002 a new edition of its manual *Mental Retardation: Definition, Classification and Systems of Supports.* Several dimensions of mental retardation are described, which might also serve as an outline for its assessment:.

Dimension I: Intellectual abilities
Dimension II: Adaptive behavior (Conceptual, social and practical skills)
Dimension III: Participation, interactions and social roles.
Dimension IV: Health (physical health, mental health, etiological factors).
Dimension V: Context (environments and culture).

This is a comprehensive description of the person's current environment: its nature, strengths, and weaknesses, supports for person's development and well-being (including factors such as poverty, family and its attitudes, availability of education and other services).

In all aspects of the assessment, attention should be paid both to the strengths as well as to the weaknesses and the impairments.

Biomedical Etiological Assessment of Mental Retardation

Mental retardation associated with syndromes and disorders with obvious phenotypical features is usually recognized earliest, such as in the case of Down syndrome. The diagnosis is then confirmed by chromosomal or other appropriate laboratory studies. If there was a suspicion of a family's risk for a genetic disorder before the birth (such as through prior genetic counseling), appropriate studies are performed in the neonatal period. Some cases of congenital mental retardation (e.g., PKU) are discovered in the course of routine neonatal screening. Newborns with perinatal risk factors like prematurity and asphyxia should be followed up closely for later manifestations of developmental delay. Other children might come to medical attention because of a delay in achieving developmental milestones or regression in a previously normal developmental pattern. Finally, many children with mental retardation will be referred for diagnostic assessment when they reach school age because of failure in academic learning.

Elements of Biomedical Assessment

The scheme for assessing the etiology of mental retardation is summarized in Figure 24.2. This work-up has been used by Finnish physicians for 20 years (Wilska and Kaski, 1999).

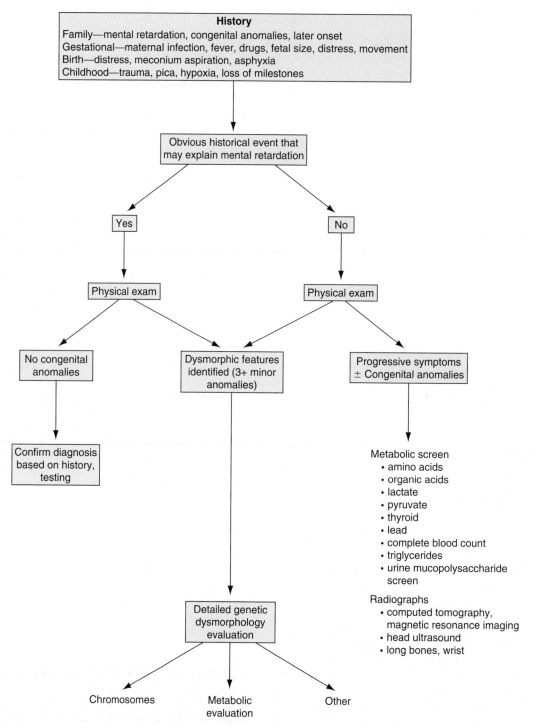

Figure 24.2 *Diagnostic approach to mental retardation of all ages. (Source: Szymanski LS and Kaplan [1991] Mental retardation. Reprinted with permission from the Text book of Child and Adolescent Psychiatry, p. 157. Weiner JM (ed). Copyright 1991, American Psychiatric Press.)*

Overall Goals of Treatment of Mental Retardation

Mental retardation is a functional disability: thus, the goal of treatment should be to reduce or eliminate the disability. There are three aspects to the treatment:

1. Treatment of the underlying disorder that is causative of mental retardation (e.g., phenylketonuria – PKU).
2. Treatment of the comorbid disorders that add to the functional disability, whether physical or mental.
3. Interventions targeted at the functional disability of the mental retardation itself: educational, habilitative and supportive approaches depending on the person's individualized needs.

The current approach to the services for persons with mental retardation is based on the following principles:

1. Inclusion into normal aspects of society and opportunities for success
2. Right to community living
3. Education and training for all children
4. Employment of adults in the community
5. Use of normal community services and facilities
6. Advocacy and appropriate protective measures.

Variations in Presentation

There is no evidence that mental disorders seen in persons who have mental retardation are basically different from mental disorders seen in the general population. However, the clinical manifestations may be modified by many factors that include: cognitive impairment; communication skills; associated sensory, motor, and other disabilities; environment; life experiences and circumstances. The most important of these factors is the presence or absence of verbal language. This is to be expected since many if not most of current diagnostic criteria of mental disorders are based on a patient's verbal productions. For instance, it might be impossible to recognize the presence of thought disorder in a nonverbal person (similar problems are encountered with young children).

Behavior Disorders

A common reason for referral for psychiatric consultation is to determine whether a person with mental retardation has "a behavior disorder or a mental disorder". The DSM-IV does not have the diagnostic category of "behavior disorder", although it is included in the ICD-10 (World Health Organization, 1992).

Although there is no clear definition of "behavior disorder", it is usually meant to refer to a behavioral problem that is severe enough to warrant intervention, but which is not a part of diagnosable mental disorder. It is often applied to a deliberate misbehavior, learned response and "attention-getting" behavior. However, in the clinical presentation of every defined mental disorder, there might be elements of learned behavior, for example, caused by the responses of persons in the patient's environment. The danger of such ill-defined, nonspecific category is that clinicians faced with a difficult case might be tempted to use it, rather than attempt to make a more specific diagnosis that might lead to a more focused treatment. Thus, it is preferable to avoid dichotomizing abnormal behaviors into "behavior" and "mental" disorders, but rather to try to decide to which mental disorder the behavioral manifestations form a part (Szymanski,

1994). Possibly "behavior disorder" could be employed to denote a maladaptive behavior that is clearly a function of situation and environment, and not primarily the individual. A commonly seen example might be an individual living in a large residential institution who, in a well-staffed workshop, is very cooperative, happy and hardworking, but becomes irritable, negativistic, even aggressive in the afternoon, when he returns to the overcrowded and understaffed ward where he lives. A maladaptive behavior may also serve as a form of communication if the person has poor language skills or when the carers do not respond to other attempts to communicate. In any case, it is essential that a comprehensive psychiatric diagnostic assessment be made to ensure that the behavior in question is not a part of a diagnosable mental disorder.

Assessment

Special Issues in the Psychiatric Assessment of Persons with Mental Retardation

The basic principles of the psychiatric diagnostic assessment of persons who have mental retardation are the same as those for persons who do not have mental retardation. However, the clinical approaches may have to be modified. The scope of the assessment might have to take into account multiple needs and problems and, in addition, these individuals depend on multiple providers for multiple services. The clinical techniques have to be modified according to the patient's discrete developmental levels in various domains, and in particular, communication skills (Szymanski, 1980). In accordance with the principle of biopsychosocial integration, all factors and their mutual interaction and contribution to the patient's problems and general functioning must be considered. Thus, the presenting problems must be assessed in the comprehensive context of a patient's abilities and disabilities and not as an isolated issue (Szymanski and Crocker, 1989).

Approaches to Obtaining a History

All involved caregivers should be interviewed if possible (parents, teachers, direct care workers, supervisors in workshops). Direct care staff members (e.g., from the group home and workshop supervisors) are particularly important because they can provide a firsthand description of a person's behavior. Exploring the following areas is important.

> Reasons for Current Referral
> Behavioral Symptoms
> Medication History
> General History
> Nature of the Disability
> Medical History
> Past and Current Services
> Milieu Events
> The Family

Approaches to the Patient's Interview

The way in which the patient's interview is approached will depend on the patient's communication skills and cooperation and might range from an age-appropriate verbal interview to observation only. The communication skills have to be explored first through brief, noncommittal conversation and questioning of the caregivers. If necessary, the caregivers might be used as interpreters of the patient's poorly intelligible speech or sign language. Directiveness and structure are often necessary to help the patient focus, but leading questions or suppression of spontaneous expression must be avoided. While firm and clear behavioral limits may have to be established at the interview's onset if necessary, a great deal of support is needed. Noncondescending verbal and social reinforcement, as appropriate for developmental age, will let the patient know that the interviewer is appreciative of her or his abilities. The patients should be approached respectfully – if possible, in a manner appropriate to the chronological age – and not as children. However, communication with them should be on the level they can understand, and their understanding should be ascertained. For instance, persons with mental retardation are afraid to be perceived as inadequate and instead of saying that they did not understand the question, they tend to agree with the interviewer's last statement. Thus, asking open-ended questions is preferable to giving a choice of answers. For the same reason structured mental-status type of questions might be counter-productive. Leading questions should be avoided. One should explore the patient's self-image, including understanding of his or her own disability as well as strengths.

Nonverbal interviewing techniques include behavioral observations, spontaneous and directed (structured) play (as developmentally and age appropriate), and other structured tasks.

Evaluation of Clinical Data

The clinical observations should be interpreted in light of a patient's life experiences, learning, understanding and communication level. The global IQ or overall mental age alone is not a good guide here. In particular, the psychiatrist should:

1. Assess clinical presentation in light of the patient's communication ability, cognitive level, associated disabilities (e.g., sensory), life experiences, environmental factors and cultural background. One should differentiate between behaviors appropriate for an earlier age and those that are pathological in any age (e.g., true hallucinations). Not all disruptive behaviors are an expression of a mental disorder: for example, an overworked staff might promote aggressive acting out by attending to the patients only when they become aggressive. However, one should not simply explain all such behaviors as attention-seeking behaviors. Conversely, persons who do not manifest disruptive behaviors might have a mental disorder, for example, a depressed individual who is considered behaving well because he is very quiet.
2. Obtain, if needed, evaluations and consultations with other disciplines, for example, language pathologists, psychologists and neurologists.
3. Assess and understand the dynamic, ongoing transactional relationships among the various factors contributing to the person's development (see Figure 24.1).
4. Try to make a formal Axis I and/or Axis II DSM-IV diagnosis (besides mental retardation) whenever clinically justified. The diagnostic criteria can usually be adapted to the patient's developmental level, just as one does with child patients). However, diagnosis does not mean listing the disorder's code and name only. To be constructive, the diagnostic statement should include description of strengths, impairments, and need for supports and services in each discrete domain of the individual's functioning, as well as in the environment (community and family). It should not merely copy the diagnostic criteria but describe how they are satisfied in the particular case by history and clinical observation, as well as why other diagnoses in the differential are ruled out.

Aggression

"Aggression" to people or property (destructiveness) is one of the most frequent reasons (if not the most frequent) for referring persons with mental retardation to a psychiatrist. On closer investigation, the actual behavior ranges from occasional swearing (verbal aggression) to serious violence (Harris, 1995). Whether a particular behavior is called aggression (except for clear physical aggression) depends on the caregiver's perception. Thus, in obtaining the history it is necessary to obtain a concrete description of the behavior in question, preferably from several informants. Prolonged direct observation of the patient may be necessary to resolve unclear cases. There is no single entity called aggression in this population that would have one explanation. It would be a mistake to talk about a single treatment for aggression (except for symptomatic emergency measures). Psychiatrists are often asked how they treat aggression in persons with mental retardation. The answer is, of course, that it is done in the same manner as in persons without mental retardation: an accurate diagnostic assessment comes first. Different factors must be considered in assessing the cause of aggressive behavior (Harris, 1995). It might be associated with a defined mental disorder, for example, aggression following a command hallucination, paranoid delusion, anxiety, borderline or antisocial personality, or depression. The factor of learning will reinforce aggressive behavior if it brings a desired response by the caregivers. A pathological brain condition, such as rage attacks after brain trauma or associated with temporo-limbic seizure disorder, may also lead to aggression. Often, several causative factors are involved, all of which require evaluation and intervention.

The DSM-IV-TR has a category of intermittent explosive disorder that can be used provided that another mental disorder has been ruled out as the cause of the aggressive behavior.

Overall Goals of Psychiatric Treatment of Persons with Mental Retardation

The most common mistake made by mental health clinicians treating persons with mental retardation is to consider suppression (usually with medications) of single problems (as a rule disruptive behaviors) as the only goal of treatment. This approach used to be the rule in the past when people with mental retardation were not expected to achieve any measure of independence and keeping them docile was the goal. Lately such approaches are reemerging, partly related to the insurer's pressure to achieve a fast and inexpensive symptomatic improvement, even if short lived.

The goal of any form of psychiatric treatment of persons with mental retardation is to contribute to this sense of satisfaction with one's own life, or happiness, in the context of a comprehensive treatment program. Suppression of behaviors inconvenient to caregivers is not enough, especially if they are a response to an inadequate habilitation program and the treatment (usually medications) is used in lieu of such program. Furthermore, medications may suppress a person's functioning through side effects such as drowsiness. The mental health clinician should not assume that "nonpsychiatric" problems are taken care of by someone else, but should take an active part in the team's assessment of various factors contributing to the clinical presentation, as well as the person's need for various supports. This is not to say that the psychiatrist should be in charge of behavioral modification or vocational rehabilitation, but that these approaches should be closely coordinated with specific psychiatric treatments and should be targeted toward the common therapeutic goal.

Prerequisites for a Successful Treatment Program

- Comprehensive diagnostic understanding
- Developing goals of treatment
- Developing treatment priorities
- Monitoring treatment results
- Avoidance of indefinite treatment
- Team collaboration

Clinical Vignette

Barbara was diagnosed at 3 years of age with severe mental retardation due to marked delay in her global development. Exhaustive genetic evaluation failed to clarify its etiology. She never developed expressive speech, but understood simple commands and knew about 30 signs. She lived with her very supportive parents, attended special classes and was a friendly, well-related and pleasant person. At 17 years of age she became gradually withdrawn, cried often, did not enjoy car rides with her parents (previously her favorite activity), lost appetite and weight, and slept poorly. When she was pressed to complete school tasks she became aggressive, prompting psychiatric referral. She was diagnosed with a major depressive episode and was put on imipramine. Over the next 2 months she gradually improved. Her appetite returned, she became cooperative and slept better. However, in the third month she again developed insomnia, roamed the house at night singing or screaming, was hyperactive, laughed for no obvious reason, and became aggressive if told to go to sleep. Detailed medical evaluation failed to disclose any general medical condition. There was no history of traumatic environmental events. She was diagnosed as having a psychotic episode and treated with risperidone. She improved dramatically at first, but in a month she was where she started; presenting with the same symptoms that led initially to the diagnosis of depression. This time a diagnosis of bipolar disorder NOS was made and she was treated with carbamazepine. She improved rapidly. Her mood stabilized, she slept and ate well, again became cooperative at school and home and returned to her "old self".

Principles of the Use of Psychotropic Drugs in Persons with Mental Retardation

This outline is based largely on an excellent review of Kalachnik and coworkers (1998), Rinck (1998), as well as on the American Academy of Child and Adolescent Psychiatry (1999), and the Health Care Financing Administration (1997).

Purpose of Drug Use

These drugs are used to treat a diagnosed mental disorder toward the goal of maximizing a person's quality of life. They should not be used merely to suppress a single, objectionable behavior without regard to the effect on a person's global adjustment, functioning and quality of life. They cannot be used as punishment, for staff convenience (such as in understaffed facilities), in lieu of appropriate habilitative program (if such is unavailable), or in dosages that interfere with such programs and with a person's quality of life (Rinck, 1998, p. 52).

Context of Drug Use

These drugs are always used as part of a comprehensive, treatment/habilitation program designed and supervised by an interdisciplinary team of which the psychiatric clinician is an integral part. They should not be prescribed merely in brief "psychopharmacology consultation" or "medication review", in isolation from other aspects of the treatment.

Prerequisites for Drug Use

1. Comprehensive psychiatric diagnostic assessment, following the guidelines described earlier (see also Figure 24.1), and resulting in a psychiatric diagnosis.
2. Presence of a comprehensive treatment plan and evidence that less intrusive measures have not been effective (such as behavior modification, psychotherapies, milieu supports, etc.).
3. Comprehensive evaluation to rule out medical conditions that could have caused the presenting symptoms.
4. Existence of a reliable system to collect behavioral data individualized to the particular patient that measures occurrence of symptoms considered an index of the person's mental disorder. This should also provide reliable baseline data and functional analysis of behavior that would assess the influence of immediate and more remote antecedents and consequences of the patient's behaviors and other symptoms.
5. Satisfaction of all relevant regulatory and legal requirements, especially obtaining informed consent of the patient and/or legal guardian.

Follow-up on Drug Effectiveness

1. The members of the interdisciplinary treatment team should follow the patient's progress regularly (at least quarterly), based on changes in individualized index behaviors, symptoms, general adjustment, functioning and well-being. Presence of side effects and their findings should be communicated among the members of the team. Behavioral changes should be documented by reliable data. The follow-up should include a direct psychiatric interview and/or observation of the patient. The implementation of all aspects of the treatment program and not just the medications should be monitored and adjusted as needed to ensure that medications are not used in lieu of, but concurrently with, a habilitation program.
2. The medication should be tried at an effective dose for an adequate period of time. If there is no clear evidence of effectiveness it should be discontinued appropriately. It should be kept in mind that "ups and downs" are to be expected, such as in reaction to environmental and physical stressors common in the lives of these patients. Medication effectiveness

should therefore be judged by a pattern evident over reasonable period of time and not by one-point observations. For the same reason, preset dosage schedules linking dosage changes to specific frequencies of index behaviors are impractical. Multiple medications should be tried only if there is evidence that a combination is known to be more effective than a single medication.

Dosages and Discontinuation

1. The optimal dosage is the lowest one that achieves the best a compromise between improving the patient's quality of life and side effects.
2. A trial of dose reduction and possibly discontinuation should be regularly considered but should be implemented only if not contraindicated clinically. Discontinuation, if attempted, should be gradual, and it may need a prolonged period depending on the type of medication and expected withdrawal effects. It is essential that all involved caregivers be aware of the possibility of such effects and be ready to deal with them, rather than demand immediate cessation of the discontinuation trial (this is particularly important with antipsychotics. As-needed (.3.prn) use of the medication is best avoided to prevent unnecessary use, or limited to clear situations, such as premedication prior to medical tests if stressful for the patient.

Monitoring Side Effects

Side effects should be monitored regularly through direct examination (especially important with nonverbal persons), laboratory tests, tardive dyskinesia examination, and so on, as appropriate for the particular drug. Possible drug interactions should be monitored as these patients are often on multiple medications.

Psychosocial Interventions

Programmatic and Educational Approaches

The goal of these interventions is to provide a proper living and programmatic environment. For instance, certain persons easily become over-stimulated, anxious and disruptive in noisy and confused large workshops; arranging for a smaller and quieter workroom is preferable to a prescription for a neuroleptic. The vocational and educational program should be individualized and focus on developing the person's strengths and providing an opportunity for success. In turn, this will lead to results such as an improvement in self-image. Many persons with severe mental retardation are placed in prevocational training indefinitely, for example, screwing or unscrewing nuts and bolts, although no one expects them ever to be employed on an assembly line. They often engage in a struggle with caregivers because of their noncompliance and may resort to aggression, which leads to removal for a "time out" and thus avoidance of a boring task. Creating a more suitable task – even such as making rounds of the workshop to collect or deliver materials – might be more interesting and appropriate. Functional analysis of behavior is an invaluable guide to these interventions. As discussed previously, such approaches should be explored prior to resorting to use of medications for disruptive behaviors.

Psychotherapies

Psychotherapy in this population is not different in nature from psychotherapy in persons with average intelligence and is similar to treating children, inasmuch as in both cases the techniques and the therapist have to adapt to the developmental needs of the patient. The treatment should be driven by the patient's needs and responses and not by the therapist's theoretical orientation. The indications are: the presence of concerns and conflicts, especially about oneself; impairments in interpersonal skills; or other mental disturbances that are known to improve through psychotherapy. The prerequisites include communication skills permitting a meaningful interchange with the therapist, an ability to develop even a minimal relationship, and the availability of a trained, experienced and unprejudiced therapist who is comfortable working in a team setting.

Behavioral Treatment

This treatment should optimally use rewards which should be age appropriate, preferably social, and the frequency of rewarding should be adapted to a person's cognitive level, so that he or she can understand why they are given. Consistency and generalization among different settings are essential. Thus, if such techniques are successfully used at the school, the family or other caregivers should be trained to use them at home as well. The focus should not be on elimination of objectionable behaviors only but on teaching appropriate replacement behaviors. Aversive techniques involving active punishment (electric shocks, spraying of noxious substances into a person's face) are not used except in a few controversial settings. There is a professional consensus that these techniques should not be used at all, or only when all other techniques have failed and the patient's behavior poses severe danger to herself or himself or to others (such as intractable SIB). Even then, these techniques should be used only if proved effective and for a limited time.

Psychiatrist–Patient Relationship: Models of Delivery of Psychiatric Services

The psychiatric care of persons with mental retardation has often followed a path different from the care provided to the general population. A common service model has been the medication clinic, in which the psychiatrist is given little, if any, time to examine the patient and to interview the caregivers. Instead, behavioral information, which is often brief and sketchy, is presented by caregivers and focuses primarily on disruptive behaviors. The psychiatrist is expected to prescribe medications and has no voice in, or knowledge of, other interventions that might be used. In some cases, the psychiatrist does the actual prescribing; in others, the psychiatrist serves as a consultant to primary physicians who may or may not follow the recommendations given. This model is obviously inadequate, even if there is another professional providing psychotherapy or behavioral therapy. It also exposes the psychiatrist to legal responsibility (Woodward *et al.*, 1993). This model has been used in institutions, especially to save on the expense of having a staff psychiatrist to provide adequate services.

The proper psychiatric care of persons with mental retardation is actually more time-consuming than the care of persons without mental retardation because of the multifactor nature of the treatment described previously. To understand the patient's clinical presentation and provide the input necessary to all relevant aspects of treatment, the psychiatrist has to have adequate time to interview all involved caregivers, observe and interview the patient, make a home or program visit if necessary, and discuss the recommendation with all involved. Thus, the interdisciplinary team approach is necessary. It might not be realistic for all patients seen in the community, but it should be followed in all treatment-resistant cases and in residential facilities where, as a rule, there are more difficult patients (Szymanski *et al.*, 1980; Szymanski and Leaverton, 1980). In most cases in the community, if a team forges a good working relationship and regular communication, exchange of information and coordination via e-mail or telephone might be sufficiently productive. Some states have developed successful models of such coordinated care (that provide for health, housing, vocational and social services) for persons who have both mental retardation and mental illness (Polgar *et al.*, 2000). In all situations, psychiatrists will use their knowledge and training in biological and behavioral aspects of medicine to help other professionals synthesize the biopsychosocial aspects of a patient's clinical presentation and treatment program.

Comparison of DSM-IV/ICD-10 Diagnostic Criteria

The methods of defining the levels of severity differs slightly between the two systems. The ICD-10 Diagnostic Criteria for Research define the levels using exact cutoff scores: Mild is defined as 50 to 69, Moderate is defined as 35 to 49, Severe is defined as 20 to 34, and Profound is defined as below 20. In contrast, DSM-IV-TR provides somewhat greater flexibility in relating severity to a given IQ score by defining severity levels using overlapping scores (i.e., Mild is 50–55, Moderate is 35–40 to 50–55, Severe is 20–25 to 35–40, and Profound is below 20–25). Within the overlapping range, the severity is determined by the level of adaptive functioning.

References

American Academy of Child and Adolescent Psychiatry (1999) Practice parameters for the assessment and treatment of children, adolescents and adults with mental retardation and comorbid mental disorders. *J Am Acad Child Adolesc Psychiatr* 38(Suppl), 12.

American Psychiatric Association (2000) *Diagnostic and Statistical Manual of Mental Disorders*, 4th edn., Text Rev. APA, Washington DC.

Harris J (1995) *Developmental Neuropsychiatry.* Oxford University Press, New York, pp. 463–486.

Health Care Financing Administration (1997) Psychopharmacological Medications: Safety Precautions for Persons with Developmental Disabilities. Health Care Financing Administration, Washington DC.

Kalachnik JE, Levanthal BL, James DH *et al.* (1998) Guidelines for the use of psychotropic medication, in *Psychotropic Medications and Developmental Disabilities: The International Consensus Handbook* (eds Reiss S and Aman MG). Ohio State University Nisonger Center, pp. 45–72.

Massey PS and McDermott S (1995) State-specific rates of mental retardation – United States, 1993. *MMWR* 45, 61–65.

McLaren J and Bryson SE (1987) Review of recent epidemiological studies of mental retardation: Prevalence, associated disorders, and etiology. *Am J Ment Retard* 92, 243–254.

Polgar MF, Johnsen MC, Starrett BE *et al.* (2000) New patterns of community care: Coordinated services for dually diagnosed adults in North Carolina. *J Health Hum Serv Admin* 23, 50–64.

Rinck C (1998) Epidemiology and psychoactive medication, in *Psychotropic Medications and Developmental Disabilities: The International Consensus Handbook.* (eds Reiss S and Aman MG). Ohio State University Nisonger Center, pp. 31–44.

Szymanski LS (1980) Psychiatric diagnosis of retarded persons, in *Emotional Disorders of Mentally Retarded Persons* (eds Szymanski LS and Tanguay PE). University Park Press, Baltimore, pp. 60–81.

Szymanski LS (1994) Mental retardation and mental health: Concepts, aetiology and incidence, in *Mental Health in Mental Retardation: Recent Advances and Practices*, (ed Bouras N). Cambridge University Press, Cambridge, pp. 19–33.

Szymanski LS and Crocker AC (1989) Mental retardation, in *Comprehensive Textbook of Psychiatry*, Vol. V (eds Kaplan HI and Sadock BJ). Williams & Wilkins, Baltimore.

Szymanski LS and Leaverton DR (1980) Mental health consultations to educational programs for retarded persons, in *Emotional Disorders of Mentally Retarded Persons* (eds Szymanski LS and Tanguay PE). University Park Press, Baltimore, pp. 244–253.

Szymanski LS, Eissner BA and Rosefsky QB (1980) Mental Health consultations to residential facilities for retarded person, in *Emotional Disorders of Mentally Retarded Persons* (eds Szymanski LS and Tanguay PE). University Park Press, Baltimore, pp. 255–273.

Wilska M and Kaski M (1999) Aetiology of intellectual disability – The Finnish classification: Development of a method to incorporate WHO ICD-10 coding. *J Intellect Disabil Res* 43, 242–250.

Woodward B, Duckworth KS and Gutheil TG (1993) The pharmacotherapist psychotherapist collaboration. *Rev Psychiatr* 12, 631–649.

World Health Organization (1992) *ICD-10 Classification of Mental and Behavioural Disorders – Clinical Description and Diagnostic Guidelines.* WHO, Geneva.

Childhood Disorders: Learning and Motor Skills Disorders

For children and adolescents, school is their "workplace". Successful school performance is essential for psychological growth and development. Social competency and social skills are developed and then shaped within the family and in the school but practiced and mastered in the school. The development of self-image and self-esteem is based on successes in school. Feedback from the school concerning academic performance and social interactions influences the parents' image of their child or adolescent. Thus, if something interferes with success in school, the impact will affect the emotional, social and family functioning of a child or adolescent.

Academic performance requires the integrated interactions of the cognitive, motor and language functions of the brain. As detailed in the *Diagnostic and Statistical Manual of Mental Disorders*, Fourth Edition (DSM-IV), if brain dysfunction results in cognitive difficulties, it is called a learning disorder; in motor difficulties, a motor skills disorder; and in language difficulties, a language disorder. This chapter focuses on the learning disorders and motor skills disorders.

Key for the mental health professional is the understanding that the underlying neurological dysfunctions that result in learning disorders and motor skills disorder have an impact on more than academic performance. These disabilities affect every aspect of the individual's life during each stage of psychosocial development (Silver, 1989, 1993b).

Definitions

Public education laws use the term learning disabilities. DSM-IV uses the terms learning disorders and motor skills disorder. It is helpful to understand that these terms reflect the diagnostic system used but refer to the same set of difficulties.

Public school systems use the federal definition based on Public Law 94–142, Education for All Handicapped Children, and its revision, Public Law 101–476, Individuals with Disabilities Education Act. In the latter, a learning disability is defined by the following inclusionary and exclusionary criteria:

Specific learning disabilities means a disorder in one or more of the basic psychological processes involved in understanding or in using language, spoken or written, which may manifest itself in an imperfect ability to listen, think, speak, read, write, spell, or to do mathematical calculations. The term includes such conditions as perceptual handicaps, brain injury, minimal brain dysfunction, dyslexia, and developmental aphasia. The term does not include children who have learning problems which

are primarily the result of visual, hearing, or motor handicaps, of mental retardation, of emotional disturbance, or of environmental, cultural, or economic disadvantage.

DSM-IV-TR Criteria

The criteria in DSM-IV-TR for establishing the diagnosis of a learning disorder are shown as a summary of three criteria sets. For each of these diagnostic categories, the criteria in DSM-IV-TR is that if a general medical (e.g., neurological) condition or sensory deficit is present, the disorder should be coded on Axis III.

DSM-IV-TR Criteria

Learning Disorders

A. Academic achievement (i.e., reading, mathematics, or written expression), as measured by individually administered standardized tests, is substantially below that expected given the person's chronological age, measured intelligence and age-appropriate education.

B. The disturbance in Criterion A significantly interferes with academic achievement or activities of daily living.

C. If sensory deficit is present, the difficulties are in excess of those usually associated with it.

Coding Note: If a general medical (e.g., neurological) condition or sensory deficit is present, code the condition on Axis III.

Reprinted from DSM-IV Guidebook (1995) Frances A, First MB, Pincus HA. American Psychiatric Press Inc, Washington, DC, p. 384.

Educational Criteria

The most recent federal guidelines for determining whether a student in a public school is eligible for special programs for learning disabilities list four criteria (Silver and Hagin, 1992):

1. Documented evidence indicating that general education has been attempted and found to be ineffective in meeting the student's educational needs.
2. Evidence of a disorder in one or more of the basic psychological processes required for learning. A psychological process is a set of mental operations that transform, access, or manipulate information. The disorder is relatively enduring and

Essentials of Psychiatry   Jerald Kay and Allan Tasman
© 2006 John Wiley & Sons, Ltd.

limits ability to perform specific academic or developmental learning tasks. It may be manifested differently at different developmental levels.

3. Evidence of academic achievement significantly below the student's level of intellectual function (a difference of 1.5 to 1.75 standard deviations between achievement and intellectual functioning is considered significant) on basic reading skills, reading comprehension, mathematical calculation, mathematical reasoning, or written expression.

4. Evidence that the learning problems are not due primarily to other handicapping conditions (i.e., impairment of visual acuity or auditory acuity, physical impairment, emotional handicap, mental retardation, cultural differences, or environmental deprivation).

The presence of a central nervous system processing deficit is essential for the diagnosis of a learning disability. A child might meet the discrepancy criteria, but without central processing deficits in functions required for learning, he or she is not considered to have a learning disability. The question of the significant discrepancy between potential and actual achievement determines eligibility for services. Different school systems use different models for determining the extent of discrepancy (Silver and Hagin, 1992, 1993).

Diagnosis of a Learning Disorder or Motor Skills Disorder

If a child or adolescent is experiencing academic difficulty, she or he would normally be referred to the special education professionals within the school system. However, the student with academic difficulties often presents with emotional or behavior problems and is more likely to be referred to a mental health professional. It is critical to understand this potential referral bias. This mental health professional must clarify whether the observed emotional, social, or family problems are causing the academic difficulties or whether they are a consequence of the academic difficulties and the resulting frustrations and failures experienced by the individual, the teacher and the parents (Silver, 1989, 1993b, 1998; Bender, 1987; Hunt and Cohen, 1984; Valletutti, 1983).

The evaluation of a child or adolescent with academic difficulties and emotional or behavior problems includes a comprehensive assessment of the presenting emotional, behavior, social, or family problems as well as a mental status examination. The psychiatrist should obtain information from the child or adolescent, parents, teachers and other education professionals to help clarify whether there might be a learning disorder or a motor skills disorder and whether further psychological or educational studies are needed. Descriptions by teachers, parents and the child or adolescent being evaluated will give the psychiatrist clues that there might be one of the learning disorders or a motor skills disorder.

Children who experience problems in reading typically have difficulty in decoding the letter-sound associations involved in phonic analysis (Rourke and Strang, 1983). As a result, they may read in a disjointed manner, knowing a few words on sight and stumbling across other unfamiliar words. They may guess. If they have difficulty with visual tracking, they may skip words or lines. If comprehension is a problem, they report that they have to read material over and over before they understand.

Children with mathematical difficulties may have problems learning math concepts or retaining this information. They may make "careless mistakes" when doing calculations. Math is a written language in that one is graded on what is put on paper. Thus, problems with visual-spatial tasks or with sequencing might interfere with producing on paper what is known. A problem may not be completed or steps skipped. They might have difficulty shifting from one operation to the next and, as a result, add when they should subtract. A visual–spatial difficulty might result in misaligned columns or rows, or decimals put in the wrong place.

Children who have difficulties with writing may have a problem with handwriting. They grasp the pencil or pen differently and tightly. They write slowly, and their hands get tired. Often, they prefer printing rather than cursive writing. Most also have problems with the language of writing. They have difficulty with spelling, often spelling phonetically. They may have difficulty with grammar, punctuation and capitalization (Poplin *et al.*, 1980).

Many if not most students with a learning disorder also have difficulties with memory or organization. The child or adolescent with a memory problem has difficulty following multistep directions or reads a chapter in a book but forgets what was read. Others might have sequencing problems, performing instructions out of order. In speaking or writing, the facts may come out but in the wrong sequence. Students with organizational difficulties may not be able to organize their life (notebook, locker, desk, bedroom); they forget things or lose things; they have difficulty with time planning; or they have difficulty using parts of information from a whole concept or putting parts of information together into a whole concept.

Children and adolescents with a developmental coordination disorder may show evidence of gross motor or fine motor difficulties. The gross motor problems might result in difficulty with walking, running, jumping, or climbing. The fine motor problems may result in difficulty with buttoning, zipping, tying, holding a pencil or pen or crayon, arts and crafts activities, or handwriting. Both gross and fine motor difficulties may result in the individual performing poorly in certain sports activities.

Ostrander (1993) and Silver (1993a) suggested a set of "systems review"-type questions (Table 25.1) to be used during an interview with parents or the child or adolescent with academic difficulties suspected of having a learning disorder (learning disability) or a developmental coordination disorder. These questions focus both on the specific areas of skills and on the possible underlying processing problems.

Evaluation of the Child or Adolescent

Difficulties in academic performance of children or adolescents can be related to a range of psychiatric, medical, or cognitive factors. To determine best the primary source of academic difficulties, the evaluation should involve a comprehensive examination of these areas. The psychiatric evaluation should clarify whether there is a psychopathological process. If one is present, it is useful first to determine whether the problems relate to a disruptive behavior disorder or to another psychiatric disorder. In particular, the disruptive behavior disorders have high comorbidity with academic difficulties. A full assessment should clarify whether a disruptive behavior disorder is causing the difficulty with academic performance or is secondary to this difficulty. Disruptive behavior disorders can result in the student being unavailable for learning or being so disruptive as to require his/her removal from traditional learning environments. The frustration and failures caused by a learning disorder can be manifested by a disruptive behavior disorder. In some cases, the disruptive behavior disorder coexists with the learning

Table 25.1   Screening Questions

Reading

Do you like to read?
Can you sound out words as well as your classmates can?
Do you know the word on sight, or not at all?
Do you skip words or lines?
Does it take you longer than other children to read?
Can you remember what you read?

Mathematics

Do you know the basic facts in addition, subtraction, multiplication and division?
Do you often add when you should subtract or multiply?
Do you often forget some of the steps when doing mathematics problems?
Do you often make careless errors?
Is your mathematics homework messy?

Writing

How is your handwriting? Can people read it?
Can you write fast enough?
How is your spelling? When you make spelling mistakes, can other people figure out what word you were trying to spell?
Do you make many mistakes in capitalization, punctuation, or grammar?

Sequencing

When you speak or write, do you sometimes have difficulty getting everything in the right order or do you start in the middle, go to the beginning, then jump to the end?
Can you name the months of the year? (Let child do.) Fine, now what comes after August? (Ask how he or she got the answer. Was it necessary to return to January and count up?)
Do you have difficulty using the alphabet when using a dictionary? Do you have to return to "a" often to know whether the next letter is above or below the letter you are on?

Abstraction

Do you understand jokes when your friends tell them?
Do you sometimes get confused when people seem to say something, yet they tell you they meant something, else?

Organization

What does your notebook look like? Is it a mess with papers in the wrong place or falling out?
What about your desk? Your locker? Your bedroom?
Do you have difficulty organizing your thoughts or the facts you are learning into a whole concept so that you can learn it?
Do you find that you can read a chapter and answer the questions at the end of the chapter but that you are still not sure what the chapter is about?

Memory

Do you find that you can learn something at night and then go to school the next day and forget what you have learned?
When talking, do you sometimes know what you want to say but halfway through you forget what you are saying? If so, do you cover up by saying things like "Oh, forget it" or "It's not important"?

Language

When the teacher is speaking in class, do you have trouble understanding or keeping up?
Do you sometimes misunderstand people and therefore give the wrong answer?
When people are talking, do you find that you have to concentrate so hard on what they say that you sometimes fall behind and have to skip quickly to what they are saying now to keep up?
Does this sometimes cause you to get lost in class?
Do you sometimes have trouble getting your thoughts organized when you speak?
Do you have a problem finding the word you want to use?

Motor

Do you feel that you can run, jump and climb as well as your friends can?
Would you describe yourself as clumsy?
Do you find that you often knock things over or bump into things?
Do you have difficulty with dressing, especially with buttoning, zipping, tying? How about cutting food and eating?
In sports do you have difficulty with throwing, hitting and catching a ball?
How would you describe your handwriting? Do you hold your pencil or pen differently from others? Does your hand get tired? Do you write slower than you need to in class?

Reprinted from Ostrander R (1993) Clinical observations suggesting a learning disability. *Child Adolesc Psychiatr Clin N Am* 2, 249–263. Copyright 1993, with permission from Elsevier.

disorder and the relation is less clear. Children and adolescents with attention-deficit/hyperactivity disorder (ADHD) have particular difficulty maintaining attention, and possibly with processing information. As a result, the same variables that have an impact on their attention also have an impact on their ability to learn. In such instances, they may have a learning disorder and ADHD.

Internalizing disorders such as depression or anxiety may result in an uncharacteristic disinterest in or avoidance of school expectations. If one of the internalizing disorders is present, it is important to clarify whether it is secondary or primary to the academic difficulty. Cognitive and language deficits as well as social skills deficits are often associated with learning disorders and can contribute to a dysphoric or anxious presentation.

The medical evaluation is necessary to explore the influence of health factors on the individual's availability and ability to learn. Problems in acquiring academic content can be significantly affected by most visual or hearing deficits. Generally poor health can influence the stamina, motivation and concentration needed to focus adequately on academic demands. Medications used for any purpose might cause sedation or other side effects that may affect the child's ability to learn. Early developmental insults can result in global or focal deficits in neurological development. Undiagnosed seizures, especially petit mal and partial complex seizures, can result in difficulties in general cognitive functioning, specific deficits in memory and problems with attention.

The evaluation of cognitive, academic and neuropsychological functioning is critical to any assessment of learning problems. Results of this psychoeducational assessment will indicate the parameters of the individual's academic and cognitive liabilities while identifying her or his assets. In some instances, borderline cognitive development or mental retardation may be the primary explanation for learning difficulties. Developmental delays are particularly evident with a preschool child; rapid and uneven developmental changes can lead to considerable variability in findings derived by measures of intellectual functioning. If any of the clinical evaluations yield results suggestive of a learning disorder, a more involved psychoeducational assessment is needed. An appropriate psychoeducational evaluation will reveal the magnitude of the child's learning difficulties as well as the nature of the child's cognitive assets and deficits. From this understanding, appropriate interventions can be designed and special accommodations can be initiated.

A family evaluation is an integral part of evaluation and must include an assessment of the parents and of the entire family. The first clinical question is whether the family is functional or dysfunctional. If the family is largely functional, there may be "normal" parenting issues that may be contributing to the child's difficulty.

A normal parenting issue may be their lack of time or energy to address the child's academic difficulties.

Environmental and Cultural Assessment

Learning problems are attributed to cognitive deficits or behavior problems in the child or adolescent. Environmental factors involving the school or community, however, can also contribute to academic difficulties. Thus, the psychiatrist should be aware of how social, cultural, or institutional structures can influence learning.

A child or adolescent with specific needs may be further impaired because of a limited range of services offered by the school system.

Social Problems

The learning disabilities that result in learning disorders or motor skills disorder may directly contribute to peer problems by interfering with success in doing activities required to interact with certain age groups (e.g., visual perception and visual–motor problems interfering with ability quickly to do such eye–hand activities as catching, hitting, or throwing a ball).

Many children and adolescents with learning disorders have difficulty learning social skills and being socially competent (Hazel and Schumaker, 1988). These individuals do not pick up such social cues as facial expressions, tone of voice, or body language and therefore do not adapt their behaviors appropriately. Rourke (1987, 1988, 1989) and Rourke and Fuerst (1991), using the definition of learning disabilities, identified a specific subtype of learning disabilities, called nonverbal learning disabilities. These students do not have the difficulties with interpersonal interactions found in pervasive developmental disorders. This pattern of learning disabilities includes deficits in tactile perception, visual perception, complex psychomotor tasks and accommodation to novel material as well as difficulty in simple motor skills, auditory perception and mastery of rote material. A small subset of these students show difficulty in social and emotional functioning that includes a predisposition toward adolescent and adult depression and suicide risk (Rourke and Fuerst, 1991).

Other Psychiatric or Medical Disorders

The first neurologically based disorder recognized as frequently associated with a learning disability (learning disorder) was ADHD (Silver, 1981; Halperin *et al.*, 1984). Studies suggest that there is a continuum of disorders associated with neurological dysfunction that are often found together. Thus, when one is diagnosed, the others must be considered in the diagnostic process.

The specific constructs for understanding the probable cognitive and language bases for the specific learning disorders and motor skills disorder are discussed under each subtype in the section on treatment. The premise is that there are neurologically based processing problems that result in the disabilities.

Clinical Vignette 1

Billy started first grade and did not do well. He did not master the early skills of reading and writing. The school decision was to have him repeat first grade. He did not make much more progress during his second year in first grade. Because of his age, he was promoted to second grade. He struggled through this year but fell further and further behind. When he entered third grade, he was overwhelmed. He knew that he was a year older than the other students. He was unable to do the work in class or at home and felt frustrated and stupid. Soon, he began to clown around in class and to get into fights with the other students.

Two other things happened during this third-grade year. First, his teacher became frustrated. She was trying to help him learn and he was not making progress. He was disrupting the class and preventing her from teaching the other children. The teacher handled her frustration by blaming it on the parents. She began to call them.

Clinical Vignette 1 *continued*

"Billy is not completing his schoolwork." "His homework is incorrect." "He is teasing and fighting with the other children." She seemed to be saying to the parents, "Do something. Fix your kid." She did not realize that the parents were just as confused and frustrated as the teacher. Secondly, the parents began to disagree on parenting decisions. One felt that the best way to help Billy was to be firm and strict, and the other felt that the best way was to be understanding and permissive. They began to argue with each other and became less available to support each other.

Finally, the principal asked the parents to come to school. They were informed that Billy was not making academic progress. They were also told that the reason for his failure was that he was emotionally disturbed because of the marital conflicts. The parents were encouraged to see a mental health professional.

This psychiatrist noted that Billy had difficulty with reading, reading comprehension, handwriting and written language. He found Billy to be frustrated with a poor self-image and low self-esteem. The parents seemed to be competent people who were also frustrated with Billy's difficulties. A full psychoeducational testing was requested. The results showed Billy to be of above-average ability but with significant learning disabilities.

The psychiatrist concluded that the primary diagnosis was the learning disability. The emotional, behavioral, social and family problems were secondary to the frustrations and failures experienced by Billy, his parents and his teacher. By working with the family, he helped to get Billy identified as having a disability and to obtain the necessary services to help him. His behavior problems diminished and then ceased.

Treatment

Treatment is directed at the underlying disabilities by use of educational interventions. Psychological interventions are also directed at any existing emotional, social, or family difficulties. In addition, social skills training may be helpful.

Educational Interventions

The goal of special educational interventions is to help children and adolescents overcome or compensate for their learning disorders or motor skills disorder so that they can succeed in school. These efforts involve remedial and compensatory approaches and use a multisensory approach that facilitates building on all areas of strength while compensating for any areas of weakness. These efforts are to be provided in as close to a regular classroom setting as possible. It is essential that the classroom teacher knows how best to adapt the classroom, curriculum and teaching style to accommodate each student's areas of difficulty.

Psychotherapeutic Interventions

Learning disorders affect all aspects of the child's or adolescent's life. The same processing problems that interfere with reading, writing, mathematics and language may interfere with communicating with peers and family, with success in sports and

activities, and with such daily life skills as dressing oneself or cutting food (Silver, 1993b).

Lack of success in school can lead to a poor self-image and low self-esteem (Black, 1974; Bryan and Pearl, 1979; Rogers and Saklofske, 1985; Shaw *et al.* 1982). These individuals might feel that they have minimal control over their life and compensate by trying to be in more control (Silver, 1993c). Some individuals may become anxious or depressed, or a disruptive behavior disorder may develop.

Genetic and family studies show that in about 40% of children and adolescents with learning disabilities (learning disorders), there is a familial pattern (Johnson, 1988). Thus, from an early identification perspective, each sibling must be considered as possibly having a learning disorder. Also, there is a 40% likelihood that one of the parents may also have a learning disorder. This parent may not have known of this problem. If this is true, the parent for the first time may be able to understand a lifetime of difficulties or underachievement. Further, when the psychiatrist offers suggestions for this parent, the parent's areas of difficulty must be considered. Do not ask a mother to be more organized when she has been just as disorganized as her child all of her life.

Some children or adolescents may need specific individual, behavioral, group, or family therapy. If so, it is critical that the therapist understand the impact that the learning disorder has had on the individual and how these disabilities might affect the process of therapy (Silver, 1993a). As noted earlier, many students with a learning disorder have difficulties with peers and social skills problems. Social skills training might be helpful.

Use of Medications

No medication has been found to be effective for treating the learning disorders or motor skills disorder. If the individual with these disorders also has ADHD, it is important that medication be used to minimize the hyperactivity, distractibility, or impulsivity so that the student can be available for learning.

Comparison of DSM-IV/ICD-10 Diagnostic Criteria

In ICD-10, DSM-IV-TR Reading Disorder is referred to as "Specific Reading Disorder" and DSM-IV-TR Mathematics Disorders as "Specific Disorder of Arithmetic Skills". For both of these learning skills disorders, the ICD-10 Diagnostic Criteria for Research suggest that the cutoff be two standard deviations below the expected level of reading achievement and mathematics achievement respectively. In contrast, DSM-IV-TR does not specify a score cutoff, instead recommending that the score be "substantially below that expected given the person's chronological age, measured intelligence, and age-appropriate education". Furthermore, in contrast to DSM-IV-TR which permits both to be diagnosed of present, ICD-10 Reading Disorder takes precedence over Mathematics Disorder so that if criteria are met for both, only Reading Disorder is diagnosed.

ICD-10 does not include a Disorder of Written Expression (as in DSM-IV-TR), but instead includes a Specific Spelling Disorder. DSM-IV-TR includes spelling problems as part of the definition of Disorder of Written Expression but requires writing problems in addition to spelling in order to warrant this diagnosis.

Finally, DSM-IV-TR Coordination Disorder is referred to as "Specific Developmental Disorder of motor function" in ICD-10. Furthermore, the ICD-10 Diagnostic Criteria for

Research suggest that the cutoff be two standard deviations below the expected level on a standardized test of fine or gross motor coordination.

References

Bender WN (1987) Secondary personality and behavioral problems in adolescents with learning disabilities. *J Learn Disabil* 20, 280–285.

Black FW (1974) Self-concept as related to achievement and age in learning disabled children. *Child Dev* 45, 1137–1140.

Bryan T and Pearl R (1979) Self-concept and locus of control of learning disabled children. *J Clin Child Psychol* 8, 223–226.

Halperin JM, Gittelman R, Klein DF *et al.* (1984) Reading-disabled hyperactive children: A distinct subgroup of attention deficit disorder with hyperactivity. *J Abnorm Child Psychol* 12, 1–14.

Hazel JS and Schumaker JB (1988) Social skills and learning disabilities: Current issues and recommendations for future research, in *Learning Disabilities: Proceedings of the National Conference* (eds Kavanagh JF and Truss TJ). York Press, Parkton, MD, pp. 293–344.

Hunt RD and Cohen DJ (1984) Psychiatric aspects of learning difficulties. *Pediatr Clin N Am* 31, 471–497.

Johnson DJ (1988) Review of research on specific reading, writing, and mathematics disorders, in *Learning Disabilities: Proceedings of the National Conference* (eds Kavanagh JF and Truss TJ). York Press, Parkton, MD, pp. 79–163.

Ostrander R (1993) Clinical observations suggesting a learning disability. *Child Adolesc Psychiatr Clin N Am* 2, 249–263.

Poplin M, Gray R *et al.* (1980) A comparison of components of written expression abilities in learning disabled and non-learning disabled students at three grade levels. *Learn Disabbil Q* 3, 46–53.

Rogers H and Saklofske DH (1985) Self-concepts, locus of control and performance expectations of learning disabled students. *J Learn Disabil* 18, 244–267.

Rourke BP (1987) Syndrome of nonverbal learning disabilities: The final common pathway of white-matter disease/dysfunction? *Clin Neuropsychol* 1, 209–234.

Rourke BP (1988) Socioemotional disturbances of learning disabled children. *J Consult Clin Psychol* 56, 801–810.

Rourke BP (1989) *Nonverbal Learning Disabilities: The Syndrome and the Model.* Guilford Press, New York.

Rourke BP and Fuerst DR (1991) *Learning Disabilities and Psychosocial Functioning: A Neuropsychological Perspective.* Guilford Press, New York.

Rourke BP and Strang JD (1983) Subtypes of reading and arithmetical disabilities: A neuropsychological analysis, in *Developmental Neuropsychiatry* (ed Rutter M). Guilford Press, New York, pp. 473–488.

Shaw L, Levine MD and Belfer M (1982) Developmental double jeopardy: A study of clumsiness and self-esteem in children with learning problems. *Dev Behav Pediatr* 3, 191–196.

Silver AA and Hagin RA (1992) *Disorders of Learning in Childhood.* John Wiley, New York, pp. 23–42.

Silver AA and Hagin RA (1993) The educational diagnostic process. *Child Adolesc Psychiatr Clin N Am* 2, 265–281.

Silver LB (1981) The relationship between learning disabilities, hyperactivity, distractibility, and behavioral problems. *J Am Acad Child Psychiatr* 20, 385–397.

Silver LB (1989) Psychological and family problems associated with learning disabilities: Assessment and intervention. *J Am Acad Child Adolesc Psychiatr* 28, 319–325.

Silver LB (1993a) Psychological interventions and therapies for children and adolescents with learning disabilities. *Child Adolesc Psychiatr Clin N Am* 2, 323–337.

Silver LB (1993b) The secondary emotional, social, and family problems found with children and adolescents with learning disabilities. *Child Adolesc Psychiatr Clin N Am* 2, 295–308.

Silver LB (1993c) Introduction and overview to the clinical concepts of learning disabilities. *Child Adolesc Psychiatr Clin N Am* 2, 181–192.

Silver LB (1998) *The Misunderstood Child. A Guide for Parents of Children with Learning Disabilities*, 3rd edn. Random House/Times Books, New York.

Valletutti P (1983) The social and emotional problems of children with learning disabilities. *Learn Disabil* 2, 17–29.

26 Childhood Disorders: Communication Disorders

Definitions

Psychiatric practice depends upon communication and language. Language and or learning disorders have been linked in the past, but in DSM-IV-TR (American Psychiatric Association, 2000) they are regarded as separate although often associated conditions. This section covers: Expressive Language Disorder, Mixed Receptive-Expressive Language Disorders, Phonological Disorder, Stuttering and Communication Disorder NOS. These disorders share many common features, as noted in Table 26.1. They are defined by criteria in DSM-IV-TR. In all cases a test score or assessment measure alone does not define these conditions. An individual must also experience social, academic or occupational difficulties directly related to the condition.

DSM-IV-TR does not consider receptive language disorders in isolation. Receptive language disorders in children seldom, if ever, can occur without concurrent (and perhaps resultant) problems with expression. This is in direct contrast with such entities as Wernicke's aphasia in adults, which affect reception alone.

Table 26.1	Features Common to All Communication Disorders

Inadequate development of some aspect of communication
Absence (in developmental types) of any demonstrable causes of physical disorder, neurological disorder, global mental retardation, or severe environmental deprivation
Onset in childhood
Long duration
Clinical features resembling the functional levels of younger normal children
Impairments in adaptive functioning, especially in school
Tendency to occur in families
Predisposition toward boys
Multiple presumed etiological factors
Increased prevalence in younger age range
Diagnosis requiring a range of standardized techniques
Tendency toward certain specific associated problems, such as attention-deficit/hyperactivity disorder
Wide range of subtypes and severity

Adapted from Baker L (1990) Specific communication disorders, in *Psychiatric Disorders in Children and Adolescents* (eds Garfinkel BD, Carlson GA and Weller EB). Copyright 1990, with permission from Elsevier.

Essentials of Psychiatry   Jerald Kay and Allan Tasman
© 2006 John Wiley & Sons, Ltd.

Outside of DSM-IV-TR, the term "phonologic disorder" may refer to a condition characterized by difficulty in generating sound combinations, as for example in the case of laryngeal dysfunction.

Epidemiology

Prevalence

Prevalences varying from 1 to 13% have been reported for language disorders, and numbers as high as 32% for speech disorders (Baker, 1990). In development of the DSM-IV-TR, researchers found that:

- Acquired language disorders appear less common than the developmental types.
- 3–7% of all children were suspected of having a developmental Expressive Language Disorder.
- Mixed Expressive – Receptive Language Disorder appears in up to 3% of school-age children.
- Phonological Disorder occurs in approximately 2% of six and seven-year olds, falling to 0.5% by age 17.
- Stuttering occurs in approximately 1% of children 10 and younger, declining to 0.8% in later adolescence.
- All of these conditions have a male to female predominance; that of stuttering is as high as 3 : 1.

Comorbidity

General

Cantwell and Baker (1991) demonstrated that approximately half of the children with a speech or language disorder have some other definable Axis I clinical disorder. Similarly, among children with a psychiatric diagnosis first made, there is a remarkably increased likelihood of speech and language disorders, which often go undetected. Beitchman (1985) found more than four times the prevalence of psychiatric illness in kindergartners with communication disorders compared with nondisordered children. Cantwell and Baker also found that psychiatric illness in their population was associated with greater severity of communication problems.

Conversely, the presence of communication disorders may be associated with increased severity of some psychiatric conditions, most notably the Disruptive Behavior Disorders. Physicians must recognize that these disorders do not occur in an isolated context.

Expressive Language Disorder and Mixed Receptive-expressive Language Disorder

Phonological Disorder and Learning Disorders are common among children with this disorder. Other neurodevelopmental conditions are also seen, such as motor delays, coordination disorders and enuresis, although the rate of association is uncertain. These disorders and the stresses they create frequently lead to Adjustment Disorders and social withdrawal. Cantwell and Baker (1991) found that the most common psychiatric disorder among children with communication disorders overall was Attention Deficit Hyperactivity Disorder (ADHD), representing 19% of their sample of 600 children referred for a communication evaluation. Some authors have speculated that ADHD may be concordant with an entity known as Central Auditory Processing Disorder (CAPD), which refers to deficits in the processing of audible signals, and which can be subsumed under the DSM-IV language disorders. A total concordance is unlikely, but Riccio *et al.* (1994) suggest that 50% of children with CAPD also have ADHD.

Phonologic Disorder

Children with this problem may have clear causal factors, such as anatomic, neurological, or cognitive disorders, although most do not. They do have a higher prevalence of language disorders, with all their associated problems, than do normal controls. They appear more likely to have ADHD, though probably not as commonly as do children with language disorders. Children with Phonological Disorders, especially when associated with stuttering or hyperactivity, are prone to social discrimination and isolation, with subsequent consequences.

Stuttering

Other communication disorders are more frequently reported in those with stuttering than in normal controls. Stuttering is frequently accompanied by many linguistic mechanisms and social maneuvers to avoid its manifestation, and is often exacerbated by anxiety or stress. Persons with stuttering face social discrimination. They have been mocked in drama and cinema (including cartoons) for centuries, and all too often are regarded as intellectually impaired.

Etiology and Pathophysiology

Genetic Influences

No clear mechanisms of genetic transmission have been elucidated, but a number of instances of family aggregation have been reported. At least one of these (Gopnik and Crago, 1991) suggested the presence of a single dominant autosomal gene. Tomblin (1989) reported increased concordance of language disorders among siblings. An increasing number of family studies now suggest that these disorders are familial, including the Twins Early Development Study (TEDS) in the United Kingdom (Plomin and Dale, 2000). These reports cannot absolutely prove any genetic hypothesis but are provocative and suggest a polygenetic basis.

A genetic basis for stuttering has been proposed for many years. The Yale Family Study of Stuttering suggested that 15% of first degree relatives of probands are affected at some time in their lives (Kidd, 1983).

Pathophysiologic influences

Neurophysiological Factors

Communication disorders arise from at least three interrelated sets of factors: neurophysiologic (including structural), cognitive-perceptual and environmental. However, the great majority of children with communication disorders exhibit no specific CNS damage, and thus minimal or subclinical damage has been postulated. The relative frequency of "soft" neurologic signs and lateral dominance problems in this population provokes this speculation. However, no clear neurophysiologic mechanisms or pathology can be correlated with these disorders. Some interesting findings are emerging, including suggested anatomical differences in the left cerebral cortex in stuttering, prenatal alcohol exposure and the physical sequelae of abuse and neglect.

Cognitive and Perceptual Factors

Perceptual hypotheses relate communication disorders to various deficits in the reception, acquisition, processing, storage, or recall of different elements of communication. Table 26.2 notes various perceptual deficits that have been implicated, including auditory

Table 26.2	Hypotheses About Influencing Factors in Communication Disorders
Types of Hypotheses	Specific Hypotheses
Neurological impairments	Specific localizable brain damage
	Subclinical (minimal) brain damage
Perceptual deficits	Deficits in auditory discrimination
	Deficits in auditory attention
	Deficits in auditory figure-ground
	Deficits in auditory memory
	Deficits in auditory–visual association
	Deficits in the processing of specific linguistic units
Cognitive deficits	Deficits in symbolic or concept development
	Deficits in anticipatory imagery
	Deficits in sorting or categorizing
	Deficits in hierarchical processing
Environmental factors	Inadequate parent–child interaction
	Socioeconomic factors (large family size, lower social class, late birth order, environmental deprivation)
	Medical factors (e.g., prematurity, history of recurrent otitis media)
Multifactorial etiology	Combinations of all of the above

Adapted from Baker L (1990) Specific communication disorders, in *Psychiatric Disorders in Children and Adolescents* (eds Garfinkel BD, Carlson GA and Weller EB). Copyright 1990, with permission from Elsevier.

discrimination, attention, memory and visual association. More purely cognitive hypotheses have also been proposed, involving deficits in symbolization, categorizing, hierarchical processing and related areas. Some authors (Friel-Patti, 1992; Helmuth, 2001) propose that there are certain language-specific cognitive deficits. The special phenomenology of stuttering suggests the possibility of dyssynchrony between phonation and articulation, as reported by Perkins (2001).

Environmental Factors

This category refers both to the psychosocial environment of the child and to general medical factors such as perinatal complications or recurrent otitis media.

The relationship of socioeconomic status to the occurrence of communication disorders is uncertain. Variables such as class, family size, income and birth order all clearly affect the amount of verbal interaction children receive and have been implicated. The association between the exacerbation of stuttering and stress is well known, although work in this area has frequently confounded predisposing, triggering and maintaining factors.

Review of these influences reveals a considerable amount of overlap, and clinical observation seldom if ever suggests a unitary causality of Communication Disorders in real patients.

Diagnosis

Phenomenology

Expressive Language Disorder

This condition varies with age and severity. Vocabulary, word-finding, sentence length, variety of expression and grammatical complexity may all be reduced. Most children with the developmental subtype of this disorder demonstrate delayed language development. Often auxiliary words or prepositions are omitted, resulting in telegraphic speech: "he was going to school" becomes "he going school". Word order may be garbled: "Him like too me" for "I like him, too". Words or phrases may be repeated to the degree that speech may be echolalic, perseverative, or both. Conversation may be tangential, with sudden inappropriate changes of topic, or conversely, perseveration. Pragmatic difficulties, such as in initiating or terminating conversations, are seen, as is avoidance of conversation. These children frequently are regarded as socially inappropriate or inept, and at times may be suspected of having a formal thought disorder or a Pervasive Developmental Disorder. They frequently have academic problems because of their difficulty in responding verbally to exercises. They may have motor coordination problems and various other neurodevelopmental abnormalities, documented upon neurological examination, EEG, or neuroimaging, although no consistent patterns are seen.

Mixed Receptive-expressive Language Disorder

Children with this disorder may have all the problems of Expressive Language Disorder. In addition, they do not understand all that they hear. The deficits may be mild or severe, and at times deceptively subtle, since patients may conceal them or avoid interaction. All areas and levels of language comprehension may be disturbed. Thus the child may not understand speech that is rapid, certain words or categories of words, such as abstract quantities, or types of statements, such as conditional clauses. These children may seem not to hear or attend, or to misbehave by not following commands correctly. At times, when conversation is redirected to them in a slower or more concise fashion, they may understand and respond belatedly, and thereby be accused of willful avoidance. More severely impaired children may not follow the rules of syntax or word order, and thus confuse subjects and objects or questions and declarations. Often in more severe cases, disabilities may be multiple and pervasive, affecting processing, recall and association. Such deficits have immense social consequences.

Phonologic Disorders

This category is characterized by persistent errors in the production of speech. These include omission, substitution or distortion of sounds. Omissions include single or multiple sounds: "I go o coo o the but" (I go to school on the bus); or "I re a boo" (I read a book). Substitutions include w/l, t/s, w/r, and d/g: "I taw a wittle wed wadio. It pwayed dood music". Lisping, the frontal or lateral misarticulation of sibilants, is a common distortion. Defects in the order of sounds or insertions of extraneous sounds may also be heard: "catht" for "cats". The occurrence of these errors is persistent but not constant. Usually only some sounds are affected. Some articulation errors are expected in early childhood, especially involving sounds that are usually mastered at a later age (in English, /l/, /r/, /s/, /z/, /th/, /ch/); these errors are not regarded as pathological unless they persist and result in adverse consequences to the individual. Ninety percent or more of children have mastered the more difficult sounds by age 6 to 8.

Stuttering

Stuttering is the most easily recognized communication disorder. It varies in severity among individuals. It may vary over time and circumstance. It is typically more severe when the affected child is stressed or anxious, and especially when communication is expected. Because of its often gradual onset, children are at first frequently not aware of its presence. Over time they may become more anxious and withdraw from conversation, as the degree of social discrimination they experience increases. Stuttering may be accompanied by various movements which may seem either to express or discharge anxiety, such as blinking, grimacing, or hyperventilation. Children who stutter may sing or talk to themselves without difficulty. Sometimes children may attempt to stop stuttering by slowing down or pausing in their speech; but this is frequently unsuccessful and leads to an exacerbation. Thus a pattern of habitual fear and avoidance emerges.

Communication Disorder Not Otherwise Specified

This category, used to include disorders that do not fit the criteria for any of the other Communication Disorders, is generally used only to describe disorders of voice, including pitch, intonation, volume, or resonance. Hyponasality is characterized by the "adenoidal" speech simulated by speaking with the nose pinched. Hypernasality, secondary to velopharyngeal insufficiency, may be associated with serious voice problems. Air escapes into the nasal cavity, resulting in nasal air emission, snorting or a nasal grimace during speech.

Assessment

Interview and Observation

The psychiatrist seeing children must be familiar with normal milestones of speech and language development and ask the parents or guardians about the child's speech and language, both past and current. Much can be learned from even a few questions: Does the child seem to hear and understand what is being said? Does the child require visual prompts? Does the child in fact use spoken language to communicate? How long and complicated are his sentences? Does the child "make sense" to outsiders? Can she be clearly understood, even by strangers? Which sounds does the child find difficult? Does the child use unusual volume, pitch, or nasality? Does he observe the rules of conversation? Parent–child communication should also be observed.

For younger children, assessment may best be carried out in a play situation. Rutter (1987) recommends that the clinician assess inner language, comprehension, production, phonation and pragmatics. Inner language means symbolization, which may be observed in the child's representational use of play materials. Comprehension is assessed through conversation and the use of developmentally appropriate questions and commands, especially with nonverbal augments or prompts. The clinician should note how well a child can follow and draw inferences from a conversation. Production refers to speech, its fluency and intelligibility. Pragmatics are those aspects of language that render it useful for social communication beyond the most concrete level. Does the child appreciate the nuances of her partner's conversation, as, for example, when they signal beginnings and endings of conversations, topic changes, or the patient's turn to talk? Pragmatic language involves nonverbal elements. Deficiencies in this area impair abstraction and may render the individual almost "robot-like".

In all cases, observations should be made in as relaxed a fashion as possible, avoiding interrogation or rote exercises. If a child fails to communicate a given item, necessary help, including nonverbal prompts, should be offered, so that the child has the experience of success. A sense of failure will stifle communication.

All of the phenomena seen in a clinical interview may also be pursued in school settings, and teacher input is essential in the evaluation of these children.

Developmental and Cultural Influences

The need for a clinician to be aware of normal developmental expectations has been cited. Special sensitivity must be exercised for the range of accents, dialects and conversational styles encountered. English is spoken in an extraordinary range of patterns even within each dialect group. It is essential that one does not pathologize differences in intonation or dialect. Many American children grow up in multilingual environments, and speak with a synthesis of languages, especially during their preschool years. Finally, children of minority groups who have suffered social discrimination and children who live in physically dangerous environments may necessarily be cautious and less forthcoming with language; this may be adaptive in some cases and not a disorder at all.

Differential Diagnosis

Expressive Language Disorders and Mixed Receptive-expressive Disorders

These disorders are distinguished from each other by the presence or absence of receptive problems. Children with autism may have any or all of the characteristics of the language disorders. However, they have many additional problems

Clinical Vignette 1 Phonation Disorder

RD presented as a 5-year-old girl, the only child of professional parents who had attempted for many years prior to her birth to conceive a child. Her birth was received with joy and relief, and her parents admitted to having indulged her, even by their privileged standards. Her developmental history was unremarkable, except for some slight delay in toilet training compared with her agemates. She received appropriate well-child care, and had no major illnesses or injuries. Her adjustment to preschool was considered appropriate when she entered at age 3, and she got along well with the other children for 2 years. She enjoyed the preschool, where individuality was accepted and encouraged. Her parents sought psychiatric evaluation for her after she reported being fearful about returning to school. When her parents questioned her, she stated that new children had come to her school for kindergarten and they were teasing her. The teacher informed the parents that new students were in fact present, but that no teasing had been observed. Upon evaluation, a picture emerged of concerned parents who were sensitive to their child's emotional state, and had sought to remedy their inexperience with children through a great deal of study and inquiry. RD appeared initially as a somewhat anxious child, who separated from her mother with mild trepidation, but who soon relaxed with the psychiatrist. She was able to relate openly, gave no evidence of a major thought or affective disorder, and seemed to be of average intelligence. She exhibited a number of articulation errors, substituting /w/ for /l/ and /r/, and /th/ for /s/, and omitting or dropping a number of closing sounds. She stated that she was shocked at the comments of her new classmates that her speech was infantile. These children were as of yet unaccustomed to the uncritical atmosphere of the school. She had never thought that her speech was unusual, nor had her parents who believed it was normal for a child of her age. The teacher explained that she had noticed some errors in RD's speech, but did not wish to offend her or her parents by pointing them out. The psychiatrist intervened by helping the child to understand that some children adopted "grown-up" speech later than others, and that her progress could be assisted by a helping adult. He referred the family to a speech and language pathologist, whose session the parents described to the child as a "conversation party". The psychiatrist worked with the parents in joint brief focal psychotherapy, addressing issues related to the parents' sense of failure because of their child's problem and their delay in recognizing it. After 6 months, RD's speech had improved and was accepted as normal by her classmates. By age 9 her speech was regarded as entirely normal by her parents and teachers and she was functioning well in all spheres. However, she continued to have subtle phonological findings as an adolescent.

including the use of language in a restricted and often stereotypic fashion, rather than for communicative purposes. They also have difficulties with a wider range of interactions with persons and objects in their environment, and exhibit a restricted range of behaviors. The language impairments of mental retardation, oral-motor deficits, or environmental deprivation are not diagnosed in this category unless they are well in excess of what is expected. Language impairment due to environmental deprivation tends to improve dramatically with environmental improvement. Sensory deficits, especially hearing impairment, may restrict language development. Any indication of potential hearing impairment, no matter how tenuous, should prompt a referral for an audiologic evaluation. Obviously, hearing and language disorders can and do coexist. Some children develop an acquired aphasia as a complication of general medical illness. This condition is usually temporary; only if it persists beyond the acute course of the medical illness is a language disorder diagnosed. A very severe acquired language disorder is seen in Landau-Kleffner Syndrome (acquired epileptic aphasia), accompanied by seizures and other CNS dysfunctions, and usually occurring between the ages of three and nine.

Phonological Disorder and Stuttering

The conditions should be distinguished from normal dysfluencies in young children. For example, misarticulation of some sounds, such as /l/, /r/, /s/, /z/, /th/, and /ch/, is common among preschoolers and resolves with age. As with the language disorders, these diagnoses are given in the case of motor of sensory deficit,

mental retardation, or environmental deprivation only if the disorder is much more severe than expected in these conditions. Problems limited to voice alone are included under Communication Disorder NOS.

Formal Speech and Language Assessment

A number of instruments are available for the assessment of communication. Some of these are listed in Table 26.3. Most are beyond the training of physicians, whose most important contributions are interview skills and medical assessment; but a familiarity with them can help the physician develop a repertoire and knowledge of screening measures. Because of the complex comorbidity of these disorders, they are often best assessed by an interdisciplinary team (McKirdy, 1985; Klykylo, 2005). The team's activities are usually coordinated by a case manager, often a pediatrician or a child and adolescent psychiatrist. Often the team includes an audiologist, a psychologist, medical specialists including pediatric neurologists and otorhinolaryngolists, an educational specialist or liaison special educator, and a speech and language pathologist.

The speech and language pathologist (SLP) has a graduate professional degree and should be certified by The American

Table 26.3 Language Tests		
Tests	Ages	Functions Assessed
Language Tests		
Sequenced Inventory of Communication Development (SICD)	0–4–4–0	Sound discrimination, auditory memory, receptive and expressive language
Test of Early Language Development (TELD)	3–0–7–11	Receptive and expressive language; oral and pointing responses
Test of Language Development (TOLD)	4–0–9–0	Auditory discrimination and memory, receptive and expressive language; oral and pointing responses
Test of Adolescent Language (TOAL)	11–0–17–5	Receptive and expressive language; oral and written responses
Clinical Evaluation of Language Function (CELF)	5–0–17–0	Screening test for auditory memory, receptive and expressive language; oral responses
Fluharty Preschool Speech and Language Screening Test	2–0–6–0	Screening test for articulation and language disorder
Tests of Specific Functions		
Peabody Picture Vocabulary Test (PPVT)	1–9–18–0	Receptive auditory vocabulary; pointing to pictures
Token Test	3–0–12–0	Receptive auditory syntax; following verbal instructions
Goldman-Fristoe-Woodcock Auditory Selective Attention Test	3–0–12–0	Auditory memory; pointing to pictures
Goldman-Fristoe-Woodcock Test of Auditory Discrimination	3–0–adult	Auditory discrimination of words; pointing to pictures
Expressive One-Word Vocabulary Test (EOWVT)	3–0–12–0	Expressive vocabulary; picture naming
Arizona Articulation Proficiency Scale	3–0–11–0	Speech articulation; picture naming

Source: Feinstein C and Aldershof A (1991) Developmental disorders of learning and language, in *Textbook of Child and Adolescent Psychiatry* (ed Wiener JM). American Psychiatric Press, Washington DC.

Speech, Language and Hearing Association (ASHA). The SLP uses a combination of interview techniques, behavioral observations and standardized instruments to identify Communication Disorders, as well as patterns of communication that are not pathologic. The assessment of an SLP is usually the definitive measure of the presence or absence of a Communication Disorder. Families may consult an SLP directly or be referred by other clinicians. The responsibility of psychiatrists and other professionals in this process is simple and straightforward: any suspicion of any communication problem in any patient should prompt referral to a qualified SLP. Even when a disorder appears to be limited and benign, communication evaluation by an SLP can disclose subtle impairments that could have profound consequences. Table 26.4 lists indication for referral.

Course and Natural History

Expressive and Mixed Receptive-expressive Language Disorders

Contrary to some popular beliefs, language disorders do not usually spontaneously resolve. In general, the course of these disorders is lengthy, and the more severe disorders are usually the more persistent. Language disorders of the developmental type generally appear gradually early in life, while those secondary to other medical illnesses tend to occur more precipitously and at any age. In the case of Expressive Language Disorder, DSM-IV-TR reports that most children with this condition acquire more or less normal language abilities by late adolescence, but that subtle deficits may persist. In the case of Mixed Receptive-expressive

---

Table 26.4   Indications for Referral for Communication Evaluation

Language

- The child does not use any single words by 16–18 mo.
- At 18 months, the child cannot follow simple instructions such as "Give me your shoe", or cannot point to body parts or common objects following a verbal request.
- The child does not combine words for short utterances by the age of 2.
- The child does not communicate with complete sentences by the age of 3.
- At 3, the child echoes parts of questions or commands rather than responding appropriately. For example, when asked "What's your name?" The child responds, "Your name".
- Sentence structures are still short and noticeably defective at the age of 4.
- At 4, the child uses words incorrectly, or frequently substitutes an associative word for the intended word. For example, the child may say "cut" for "scissors" or "dog" for "cow".

Articulation

- The child does not babble using consonant sounds (particularly b, m, d, and n) by 8 or 9 mo of age.
- The child uses mostly vowel sounds and gestures for communication after 18 mo.
- The speech is usually unintelligible at the age of 3.
- The child frequently omits consonants in words at the age of 3.
- The speech is difficult to understand at the age of 4.
- At the age of 6, the child is still unable to produce many sounds.
- The child is omitting, substituting, or distorting any sounds after the age of 7.
- The child is embarrassed or disturbed by his speech at any age.

Voice

- The voice is hoarse, harsh, breathy, or of poor quality.
- The voice is always too loud or too soft.
- The pitch is inappropriate for the child's age or sex.
- Pitch breaks occur frequently.
- The voice is hyponasal or hypernasal.
- There is nasal air emission, a nasal "rustle", snorting, or a nasal grimace during speech.

Stuttering

- The parents have expressed a concern about stuttering.
- The child has an abnormal number of repetitions, hesitations, prolongations, blocks, or disruptions in the natural flow of speech.
- The child exhibits tension during speech.
- The child avoids speaking situations due to a fear of stuttering.
- The child considers himself to be a stutterer.

Source: Feinstein C and Aldershof A (1991) Developmental disorders of learning and language, in *Textbook of Child and Adolescent Psychiatry* (ed Wiener JM). American Psychiatric Press, Washington DC.

Language Disorders only a minority of children are free of communication problems in adulthood. Even when their communication skills seem grossly normal, subtle deficits may persist, and they may experience educational difficulties. The prognosis for individuals with acquired language disorders often depends upon the severity of injury or illness, as well as their premorbid state.

Phonation Disorder

The course of Phonation Disorder is much more encouraging than those of other communication disorders. Milder cases may not be discovered until the child starts school. These cases often recover spontaneously, especially if the child does not encounter adverse psychosocial consequences because of his speech. Severe cases associated with anatomic malformations may at times require surgical intervention. Between these two extremes are children who gradually improve, often to the point of total remission, and whose improvement may be accelerated by speech therapy.

Stuttering

Stuttering usually appears in early childhood, at as early as two years of age and frequently around five, with a typically gradual onset. A study by Yairi *et al.* (1993) suggested that often early-appearing stuttering takes on a moderate to severe form. Children are generally not aware of this condition in themselves until it is pointed out to them by others. The disorder can wax and wane during childhood. By early adolescence, it abates spontaneously in some cases, and from 60 to 80% of individuals eventually recover totally or to a major extent. DSM-IV-TR asserts that spontaneous recovery typically occurs before the age of 16. Stuttering may persist into adulthood, often leading to adverse social and occupational consequences.

Treatment

Speech and Language Therapy

Speech and language therapy typically has three major goals:

- the development of communication skills with concurrent remediation of deficits;
- the development of alternative or augmentative communication strategies, where required; and
- the social habilitation of the individual with regard to communication.

The speech and language pathologist plays the most direct role in treatment of these conditions. SLPs employ a wide range of techniques with children that require both science and art. As in child psychotherapy, the participation of parents is necessary. Parent–infant work involves demonstration and modeling of language-stimulation techniques. Individual therapy can usually be begun by three years of age, and early initiation of therapy is frequently recommended. Individual sessions can include formal exercises along with seemingly less structured but nonetheless carefully directed verbal and play interactions. Group therapy can also be used, especially in the development of language skills applied to a social context; but it should not be regarded as a low-budget substitute for individual treatment. Treatment requires regular reassessment, ongoing support to parents and regular reconsultation with other professionals.

The need for clinicians to avoid regarding variations in accent and dialect as pathologic has been cited. Very little empirical literature on cultural variations in communication therapy is extant. McCrary (1992) and others have pointed out the need for cultural sensitivity in treatment, citing the efforts of ASHA in this area.

The treatment of stuttering addresses both the mechanics of speech and associated attitudinal and affective patterns. Guitar (1985) notes that therapists attempt to modify speech rhythm and speed, leading subjects to regularize rhythm and, as a temporary measure, prolong their speech. Treatment also addresses respiration, airflow and "gentle" onset of phonation. Success rates for various treatments of up to 70% have been reported, though with varying follow-up periods and relapse rates. Some speech and language pathologists specialize in the treatment of this disorder.

The Role of the Psychiatrist

Children with these disorders may present for treatment of psychiatric disorders based on or related to communication problems. Thus, the psychiatrist may in the first place be a case finder or case manager, facilitating the evaluation and treatment of these disorders by a multidisciplinary team. The psychiatric comorbidity of these disorders will necessitate the psychiatrist's involvement on many levels, both as a clinician primarily treating a child, and as a therapist, counselor, and agent of advice and support for the entire family.

Individual and family psychotherapy may be a useful augment in reducing the stress these children encounter, even though psychotherapy does not directly address language disorders. The psychotherapist must, in any event, be sensitive to the manner in which communication disorders can affect or interfere with the therapeutic process. Nonverbal augments or prompts should be sensitively provided children who need them.

The role of psychotropic medication in the management of these disorders is mainly limited to the treatment of comorbid psychiatric problems according to standard practices. From time to time, some interest in the use of drugs specifically for these conditions has arisen. The author has received occasional reports of treatment of stuttering in the past with tricyclic antidepressants and, more recently, selective serotonin re-uptake inhibitors. The rationale for these treatments appears to be a hypothetical connection between stuttering and similar compulsive behaviors. These accounts are provocative but do not suggest any real indication for these medications for stuttering alone.

Outcome

Outcome studies of communication therapy, especially for the language disorders, have often been complicated by multiple theories of language development, diagnostic and methodologic variations, lack of standardization of therapeutic techniques, and comorbidity. Thus the literature in this area is relatively sparse and not always conclusive. Nonresponse to initial treatment may be common, requiring patience and persistence. It is important to note in assessing these issues that, even when communication therapy does not lead to apparent improvements in language beyond developmental improvements, it may still facilitate the child's use of extant language for environmental and self-control.

Academic Comorbidity and Outcome

Not surprisingly, children with communication disorders, especially language disorders, are academically vulnerable. Bashir and Scavuzzo (1992) suggest that this vulnerability arises from the persistence of these disorders in the face of the continuing need for language in school. Even if a language disorder has been remediated, children may have failed in the meantime; and it is immensely hard for many children in many schools to succeed again, once they have failed for any reason. A further complication is the comorbidity of Learning Disorders in these children. Of children with language disorders 50% to 75% will have persistent academic problems. They tend to learn less at any given time and learn more slowly than their peers. These children need ongoing comprehensive special educational services and regular re-evaluation of their educational needs.

Children with Phonologic Disorder may also have persistent problems. These are generally less severe than those of language-disordered children, unless both types of disorders are present. Lewis and Fairbairn (1992) reported mild but persistent problems with reading and spelling in individuals with phonologic disorder, even into young adulthood. Subjects tended to improve steadily over time however. Although most of the subjects and all of the adolescents and adults were considered normal speakers, they tended to show subtle phonologic problems on specialized tests. Again, children with an associated language disorder fared less well.

The academic and social consequences of these conditions, as well as their psychiatric comorbidities, require the clinician to be sensitive to their presence and diligent in their remediation.

Comparison of DSM-IV/ICD-10 Diagnostic Criteria

Regarding expressive language disorder, the ICD-10 Diagnostic Criteria for Research suggest specific cutoffs for the expressive language scores: 2 standard deviations below the expected level and 1 standard deviation below nonverbal IQ. Furthermore, in contrast to DSM-IV-TR, the diagnosis cannot be made if there are any neurological, sensory, or physical impairments that directly affect the use of spoken language or if there is mental retardation.

For DSM-IV-TR mixed receptive expressive language disorder, the corresponding ICD-10 disorder is "receptive language disorder". In contrast to DSM-IV which specifies both expressive and receptive language difficulties because these generally occur together, the ICD-10 definition only mentions deviations in language comprehension. As with expressive language disorder, the ICD-10 Diagnostic Criteria for Research suggest a cutoff of receptive language scores of 2 standard deviations below the expected level and 1 standard deviation below nonverbal IQ. Furthermore, in contrast to DSM-IV-TR, the diagnosis cannot be made if there are any neurological, sensory, or physical impairments that directly affect receptive language or if there is mental retardation.

As compared with DSM-IV-TR phonological disorder, in which no mention is made in place of the ICD-10 Diagnostic Criteria for Research suggest that articulation skills, as assessed on standardized tests, be 2 standard deviations below the expected level and 1 standard deviation below nonverbal IQ. Furthermore, in contrast to DSM-IV-TR, the diagnosis cannot be made if there are any neurological, sensory, or physical impairments that directly affect receptive language or if there is mental retardation.

Regarding stuttering, in contrast to DSM-IV-TR which establishes clinical significance based on interference with academic or occupational achievement or with social communication, the ICD-10 Diagnostic Criteria for Research establish clinical significance by requiring a minimum duration of at least 3 months.

References

American Psychiatric Association (2000) *Diagnostic and Statistical Manual of Mental Disorders*, 4th edn., Text Rev. APA, Washington DC.

Baker L (1990) Specific communication disorders, in *Psychiatric Disorders in Children and Adolescents* (eds Garfinkel BD, Carlson GA, and Weller EB). WB Saunders, Philadelphia, pp. 257–270.

Bashir AS and Scavuzzo A (1992) Children with language disorders: Natural history and academic success. *J Learn Disabil* 25(1), 53–65.

Beitchman JH (1985) Speech and language impairment and psychiatric risk: Toward a model of neurodevelopmental immaturity. *Psychiatr Clin N Am* 8, 721–735.

Cantwell DP and Baker L (1991) *Psychiatric and Developmental Disorders in Children with Communication Disorder.* American Psychiatric Press, Washington DC.

Feinstein C and Aldershof A (1991) Developmental disorders of learning and language, in *Textbook of Child and Adolescent Psychiatry* (ed Wiener JM). American Psychiatric Press, Washington DC.

Friel-Patti S (1992) Research in language disorders: What do we know and where are we going? *Folia Phoniatr* 44, 126–142.

Gopnik M and Crago MB (1991) Familial aggregation of a developmental language disorder. *Cognition* 39, 1–50.

Guitar B (1985) Stammering and stuttering, in *The Clinical Guide to Child Psychiatry* (eds Shaffer D, Ehrhardt AA and Greenhill L). Free Press, New York, pp. 97–109.

Helmuth L (2001) From the mouths (and hands) of babes. *Science* 293, 1758–1759.

Kidd K (1983) Genetic aspects of speech and language disorders, in *Genetic Aspects of Speech and Language Disorders* (eds Ludlow C and Cooper J). Academic Press, New York, pp. 197–213.

Klykylo W (2003) Childhood disorders: communication disorders, in *Psychiatry*, 2nd edn (eds Tasman A, Kay J and Lieberman J). Wiley and Sons, London, pp. 743–756.

Lewis BA and Fairbairn L (1992) Residual effects of preschool phonology disorders in grade school, adolescence, and adulthood. *J Speech Hear Res* 35, 819–831.

McCrary MB (1992) Urban multicultural trauma patients. *ASLHA* 34(4), 37–40, 42.

McKirdy LS (1985) Childhood language disorders, in *The Clinical Guide to Child Psychiatry* (eds Shaffer D, Ehrhardt AA and Greenhill L). Free Press, New York, pp. 79–96.

Perkins WH (2001) Stuttering: A matter of bad timing. *Science* 294, 786.

Plomin R and Dale PS (2000) Speech and language impairments in children: Causes, characteristics, intervention, and outcome, in *Speech and Language Impairments in Children* (eds Bishop DVM and Leonard BE). Psychology Press, Hove, East Coast Sussex, pp. 35–51.

Riccio CA, Hynd GW, Morris MJ et al. (1994) Comorbidity of central auditory processing disorder and attention-deficit hyperactivity disorder. *J Am Acad Child Adolesc Psychiatr* 33(6), 849–857.

Rutter M (1987) Assessment objectives and principles, in *Language Development and Disorders* (eds Yule W and Rutter M). JB Lippincott, Philadelphia.

Tomblin JB (1989) Familial concentration of developmental language impairment. *J Speech Hear Disord* 54, 287–295.

Yairi E, Ambrose NG and Niermann R (1993) The early months of stuttering: A developmental study. *J Speech Hear Res* 36, 521–528.

CHAPTER

27

Childhood Disorders: The Autism Spectrum Disorders

Definition

The autism spectrum disorders (ASDs) are a group of neurodevelopmental syndromes characterized by disturbances in social interactions, language and communication, and the presence of stereotyped behaviors and interests. Diagnoses include autistic disorder, Rett's disorder, childhood disintegrative disorder, Asperger's disorder and pervasive developmental disorder not otherwise specified (PDD NOS) (Table 27.1).

History

The contemporary conceptualization of ASD began with Leo Kanner's (1943) description of 11 children with "fascinating peculiarities" that he labeled **early infantile autism**. Kanner noted the lack of social relatedness in these children, including their seeming not to acknowledge the presence of others and their difficulties in recognizing the feelings of others. These children had language irregularities that included a paucity of communicative speech, echolalia and pronoun reversal. Kanner also described their need for sameness and routines, and their engagement in rituals and repetitive activities. The following year, Asperger (1944) described a similar syndrome, but this group had more language and communication skills than the patients reported by Kanner. Asperger called this collection of symptoms **autistic psychopathy**, now referred to as Asperger's disorder.

More recently, the ASDs have been conceptualized as a spectrum of conditions that are related by the common features of the disorders: difficulties in social interactions and use of language, and restricted interests and repetitive behaviors. Despite the enormous heterogeneity evident in this area, there is increasing evidence that conceptualizing these disorders as a spectrum is useful and valid.

Phenomenology

ASDs are notoriously heterogeneous in their presentation: there may be variability in the particular symptoms manifested in any individual at a given point in time and there may be significant levels of comorbidity. Accurate diagnosis requires that the clinician looks for the particular symptoms and signs that characterize it: peculiar and deficient modes of social interaction, deficits in communication and the focused behaviors and interests.

Many consider the disturbance of social development, including difficulty in developing meaningful attachments and interpersonal reciprocity, to be the central impairment in ASD. While many children with ASD will seem aloof and unattached to their parents, many will display age-appropriate separation anxiety. Typically, a child with autistic disorder has abnormal patterns of eye contact and facial expression. When compared with normal children, children with autism fail consistently to maintain eye contact or vary facial expression to establish social. These children seem to have considerable difficulty effectively coordinating social cues. They have difficulty demonstrating empathy or perceiving or anticipating others' moods or responses The child with ASD often acts in a socially inappropriate manner or lacks the social responsiveness needed to succeed in social settings, leading to difficulty in the development of close, meaningful relationships. Some children with ASD eventually develop warm, friendly relationships with family while their relationships with peers lag behind considerably, and these deficits typically persist across time.

It is estimated that only about half of children with autistic disorder develop functional speech. If autistic children do begin to speak, their babble is frequently decreased in quantity and lacking in vocal experimentation. When children with autistic disorder do acquire some speech, it is often peculiar and lacking in social perspective. Some children with autistic disorder are even loquacious, although their speech tends to be repetitious and self-directed rather than aimed at maintaining a reciprocal dialogue. People with autistic disorder commonly make use of stereotyped speech, including immediate and delayed echolalia, pronoun reversal and neologisms. Speech usage is often idiosyncratic, may consist of concrete and poorly constructed grammar, may not be used to convey social meaning, and is often literal, lacking in inference, and lacking in imagination. The delivery of speech is frequently abnormal with atypical tone, pitch and cadence. Paradoxically, children with autistic disorder often have echolalia, in which prosody and other aspects of speech are frequently imitated verbatim.

Individuals with autistic disorder routinely engage in unusual patterns of behavior. Most people with ASD also resist or have significant difficulty with new experiences or transitions. They are commonly resistant to changes in their environment. They often repeatedly perform stereotyped motor acts such as hand clapping or flapping, or peculiar finger movements. These movements frequently occur at the periphery of their vision near their own face. Some children with autistic disorder engage in self-injurious behaviors including biting or striking themselves or banging their heads. This is most likely to occur with severe or profound mental retardation but is also seen in children with autistic disorder without mental retardation. Their play only occasionally involves traditional toys, and objects may be used in

Essentials of Psychiatry Jerald Kay and Allan Tasman
© 2006 John Wiley & Sons, Ltd.

Table 27.1   Comparison of Domains of Diagnostic Criteria for Pervasive Developmental Disorders

	Autistic Disorder	Rett's Disorder	Childhood Disintegrative Disorder	Asperger's Disorder	Pervasive Developmental Disorder NOS
Age at onset	Delays social interaction, language, or play by age or abnormal functioning in 3 yr	Apparently normal prenatal development. Apparently normal motor development for first 5 mo. Deceleration of head growth between ages 5 and 48 mo	Apparently normal development for at least the first 2 yr. Clinically significant loss of previously acquired skills before age 10 yr	No language, cognitive development, or clinically significant delay in development of age-appropriate self-help skills, adaptive behavior, and curiosity about the environment in childhood	Category pervasive impairment in social interaction, and used in cases of communication, with presence of stereotyped behaviors or interests when criteria are not met for a specific disorder
Social interaction	Qualitative least two interaction, as manifested by at impairment in social of the following: • Marked impairment in the use of multiple nonverbal behaviors (e.g., eye-to-eye gaze) • Failure to develop peer relationships appropriate to developmental level • Lack of spontaneous seeking to share enjoyment with other people • Lack of social or emotional reciprocity	Loss in the course (although often social of social engagement early interaction develops later)	Same with loss of social skills (previously acquired) as autistic disorder along	Same as autistic disorder	
Communication	Qualitative communication as manifested by at least one of the impairments of following: • Delay in, or total lack of, the development of spoken language	Severely and receptive language development and severe impaired expressive psychomotor retardation	Same with loss of expressive or receptive as autistic disorder along language previously acquired	No language clinically significant delay in	

Continues

Table 27.1 Comparison of Domains of Diagnostic Criteria for Pervasive Developmental Disorders *Continued*

	Autistic Disorder	Rett's Disorder	Childhood Disintegrative Disorder	Asperger's Disorder	Pervasive Developmental Disorder NOS
	• Marked impairment in initiating or sustaining a conversation with others, in individuals with adequate speech • Stereotyped and repetitive use of language or idiosyncratic language • Lack of varied, spontaneous make-believe, or imitative play				
Behavior	Restricted, stereotyped patterns of behavior, as manifested by one repetitive, and of the following: • Preoccupation with one or more stereotyped or restricted patterns of interest • Adherence to nonfunctional routines or rituals • Stereotyped and repetitive motor mannerisms • Persistent preoccupation with parts of objects	Loss purposeful hand of previously acquired movement Appearance of poorly coordinated gait or trunk movements	Same with loss of bowel or bladder control, as autistic disorder along play, motor skills previously acquired	Same as autistic disorder	
Exclusions	Disturbance by not better accounted for Rett's disorder or childhood disintegrative disorder		Disturbance accounted for by another PDD or schizophrenia not better	Criteria PDD or schizophrenia are not met for another	

Data from American Psychiatric Association (1994) *Diagnostic and Statistical Manual of Mental Disorders*, 4th edn. Copyright, American Psychiatric Association, Washington DC.

ways other than intended (for instance, a doll is used as a hammer), and there is a paucity of make-believe play. Individuals with autistic disorder seem to have unusual sensitivity to some sensory experiences, particularly specific sounds.

Other problems in ASD include impair ment in "joint attention", the sharing or mutual focus on an object or event by two or more people, and the ability to shift attention when the social situation calls for it. Many children with ASD also have symptoms of hyperactivity and difficulty sustaining attention, but these should be distinguished from the joint attentional dysfunction found in all patients with autistic disorder. Examples of joint attention include social exchanges that require pointing, referential gaze and gestures showing interest.

Children with Asperger's disorder begin to speak at about the same time as other children do and eventually gain a full complement of language and syntax. However, they display unusual use of pronouns, continuous repetition of certain words or phrases, and exhaustive focus of speech on particular topics. These children have difficulty in social reciprocity, engage in repetitive play and focus on certain interests excessively. Thus, the predominant differentiating feature between autistic disorder and Asperger's disorder is that those with Asperger's disorder do not have a delay in general (i.e., nonsocial) language development.

Rett's disorder is a developmental disorder that preferentially strikes girls and differs substantially from autistic disorder past the toddler stage. The disorder was first described by Rett when 22 patients were reported in 1966 (Rett, 1966). Typically, a child with Rett's disorder has an uneventful prenatal and perinatal course that continues through at least the first 6 months. With onset of the classic form of the disease, there is deceleration of head growth, usually between 5 months and 4 years of age. In toddlerhood, the manifestations can be similar to autistic disorder in which there is frequently impairment in language and social development, along with the presence of stereotyped motor movements. In particular, there is a loss of acquired language, restricted interest in social contact or interactions, and the start of handwringing, clapping, or tapping in the midline of the body. This type of activity begins after purposeful hand movement is lost. Serious psychomotor retardation sets in as well as receptive and expressive language impairments. Between the ages of 1 and 4 years, truncal apraxia and gait apraxia typically ensue. Since the vast majority of Rett's disorder cases have mutations in *MECP2*, it has been possible to confirm that many variants of Rett's disorder, including those with preserved ambulation and preserved speech, are due to mutations in the same gene (Amir *et al.*, 1999; Kim and Cook, 2000).

Childhood disintegrative disorder and autistic disorder share some similar deficits in social interaction and communication as well as repetitive behaviors. However, the symptoms of childhood disintegrative disorder appear abruptly or in the period of a few months' time after 2 years or more of normal development. There is generally no prior serious illness or insult, although a few cases have been linked to certain brain ailments such as measles, encephalitis, leukodystrophies, or other diseases. With the onset of childhood disintegrative disorder, the child loses previously mastered cognitive, language and motor skills and regresses to such a degree that there is loss of bowel and bladder control (Volkmar and Cohen, 1989). Children with childhood disintegrative disorder tend to lose abilities that would normally allow them to take care of themselves, and their motor activity contains fewer complex, repetitive behaviors

than autistic disorder. Some children with this disorder experience regression that occurs for a time and then becomes stable. Another group of children has a poorer outcome, with onset of focal neurological findings and seizures in the face of a worsening course and greater motor impairment. The majority of children with this disorder deteriorate to a severe level of mental retardation; a few retain selected abilities in specific areas. Differential diagnosis of childhood disintegrative disorder requires obtaining a particularly thorough developmental history, history of course of illness and an extensive neurological evaluation and testing.

PDD NOS or atypical autism should be reserved for cases in which there are qualitative impairments in reciprocal social development, and either communication or imaginative and flexible interests are met, but not full criteria for a specific PDD.

Etiology and Pathophysiology

Currently, the precise etiology and pathogenesis of ASDs are unknown. Strong evidence for genetic bases for the disorders, along with the advent of sophisticated genetic techniques, has led to a shift toward looking for the genetic underpinnings in the disorder. Most contemporary etiological theories strongly suggest a genetic or other early neurodevelopmental disruption with overt clinical manifestations potentially modified by social or environmental experiences.

Biochemical Findings in ASD

Serotonin dysfunction has been implicated as a possible factor in the genesis of autistic disorder since the finding of significantly elevated whole blood 5-HT in these patients. Hyperserotonemia is a robust finding in autistic disorder and has been consistently replicated.

In nonautistic children, serotonin synthesis capacity, as measured by positron emission tomography (PET), is more than 200% adult levels until the age of 5, when it begins to decline toward adult levels; in autistic children, however, serotonin synthesis capacity has been shown to increase gradually between the ages of 2 and 15, reaching a level of 1.5 times normal adult levels (Chugani *et al.*, 1999). In related studies others have shown that platelet serotonin levels appear to stabilize after the age of 12 (Ritvo *et al.*, 1971).

Hyperserotonemia in autistic disorder appears to have a familial component Several studies have shown that whole blood serotonin levels have a positive correlation between probands with autism and their parents and siblings (Leventhal *et al.*, 1990). Additionally, individuals with autism who have siblings with autism have higher platelet serotonin than autistic subjects without an autistic sibling, suggesting that hyperserotonemia may be an indicator of autism with a higher risk of sibling recurrence (Cook and Leventhal, 1996).

It is clear that it is serotonin within platelets that is responsible for the findings of increased whole blood hyperserotonemia. More than 99% of whole blood serotonin is contained in platelets, and platelet-poor plasma ultrafiltrate serotonin levels are not elevated in subjects with hyperserotonemia. This suggests that patients with autism exhibit either increased serotonergic uptake in platelets, or decreased serotonergic release from platelets, leading to an increased steady-state level of serotonin. There is evidence for a positive correlation between platelet serotonin levels and the rate of platelet serotonin transport.

Neuropathological Findings in ASD

Some investigators have found evidence for differences in the hippocampus and amygdala. While noting no gross abnormalities in their study of the brains of six autistic individuals, they have noted increased cell packing and diminished neuronal size in the hippocampus and some nuclei in the amygdala. They also found decreased complexity and extent of dendritic arbors in hippocampal pyramidal cells. They speculated that such lesions might produce changes in behavior similar to those with Klüver Bucy Syndrome (hyperexploratory behavior, severe impairment of social interaction) and some cases of limbic injuries leading to memory loss (and a subsequent "rigidly specific habit memory system"). Others (Bachevalier, 1994) have suggested that such changes might result in difficulty in assigning affective significance to social stimuli.

A number of investigators have noted loss of cerebellar Purkinje cells as well as changes in neurons of the deep cerebellar nuclei. Such findings have led to the hypothesis that these lesions could affect selective attention, in particular leading to stimulus overselectivity and difficulties in shifting attention.

Functional Neuroimaging Findings in ASD

Haznedar and colleagues (1997) found reductions in portions of the right anterior cingulate during a word list learning task, and Schifter (1994) found hypometabolism in many brain regions during a resting state PET scan of autistic children with both mental retardation and seizure disorders. Chugani and colleagues (1996) conducted PET scans on patients with infantile spasms, and found that 10 of 14 children that had bitemporal hypometabolism met criteria for ASD at a later follow-up. Using PET and functional magnetic resonance imaging, Muller and colleagues (1998) showed that a small group of high functioning ASD adults had reversal of the usual left hemisphere dominance when listening to sentences.

Chugani and colleagues (1997) scanned autistic children utilizing an analog of tryptophan to act as a tracer in order to look at serotonin synthesis in the brain. She found asymmetries in serotonin synthesis in many of the autistic subjects. She also found that the global cerebral serotonin synthesis capacity of ASD children tended to increase with age (versus control subjects that show a steady decrease with age towards adult levels). Similar methods using a tracer to look at dopamine storage and metabolism have revealed that accumulation of this tracer was significantly reduced in the anterior medial prefrontal cortex compared with controls.

Genetics and ASD

ASD has a relatively low prevalence of approximately two per 1000, yet the recurrence risk to siblings is 4 to 5%. Concordance in monozygotic twin pairs has ranged from 60 to 90%, while dizygotic twin pairs in these studies have generally found a concordance similar to that found in siblings of affected children. Even these concordance numbers are likely underestimates of the genetic contribution, since many pairs discordant for autistic disorder were concordant for another ASD. When considered as a spectrum disorder, twin studies suggest that at least 92% of monozygotic twin pairs are concordant for at least milder but similar deficits in the social and communication realms (compared with a 10% rate in these studies for dizygotic twin pairs).

Table 27.2	Chromosomal Abnormalities Associated with Autistic Disorder or Other Pervasive Developmental Disorders

Fragile X syndrome (trinucleotide expansion at Xq27.3)
Down's syndrome (trisomy 21)
Prader-Willi syndrome (deletion or maternal isodisomy of chromosome 15)
Marker chromosome
Duplication of 15q11–13

ASD is currently thought to be a complex genetic disorder. The varying strength of the contributions of different loci is likely also to be responsible for the genetic heterogeneity that characterizes ASD. In ASD, findings so far suggest a disease process with greater than 10, and perhaps as many as 100 loci.

Chromosomal abnormalities have provided some clues as to where some of these susceptibility genes may be (Table 27.2). The most common chromosomal abnormality associated with ASD has been in a region of chromosome 15 (15q11–13). These abnormalities usually involve either an interstitial duplication or a supernumerary pseudodicentric chromosome (an extra chromosome with two centromeres; "pseudo" refers to the fact that only one centromere can be active).

Linkage studies have shown evidence of linkage in several polymorphisms in the area of chromosome 15 noted above, including the gamma-aminobutyric acid receptor subunit gene (*GABRB3*) and transmission disequilibrium for markers in *GABRB3* has also been found. Most recently, evidence of transmission disequilibrium was found to peak at another region of the serotonin transporter gene, supporting evidence of involvement of the gene, but not specifically the *5HTTLPR* variant (Kim *et al.*, 2002).

There has been significant progress in terms of identifying the genetic basis of Rett's syndrome. Mutations in the gene (*MECP2*) encoding X-linked methyl-CpG-binding protein 2 (MeCP2) have been identified as the cause of more than 80% of classic cases of Rett's syndrome.

Autistic Disorder and MMR Vaccinations

Some have suggested that there is a variant of ASD called **autistic enterocolitis** that involves developmental regression and gastrointestinal symptoms, and that this variant is a consequence of measles–mumps–rubella (MMR) immunization. This hypothesis, which has been postulated to account for the rise in the number of cases of ASD, suggests that there are specific biological findings in these children that result from a persistent measles viral infection. At the current time, investigations into this hypothesis have shown no relationship between MMR vaccinations and the development of ASD; this lack of evidence argues against changes in MMR vaccination programs.

Assessment and Differential Diagnosis

The diagnosis of ASD first involves completing a comprehensive psychiatric examination (Table 27.3). The clinician should obtain a full developmental history, including all information regarding pregnancy and delivery. While questioning about neonatal development, particular attention should be paid to

Table 27.3	**Suggested Work-up for Children and Adults with Autistic Disorder or Other Pervasive Developmental Disorders**

History
   Particular attention to
      Developmental phases of language, social interactions, play
      Family history of psychiatric and neurological disease
Physical examination
   Thorough physical examination including a search for
      Neurological problems
      Cardiac problems
      Congenital anomalies
      Skin lesions or abnormalities
      Dysmorphology
Psychological evaluation
   Autism Diagnostic Interview-revised
   Autism Diagnostic Observation Schedule
   Cognitive testing (e.g., Differential Abilities Scales)
   Vineland Adaptive Behavior Scales
Speech and language evaluation
Audiological evaluation
Visual acuity evaluation

social, communicative and motor milestones. The clinician needs to understand fully the child's adaptive skills, including which tasks can be undertaken independently, including grooming skills, feeding skills and the ability to self-initiate. There should be a sense of the child's vocabulary, receptive and expressive language skills, articulation and pragmatic communication. A full medical history should be obtained, and should include queries regarding any hearing or vision problems, any history of seizures and information regarding the use of any medications.

Because these children dislike novelty, the first visit to the clinician's office is sometimes an anxiety-provoking undertaking. It is not unusual (and is in fact helpful diagnostically) to allow a child with ASD to extensively explore the clinician's office, looking under desks or opening drawers, in an attempt to become familiar with the surroundings. Some children will appear shy and self-absorbed. It is ideal if the clinician can arrange an opportunity to see the child in another environment in addition to the office. Observation of the child interacting with the parents and siblings is helpful in understanding modes of interaction and social skills. If the child is having difficulty, it is usually preferable, especially on the first visit, to allow the parents to intervene. This will allow the clinician to see how (effectively) the family responds to this distress, and how the child responds to the efforts of caregivers to soothe the child. During observation, the clinician needs to assess social interaction, communication, unusual behaviors and all other information in the context of developmental level.

A full physical examination should be undertaken including observations for dysmorphic features and unusual dermatologic lesions. The clinician must maintain a high suspicion for seizures in this population, both when taking the history and during the examination. A full neurological examination should be made with an emphasis on motor impairments. A Wood's light examination for hypopigmented lesions consistent with tuberous sclerosis should be made.

There are no diagnostic laboratory tests for ASD. If the child has not had routine tests (blood count, liver function tests, thyroid, lead level, etc.), these should be completed, as with any child. Patients with mental retardation or dysmorphology should have chromosomal analysis performed. Fragile X testing and fluorescent in situ hybridization (FISH) studies for possible interstitial duplication of 15q11–13 should be suggested after consultation with the family. There should be a low threshold for ordering an electroencephalogram (EEG), and one should always be ordered in the context of unusual movements, regressive behavior, regressive loss of previously acquired sleep, or in the face of unusually poor sleep. Structural brain imaging (i.e., MRI) should take place only if the physical examination or history suggests that a treatable lesion is present. Carried out routinely, these scans have a very low clinical yield, are quite expensive, and in this population often require anesthesia, a seemingly unnecessary risk. Consultative services should be utilized as needed with pediatric neurologists and geneticists. Difficulties with motor development will often mean a referral to an occupational and/or physical therapist. Children with Rett's syndrome will often require referral to neurologists and developmental pediatricians.

All children with autism require a careful language assessment that may include hearing testing and assessment of expressive and receptive, verbal and nonverbal language. Speech and language therapists trained to work with this population are an essential part of the assessment team.

Children with ASD should have a neuropsychological assessment at the time of initial assessment and at periodic intervals thereafter. The initial evaluation helps establish the diagnosis and a baseline level of functioning. Additionally, it can be utilized to make the appropriate adjustments in the child's educational plan. The later evaluations serve to chart progress, evaluate the success of (pharmacological, behavioral and academic) interventions, and to assess for possible regression in particular areas.

While there are many rating scales and structured interviews to assist in making the diagnosis of ASD, the current gold standard in diagnostic assessment is the autism diagnostic observation schedule-generic (ADOS-G) (Lord *et al.*, 2000). This is often given with the autism diagnostic inventory-revised (ADI-R) (Lord *et al.*, 1994), which is a comprehensive, clinician-administered interview of the patient's primary caregiver and covers most developmental and behavioral aspects of autism. The ADI/ADOS combination is now established as a reliable and valid method for making the diagnosis of ASD.

Differential Diagnosis

There may initially be some difficulty in differentiating ASD from other syndromes (Table 27.4), especially in the context of considerable comorbidity. Mental retardation commonly occurs in ASD, and children with mental retardation may present with stereotyped movements or obsessiveness. However, the child with mental retardation and not with ASD will have social and communicative skills commensurate with their level of overall development.

Differentiating ASD from childhood schizophrenia is not usually difficult. The onset of psychosis in childhood is extraordinarily rare, and hallucinations and delusions are not a part of the ASD picture. It is important not to diagnose some of the atypical features in ASD as psychotic and equally important to recognize that verbal patients with ASD have impaired language that should not be confused with schizophrenia. Selective mutism

Table 27.4	Differential Diagnosis of Autistic Disorder and Other Pervasive Developmental Disorders

Developmental language disorder
Mental retardation
Acquired epileptic aphasia (Landau-Kleffner's syndrome)
Fragile X syndrome
Schizophrenia
Selective mutism
Psychosocial deprivation
Hearing impairment
Visual impairment
Traumatic brain injury
Dementia
Metabolic disorders (inborn errors of metabolism, e.g., phenylketonuria)

can be differentiated by the child's ability to interact normally in some environments.

Children exposed to severe neglect can sometimes present with symptoms that look like ASD, but these symptoms will usually show dramatic improvement when the child is in a more appropriate environment.

Perhaps the most difficult differentiation is in a child with severe obsessive–compulsive disorder (OCD) who also has unusual interests and is inflexible to changes in routines or transitions to a new activity. It is even further complicated if attentional problems coexist. In these cases, it is important to emphasize the social difficulties of children with ASD; even if the child with OCD is difficult interpersonally, his or her ability to maintain eye contact, interpret social situations and emotions and otherwise interact socially is relatively preserved.

Epidemiology and Comorbidity

Large scale epidemiologic studies of early childhood onset neuropsychiatric disorder simply have not been undertaken thus making prevalence rates of many pediatric onset disorders relatively obscure. It is also worth noting that disorders that are relatively uncommon pose particular problems when it comes to the ascertainment of prevalence rates.

Increased awareness of ASD through laudable efforts at better education of mental health workers, pediatricians and school personnel has led to better (and earlier) identification of the core symptoms that had previously gone undiagnosed.

While there is no definitive way to know what accounts for the rise in ASD (and an increase due to, for instance, an environmental insult cannot be ruled out), the current informed consensus is that this increased prevalence rate reflects better recognition and detection together with more inclusive diagnostic definitions.

Boys are affected with ASD more than girls in a 4 : 1 ratio. The exception is Rett's disorder, which is found almost exclusively in females. Interestingly, the gender ratio in ASD increases when cases with mental retardation are excluded to about 6 : 1, and decreases to approximately 1.7 : 1 when only cases with moderate to severe mental retardation are considered.

The prevalence rates of ASD do not appear to be influenced by immigrant status or socioeconomic status.

With the exception of childhood disintegrative disorder (in which all affected children are mentally retarded), there is wide individual variability in intellectual functioning in ASD. Only about 20 to 25% of children with ASD have an IQ over 70, with 30 to 35% having mild to moderate mental retardation, and 40 to 45% having severe to profound mental retardation. However, with more intensive case-finding (i.e., less dependence on mental retardation for referral), the number of patients with ASD who have an IQ over 70 may be as high as 50%. Follow-up studies suggest that IQ levels tend to be constant from the time of diagnosis (when over 5 years old at the time of diagnosis) and are stable over time, and thus are thought to be important predictors of outcome. Particular cognitive deficits are seen in language, abstraction, sequencing and coding operations, while visual–spatial skills are often a relative strength (Lord et al; 1997, Rutter 1983).

Course

Retrospective analysis of some children reveals deficits in the first year of life while those with less severe symptoms may not be diagnosed until their first years of school or, in the case of higher functioning persons with ASD, even later. It is not uncommon (15–22%) for deterioration in functioning with the onset of puberty, characterized by mood lability, aggressiveness and hyperactivity. It has also been suggested that low IQ, female sex, epilepsy and family history of mood difficulties may be risk factors for this pubertal deterioration. Others have reported that some individuals with ASD improve during their teen years.

Episodes of depression are common for patients with ASD in their teens, especially among those with Asperger's syndrome. It has been hypothesized that this may be a function of these patients' better recognition of their social inadequacies. This may also lead to subsequent demoralization and dysphoria.

Epilepsy presents in a bimodal fashion, with many children first experiencing seizures before starting school, and another group having their onset at the time of puberty; overall, 25 to 30% of patients will experience seizures before the age of 30. It should be noted that there is an inverse correlation between the incidence of seizures and cognitive level.

Long-term follow-up studies predict for a poor or very poor long-term outcome for up to 75% of cases, and a good outcome (using social life, and school or vocational functioning as outcome measures) in only 5 to 15%. It appears that IQ is the best predictor of outcome. There is wide variability in final outcome, with most patients with low IQs unable to live independently, and with many high functioning patients able to work (sometimes very successfully) and live independently, as well as raise children.

Treatment

Nonpharmacological and Behavioral Treatments

Developing a comprehensive individual intervention program for a child with ASD is a daunting task for the child's parents (Figure 27.1). Each child is unique, with a different set of difficulties, as well as strengths. The child's primary physician must work with the parents to help make this task less overwhelming. The physician can anticipate being asked about a wide array of alternative treatments being offered in the community, which vary enormously in their claims, in the integrity of those making the

Identification of developmental delay by caretaker

↓↓
↓↓

Evaluation by pediatrician

↓↓
↓↓ Referral for specialty testing
↓↓

ADOS, ADI, measures of intellectual functioning and daily functioning, full physical, history, and labs

↓↓
↓↓ Autism spectrum disorder established
↓↓

Initiation of treatment includes:

1. Implementing changes in the child's academic program including relevant changes in the curriculum in order to tailor it to the child's specific needs, as well as probable speech, occupational, and physical therapy.

2. The use of behavioral programs in order to improve social and communication difficulties as well as address negative behaviors.

3. Examination of any symptoms that may be potential target symptoms for a pharmacological intervention.

Figure 27.1 *An example of the typical progression from identification, to evaluation, to treatment of a child with ASD (ADOS, Autism Diagnostic Observation Schedule; ADI, Autism Diagnostic Inventory).*

claims, and in their ultimate safety and utility. The physician who immediately and outright and pejoratively dismisses these alternatives as useless is not helpful to the child or his family (the exception being dangerous or cost-prohibitive prospective treatments). Rather, it is helpful to listen and then educate the family, at a level commensurate with their sophistication, about how to analyze and interpret claims and science underlying these treatments.

Autistic disorder is recognized as a chronic disorder with a changing course requiring a long-term course of treatment that includes the necessity of an intervention with various treatments at different times. At the present time, most treatments for the ASDs are symptom directed. Given that there is no current cure for autistic disorder or the other ASD, goals of treatment should encompass short-term and long-term needs of the individual and his or her family (Table 27.5).

Every attempt should be made to achieve treatment goals on a community-based environment since institutionalization may hinder a child's ability to learn means of functioning and adapting in typical social settings. Community-based treatment can usually be maintained, except in times of extreme stress or need, during which time a child (and family) might benefit from respite care or brief hospitalization. Effective treatment often entails setting appropriate expectations for the child and adjusting the child's environment to foster success.

Approach to Treatment

Because the autistic individual often requires diverse treatments and services simultaneously, the role of the primary physician is to be the coordinator of services. Frequent visits with the child and the child's caretakers initially allow the physician to assess the individual needs of the child while establishing a therapeutic alliance. An effective approach often calls for the services of a number of professionals working in a multidisciplinary fashion. This group may include psychiatrists, pediatricians, pediatric neurologists, psychologists, special educators, speech and language therapists social workers, and other specialized therapists (Table 27.6).

Table 27.5 Goals for Treatment
Advancement of normal development, particularly regarding cognition, language and socialization
Promotion of learning and problem solving
Reduction of behaviors that impede learning
Assistance of families coping with autistic disorder
Treatment of comorbid psychiatric disorders

Table 27.6 Summary of Treatment Principles
Psychosocial interventions
Educational
Curricula that target communication
Behavioral techniques
Structured milieu
Vocational interventions such as speech training and placement: other specialized and language therapy, physical therapy and occupational therapy
Social skills training
Individual psychotherapy for high-functioning individuals
Medical Interventions
Cohesive physician–patient relationship
Supportive measures with families coping with autistic disorder
Behavioral treatment
Pharmacotherapy to address problem signs and symptoms

There is significant controversy over what particular forms of therapy are best for children with ASD. Some of this controversy is a result of claims of children making dramatic improvements with some of these therapies.

The most successful interventions use a variety of positive reinforcement schedules to enhance the desired behaviors and extinguish undesirable behaviors. Discrete trial training, an operant conditioning model, is particularly useful in this regard. Generalization of skills from the behavioral training environment to other settings is a key to success. Applied behavioral analysis (ABA) uses careful assessment of adaptive and maladaptive behaviors and specific interventions addressing each behavior and children receiving ABA have shown significant improvement in a number of areas, including IQ, visual–spatial skills, language, and academics (Smith *et al.* 2001).

Problem Behaviors

A prerequisite to putting a behavioral plan in place with a child with ASD is to identify the problem behaviors. These behaviors often include interfering repetitive actions, self-injurious behaviors, or aggression. While there is little difficulty in identifying these highly visible behaviors, what is much more difficult is 1) determining the antecedents to these behaviors and 2) knowing what constitutes an appropriate reaction or consequence to these behaviors on the part of the caregiver.

To determine the antecedent is often extraordinarily difficult, since it is often not apparent exactly what happened in the environment that stimulated the behavior. This is particularly true if the behavior is chronic and has developed some autonomous function (i.e., no longer a stimulus–response event). To make things more complicated, it could be internal perception or meaning of what happened in a child with autism (poor language and socially nonresponsive) that may have initiated the behavior. For example, imagine a nonverbal child frustrated by his inability to continue a mental routine created by a teacher insisting that the child orient himself to a school task like sitting in reading circle. Further, assume that the child does not have a repertoire of appropriate social responses, and instead responds by biting the teacher on the arm. It will be very difficult for the teacher to know that the child was in the middle of a mental routine and not able to communicate his distress verbally, thus leading to the inappropriate behavior. It takes time and attention to understand these events processes in children with ASD. Once they are clear, appropriate behavioral intervention is possible.

Durand and Carr (1991) attempted to determine the function of problem behaviors in children with ASD. They concluded that most behaviors could be classified as:

1. a need for help;
2. a desire to escape a stressful situation;
3. a desire to obtain an object;
4. an attempt to protest unwanted events;
5. an attempt to obtain stimulation or attention.

There are scales available to help caretakers determine the primary functions behind typical problem behaviors. Despite the notorious difficulty in determining the function of a problem behavior in these children, if the function(s) can be identified, a behavioral intervention will likely be successful in diminishing the atypical, maladaptive behavior and enhance overall adaptation and behavioral functioning.

Obsessions and Rituals

Children with ASD often engage in rituals and routines which appear to be an attempt to relieve anxiety and/or to exert control over their environment. The key to success is a gradual shaping of the behavior rather than dramatic expectations and harsh consequences. One should begin intervention by evaluating possible, underlying stimuli or predisposing factors for the behavior. Strategies include determining when, where and for how long an activity can take place. Additional strategies include making environmental changes that reduce anxiety and even ignoring behaviors that do not create undue problems. Adjunct pharmacological intervention is often helpful.

Communication Therapy

Up to 50% of children with ASD will not acquire useful language. For those with some but not fully intact language skills, speech therapy is an important part of therapeutic and academic planning. An emphasis on the social use of language is often helpful, and when the child can articulate some of his or her needs, there is often a reduction in problem behaviors.

Longitudinal studies indicate that children who have not acquired useful language by the age of 7 usually have longstanding verbal communication difficulties. For these children, it is often helpful to devise an alternative means of communication: sign language or use of augmentative communication devices such as computers and picture exchange communication systems or PECS. PECS involves the use of photographs or line drawings on cards. The child then points to or hands the appropriate card or cards to another person in order to effect communication. Once again, children are encouraged to use verbalization, when possible, in conjunction with sharing the cards (Erdmann *et al.*, 1996). Irrespective of the technique used, establishing a consistent method of communication is central to the treatment of individuals with ASD.

Social Interaction Therapy

Children and adults with ASD lack many of the innate and learned social skills, especially reciprocal social interactions, that most people simply take for granted. Maintaining appropriate interpersonal distance, spontaneously initiating conversation, participating in reciprocal social exchange and other facets of complex social interaction are not easily incorporated in the routine behaviors and activities of individuals with ASDs. Subtlety and changing complexity of social interaction as well as the innateness of many social skills is a central part of daily life and a key to successful adaptation for typically functioning individuals. Helping individuals with ASDs address these challenges is difficult but also critical for enhancing overall functioning.

Odom and Strain (1986) identified the three primary techniques that can be effectively utilized:

1. Proximity. Establish proximity refers to the fact that it is very helpful to have the child with ASD near other children in the environment. The mere proximity increases the likelihood of interaction and imitation as well as positive social reinforcement.
2. Use. The use of prompts relates to have specific prompts and reinforcement cues to use previously learned behaviors in social settings (e.g., "Raise your hand if you have a question"). Attention to reinforcement means that even a less than fully competent attempt at appropriate social behavior, even if response to a prompt, receive clear and effective reinforcement

when it occurs (e.g., calling on the child promptly when he raises his hand to ask a question and also saying "You did a good job when you raised your hand to ask the question").

Encourage peer initiation is helpful to train peers who are likely to interact with the child or adult with ASD in techniques for initiating social contact. For many individuals, this means explaining the disability and dealing with fears or biases. For others, it may mean encouraging them to persist in their attempts at engagement, even in the face of limited, inappropriate, or inadequate responses.

Academic Needs

Academic resources and placement are important components in the child's overall treatment. First and foremost, schools are where children go to acquire social skills and acquaintances, as well as academic skills. Secondly, schools often have a variety of skilled professionals who are trained to provide necessary services for the individual with ASD. And, finally, in the USA, all public schools have a statutory obligation to provide all children (even those with disabilities) with a free and appropriate education in the least restrictive environment.

Previously, children with ASD had been put in alternative settings, but more recently there has been increased interest in maintaining many ASD children in regular classroom settings. Studies seem to indicate that ASD children in regular classrooms have increased social interaction, a larger social network and have more advanced individualized education plan goals later in their academic careers (Fryxell and Kennedy, 1995). Whether a child is fully or partially included in a regular classroom or placed in a self-contained setting, each ASD child will need to have an individualized plan of care that carefully and specifically articulates goals and the techniques to be used to reach those goals. In addition, specific measures of goal attainment and regular review of the plan should be a part of this important intervention. In order to establish these goals and plans, a full assessment of the child's strengths and weaknesses must be completed through the efforts of numerous skilled professionals. Educational plans must incorporate academic, social and behavioral goals.

Pharmacotherapy

At this time, there are no pharmacological agents with US Food and Drug Administration (FDA)-approved labeling specific for the treatment of ASD in either children or adults. Many of the symptoms commonly seen in ASD (rituals, aggressive behavior and hyperactivity) are also commonly seen in children, adolescents and adults with mental retardation but without a PDD. Some of the pharmacological strategies for the treatment of autistic disorder have been extrapolated from studies of related conditions, largely in adults, but including attention-deficit/hyperactivity disorder and OCD. Clinicians and families should be reminded before any treatment is initiated that:

- Current treatments target symptoms.
- Current treatments do not target a specific etiological mechanism for ASD.
- Anecdotal reports do not establish efficacy, effectiveness, or safety for any treatment.
- Controlled, double-blind trials (preferably with replication) are the contemporary standard for determining if a treatment is safe and appropriate.
- All treatments have side effects.

Before specific pharmacological agents are discussed, it must be stressed that one should not use psychopharmacological agents with the expectation that they will cure children with autistic disorder as many parents and teachers of children with autistic disorder expect medication to eliminate core social, cognitive and communication dysfunction. There is no pharmacological substitute for appropriate educational, behavioral, psychotherapeutic, vocational and recreational programming. It is essential to remember and to remind parents, teachers and others that medication should always be seen as an adjunct to these core interventions that address the developmental challenges associated with these disorders.

Because many individuals with ASD have impairments in language and social communication, the use of rating scales becomes an essential part of the treatment. Standard rating scales provide the pharmacotherapist with a framework in which to assess response to medication and a relatively straightforward way to collect standard information about the patient's functioning in a variety of settings. The Aberrant Behavior Checklist – Community Version (Aman, 1994) covers many target symptom areas for most patients with ASD. Although rating scales cannot replace careful clinical examination of the patient and interviews with parents and teachers, they may be graphed next to dosages of medications to assist in treatment planning in response to the patient's clinical condition. This is often not only helpful in making clinical decisions but also gives families and service providers a concrete sense of how a treatment is progressing.

The use of medications to treat autistic disorder and other ASDs appears to have significant potential as an adjunct to educational, environmental and social interventions. It is a reasonable goal for the pharmacotherapist to adopt the judicious use of psychopharmacological agents to assist in alleviating symptoms that have been found to respond to pharmacological intervention (Table 27.7). This focus on facilitating adaptation requires attention to five important principles:

1. Environmental manipulations, including behavioral treatment, may be as effective as, if not more effective than, medication for selected symptomatic treatment.
2. It is essential that the living arrangement for the individual must ensure safe and consistent administration and monitoring of the medication to be used.
3. Individuals with autistic disorder and other ASDs often have other DSM-IV-TR Axis I disorders. If a comorbid DSM-IV-TR Axis I disorder is present, standard treatment for that disorder should be initiated first.
4. Medication should be selected on the basis of potential effects on target symptoms and there should be an established way of specifically monitoring the response to the treatment over time.

Table 27.7 Summary of Pharmacotherapy Principles
Psychosocial interventions should accompany medication treatment.
The individual's living arrangement must ensure safe, consistent administration of medications.
Maintain a high index of suspicion for comorbid disorders and treat these appropriately.
Establish a means of monitoring effects of medications on symptoms over time.
Assess the risk/benefit ratio of starting medications and educate the patient and family about these.

5. A careful assessment of the risk/benefit ratio must be made before initiating treatment and, to the extent possible, the patient's caretakers and the patient must understand the risks and benefits of the treatment.

Potent Serotonin Transporter Inhibitors

This class of agents includes selective serotonin reuptake inhibitors (SSRIs) as well as the less selective but potent clomipramine, a tricyclic antidepressant (Table 27.8). This group of medications is most effective when insistence on routines or rituals are present to the point of manifest anxiety or aggression in response to interruption of the routines or rituals, or after the onset of another disorder such as major depressive disorder or OCD. The common side effects associated with SSRIs are motor restlessness, insomnia, elation, irritability and decreased appetite. Because many of these symptoms may be present in the often cyclical natural course of ASD before the medication is initiated, the emergence of new symptoms, a different quality of the symptoms, and occurrence of these symptoms in a new cluster are clues that the symptoms are side effects of medication rather than part of the natural course of the disorder.

Stimulants

Small but significant reductions in inattention and hyperactivity ratings may be seen in children with autistic disorder in response to stimulants such as methylphenidate and dextroamphetamine.

| Table 27.8 | Psychopharmacological Approach to Presenting Symptoms in Pervasive Developmental Disorders |

Rituals, Compulsions, Irritability

Potent serotonin transporter inhibitors
  Selective serotonin reuptake inhibitor
    Fluoxetine 5–80 mg/d in a single dose
    Paroxetine 2.5–50 mg/d in one or two divided doses
    Sertraline 25–200 mg/d in one or two divided doses
    Fluvoxamine 25–300 mg/d in two or three divided doses
    Citalopram 5–40 mg/d in a single or two divided doses
  Tricyclic antidepressants
    Clomipramine 25–250 mg/d in one or two divided doses

Hyperactivity, Distractibility, Impulsivity

Stimulant medications
  Methylphenidate 5–60 mg/d in three to five divided doses
  Dextroamphetamine 5–60 mg/d in three to five divided doses
Clonidine 0.05–0.3 mg/d in one to three divided doses or by transdermal skin patch
Naltrexone 0.5–2.0 mg/kg/d in a single dose

Aggression, Irritability

Sympatholytics
  Propranolol 20–400 mg/d in three to four divided doses
  Nadolol 40–400 mg/d in a single dose
Anticonvulsants
  Carbamazepine to a blood level of 4–12 ng/mL
  Valproate to a blood level of 50–100 ng/mL
Lithium to a serum level of 0.8–1.2 mEq/L
Neuroleptics
Naltrexone 0.5–2.0 mg/kg/d in a single dose

In a placebo-controlled crossover study, eight of 13 subjects showed a reduction of at least 50% on methylphenidate (Handen *et al.*, 2000). However, stereotypies may worsen, so drug trials for the individual patient must always be assessed to determine whether the therapeutic effects outweigh side effects. A key distinction in assessing attentional problems of children with ASD is the distinction between poor sustained attention (characteristic of children with attention-deficit/hyperactivity disorder) and poor joint attention (characteristic of children with autistic disorder). Problems in joint attention require educational and behavioral interventions or treatment of rituals with an SSRI. Problems in maintenance of attention of the type seen in attention-deficit/hyperactivity disorder are more likely to respond to stimulants.

Sympatholytics

The alpha-2-adrenergic receptor agonist clonidine reduced irritability as well as hyperactivity and impulsivity in two double-blind, placebo-controlled trials. However, tolerance developed several months after initiation of the treatment in each child who was treated long term but may have been reduced in several cases by administering clonidine in the morning and then 6 to 8 hours later with a 16- to 18-hour interval between the last dose of one day and the first dose of the next day. If tolerance does develop, the dose should not be increased because tolerance to sedation does not occur, and sedation may lead to increased aggression due to disinhibition or decreased cognitive control of impulses. Adrenergic receptor antagonists, such as propranolol and naldolol, have not been tested in double-blind trials in ASD. However, open trials have reported the use of these medications in the treatment of aggression and impulsivity in developmental disorders including autistic disorder.

Neuroleptics

Typical Neuroleptics

Because they were among the first modern psychopharmacological agents, typical neuroleptics have been among the most extensively studied drugs in autistic disorder. Trifluoperazine, thioridazine, haloperidol and pimozide have been studied in double-blind, controlled trials lasting from 2 to 6 months. Reduction of fidgetiness, interpersonal withdrawal, speech deviance and stereotypes has been documented in response to these. However, patients with autistic disorder are as vulnerable to potentially irreversible tardive dyskinesia as any other group of young patients. Owing to the often earlier age at initiation of pharmacotherapy, patients with ASD treated with typical neuroleptics may be at higher risk because of the potential increased lifetime exposure of medication limiting their routine use in the care of patients with ASD, especially as first-line treatments.

Atypical Neuroleptics

Because of the positive response of many children with autistic disorder to typical neuroleptics, similar medications with reduced risk of tardive dyskinesia must be considered. In addition, atypical neuroleptics are often effective in treating the negative symptoms of schizophrenia, which seem similar to several of the social deficits in autistic disorder. Both risperidone and olanzapine have shown promise in open label trials in reducing hyperactivity, impulsivity, aggressiveness and obsessive preoccupations. A double-blind, placebo-controlled study found risperidone to be more effective than placebo in the treatment of repetitive behavior, aggression and irritability (McDougle *et al.*, 1998).

Anticonvulsants

Because 25 to 33% of patients with autistic disorder have seizures, the psychopharmacological management of patients with autistic disorder or other ASD must take into consideration the past or current history of epilepsy and the potential role of anticonvulsants. In an open trial of divalproex, 10 of 14 patients responded favorably, showing improvements in affective stability, impulsivity and aggression (Hollander *et al.*, 2001). Because barbiturates have been associated with hyperactivity, depression and cognitive impairment, they should be changed to an alternative drug, depending on the seizure and avoided when possible. In addition, phenytoin (Dilantin) is sedating and can cause hypertrophy of the gums and hirsutism, which may contribute to the social challenges for people with autistic disorder. Carbamazepine and valproate may have positive psychotropic effects, particularly when cyclical irritability, insomnia and hyperactivity are present.

Naltrexone

Double-blind trials have demonstrated that naltrexone, an opiate antagonist, has little efficacy in treating the core social and cognitive symptoms of autistic. While the use of naltrexone as a specific treatment for autistic disorder no longer seems to be likely, it may have a role in the treatment of self-injurious behavior, although the controlled data are equivocal. Controlled trials have shown a modest reduction in symptoms of hyperactivity and restlessness sometimes associated with autistic disorder. Potential side effects include nausea and vomiting. Naltrexone may have an adverse effect on the outcome of Rett's disorder on the basis of a relatively large, randomized, double-blind, placebo-controlled trial (Percy *et al.*, 1994).

Lithium

Adolescents and adults with autistic disorder often exhibit symptoms in a cyclic manner and so there is much interest in how these patients might respond to agents typically used in bipolar disorder. A single open trial of lithium revealed no significant improvement in symptoms in patients with autistic disorder without bipolar disorder (Campbell *et al.*, 1972).

Anxiolytics

Benzodiazepines have not been studied systematically in children and adolescents with autistic disorder. However, their use to reduce anxiety in short-term treatment, such as before dental procedures, is similar to their use in management of anxiety in people without a PDD. One open label study has found a decrease in anxiety and irritability in patients receiving the anxiolytic buspirone (Buitelaar *et al.*, 1998).

Glutamatergic Antagonists

Interest in these agents has been sparked by the hypothesis that ASDs may be a disorder of hypoglutaminergic activity. In a double-blind, placebo-controlled study of the glutamatergic antagonist amantadine hydrochloride, there were substantial improvements in clinician-rated hyperactivity and irritability, although parental reports did not reach statistical significance (King *et al.*, 2001).

Other Treatments

Pyridoxine, the water-soluble essential vitamin B_6, has been used extensively as a pharmacological treatment in autistic disorder. In the doses used for autistic disorder, it is not being used as a cofactor for normally regulated enzyme function or as a vitamin; rather, it is used to modulate the function of neurotransmitter enzymes, such as tryptophan hydroxylase and tyrosine hydroxylase. Recent reviews have concluded that there are little data to support the claim that vitamin B_6 improves developmental course. The same is true for using fenfluramine, naloxone and secretin.

Comparison of DSM-IV/ICD-10 Diagnostic Criteria

The DSM-IV and ICD-10 item sets and diagnostic algorithms for autistic disorder are almost identical. However, the ICD-10 exclusion criterion is considerably more broad, requiring that a number of other disorders should be considered instead (e.g., early-onset schizophrenia, mental retardation with an associated emotional or behavioral disorder). In ICD-10, this disorder is referred to as childhood autism.

The DSM-IV and ICD-10 item sets and diagnostic algorithms for Rett's disorder and Asperger's disorder are almost identical. In ICD-10, these disorders are referred to as Rett's syndrome and Asperger's syndrome respectively.

Regarding childhood disintegrative disorder, the DSM-IV and ICD-10 item sets and diagnostic algorithms are identical except for the C criterion, in which ICD-10 also allows for a "general loss of interest in objects and the environment". In ICD-10, this disorder is referred to as other childhood disintegrative disorder.

References

Aman M (1994) *Aberrant Behavior Checklist—Community*. Slosson Educational Publications, East Aurora, NY.

Amir RE, Van den Veyver IB, Wan M *et al.* (1999) Rett syndrome is caused by mutations in X-linked MECP2, encoding methyl-CpG-binding protein 2. *Nat Genet* 23, 185–188.

Asperger H (1944) Die "Autistischen Psychopathen" kindesalter. *Arch Psychiatr Nervenkr* 117, 76–136.

Bachevalier J (1994) Medial temporal lobe structures and autism: A review of clinical and experimental findings. *Neuropsychologia* 32, 627–648.

Buitelaar JK, Willemsen-Swinkels S and Van Engeland H (1998) Naltrexone in children with autism. *J Am Acad Child Adolesc Psychiatr* 37, 800–802.

Campbell M, Fish B, Korein J *et al.* (1972) Lithium and chlorpromazine: A controlled crossover study of hyperactive severely disturbed young children. *J Aut Child Schizophr* 2, 234–263.

Chugani DC, Muzik O, Rothermel R *et al.* (1997) Altered serotonin synthesis in the dentatothalamocortical pathway in autistic boys. *Ann Neurol* 42, 666–669.

Chugani HT, Da Silva E and Chugani DC (1996) Infantile spasms: III. Prognostic implications of bitemporal hypometabolism on positron emission tomography. *Ann Neurol* 39, 643–649.

Cook E and Leventhal B (1996) The serotonin system in autism. *Curr Opin Pediatr* 8, 348–354.

Durand VM and Carr EG (1991) Functional communication training to reduce challenging behavior: Maintenance and application in new settings. *J Appl Behav Anal* 24, 251–264.

Erdmann J, Shimron-Abarbanell D, Rietschel M *et al.* (1996) Systematic screening for mutations in the human serotonin-2A (5-HT_{2A}) receptor gene: Identification of two naturally occurring receptor variants and association analysis in schizophrenia. *Hum Genet* 97, 614–619.

Fryxell D and Kennedy CH (1995) Placement along the continuum of services and its impact on students' social relationships. *J Assoc Pers Severe Handicaps* 20, 259–269.

Handen BL, Johnson CR and Lubetsky M (2000) Efficacy of methylphenidate among children with autism and symptoms of attention-deficit hyperactivity disorder. *J Aut Dev Disord* 30, 245–255.

Haznedar MM, Buchsbaum MS, Metzger M *et al.* (1997) Anterior cingulated gyrus volume and glucose metabolism in autistic disorder. *Am J Psychiatric* 154, 1047–1050.

Hollander E, Dolgoff-Kaspar R, Cartwright C *et al.* (2001) An open trial of divalproex sodium in autism spectrum disorders. *J Clin Psychiatr* 62, 530–534.

Kanner L (1943) Autistic disturbances of affective contact. *Nerv Child* 2, 217–250.

Kim SJ and Cook EH Jr. (2000) Novel de novo nonsense mutation of MECP2 in a patient with Rett syndrome. *Hum Mutat (Online)* 15, 382–383.

Kim S-J, Cox N, Courchesne R *et al.* (2002) Transmission disequilibrium mapping in the serotonin transporter gene (SLC6A4) region in autistic disorder. *Mol Psychiatr* 7(3), 278–288.

King B, Wright D, Handen B *et al.* (2001) A double-blind, placebo-controlled study of amantidine hydrochloride in the treatment of children with autistic disorder. *J Am Acad Child Adolesc Psychiatr* 40, 658–665.

Leventhal BL, Cook EH Jr., Morford M *et al.* (1990) Relationships of whole blood serotonin and plasma norepinephrine within families. *J Aut Dev Disord* 20, 499–511.

Lord C, Rutter M and Le Couteur A (1994) Autistism diagnostic interview-revised: A revised version of a diagnostic interview for caregivers of individuals with possible pervasive development disorders. *J Aut Dev Disord* 24, 659–685.

Lord C, Pickles A, McLennan J, *et al.* (1997) Diagnosing autism: Analyses of data from the autism diagnostic interview. *J Aut Dev Disord* 27, 501–517.

Lord C, Risi S, Lambrecht L *et al.* (2000) The autism diagnostic observation schedule-generic: A standard measure of social and communication deficits associated with the spectrum of autism. *J Aut Dev Disord* 30, 205–223.

McDougle CJ, Holmes JP, Carlson DC *et al.* (1998) A double-blind, placebo-controlled study of risperidone in adults with autistic disorder and other pervasive developmental disorders. *Arch Gen Psychiatr* 55, 633–641.

Muller RA, Chugani DC, Behen ME *et al.* (1998) Impairment of dentato-thalamo-cortical pathway in autistic men: Language activation data from positron emission tomography. *Neurosci Lett* 245, 1–4.

Odom SL and Strain PS (1986) A comparison of peer-initiation and teacher–antecedent interventions for promoting reciprocal social interaction of autistic preschoolers. *J Appl Behav Anal* 19, 59–71.

Percy AK, Glaze DG, Schultz RJ *et al.* (1994) Rett syndrome: Controlled study of an oral opiate antagonist, naltrexone. *Ann Neurol* 35, 464–470.

Rett A (1966) On an until now unknown disease of a congenital metabolic disorder. *Krankenschwester* 19, 121–122.

Ritvo E, Yuwiler A, Geller E *et al.* (1971) Maturational changes in blood serotonin levels and platelet counts. *Biochem Med* 5, 90–96.

Rutter M (1983) Cognitive deficits in the pathogenesis of autism. *J Child Psychol Psychiatr* 24, 513–532.

Smith T, Groen AD and Wynn JW (2001) Randomized trial of early intervention for children with pervasive developmental disorder. *Am J Ment Retard* 105(4), 269–285.

Volkmar F and Cohen D (1989) Disintegrative disorder or "late onset" autism. *J Child Psychol Psychiatr* 30, 717–724.

CHAPTER

28 Childhood Disorders: Attention-deficit and Disruptive Behavior Disorders

Introduction

Attention-deficit/hyperactivity disorder (ADHD), conduct disorder (CD) and oppositional defiant disorder (ODD) form the attention-deficit and disruptive behavior disorders (AD-DBDs) in DSM-IV-TR (American Psychiatric Association, 2000). As a group, these are the most common disorders of childhood and among the most researched areas of childhood psychopathology. There is also increasing recognition that these disorders continue into adulthood.

Children with ADHD are challenged in their ability to modulate impulsivity, hyperactivity and inattention. Some children, however, can present with either predominate hyperactivity or inattention, the latter more likely to go undiagnosed since they are often less disruptive within the classroom. To establish the diagnosis of ADHD, DSM-IV TR requires that children must have, before the age of seven, at least six signs of hyperactivity/impulsivity and an equal number of signs demonstrating inattention. Children often are diagnosed after the age of seven, however, a carefully elicited history generally reveals symptoms of ADHD earlier in the child's development that clearly distinguish them from their peers. Functional impairment must be present in at least two sectors of the child's life. For younger children, problems at home and at school are the rule. Common symptoms include hyperactivity, as manifested by fidgetiness, excessive talking, inability to participate in leisure activities quietly, inability to remain seated in the classroom or social settings, frequent inappropriate running or climbing, Teachers and parents describe children with ADHD as "always on the go" or seem to be "driven by a motor".

The essential feature of CD is a repetitive and persistent pattern of behavior in which the basic rights of others or major age appropriate societal norms or rules are violated. Behaviors are categorized within the following four groups:

- destruction of property;
- theft and or deceitfulness;
- serious violations of rules;
- aggression directed at animals and people.

Similar to ADHD, symptoms of CD are seen in more than one setting and cause significant impairment in functioning. The diagnosis of CD requires that symptoms be present for at least one year, with one or more symptoms occurring within the previous six months. Adults with conduct problems, whose behavior does not meet criteria for antisocial personality disorder, may have symptoms that meet criteria for CD and thus qualify for the diagnosis. Subtypes of CD are determined on the basis of age of onset. The childhood onset subtype is diagnosed in children who show at least one of the behaviors before the age of 10 years, while the adolescent onset subtype is characterized by the absence of any CD behaviors before 10 years of age.

The essential feature of ODD is a recurrent pattern of negativistic, defiant, disobedient and hostile behavior toward authority figures that persists for at least 6 months and results in social and academic impairment. Typical behaviors include excessive:

- anger;
- vindictiveness;
- arguing with and disobeying adults;
- loss of temper;
- annoying others;
- blaming of others for poor behavior and mistakes.

The rationale for grouping ADHD, CD and ODD is that similar areas of difficulty are present in children with these disorders. Academic difficulties, poor social skills and overrepresentation of boys are among the shared characteristics. Further, the three disorders demonstrate a commonality of core symptoms, with impulsivity being prominent in all three conditions. Not surprisingly, there is a high degree of comorbidity among the three disorders. In part related to this, there has been extensive debate as to whether these conditions are truly distinct from each other. While there is now a consensus that ADHD and CD are separable diagnoses with distinct correlates and outcome, the relationship of ODD to both disorders is less clear.

Epidemiology

While DSM-IV-TR estimates the prevalence rates for ADHD to range from 2 to 7% in school-age, rates as high as 17.1% have been reported in community surveys (Cohen *et al.*, 1993). Rates for CD have been estimated to be as low as 0.9% for school-age children but as high as 8.7% in adolescents. The overall prevalence of ODD varies across studies from 5.7 to 9.9%.

In school-age children, boys have higher rates than girls for all three disorders. In clinic settings, the ratio of boys to girls is about 9:1, but in community samples, this decreases to approximately 3:1. Furthermore, teachers tend to identify fewer girls than boys as having ADHD symptoms. The combined type of ADHD is the most common subtype in both genders. However, in the predominantly hyperactive–impulsive subtype of ADHD, the male to female ratio is approximately 4 : 1 while in the predominantly inattentive subtype the ratio falls to 2 : 1. In general, prevalence declines with age, but follow-up studies of children and adolescents indicate that the disorder frequently persists into adulthood. Longitudinal studies have reported rates of childhood cases that persist into adulthood to range from 4 to 75%. Factors that appear to predict the persistence of ADHD into adulthood include a positive family history for ADHD and the presence of psychiatric comorbidity, particularly aggression.

Among the AD-DBDs, approximately 90% of children with CD would also meet the criteria for ODD. Furthermore, 40% of children with ADHD also have ODD and 40% of children with ODD have ADHD. In terms of the comorbidity of the AD-DBD group with other diagnostic categories, it has been estimated that 15 to 20% of children with ADHD have comorbid mood disorders, 20 to 25% have anxiety disorders and 6 to 20% have learning disabilities. Other conditions which may occur comorbidly with the AD-DBDs include Tourette's disorder (TD), drug and alcohol abuse or dependence and mental retardation.

Etiology

There is no single etiology for any of the AD-DBDs. It is likely that each of these disorders is heterogeneous. Nevertheless, a variety of studies using neurochemical markers, family-genetic analyses, patterns of comorbidity, and family studies have begun to delineate more homogeneous groups.

Neurobiology

Attention-deficit Hyperactivity Disorder (ADHD)

ADHD pathophysiologic research has focused on neural circuits centered in the prefrontal cortex and striatum, as well as on the brain stem catecholamine systems that innervate these circuits.

The prefrontal cortex and the striatum are part of a complex neural system that mediates inhibitory control processes. The prefrontal cortex receives higher-order sensory input and inhibits the processing of irrelevant sensory stimuli through reciprocal connections with temporal and parietal association cortices. In turn, the prefrontal cortex exerts inhibitory control over motor functions through well-organized connections with the caudate nucleus, and indirectly with the globus pallidus. The globus pallidus feeds back to the prefrontal cortex via thalamic nuclei. Emerging data from neuroimaging studies suggest that impairments in these prefrontal–striatal regions play a central role in the pathophysiology of ADHD.

Morphological studies using magnetic resonance imaging (MRI) have identified a smaller right prefrontal cortex, caudate nucleus and globus pallidus in children with ADHD which suggests that ADHD may be associated with fewer prefrontal corticostriatal fibers and less pallidal feedback to prefrontal regions. In addition, reduced area in the corresponding anterior genu region of the corpus callosum in children with ADHD indicates the presence of fewer inter-hemispheric fibers in prefrontal regions. Anomalies have also been found in ADHD in regions that project to the prefrontal cortex, including in the parietal–occipital region (i.e., reduced white matter) and the cerebellum (i.e., smaller posterior vermis). The latter findings raise the possibility that brain anomalies in ADHD extend beyond the prefrontal cortex and striatum to the posterior and subcortical regions that innervate these frontal circuits.

Studies with single photon emission computerized tomography (SPECT) and positron emission tomography (PET) have reported lower basal activity in the prefrontal cortex and striatum of children (Zametkin et al., 1990), but not adolescents with ADHD (Zametkin et al., 1993). More recent studies employing functional MRI (fMRI) have tentatively linked altered prefrontal–striatal activation with deficits in inhibitory control. Reduced striatal activation during response inhibition tasks has been consistently reported in children and adolescents with ADHD. However, prefrontal activation during the same tasks was enhanced in children, but reduced in adolescents with the disorder. Normal age-related declines in prefrontal activation may account for the disparate findings.

The fact that virtually all medications that are efficacious in ADHD affect noradrenaline (NA) and dopamine (DA) transmission strongly suggest that perturbations of these catecholamine inputs play a significant role in the pathophysiology of ADHD, although studies of catecholamine function in ADHD have yielded highly inconsistent findings (Zametkin and Rapoport, 1987). Only more recent studies that used central indices of catecholamine function or that examined more homogeneous subgroups of children with ADHD have provided evidence of DA and NA dysfunction associated with ADHD. For example, cerebrospinal (CSF) levels of the DA metabolite homovanillic acid were positively correlated with ratings of hyperactivity and stimulant response in boys with ADHD (Castellanos et al., 1996). Further, dividing boys with ADHD based on the presence or absence of reading disabilities revealed differences in plasma levels of the NA metabolite 3-methoxy-4-hydroxy-phenylglycol (MHPG) that correlated with differences in clinical characteristics (Halperin et al., 1997).

A promising recent development has been the use of PET and SPECT imaging in combination with DA-selective radiotracers to examine localized DA function in vivo. These studies have revealed preliminary evidence of increased striatal DA transporter binding in adults with ADHD (Dougherty et al., 1999; Krause et al., 2000) and altered DA synthesis in the prefrontal cortex and right midbrain of children and adults with ADHD. These data point to localized DA deficits in the nigrostriatal and mesocortical fiber systems in ADHD.

Conduct Disorder (CD)

The neurobiologic basis of CD has focused primarily on the neurochemical substrates of aggressive behaviors. An early body of literature pointed to a role for reduced noradrenergic function. Several studies found negative correlations between plasma and CSF concentrations of MHPG and aggression and conduct problems (Kruesi et al., 1990; Rogeness et al., 1987). Children with CD were also reported to exhibit low activity of the enzyme dopamine-beta-hydroxylase, which converts DA into NA. These data suggest that NA dysfunction may play a role in aggression through its involvement in the regulation of behavioral arousal.

More recent research has focused on the role of central serotonergic (5-HT) function in aggression and antisocial behavior (Markowitz and Coccaro, 1995). Aggressive and antisocial adults have consistently been shown to have reduced CSF levels of 5-HT metabolites and blunted responses to 5-HT challenge agents. Studies examining central 5-HT function in aggressive children have had mixed results. Reduced central 5-HT function is associated with numerous risk factors for persistence in aggressive children, including affective lability, adverse child-rearing and parental history of aggression.

Genetics

Research data support the familial transmission of ADHD and CD and suggest that these disorders may share common familial vulnerabilities (Biederman *et al.*, 1992). Estimates of heritability range from 60 to 80% for ADHD (Sherman *et al.*, 1997) and from 30 to 70% for CD (Slutske *et al.*, 1997).

Newer molecular genetic studies have identified a number of individual genes as potential candidate genes in the AD-DBDs. Evidence of altered DA activity in ADHD has focused on the search for candidate genes among DA system genes, including the DA D2, DA D4 and DA D5 receptor genes and the DA transporter gene (DAT1; with the strongest evidence for the 7-repeat allele of DRD4 (Swanson *et al.*, 1998), which mediates a blunted intracellular response to DA, and the 10-repeat allele of DAT1 (Daly *et al.*, 1999), which is linked to elevated DA reuptake. Preliminary data have also linked the 10-repeat allele of DAT1 with poor response to methylphenidate (Winsberg and Comings, 1999), which acts primarily by inhibiting the DA transporter in the striatum.

Several 5-HT system genes have been identified as candidates for study in CD. These include the genes encoding the enzymes tryptophan hydroxylase (TPH)) and monoamine oxidase A (MAOA), which are involved in the synthesis and metabolism of 5-HT, respectively.

Environmental Factors

Twin studies have provided some of the strongest evidence implicating environmental factors in the etiology of the AD-DBDs. These studies indicate that a moderate-to-significant proportion of the susceptibility to AD-DBDs is accounted for by nonshared factors. Nonshared factors have their greatest effect in CD (Slutske *et al.*, 1997); and are less important contributors to ADHD (Sherman *et al.*, 1997). Examples of nonshared factors include low verbal intelligence, poor school performance, difficult temperament inflated self-esteem and biological events, such as perinatal insults and head trauma. Among the most salient risk factors for CD is the presence of early ODD and ADHD (Hinshaw, 1987).

Shared family, peer and neighborhood risk factors also play a role in the etiology of ODD and CD, and to a lesser degree of ADHD. These so-called adversity factors include large sibships, families that have experienced separation, single-parent households, child neglect, parental conflict and poverty. Parental child-rearing practices, such as harsh physical discipline and poor supervision, have also been implicated in ODD and CD. However, the most salient familial risk factor for CD is parental criminality which likely has both environmental and genetic components. Delinquent peer membership and repeated victimization by peers also add to the etiology of CD and aggression. Finally, residing in a neighborhood with high rates of crime, poverty and/or unemployment is associated with an earlier onset of CD. These factors seem to operate in an additive fashion, with the probability of CD increasing linearly with the aggregation of risk factors (Rutter *et al.*, 1975).

Course and Natural History

Some behaviors characteristic of the AD-DBDs are observable as early as the preschool years. Hyperactive behaviors such as "moves too much during sleep" have been reported as early as age one and a half years, followed by the appearance of "difficulty playing quietly"

and "excessive climbing/running" by age 3 years. Attentional problems are usually reported after hyperactivity. However, it is likely that these problems are present from early on but are not reported until the child enters school, when there are increased environmental and cognitive demands. Hyperactivity and attentional problems emerge gradually and may overlap with the emergence of oppositional behaviors. Many individuals with ADHD continue to have attentional, behavioral and emotional problems well into adolescence and adulthood. Typically, adults with ADHD are less overtly overactive, although they may retain a subjective sense of restlessness. Impairment in these adults is more often a result of inattention, disorganization and impulsive behavior.

During the preschool years, transient oppositional behavior is very common. However, when the oppositionality is of a persistent nature and lasts beyond the preschool years, the escalation to more disruptive behaviors is more likely. In most oppositional children, who are usually not physically aggressive, oppositional behaviors peak around age 8 years and decline beyond that. In a second group of children, delinquent behaviors follow the onset of oppositional behaviors. Early physical aggression is a key predictor of this latter trajectory, with physically aggressive children being more likely to progress from early oppositional behaviors to more severe and disabling conduct problems. Coexistent ADHD tends to speed this escalation to more severe conduct problems and the development of antisocial personality disorder in adulthood.

Generally, conduct problems first appear in middle childhood. The progression of conduct problems is from rule violations, such as poor school attendance, to aggression toward animals and people. In males, the progression to more serious forms of conduct problems, such as rape or mugging, generally emerge after age 13 years (Loeber, 1990). A different group of children show conduct problems for the first time during adolescence, without preexisting oppositional or aggressive behaviors. This latter group tends to have disorders that are transient and nonaggressive. When conduct disorder is seen in adolescence for the first time, the problems tend to diminish by adulthood. However, if conduct disorder is present from middle childhood, there is a much greater degree of persistence of aggression through adulthood and often a history of arrests and/or incarceration.

Considerable data indicate that a subgroup of hyperactive children show high rates of delinquency and substance abuse during adolescence, and this continues into adulthood. However, it is likely due to the comorbidity with conduct disorder or bipolar disorder that higher rates of substance abuse are found in adolescents with ADHD. Families of these children tend to be less stable, have higher divorce rates and move more frequently. First degree relatives have been found to have higher rates of antisocial behaviors, substance abuse and depression The difficulties experienced by these adolescents and adults include poor self-esteem, difficulty in interpersonal relationships, difficulties in holding onto jobs, as well as assault and armed robbery in a minority of cases (Hechtman *et al.*, 1981).

Assessment

The clinical evaluation of a child with possible AD-DBD requires a multisource, multimethod approach. In addition to clinical interviews of parents and children, supplemental information may be obtained from school reports, rating scales completed by teachers and parents, neuropsychological test data and direct observations of the child. Generally, adults are considered to be the best informants of disruptive behaviors, although children and adolescents may provide important data regarding internalizing symptoms and some infrequent behavior problems, such as antisocial acts (American Academy of Child and Adolescent Psychiatry, 1997; Barkley *et al.*, 1991; Loeber *et al.*, 1991).

Rating Scales

Rating scales facilitate the systematic acquisition of information about the child's behavior in different settings in a cost-effective manner. Most are standardized and provide scores that are norm-referenced by age and gender. The systematic use of these instruments ensures that a complete set of specific behaviors is assessed at different points in time, enabling comparisons over the course of treatment. Teacher and parent rating scales are complimentary because they yield data from different situations. Parents are knowledgeable about their child's day-to-day behavior, and present information related to the child's behavior at home and his/her interaction with siblings. Teachers are often a valuable source of information regarding attentional problems and disruptive behaviors in a classroom setting.

The most commonly used rating scales are the Conners (1998a, 1998b), and the Achenbach (1991a, 1991b) scales, which are available in parent and teacher versions. The Conners Teachers Rating Scale – Revised (CTRS-R) is a 28-item scale that is normed for children from 3 to 17 years of age and is sensitive to medication effects. The Conners Parent Rating Scale (CPRS-R) contains 48 items is also sensitive to treatment effects and can differentiate groups of ADHD children from normals. The Child Behavior Checklist (CBCL) assesses a broad range of behavioral problems and is useful with children from ages 4 to 16 years. The CBCL is also available in a more recently developed Teacher Report Form (Achenbach, 1991b), which is similar to the parent form and applicable for children aged 4 to 18 years.

Rating scales have several limitations, and diagnoses should not be made on the bases of these data alone. It has been consistently found that elevations on discrete scale factors do not necessarily coincide with specific psychiatric disorders.

Interviews

Interviews with children and their parents form the core of the clinical evaluation. It is essential that the interviewer directly enquire about all symptoms of ADHD and common comorbidities, and therefore some structured questioning is usually required.

A number of structured and semistructured diagnostic interviews are currently available for use with children, including the Diagnostic Interview Schedule for Children (DISC-II), the Diagnostic Interview for Children and Adolescents (DICA), the Schedule for Affective Disorders and Schizophrenia for School Aged Children (K-SADS), the Child and Adolescent Psychiatric Assessment (CAPA), the Child Assessment Schedule (CAS) and the Diagnostic Interview Schedule for Children (DISC). Among the AD-DBDs, it has been found that CD often has better reliability and validity coefficients than ADHD.

Psychological/Psychometric Evaluation

Psychological and cognitive test performance is generally not required to determine the presence of an AD-DBD. Nevertheless, because the AD-DBDs are frequently associated with learning problems, neuropsychological testing may be indicated, particularly when assessment of cognitive functioning is required. Information from a neuropsychological and/or educational evaluation can often be used to supplement the clinical evaluation by providing an understanding of the individual child's level of cognitive and attentional functioning, as well as screening for suspected mental retardation and various learning disabilities.

Other psychometric measures include computerized continuous performance tests (CPTs), of which there are many varieties. Recent interest in creating developmentally appropriate measures of AD-DBDs symptom domains for preschoolers has led to the development of CPTs for use in this population (Harper and Ottinger, 1992). While CPTs have been found to differentiate children with ADHD from normals, their ability to differentiate ADHD from other clinical groups is less clear, and there is little evidence that they are able to identify individuals with enough precision to be useful as diagnostic instruments.

Objective measures of activity level, such as stabilometric chairs, wrist actometers and solid state actigraphs, have also been used in the assessment of ADHD. Although these devices provide a judgment-free assessment of activity level, their validity, as assessed by correlations with ratings of behavior, has been inconsistent. At the present time, it is suggested that these measures not be used to diagnose clinical syndromes.

Observational Measures

Several studies have used direct behavioral observation in the assessment of the AD-DBDs. In a structured playroom setting, measures include counting the number of times a child crosses grids marked on the floor, recording the number of toys touched, the amount of time played with each toy and the amount of time the child spends focused on a particular task. In the school setting, typical measures include monitoring the amount of time the child spends on-task, remains in his/her seat and so on. These observational measures have consistently been found to differentiate ADHD children from normals, although their utility in discriminating among clinical groups is less clear.

Laboratory Measures

At the present time, there are no laboratory measures that can serve as diagnostic tools for AD-DBDs. Similarly, findings from neuroimaging studies have neither been consistent enough nor specific enough to warrant their use as diagnostic tools.

Other Domains of Functioning

Many children with AD-DBDs have impaired social skills and consequently experience difficulties with peer relationships. Data suggest that both hyperactivity and aggression often lead to peer rejection, which may occur as early as the preschool. The level of hyperactivity, age of onset of aggression and the developmental level of the child, all affect the extent of peer rejection experienced. Information regarding social adjustment is crucial in treatment planning, since increased impairment in social and school function is predictive of poor outcome.

Parent–child interactions also play a role in the maintenance of disruptive behaviors, poor social skills, the presence of internalizing symptoms and response to treatment. It has been noted that robust reductions in negative and ineffective parenting practices at home mediate improvement in children's social skills in the school setting (Hinshaw *et al.*, 2000).

Differential Diagnoses

Proper differential diagnosis of ADHD, CD and ODD requires not only discrimination among the three disorders, but also from a wide range of other psychiatric, developmental and medical conditions. ADHD can be conceptualized as a cognitive/developmental disorder, with an earlier age of onset than CD. ADHD children more frequently show deficits on measures of attentional and cognitive function, have increased motor activity and greater neurodevelopmental abnormalities. In contrast, CD children tend to be characterized by higher levels of aggression and greater familial dysfunction.

A significant proportion of children present with symptoms of both ADHD and CD, and both conditions should be diagnosed when this occurs. Comorbid ADHD and CD is consistently reported to be more disabling with poorer long-term outcome than either disorder alone. These children show persistantly increased levels of aggressive behaviors at an early age. This is in contrast to the more typical episodic course seen in children who have CD alone.

It appears that among children with ADHD, those who are most hyperactive/impulsive are at greatest risk for developing ODD. ODD symptoms, such as "loses temper", "actively defies", and "swears", are less characteristic of children with ADHD. In general, the onset of ODD symptoms peaks by age 8 years and shows a declining course thereafter, while hyperactivity and attentional problems appear at a much earlier age and often persist, although the levels of inattentiveness and/or hyperactivity often decrease with age.

A diagnosis of CD supersedes ODD since approximately 90% of children with CD would also meet criteria for ODD, and some question whether they represent a spectrum of severity or distinct diagnoses. Although the majority of ODD children will not develop CD, in some cases ODD appears to represent a developmental precursor of CD. In cases where ODD precedes CD, the onset of CD is typically before age 10 years (childhood onset CD). In children who have the onset of CD after age 10 years, symptoms of ODD and ADHD are usually not present during early childhood. It has been shown that children with ODD demonstrate lower degrees of impairment and are more socially competent as compared with children with CD. Furthermore, children with CD come from less advantaged families, and have greater conflict with school and judicial systems as compared with children with ODD.

Mood and anxiety disorders, learning disorders, mental retardation, pervasive developmental disorders, organic mental disorders and psychotic disorders may all present with impairment of attention, as well as hyperactive/impulsive behaviors. The diagnosis of ADHD in DSM-IV requires that the symptoms of inattention/cognitive disorganization and impulsivity/hyperactivity are not better accounted for by one of the above conditions. Differentiating ADHD from bipolar disorder in childhood is complicated by the low base rate of bipolar disorder and the variability in clinical presentation. A positive family history of bipolar disorder is especially helpful in diagnosing bipolar disorder in children. In addition, a variety of medical conditions such as epilepsy, Tourette's disorder, thyroid disease, postinfectious and/or post traumatic encephalopathy and sensory impairments can present with symptoms similar to ADHD and must also be considered. Finally, many medications which are prescribed to children can mimic ADHD symptomatology. Examples include anticonvulsants (e.g., phenobarbital), antihistamines, decongestants, bronchodilators (e.g., theophylline) and systemic steroids.

Treatment

Given the heterogeneity of the three disorders that make-up the AD-DBDs, the wide ranging effects of the disruptive behaviors, the high rates of comorbidity and the presence of associated features such as learning disabilities, multimodal treatments (i.e., psychopharmacologic and psychosocial) are almost always warranted. Nevertheless, good response can be achieved with either treatment alone in certain instances (e.g., medication treatment for uncomplicated ADHD or ADHD + ODD; psychosocial treatment for ADHD + anxiety disorder) (MTA Cooperative Group, 1999a, 1999b). A diagnosis of ODD without any comorbid condition will usually be responsive to behavioral intervention without medication. Similarly, treatment of children with CD without comorbidity usually involves psychosocial interventions with the possibility of augmenting treatment with one of several pharmacological agents. In contrast, comorbid ADHD + CD almost always requires medication, and medication response is augmented if psychosocial treatment is offered concomitantly (Jensen *et al.*, 2001).

Psychopharmacology

Psychopharmacological treatments of the AD-DBDs can be traced to 1930s when benzedrine was successfully used to treat a heterogeneous group of behaviorally disturbed children and adolescents. Psychostimulants remain the medication of choice for the majority of children with ADHD. They have been studied in literally hundreds of controlled trials in all age groups, have documented safety and are now available in extended release preparations that are easy to use and decrease the potential for stigma associated with school administration that previously plagued children and families with ADHD. However, several other currently available medications have demonstrated efficacy for ADHD and are often used off-label to treat this condition. They offer useful alternatives for those who are stimulant nonresponders, or for whom stimulants may be contraindicated.

Psychostimulants

Methylphenidate (MPH), dextroamphetamine (DEX) and mixture of amphetamine salts (MAS) (which is a mixture of several amphetamine compounds, 75% of which is DEX) have all been shown to be effective in treating ADHD. Of these, MPH is the most often prescribed and accounts for approximately 60% of stimulant use in the USA. MAS has become a popular alternative to MPH, and despite slight differences in mechanism of action, profiles of response and adverse effects, there are no strong data to indicate that any one stimulant preparation is substantially more effective or better tolerated than any other. Despite these similarities, there are sometimes differences in individual response profiles, which demonstrate that one preparation may be substantially better than the others for a particular individual.

The stimulants produce significant improvement in attention, hyperactivity, impulse control and aggressiveness, leading to better organization of behavior, task completion and self-regulation. There is fairly robust improvement in social skills, as evidenced by peer ratings, and parent and teacher ratings of social function. There is also improvement in academic productivity, although change in actual academic performance has been more difficult to demonstrate. Although most data with stimulants have been obtained in samples of school-age children with ADHD, there is increasing recognition that stimulants can be used successfully across the lifespan (Spencer *et al.*, 2001).

The decision to prescribe psychostimulant medication is best undertaken following a comprehensive assessment, with full consideration given to the range of pharmacologic and nonpharmacologic treatment options which are available. Prior to a trial with any of the stimulants, baseline data should be obtained, including general medical status, and more specific evaluations of height, weight, blood pressure and a complete blood count.

The past several years have seen a veritable explosion in the number of stimulant treatment options for individuals with ADHD. Most of the attention has focused on development of sustained release preparations, which eliminate the need to take medication several times over the course of the day, and to provide a more consistent profile of delivery. This has the added benefit of decreasing the need for in-school dosing, and along with it the potential for stigmatization of children with ADHD and diversion of medication. Both MPH and MAS are now available in preparations formulated to last 12 hours. MPH is also available in two new delivery forms that are each intended to last 8 hours A new immediate-release stimulant treatment, d-MPH (the active stereoisomer of MPH), has also recently come on the market.

The decision regarding which stimulant to select is best determined by considering properties intrinsic to the different medications – such as duration of activity and adverse effect profile – as well as the individual circumstances of the patient (e.g., when is peak medication level needed most, what is the individual's lifestyle, etc.). Nonresponders to one medication may respond well to another, since their mechanisms of action are not identical, and if there is not adequate response to one stimulant medication, another should be tried.

Increasingly, MPH is given in its long-acting forms as a first-line approach. The usual starting dose for Concerta (12-hour formulation) is 18 mg, which is equivalent to 5 mg IR-MPH administered three times daily, and may be increased 18 mg at a time. Various forms and strengths of intermediate-release MPH are also available. Immediate-release (IR) MPH can be used as a primary therapeutic agent, given in either b.i.d. or t.i.d. dosing schedules, however, its niche increasingly is to supplement the longer-acting preparations, either to achieve more rapid onset of effect or to extend duration of action. When IR-MPH is used as a primary option, the usual starting dose is 5 mg. The dose is then increased in 5 mg increments. The upper recommended dose for MPH is 60 mg, although use of higher doses may be required in certain cases.

MAS and DEX can often be administered in a similar manner to MPH, and also come in a variety of IR and extended release formulations. Adderall XR (MAS) is the only amphetamine preparation formulated to act for 12 hours. Brand Adderall or generic MAS are also available in a shorter acting form that lasts approximately 5 to 6 hours. DEX is available in both a spansule, with duration of activity comparable to the shorter acting MAS, and an IR preparation, which lasts approximately 4 hours. A recent study found that DEX spansule and MAS have comparable efficacy and duration. DEX and MAS are more potent than MPH, so the initial starting dose and upper dose limit are lower. The recommended dosage range for DEX is 2.5 to 40 mg. Although DEX has a somewhat longer half-life than MPH, a t.i.d. schedule is still often required.

Adverse effects (AE) of stimulants are generally mild, but occasionally can become problematic. The most commonly observed AEs include headache, abdominal pain, decreased appetite (with or without weight loss) and initial insomnia. There are slight increases in pulse and BP, which are not very meaningful at the group level, but can take on greater significance for particular individuals. Affective changes, including blunted affect, irritability and mood lability, can also be seen, either at peak dose or when the dose wears off. Use of longer acting psychostimulants tends to minimize mood lability and other AEs that are often considered to be a reflection of the on–off effects which are more frequently seen with IR preparations. Motor or vocal tics can develop. However, there has been a convergence of evidence that stimulant treatment does not necessarily exacerbate tics, and even some suggestions that these conditions are relatively independent. There has been some concern that stimulants can precipitate psychotic symptoms such as hallucinations, although this is very rare and almost always seen as a reflection of excessive dosing or use in individuals with disorders other than ADHD (e.g., psychotic disorders).

Atomoxetine

Atomoxetine is a new medication with highly potent and selective activity to block the noradrenergic transporter. It is structurally distinct from both the stimulants and the tricyclic antidepressants and has been studied extensively in both children and adults. Atomoxetine was shown to be effective in reducing both inattentive and hyperactive/impulsive symptoms over a 9-week period in a sample of children and adolescents. Doses of 0.5 mg/kg, 1.2 mg/kg and 1.8 mg/kg were studied. All doses had treatment effects that were different from placebo, with treatment effects seen at the first postmedication treatment visit, but the highest degree of improvement was found in the 1.2 mg/kg and the 1.8 mg/kg groups. The medication also produced change in functional measures as well as ADHD symptoms, with the greatest degree of change in the 1.8 mg/kg group.

Atomoxetine can be administered on either a twice daily or once daily schedule, even though that its half-life in the overwhelming majority of individuals is 4 hours. Despite this fact, therapeutic benefit seems to be maintained over the full day. Adverse effects with atomoxetine have been relatively mild, with decreased appetite and a small increase in pulse and BP being the two most consistent findings. Because it is not a stimulant, and because its effects are highly selective for noradrenaline and not dopamine, atomoxetine is thought not to have abuse potential.

Tricyclic Antidepressants

The noradrenergic tricyclic antidepressants, principally imipramine and desipramine, have been the most extensively studied and, until the mid-1990s, were the most often prescribed nonstimulant medication for individuals with ADHD. For desipramine, doses between 2.5 and 5 mg/kg/day have been recommended. In the case of both of these medications, cardiac side effects are of concern and premedication work-up must include at least an ECG. Tachycardia and postural hypotension are commonly seen, but are not often problematic. Prolongation of the PR and QT intervals may be a greater source of concern and should be reviewed with a pediatric cardiologist. The decision to prescribe tricyclics for ADHD children must be made with the knowledge that several sudden deaths have been reported in children taking desipramine. Although it has been argued that data do not support the conclusion and that tricyclics have a high degree of cardiovascular toxicity in children, proper informed consent should be obtained. It should also be noted that neither imipramine nor desipramine is FDA approved for the treatment of ADHD children.

Other Antidepressants

Bupropion and venlafaxine have been studied for their potential utility in the AD-DBDs. Investigations of bupropion in ADHD have demonstrated the effectiveness of the medication compared with placebo, but not as effective as stimulants. In contrast to this latter finding, others have found bupropion to be as effective as methylphenidate.

There are similar but more preliminary data indicating that venlafaxine might be useful for ADHD. Significant improvements in attention, concentration and other cognitive functions have been reported in volunteers. Open label studies of adults with ADHD also found venlafaxine to be effective. The most common side effects reported were nausea and sedation. An open label study in 8- to 17-year-old subjects found significant reductions in impulsivity and hyperactivity as rated by parents.

Sertonin Reuptake Inhibitors

Although there have been no studies using SSRIs in ADHD and comorbid CD/ODD, these medications are of some interest in light of recent findings implicating serotonergic mechanisms in aggression and reported utility of fluoxetine in treating adults with impulsive aggression. At present, there are no controlled trials to support the efficacy of the SSRIs for the core symptoms of ADHD, and their role in treating comorbid ADHD and CD/ODD is inferential only.

Alpha-2-adrenergic Agonists

Since the mid-1980s, there has been considerable interest in the use of alpha-2-adrenergic agonists in the treatment of ADHD Initial studies were conducted with clonidine, but the more specific alpha-2 agent guanfacine has recently been the focus of investigation. The alpha-2 agonists are reportedly most effective in treating symptoms of hyperactivity, impulsivity and aggression in children with ADHD. Effects on attentional symptoms have been less clear, although a recent study found that guanfacine treatment was associated with improved ratings and CPT measures of attention (Scahill *et al.*, 2001). Because of their role in treating overarousal and aggression, the alpha-2 agonists seem ideally suited for use in children with comorbid ODD/CD/aggression. They have been effective in treating ADHD patients who either have diagnosed tic disorders, or are at increased risk of developing them, such as those children with a positive family history of tics. This is particularly important, since as many as 40 to 60% of patients with Tourette's syndrome seen in psychiatric settings have significant behavior problems. Although the alpha-2 agonists may be less effective than stimulants in the treatment of ADHD, they may be particularly useful in individuals whose tics worsen on a stimulant medication. These agonists have also been used in combination with a stimulant. However, there have been safety considerations involving this combination. These are primarily involving the possibility of additive risk of rebound hypertension of alpha-2 agonists with the mild increase in pulse and blood pressure from stimulants.

Clonidine has a gradual onset of action which may be related to the time required for receptor down regulation. The usual dose ranges from 0.05 to 0.3 mg/day, often in a three times a day dosing schedule. One of the advantages is that it can be used to treat the initial insomnia, which sometimes results from late afternoon stimulant. Clonidine is available in both tablet form and a depot skin patch preparation. The latter provides sustained coverage for one week, and may be particularly useful for treating children with ADHD whose behavior is characterized

by a variable pattern of extreme lability, especially in the early morning, before stimulants and oral clonidine take effect. Guanfacine comes only in an oral preparation. Guanfacine tablets are of 1.0 mg strength, so care must be taken not to confuse the different doses for clonidine and guanfacine. Since guanfacine has a somewhat longer half-life than clonidine, it can often be given in a two or three times a day dosing schedule.

The most common side effect of the alpha-2 medications is sedation, although this tends to decrease after several weeks. Dry mouth, nausea and photophobia are among the other adverse effects reported. At high doses, hypotension and dizziness are also possible. The skin patch often causes local pruritic dermatitis. Glucose tolerance may decrease, especially in those at risk for diabetes. It is important carefully to evaluate cardiovascular function when using the alpha-2 agonists, especially when used in combination with stimulants treatment as noted earlier. Additionally, there have been reports of sudden death in three cases treated with the combination of clonidine and methylphenidate, although a review of this situation by the FDA concluded these unfortunate events were not attributable to the combination. However, careful monitoring is required. Since clonidine is not FDA approved for use in ADHD, informed consent should clearly indicate that this is an "off-label" treatment.

Other Agents

Lithium has been found to be effective in well-designed studies of aggressive children, impulsive–aggressive adolescents and young adult delinquents, although there are some questions regarding the magnitude of effect. Antiepileptic medications have also been used in the treatment of behavior problems characterized by aggressiveness and impulsivity. Carbamezapine is considered an effective treatment for aggression in children, but more recent findings have tempered the initial enthusiasm. Sodium valproate is another antiepileptic shown to be effective in the treatment of chronic temper outbursts and mood. Although valproate has been used for the treatment of aggressive patients for over a decade, very few published reports have used a controlled design.

Neuroleptic medications have also been used in the treatment of the AD-DBDs, principally to treat children with severe behavioral problems characterized by aggression and combativeness. Although older neuroleptics such as chlorpromazine, thioridazine and halperidol are FDA approved for the treatment of severe behavior problems in children, they are infrequently used at present. Recently, there has been more interest in the atypical neuroleptic risperidone. In a double blind placebo controlled study, risperidone was found to be superior to placebo in ameliorating aggression in youths with conduct disorder (Findling *et al.*, 2000).

During the course of the last few years, there has been a remarkable increase in the number of medications that are used in the treatment of ADHD and CD. It is important to keep in mind that the majority of the medications are not approved by the FDA for specific use in ADHD and/or CD and as such their use for these two disorders continues to be "off-label". Less than optimal treatment is likely to result in inadequate or partial improvement, as demonstrated in the community standard group of the multimodal treatment study of children with ADHD (i.e., MTA), which is discussed in more detail below. In order to reduce this variability in treatment practices, recently there have been attempts to develop treatment algorithms. The purpose of such algorithms is to integrate relevant research findings and clinical experience in the development of medication decision trees. Recently, an expert panel has reported on the development and implementation of an algorithm for the treatment of ADHD and its common comorbid conditions (Pliszka *et al.*, 2000a, 2000b).

Psychosocial Interventions

Among the systematically studied psychosocial interventions found to be useful are home-based interventions/parent training, classroom-based behavior modifications, social skills training and intensive summer treatment programs. Since family, peer and school interactions are important in the morbidity and maintenance of these disorders, it is important to utilize psychosocial treatments to target each of these areas. In contrast to these more structured techniques, individual play therapy with children is generally ineffective in decreasing problem behaviors of the AD-DBDs.

Behavior therapy (BT) relies primarily on training parents and/or teachers to be the agents of change. The focus is on decreasing the frequency of problematic behaviors and/or increasing the rate of desirable behaviors. Parent management training is one of the most common techniques and consists of group and individual sessions with parents in order to offer psychoeducational intervention and to teach the principles and implementation of behavioral programs. Consultation with classroom teachers to set up parallel behavioral programs in the school is also an important adjunct to this treatment. When effective, some parent-based interventions have resulted in benefits that have generalized for periods of over a year. Among the limitations of this technique are the labor-intensive nature of the interventions, nongeneralizability to nontargeted behaviors, and the fact that effectiveness depends upon the competence and willingness of parents and teachers to carry out the behavioral programs.

Another aspect of BT is contingency management (CM), which is implemented directly with the child in the setting in which the problem behaviors occur. CM programs use both reward procedures and negative consequences, such as time-out and response cost or "punishments". In some situations, maintenance of appropriate behavior following withdrawal of contingencies is better for a negative consequence than for a reward. Similarly to BT, CM approaches are extremely labor-intensive and questions regarding their generalizability remain.

Cognitive–behavioral approaches (CBT) are based on the premise that the difficulties experienced by children with AD-DBDs are a result of deficient self-control and problem-solving skills, or that changes in these domains of function can override other deficits. Examples of CBT include training in self-monitoring, anger control and self-reinforcement. Study results have been mixed, although some CBT procedures, such as anger control, have shown more consistent success.

Short-term gains from psychosocial interventions are often limited to the period during which the programs are actually in effect. Additional problems in implementation include the unwillingness of many teachers to use behavioral programs and the fact that as many as half the parents discontinue parent training due to their labor-intensive nature. However, it is important to note that in the MTA study, the presence of anxiety (as reported by parents on the DISC interview) moderated the outcome of treatment, such that psychosocial interventions were more efficacious than medication alone in children with ADHD who also had symptoms of anxiety (March *et al.*, 2000).

The MTA Study

The multimodal treatment study of children with ADHD (MTA) was a landmark multisite clinical trial, conducted at six performance sites across the USA and Canada, that examined the comparative response to 14 months of medication and psychosocial treatments, administered alone or together, in 579 7- to 9-year-old children with combined subtype ADHD. The principal objectives of the study were to determine the relative effectiveness of the three active treatments in comparison to one another, and in comparison with community standard care.

The treatment arms were not individual treatments but rather combinations of treatments, or treatment algorithms. Children treated in the medication arm began with a controlled trial of MPH given three times a day, and, if this was not effective, could go on to receive other treatments, such as DEX or other stimulant or nonstimulant medications. The psychosocial arm consisted of a variety of interventions, including an intense parent behavior management training program which trained parents to use behavioral techniques such as contingency management, ongoing consultation to the classroom teacher, a summer treatment program and a paraprofessional program. In the latter program, an aide was placed in each child's classroom for half day each day for 3 months. The combined treatment was the combination of all medication and psychosocial interventions. Finally, the community standard group received evaluations as part of the study, but was treated by community providers of their own choosing outside the study.

Results of the 14-month intent-to-treat analyses indicated that, for ADHD symptoms, treatments that included medication performed better than other treatments in reducing ADHD symptoms (MTA Cooperative Group, 1999). For nonADHD symptoms, only combined treatment was statistically superior to the community standard care, although it was not different from the medication group. Children with comorbid ADHD and anxiety disorders tended to have a relatively better response to the psychosocial treatment administered alone as compared with those without comorbid anxiety. Medication was as effective in treating comorbid ADHD and anxiety as it was in the group with ADHD only. Lower effectiveness was seen in the community standard group, despite the fact that two-thirds of the community-treated children received medication at some time over the 14-month period of the study.

Impact of Comorbidity on Treatment

Studies of stimulant treatment have shown that ADHD children with and without aggression respond equally well to MPH treatment in terms of ADHD symptoms. Research examining whether aggression in ADHD children can be treated with psychostimulants has mainly yielded positive findings. Finally, one study found that some covert, nonaggressive symptoms (e.g., stealing) were also decreased in ADHD children (independent of comorbidity) following treatment with MPH (Hinshaw *et al.*, 1992). Treatment of comorbid ADHD and CD/ODD in the MTA study was superior when medication was used, although the best outcome was seen with combined treatment (Jensen *et al.*, 2001).

While it is now clear that stimulant treatment can improve performance on a wide array of cognitive measures, treatment of comorbid learning disabilities requires direct, nonpharmacological, academic interventions. There has been some concern regarding the possible dissociation of cognitive and behavioral effects of stimulant medication. One landmark study found that optimal cognitive performance was achieved at low doses (i.e., 0.3 mg/kg) while optimal behavioral function was achieved at high doses (i.e., 1.0 mg/kg), with an accompanying decline in cognitive function at the higher dose (Sprague and Sleator, 1977). However, other investigators have reported a linear rather than a curvilinear dose–response curve for both behavioral and cognitive functions and have therefore not supported the previously hypothesized "cognitive toxicity".

In contrast to studies in children with ADHD who are aggressive, studies of stimulant response in ADHD children with comorbid anxiety have produced somewhat inconsistent findings. Recent studies have found that medication is equally effective in comorbid ADHD and anxiety disorders. Other studies have found that children with ADHD and anxiety respond as well as those without comorbid anxiety to the antidepressant DMI (Biederman et al., 1993).

Conclusion

The AD-DBDs are a group of disorders that together account for the majority of referrals to child and adolescent psychiatry services. They represent a significant public health problem in terms of morbidity, and have substantial risk for poor outcome in adolescence and adulthood. In recent years, there has been considerable progress in more precisely elucidating the clinical presentation as well as the genetic and neurobiological bases of these disorders. One important confound that has made these endeavors difficult has been the frequency and variety of comorbid conditions and the potential impact of comorbidity on natural history and treatment response. A variety of pharmacological and psychosocial interventions have been found to provide success over the short term, and increasingly data indicate that treatment effects can be maintained over more extended periods of time. This is an important finding because successful treatment of the AD-DBDs often requires long-term treatment using multiple modalities.

Comparison of DSM-IV/ICD-10 Diagnostic Criteria

For attention-deficit/hyperactivity disorder, the item set chosen for the ICD-10 Diagnostic Criteria for Research is almost identical to the items in the DSM-IV-TR criteria set but the algorithm is quite different resulting in a more narrowly defined ICD-10 category. Specifically, whereas the DSM-IV-TR algorithm requires either six inattention items or six hyperactive/impulsive items, the ICD-10 Diagnostic Criteria for Research requires at least six inattention items, at least three hyperactive items, and at least one impulsive item. Instead of subtyping the disorder based on the predominant type, ICD-10 subspecifies the condition based on whether criteria are also met for a conduct disorder.

Although formatted quite differently, the DSM-IV-TR and ICD-10 item sets and diagnostic algorithms for Conduct Disorder are almost identical. Although ICD-10 provides a list of 23 items (in contrast to the 15 included in the DSM-IV-TR criteria for conduct disorder), only the last 15 items count towards a diagnosis of conduct disorder. Although the first eight items on the conduct disorder list are identical to the DSM-IV-TR items for oppositional disorder, ICD-10 oppositional defiant disorder can be considerably more severe because up to two of the items can be drawn from the 15 items that comprise the conduct disorder item set.

References

Achenbach TM (1991a) *Integrative Guide for the 1991 CBCL/4-18, YSR, and TRF Profiles.* Department of Psychiatry, University of Vermont, Burlington, VT.

Achenbach TM (1991b) *Manual for the Teacher's Report Form and 1991 Profile.* University of Vermont, Department of Psychiatry, Burlington, VT.

American Academy of Child and Adolescent Psychiatry (1997) Practice parameters for the assessment and treatment of children, adolescents, and adults with attention-deficit/hyperactivity disorder. *J Am Acad Child Adolesc Psychiatr* 36, 85S–121S.

American Psychiatric Association (2000) *Diagnostic and Statistical Manual of Mental Disorders*, 4th edn. Text Rev (DSM-IV-TR). APA, Washington DC.

Barkley RA, Anastopolous AD, Guevremont DC et al. (1991) Adolescents with ADHD: Patterns of behavioral adjustment, academic functioning and treatment utilization. *J Am Acad Child Adolesc Psychiatr* 30, 752–761.

Biederman J, Faraone SV, Keenan K et al. (1992) Further evidence for family-genetic risk factors in attention-deficit hyperactivity disorder. Patterns of comorbidity in probands and relatives in psychiatrically and pediatrically referred samples. *Arch Gen Psychiatr* 49, 728–738.

Biederman J, Baldessarini RJ, Wright V et al. (1993) A double blind placebo-controlled study of desipramine in the treatment of attention deficit disorder. III. Lack of impact of comorbidity and family history factors on clinical response. *J Am Acad Child Adolesc Psychiatr* 32, 199–204.

Castellanos FX, Elia J, Kruesi MJ et al. (1996) Cerebrospinal fluid homovanillic acid predicts behavioral response to stimulants in 45 boys with attention-deficit/hyperactivity disorder. *Neuropsychopharmacology* 14, 125–137.

Cohen P, Cohen J, Kasen S et al. (1993) An epidemiological study of disorders in late childhood and adolescence. I. Age- and gender-specific prevalence. *J Child Psychol Psychiatr* 34, 851–867.

Conners CK, Sitarenios G, Parker JDA et al. (1998a) The Revised Conners' Parent Rating Scale (CPRS-R): Factor structure, reliability, and criterion validity. *J Abnorm Child Psychol* 26, 257–268.

Conners CK, Sitarenios G, Parker JDA et al. (1998b) Revision and Restandardization of the Conners Teacher Rating Scale (CTRS-R): Factor structure, reliability, and criterion validity. *J Abnorm Child Psychol* 26, 279–291.

Daly G, Hawi Z, Fitzgerald M et al. (1999) Mapping susceptibility loci in attention-deficit hyperactivity disorder: Preferential transmission of parental alleles at DAT1, DBH and DRD5 to affected children. *Mol Psychiatr* 4, 192–196.

Dougherty DD, Bonab AA, Spencer TJ et al. (1999) Dopamine transporter density in patients with attention-deficit hyperactivity disorder. *Lancet* 354, 2132–2133.

Findling RL, McNamara NK, Branicky LA et al. (2000) A double-blind pilot study of risperidone in the treatment of conduct disorder. *J Am Acad Child Adolesc Psychiatr* 39, 509–516.

Halperin JM, Newcorn JH, Koda VH et al. (1997) Noradrenergic mechanisms in ADHD children with and without reading disabilities: A replication and extension. *J Am Acad Child Adolesc Psychiatr* 36, 1688–1697.

Harper GW and Ottinger DR (1992) The performance of hyperactive and control preschoolers on a new computerized measure of visual vigilance: The preschool vigilance task. *J Child Psychol Psychiatr* 33, 1365–1372.

Hechtman L, Weiss G, Perlman T et al. (1981) Hyperactives as young adults: Various clinical outcomes. *Adolesc Psychiatr* 9, 295–306.

Hinshaw SP (1987) On the distinction between attentional-deficits/hyperactivity and conduct problems/aggression in child psychopathology. *Psychol Bull* 101, 443–463.

Hinshaw SP, Heller T and McHale JP (1992) Covert antisocial behavior in boys with attention-deficit hyperactivity disorder: External validation and effects of methylphenidate. *J Consult Clin Psychol* 60, 274–281.

Hinshaw SP, Owens EB, Wells KC *et al.* (2000) Family processes and treatment outcome in the MTA: Negative/ineffective parenting practices in relation to multimodal treatment. *J Abnorm Child Psychol* 28, 555–568.

Jensen PS, Hinshaw SP, Kraemer HC *et al.* (2001) ADHD comorbidity findings from the MTA study: Comparing comorbid subgroups. *J Am Acad Child Adolesc Psychiatr* 40, 147–158.

Krause K-H, Dresel SH, Krause J *et al.* (2000) Increased striatal dopamine transporter in adult patients with attention-deficit hyperactivity disorder: Effects of methylphenidate as measured by single photon emission computed tomography. *Neurosci Lett* 285, 107–110.

Kruesi MJ, Rapoport JL, Hamburger SD *et al.* (1990) Cerebrospinal fluid monoamine metabolites, aggression, and impulsivity in disruptive behavior disorders of children and adolescents. *Arch Gen Psychiatr* 47, 419–426.

Loeber R (1990) Developmental and risk factors of juvenile antisocial behavior and delinquency. *Clin Psychol Rev* 10, 1–41.

Loeber R, Green SM, Lahey BB *et al.* (1991) Differences and similarities between children, mothers and teachers as informants on disruptive child behavior. *J Abnorm Child Psychol* 19, 75–95.

March JS, Swanson JM, Arnold LE *et al.* (2000) Anxiety as a predictor and outcome variable in the multimodal treatment study of children with ADHD (MTA). *J Abnorm Child Psychol* 28, 527–541.

Markowitz PI and Coccaro EF (1995) Biological studies of impulsivity aggression, and suicidal behavior, in *Impulsivity and Aggression* (eds Hollander E and Stein D). John Wiley, Chichester, pp. 71–91.

MTA Cooperative Group (1999a) A 14-month randomized clinical trial of treatment strategies for attention-deficit/hyperactivity disorder: The Multimodal Treatment Study of children with ADHD. *Arch Gen Psychiatr* 56, 1073–1086.

MTA Cooperative Group (1999b) Moderators and mediators of treatment response for children with attention-deficit/hyperactivity disorder: The Multimodal Treatment Study of children with attention-deficit/ hyperactivitydisorder. *Arch Gen Psychiatr* 56, 1088–1096.

Pliszka SR, Greenhill LL, Crismon ML *et al.* (2000a) The Texas Children's Medication Algorithm Project: Report of the Texas Consensus Conference Panel on Medication Treatment of Childhood Attention-Deficit/Hyperactivity Disorder. Part I. Attention-deficit/hyperactivity disorder. *J Am Acad Child Adolesc Psychiatr* 39, 908–919.

Pliszka SR, Greenhill LL, Crismon ML *et al.* (2000b) The Texas Children's Medication Algorithm Project: Report of the Texas Consensus Conference Panel on Medication Treatment of Childhood Attention-Deficit/Hyperactivity Disorder. Part II. Tactics. Attention-deficit/hyperactivity disorder. *J Am Acad Child Adolesc Psychiatr* 39, 920–927.

Rogeness GA, Javors MA, Maas JW *et al.* (1987) Plasma dopamine-b-hydroxylase, HVA, MHPG, and conduct disorder in emotionally disturbed boys. *Biol Psychiatr* 22, 1158–1162.

Rutter M, Cox A, Tupling C *et al.* (1975) Attainment and adjustment in two geographical areas, Vol. 1. The prevalence of psychiatric disorders. *Br J Psychiatr* 126, 493–509.

Scahill L, Chappell PB, Kim YS *et al.* (2001) A placebo-controlled study of guanfacine in the treatment of children with tic disorders and attention-deficit hyperactivity disorder. *Am J Psychiatr* 158, 1067–1074.

Sherman D, Iacono W and McGue M (1997) Attention-deficit hyperactivity disorder dimensions: A twin study of inattention and impulsivity-hyperactivity. *J Am Acad Child Adolesc Psychiatr* 36, 745–753.

Slutske WS, Heath AC, Dinwiddie SH *et al.* (1997) Modeling genetic and environmental influences in the etiology of conduct disorder: A study of 2682 adult twin pairs. *J Abnorm Psychol* 106, 266–279.

Spencer T, Biederman J, Wilens T *et al.* (2001) Efficacy of a mixed amphetamine salts compound in adults with attention-deficit/hyperactivity disorder. *Arch Gen Psychiatr* 58, 775–782.

Sprague RL and Sleator EK (1977) Methylphenidate in hyperkinetic children: Differences in dose effects on learning and social behavior. *Science* 198, 1274–1276.

Swanson JM, Sunohara GA, Kennedy JL *et al.* (1998) Association of the dopamine receptor D$_4$ (DRD4) gene with a refined phenotype of attention-deficit hyperactivity disorder (ADHD): A family-based approach. Mol Psychiatr 3, 38–41.

Winsberg BG and Comings DE (1999) Association of the dopamine transporter gene (DAT1) with poor methylphenidate response. *J Am Acad Child Adolesc Psychiatr* 38, 1474–1477.

Zametkin AJ and Rapoport JL (1987) Neurobiology of attention-deficit disorder with hyperactivity: Where have we come in 50 years? *J Am Acad Child Adolesc Psychiatr* 26, 676–686.

Zametkin AJ, Nordahl TE, Gross M *et al.* (1990) Cerebral glucose metabolism in adults with hyperactivity of childhood onset. *New Engl J Med* 323, 1361–1366.

Zametkin AJ, Liebenauer LL, Fitzgerald GA *et al.* (1993) Brain metabolism in teenagers with attention-deficit hyperactivity disorder. *Arch Gen Psychiatr* 50, 333–340.

Childhood Disorders: Feeding and Other Disorders of Infancy or Early Childhood

In the literature, the term "feeding disorder" generally encompasses a variety of conditions ranging from problem behaviors during feeding – poor appetite, food refusal, food selectivity, food avoidance, and pica to rumination and vomiting – and is generally used to emphasize the dyadic nature of eating problems in infants and young children. Feeding disorder cannot be attributed to a medical condition and appears most often during the first year of life and before the age of six. Its hallmarks are the failure to eat with resultant inability to gain weight or a significant weight loss for at least one month.

Some authors have used various diagnostic methods and assigned different labels to address the heterogeneity of feeding problems associated with failure to thrive. The pediatric literature has focused primarily on failure to thrive as a diagnostic label. The term "failure to thrive" describes infants and young children who demonstrate failure in physical growth, often associated with delay of social and motor development.

Because of the diversity of feeding disorders associated with failure to thrive and the lack of a subclassification of feeding disorder as defined in DSM-IV-TR, Chatoor proposed a classification of feeding disorders based on the definition of psychiatric disorders. A psychiatric disorder has three properties: it is a limited syndrome with possible links to etiological and pathophysiological factors; the use of treatment depends on proper diagnosis; and the diagnosis is linked to prognosis. Considering these criteria, five different feeding disorders will be described. The first three feeding disorders are associated with various developmental stages. In addition, two feeding disorders are described that are not linked to specific developmental stages: 1) sensory food aversions, a common feeding disorder which becomes evident during the introduction of different milks, baby food, or table food with various tastes and consistencies, and 2) post traumatic feeding disorder, which is characterized by an acute disruption in the regulation of eating and can occur at various ages and stages of feeding development.

Epidemiology

It is estimated that up to 25% of otherwise normally developing infants and up to 80% of those with developmental handicaps have feeding problems including food refusal, eating "too little" or "too much", restricted food preferences, delay in self-feeding, objectionable mealtime behaviors and bizarre food habits. It has also been reported that 1 to 2% of infants under 1 year of age demonstrate severe food refusal and poor growth.

Course and Natural History

Those infants who at 3 to 12 months of age are identified for refusal to eat for at least 4 weeks with no apparent medical cause have significantly more problems in eating patterns, behavior and growth, and are more susceptible to infection at 2 and 4 years of age. A study by Marchi and Cohen (1990), who observed a sample of more than 800 children for a 10-year period from early childhood to late childhood–adolescence, found that feeding problems in young children were stable over time. They reported that gastrointestinal symptoms and picky eating during early childhood correlated with anorectic behavior during adolescence, while problem behaviors during mealtime and pica early in life were associated with bulimia nervosa during the adolescent years.

Etiology

Hampering our understanding of the etiology, symptoms and treatment of specific feeding disorders are the lack of a standard classification, overlap between feeding disorders and failure to thrive, and the tendency of investigators to address different aspects of the disorders while using differing criteria and methodologies. To clarify the specificity in etiology and its implication for treatment, each feeding disorder as defined by Chatoor and colleagues (1985) is discussed separately.

Diagnosis

The diagnostic assessment of feeding disorders should include assessment of the infant's temperament characteristics; the infant's medical, developmental and feeding history; the caretaker's psychological functioning and past history, socioeconomic background, stressors and social support system; and the relationship of the infant and his or her primary caretakers during feeding and play.

Treatment

Treatment begins with the first contact with the infant and his or her caregivers. The establishment of a therapeutic alliance with the caregivers is critical to any successful treatment. The diagnostic evaluation needs to identify the specific dynamics of each feeding disorder in order to develop a specific treatment plan. This is discussed in more detail for each feeding disorder.

Essentials of Psychiatry Jerald Kay and Allan Tasman
© 2006 John Wiley & Sons, Ltd.

Feeding Disorder of State Regulation

Diagnostic Criteria

A. Has difficulty reaching and maintaining a calm state of alertness for feeding; is either too sleepy or too agitated and/or distressed to feed.
B. The feeding difficulties start in the newborn period.
C. Shows significant failure to gain weight or exhibits weight loss.

Epidemiology

The most frequently used label in the pediatric literature for excessive crying in young infants is colic, which is reported to occur at rates varying from 5 to 19%. Colic is usually defined as crying for more than 3 hours per day, and frequently colic is associated with feeding difficulties during the crying periods. However, a feeding disorder of state regulation should be considered only in more severe cases of colic when it is associated with growth failure.

Etiology

Both infant and maternal characteristics appear to contribute to the difficulties in the regulation of feeding. After birth, the infant needs to establish regular rhythms of sleep and wakefulness, and of feeding and elimination. In order to feed successfully, the infant needs to reach a state of calm alertness. However, some infants may be too irritable or too difficult to awaken for feedings.

Clinical Vignette 1

Jeff is a 3-month-old baby who was brought into the hospital by his 17-year-old mother and his grandmother because of feeding difficulties and lack of appropriate weight gain starting at birth. On physical examination, he appeared weak and had poor muscle tone but otherwise had no signs of physical illness. His weight was 6 pounds and 9 ounces, which was only 4 ounces above birth weight. The history revealed that Jeff's mother had an uncomplicated pregnancy and delivery. She was a senior in high school and had missed only a few weeks of school before the delivery of Jeff and 6 weeks thereafter. The mother and her three younger siblings lived with their mother. The father of the infant and the father of the mother were out of the picture. The mother and the grandmother shared taking care of Jeff. They reported that, at times, Jeff would be irritable and difficult to calm for feedings. At other times, particularly in recent weeks, he would be so sleepy that it was difficult to waken him enough to feed. Both mother and grandmother appeared distressed about Jeff's feeding difficulties.

The mother admitted that the pregnancy with Jeff was unplanned and that she broke up with Jeff's father soon after she found out that she was pregnant. She had felt anxious throughout the pregnancy because she worried about the baby's future and her own. When she returned to school several weeks ago, she had difficulty concentrating and had done poorly on her grades. In recent weeks, she had difficulty sleeping at night, had felt weak during the day, had been eating poorly and had lost some weight herself. Despite having a good relationship with her mother, she felt lonely and isolated from her peers.

Mother–infant interactions during feeding revealed a sad young mother who gently tried to awaken her lethargic infant by rubbing his hands and feet. When unsuccessful, she held his little body upright. This resulted in the infant's head dropping backward abruptly. He was startled and cried loudly. When the mother successfully calmed the infant, he went right back to sleep without drinking from the bottle. The mother looked despondent and helpless.

Diagnostic Impression

It appeared that the infant's difficulty in regulating his state, being either too irritable to calm for feedings or too lethargic to awaken for feedings, together with the mother's anxiety and inexperience had resulted in a vicious cycle, leading to increasing depression in the mother and a severe feeding disorder of state regulation in the infant.

Treatment

Because of his poor nutritional state and his lethargy, Jeff was hospitalized. For a few days, he was given nasogastric tube feedings to supplement his poor oral intake. He was assigned a primary care nurse who was experienced in feeding babies. She would take him into a quiet room on the unit for feedings and gradually increase the physical stimulation to arouse him enough to be interested in drinking from the bottle. If she moved too quickly, he would start to cry and could not be fed. After a week of increasingly successful feedings, both the mother and the grandmother were invited to observe the feedings and were later coached by the nurse to take over the feedings themselves.

At the same time, while the nurse was working with Jeff, a psychiatric resident met regularly with the mother to address her feelings of anxiety and depression. Because of the severity of her depression, the mother was prescribed an antidepressant to which she responded well. When the mother began to sleep better and Jeff became more lively and responsive, she was able to deal with him more effectively. She enjoyed the positive reinforcement by the nurse, who tutored her in how to stimulate Jeff to reach a state of calm alertness that allowed him to feed successfully.

After 3 weeks, both mother and infant had made sufficient gains to be discharged from the hospital. Back at their home, Jeff and his mother were visited weekly by a home care nurse and the mother continued in psychotherapy and pharmacotherapy with the psychiatric resident for the next 7 months. Jeff developed into an engaging little boy who continued to be vulnerable to changes in his caretaking environment, manifested by irritability and poor feeding. His mother recovered from her depression and graduated successfully from high school.

Other infants may tire quickly or become distracted during feeding and terminate feedings without taking in adequate amounts of milk to grow. Some mothers learn to compensate for these vulnerabilities by adjusting the environment and the degree of stimulation of the infant during feeding. However, other mothers become anxious, fatigued, or depressed, and consequently they inadvertently intensify the feeding difficulties of their infants.

Diagnosis

Young infants who present with feeding difficulties and growth failure dating to the postnatal period need to be considered for the diagnosis of a feeding disorder of state regulation. The evaluation should begin by obtaining a history of the mother's pregnancy and delivery and a report of the infant's history of feeding, development and medical illnesses that might contribute to the feeding problems. In addition, the mother's functioning and her social support system need to be explored. Most important, the mother and her infant should be observed during feeding and during play to assess the infant's special characteristics, the infant's regulation of state and feeding behavior, and the mother's ability to read the infant's signals and to respond to them in a contingent way.

Course and Natural History

During the first few months of life, the foundation for the regulation of feeding, sleep and emotions is laid. Infants with feeding problems during these early months usually trigger anxiety in their mothers and tend to have difficulties in self-regulation during the transition to self-feeding in the second year of life.

Treatment

Treatment can be directed toward the infant, toward the mother, and toward the mother–infant interaction. In severe cases, if the infant's growth is seriously impaired, nasogastric tube feeding might have to be used to supplement oral feedings in an infant who tires quickly. This will allow an anxious mother to relax because her infant is receiving adequate nutrition to grow. Subsequently, a more relaxed mother can tune into her infant more readily and break the cycle of dyadic escalation of tension during feedings.

On the other hand, the intervention might have to be directed primarily toward the mother to treat her anxiety, fatigue, or depression to enable her to be more effective in dealing with her infant. In addition, most mothers can be helped by assisting them in problem solving in how to facilitate a feeding environment that provides the optimal amount of stimulation for their vulnerable infants. Videotaping the feeding and observing the tape together with the mother can heighten her awareness of the infant's reactions during feeding and enhance her ability to read the infant's cues. The therapist can then engage the mother in a dialogue on how to respond to the infant's cues most effectively.

Feeding Disorder of Poor Care Giver–Infant Reciprocity

Diagnostic Criteria

A. Shows a lack of developmentally appropriate signs of social reciprocity (e.g., visual engagement, smiling, or babbling) with the primary caregiver during feeding.

B. Onset under 1 year of age.

C. Shows significant growth deficiency.

D. The growth deficiency and lack of engagement with the primary caregiver are not due solely to a physical disorder, or a pervasive developmental disorder.

This feeding disorder has been referred to in the early literature as maternal deprivation, deprivation dwarfism and psychosocial deprivation. The growth failure and developmental delay of these infants were considered a consequence of a continuum of neglect and/or maltreatment of the child leading to insecure attachment to the caregiver.

Epidemiology

It is difficult to assess how commonly this feeding disorder occurs. However, there appears to be an increased prevalence of cases in the lower socioeconomic classes, as noted by Chatoor and colleagues (1997).

Etiology

Much has been written about mothers whose infants fail to thrive and appear to have a disorder of reciprocity. They are frequently described as suffering from character disorder, affective illness, alcohol abuse and drug abuse. Early research suggested that the highest risk exists when the mother's needs take precedence over those of the infant, and that difficulties of these mothers in nurturing their infants stem from the unmet needs of the mothers during their own childhood.

Family problems and distressed marital relationships have been reported in a number of noncontrolled and controlled studies of failure to thrive. In addition, socially adverse living conditions, poverty and unemployment are reported to be more prevalent in these families of infants with failure to thrive.

Between 45 to 93% of the infants with failure to thrive are insecurely attached. Mothers of infants with failure to thrive are more likely to be classified as insecurely attached to their own parents, as measured by the Adult Attachment Interview (Main and Goldwyn, 1991).

The growth failure of these infants with poor caregiver–infant reciprocity appears to be a critical manifestation of a failed relationship between a mother and her infant during the first year of life, when the foundation for mutual engagement and attachment is usually laid. A transgenerational pattern of insecure attachment appears to be at the root of the mother's difficulty to engage with her infant and leads to a lack of emotional and physical nurturance of the infant.

Diagnosis

Most of these infants are not brought for pediatric well-baby care but present to the emergency department because of an acute illness, when their poor nutritional state draws the attention of pediatricians. Because of their severe failure to thrive, these infants frequently require hospitalization. During the hospitalization, the psychiatric consultant is usually called in to assist in the diagnosis and treatment of the infant's growth and developmental problems. The evaluation should include an assessment of the infant's feeding, developmental and health history, including any changes in the infant's behavior during the hospitalization. In addition, the mother's pregnancy, delivery, family situation and social support need to be thoroughly explored. A mental status examination of the mother should be performed to rule out severe psychiatric illness, particularly whether she suffers from depression or is abusing alcohol or drugs.

Many of these mothers are elusive and avoidant of any contact with professionals. Consequently, the observation of mother–infant interactions may have to be obtained indirectly, through the report of other professionals who admitted the infant to the hospital.

Infants with feeding disorders of poor mother–infant reciprocity characteristically feed poorly, avoid eye contact and are weak in the first few days of hospitalization. When picked up, they might scissor their legs and hold up their arms in a surrender posture to balance their heads, which seem too heavy for their little weak bodies. They usually do not cuddle like healthy well-fed infants, rather they keep their legs drawn up or appear hypotonic, like rag dolls. However, these infants appear to blossom under the tender care of a primary care nurse who engages with them during feeding and plays with them. They become increasingly responsive, begin to smile, feed hungrily and gain weight. These striking changes in behavior of these young infants when they are fed and attended to by a nurturing caretaker are characteristic of a feeding disorder of poor mother–infant reciprocity and differentiate these infants from infants with organic problems that have resulted in growth failure and developmental delays.

Course and Natural History

Because of an inconsistent definition of failure to thrive, it is not clear whether all of these infants suffered from a feeding disorder of poor mother–infant reciprocity. In general, nonorganic failure to thrive during infancy has been associated with later cognitive and behavioral problems. Hufton and Oates (1977) reported that of 21 children who had been diagnosed with nonorganic failure to thrive during infancy, at the age of 6 years, half of the children had abnormal personalities and two-thirds had a delayed reading age.

Treatment

Various treatment approaches have been proposed, ranging from home-based interventions to hospitalization in severe cases Because of the complexity of the issues involved in the etiology of nonorganic failure to thrive, most psychiatrists and researchers suggest that multiple and case-specific interventions may be required. An outpatient approach appears to be safe in cases of mild neglect when there is no evidence of deprivational behavior on the part of the mother, the infant is older than 12 months, and the parents have a support system and have sought medical care for previous sickness. Immediate hospitalization of young infants with neglectful failure to thrive is indicated if it is associated with non-accidental trauma; if the degree of failure to thrive is considered severe; if there is serious hygiene neglect; if the mother appears severely disturbed, abusing drugs or alcohol; if the mother lives in a chaotic lifestyle and appears overwhelmed with stresses; or if the mother–infant interaction appears angry and uncaring.

During the hospitalization it is most important to assign a primary care nurse who can be warm and nurturing to woo the infant into a mutual relationship. Improvement of the infant's health and affective availability can then be used to engage the mother with her infant and in the treatment process. Recovery from growth failure does not indicate that the parent–child relationship is adequate. The mother's ability to engage her infant and to participate in the treatment process has to be at the core of the treatment plan. The degree of parental awareness and cooperation is predictive of outcome for failure to thrive.

Because these mothers frequently present with a variety of psychological and social disturbances, their problems need to be explored while nutritional, emotional and developmental rehabilitation goes on with the infant. It is important to look for and identify any positive behavior a mother shows toward her infant and to use it as a building block to bolster her competence and interest in her infant. Nurturance of the mother is the first critical step in the treatment to facilitate her potential to nurture her infant. Moreover, the family can serve as a stress-buffering or stress-producing system. The hospitalization of the infant provides a critical time to assess whether the infant needs to be placed in alternative care. In some situations of severe neglect or associated abuse, the case needs to be reported to protective services, which at times can be instrumental in mobilizing the family or in finding foster care.

Discharge from the hospital is a critical time when all services need to be in place to ensure appropriate follow-through of the treatment plan for these vulnerable infants. For some infants, daycare in a nurturing environment will give the mother an opportunity to pursue some of her own interests and needs as well as to make the time with her infant more special and enjoyable. Visits by a home care nurse or regular treatment sessions in the home by a social worker are some of the alternatives to consider because many of these mothers struggle with coming to therapy in an office setting. Because of the complexity of the problems involved in the etiology of this feeding disorder, a flexible multidisciplinary approach that is coordinated by the primary therapist is usually most effective.

Infantile Anorexia

Diagnostic Criteria

A. Refusal to eat adequate amounts of food for at least 1 month.
B. Onset of the food refusal under 3 years of age, most commonly during the transition to spoon- and self-feeding.
C. Does not communicate hunger signals, lacks interest in food, but shows strong interest in exploration and/or interaction with caregiver.
D. Shows significant growth deficiency.
E. The food refusal did not follow a traumatic event.
F. The food refusal is not due to an underlying medical illness.

Epidemiology

A study from Sweden reported that 1 to 2% of infants younger than 1 year of age had severe feeding problems associated with refusal to eat or vomiting, resulting in poor weight gain. At 4 years, 71% of those with food refusal were reported by their parents as still having feeding problems (Dahl and Sundelin, 1992). The disorder seems to be equally as common among boys and girls of all racial backgrounds and appears most commonly in the middle and upper middle class.

Etiology

Chatoor and colleagues (2000) tested a transactional model for the understanding of infantile anorexia by which certain characteristics of the infant combine with certain vulnerabilities in the mother to bring out negative responses and conflict in their interactions. They also found that infants with infantile anorexia were rated higher by their mothers on temperament difficulty, irregularity of feeding and sleeping patterns, negativity, dependence and unstoppable behaviors than were healthy eaters. The mothers of children with infantile anorexia were found to demonstrate more attachment insecurity to their own parents. The mothers' attachment insecurity frequently stemmed from extremes of parental discipline in the form of parental over control or emotional unavailability while they were growing up. The infants' temperament characteristics, their mothers' insecure attachment to their own parents, and the mothers' drive to be thin themselves correlated significantly with mother–infant conflict during feeding.

It is helpful to look at infantile anorexia from a developmental perspective. Between 9 and 18 months of age, the general developmental task of separation and individuation takes on special significance in the feeding relationship. Issues of autonomy versus dependency must be worked out in the dyad, particularly during the transition to self-feeding. If the mother is able to read the infant's signals correctly and responds contingently, the infant will learn to differentiate physiological feelings of hunger and fullness from emotional experiences such as anger, frustration, or the wish for attention. In this case, the infant's food intake will be internally regulated through physiological cues of hunger and satiety. On the other hand, if the mother is insecure in how to interpret the infant's cues and responds in a noncontingent way, the infant will learn to associate feeding with negative or positive emotional experiences. Consequently, infants who are irregular and whose cues are difficult to read, and mothers who are insecure in how to interpret their infants' cues and respond in an inconsistent and noncontingent way, will develop conflict during feeding, and the infant will fail to develop internal regulation of eating.

Diagnosis

Infants with this feeding disorder are usually referred for a psychiatric evaluation due to food refusal and growth failure. The infants' food refusal usually becomes of concern between 6 months and 3 years, most commonly between 9 and 18 months of age, during the transition to spoon- and self-feeding. However, some parents report that even during the first few months of life, these infants were easily distracted by external stimuli and became disinterested in feeding. Then, the mothers were able to compensate for the infants' poor feeding by feeding them more frequently. However, by the end of the first year when infants are transitioned to spoon- and self-feeding, these infants take only a few bites and want to get out of the high chair to play. Most parents report that these infants hardly show any signals of hunger and seem more interested in exploring and playing than eating. Usually, the parents become increasingly worried about their infants' poor food intake and try to increase their infants' eating by coaxing, distracting, offering different food, feeding during play, feeding at night, threatening and even force-feeding their infants. However, most parents report that these methods worked only temporarily, if at all, and that their infants continued to eat poorly in spite of all their efforts.

The diagnostic evaluation of this feeding disorder should include the infant's feeding, developmental and health history, and the observation of mother and infant during feeding. In addition to the infant's history, the mother's perception of her infant's temperament, her family situation, her childhood background, and her own eating habits and attitude toward limit setting need to be explored.

Course and Natural History

Initially, infants with this feeding disorder fail to gain adequate weight. After several weeks or months of poor food intake, their linear growth slows down and they develop chronic malnutrition. In most cases their heads continue to grow at a normal rate. As the children grow older, their bodies appear small and thin, but their head size and brain development appear to progress at a normal rate.

Treatment

The psychotherapeutic intervention is based on the developmental psychopathological model of infantile anorexia as outlined in the section on etiology. The major goal of the intervention is to "facilitate internal regulation of eating" by the infant. The intervention consists of three components:

1. Assess and then explain the infant's special temperamental characteristics and developmental conflicts to the mother to help her understand the lack of expected hunger cues and the infant's struggle for control during the feeding situation.
2. Explore the mother's upbringing and the effect it has had on the parenting of her infant to help the mother understand her conflicts and difficulties in regard to limit setting.
3. Explain the concept of internal versus external regulation of eating. Help the mother to develop mealtime routines that facilitate the infant's awareness of hunger, leading to internal regulation of eating, improved food intake and growth. In addition, coach the parents to set limits to the infant's behaviors that interfere with eating. These feeding guidelines include:
   a. Schedule meals and snacks at regular 3- to 4-hour intervals and do not allow the infant to snack or drink from the bottle or breast in between.
   b. Limit meal duration to 30 minutes.
   c. Praise the infant for self-feeding but stay emotionally neutral whether the infant eats little or a lot.
   d. Do not use distracting toys or television during feedings.
   e. Eliminate desserts or sweets as a reward at the end of the meal; rather integrate them into regular meals and snacks.
   f. Put the infant in "time-out" for inappropriate behaviors during feeding (e.g., throwing the spoon or food, climbing out of the high chair).

These three steps in the treatment are best accomplished in three sessions lasting 2 to 3 hours each and grouped close together within a 2- to 3-week period. The intensity of this brief intervention facilitates a close therapeutic alliance between the therapist and the mother and gives the mother the opportunity to experience the support she needs to make major changes in her interactions with her infant.

Giving the mother the choice as to who in the family (or anyone else) should be included in the therapeutic process, and at what point, is part of putting the mother in control. Because many of these mothers have felt helpless as children and ineffective as parents, the empowerment of the mother is critical to the success of the treatment.

Sensory Food Aversions

Diagnostic Criteria

A. Consistently refuses to eat specific foods with specific tastes, textures, and/or smells.
B. Onset of the food refusal during the introduction of a different type of food (different milk, different baby food, or different table food).
C. Eats without difficulty when offered preferred foods.
D. The food refusal has resulted in specific nutritional deficiencies and/or delay in oral motor development.

Epidemiology

Sensory food aversions are a common problem among toddlers. A survey of 1523 parents of toddlers ranging in age from 12 to 36 months found that 20% of the parents indicated that their toddlers were eating only a few types of food "often" or "always", and 6% of the same parents were indicating that they worried "often" or "always" that their children were not eating enough to grow.

Etiology

Several studies indicate that genetic predisposition as well as environment affect toddlers' food preferences, though empirical studies have not explored the origins of selective food refusal in infants and toddlers. Some individuals avoid particular foods because they find their taste and/or odor too aversive. Parents with extreme taste sensitivities may offer a restricted range of foods to their children and model eating only certain foods that they like. Limited exposure to a variety of foods may enhance the toddlers' food selectivity.

Diagnosis

Sensory food aversions occur along a spectrum of severity. Some children refuse to eat only a few types of food, making it possible for the parents to accommodate the child's food preferences. Others may refuse most foods, disrupt family meals and cause serious parental concern about the children's nutrition. The diagnosis of a feeding disorder should only be made if the food selectivity results in nutritional deficiencies, and/or has led to oral motor delay.

Sensory food aversions become apparent when infants are introduced to a different milk, to baby food, or to table food with a variety of tastes and textures. Usually, when foods that are aversive to the infant are placed in the infant's mouth, the infant's reactions range from grimacing to gagging, vomiting, or spitting out the food. After an initial aversive reaction, the infants usually refuse to continue eating that particular food, becoming distressed if forced to do so, and may generalize their reluctance to eat one food to other foods with similar characteristics.

If infants refuse many foods or whole food groups, their limited diet may lead to specific nutritional deficiencies, and they will experience delay in their oral motor development due to lack of practice with chewing. In addition, the children's refusal to eat a variety of foods frequently leads to family conflict at mealtime, and puts a strain on the child and the family in social situations outside the home.

The evaluation of infants and young children with sensory food aversions should address how many foods the child consistently refuses and how many foods he/she usually accepts. A nutritional assessment needs to look not only at the anthropometric measures of the child to rule out acute and/or chronic malnutrition, but needs to address whether the child may lack adequate intake of vitamins, zinc, iron and/or protein. In addition, an oral motor assessment needs to determine whether the child has fallen behind in this area of development. Delayed oral motor development will limit the kind of foods the child should be offered in order to prevent choking, and may be associated with a delay in speech development. In addition, the parents' food preferences during childhood and adulthood should be explored to assess whether the parents may be limited in the variety of foods they offer their child. Additional, nonfood hypersensitivities should also be explored.

Course and Natural History

No longitudinal data are available outlining the course of this feeding disorder. Sensory food aversions begin to show in about 10% of toddlers between 12 and 18 months of age, but then increase to 20% and stay around that frequency until 3 years of age. Older children with sensory food aversions may experience social anxiety when their peers become aware that they eat only certain foods, and some children avoid social situations that include eating.

Treatment

In young infants (4–7 months of age), a few repeated exposures to new foods enhance the infants' acceptance not only of that food but also of other similar foods. However, this changes in the second year of life, when the acceptance of new foods only increased significantly after 10 or more exposures to those same foods It appears that novel flavors become more preferred after repeated pairing with high caloric carbohydrates versus low caloric carbohydrates.

It is useful to introduce a variety of foods during the first year of life when infants in general are less discriminating in their food preferences. However, if infants show strong aversive reactions (e.g., gagging or vomiting) early on when offered a certain food, it is advisable to give up on that particular food and not offer it again. If the infant shows a less severe reaction (e.g., grimaces or wants to spit out a new food) it is also best to stop offering the new food during that feeding, but introduce it again after a few days in a small amount and paired with some other food that the infant likes, increasing the amounts of the new food very gradually until the infant appears comfortable with it.

For toddlers, the challenge remains how to keep them interested in trying new foods after they have had aversive experiences with some foods. Coercive techniques, for example, threatening children to sit at the table until they finish eating everything on their plate or depriving them of certain privileges, have a significant negative effect. On the other hand, toddlers are very responsive to modeling by their parents. Toddlers are more willing to try a new food if they can observe their parents eating it without being offered. If they ask for their parents' food, it is best to give them only a small amount while saying that they can have more if they like the food. If the parents stay neutral as to whether the toddler likes the food or not, toddlers remain neutral as well and do not appear to become scared of trying new foods. However, once children fear to try new foods, their diet becomes more and more limited and, by 3 years of age, most young children are not swayed by what their parents eat. Some young children like to imitate their peers and may be willing to eat new foods in a preschool setting; however, others become anxious in social situations and try to avoid eating with others.

Post Traumatic Feeding Disorder

Diagnostic Criteria

A. Food refusal follows a traumatic event or repeated traumatic insults to the oropharynx or gastrointestinal tract (e.g., choking, severe vomiting, reflux, insertion of nasogastric or endotracheal tubes, suctioning) that trigger intense distress in the infant.

B. Consistent refusal to eat manifests in one of the following ways:

1. Refuses to drink from the bottle, but may accept food offered by spoon (although consistently refuses to drink from the bottle when awake, may drink from the bottle when sleepy or asleep).
2. Refuses solid food, but may accept the bottle.
3. Refuses all oral feedings.

C. Reminders of the traumatic event(s) cause distress as manifested by one or more of the following:

1. Shows anticipatory distress when positioned for feeding.
2. Shows intense resistance when approached with bottle or food.
3. Shows intense resistance to swallow food placed in the infant's mouth.

D. The food refusal poses an acute or long-term threat to the child's nutrition.

Epidemiology

Although no studies on the prevalence of this disorder are available, it appears that the occurrence of this feeding disorder has been increasing because of the growing number of infants with complex medical problems who survive.

Etiology

Although it is difficult to say what the inner experience of a young infant might be, the affective and behavioral expressions of infants provide a window to their inner life. In a study of infants diagnosed with post traumatic feeding disorder, also including a control group of healthy eaters and a group of anorectic infants matched by age, sex, race and socioeconomic background, conflict in mother–infant interactions during feeding was present in both feeding-disordered groups. However, only those subjects with a post traumatic feeding disorder demonstrated intense pre-oral and intraoral feeding resistance. They appeared distressed, cried and pushed the food away in anticipation of being fed, and kept solid food in their cheeks or spat it out if the mothers were able to place any food in their mouths. The mothers usually reported that these defensive behaviors started abruptly after the infant experienced severe vomiting, gagging, or choking or underwent invasive manipulation of the oropharynx (e.g., insertion of feeding and endotracheal tubes or vigorous suctioning).

Diagnosis and Differential Diagnosis

This feeding disorder is characterized by the infant's consistent refusal either to drink from the bottle or to eat any solid foods, and in most severe cases, by the infant's refusal to eat at all. Depending on the mode of feeding that the infants appear to associate with the traumatic event(s), some refuse to eat solids, but will continue to drink from the bottle, whereas others may refuse to drink from the bottle, but are willing to eat solids. Some infants may put baby food in their mouths, but then spit out any food that has any little lumps in it. Most infants get stuck in these food patterns and may lose weight or lack certain nutrients because of their limited diet.

Reminders of the traumatic event(s) (e.g., the bottle, the bib, or the high chair) may cause intense distress for some infants, whereby they become fearful when they are positioned for feedings and/or presented with feeding utensils and food. They resist being fed by crying, arching and refusing to open their mouths. If food is placed in their mouths, they intensely resist swallowing.

They may gag or vomit, let the food drop out, actively spit the food out, or store the food in their cheeks and spit it out later. The fear of eating seems to override any awareness of hunger. Therefore, infants who refuse all foods, including liquids and solids, require acute intervention due to dehydration and starvation.

In addition to a thorough history about the onset of the infant's food refusal and the medical and developmental history, the observation of the infant and mother during feeding is critical for understanding this feeding disorder and differentiating it from infantile anorexia and from sensory food aversions. It is helpful to ask the mother to bring a variety of foods, including those that the infant refuses and those that he or she accepts. Infants with a post traumatic feeding disorder characteristically appear engaged and comfortable with their mothers as long as the feared food is out of sight. Some infants begin to show distress when they are placed in the high chair and they struggle to get away. In less severe cases, the infant might allow the food to go into the mouth but then spit it out and show distress only when urged to swallow. This anticipatory fear of food differentiates infants with a post traumatic feeding disorder from anorectic infants, whose food refusal appears random and related to issues of control in the relationship with the mothers. Toddlers with sensory aversions to certain types of food might also show distress when urged to eat these foods. However, their mothers do not remember a traumatic event that seemed to trigger the food refusal behaviors.

Course and Natural History

Most infants seem to get locked into their food refusal patterns. The more anxiously the parents react to the infant's food refusal, the more anxious the infants appear to become, with the parent and the infant feeding off each other's anxiety. Individual case studies indicate that some of these infants depend for years on gastrostomy feedings to survive. Others may live on milk and puréed food until school age, when the social embarrassment of their eating behavior urges the parents to seek help.

Treatment

Because of the complexity of many of these cases, a multidisciplinary team (consisting of a pediatrician or gastroenterologist, a psychiatrist or psychologist, a social worker, an occupational therapist or hearing and speech specialist, a nutritionist and a specially trained nurse to serve as team coordinators) is best equipped to meet all the needs of these infants and their parents.

Before any psychiatric treatment can be successfully initiated, the medical and nutritional needs of the infant need to be addressed. In severe cases of total food refusal, it is important to act quickly to maintain the infant's hydration. The medical and psychiatric team members must work together to assess whether temporary nasogastric tube feedings are indicated or whether plans for a gastrostomy should be made. Unfortunately, the repeated insertion of nasogastric feeding tubes can intensify a post traumatic feeding disorder, and an infant in a labile medical condition can take months if not years to recover.

The psychiatric treatment of this feeding disorder involves a desensitization of the infant to overcome the anticipatory anxiety about eating and return to internal regulation of eating in response to hunger and satiety. It is most important to help the parents understand the dynamics of a post traumatic feeding disorder so that they can recognize the infant's anticipatory anxiety and become active participants in the treatment. After identification of triggers of anticipatory anxiety (e.g., the sight of the high chair, the bottle, or certain types of food), a desensitization by gradual exposure can be initiated or a more rapid desensitization through more intensive behavioral techniques can be implemented.

With both techniques, it is important to have a professional assess the infant's oral motor coordination because many infants who refuse to eat for extended periods fall behind in their oral motor development due to lack of practice. The rapid introduction of table food to a child who has delayed oral motor skills may lead to choking, thereby creating a setback to the desensitization process.

During the desensitization process, the infant has to be reinforced for swallowing the food. This behavioral manipulation of the infant's eating frequently leads to external regulation of eating in response to the reinforcers. Once the infant has become comfortable with eating, it is important to phase out these external reinforcers to allow the infant to regain internal regulation of eating in response to hunger and fullness. This can be a difficult transition because many infants gain control over their parent's emotions by eating or not eating. The techniques described under infantile anorexia – the implementation of the feeding guidelines contained in step 3 – can be helpful in making this transition.

As summarized in Figure 29.1, each of these five feeding disorders presents with specific symptom patterns and characteristic mother–infant interactions, which help to diagnose and differentiate the various feeding disorders. The correct diagnosis is critical because a treatment that is helpful for one feeding disorder may be ineffective or even worsen another feeding disorder. For example, infants with infantile anorexia become more aware of their hunger cues and feed better if fed only every

4 hours without being offered food or liquids in between meals. However, an infant with post traumatic feeding disorder who is afraid of eating will not accept food regardless of how long he or she has been kept without feeding. On the other hand, behavioral techniques that help extinguish fear-based food refusal in a post traumatic feeding disorder further distract an infant with infantile anorexia and further interfere with the awareness of hunger.

Rumination Disorder

Definition

Rumination disorder is characterized by the repeated regurgitation and rechewing of food occurring for at least one month with prior normal functioning. As in the case of feeding disorder of infancy and early childhood, these behaviors cannot be the result of a medical condition affecting the gastrointestinal tract. Similarly, this diagnosis is not made in the presence of anorexia nervosa or bulimia nervosa.

Epidemiology and Etiology

Rumination disorder appears to be uncommon, occurring more often in boys than in girls and also in individuals with mental retardation.

Several authors have attributed rumination to an unsatisfactory mother–infant relationship, (including neglect or lack of stimulation, and sometimes to stressful life situations of the

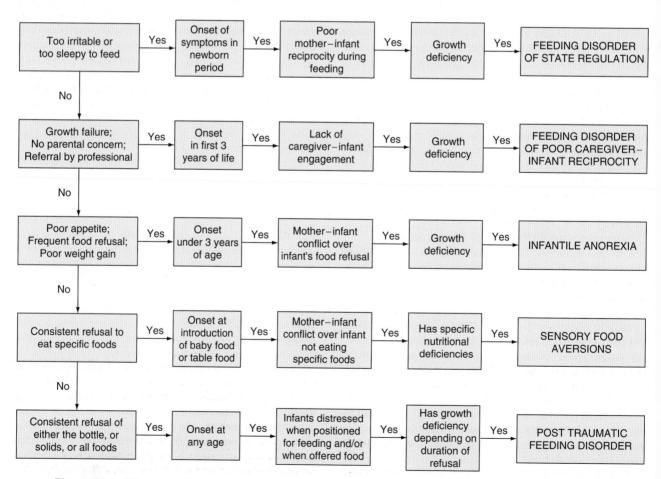

Figure 29.1 *Diagnostic decision tree for differential diagnosis of feeding disorders of infancy or early childhood.*

parent. Others have considered rumination a learned behavior that is maintained by special attention by the caregivers to the child's rumination and, consequently, the rumination has to be unlearned by counter conditioning. Rumination can be seen along a continuum: a patient may have gastrointestinal disease, such as hiatal hernia or reflux, and little psychiatric illness in the mother–infant relationship at one end of the spectrum; or the converse, a patient might have no reflux and severe psychiatric illness in the mother–infant relationship at the other end of the spectrum. Reflux or a temporary illness associated with vomiting frequently precedes the rumination. At some point, the infant seems to learn to initiate vomiting and turn it into rumination to achieve self-regulation. It appears that in circumstances in which the infant fails to elicit or loses either caring attention or tension-relieving responses from the caretaker, the infant resorts to rumination as a means of self-soothing and relief of tension.

Diagnosis

Most frequently, infants who ruminate come to the attention of professionals because of "frequent vomiting" and weight loss. Some infants ruminate primarily during the transition to sleep when left alone, and their ruminatory activity might not be readily observed. However, these infants are frequently found in a puddle of vomitus, which should raise suspicion of rumination. Other infants can be observed to posture with the back arched, to put the thumb or whole hand into the mouth, or to suck on the tongue rhythmically to initiate the regurgitation of food. Most of the regurgitated food is initially vomited, but gradually the infant appears to learn to hold more of the food in the mouth to rechew and reswallow. "Experienced" ruminators appear to be able to bring up food through repeated tongue movements. They learn to rechew and reswallow the food without losing any of it. Their rumination can be inferred only from the movements of their cheeks and foul oral odor because of the frequent regurgitation.

In addition to taking a thorough medical history, it is important to explore the onset of vomiting and the social context under which the symptoms developed. An acute medical illness or a stressor in the parents' life is frequently associated with the onset of vomiting.

When exploring the stressors in the mother–infant relationship, one needs to be careful neither to alienate the mother nor to add additional stress to the relationship. It is best to observe the infant in various situations with the mother, with other caretakers and alone in the crib during the transition to sleep. These observations will help in understanding the severity of the rumination, and whether it is situational or pervasive. In addition to assessing the rumination in the infant, the mother–infant relationship and the mother's life circumstances need to be evaluated because the mother's ability to soothe and to stimulate her infant is critical for successful intervention.

Course and Natural History

The onset of rumination is frequently in the first year of life except in individuals with developmental delays, in whom the disorder may occur during later years. Rumination has also been reported to occur in adults with normal intelligence and in association with bulimia nervosa. In some infants and children, the disorder is believed to remit, however, electrolyte imbalance, weight loss, dehydration and death have been reported to result from rumination, and rumination should always be taken seriously.

Treatment

Diverse theories of etiology have resulted in various proposed methods of treatment. Besides surgical intervention to prevent reflux and the early use of mechanical restraints, treatment has been primarily behavioral or psychodynamic or a combination of both.

On the basis of the assumption that rumination is a learned habit reinforced by increased attention for regurgitation, unlearning by counter conditioning has been suggested. Some authors have used electric shock after other methods had failed. A number of alternative procedures of punishment, such as aversive taste stimuli (lemon juice or hot sauce), have been developed. There are difficulties in the use of aversive taste stimuli as punishment. Frequently, the infants are out of reach of the caretakers when they ruminate; consequently, the use of lemon juice or hot sauce is inconsistent, and this delays learning. Some infants appear to become adapted to these aversive taste stimuli. These authors suggest scolding the infant by shouting "No", placing the infant down, and leaving the room for 2 minutes immediately on initiation of rumination by the infant. If the infant is not ruminating on the caretaker's return, he or she is to be picked up, washed and played with as a reward.

There may be two behavioral causes of rumination: 1) reward learning through increased attention for regurgitation, and 2) social deprivation. Whereas punishment with time-out may be necessary for the first type, holding the child for 10 to 15 minutes before, during and after meals is the treatment of choice for the second type. A psychodynamic approach based on the assumption that rumination results from a disturbance in the mother–infant relationship has been advocated. Mothers of ruminating infants are frequently found to be overwhelmed by their personal lives, which make them unavailable or tense in their relationship with their infants. Psychotherapy for the mother and environmental changes that produce enhanced mothering have been proposed.

After an understanding of the mother's situation has been gained, treatment is best individualized by use of a combination of psychodynamic and behavioral interventions to enhance the mother–infant relationship in general, and to address the symptom of rumination in particular.

Pica

Definition

Pica refers to behaviorally and culturally inappropriate eating of nonnutritional substances for at least 4 weeks. It is most often associated with poverty related nutritional deficiencies and mental retardation.

Epidemiology

Pica is a common, but frequently missed problem. The onset of pica is usually during the toddler age between 12 and 24 months. Because infants commonly mouth objects, it is difficult to make the diagnosis in young infants. Estimates of the prevalence of pica among institutionalized mentally retarded individuals range from 10 to 33%.

Children with pica are more susceptible to malnutrition, anemia, diarrhea or constipation, and worm infestation. It has been noted that pica is highest in a group of children hospitalized for accidental poisoning and that more than 60% of mothers with children with pica have pica themselves.

Etiology

Organic, psychodynamic, socioeconomic and cultural factors have been implicated in the cause of this disorder. Some authors have suggested that inadequate dietary intake of iron and calcium leading to abnormal cravings may induce pica. Other authors have implicated psychosocial stress, maternal deprivation, parental neglect and abuse, and disorganized and impoverished family situations in the etiology of pica. In certain population groups, cultural acceptance of pica has been considered an important factor in the etiology of this disorder as well.

Most helpful clinically is a multifactorial etiology, whereby constitutional, developmental, familial, socioeconomic and cultural factors interact with each other. Children who engage in pica often experience frequent separations from one or both parents followed by replacement of rapidly changing, inadequate caretakers who seemed to encourage oral gratification in response to the child's distress. These children show a high degree of other oral activities (e.g., thumb-sucking or nail-biting) and may be seeking gratification caused by the lack of parental availability and nurture.

Diagnosis

Because mouthing of objects is still common in toddlers between 1 and 2 years, the diagnosis of pica should be made only if the behavior is persistent and inappropriate for the child's developmental level. The diagnosis of pica should be explored in children with accidental poisoning, with lead intoxication, or with worm infestation. Young children with signs of malnutrition or iron deficiency should also be considered for the diagnosis of pica.

The assessment should include the history of the child's development in general, and feeding in particular. Special attention should be given to other oral activities that the child may use for self-soothing and relief of tension. In addition, the home environment and the parents' relationship with each other and with the child need to be explored to assess the parents' availability to nurture and supervise the child. Above all, mother and child should be observed during a meal and during play to gain a better understanding of their relationship and how the symptoms of pica can be understood in the context of that relationship.

If the diagnosis of pica is established, it is critical that the child undergo a thorough physical examination to rule out any of the complications associated with this disorder, such as nutritional deficiencies (especially iron deficiency), lead poisoning, intestinal infections (toxoplasmosis or intestinal parasites), or gastrointestinal bezoars.

Course and Natural History

In many instances, the disorder is believed to be self-limited and to remit spontaneously after a few months. However, there may be a developmental impact of the disorder in some children. For example, younger children may be somewhat retarded in the use of their speech and show conflicts about their dependency needs and aggressive feelings. Adolescents may evidence some degree of depression, borderline personality disorders, other forms of disturbed oral activities and the use of tobacco, alcohol, or drugs. There may be a strong relationship between pica in childhood and symptoms of bulimia nervosa in adolescence.

Treatment

In treating pica, one must consider the various factors that appear to contribute to the development of pica as well as its complications. It is important to treat the child medically while addressing the psychosocial needs of the child's family as well. The mothers need to be made aware of the dangers of pica and should be enlisted in providing a childproof environment. This might include removing lead from paint in old substandard housing units or instituting anthelmintic therapy for family pets. A psychoeducational treatment approach that, in addition to teaching the mothers the dangers of pica, would also provide social support to help them become more available to their children is preferable.

Comparison of DSM-IV/ICD-10 Diagnostic Criteria

In contrast to DSM-IV-TR, which allows the diagnosis of pica to be made in the presence of other mental disorders if it is sufficiently severe to warrant independent clinical attention, the ICD-10 Diagnostic Criteria for Research for Pica exclude this diagnosis in the presence of any other mental disorder (except mental retardation). ICD-10 does not have a separate category for rumination disorder. Instead it includes this DSM-IV-TR category within its definition of Feeding Disorder of Infancy and Childhood which combines rumination with the persistent failure to eat adequately.

References

American Psychiatric Association (2000) *Diagnostic and Statistical Manual of Mental Disorders*, 4th edn, Text Revision.

Chatoor I, Dickson L, Schaefer S *et al.* (1985) A developmental classification of feeding disorders associated with failure to thrive: Diagnosis and treatment, in *New Directions in Failure to Thrive: Research and Clinical Practice* (ed Drotar D). Plenum Press, New York, pp. 235–238.

Chatoor I, Getson P, Menvielle E *et al.* (1997) A feeding scale for research and clinical practice to assess mother–infant interactions in the first three years of life. *Inf Ment Health J* 18, 76–91.

Chatoor I, Ganiban J, Hirsch R *et al.* (2000) Maternal characteristics and toddler temperament in infantile anorexia. *J Am Acad Child Adolesc Psychiatr* 39, 743–751.

Dahl M and Sundelin C (1992) Feeding problems in an affluent society: Follow-up at 4 years of age in children with early refusal to eat. *Acta Paediatr Scand* 81, 575–579.

Hufton IW and Oates RK (1977) Nonorganic failure to thrive: A long-term follow-up. *Pediatrics* 59, 73–77.

Main M and Goldwyn R (1991) *The Adult Attachment Interview Classification System*. Department of Psychology, University of California, Berkeley.

Marchi M and Cohen P (1990) Early childhood eating behaviors and adolescent eating disorders. *J Am Acad Child Adolesc Psychiatr* 29, 112–117.

Childhood Disorders: Tic Disorders

Phenomenology and Diagnostic Criteria

The cardinal features of Tourette's disorder and the other tic disorders are motor and vocal tics. Motor tics are usually brief, rapid and stereotyped movements, but can also be slower, more rhythmical, or even dystonic in nature. Simple motor tics are movements of individual muscle groups and include brief movements such as eye blinking, head shaking and shoulder shrugging. Complex motor tics involve multiple muscle groups, such as a simultaneous eye deviation, head turn and shoulder shrug. Some complex tics appear more purposeful, such as stereotyped hopping, touching, rubbing, or obscene gestures (copropraxia). Vocal tics are usually brief, staccato-like sounds, but can also be words or phrases. Simple vocal tics, often caused by the forceful movement of air through the nose and mouth, include sniffing, throat clearing, grunting, or barking-type sounds. Complex vocal tics usually include words, phrases, or the repetition of one's own words (palilalia) or the words of others (echolalia). Coprolalia (repetition of obscene phrases), often incorrectly considered essential for the diagnosis of Tourette's disorder, is an uncommon symptom with only 2 to 6% of Tourette's disorder cases so affected.

Tics most often begin early in childhood, wax and wane in severity, and change in character and quality over time. Tics are exacerbated by excitement and tension, and can attenuate during periods of focused, productive activity and sleep. Tics are involuntary, yet because they are briefly suppressible or can be triggered by environmental stimuli, they may appear as volitional acts. Patients describe tension developing if a tic is resisted, which only subsides by completion of the tic. In some individuals, tics are preceded or provoked by a thought or physical sensation referred to as a premonitory urge.

Diagnostic Criteria for the Tic Disorders

There are four diagnostic categories included in the tic disorders section of the *Diagnostic and Statistical Manual of Mental Disorders*: Fourth Edition (DSM-IV) (American Psychiatric Association, 1994): 1) Tourette's disorder; 2) chronic motor or vocal tic disorder (CT); 3) transient tic disorder; and 4) tic disorder not otherwise specified, which is a residual category for tic disorders not meeting the duration or age criteria of the other categories. In general, diagnostic decisions are based on whether both motor and phonic tics are present, duration of time affected with tics, age at onset, lack of another medical cause for the tics, and the presence of impairment.

DSM-IV-TR Criteria 307.23

Tourette's Disorder

A. Both multiple motor and one or more vocal tics have been present at some time during the illness, although not necessarily concurrently. (A **tic** is a sudden, rapid, recurrent, nonrhythmic, stereotyped motor movement or vocalization.)

B. The tics occur many times a day (usually in bouts) nearly every day or intermittently throughout a period of more than 1 year, and during this period there was never a tic-free period of more than three consecutive months.

C. The disturbance causes marked distress or significant impairment in social, occupational, or other important areas of functioning.

D. The onset is before age 18 years.

E. The disturbance is not due to the direct physiological effects of a substance (e.g., stimulants) or a general medical condition (e.g., Huntington's disease or postviral encephalitis).

Reprinted with permission from the *Diagnostic and Statistical Manual of Mental Disorders*, Fourth Edition, Text Revision. Copyright 2000 American Psychiatric Association.

Epidemiology

Incidence and Prevalence

Tic disorders appear to be common (>1 : 100), whereas Tourette's disorder is less common (5 : 10 000. In general, tic disorders occur more frequently in children than adults. People with mild tic disorders are much more common that those with severe, complex symptoms. Also people with tic disorders may present for clinical attention with tics, but tics may not end up as the focus of clinical attention as comorbid conditions are often more impairing than the tics themselves. Given these realities, the numbers of adults with persistent and severely impairing tics that warrant tic-suppressing medication is probably very small and may still be considered rare. More common are those adults with mild to moderate Tourette's disorder who come to clinical attention not only because of tics, but also because of comorbid psychiatric

Chronic Motor or Vocal Tic Disorder

A. Single or multiple motor or vocal tics (i.e., sudden, rapid, recurrent, nonrhythmic, stereotyped motor movements or vocalizations), but not both, have been present at some time during the illness.

B. The tics occur many times a day nearly every day or intermittently throughout a period of more than 1 year, and during this period there was never a tic-free period of more than three consecutive months.

C. The disturbance causes marked distress or significant impairment in social, occupational, or other important areas of functioning.

D. The onset is before age 18 years.

E. The disturbance is not due to the direct physiological effects of a substance (e.g., stimulants) or a general medical condition (e.g., Huntington's disease or postviral encephalitis).

F. Criteria have never been met for Tourette's disorder.

Reprinted with permission from the *Diagnostic and Statistical Manual of Mental Disorders*, Fourth Edition, Text Revision. Copyright 2000 American Psychiatric Association.

Transient Tic Disorder

A. Single or multiple motor and/or vocal tics (i.e., sudden, rapid, recurrent, nonrhythmic, stereotyped motor movements or vocalizations).

B. The tics occur many times a day, nearly every day for at least 4 weeks, but for no longer than 12 consecutive months.

C. The disturbance causes marked distress or significant impairment in social, occupational, or other important areas of functioning.

D. The onset is before age 18 years.

E. The disturbance is not due to the direct physiological effects of a substance (e.g., stimulants) or a general medical condition (e.g., Huntington's disease or postviral encephalitis).

F. Criteria have never been met for Tourette's disorder or chronic motor or vocal tic disorder.

Specify if:

Single episode or **recurrent**.

Reprinted with permission from the *Diagnostic and Statistical Manual of Mental Disorders*, Fourth Edition, Text Revision. Copyright 2000 American Psychiatric Association.

disorders. Perhaps most common are those adults with mild tics, with and without comorbid symptoms that do not come to clinical attention at all. A similar pattern is seen in children, with fewer children presenting with severe tics warranting tic suppression than children with mild to moderate tics and comorbid psychiatric disorders. Perhaps the most common are those children with transient tics that are not impairing and without comorbid conditions who may never come to clinical attention.

Frequently Cooccurring Symptoms or Disorders

Cooccurring problems can be more disabling than tics and are often the reason people with tics come to clinical attention. Difficulties with mood, impulse control, obsessive–compulsive behaviors, anxiety, attention and learning problems, and conduct problems are common. In some patients, these problems reach diagnosable proportions, but in many others, they are less severe and do not fulfill diagnostic criteria. The most frequent cooccurring disorders are attention-deficit/hyperactivity disorder (ADHD; 50–60%) and obsessive–compulsive disorder (OCD; 30–70%). The exact relationship of these problems to Tourette's disorder is controversial.

Attention-deficit/Hyperactivity Disorder

Upward of 50% of clinically ascertained children and adolescents with Tourette's disorder may be affected with problems of attention, concentration, activity level, or impulse. In community-based epidemiological samples of subjects with Tourette's disorder, the estimated frequency of ADHD is lower (8–41%) than in clinic populations (Apter *et al.*, 1993). In the epidemiological study with the lowest prevalence estimate of ADHD in Tourette's disorder (8%), subjects were 16 to 17 years of age, and the assessment of ADHD focused on current affected status (point prevalence), not lifetime diagnosis (Apter *et al.*, 1993). Even though the point prevalence of ADHD was more than twice than that seen in the general population, factors such as the age of the sample and examination for current status probably led to an underestimate of ADHD in Tourette's disorder.

Obsessive–Compulsive Symptoms

Obsessions and compulsions are stereotyped, persistent, and intrusive thoughts and behaviors that are experienced as senseless. Because these thoughts and behaviors can be common in the general population, persons are considered "disordered" only when the obsessions or compulsions become severe, disabling, or time-consuming. Obsessions that are commonly seen in OCD include fears of contamination, fears of harm coming to oneself or others, scrupulosity, fear of losing control of one's impulses, counting, fear of losing things, fear of being unable to remember, or experiencing images of terrible things happening. Compulsions commonly seen in OCD include repeated or stereotyped washing and grooming rituals; repeated checking of locks, switches, or doors; and repetition of other senseless rituals.

Differences in clinical phenomenology have been noted in studies of obsessions and compulsions in patients with Tourette's disorder compared with patients with OCD (without Tourette's disorder). Patients with Tourette's disorder have greater concern with physical symmetry, evenness, and exactness, which are often described as "just right" phenomena and concerns with impulse control. In contrast, patients with OCD have more frequent concerns regarding contamination and more cleaning and grooming rituals than do patients with Tourette's disorder. Also, the absolute number of independent concerns appears to be greater in patients with Tourette's disorder than in patients with OCD. Patients with OCD more often have a single concern around which their symptoms coalesce, such as contamination.

In contrast, patients with Tourette's disorder may have multiple concerns, such as symmetry, violent or sexual images or urges, worries about losing control, or counting. Some investigators have argued that the obsessions and compulsions in Tourette's disorders are more sensory–motor in character, whereas those in OCD are more cognitive and affective.

Relationship of the Commonly Cooccurring Symptoms and Conditions with Tourette's Disorder

Some studies support a broad Tourette's disorder phenotype that include commonly cooccurring comorbid conditions, whereas others identify a more circumscribed phenotype and define Tourette's disorder consistent with DSM-IV diagnosis – impairing multiple motor and vocal tics of 1-year duration. The outcome of this controversy has implications for treatment, but also for the definition of what Tourette's disorder is. For example, for people with Tourette's disorder and multiple comorbid conditions a simple moniker – Tourette's disorder – can simplify a very complex situation. For example, some parents have noted that it is difficult for them to conceptualize their child as having Tourette's disorder, OCD, ADHD, major depressive disorder and a learning disorder and prefer to use Tourette's disorder as a way to simplify the complexity in their own minds and in the minds of others. On the other hand people with Tourette's disorder but without multiple comorbidities may not be appropriately understood or treated if it is assumed that the Tourette's disorder label means tics plus a variety of other psychiatric disorders.

For clinical purposes we recommend that clinicians use a narrow conceptualization of Tourette's disorder and describe other problems as they may or may not occur. In this way each individual will carry diagnoses or problems that can be specifically described and appropriately addressed.

In the available research studies there is general agreement that chronic vocal or motor tics are a milder form of Tourette's disorder and that some forms of OCD are an alternative expression of the Tourette's disorder genetic diathesis. ADHD is very common in clinically ascertained subjects with Tourette's disorder, but may not be as uniformly present in community samples of people with Tourette's disorder. Within the literature, there are two major hypotheses regarding the relationship of Tourette's disorder to cooccurring disorders:

1) The putative Tourette's disorder gene is responsible for Tourette's disorder, CT, OCD and some forms of ADHD in Tourette's disorder probands and their families. Other disorders that commonly cooccur in Tourette's disorder subjects are not associated with Tourette's disorder and are not part of the Tourette's disorder phenotype. The cooccurrence of these other disorders with Tourette's disorder reflects either ascertainment bias in the sample or the development of disorders secondary to living with Tourette's disorder.
2) The putative Tourette's disorder gene is responsible for Tourette's disorder and the frequently associated psychiatric and behavioral problems seen in Tourette's disorder subjects.

Etiology

Genetics

Comparison of the concordance rates for Tourette's disorder in monozygotic and dizygotic twins identifies Tourette's disorder as an inherited condition. The twin studies, however, are unable to identify a particular mode of genetic transmission or to identify the breadth of the clinical phenotype. To answer these questions, other research methods are required. Segregation analyses of family study data have been used to identify the pattern of genetic transmission and alternative phenotypes of the Tourette's disorder genetic diathesis. Linkage studies of Tourette's disorder based on the assumption of Tourette's disorder as an autosomal dominant condition have been undertaken but to date have not been successful. Candidate gene studies based on the neurotransmitter hypotheses of the etiology of Tourette's disorder have also not been successful in identifying the Tourette's disorder gene(s). Recently, a large federally funded sibpairs study of Tourette's disorder has published encouraging results.

Twin Studies

Evidence from twin studies suggests an important role for both genetic and nongenetic factors in the development of Tourette's disorder. Two large twin studies have shown high concordance rates in monozygotic twins for Tourette's disorder (both twins have Tourette's disorder) and for tic disorders (one twin has Tourette's disorder, the other has tics but not Tourette's disorder). In both of the studies, the concordance rate for Tourette's disorder in monozygotic twins was more than 50%. When the concordance rates were calculated for the presence of any tic disorder, they approached 100%. By comparing the concordance rates of monozygotic twins with dizygotic twins, one can separate the role of genetic factors from other environmental factors. In the one study in which such a comparison was done, the concordance rate for Tourette's disorder in monozygotic twins was significantly higher than the concordance rate in dizygotic twins (Price et al., 1985), further suggesting a powerful role for genetics in Tourette's disorder.

Pathophysiology

In Tourette's disorder, the complex clinical presentation suggests several neuroanatomical sites of disease as well as neurochemical substrates including the basal ganglia and their interconnections with the frontal cortex and limbic system. Abnormalities in these structures could readily cause the wide variety of motor, sensory–motor, cognitive and affective symptoms seen in patients with Tourette's disorder. The complex phenotypic presentation seen in Tourette's disorder could also be produced by a neurochemical abnormality at various locations within this circuitry. Reports of group A beta-hemolytic streptococcus-related antineuronal antibodies being associated with the development or exacerbation of tics and OCD suggest a role for infectious agents and autoimmune processes in the etiology of these complex disorders.

Anatomical and Biological Abnormalities

Neuroanatomical Abnormalities in Tourette's Disorder

Increasingly sophisticated imaging methods, such as volumetric magnetic resonance imaging (MRI) and functional neuroimaging, have identified subtle abnormalities in the basal ganglia and its interconnections with cortical and limbic regions of the brain.

Two volumetric magnetic resonance studies identified the absence of the usual left–right asymmetry in the basal ganglia, leading to speculation of hypoplasia or atrophy of the left basal ganglia in Tourette's disorder. Areas associated with tic suppression may reflect brain areas involved in central nervous system disinhibition and ultimately tic symptoms. Functional neuroimaging studies, such as single-photon emission computed tomography, have identified decreased blood flow to the basal ganglia, specifically the left lenticular region. Positron emission tomography identified similar decrements of glucose use in the basal ganglia. Areas associated with increased functioning in Tourette's disorder include the midbrain, lateral premotor and supplemental motor cortexes and areas associated with sensorimotor, executive and paralimbic functioning. Areas associated with decreased functioning include the circuitry involving the caudate and thalamus, and their interconnections with the cortical and limbic areas.

Neurochemical Abnormalities

A number of neurochemical abnormalities have been proposed in Tourette's disorder, in large part on the basis of responsiveness of symptoms to specific pharmacological agents. Tic suppression with dopamine blockers such as haloperidol and beta-adrenergic agonists such as clonidine have implicated the dopamine–acetylcholine and adrenergic systems, respectively. The serotonin system has been implicated because of the association of Tourette's disorder with OCD and the positive therapeutic effect of serotonin reuptake inhibitors in OCD.

Other Biological Causes

In several reports the development of tics as well as obsessive–compulsive symptoms in children and adolescents has been associated in time with group A beta-hemolytic streptococcal infection. The underlying mechanism is proposed to be similar to that involved in the development of Sydenham's chorea, in which antibodies developed in the course of infection cross-react with basal ganglia tissues, resulting in the characteristic choreiform movement disorder of Sydenham's. Case reports have described subjects with the abrupt onset or exacerbation in symptoms occurring in parallel with antibody increases and with MRI changes in caudate size. These cases have been given the acronym PANDAS for Pediatric Autoimmune Neuropsychiatric Disorders Associated with Streptococcal Infection. These preliminary findings link the development of a movement disorder and psychiatric symptoms to an infectious agent and autoimmune processes, and suggest new and alternative treatments including the potential for vaccines for Tourette's disorder and OCD, though the possibility of chance association is high given that tics, obsessive–compulsive symptoms and streptococcal infections are common events in childhood.

Environmental Causes of Tourette's Disorder

To date, studies have not identified any specific factors that cause Tourette's disorder, yet it is increasingly clear that environmental factors have an impact on tic severity and, perhaps, even on the types of symptoms expressed. Clinical wisdom suggests that tic severity increases in response to stressful (e.g., examinations) or exciting life experiences (e.g., amusement parks). It is also not uncommon for persons with Tourette's disorder to be able to identify a particular environmental stimulus that initiated either a bout of symptoms or a new tic symptom.

Environmental factors associated with increases in symptom severity can occur early in development, including prenatal (intrauterine) development. In a study comparing groups of Tourette's disorder subjects with severe versus mild tics, protracted vomiting by a subject's mother during her pregnancy with the subject was a risk factor for increased tic severity (Leckman et al., 1990). Because of the male preponderance of Tourette's disorder, it has been postulated that intrauterine exposure to androgenic hormones may be a factor in the development of tics and in

tic severity. An open-label study of flutamide, an antiandrogenic hormone, identified significant but transient tic reduction in adult men, suggesting at least a partial role for sex hormones in tic severity (Peterson et al., 1994). Family-genetic and twin studies have also been useful for identifying factors associated with tic severity and have found an association between birth weight and tic severity suggesting that differences in intrauterine environment may be associated with tic severity.

Psychosocial Aspects of Tourette's Disorder

Although psychosocial issues do not play a large etiological role in the development of tic disorders they do play a major role in adaptation and impairment and are often the focus of treatment and rehabilitative efforts. Clinical work that involves the family, friends, school and workplace is often the bedrock of treatment in a patient with Tourette's disorder.

Children

For children with Tourette's disorder, the onset of symptoms occurs early in development and directly affects family life and relationships with peers and schoolmates. The diagnostic label of Tourette's disorder can be helpful for understanding the nature of a youngster's problems and can communicate the need to protect the youngster from excessive adversity. The diagnostic label can, however, be a problem. There is a tension between protecting a child with Tourette's disorder from adversity while ensuring that the child encounters and masters life's challenges. With too much protection, a child may run the risk of not developing a strong and complex identity adequate for the rigors of adult life. Support from parents for mastering the challenges of development is key to long-term functioning of children with Tourette's disorder.

Young Adults

The transition to adulthood is difficult enough for most young people, but young adults with Tourette's disorder have a particular challenge. The transition to adulthood often occurs when an important component of their early experience and identity (i.e., Tourette's disorder) begins to show some improvement. Young adults most vulnerable during this transition are those who, as a result of their Tourette's disorder, did not develop the foundations of an adult identity as a child. These adults often face the rigors of adult life without the necessary skills to manage, but also without the presence of tic symptoms of sufficient severity to explain their impairment.

Adults

Today's adult with Tourette's disorder belongs to a different cohort than today's child with Tourette's disorder. Most adults with Tourette's disorder were not diagnosed in childhood. They did not have the "protection" of the diagnosis and often experienced significant confusion, isolation and discrimination. Some adults with Tourette's disorder have significant anger, resentment and distrust related to their early life experiences including ineffective treatments, which can have an impact on current functioning. Many adults who appear to function well in spite of their Tourette's disorder may be doing so at an emotional cost.

Diagnosis

Clinical Presentation

Before the 1980s, only people with the most severe and clinically obvious tics were diagnosed with Tourette's disorder. The majority of these patients were adults who pursued care and were correctly diagnosed only when their tic symptoms were disabling and when classic symptoms such as coprolalia were present. Adults with milder tics generally did not pursue care and may have been stigmatized without the awareness of the cause of their movements. Children with tics were not identified at all or were identified as having other behavioral or psychiatric difficulties. Increasingly, as medical professionals and the public became more knowledgeable about tic disorders, psychiatrists began to see children at younger ages and with milder symptoms. Today, psychiatrists sometimes become involved even when the tics themselves are not obvious or even disabling. In today's clinical practice, the challenge is often not the treatment of the tics but identification of cooccurring and often more disabling psychiatric, behavioral, family and school problems.

More than half of families who finally pursue expert consultation find out about tic disorders from news articles or television. Many parents describe as their worst fear that their child's mild tic disorder is the beginning of a permanent neuropsychiatric disorder with a deteriorating course. Other children are identified during evaluation for other problems, such as ADHD. When the diagnosis of Tourette's disorder is made as part of an evaluation for other problems, it can be particularly difficult for the family and the patient to cope with the additional and unexpected diagnosis. Clearly, at the time of the evaluation, the patient and family are often frightened and require considerable psychological support.

Some children with tics, who present directly to a neurologist or a psychiatrist for an evaluation, may have a parent who has been diagnosed with a tic disorder. In this context, children can present early in the course of their disorder, often before a clear diagnosis can be made. The parents of these children were often diagnosed with tics late in their life or experienced significant duress from their symptoms and want their child to have a better experience.

Assessment

Tic Severity

Clinical assessment of the tic disorders begins with identification of the specific movements and sounds. It is also important to identify the severity of and impairment caused by the tics. A number of structured and semistructured instruments are available for the identification of tics and the rating of tic. Knowledge of the basic clinical parameters of tics and the course of illness dictates the evaluation. Questioning patients and their families about the presence of simple and complex movements in muscle groups from head to toe is a good beginning. Because vocal tics usually follow the development of motor tics, questions about the presence of simple sounds is next. Inquiring about the presence of complex vocal tics completes the tic inventory. It is helpful to elucidate other aspects of tic severity, such as the absolute number of tics; the frequency, forcefulness and intrusiveness of the symptoms; the ability of the patient successfully to suppress the tics; and how noticeable the tics are to others. It is also important to know whether premonitory sensory or cognitive experiences are a component of specific tics because these intrusive experiences may disrupt functioning more than the tics themselves. Although the waxing and waning nature of the tics and the replacement of one tic with another do not directly affect severity, identifying the characteristic course of illness is important for diagnostic confidence.

Last, it is important to assess the impairment due to the tics themselves. Whereas tic severity is frequently correlated with overall impairment, it is not uncommon to identify patients in whom tic severity and impairment are not correlated. Patients who experience more impairment than their tic symptoms apparently warrant are a particular clinical challenge. A number of clinical features of tics are associated with impairment:

- Large, disruptive, or painful motor movements;
- Vocalizations that call attention to the patient;
- Premonitory sensations or cognitions that intrude into consciousness;
- Tics that are socially unacceptable.

Associated Cooccurring Conditions

Whereas tic severity and impairment are often correlated, many patients with mild tics are most impaired by the comorbid conditions ADHD, OCD and Learning Disorders. An adequate assessment of these conditions is part of any comprehensive evaluation. The assessment of tic-related obsessive–compulsive symptoms, for example, touching, tapping, rubbing, "evening up", repeating actions, stereotypical self-mutilation, staring, echolalia and palilalia, although often omitted from the traditional psychiatric and neurological review of symptoms, should always be part of the routine evaluation of patients with tics, OCD, or ADHD.

Psychosocial Issues

Psychosocial issues can play a role in tic severity and in overall adaptation and impairment. Assessment of family, peer and school support for the youngster (adequate protection) along with assessment for the presence of opportunities to be intellectually, physically and socially challenged is important. The balance between protection and challenge in children is critical for long-term development. An environment that is too protective decreases opportunities for building skills. An environment that is too challenging can lead to frustration, anger and maladaptive coping.

Physical Examination Findings

Tic assessment requires a careful evaluation of observable tic symptoms. Interestingly, the absence of tic symptoms during an evaluation, in spite of the parent's or patient's report, is not uncommon and should not necessarily lead to clinical doubt. Occasionally, an additional clinical observer (e.g. nurse or medical student) may identify tics more readily than the psychiatrist conducting the evaluation. Other than the observation of tics in the interview, there are no pathognomonic physical examination findings. Patients with Tourette's disorder have been noted to have nonfocal and nonspecific subtle neurological findings ("soft" signs). If tic suppression with neuroleptic agents is considered, a more structured method of documenting the complex movements that are part of the pretreatment baseline evaluation is useful for following the progression of the disease and for subsequent assessment for neuroleptic-induced movements.

Differential Diagnosis

Differential Diagnosis of Tics

Tics have many characteristics that differentiate them from the other movement disorders. Perhaps most important to "ruling in"

Jankovic J (1992) Diagnosis and classification of tics and Tourette syndrome. Adv Neurol 58, 7–14. Reprinted with permission from Lipincott William & Wilkins.

tics as a diagnostic possibility is the childhood history of simple motor tics in the face. Other movement disorders do not have a similar pattern of movement onset or location. There are atypical presentations of tic disorders that may resemble other movement disorders, but these would be unusual and would probably require a consultation with a movement disorders expert.

Movement disorders such as chorea and dystonia are continuous movements and can be distinguished from tics, which are intermittent. Paroxysmal dyskinesias, although episodic, are more often characterized by choreiform and dystonic movements, which are different from tics. Myoclonic movements and exaggerated startle responses are also intermittent movements but are usually large-muscle movements that occur in response to a patient-specific stimulus. Complex tics can be more difficult to differentiate from other complex movements such as mannerisms, gestures, or stereotypies. In a person with clear-cut motor tics, it may be difficult to differentiate a complex motor tic from a "camouflaged" tic (making a simple tic appear to be a purposeful action, e.g., an upward hand movement that the person turns into a hair smoothing gesture), mannerism, gesture, or stereotypy. Mannerisms or gestures are often not impairing; stereotypies tend to occur exclusively in children and adults with developmental disabilities and mental retardation (Jankovic, 1992).

It is also possible to have a tic disorder and another movement disorder. For example, tic movements can cooccur with dystonia. Similarly, it is not uncommon in tertiary referral centers to see developmentally disabled children and adults with both tics and stereotypes.

Course and Natural History

In Tourette's disorder, tic symptoms usually begin in childhood; mean age at onset is 7 years. Motor tics of the eyes and face are the most common and earliest presenting symptoms. In many patients, the motor tics remain isolated in the face. When motor tics do progress, there is a tendency for additional tics to present sequentially from the head and face to the neck, shoulders, trunk and extremities. Vocal tics tend to follow the development of motor tics. Complex tics of both types tend to follow the development of simple tics. Longitudinal studies suggest that tic severity is greatest in most patients during the latency and early teenage years. Most patients experience a decline in tic severity as they get older and only a small percentage of patients (10%) experience a severe or deteriorating course.

Table 30.1 Goals of Treatment

Educate the patient and family about tic disorders.
Define the cooccurring disorders.
Creative a hierarchy of the clinically impairing conditions.
Treat the impairing conditions using somatic, psychological and rehabilitative approaches.
Aid in creating a supportive yet challenging psychosocial milieu.

Obsessive–compulsive symptoms in persons with Tourette's disorder generally begin somewhat later than ADHD and tics and may actually progress differentially from tic symptoms. Tic symptoms tend to improve into adulthood; obsessive–compulsive symptoms may actually increase in severity. Long-term studies of the course of obsessive–compulsive symptoms in persons with Tourette's disorder have not been made. The course of ADHD symptoms is similar in persons with and without Tourette's disorder.

Standard Approaches to Treatment

Educate the Patient and Family

The initiation of treatment can be a delicate process, given the difficulties patients and their families experience before finding appropriate care. Most families are frightened about their child's having a neuropsychiatric disorder and envision a grim prognosis. After the evaluation is completed, often in the first session, general education of the patient and family about the course of the tic disorder is essential (Table 30.1). Most patients and families are relieved to hear that the majority of persons with tics have consistent improvement in tic severity as they move through their teenage years and into adulthood. They are also pleased to hear that tic symptoms are not inherently impairing.

Identify Cooccurring Disorders

Identifying whether ADHD, LD and OCD are present is especially important because they are often the more common impairing conditions in these children. One of the major pitfalls of treatment of patients with Tourette's disorder is to pursue tic suppression to the exclusion of the treatment of other cooccurring conditions that are present and possibly more impairing.

Create a Hierarchy of the Clinically Impairing Conditions

Most psychiatrists, as part of their formulation, create some clinical hierarchy; yet in Tourette's disorder, with the multitude of often complex problems, it is essential that a conscious effort be made to formulate, organize and create hierarchies for treatment. For example children with moderate tics and separation anxiety with school refusal should be considered for a treatment with selective serotonin reuptake inhibitor (SSRI) for their separation anxiety rather than neuroleptics for tic suppression (The Research Unit on Pediatric Psychopharmacology Anxiety Study Group, 2001). It is possible with successful treatment of the anxiety disorder that patient may also experience a reduction in tic severity also.

Treat the Impairing Conditions

Tic Suppression: Pharmacological

The goal of pharmacological treatment is the reduction of tic severity, not necessarily the elimination of tics. Haloperidol has been used effectively to suppress motor and phonic tics for more than 30 years. Since that time, a number of other neuroleptic agents have also been identified as useful in tic suppression, including fluphenazine and pimozide. In Europe, the substituted benzamides, sulpiride and tiapride, and the nonneuroleptic tetrabenazine have also been shown to be useful. As new neuroleptic agents become available, clinical trials for tic suppression invariably occur. Preliminary results with risperidone have been mixed, whereas trials with clozapine are more uniformly negative. The major drawback with neuroleptic agents is the frequent and significant side effects, which often preclude continued use of the medication.

Haloperidol

Haloperidol is a high-potency neuroleptic that preferentially blocks dopamine D_2 receptors. Historically, haloperidol has been the most frequently used medication for tic suppression. It is effective in a clear majority of patients, although relatively few patients are willing to tolerate the side effects to obtain the tic-suppressing benefits. Neuroleptics are often effective at low doses, and low doses minimize side effects. For haloperidol, doses in the range of 0.5 to 2.0 mg/day are usually adequate. Starting dosages are low (0.25–0.5 mg/day), with small increases in dose (0.25–0.5 mg/day) every 5 to 7 days. Most often the medication is given at bedtime, but with low doses, some patients may require twice-a-day dosing for good tic control.

Side effects with all neuroleptics are common and include sedation, acute dystonic reactions, extrapyramidal symptoms including akathisia, weight gain, cognitive dulling and the common anticholinergic side effects. There have also been reports of subtle, difficult to recognize side effects with neuroleptics, including clinical depression, separation anxiety, panic attacks and school avoidance.

Dosage reduction is the most prudent response to side effects, although the addition of medications such as benztropine for the extrapyramidal symptoms can be useful. Dosage reduction in those children with Tourette's disorder who have been administered neuroleptics long term may be complicated by withdrawal dyskinesias and significant tic worsening or rebound. Withdrawal dyskinesias are choreoathetoid movements of the orofacial region, trunk and extremities that appear after neuroleptic discontinuation or dosage reduction and tend to resolve in 1 to 3 months. Tic worsening even above pretreatment baseline level (i.e., rebound) can last up to 1 to 3 months after discontinuation or dosage reduction. Tardive dyskinesia, which is similar in character to withdrawal dyskinesia, most often develops during the course of treatment or is "unmasked" with dosage reductions. Rarely have cases of tardive dyskinesia been reported to occur in patients with Tourette's disorder.

Fluphenazine

Whereas fluphenazine has never undergone controlled trials, clinical experience suggests that it has somewhat fewer side effects than haloperidol. Fluphenazine has both dopamine D_1 and D_2 receptor-blocking activity, and the side effect profile is similar to that of haloperidol. Fluphenazine is slightly less potent than haloperidol so that starting doses are somewhat higher (0.5–1 mg/day), as are treatment doses (3–5 mg/day).

Pimozide

Pimozide is a potent and specific blocker of dopamine D_2 receptors. Its side-effect profile is generally similar to that of the other neuroleptics, although it has fewer sedative and extrapyramidal side effects than haloperidol. In contrast to either haloperidol or fluphenazine, pimozide has calcium channel blocking properties that affect cardiac conduction, as evidenced by changes in the electrocardiogram. The coadministration of other medications that affect cardiac conduction, such as the tricyclic antidepressants (TCAs), is generally contraindicated. Baseline and follow-up electrocardiograms are important for adequate management of patients.

Beginning treatment with a dose of 1 mg/day is prudent, although with pimozide's long half-life, every-other-day dosing can be used to decrease the effective daily dose. Increases of up to 1 mg/day can occur every 5 to 7 days until symptoms are controlled. Most patients experience clinical benefit with few side effects with doses of 1 to 4 mg/day. Higher doses can be associated with more side effects. In a comparison of pimozide, haloperidol and no drug in patients with Tourette's disorder and ADHD, pimozide at 1 to 4 mg/day was useful in decreasing tics and improving some aspects of cognition that are commonly impaired in ADHD (Sallee and Rock 1994). The potential to have impact on both Tourette's disorder and ADHD symptoms with a single drug is a clear advantage that pimozide may have over other neuroleptics.

Atypical Neuroleptics

The atypical neuroleptics appear to have replaced the standard neuroleptics as the mainstay of treatment for the psychotic disorders. Given the potentially lower risk for tardive dyskinesia with these agents, their efficacy has been assessed for tic suppression in patients with Tourette's disorder. To date there are only small controlled or open trials to guide the clinician in the use of these agents. Clozapine does not appear to be effective as a tic-suppressing agent and its hematological side effects preclude its use. Risperidone has been effective in reducing tic symptoms severity in one controlled trial (Dion et al., 2002) and may have the added benefit of augmenting SSRIs in treating tic-related OCD.

Olanzapine in low doses does not appear to have the same tic-suppressing power as the typical neuroleptics which may be related to olanzapine's relatively weak dopamine D_2 blocking activity. Side effects, especially weight gain, have dampened the enthusiasm for the atypicals risperidone, olanzapine and quetiapine. In one of the larger placebo-controlled trials ($N = 56$) of the new neuroleptics, ziprasidone was found to be effective in reducing tic symptoms. The mean dose was low 28 ± 10 mg/day. There were few side effects including a low incidence of weight gain (Gilbert et al., 2000).

Clonidine and Guanfacine

Whereas controlled trials have shown that some patients benefit with symptom reduction, the overall effect of clonidine for tic suppression and ADHD is more modest than that achieved with the "gold standards" (haloperidol and the stimulants, respectively) for these conditions (Goetz, 1993). Given clonidine's mild side-effect profile, it is often the first drug used for tic suppression, especially in those children with Tourette's disorder and ADHD. Treatment is initiated at 0.025 mg/day and increased in increments of 0.025 to 0.05 mg/day every 3 to 5 days or as side effects (sedation) allow. Usual effective treatment doses are in the range of 0.1 to 0.3 mg/day and are given in divided doses (4–6 hours apart). Higher doses are associated with side effects, primarily sedation, and are not necessarily more effective. The onset of action is slower for tic suppression (3–6 weeks) than for ADHD symptoms. Side effects, in addition to sedation, include irritability, headaches, decreased salivation, and hypotension and dizziness at higher doses. Interestingly, owing to clonidine's short half-life, some patients experience mild withdrawal symptoms between doses. More severe rebound in autonomic activity and tics can occur if the medication is discontinued abruptly. Some patients find that clonidine in the transdermal patch form provides a more stable clinical effect and avoids multiple doses each day. Children are usually stabilized on oral doses before they are switched to the patch. A rash at the site of the patch is a common, but manageable, complication of treatment.

Guanfacine is an alpha-2-adrenergic agonist that potentially offers greater benefit than clonidine because of differences in site of action, side effects and duration of action. In nonhuman primates, guanfacine appears to bind preferentially with alpha-2-adrenergic receptors in prefrontal cortical regions associated with attentional and organizational functions. Guanfacine's long half-life offers the advantage of twice-a-day dosing, which is more convenient than the multiple dosing required with clonidine. In a randomized, placebo-controlled trial ($N = 31$) of children with tics and ADHD, guanfacine in doses up to 0.3 mg/day had an average 31% reduction in tic severity compared with no reduction on placebo. Clinically the effect on tics is less than would be expected on neuroleptics (Scahill et al., 2001).

Benzodiazepines

Benzodiazepines can be useful in decreasing comorbid anxiety in patients with Tourette's disorder. In addition, clonazepam appears also to be useful in selected patients for tic reduction. Often, doses of 3 to 6 mg/day may be necessary for tic reduction. Because sedation is a significant side effect at these dosages, an extended titration phase of 3 to 6 months may be necessary. Similarly, a slow taper is required to avoid withdrawal symptoms.

Pergolide

Agonist activity on presynaptic dopamine neurons results in decrease dopamine release and may therefore result in decreased tic severity in people with Tourette's disorder. To exploit this finding a number of small open trials of dopamine agonists and a small controlled trial of pergolide ($N = 24$) have been conducted. Pergolide, a mixed D_1–D_2–D_3 dopamine agonist often used for restless leg syndrome, was found to be superior to placebo in reducing tic severity and was associated with few adverse events (Gilbert et al., 2000). Doses used were low as higher doses may be associated with dopamine agonist effects postsynaptically.

Baclofen

Baclofen, a muscle relaxant, is GABA-B receptor agonist that acts presynaptically to inhibit the release of excitatory amino acids such as glutamate. In a small placebo controlled crossover trial ($N = 10$) baclofen 20 mg t.i.d. was not found to be effective in reducing tic severity but did appear to have an effect on tic-related impairment (Singer et al., 2001).

Infection and Autoimmune-based Treatments

Several treatment studies have been undertaken based on the hypothesis that some forms of Tourette's disorder or OCD may be related to streptococcal infection. Based on the beneficial effects of penicillin prophylaxis in preventing recurrences of rheumatic fever, a similar strategy was employed in subjects meeting criteria for PANDAS (Garvey et al., 1999). The study was limited by a number of flaws and although the concept of prophylaxis is compelling, special design considerations will be required in future studies.

After small open trials with the immunomodulatory treatments such as plasma exchange or intravenous immunoglobulin (IVIG), a larger trial comparing these methods to sham IVIG was undertaken. Children meeting criteria for PANDAS ($N = 30$) were randomly assigned (1 : 1 : 1) to treatment with plasma exchange (five single-volume exchanges over 2 weeks), IVIG (1 g/kg daily on two consecutive days), or placebo (saline solution given in the same manner as IVIG) and subjects were reported as doing well at 1 year (Lougee et al., 2000). Although this study is encouraging there are a number of methodological problems including lack of a placebo control for plasma exchange and inclusion of uncontrolled subjects in outcome analysis after the first month. These findings do support ongoing investigation of these treatment methods but given the cost, risk and highly experimental nature of these treatments it is recommended that patients obtain these treatments only in the context of ongoing clinical investigations of these treatments at major medical research centers (for further information, see http://intramural.nimh.nih.gov/research/pdn/web.htm).

Tic Suppression: Nonpharmacological

The behavioral technique shown to be most effective is habit reversal training. For Tourette's disorder, habit reversal training is the use of a competing muscle contraction or behavioral response that opposes the tic movement. This method is usually combined with relaxation training, self-monitoring, awareness training and positive reinforcement. In the few published studies of habit reversal training, there were marked overall reductions in tic frequency. Treatment averaged 20 training sessions during an 8- to 11-month period. Marked tic reduction was noted at 3 to 4 months. Interestingly, urges or sensations experienced before the tic movements also decreased with behavioral treatment (Azrin and Peterson, 1990).

Psychosocial Treatments

There are no published systematic studies of psychosocial interventions for patients with Tourette's disorder. Most treatment efforts are based on a combination of traditional psychosocial interventions and clinical judgment.

Education

Perhaps the most useful psychosocial and educational intervention is to make the patient aware of the Tourette Syndrome Association, both national and local chapters. This and other self-help groups can be useful as a source of support and education for patients, families and psychiatrists.

Therapy

Individual psychotherapy can be useful for support, development of awareness, or addressing personal and interpersonal problems more effectively. Family therapy can be useful when families have problems adjusting, functioning and communicating. Although most families do well, some families have difficulties understanding the involuntary nature of tics and may punish their children for their tics, even after diagnosis and education. Alternatively, some families have more behavior difficulties with their children after diagnosis than before. Many parents of children with Tourette's disorder inadvertently lower general behavior expectations because of confusion about what behaviors are and are not tics, or because of the parents' desire not to add any additional stress to the youngster's life. Also, with confusion in the field regarding the scope of problems in Tourette's disorder, some parents see all maladaptive behaviors as involuntary and do not hold their children responsible for their behaviors. For children with Tourette's disorder to do well, they need support from their family to develop effective self-control in areas not affected by Tourette's disorder so that optimal adaptation can occur.

In newly diagnosed adults, psychotherapy oriented toward adequate adjustment to the diagnosis is important but not always easy. Adult patients frequently experience a mixture of relief to be finally diagnosed, with anger and resentment related to their past experiences with discrimination or inadequate medical care. Severely affected adults may also need psychotherapy to deal with the psychological and psychosocial difficulties related to having a chronic illness.

Other Psychosocial Interventions

For children, active intervention at school is essential to create a supportive yet challenging academic and social environment. Efforts to educate teachers, principals and other students can result in increased awareness of Tourette's disorder and tolerance for the child's symptoms.

Many young adults are finding Tourette's disorder support and social groups important for interpersonal contact and continued adult development. Efforts to keep people with Tourette's disorder working are important, as are rehabilitation efforts for those who are not working. Finding housing and obtaining disability or public assistance may be necessary for the most disabled patients with Tourette's disorder.

Genetic Counseling

One question commonly asked by young adults with Tourette's disorder is their risk for having a child with Tourette's disorder. Given the fact that many who present for clinical attention with Tourette's disorder have comorbid conditions, genetic counseling of people with Tourette's syndrome should include not only the risk for Tourette's disorder but also the risk for other neuropsychiatric problems such as ADHD or OCD that may be part of the young person's history. In addition, because the base rate of neuropsychiatric disorders is high, it is not uncommon for spouses of people with Tourette's disorder to have a neuropsychiatric disorder. In providing counseling to these couples it is important that genetic counseling be conducted not just about Tourette syndrome, but about the other conditions that occur as part of the young couple's history.

Treatment of Cooccurring Psychiatric Disorders in Tourette's Disorder

Treatment of Attention-deficit/Hyperactivity Disorder

Nonpharmacological Approaches

The nonpharmacological approaches to ADHD in Tourette's disorder are similar to approaches in children without Tourette's disorder. The presence both at home and at school of a structured environment, consistent behavioral management, and a generally positive, rewarding atmosphere can produce significant improvement in ADHD symptoms. Increasingly, there are specific programs for children with ADHD that go beyond basic positive programming and include more intensive and specific behavioral approaches.

Pharmacological Treatments

The two major difficulties in the treatment of ADHD in Tourette's disorder are the risk of side effects from the stimulants and desipramine, arguably the most potent treatment agents for ADHD and the lack of adequate alternatives.

Stimulants

In the early 1970s, a number of reports of induction or exacerbation of tics by stimulant medications raised concerns about the role of stimulants as a cause of Tourette's disorder. At that time, the concern was that stimulants could be causing tics *de novo* or that increases in tic severity would endure even if stimulant medications were discontinued. Concurrent with these reports, other authors noted that tic induction or exacerbation was relatively infrequent and that the beneficial effects in some patients with Tourette's disorder outweighed any negative impact on tic severity.

As a result, stimulants have been used infrequently for ADHD in Tourette's disorder. However, results of short-term and long-term double-blind, placebo-controlled trials with stimulants in Tourette's disorder are positive and support a role for stimulants in some patients with Tourette's disorder plus ADHD. Increasingly, psychiatrists are cautiously, and with fully informed consent, using stimulant medication in selected children and adolescents with Tourette's disorder and ADHD. In the patient in whom tics are increased by stimulants, combined treatment with stimulants and tic-suppressing agents can be used.

More recently, in a large ($N = 136$) multicenter double-blind, placebo-controlled trial, children with ADHD and a chronic tic disorder were randomly assigned to clonidine alone, methylphenidate alone, clonidine plus methylphenidate or placebo for the treatment of their ADHD. The results suggest that the active treatments were superior to placebo, with the combination treatment being the most effective. With respect to worsening of tic severity the percentage of children with worsening of tics was similar in each of the medication conditions including placebo. For methylphenidate, 20% reported tic increases compared with 26% on clonidine alone and 22% on placebo. Interestingly tic severity lessened in all active treatment groups even in the methylphenidate group. Other side effects were predictable with sedation commonly associated with clonidine treatment (The Tourette Syndrome Study Group, 2002). Given the controversy regarding the coadministration of clonidine and methylphenidate it is important to note the absence of cardiac toxicity in children on combined medication.

Given the above, informed consent prior to initiating stimulant medication should include information regarding the risks for new onset of tics or tic exacerbations. In Table 30.2 is a listing of topics that might be useful to address during informed consent. This listing is not intended to be a comprehensive or exhaustive.

Desipramine

Desipramine is a TCA with prominent noradrenergic activity that has been noted to improve attention and concentration in children and adolescents with ADHD and Tourette's disorder plus ADHD. Symptom improvement is often significant with lower doses than needed for depression. Side effects are generally limited. The cardiac side effects of increased heart rate and elevation in blood pressure are usually not clinically significant; however, reports

Table 30.2 Informed Consent for Stimulants

- Parent education about the complexity of presentation and relevant information about ADHD and tics.
  - Tics go up and down, usually tics increase with excitement and stress and go down with calm, focused activity. Such changes will likely continue to occur while on stimulants.
  - Predictable exacerbation each year – starting and ending school, winter holidays, vacations, parties, etc.
  - Over the lifetime tics tend to decrease in mid to late teens.

- Risk of stimulants for tic exacerbation
  - Controlled trials demonstrate that tics go up, go down, or stay the same with stimulant treatment. In approximately 20% of children tics will increase regardless of treatment medication or placebo. There is no clear association as previously thought.
  - Longer-term studies suggest that when tics do appear to increase on stimulants there is a reasonable chance they are reversible with discontinuation of stimulant medication.
  - It is possible that there is greater risk in younger children than teens.
- Parents have to understand the following: "If you are willing, you need to understand that your kid's tics may go up and not come down with medication treatment. Or if there are no tics now that tics may start and continue. This is very unfortunate it could be related to medication but it might have been his time for his tics either to begin or worsen".
- Doctors should understand the following: Do not start if parents are not really prepared. It is better for parents to make a risk–benefits decision after gaining knowledge, experience and perspective while under your care.

of sudden death in children and adolescents taking desipramine have resulted in marked reductions nationally in the use of desipramine in children and adolescents.

Nortriptyline

Given the concern about the cardiac effects of desipramine, TCAs such as nortriptyline have been used for the treatment of ADHD. The only available report, a chart review, assessed the effect of nortriptyline in children and adolescents with Tourette's disorder plus ADHD. The majority of subjects experienced moderate to marked improvement in both ADHD and tics (Wilens *et al.*, 1993). Although the concern regarding sudden death is less with nortriptyline than with desipramine, it is prudent to obtain baseline and follow-up electrocardiograms.

Clonidine and Guanfacine

Data supporting the efficacy of these agents has been limited to open trial or small controlled trials. In the largest trial to date subjects ($N = 34$; mean age of 10.4 years) were randomly assigned to 8 weeks of guanfacine or placebo. Guanfacine was superior to placebo (37 versus 8%) in reduction of the total score on the teacher-rated ADHD Rating Scale and significant differences were also observed in omission and commission errors on a continuous performance test (Scahill *et al.*, 2001).

Selective Noradrenergic Reuptake Inhibitors (SNRIs)

One SNRI has recently been approved for the treatment of ADHD in children and one is under FDA review for major depression. Atomoxetine has been demonstrated to be effective and approved for use in children and adults with ADHD. Given its mechanism of action it is possible that atomoxetine could improve ADHD symptoms without exacerbating tic symptoms. Studies are currently underway. Similarly reboxetine, which has an indication in Europe for depression, may be useful for ADHD in people with tics disorders.

Treatment of Obsessive–Compulsive Disorder

Nonpharmacological Approaches

The positive role of cognitive–behavioral treatments of OCD is well established in adults. Most reports of nonpharmacological treatment of OCD in children and adolescents are case studies. Only one report has a sufficient sample size and a protocol-driven, cognitive–behavioral treatment regimen to begin to establish the possible role of such treatment in children and adolescents with OCD. There are no specific reports of cognitive–behavioral treatment or other nonpharmacological treatments of OCD in adults or children with Tourette's disorder. Given the success of cognitive–behavioral treatment in OCD, it is likely that patients with Tourette's disorder and OCD will also be able to benefit from cognitive–behavioral treatment.

Pharmacological Treatments

The number of agents available for the treatment of OCD in patients with and without Tourette's disorder is increasing. Currently available agents include the TCA clomipramine and the specific serotonin reuptake inhibitors fluoxetine, sertraline, paroxetine, fluvoxamine and citalopram. Even though only a few of these agents have a specific indication for OCD (clomipramine and fluvoxamine), others may be effective in OCD given their serotoninergic activity. The choice of agent depends on the side-effect profile, the potential drug interactions and the psychiatrist's familiarity with the drug.

With the exception of clomipramine, all of the available agents have mild and somewhat similar side-effect profiles. Drug interaction issues must be taken into account, especially in children with complex presentations or multiple medical conditions given the increased possibility of multiple drug regimens. The reports of elevated TCA levels in patients receiving TCA and fluoxetine are good examples of unforeseen drug interactions with the specific serotonin reuptake inhibitors.

Increasingly, augmentation strategies are pursued in patients with OCD and with Tourette's disorder plus OCD, when clinical symptoms remain after initial treatment. A number of strategies have been used, including augmentation with lithium, neuroleptics, buspirone, clonazepam, liothyronine sodium (T3) and fenfluramine. Although positive outcomes of these strategies have been reported in open trials, only neuroleptic augmentation has shown to be of any benefit in controlled trials. Interestingly, controlled trials of haloperidol combined with specific serotonin reuptake inhibitors in patients with Tourette's disorder and OCD demonstrated improvement in both tic and OCD symptoms.

Treatment-refractory Cases

Strategies for approaching two types of treatment-refractory symptoms are discussed here: 1) patients who are truly treatment-refractory with severe and impairing symptoms of Tourette's disorder and OCD, despite conventional and heroic treatments, and 2) patients, often children, who are clinically complex and enigmatic, and whose impairment is disproportionally greater than their tic, obsessive–compulsive, or ADHD symptoms would suggest.

Treatment-refractory Tics

Perhaps the most important "treatment" in patients with severe incapacitating tics is a full clinical reevaluation to assess the adequacy of previous evaluations and treatment efforts. It is not uncommon for treatment-refractory patients to have had inadequate evaluations and treatment trials.

Two alternative treatment strategies are available for truly treatment-refractory tics. When a single tic or a few tics are refractory and impairing, the injection of botulinum toxin into the specific muscle group can be helpful. This strategy is most useful for painful, dystonic tics. Treatment has a long duration of action, but the effect does decrease in 2 to 4 months, and repeated injections may be necessary. Specific side effects are few, other than weakness in the affected muscle. Some patients reported the loss of the premonitory sensation with their botulinum toxin treatment. For the psychiatrist, it is essential to work with a neurologist experienced in using botulinum toxin.

There have been reports in the literature and the media concerning the use of neurosurgical approaches for the treatment of refractory tics. To date, the optimal size and location of the surgical treatment lesions are not known. There are no well-controlled trials, although some data are available from patients with OCD and tics who were treated for OCD. In these patients, the impact on tic severity was mixed. Because these approaches are particularly controversial, it is important, before considering neurosurgical approaches, to complete a detailed and exhaustive reevaluation to determine whether all other treatment options are exhausted. It is also important that patients who pursue neurosurgical approaches consider centers of clinical excellence where controlled treatment trials are ongoing.

Treatment-refractory Obsessive–Compulsive Disorder

A similarly thorough and exhaustive reevaluation is critical for patients with Tourette's disorder plus OCD who present as treatment-refractory. Diagnostic reevaluation focuses on whether other psychiatric disorders are present and disabling and whether the current hierarchy of clinical disability considers all conditions.

Pharmacological reevaluation is especially critical because there are an increasing number of new medications and potential medication combinations. Rather than repeated change from one antiobsessional agent to another, consideration can be given to augmentation strategies, because they take less time than changing agents and may offer synergistic benefits. Low-dose neuroleptic augmentation is the best first choice; controlled trials support the use of low-dose neuroleptics for augmentation of serotonin reuptake inhibitors in OCD. Lithium and T3 are proven, effective augmenters of antidepressants for depression, yet neither is proven effective in OCD. Because of the frequent overlap of OCD and major depression, lithium or T3 augmentation may be the next best choice.

Treatment-refractory or malignant OCD has been the psychiatric disorder most frequently treated with neurosurgical interventions in the modern era. Whereas it is a major treatment intervention, the surgical approaches are somewhat better defined, and the outcome in severe cases is often positive. Also, medical centers are available that specialize in the presurgical work-up and the neurosurgical procedure.

Clinically Complex Patients

Clinically complex patients may be severely impaired without having severe tic or OCD symptoms. The clinically complex patient is often a diagnostic dilemma with additional diagnoses complicating the clinical picture. In addition, patients can become clinically complex when otherwise straightforward treatments are a challenge to implement.

Diagnosis

In clinically complex patients, the diagnostic challenge is not an accurate assessment of tics, ADHD, obsessive–compulsive symptoms, or LDs, although this is important. In clinically complex patients, the diagnostic goal is to identify what other conditions or factors may be present that make the current treatment approaches difficult.

From a strictly diagnostic point of view, it is the additional psychiatric conditions beyond Tourette's disorder, OCD, ADHD and LDs that often escape clinical observation and result in diagnostic dilemmas and treatment failures.

Treatment Implementation

Clinical problems occur when the treating psychiatrist does not have access to critical information or is not in control of the treatment process. Traditionally, psychiatrists develop a relationship with the patient and the other major figures in the patient's life. Given the current clinical climate, a comprehensive level of involvement can be overwhelming and enormously time-consuming for the psychiatrist. Because it is increasingly difficult for the psychiatrist to be as involved as necessary, problems with poorly coordinated team efforts and the psychiatrist's lack of awareness of important clinical issues can have a negative impact on the treatment of a patient.

Psychiatrists who work with children and adolescents may wish to consider changes in their treatment approaches to these patients. Experience in tertiary care centers suggests that expanded time with the parents is a critically important and efficient approach to care. Psychiatrists who form a treatment partnership with families, respecting and addressing their concerns, educating them about Tourette's disorder, training them to evaluate and manage complex behaviors, and empowering them to be an effective advocate for their child, are providing good care. In working directly with families, the collection of important information regarding the family's and patient's functioning is direct and regular, and often small interventions can produce changes in family functioning that have a positive ripple effect throughout the life of the child.

Pharmacological Treatment Dilemmas

It is often difficult to obtain accurate information regarding side effects and treatment response in child patients. Parents, children and psychiatrists, in spite of a good collaborative effort, may have different understandings of the target symptoms, side-effect profile, and what constitutes a positive clinical response. This ambiguity makes any but the most robust clinical responses difficult to observe. Again, experience at tertiary referral centers suggests that the lack of a clinical response to medication in complex patients may often be related to inadequate monitoring of medicine effects and inadequate treatment trials.

Clinically complex patients may not have a robust response to a single medication but may require multiple medication trials to identify which medications offer the most benefit, and in which combination. Sequential treatment trials are difficult for all involved, especially children and families, who are often looking for a single powerful intervention. With the added complexity of treatment, there is the added risk of confusion and the need for an excellent psychiatrist–patient–family relationship. In those cases in which the relationship is not optimal, it is possible that a patient may not have the maximal clinical benefit of pharmacological interventions.

With increasing numbers of available psychotropic medications, psychiatrists become increasingly less experienced with the range of clinical effects and side effects in individual medications. In clinically complex patients, the prescription of unfamiliar medications may be necessary but may add to the risk that a trial will be discontinued prematurely because of doubt about a side effect. In addition, unusual side effects, such as the apathy or disinhibition syndromes seen with some patients receiving the specific serotonin reuptake inhibitors, may go unnoticed and add to clinical morbidity.

Whereas pharmacological interventions offer great promise, clinical experience suggests that excellent diagnostic skills, good relationships with the patient and family, time, and a keen eye for effects and side effects are necessary for benefits to be realized. Less intensive efforts may make patients appear more complex than necessary.

Comparison of DSM-IV/ICD-10 Diagnostic Criteria

The ICD-10 and DSM-IV-TR criteria sets for the tic disorders are almost identical.

References

American Psychiatric Association (2000). *Diagnostic and Statistical Manual of Mental Disorders*, 4th edn, Text Revision.

American Psychiatric Association (1994) *Diagnostic and Statistical Manual of Mental Disorders*, 4th edn. APA, Washington DC.

Apter A, Pauls DL, Bleich A *et al.* (1993) An epidemiologic study of Gilles de la Tourette's syndrome in Israel. *Arch Gen Psychiatr* 50, 734–738.

Azrin NH and Peterson AL (1990) Treatment of Tourette syndrome by habit reversal: A waiting list control group comparison. *Behav Ther* 21, 305–318.

Dion Y, Annable L, Sandor P *et al.* (2002) Risperidone in the treatment of tourette syndrome: A double-blind, placebo-controlled trial. *J Clin Psychopharmacol* 22(1), 31–39.

Garvey MA, Perlmutter SJ, Allen AJ *et al.* (1999) A pilot study of penicillin prophylaxis for neuropsychiatric exacerbations triggered by streptococcal infections. *Biol Psychiatr* 45(12), 1564–1571.

Gilbert DL, Sethuraman G, Sine L *et al.* (2000) Tourette's syndrome improvement with pergolide in a randomized, double-blind, crossover trial. *Neurology* 54(6), 1310–1315.

Goetz CG (1993) Clonidine, in *Handbook of Tourette's Syndrome and Related Tic and Behavioral Disorders* (ed Kurlan R). Marcel Dekker, New York, pp. 377–388.

Jankovic J (1992) Diagnosis and classification of tics and Tourette syndrome. *Adv Neurol* 58, 7–14.

Leckman JF, Dolnansky ES, Hardin MT *et al.* (1990) Perinatal factors in the expression of Tourette syndrome: An exploratory study. *J Am Acad Child Adolesc Psychiatr* 29, 220–226.

Lougee L, Perlmutter SJ, Nicolson R *et al.* (2000) Psychiatric disorders in first-degree relatives of children with pediatric autoimmune neuropsychiatric disorders associated with streptococcal infections (PANDAS). *J Am Acad Child Adolesc Psychiatr* 39(9), 1120–1126.

Peterson BS, Leckman JF, Scahill L *et al.* (1994) Steroid hormones and Tourette's syndrome: Early experience with antiandrogen therapy. *J Clin Psychopharmacol* 14, 131–135.

Price RA, Kidd K, Cohen DJ *et al.* (1985) A twin study of Tourette syndrome. *Arch Gen Psychiatr* 42, 815–820.

Sallee FR and Rock CM (1994) Effects of pimozide on cognition in children with Tourette syndrome: Interaction with comorbid attention deficit hyperactivity disorder. *Acta Psychiatr Scand* 90, 4–9.

Scahill L, Chappell PB, Kim YS *et al.* (2001) A placebo-controlled study of guanfacine in the treatment of children with tic disorders and attention-deficit hyperactivity disorder. *Am J Psychiatr* 158(7), 1067–1074.

Singer HS, Wendlandt J, Krieger M *et al.* (2001) Baclofen treatment in Tourette syndrome: A double-blind, placebo-controlled, crossover trial. *Neurology* 56(5), 599–604.

The Research Unit on Pediatric Psychopharmacology Anxiety Study Group (2001). Fluvoxamine for the treatment of anxiety disorders in children and adolescents. *N Engl J Med* 344(17), 1279–1285.

The Tourette Syndrome Study Group (2002) Treatment of ADHD in children with tics: A randomized controlled trial. *Neurology* 58(4), 527–536.

Wilens TE, Biederman J, Geist DE *et al.* (1993) Nortriptyline in the treatment of ADHD: A chart review of 58 cases. *J Am Acad Child Adolesc Psychiatr* 32, 343–349.

31 Childhood Disorders: Elimination Disorders and Childhood Anxiety Disorders

Enuresis

Definition

Functional enuresis is usually defined as the intentional or involuntary passage of urine into bed or clothes in the absence of any identified physical abnormality in children older than 4 years of age. It is often associated with psychiatric disorder and enuretic children are frequently referred to mental health services for treatment.

Course and Natural History

The acquisition of urinary continence at night is the end stage of a fairly consistent developmental sequence. Bowel control during sleep marks the beginning of this process and is followed by bowel control during waking hours, bladder control during the day, and finally night-time bladder control. Most children achieve this final stage by the age of 36 months. With increasing age, the likelihood of spontaneous recovery from enuresis decreases. The chronic nature of the condition is further shown in the study by Rutter and colleagues (1973), in which only 1.5% of 5-year-old bed-wetters became dry during the next 2 years.

Enuresis (Not Due to a Medical Condition)
This disorder is characterized by the repeated voiding of urine into clothes or bed at the age of 5 (chronicalogically or developmentally) or older for a period of at least twice weekly over three months. Enuresis reflects a significant emotional distress or impairment in social, academic or other important ares of functioning. Enuresis may be either diurnal (during waking hours) or nocturnal (during night-time sleep) or a combination of both.

Nocturnal enuresis is as common in boys as girls until the age of 5 years, but by age 11 years, boys outnumber girls 2 : 1. Not until the age of 8 years do boys achieve the same levels of night-time continence that are seen in girls by the age of 5 years, probably due to slower physiological maturation in boys. In addition, the increased incidence of secondary enuresis (occurring after an initial 1-year period of acquired continence) in boys further affects the sex ratio seen in later childhood. Daytime enuresis occurs more commonly in girls and is associated with higher rates of psychiatric disturbance.

Etiology and Pathophysiology

Possible biological factors include a structural pathological condition or infection of the urinary tract (or both), low functional bladder capacity, abnormal antidiuretic hormone secretion, abnormal depth of sleep, genetic predisposition and developmental delay. Evidence has also been found for sympathetic hyperactivity and delayed organ maturation as seen by delay in ossification.

Obstructive lesions of the urinary outflow tract, which can cause urinary tract infection (UTI) as well as enuresis, have been thought to be important, with a high prevalence of such abnormalities seen in enuretic children referred to urologic clinics. This degree of association is not seen at less specialized pediatric centers, however, and most studies linking urinary outflow obstruction to enuresis are methodologically flawed (Shaffer *et al.*, 1979). Structural causes for enuresis should be considered the exception rather than the rule.

UTI has been found to occur frequently in children, especially girls and a large proportion (85%) of them have been shown to have nocturnal enuresis. Also, in 10% of bedwetting girls, urinalysis results show evidence of bacterial infection. The consensus is that as treating the infection rarely stops the bedwetting, UTI is probably a result rather than a cause of enuresis.

The concept that children with enuresis have low functional bladder capacities has been widely promoted. Shaffer and colleagues (1984) found a functional bladder capacity one standard deviation lower than expected in 55% of a sample of enuretic children in school clinics. Although low functional capacity may predispose the child to enuresis, successful behavioral treatment does not appear to increase that capacity, rather the sensation of a full (small) bladder promotes waking to pass urine so that enuresis does not occur. Reduction of nocturnal secretion of antidiuretic hormone (ADH) has been described in a small number of children with enuresis, causing excessive amounts of dilute urine to be produced during the night and overwhelming bladder capacity. Several mechanisms are associated with enuresis, including increased nocturnal urine volume, small nocturnal functional bladder capacity, increased spontaneous bladder contractions, and the inability to arouse to the stimulus of a large and/or contracting bladder. This may identify two main groups of children with enuresis: those who demonstrate nocturnal spontaneous bladder contractions (detrusor dependent enuresis) and those with nocturnal polyuria (volume dependent enuresis).

Approximately 70% of children with nocturnal enuresis have a first-degree relative who also has or has had nocturnal enuresis. Twin studies have shown greater monozygotic (68%) than dizygotic (36%) concordance. An association between enuresis and early delays in motor, language and social development has been noted in both prospective community samples and a large retrospective study of clinical subjects (Steinhausen and Gobel, 1989). Genetic factors are probably the most important in the etiology of nocturnal enuresis but somatic and psychosocial environmental factors have a major modulatory effect. Most commonly, nocturnal enuresis is inherited via an autosomal dominant mode of transmission with high penetrance (90%). However, a third of all cases are sporadic. Four gene loci associated with nocturnal enuresis have been identified but the existence of others is presumed (locus heterogeneity). Other psychosocial correlates described include delayed toilet training, low socioeconomic class, stress events and other child psychiatric disorders. Stress events seem to be more clearly associated with secondary enuresis. Reported events include the birth of a younger, early hospitalizations and head injury (Chadwick, 1985).

Psychiatric disorder occurs more frequently in enuretic children than in other children, although no specific types have been identified (Mikkelsen and Rapoport, 1980). The relative frequency of disorder ranges from two to six times that in the general population and is more frequent in girls, in children who also have diurnal enuresis and in children with secondary enuresis.

There is little evidence that enuresis is a symptom of underlying disorder because psychotherapy is ineffective in reducing enuresis, anxiolytic drugs have no antienuretic effect, tricyclic antidepressants exert their therapeutic effect independent of the child's mood, and purely symptomatic therapies, such as the bell and pad, are equally effective in disturbed and nondisturbed children. A further explanation for the association is that enuresis, a distressing and stigmatizing affliction, may cause the psychiatric disorder. However, although some studies have shown that enuretic children who undergo treatment become happier and have greater self-esteem, other studies show that psychiatric symptoms do not appear to lessen in children who are successful with a night alarm. A final possibility is that enuresis and psychiatric disorder are both the result of joint etiological factors such as low socioeconomic status, institutional care, large sibships, parental delinquency, and early and repeated disruptions of maternal care. Shared biological factors may also be important in that delayed motor, speech and pubertal development, already shown to be associated with enuresis, have proven to be more frequent in disturbed enuretic children than in those without psychiatric disorder.

Diagnosis and Differential Diagnosis

The presence or absence of conditions often seen in association with enuresis should be assessed and ruled out as appropriate (Figure 31.1). Other causes of nocturnal incontinence should be excluded, for example, those leading to polyuria (diabetes mellitus, renal disease, diabetes insipidus) and, rarely, nocturnal epilepsy.

Assessment

History

Information on the frequency, periodicity and duration of symptoms is needed to make the diagnosis and distinguish functional enuresis from sporadic seizure-associated enuresis. If there is diurnal enuresis, an additional treatment plan is required. A family history of enuresis increases the likelihood of a diagnosis of functional enuresis and may explain a later age at which children are presented for treatment. Projective identification by the affected parent–whereby the parent does not separate feelings about himself having the diagnosis and the current experience of the affected child–may further hinder treatment. For subjects

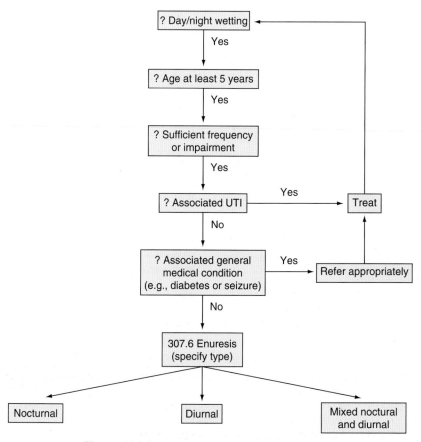

Figure 31.1 *Diagnostic decision tree for enuresis.*

with secondary enuresis, precipitating factors should be elicited, although such efforts often represent an attempt to assign meaning after the event.

Questions that are useful in obtaining information for treatment planning include "Why is this a problem?" and "Why does this need treatment now?" because these factors may influence the choice of treatment (is a rapid effect needed?) or point to other pressures or restrictions on therapy. It is important to inquire about previous management strategies used at home, for example, fluid restriction, nightlifting (getting the child out of bed to take to the toilet in an often semi-asleep state), rewards and punishments. Parents often come with the assertion that they have tried everything and that nothing has helped. Examining the reasons for failure of simple strategies is useful for ensuring that more sophisticated treatments do not befall the same fate. There is little evidence that fluid restriction is useful, although nightlifting may be beneficial for the large number of children who never reach professional attention. Rewards are usually material and are given only for unreasonably high performance levels, with the delay between action and reward being too long. Physical punishment and verbal chastisements, ineffective at best, may well maintain the enuresis. Punishment is often too harsh and tends to be applied inconsistently depending on parental mood. If specific treatments have been prescribed, either behavioral or pharmacological, it is important to discover the reasons they may have failed.

Mental Status Examination

The child's views and any misconceptions that he or she may have about the enuresis, its causes and its treatment should be fully explored. Asking the child for three wishes may help determine whether the enuresis is a concern to the child. This may unmask marked embarrassment or guilt from behind a facade of denial about the problem and can be educational for parents who believe their children could stop wetting "if only they wanted to or tried harder". Pictures drawn by the child that describe how the child views himself or herself when enuresis is a problem and when it is not appropriate for younger children and can graphically illustrate the misery experienced by children with enuresis.

Physical Examination

All children should have a routine physical examination, with particular emphasis placed on detection of congenital malformations indicative of urogenital abnormalities. A midstream specimen of urine should be examined for the presence of infection. Radiological or further medical investigation is indicated only in the presence of infected urine, enuresis with symptoms suggestive of recurrent UTI (frequency, urgency and dysuria), or polyuria.

Treatment

Practical management for nocturnal enuresis is presented in Table 31.1.

Table 31.1	Practical Management of Nocturnal Enuresis
Stage 1	**Assessment**
	Obtain history: frequency, periodicity and duration of wetting. Why is this a problem? Why now? Mental status: views and misconceptions (parent and child). Discover reasons for previous failure or failures. Perform routine physical examination (any minor congenital abnormalities?). Midstream specimen of urine must be obtained. Radiology and further physical investigation is needed only if symptoms or evidence of urinary tract infection (dysuria and frequency or positive culture results) or polyuria.
Stage 2	**Advice**
	Education that enuresis is common and not deliberate. Aim to reduce punitive behavior. Transmit optimism: however, anticipate disappointment at no instant cure. Preview the stepwise recovery and warn of the possibility of relapse.
Stage 3	**Baseline**
	Use star chart. Focus on positive achievements (be creative). Examine the effect of simple interventions (e.g., lifting)
Stage 4	**Night Alarm**
	First-line management unless important to obtain rapid short-term effect. Demonstrate night alarm equipment in the office. Telephone follow-up within a few days of commencing therapy.
	Or
	Drug Therapy
	If rapid suppression of wetting is needed (e.g., before vacation or camp, to defuse aggressive or hostile situation between child and parents and siblings). When family has proved incapable of using the equipment. After failure or multiple relapses. Medication of choice: DDAVP (Desmopressin) 20–40 µg at night

The overall goals of treatment can depend on the reason for referral. Commonly, the child is brought to the physician before some planned activity, for example, a family vacation or a trip to camp, and the need is for a rapid (e.g., pharmacological) short-term therapy. A gradual behavioral approach would not likely meet with much approval even though it may offer a chance for a permanent cessation of wetting.

Standard Treatment

About 10% of children have a reduction in the number of wet nights after a single visit to a clinician in which the only intervention was the recording of baseline wetting frequency and simple reassurance. Such reassurance should make clear that enuresis is a biological condition that is made worse by stress and that may be associated in a noncausal way with other psychiatric disorders. Younger children can be told that their problem is shared by many others of the same age. The excellent prognosis for patients who comply with therapy should be stressed. Recording the frequency of enuresis can be achieved by using a simple star chart. This is most effective if performed by the child, who records each dry night with a star. The completed chart is then shown to the parents on a daily basis, and they can provide appropriate praise and reinforcement.

Waking and Fluid Restriction

Although systematic studies have failed to show any effect of these interventions with enuretic inpatients, it may be that these strategies work for the majority of enuretic children who are not referred for treatment.

Surgery

Based on the premise that enuresis is causally associated with outflow tract obstruction, various surgical procedures have been advocated, for example, urethral dilatation, meatotomy, cystoplasty and bladder neck repair. This cannot be supported because, in addition to the dubious concept of outflow tract obstruction per se, the surgery does not alter the urodynamics of the bladder. Reported positive treatment effects are slight (no controlled studies exist), and there remains a significant potential for adverse effects (urinary incontinence, epididymitis and aspermia).

Pharmacotherapy

Although it has been repeatedly demonstrated that temporary suppression rather than cure of enuresis is the usual outcome of drug therapy, it remains the most widely prescribed treatment in the USA. Four classes of drugs have principally been employed: synthetic antidiuretic hormones, tricyclic antidepressants, stimulants and anticholinergic agents.

Synthetic Antidiuretic Hormone   A number of randomized double-blind placebo-controlled trials (RCT) have shown that the synthetic vasopeptide DDAVP (desmopressin) is effective in enuresis. The drug is usually administered intranasally, although oral preparations of equal efficacy have been developed (equivalent oral dose is 10 times the intranasal dose). Almost 50% of children are able to stop wetting completely with a single nightly dose of 20 to 40 µg of DDAVP given intranasally. A further 40% are afforded a significant reduction in the frequency of enuresis with this treatment. As with tricyclic antidepressants, however, when treatment is stopped, the vast majority of individuals relapse. Side effects of this medication include nasal pain and con-

gestion, headache, nausea and abdominal pain. Serious problems of water intoxication, hyponatremia and seizures are rare. It is important to be aware that intranasal absorption is reduced when the patient has a cold or allergic rhinitis. The mode of action of desmopressin is unknown. It may reduce the production of night-time urine to an amount less than the (low) functional volume of the enuretic bladder, thereby eliminating the urge to micturate. With regard to identifying those most likely to respond to DDAVP treatment, it has been found that those most likely to be permanently dry are infrequent wetting older children who respond to lower dose (20 µg) desmopressin.

Tricyclic Antidepressants   The short-term effectiveness of imipramine and other related antidepressants has also been demonstrated via many RCTs. Imipramine reduces the frequency of enuresis in about 85% of bed-wetters and eliminates enuresis in about 30% of these individuals. Night-time doses of 1 to 2.5 mg/kg are usually effective and a therapeutic effect is usually evident in the first week of treatment. Relapse after withdrawal of medication is almost inevitable, so that 3 months after the cessation of tricyclic antidepressants, nearly all patients will again have enuresis at pretreatment levels. Side effects are common and include dry mouth, dizziness, postural hypotension, headache and constipation. Toxicity after accidental ingestion or overdose is a serious consideration, causing cardiac effects, including arrhythmias and conduction defects, convulsions, hallucinations and ataxia. Concern has been expressed about the possibility of sudden death (presumably caused by arrhythmia) in children taking tricyclic drugs. The mode of action for tricyclic antidepressants is unclear, although one observation is that tricyclic agents seem to increase functional bladder volumes possibly resulting from noradrenergic reuptake inhibition.

Stimulant Medication   Sympathomimetic stimulants such as dexamphetamine have been used to reduce the depth of sleep in children with enuresis; but because there is no evidence that enuresis is related to abnormally deep sleep, their lack of effectiveness in stopping bed-wetting is no surprise. Used in combination with behavioral therapy, there is some evidence that stimulants can accentuate the learning of nocturnal continence.

Anticholinergic Drugs   Drugs such as propantheline, oxybutynin and terodiline can reduce the frequency of voiding in individuals with neurogenic bladders, reduce urgency and increase functional bladder capacity. There is no evidence, however, that these anticholinergic drugs are effective in bed-wetting, although they may have a role in diurnal enuresis. Side effects are frequent and include dry mouth, blurred vision, headache, nausea and constipation.

Psychosocial Treatments

The night alarm was first used in children with enuresis in the 1930s. This system used two electrodes separated by a device (e.g., bedding) connected to an alarm. When the child wet the bed, the urine completed the electrical circuit, sounded the alarm and the child awoke. All current night alarm systems are merely refinements on this original design. A vibrating pad beneath the pillow can be used instead of a bell or buzzer, or the electrodes can be incorporated into a single unit or can be miniaturized so that they can be attached to night (or day) clothing. With treatment, full cessation of enuresis can be expected in 80% of cases. Reported cure rates (defined as a minimum of

14 consecutive dry nights) have ranged from 50 to 100%. The main problem with this form of enuretic treatment, however, is that cure is usually achieved only within the second month of treatment. This factor may influence clinicians to prescribe pharmacological treatments that, although more immediately gratifying, do not offer any real prospect of cure. It has been suggested that adjuvant therapy with methamphetamine or desmopressin will reduce the amount of time before continence is achieved. Using a louder auditory stimulus or using the body-worn alarm may also improve the speed of treatment response. Factors associated with delayed acquisition of continence include failure of the child to wake with the alarm, maternal anxiety and a disturbed home environment, although no influence has been seen regarding the age of the child or the initial wetting frequency.

A further consequence of the delayed response to a night alarm is premature termination occurring in as many as 48% of cases and is more common in families that have made little previous effort to treat the problem, in families that are negative or intolerant of bed-wetting, and in children who have other behavioral problems. Compliance-reducing factors also include failure to understand or follow the instructions, failure of the child to awaken, and frequent false alarms. The only reported side effect of treatment with the night alarm is "buzzer ulcers" caused by the child lying in a pool of ionized urine. This problem has been eliminated with modern transistorized alarms that do not employ a continuous, relatively high voltage across the electrodes to detect enuresis.

Relapse after successful treatment, if it occurs, will usually take place within the first 6 months after cessation of treatment. It is reported that approximately one-third of children relapse; however, no clear predictors of relapse have been identified.

Table 31.2 presents various remedies for night alarm problems.

Ultrasonic Bladder Volume Alarm

Although the traditional enuresis alarm has good potential for a permanent cure, the child is mostly wet during treatment. Furthermore, the moisture alarm requires that the child make the somewhat remote association between the alarm event and a full bladder after the bladder has emptied. In an exploratory study (Pretlow, 1999), a new approach to treating nocturnal enuresis was investigated using a miniature bladder volume measurement instrument during sleep. In this, an alarm sounded when bladder volume reached 80% of the typical enuretic volume. Two groups were studied. Group 1 used the night-time device alone; group 2, in addition, had supplementary daytime bladder retention training (aiming to increase functional capacity). In groups 1 and 2 the mean dryness rate before study initiation versus during the study was 32.9 and 9.3% versus 88.7 and 82.1%, respectively. Night-time bladder capacity increased 69% in group 1 and 78% in group 2, while the cure rate was 55% (mean treatment period 10.5 months) and 60% (mean treatment period 7.2 months), respectively.

Acupuncture

The efficacy of traditional Chinese acupuncture has been studied (Serel et al., 2001) in a small ($n = 50$) clinical sample. It was reported that within 6 months, 86% of patients were completely dry and a further 10% of patients were dry on at least 80% of

Table 31.2	Problem Solving for the Night Alarm *If...*
Bell "does not work"	Check position, connections and batteries. If using separating sheet, check that it is porous. Check that child is not turning off equipment. Place alarm out of easy reach.
Child does not wake	Make alarm louder. Parent should wake child.
Child does not become dry	Ensure compliance. Ensure that child responds promptly. Use adjuvant DDAVP or dextroamphetamine. Ensure that child has role (e.g., change own bed-sheets) after alarm.
False alarms	Ensure that separating sheet is big enough, not soiled and will insulate. Use thicker nightclothes.
Relapse	Repeat treatment. Consider over learning after response to re-treatment.

nights. Relapse rates appeared better than with psychopharmacologic agents.

Summary

There were approximately 22 randomized trials conducted between 1985 and 1997 involving 1100 children treated pharmacologically or behaviorally for primary nocturnal enuresis. The quality of many of these trials is poor with very few trials comparing drugs with each other, or drugs with alarms or other behavioral interventions, and few having adequate follow-up periods. Desmopressin and tricyclics appeared equally effective while on treatment, but this effect was not sustained after treatment stopped. It is clear that further comparisons between drug and behavioral treatments are needed, and should include relapse rates after treatment is finished.

Assessment and Management of Diurnal Enuresis

Daytime enuresis, although it can occur together with night-time enuresis, has a different pattern of associations and responds to different methods of treatment. It is much more likely to be associated with urinary tract abnormalities and to be comorbid with other psychiatric disorders. As a result, a more detailed and focused medical and psychiatric evaluation is indicated. Urine should be checked repeatedly for infection, and the threshold for ordering ultrasonographical visualization of the urological system should be low. The history may make it apparent that the daytime wetting is situation specific. For example, school-based enuresis in a child who is too timid to ask to use the bathroom could be alleviated by the teacher's tactfully reminding the child to go to the bathroom at regular intervals.

Observation of children with diurnal enuresis has established that they do experience an urge to pass urine before micturition but that either this urge is ignored or the warning comes too late to be of any use because of an "irritable bladder". Therefore, treatment strategies are based on establishing a pattern of toileting before the times that diurnal enuresis is likely to occur (usually between 12 noon and 5 pm) and using positive reinforcement to promote regular use of the bathroom.

Portable systems that can be worn on the body and use a sensor in the underwear as well as an alarm that can be worn on the wrist have been developed. Studies have shown no significant differences between the wetness alarm and the simple timed alarm. The easiest therapeutic alternative, therefore, is to buy the child a digital watch with a countdown alarm timer.

Unlike nocturnal enuresis, drug treatment with tricyclic antidepressants such as imipramine is ineffective, whereas the use of anticholinergic agents such as oxybutynin and terodiline shows a therapeutic impact on the frequency of daytime enuresis.

Encopresis

Definition

Encopresis is usually defined as the intentional or involuntary passage of stool into inappropriate places in the absence of any identified physical abnormality in children older than 4 years. It may not be attributable to a medical condition and must occur at least monthly for a period of three months. The distinction is drawn between encopresis with constipation (retention with overflow based on history or physical examination) and encopresis without constipation. Other classification schemes include making a primary–secondary distinction (based on having a 1-year period of continence) or soiling with fluid or normal feces.

Course and Natural History

Less than one-third of children in the USA have completed toilet training by the age of 2 years with a mean age of 27.7 months. Bowel control is usually achieved before bladder control.

The age cutoff for "normality" is set at 4 years, the age at which 95% of children have acquired fecal continence (Stein and Susser, 1967). As with urinary continence, girls achieve bowel control earlier than boys.

Epidemiology

The overall prevalence of encopresis in 7- and 8-year-old children has been shown to be 1.5%, with boys (2.3%) affected more commonly than girls (0.7%). There was a steadily rising likelihood of continence with increasing age, until by age 16 years the reported prevalence was almost zero. Rutter and coworkers (1970) reported a rate of 1% in 10- to 12-year-old children, with a strong (5 : 1) male/female ratio. Retrospective study of clinic-referred encopretic children has shown that 40% of cases are primary (true failure to gain control), with a mean age of 6.7 years, and 60% of cases are secondary, with a mean age of 8 years (Levine, 1975). Eighty percent of patients were constipated, with no difference in this feature seen between primary and secondary subtypes.

Etiology and Pathophysiology

Within the first year of life, children can show a tendency toward constipation, with concordance for constipation being six times

---

Clinical Vignette 1

John, an 8-year-old boy, was the sixth child in a sibship. He was brought by his mother for treatment of nocturnal enuresis which was occurring on average five times a week, with no particular pattern. Two of his elder brothers had also wet the bed until the age of 10 and 13 years, respectively, as had his biological father who was no longer living with the family. The mother had become exasperated with John's wetting and had begun punishing him by forcing him to wash his bedclothes by hand every morning before school. His brothers made fun of him, and peers at school avoided him because he frequently came to school still smelling of stale urine. He was not allowed to have anything to drink after 6 pm, and a star chart was currently being used without much success. No praise was given for the two dry nights per week because his mother was convinced that this meant the enuresis was deliberate. John drew a picture describing the terror and anxiety of having a wet night. His three wishes were to stop wetting, to get a Nintendo machine of his own and to find a real dinosaur fossil.

The initial management included an explanation of the condition, microbiological analysis of a midstream specimen of urine and instructions on baseline recording using the star chart. Overt punishments were eliminated, although John was expected to help change his sheets, and effort was expended in trying to help his mother praise him for the dry nights he was able to achieve. After a 2-week baseline period, urinalysis results came back negative and the frequency of enuresis remained at four to five nights per week. John and his mother were instructed in the use of a night alarm and were telephoned 2 days later to check on any problems. It appeared that John was not waking with the buzzer, and they were instructed to place the alarm unit on an old cookie tin to amplify the sound. Dry nights were recorded on John's chart, with verbal praise after each one.

An initial target of three dry nights per week was set, with the promise of a trip to the movies for John and the two brothers who shared a bedroom with him. This was achieved the first week, although it took a further 6 weeks before he went a full week without a wet bed. After 2 weeks of continence, the restriction on night-time fluids was relaxed without incident. Six months later he remained dry, and school and home relationships were markedly improved.

---

more frequent in monozygotic than in dizygotic twins. Fecal retention and reduced stool frequency between 12 and 24 months of age can predict later encopresis. Encopretic children with constipation and overflow are found to have rectal and colonic distention, massive impaction with hard feces and a number of specific abnormalities of anorectal physiology. These abnormalities, which may be primary or secondary to constipation, include elevated anal resting tone, decreased anorectal motility and weakness of the internal anal sphincter, and dysfunction of the external anal sphincter. Encopresis may occur after an acute episode of constipation following illness or a change in diet. In addition to the pain caused by attempts to pass an extremely hard stool, a number of specific painful perianal conditions such as anal fissure can lead to stool withholding and later fecal soiling. Stressful events such as the birth of a sibling or attending a new school have been associated with up to 25% of cases of secondary encopresis. In nonretentive encopresis, the main theories center on faulty toilet training. Stress during the training period, coercive toileting leading to anxiety and "pot phobia", and failure to learn or to have been taught the appropriate behavior have all been implicated. True fecal urgency, which may have a physiological or pathological basis, may also be important in a small proportion of cases (Woodmansey, 1967).

Diagnosis and Differential Diagnosis

The main efforts during the diagnostic process are to establish the presence or absence of constipation and, to a lesser extent, distinguish continuous (primary) from discontinuous (secondary) soiling (Figure 31.2). Taylor and Hersov (1994) listed three types of identifiable encopresis in children: 1) it is known that the child can control defecation, but she or he chooses to defecate in inappropriate places; 2) there is true failure to gain bowel control, and the child is unaware of or unable to control soiling; and 3) soiling is due to excessively fluid feces, whether from constipation and overflow, physical disease, or anxiety. In practice, there is frequently overlap among types or progression from one to another. Unlike enuresis, fecal soiling rarely occurs at night or during sleep, and if present, is indicative of a poor prognosis. Soiling due to anal masturbation has been reported, although this causes staining of the sheets rather than full stools in the bedclothes.

Phenomenology

In the first group, in which bowel control has been established, the stool may be soft or normal (but different from fluid-type feces seen in overflow). Soiling due to acute stress events (e.g.,

the birth of a sibling, a change of school, or parental separation) is usually brief once the stress has abated, given a stable home environment and sensible management. In more severe pathological family situations, including punitive management or frank physical or sexual abuse (Boon, 1991), the feces may be deposited in places deliberately to cause anger or irritation, or there may be associated smearing of feces on furniture and walls. Other covert aggressive antisocial acts may be evident, with considerable denial by the child of the magnitude or seriousness of the problem.

In the second group, in which there is failure to learn bowel control, a nonfluid stool is deposited fairly randomly in clothes, at home and at school. There may be conditions such as mental retardation or specific developmental delay, spina bifida, or cerebral palsy that impair the ability to recognize the need to defecate and the appropriate skills needed to defer this function until a socially appropriate time and location. In the absence of low IQ or pathological physical condition, patients have been reported as having associated enuresis, academic skills problems and antisocial behavior. They present to pediatricians primarily and are usually younger (age 4–6 years) than other encopretic individuals. It is thought that this type of soiling is considerably more common in socially disadvantaged, disorganized families because of stressful, faulty or inconsistent training.

In the third group, excessively fluid feces are passed, which may result from conditions that cause true diarrhea (e.g., ulcerative colitis) or, much more frequently, from constipation with overflow causing spurious diarrhea. A history of retention, either willful or in response to pain, is prominent in the early days of this form of encopresis, although later it may be less apparent because of fecal overflow. Behavior such as squatting on the heels to prevent defecation or marked anxiety about the prospect of

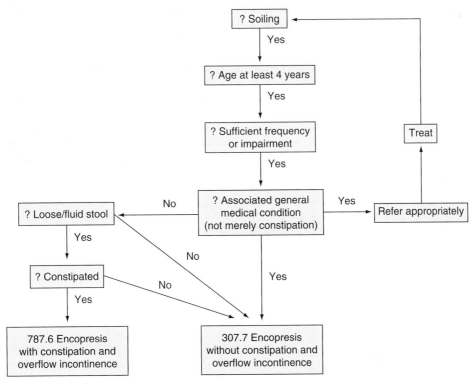

Figure 31.2 *Diagnostic decision for encopresis.*

using the toilet (although rarely amounting to true phobic avoidance) may be described.

Issues and Further Assessment

The comprehensive assessment process should include a medical evaluation, psychiatric and family interviews, and a systematic behavioral recording.

The medical evaluation comprises a history, review of systems, physical examination, and appropriate hematological and radiological tests. Although the vast majority of patients with encopresis are medically normal, a small proportion have pathological features of etiological significance. Physical causes of encopresis without retention include inflammatory bowel disease (e.g., ulcerative colitis, Crohn's disease), central nervous system disorders, sensory disorders of the anorectal region or pelvic floor muscles (e.g., spina bifida, cerebral palsy). Organic causes of encopresis with retention include Hirschsprung's disease (aganglionosis in intermuscular and submucous plexuses of the large bowel extending proximally from the anus), neurogenic megacolon, hypothyroidism, hypercalcemia, chronic codeine or laxative usage, anorectal stenosis and fissure. It should also be remembered that these conditions rarely have their first presentation with encopresis alone.

The physical assessment should include an abdominal and rectal examination, although a plain abdominal radiograph is the most reliable way to determine the presence of fecal impaction. Anorectal manometry should be considered in the investigation of children with severe constipation and chronic soiling, especially those in whom Hirschsprung's disease is suspected.

Psychiatric and family interviews should include a developmental history and a behavioral history of encopresis (antecedents, behavior and consequences). Specific areas of stress, acute or chronic, affecting the child or family, or both, should be discovered. Associated psychopathological conditions are more commonly found in the older child, in secondary encopresis, and when soiling occurs not only in clothes. Anxiety surrounding toileting may indicate pot phobia, coercive toileting, or a history of painful defecation. A history should be obtained of the parents' previous attempts at treatment together with previously prescribed therapy so that reasons for previous failure can be identified and anticipated in future treatment planning.

Treatment

Practical management for encopresis is presented in Table 31.3.

Standard Treatment

The principal approach to treatment is predicated on the results of the evaluation and the clinical category assigned. This differentiates between the need to establish a regular toileting procedure in patients in whom there has been a failure to learn this social behavior and the need to address a psychiatric disorder, parent–child relationship difficulties, or other stresses in the child who exhibits loss of this previously acquired skill in association with these factors. In both cases, analysis of the soiling behavior may identify reinforcing factors important in maintaining dysfunction. Detection of significant constipation will, in addition, provide an indication for adjuvant laxative therapy.

Behavioral Treatments

Behavioral therapy is the mainstay of treatment for encopresis. In the younger child who has been toilet trained, this focuses on practical elimination skills, for example, visiting the toilet after

Table 31.3   Practical Management of Encopresis

Stage 1	Assessment
	Whether primary or secondary.
	Is there physical cause?
	Presence or absence of constipation.
	Presence or absence of acute stress.
	Presence or absence of psychiatric disorder including phobic symptoms or smearing.
	ABC (antecedents, behavior, consequences) of encopresis including secondary gain.
	Discover reasons for previous failure or failures.
Stage 2	**Advice**
	Education regarding diet, constipation and toileting.
	Aim to reduce punitive or coercive behavior.
	Transmit optimism; however, anticipate disappointment at no instant cure.
	Preview the stepwise recovery and warn of the possibility of relapse.
Stage 3	**Toileting**
	Baseline observation using star chart.
	Focus on positive achievements, e.g., toileting, rather than soiling.
	High-fiber diet (try bran in soup, milk shakes).
	Toilet after meals, 15 min maximum.
	Check that adequately rising intra-abdominal pressure is present.
	Graded exposure scheme if "pot phobic".
	with
	Laxatives
	Indicated if physical examination or abdominal radiograph shows fecal loading.
	Medication of choice: Senokot syrup (senna) up to 10 mL b.i.d., lactulose syrup up to 30 mL (20 mg) b.i.d.
	Dosage will be reduced over time; titrate with bowel frequency.
	Enemas
	Microenema (e.g., bisacodyl, 30 mL) if the bowel is excessively loaded with rock-like feces.
Stage 4	**Biofeedback**
	Consider after relapse or failure to respond to toileting or laxatives.

each meal, staying there for a maximum of 15 minutes, using muscles to increase intra-abdominal pressure and cleaning oneself adequately afterward. Parents or caretakers, or both, need to be educated in making the toilet a pleasant place to visit and should stay with the younger child, giving encouragement and praise for appropriate effort. Small children whose legs may dangle above the floor should be provided with a step against which to brace when straining. Initially, a warm bath before using the toilet may relax the anxious child and make it easier to pass stool. Systematic recording of positive toileting behavior, not necessarily being clean (depending on the level of baseline behavior), should be performed with a personal star chart. For the child with severe anxiety about sitting on the toilet, a graded exposure scheme may be indicated.

Role of the Family in Treatment

Removing the child's and family's attention from the encopresis alone and focusing onto noticing, recording and rewarding positive behavior often defuses tension and hostility and provides the opportunity for therapeutic improvement. Identifying and eliminating sources of secondary gain, whereby soiling is reinforced by parental (or other individuals') actions and attention, even if negative or punitive, make positive efforts more fruitful. Some investigators advocate mild punishment techniques, such as requiring the child to clean his or her own clothes after soiling, although care must be taken to prevent this from becoming too punitive. In certain settings, particularly school, attempts are made to prevent soiling by extremely frequent toileting that, although keeping the child clean, does not promote and may even hinder the acquisition of a regular bowel habit. Formal therapy, either individual or family based, is indicated in only a minority of patients with an associated psychiatric disorder, marked behavioral disturbance, or clear remediable family or social stresses.

Physical Treatments

In patients with retention leading to constipation and overflow, medical management is nearly always required, although it is usually with oral laxatives or microenemas alone. The use of more intrusive and invasive colonic and rectal washout or surgical disimpaction procedures is nearly always the result of the clinician's impatience rather than true clinical need.

Uncontrolled studies of combined treatment with behavioral therapy and laxatives reported marked improvement in symptoms (not cure) in approximately 70 to 80% of patients. A more recent controlled randomized trial (Nolan et al., 1991) comparing behavioral therapy in retentive primary encopresis with and without laxatives showed that at 12-month follow-up, 51% of the combined treatment (laxative plus behavioral therapy) group had achieved remission (at least one 4-week period with no soiling episodes), compared with 36% of the behavioral therapy only group ($P = 0.08$). Partial remission (soiling no more than once a week) was achieved in 63% of patients with combined therapy versus 43% with behavioral therapy alone ($P = 0.02$). Patients receiving laxatives achieved remission significantly sooner, and the difference in the Kaplan–Meier remission curves was most striking in the first 30 weeks of follow-up ($P = 0.012$). When patients who were not compliant with the toileting program were removed from the analysis, however, the advantage of combined therapy was not significant. These results must also be viewed in light of a 50% spontaneous remission rate at 2 years reported in some studies.

Biofeedback Therapy

The finding that some children with treatment-resistant retentive encopresis involuntarily contract the muscles of the pelvic floor and the external anal sphincter, effectively impeding passage of stool, has led to efforts to use biofeedback in this instance. It has similarly been reported that as few as six sessions of biofeedback therapy can lead to a significant reduction in symptom frequency for as many as 86% of previously treatment-resistant patients (Loening-Baucke, 1995). It is possible, however, that biofeedback is principally of benefit to nonretentive chronic soilers (van Ginkel et al., 2000).

Other Disorders Specific to Children and Adolescents

Separation Anxiety Disorder

Definition

Separation anxiety disorder is typified by developmentally inappropriate and excessive anxiety concerning separation from home or attachment figures. This diagnosis is included within the child and adolescent disorders because, although adults may have separation problems/symptoms, a diagnosis of separation anxiety disorder is not made in adulthood. The onset of this disorder, therefore, must be prior to the age of 18 years. Symptoms (a minimum of three) must be present for at least four weeks and cause significant distress or impairment in social or academic functioning. Excessive and developmentally inappropriate levels of anxiety are manifested by the following behaviors:

- Fears and worry about losing, or about harm befalling significant attachment figures.
- Recurrent and intense distress when leaving home or attachment figures.
- Reluctance or refusal to attend school.
- Excessive worry about separation from an attachment figure through getting lost or kidnapped.
- Inability to feel comfortable being alone without the presence of attachment figures or other adults.
- Difficulty in sleeping without being in the presence of an attachment figure.
- Frequent anxiety dreams about separation.
- Repeated complaints of symptom such as nausea, vomiting, stomach aches, headaches, prior to threatened separation from an attachment figure.

The diagnosis of early onset separation anxiety disorder is made when symptoms appear prior to the age of six years.

Natural History and Course

The community prevalence of SAD is generally estimated to be around 4% in children and young adolescents; it decreases in prevalence from childhood through adolescence. Amongst clinically referred subjects (aged 5–18 years) with anxiety disorders, separation anxiety disorder was found to be the most frequently occurring disorder, with a lifetime prevalence of 44.7%. The age of onset has been reported to be 4 to 7 years, with earlier onset being associated with clinical status and comorbidity (Biederman et al., 1997). Separation anxiety, particularly in younger samples, is found more frequently in girls than boys: a ratio as high as 2.5:1. In a 3- to 4-year prospective study (Last et al., 1996) of subjects with anxiety disorders, 29% of children had separation anxiety disorder (21% had SAD as their primary diagnosis) at baseline. On follow-up, 92% of children previously diagnosed with SAD no longer had symptoms that met full criteria for SAD, although 25% had developed a new disorder, most frequently a depressive disorder. Finding that 50% of adult panic patients had experienced separation anxiety during childhood, it has been hypothesized that separation anxiety may be a childhood precursor to adult panic disorder and agoraphobia.

Etiology and Pathophysiology

Sensitivity to suffocation cues, important in the carbon dioxide (CO_2) challenge paradigm in panic disorder and respiratory response, may differentiate children with anxiety disorder, and separation anxiety in particular, from children without an anxiety disorder. Inhalation of air containing raised CO_2 concentration results in increased catecholamine release throughout the body and perceived anxiety. This response appears mediated via the locus coeruleus, a group of norepinephrine-containing neurons originating in the pons and projecting to all major brain areas. The locus coeruleus forms part of the reticular activating system (RAS) and functions to regulate noradrenergic tone and activity. Hypothalamic and thalamic nuclei also play a role in the perception of and response to external threats. They act by transmitting arousal information from the RAS to limbic and cortical areas involved in sensory integration and perception. The thalamus is thought to have a role in the perception of anxiety, whereas the hypothalamic nuclei mediate the response by the neuroendocrine system. Urinary cortisol has been shown to be raised (indicative of HPA overactivity) in infants aged 1 year who demonstrated extreme distress when separated from their primary attachment figure.

Separation anxiety, when developmentally appropriate, is seen via attachment theory as an adaptive response that infants use to enhance proximity to their caregivers. In this, when the infant has adequate proximity to the caregiver in a given context, attachment behaviors (separation anxiety symptoms) subside and are replaced by alternate behaviors. On the basis of their response to various experimental paradigms, infants can be categorized into having different types of attachment. Although the nosology of attachment has varied, the most frequently described type of pathological attachment is known as "insecure attachment". Excessive distress on separation evinced by insecurely attached infants appears to be the earliest manifestation of separation anxiety disorder, but this pattern is not specific, in that it can be the precursor of other types of anxiety (e.g., social phobia/avoidant disorder, panic disorder) in childhood and adolescence.

Diagnosis and Differential Diagnosis

The assessment strategy will depend upon the child's age, symptom profile, the sources of available information and the purpose of the assessment. As discussed above, separation anxiety is normal at some ages and is maximal around 14 months of age. The most prevalent symptoms in young children (aged 5–8 years) are worry about losing or about possible harm to an attachment figure, and reluctance or refusal to go to school. Children aged 9 to 12 years most frequently reported recurrent excessive distress when separated from home or attachment figures, whereas adolescents (aged 13–16 years) had physical symptoms on school days. More symptoms were reported with decreasing age.

The usual unstructured clinical interview can, in view of its poor reliability and variable symptom coverage, be supplemented by standardized diagnostic interviews such as the Diagnostic Interview Schedule for Children (DISC) or the Anxiety

Disorder Interview Schedule (ADIS) which have shown acceptable test–retest reliability and validity. In addition, there are a large number of self-report questionnaires that can assess children's fears and anxieties, either to detect anxiety disorders in community samples or to distinguish between different anxiety disorders in clinically referred children. The most useful of these are the Multidimensional Anxiety Scale for Children (MASC) (March et al., 1997) and the Screen for Child Anxiety Related Emotional Disorders (SCARED) (Birmaher et al., 1997). These have been shown to have good test–retest reliability, internal consistency and can differentiate not only anxious children from nonanxious children but also distinguish specific anxiety disorders from each other. Particularly with younger children, there is value to direct observation of the child either in determining the diagnosis or in behavioral analysis.

Other issues in assessment of separation anxiety include: the relative value of information from differing methodologies, how to integrate information from separate informants, and also the cultural validity of most measures of anxiety Differential diagnoses to consider include generalized anxiety disorder (GAD), where the anxiety is more free-floating, less situation-specific and occurs independent of separation from the primary attachment figure. Children with social phobia will display a fear of social situations where they may be the object of public scrutiny. This anxiety may be ameliorated by the presence of a familiar person but will not occur exclusively when the attachment figure is absent, as with separation anxiety.

School refusal has long been associated with separation anxiety disorder, though this relationship holds mainly for younger children when school nonattendance is most closely linked to fear of separation, whereas in adolescents fear of school and social-evaluative situations is more typical. It is important in the assessment of school nonattendance, a frequent impairment associated with SAD, to distinguish anxiety-related school refusal from conduct disorder–related truancy. Typically the school-refusing child will stay at home or with parents, whereas the truanting child will go off with peers. In the presence of school refusal, a useful approach (Kearney and Silverman, 1999) is to attempt to categorize the behavior as fulfilling one of the four following functions:

1. Avoidance of stimuli provoking specific fearfulness or anxiety (e.g., separation).
2. Escape from aversive social or evaluative situations (e.g., social phobia).
3. Attention-getting behavior (e.g., physical complaints/tantrums).
4. Positive tangible reinforcement (e.g., parental collusion).

Treatment

Following a good behavioral and functional analysis, the most frequently employed clinical approach to the treatment of separation anxiety and school refusal is behavioral. The principles of systematic desensitization to feared objects or situations will be employed, gradually increasing the amount of separation that can be tolerated in a graduated fashion. Systematic desensitization usually has three components. First, a response, incompatible with anxiety (relaxation techniques), is taught. The second component is the collaborative construction of a hierarchy of feared situations. These will range from the very mild (producing mild disquiet) to the most anxiety provoking (avoided at all costs!). It is important to include a great deal of specificity in describing these situations including the duration spent in the feared situation, the degree to which others are involved, and the distance from home/attachment figure. After ranking these feared situations, the final component of treatment is the regular progression of exposure to feared situations whilst employing anxiety management techniques. It is important that the child is allowed to exercise some control over the speed with which new settings are experienced. The avoidance of reinforcement of unwanted behaviors and the promotion of fear-coping strategies is similarly important.

In the particular example of school refusal associated with separation anxiety, it is important to encourage an early return to school so that secondary impairments (academic failure and social isolation) are minimized. Generally, if the period of absence has been less than 2 months then return is very often successful.

In older subjects, cognitive approaches may be more successful than the primary behavior strategies usually employed with younger children. Cognitive approaches postulate that the child's maladaptive thoughts, beliefs and attitudes (schema) cause or maintain the experience of anxiety. Treatment consists of identifying negative self-statements ("I can't ever do this") or external beliefs ("If I'm not there my Mom won't be able to cope"), and replacing them with more adaptive beliefs.

Pharmacological treatment studies of separation anxiety similarly have tended to focus on samples with school refusal behavior and various diagnostic status and/or comorbidity. Early studies used imipramine or clomipramine with varying success. Considering safety and efficacy, the SSRIs appear to be the first-line treatment for separation anxiety disorder, but more studies are needed to confirm preliminary results. Tricyclic antidepressants and benzodiazepines may be considered when the child has not responded to SSRIs or when adverse effects have exceeded benefits. There is some evidence that treatments can be additive or synergistic. Alternatively, when combining drug and psychosocial treatments, a lower dose of one or both may be possible, with a resultant decrease in expense, inconvenience, or adverse events. Drug effects are often seen sooner than those due to exposure-based therapy, though it is hoped that the slower to emerge benefits of therapy may be more long lasting.

Selective Mutism

Definition
The essential feature of selective mutism is the persistent failure for at least one month (but not limited to the first month after the start of school) to speak in specific social situations where speaking is expected, despite speaking in other situations (most commonly in the home). Children with this disorder become impaired in social and educational settings. Selective mutism must not be diagnosed when there is a lack of knowledge or comfort speaking, for example, when a child is an immigrant.

Epidemiology
Previously referred to as **elective mutism**, in DSM-IV-TR the condition was renamed **selective mutism**, so as to be less judgmental. The prevalence is usually reported as 0.6 to seven per 1000, with higher incidence in females rather than males. When subjects failing to speak in the first few weeks of school (a DSM-IV-TR requirement) are excluded, rates do not exceed two per

1000. Onset is usually in the preschool years, but the peak age of presentation and diagnosis is between 6 and 8 years. A high incidence of insidious onset of refusal to speak with anyone except family members is reported. The other typical picture is one of acute onset of mutism on starting school.

Etiology
Three basic theories have been proposed to explain the etiology of selective mutism: children who are negative, oppositional and controlling; traumatized children; and children who have severe anxiety, chiefly social phobia. Although early psychodynamic theorists described an enmeshed relationship between mother and child, the father being distant and ineffectual, and a conflicted relationship between the parents, the only two controlled studies of selective mutism did not find family functioning worse compared with the families of other emotionally disturbed children (Kolvin and Fundudis, 1981; Wilkins, 1985). Associated features include a history of delayed speech and articulation problems, and possibly increased incidence of enuresis and/or encopresis. There may be a family history of general shyness, or of elevated levels of anxiety in the parents.

Assessment
Prior to making a diagnosis of selective mutism, a comprehensive evaluation should be conducted to rule out other explanations for mutism and to assess important comorbid factors. For obvious reasons, the parental interview will form the mainstay of evaluation but, as discussed below, direct observation (and interview if it is possible) of the child can afford important diagnostic information important to obtain information of the nature of the onset (insidious or sudden), any uncharacteristic features (i.e., not talking to family members, abrupt cessation of speech in one setting, absence of communication in all settings) suggestive of other neurological or psychiatric disorders (e.g., pervasive developmental disorders, acquired aphasias), and any history of neurological insult/injury, developmental delays, or atypical language and/or speech. The assessment should also include the degree to which nonverbal communication or non-face-to-face communication is possible, the presence of anxiety symptoms in areas other than speaking, social and behavioral inhibition, medical history including ear infections and hearing deficiencies. Parents will be able to give information on where and to whom the child will speak, the child's speech and language complexity at home, articulation problems, use of nonverbal communication (e.g., gestures), any history of speech and language delays, and the possible importance of bilingualism (where primary language is not English). It can be useful to have the parents provide an audiotape of the child speaking at home. The child evaluation can assess the presence of anxiety and social inhibition (willingness to communication through gesture or drawing). Physical examination of oral sensory and motor ability may provide evidence of neurological problems (i.e., drooling, asymmetry, orofacial weakness, abnormal gag reflex, impaired sucking or swallowing). Specialist audiometry (pure tone and speech stimuli as well as tympanometry and acoustic reflex testing) may provide evidence of hearing and/or middle ear problems that can have a significant effect on speech and language development. Cognitive abilities may be difficult to assess, but the performance section of the WISC-R or Raven's Progressive Matrices as well as the Peabody Picture Vocabulary Test may be useful in the nonverbal child.

Treatment

Treatment has long been regarded as difficult and the prognosis poor. Approaches have included behavioral therapy, family therapy, speech therapy and, more recently, pharmacological agents. Unfortunately most published studies are single case reports, with very few controlled studies.

Behavioral treatment focuses on mutism as a means of getting attention and/or escaping from anxiety. A controlled study (Calhoun and Koenig, 1973) of eight subjects with random assignment to treatment (teacher and peer reinforcement of verbal behavior) or control showed significant increases in mean number of vocalizations after 5 weeks of treatment. These gains were not, however, maintained at 12-month follow-up. Other techniques have included graded exposure, shaping and modeling. The goal of a treatment program should be to decrease the anxiety associated with speaking whilst encouraging the child to interact verbally.

Regarding pharmacotherapy, the use of SSRI medication in cases of selective mutism with associated anxiety (principally social phobia) has promise. An open trial of 21 children using a mean dose of 28.1 mg/day of fluoextine showed improvement in 76% of cases (Dummit *et al.*, 1996). A placebo-controlled double-blind study showed mixed results, though both groups remained highly symptomatic. More chronic (>14 weeks) treatment was recommended (Black and Uhde, 1994).

Comparison of DSM-IV/ICD-10 Diagnostic Criteria

In contrast to DSM-IV-TR which establishes a minimum duration of 3 months for encopresis, the ICD-10 Diagnostic Criteria for Research has set a minimum duration of 6 months. In ICD-10, this disorder is referred to as "Nonorganic Encopresis".

For enuresis, the ICD-10 Diagnostic Criteria for Research have a different frequency threshold: at least twice a month in children aged under 7 years and at least once a month in children aged 7 years or more. In contrast, DSM-IV-TR requires either a frequency of twice a week for at least three consecutive months (regardless of age) or else the presence of clinically significant distress or impairment. Furthermore, ICD-10 includes a very strict exclusion criterion, preventing a diagnosis of enuresis to be made if there is any evidence of another mental disorder. In ICD-10, this disorder is referred to as "nonorganic enuresis".

For separation anxiety disorder, the DSM-IV-TR and ICD-10 symptom items are almost identical. The ICD-10 Diagnostic Criteria for Research are narrower in that the age of onset must be before the age of six years and the diagnosis cannot be made if the presentation is "part of a broader disturbance of emotions, conduct, or personality". The DSM-IV-TR criteria and ICD-10 Diagnostic Criteria for Research for selective mutism are almost identical. In ICD-10, the disorder is referred to as "elective mutism".

References

Biederman J, Faraone SV, Marrs A *et al.* (1997) Panic disorder and agoraphobia in consecutively referred children and adolescents. *J Am Acad Child Adolesc Psychiatr* 36, 214–223.

Birmaher B, Khertarpal S, Brent D *et al.* (1997) The Screen for Child Anxiety Related Emotional Disorders (SCARED): Scale construction and psychometric characteristics. *J Am Acad Child Adolesc Psychiatr* 36, 545–553.

Black B and Uhde TW (1994) Treatment of elective mutism with fluoxetine: A double-blind placebo-controlled study. *J Am Acad Child Adolesc Psychiatr* 33, 1000–1006.

Boon F (1991) Encopresis and sexual assault. *J Am Acad Child Adolesc Psychiatr* 30, 479–482.

Calhoun J and Koenig KP (1973) Classroom modification of elective mutism. *Behav Ther* 4, 700–702.

Chadwick O (1985) Psychological sequelae of head injury in children. *Dev Med Child Neurol* 27, 69–79.

Dummit ES, Klein RG, Tancer NK *et al.* (1996) Fluoxetine treatment of children with selective mutism: An open trial. *J Am Acad Child Adolesc Psychiatr* 35, 615–621.

Kearney CA and Silverman WK (1999) Functionally-based prescriptive and nonprescriptive treatment for children and adolescents with school refusal behavior. *Behav Ther* 30, 673–695.

Kolvin I and Fundudis T (1981) Elective mute children: Psychological development and background factors. *J Child Psychol Psychiatr* 22, 219–232.

Last CG, Perrin S, Hersen M *et al.* (1996) A prospective study of childhood anxiety disorders. *J Am Acad Child Adolesc Psychiatr* 35, 1502–1510.

Levine MD (1975) Children with encopresis: A descriptive analysis. *Pediatrics* 56, 412–416.

Loening-Baucke VA (1995) Biofeedback treatment for chronic constipation and encopresis in childhood: Long-term outcome. *Pediatrics* 96, 105–110.

March JS, Parker JDA, Sullivan K *et al.* (1997) The Multidimensional Anxiety Scale for Children (MASC): Factor structure, reliability and validity. *J Am Acad Child Adolesc Psychiatr* 36, 554–565.

Mikkelsen EJ and Rapoport JL (1980) Enuresis: Psychopathology sleep stage and drug response. *Urol Clin N Am* 7, 361–377.

Nolan T, Debelle G, Oberklaid F *et al.* (1991) Randomised trial of laxatives in treatment of childhood encopresis. *Lancet* 338, 523–527.

Pretlow RA (1999) Treatment of nocturnal enuresis with an ultrasound bladder volume controlled alarm device. *J Urol* 162, 1224–1228.

Rutter M, Tizard J and Whitmore K (eds) (1970) *Education, Health and Behavior.* Longman, London.

Rutter ML, Yule W and Graham PJ (1973) Enuresis and behavioral deviance: Some epidemiological considerations in *Bladder Control and Enuresis. Clinics in Developmental Medicine*, Nos. 48/49. (eds Kolvin I, MacKeith R, and Meadow SR). Heinemann/Spastics International Medical Publications, London, pp. 137–147.

Serel TA, Perk H, Koyuncuoglu HR *et al.* (2001) Acupuncture therapy in the management of persistent primary nocturnal enuresis – preliminary results. *Scand J Urol Nephrol* 35(1), 40–43.

Shaffer D, Stephenson JD and Thomas DV (1979) Some effects of imipramine on micturition and their relevance to their antienuretic activity. *Neuropharmacology* 18, 33–37.

Shaffer D, Gardner A and Hedge B (1984) Behavior and bladder disturbance in enuretic children: A rational classification of a common disorder. *Dev Med Child Neurol* 26, 781–792.

Stein Z and Susser M (1967) Social factors in the development of sphincter control. *Dev Med Child Neurol* 9, 692–700.

Steinhausen HC and Gobel D (1989) Enuresis in child psychiatric clinic patients. *J Am Acad Child Adolesc Psychiatr* 28, 279–281.

Taylor E and Hersov L (1994) Fecal soiling, in *Child and Adolescent Psychiatry: Modern Approaches*, 3rd edn. (eds Rutter M, Taylor E, Hersov L *et al.*) Blackwell Scientific, London.

van Ginkel R, Benninga MA, Blommaart PJ *et al.* (2000) Lack of benefit of laxatives as adjunctive therapy for functional nonretentive fecal soiling in children. *J Pediatr* 137(6), 808–813.

Wilkins R (1985) A comparison of elective mutism and emotional disorders in children. *Br J Psychiatr* 146, 198–203.

Woodmansey AC (1967) Emotion and the motions: An inquiry into the causes and prevention of functional disorders of defecation. *Br J Med Psychol* 40, 207–223.

32 Delirium and Dementia

This chapter reviews dementia, delirium, amnestic and other cognitive disorders. Traditionally, these conditions have been classified as organic brain disorders to distinguish them from such diseases as schizophrenia, mania and major depressive disorder, the so-called functional disorders. With the publication of the DSM-IV, the distinction between functional and organic disorders was eliminated. Significant research into the neurobiological aspects of psychiatric disorders and the utilization of sophisticated neurodiagnostic tests such as positron emission tomographic scanning in individuals with schizophrenia led to the inescapable conclusion that every psychiatric condition has a biological component. Thus the term functional became obsolete and even misleading.

The conditions formerly called organic are classified in DSM-IV into three groupings: 1) delirium, dementia, and amnestic and other cognitive disorders; 2) mental disorders due to a general medical condition; and 3) substance-related disorders (American Psychiatric Association, 1994). Delirium, dementia and amnestic disorders are classified as cognitive because they feature impairment in such parameters as memory, language, or attention as a cardinal symptom. Each of these three major cognitive disorders is subdivided into categories that ascribe the etiology of the disorder to a general medical condition, the persisting effects of a substance, or multiple etiologies. A "not otherwise specified" category is included for each disorder (American Psychiatric Association, 1994).

In the case of delirium, the primary disturbance is in the level of consciousness with associated impairments in orientation, memory, judgment and attention. Dementia features cognitive deficits in memory, language and intellect. The amnestic disorder is characterized by impairment in memory in the absence of clouded consciousness or other noteworthy cognitive dysfunction. In general, the cognitive disorders should represent a decline from a previous higher level of function, of either acute (delirium) or insidious (dementia) onset, and should interfere with the patient's social or occupational functioning (American Psychiatric Association, 1994).

Dementia, Delirium and Other Cognitive Disorders

Dementia

Dementia is defined in DSM-IV as a series of disorders characterized by the development of multiple cognitive deficits (including memory impairment) that are due to the direct physiological effects of a general medical condition, the persisting effects of a substance, or multiple etiologies (e.g., the combined effects of a metabolic and a degenerative disorder) (American Psychiatric Association, 1994). The disorders constituting the dementias share a common symptom presentation and are identified and classified on the basis of etiology. The cognitive deficits exhibited in these disorders must be of significant severity to interfere with either occupational functioning or the individual's usual social activities or relationships. In addition, the observed deficits must represent a decline from a higher level of function and not be the consequence of a delirium. A delirium can be superimposed on a dementia, however, and both can be diagnosed if the dementia is observed when the delirium is not in evidence. Dementia typically is chronic and occurs in the presence of a clear sensorium. If clouding of consciousness occurs, the diagnosis of delirium should be considered. The DSM-IV classification of dementia is reviewed in Table 32.1.

Epidemiology

The prevalence of dementias is not precisely known. Estimates vary depending on the age range of the population studied and whether the individuals sampled were in the general community, acute care facilities, or long-term nursing institutions. A review of 47 surveys of dementia conducted between 1934 and 1985 indicated that the prevalence of dementia increased exponentially by age, doubling every 5 years up to age 95 years, and that this condition was equally distributed among men and women, with Alzheimer's dementia (AD) much more common in women (Slaby and Erle, 1993). A National Institute of Mental Health Multisite Epidemiological Catchment Area study revealed a 6-month prevalence rate for mild dementia of 11.5 to 18.4% for persons older than 65 years living in the community (Kallmann, 1989). The rate for severe dementia was higher for the institutionalized elderly: 15% of the elderly in retirement communities, 30% of nursing home residents and 54% of the elderly in state hospitals (Cummings and Benson, 1983).

Studies suggest that the fastest growing segment of the US population consists of persons older than the age of 85 years, 15% of whom are demented (Henderson, 1990). Half of the US population currently lives to the age of 75 years and one quarter lives to the age of 85 (Berg *et al.*, 1994). A study of 2000 consecutive admissions to a general medical hospital revealed that 9% were demented and, among those, 41% were also delirious on admission (Erkinjuntii *et al.*, 1986). The cost of providing care for demented patients exceeds $100 billion annually (about 10% of all health care expenditures), and the average cost to families in 1990 was $18 000 a year (Berg *et al.*, 1994).

Essentials of Psychiatry Jerald Kay and Allan Tasman
© 2006 John Wiley & Sons, Ltd.

Table 32.1	DSM-IV Classification of Dementia

Dementia of the Alzheimer type
    Early onset vs. late onset
    Uncomplicated
    With delirium
    With delusions
    With depressed mood
Vascular dementia
    Uncomplicated
    With delirium
    With delusions
    With depressed mood
Dementia due to head trauma
Dementia due to Parkinson's disease
Dementia due to HIV disease
Dementia due to Huntington's disease
Dementia due to Pick's disease
Dementia due to Creutzfeldt–Jakob disease
Dementia due to other general medical conditions (e.g.,
    neurosyphilis, normal-pressure hydrocephalus)
Substance-induced persisting dementia
Dementia due to multiple etiologies
Dementia not otherwise specified

Reprinted with permission from the *Diagnostic and Statistical Manual of Mental Disorders*, Fourth Edition. Copyright 1994 American Psychiatric Association.

Clinical Features

Essential to the diagnosis of dementia is the presence of cognitive deficits that include memory impairment and at least one of the following abnormalities of cognition: aphasia, agnosia, apraxia, or a disturbance in executive function (American Psychiatric Association, 1994). Memory function is divided into three compartments that can easily be evaluated during a mental status examination. These are immediate recall (primary memory), recent (secondary) memory and remote (tertiary) memory. Primary memory is characterized by a limited capacity, rapid accessibility and a duration of seconds to a minute (Karp, 1984). The anatomic site of destruction of primary memory is the reticular activating system, and the principal activity of the primary memory is the registration of new information. Primary memory is generally tested by asking the individual to repeat immediately a series of numbers in the order given. For instance, if the examiner mentions the numbers 1–2–3, the patient should be able to repeat them in the same order. This loss of ability to register new information accounts in part for the confusion and frustration the demented patient feels when confronted with unexpected changes in daily routine. Secondary memory has a much larger capacity than primary memory, a duration of minutes to years, and relatively slow accessibility. The anatomic site of dysfunction for secondary memory is the limbic system, and individuals with a lesion in this area may have little difficulty repeating digits immediately, but show rapid decay of these new memories. In minutes, the patient with limbic involvement may be totally unable to recall the digits or even remember that a test has been administered (Karp, 1984). Thus, secondary memory represents the retention and recall of information that has been previously registered by primary memory. Clinically, secondary memory is tested by having the individual repeat three objects after

having been distracted (usually by the examiner's continuation of the Mental Status Examination) for 3 to 5 minutes. Like primary memory, secondary recall is often impaired in dementia. Often if the examiner gives the demented patient a clue (such as "one of the objects you missed was a color"), the patient correctly identifies the object. If this occurs the memory testing should be scored as "three out of three with a cue", which is considered to be a slight impairment. Giving clues to the demented patient with a primary memory loss is pointless, because the memories were never registered. Wernicke–Korsakoff syndrome is an example of a condition in which primary memory may be intact while secondary recall is impaired.

Tertiary (remote) memory has a capacity that is probably unlimited, and such memories are often permanently retained. Access to tertiary memories is slow, and the anatomical dysfunction in tertiary memory loss is in the association cortex (Karp, 1984). In the early stages of dementia, tertiary memory is generally intact. It is tested by instructing the individual to remember personal information or past material. The personal significance of the information often influences the patient's ability to remember it. For example, a woman who worked for many years as a seamstress might remember many details related to that occupation, but could not recall the names of past presidents or three large cities in the USA. Thus, a patient's inability to remember highly significant past material is an ominous finding. Collateral data from informants is essential in the proper assessment of memory function. In summary, primary and secondary memories are most likely to be impaired in dementia, with tertiary memory often spared until late in the course of the disease.

In addition to defects in memory, patients with dementia often exhibit impairments in language, recognition, object naming and motor skills. Aphasia is an abnormality of language that often occurs in vascular dementias involving the dominant hemisphere. Because this hemisphere controls verbal, written and sign language, these patients may have significant problems interacting with people in their environment. Patients with dementia and aphasia may exhibit paucity of speech, poor articulation and a telegraphic pattern of speech (nonfluent, Broca's aphasia). This form of aphasia generally involves the middle cerebral artery with resultant paresis of the right arm and lower face. Despite faulty communication skills, patients having dementia with nonfluent aphasia have normal comprehension and awareness of their language impairment. As a result, such patients often present with significant depression, anxiety and frustration.

By contrast, patients having dementia with fluent (Wernicke's) aphasia may be quite verbose and articulate, but much of the language is nonsensical and rife with such paraphasias as neologisms and clang (rhyming) associations. Whereas nonfluent aphasias are usually associated with discrete lesions, fluent aphasia can result from such diffuse conditions as dementia of the Alzheimer type. More commonly, fluent aphasias occur in conjunction with vascular dementia secondary to temporal or parietal lobe CVA. Because the demented patients with fluent aphasia have impaired comprehension, they may seem apathetic and unconcerned with their language deficits if they are, in fact, aware of them at all. They do not generally display the emotional distress of patients with dementia and nonfluent aphasia (Table 32.2).

Patients with dementia may also lose their ability to recognize. Agnosia is a feature of a dominant hemisphere lesion and involves altered perception in which, despite normal sensations, intellect and language, the patient cannot recognize objects. This

Table 32.2	**Classification of Aphasias**		
Type	Language	Comprehension	Motor
Wernicke's (receptive)	Impaired Articulate Paraphasias	Impaired	Normal
Broca's (expressive)	Nonfluent Sparse Telegraphic Inarticulate	Intact	Right hemiparesis
Global	Nonfluent Mute	Impaired	Variable right hemiplegia

is in contrast to aphasia in which the patient with dementia may not be able to name objects, but can recognize them. The type of agnosia depends on the area of the sensory cortex that is involved. Some demented patients with severe visual agnosia cannot name objects presented, match them to samples, or point to objects named by the examiner. Other patients may present with auditory agnosia and be unable to localize or distinguish such sounds as the ringing of a telephone. A minority of demented patients may exhibit astereognosis, inability to identify an object by palpation. Demented patients may also lose their ability to carry out selected motor activities despite intact motor abilities, sensory function and comprehension of the assigned task (apraxia). Affected patients cannot perform such activities as brushing their teeth, chewing food, or waving good-bye when asked to do so.

The two most common forms of apraxia in demented patients are ideational and gait apraxia. Ideational apraxia is the inability to perform motor activities that require sequential steps and results from a lesion involving both frontal lobes or the complete cerebrum. Gait apraxia, often seen in such conditions as normal-pressure hydrocephalus, is the inability to perform various motions of ambulation. It also results from conditions that diffusely affect the cerebrum. Impairment of executive function is the ability to think abstractly, plan, initiate and end complex behavior. On Mental Status Examination, patients with dementia display problems coping with new tasks. Such activities as subtracting serial sevens may be impaired.

Obviously, aphasia, agnosia, apraxia and impairment of executive function can seriously impede the ability of the demented patients to interact with their environment. An appropriate mental status examination of the patient with suspected dementia should include screening for the presence of these abnormalities.

Associated Features and Behavior

In addition to the diagnostic features already mentioned, patients with dementia display other identifying features that often prove problematic. Poor insight and poor judgment are common in dementia and often cause patients to engage in potentially dangerous activities or make unrealistic and grandiose plans for the future. Visual–spatial functioning may be impaired, and if patients have the ability to construct a plan and carry it out, suicide attempts can occur. More common is unintentional self-harm resulting from carelessness, undue familiarity with strangers, and disregard for the accepted rules of conduct.

Emotional lability, as seen in pseudobulbar palsy after cerebral injury, can be particularly frustrating for caregivers, as are occasional psychotic features such as delusions and hallucinations. Changes in their environment and daily routine can be particularly distressing for demented patients, and their frustration can be manifested by violent behavior.

Course

The course of a particular dementia is influenced by its etiology. Although historically the dementias have been considered progressive and irreversible, there is, in fact, significant variation in the course of individual dementias. The disorder can be progressive, static, or remitting (American Psychiatric Association, 1994). In addition to the etiology, factors that influence the course of the dementia include: 1) the time span between the onset and the initiation of prescribed treatment, 2) the degree of reversibility of the particular dementia, 3) the presence of comorbid psychiatric disorders, and 4) the level of psychosocial support. The previous distinction between treatable and untreatable dementias has been replaced by the concepts of reversible, irreversible and arrestable dementias. Most reversible cases of dementia are associated with shorter duration of symptoms, mild cognitive impairment and superimposed delirium. Specifically, the dementias caused by drugs, depression and metabolic disorders are most likely to be reversible. Other conditions such as normal pressure hydrocephalous, subdural hematomas and tertiary syphilis are more commonly arrestable.

Although potentially reversible dementias should be aggressively investigated, in reality, only 8% of dementias are partially reversible and about 3% fully reversible (Kaufman, 1990b). There is some evidence to suggest that early treatment of demented patients, particularly those with Alzheimer's type, with such agents as donepezil, which acts as an inhibitor of acetylcholinesterase, and galanthamine may slow the rate of progression of the dementia.

Differential Diagnosis

Memory impairment occurs in a variety of conditions including delirium, amnestic disorders and depression (American Psychiatric Association, 1994). In delirium, the onset of altered memory is acute and the pattern typically fluctuates (waxing and waning) with increased proclivity for confusion during the night. Delirium is more likely to feature autonomic hyperactivity and alterations in level of consciousness. In some cases a dementia can have a superimposed delirium (Figure 32.1).

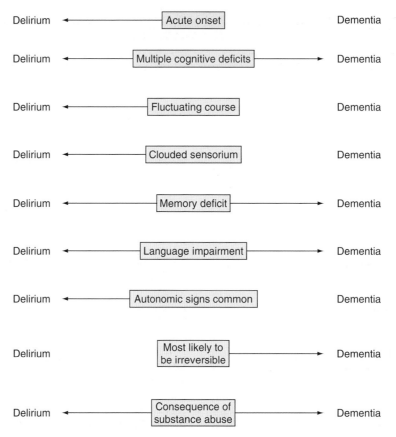

Figure 32.1   *Differentiation of delirium and dementia.*

Patients with major depressive disorder often complain of lapses in memory and judgment, poor concentration and seemingly diminished intellectual capacity. Often these symptoms are mistakenly diagnosed as dementia, especially in elderly patients. A thorough medical history and mental status examination focusing on such symptoms as hopelessness, crying episodes and unrealistic guilt, in conjunction with a family history of depression, can be diagnostically beneficial. The term **pseudodementia** has been used to denote cognitive impairment secondary to a functional psychiatric disorder, most commonly depression (Korvath *et al.*, 1989). In comparison with demented patients, those with depressive pseudodementia exhibit better insight regarding their cognitive dysfunction, are more likely to give "I don't know" answers, and may exhibit neurovegetative signs of depression. Pharmacological treatment of the depression should improve the cognitive dysfunction as well. Because of the rapid onset of their antidepressant action, the use of psychostimulants (methylphenidate, dextroamphetamine) to differentiate between dementia and pseudodementia has been advocated by some authors (Frierson *et al.*, 1991). Some authors have proposed abandonment of the term pseudodementia, suggesting that most patients so diagnosed have both genuine dementia and a superimposed affective disorder (Figure 32.2).

An amnestic disorder also presents with a significant memory deficit, but without the other associated features such as aphasia, agnosia and apraxia. If cognitive impairment occurs only in the context of drug use, substance intoxication or substance withdrawal is the appropriate diagnosis. Although mental retardation implies below average intellect and subsequent impairment in other areas of function, the onset is before 18 years

of age and abnormalities of memory do not always occur. Mental retardation must be considered in the differential diagnosis of dementias of childhood and adolescence along with such disorders as Wilson's disease (hepatolenticular degeneration), lead intoxication, subacute sclerosing panencephalitis, HIV spectrum disorders and substance abuse, particularly abuse of inhalants. If an individual develops dementia before age 18 years and has an IQ in the mentally retarded range (i.e., below 70), an additional diagnosis of mental retardation may be justified.

Patients with schizophrenia may also exhibit a variety of cognitive abnormalities, but this condition also has an early onset, a distinctive constellation of other symptoms (e.g., delusions, hallucinations, disorganized speech), and does not result from a medical condition or the persisting effects of a substance. Factitious disorder and malingering must be distinguished from dementia. The patient with factitious disorder and psychological symptoms may have some apparent cognitive deficits reminiscent of a dementia.

Dementia must also be distinguished from age-related cognitive decline (also known as benign senescence). Only when such changes exceed the level of altered function to be expected for the patient's age is the diagnosis of dementia warranted (American Psychiatric Association, 1994).

Physical and Neurological Examinations in Dementia

The physical examination may offer clues to the etiology of the dementia; however, in the elderly, one must be aware of the normal changes associated with aging and differentiate them from signs of dementia. Often the specific physical examination

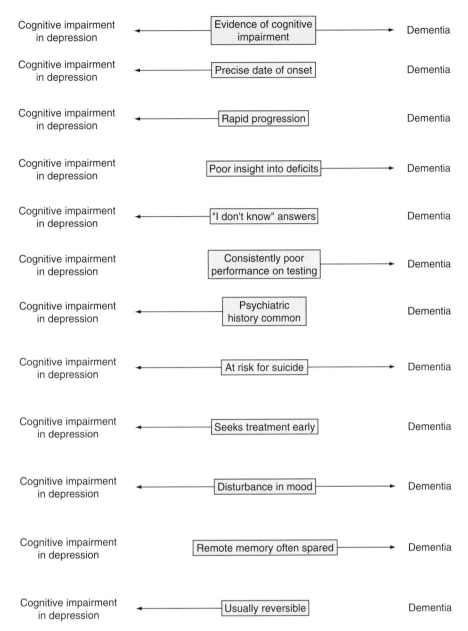

Cognitive impairment in depression	←	Evidence of cognitive impairment	→	Dementia
Cognitive impairment in depression	←	Precise date of onset		Dementia
Cognitive impairment in depression		Rapid progression		Dementia
Cognitive impairment in depression		Poor insight into deficits	→	Dementia
Cognitive impairment in depression	←	"I don't know" answers		Dementia
Cognitive impairment in depression		Consistently poor performance on testing	→	Dementia
Cognitive impairment in depression	←	Psychiatric history common		Dementia
Cognitive impairment in depression	←	At risk for suicide	→	Dementia
Cognitive impairment in depression	←	Seeks treatment early		Dementia
Cognitive impairment in depression	←	Disturbance in mood	→	Dementia
Cognitive impairment in depression		Remote memory often spared	→	Dementia
Cognitive impairment in depression	←	Usually reversible		Dementia

Figure 32.2 *Differential diagnosis of dementia and cognitive impairment in depression.*

findings indicate the area of the central nervous system affected by the etiological process. Parietal lobe dysfunction is suggested by such symptoms as astereognosis, constructional apraxia, anosognosia and problems with two-point discrimination (Kaufman, 1990a). The dominant hemisphere parietal lobe is also involved in Gerstmann's syndrome, which includes agraphia, acalculia, finger agnosia and right–left confusion.

Reflex changes such as hyperactive deep tendon reflexes, Babinski's reflex and hyperactive jaw jerk are indicative of cerebral injury. However, primitive reflexes such as the palmar–mental reflex (tested by repeatedly scratching the base of the patient's thumb, with a positive response being slight downward movement of the lower lip and jaw), which occurs in 60% of normal elderly people, and the snout reflex, seen in a third of elderly patients, are not diagnostically reliable for dementia (Wolfson and Katzman, 1983).

Ocular findings such as nystagmus (as in brain stem lesions), ophthalmoplegia (Wernicke–Korsakoff syndrome), anisocoria,

papilledema (hypertensive encephalopathy), cortical blindness (Anton's syndrome), visual field losses (CVA hemianopia), Kayser–Fleischer rings (Wilson's disease) and Argyll Robertson pupils (syphilis, diabetic neuropathy) can offer valuable clues to the etiology of the cognitive deficit (Victor and Adams, 1974).

Movement disorders including tremors (Parkinson's disease, drug intoxication, cerebellar dysfunction, Wilson's disease), chorea (Huntington's disease, other basal ganglia lesions), myoclonus (subacute sclerosing panencephalitis, Creutzfeldt–Jakob disease, Alzheimer's disease, anoxia) and asterixis (hepatic disease, uremia, hypoxia, carbon dioxide retention) should be noted.

Gait disturbances, principally apraxia (normal-pressure hydrocephalus, inhalant abuse, cerebellar dysfunction) and peripheral neuropathy (Korsakoff's syndrome, neurosyphilis, heavy metal intoxication, solvent abuse, isoniazid or phenytoin toxicity, vitamin deficiencies and HIV spectrum illnesses), are

Table 32.3	Physical Signs Associated With Dementia or Delirium

Physical Sign	Condition
Myoclonus	Creutzfeldt–Jakob disease
	Subacute sclerosing panencephalitis
	Postanoxia
	Alzheimer's disease (10%)
	AIDS dementia
	Uremia
	Penicillin intoxication
	Meperidine toxicity
Asterixis	Hepatic encephalopathy
	Uremia
	Hypoxia
Chorea	Huntington's disease
	Wilson's disease
	Hypocalcemia
	Hypothyroidism
	Hepatic encephalopathy
	Oral contraceptives
	Systemic lupus erythematosus
	Carbon monoxide poisoning
	Toxoplasmosis
	Pertussis, diphtheria
Peripheral neuropathy	Wernicke–Korsakoff syndrome
	Neurosyphilis
	Heavy metal intoxication
	Organic solvent exposure
	Vitamin B$_{12}$ deficiency
	Medications: isoniazid, phenytoin

Table 32.4	Evaluation of Dementia

Medical history and physical examination
Family interview
Routine laboratory
   Chemistry (SMA 20)
   Urinalysis
   Hematology (complete blood count)
Other routine tests
   Chest radiography
   Electrocardiography
Specialized laboratory
   Thyroid functions
   VDRL (fluorescent treponemal antibody screen if indicated)
   Drug screen
   Vitamin B$_{12}$ and folate levels
   Cerebrospinal fluid analysis (if indicated)
   HIV testing (if indicated)
Other studies
   Computed tomography or magnetic resonance imaging
   Electroencephalography

also common in dementia. Extrapyramidal symptoms in the absence of antipsychotics may indicate substance abuse, especially phencyclidine abuse, or basal ganglia disease. Although the many and varied physical findings of dementia are too numerous to mention here in any detail, it should be obvious that the physical examination is an invaluable tool in the assessment of dementia (Table 32.3).

Mental Status Examination

The findings on the Mental Status Examination vary depending on the etiology of the dementia. Some common abnormalities have been discussed previously (see earlier section on clinical features). In general, symptoms seen on the Mental Status Examination, whatever the etiology, are related to the location and extent of brain injury, individual adaptation to the dysfunction, premorbid coping skills and psychopathology, and concurrent medical illness.

Disturbance of memory, especially primary and secondary memory, is the most significant abnormality. Confabulation may be present as the patient attempts to minimize the memory impairment. Disorientation and altered levels of consciousness may occur, but are generally not seen in the early stages of dementia uncomplicated by delirium. Affect may be affected as in the masked facies of Parkinson's disease and the expansive affect

and labile mood of pseudobulbar palsy after cerebral injury. The affect of patients with hepatic encephalopathy is often described as blunted and apathetic. Lack of inhibition leading to such behavior as exposing oneself is common, and some conditions such as tertiary syphilis and untoward effects of some medication can precipitate mania. The Mental Status Examination, in conjunction with a complete medical history from the patient and informants and an adequate physical examination, is essential in the evaluation and differential diagnosis of dementia (Table 32.4).

Degenerative Causes of Dementia

Dementia of the Alzheimer Type

Historical Perspective

In 1906 Alois Alzheimer reported a case of presenile dementia in a 51-year-old woman who displayed progressive memory loss and disorientation.

Two years earlier, Alzheimer had written of miliary plaque formations that often appeared in the brains of patients with senile dementia. He and his coworkers subsequently described neurofibrillary changes and granulovacuolar degeneration in senile and presenile dementia (Bick, 1994). Almost 90 years later, Alzheimer's disease is the most common form of dementia and remains a major focus of scientific investigation.

Epidemiology

Alzheimer's disease is the most common cause of dementia, accounting for 55 to 65% of all cases. There were fewer than 3 million cases diagnosed in the USA in 1980, but the Census Bureau predicted that there will be more than 10 million American citizens with Alzheimer's disease by the year 2050. Prevalence of the disease doubles with every 5 years between the ages of 65 and 85 years. Onset of symptoms occurs after the age of 40 years in 96% of cases.

DSM-IV-TR Criteria 294

Dementia of the Alzheimer Type

A. The development of multiple cognitive deficits manifested by both

 (1) memory impairment (impaired ability to learn new information or to recall previously learned information)

 (2) one (or more) of the following cognitive disturbances:

  (a) aphasia (language disturbance)

  (b) apraxia (impaired ability to carry out motor activities despite intact motor function)

  (c) agnosia (failure to recognize or identify objects despite intact sensory function)

  (d) disturbance in executive functioning (i.e., planning, organizing, sequencing, abstracting)

B. The cognitive deficits in criteria A1 and A2 each cause significant impairment in social or occupational functioning and represent a significant decline from a previous level of functioning.

C. The course is characterized by gradual onset and continuing cognitive decline.

D. The cognitive deficits in criteria A1 and A2 are not due to any of the following:

 (1) other central nervous system conditions that cause progressive deficits in memory and cognition (e.g., cerebrovascular disease, Parkinson's disease, Huntington's disease, subdural hematoma, normal-pressure hydrocephalus, brain tumor)

 (2) systemic conditions that are known to cause dementia (e.g., hypothyroidism, vitamin B_{12} or folic acid deficiency, niacin deficiency, hypercalcemia, neurosyphilis, HIV infection)

 (3) substance-induced conditions

E. The deficits do not occur exclusively during the course of a delirium.

F. The disturbance is not better accounted for by another Axis I disorder (e.g., major depressive disorder, schizophrenia).

Code based on type of onset and predominant features:

With early onset: if onset is at age 65 years or below
 294.11 With delirium: if delirium is superimposed on the dementia

 294.12 With delusions: if delusions are the predominant feature

 294.13 With depressed mood: if depressed mood (including presentations that meet full symptom criteria for a major depressive episode) is the predominant feature. A separate diagnosis of mood disorder due to a general medical condition is not given.

 294.10 Uncomplicated: if none of the above predominates in the current clinical presentation

With late onset: if onset is after age 65 years
 294.3 With delirium: if delirium is superimposed on the dementia

 294.20 With delusions: if delusions are the predominant feature

 294.21 With depressed mood: if depressed mood (including presentations that meet full symptom criteria for a major depressive episode) is the predominant feature. A separate diagnosis of mood disorder due to a general medical condition is not given.

 294.0 Uncomplicated: if none of the above predominates in the current clinical presentation

Specify if:

With behavioral disturbance

Coding note: Also code 331.0 Alzheimer's disease on Axis III.

Reprinted with permission from the *Diagnostic and Statistical Manual of Mental Disorders*, Fourth Edition, Text Revision. Copyright 2000 American Psychiatric Association.

Some authors separate Alzheimer's disease into senile and presenile forms, but the two disorders represent the same pathological process. Significantly, however, early-onset (that is, onset before the age of 65) Alzheimer's disease is associated with a more rapid course than later-onset disease.

Alzheimer's disease affects women three times as often as men, for unknown reasons. Furthermore, at least one study suggests that dementia, including Alzheimer's, is more common in black than in white American women (Heyman *et al.*, 1991). Comparison of population studies in diverse countries shows strikingly similar prevalence rates. Longitudinal studies have revealed the importance of family history as a risk factor; however, no consistent genetic pattern has been established. For Alzheimer's alone, the probability of developing dementia

if a first-degree relative (parent or sibling) is afflicted is four times greater than that of the general population, and if two or more first-degree relatives have the disease the risk is increased eightfold compared with a normal sample of US citizens. Among monozygotic twins 43% are concordant for the disorder, compared with only 8% of dizygotic twins.

In addition to age, gender and family history, the presence of Down syndrome, a history of head trauma and a low level of education have been proposed as risk factors. Most studies concur that individuals with trisomy 21 develop the features of AD by age 35 years; however, studies have looked at the possibility that families with a member who has AD are more likely to produce offspring with Down syndrome and have had inconclusive results. Significant head injury, as either a single incident or a chronic occurrence as in sports injuries, increases the risk of developing Alzheimer's by a factor of 2. An uneducated person older than 75 years is about twice as likely to develop dementia as one who has 8 years or more schooling, leading to the speculation that the cognitive processes involved in obtaining an education may be partially protective. Risk factors found in some but not all studies include myocardial ischemia in the elderly, having a child at 40 years or older, and exposure to aluminum (Katzman and Kawas, 1994).

Pathology

The etiology and pathogenesis of Alzheimer's disease are unknown. Multiple agents and pathways are probably involved in this disorder. Many hypotheses have been proposed regarding the cause and progression of Alzheimer's disease including genetic factors, slow or unconventional viruses, defective membrane metabolism, endogenous toxins, autoimmune disorders and neurotoxicity of such trace elements as aluminum and mercury.

The brains of patients with Alzheimer's disease contain many senile plaques, neurofibrillary tangles and Hirano's bodies (Figures 32.3 and 32.4). There is degeneration of nerve cells, but the significant atrophy seen on neurodiagnostic examination may be more the result of shrinkage of neurons and loss of dendritic spines than of actual neuronal loss (Wolf, 1980). The atrophy is most apparent in the associational cortex areas, and early decay on the primary motor and sensory areas are relatively spared (Figures 32.5 and 32.6). Significant degenerative changes in neurons are seen in the hippocampus, locus ceruleus and nucleus basalis of Mynert. With advancing disease, these changes, in effect, separate the hippocampus from the remainder of the brain. Initially, the parietal and temporal regions are most affected by plaques and tangles, accounting for the memory impairment and parietal lobe–associated syndromes (some apraxias, hemi-attention, anosognosia, Gerstmann's syndrome) occasionally associated with Alzheimer's disease. Neurofibrillary tangles do not correlate with the severity of

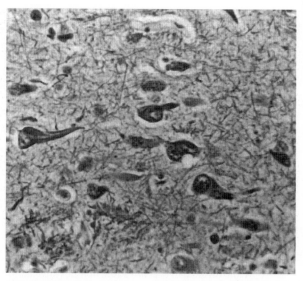

Figure 32.4 *Intraneuronal neurofibrillary tangles with neuritic plaques in a patient with Alzheimer's disease. (Courtesy of Joseph Parker, MD, Duke University Medical Center, Durham, NC.)*

the dementia; however, the concentration of neuritic plaques is directly associated with the severity of the disease (Kaufman, 1990a).

Neurochemically, the brains of patients with Alzheimer's disease exhibit significant cholinergic abnormalities (Kaufman, 1990b). There is a profound decrease in acetylcholine (ACh) in almost all patients, as well as decreased immunological activity of somatostatin- and corticotropin-releasing factors (Kaufman, 1990b). The enzyme required for ACh synthesis, choline acetyltransferase, is also greatly reduced. Other studies suggest involvement of noradrenergic and serotonergic systems in later-onset disease and diminished gamma-aminobutyric acid (GABA) (Kaufman, 1990b). Specifically, the noradrenergic deficiencies seen in younger patients may be connected to changes in the locus coeruleus, and abnormalities of serotonin to effects

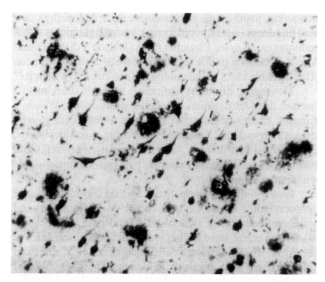

Figure 32.3 *Numerous neuritic plaques and neurofibrillary tangles in a patient with Alzheimer's disease. (Courtesy of Joseph Parker, MD, Duke University Medical Center, Durham, NC.)*

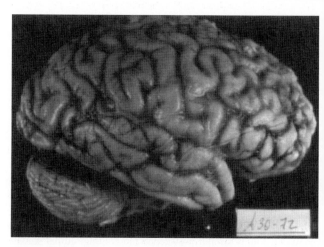

Figure 32.5 *Gross specimen showing prominent frontal lobe atrophy in a patient with Alzheimer's disease. (Courtesy of Joseph Parker, MD, Duke University Medical Center, Durham, NC.)*

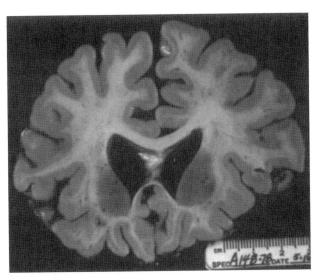

Figure 32.6 *Cortical and white matter atrophy. (Courtesy of Joseph Parker, MD, Duke University Medical Center, Durham, NC.)*

on the raphe nuclei (Korvath *et al.*, 1989). The serotoninergic neurons of the raphe nuclei in patients with Alzheimer's disease contain six to 39 times as many neurofibrillary tangles as those of age-appropriate control subjects, and noradrenergic neurons from the locus ceruleus of patients with Alzheimer's disease show neuronal loss of 40 to 80%. Unfortunately, despite these observed neurochemical abnormalities, neurotransmitter-related treatment with cholinergic and GABAergic agents has proved largely unsuccessful.

Although the involvement of cholinergic transmission along the hippocampus and nucleus basalis is essential to the ability to learn new information, it seems that many of the symptoms of Alzheimer's disease are not explainable solely on the basis of cholinergic abnormalities. Thus, investigators have examined a number of other potential etiological or contributory agents. Some researchers have investigated the role of beta-amyloid protein in Alzheimer's disease, and some assert that this material, a significant component of all plaques, is a major contributor to the neurodegenerative changes in the disease as both an initiator and a promotor of the disease. Supporting this assertion are genetic studies of families with inheritable forms of presenile dementia, which show that disease occurrence is linked to mutations involving beta-amyloid-related systems (Kidd, 1963). This hypothesis targets the protein found in senile plaques; other investigators have focused on the neurofibrillary tangles and the identification of a major component of its helical filament, the tau protein. Specifically, these researchers analyzed the possibility that modification of tau protein, predominantly by phosphorylation, is an important feature of AD.

Aluminum, the third most common element in the universe, is absorbed from the gastrointestinal tract, lungs, nasal passage and skin. Crapper and Dalton (1972) reported increased aluminum in the brain of patients with Alzheimer's disease, with about a quarter of such samples showing concentrations three standard deviations above the control values. Other studies of bulk brain aluminum in patients with Alzheimer's disease have shown no such elevation. The current consensus appears to be that although aluminum and other

elements such as iron and mercury might accelerate neuronal degeneration in AD, these elements are not primary etiological agents. The role of genetic factors in the development of AD has received increased attention as the role of the apolipoprotein (APO) E4 allele as a major genetic susceptibility risk factor has been confirmed by numerous studies (Katzman, 1994). Corder and colleagues (1993) studied 234 members of 42 families with late-onset AD. Of 95 affected members, 80% had the E4 allele, compared with 26% in the general population (Corder *et al.*, 1993). Furthermore, in these families, 91% of those homozygous for E4 had developed Alzheimer's disease by 80 years of age – evidence that the APO E E4 allele is causing these familial cases (Corder *et al.*, 1993). In a study of 176 autopsy specimens of confirmed AD, Schmechel and coworkers in 1993 found that 65% of patients carried at least one APO E E4 gene. Examination of all such studies indicates that between 25 and 40% of AD cases can be attributable to this marker, making its presence one of the most common risk factors yet discovered for AD.

Finally, several studies suggest that changes in membrane function, metabolism and morphology are involved in the pathology of AD. Nonetheless, the basic molecular defect responsible for AD dementia has not been defined.

The neuropathology of Alzheimer's disease should be compared with the normal neuropathic effects of aging. These include the following:

1. The leptomeninges become more fibrotic and are more adherent to the brain surface with increased opacity.
2. The ventricles show slight to moderate enlargement that increases with the passage of time.
3. The distance between the dura and the brain is increased.
4. Sulci widen and gyri become narrower.
5. The number of neurons decreases slightly.
6. The weight of the brain decreases in the fourth and fifth decades, with significant decrease by the age of 80 years.
7. Neurofibrillary tangles and senile plaques occur in virtually every elderly individual by the 10th decade of life (Berg *et al.*, 1994).

Laboratory and Radiological Findings

The role of laboratory determinations in the evaluation for AD is to exclude other causes of dementia, especially those that may prove reversible or arrestable. Before death, AD is largely a diagnosis of exclusion. Throughout the course of this disorder, laboratory values are essentially normal. Some nonspecific changes may occur, but electroencephalography and lumbar puncture are not diagnostic. As the disease progresses, computed tomography (CT) and magnetic resonance imaging (MRI) may show atrophy in the cerebral cortex and hydrocephalus *ex vacuo* MRI may show nonspecific alteration of white matter (leukoariosis), and eventually the electroencephalogram (EEG) shows diffuse background slowing.

Pneumoencephalography has demonstrated enlarged ventricles and widening of cortical sulci in Alzheimer's disease, and positron emission tomography in the later stages shows decreased cerebral oxygen and glucose metabolism in the frontal lobes. At present, in the work-up of a patient with a slowly progressive dementia, a good family history, physical examination, and laboratory and radiographic tests to rule out other causes of dementia, are the most effective tools in the diagnosis of Alzheimer's disease.

Clinical Features

The course and clinical features of AD parallel those discussed for dementia in general. Typically, the early course of AD is difficult to ascertain because the patient is usually an unreliable informant, and the early signs may be so subtle as to go unnoticed even by the patient's closest associates. These early features include impaired memory, difficulty with problem solving, preoccupation with long past events, decreased spontaneity, and an inability to respond to the environment with the patient's usual speed and accuracy. Patients may forget names, misplace household items, or forget what they were about to do. Often the individuals have insight into these memory deficits and occasionally convey their concerns to family members. Such responses as "You're just getting older", and "I do that sometimes myself" are common from these family members and as a result the patient becomes depressed, which can further affect cognitive functioning. Anomia, or difficulty with word finding, is common in this middle stage of Alzheimer's disease. Eventually the patient develops schemes, word associations and excuses ("I never was very good in math") to assist in retention and cover up deficits. The patient may also employ family members as a surrogate memory (Karp, 1984).

Because memory loss is usually most obvious for newly acquired material, the patient tries to avoid unfamiliar activities. Typically, the patient is seen by the physician when confusion, aggression, wandering, or some other socially undesirable behavior ensues. At that time, disorders of perception and language may appear. The patient often turns to a spouse to answer questions posed during the history taking. By this time the affected individual has lost insight into his or her dementia and abandons attempts to compensate for memory loss. Finally, in the late stage of Alzheimer's disease, physical and cognitive effects are marked. Disorders of gait, extremity paresis and paralysis, seizures, peripheral neuropathy, extrapyramidal signs and urinary incontinence are seen, and the patient is often no longer ambulatory. The aimless wandering of the middle stage has been replaced by a mute, bedridden state and decorticate posture. Myoclonus occasionally occurs. Significantly, affective disturbances remain a distinct possibility throughout the course of the illness. AD progresses at a slow pace for 8 to 10 years to a state of complete helplessness.

Treatment

The two principles of management in AD are to treat what is treatable without aggravating existing symptoms and to support caregivers, who are also victims of this disease. Despite the significant decrease in ACh and choline acetyltransferase in Alzheimer's disease, treatments based on the cholinergic hypothesis have been unsuccessful (Kaufman, 1990a) Because vasopressin levels are slightly decreased in the hippocampus of patients with Alzheimer's disease and somatostatin is adversely affected as well, attempts were made to replace these agents with little effect. In the belief that improving blood flow might be of benefit, such agents as the metabolic enhancer and vasodilator ergoloid mesylates (Hydergine) (an ergot alkaloid) were tried. Hydergine did seem to have some benefit; however, these effects may have been related to its mild antidepressant action. Onset of action of any beneficial effects of Hydergine was quite long. Corticotropin release is promoted by corticotropin-releasing factor, which is decreased in patients with AD, but clinical trials with corticotropin were disappointing. Despite lackluster effects of physostigmine, a second cholinesterase inhibitor has shown promise. Tetrahydroaminoacridine (tacrine) produced significant

cognitive improvement in 16 of 17 patients with AD in an early study (Summers *et al.*, 1986). Subsequent studies have been less impressive, but significant improvement in a number of scales measuring cognitive performance illustrated the benefit of this agent for some patients. Side effects, particularly hepatic and cholinergic, were noted; however, in 1993 the US Food and Drug Administration (USFDA) approved of tacrine for the treatment of AD. Donepezil, an inhibitor of acetylcholinesterase, has also been utilized in an attempt to enhance cholinergic function by inhibiting its breakdown. This agent must be given early in the course of the dementia.

Whereas much attention has been focused on research aimed at understanding and altering the pathogenesis of AD, less work has been done regarding appropriate pharmacotherapy of the varied psychological manifestations of the disease. Depression is often associated with AD. If antidepressant medication is to be used, low doses (about one-third to one-half of the usual initial dose) are advised and only agents with minimal anticholinergic activity should be employed. Appropriate choices would be the selective serotonin reuptake inhibitors such as paroxetine, fluoxetine, sertraline and citalopram. Sertraline and citalopram are least likely to cause drug–drug interactions. Even these agents have the potential to increase confusion in Alzheimer's patients. Agents such as trazodone and mirtazapine have occasionally been employed because of their sedating properties. If tricyclic antidepressants are used, the secondary amines (desipramine, nortriptyline) are recommended over the tertiary ones (amitriptyline, doxepin). Careful attention to the possible side effects of these agents, particularly orthostatic hypotension, lowering of the seizure threshold, excessive fatigue, urinary retention, constipation, confusion and accelerated memory impairment, is suggested. Most clinicians now feel that tricyclic antidepressants are inappropriate for this patient population.

Anxiety and psychosis, particularly paranoid delusions, are common in AD. Benzodiazepines can be disinhibiting in such patients and may exacerbate confusion. They should be avoided if possible. If minor tranquilizers are required, agents with a shorter duration of action (e.g., lorazepam, oxazepam) are preferred. Antipsychotic medications with high anticholinergic potential (thioridazine, chlorpromazine) may also affect memory adversely. While these agents have been favored in the past because of their tendency to produce sedation, newer agents such as olanzepine, risperdone, quetiapine and ziprasidone, have been reported to have lower incidences of neuroleptic-related side effects. Haloperidol has less anticholinergic activity but has a greater tendency toward extrapyramidal effects. These agents will be discussed in more detail in the consideration of management of delirious states. In summary, the psychopharmacological management of AD is designed to ameliorate cognitive deficits, if possible, control agitated, psychotic and dangerous behavior, and treat any underlying psychiatric disorder (e.g., major depressive disorder) that might be comorbid with dementia. The appropriate management of AD entails more than psychopharmacological intervention. Other elements of the treatment plan should be environmental manipulation and support for the family.

In the attempt to maintain patients with Alzheimer's disease in their homes for as long as possible, some adjustments of their environment are important. Written daily reminders can be helpful in the performance of daily activities. Prominent clocks, calendars and windows are important. An effort should be made to minimize changes in the patient's daily activities and environment. Repeated demonstrations of how to lock doors and windows and operate appliances are helpful, and arranging for rapid dialing of essential telephone numbers can be useful. Maintaining adequate hydration, nutrition, exercise and cleanliness is essential. The family of the patient with Alzheimer's disease is also a victim of the disease. Family members must watch the gradual deterioration of the patient and accept that a significant part of their own lives must be devoted to the care of the individual. Difficult decisions about institutionalization and termination of life support are distinct possibilities, and the patients often turn their anger and paranoia toward the caregiver. Education is a valuable treatment tool for families. Information about the disease and peer support are available through Alzheimer's associations, and many such agencies provide family members with a companion for the patient to allow the family some time away. (The National Alzheimer's Education and Referral Service can be accessed by calling 1-800-621-0379.) Many studies suggest that the primary reason for institutionalization of these patients is the tremendous burden of care they pose for their families. Aimless wandering seems to be a particularly disturbing behavior. Unfortunately, the unfamiliar surroundings of a nursing home often increase the patient's level of confusion and anxiety. For these reasons, family members are at risk for depression, anxiety disorders, insomnia and a variety of other psychological manifestations. Should these occur, they should be promptly treated.

Dementia Due to Pick's Disease

Pick's disease is a rare form of progressive dementia clinically indistinguishable from Alzheimer's disease. It is about one-fifth as common as AD. Pick's disease occurs in the sixth and seventh decades of life and has a duration that varies from 2 to 15 years. It has a strong familial tendency, but definite genetic pattern has not been established. ACh levels are reduced.

The pathology of Pick's disease involves prominent changes (e.g., sclerosis, atrophy) in the frontal and temporal lobes (Figure 32.7). The parietal and occipital lobes are spared. Alzheimer himself noted the argentophilic (staining silver) intraneuronal inclusion in Pick's bodies.

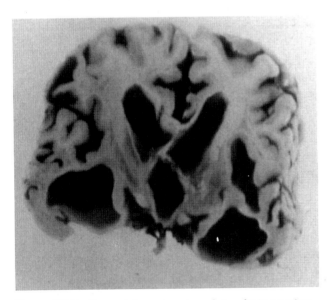

Figure 32.7 *Severe lobar sclerosis and atrophy in a patient with Pick's disease. (Courtesy of Joseph Parker, MD, Duke University Medical Center, Durham, NC.)*

The clinical features of Pick's disease are quite similar to those of Alzheimer's disease, and since neither condition is curable, an elaborate differential diagnosis is unnecessary. Because of parietal sparing, such features as apraxia and agnosia are less common in Pick's disease, and visual–spatial ability, often impaired in Alzheimer's disease, is preserved (Kaufman, 1990b). Given the prominent changes in the frontal lobe, disinhibited behavior, loss of social constraints and lack of concern about appearance and matters of personal hygiene occur relatively early in Pick's disease. Such speech disorders as echolalia and logorrhea are common, and patients with Pick's disease are more likely to develop Klüver–Bucy syndrome (orality, hyperphagia, hypersexuality, placidity) indicative of damage to the temporal lobes. Significant memory impairment may occur relatively late in the course, and eventually the patient becomes listless, mute, and ultimately decerebrate and comatose. Like Alzheimer's disease, the treatment of Pick's disease is symptomatic.

Dementia Due to Parkinson's Disease

Although dementia rarely occurs as an initial symptom of Parkinson's disease, it is found in nearly 40% of such patients older than 70 years of age. Approximately 1 million people in the USA have the disease, with 50 000 new cases being diagnosed each year. The prevalence for persons over 60 is 1%. The disease results from loss of dopamine production in the basal ganglia, and can be idiopathic or postencephalitic. Usually the patient is 50 years of age or older, and unlike Alzheimer's and Pick's dementias, this disease occurs slightly more often in men (Berg *et al.*, 1994). Dementia most commonly occurs in cases of Parkinson's disease in which the decline has been rapid and response to anticholinergics has been poor.

The pathology of Parkinson's disease involves depigmentation of the so-called pigmented nuclei of the brain (**locus coeruleus, substantia nigra**). These nuclei then contain eosinophilic Lewy bodies. As in Alzheimer's disease the cerebral cortex of many of these patients contains many senile plaques and neurofibrillary tangles, loss of neurons, and decreased concentrations of choline acetyltransferase. Patients with parkinsonian dementia also have reduced choline acetyltransferase in the cerebral cortex and substantia nigra.

The clinical features of Parkinson's disease are well described, with the cardinal triad being tremor, rigidity and bradykinesia. Associated features include postural instability, a festinating gait, micrographia, seborrhea, urinary changes, constipation, hypophonia and an expressionless facial countenance. The tremor in Parkinson's disease has a regular rate and is most prominent when the patient is sitting with arms supported; it has therefore been described as intention tremors. Paranoid delusions and visual hallucinations may occur, but auditory hallucinations are rare. Antipsychotics with low incidence of extrapyramidal symptoms such as quetiapine, olanzepine, and ziprasidone are The pharmacological treatment of Parkinson's disease recommended. involves the use of a number of types of medication and ziprasidone are recommended. These include selegiline a selective monoamine oxidase inhibitor, levodopa, other dopamine agonists (pramipexole, bromocriptine, pergolide mesylate, amantadine), and various anticholinergic agents (benztropine). Selegiline should not be given to patients on antidepressant medication as there is a risk that dopaminergic agents may activate psychosis or mania and that anticholinergic drugs may increase confusion. When discontinuing levodopa after a long course of treatment, the drug should be tapered so as to prevent a discontinuation syndrome similar in nature to the neuroleptic malignant syndrome. Some medications (metoclopramide, droperidol, several antipsychotics) may produce parkinsonian features such as masked facies, sparsity of speech and tremor, and in those cases the appropriate course of treatment is to discontinue the offending medication. Several researchers are looking into the possibility of using embryonic stem cells implants as treatment for Parkinson's disease and several other conditions.

Dementia Due to Huntington's Disease

Dementia is also a characteristic of Huntington's disease, an autosomal dominant inheritable condition localized to chromosome 4. Unfortunately, this condition does not become apparent until age 35 to 45 years, usually after childbearing has occurred. Fifty percent of offspring are affected. There is also a juvenile form of the disease. Huntington's disease affects about four in 100 000 people, making it a significant cause of dementia in middle-aged adults.

The pathology of Huntington's disease involves selective destruction in the caudate and putamen. In the caudate nuclei, GABA concentrations are reduced to 50% of normal. The frontal lobes of the cerebral cortex are also involved, but GABA and choline acetyltransferase concentrations in the cortex are normal.

The most noticeable clinical feature of Huntington's disease is the movement disorder, which involves both choreiform movements (frequent movements that cause a jerking motion of the body) and athetosis (slow writhing movements). In the juvenile form of Huntington's disease, which represents about 3% of all cases, the chorea is replaced by dystonia, akinesia and rigidity, and the course of the disease is more rapid than in the adult form. In the early stages of the disease, the chorea is not as noticeable and may be disguised by the patient by making the movements seem purposeful.

The dementia typically begins 1 year before or 1 year after the chorea and, unlike patients with other dementias, patients with Huntington's disease are often well aware of their deteriorating mentation. This may be a factor in the high rates of suicide and alcoholism associated with this condition. Although attempts have been made to increase ACh and GABA concentrations in these patients, such pharmacological interventions have been unsuccessful, and the dementia in untreatable. Genetic counseling is indicated.

Vascular Dementia

Vascular dementia usually results from multiple CVAs or one significant CVA. It is generally considered the second most common cause of dementia after Alzheimer's disease, accounting for about 10% of all cases. Men are twice as likely as women to be diagnosed with this condition. Vascular dementia is characterized by a stepwise progression of cognitive deterioration with accompanying lateralizing signs. It is always associated with evidence of systemic hypertension and usually involves renal and cardiac abnormalities. Risk factors for the development of a vascular dementia include those generally associated with obstructive coronary artery disease, including obesity, hypercholesterolemia, smoking, hypertension, stress and lack of exercise. The actual incidence of vascular dementia has decreased somewhat with better standards of care, improved diagnostic techniques and lifestyle changes.

DSM-IV-TR Criteria 290.4x

Vascular Dementia

A. The development of multiple cognitive deficits manifested by both

  (1) memory impairment (impaired ability to learn new information or to recall previously learned information)

  (2) one (or more) of the following cognitive disturbances:

    (a) aphasia (language disturbance)

    (b) apraxia (impaired ability to carry out motor activities despite intact motor function)

    (c) agnosia (failure to recognize or identify objects despite intact sensory function)

    (d) disturbance in executive functioning (i.e., planning, organizing, sequencing, abstracting)

B. The cognitive deficits in criteria A1 and A2 each cause B. significant impairment in social or occupational functioning and represent a significant decline from a previous level of functioning.

C. Focal neurological signs and symptoms (e.g., exaggeration of. deep tendon reflexes, extensorplantar response, pseudobulbar palsy, gait weakness of an extremity) or laboratory evidence abnormalities,

D. indicative of cerebrovascular disease (e.g., multiple infarctions involving cortex and underlying white matter) that are judged to be etiologically related to the disturbance.

The deficits do not occur exclusively during the course of a delirium.

Code based on predominant features:

290.41 With delirium: if delirium is superimposed on the dementia

290.42 With delusions: if delusions are the predominant feature

390.43 With depressed mood: if depressed mood (including presentations that meet full symptom criteria for a major depressive episode) is the predominant feature. A separate diagnosis of mood disorder due to a general medical condition is not given.

209.40 Uncomplicated: if none of the above predominates in the current clinical presentation

Specify if:

With behavioral disturbance

Coding note: Also code cerebrovascular condition on Axis III.

Reprinted with permission from the *Diagnostic and Statistical Manual of Mental Disorders*, Fourth Edition, Text Revision. Copyright 2000 American Psychiatric Association.

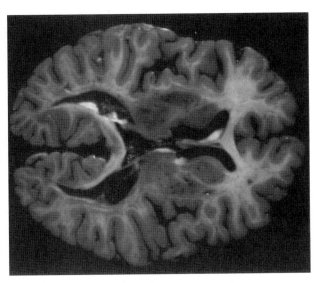

Figure 32.8 *Multiple lucencies in basal nuclei with reduced white matter in vascular dementia. (Courtesy of Joseph Parker, MD, Duke University Medical Center, Durham, NC.)*

Clinical Features

Vascular dementia is characterized by the early appearance of localizing neurological signs. Spasticity, hemiparesis, ataxia and pseudobulbar palsy are common. Pseudobulbar palsy is associated with injury to the frontal lobes and results in impairment of the corticobulbar tracts. It is characterized by extreme emotional lability, abnormal speech cadence, dysphagia, hyperactive jaw jerk, hyperactive deep tendon reflexes and Babinski's reflex. CT, MRI and gross specimens show cerebral atrophy and infarctions, with the radiological procedures showing multiple lucencies and the gross specimens revealing distinct white matter lesions (Figure 32.8). The EEG is abnormal but nonspecific, and positron emission tomography reveals hypometabolic areas. Vascular dementia is differentiated from AD on the basis of its mode of progression, early appearance of neurological signs, and radiographical evidence of cerebral ischemia.

Treatment

Primary prevention and secondary prevention are important in the treatment of cerebrovascular disorders. Lifestyle changes are effective in arresting the progress of the disease; however, no known pharmacological treatment can reverse the effects of a completed stroke. Such interventions as anticoagulants for frequent transient ischemic attacks after a hemorrhagic lesion have been investigated but excluded; aspirin for decreasing platelet aggregation, and surgical removal of obstructing plaques probably do not reverse the mental state. Depression occurs in 50 to 60% of patients with CVAs and responds to traditional antidepressants. Tricyclic antidepressants, such as amitriptyline, in less than antidepressant doses, improve both CVA depression and pseudobulbar palsy. Physical rehabilitation is essential and often results in an improvement in mood and outlook.

Infectious Causes of Dementia

Subacute Sclerosing Panencephalitis

Subacute sclerosing panencephalitis is an infectious cause of dementia that usually appears in childhood. The average age at onset is 10 years, and most patients are male and live in rural areas. It is diagnosed on the basis of periodic complexes on the EEG and an elevated measles titer in the cerebrospinal fluid (CSF). The CT scan shows cerebral atrophy and dilated ventricles. Myoclonus and dementia are prominent features.

It has been postulated that a mutant measles virus is the infectious agent, based on the high CSF measles antibody titer and the fact that the disease is virtually nonexistent in children who have been vaccinated for measles. Affected patients show an insidious onset of impairment of cognition usually preceded by behavioral problems.

Creutzfeldt–Jakob Disease

This disease has received intense scientific scrutiny. The primary features of Creutzfeldt–Jakob disease are dementia, basal ganglia and cerebellar dysfunction, myoclonus, upper motor neuron lesions and rapid progression to stupor, coma, and death in a matter of months. The disease generally affects people 65 years of age or older, with a duration of 1 month to 6 years and an average life span after disease onset of 15 months (Karp, 1984). The clinical and pathological features of Creutzfeldt–Jakob have been produced experimentally by injecting animals with brain tissue from affected adults. It has unknowingly been transferred to humans by organ transplantation, cerebral electrodes and pituitary growth hormone. These incidents, although tragic, illustrated the infectious nature of this condition, and the agent of transmission is believed to be a prion-containing protein (not DNA or RNA). These prions have been detected in the cerebral cortex of autopsy specimens of both patients with Creutzfeldt–Jakob disease and victims of kuru, a fatal disease transmitted by cannibalism (Kaplan *et al.*, 1994; Prusiner, 1987). Slow viruses have also been implicated as infectious agents in kuru. Creutzfeldt–Jakob has been accidentally transferred to humans by corneal and pituitary gland transplantation, electroencephalogram electrodes, and ingesting meat infected with the disease (mad cow disease).

The memory loss in Creutzfeldt–Jakob disease involves all phases of memory, with recent (secondary) memory being the most impaired. Personality changes, immature behavior and paranoia are early signs, and virtually every aspect of brain functioning can be involved. Motor disorders including rigidity, incoordination, paresis and ataxia usually follow.

As with subacute sclerosing panencephalitis, the EEG in Creutzfeldt–Jakob disease shows periodic complexes and biopsy specimens that reveal a characteristic spongiform encephalopathy and occasional amyloid plaques.

Acquired Immunodeficiency Syndrome

The CDC reports that as of June 1, 2001, 793 026 individuals had been diagnosed as having AIDS, with over 134 000 women included in that total. Nine thousand children under age 13 years have been diagnosed. Deaths from AIDS-related illnesses have reached 458 000. Worldwide, about 40 million people, including 3 million children, have AIDS. Forty-eight percent of the worldwide cases are women, and 95% of AIDS cases are in undeveloped countries (AIDS Surveillance Report, 2002). The number of people infected is postulated to be as much as 50 to 100 times the number of people diagnosed with AIDS, and 80 to 90% of people infected have not been tested.

In the developed countries, the death rate from AIDS has been on the decline since the advent of new medication regimens utilizing traditional antiretrovirals and the newer protease inhibitors. These medication cocktails have also decreased the incidence of AIDS dementia complex, so that physicians are now more likely to see AIDS-related delirium secondary to infection, metabolic disarray and medication rather than traditional AIDS dementia.

In the truest sense, AIDS is not a disease but an increased susceptibility to a variety of diseases caused by loss of immunocompetence. It results from infection with HIV, a retrovirus that attaches to the CD4 molecule on the surface of the T4 (thymus-derived) lymphocyte. Then, using reverse transcriptase, the virus reverses the usual sequence of genetic information and becomes integrated into the host cell's DNA. The ultimate result is destruction of the T4 cell, replication of the virus, a defect in cell-mediated immunity and the development of various opportunistic infections and neoplasms.

The epidemiology of HIV spectrum diseases has changed significantly in the 16 years since its identification. Initially, homosexual and bisexual men with multiple partners were the highest-risk group. Intravenous drug abusers and recipients of tainted blood products were soon added to high-risk groups. In the 1990s, the number of new infections among homosexual men decreased significantly and rates for women, intravenous drug abusers who shared contaminated needles, and infants born to infected mothers increased significantly. Intravenous drug abusers, regardless of sexual orientation, represent the fastest growing population of the newly infected people. Conversely, instances of transmission by blood products have decreased since the development of laboratory testing for HIV antibodies. The CDC has now established a reactive HIV antibody screen, presence of an opportunistic condition, and a CD4$^+$ cell count of 200 or less (normal being 1000–1500) as criteria for the diagnosis of AIDS.

AIDS is now best considered as part of the spectrum of HIV infection. There are four stages of infection.

Stage 1: Acute Infection: Most infected persons remember no signs or symptoms at the time of the initial infection. The acute syndrome follows infection by 4 to 6 weeks and is characterized by fevers, rigors, muscle aches, maculopapular rash, diarrhea and abdominal cramps. These symptoms, often mistaken for those of influenza, resolve spontaneously after 2 to 3 weeks.

Stage 2: Asymptomatic carrier: This stage follows the acute infection. The patient is without symptoms for a variable amount of time. The mean symptom-free period has increased significantly since the disease was first identified and is now about 10 years. Most of the estimated 2 million infected Americans are at this stage. Even though these individuals are asymptomatic, they are carriers of the disease and can infect others.

Stage 3: Generalized adenopathy: In older terminology, this stage was referred to as the AIDS-related complex. It is characterized by palpable lymph nodes that persist for longer than 3 months. These nodes must be outside the inguinal area and due to no other condition except HIV.

Stage 4: Other diseases:

1. Constitutional symptoms such as lingering fever, wasting syndromes and intractable diarrhea.
2. Secondary infections including *P. carinii* pneumonia, cytomegalovirus retinitis, parasitic colitis, and oral esophageal thrush.
3. Secondary neoplasms such as Kaposi's sarcoma and B-cell lymphomas.
4. Neurological diseases (AIDS dementia complex).

Thus, the diagnosis of AIDS is made when an infected individual develops either a CD4$^+$ cell count of less than 200 or a certain condition listed in the stages.

Dementia Due to HIV Diseases

Initially, the behavioral abnormalities observed in HIV-positive patients were attributed to the emotional reaction to the disease. Subsequent investigations demonstrated that neurological complications occur in 40 to 45% of patients with AIDS, and in about 10% of cases neurological signs are the first feature of the disease (Berg *et al.*, 1994). The neurological signs present in AIDS are believed to be related to both the direct effects of the virus on cells (such as macrophages) that enter the central nervous system and the neurological conditions that opportunistically affect these patients. Ho and colleagues (1987) reported that 90% of the brains of AIDS patients examined showed neuropathological abnormalities. AIDS dementia must be considered in the differential diagnosis of dementia in older patients, because about 10% of AIDS patients are older than 50 years of age.

Patients with AIDS dementia present with impairments of cognitive, behavioral and motor systems. The cognitive disorders include memory impairment, confusion and poor concentration. Behavioral features include apathy, reclusivity, anhedonia, depression, delusions, and hallucinations. Motor symptoms include incoordination, lower extremity paresis, unsteadiness, and difficulty with fine motor movements like handwriting and buttoning clothes. As the disease progresses, parkinsonism and myoclonus develop.

Localizing signs such as tremors, focal seizures, abnormal reflexes and hemiparesis can result. The protozoan *Toxoplasma gondii* commonly infects the central nervous system and can be diagnosed by CT or by increased toxoplasmosis antibody titers. Discrete cerebral lesions are also produced by fungi such as *Candida* and *Aspergillus*, *Mycobacterium tuberculosis*, and viruses such as cytomegalovirus and papovavirus. Papovavirus causes progressive multifocal leukoencephalopathy. Tertiary syphilis has increased significantly since the advent of AIDS, and neoplasms such as lymphomas, metastatic Kaposi's sarcoma and gliomas are also causes of AIDS dementia.

Many confounding factors can increase cognitive dysfunction in AIDS, including a high incidence of drug and alcohol abuse; medications such as histamine H$_2$ receptor antagonists (cimetidine), corticosteroids, narcotics and antiviral drugs (e.g., zidovudine [formerly azidothymidine, AZT]) that increase confusion; and coexistent depression (Table 32.5).

The CT scan shows cerebral atrophy and MRI reveals nonspecific white matter abnormalities (Kaufman, 1990b). Neoplasms and lesions such as toxoplasmosis are also visible. Lumbar puncture reveals a pleocytosis and elevated protein levels, and autopsy demonstrates an atrophic brain with demyelination, multinuclear giant cells and gliosis of the cerebral cortex (Kaufman, 1990b).

Treatment

The increase in life span of patients affected by HIV is directly related to improvements in treating the opportunistic conditions that occur. Aerosol pentamidine as prophylaxis for *P. carinii*

Table 32.5   Neuropsychiatric Effects of AIDS-related Drugs

Drug	Use	Effect
Ketoconazole	Antifungal	Severe depression Suicidality (rare)
Foscarnet	Cytomegalovirus retinitis Herpes	Depression Confusion
Ganciclovir	Cytomegalovirus retinitis	Anxiety Psychosis
Bactrim	*Pneumocystis* pneumonia	Hallucinations Depression Apathy
Pentamidine	*Pneumocystis* pneumonia	Delirium Hallucinations
Interferon alpha	Cancer	Depression
Rifampin	Tuberculosis	Delirium Behavioral changes
Isoniazid	Tuberculosis	Memory disturbance Psychosis
Dronabinol (Marinol)	Appetite stimulant Wasting syndrome Nausea	Depression Anxiety Psychosis Euphoria
Zalcitabine (DDC)	Antiviral	Psychosis Amnesia Confusion Depersonalization Depression Mania Suicidality Mood swings
Didanosine	Antiviral	Anxiety
Zidovudine (AZT)	Antiviral	Confusion, mania Depression, anxiety

pneumonia and ganciclovir for cytomegalovirus retinitis are examples of effective intervention. The use of antiviral agents has generated some controversy. Zidovudine, the first antiviral treatment for AIDS approved by the USFDA, increased or stabilized CD4$^+$ cell concentrations in early studies. Later investigations revealed that zidovudine has a narrow window of effectiveness and may not be appropriate immediately after such exposure as a needle stick. Side effects of zidovudine include blood dyscrasias, peripheral neuropathy, seizures, lymphomas, confusion, anxiety, mania and a Wernicke–Korsakoff type of picture (Kaufman, 1990b).

Studies suggest that administration of zidovudine to HIV-positive patients during pregnancy, intravenously during delivery, and to the neonate for 6 weeks after birth can decrease the percentage of infants who seroconvert from 30% to as low as 10%. However, results of studies of the effectiveness of zidovudine in children already HIV-positive have been disappointing. Subsequent antiviral agents such as dideoxyinosine and dideoxycytidine (DDC) have been associated with painful neuropathy

and pancreatic disorders. DDC in particular can produce serious neuropsychiatric complications. Combined therapy with two antiviral agents may be more effective than single-drug therapy. Many pharmaceutical companies are combining two antivirals into a single pill, and the development of protease inhibitor agents such as indinavir and nelfinavir have been especially effective in retarding the progression of the disease. The treatment of neuropsychiatric disorders in AIDS involves utilizing agents that are least likely to interfere with other medications prescribed, or to exacerbate the symptoms of the disease. AIDS-related depression has responded well to the selective serotonin reuptake inhibitors (SSRIs) and to psychostimulants. Some HIV drugs can have interactions with SSRIs, particularly ritonavir and the SSRIs themselves, especially paroxetine and fluoxetine can interact with other agents the HIV patient may have been prescribed, such as antiarrhythmics, benzodiazepines and anticonvulsants by inhibiting the cytochrome P-450 enzyme system. Some individuals have suggested that citalopram is less likely to inhibit this enzyme system. Careful attention to drug–drug interactions, using lower starting doses of certain psychiatric drugs, and monitoring of blood levels of affected medications are recommended. Among the psychostimulants, methylphenidate is preferred to dextroamphetamine because of the latter's tendency to produce dyskinesias. Use of stimulants for treating patients with a history of substance abuse is not recommended. Anticholingeric agents have a number of side effects such as mydriasis, decreased gastrointestinal motility and postural hypotension. However, low dose tricyclic antidepressants are often used for their sedative, analgesic and appetite stimulant properties. Most antidepressants and some mood stabilizers and antipsychotics can cause bone marrow suppression so they should be used with care, and hematologic parameters routinely monitored. Lithium carbonate, which produces a leukocytosis, may be of benefit in recurrent unipolar and treatment resistant depression, but may potentiate AIDS-related diarrhea. Many of the drugs used to treat AIDS-related conditions may produce untoward psychiatric effects. Depression has been well documented as a side effect of indinavir and nelfinavir has been associated with anxiety, depression, mood lability and even suicidality. St John's Wort may decrease the concentration of many of the protease inhibitors and is therefore contraindicated in patients taking these agents. In summary, AIDS dementia is best treated by identifying the associated medical condition, instituting appropriate therapy and managing behavior in the interim.

Neurosyphilis

The rise of AIDS in the 1980s and 1990s has led to an increase in the number of diagnosed cases of neurosyphilis.

Late syphilis consists of ongoing inflammatory disease most likely in the aorta or nervous system (neurosyphilis), the latter occurring in about 10% of patients. The neurosyphilis of the late stage can consist of 1) asymptomatic neurosyphilis, 2) meningovascular syphilis, and 3) parenchymal neurosyphilis which has two forms. One form of parenchymal neurosyphilis consists of general paresis, which occurs about 20 years after infection and includes cognitive impairment, myoclonus, dysarthria, personality changes, irritability, psychosis, grandiosity and mania. Untreated general paresis leaves the patient a helpless invalid. The second form of parenchymal neurosyphilis is **tabes dorsalis** with onset 25 to 30 years after initial infection. Tabes features loss of position and vibratory sense, areflexia in lower extremities, chronic pain, ataxia and incontinence.

The original screening test for syphilis is the venereal disease research laboratory (VDRL) test. This test has a significant false-positive rate, especially in the elderly and in patients with addictions and autoimmune disorders (Kaufman, 1990b). The VDRL test may revert to negative after a number of years, and 20 to 30% of patients in the stage of late syphilis have a negative (nonreactive) VDRL result. A more specific test is the fluorescent treponemal antibody screen, which is positive 95% of the time in neurosyphilis. The false-positive rate for the fluorescent treponemal antibody screen is extremely low, and reversion to a nonreactive state is unlikely. In addition to a positive VDRL result, the CSF in patients with neurosyphilis generally shows pleocytosis.

Dementia secondary to neurosyphilis produces various physical findings in advanced cases. These may include dysarthria, Babinski's reflex, tremor, Argyll Robertson pupils, myelitis and optic atrophy. Although notorious, delusions of grandeur in neurosyphilis are rare. A reactive CSF VDRL result or a positive serum fluorescent treponemal antibody result in a patient with neurological symptoms who cannot document treatment should be treated with appropriate therapy. Penicillin often improves cognitive deficits and corrects CSF abnormalities, but complete recovery is rare.

Dementia Due to Head Trauma

Head trauma is the leading cause of brain injury for children and young adults. It is estimated that more than 7 million head injuries and 500 000 hospital admissions related to the same cause occur in the USA annually. Traumatic head injuries result in concussions, contusions, or open head injuries, and the physical examination often reveals such features as blood behind the tympanic membranes (Battle's sign), infraorbital ecchymosis and pupillary abnormalities. The psychiatric manifestations of an acute brain injury are generally classified as a delirium or amnestic disorder; however, head trauma-induced delirious states often merge into a chronic dementia.

A single head injury may result in a postconcussional syndrome with resultant memory impairment, alterations in mood and personality, hyperacusis, headaches, easy fatigability, anxiety, belligerent behavior and dizziness. Alcohol abuse, postural hypotension and gait disturbances are often associated with head injuries that result in dementia.

Substance-induced Persisting Dementia

In instances in which the features of dementia result from central nervous system effects of a medication, toxin, or drug of abuse (including alcohol), the diagnosis of dementia due to the persisting effects of a substance should be made (American Psychiatric Association, 1994). The most common dementias in this category are those associated with alcohol abuse, accounting for about 10% of all dementias. The diagnosis of alcohol abuse dementia requires that the cognitive changes persist after the cessation of alcohol use and are not the result of changes in mentation associated with early abstinence, amnestic episodes (blackouts), or Wernicke–Korsakoff syndrome. In addition to various nutritional deficiencies and the toxic effects of alcohol itself, alcohol abusers are more prone to develop dementia as a result of head trauma and chronic hepatic encephalopathy.

Alcohol-induced Dementia

Epidemiology

Severe alcohol dependence is the third leading cause of dementia. Alcohol-induced dementia is a relatively late occurrence, generally following 15 to 20 years of heavy drinking. Dementia is more common in individuals with alcoholism who are malnourished. The CT scan shows cortical atrophy and ventricular dilatation after about 10 years with neuronal loss, pigmentary degeneration and glial proliferation. The frontal lobes are the most affected, followed by parietal and temporal areas. The amount of deterioration is related to age, number of episodes of heavy drinking and total amount of alcohol consumed over time.

Clinical Features

Alcohol-induced dementia, secondary to the toxic effects of alcohol, develops insidiously and often presents initially with changes in personality. Increasing memory loss, worsening cognitive processing and concrete thinking follow. The dementia may be affected by periodic superimposed delirious states including those caused by recurrent use of alcohol and cross-sensitive drugs, respiratory disease related to smoking, central nervous system

Treatment

The presence of dementia makes the treatment of alcoholism more difficult. Most treatment programs depend on education about substance abuse, working the 12 steps, some degree of sociability, and such relatively abstract concepts as secondary gratification and a higher power. Such treatment programs are often reluctant to engage in the painstaking repetition that patients with alcohol-induced dementia often require. These patients may become frustrated in peer support groups such as Alcoholics Anonymous. Despite these obstacles, patients with alcoholism who complete a treatment program and remain sober do have some improvement in their mental state. There is an initial improvement that peaks at 3 to 4 weeks, followed by a slow but steady improvement detected at 6 to 8 months. In general, the presence of a cognitive deficit (dementia) dictates an alcohol treatment program that is behavior based, concrete, structured, supportive and repetitive.

Other Substances

Many other agents can produce dementia as a result of their persisting effects. Exposure to such heavy metals as mercury and bromide, chronic contact with various insecticides, and use of various classes of drugs of abuse may produce dementia. In particular, the abuse of organic solvents (inhalants) has been associated with neurological changes. The inhalants are generally classified as anesthetics (halothane, chloroform, ether, nitrous oxide), solvents (gasoline, paint thinner, antifreeze, kerosene, carbon tetrachloride), aerosols (insecticides, deodorants, hair sprays) and nitrites (amyl nitrite). The solvent category is particularly toxic to the brain. In addition, acute anoxia may result from the common practice of inhaling a substance with a plastic bag around the head. Such neurological findings as peripheral neuropathy, paresis, paresthesias, areflexia, seizures, signs of cerebellar damage and Babinski's sign are common. Although the cerebellum is often involved, any area of the cerebral cortex may be affected (Table 32.7).

Dementia Due to Other General Medical Conditions

Normal-pressure Hydrocephalus

Normal-pressure hydrocephalus is generally considered the fifth leading cause of dementia after Alzheimer's, vascular, alcohol-related, and AIDS dementias. Long considered reversible but often merely arrestable, normal-pressure hydrocephalus is a syndrome consisting of dementia, urinary incontinence and gait apraxia. It results from subarachnoid hemorrhage, meningitis, or trauma that impedes CSF absorption. Unlike other dementias, the dementia caused by normal-pressure hydrocephalus has physical effects that often overshadow the mental effects. Psychomotor retardation, marked gait disturbances and, in severe cases, complete incontinence of urine occur. A cisternogram is often helpful in the diagnosis, and CT and MRI show ventricular dilatation without cerebral atrophy. CSF analysis reveals a normal opening pressure, and glucose and protein determinations are within the normal range.

   The hydrocephalus can be relieved by insertion of a shunt into the lateral ventricle to drain CSF into the chest or abdominal cavity, where it is absorbed. Clinical improvement with shunting approaches 50% with a neurosurgical complication rate of 13 to 25%. Infection remains the most common complication.

DSM-IV-TR Criteria

Substance-induced Persisting Dementia

A. The development of multiple cognitive deficits manifested by both

   (1) memory impairment (impaired ability to learn new information or to recall previously learned information)

   (2) one (or more) of the following cognitive disturbances:

   (a) aphasia (language disturbance)

   (b) apraxia (impaired ability to carry out motor activities despite intact motor function)

   (c) agnosia (failure to recognize or identify objects despite intact sensory function)

   (d) disturbance in executive functioning (i.e., planning, organizing, sequencing, abstracting)

B. The cognitive deficits in criteria A1 and A2 each cause significant impairment in social or occupational functioning and represent a significant decline from a previous level of functioning.

C. The deficits do not occur exclusively during the course of a delirium and persist beyond the usual duration of substance intoxication or withdrawal.

D. There is evidence from the history, physical examination, or laboratory findings that the deficits are etiologically related to the persisting effects of substance use (e.g., a drug of abuse, a medication).

Code: [specific substance]–induced persisting dementia:

   (291.2 alcohol; 292.82 inhalant; 292.82 sedative, hypnotic, or anxiolytic; 292.82 other [or unknown] substance)

Reprinted with permission from the *Diagnostic and Statistical Manual of Mental Disorders*, Fourth Edition, Text Revision.Copyright 2000 American Psychiatric Association.

---

hemorrhage secondary to trauma, chronic hypoxia related to recurrent seizure activity, folic acid deficiency and higher rates of some neoplasms among those with alcoholism (Table 32.6).

Table 32.6	Central Nervous System Sequelae of Alcohol Abuse

Blackouts
Dementia
Marchiafava–Bignami disease
Wernicke–Korsakoff syndrome
Hepatic encephalopathy
Delirium tremens
Withdrawal seizures
Episodic dyscontrol (pathological intoxication)
Alcoholic hallucinosis
Head injury

Table 32.7	Neurological Effects of Selected Inhalants	
Agent	Use	Effect
n-Hexane	Organic solvent	Peripheral neuropathy
Methyl butyl ketone	Paint thinner	Polyneuropathy
Toluene	Paint thinner	Cognitive dysfunction Cerebellar ataxia Optic neuropathy loss Sensorineural hearing Dementia
Trichloroethylene	Metal degreasing Extracting oils	Trigeminal neuropathy
Methylene chloride	Paint stripping, propellant Aerosol	Carbon monoxide poisoning Hypoxic encephalopathy
1,1,1-trichloroethane	Solvent Industrial degreasing	Cerebral hypoxia

Wilson's Disease

Hepatolenticular degeneration (Wilson's disease) is an inherited autosomal recessive condition associated with dementia, hepatic dysfunction and a movement disorder. Localized to chromosome 13, this disorder features copper deposits in the liver, brain and cornea. Symptoms begin in adolescence to the early twenties and cases are often seen in younger children. Wilson's disease should be considered along with Huntington's disease, AIDS dementia, substance abuse dementia, head trauma and subacute sclerosing panencephalitis in the differential diagnosis of dementia that presents in adolescence and early adulthood. Personality, mood and thought disorders are common, and physical findings include a wing-beating tremor, rigidity, akinesia, dystonia and the pathognomonic Kayser–Fleischer ring around the cornea. Wilson's disease can mimic other conditions including Huntington's disease, Parkinson's disease, atypical psychosis and neuroleptic-induced dystonia. Slit-lamp ocular examination, abnormal liver function tests and markedly decreased serum ceruloplasmin levels are diagnostic. Chelating agents such as penicillamine, if administered early, can reverse central nervous system and nonneurological findings in about 50% of cases.

Other Medical Conditions

In addition to the conditions mentioned previously, other medical illnesses can be associated with dementia. These include endocrine disorders (hypothyroidism, hypoparathyroidism), chronic metabolic conditions (hypocalcemia, hypoglycemia), nutritional deficiencies (thiamine, niacin, vitamin B_{12}), structural lesions (brain tumors, subdural hematomas) and multiple sclerosis.

Treatment of Dementia

Most of the treatment strategies for dementia have been discussed previously (see treatment of dementia of the Alzheimer type). In summary, the management of dementia involves 1) identification and, if possible, correction of the underlying cause; 2) environmental manipulation to reorient the patient; 3) intervention with the family by means of education, peer support, providing access to community organizations, discussing powers of attorney, living wills, and institutionalization if appropriate, and arranging therapy if indicated; and 4) pharmacological management of psychiatric symptoms and behavior. Low dose antipsychotics with minimal anticholinergic potential and occasionally short-acting benzodiazepines (e.g., lorazepam) are the drugs of choice. Because depression occasionally accompanies dementia, pharmacotherapy with antidepressants of low anticholineric and hypotensive potential is often indicated. For patients with dementia, secondary to drug or alcohol abuse, appropriate referral for rehabilitation is essential.

Delirium

Delirium (also known as acute confusional state, toxic metabolic encephalopathy) is the behavioral response to widespread disturbances in cerebral metabolism. Like dementia, delirium is not a disease but a syndrome with many possible causes that result in a similar constellation of symptoms. DSM-IV-TR describes five categories of delirium based on etiology. These include delirium due to a general medical condition, substance intoxication, withdrawl delirium, delirium due to muttiple etiologies and delirium not otherwise specified.

Epidemiology

The overall prevalence of delirium in the community is low, but delirium is common in hospitalized patients. Lipowski (Saito, 1987) reported studies of elderly patients and suggested that about 40% of them admitted to general medical wards showed signs of delirium at some point during the hospitalization. Because of the increasing numbers of elderly in this country and the influence of life-extending technology, the population of hospitalized elderly is rising; and so is the prevalence of delirium. The intensive care unit, geriatric psychiatry ward, emergency department, alcohol treatment units and oncology wards have particularly high rates of delirium. Massie and colleagues (Lipowski, 1987) reported that 85% of terminally ill patients studied had symptoms that met criteria for delirium, as did 100% of postcardiotomy patients in a study by Theobald (Lipowski, 1989). Overall, it is estimated that 10% of hospitalized patients are delirious at any particular point in time.

Predisposing factors in the development of delirium include old age, young age (children), previous brain damage, prior episodes of delirium, malnutrition, sensory impairment (especially vision) and alcohol dependence. In general, the mortality and morbidity of any serious disease are doubled if delirium ensues. The risk of dying after a delirious episode is greatest in the first two years after the illness, with a higher risk of death from heart disease and cancer in women and from pneumonia in men. Overall, the 3-month mortality rate for persons who have an episode of delirium is about 28%, and the 1-year mortality rate for such patients may be as high as 50%.

Dementia due to Other General Medical Conditions

A. The development of multiple cognitive deficits manifested by both

   (1) memory impairment (impaired ability to learn new information or to recall previously learned information)

   (2) one (or more) of the following cognitive disturbances:

   (a) aphasia (language disturbance)

   (b) apraxia (impaired ability to carry out motor activities despite intact motor function)

   (c) agnosia (failure to recognize or identify objects despite intact sensory function)

   (d) disturbance in executive functioning (i.e., planning, organizing, sequencing, abstracting)

B. The cognitive deficits in criteria A1 and A2 each cause. significant impairment in social or occupational functioning and represent a significant decline from a previous level of functioning.

C. There is evidence from the history, physical examination, or laboratory findings that the disturbance is the direct physiological consequence of one of the general medical conditions listed below.

D. The deficits do not occur exclusively during the course of a delirium.

294.9 Dementia due to HIV Disease

Coding note: Also code 043.1 HIV infection affecting central nervous system on Axis III.

294.1 Dementia due to Head Trauma

Coding note: Also code 854.00 head injury on Axis III.

294.1 Dementia due to Parkinson's Disease

Coding note: Also code 332.0 Parkinson's disease on Axis III.

294.1 Dementia due to Huntington's Disease

Coding note: Also code 333.4 Huntington's disease on Axis III.

290.10 Dementia due to Pick's Disease

Coding note: Also code 331.1 Pick's disease on Axis III.

290.10 Dementia due to Creutzfeldt–Jakob Disease

Coding note: Also code 046.1 Creutzfeldt–Jakob disease on Axis III.

294.1 Dementia due to…[Indicate the General Medical Condition Not Listed Above]

For example, normal-pressure hydrocephalus, hypothyroidism, brain tumor, vitamin B_{12} deficiency, intracranial radiation

Coding note: Also code the general medical condition on Axis III.

Reprinted with permission from the *Diagnostic and Statistical Manual of Mental Disorders*, Fourth Edition, Text Revision. Copyright 2000 American Psychiatric Association. Table 32.8 summarize the causes of dementia.

Pathophysiology

ACh is the primary neurotransmitter believed to be involved in delirium, and the primary neuroanatomical site involved is the reticular formation. Thus, one of the frequent causes of delirium is the use of drugs with high anticholinergic potential. As the principal site of regulation of arousal and attention, the reticular formation and its neuroanatomical connections play a major role in the symptoms of delirium. The major pathway involved in delirium is the dorsal tegmental pathway projecting from the mesencephalic reticular formation to the tectum and the thalamus.

Clinical Features

According to DSM-IV-TR, the primary feature of delirium is a diminished clarity of awareness of the environment (American Psychiatric Association, 1994). Symptoms of delirium are characteristically global, of acute onset, fluctuating and of relatively brief duration. In most cases of delirium, an often overlooked prodrome of altered sleep patterns, unexplained fatigue, fluctuating mood, sleep phobia, restlessness, anxiety and nightmares occurs. A review of nursing notes for the days before the recognized onset of delirium often illustrates early warning signs of the condition.

Several investigators have divided the clinical features of delirium into abnormalities of 1) arousal, 2) language and cognition, 3) perception, 4) orientation, 5) mood, 6) sleep and wakefulness, and 7) neurological functioning (Kaplan *et al.*, 1994).

The state of arousal in delirious patients may be increased or decreased. Some patients exhibit marked restlessness, heightened startle, hypervigilance and increased alertness. This pattern is often seen in states of withdrawal from depressive substances (e.g., alcohol) or intoxication by stimulants (phencyclidine, amphetamine, lysergic acid diethylamide). Patients with increased arousal often have such concomitant autonomic signs as pallor, sweating, tachycardia, mydriasis, hyperthermia, piloerection and gastrointestinal distress. These patients often require sedation with neuroleptics or benzodiazepines. Hypoactive arousal states such as those occasionally seen in hepatic encephalopathy and hypercapnia are often initially perceived as depressed or demented states. The clinical course of delirium in any particular patient may include both increased and decreased arousal states. Many such individuals display daytime sedation with nocturnal agitation and behavioral problems (sundowning).

Perceptual abnormalities in delirium represent an inability to discriminate sensory stimuli and to integrate current perceptions with past experiences. Consequently, patients tend to personalize events, conversations and so forth that do not directly pertain to them, become obsessed with irrelevant stimuli and misinterpret objects in their environment. The misinterpretations generally take the form of auditory and visual illusions. Patients with auditory illusions, for example, might hear the sound of leaves rustling and perceive it as someone whispering

Table 32.8	Causes of Dementia

Vascular
   Multiinfarct
   CVA
   Binswanger's disease
Degenerative
   Alzheimer's disease
   Pick's disease
   Huntington's disease
   Parkinson's disease
Toxic
   Medications
   Alcohol
   Poisons
   Inhalants
   Heavy metals
Infectious
   HIV spectrum illness
   Neurosyphilis
   Creutzfeldt–Jakob disease
   Kuru
   Subacute sclerosing panencephalitis
Metabolic
   Chronic hypoglycemia
   Electrolyte imbalances
   Vitamin deficiencies
Endocrine
   Thyroid abnormalities
   Parathyroid abnormalities
Trauma
   Single head injury
   Dementia pugilistica
Neoplastic
   Primary brain tumor
   Metastatic brain tumor

DSM-IV-TR Criteria 290.0

Delirium due to … [Indicate the General Medical Condition]

A. Disturbance of consciousness (i.e., reduced clarity of awareness of the environment) with reduced ability to focus, sustain, or shift attention.

B. A change in cognition (such as memory deficit, disorientation, language disturbance) or the development of a perceptual disturbance that is not better accounted for by a preexisting, established, or evolving dementia.

C. The disturbance develops over a short period of time (usually hours to days) and tends to fluctuate during the course of the day.

D. There is evidence from the history, physical examination, or laboratory findings that the disturbance is caused by the direct physiological consequences of a general medical condition.

Coding note: If delirium is superimposed on a preexisting dementia of the Alzheimer's type or vascular dementia, indicate the delirium by coding the appropriate subtype of the dementia, e.g., 290.3 dementia of the Alzheimer's type, with late onset, with delirium.

Coding note: Include the name of the general medical condition on Axis I, e.g., 293.0 delirium due to hepatic encephalopathy; also code the general medical condition on Axis III.

Reprinted with permission from the *Diagnostic and Statistical Manual of Mental Disorders*, Fourth Edition, Text Revision. Copyright 2000 American Psychiatric Association.

about them. Paranoia and sleep phobia may result. Typical visual illusions are that intravenous tubing is a snake or worm crawling into the skin, or that a respirator is a truck or farm vehicle about to collide with the patient. The former auditory illusion may lead to tactile hallucinations, but the most common hallucinations in delirium are visual and auditory.

     Orientation is often abnormal in delirium. Disorientation in particular seems to follow a fluctuating course, with patients unable to answer questions about orientation in the morning, yet fully oriented by the afternoon. Orientation to time, place, person and situation should be evaluated in the delirious patient. Generally, orientation to time is the sphere most likely impaired, with orientation to person usually preserved. Orientation to significant people (parents, children) should also be tested. Disorientation to self is rare and indicates significant impairment. The examiner should always reorient patients who do not perform well on any portion of the orientation testing of the mental status examination, and serial testing of orientation on subsequent days is important.

Language and Cognition

Patients with delirium frequently have abnormal production and comprehension of speech. Nonsensical rambling and incoherent

speech may occur. Other patients may be completely mute. Memory may be impaired, especially primary and secondary memory. Remote memory may be preserved, although the patient may have difficulty distinguishing the present from the distant past.

Mood

Patients with delirium are susceptible to rapid fluctuations in mood. Unprovoked anger and rage reactions occasionally occur and may lead to attacks on hospital staff. Fear is a common emotion and may lead to increased vigilance and an unwillingness to sleep because of increased vulnerability during somnolence. Apathy, such as that seen in hepatic encephalopathy, depression, use of certain medications (e.g., sulfamethoxazole [Bactrim]) and frontal lobe syndromes, is common as is euphoria secondary to medications (e.g., corticosteroids, DDC, zidovudine) and drugs of abuse (phencyclidine, inhalants).

Neurological Symptoms

Neurological symptoms often occur in delirium. These include dysphagia as seen after a CVA, tremor, asterixis (hepatic encephalopathy, hypoxia, uremia), poor coordination, gait apraxia, frontal release signs (grasp, suck), choreiform movements, seizures, Babinski's sign and dysarthria. Focal neurological signs occur less frequently.

Sleep–Wakefulness Disturbances

Sleeping patterns of delirious patients are usually abnormal. During the day they can be hypersomnolent, often falling asleep in midsentence, whereas at night they are combative and restless. Sleep is generally fragmented, and vivid nightmares are common. Some patients may become hypervigilant and develop a sleep phobia because of concern that something untoward may occur while they sleep.

Causes of Delirium

The cause of delirium may lie in intracranial processes, extracranial ones, or a combination of the two. The most common etiological factors are as follows (Francis *et al.*, 1990).

Infection Induced

Infection is a common cause of delirium in hospitalized patients and typically, infected patients will display abnormalities in hematology and serology. Vital signs are noted except in persons (elderly, chronic alcohol abusers, chemotherapy patients, those with HIV spectrum disease) who may not be able to mount the typical response. Bacteremic septicemia (especially that caused by gram-negative bacteria), pneumonia, encephalitis and meningitis are common offenders. The elderly are particularly susceptible to delirium secondary to urinary tract infections.

Metabolic and Endocrine Disturbances

Metabolic causes of delirium include hypoglycemia, electrolyte disturbances and vitamin deficiency states. The most common endocrine causes are hyperfunction and hypofunction of the thyroid, adrenal, pancreas, pituitary and parathyroid. Metabolic causes may involve consequences of diseases of particular organs, such as hepatic encephalopathy resulting from liver disease, uremic encephalopathy and postdialysis delirium resulting from kidney dysfunction, and carbon dioxide macrosis and hypoxia resulting from lung disease. The metabolic disturbance or endocrinopathy must be known to induce changes in mental status and must be confirmed by laboratory determinations or physical examination, and the temporal course of the confusion should coincide with the disturbance (Francis *et al.*, 1990). In some individuals, particularly the elderly, brain injured and demented, there may be a significant lag time between correction of metabolic parameters and improvement in mental state.

Low-perfusion States

Any condition that decreases effective cerebral perfusion can cause delirium. Common offenders are hypovolemia, congestive heart failure and other causes of decreased stroke volume such as arrhythmias and anemia, which decreases oxygen binding. Maintenance of fluid balance and strict measuring of intake and output are essential in delirious states.

Intracranial Causes

Intracranial causes of delirium include head trauma, especially involving loss of consciousness, postconcussive states and hemorrhage; brain infections; neoplasms; and such vascular abnormalities as CVAs, subarachnoid hemorrhage, transient ischemic attacks and hypertensive encephalopathy.

Postoperative States

Postoperative causes of delirium may include infection, atelectasis, postpump confusion from maintenance on a heart–lung machine, lingering effects of anesthesia, thrombotic and embolic phenomena, and adverse reactions to postoperative analgesia. General surgery in an elderly patient has been reported to be followed by delirium in 10 to 14% of cases and may reach 50% after surgery for hip fracture (Lipowski, 1989).

Sensory and Environmental Changes

Many clinicians underestimate the disorienting potential of an unfamiliar environment. The elderly are especially prone to develop environment-related confusion in the hospital. Individuals with preexisting dementia, who may have learned to compensate for cognitive deficits at home, often become delirious once hospitalized. In addition, the nature of the intensive care unit often lends itself to periods of high sensory stimulation (as during a "code") or low sensory input, as occurs at night. Often, patients use such external events as dispensing medication, mealtimes, presence of housekeeping staff, and physicians' rounds to mark the passage of time. These parameters are often absent at night, leading to increased rates of confusion during night-time hours. Often, manipulating the patient's environment (see section on treatment) or removing the patient from the intensive care unit can be therapeutic.

Substance Intoxication Delirium

The list of medications that can produce the delirious state is extensive (Table 32.9). The more common ones include such antihypertensives as methyldopa and reserpine, histamine (H_2) receptor antagonists (cimetidine), corticosteroids, antidepressants, narcotics (especially opioid) and nonsteroidal analgesics, lithium carbonate, digitalis, baclofen, anticonvulsants, antiarrhythmics, colchicine, bronchodilators, benzodiazepines, sedative-hypnotics and anticholinergics. Of the narcotic analgesics, meperidine can produce an agitated delirium with tremors, seizures and myoclonus. These features are attributed to its active metabolite normeperidine, which has potent stimulant and anticholinergic properties and accumulates with repeated intravenous dosing. In general, adverse effects of narcotics are more common in those who have never received such agents before (the narcotically naive) or who have a history of a similar response to narcotics.

Table 32.9 Selected Drugs Associated with Delirium	
Antihypertensives	Indomethacin
Amphotericin B	Ketamine
Antispasmodics	Levodopa
Antituberculous agents	Lidocaine
Baclofen	Lithium
Barbiturates	Meperidine
Cimetidine	Morphine
Corticosteroids	Procainamide
Colchicine	Pentamidine
Contrast media	Tricyclic antidepressants
Digitalis	Zalcitabine (DDC)
Ephedrine	Zidovudine (AZT)

DSM-IV-TR Criteria

Substance Intoxication Delirium

A. Disturbance of consciousness (i.e., reduced clarity of awareness of the environment) with reduced ability to focus, sustain, or shift attention.

B. A change in cognition (such as memory deficit, disorientation, language disturbance) or the development of a perceptual disturbance that is not better accounted for by a preexisting, established, or evolving dementia.

C. The disturbance develops over a short period of time (usually hours to days) and tends to fluctuate during the course of the day.

D. There is evidence from the history, physical examination, or laboratory findings of either (1) or (2):

   (1) the symptoms in criteria A and B developed during substance intoxication

   (2) medication use is etiologically related to the disturbance

Note: This diagnosis should be made instead of a diagnosis of substance intoxication only when the cognitive symptoms are in excess of those usually associated with the intoxication syndrome and when the symptoms are sufficiently severe to warrant independent clinical attention.

Note: The diagnosis should be recorded as substance-induced delirium if related to medication use.

Code: [specific substance] intoxication delirium:

(291.0 alcohol; 292.81 amphetamine [or amphetamine-like substance]; 292.81 cannabis; 292.81 cocaine; 292.81 hallucinogen; 292.81 inhalant; 292.81 opioid; 292.81 phencyclidine [or phencyclidine-like substance]; 292.81 sedative, hypnotic, or anxiolytic; 292.81 other [or unknown] substance [e.g., cimetidine, digitalis, benztropine])

Reprinted with permission from the *Diagnostic and Statistical Manual of Mental Disorders*, Fourth Edition, Text Revision. Copyright 2000 American Psychiatric Association.

Lithium-induced delirium occurs at blood levels greater than 1.5 mEq/L and is associated with early features of lethargy, stuttering and muscle fasciculations. The delirium may take as long as 2 weeks to resolve even after lithium has been discontinued, and other neurological signs such as stupor and seizures commonly occur. Maintenance of fluid and electrolyte balance is essential in lithium-induced delirium. Facilitation of excretion with such agents as aminophylline and acetazolamide helps, but hemodialysis is often required.

Principles to remember in cases of drug-induced delirium include the facts that 1) blood levels of possibly offending agents are helpful and should be obtained, but many persons can become delirious at therapeutic levels of the drug, 2) drug-induced delirium may be the result of drug interactions and polypharmacy and not the result of a single agent, 3) over-the-counter medications and preparations (e.g., agents containing caffeine or phenyl-propanolamine) should also be considered, and 4) delirium can be caused by the combination of drugs of abuse and prescribed medications (e.g., cocaine and dopaminergic antidepressants).

The list of drugs of abuse that can produce delirium is extensive. Some such agents have enjoyed resurgence after years of declining usage. These include lysergic acid diethylamide, psilocybin (hallucinogenic mushrooms), heroin and amphetamines. Other agents include barbiturates, cannabis (especially dependent on setting, experience of the user and whether it is laced with phencyclidine ["superweed"] or heroin), jimsonweed (highly anticholinergic) and mescaline. In cases in which intravenous use of drugs is suspected, HIV spectrum illness must be ruled out as an etiological agent for delirium.

The physical examination of a patient with suspected illicit drug-induced delirium may reveal sclerosed veins, "pop" scars caused by subcutaneous injection of agents, pale and atrophic nasal mucosa resulting from intranasal use of cocaine, injected conjunctiva and pupillary changes. Toxicological screens are helpful but may not be available on an emergency basis.

Substance Withdrawal Delirium

Alcohol and certain sedating drugs can produce a withdrawal delirium when their use is abruptly discontinued or significantly reduced. Withdrawal delirium requires a history of use of a potentially addicting agent for a sufficient amount of time to produce dependence. It is associated with such typical physical findings as abnormal vital signs, pupillary changes, tremor, diaphoresis, nausea and vomiting, and diarrhea. Patients generally

DSM-IV-TR Criteria

Substance Withdrawal Delirium

A. Disturbance of consciousness (i.e., reduced clarity of awareness of the environment) with reduced ability to focus, sustain, or shift attention.

B. A change in cognition (such as memory deficit, disorientation, language disturbance) or the development of a perceptual disturbance that is not better accounted for by a preexisting, established, or evolving dementia.

C. The disturbance develops over a short period of time (usually hours to days) and tends to fluctuate during the course of the day.

D. There is evidence from the history, physical examination, or laboratory findings that the symptoms in criteria A and B developed during, or shortly after, a withdrawal syndrome.

Note: This diagnosis should be made instead of a diagnosis of substance withdrawal only when the cognitive symptoms are in excess of those usually associated with the withdrawal syndrome and when the symptoms are sufficiently severe to warrant independent clinical attention.

Code: [specific substance] withdrawal delirium:
(291.0 alcohol; 292.81 sedative, hypnotic, or anxiolytic; 292.81 other [or unknown] substance)

Reprinted with permission from the *Diagnostic and Statistical Manual of Mental Disorders*, Fourth Edition, Text Revision. Copyright 2000 American Psychiatric Association.

Table 32.10	Causes of Delirium

Medication effect or interaction
Substance intoxication or withdrawal
Infection
Head injury
Metabolic disarray
    Acid–base imbalance
    Dehydration
    Malnutrition
    Electrolyte imbalance
    Blood glucose abnormality
    Carbon dioxide narcosis
    Uremic encephalopathy
    Hepatic encephalopathy
Cerebrovascular insufficiency
    Congestive heart failure
    Hypovolemia
    Arrhythmias
    Severe anemia
    Transient ischemia
    Acute CVA
Endocrine dysfunction
Postoperative states
    Postcardiotomy delirium
Environmental factors
    Intensive care unit psychosis
Sleep deprivation

complain of abdominal and leg cramps, insomnia, nightmares, chills, hallucinations (especially visual) and a general feeling of "wanting to jump out of my skin". Some varieties of drug withdrawal, although uncomfortable, are not life threatening (e.g., opioid withdrawal). Others such as alcohol withdrawal delirium are potentially fatal. Withdrawal delirium is much more common in hospitalized patients than in patients living in the community. The incidence of delirium tremens, for example, is found in 1% of all alcoholics, but in 5% of hospitalized alcohol abusers. Improvement of the delirium occurs when the offending agent is reintroduced or a cross-sensitive drug (e.g., a benzodiazepine for alcohol withdrawal) is employed. The causes of delirium are summarized in Table 32.10).

Diagnosis

Appropriate workup of delirious patients includes a complete physical status, mental status and neurological examination.

History taking from the patient, any available family, previous physicians, the old chart and the patient's current nurse is essential. Previous delirious states, etiologies identified in the past and interventions that proved effective should be elucidated. The appropriate evaluation of the delirious patient is reviewed in Figure 32.9

Differential Diagnosis

Delirium must be differentiated from dementia because the two conditions may have different prognoses. In contrast to the changes in dementia, those in delirium have an acute onset. The symptoms in dementia tend to be relatively stable over time, whereas clinical features of delirium display wide fluctuation with periods of relative lucidity. Clouding of consciousness is an essential feature of delirium, but demented patients are usually alert. Attention and orientation are more commonly disturbed in delirium, although the latter can become impaired in advanced dementia. Perception abnormalities, alterations in the sleep–wakefulness cycle, and abnormalities of speech are more common in delirium. Most important, a delirium is more likely to be reversible than is a dementia.

Delirium and dementia can occur simultaneously; in fact, the presence of dementia is a risk factor for delirium. Some studies suggest that about 30% of hospitalized patients with dementia have a superimposed delirium.

Delirium must often be differentiated from psychotic states related to such conditions as schizophrenia or mania and factitious disorders with psychological symptoms or malingering. Generally, the psychotic features of schizophrenia are more constant and better organized than are those in delirium, and patients with schizophrenia seldom have the clouding of consciousness seen in delirium. The "psychosis" of patients with factitious disorder or malingering is inconsistent, and these persons do not exhibit many of the associated features of delirium. Apathetic and lethargic patients with delirium may occasionally resemble depressed individuals, but tests such as EEG distinguish between the two. The EEG demonstrates diffuse slowing in most delirious states, except for the low-amplitude, fast activity EEG pattern seen in alcohol withdrawal. The EEG in a functional depression or psychosis is normal.

Management

Once delirium has been diagnosed, the etiological agent must be identified and treated. For the elderly, the first step generally involves discontinuing or reducing the dosage of potentially offending medications. Some delirious states can be reversed with medication, as in the case of physostigmine administration for anticholinergic delirium. However, most responses are not as immediate, and attention must be directed toward protecting the patient from unintentional self-harm, managing agitated and psychotic behavior, and manipulating the environment to minimize additional impairment. Supportive therapy should include fluid and electrolyte maintenance and provision of adequate nutrition. Reorienting the patient is essential and is best accomplished in a well-lit room with a window, clock and visible wall calendar. Familiar objects from home such as a stuffed animal, favorite blanket, or photographs are helpful. Patients who respond incorrectly to questions of orientation should be provided with the correct answers. Because these individuals often see many consultants, physicians should introduce themselves and state their purpose for coming at every visit. Physicians must take into account that impairments of vision and hearing can produce confusional states, and the provision of appropriate prosthetic devices may be beneficial. Around-the-clock accompaniment by hospital-provided "sitters" or family members may be required (see Table 32.11).

Despite these conservative interventions, the delirious patient often requires pharmacological intervention. The liaison psychiatrist is the most appropriate person to recommend such treatment. The drug of choice for the agitated delirious patients has traditionally been haloperidol. It is particularly beneficial when given by the intravenous route and some authors have reported using dosages as high as 260 mg/day without adverse effect. Extrapyramidal symptoms may be less common with haloperidol administered intravenously as opposed to orally and intramuscularly. In general, doses in the range of 0.5 to 5 mg intravenously

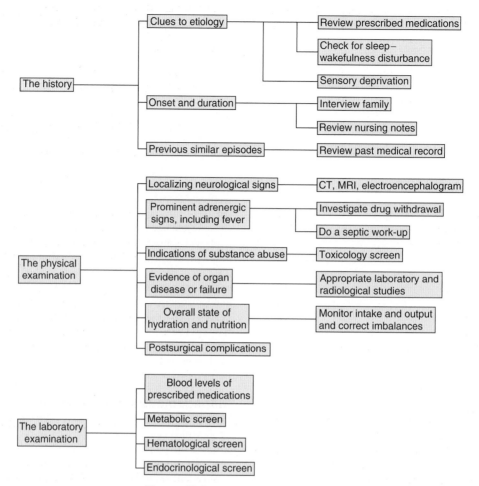

Figure 32.9 *Evaluation of delirium.*

are used, with the frequency of administration depending on a variety of factors including the patient's age. An electrocardiogram should be obtained before administering haloperidol. If the QT interval is greater than 450, use of intravenous haloperidol can precipitate an abnormal cardiac rhythm known as **Torsades de pointes**. Lorazepam has also been proven effective in doses of 0.5 to 2 mg intravenously. Some authors have suggested that haloperidol and lorazepam act synergistically when given to the agitated delirious patient. If the delirium is secondary to drug or alcohol abuse, benzodiazepines or clonidine should be used.

Table 32.11	Managing the Delirious Patient

Identify and correct the underlying cause.
Protect the patient from unintentional self-harm.
Stabilize the level of sensory input.
Reorient patient as often as possible.
Employ objects from the patient's home environment.
Provide supportive therapy (fever control, hydration).
Streamline medications.
Correct sleep deprivation.
Manage behavior with appropriate pharmacotherapy.
Address postdelirium guilt and shame for behavior that occurred during confusion.

For patients who are mildly agitated or amenable to taking medications by mouth, oral haloperidol or lorazepam is appropriate. Recent studies have advocated the use of newer atypical antipsychotics for management of behavior and psychotic features in delirium. Such agents as quetiapine, olanzapine, and risperdal and ziprasidone have been used successfully to treat delirium. Newer agents may have lower incidences of dystonias and dyskinesias, but still carry the risk of QT interval prolongation, particularly in patients with electrolyte abnormalities. Quetiapine and olanzapine are quite sedating, and occasionally a combination of bedtime olanzapine and "as needed" haloperidol is utilized. Olanzapine may raise blood glucose levels and precipitate weight gain, but is available as a Zydis preparation, which is absorbed through the oral mucosa and can therefore be given to patients who are unable to take medications by mouth. A parenteral form of ziprasidone is also available. Whatever antipsychotic is chosen, the patient should be carefully monitored for muscle rigidity, unexplained fever, tremor and other warning signs of neuroleptic side effects.

Outcome of Delirium

After elimination of the cause of the delirium, the symptoms gradually recede within 3 to 7 days. Some symptoms in certain populations may take weeks to resolve. The age of the patient and the period of time during which the patient was delirious affect the symptom resolution time. In general, the patient has a spotty memory for events that occurred during delirium. These remembrances are reinforced by comments from the staff ("You're not as confused today"), or the presence of a sitter, or use of wrist restraints. Patient should be reassured that they were not responsible for their behavior while delirious, and that no one hates or resents them for the behavior they may have exhibited. As mentioned earlier, delirious patients have an increased risk of mortality in the year following their first episode. Patients with underlying dementia show residual cognitive impairment after resolution of delirium, and it has been suggested that a delirium may merge into a dementia (Kaplan *et al.*, 1994).

Amnestic Disorders

The amnestic disorders are characterized by a disturbance in memory related to the direct effects of a general medical condition or the persisting effects of a substance (American Psychiatric Association, 1994). The impairment should interfere with social and occupational functioning and represent a significant decline from the previous level of functioning. The amnestic disorders are differentiated on the basis of the etiology of the memory loss. These disorders should not be diagnosed if the memory deficit is a feature of a dissociative disorder, is associated with dementia, or occurs in the presence of clouded sensorium, as in delirium. Amnestic disorders are predominately comprised of those caused by a general medical condition or those whose etiology is substance-induced.

Epidemiology

The exact prevalence and incidence of the amnestic disorders are unknown (Kaplan *et al.*, 1994). Memory disturbances related to specific conditions such as alcohol dependence and head trauma have been studied and these appear to be the two most common causes of amnestic disorders. Kaplan and coworkers (Torres *et al.*, 2001) reported that in the hospital setting the incidence of alcohol-induced amnestic disorders is decreasing while that of amnestic disorders, secondary to head trauma, is on the rise. This may be related to rigorous efforts by hospital personnel to decrease the incidence of iatrogenic amnestic disorder by giving thiamine before glucose is administered to a patient with chronic alcohol dependence and nutritional deficiencies.

Etiology

Amnesia results from generally bilateral damage to the areas of the brain involved in memory. The areas and structures so involved include the dorsomedial and midline thalamic nuclei, such temporal lobe-associated structures as the hippocampus, amygdala and mamillary bodies. The left hemisphere may be more important than the right in the occurrence of memory disorders. Frontal lobe involvement may be responsible for such commonly seen symptoms as apathy and confabulation.

The specific causes of amnestic disorders include 1) systemic medical conditions such as thiamine deficiency; 2) brain conditions, including seizures, cerebral neoplasms, head injury, hypoxia, carbon monoxide poisoning, surgical ablation of temporal lobes, electroconvulsive therapy and multiple sclerosis; 3) altered blood flow in the vertebral vascular system, as in transient global amnesia; and 4) effects of a substance (drug or alcohol use and exposure to toxins).

Conditions that affect the temporal lobes such as herpes infection and Kluver–Bucy syndrome can produce amnesia. Among drugs that can cause amnestic disorders, triazolam has received the most attention, but all benzodiazepines can produce

---

DSM-IV-TR Criteria 294.0

Amnestic Disorder

A. The development of memory impairment as manifested by impairment in the ability to learn new information or the inability to recall previously learned information.

B. The memory disturbance causes significant impairment in social or occupational functioning and represents a significant decline from a previous level of functioning.

C. The memory disturbance does not occur exclusively during the course of a delirium or a dementia.

D. There is evidence from the history, physical examination, or laboratory findings that the disturbance is the direct physiological consequence of a **general medical condition** (including physical trauma).

Or

D. D. There is evidence from the history, physical examination, or laboratory findings that the memory disturbance is etiologically related to the **persisting effects of substance use** (e.g., a drug of abuse, a medication).

Specify if:

Transient: if memory impairment lasts for 1 month or less

Chronic: if memory impairment lasts for more than 1 month

Coding note: Include the name of the general medical condition on Axis I, e.g., 294.0 amnestic disorder due to head trauma; also code the general medical condition on Axis III.

Or

Coding note:[specific substance]-induced persisting amnestic disorder:

(291.1 alcohol;292.83 sedative, hypnotic, or anxiolytic;292.83 [or unknown substance)

Reprinted with permission from the *Diagnostic and Statistical Manual of Mental Disorders*, Fourth Edition, Text Revision.Copyright 2000 American Psychiatric Association.

---

memory impairment, with the dose utilized being the determining factor (Kirk *et al.*, 1990) (Table 32.12).

Clinical Features

Patients with amnestic disorder have impaired ability to learn new information (anterograde amnesia) or cannot remember material previously learned (retrograde amnesia). Memory for the event that produced the deficit (e.g., a head injury in a motor vehicle accident) may also be impaired.

Remote recall (tertiary memory) is generally good, so patients may be able to relate accurately incidents that occurred during childhood but not remember what they had for breakfast. As illustrated by such conditions as thiamine amnestic syndrome, immediate memory is often preserved. In some instances, disorientation to time and place may occur, but disorientation to person is unusual.

Table 32.12	Causes of Amnestic Disorders

Types simplex encephalopathy
Substance-induced (alcohol) blackouts
Wernicke–Korsakoff syndrome
Multiple sclerosis
Klüver–Bucy syndrome
Electroconvulsive therapy
Seizures
Head trauma
Carbon monoxide poisoning
Metabolic
   Hypoxia
   Hypoglycemia
Medications
   Triazolam
   Barbiturates (thiopental sodium)
   Diltiazem (Cardizem)
   Zalcitabine (DDC)
Cerebrovascular disorders

The onset of the amnesia is determined by the precipitant and may be acute as in head injury or insidious as in poor nutritional states. DSM-IV characterizes short-duration amnestic disorder as lasting less than 1 month and long-duration disorder lasting 1 month or longer. Often individuals lack insight into the memory deficit and vehemently insist that their inaccurate responses on a Mental Status Examination are correct.

Selected Amnestic Disorders

Blackouts

Blackouts are periods of amnesia for events that occur during heavy drinking (Tarter and Schneider, 1976). Typically, a person awakens the morning after consumption and does not remember what happened the night before. Unlike delirium tremens, which is related to chronicity of alcohol abuse, blackouts are more a measure of the amount of alcohol consumed at any one time. Thus, blackouts are common in binge pattern drinkers and may occur the first time a person ingests a large amount of alcohol. Blackouts are generally transient phenomena, but some patients may continue to have blackouts for weeks even after they have stopped using alcohol. These memory lapses are similar to blackouts experienced while using alcohol. With continued sobriety, the blackouts should end, but information forgotten during past blackouts is never remembered. Blackouts may also be produced by agents with cross-sensitivity to alcohol, such as benzodiazepines. Blackouts should not be confused with alcohol-induced dementia, which presents with cortical atrophy on CT scans, associated features of dementia and a usually irreversible course.

Korsakoff's Syndrome

Korsakoff's syndrome is an amnestic disorder caused by thiamine deficiency. Although generally associated with alcohol abuse, it can occur in other malnourished states such as marasmus, gastric carcinoma and HIV spectrum disease (Reulen *et al.*, 1985; Victor, 1987). This syndrome is usually associated with Wernicke's encephalopathy, which involves ophthalmoplegia,

ataxia and confusion. Korsakoff's syndrome is often associated with a neuropathy and occurs in about 85% of untreated patients with Wernicke's disease (Kaplan *et al.*, 1994). Complete recovery from Korsakoff's syndrome is rare.

Head Injury

Head injuries can produce a wide variety of neurological and psychiatric disorders, even in the absence of radiological evidence of structural damage. Delirium, dementia, mood disturbances, behavioral disinhibition, alterations of personality and amnestic disorders may result (Torres *et al.*, 2001). Amnesia in head injury is for events preceding the incident and the incident itself, leading some physicians to consider these patients as having factitious disorders or being malingerers. The eventual duration of the amnesia is related to the degree of memory recovery that occurs in the first few days after the injury. Amnesia after head injury has become a popular plot device in novels and motion pictures, many of which are depictions that erroneously suggest that a second blow to the head is curative

Differential Diagnosis

Amnestic disorders must be differentiated from the less disruptive changes in memory that occur in normal aging, the memory impairment that is accompanied by other cognitive deficits in dementia, the amnesia that might occur with clouded consciousness in delirium, the stress-induced impairment in recall seen in dissociative disorders, and the inconsistent amnestic deficits seen in factitious disorder and malingering.

Treatment

As in delirium and dementia, the primary goal in the amnestic disorders is to discover and treat the underlying cause. Because some of these causes of amnestic disorder are associated with dangerous self-damaging behavior (e.g., suicide attempts by hanging, carbon monoxide poisoning, deliberate motor vehicle accidents, self-inflicted gunshot wounds to the head and chronic alcohol abuse), some form of psychiatric involvement is often necessary. In the hospital, continuous reorientation by means of verbal redirection, clocks and calendars can allay the patient's fears. Supportive individual psychotherapy and family counseling are beneficial.

References

AIDS Surveillance Report (2002) Centers for Disease Control, February.

American Psychiatric Association (1994) *Diagnostic and Statistical Manual of Mental Disorders*, 4th edn. APA, Washington DC, pp. 123–174.

Berg R, Franzen M and Wedding D (1994) Neurological disorders, in *screening for Brain Impairment*, 2nd edn. Springer-Verlag, New York.

Bick KL (1994) Early story of Alzheimer's disease, in *Alzheimer's Disease* (eds Terry RD, Katzman R and Bick KL). Raven Press, New York.

Corder EH, Saunder AM, Strittmatten WJ *et al.* (1993) Gene dose of apolipoprotein E type 4 allele and the risk of Alzheimer's disease in late onset families. *Science* 261, 921–923.

Crapper DR and Dalton AJ (1972) Alterations in short term retention, conditioned avoidance response, acquisition and motivation following aluminum-induced neurofibrillary degeneration. *Physiol Behav* 10, 925–933.

Cummings JL and Benson DF (1983) *Dementia: A Clinical Approach*. Butterworth, Boston.

Erkinjuntii T, Wikstrom J, Paolo J *et al.* (1986) Evaluation of 2000 consecutive admissions. *Arch Intern Med* 146, 1923–1926.

Francis J, Martin D and Kapoor W (1990) A prospective study of delirium in hospitalized elderly. *JAMA* 263, 1097–1101.

Frierson RL, Wey JJ and Tabler JB (1991) Psychostimulants for depression in the medically ill. *Am Fam Phys* 43, 163–170.

Henderson AS (1990) Epidemiology of dementia disorders. *Adv Neurol* 51, 15–25.

Heyman A, Fillenbaum G, Prosnitz B *et al.* (1991) Estimated prevalence of dementia among elderly black and white community residents. *Arch Neurol* 48, 594–599.

Ho D, Bredesen DE, Vinters HV *et al.* (1987) AIDS dementia complex. *Ann Intern Med* 2, 400–409.

Kallmann MH (1989) Mental status assessment in the elderly. *Prim Care* 16, 329–347.

Kaplan H, Sadock B and Grebb J (1994) *Kaplan and Sadock's Synopsis of Psychiatry,* 7th edn. Williams & Wilkins, Baltimore.

Karp H (1984) Dementia in adults, in *Clinical Neurology*, Vol. 3 (eds Baker AB and Baker LH). Harper & Row, New York, pp. 1–32.

Katzman R and Kawas C (1994) Epidemiology of dementia and Alzheimer's disease, in *Alzheimer's Disease* (eds Terry RD, Katzman R and Bick KL). Raven Press, New York, pp. 105–123.

Kaufman D (1990a) Aphasia and related disorders, in *Clinical Neurology for Psychiatrists*. WB Saunders, Philadelphia, pp. 146–171.

Kaufman D (1990b) Dementia, in *Clinical Neurology for Psychiatrists*. WB Saunders, Philadelphia, pp. 107–146.

Kidd M (1963) Paired helical filaments in electron microscopy of Alzheimer's disease. *Nature* 197, 192–193.

Kirk T, Roache JD and Griffiths RR (1990) Dose–response evaluation of the amnestic effects of triazolam and pentobarbital in normal subjects. *J Clin Psychopharmacol* 10, 160–167.

Korvath T, Siever L, Mohs R *et al.* (1989) Organic mental syndromes and disorders, in *Comprehensive Textbook of Psychiatry* V, Vol. I (eds Kaplan H and Sadock B). Williams & Wilkins, Baltimore, pp. 599–642.

Lipowski ZJ (1987) Delirium (acute confusional states). *JAMA* 258, 1789–1792.

Lipowski ZJ (1989) Delirium in the elderly patient. *New Engl J Med* 320, 578–582.

Prusiner SB (1987) Prions and neurodegenerative diseases. *New Engl J Medicine* 317, 1571.

Reulen JB, Girard DE and Cooney TG (1985) Wernicke's encephalopathy. *New Engl J Med* 312, 1035–1039.

Saito T (1987) Presenting symptoms and natural history of Wilson's disease. *Eur J Pediatr* 146, 261–265.

Slaby AE and Erle SR (1993) Dementia and delirium, in *Psychiatric Care of the Medical Patient* (ed Stoudemire A). Oxford University Press, New York, pp. 415–455.

Summers WK, Majorski LV, March GM *et al.* (1986) Oral tetrahydroaminoacridine in long term treatment of senile dementia, Alzheimer type. *New Engl J Med* 315, 1241–1245.

Tarter RE and Schneider DU (1976) Blackouts: Relationship with memory capacity and alcoholism history. *Arch Gen Psychiatr* 33, 1492–1495.

Torres R, Mittal D and Kennedy R (2001) Use of quetiapine in delirium. *Psychosomatics* 42, 347–349.

Victor M (1987) *The Wernicke–Korsakoff Syndrome*, 2nd edn. FA Davis, Philadelphia.

Victor M and Adams RD (1974) Common disturbances of vision, ocular movement, and hearing, in *Harrison's Principles of Internal Medicine*, Vol. I, 7th edn. Wintrobe MM, Thron GW, and Adams RD (eds). McGraw-Hill, New York, pp. 100–110.

Wolf JK (1980) *Practical Clinical Neurology*. Medical Examination Publishing, Garden City, NY.

Wolfson LI and Katzman R (1983) The neurological consultation at age 80, in *Neurology of Aging* (eds Katzman R and Terry RD). FA Davis, Philadelphia, pp. 221–244.

Mental Disorders Due to a General Medical Condition

Introduction

This chapter deals with disorders characterized by mental symptoms which occur due to the direct physiological effect of a general medical condition. In evaluating patients with mental symptoms of any sort, one of the first questions to ask is whether those symptoms are occurring as part of a primary psychiatric disorder or are caused by a general medical condition, and Figure 33.1 presents a decision tree designed to help in making this decision. The first step is to review the history, physical examination and laboratory tests to see if there is evidence for the presence of a general medical disorder that could plausibly cause the mental symptoms in question. In making this determination, one looks not only for a temporal correlation (e.g., the onset of a psychosis shortly after starting or increasing the dose of a medication), but also keeps in mind well-documented associations between certain mental symptoms (e.g., depression) and certain general medical conditions (e.g., Cushing's syndrome). If it appears, at this point, that the mental symptoms could indeed be occurring secondary to a general medical condition, the next step involves determining whether or not these symptoms could be better accounted for by a primary psychiatric disorder. For example, consider the case of a 45-year-old man with a history of recurrent major depression, currently euthymic, who begins a course of steroids for asthma and then, within a week, becomes depressed. The steroids are stopped but the depression continues. In this case, if the depression had cleared shortly after stopping the steroids, one might make the case that the depression occurred secondary to the steroid treatment; the persistence of the symptoms, however, argues strongly that this depression represents rather a recurrence of the major depression.

Once it appears that the mental symptoms in question could well directly result from a general medical condition and could not be better accounted for by a primary psychiatric disorder, then it remains to classify these symptoms into one of the specific types noted in Figure 33.1, and to proceed to the appropriate section below. There is also, at the end of the decision tree, a residual category for "unspecified" mental symptoms, and in this chapter two such syndromes, not uncommonly found in consult-liaison work, are included, namely pseudobulbar palsy and the Klüver–Bucy syndrome.

In caring for patients with mental disorders due to a general medical condition, the question arises as to whether or not symptomatic treatment for these mental symptoms should be offered. First, one must determine whether the mental symptoms demand emergent treatment. Consider, for example, a postictal psychosis characterized by delusions of persecution which prompt the patient

to become assaultive: here, even though the condition itself will eventually resolve spontaneously, symptomatic treatment of the psychosis is required to protect the patient or others. In cases where the mental symptoms do not present an emergency, one looks to whether the underlying general medical condition is treatable or not. For example, in the case of psychosis due to Huntington's disease, as the underlying condition is not treatable, one generally proceeds directly to symptomatic treatment. In cases where the underlying condition is treatable, then one must make a judgment as to whether, with treatment of the underlying general medical condition, the mental symptoms will resolve at a clinically acceptable rate. Consider, for example, a patient with anxiety due to hyperthyroidism who has just begun treatment with an antithyroid drug. In such a case, the decision as to whether to offer a benzodiazepine as symptomatic treatment for the anxiety depends not only on the severity and tolerability of the anxiety, but also on the expected time required for the antithyroid drug to resolve the hyperthyroidism: here, clearly, considerable clinical judgment is required.

Psychotic Disorder Due to a General Medical Condition

Definition

A psychotic disorder due to a general medical condition is characterized clinically by hallucinations or delusions occurring in a clear sensorium, without any associated decrement in intellectual abilities. Furthermore, one must be able to demonstrate, by history, physical examination or laboratory findings, that the psychosis is occurring on the basis of a general medical disorder.

Etiology and Pathophysiology

Of all the causes of psychosis, the most commonly encountered are three primary psychiatric disorders, namely, schizophrenia, schizoaffective disorder and delusional disorder, each of these being covered elsewhere in this text. Table 33.1 lists the various secondary causes of psychosis dividing them into those occurring **secondary to precipitants** (e.g., medications), those occurring **secondary to diseases with distinctive features** (e.g., the chorea of Huntington's disease) and finally a group occurring **secondary to miscellaneous causes** (e.g., cerebral tumors).

Psychosis occurring **secondary to precipitants** is perhaps the most common form of secondary psychosis. Among the various possible precipitants, substances, that is to say, drugs of abuse, are perhaps the most common, but these are treated in the

Essentials of Psychiatry   Jerald Kay and Allan Tasman
© 2006 John Wiley & Sons, Ltd.

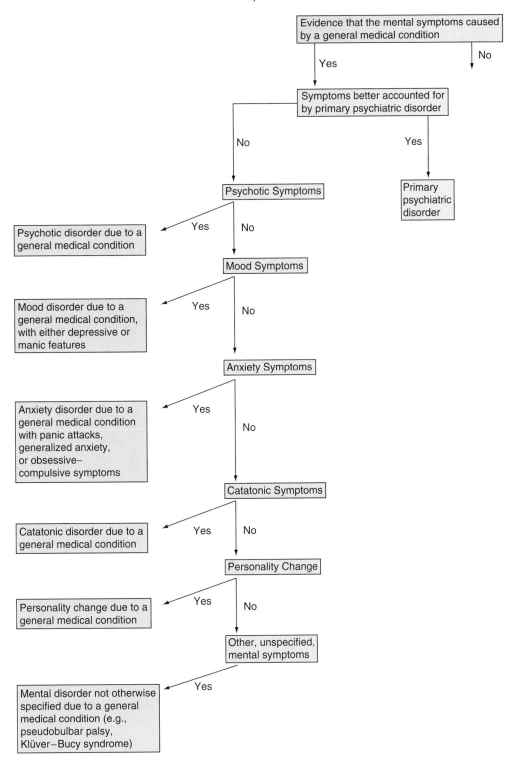

Figure 33.1 *Diagnostic decision tree.*

chapters on stimulants, hallucinogens, phencyclidine, cannabis and alcohol. After drugs of abuse, various medications are the next most common precipitants, and of the medications listed in Table 33.1, the most problematic are the neuroleptics themselves. It appears that in a very small minority of patients treated chronically with neuroleptics, a "supersensitivity psychosis" (or, as it has also been called, on analogy with tardive dyskinesia, "tardive psychosis") may occur. Making such a diagnosis in the case of patients with schizophrenia may be difficult, as one may well say that any increase in psychotic symptoms, rather than evidence for a supersensitivity psychosis, may merely represent an exacerbation of the schizophrenia; in the case of patients treated with antipsychotics for other conditions (e.g. Tourette's syndrome), however, the appearance of a psychosis is far more suggestive, as it could not be accounted for on the basis of the disease for which the neuroleptic was prescribed. Dopaminergic drugs capable

Table 33.1	Causes of Psychosis Due to a General Medical Condition

Secondary to Precipitants

Medications
  Neuroleptics (supersensitivity psychosis)
  Dopaminergic drugs
  Disulfiram
  Sympathomimetics
  Bupropion
  Fluoxetine
  Baclofen (upon discontinuation)
Other precipitants
  Postencephalitic psychosis
  Posthead trauma

Secondary to Diseases with Distinctive Features

Associated with epilepsy
  Ictal psychosis
  Postictal psychosis
  Psychosis of forced normalization
  Chronic interictal psychosis
Encephalitic onset
  Herpes simplex encephalitis
  Encephalitis lethargica
  Infectious mononucleosis With other specific features:
With other specific features:
  Huntington's disease (chorea)
  Sydenham's chorea
  Chorea gravidarum
  Manganism (parkinsonism)

Creutzfeldt–Jakob disease (myoclonus)
Hashimoto's encephalopathy (myoclonus)
Wilson's disease (various abnormal involuntary movements)
AIDS (thrush, *Pneumocystis* pneumonia)
Systemic lupus erythematosus (arthralgia, rash, pericarditis, pleurisy)
Hyperthyroidism (tremor, tachycardia)
Hypothyroidism (cold intolerance, voice change, constipation, hair loss, myxedema)
Cushing's syndrome ("Cushingoid" habitus, e.g., "moon" facies)
Adrenocortical insufficiency (abdominal complaints and dizziness)
Hepatic porphyria (abdominal pain)
Autosomal dominant cerebellar ataxia
Dentatorubropallidoluysian atrophy (ataxia)
Prader–Willi syndrome (massive obesity)

Secondary to Miscellaneous Causes

Cerebral tumors
Cerebral infarction
Multiple sclerosis
Neurosyphilis
Vitamin B_{12} deficiency
Metachromatic leukodystrophy
Subacute sclerosing panencephalitis
Fahr's syndrome
Thalamic degeneration
Velo–cardio–facial syndrome

---

of causing a psychosis include levodopa itself, and such direct-acting dopamine agonists as bromocriptine and lergotrile. The other medications noted in Table 33.1 only very rarely cause a psychosis.

Of the various encephalitidies which may have a psychosis as a sequela, the most classic is encephalitis lethargica (von Economo's disease), a disease which, though no longer occurring in epidemic form, may still be seen sporadically.

Of the psychoses **secondary to diseases with distinctive features**, the psychoses of epilepsy are by far the most important, and these may be ictal, postictal, or interictal. Ictal psychoses represent complex partial seizures and are immediately suggested by their exquisitely paroxysmal onset. Postictal psychoses are typically preceded by a "flurry" of grand mal or complex partial seizures and, importantly, are separated from the last of this "flurry" of seizures by a "lucid" interval lasting from hours to days. Interictal psychoses appear in one of two forms, namely, the psychosis of forced normalization and the chronic interictal psychosis. The psychosis of forced normalization appears when anticonvulsants have not only stopped seizures but have essentially "normalized" the EEG: a disappearance of the psychosis with the resumption of seizure activity secures the diagnosis. The chronic interictal psychosis, often characterized by delusions of persecution and reference and auditory hallucinations, appears subacutely, over weeks or months, in patients with longstanding, uncontrolled grand mal or complex partial seizures.

Encephalitic psychoses are suggested by such typical "encephalitic" features such as headache, lethargy and fever. Prompt diagnosis is critical, especially in the case of herpes simplex encephalitis, given its treatability.

The other specific features listed in Table 33.1 are fairly straightforward. In the past, the differential between Huntington's disease and schizophrenia complicated by tardive dyskinesia was difficult; today, the availability of genetic testing has greatly simplified this diagnostic task.

Of the **miscellaneous causes** capable of causing psychosis, cerebral tumors are perhaps the most important, with psychosis being noted with tumors of the frontal lobe, corpus callosum and temporal lobe. Suggestive clinical evidence for such a cause includes prominent headache, seizures, or certain focal signs, such as aphasia. Cerebral infarction is likewise an important cause, and is suggested not only by accompanying focal signs, but also by its acute onset: infarction of the frontal lobe, temporo-parietal and thalamus have all been implicated. Neurosyphilis should never be forgotten as a differential possibility in cases of psychosis of obscure origin, and an FTA (Fluorescent Treponemal Antibody) is appropriate in such cases. Vitamin B_{12} deficiency, likewise, should be borne in mind, especially as this may present with psychosis without any evidence of spinal cord or hematologic involvement. The remaining disorders listed in Table 33.1 are extremely rare causes of psychosis, and represent the "zebras" of this differential listing. Among these "zebras", however, one is of particular interest, namely velo–cardio–facial syndrome. This genetic disorder, characterized by cleft palate, cardiovascular malformations and dysmorphic facies (micrognathia and prominent nose), and, often, mental retardation, also appears, in

DSM-IV-TR Criteria 293.xx

Psychotic Disorder Due to ... [*Indicate the General Medical Condition*]

A. Prominent hallucinations or delusions.

B. There is evidence from the history, physical examination, or laboratory findings that the disturbance is the direct physiological consequence of a general medical condition.

C. The disturbance is not better accounted for by another mental disorder.

D. The disturbance does not occur exclusively during the course of a delirium.

Code based on predominant symptom:

.81 With Delusions: if delusions are the predominant symptom

.82 With Hallucinations: if hallucinations are the predominant symptom

Coding note: Include the name of the general medical condition on Axis I. e.g., 293.81 Psychotic Disorder Due to Malignant Lung Neoplasm. With Delusions: also code the general medical condition on Axis III (see Appendix G for codes).

Coding note: If delusions are part of a preexisting dementia, indicate the delusions by coding the appropriate subtype of the dementia if one is available e.g., 290.20 Dementia of the Alzheimer's Type. With Late Onset. With Delusions.

Reprinted with permission from the *Diagnostic and Statistical Manual of Mental Disorders*, Fourth Edition, Text Revision. Copyright 2000 American Psychiatric Association.

a substantial minority of cases, to cause a psychosis phenotypically very similar to that caused by schizophrenia.

Assessment and Differential Diagnosis

As noted earlier, psychotic disorder due to a general medical condition is a disorder which by definition occurs in a clear sensorium, without any associated decrement in intellectual abilities: both delirium and dementia are commonly accompanied by hallucinations and delusions, but these conditions are clearly distinguished from psychotic disorder due to a general medical condition by the presence of confusion or significant intellectual deficits. When these features are present, one should proceed to the differential for delirium and dementia described in Chapter 32 of this book (see DSM-IV criteria).

In most cases, a thorough history and physical examination will disclose evidence of the underlying cause of the psychosis in question. In those cases, however, where the patient's symptomatology is atypical for one of the primary causes of psychosis (e.g., schizophrenia), yet the history and physical examination fail to disclose clear evidence for another cause, a "laboratory screen," as listed in Table 33.2, may be appropriate. Clearly, one does not order all these tests at once, but begins with

Table 33.2	A "Laboratory Screen" for Secondary Psychosis

Serum or urine drug screen
Testosterone level (reduced in anabolic steroid abusers)
Red blood cell mean corpuscular volume (elevated in alcoholism and many cases of B_{12} deficiency)
Liver transaminases (elevated in alcoholism)
HIV testing
FTA
B_{12} levels (or, for increased sensitivity, plasma methylmalonic acid and homocysteine levels)
ANA
Antithyroid antibodies (present in Hashimoto's encephalopathy)
Thyroid profile with TSH
Cortisol and ACTH levels and 24-hour urine for free cortisol
Copper and ceruloplasmin levels
MRI
EEG
Lumbar puncture

those most likely, given the overall clinical picture, to be most informative.

Epidemiology and Comorbidity

The overwhelming majority of patients with a chronic psychosis have one of the primary disorders, that is, schizophrenia, schizoaffective disorder or delusional disorder: secondary causes of psychosis are relatively uncommon.

Course

This is determined by the underlying cause. For example, whereas a psychosis occurring secondary to a medication, such as a dopaminergic drug, generally clears within days of discontinuation of the drug, the psychosis due to a chronic condition, such as Huntington's disease, is likewise chronic.

Treatment

Treatment, if possible, is directed at the underlying cause. In those cases where such treatment is unavailable or ineffective, or where control of the psychosis is emergently required, neuroleptics are indicated. Although conventional neuroleptics, such as haloperidol, have long been used successfully, newer atypical agents, such as olanzapine or risperidone, may be better tolerated. In general, it is best to start with a low dose (e.g., 2.5 mg of haloperidol, 5 mg olanzapine or 1 mg of risperidone) with incremental increases, if necessary, performed slowly.

Mood Disorder Due to a General Medical Condition

Mood disorders due to general medical conditions may occur either with depressive features or manic features, and each is covered in turn.

Table 33.3   Causes of Depression Due to a General Medical Condition

Secondary to Precipitants

Medications
  Propranolol
  Interferon
  ACTH
  Prednisone
  Reserpine
  Alpha-methyldopa
  Nifedipine
  Ranitidine
  Bismuth subsalicylate
  Pimozide
  Subdermal estrogen/progestin
Anticholinergic withdrawal ("cholinergic rebound")
Poststroke depression
Head trauma
Whiplash

Secondary to Diseases with Distinctive Features

Hypothyroidism (hair loss, dry skin, voice change)
Hyperthyroidism (weight loss with **increased** appetite, tachycardia, and, in the elderly, atrial fibrillation or congestive heart failure)
Cushing's syndrome (moon facies, hirsutism, acne, "buffalo hump", abdominal striae)
Chronic adrenocortical insufficiency (nausea, vomiting, abdominal pain, postural dizziness)
Obstructive sleep apnea (severe snoring)

Multiple sclerosis (various focal findings)
Down syndrome
Epilepsy
  Ictal depression
  Chronic interictal depression

Occurring as Part of Certain Neurodegenerative or Dementing Disorders

Alzheimer's disease
Multi-infarct dementia
Diffuse Lewy body disease
Parkinson's disease
Fahr's syndrome
Tertiary neurosyphilis
Limbic encephalitis

Miscellaneous or Rare Causes

Cerebral tumors
Hydrocephalus
Pancreatic cancer
New-variant Creutzfeldt–Jakob disease
Hyperparathyroidism
Systemic lupus erythematosus
Pernicious anemia
Pellagra
Lead encephalopathy
Hyperaldosteronism

Mood disorder with Depressive Features

Definition

A mood disorder secondary to a general medical condition with depressive features is characterized by a prominent and persistent depressed mood or loss of interest, and by the presence of evidence, from the history, physical examination or laboratory tests, of a general medical condition capable of causing such a disturbance. Although other depressive symptoms (e.g., lack of energy, sleep disturbance, appetite change or psychomotor change) may be present, they are not necessary for the diagnosis.

Etiology and Pathophysiology

The overwhelming majority of cases of depression occur as part of one of the primary mood disorders, including major depressive disorder, dysthymic disorder, bipolar disorder, cyclothymic disorder, or premenstrual dysphoric disorder, all of which are covered elsewhere in this text. The various secondary causes of depression are listed in Table 33.3.

In utilizing Table 33.3, the first question to ask is whether the depression could be **secondary to precipitants**. Of the various possible precipitants, substances of abuse (e.g., as seen in alcoholism or during stimulant withdrawal) are very common causes, and these are treated in their respective chapters. Medications are particularly important, however it must be borne in mind that most patients are able to take the medications listed in Table 33.3 without untoward effect: consequently, before ascribing a depression to any medication it is critical to demonstrate

that the depression did not begin before the medication was begun and, ideally, to demonstrate that the depression resolved after the medication was discontinued. Anticholinergic withdrawal may occur within days after abrupt discontinuation of highly anticholinergic medications, such as benztropine or certain tricyclic antidepressants, and is characterized by depressed mood, malaise, insomnia and gastrointestinal symptoms such as nausea, vomiting, abdominal cramping and diarrhea. Poststroke depression is not uncommon, and may be more likely when the anterior portion of the left frontal lobe is involved; although spontaneous remission within a year is the rule, depressive symptoms, in the meantime, may be quite severe. Both head trauma and whiplash injuries may be followed by depressive symptoms in close to half of all cases.

Depression may occur **secondary to diseases with distinctive features**, and keeping such features in mind whenever evaluating depressed patients will lead to a gratifying number of diagnostic "pick-ups". These features are noted in Table 33.3, and are for the most part self-explanatory; depression associated with epilepsy, however, may merit some further discussion. Ictal depressions are, in fact, simple partial seizures whose symptomatology is for the most part restricted to affective changes. The diagnosis of ictal depression is suggested by the paroxysmal onset of depression (literally over seconds): although such simple partial seizures may last only minutes, longer durations, up to months, have also been reported. Interictal depressions, rather than occurring secondary to paroxysmal electrical activity within the brain, occur as a result of long-lasting changes in neuronal

Mood Disorder Due to ... [*Indicate the General Medical Condition*]

A. A prominent and persistent disturbance in mood predominates in the clinical picture, and is characterized by either (or both) of the following:

(1) depressed mood or markedly diminished interest or pleasure in all, or almost all, activities.

(2) elevated, expansive, or irritable mood.

B. There is evidence from the history, physical examination, or laboratory findings that the disturbance is the direct physiological consequence of a general medical condition.

C. The disturbance is not better accounted for by another mental disorder (e.g., Adjustment Disorder With Depressed Mood in response to the stress of having a general medical condition).

D. The disturbance does not occur exclusively during the course of a delirium.

E. The symptoms cause clinically significant distress or impairment in social, occupational, or other important areas of functioning.

Specify type:

With Depressive Features: if the predominant mood is depressed but the full criteria are not met for a Major Depressive Episode

With Major Depressive-Like Episode: if the full criteria are met (except Criterion D) for a Major Depressive Episode (see p. 327)

With Manic Features: if the predominant mood is elevated, euphoric, or irritable

With Mixed Features: if the symptoms of both mania and depression are present but neither predominates

Coding note: Include the name of the general medical condition on Axis I. e.g., 293.83 Mood Disorder Due to Hypothyroidism. With Depressive Features: also code the general medical condition on Axis III (see Appendix G for codes).

Coding note: If depressive symptoms occur as part of a preexisting dementia, indicate the depressive symptoms by coding the appropriate subtype of the dementia if one is available, e.g., 290.21 Dementia of the Alzheimer's Type. With Late Onset. With Depressed Mood.

activity, perhaps related to "kindling" within the limbic system, in patients with chronically recurrent seizures, either grand mal or, more especially, complex partial (Indaco *et al.*, 1992; Perini *et al.*, 1996). Such interictal depressions are of gradual onset and are chronic.

Depression **occurring as part of certain neurodegenerative or dementing disorders** is immediately suggested by the presence of other symptoms of these disorders, such as dementia or distinctive physical findings, for example, parkinsonism.

The **miscellaneous or rare causes** represent, for the most part, the "zebras" in the differential for depression, and should be considered when, despite a thorough investigation, the diagnosis of a particular case of depression remains unclear.

Assessment and Differential Diagnosis

Although the foregoing list of possible causes of depression due to a general medical condition is long, utilizing it in the clinical evaluation of depressed patients need not be burdensome. Evidence for most of the **precipitants, diseases with distinctive features** and **neurodegenerative or dementing disorders** will be uncovered in the course of a standard interview and examination and, after using the list a few times, the physician will immediately recognize their diagnostic relevance. The **miscellaneous or rare** "zebras," as with zebras in any other branch of medicine, are only considered when one is at the end of one's diagnostic rope, a situation often reached when patients fail to respond to treatment which, if the diagnosis were correct, should have led to relief, but did not.

Epidemiology and Comorbidity

Depression is the most common of psychiatric symptoms and although, as noted earlier, the vast majority of cases of depression occur as part of one of the primary depressive disorders (most commonly major depressive disorder), depressions due to a general medical condition, in certain settings, should nevertheless, by virtue of their frequency, receive prime diagnostic consideration. Examples include treatment with ACTH or prednisone as in multiple sclerosis or collagen–vascular diseases and cases of cerebral infarction involving the left frontal area.

Course

Most medication-induced depressions begin to clear within days of discontinuation of the offending medication; depression as part of withdrawal from stimulants or anabolic steroids clears within days or weeks, and from anticholinergics, within days. Post-stroke depression, as noted above, typically remits within a year. The course of depression secondary to head trauma or whiplash is generally prolonged, though quite variable. Most of the other conditions or disorders in the list are chronic, and depression occurring secondary to them likewise tends to be chronic: exceptions include depression in multiple sclerosis, which may have a relapsing and remitting course, corresponding to the appearance and disappearance of appropriately situated plaques.

Treatment

Treatment efforts should be directed at relieving, if possible, the underlying cause. When this is not possible, antidepressants should be considered. Controlled studies have demonstrated the effectiveness of both nortriptyline (Robinson *et al.*, 2000) and citalopram (Anderson *et al.*, 1994) for poststroke depression, and nortriptyline for depression seen in Parkinson's disease (Anderson *et al.*, 1980). For other secondary depressions, citalopram is probably a good choice, given its benign side-effect profile and notable lack of drug–drug interactions; nortriptyline should be used with caution in patients with cardiac conduction defects (as it may prolong conduction time) and in those at risk for seizures as in head trauma as this agent may also lower the seizure threshold.

Table 33.4   Causes of Mania Due to a General Medical Condition

Secondary to Precipitants

Medications
  Corticosteroids or adrenocorticoptrophic hormone
  Levodopa
  Zidovudine
  Oral contraceptives
  Isoniazid
  Buspirone
  Procyclidine
  Procarbazine
  Propafeone
  Baclofen, upon discontinuation after long-term use
  Reserpine upon discontinuation after long-term use
  Methyldopa upon discontinuation after long-term use
Closed head injury
Hemodialysis
Encephalitis
Aspartame
Metrizamide

Secondary to Diseases with Distinctive Features

Hyperthyroidism (proptosis, tremor, tachycardia)
Cushing's syndrome (moon facies, hirsutism, acne, "buffalo hump", abdominal striae)

Multiple sclerosis (various focal findings)
Cerebral infarction (sudden onset with associated localizing signs)
Sydenham's chorea
Chorea gravidarum
Hepatic encephalopathy (asterixis, delirium)
Uremia (asterixis, delirium)
Epilepsy
  Ictal mania
  Postictal mania

Occurring as Part of Certain Neurodegenerative or Dementing Diseases

Alzheimer's disease
Neurosyphilis
Huntington's disease
Creutzfeldt–Jakob disease

Miscellaneous or Rare Causes

Cerebral tumors
Systemic lupus erythematosus
Vitamin B_{12} deficiency
Metachromatic leukodystrophy
Adrenoleukodystrophy
Tuberous sclerosis

Mood Disorder with Manic Features

Definition

Mood disorder due to a general medical condition with manic features is characterized by a prominent and persistently elevated, expansive or irritable mood which, on the basis of the history, physical or laboratory examinations can be attributed to an underlying general medical condition. Other manic symptoms, such as increased energy, decreased need for sleep, hyperactivity, distractibility, pressured speech and flight of ideas, may or may not be present.

Etiology and Pathophysiology

The vast majority of cases of sustained, elevated or irritable mood occur as part of four primary disorders, namely bipolar I disorder, bipolar II disorder, cyclothymic disorder and schizoaffective disorder (bipolar type). Cases of elevated or irritable mood secondary to other causes (e.g., secondary to treatment with corticosteroids) are much less common. Table 33.4 lists secondary causes of elevated or irritable mood, with these causes divided into categories designed to facilitate the task of differential diagnosis.

In utilizing Table 33.4, the first step is to determine whether the mania could be **secondary to precipitants**. Substance-induced mood disorder related to drugs of abuse is covered in the relevant substance-related disorders chapters in this textbook. Of the precipitating factors listed in Table 33.4, medications are the most common offenders. Before, however, attributing the mania to one of these medications, it is critical to demonstrate that the mania occurred only after initiation of that medication; ideally, one would also want to show that the

mania spontaneously resolved subsequent to the medication's discontinuation. Of the medications listed, corticosteroids, such as prednisone, are likely to cause mania, with the likelihood increasing in direct proportion to dose: in one study (Wolkowitz *et al.*, 1990), 80 mg of prednisone produced mania within five days in 75% of subjects. Levodopa is the next most likely cause, and in the case of levodopa the induced mania may be so pleasurable that some patients have ended up abusing the drug (Giovannoni *et al.*, 2000). Anabolic steroid abuse may cause an irritable mania, and such a syndrome occurring in a "bulked up" patients should prompt a search for other clinical evidence of abuse, such as gynecomastia and testicular atrophy. Closed head injury may be followed by mania either directly upon emergence from postcoma delirium, or after an interval of months. Hemodialysis may cause mania, and in one case (Jack *et al.*, 1983) mania occurred as the presenting sign of an eventual dialysis dementia. Encephalitis may cause mania, as, for example, in postinfectious encephalomyelitis, with the correct diagnosis eventually being suggested by more typical signs such as delirium or seizures. Encephalitis lethargica (Von Economo's disease; European Sleeping Sickness) may also be at fault, with the diagnosis suggested by classic signs such as sleep reversal or oculomotor paralyses.

Mania occurring **secondary to disease with distinctive features** is immediately suggested by these features, as listed in Table 33.4. Some elaboration may be in order regarding mania secondary to cerebral infarction. This cause, of course, is suggested by the sudden onset of the clinical disturbance, with the mania being accompanied by various other more or less localizing signs: what is most remarkable here is the variety of structures which, if infarcted, may be followed by mania.

Thus, mania has been noted with infarction of the midbrain, thalamus (either on the right side or bilaterally, anterior limb of the internal capsule and adjacent caudate on the right, and subcortical white matter or cortical infarction on the right in the frontoparietal or temporal areas. Mania associated with epilepsy may also deserve additional comment. Ictal mania is characterized by its paroxysmal onset, over seconds and the diagnosis of postictal mania is suggested when mania occurs shortly after a "flurry" of grand mal or complex partial seizures.

Mania **occurring as part of certain neurodegenerative or dementing diseases** is suggested, in general, by a concurrent dementia, and in most cases the mania plays only a minor role in the overall clinical pictures. Neurosyphilis, however, is an exception to this rule, for in patients with general paresis of the insane (dementia paralytica) mania may dominate the picture.

Of the **miscellaneous or rare causes** of mania, cerebral tumors are the most important to keep in mind, with mania being noted with tumors of the midbrain, tumors compressing the hypothalamus, e.g., a craniopharyngioma or a pituitary adenoma, and tumors of the right thalamus, right cingulate gyrus or one or both frontal lobes.

Assessment and Differential Diagnosis

In most cases of mania **secondary to precipitants**, the cause (e.g., treatment with high dose prednisone) is fairly straightforward; in cases **secondary to diseases with distinctive features** or **occurring as part of certain neurodegenerative or dementing diseases**, the cause is generally readily discernible if the clinician is alert to the telltale distinctive features (e.g., a Cushingoid habitus) and to the presence of dementia indicating one of the dementing disorders listed in Table 33.4. The **miscellaneous or rare causes** represent the "zebras" in the differential of secondary mania, and are generally only resorted to when other investigations prove unrewarding.

As a rule, it is very rare for mania to constitute the initial presentation of any of the disease or disorders listed in Table 33.4; thus, other evidence of their presence will become evident during the routine history and physical examination. Exceptions to the rule include neurosyphilis, vitamin B_{12} deficiency and Creutzfeldt–Jakob disease, however in all these cases continued observation will eventually disclose the appearance of other evidence suggestive of the correct diagnosis.

It must always be kept in mind that certain medications (e.g., antidepressants) may precipitate mania in patients with bipolar disorder: in such cases, history will reveal earlier episodes of either depression, or mania, or both and such cases of mania should not be considered secondary.

Epidemiology and comorbidity

Relative to cases of primary mania (e.g., bipolar disorder), secondary mania is relatively rare. In certain settings, however, secondary mania may be so common as to merit a "top" position on the differential diagnosis; a prime example would be when prednisone is used in high doses, as in the treatment of multiple sclerosis or rheumatoid arthritis.

Course

Most cases of medication-induced mania begin to clear in a matter of days; for other causes, the course of the mania generally reflects the course of the underlying disease.

Treatment

Treatment, if possible, is directed at the underlying cause. In cases where such etiologic treatment is not possible, or not rapidly effective enough, pharmacologic measures are in order. Mood stabilizers, such as lithium or divalproex used in a fashion similar to that for the treatment of mania occurring in bipolar disorder, are commonly used: both lithium and divalproex are effective in the prophylaxis of mania occurring secondary to prednisone; case reports also support the use of lithium for mania secondary to zidovudine and divalproex for mania secondary to closed head injury. As between lithium and divalproex, in cases where there is a risk for seizures (e.g., head injury, encephalitis, stroke or tumors), divalproex clearly is preferable.

Clinical Vignette 1

Liebson (2000) reported the case of a 53-year-old man with a right thalamic hemorrhage, who presented with headache and left-sided hemiparesis and hemianesthesia. Four days later he displayed signficant anosognosia for his hemiparesis; more remarkable, however, was the change in his mood. One week after the stroke his "mood was remarkably cheerful and optimistic...he was noted to praise extravagantly the hospital food, and the nurses found him 'talkative'. When he arrived on our ward 11 days after the stroke he was flirtatious with female staff and boasted of having fathered 64 children. His girlfriend was surprised when he kissed her in front of the staff because he had never publicly displayed affection before. He reported excellent energy and expansively invited all the staff to his home for Thanksgiving...The mania resolved gradually over a 10-week period after (the) stroke".

In cases where emergent treatment is required, before lithium or divalproex could have a chance to become effective, oral or intramuscular lorazepam or haloperidol (in doses of 2 mg and 5 mg, respectively) may be utilized, again much as in the treatment of mania in bipolar disorder.

Anxiety Disorder Due to a General Medical Condition with Panic Attacks or with Generalized Anxiety

Definition

Pathologic anxiety secondary to a general medical condition may occur in the form of well-circumscribed and transient panic attacks or in a generalized, more chronic form. As the differential diagnoses for these two forms of anxiety are quite different, it is critical clearly to distinguish between them.

Panic attacks have an acute or paroxysmal onset, and are characterized by typically intense anxiety or fear which is accompanied by various "autonomic" signs and symptoms, such as tremor, diaphoresis and palpitations. Symptoms rapidly crescendo over seconds or minutes and in most cases the attack will clear within anywhere from minutes up to a half-hour. Although attacks tend to be similar one to another in the same patient, there is substantial interpatient variability in the symptoms seen.

Generalized anxiety tends to be of subacute or gradual onset, and may last for long periods of time, anywhere from days to

Table 33.5	Causes of Panic Attacks Due to a General Medical Condition

Partial seizures
Paroxysmal atrial tachycardia
Hypoglycemia
Angina or acute myocardial infarction
Pulmonary embolus
Acute asthmatic attack
Pheochromocytoma
Parkinson's disease

months, depending on the underlying cause. Here, some patients, rather than complaining of feeling anxious *per se*, may complain of being worried, tense or ill at ease. Autonomic symptoms tend not to be as severe or prominent as those seen in panic attacks: shakiness, palpitations (or tachycardia) and diaphoresis are perhaps most common.

Etiology and Pathophysiology

Panic attacks are most commonly seen in one of the primary anxiety disorders, namely, panic disorder, agoraphobia, specific phobia, social phobia, obsessive–compulsive disorder or post traumatic stress disorder, all of which are covered elsewhere in this book. The causes of secondary panic attacks are listed in Table 33.5. Substance-induced anxiety disorder related to drugs of abuse (e.g., cannibis, LSD) is covered in the relevant substance-related disorders chapters in this textbook. Partial seizures and paroxysmal atrial tachycardia are both characterized by their exquisitely paroxysmal onset, over a second or two; in addition, paroxysmal atrial tachycardia is distinguished by the prominence of the tachycardia and by an ability, in many cases, to terminate the attack with a Valsalva maneuver. Hypoglycemia is often suspected as a cause of anxiety, but before the diagnosis is accepted, one must demonstrate the presence of "Whipple's triad": hypoglycemia (blood glucose $\leq$45 mg/dL), typical symptoms, and the relief of those symptoms with glucose. Angina or acute myocardial infarction can present with a panic attack, with the diagnosis being suggested by the clinical setting, for example, multiple cardiac risk factors. A pulmonary embolus, at the moment of its lodgment in a pulmonary artery, may also present with a panic attack, and again here the correct diagnosis is suggested by the clinical setting, for example, situations, such as prolonged immobilization, which favor deep venous thrombosis. Acute asthmatic attacks are suggested by wheezing, and pheochromocytoma by associated hypertension. Parkinson's disease patients treated with levodopa may experience panic attacks during "off" periods.

Generalized anxiety is most commonly seen in the primary psychiatric disorder, generalized anxiety disorder, and is discussed elsewhere in this book. The secondary causes of generalized anxiety are listed in Table 33.6. Sympathomimetics and theophylline, as used in asthma and COPD, are frequent causes, as are many of the antidepressants. Hyperthyroidism is suggested by heat intolerance and proptosis, and Cushing's syndrome by the typical Cushingoid habitus (i.e., moon facies, hirsutism, acne, "buffalo hump" and abdominal striae). Hypocalcemia may be suggested by a history of seizures or tetany. Both chronic obstructive pulmonary disease and congestive heart failure are suggested by marked dyspnea. Stroke and severe head trauma may be followed by chronic anxiety, but this is seen in only a minority of these patients.

DSM-IV-TR Criteria 293.89

Anxiety Disorder Due to ... [Indicate the General Medical Condition]

A. Prominent anxiety, Panic Attacks, or obsessions or compulsions predominate in the clinical picture.

B. There is evidence from the history, physical examination, or laboratory findings that the disturbance is the direct physiological consequence of a general medical condition.

C. The disturbance is not better accounted for by another mental disorder (e.g., Adjustment Disorder With Anxiety in which the stressor is a serious general medical condition).

D. The disturbance does not occur exclusively during the course of a delirium.

E. The disturbance causes clinically significant distress or impairment in social, occupational, or other important areas of functioning.

Specify if:

With Generalized Anxiety: if excessive anxiety or worry about a number of events or activities predominates in the clinical presentation

With Panic Attacks: if Panic Attacks (see p. 395) predominate in the clinical presentation

With Obsessive–Compulsive Symptoms: if obsessions or compulsions predominate in the clinical presentation

Coding note: Include the name of the general medical condition on Axis I, e.g., 293.89 Anxiety Disorder Due to Pheochromocytoma. With Generalized Anxiety; also code the general medical condition on Axis III (see Appendix G for codes).

Reprinted with permission from the *Diagnostic and Statistical Manual of Mental Disorders*, Fourth Edition, Text Revision. Copyright 2000 American Psychiatric Association.

Assessment and Differential Diagnosis

Should one be fortunate enough to observe a patient during the panic attack, it is critical, in addition to carefully noting the specific symptoms of the attack, to obtain vital signs, auscultate the

Table 33.6	Causes of Generalized Anxiety Due to a General Medical Condition

Sympathomimetics
Theophylline
Various antidepressants (tricyclics, SSRIs, etc.)
Hyperthyroidism
Cushing's syndrome
Hypocalcemia
Chronic obstructive pulmonary disease
Congestive heart failure
Poststroke
Posthead trauma

heart and lungs, perform an EKG, and obtain blood for glucose and toxicology.

In evaluating a patient who complains of chronic anxiety, it is important, before deciding that this is, indeed, a case of pathologic generalized anxiety, first to determine whether or not the patient has a depression, whether it be primary or secondary: depression is often accompanied by anxiety, and such anxiety clears upon adequate treatment of the depression. Assuming that the patient, however, is not depressed, a work-up should include the following: auscultation of the heart and lungs; CBC and liver enzymes (looking for the telltale "alcoholic" combination of an elevated mean corpuscular volume and elevated transaminases); thyroid profile; cortisol level and calcium level.

Epidemiology and Comorbidity
Although epidemiologic studies are lacking, the clinical impression is that anxiety secondary to a general medical condition is common.

Course
This is determined by the underlying cause.

Treatment
Treatment is directed at the underlying cause, and this is sufficient for all cases of secondary panic attacks and most cases of secondary generalized anxiety: exceptions include poststroke and posthead trauma anxiety, and in these cases benzodiazepines have been used with success.

Mood Disorder with Obsessive–Compulsive Symptoms

Definition
Obsessions consist of unwanted, and generally anxiety-provoking, thoughts, images or ideas which repeatedly come to mind despite patients' attempts to stop them. Allied to this are compulsions, which consist of anxious urges to do or undo things, urges which, if resisted, are followed by rapidly increasing anxiety which can often only be relieved by giving into the compulsion to act. The acts themselves which the patients feel compelled to perform are often linked to an apprehension on the patients' part that they have done something that they ought not to have done or have left undone something which they ought to have done. Thus, one may feel compelled repeatedly to subject the hands to washing to be sure that all germs have been removed, or repeatedly to go back and check on the gas to be sure that it had been turned off.

Etiology and Pathophysiology
In the vast majority of cases, obsessions and compulsions occur as part of certain primary psychiatric disorders, including obsessive–compulsive disorder, depression, schizophrenia and Tourette's syndrome. Those rare instances where obsessions and compulsions are secondary to a general medical condition or medication are listed in Table 33.7.

In most cases, these causes of secondary obsessions or compulsions are readily discerned, as for example, a history of encephalitis, anoxia, closed head injury or treatment with clozapine. Sydenham's chorea is immediately suggested by the appearance of chorea, however, it must be borne in mind that obsessions and compulsions may constitute the presentation of Sydenham's chorea, with the appearance of chorea being delayed for days

Table 33.7	Causes of Obsessions and Compulsions Due to a General Medical Condition

Postencephalitic
Postanoxic
Postclosed head injury
Clozapine
Sydenham's chorea
Huntington's disease
Simple partial seizures
Infarction of the basal ganglia or right parietal lobe
Fahr's syndrome

(Swedo *et al.*, 1989). Ictal obsessions or compulsions, constituting the sole clinical manifestation of a simple partial seizure, may, in themselves, be indistinguishable from the obsessions and compulsions seen in obsessive–compulsive disorder, but are suggested by a history of other seizure types, for example, complex partial or grand mal seizures. Infarction of the basal ganglia or parietal lobe is suggested by the subacute onset of obsessions or compulsions accompanied by "neighborhood" symptoms such as abnormal movements or unilateral sensory changes. Fahr's syndrome, unlike the foregoing, may be an elusive diagnosis, only suggested perhaps when CT imaging incidentally reveals calcification of the basal ganglia.

Assessment and Differential Diagnosis
Most causes of secondary obsessions and compulsions are picked up on the routine history and physical examination, with the possible exception of ictal cases, and here it is critical to make a close inquiry as to a history of other seizure types: ictal EEGs are not reliable here, as they are often normal in the case of simple partial seizures. In doubtful cases a "diagnosis by treatment response" to a trial of an anticonvulsant may be appropriate.

Epidemiology and Comorbidity
As noted earlier, secondary obsessions and compulsions are relatively rare.

Course
Although the course of obsessions and compulsions due to fixed lesions, such as those seen with head trauma or cerebral infarction tends to be chronic, some spontaneous recovery may be anticipated over the following months to a year.

Treatment
When treatment of the underlying cause is not possible, a trial of an SSRI, as used for obsessive–compulsive disorder, might be appropriate.

Mental Conditions Due to a General Medical Disorder not Elsewhere Classified

Catatonic Disorder Due to a General Medical Condition

Definition
Catatonia exists in two subtypes, namely, stuporous catatonia (also known as the akinetic or "retarded" subtype) and excited catatonia, and each will be described in turn.

Stuporous catatonia is characterized by varying combinations of mutism, immobility and waxy flexibility; associated features include posturing, negativism, automatic obedience and "echo" phenomena. Mutism ranges from complete to partial: some patients may mumble or perhaps utter brief, often incomprehensible, phrases. Immobility, likewise, ranges in severity: some patients may lie in bed for long periods, neither moving, blinking or even swallowing; others may make brief movements, perhaps to pull at a piece of clothing or to assume a different posture. Waxy flexibility, also known by its Latin name, *cerea flexibilitas*, is characterized by a more or less severe "lead pipe" rigidity combined with a remarkable tendency for the limbs to stay in whatever position they are placed, regardless of whether the patient is asked to maintain that position or not. Posturing is said to occur when patients spontaneously assume more or less bizarre postures, which are then maintained: one patient crouched low with his arm wrapped over his head, another stood with one arm raised high and the other stuffed inside his belt. Negativism entails a mulish, intractable and automatic resistance to whatever is expected, and may be either "passive" or "active". Passively negativistic patients simply fail to do what is asked or expected: if clothes are laid out they will not dress; if asked to eat or take pills, their lips remain frozen shut. Active negativism manifests in doing the opposite of what is expected: if asked to come into the office, the patient may back into the hallway or if asked to open the eyes wide to allow for easier examination, they may cramp the eyes closed. Automatic obedience, as may be suspected, represents the opposite of negativism, with affected patients doing exactly what they are told, even should it place them in danger. Echo phenomena represent a kind of automatic obedience: in echolalia patients simply repeat what they hear and in echopraxia they mimic the gestures and activity of the examiner.

It should be noted that in negativism, automatic obedience and echo phenomena there is nothing natural or fluid about the patient's behavior. To the contrary, movements are often awkward, wooden and tinged with the bizarre.

Excited catatonia manifests with varying degrees of bizarre, frenzied and purposeless behavior. Such patients typically keep to themselves: one marched in place, all the while chanting and gesticulating; another tore at his hair and clothing, broke plates in a corner then crawled under the bed where he muttered and thrashed his arms.

Etiology and Pathophysiology

Stuporous catatonia, in the majority of cases, occurs as part of such primary psychiatric disorders as schizophrenia or a depressive episode of either major depression or bipolar disorder, and these are discussed elsewhere in this text. The causes of catatonia due to a general medical condition or medications are listed in Table 33.8.

Stuporous catatonia occurring in association with epilepsy is often suggested by a history of grand mal or complex partial seizures. Ictal catatonia is further suggested by its exquisitely paroxysmal onset, and postictal catatonia by an immediately preceding "flurry" of grand mal or complex partial seizures. Psychosis of forced normalization is an interictal condition distinguished by the appearance of symptoms subsequent to effective control of seizures. The chronic interictal psychosis is also, as suggested by the name, an interictal condition which, however, appears not after seizures are controlled but rather in the setting of ongoing, chronic uncontrolled epilepsy. Of medications capable of causing catatonia, neuroleptics are by far the most common. Viral

---

DSM-IV-TR Criteria 293.89

Catatonic Disorder Due to... [*Indicate the General Medical Condition*]

A. The presence of catatonia as manifested by motoric immobility, excessive motor activity (that is apparently purposeless and not influenced by external stimuli), extreme negativism or mutism, peculiarities of voluntary movement, or echolalia or echopraxia.

B. There is evidence from the history, physical examination, or laboratory findings that the disturbance is the direct physiological consequence of a general medical condition.

C. The disturbance is not better accounted for by another mental disorder (e.g., a Manic Episode).

D. The disturbance does not occur exclusively during the course of a delirium.

Coding note: Include the name of the general medical condition on Axis I. e.g., 293.89 Catatonic Disorder Due to Hepatic Encephalopathy: also code the general medical condition on Axis III (see Appendix G for codes).

Reprinted with permission from the *Diagnostic and Statistical Manual of Mental Disorders*, Fourth Edition, Text Revision. Copyright 2000 American Psychiatric Association.

Table 33.8 Causes of Catatonia Due to a General Medical Condition

Stuporous Catatonia

Associated with epilepsy
  Ictal catatonia
  Postictal catatonia
  Psychosis of forced normalization
  Chronic interictal psychosis
Medication
  Neuroleptics
  Disulfiram
  Benzodiazepine withdrawal
Viral encephalitis
Herpes simplex encephalitis
Encephalitis lethargica
Focal lesions, especially of the frontal lobes Focal lesions, especially of the frontal lobes
Miscellaneous conditions
  Hepatic encephalopathy
  Limbic encephalitis
  Systemic lupus erythematosus
  Lyme disease, in stage III
  Subacute sclerosing panencephalitis, in stage I
  Tay–Sachs disease
  Thrombotic thrombocytopenic purpura

Excited Catatonia

Viral encephalitis

encephalitis is suggested by concurrent fever and headache: herpes simplex encephalitis should always be considered in such cases, given its treatability; further it must be kept in mind that although encephalitis lethargica no longer occurs in epidemics, sporadic cases do still occur. Focal lesions capable of causing catatonia are typically found in the medial or inferior portions of the frontal lobes. The miscellaneous conditions listed are all quite rare causes of catatonia.

Excited catatonia, in the vast majority of cases, is caused by either schizophrenia or bipolar disorder (during a manic episode): only rarely is it seen due to a general medical condition, as for example, a viral encephalitis.

Assessment and Differential Diagnosis

Stuporous catatonia must be distinguished from akinetic mutism and from stupor of other causes. Akinetic mutes appear quite similar to immobile and mute catatonics: akinetic mutes, however, lack such signs as waxy flexibility, posturing and negativism, all of which are typically seen in catatonia. Stupor of other causes is readily distinguished from catatonic stupor by the salient fact that catatonics remain alert, in stark contrast with the somnolence or decreased level of consciousness seen in all other forms of stupor.

Excited catatonia must be distinguished from mania. Mania is typified by hyperactivity, which at times may be quite frenzied: the difference with catatonia is that patients with mania want to be involved, whereas those with catatonia keep to themselves; as Kraepelin (Bear *et al.*, 1982) noted, in catatonia "the excitement, even when extremely violent, frequently takes place within the *smallest space* .... The patients have not as a rule any tendency to influence their surroundings, but their restlessness exhausts itself in wholly aimless activity…".

Epidemiology and Comorbidity

Stuporous catatonia due to a general medical condition overall is, in general, a rare condition.

Course

This is determined by the course of the underlying cause.

Treatment

In addition to treating, if possible, the underlying cause, catatonia may be symptomatically relieved by lorazepam given parenterally in a dose of 2 mg; in severe cases wherein lorazepam is not sufficiently effective and the patient is at immediate risk, consideration should be given to emergency ECT, which is typically dramatically effective, generally bringing relief after but a few treatments.

Personality Change Due to a General Medical Condition

Definition

The personality of an adult represents a coalescence of various personality traits present in childhood and adolescence, and is generally quite enduring and resistant to change. Thus, the appearance of a significant change in an adult's personality is an ominous clinical sign and indicates the presence of intracranial pathology. Patients themselves may not be aware of the change, however to others, who have known the patient over time, the change is often quite obvious: such observers often note that the patient is "not himself" anymore.

DSM-IV-TR Criteria 310.1

Personality Change Due to … [*Indicate the General Medical Condition*]

A. A persistent personality disturbance that represents a change from the individual's previous characteristic personality pattern. (In children, the disturbance involves a marked deviation from normal development or a significant change in the child's usual behavior patterns lasting at least 1 year).

B. There is evidence from the history, physical examination, or laboratory findings that the disturbance is the direct physiological consequence of a general medical condition.

C. The disturbance is not better accounted for by another mental disorder (including other Mental Disorders Due to a General Medical Condition).

D. The disturbance does not occur exclusively during the course of a delirium and does not meet criteria for a dementia.

E. The disturbance causes clinically significant distress or impairment in social, occupational, or other important areas of functioning.

Specify type:

Labile Type: if the predominant feature is affective lability

Disinhibited Type: if the predominant feature is poor impulse control as evidenced by sexual indiscretions, etc.

Aggressive Type: if the predominant feature is aggressive behavior

Apathetic Type: if the predominant feature is marked apathy and indifference

Paranoid Type: if the predominant feature is suspiciousness or paranoid ideation

Other Type: if the predominant feature is not one of the above, e.g., personality change associated with a seizure disorder

Combined Type: if more than one feature predominates in the clinical picture

Unspecified Type

Coding note: Include the name of the general medical condition on Axis I, e.g., 310.1 Personality Change Due to Temporal Lobe Epilepsy: also code the general medical condition on Axis III (see Appendix G for codes).

Reprinted with permission from the *Diagnostic and Statistical Manual of Mental Disorders*, Fourth Edition, Text Revision. Copyright 2000 American Psychiatric Association.

In most cases, the change is nonspecific in nature: there may be either a gross exaggeration of hitherto minor aspects of the patient's personality or the appearance of a personality trait quite uncharacteristic for the patient. Traits commonly seen in a personality change, as noted in DSM-IV-TR, include lability, disinhibition, aggressiveness, apathy, or suspiciousness.

In addition to these nonspecific changes, there are two specific syndromes which, though not listed in DSM-IV-TR, are well-described in the literature, namely, the **frontal lobe syndrome** and the **interictal personality syndrome** (also known as the "Geschwind syndrome").

The **frontal lobe syndrome** is characterized by a variable mixture of disinhibition, affective changes, perseveration and abulia. Disinhibition manifests with an overall coarsening of behavior. Attention to manners and social nuances is lost: patients may eat with gluttony, make coarse and crude jokes, and may engage in unwelcome and inappropriate sexual behavior, perhaps by propositioning much younger individuals or masturbating in public. Affective changes tend toward a silly, noninfectious euphoria; depression, however, may also be seen. Perseveration presents with a tendency to persist in whatever task is currently at hand, and patients may repeatedly button and unbutton clothing, open and close a drawer or ask the same question again and again. Abulia is characterized by an absence of desires, urges or interests, and such patients, being undisturbed by such phenomena, may be content to sit placidly for indefinite periods of time. Importantly, such abulic patients are not depressed, nor are they incapable of activity: indeed, with active supervision they may be able to complete tasks; however, once supervision stops, so too do the patients, as they lapse back into quietude.

The **interictal personality syndrome**, a controversial entity (Bear *et al.*, 1982; Rodin and Schmaltz, 1984) is said to occur as a complication of longstanding uncontrolled epilepsy, with repeated grand mal or complex partial seizures. The cardinal characteristic of this syndrome is what is known as "viscosity", or, somewhat more colloquially, "stickiness". Here, patients seem unable to let go or diverge from the current emotion or train of thought: existing affects persist long after the situation which occasioned them, and a given train of thought tends to extend itself indefinitely into a long-winded and verbose circumstantiality or tangentiality. This viscosity of thought may also appear in written expression as patients display "hypergraphia", producing long and rambling letters or diaries. The inability to "let go" may even extend to such simple acts as shaking hands, such that others may literally have to extract their hand to end the handshake. The content of the patient's viscous speech and writing generally also changes, and tends toward mystical or abstruse philosophical speculations. Finally, there is also a tendency to hyposexuality, with an overall decrease in libido (Blumer, 1970).

Etiology and Pathophysiology

A personality change is not uncommonly seen as the prodrome to schizophrenia, however in such cases the eventual appearance of the typical psychosis will indicate the correct diagnosis.

Personality change of the nonspecific or of the frontal lobe type, as noted in Table 33.9, may occur **secondary to precipitants** (e.g., closed head injury), **secondary to cerebral tumors** (especially those of the frontal or temporal lobes) or **as part of certain neurodegenerative or dementing disorders**. Finally, there is a group of **miscellaneous causes**. In Table 33.9, those disorders or diseases which are particularly prone to cause a personality change of the frontal lobe type are indicated by an asterisk. The interictal personality syndrome occurs only in the setting of chronic repeated grand mal or complex partial seizures, and may represent microanatomic changes in the limbic system which have been "kindled" by the repeated seizures (Adamec and Stark-Adamec, 1983; Bear, 1979).

Table 33.9	Causes of Personality Change of the Nonspecific or Frontal Lobe Type

Secondary to Precipitants

Closed head injury
Head trauma with subdural hematoma
Postviral encephalitis
Gunshot wounds
Cerebral infarction
Secondary to Cerebral Tumors
Frontal lobe*
Corpus callosum*
Temporal lobe

Occurring as Part of Certain Neurodegenerative or Dementing Disorders

Pick's disease*
Fronto-temporal dementia*
Alzheimer's disease*
Amyotrophic lateral sclerosis*
Progressive supranuclear palsy*
Cortico-basal ganglionic degeneration*
Multiple system atrophy*
Huntington's disease
Wilson's disease
Lacunar syndrome* (Ishii *et al.*, 1986)
Normal pressure hydrocephalus
AIDS
Neurosyphilis
Creutzfeldt–Jakob disease

Miscellaneous Causes

Granulomatous angiitis
Vitamin B_{12} deficiency
Limbic encephalitis
Metachromatic leukodystrophy
Adrenoleukodystrophy
Mercury intoxication
Manganism

*Particularly likely to cause a frontal lobe syndrome.

In the case of personality change occurring **secondary to precipitants**, the etiology is fairly obvious; an exception might be cerebral infarction, but here the acute onset and the presence of "neighborhood" symptoms are suggestive. In addition to infarction of the frontal lobe, personality change has also been noted with infarction of the caudate nucleus and of the thalamus.

Personality change occurring **secondary to cerebral tumors** may not be accompanied by any distinctive features, and indeed a personality change may be the only clinical evidence of a tumor for a prolonged period of time.

Personality change **occurring as part of certain neurodegenerative or dementing disorders** deserves special mention, for in many instances the underlying disorder may present with a personality change; this is particularly the case with Pick's disease, fronto-temporal dementia and Alzheimer's disease. The inclusion of amyotrophic lateral sclerosis here may be surprising to some, but it is very clear that, albeit in a small minority, cerebral symptoms may not only dominate the early course of ALS, but may even constitute the presentation of the disease. In the case of the other neurodegenerative disorders (i.e., progressive supranuclear palsy, cortico–basal ganglionic degeneration, multiple system atrophy, Huntington's disease and Wilson's disease) a personality change, if present, is typically accompanied by abnormal involuntary movements of one sort or other, such as parkinsonism, ataxia or chorea. The lacunar syndrome, occurring secondary to multiple lacunar infarctions affecting the thalamus, internal capsule or basal ganglia, deserves special mention as it very commonly causes a personality change of the frontal lobe type by interrupting the connections between the thalamus or basal ganglia and the frontal lobe. Normal pressure hydrocephalus is an important diagnosis to keep in mind, as the condition is treatable: other suggestive symptoms include a broad-based shuffling gait and urinary urgency or incontinence. AIDS should be suspected whenever a personality change is accompanied by clinical phenomena suggestive of immunodeficiency, such as thrush. Neurosyphilis may present with a personality change characterized by slovenliness and disinhibition. Creutzfeldt–Jakob disease may also present with a personality change, and this appears particularly likely with the "new variant" type: the eventual appearance of myoclonus suggests the correct diagnosis.

The **miscellaneous causes** represent the diagnostic "zebras" in the differential for personality change. Of them two deserve comment, given their treatability: granulomatous angiitis is suggested by prominent headache, and vitamin B_{12} deficiency by the presence of macrocytosis or a sensory polyneuropathy.

Assessment and Differential Diagnosis

Personality change must be clearly distinguished from a personality disorder. The personality disorders (e.g., antisocial personality disorder, borderline personality disorder), all discussed elsewhere in this book, do not represent a change in the patient's personality but rather have been present in a lifelong fashion. In gathering a history on a patient with a personality change, one finds a more or less distinct time when the "change" occurred; by contrast, in evaluating a patient with a personality disorder, one can trace the personality traits in question in a more or less seamless fashion back into adolescence, or earlier.

The frontal lobe syndrome, at times, may present further diagnostic questions, raising the possibility of either mania, when euphoria is prominent, or depression, when abulia is at the forefront. Mania is distinguished by the quality of the euphoria, which tends to be full and infectious in contrast with the silly, shallow and noninfectious euphoria of the frontal lobe syndrome. Depression may be distinguished by the quality of the patients' experience: depressed patients definitely feel something, whether it be a depressed mood or simply a weighty sense of oppression. By contrast, the patient with abulia generally feels nothing: the "mental horizon" is clear and undisturbed by any dysphoria or unpleasantness.

MRI scanning is diagnostic in most cases: where this is uninformative, further testing is dictated by one's clinical suspicions (e.g., HIV testing).

The interictal personality syndrome must be distinguished from a personality change occurring secondary to a slowly growing tumor of the temporal lobe. In some cases, very small tumors, which may escape detection by routine MRI scanning, may cause epilepsy, and then, with continued growth, also cause a personality change. Thus, in the case of a patient with epilepsy who develops a personality change, the diagnosis of the interictal personality syndrome should not be made until a tumor has been ruled out by repeat MRI scanning.

Epidemiology and Comorbidity

Personality change is common, and is seen with especial frequency after closed head injury and as a prodrome to the dementia occurring with such neurodegenerative disorders as Pick's disease, fronto-temporal dementia and Alzheimer's disease.

Course

This is determined by the underlying cause; in the case of the interictal personality syndrome it appears that symptoms persist even if seizure control is obtained.

Treatment

Treatment, if possible, is directed at the underlying cause. Mood stabilizers (i.e., lithium, carbamazepine or divalproex) may be helpful for lability, impulsivity and irritability; propranoalol, in high dose, may also have some effect on irritability. Neuroleptics (e.g., olanzapine, risperidone, haloperidol) may be helpful when suspiciousness or disinhibition are prominent. Antidepressants (e.g., an SSRI) may relieve depressive symptoms. Regardless of which agent is chosen, it is prudent, given the general medical condition of many of these patients, to "start low and go slow". In many cases, some degree of supervision will be required.

Mental Disorder not Otherwise Specified Due to a General Medical Condition

This is a residual category in DSM-IV for those clinical situations in which the mental disorder occurring secondary to a general medical condition does not fall into one of the specific categories described earlier. Of these various disorders, two are worthy of detailed description, namely, pseudobulbar palsy and the Klüver–Bucy syndrome. Both disorders are commonly seen in dementia clinics, and their occurrence often prompts a request for psychiatric consultation.

Pseudobulbar Palsy

Definition

When fully developed, this syndrome is characterized by emotional incontinence (also known as "pathological laughing and crying"), dysarthria, dysphagia, a brisk jaw-jerk and gag reflex, and difficulty in protruding the tongue.

The most remarkable aspect of the syndrome is the emotional incontinence. Here, patients experience uncontrollable paroxysms of laughter or crying, often in response to minor stimuli, such as the approach of the physician to the bedside (Lieberman and Benson, 1977). Importantly, despite the strength of these outbursts, patients do not experience any corresponding sense of mirth or sadness; some may attempt to stop the emotional display, only to become acutely distressed at their inability to do so: one patient, who experienced "gales

Table 33.10	Causes of Pseudobulbar Palsy
Vascular Disorders	
Large vessel cortical infarctions	
Subcortical lacunar infarctions	
Binswanger's disease	
CADASIL	
Certain Neurodegenerative Disorders	
Amyotrophic lateral sclerosis	
Progressive supranuclear palsy	
Alzheimer's disease	
Miscellaneous Causes	
Cerebral tumors	
Closed head injury	
Multiple sclerosis	
Behçet's syndrome	

of laughter" whenever he attempted to speak, "felt foolish and ashamed, and had tears in his eyes because he could not 'control the laughter' " (Davison and Kelman, 1939). Some may go out of their way to avoid having these paroxysms. In one case, described by Wilson (1924), the patient "used to walk about the hospital with his eyes glued to the ground (because) if he so much as raised them to meet anyone else's gaze he was immediately overcome by compulsory laughter, which sometimes lasted for 4 or 5 minutes".

Etiology and Pathophysiology

Pseudobulbar palsy results from bilateral interruption of corticobulbar fibers, with this interruption occurring anywhere from the cortex through the centrum semiovale to the internal capsule and down to the midbrain and pons. Thus "released" from upper motor neuron control, the bulbar nuclei act reflexively, creating, in a sense, a kind of "spasticity" of emotional display. The various disorders capable of causing such a bilateral interruption are listed in Table 33.10.

Vascular disorders are by far the most common cause of bilateral interruption of the corticobulbar tracts, as may be seen with infarctions of the cortex or with lacunar infarctions in the corona radiata or internal capsule. Although in some cases it appears that the syndrome occurs after only one stroke, further investigation typically reveals evidence of a preexisting lesion on the contralateral side, a lesion which had been clinically "silent" (Besson *et al.*, 1991). Other vascular causes include Binswanger's disease, characterized by diffuse white matter damage in the centrum semiovale, and CADASIL (Cerebral Autosomal Dominant Arteriopathy with Subcortical Infarcts and Leukoencephalopathy), characterized by both subcortical infarctions and a widespread leukoencephalopathy.

Of the **neurodegenerative disorders** associated with pseudobulbar palsy, the most prominent is amyotrophic lateral sclerosis, wherein approximately one-half of patients are eventually so affected (Gallagher, 1989).

Of the **miscellaneous causes**, cerebral tumors which bilaterally compress or invade the brainstem are particularly important.

Assessment and Differential Diagnosis

The diagnosis should be suspected whenever patients present with exaggerated and uncontrollable emotional displays. Lability of affect, as may be seen in mania, is ruled out by the fact that the labile patient, while displaying the affect, also experiences a congruent emotional feeling: by contrast, in emotional incontinence the patient often feels nothing, except perhaps consternation at the unmotivated and uncontrollable emotional display. Inappropriate affect, as may be seen in schizophrenia, is similar to emotional incontinence in that patients with schizophrenia may not experience any corresponding feeling: in schizophrenia, however, one sees other accompanying symptoms, such as mannerisms, hallucinations and delusions, symptoms which are absent in pseudobulbar palsy. "Emotionalism", as may be seen after strokes, may suggest the diagnosis, especially given the clinical setting, however here, as with lability, patients also experience a concurrent feeling that is congruent with the emotional display.

Findings on the neurologic examination are also helpful. Bilateral interruption of corticobulbar tracts, as noted above, typically leads to cranial nerve dysfunction with dysarthria, dysphagia and brisk jaw-jerk and gag reflexes. Given the proximity of the corticospinal tracts, one often also finds evidence of long-tract damage, such as hemiplegia or Babinski signs.

MRI scanning is generally diagnostic in cases secondary to vascular lesions, tumors and multiple sclerosis. Amyotrophic lateral sclerosis is suggested by the gradual progression of upper and lower motor neuron signs and symptoms; progressive supranuclear palsy by the presence of parkinsonism and supranuclear gaze palsy, and Alzheimer's disease by the long history of a gradually progressive dementia.

Epidemiology and Comorbidity

Pseudobulbar palsy is not uncommon: as noted above, it is found in almost half of patients with amyotrophic lateral sclerosis. It may also be seen in a much smaller, but still clinically significant, proportion of patients with vascular lesions, Alzheimer's disease and multiple sclerosis.

Course

The overall course of the syndrome reflects the course of the etiologic disorder. The appearance of dysphagia, however, is an ominous sign, carrying, as it does, the risk of aspiration.

Treatment

In addition to treating, if possible, the underlying cause, various medications may be used to reduce the severity of the emotional incontinence, including tricyclics and SSRIs. Among the tricyclics, both amitriptyline (in doses of 50–75 mg) and nortriptyline (in doses up to 100 mg) are effective, with nortriptyline generally better tolerated. Of the SSRIs, citalopram, in a dose of 20 mg, was effective, and there are also case reports of the effectiveness of paroxetine, sertraline and fluoxetine (Seliger and Hornstein, 1989). Overall, it is probably best to begin with an SSRI, and to hold nortriptyline in reserve.

Klüver–Bucy Syndrome

Definition

In 1939, Klüver and Bucy (1939) noted some striking behavioral changes in monkeys which had been subjected to bilateral temporal lobectomy, and in so doing described the syndrome that now bears their names. The full syndrome is characterized by hypermetamorphosis (excessive tendency to take notice and attend and react to every visual stimulus), agnosia, hyperorality, emotional placidity and hypersexuality. Some examples of the syndrome in humans follow.

The first example demonstrates hypersexuality, hyperorality, agnosia and emotional placidity. The patient was a 31-year-old woman, who, after recovering from a herpes simplex encephalitis, "made inappropriate sexual advances to female attendants, both manually and orally. At home, she was constantly chewing and swallowing, and all objects within reach were placed in her mouth… including toilet paper and faeces… Her affect was characterized by passivity and a pet-like compliance with those attending her" (Lilly *et al.*, 1983).

The second example provides examples of hypermetamorphosis, hyperorality, agnosia and hypersexuality. The patient, a 58-year-old man who had suffered from Alzheimer's disease for 6 years, "spent much of his time examining ordinary objects such as the doorstep, ashtrays, or spots on the floor. He placed many objects in his mouth and occasionally ate soil from plant containers… he rubbed his genitals so frequently that he developed an excoriation on the shaft of his penis" (Lilly *et al.*, 1983).

Finally, there is the case of a 46-year-old man, who, during a complex partial seizure, "was observed grabbing for objects on his bedside table, and he masturbated in front of the nursing staff. He also placed objects in his mouth, chewed on tissue paper, and attempted to drink from his urine container" (Nakada *et al.*, 1984). Here, there are hypermetamorphosis, hypersexuality, hyperorality and agnosia.

Etiology and Pathophysiology

The various causes of the Klüver–Bucy syndrome are listed in Table 33.11: in each case, bilateral damage or dysfunction of the temporal lobes has occurred. The mechanism of such bilateral damage in the case of precipitants is fairly straightforward. The neurodegenerative disorders listed have a predilection for the temporal lobes, and this is particularly the case in Pick's dis-

Table 33.11 Causes of The Klüver–Bucy Syndrome
Secondary to Precipitants
Bilateral temporal lobectomy
Head trauma with bilateral damage to temporal lobes
Herpes simplex encephalitis
Status epilepticus
Heat stroke
Occurring as Part of Certain Neurodegenerative Disorders
Pick's disease
Fronto-temporal dementia
Alzheimer's disease
Miscellaneous Causes
Ictal
Postictal
Adrenoleukodystrophy

ease and fronto-temporal dementia. Indeed, the appearance of the Klüver–Bucy syndrome early in the course of a dementia is a significant diagnostic clue to one of these two disorders; in the case of Alzheimer's disease, the syndrome, if it does occur, is generally seen only late in the course. Of the miscellaneous causes, an ictal Klüver–Bucy syndrome is suggested by its exquisitely paroxysmal onset and by the occurrence of other symptoms typical for a complex partial seizure, such as confusion, and a postictal Klüver–Bucy syndrome by the history of an immediately preceding generalized seizure. Adrenoleukodystrophy, the last in the list, is an extremely rare cause of the Klüver–Bucy syndrome.

Assessment and Differential Diagnosis

The combination of hyperorality and hypersexuality often brings the patient to medical attention: although the full syndrome presents little diagnostic difficulty, as it is not mimicked by any other condition, partial syndromes, consisting primarily of hypermetamorphosis and hypersexuality, may suggest mania. The differential rests on the presence or absence of pressured speech and activity, findings typical of mania but absent in the Klüver–Bucy syndrome.

Epidemiology and Comorbidity

The full Klüver–Bucy syndrome is, overall, rare; in dementia clinics, however, full or partial Klüver–Bucy syndromes are commonly seen.

Course

The course depends on the underlying cause; in some cases, the syndrome itself may have a fatal outcome, as in the following clinical vignette.

Treatment

The underlying cause, if possible, is treated. In chronic cases, neuroleptics have been reported to be helpful; there are, however, no controlled studies.

Comparison of DSM-IV/ICD-10 Diagnostic Criteria

The DSM-IV-TR Category Psychotic Disorder Due to a General Medical Condition is referred to in ICD-10 as "organic hallucinosis" or "organic delusional disorder" depending on the type of presenting symptom.

In contrast to DSM-IV-TR which requires clinically significant mood symptoms of any type, the ICD-10 Diagnostic Criteria for Research for Mood Disorder Due to a General Medical Condition require that the full symptomatic and duration criteria be met for a hypomanic, manic, or major depressive episode. This disorder is referred in ICD-10 as "organic mood disorder". Also in contrast to DSM-IV-TR which requires anxiety symptoms of any type, the ICD-10 Diagnostic Criteria for Research for Anxiety Disorder Due to a General Medical Condition require that the clinical picture meet full symptomatic and duration criteria for panic disorder or generalized anxiety disorder.

For catatonic disorder due to a general medical condition, the ICD-10 Diagnostic Criteria for Research are more narrowly defined than the criteria in DSM-IV-TR by virtue of requiring both catatonic stupor/negativism "and" excitement and that there be a rapid alternation of stupor and excitement. In ICD-10, this disorder is referred to as "organic catatonic disorder".

The DSM-IV-TR category of Personality Change Due to a General Medical Condition corresponds to two ICD-10 categories: "organic personality disorder" and "organic emotionally labile disorder". The ICD-10 Diagnostic Criteria for Research for Organic Personality Disorder are probably more narrowly defined in that "at least three" features characteristic of a personality change are required.

References

Adamec DE and Stark-Adamec C (1983) Limbic kindling in animal behavior: Implications for human psychopathology associated with complex partial seizures. *Biol Psychiatr* 18, 269–274.

Anderson G, Vestergaard K and Lauritzen L (1994) Effective treatment of poststroke depression with the selective serotonin reuptake inhibitor citalopram. *Stroke* 25, 1099–1104.

Anderson J, Aabro E, Gulmann N et al. (1980) Antidepressive treatment in Parkinson's disease: A controlled trail of the effect of nortriptyline in patients with Parkinson's disease treated with 1-dopa. *Acta Neurol Scand* 62, 210–219.

Bear D, Levin K, Blumer D et al. (1982) Interictal behavior in hospitalized temporal lobe epileptics: Relationship to idiopathic psychiatric syndrome. *J Neurol Neurosurg Psychiatr* 45, 481–488.

Bear DM (1979) Temporal lobe epilepsy: A syndrome of sensory–limbic hyperconnection. *Cortex* 15, 357–369.

Besson G, Bogousslavsky J, Regli F et al. (1991) Acute pseudobulbar or suprabulbar palsy. *Arch Neurol* 48, 501–507.

Blumer D (1970) Hypersexual episodes in temporal lobe epilepsy. *Am J Psychiatr* 126, 1099–1106.

Davison C and Kelman H (1939) Pathologic laughing and crying. *Arch Neurol Psychiatr* 42, 595–643.

Gallagher JP (1989) Pathologic laughter and crying in ALS: A search for their origin. *Acta Neurol Scand* 80, 114–117.

Giovannoni G, O'Sullivan JD, Turner K et al. (2000) Hedonistic homeostatic dysregulation in patients with Parkinson's disease on dopamine replacement therapies. *J Neurol Neurosurg Psychiatry* 68, 423–428.

Indaco A, Carrieri PB, Nappi C et al. (1992) Interictal depression in epilepsy. *Epilepsy Res* 12, 45–50.

Ishii N, Nishihara Y and Imamura T (1986) Why do frontal lobe symptoms predominate in vascular dementia with lacunes? *Neurology* 36, 340–345.

Jack RA, Rivers-Bulkeley NT and Rabin PL (1983) Single case study: Secondary mania as a presentation of progressive dialysis encephalopathy. *J Nerv Ment Dis* 171, 193–195.

Klüver H and Bucy PC (1939) Preliminary analysis of functions of the temporal lobes in monkeys. *Arch Neurol Psychiatr* 42, 979–1000.

Lieberman A and Benson DF (1977) Control of emotional expression in pseudobulbar palsy. *Arch Neurol* 34, 717–719.

Liebson E (2000) Anosognosia and mania associated with right thalamic hemorrhage. JH *Neurol Neurosurg Psychiatry* 68, 107–108.

Lilly R, Cummings JL, Benson DF et al. (1983) The human Klüver–Bucy syndrome. *Neurology* 33, 1141–1145.

Nakada T, Lee H, Kwee IL et al. (1984) Epileptic Klüver–Bucy syndrome: Case report. *J Clin Psychiatr* 45, 87–88.

Perini GI, Tosin C, Carraro C et al. (1996) Interictal mood and personality disorders in temporal lobe epilepsy and juvenile myoclonic epilepsy. *J Neurol Neurosurg Psychiatr* 61, 601–605.

Robinson RG, Schultz SK, Castillo C et al. (2000) Nortriptyline versus fluoxetine in the treatment of depression and in short-term recovery after stroke: A placebo-controlled, double-blind study. *Am J Psychiatr* 157, 351–359.

Rodin E and Schmaltz S (1984) The Bear–Fedio personality inventory and temporal lobe epilepsy. *Neurology* 34, 591–596.

Seliger GM and Hornstein A (1989) Serotonin, fluoxetine and pseudobulbar affect. *Neurology* 39, 1400.

Swedo SE, Rapoport JL, Cheslow DL, et al. (1989) High prevalence of obsessive-compulsive symptoms in patients with Sydenham's chorea. *Am J Psychiatr* 146, 246–249.

Wilson SAK (1924) Some problems in neurology. No. II. Pathological laughing and crying. *J Neurol Psychopathol* 4, 299–333.

Wolkowitz OM, Rubinow D, Doran AR et al. (1990) Prednisone effects on neurochemistry and behavior. *Arch Gen Psychiatr* 47, 963–968.

34 General Approaches to Substance and Polydrug Use Disorders

Definition

Substance Abuse and Dependence

The definitions of substance abuse and dependence are based on the dependence syndrome of Griffith Edwards (Edwards and Gross, 1976). Substance abuse is a maladaptive pattern of substance use leading to significant adverse consequences manifested by psychosocial, medical, or legal problems or use in situations in which it is physically hazardous that must recur during a 12-month period. Since a diagnosis of substance dependence preempts a diagnosis of abuse, tolerance, withdrawal and compulsive use are generally not present in individuals with a diagnosis of substance abuse. Since caffeine and nicotine generally do not cause psychosocial or legal problems and since it is not physically hazardous to use caffeine and nicotine, a diagnosis of abuse does not apply to these substances. The two abuse criteria focusing on legal and interpersonal problems are not among the dependence criteria. In the following chapters on substance abuse, readers will be referred to the DSM-IV TR criteria presented in this chapter as the outlines for specific disorders.

Substance Intoxication

Substance intoxication is a reversible substance-specific syndrome with maladaptive behavioral or psychological changes developing during or shortly after using the substance. It does not apply to nicotine. Recent use can be documented by a history or toxicological screening of body fluids (urine or blood). Different substances may produce similar or identical syndromes and, in polydrug users, intoxication may involve a complex mixture of disturbed perceptions, judgment and behavior that can vary in severity and duration according to the setting in which the substances were taken. Physiological intoxication is not in and of itself necessarily maladaptive and would not justify a diagnosis of the DSM-IV-TR category substance intoxication. For example, caffeine-induced tachycardia with no maladaptive behavior does not meet the criteria for substance intoxication.

Substance Withdrawal

Substance withdrawal is a syndrome due to cessation of, or reduction in, heavy and prolonged substance use. It causes clinically significant impairment or distress and is usually associated with substance dependence. Most often the symptoms of withdrawal

---

DSM-IV-TR Criteria

Substance Abuse

A. A maladaptive pattern of substance use leading to clinically significant impairment or distress, as manifested by one (or more) of the following, occurring within a 12-month period:

(1) recurrent substance use resulting in a failure to fulfill major role obligations at work, school, or home (e.g., repeated absences or poor work performance related to substance use; substance-related absences, suspensions, or expulsions from school; neglect of children or household)

(2) recurrent substance use in situations in which it is physically hazardous (e.g., driving an automobile or operating a machine when impaired by substance use)

(3) recurrent substance-related legal problems (e.g., arrests for substance-related disorderly conduct)

(4) continued substance use despite having persistent or recurrent social or interpersonal problems caused or exacerbated by the effects of the substance (e.g., arguments with spouse about consequences of intoxication, physical fights)

B. The symptoms have never met the criteria for substance dependence for this class of substance.

Reprinted with permission from the *Diagnostic and Statistical Manual of Mental Disorders*, Fourth Edition, Text Revision. Copyright 2000 American Psychiatric Association.

---

are the opposite of intoxication with that substance. The withdrawal syndrome usually lasts several days to 2 weeks.

Etiology and Pathophysiology

The cause of substance addiction depends on a variety of biological, psychological and social factors. Biological factors can include genetic predisposition as well as neurobiological

Essentials of Psychiatry   Jerald Kay and Allan Tasman
© 2006 John Wiley & Sons, Ltd.

DSM-IV-TR Criteria

Substance Intoxication

A. The development of a reversible substance-specific syndrome due to recent ingestion of (or exposure to) a substance. Note: Different substances may produce similar or identical syndromes.

B. Clinically significant maladaptive behavioral or psychological changes that are due to the effect of the substance on the central nervous system (e.g., belligerence, mood lability, cognitive impairment, impaired judgment, impaired social or occupational functioning) and develop during or shortly after use of the substance.

C. The symptoms are not due to a general medical condition and are not better accounted for by another mental disorder.

Reprinted with permission from the *Diagnostic and Statistical Manual of Mental Disorders*, Fourth Edition, Text Revsion. Copyright 2000 American Psychiatric Association.

DSM-IV-TR Criteria

Substance Withdrawal

A. The development of a substance-specific syndrome due to the cessation of (or reduction in) substance use that has been heavy and prolonged.

B. The substance-specific syndrome causes clinically significant distress or impairment in social, occupational, or other important areas of functioning.

C. The symptoms are not due to a general medical condition and are not better accounted for by another mental disorder.

Reprinted with permission from the *Diagnostic and Statistical Manual of Mental Disorders*, Fourth Edition, Text Revsion. Copyright 2000 American Psychiatric Association.

substrates for positive and negative reinforcement by abused substances (Nestler, 2000). Family genetic studies have found rates of substance dependence three to four times higher in identical twins than in dizygotic twins (Cloninger, 1999). Although no single biological marker or specific genetic defect has been confirmed, work has suggested that some alleles associated with variations in the dopamine receptor may be more common in substance-dependent individuals than in those who are not dependent. Similarly, risk factor studies have found that the sons of individuals suffering from alcoholism have a general hyporesponsiveness to alcohol and sedative drugs, when compared with the sons of individuals without alcoholism.

Psychological factors related to etiology include high rates of depressive disorders and sensation seeking, which are found in substance addiction. The association of sensation seeking with substance addiction suggests not only that drugs enhance pleasant sensations, such as a high, but also that abused drugs may provide potential control of aggressive impulses. Whether abused drugs

serve as self-medication for individuals with these psychological disturbances (e.g., depression and impulsivity) has not been resolved clearly because the age at onset for major psychiatric disorders, such as depression, is older than the age at onset for substance abuse and dependence (Khantzian, 1985). Childhood precursors of substance abuse and dependence, including shy and aggressive behaviors, can also be precursors of later depressive disorders as well as of antisocial personality disorder – the adult expression of aggressive impulsivity.

Finally, social factors, including peer and family influences, which are not dependent on genetic inheritance, are important in leading to initial drug exposure. Kandel (1975) has conducted longitudinal studies of "gateway drug" usage by adolescents, and these original concepts have been expanded over the last 25 years to recognize their treatment implications. These gateway drugs are tobacco, alcohol and marijuana. Adolescents who begin using gateway drugs in their early teens are more likely to have substance dependence in their twenties than are adolescents who begin use in their late teens. Delaying the initiation of these gateway drugs and their associated intoxication by 1 to 2 years substantially decreases the later risk of the development of substance dependence. This association between early gateway drug use and later dependence may be related to the relatively higher rates of conduct disorder and failure to complete school in those who acquire a substance-related disorder in early adolescence. Life stressors related to peers and family are also possible causative factors in substance dependence and their associated comorbid psychiatric disorders.

Special Issues in the Psychiatric Examination

Two special issues in the psychiatric examination of substance dependence include 1) the source of information when obtaining the history of the substance abuse, and 2) the management of aberrant behaviors. Information about a patient's substance abuse history can be provided not only by the patient but also by employers, family members and school officials. When patients self-report the amount of substance abused, there is a tendency to underreport the severity and duration of abuse, particularly if the patient is being referred to treatment by an outside source such as the family, the employer, or the legal system. Objective verification of the exact amount of substance use is sometimes difficult but the critical issues in arriving at a diagnosis of substance dependence do not depend on the precise amount of substance abused. Tolerance and withdrawal can be assessed independently by using tests such as the naloxone challenge and the barbiturate tolerance test. In general, significant others' estimates of the amount of drug use by the patient can be a good source of data. Thus, the initial evaluation of substance abuse and dependence may involve a wider range of interviews than would occur with many other types of psychiatric patients.

Aberrant behaviors potentially requiring management include intoxication, violence, suicide, impaired cognitive functioning and uncontrolled affective displays. The evaluation of an intoxicated substance abuser can address only a limited number of issues. These issues are primarily related to the safety of the substance abuser and other individuals who may be affected by his or her actions. Thus, a medical evaluation for signs of overdose or major cognitive impairment is critical, with consideration of detaining the patient for several hours or even days if severe complications are evident. Intoxication with sedating drugs such

DSM-IV-TR Criteria

Substance Dependence

A maladaptive pattern of substance use, leading to clinically significant impairment or distress, as manifested by three (or more) of the following, occurring at any time in the same 12-month period:

(1) tolerance, as defined by either of the following:

    (a) a need for markedly increased amounts of the substance to achieve intoxication or desired effect

    (b) markedly diminished effect with continued use of the same amount of the substance

(2) withdrawal, as manifested by either of the following:

    (a) the characteristic withdrawal syndrome for the substance (refer to criteria A and B of the criteria sets for withdrawal from the specific substances)

    (b) the same (or a closely related) substance is taken to relieve or avoid withdrawal symptoms

(3) the substance is often taken in larger amounts or over a longer period than was intended

(4) there is a persistent desire or unsuccessful effort to cut down or control substance use

(5) a great deal of time is spent in activities necessary to obtain the substance (e.g., visiting multiple doctors or driving long distances), use the substance (e.g., chain-smoking), or recover from its effects

(6) important social, occupational, or recreational activities are given up or reduced because of substance use

(7) the substance use is continued despite knowledge of having a persistent or recurrent physical or psychological problem that is likely to have been caused or exacerbated by the substance (e.g., current cocaine use despite recognition of cocaine-induced depression, or continued drinking despite recognition that an ulcer was made worse by alcohol consumption)

Specify if:

With physiological dependence: evidence of tolerance or withdrawal (i.e., either item 1 or 2 is present)

Without physiological dependence: no evidence of tolerance or withdrawal (i.e., neither item 1 nor 2 is present)

Course specifiers (see text for definitions):

Early full remission

Early partial remission

Sustained full remission

Sustained partial remission

On agonist therapyIn a controlled environment

Reprinted with permission from the *Diagnostic and Statistical Manual of Mental Disorders*, Fourth Edition, Text Revision. Copyright 2000 American Psychiatric Association.

as alcohol can lead to significant motor and cognitive impairment, which would have an impact on a patient's capacity to drive a motor vehicle. When a patient drives a car to an evaluation and is obviously intoxicated, the psychiatrist has an obligation to prevent the patient from getting back into the driver's seat of that vehicle until the effects of that drug intoxication have worn off. This may involve contacting the police to restrain the patient from driving at least temporarily. Similar issues of police restraint can arise when an intoxicated patient becomes violent and has threatened to harm his or her employers or family members. Judgment and impulse control may be substantially affected by abused drugs, but these effects may be temporary, and a short-term preventive intervention may be sufficient to avert substantial harm to the patient or others.

    Temporary suicidal behavior may be encountered in a variety of substance addictions, particularly those with alcohol and stimulants. Suicidal ideation may be intense but may clear within hours. During the evaluation session, it is important to elicit the precipitants that led the patient to seek treatment at this time and to keep the evaluation focused on specific data needed for the evaluation of substance dependence, its medical complications and any comorbid psychiatric disorders. Many patients spend a great deal of time detailing their drug-abusing careers, but in general these stories do not provide useful material for the evaluation or for future psychotherapeutic interventions. Similarly, the evaluation should not become focused on the affective aspects of a patient's recent life because affect is frequently used as a defense to avoid discussing issues of more immediate relevance such as precipitants or to act as a pretext for obtaining benzodiazepines or other anti-anxiety agents from the physician. Abused substances have generally been a way of managing affect and these patients need to develop alternative coping strategies.

Course and Natural History

The natural history of substance dependence characteristically follows the course of a chronic relapsing disorder, although a large number of individuals who experiment with potentially abusable drugs in adolescence do not go on to acquire dependence. The initial phase of the natural history of experimenting with drugs has been well described in studies by Kandel (1975), who has used the concept of gateway drug use and its evolution into more serious drug dependence during adolescence and the early twenties. The later phases of dependence are characterized in the 20- to 30-year follow-up studies of individuals with alcoholism and those with opioid addiction by Vaillant (1988, 1983) and Laub and Vaillant (2000). He has documented the natural history after age 20 years in delinquent boys, which is most closely synonymous with having lifetime conduct disorder using DSM-IV-TR criteria, and found high mortality rates by age 40 years in those delinquent boys who later become substance users. In his most recent studies following 475 delinquent boys and 456 matched nondelinquent comparison boys from age 14 years until age 65 years he found that 13% of the delinquent and only 6% ($N = 28$) of the nondelinquent subjects died unnatural deaths. These deaths were significantly associated with abuse of alcohol during adulthood and childhood delinquency, and these two factors completely accounted for the other associations of adult crime, dysfunctional home environment and poor education with the increased mortality. Thus, abusing substances may have a critical impact on later health, but having a conduct disorder as a child increases this risk, perhaps due to related behaviors such as unwillingness to seek out appropriate health care. Clearly, these studies open more questions about the interaction of substance abuse and childhood behaviors that may not include substance abuse.

Population surveys, such as the high school senior surveys and National Institute on Drug Abuse household survey (Wallace *et al.*, 1999), have provided repeated cross-sectional data on changing trends in substance use and its associated problems. These surveys have increasingly recognized cultural differences in the course of drug use. Individuals with substance dependence also have been followed up in a variety of longitudinal treatment studies such as the Drug Abuse Treatment Outcome Studies (DATOS) (Flynn *et al.*, 1999; Simpson *et al.*, 1999). These surveys and treatment follow-up studies provide indications of how the natural history of substance abuse changes over the course of several decades. In contrast to most medical disorders, substance abuse and dependence differs because the substances of abuse change over time as epidemics come and go and as new drugs, such as the "designer drugs", are developed. The natural history of abuse and dependence on these new substances can be unique, with patterns of sustained low-level use, such as with methylenedioxymethamphetamine (Ectasy), or associated social phenomena, such as parkinsonism in abusers of fentanyl-related designer drugs. Thus, the natural history of substance abuse and dependence is determined by the type of substance used and, for polysubstance dependence, can be complicated by changing secular trends and epidemics lasting from months to decades.

Other Substance Use Disorders: Anabolic Steroids

This group of substance-induced conditions most notably includes anabolic steroids and nitrite inhalants. Both have psychoactive effects and can have consequences for the individual and broad public health, which suggest that future research may lead to their inclusion in DSM-V as separate disorders.

In 1988, a survey of male high school seniors showed that anabolic steroids had a lifetime use rate of 6.6% (Buckley *et al.*, 1988). Thus, by the late 1980s, widespread abuse of anabolic steroids was occurring among males as well as females. Multiple types of steroid derivatives were being used in order to make the lipid soluble steroids more water soluble and easier to administer than the intramuscular injections that were typically required. Because of this abuse, anabolic steroids were added to Schedule III of the Controlled Substances Act in 1990.

The clinical effects of anabolic steroids are related to a typical "cycle" 4 to 18 weeks on steroids and 1 month to 1 year off. While taking the steroids, the primary effects sought by abusers are increasing muscle mass and strength and not euphoria. In the context of an adequate diet and significant physical activity, these individuals appear quite healthy and they are unlikely to appear for treatment of their anabolic steroid abuse. However, some of the adverse cardiovascular, hepatic and musculoskeletal effects of steroids as well as virilization in women may bring these users to medical attention. Severe cases of acne can also bring some adolescents to medical attention. Abuse of other psychoactive drugs may occur in up to a third of these steroid users, but generally is relatively low compared with other substance abusers.

Heavy use can increase aggression, change libido and sexual functions, and induce mood changes with occasional psychotic features (Brower *et al.*, 1991; Su *et al.*, 1993). In studies comparing doses of 40 to 240 mg/day of methyltestosterone in a double-blind inpatient trial, irritability, mood swings, violent feelings and hostility were greater during the high dose period than at baseline. The tendency of Androgenic steroids to provoke aggression and irritability has raised concerns about violence towards family members by abusers. Prospective trials have reported mood disturbances in over 50% of body builders using anabolic steroids, as well as cognitive impairment including distractibility, forgetfulness and confusion.

Dependence symptoms have included a withdrawal syndrome with common symptoms being fatigue, depressed mood and desire to take more steroids. Other common dependence symptoms are using the substance more than intended, continuing to use steroids despite problems worsened by its use and the excessive spending of time relating to obtaining steroids. Because few clinical laboratories are equipped to conduct steroid tests and these tests are quite expensive, these signs of dependence and some common laboratory abnormalities are usually used to access the diagnosis.

Anabolic steroid abuse leads to hypertrophied muscles, acne, oily skin, needle punctures over large muscles, hirsutism in females and gynecomastia in males. Heavy users can also develop edema and jaundice. Common laboratory abnormalities include elevated hemoglobin and hematocrit, elevated low density lipoprotein cholesterol, elevated liver function tests and reduced luteinizing hormone levels.

Mental health professionals may have these patients come to their attention due to the excessive aggression, loss of sexual ability, or mood disturbances. Treatment approaches are generally symptomatically oriented towards controlling the depressed mood and the psychotic features, but longer-term interventions such as peer counseling by former body builders and group support may be of value for these users.

Comparison of DSM-IV/ICD-10 Diagnostic Criteria

The ICD-10 Diagnostic Criteria for Research for Substance Dependence are close, but not identical, to the DSM-IV-TR criteria. ICD-10 has included all seven of the DSM-IV-TR items but condenses these into five criteria and adds a sixth item tapping drug-craving behavior. Furthermore, the method for establishing clinical significance differs in the two systems. DSM-IV-TR specifies that there be a maladaptive pattern of substance use leading to clinically significant impairment or distress whereas the ICD-10 Diagnostic Criteria for Research indicate either a one month duration or repeated occurrences within a 12 month period.

The ICD-10 Diagnostic Criteria for Research corresponding to Substance Abuse is less specific than the criteria in DSM-IV-TR, requiring that there be "clear evidence that substance use was responsible for (or substantially contributed to) physical or psychological harm, including impaired judgment or dysfunctional behavior, which may lead to disability or have adverse consequences for interpersonal relationships". In ICD-10, this disorder is referred to as "Harmful Use".

The ICD-10 Diagnostic Criteria for Research for Intoxication are nearly equivalent to the DSM-IV-TR criteria. However, in contrast to the DSM-IV-TR definition of Withdrawal which specifies that the withdrawal symptoms cause clinically significant distress or impairment, the ICD-10 Diagnostic Criteria for Research for Withdrawal indicates only the presence of characteristic signs and symptoms.

References

Brower KJ, Blow FC, Young JP *et al.* (1991) Symptoms and correlates of anabolic-androgenic steroid dependence. *Br J Addict* 86(6), 759–768.

Buckley WE, Yesalis CE, Freidl KE *et al.* (1988) Estimated prevalence of anabolic steroid use among male high school seniors. *J Am Med Assoc* 260(23), 3441–3445.

Cloninger CR (1999) Genetics of substance abuse, in *Textbook of Substance Abuse Treatment*, 2nd edn, Galanter M and Kleber H (eds). American Psychiatric Press, Washington DC, pp. 59–66.

Edwards G and Gross MM (1976) Alcohol dependence: Provisional description of the clinical syndrome. *Br Med J* 1, 1058–1061.

Flynn PM, Kristiansen PL, Porto JV *et al.* (1999) Costs and benefits of treatment for cocaine addiction in DATOS. *Drug Alcohol Depend* 57(2), 167–174.

Kandel DB (1975) Stages in adolescent involvement in drug use. *Science* 190, 912–914.

Khantzian EJ (1985) The self-medication hypothesis of addictive disorders: Focus on heroin and cocaine dependence. *Am J Psychiatr* 142, 1259–1264.

Laub JH and Vaillant GE (2000) Delinquency and mortality: A 50-year follow-up study of 1000 delinquent and nondelinquent boys. *Am J Psychiatr* 157(1), 96–102.

Nestler EJ (2000) Genes and addiction. *Nat Genet* 26, 277–281.

Simpson DD, Joe GW, Fletcher BW *et al.* (1999) A national evaluation of treatment outcomes for cocaine dependence. *Arch Gen Psychiatr* 56(6), 507–514.

Su TP, Pagliaro M, Schmidt PJ *et al.* (1993) Neuropsychiatric effects of anabolic steroids in male normal volunteers. *J Am Med Assoc* 269(21), 2760–2764.

Vaillant GE (1983) *Natural History of Alcoholism*. Harvard University Press, Cambridge, MA.

Vaillant GE (1988) What can long-term follow-up teach us about relapse and prevention of relapse in addiction? *Br J Addict* 83, 1147–1157.

Wallace JM Jr., Forman TA, Guthrie BJ *et al.* (1999) The epidemiology of alcohol, tobacco and other drug use among black youth. *J Stud Alcohol* 60(6), 800–809.

Substance Abuse: Alcohol Use Disorders

Definition

Alcohol consumption occurs along a continuum, with considerable variability in drinking patterns among individuals. There is no sharp demarcation between "social" or "moderate" drinking and "problem" or "harmful" drinking. It is clear, however, that as average alcohol consumption and frequency of intoxication increase, so does the incidence of medical and psychosocial problems. The focus of this chapter is the alcohol use disorders which include alcohol abuse and alcohol dependence.

The most visible group of people affected by alcohol problems are those who have developed a syndrome of alcohol dependence and who are commonly referred to as alcoholics. In this chapter, the term alcoholic is applied specifically to those individuals with alcohol dependence. A less prominent group consists of those persons who experience problems with their drinking but who are not dependent on alcohol. These individuals are variously termed alcohol abusers, problem drinkers and harmful drinkers. These two "worlds" of alcohol problems may require different approaches to diagnosis and clinical management.

Etiology and Pathophysiology

Alcoholism is a complex, multifaceted disorder which has long been recognized to run in families. There is substantial evidence from twin research and adoption studies that a major genetic component is operative in the development of alcoholism. Nonetheless, the disorder is etiologically complex, with a variety of other vulnerability factors. It has been estimated that there is a sevenfold risk of alcoholism in first-degree relatives of alcohol-dependent individuals, with male relatives of male alcohol-dependent individuals having the greatest risk for the disorder. However, the majority of alcohol-dependent individuals do not have a first-degree relative who is alcohol dependent. This underscores the fact that the risk for alcohol dependence is also determined by environmental factors, which may interact in complex ways with genetics. In addition to studying genetic contributions to alcoholism, another approach to understanding the etiology of alcoholism is to identify distinct subtypes of alcoholics. The best known of these typologies is the Type 1/Type 2 distinction developed by Cloninger and colleagues (1981) from studies of adopted sons of Swedish alcoholics (see Table 35.1).

Type 1 alcoholics are characterized by the late onset of problem drinking, rapid development of behavioral tolerance to alcohol, prominent guilt and anxiety related to drinking, and infrequent fighting and arrests when drinking. Cloninger also termed this

Table 35.1	Cloninger's Alcoholism Typology	
	Type 1	Type 2
Onset of problem drinking	Late onset	Early onset
Tolerance	Rapid development of behavioral tolerance	Not specified
Mood issues	Prominent guilt and anxiety about drinking	Absence of guilt and anxiety about drinking
Personality traits	High reward dependence High harm avoidance Low novelty seeking	Low reward dependence Low harm avoidance High novelty seeking

Source: Adapted from Cloninger CR, Bohman M and Sigvardsson S (1981) Inheritance of alcohol abuse: Cross-fostering analysis of adopted men. *Arch Gen Psychiatr* 38, 861–868. Copyright 1981 American Medical Association

subtype "milieu-limited", which emphasizes the etiologic role of environmental factors. In contrast, Type 2 alcoholics are characterized by early onset of an inability to abstain from alcohol, frequent fighting and arrests when drinking, and the absence of guilt and fear concerning drinking. Cloninger postulated that transmission of alcoholism in Type 2 alcoholics was from fathers to sons, hence term the **male-limited** alcoholism. Differences in the two subtypes are thought to result from differences in three basic personality (i.e., temperament) traits, each of which has a unique neurochemical and genetic substrate. Type 1 alcoholics are characterized by high reward dependence, high harm avoidance and low novelty seeking. In contrast, Type 2 alcoholics are characterized by high novelty seeking, low harm avoidance and low reward dependence.

Cloninger also hypothesized that specific neurotransmitter systems underlie personality structure. Specifically, dopamine is hypothesized to modulate novelty seeking, which is characterized by frequent exploratory behavior and intensely pleasurable responses to novel stimuli. Serotonin is hypothesized to modulate harm avoidance, which is a tendency to respond intensely to aversive stimuli and their conditioned signals. Finally, norepinephrine

Essentials of Psychiatry   Jerald Kay and Allan Tasman
© 2006 John Wiley & Sons, Ltd.

is hypothesized to modulate reward dependence or the resistance to extinction of previously rewarded behavior. Although Cloninger's typology has generated substantial research, studies have failed to provide empirical support for this tridimensional personality scheme and other aspects of the classification (Glenn and Nixon, 1991; Schuckit *et al.*, 1990; Sannibale and Hall, 1998; Vaillant, 1994).

Implicit in the subtyping theories that have been developed to explain different clinical varieties of alcoholism is the notion that there are a variety of plausible etiological factors in addition to or mediated by genetic predisposition. Three such factors are pharmacological vulnerability, affective dysregulation and personality disorder. The evidence for pharmacological vulnerability as an etiological factor is based on studies showing reduced sensitivity to the effects of alcohol in adult children of alcoholics (Schuckit and Smith, 1996; Pollock, 1992). Other evidence comes from research on the effects of the alcohol metabolizing enzymes aldehyde dehydrogenase and alcohol dehydrogenase polymorphisms in individuals of Asian ancestry in which aversive reactions to the effects of alcohol are associated with reduced risk of alcohol dependence (Thomasson *et al.*, 1993). A second etiological factor is affect dysregulation, which proposes that alcoholism is caused by repeated use of alcohol to "self-medicate" negative affective states such as anxiety and depression. This theory is supported by research indicating strong associations between alcohol problems, mood disorders and life stress (Schuckit, 1985). The third etiological factor that has received considerable research support is deviance proneness or behavioral undercontrol, as indicated by hyperactivity, distractibility, sensation seeking, impulsivity, difficult temperament and conduct disorder. These conditions are hypothesized to contribute to school failure and association with deviant peers, which then provide a context for heavy drinking and drug use (Sher and Trull, 1994).

In summary, despite considerable progress in the identification of risk factors for alcoholism, the interactions among genetic, familial, psychological, interpersonal and environmental influences remain so complex that there is little consensus about etiology at this time.

Pathophysiology

Neuropharmacology

Taken in large doses, alcohol is considered to have anesthetic or depressive properties. It also has the ability to elicit euphoria when administered in small doses to susceptible persons (Begleiter and Porjesz, 1999). This phenomenon appears to be mediated by direct activation by alcohol of the mesolimbic dopaminergic circuit, particularly the ventral tegmental area (VTA) and the nucleus accumbens (NAc). Anxiolysis and relaxation also appear to be part of the spectrum of the rewarding effects of alcohol, though these effects appear to be mediated by activation of the GABAergic neurotransmitter system.

In contrast to other addictive substances (e.g., nicotine, cocaine and opioids) and despite its significant effect on dopaminergic neurotransmission, the existence of specific alcohol binding sites on neuronal membranes has not been conclusively established. The lack of an alcohol receptor has led to the hypothesis that some alcohol effects, particularly those observed when it is administered at large doses, may be explained by disturbances in fluidity of the bi-layer lipid neuronal membrane. Changes in fluidity of neuronal membranes may affect the structure and function

of neurotransmitter receptors and ion channels. However, this hypothesis has failed to explain alcohol-rewarding effects that occur at lower doses.

On the other hand, alcohol administration appears to have effects across the major neurotransmitter systems (i.e., opioidergic, serotonergic, GABAergic and glutamatergic). These systems are affected by both acute and chronic alcohol administration. They appear to play a major role in mediating the rewarding effects of alcohol by modulating the firing of dopaminergic neurons in the VTA and the release of dopamine in the NAc.

Assessment and Differential Diagnosis

Phenomenology and Variations in Presentation

The DSM-IV-TR diagnosis of **alcohol dependence** is given when three or more of the seven criteria are present (see DSM-IV-TR for alcohol dependence). Because physiological dependence is associated with greater potential for acute medical problems (particularly acute alcohol withdrawal), the first criteria to be

---

DSM-IV-TR Criteria 303.90

Alcohol Dependence

A maladaptive pattern of drinking as manifested by three or more of the following during a 12-month period:

1. Tolerance, that is, either:

a. a need for markedly more alcohol to achieve intoxication

b. markedly diminished effect despite continued consumption of the same amount of alcohol

2. Withdrawal, that is, either:

a. two or more signs or symptoms (autonomic hyperactivity, tremor, insomnia, nausea or vomiting, transient illusions or hallucinations, psychomotor agitation, anxiety, grand mal seizures) within several hours of stopping or reducing heavy, prolonged drinking (bconsuming) alcohol or a related substance (e.g., benzodiazepines) to relieve or avoid withdrawal symptoms

3. Alcohol is often consumed in larger amounts or over a longer period than was intended

4. There is a persistent desire to cut down or control drinking

5. A great deal of time is spent in drinking or recovering from drinking

6 Important social, occupational, or recreational activities are given up or reduced because of drinking

7. Drinking is continued despite knowledge of having a persistent or recurrent physical or psychological problem that is likely to have been caused or exacerbated by alcohol.

Reprinted with permission from the *Diagnostic and Statistical Manual of Mental Disorders*, Fourth Edition, Text Revision. Copyright 2000 American Psychiatric Association.

considered are tolerance and withdrawal. The remaining criteria reflect behavioral and cognitive dimensions: a) impaired control (i.e., alcohol is consumed in larger amounts or over a longer period of time than was intended; there is a persistent desire or unsuccessful efforts to cut down or control drinking; the individual continues to drink despite knowledge of a persistent or recurrent physical or psychological problem), and b) increase salience of alcohol (i.e., a great deal of time spent drinking or recovering from its effects; important social, occupational, or recreational activities are given up or reduced due to drinking).

Once a diagnosis of alcohol dependence is given, a specification is made concerning course. **Early remission** is used if no criteria (**full remission**) or fewer than three symptoms (**partial remission**) of alcohol dependence are present for at least 1 month, but less than 12 months. **Sustained remission** is used if no symptoms (**full remission**) or fewer than three symptoms (**partial remission**) of alcohol dependence are present for at least 12 months. Finally, if the individual is in a setting in which he or she has no access to alcohol, the course specifier **in a controlled environment** is added.

Alcohol abuse is considered to be present only if the individual's drinking pattern has never met criteria for alcohol dependence and he or she demonstrates a pattern of drinking that leads to clinically significant impairment or distress, as evidenced by one or more of the four criteria in DSM-IV for alcohol abuse.

In addition to alcohol abuse and dependence, there is another important group of alcohol-related disorders described in DSM-IV as alcohol-induced disorders. These will be described briefly before returning to a discussion of assessment issues.

Alcohol Intoxication

A DSM-IV diagnosis of alcohol intoxication is given when, shortly after alcohol consumption, there are maladaptive behaviors such as aggression or inappropriate sexual behavior, or there are psychological changes such as labile mood and impaired judgment. Clinical signs indicative of alcohol intoxication include slurred speech, lack of coordination, unsteady gait, nystagmus, impairment of attention and memory and, in the most severe cases, stupor and coma. Alcohol intoxication may also present with severe disturbances in consciousness and cognition (alcohol intoxication delirium), especially when large amounts of alcohol have been ingested or after alcoholic intoxication has been sustained for extended periods. Usually, this condition subsides shortly after alcohol intoxication ends. Physical and mental status examinations accompanied by analysis of blood and urine allow the clinician to rule out general medical conditions or psychiatric disorders mimicking this condition. In this regard, urine toxicology is a valuable tool in ruling out intoxication with benzodiazepines, barbiturates, or other sedatives that can present with a similar clinical picture. Collateral information from relatives or friends confirming the ingestion of alcohol is also useful, and should be actively pursued by the clinician. The blood alcohol level (BAL) is frequently used as a measure of alcohol intoxication, although this measure is less reliable in persons with a high degree of tolerance to alcohol. Alcohol is metabolized in the average adult at a rate of 1 oz or 7 to 10 g/hour. When this clearance rate is surpassed, signs of alcohol intoxication begin to appear. During the ascending limb of the BAL curve, euphoria, anxiolysis and mild deficits in coordination, attention and cognition can be observed at levels between 0.01 and 0.10%. Marked deficits in coordination and psychomotor skills, decreased attention, ataxia, impaired judgment, slurred speech and mood lability can be observed at a greater BAL. Severe intoxication, characterized by lack of coordination, incoherent thoughts, confusion, nausea and vomiting can be observed at BALs between 0.20 and 0.30. However, at these levels some heavy drinking individuals who have developed tolerance to the effects of alcohol may not appear intoxicated and may perform well on psychomotor or cognitive tasks. Stupor and loss of consciousness often occur when the BAL is between 0.30 and 0.40. Beyond this level, coma, respiratory depression and death are possible outcomes. It should also be noted that alcohol intoxication is often associated with toxicity and overdose with other drugs, particularly those with depressant effects on the CNS.

Alcohol Withdrawal

Alcohol withdrawal is a condition that follows a reduction in alcohol consumption or an abrupt cessation of drinking in alcohol-dependent individuals. In addition to significant distress, alcohol withdrawal is also associated with impairment of social, occupational and other areas of functioning. Uncomplicated cases of alcohol withdrawal are characterized by signs and symptoms of autonomic hyperactivity, and may include increased heart rate, increased blood pressure, hyperthermia, diaphoresis, tremor, nausea, vomiting, insomnia and anxiety. Onset of symptoms of uncomplicated alcohol withdrawal usually occurs between 4 and 12 hours following the last drink. Symptom severity tends to peak around the second day, usually subsiding by the fourth or fifth day of abstinence. After this period, less severe anxiety, insomnia and autonomic symptoms may persist for a few weeks, with some individuals experiencing a protracted alcohol-withdrawal syndrome up to 5 or 6 months after cessation of drinking. A small but significant number of alcohol-dependent individuals (10%) can experience complicated alcohol-withdrawal episodes. Alcohol-withdrawal delirium (also known as delirium tremens) can occur in 5% of the cases, usually between 36 and 72 hours following alcohol cessation. In addition to signs of autonomic hyperactivity, this condition is characterized by illusions, auditory, visual, or tactile hallucinations, psychomotor agitation, fluctuating cloudiness of consciousness and disorientation. Grand-mal seizures associated with alcohol-withdrawal occur in 3 to 5% of the cases, typically within the first 48 hours following reduction or cessation of drinking. In both instances of complicated alcohol withdrawal, lack or delay in instituting proper treatment is associated with an increased mortality rate. Prior history of delirium tremens and/or alcohol-withdrawal seizures, older age, poor nutritional status, comorbid medical conditions and history of high tolerance to alcohol are predictors of increased severity of alcohol withdrawal.

Alcohol-induced Persisting Amnestic Disorder

Continuous heavy alcohol consumption can lead to several neurological deficits caused by thiamin deficiency. Among them, alcohol-induced persisting amnestic disorder (AIPAD, also known as a Korsakoff's psychosis, due to the fantastic confabulatory stories described by patients suffering this condition) is prominent. Profound deficits in anterograde memory and some deficits in retrograde memory characterize this condition. Patients cannot retain or learn new information and experience profound disorientation to time and place. The severity of anterograde memory deficits typically leads Korsakoff's patients, who are unaware of their deficit, to reconstruct forgotten events by confabulating. Korsakoff's amnestic disorder is usually preceded by several episode of Wernicke's encephalopathy, characterized by confusion, ataxia, nystagmus and gaze palsies. When this condition subsides, the characteristic memory deficits of Korsakoff's psychosis become prominent.

Cessation of drinking can lead to an improvement in memory with approximately 20% of the cases demonstrating complete recovery. However, in most cases memory deficits remain unchanged, and in some instances long-term care is needed despite sobriety.

Alcohol-induced Persisting Dementia

Continuous heavy drinking is also associated with progressive and gradual development of multiple cognitive deficits characterized by memory impairment, apraxia, agnosia, or disturbances in executive functioning. These deficits cause serious impairment in social and occupational functioning and persist beyond the duration of alcohol intoxication and alcohol withdrawal. History, physical exam and laboratory tests should be utilized to determine whether these deficits are etiologically related to the toxic effects of alcohol use. Other factors associated with this condition are poor nutritional status and vitamin deficiencies, as well as history of head trauma. It is believed that this condition is associated with the repeated occurrence of Wernicke's encephalopathy. Atrophy of frontal lobes and increased ventricular size have been described in this condition. Continuous alcohol consumption exacerbates the dementia, whereas drinking cessation is associated with improvement and even recovery of cognitive deficits.

Alcohol-induced Mood Disorder

Alcohol-induced mood disorder (AIMD), characterized by depressed mood and anhedonia, as well as elevated, expansive, or irritable mood, frequently develops as a consequence of heavy drinking. Onset of symptoms can occur during episodes of alcohol intoxication or withdrawal, and may resemble a primary major depressive, manic, hypomanic, or a mixed episode. In contrast to the dysphoria and lack of energy observed during episodes of alcohol withdrawal, severity and duration of alcohol-induced mood symptoms is greater than is usually expected, warranting independent attention by the clinician. Although mood disturbances are common among alcoholic patients entering treatment (80%), alcohol-induced mood symptoms tend to subside within 2 to 4 weeks following alcohol cessation. Evidence that the mood disturbances are not better explained by a primary mood disorder should be sought by the clinician. Evidence suggesting a primary mood disorder includes onset of mood symptoms preceding onset of alcohol abuse and persistence of mood symptoms after alcohol cessation or during extended periods of abstinence. Regardless of the primary or secondary nature of mood symptoms, given the high prevalence of suicide among alcoholics, clinicians should closely monitor the patient for emerging suicidal thoughts, implementing more intensive treatment (discussed later) if necessary.

Alcohol-induced Anxiety Disorder

Although alcohol has anxyolitic properties at low doses, heavy alcohol consumption can induce prominent anxiety symptoms. Alcohol-induced anxiety (AIA) symptoms more commonly include generalized anxiety symptoms, panic attacks and phobias. In order to establish this diagnosis, clinicians must rule out other general medical conditions or psychiatric disorders that can mimic this problem. AIA may develop during alcohol intoxication or withdrawal, but its severity and duration are typically worse than the anxiety normally observed during the course of these conditions. An onset of drinking preceding the anxiety syndrome, and improvement or remission of anxiety during periods of abstinence, suggest AIAD. Monitoring the course of these symptoms for several weeks after alcohol cessation can be useful in determining their nature. Usually, a substantial improvement of anxiety will be observed during this period, suggesting a direct relationship of anxiety to alcohol. In some cases, a full remission of symptoms is not observed until after 3 to 4 weeks of abstinence.

Alcohol-induced Psychotic Disorder

This disorder is characterized by prominent hallucinations or delusions that are judged by the clinician to be due to the effects of alcohol. The psychotic symptoms usually occur within a month of an alcohol intoxication or withdrawal episode, and the patient is characteristically fully alert and oriented, lacking insight that these symptoms are alcohol-induced. Although onset of psychotic symptoms can occur during or shortly after alcohol intoxication, delirium or alcohol withdrawal delirium, alcohol-induced hallucinations, and/or delusions do not occur exclusively during the course of these conditions. Evidence that hallucinations and delusions are not part of a primary psychotic disorder include: atypical or late age of onset of psychotic symptoms, onset of alcohol drinking preceding the onset of psychiatric symptoms, and remission of psychotic episodes during extended periods of abstinence. Usually, alcohol-induced psychotic symptoms tend to subside within a few weeks of abstinence, although in a subset of patients psychotic symptoms can become chronic, requiring long-term treatment with antipsychotic medication. In these cases clinicians are obligated to consider a schizophrenic or a delusional disorder as part of the differential diagnosis.

Alcohol-induced Sleep Disorder

Heavy alcohol consumption can be associated with a prominent disturbance of sleep. At intoxicating BALs, especially when blood alcohol levels are declining, sedation and sleepiness can be observed. Alcohol intoxication induces an increase in nonrapid eye movement (NREM) sleep, whereas rapid eye movement (REM) sleep density decreases. Subsequently, there is an increase in wakefulness, restless sleep, and vivid dreams or nightmares related to a reduction in NREM sleep and a rebound in REM sleep density. During alcohol withdrawal, sleep is fragmented and discontinuous with an increase in REM sleep. After withdrawal, patients frequently complain of sleep difficulties and may experience superficial and fragmented sleep for months or years.

In contrast to the primary sleep disorders (PSD), alcohol-induced sleep disorder (AISD) is characterized by an onset of drinking preceding the sleep disturbance and by remission of symptoms during the course of sustained abstinence. AISD can occur during the course of a typical alcohol intoxication or alcohol withdrawal episode. However, duration and severity of the sleep disturbances exceed those typically observed during these conditions. Given that protracted alcohol-withdrawal symptoms are frequent among abstinent alcoholics, onset of AISD can occur up to 4 weeks after initiation of alcohol abstinence. History of a previous PSD and/or persistence of sleep disturbances for more than 4 weeks following intoxication or acute withdrawal are highly suggestive of a PSD. Differential diagnosis is complicated by the fact that heavy alcohol consumption can cooccur and exacerbate other psychiatric disorders that present with sleep disturbances (e.g., mood disorders, anxiety). Alcohol consumption can also intensify other sleep problems such as narcolepsy or breathing-related sleep disorders BRSD.

Alcohol-induced Sexual Dysfunction

Although small doses of alcohol in healthy individuals appear to enhance sexual receptivity in women and facilitate arousal to erotic stimuli in men, continuous and/or heavy drinking may cause significant sexual impairment. Alcohol-induced sexual dysfunction is characterized by impaired desire, impaired arousal and impaired orgasm, or sexual pain. It is also associated with marked distress or interpersonal conflicts. Onset of these impairments usually occurs during alcohol intoxication but duration of symptoms exceeds the uncomplicated course of alcohol intoxication. Symptoms usually subside after 3 to 4 weeks of alcohol abstinence. Persistence of symptoms beyond this time may suggest a primary sexual dysfunction (PSD) or a sexual dysfunction due to the medical complications of alcoholism (e.g., neuropathy, alcoholic-liver disease). Onset of a recurrent sexual dysfunction preceding the onset of alcohol abuse also suggests a primary disorder. Use of other substances, particularly those prescribed for the treatment of alcohol withdrawal such as benzodiazepines or barbiturates, should be ruled out as a cause of the sexual dysfunction.

Assessment of Alcohol Use Disorders

Comprehensive assessment provides the basis for an individualized plan of treatment. Depending upon the severity of alcohol dependence, the nature of comorbid medical and psychiatric pathology, the presence of social supports, and evidence of previous response to treatment, decisions can be made concerning the most appropriate intensity, setting and modality of treatment.

Although denial of alcohol-related problems is legendary among alcoholics, there is substantial evidence that a valid alcohol history can be obtained, given adequate assessment procedures and the right conditions. A complete alcohol history should include specific questions concerning average alcohol consumption, maximal consumption per drinking occasion, frequency of heavy drinking occasions and drinking-related social problems (e.g., objections raised by family members, friends, or people at work), legal problems (including arrests or near-arrests for driving while intoxicated [DWI]), psychiatric symptoms (e.g., precipitation or exacerbation of mood or anxiety symptoms), and alcohol-related medical problems (e.g., alcoholic gastritis or pancreatitis).

It is crucial that questions concerning alcohol consumption and related problems be asked nonjudgmentally in order to enhance the likelihood of accurate reporting. The optimal approach to history-taking in the substance abuse patient includes reassuring the patient that information provided will be kept confidential. The interview begins with questions that are least likely to make the patient defensive (e.g., a review of systems or psychiatric symptoms, without relating these to alcohol use), and beginning questions with **How**, rather than with **Why**, to reduce the appearance of being judgmental (Schottenfeld, 1994).

Screening

Systematic clinical assessment often begins with routine screening to identify active cases, as well as persons at risk. During the past 25 years a number of self-report screening tests have been developed to identify alcoholics as well as persons at risk of alcohol problems. The Michigan Alcoholism Screening Test (MAST), developed by Selzer (1971), is one of the most often cited instruments. It contains 25 items that ask about drinking habits, as well as social, occupational and interpersonal problems associated with excessive drinking. A total score is calculated, placing the individual along a continuum from "nonalcohol dependent" to "definitely alcohol dependent". There are several shortened versions of the MAST (e.g., the 10-item Brief MAST, the 13-item Short MAST and the 35-item Self-Administered Alcohol Screening Test – SAAST). Perhaps the most widely used alcohol screening test is the CAGE (Ewing, 1984), which contains only four questions: 1) Have you ever felt you ought to **Cut** (the "C" in CAGE) down on your drinking? 2) Have people **Annoyed** (A) you by criticizing your drinking? 3) Have you ever felt bad or **Guilty** (G) about your drinking? 4) Have you ever had a drink first thing in the morning to steady your nerves or get rid of a hangover that is, an **Eye** opener (E)? Reliability and validity studies of this test have been conducted in diverse samples (e.g., psychiatric inpatients, ambulatory medical patients, prenatal clinics), with generally acceptable levels of sensitivity. The Alcohol Use Disorders Identification Test (AUDIT) (Saunders *et al.*, 1993; Babor), a 10-item screening instrument, may be used as the first step in a comprehensive and sequential alcohol use history. The AUDIT (Table 35.2) covers the domains of alcohol consumption, symptoms of alcohol dependence and alcohol-related consequences. It has been shown to be sensitive and specific in discriminating alcoholics from nonalcoholics, and is superior to the MAST in identifying hazardous drinkers, that is, those heavy drinkers who have not yet experienced serious harm from their drinking (Bohn *et al.*, 1995). The AUDIT total score increases with the severity of alcohol dependence and related problems, and can be used as part of a comprehensive approach to early identification and patient placement. Because the misuse of both prescribed and illicit

Table 35.2	Alcohol Use Disorders Identification Test				

1. How often do you have a drink containing alcohol?

Never (0)	Monthly or less (1)	Two to four (2) times a month	Two or three (3) times a week	Four or more (4) times a week

2.* How many drinks containing alcohol do you have on a typical day when you are drinking? [Code number of standard drinks]

1 or 2 (0)	3 or 4 (1)	5 or 6 (2)	7 or 8 (3)	10 or more (4)

3. How often do you have six or more drinks on one occasion?

Never (0)	Less than (1) monthly	Monthly (2)	Weekly (3)	Daily or almost (4) daily

4. How often during the last year have you found that you were not able to stop drinking once you had started?

Never (0)	Less than (1) monthly	Monthly (2)	Weekly (3)	Daily or almost (4) daily

5. How often during the last year have you failed to do what was normally expected from you because of drinking?

Never (0)	Less than (1) monthly	Monthly (2)	Weekly (3)	Daily or almost (4) daily

6. How often during the last year have you needed a first drink in the morning to get yourself going after a heavy drinking session?

Never (0)	Less than (1) monthly	Monthly (2)	Weekly (3)	Daily or almost (4) daily

7. How often during the last year have you had a feeling of guilt or remorse after drinking?

Never (0)	Less than (1) monthly	Monthly (2)	Weekly (3)	Daily or almost (4) daily

8. How often during the last year have you been unable to remember what happened the night before because you had been drinking

Never (0)	Less than (1) monthly	Monthly (2)	Weekly (3)	Daily or almost (4) daily

9. Have you or someone else been injured as a result of your drinking?

No (0)	Yes, but not in (2) the last year	Yes, during the (4) last year

10. Has a relative or friend or a physician or other health care worker been concerned about your drinking or suggested you cut down?

No (0)	Yes, but not in (2) the last year	Yes, during the (4) last year

Record sum of individual item scores here _____.

*In determining the response categories, it has been assumed that one "drink" contains 10 g of alcohol.

drugs is common among alcoholics, screening should include other psychoactive substances, including tobacco products.

Psychiatric History and Examination

Diagnostic assessment in specialized treatment facilities, such as detoxification centers, residential programs, partial hospital programs and outpatient clinics, should be conducted with a standard interview schedule. If it is not possible to use a complete psychiatric interview, such as the Composite International Diagnostic Interview (CIDI) or the Structured Clinical Interview for DSM (SCID), then the alcohol sections of these interviews should be used. Given the lack of reliability in unstructured clinical diagnosis, it is imperative that programs specializing in the treatment of alcohol dependence use a structured interview to conduct and report their diagnostic evaluations.

An important purpose of clinical assessment is to obtain an estimate of illness severity. The number of DSM symptoms obtained using a structured interview can serve this purpose or the total score on the AUDIT screening test.

Assessment of psychological function should focus on measures of depression, anxiety and more global psychological distress. Instruments that are generally reliable, valid and accept-

able in a variety of health care settings include the Beck Depression Inventory and the Symptom Checklist 90-Revised One subscale of the ASI assesses overall psychiatric severity, including number of inpatient and outpatient treatment episodes, medication status, and lifetime and current symptomatology.

There has been considerable attention devoted to the role of motivation and patient readiness to change, as critical ingredients in treatment planning for alcoholics. The University of Rhode Island Change Assessment Scale (URICA) is a 32-item questionnaire designed to measure the stages of change across diverse problem behaviors. The URICA score profiles have been used to predict treatment response in research on addictive behaviors such as smoking and alcoholism. The readiness to change questionnaire (RCQ) (I is a short 12-item instrument developed for the same purpose.

Relevant Physical Examination and Laboratory Findings

Medical illness is a common consequence of heavy drinking and may be present in the absence of physical dependence. Early in the course individuals with alcoholism may show no physical or laboratory abnormalities. But as it progresses, it is widely manifested throughout most organ systems. A thorough physical examination is indicated if, in the history, there is evidence of medical problems. The physical examination provides essential information about the presence and extent of end-organ damage, and should be focused on the systems most vulnerable to developing alcohol-related pathology: the cardiovascular system, the gastrointestinal system, and the central and peripheral nervous systems. The physician should also be alert to other acute alcohol-related signs, including alcohol withdrawal or delirium, intoxication or withdrawal from other drugs, and the acute presentation of psychiatric symptomatology. Other systemic or nonspecific health problems associated with alcoholism include malnutrition, muscle wasting, neuritis, specific vitamin deficiencies, infectious diseases (such as tuberculosis, dermatitis, pediculosis, and hepatitis) and trauma secondary to fights and accidents.

Laboratory testing can assist the clinician in providing objective, nonjudgmental feedback to alcoholic patients on the negative physical consequences of excessive drinking. Laboratory determinations should be repeated biweekly at the initial phase of treatment, and monthly during the aftercare. Results should be graphically presented to the patient in an easy-to-comprehend format with reference to normal values. This allows the patient to appreciate the declining and eventual stabilization of laboratory indexes thereby enhancing his/her motivation to maintain sobriety.

Laboratory tests can also help to detect relapse to the extent they are sensitive to heavy drinking. Early identification of relapse can prevent the reinstatement of alcohol dependence. It can diminish adverse consequences of heavy drinking by promoting modifications to the original treatment plan and by prompting more aggressive therapeutic interventions. Finally, laboratory markers of drinking can be used to evaluate effectiveness of specific therapeutic interventions and provide funding agencies with objective treatment outcome information.

Several laboratory tests, particularly those related to hepatic function (e.g., serum transaminases, bilirubin, prothrombin time and partial thromboplastin time) have been commonly used by clinicians. Other laboratory tests (e.g., gamma-glutamyl transpeptidase [GGTP], mean corpuscular volume [MCV]) of erythrocytes can be used as objective indicators of heavy drinking. Elevation in GGTP occurs in approximately three-fourths of alcoholics before there is clinical evidence of liver disease. It is often considered to be the earliest indication of heavy alcohol consumption and is widely available clinically. GGTP levels usually return to normal limits after 4 to 5 weeks of abstinence. As with GGTP, elevations of the transaminases serum glutamic oxaloacetic transaminase (SGOT) and serum glutamic pyruvic transaminase (SGPT) are common in other liver diseases. However, elevations in the transaminases are less sensitive indicators of heavy drinking, with SGOT being elevated in 32 to 77% of alcoholics, while elevations in SGPT have been observed in 50% of alcoholics. In contrast to the use of absolute values of SGPT and SGOT, the ratio of SGPT to SGOT may provide a more accurate indicator of heavy drinking. A ratio greater than 2 is more likely to be related to heavy alcohol consumption whereas a ratio below 1 would suggest a different etiology. Elevation of MCV, which has also been associated with folate deficiency, is more prominent in alcoholics, especially among those who are smokers. Though MCV can assist clinicians in identifying patients who are drinking excessively, particularly when this marker is used in combination with GGTP or carbohydrate-deficient transferrin (CDT), this is not an efficient indicator of relapse because of the 2- to 4-month period of abstinence that is needed for its normalization.

CDT is more sensitive than most routine laboratory tests for the identification of heavy alcohol consumption. In contrast to GGTP, CDT elevations are associated with few conditions other than heavy drinking. CDT and GGTP appear to identify two different subsets of alcoholic patients. Elevations in GGTP values detect alcoholics with hepatic damage secondary to heavy drinking, whereas CDT appears to be more directly related to heavy drinking. Whenever possible, CDT and GGTP should be used together by classifying as a case individuals who have elevated scores in either test. This approach increases the likelihood of identifying individuals experiencing alcohol use disorders. CDT appears to detect relapse to heavy drinking among patients in alcohol treatment more accurately than other laboratory tests.

In a clinical setting where laboratory results are generally not immediately available, the alcohol breath test, which measures the amount of alcohol in expired air (providing an estimate of venous ethanol concentration), is valuable. Although its accuracy depends on the patient's cooperation (which in an intoxicated patient is often problematic), the alcohol breath test can be a reliable and inexpensive method for assessing recent alcohol consumption. Venous blood levels should be obtained if dangerously high levels of intoxication are suspected, when a patient is comatose, or for medical–legal purposes. A BAL greater than 150 mg/dL in a patient showing no signs of intoxication (i.e., no dysarthria, motor incoordination, gait ataxia, nystagmus, or impaired attention) can be interpreted to reflect physiological tolerance. In nontolerant individuals, a BAL in excess of 400 mg/dL can result in death, and 300 mg/dL indicates a need for emergency care.

Another laboratory evaluation that is indicated in alcoholics is a urine toxicology screen. To identify drug use that the patient may not recognize or which he or she denies is a problem, the screen should include opiates, cocaine, cannabis and benzodiazepines. Routine urinalysis, blood chemistries, hepatitis profile, complete blood count and serologic test for syphilis and (for the female patient) serum testing for pregnancy should also be obtained.

Gender and Developmental Presentations

There are substantial differences in the prevalence of alcoholism among different gender, age and racial/cultural groups. Unfortunately, the high prevalence among young adult and middle-aged males often leads to inadequate consideration of the possibility that women and the elderly may drink excessively.

Women

Women are more likely to abstain from alcohol, and if they do drink, they are more likely to consume less alcohol than men. Nevertheless, in comparison to men, problem drinking among women is more likely to be associated with negative mood states, particularly depression, anxiety and somatic symptoms. Alcoholic women identify negative emotions and interpersonal conflicts as antecedents of a relapse to drinking more frequently than men and substance-dependent women more frequently report depressive and anxiety symptoms as motivators for treatment. This is consistent with epidemiological and clinical studies which show that women who are diagnosed with alcohol or drug dependence experience higher rates of mood and anxiety disorders than their male counterparts. Furthermore, it is more common among women that mood and anxiety disorders precede the onset of substance use and dependence. Alcoholic women have a **Negative profile** of situations surrounding their alcohol use, characterized by solitary drinking and greater severity of alcohol dependence, whereas alcoholic men tend to have a **Positive profile**, characterized by social drinking and drinking in the context of positive emotions. Studies comparing male and female alcoholics have found that women are significantly older than men when a variety of alcohol-related milestones occur, including regular drunkenness, loss of control over drinking, first drinking problems, drinking to relieve withdrawal symptoms, first attempt to stop drinking and realization that alcohol use is a problem. These studies have also found that women exhibit more rapid progression than men between the time of first regular intoxication and first treatment (Randall *et al.*, 1999).

Despite drinking for fewer years at lower levels, women have an increased sensitivity to toxic effects of alcohol on body organs. Alcoholic women are more likely to develop liver damage and, in general, alcoholic liver diseases tend to progress faster among women than men. The five-year mortality rate among alcoholic women is almost twice the mortality rate of alcoholic men. Alcoholic women diagnosed with alcoholic liver disease die almost a decade younger than alcoholic men. Alcoholic women appear to be more susceptible to alcohol-induced brain damage, evidenced by greater widening of the cerebral sulci and fissures in CT scans of the brain, as well as poorer performance in cognitive testing. The concept of "telescoping" has been used to describe the course of symptom progression observed among women who, despite beginning heavy drinking later than men, experience alcohol-related problems and seek treatment sooner than men.

Since alcohol is distributed in the aqueous phase, greater body fat composition among women reduces the volume of distribution. This, combined with smaller average body mass, translates into higher BALs for women in response to a specified level of alcohol consumption. In addition, less first-pass metabolism due to less gastric oxidation of ethanol may also contribute to the higher blood levels obtained by women following an equivalent dose of ethanol. Compared with men, women with alcohol problems are also at greater risk of comorbid drug abuse/dependence. Perhaps as a consequence of these differences, women alcoholics who seek treatment do so earlier in the course of the disorder than do men.

Since heavy drinking among women is most prevalent during the child bearing years, it has important public health implications for prenatal alcohol exposure and possible fetal alcohol effects. A variety of adverse outcomes have been related to heavy drinking in pregnant women, although the minimum amount of alcohol and the pattern of consumption necessary to produce such effects are not known. Heavy drinking in pregnant women may produce malnutrition in both the mother and the fetus, as well as spontaneous abortion, preterm delivery and intrauterine growth retardation. Alcohol-related birth defects (ARBDs) are estimated to occur in as many as 1 in 100 live births The most severe manifestation of ARBDs is fetal alcohol syndrome (FAS), a constellation of morphological and developmental defects resulting from high-dose prenatal alcohol exposure. FAS is estimated to occur in 1 in 1000 to 1 in 300 live births. Prenatal or postnatal growth retardation, CNS involvement and characteristic facial dysmorphology are necessary for a diagnosis of FAS.

Since ARBDs can be avoided, the evaluation of pregnant patients should routinely include questions about alcohol and other substance use. Routine screening with an instrument such as the AUDIT, or the T-ACE (Chang, 2001), supplemented by questions concerning drug use, may also be useful with pregnant women. Those pregnant women who are identified as heavy drinkers or drug users should be designated as "high risk" and provided with specialized, comprehensive perinatal care, including rehabilitation and appropriate attention to related psychosocial disabilities.

Adolescents

There are a number of features that distinguish adolescents with alcohol abuse/dependence from adult alcoholics. As might be expected, adolescents have comparatively short histories of heavy drinking. A corollary to this is the rarity of physiological dependence on alcohol and alcohol-related medical complications among adolescents. Nonetheless, abuse of alcohol and drugs contributes in important ways to morbidity and mortality in adolescents, the leading causes of which are motor vehicle accidents, homicide and suicide. The values and behavior of the adolescent's peer group are important elements in the evaluation of alcohol use and abuse in the adolescent. The evaluation of adolescents with an alcohol disorder must also take into account other prominent developmental issues that characterize adolescence, including the conflict inherent in asserting one's independence from the family.

A number of instruments have been developed for the assessment of substance use symptoms and disorders in adolescents (Kaminer, 1994). As is generally true in dealing with adolescents, given their economic and emotional dependence, whenever possible a thorough family evaluation is important for understanding the adolescent's substance use and related problems.

The Elderly

Although heavy drinking is less prevalent in the elderly, it is nonetheless an important source of morbidity in this group. Elderly alcoholics suffer from more chronic medical problems and poorer psychosocial functioning than elderly nonalcoholics. The increased use of prescription medications in the elderly increases the potential for adverse pharmacokinetic interactions with alcohol. In addition, decreased cognitive functioning associated with heavy alcohol use can increase medication errors and noncompliance in this group.

The manifestations of alcoholism in the elderly are often more subtle and nonspecific than those observed in younger individuals. Because self-reported alcohol consumption may be particularly unreliable in the elderly, other sources of information such as family and neighbors should be used to identify heavy drinkers. The following areas should be systematically evaluated in the elderly when heavy drinking has been identified: untreated medical illness, prescription drug abuse, psychiatric comorbidity, cognitive impairment, functional assessment and need for social services.

Similar to the approach used with younger adults, alcoholism in the elderly has been classified by age of onset. It has been estimated that about two-thirds of elderly alcoholics began heavy drinking prior to age 60, while the remaining one-third began heavy drinking after the age of 60. Late-onset alcoholism appears to be more common among women and people of higher socioeconomic status and is less frequently associated with a family history of alcoholism. As might be expected, older alcoholics with early-onset alcoholism also have more alcohol-related medical and psychosocial problems and are more likely to require alcoholism treatment.

Epidemiology and Comorbidity

Patterns of Drinking and Types of Alcohol Problems in the USA

The majority (85.8%) of the US population aged 18 year and older has used alcohol in their lifetime, although only half (50.0%)

report current drinking. The highest rates of current use are among young adults aged 18 to 25 years, with males predominating. NonHispanic whites have the highest prevalence of drinking (89.3% lifetime use and 53.7% past month use), while Asians are least likely to drink (62.7% lifetime and 33.4% current). The prevalence of drinking is positively associated with education level; persons with less than a high school education are almost half as likely to report past month drinking as college graduates (33.5% compared with 62.6%).

More than 1 in 5 persons aged 18 years and older (21.4%) reported binge drinking in the past month, and more than 1 in 20 (6.1%) reported heavy alcohol use. Consistent with the prevalence of drinking, both binge and heavy drinking are more likely to be found among young adults and males. Compared with women, men are twice as likely to binge drink (defined as five or more drinks per occasion) and are four times more likely to be heavy drinkers. Asians, followed by blacks, have the lowest levels of binge drinking (11.6 and 18%, respectively); Hispanics and those reporting a mixed racial background have the highest prevalence of binge drinking (23.5 and 23.1% respectively). Heavy drinking is most often reported by those with multiple racial backgrounds (8.9%), followed by nonHispanic whites (6.5%). In contrast to the demographic correlates of any alcohol use, binge drinking and heavy alcohol use appear to have a curvilinear relationship with education level. The lowest levels of binge and heavy problem drinking are found among those with the least and most education.

Several large-scale community studies conducted since 1980 have provided estimates of the lifetime and past year prevalence of alcohol use disorders in the general population. For example, the National Comorbidity Study (NCS), a representative household survey of 8098 persons aged 15 to 54 years that was conducted between 1990 and 1992, assessed lifetime and past-year alcohol disorders using DSM-III-R criteria. The NCS estimated that the lifetime prevalence of alcohol abuse and alcohol dependence for adults 18 to 54 years old were 9.4 and 14.1%, respectively, indicating that more than one-in-five young to middle-aged adults in the USA have had a pattern of alcohol use that met criteria for lifetime alcohol disorder. The prevalences of alcohol abuse and dependence during the 12 months preceding the interview were 2.5 and 4.4%, respectively.

Narrow and colleagues (2002) applied "clinically significant" criteria to the NCS data to determine the percentage of the population who were in need of treatment, more in keeping with DSM-IV diagnostic guidelines. The revised estimates of the 12-month prevalence of clinically significant alcohol disorder is 5.2% for adults in the USA (including 6.5% of adults aged 18–54 years and 2% of adults aged 55 years or older).

Differences in the rates of disorder across the various studies have been attributed to differences in diagnostic criteria, age ranges of the samples and sampling approaches. Regardless of the differences, it should be noted that all of these studies are based on self-reports of drinking behavior and are likely to be conservative estimates of the prevalence of problem drinking due to underreporting.

Analyses of national prevalence data show that disorder rates vary by gender, age, race, ethnicity, socioeconomic status and geographic location. The prevalence of alcohol disorder is consistently found to be higher among men than women, often at a ratio of two to one or greater Substance Abuse and Mental Health Services Administration, 2000). Evidence suggests, however, that the gender differential has narrowed among more recent cohorts of young adults, in part due to an increased likelihood of early onset drinking among women and the subsequent emergence of drinking problems. The highest prevalence rates of alcohol abuse and dependence occur among young adults, with a gradual decline associated with increasing age. The highest rates of past year dependence were found among those identifying their racial/ethnic background as "multiple race" (9%). There is a negative association between education level and alcohol dependence and 1-year alcohol dependence risk is highest among the unemployed). Urban residence is associated with higher rates of alcohol dependence.

Adverse consequences of drinking include a variety of social, legal and medical problems. Overall, alcohol-related mortality in 1988 totaled 107 800 deaths, or about 5% of all deaths in the USA, putting it among the top four causes of death. Of alcohol-related deaths, approximately 17% were directly attributable to alcohol, 38% resulted from diseases indirectly attributable to alcohol and 45% were attributable to alcohol-related traumatic injury (US Department of Health and Human Service, 1994). Alcohol-related mortality declined during the last few decades of the 20th century.

Alcohol-related morbidity is manifested in virtually all organ systems. The primary chronic health hazard associated with heavy drinking is cirrhosis of the liver, which in 1988 was the ninth leading cause of death in the USA. Although the percentage of drivers in fatal crashes with BALs in excess of the legal limit has declined in recent years, alcohol intoxication remains a major contributor to this and other types of accidental injury, as well as to suicide and homicide. In addition, heavy drinking has been implicated in such health conditions as FAS, esophageal cancer, chronic pancreatitis, nutritional deficiencies, cardiomyopathy, hypertension and neurological problems. The social consequences of alcohol abuse and dependence are equally serious, with heavy drinking contributing to a variety of family, work and legal problems. The economic impact of alcoholism is substantial. Alcohol abuse and dependence contribute to unemployment, reduced productivity in the workplace and crime, as well as increased costs for health care. It has been estimated that the nonhealth related costs associated with alcohol abuse reached approximately $13 billion in 1992, owing in part to costs associated with crime committed while under the influence of alcohol. In summary, the annual cost of heavy drinking and alcohol-related disorders in the USA (both in dollars and in suffering) is enormous. Successful efforts to reduce the burden of illness attributable to alcohol could produce substantial reductions in the social, economic and personal costs of alcohol-related problems.

Psychiatric Comorbidity in Individuals with an Alcohol Use Disorder

High rates of comorbid psychiatric disorders have been found in both clinical and community samples of alcohol-dependent individuals. These studies show a consistent association between alcohol abuse/dependence and a variety of other psychiatric symptoms and disorders. The Epidemiological Catchment Area (ECA) study, for example, revealed that 36.6% of those with a lifetime alcohol use disorder received at least one other psychiatric diagnosis, which is nearly double the rate for community respondents with no lifetime alcohol disorder (Regier et al., 1990). The evidence from the NCS study showed that cooccurring disorder is more likely with alcohol dependence than alcohol abuse (Kessler et al., 1997). Among individuals with one or more psychiatric disorders, 22.3% also had a lifetime alcohol disorder, substantially greater than the overall lifetime prevalence of alcohol abuse/dependence (13.5%). Women diagnosed with an alcohol disorder appear to be at greater risk for a comorbid psychiatric disorder. The NCS found that 72% of females with a lifetime alcohol abuse diagnosis had experienced one or more cooccurring psychiatric disorders, compared with 57% of men who had a lifetime history of alcohol abuse. While the prevalence of comorbid disorders was greater with alcohol dependence, the gender differential was smaller: 86% of women and 78% of men with lifetime alcohol dependency had had other lifetime DSM-III-R disorders.

The most frequent cooccurring diagnoses are for other drug use disorders, conduct disorder, antisocial personality disorder, anxiety disorders and affective disorders. The relative risks for different types of disorder vary somewhat by gender. Among women, anxiety and affective disorders are the most common cooccurring disorders. Among men with a history of alcohol abuse or dependence, drug disorders and conduct disorder account for the largest proportion of comorbid cases.

Both community and clinical studies underscore the importance of ASPD and drug abuse/ dependence as comorbid diagnoses in individuals with an alcohol disorder. The odds ratios obtained for these disorders in community studies indicate that these associations are elevated not only as a function of greater treatment-seeking behavior in affected individuals, but also because of potential commonalities in the etiology and development of alcohol abuse/dependence. That is, genetic and/or psychosocial risk factors for the development of ASPD are likely to overlap with factors that increase risk for alcohol and drug use disorders. Similarly, the risk factors for alcohol and drug use disorders may overlap with those for schizophrenia and bipolar disorder. In contrast, although anxiety disorders and depression are highly prevalent in clinical samples of alcohol-dependent individuals, their association with alcohol dependence appears largely due to chance, since these disorders are also highly prevalent in the general population.

Given a high rate of psychiatric comorbidity, it is axiomatic that a careful psychiatric assessment be conducted in patients being seen for alcohol treatment, and that alcohol use and associated problems be evaluated in patients being seen primarily for other psychiatric conditions. Because the presence of comorbid disorders may have important implications for the development of alcoholism and its prognosis, the assessment of comorbid psychopathology is an essential element in the clinical evaluation. When comorbid diagnoses are present, an effort should be made to ascertain the order of onset of each disorder since treatment and prognosis may follow from such information.

Course and Natural History

Schuckit and colleagues (1993) found that the symptoms of alcohol dependence appear in the following sequence in a sample of male veteran alcoholics: heavy drinking during the late twenties; interference with functioning in multiple life areas during their early thirties; loss of control, followed by an intensification of social and work-related problems, and onset of medical consequences in the mid- to late thirties; and severe long-term consequences by the late thirties and early forties. However, as mentioned above, women appear to experience many of these milestones at a later age than men. The study by Schuckit and colleagues showed no effect of onset age, family history of alcoholism, or comorbid psychiatric diagnoses on the order of symptom appearance. However, other features defining the course of alcoholism, particularly the response to treatment, vary as a function of patient-related variables, including age of onset, severity of alcohol dependence and comorbid psychiatric disorders. There is consistent evidence that early age of onset is a predictor of greater severity of alcoholism and a poorer response to treatment.

Although a number of studies have shown that patients experience substantial improvement during the year following alcoholism treatment (Lindstrom, 1992), Vaillant (1983) found that treatment had minimal effects on long-term outcome. More long-term treatment outcome studies are needed to examine the impact of different kinds of alcoholism treatment on the course of the disorder. Additional studies are also needed to clarify both the prognostic significance of patient-related variables, including comorbid psychiatric disorders, and their interaction with different kinds of treatment.

Treatment

Goals, Setting and Costs of Treatment

When a determination has been made that an individual is drinking excessively, the nature, setting and intensity of the intervention must be determined in order to address the specific treatment needs of the patient. Among heavy drinkers without evidence of alcohol dependence, a brief intervention aimed at the reduction of drinking may suffice. In contrast, among alcoholics, there are typically a variety of associated disabilities, so it is necessary to address both the excessive drinking **and** problems related to it. Consequently, alcoholism treatment is best conceived of as multimodal. Table 35.3 provides an overview of the goals of alcoholism treatment. It should be noted that while total abstinence is a primary goal of treatment for persons with alcohol dependence, moderate drinking can be considered as a goal for persons with alcohol abuse.

Figure 35.1 describes a process for the management of patients with alcohol abuse and dependence. The algorithm is written from the perspective of a community-based or consultation/liaison psychiatrist who does not necessarily have specialized training in addiction medicine. Following the initial

Table 35.3 Goals of Alcoholism Treatment
Promote complete abstinence from alcohol.
Stabilize acute medical (including alcohol withdrawal) and psychiatric conditions, as needed.
Increase motivation for recovery.
Initiate treatment for chronic medical and psychiatric conditions, as needed.
Assist the patient in locating suitable housing (e.g., moving from a setting in which drinking is widespread), as needed.
Enlist social support for recovery (e.g., introduce to 12-step programs and, when possible, help the patient to repair damaged marital and other family relationships).
Enhance coping and relapse prevention skills (including social skills, identification and avoidance of high-risk situations).
Improve occupational functioning.
Promote maintenance of recovery through ongoing participation in structured treatment or self-help groups.

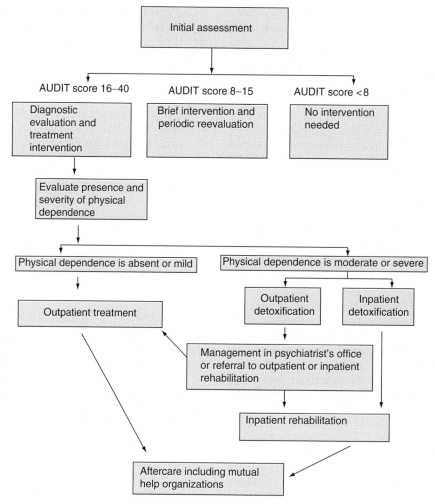

Figure 35.1   *Algorithm for the identification and management of patients with alcohol abuse and dependence.*

assessment, using a screening test like the CAGE or AUDIT, the patient is referred to either a diagnostic evaluation with a likely treatment recommendation or a brief intervention with further monitoring. Brief interventions are characterized by their low intensity and short duration. They typically consist of one to three sessions of counseling and education. They are intended to provide early intervention, before or soon after the onset of alcohol-related problems. Brief interventions seek to motivate high risk drinkers to moderate their alcohol consumption, rather than promote total abstinence with specialized treatment techniques. They are simple enough to be delivered by primary care practitioners and are especially appropriate for psychiatric patients whose at-risk drinking meets criteria for alcohol abuse rather than dependence.

If the patient's screening results and diagnostic evaluation provide evidence of alcohol dependence, the next step is to differentiate between mild and more severe levels of physical dependence to determine the need for detoxification. If withdrawal risk is low, the patient may be referred directly to outpatient therapy. If the withdrawal risk is moderate or high, outpatient or inpatient detoxification is indicated.

There are a number of potentially life-threatening conditions for which alcoholics are at increased risk. The presence of any of the following requires immediate attention: acute alco-

hol withdrawal (with the potential for seizures and delirium tremens), serious medical or surgical disease (e.g., acute pancreatitis, bleeding esophageal varices) and serious psychiatric illness (e.g., psychosis, suicidal intent). In the presence of any of these emergent conditions, acute stabilization should be the first priority of treatment.

The presence of complicating medical or psychiatric conditions is an important determinant of whether detoxification and rehabilitation are initiated in an inpatient or an outpatient setting. Other considerations are the alcoholic's current living circumstances and social support network. Women with children are sometimes unwilling to enter residential treatment unless their family needs are taken care of. Homeless people may be eager to enter residential treatment even when their medical or psychiatric condition does not warrant it.

In the alcoholic patient whose condition is stabilized or in the patient without these complicating features, the major focus should be on the establishment of a therapeutic alliance, which provides the context within which rehabilitation can occur. The presence of a trusting relationship facilitates the patient's acknowledgement of alcohol-related problems and encourages open consideration of different treatment options. In addition to participation in structured rehabilitation treatment, the patient should be made aware of the widespread availability of Alcoholics Anonymous (AA) and the wide diversity of its membership.

Residential settings include hospital-based rehabilitation programs, freestanding units and psychiatric units. With the growth of managed care in the 1990s, there has been a dramatic reduction in the average length of stay for residential treatment and a shift in emphasis to less costly outpatient treatment settings. There is no consistent evidence that intensive or inpatient residential treatment provides more benefit than less intensive outpatient treatment, but for certain kinds of patients residential treatment may have advantages (Finney and Monahan, 1996). In many populations, outpatient programs produce results comparable to those of inpatient programs.

Another approach to patient placement and treatment matching is based on the notion that patients should initially be matched to the least intensive level of care that is appropriate, and then stepped up to more intensive treatment settings if they do not respond.

Despite treatment, some alcoholics relapse repeatedly. For many emergency department personnel, the multiple recidivist alcoholic has come to personify the disorder. For clinicians involved in the delivery of alcoholism rehabilitation services, these individuals' apparent unresponsiveness to treatment may contribute to frustration and a sense of futility. Presently, long-term residential treatment appears to be the only option for alcoholics who do not respond to more limited efforts at rehabilitation. Unfortunately, the availability of such care in many states is limited as a consequence of the effort to deinstitutionalize psychiatric patients.

Finally, the importance of continuing care by means of aftercare groups, and other mutual help organizations cannot be overestimated. The value of these resources as well as the newer pharmacological and nonpharmacological interventions developed in the past two decades are discussed in subsequent sections of this chapter.

The Management of Alcohol Withdrawal

An important initial intervention for a substantial number of alcohol-dependent patients is the management of alcohol withdrawal through detoxification. The objectives in treating alcohol withdrawal are the relief of discomfort, prevention or treatment of complications, and preparation for rehabilitation. Successful management of the alcohol withdrawal syndrome provides a basis for subsequent efforts at rehabilitation.

Careful screening for concurrent medical problems is an important element in detoxification. Administration of thiamine (50–100 mg by mouth or IM) and multivitamins is a low-cost, low-risk intervention for the prophylaxis and treatment of alcohol-related neurological disturbances. Good supportive care and treatment of concurrent illness, including fluid and electrolyte repletion, are essential.

Social detoxification, which involves the nonpharmacological treatment of alcohol withdrawal, has been shown to be effective. It consists of frequent reassurance, reality orientation, monitoring of vital signs, personal attention and general nursing care. Social detoxification is most appropriate for patients in mild-to-moderate withdrawal. Increasingly, detoxification is being done on an ambulatory basis, which is much less costly than inpatient detoxification Inpatient detoxification is indicated for serious medical or surgical illness, and for those individuals with a past history of adverse withdrawal reactions or with current evidence of more serious withdrawal (e.g., delirium tremens).

A variety of medications have been used for the treatment of alcohol withdrawal. However, due to their favorable side-effect profile, the benzodiazepines have largely supplanted all other medications. Although any benzodiazepine will suppress alcohol withdrawal symptoms, diazepam and chlordiazepoxide are often used, since they are metabolized to long-acting compounds, which in effect are self-tapering. Because metabolism of these drugs is hepatic, impaired liver function may complicate their use. Oxazepam and lorazepam are not oxidized to long-acting metabolites and thus carry less risk of accumulation.

Although carbamazepine appears useful as a primary treatment of withdrawal the liver dysfunction that is common in alcoholics may affect its metabolism, which makes careful blood level monitoring necessary. Antipsychotics are not indicated for the treatment of withdrawal except in those instances where hallucinations or severe agitation are present, in which case they should be added to a benzodiazepine. In addition to their potential to produce extrapyramidal side effects, antipsychotics lower seizure threshold, which may be particularly problematic during alcohol withdrawal.

Therapeutic Modalities: Nonpharmacological

A variety of treatment components are delivered within the context of rehabilitation services. In many programs a combination of therapeutic interventions is provided to all clients, based on the assumption that multiple components have a greater chance of meeting at least some of each client's needs. Therapeutic approaches most often employed in both residential and outpatient programs include behavior therapy, group therapy, family treatment and pharmacotherapy. Regarding specific treatment modalities, the weight of evidence suggests that behavioral treatments are likely to be more effective than insight-oriented or family therapies.

Nevertheless, recent research also indicates that Twelve Step Facilitation, which is based on the principles of AA, is as effective as more theory-based therapies.

Cognitive and behavior therapies are among the most investigated theory-based treatments. Behavioral elements most frequently employed in treatment programs are relapse prevention, social skills and assertiveness training, contingency management, deep muscle relaxation, self-control training and cognitive restructuring. Behavior therapists stress the importance of teaching new, adaptive skills designed to alter the conditions that precipitate and reinforce drinking, as well as developing alternative ways of coping with persons, events and feelings that serve to maintain drinking. A number of studies have demonstrated the benefits of teaching social and other coping skills. Patients who received skills training attended aftercare more regularly and they had less severe (though no less frequent) relapses than patients in control groups. These and other trials of cognitive–behavioral treatments have provided the empirical basis for elaboration of a generalized relapse prevention strategy.

In addition to specific treatment for alcoholic couples or families, self-help groups for family members of alcoholics have grown substantially. Al-Anon, although not formally affiliated with AA, shares the structure and many of the tenets of the 12 Steps of AA. Al-Anon and AA meetings are often held jointly. Alateen groups, sponsored by Al-Anon for children of alcoholics, are available as well.

Therapeutic Modalities: Pharmacological

Although the benzodiazepines have played a key role in the treatment of alcohol withdrawal, pharmacotherapy has not yet had a demonstrable effect on other aspects of alcoholism treatment. Disulfiram, an alcohol-sensitizing drug, has been approved for clinical use in the USA since the 1940s, but it has not been widely prescribed. During the past decade, however, medications have begun to play a more important role both in the treatment of comorbid psychiatric disorders in alcoholics and in the rehabilitation of alcohol dependence. In dually diagnosed patients, medications that reduce psychiatric symptomatology may also reduce the risk of drinking. Independent of their effects on comorbid psychopathology, medications that reduce drinking may enhance the alcoholic's participation in psychosocial treatment. This rationale is similar to that underlying the combination of medications with psychotherapy in the treatment of depressive or anxiety disorders.

Alcohol-sensitizing Drugs

Medications such as disulfiram or calcium carbimide cause an unpleasant reaction when combined with alcohol. The efficacy of such drugs in the prevention or limitation of relapse in alcoholics has not been demonstrated. However, these drugs may be of utility in selected samples of alcoholics with whom special efforts are made to ensure compliance.

Disulfiram (Antabuse) is the most commonly used alcohol-sensitizing medication and the only one approved for use in the USA. When given in a single daily dose of 125 to 500 mg, disulfiram binds irreversibly to ALDH, permanently inactivating this enzyme. When alcohol is consumed, it is metabolized to acetaldehyde which accumulates due to inhibition of the enzyme that metabolizes it. Elevated levels of acetaldehyde are responsible for the aversive effects associated with the disulfiram-ethanol reaction (DER).

In addition to its effects on ALDH, disulfiram inhibits a variety of other enzymes. Disulfiram also reduces clearance rates of a number of medications. Common side effects of disulfiram include drowsiness, lethargy and fatigue. More serious adverse effects, such as optic neuritis, peripheral neuropathy and hepatotoxicity are rare. The exacerbation of psychotic symptoms in patients with schizophrenia, and occasionally their appearance in other individuals as well as the development of depression, may be linked to inhibition of the enzyme dopamine-beta-hydroxylase. As with its neuropathic effects, the psychiatric effects of disulfiram are uncommon and may only occur at higher dosages of the medication.

Disulfiram is usually given orally. Although the daily dosage prescribed in the USA has been limited to 250–500 mg/day, some patients require in excess of 1 g/day of disulfiram to reach blood levels sufficient to produce the DER. The requirement that disulfiram undergo bioactivation before it can inhibit ALDH may explain the need for a higher dosage in some patients. At the dosage that is used clinically, faulty bioactivation in some individuals may yield too low a concentration of the active metabolite to inhibit ALDH.

Given the limited efficacy of disulfiram for the prevention of relapse, it should not be used as a first line treatment for alcohol dependence. However, if a patient has not responded to other pharmacological treatments and is motivated to take disulfiram, it may be beneficial. Whenever disulfiram is prescribed patients should be warned about its hazards, including the need to avoid over-the-counter (OTC) preparations with alcohol and drugs that interact adversely with disulfiram, as well as the potential for a DER to result from alcohol used in food preparations.

The Treatment of Psychiatric Comorbidity in Alcoholics

Comorbid psychiatric disorders may contribute to the development or maintenance of heavy drinking. Efforts to treat the comorbidity may have beneficial effects on drinking outcomes. Following detoxification, many alcoholics complain of persistent anxiety, insomnia and general distress. These symptoms may last for weeks or months and may be difficult to differentiate from the emergence of diagnosable psychiatric disorders. Irrespective of their etiology, negative emotional states, including frustration, anger, anxiety, depression and boredom, have been shown to contribute to relapse in a substantial proportion of alcoholics.

A variety of medications have been employed to treat comorbid psychiatric symptoms and disorders in alcoholics. Indications for the use of these medications in alcoholics are similar to those for nonalcoholic populations, but there is added potential for adverse effects due to comorbid medical disorders and the pharmacokinetic effects of acute and chronic alcohol consumption. The use of these medications in alcoholics therefore entails additional considerations that can only be arrived at through careful psychiatric diagnosis.

Treatment of Depressive Symptoms/Disorders

Although it has been argued that most instances of postwithdrawal depression will spontaneously remit within a few days to several weeks there are still a substantial number of patients whose severe and persistent depression requires treatment. Given the superior safety profile of SSRIs, particularly in relation to risk of suicide by medication overdose, use of these drugs is preferable to the use of TCAs.

Treatment of Anxiety Symptoms/Disorders

A number of studies have shown chlordiazepoxide to be effective in the maintenance of alcoholics in long-term outpatient treatment. However, the potential for additive CNS depression produced by the concurrent use of alcohol and benzodiazepines is well recognized. Furthermore, the use of benzodiazepines may itself result in tolerance and dependence and may increase depressive symptoms. Although this concern may be exaggerated and all benzodiazepines may not be equal in their capacity to produce dependence in alcoholics the use of benzodiazepines in alcoholics is probably best limited to detoxification. Buspirone, a nonbenzodiazepine anxiolytic that is less sedating than diazepam or clorazepate, does not interact with alcohol to impair psychomotor skills, and has a low potential for abuse. When combined with appropriate psychosocial treatment, buspirone appears useful in the treatment of alcoholics with persistent anxiety. Currently, antipsychotics are indicated only in alcoholics with a coexistent psychotic disorder or for the treatment of alcoholic hallucinosis. Several placebo-controlled studies have found no advantage in the use of phenothiazines for treatment of anxiety, tension and depression following detoxification (Jaffe et al., 1992). Because of their capacity to lower seizure threshold, antipsychotics should be used with caution in this population.

Drugs that May Directly Reduce Alcohol Consumption

A number of specific neurotransmitter systems have been implicated in the control of alcohol consumption, including endogenous opioids, catecholamines, especially dopamine and serotonin. Although these systems appear to function interactively in their effects on drinking behavior, efforts to use medications to treat excessive drinking have increasingly focused on agents that have selective effects on specific neurotransmitter systems.

Opioid Antagonists

An extensive literature supports the role of opioidergic neurotransmission in the pathophysiology of alcohol consumption and related phenomena. For example, small doses of morphine increase alcohol intake in experimental animals. In contrast, opioid antagonists, such as naltrexone, decrease ethanol consumption and self-administration. Effects similar to those in animals have been reported in some, but not all, studies of naltrexone for the treatment of alcohol dependence (Kranzler and Van Kirk, 2001). The considerable variability in findings concerning the efficacy of naltrexone underscores the need to identify the circumstances under which the medication exerts its therapeutic effects. Naltrexone appears to produce a modest effect on drinking behavior among alcoholics. However, given the comparatively small overall effect of the medication, a variety of other factors, including medication compliance, the severity and chronicity of alcohol dependence, and the choice of concomitant psychotherapy, may determine whether an effect of the medication is observed.

Serotonergic Medications

5-HT has been shown consistently to exert an influence over alcohol consumption in preclinical models of drinking behavior. In contrast to this preclinical literature, data on the effects of serotonergic medications on human drinking behavior are more limited, and the results are less consistent. One explanation for the variable findings in studies of whether SSRIs reduce drinking is the diversity of study samples. The initial studies were conducted in nontreatment-seeking heavy drinkers. Subsequent studies, which have shown differential effects based on severity, suggest that SSRIs are efficacious only in subgroups of alcoholics.

Acamprosate

Acamprosate, an amino acid derivative, affects both gamma-aminobutyric acid (GABA) and excitatory amino acid (i.e., glutamate) neurotransmission (the latter effect most likely being the one that is important for its therapeutic effects in alcoholism. Together, studies involving more than 4000 patients provide consistent evidence of the efficacy of acamprosate in alcoholism rehabilitation (Kranzler and Van Kirk, 2001). Based on these findings, and the benign side-effect profile of the medication, it appears to hold considerable value for the treatment of alcohol dependence.

Summary

Considerable additional research is required before medications are likely to play a meaningful role in the postwithdrawal treatment of alcohol dependence. One currently useful strategy is the identification of comorbid psychopathology in alcoholics, with pharmacotherapy directed toward reducing both psychiatric symptoms and alcohol consumption. In addition, the opioid antagonist naltrexone, which is capable of yielding a modest effect overall in reducing drinking behavior, appears to be of consider-

able value in some individuals. Further research is required with naltrexone to determine the optimal dosage, duration of treatment and psychosocial treatment strategies with which to use the medication. The question of whether the medication is most efficacious for alcoholics with high levels of craving for alcohol remains an important one. The SSRIs fluoxetine, citalopram and sertraline may be of value in subgroups of heavy drinkers, particularly those with a later onset of problem drinking. In contrast, ondansetron may be useful in alcoholics with an early onset of problem drinking. Prospective replication of this serotonergic matching strategy is required, however, before it can be recommended for general clinical use. A camprosate could assume a prominent role in the pharmacological management of alcohol dependence in the USA.

Alcoholics Anonymous (AA) and Mutual Help Organizations

Although mutual help societies composed of recovering alcoholics are not considered a formal treatment, they are often used as a substitute, an alternative and an adjunct to treatment. Mutual help groups based on the Twelve Steps of AA have proliferated throughout the world. To the extent that AA and other mutual help groups are more numerous than outpatient treatment, they may constitute a significant resource for problem drinkers who are attempting to reduce or stop drinking.

With an estimated 87 000 groups in 150 countries, AA is by far the most widely utilized source of help for drinking problems in the USA and throughout the world. In addition, a number of self-help organizations have modeled themselves after AA, basing recovery from drug abuse, overeating, and other behavioral disorders on the 12 Steps of AA (see Table 35.4). Unfortunately, clinicians often refer patients to self-help groups such as AA without consideration of the patient's needs and without adequate monitoring of the patient's response. Not all people are willing to endorse the AA emphasis on spirituality and its disease concept of alcoholism, which requires lifelong abstinence as the only means to recovery. Greater familiarity with AA may help clinicians to identify those patients who might benefit from this approach.

Although it is regarded as one of the most useful resources for recovering alcoholics, the research literature supporting the efficacy of AA is limited. Attendance at AA tends to be correlated with long-term abstinence, but this may reflect motivation for recovery. The type of motivated alcoholic that persists with AA might do just as well with other forms of supportive therapy. In fact, the few random assignment studies that have been conducted (Walsh et al., 1991) do not indicate that AA (or similar programs) is more effective than other types of treatment.

Infrequent attempts have been made to assess the efficacy of AA using controlled research designs because of methodological challenges, such as self-selection and ethical concerns about random assignment to treatment conditions. Nevertheless, several large-scale, well designed studies (Project MATCH Research Group, 1997, 1998) suggest that AA can have an incremental effect when combined with formal treatment, and AA attendance alone may be better than no intervention.

A study of long-term outcomes of treated and untreated alcoholics (Timko et al., 2000) indicates that individuals who obtain help for a drinking problem, especially in a timely manner, have better outcomes over 8 years than those who do not receive help, but the type of help they receive (e.g., self-help or formal treatment) makes little difference in long-term outcomes.

Table 35.4   The 12 Steps of Alcoholics Anonymous

1. We admitted we were powerless over alcohol – that our lives had become unmanageable.
2. Came to believe that a Power greater than ourselves could restore us to sanity.
3. Made a decision to turn our will and our lives over to the care of God **as we understood Him**.
4. Made a searching and fearless moral inventory of ourselves.
5. Admitted to God, to ourselves, and to another human being the exact nature of our wrongs.
6. Were entirely ready to have God remove all these defects of character.
7. Humbly asked Him to remove our shortcomings.
8. Made a list of all persons we had harmed, and became willing to make amends to them all.
9. Made direct amends to such people wherever possible, except when to do so would injure them or others.
10. Continued to take personal inventory and when we were wrong, promptly admitted it.
11. Sought through prayer and meditation to improve our conscious contact with God **as we understood Him**, praying only for knowledge of His will for us and the power to carry that out.
12. Having had a spiritual awakening as the result of these steps, we tried to carry this message to alcoholics, and to practice these principles in all our affairs.

The 12 Steps are reprinted with permission of Alcoholics Anonymous World Services, Inc. Permission to reprint this material does not mean that AA has reviewed or approved the contents of this publication, nor that AA agrees with the views expressed herein. AA is a program of recovery from alcoholism. Use of the 12 Steps in connection with programs and activities that are patterned after AA but address other problems does not imply otherwise.

Special Features Influencing Treatment

Psychiatric Comorbidity

There is considerable evidence that links the outcome of alcoholism treatment to comorbid psychopathology. General measures of psychopathology, as well as the specific diagnoses of drug abuse, drug dependence, antisocial personality disorder and major depressive disorder have been shown to predict poorer outcomes in alcoholics. The extent to which treatment of concomitant psychopathology enhances alcoholism treatment outcome is unclear. Ries (1993) has distinguished among serial, parallel and integrated models for treating these disorders. The serial model involves the treatment of one disorder, followed by the treatment of the second disorder. For example, a psychotic alcoholic might first be treated on a general psychiatric unit and once his acute psychosis is controlled, transferred to an alcoholism rehabilitation program. The parallel treatment approach involves concurrent, but separate, treatment of both the psychiatric and the alcohol use disorder. The integrated model involves the treatment of both disorders in a single treatment setting at the same time. This approach requires that personnel with expertise in both the addictions and psychiatric treatment be available in a single location. Each of these approaches has advantages and disadvantages. For

example, the integrated model, while it provides the most comprehensive approach, is the most difficult and costly to configure and may, therefore, not be feasible for many treatment providers.

Demographic Features

Adolescents

Despite a paucity of controlled, age-specific treatment outcome studies of adolescents with alcohol use disorders, the need for prevention and specialized treatment for this group is clear. The literature indicates that in substance-abusing adolescents some treatment is better than no treatment, relapse rates are high, and there is no consistent support for the superiority of any single treatment modality. However, several factors have been associated with better treatment outcome: later onset of problem drinking, pretreatment attendance at school, voluntary entrance into treatment, active parental input and availability of ancillary adolescent-specific services, including those pertaining to school, recreation, vocational needs and contraception.

Because many adolescents have not yet fully developed formal operational thinking, treatment efforts should be concrete and goal-oriented. Furthermore, the clinician should consider the potential impact on treatment of other cognitive problems: learning disabilities, attention-deficit/hyperactivity disorder and other psychopathology which may previously have gone undiagnosed. Treatment of the adolescent with an alcohol use disorder also requires an appreciation of the importance of modeling, imitation and peer pressure, which are intrinsic to identity development. The use of age-appropriate support groups (e.g., Alateen) may be particularly useful in this regard.

Geriatric Patients

In addition to the high prevalence of medical problems, pharmacokinetic and pharmacodynamic variables can affect treatment outcome in elderly alcoholics. For example, Liskow and colleagues (1989) found that elderly alcoholics, despite having drunk less than younger patients during the month prior to admission, had more severe alcohol withdrawal symptomatology and required a higher dosage of chlordiazepoxide. These investigators speculated that the observed differences might delay the entry of elderly alcoholics into rehabilitation.

An important question in treating elderly alcoholics is the extent to which specialized treatment services improve outcome. Kofoed and colleagues (1987) found that patients treated in special elderly peer groups remained in treatment longer and were more likely to complete treatment than those treated in mixed-age groups. These investigators concluded that elder-specific treatment has differential therapeutic value.

Recent shifts in the demographic features of AA participants suggest that the current cohort of elderly alcoholics has less experience with self-help groups at a time when AA is attracting younger members who are more likely to have comorbid drug abuse/dependence. As a consequence, the elderly can be expected to experience increased difficulty affiliating with AA. This, along with evidence indicating an advantage for age-specific treatment in the elderly, suggests that special efforts should be made to help the elderly alcoholic locate AA meetings that include a substantial proportion of older participants. Age-appropriate AA groups may be especially beneficial to the older alcoholic who is isolated and lonely and for whom the prospect of helping others may help to combat feelings of uselessness.

Gender (Including Pregnancy)

As described above, epidemiological and clinical studies have shown that alcohol abuse and dependence have become quite common among women, as historical gender differences in drinking problems have diminished during the past 25 years. This trend has promoted greater awareness of the impact of alcohol use on women's health and the importance of gender as a potential determinant of treatment outcome. Nonetheless, the vast majority of studies related to alcohol use and its effects, including the diagnosis and treatment of alcohol dependence, have involved men.

To guide the treatment of alcoholism in women, Blume (1992) suggests that evaluation should include special attention to the identification of physical abuse, sexual abuse, medical problems, psychiatric comorbidity, the presence of alcoholism and drug abuse in spouses, and alcohol-related birth defects in children. To enable women with children to participate in treatment, the availability of child care services is critical, although it must generally be arranged independent of treatment. Blume (1992) also lists the following special treatment needs of women: information about the effects of substance use on the fetus, parenting skills, couples and family therapy, sober female role models, assertiveness training, and an awareness of sexism and its consequences. Special care must also be taken to avoid creating iatrogenic drug dependence in women (e.g., through the use of benzodiazepines to treat comorbid anxiety and depressive symptoms). While these are useful guidelines for treating alcoholic women, empirical research is needed to evaluate these and other issues more systematically.

Ethnic and Cultural Issues and Treatment

In 1991 approximately two-thirds of patients in alcoholism treatment were white, 17% were black and 12% were Hispanic. Although socioeconomic and cultural issues should be addressed in alcoholism treatment, guidelines for such treatment are based largely on common sense, rather than systematic outcome evaluation. Obviously, where language barriers exist, special efforts must be made to ensure adequate communication. Treatment providers should also be aware of their patients' traditional patterns of drinking, how drinking may be influenced by acculturation, differences among ethnic groups in their perception of alcohol-related problems, the impact of sociocultural differences between patients and providers, and how prevailing social (e.g., family) relationships can affect treatment outcome.

Conclusion

During the past 25 years significant progress has been made in the scientific study of alcoholism and its treatment. On the basis of evidence reviewed in this chapter, a number of conclusions appear warranted at this time:

1. Alcoholics are heterogeneous with respect to demographic features (e.g., age, gender, race/ethnicity), age of onset of heavy drinking, severity of alcohol dependence, comorbid psychopathology, genetic vulnerability and other prognostic factors.
2. The available evidence suggests that any treatment for alcoholism is better than no treatment. The majority of those treated demonstrate improvement, but many of these alcoholics may improve with minimal treatment.
3. The intensity of treatment has not been shown to produce pronounced differences in outcome (Moos and Moos, in press).

Similarly, medical inpatient treatment, while more costly, is not demonstrably more effective than nonmedical residential or outpatient treatment. For patients with serious comorbid medical and psychiatric disorders, medical inpatient treatment may, nonetheless, be necessary. Some evidence indicates that continuing aftercare helps to maintain abstinence following short-term intensive rehabilitation in inpatient settings.

4. There is little evidence that any one treatment approach is superior. There is some support for certain kinds of behavior therapy, but the effectiveness of AA and disulfiram seem to depend on patient characteristics and compliance. Several kinds of carefully specified and theoretically-derived therapeutic approaches show promise as a basis for a new generation of ambulatory treatments. These include the relapse prevention strategies that teach the alcoholic how to avoid high risk relapse situations, and new pharmacologic agents (e.g., naltrexone) that appear to reduce the alcoholic's risk of relapse by dampening the reinforcement potential of alcohol. Continued improvements in treatment outcome will depend upon successfully matching treatment settings and modalities to the specific needs of the individual patient.

Comparison of DSM-IV/ICD-10 Diagnostic Criteria

The ICD-10 and DSM-IV-TR criteria sets are nearly identical except for the following: The ICD-10 Diagnostic Criteria for Research for Alcohol Intoxication also lists flushed face and conjunctival injection as symptoms but does not include the DSM-IV-TR item for impairment in attention; the ICD-10 Diagnostic Criteria for Research for Alcohol Withdrawal require three symptoms from a list of 10 which includes headache and splits tachycardia and sweating into two separate items.

References

Babor TF and Higgins-Biddle JC (2001) AUDIT The Alcohol Use Disorders Identification Test: Guidelines for use in Primary Care, 2nd ed. World Health Organization, Geneva Switzerland.

Begleiter H and Porjesz B (1999) What is inherited in the predisposition toward alcoholism? A proposed model. *Alcohol Clin Exp Res* 23, 1125–1135.

Blume SB (1992) Alcohol and other drug problems in women, in *Substance Abuse: A Comprehensive Textbook*, 2nd edn. (eds Lowinson JH, Ruiz P and Millman RB). Williams & Wilkins, Philadelphia, pp. 794–807.

Bohn MJ, Babor TF and Kranzler HR (1995) The Alcohol Use Disorders Identification Test (AUDIT): Validation of a screening instrument for use in medical settings. *J Stud Alcohol* 56, 423–432.

Chang G (2001) Alcohol-screening instruments for pregnant women. *Alcohol Res Health* 25, 204–209.

Finney JW and Monahan SC (1996) The cost-effectiveness of treatment for alcoholism: A second approximation. *J Stud Alcohol* 57, 229–243.

Glenn SW and Nixon SJ (1991) Applications of Cloninger's subtypes in a female alcoholic sample. *Alcohol Clin Exp Res* 15, 851–857.

Jaffe JH, Kranzler HR and Ciraulo D (1992) Drugs used in the treatment of alcoholism, in *Medical Diagnosis and Treatment of Alcoholism*, 3rd edn. (eds Mendelson JH and Mello NK). McGraw-Hill, New York, pp. 421–461.

Kaminer Y (1994) *Adolescent Substance Abuse: A Comprehensive Guide to Theory and Practice*. Plenum Press, New York.

Kessler RC, Crum RM, Warner LA *et al.* (1997) Lifetime-cooccurrence of DSM-III-R alcohol abuse and dependence with other psychiatric disorders in the National Comorbidity Survey. *Arch Gen Psychiatr* 54, 313–321.

Kofoed LL, Tolson RL, Atkinson RM *et al.* (1987) Treatment compliance of older alcoholics: An elder-specific approach is superior to "mainstreaming". *J Stud Alcohol* 48, 47–51.

Kranzler HR and Van Kirk J (2001) Naltrexone and acamprosate in the treatment of alcoholism: A meta-analysis. *Alcohol Clin Exp Res* 25, 1335–1341.

Lindstrom L (1992) *Managing Alcoholism: Matching Clients to Treatments.* Oxford University Press, New York.

Liskow BI, Rinck C and Campbell J (1989) Alcohol withdrawal in the elderly. *J Stud Alcohol* 50, 414–421.

Moos RH and Moos BS (in press) Long-term influence of duration and intensity of treatment on previously untreated individuals with alcohol use disorders. *Addiction.*

Narrow WE, Rae DS, Robins LN *et al.* (2002) Revised prevalence estimates of mental disorders in the United States: Using a clinical significance criterion to reconcile two surveys' estimates. *Arch Gen Psychiatr* 59, 115–123.

Pollock VE (1992) Meta-analysis of subjective sensitivity to alcohol in sons of alcoholics. *Am J Psychiatr* 149, 1534–1538.

Project MATCH Research Group (1997) Matching alcoholism treatments to client heterogeneity: Project MATCH posttreatment drinking outcomes. *J Stud Alcohol* 58, 7–29.

Project MATCH Research Group (1998) Matching alcoholism treatments to client heterogeneity: Project MATCH three-year drinking outcomes. *Alcohol Clin Exp Res* 22, 1300–1311.

Randell CL, Roberts JS, Del Boca FK *et al.* (1999) Telescoping of landmark events associated with drinking: A gender comparison. *J Stud Alcohol* 60, 252–260.

Regier DA, Farmer ME, Rae DS *et al.* (1990) Comorbidity of mental disorders with alcohol and other drug abuse: Results from the Epidemiologic Catchment Area (ECA) study. *J Am Med Assoc* 264, 2511–2518.

Ries R (1993) Clinical treatment matching models for dually diagnosed patients. *Psychiatr Clin N Am* 16, 167–175.

Sannibale C and Hall W (1998) An evaluation of Cloninger's typology of alcohol abuse. *Addiction* 93, 1241–1249.

Saunders JB, Aasland OG, Babo TF *et al.* (1993) Development of the Alcohol Use Disorders Identification Test (AUDIT): WHO collaborative project on early detection of persons with harmful alcohol consumption-II. *Addiction* 88, 791–804.

Schottenfeld RS (1994) Assessment of the patient, in *Textbook of Substance Abuse Treatment* (eds Galanter M and Kleber HD). Am Psychiatric Press, Washington DC, pp. 25–33.

Schuckit MA (1985) The clinical implications of primary diagnostic groups among alcoholics. *Arch Gen Psychiatr* 42, 1043–1049.

Schuckit MA and Smith T (1996) An 8-year follow-up of 450 sons of alcoholic and control subjects. *Arch Gen Psychiatr* 53, 202–210.

Schuckit MA, Irwin M and Mahler HM (1990) Tridimensional personality questionnaire scores of sons of alcoholic and nonalcoholic fathers. *Am J Psychiatr* 147, 481–487.

Schuckit MA, Smith TL, Anthenelli R *et al.* (1993) Clinical course of alcoholism in 636 male inpatients. *Am J Psychiatr* 150, 786–792.

Selzer ML (1971) The Michigan Alcoholism Screening Test: The quest for a new diagnostic instrument, *Am J Psychiatr* 127, 1653–1658.

Sher KJ and Trull T (1994) Personality and disinhibitory psychopathology: Alcoholism and antisocial personality disorder. *J Abnormal Psychol* 203, 92–102.

Substance Abuse and Mental Health Services Administration (SAMHSA) (2000) Office of Applied Studies, National Household Survey on Drug Abuse.

Thomasson HR, Crabb DW, Edenberg HJ *et al.* (1993) Alcohol and aldehyde dehydrogenase polymorphins and alcoholism. *Behav Gen* 23, 131–136.

Timko C, Moos RH, Finney JW *et al.* (2000) Long-term outcomes of alcohol use disorders: Comparing untreated individuals with those in Alcoholics Anonymous and formal treatment. *J Stud Alcohol* 61, 529–538.

US Department of Health and Human Services (DHHS) (1994) English Special Report to the US Congress on Alcohol and Health. NIH Publication No. 94-3699

Vaillant GE (1983) *The Natural History of Alcoholism.* Harvard University Press, Cambridge, MA.

Vaillant GE (1994) Evidence that the Type 1/Type 2 dichotomy in zlcoholixm must be re-examined. Addiction 89, 1049–1057.

Walsh DC, Hingson RW, Merrigan DM *et al.* (1991) A ramdomized trial of treatment options for alcohol-abusing workers. *New Engl J Med* 325, 775–782.

Substance Abuse: Caffeine Use Disorders

Caffeine is most widely consumed psychoactive substance in the world. In North America, it is estimated that more than 80% of adults and children consume caffeine regularly. Habitual consumption of coffee, tea, or caffeinated soda drinks with meals is extermely common and may not be readily recognized as caffeine consumption. This cultural integration of caffeine use can make the recognition of psychiatric disorders associated with caffeine use particularly difficult. However, it is important for the psychiatrist to recognize the role of caffeine as a psychoactive substance capable of producing a variety of psychiatric syndromes, despite the pervasive and well-accepted use of caffeine. In this chapter, five disorders associated with caffeine use are reviewed: caffeine intoxication, caffeine withdrawal, caffeine dependence, caffeine-induced anxiety disorder and caffeine-induced sleep disorder.

Caffeine Intoxication

Definition

The *Diagnostic and Statistical Manual of Mental Disorders*, Fourth Edition, Text Revision (DSM-IV-TR) defines caffeine intoxication as a set of symptoms that develop during or shortly after caffeine use (American Psychiatric Association, 2000). There may be two kinds of presentation associated with caffeine intoxication. The first presentation is associated with the **acute** ingestion of a large amount of caffeine and represents an acute drug overdose condition. The second presentation is associated with the **chronic** consumption of large amounts of caffeine and results in a more complicated presentation.

The diagnosis of caffeine intoxication is based on the DSM-IV TR criteria of substance intoxication found in **Chapter** 34. Specifically, this disorder is diagnosed after the consumption of 250 mg of caffeine. Table 36.1 indicates the approximate caffeine content of numerous foods. This diagnosis is entertained when at least five of the following 12 signs are present and they produce significant distress not due to a general medical condition:

- nervousness
- restlessness
- insomnia
- periods of inexhaustibility
- diuresis
- excitement
- gastrointestinal disturbance
- muscle twitching

Table 36.1	Typical Caffeine Content of Foods and Medications	
Substance	Caffeine Content (mg)
Brewed coffee	100 mg/6 oz
Instant coffee	70 mg/6 oz
Esspresso	40 mg/1 oz
Decaffeinated coffee	4 mg/6 oz
Brewed tea	40 mg/6 oz
Instant tea	30 mg/6 oz
Canned or bottled tea	20 mg/12 oz
Caffeinated soda	40 mg/12 oz
Cocoa beverage	7 mg/6 oz
Chocolate milk	4 mg/6 oz
Dark chocolate	20 mg/1 oz
Milk chocolate	6 mg/1 oz
Caffeinated water	100 mg/16.9 oz
Coffee ice cream or yogurt	50 mg/8 oz
Caffeinated gum	50 mg/stick
Caffeine-containing analgesics	32–65 mg/tablet
Stimulants	100–100 mg/tablet
Weight-loss aids	40–100 mg/tablet
Sports nutrition	100 mg/tablet

American Society of Addiction Medicine. *Source*: Griffiths RR, Juliano LM and Chausmer AL (in press) Caffeine pharmacology and clinical effects, in *Principles of Addiction Medicine* (eds Graham AN, Schultz TK, Mayo-Smith M *et al.*). Chevy Chase, Maryland.

- psychomotor agitation
- flushed face
- tachycardia or cardiac arrhythmia
- rambling flow of thought and speech

Acquired Tolerance

In a person who regularly consumes caffeine, tolerance may occur to the acute effects of caffeine. Thus a sensitive person with no tolerance to caffeine might have signs and symptoms of caffeine intoxication in response to a relatively low dose of caffeine (such as 100 mg, the amount found in a typical cup of brewed coffee) (Table 36.1), whereas another person with a high daily consumption of caffeine would show no evidence of intoxication with a similar dose.

Essentials of Psychiatry Jerald Kay and Allan Tasman
© 2006 John Wiley & Sons, Ltd.

Inadvertent Overdosing

Although caffeine intoxication can occur in the context of habitual chronic consumption of high doses, probably most often it occurs after inadvertent overdosing. Examples include overdosing of intravenous caffeine to children in medical settings (e.g., for respiratory stimulating effects), excessive caffeine consumption in tablet form by students who fail to appreciate the dose being ingested (e.g., to study through the night), and the person who unknowingly consumes a highly concentrated form of caffeine (e.g., caffeinated coffee brewed with caffeine-containing water to create an especially high dose of caffeine in the coffee).

Pathophysiology

The principal cellular site of action of caffeine is the adenosine receptor, where caffeine functions as an antagonist. Adenosine produces a wide variety of physiological effects, including decreasing spontaneous electrical activity in brain, inhibiting neurotransmitter release in brain, decreasing spontaneous and operant motor activity, dilating central vasculature, producing antidiuresis, inhibiting renin release, and inhibiting gastric secretion and lipolysis. As an antagonist of adenosine many of caffeine's actions are opposite to those produced by adenosine (e.g., central nervous system stimulation, decreased cerebral blood flow, increased renin release and diuresis, increased gastric secretions and stimulation of respiration).

Assessment

The primary features of caffeine intoxication can be found in the diagnostic criteria from DSM-IV. The diagnostic decision tree for caffeine intoxication disorder, caffeine-induced anxiety disorder and caffeine-induced sleep disorder is shown in Figure 36.1. The most common symptoms reported in decreasing order of frequency are frequent urination, restlessness, insomnia, nervousness and excitement (all which were at rates greater than 20%). In addition, nearly 25% of people report heart pounding in response to high caffeine use (although this is not one of the DSM-IV criteria).

Differential Diagnosis

The diagnosis of caffeine intoxication is based on the history and clinical presentation of the patient. Ideally, the extent of caffeine exposure can also be assessed by a serum or saliva assay of the caffeine level. In the past, caffeine use has often been overlooked in patients presenting with symptoms consistent with a caffeine use disorder. However, it may be that there is presently a greater awareness of the deleterious effects of caffeine, making psychiatrists more sensitive to the inclusion of caffeine in a differential diagnosis (see Table 36.2), and patients more aware of the possible role of excessive caffeine in somatic and psychological symptoms.

Epidemiology

Despite the long history of recognition of caffeine intoxication, there is little information available about the prevalence or incidence of caffeine intoxication either in the general community or in selected populations. It appears that the incidence of caffeine intoxication in the general community is about 7% per year, and it may be higher in selected populations at greater risk for caffeine intoxication (e.g., students).

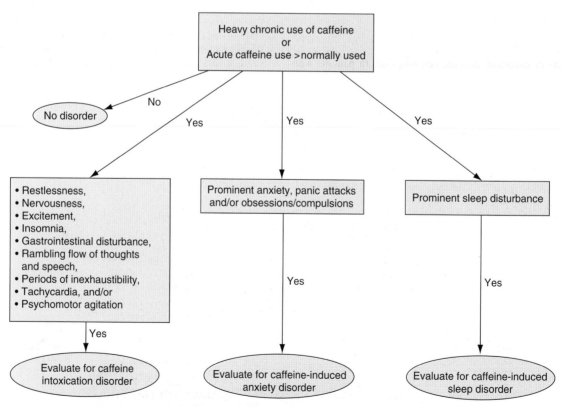

Figure 36.1   *Diagnostic decision tree for caffeine intoxication disorder, caffeine-induced anxiety disorder and caffeine-induced sleep disorder.*

Table 36.2	Differential Diagnosis of Caffeine Intoxication
Manic episode	Panic disorder
Amphetamine/cocaine intoxication	Generalized anxiety disorder
Sedative, hypnotic or anxiolytic withdrawal	Medication-induced side effect (e.g., akathisia)
Nicotine withdrawal	Sleep disorders

Table 36.3	Signs and Symptoms Associated with Caffeine Withdrawal
Headache – most common symptom
Fatigue, lethargy, sluggishness
Sleepiness, drowsiness
Dysphoric mood
Difficulty concentrating
Work difficulty, unmotivated
Depression
Anxiety
Irritability
Nausea or vomiting
Muscle aches or stiffness

Course

In the patient who is not tolerant to caffeine, acute caffeine ingestion producing caffeine intoxication is a time-limited condition that will rapidly resolve with cessation of caffeine use, consistent with the relatively short half-life of caffeine (3–6 hours).

Treatment

The first step in evaluating a patient with a possible diagnosis of caffeine intoxication is to obtain a careful history about all recent caffeine consumption. The possible use of beverages and medications – both prescription and over-the-counter (OTC) diet aids and energy pills – should be reviewed. Some beverages (e.g., caffeine-containing soft drinks) and medications (e.g., energy pills, aids to combat sleep, or diet pills) may not be recognized by the patient as containing caffeine. The amount of caffeine acutely consumed should help clarify the diagnosis of caffeine intoxication, although it is important to determine whether the patient has been chronically consuming high doses of caffeine. If this is the case, the patient may be tolerant and therefore less likely to be experiencing caffeine intoxication. However, some clinicians have reported that caffeine intoxication can occur even in the context of chronic caffeine use. The primary approach to the treatment of caffeine intoxication is to teach the patient about the effects of excessive caffeine consumption. In patients who

are resistant to accepting the role of caffeine in their presenting symptoms, it may be useful to suggest a trial-off of caffeine as both a diagnostic and a potentially therapeutic probe.

Caffeine Withdrawal

Definition

Table 36.3 lists the signs and symptoms of withdrawal. As is the case with all DSM diagnoses, this disorder implies clinically significant distress or impairment and a general medical condition must be ruled out.

Assessment

The key steps in establishing a diagnosis of caffeine withdrawal are to determine the history of the person's caffeine consumption from all dietary sources, and then establish whether there has been a significant decrease in caffeine intake. The diagnostic decision tree for caffeine dependence disorder and caffeine withdrawal disorder is shown in Figure 36.2. Caffeine withdrawal

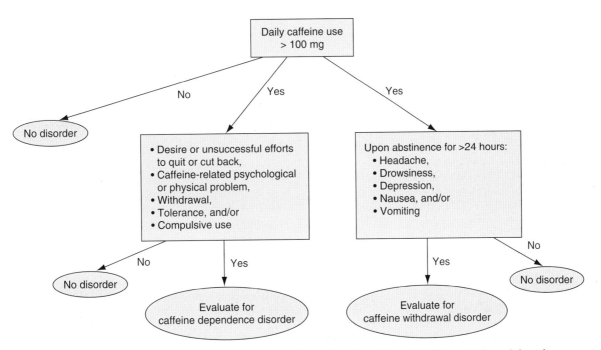

Figure 36.2 *Diagnostic decision tree for caffeine dependence disorder and caffeine withdrawal disorder.*

is probably more common than is generally recognized, and it seems there is a tendency for people to attribute the symptoms of caffeine withdrawal to other etiologies besides caffeine (e.g., having the flu, or a bad day). Caffeine withdrawal may be particularly common in medical settings where patients are required to abstain from food and fluids, such as before surgical procedures and certain diagnostic tests. In addition, caffeine withdrawal may occur in settings where the use of caffeine-containing products is restricted or banned, such as inpatient psychiatric wards.

Differential Diagnosis

Caffeine withdrawal should be considered when evaluating individuals presenting with headaches, fatigue, sleepiness, mood disturbances or impaired concentration. The differential diagnosis of caffeine withdrawal includes: viral illnesses; sinus conditions; other types of headaches such as migraine, tension, postanesthetic; other drug withdrawal states such as amphetamine or cocaine withdrawal; and idiopathic drug reactions.

Course

Caffeine withdrawal generally begins within 12 to 24 hours after discontinuing caffeine use. The peak of caffeine withdrawal generally occurs within 24 to 48 hours, and the duration of caffeine withdrawal is generally 2 days to about 1 week.

Treatment

There have been few studies attempting to address the treatment of caffeine withdrawal, although it has frequently been observed that the symptoms of caffeine withdrawal can be alleviated with the consumption of caffeine and this approach is probably best. If the medical recommendation is made to eliminate or substantially reduce caffeine consumption, then it may be useful to recommend a tapering dose schedule rather than abrupt discontinuation. Caffeine tapering (or "fading") is described in more detail in the section on "caffeine dependence".

Caffeine Dependence

Definition

This diagnosis is predicated on the DSM-IV TR criteria of substance dependence found in **Chapter** 34.

The clinical features of individuals with caffeine dependence were described in a series of 16 cases described by Strain and colleagues (1994). Most of these individuals reported physical or psychological problems from caffeine use which had prompted multiple unsuccessful attempts to cut down or quit caffeine use, often in response to physicians' recommendations. Most reported tolerance to caffeine and withdrawal when attempting to abstain completely. A double-blind withdrawal trial showed functional impairment in most cases. For the group, median daily caffeine intake was 357 mg with a wide range of 129 to 2548 mg. The preferred vehicle was almost equally divided between soft drinks and coffee.

Etiology

It is known that the consumption of caffeine may be influenced by several different factors, which are summarized below.

Caffeine Subjective Effects

Many studies have shown that caffeine in low to moderate doses (20–200 mg) produces mild positive subjective effects of increased feelings of well-being, alertness, energy, concentra-tion, self-confidence, motivation for work and desire to talk to people. The profile of positive effects with caffeine is qualitatively similar to that produced by d-amphetamine and cocaine, which may reflect a common dopaminergic mechanism of action. High doses of caffeine (e.g., 800 mg) produce negative subjective effects such as anxiety and nervousness, especially in people who are not tolerant to caffeine.

Caffeine Reinforcement

Consistent with its ability to produce mild positive subjective effects, low to moderate doses of caffeine have also been shown to function as a reinforcer in humans, that is, when given the choice under experimental conditions, some people will consistently choose to consume caffeine rather than placebo.

Caffeine Tolerance

Survey data indicate 17% of current caffeine users reported tolerance (Hughes *et al.*, 1998), whereas 75% of a group of caffeine dependent individuals reported tolerance (Strain *et al.*, 1994). Although tolerance is one of the criteria for making a diagnosis of caffeine dependence (see DSM-IV-TR criteria for substance dependence), it is not clear what role the development of tolerance may have in the development of clinical dependence upon caffeine.

Genetics and Caffeine Use

Genetic studies suggest that caffeine use problems have an underlying biological basis, part of which may be shared with other commonly abused substances. Twin studies comparing monozygotic and dizygotic twins showed heritabilities of heavy caffeine use, caffeine tolerance and caffeine withdrawal which ranged between 35 and 77% (Kendler and Prescott, 1999).

Caffeine Use and Alcoholism

The conclusion suggested by the genetic studies described above is that a common genetic factor underlies joint use of caffeine, alcohol and cigarettes. This is consistent with findings of studies on the cooccurrence of use of these three substances (Kozlowski *et al.*, 1993). A study of individuals whose pattern of caffeine use fulfilled DSM-IV diagnostic criteria for substance dependence on caffeine found that almost 60% had a past diagnosis of alcohol abuse or dependence (Strain *et al.*, 1994).

Caffeine Use and Nicotine/Cigarette Smoking

Epidemiological studies have shown that cigarette smokers consume more caffeine than nonsmokers (Swanson *et al.*, 1994).

Caffeine Use in Psychiatric Patients

Surveys of psychiatric patients (typically inpatients) have found high rates of caffeine consumption, particularly among patients with schizophrenia. Other groups at risk may include substance abusers (Russ *et al.*, 1988; Hays *et al.*, 1998) and patients with anorexia nervosa (Sours, 1983). While preliminary work suggests there may be some factors (such as heritability) that contribute to the predisposition to use caffeine, there are no studies that have examined the possible etiologic role of such factors in the development of caffeine dependence as a specific diagnosis. Caffeine dependence, like other drug dependence syndromes, in all likelihood represents the interaction of social and cultural forces, and individual histories and predispositions, operating in the context of a psychoactive substance that produces pleasant subjective effects and is reinforcing.

Assessment

Caffeine dependence may be an unrecognized condition with a higher prevalence than is generally appreciated (see Figure 36.2). Clinicians do not typically think to inquire about caffeine use and about problematic use consistent with a diagnosis of caffeine dependence. However, probing for evidence of caffeine dependence may be useful, and it would be reasonable to focus upon the DSM-IV criteria for dependence that are more appropriate for a substance that is widely available and generally culturally accepted. Thus, the clinician should probe for evidence of tolerance, withdrawal, continued use despite a doctor's recommendation that the person cut down or stop using caffeine, use despite other problems associated with caffeine, often using larger amounts or over a longer period than intended, or persistent desires and/or difficulties in decreasing or discontinuing use.

Differential Diagnosis

The diagnosis of caffeine dependence includes symptoms that can also contribute to a diagnosis of caffeine intoxication and caffeine withdrawal, and both of these conditions should be included in the differential diagnosis of a patient with possible caffeine dependence. Since intoxication and withdrawal symptoms can contribute to the diagnosis of dependence, conditions that overlap with these caffeine-related disorders should also be considered. When considering a patient for a possible diagnosis of caffeine dependence, the clinician should also consider other substance dependence syndromes – especially those related to stimulants – in the differential diagnosis.

Epidemiology

Caffeine is the most widely used mood-altering drug in the world. In North America, dietary surveys indicate that weekly or more frequent consumption of caffeine-containing foods occurs in 80 to 90% of children and adults (Gilbert, 1984; Hughes and Oliveto, 1997). In the USA, average daily caffeine consumption among caffeine consumers is 280 mg (Barone and Roberts, 1996). There is only one study of the prevalence of caffeine dependence in the general population based upon standardized diagnostic criteria (Hughes *et al.*, 1998). In this random telephone survey of residents of Vermont, 162 out of the 202 surveyed participants reported current caffeine use. Employing the generic DSM-IV criteria for dependence, 30% of the 162 current caffeine users fulfilled criteria for a diagnosis of caffeine dependence by endorsing three or more dependence criteria, with 56% endorsing the diagnostic criterion of persistent desire or unsuccessful efforts to cut down or control caffeine use, 28% endorsing using more than intended, 14% endorsing caffeine use continued despite knowledge of a physical or psychological problem likely to have been caused or exacerbated by caffeine use, 18% endorsing withdrawal and 9% endorsing tolerance. These results suggest there may be a large number of people who demonstrate symptoms consistent with a DSM-defined diagnosis of caffeine dependence.

Course

While there are no studies that have specifically examined the course and natural history of caffeine dependence, like other drug dependence syndromes caffeine dependence appears to be a chronic relapsing disorder. In the study described above by Strain and colleagues (1994), caffeine dependence participants reported recurrent efforts to discontinue caffeine use, with failures to discontinue use or frequent relapses.

Treatment

In a survey of physicians' practices, it was found that over 75% of medical specialists recommend that patients reduce or eliminate caffeine for certain conditions including anxiety, insomnia, arrhythmias, palpitations and tachycardia, esophagitis/hiatal hernia and fibrocystic disease (Hughes *et al.*, 1988). However, stopping caffeine use can be difficult for some people. For example, in the diagnostic study of caffeine dependence (Strain *et al.*, 1994), subjects reported physical conditions such as acne rosacea, pregnancy, palpitations and gastrointestinal problems that led physicians to recommend that they reduce or eliminate caffeine; all reported that they were unable to follow their doctors' recommendations.

Caffeine-induced Anxiety Disorder

Definition

In addition to the symptom of anxiety that can be a component of caffeine intoxication and caffeine withdrawal, caffeine can also produce anxiety disorder, caffeine-induced anxiety disorder (American Psychiatric Association, 2000) (see DSM-IV-TR (criteria). Although there has been no work using this specific set of diagnostic criteria, there have been several studies examining the relationship between caffeine in general, and this work is reviewed here.

Etiology and Pathophysiology

Caffeine-induced anxiety disorder by definition is etiologically related to caffeine. Caffeine's primary cellular site of action appears to be the adenosine receptor, where it functions as an antagonist.

Caffeine's Anxiety-inducing Effects in Persons with Anxiety Disorders

Several studies have examined caffeine consumption in patients with an independent anxiety disorder. Interestingly, patients with anxiety disorders generally have lower levels of caffeine consumption compared with patients without an anxiety disorder (Boulenger *et al.*, 1984; Rihs *et al.*, 1996). After the acute consumption of caffeine, self-reports by patients with anxiety disorders versus control subjects show greater anxiety scores. This suggests that some people (such as patients with an anxiety disorder) may avoid caffeine use because of anxiety effects produced by caffeine.

Assessment and Differential Diagnosis

The diagnosis of caffeine-induced anxiety disorder is based on evidence of an anxiety disorder etiologically related to caffeine (see previous diagnostic decision tree for caffeine intoxication disorder, caffeine-induced anxiety disorder and caffeine-induced sleep disorder). Other diagnostic considerations besides caffeine-induced anxiety disorder include caffeine intoxication and caffeine withdrawal, a primary anxiety disorder, and an anxiety disorder due to a general medical condition. Caffeine-induced anxiety disorder can occur in the context of caffeine intoxication or caffeine withdrawal, but the anxiety symptoms associated with the caffeine-induced anxiety disorder should be excessive

Substance-induced Anxiety Disorder

A. A prominent anxiety, panic attacks, or obsessions or compulsions predominate in the clinical picture.

B. There is evidence from the history, physical examination, or laboratory findings of either (1) or (2):

 (1) the symptoms in Criterion A developed during, or within 1 month of, substance intoxication or withdrawal

 (2) medication use is etiologically related to the disturbance

C. The disturbance is not better accounted for by an anxiety disorder that is not substance induced might include the following: The symptoms precede the onset of the substance use (or medication use); the symptoms persist for a substantial period of time (e.g., about a month) after the cessation of acute withdrawal or severe intoxication, or are substantially in excess of what would be expected given the type or amount of the substance used or the duration of use; or there is other evidence suggesting the existence of an independent nonsubstance-induced anxiety disorder (e.g., a history of recurrent nonsubstance-related episodes).

D. The disturbance does not occur exclusively during the course of a delirium.

E. The disturbance causes clinically significant distress or impairment in social, occupational, or other important areas of functioning.

Note: This diagnosis should be made instead of a diagnosis of substance intoxication or substance withdrawal only when the anxiety symptoms are in excess of those usually associated with the intoxication or withdrawal syndrome and when the anxiety symptoms are sufficiently severe to warrant independent clinical attention.

Reprinted with permission from the Diagnostic and Statistical Manual of Mental Disorders. Fourth Edition, Text Revision. Copyright 2000 American Psychiatric Association.

relative to the anxiety seen in caffeine intoxication or caffeine withdrawal. In addition to these conditions, substance-induced anxiety disorder can be produced by a variety of other psychoactive substances (e.g., cocaine).

Epidemiology and Comorbidity

There are no specific data on the prevalence or incidence of caffeine-induced anxiety disorder, and there is no information known about comorbid conditions.

Course

There is no known information on the course or natural history of caffeine-induced anxiety disorder.

Treatment

Although there are no studies on the treatment of caffeine-induced anxiety disorder, guidelines for treatment should generally follow those recommended for the treatment of caffeine

dependence (see earlier). Thus, an initial, careful assessment of caffeine consumption should be conducted, and a program of gradual decreasing caffeine use should be instituted. Abrupt cessation of caffeine use should be avoided to minimize withdrawal symptoms and to increase the likelihood of long-term compliance with the dietary change. Given the etiological role of caffeine in caffeine-induced anxiety disorder, the prudent course of treatment would avoid the use of pharmacological agents such as benzodiazepines for the treatment of the anxiety disorder until caffeine use has been eliminated. A temporary caffeine-free trial may be useful in persuading skeptical patients about the role of caffeine in their anxiety symptoms.

Caffeine-induced Sleep Disorder

Definition

Psychoactive substances can produce sleep disorders distinct from the sleep disturbances associated with intoxication or withdrawal produced by that substance. It has long been recognized that caffeine-containing products can produce sleep disturbances, primarily in the form of insomnia. The primary feature of a substance-induced sleep disorder is a sleep disturbance directly related to a psychoactive substance (see DSM-IV-TR criteria). The form of the disorder can be insomnia, hypersomnia, parasomnia, or mixed, although caffeine typically produces insomnia. In general, sleep disturbance can often be a feature of substance intoxication or withdrawal (although sleep disturbance does not typically occur with caffeine withdrawal), and caffeine-induced sleep disorder should be diagnosed in patients who are having caffeine intoxication only if the symptoms of the sleep disturbance are excessive relative to what would typically be expected.

Etiology and Pathophysiology

Caffeine's effects on sleep can depend on a variety of factors, such as the dose of caffeine ingested, the individual's tolerance to caffeine, the time between caffeine ingestion and attempted sleep onset, and the ingestion of other psychoactive substances. The effects of caffeine on various measures of sleep quality are an increasing function of dose. Caffeine administered immediately prior to bedtime or throughout the day has been shown to delay onset of sleep and rapid eye movement sleep, reduce total sleep time, alter the normal stages of sleep and decrease the reported quality of sleep.

Assessment and Differential Diagnosis

The diagnosis of a caffeine-induced sleep disorder is based on evidence of a sleep disorder etiologically related to caffeine (see diagnostic decision tree for caffeine intoxication disorder, caffeine-induced anxiety disorder and caffeine-induced sleep disorder). Although caffeine consumption may decrease with age, the elderly commonly report increased sleeping problems which may be exacerbated by caffeine (Curless et al., 1993). Occult caffeine consumption in the form of analgesic medication may produce sleep problems in the elderly (Brown et al. 1995).

Epidemiology, Comorbidity, Course and Treatment

There are no specific data on the prevalence, incidence, course, treatment, comorbidity or patterns of caffeine-induced sleep disorder.

DSM-IV-TR Criteria 292.89

Substance-induced Sleep Disorder

A. A prominent disturbance in sleep that is sufficiently severe to warrant independent clinical attention.

B. There is evidence from the history, physical examination, or laboratory findings of either (1) or (2):

(1) the symptoms in Criterion A developed during, or within 1 month of, substance intoxication or withdrawal

(2) medication use is etiologically related to the sleep disturbance

C. The disturbance is not better accounted for by a sleep disorder that is not substance induced. Evidence that the symptoms are better accounted for by a sleep disorder that is not substance induced might include the following: the symptoms precede the onset of the substance use (or medication use); the symptoms persist for a substantial period of time (e.g., about a month) after the cessation of acute withdrawal or severe intoxication, or are substantially in excess of what would be expected given the type or amount of the substance used or the duration of use; or there is other evidence that suggests the existence of an independent nonsubstance-induced sleep disorder (e.g., a history of recurrent nonsubstance-related episodes).

D. The disturbance does not occur exclusively during the course of a delirium.

E. The sleep disturbance causes clinically significant distress or impairment in social, occupational, or other important areas of functioning.

Note: This diagnosis should be made instead of a diagnosis of substance intoxication or substance withdrawal only when the sleep symptoms are in excess of those usually associated with the intoxication or withdrawal syndrome and when the symptoms are sufficiently severe to warrant independent clinical attention.

Reprinted with permission from the Diagnostic and Statistical Manual of Mental Disorders. Fourth Edition, Text Revision. Copyright 2000 American Psychiatric Association.

Comparison of DSM-IV/ICD-10 Diagnostic Criteria

ICD-10 includes caffeine-related disorders in its "Other Stimulant" class which also includes amphetamines. This results in the ICD-10 Diagnostic Criteria for Research for Caffeine Intoxication being the same as those for amphetamine intoxication.

References

American Psychiatric Association (2000) *Diagnostic and Statistical Manual of Mental Disorders*, Fourth Edition, Text Revision. APA, Washington DC.

Barone JJ and Roberts HR (1996) Caffeine consumption. *Food Chem Toxicol* 34(1), 119–129.

Boulenger JP, Uhde TW, Wolff EA 3rd *et al.* (1984) Increased sensitivity to caffeine in patients with panic disorders. Preliminary. *Arch Gen Psychiatr* 41(11), 1067–1071.

Brown SL, Salive ME, Pahor M *et al.* (1995) Occult caffeine as a sours of sleep problems in an older population. *J Am Geriatr Soc* 43(8), 860–864.

Curless R, French JM, James OF *et al.* (1993) Is caffeine a factor in subjective insomnia of elderly people? *Age Ageing* 22(1), 41–45.

Gilbert RM (1984) Caffeine consumption, in *Methylxanthine Beverages and Foods: Chemistry, Consumption, and Health Effects* (ed Spiller GA) Alan R. Liss, New York, pp. 185–213.

Hays LR, Farabee D and Miller W (1998) Caffeine and nicotine use in an addicted population. *J Addict Dis* 17(1), 47–54.

Hughes JR and Oliveto AH (1997) A systematic survey of caffeine intake in Vermont. *Exp Clin Psychopharmacol* 5(4), 393–398.

Hughes JR, Amori G and Hatsukami DK (1988) A survey of physician advice about caffeine. *J Subst Abuse* 1(1), 67–70.

Hughes JR, Oliveto AH, Liguori A *et al.* (1998) Endorsement of DSM-IV dependence criteria among caffeine users. *Grug Alcohol Depend* 52(2), 99–107.

Kendler KS and Prescott CA (1999) Caffeine intake tolerance, and withdrawal in women: A population-based twin study. *Am J Psychiatr* 156(2), 223–228.

Kozlowski LT, Henningfield JE, Keenan RM *et al.* (1993) Patterns of alcohol, cigarette, and caffeine and other drug use in two drug abusing populations. *J Subst Abuse Treat* 10(2), 171–179.

Rihs M, Muller C and Baumann P (1996) Caffeine consumption in hospitalized psychiatric patients. *Eur Arch Psychiatr Clin Neurosci* 246(2), 83–92.

Russ NW, Sturgis ET, Malcolm RJ *et al.* (1988) Abuse of caffeine in substance abusers. *J Clin Psychiatr* 49(11), 457.

Sours JA (1983) Case reports of anorexia nervosa and caffeinism. *Am J Psychiatr* 140(2), 235–236.

Strain EC, Mumford GK, Silverman K *et al.* (1994) Caffeine dependence syndrome. Evidence from case histories and experimental evaluations. *JAMA* 272(13), 1043–1048.

Swanson JA, Lee JW and Hopp JW (1994) Caffeine and nicotine: A review of their joint use and possible interactive effects in tobacco withdrawal. *Addict Behav* 19(3), 229–256.

Substance Abuse: Cannabis-related Disorders

Definition

As with other substances of abuse, the *Diagnostic and Statistical Manual of Mental Disorders*, Fourth Edition (DSM-IV-TR) distinguishes a number of different cannabis-related diagnoses, which are shown in Table 37.1. These fall into two basic groups. The first group is defined by adverse effects resulting from cannabis use; these include cannabis abuse and cannabis dependence. The category of cannabis dependence includes a number of specifers that indicate the presence or absence of physiological dependence, type of remission, and whether or not the individual has been in a controlled environment. The second set of cannabis-related disorders in DSM-IV-TR includes psychiatric syndromes presumed to be induced by cannabis. This group includes: cannabis intoxication, which is almost certainly induced by cannabis and consists of the common signs and symptoms that normally follow cannabis use; cannabis intoxication delirium, a degree of disturbance beyond that normally expected with ordinary intoxication; cannabis-induced psychotic disorder which is subdivided into categories of psychosis with delusions and psychosis with hallucinations; and cannabis-induced anxiety disorder which is also subdivided into several types as shown in Table 37.1.

Throughout the remainder of this chapter, we discuss cannabis abuse and dependence under the general heading of cannabis use disorders; cannabis intoxication, cannabis intoxication delirium, cannabis-induced psychotic disorder and cannabis-induced anxiety disorder are discussed as cannabis-induced disorders.

Cannabis: Botany and Pharmacology

Cannabis preparations, derived from the female *Cannabis sativa* plant, have been widely used for their psychotropic effects since the beginning of history. The drug is prepared in different ways in different parts of the world. The flowering tops and resin secreted by the female plant contain the highest concentrations of Δ-9-tetrahydrocannabinol (Δ-9-THC), the primary psychoactive component. Marijuana, the most common preparation, is made by drying and shredding the upper leaves, tops, stems, flowers and seeds of the plant. Hashish is a more potent preparation made by extracting and drying the resin and sometimes also the compressed flowers. Hashish oil, which is even more potent, is distilled from hashish. Marijuana and hashish can be smoked either in the form of cigarettes or by using a pipe. Hashish, hashish oil and, less commonly, marijuana can be mixed with tea or food and taken orally (Ashton, 2001; Hall and Solowij, 1998). For the

Table 37.1	Cannabis-related Disorders
Cannabis Use Disorders	
304.30	Cannabis dependence
	With physiological dependence
	Without physiological dependence
	Early full remission
	Early partial remission
	Sustained full remission
	Sustained total remission
	In a controlled environment
305.20	Cannabis abuse
Cannabis-induced Disorders	
292.89	Cannabis intoxication
	With perceptual disturbances
292.81	Cannabis intoxication delirium
292.11	Cannabis-induced psychotic disorder, with delusions
	With onset during intoxication
292.12	Cannabis-induced psychotic disorder, with hallucinations
	With onset during intoxication
292.89	Cannabis-induced anxiety disorder
	With onset during intoxication
	With generalized anxiety
	With panic attacks
	With obsessive–compulsive symptoms
	With phobic symptoms
292.9	Cannabis-related disorder not otherwise specified

remainder of this chapter we will refer to these preparations collectively as "cannabis".

Selective breeding and improved growing methods have produced cannabis plants that contain significantly higher Δ-9-THC concentrations than naturally occurring plants. Thus, although there is a great deal of variation, the potency of illicit cannabis available in the USA has increased substantially, on average, over the last 30 years (Ashton, 2001; Hall and Solowij, 1998).

Intoxication occurs within minutes after smoking cannabis and typically persists for several hours. After eating foods

Essentials of Psychiatry Jerald Kay and Allan Tasman
© 2006 John Wiley & Sons, Ltd.

containing cannabis, intoxication occurs after approximately an hour and can persist for 8 to 24 hours. The onset of intoxication after drinking cannabis steeped in tea is shorter, but not as rapid as after smoking, and has an intermediate duration of intoxication. Smoking cannabis induces intoxication more quickly than ingesting cannabis because first-pass metabolism in the liver is avoided and the combustion causes enhanced release of Δ-9-THC from pyrolysis of acids in cannabis preparations. Smoking is the predominant method of taking cannabis in most parts of the world, including the USA, probably because of the more rapid onset of action and because the potency of the drug when it is smoked is about three times that experienced when an equivalent amount is eaten (Ashton, 2001; Hall and Solowij, 1998).

Δ-9-THC and other cannabinoids are highly lipophilic and are quickly and widely distributed throughout the body. Δ-9-THC can cross the placenta and enter breast milk; it may interact with other drugs by inducing liver enzymes and competing for plasma binding sites. Δ-9-THC is metabolized in the liver by hydroxylation to at least 20 different metabolites. Some, such as 11-hydroxy-THC, are psychoactive and have half-lives exceeding 2 days. Δ-9-THC may also be conjugated to more water-soluble metabolites that are excreted predominantly into the gut where they may be reabsorbed, and also into the bile, urine, sweat and hair. Δ-9-THC is stored in adipose tissue from which it is released slowly; in regular users it can often be detected more than 30 days after the individual's last exposure to cannabis (Johnson, 1990). If an individual uses cannabis regularly, the stores of Δ-9-THC in the adipose tissue result in a constant supply of cannabinoids to the body including the brain (Ashton, 2001).

There are two types of G-protein-coupled cannabinoid receptors. CB_1 receptors are found in the lipid membranes of neurons in the central nervous system, including the cerebral cortex, basal ganglia, thalamus and brain stem, with high densities in the hippocampus, cerebellum and striatum. CB_2 receptors are found in the lipid membranes of various types of cells in the immune system. Δ-9-THC is a partial agonist, activating both CB_1 and CB_2 receptors (Hall and Solowij, 1998). Activation of cannabinoid receptors mediates the inhibitory effect of adenylate cyclase, decreasing cyclic adenosine monophosphate, and also inhibits calcium and potassium transport. Receptor activation also mediates the excitatory effect of mitogen-activated protein kinase (Ameri, 1999). The cannabinoid system plays a modulatory role in regulating many different functions including mood, motor control, perception (including pain perception), appetite, sleep, memory and cognition, reproductive function and immune response (Hall and Solowij, 1998). Δ-9-THC can potentiate the effects of alcohol, barbiturates, caffeine and amphetamines (Solomons and Neppe, 1989).

Etiology and Pathophysiology

Cannabis Use Disorders

Cannabis dependence develops as a result of repeated use of the drug, and frequency of use is one of the most important predictors of developing dependence (Chen and Kandel, 1998; Kandel and Chen, 2000). Like most other dependence-producing drugs, cannabis produces its reinforcing effects by activating the mesolimbic dopaminergic "reward" pathway, which consists of dopaminergic neurons in the ventral tegmental area (VTA) that project to the nucleus accumbens, increasing dopamine levels in the shell of the nucleus accumbens (Diana *et al.*, 1998a; Gardner,

1999; Tanda *et al.*, 1997). Naloxone, an opiate antagonist at the μ_1 opioid receptor in the VTA, blocks this increase in dopamine, which suggests that Δ-9-THC and opiates share the same mechanism of activating this pathway (Tanda *et al.*, 1997). Studies have shown that people choose higher-potency cannabis preparations over lower-potency preparations, a finding which suggests that increased potency may result in an increased risk of progression to addiction and dependence (Chait and Burke, 1994; Harder and Reitbrock, 1997).

Regular use of cannabis for periods as short as 1 to 3 weeks can produce tolerance to many of its acute physiological and psychological effects (Jones *et al.*, 1976, 1981; Jones, 1983). Such tolerance may cause some individuals to increase their use in order to continue to experience desired effects. As with other addictive drugs, discontinuation of cannabis use increases corticotropin-releasing factor (CRF) in the central amygdala and decreases dopaminergic transmission in the limbic system, resulting in withdrawal symptoms (Diana *et al.*, 1998b; Rodriguez *et al.*, 1997).

The core symptoms of cannabis withdrawal are irritability, anxiety, physical tension, and decreases in mood and appetite. Restlessness, tremors, sweating, insomnia, increased aggressiveness and very vivid dreams have also been reported (Budney *et al.*, 1999; Haney *et al.*, 1999; Kouri *et al.*, 1999; Kouri and Pope, 2000; Kaymakcalan, 1973, 1981; Tennant, 1986; Compton *et al.*, 1990; Jones *et al.*, 1976, 1981; Jones, 1983; Wiesbeck *et al.*, 1996). The symptoms of cannabis withdrawal are similar to those of opiate withdrawal, except that their intensity is milder and their course is delayed and prolonged due to the fact that cannabis is cleared from the body gradually as it is released slowly from storage in adipose tissue. Symptoms typically begin the day after last use, do not reach maximal intensity until the third day, and then resolve over the following week. The severity of the withdrawal syndrome varies considerably among individuals. In a recent study of 108 chronic, long-term cannabis users, the authors observed a number of individuals who experienced severe withdrawal symptoms which precluded their completion of the month-long abstinence period required by the study protocol, suggesting that, for at least some individuals, the withdrawal syndrome is an important factor in the development and persistence of dependence (Pope *et al.*, 2001a; Gruber *et al.*, in press). The two clinical vignettes provided at the end of the chapter describe individuals who experienced withdrawal effects from their use of cannabis.

Environment appears to play a major role in determining whether an individual will initiate cannabis use, but only a minor role in determining whether an individual will go on to develop cannabis dependence. Genetic factors, on the other hand, appear to play only a moderate role in determining whether an individual will initiate cannabis use, but a major role in determining whether an individual who initiates use will subsequently develop cannabis dependence. A study of female twins reported that genetic factors accounted for 60 to 80% of the variance in liability for cannabis dependence (Kendler and Prescott, 1998). A study of male twins reported that genetic factors contributed significantly to progression from first exposure or opportunity to use cannabis to initial use of cannabis, from initial use to use more than five times, and from use more than five times to regular use (Tsuang *et al.*, 1999). A second study of male twins reported that genetic factors were responsible for 44% and common environmental factors for only 21% of the variance in risk of developing cannabis dependence (True *et al.*, 1999).

In addition to the addictive properties of cannabis and the genetic predisposition of individuals, another possible etiology for cannabis dependence is that some individuals may be "self-medicating" themselves for underlying psychiatric symptoms. Some patients with depression, anxiety, or negative symptoms of schizophrenia report that marijuana use alleviates their symptoms (Peralta and Cuesta, 1992; Dixon *et al.*, 1991; Estroff and Gold, 1986; Warner *et al.*, 1994; Gruber *et al.*, 1996). In addition, a large portion of adolescents and young adults with cannabis dependence have reported using marijuana to self-treat anger, boredom, or lack of direction (Chen and Kandel, 1998; Gruber *et al.*, in press; Johnston *et al.* 2001; Newcombe and Bentler, 1988). An interesting finding of a longitudinal study of chronic cannabis users is that prescriptions for psychoactive medications increased as cannabis use decreased when the subjects were in their late twenties and early thirties, raising the possibility that for some individuals the prescription medications were serving the same purpose as the cannabis (Chen and Kandel, 1995, 1998). We have observed this apparent self-medication phenomenon in a number of patients with underlying depressive illness or bipolar disorder.

However, contrary to the beliefs of the users, cannabis may also contribute to the symptoms enumerated above (Miller *et al.*, 1989; Lex *et al.*, 1989; Mirin *et al.*, 1971; Chen and Kandel, 1998; Baigent *et al.*, 1995, Green and Ritter, 2000).

Cannabis-induced Disorders

The mechanism causing the euphoria experienced during cannabis intoxication is activation of the mesolimbic dopaminergic "reward" pathway, and is described in detail in the botany and pharmacology section (Diana *et al.*, 1998a; Gardner, 1999; Tanda *et al.*, 1997). The mechanisms causing the physiological signs and symptoms associated with cannabis intoxication are thought to result from the action of the cannabinoid system on other major neurotransmitter systems including the noradrenergic, cholinergic, serotonin and opioid systems (Ameri, 1999).

There are no adequate data regarding the mechanism by which cannabis intoxication delirium, cannabis-induced psychotic disorder, or cannabis-induced anxiety disorder can occur *de novo* in individuals without preexisting medical or psychiatric disorders. In a review of studies of patients with cannabis-induced psychotic disorder, it was found that most of the studies had not excluded individuals with a preexisting Axis I disorder, such as schizophrenia or a major mood disorder, which would render the individual vulnerable to psychotic symptoms even in the absence of cannabis use. At present, therefore, it seems possible that the majority of cannabis-induced psychotic or anxiety disorders represent exacerbations of preexisting DSM-IV Axis I psychiatric disorders in individuals who become intoxicated with the drug (Gruber and Pope, 1994).

Assessment and Differential Diagnosis

Cannabis-related Disorders

To diagnose any of the cannabis-related disorders, it is important to obtain a detailed history of the individual's pattern of substance abuse (including abuse not only of cannabis but of other substances) and to attempt to substantiate this report with toxicology screening for drugs of abuse. Individuals who smoke cannabis regularly can have substantial accumulations of THC in their fat stores. Thus, for weeks after cessation of smoking, de-

tectable levels of cannabinoids may be found in urine (Johnson, 1990). However, a positive response on toxicology screening for cannabinoids cannot establish any of the cannabis-related diagnoses; it is useful only as an indicator that these diagnoses should be considered.

Cannabis Dependence

It is uncommon to see patients who exhibit cannabis dependence as their only diagnosis because such individuals rarely seek treatment as they generally do not acknowledge that they have a problem and are unaware that treatment is available. However, some patients with this disorder will respond to offers for treatment because they realize that they are unable to stop use on their own and because they notice the deleterious effect of compulsive use (Roffman and Barnhart, 1987). Therefore, the diagnosis of cannabis dependence will most often be made in patients who present with other psychiatric problems, such as mood and anxiety disorders, and other substance use disorders. Another manner in which individuals with cannabis dependence may come to the attention of psychiatrists is when they are arrested for possession of the substance or some crime related to cannabis abuse, such as driving under the influence of the drug. Nevertheless, cannabis dependence is probably underdiagnosed in both psychiatric and general medical populations because it is not considered.

The diagnosis of cannabis dependence cannot be made without obtaining a history indicating that the cannabis use is impairing the patient's ability to function either physically or psychologically. Areas to inquire about include the patient's performance at work, ability to carry out social and family obligations, and physical health. It is also important to find out how much of the patient's time is spent on cannabis-related activities and whether the patient has tried unsuccessfully to stop or cut down on use in the past. Although it has been our experience that people who have used cannabis daily over a period of years almost invariably report tolerance to many of the effects of cannabis and to experience an unpleasant withdrawal state if use is discontinued, neither tolerance nor withdrawal is necessary for the diagnosis of cannabis dependence. When this diagnosis is made, it can be described further by the following specifiers: with or without physiological dependence, early full or partial remission, sustained full or partial remission, or in a controlled environment. These diagnostic distinctions must be based on the pattern of use reported by the patient.

Cannabis Abuse

Most individuals who are diagnosed with cannabis abuse have only recently started using cannabis. As with cannabis dependence, cannabis abuse is unlikely to be diagnosed unless some additional condition or circumstance brings the individual to medical attention. Teenagers often fall into this category because they spend time in supervised environments like school and home where responsible adults may intervene. Also, teenagers are more likely to have motor vehicle accidents while intoxicated because they are inexperienced drivers, and are more likely to be arrested for possession because they have a greater tendency to participate in risky behaviors of all types.

Although virtually all individuals with cannabis dependence meet the inclusion criteria for cannabis abuse, they cannot be given this diagnosis because the presence of cannabis dependence is an exclusion criterion. Undoubtedly, the vast majority of people with cannabis dependence would have been given the diagnosis of cannabis abuse until they developed dependence.

It is probable that individuals qualifying for a diagnosis of cannabis abuse will either cease use (see course section) or develop cannabis dependence. The criteria for cannabis abuse focus on adverse consequences of cannabis use that could potentially result from just a single use such as failure to fulfill obligations at work, school, or home, participating in potentially dangerous activities like driving while intoxicated with cannabis, having cannabis-related legal problems, or social or interpersonal difficulties. Even though these adverse consequences can occur following a single episode of cannabis use, the consequences must be recurrent, requiring multiple episodes of use. Since the number of episodes necessary for "recurrent" is not defined, and the pattern of use is often dependent on patient self-report, it is often difficult to distinguish between abuse and dependence. This difficulty is easier to recognize if one looks at the extremes. On one end of the continuum, a high school student who actually has only used cannabis twice, but who was unfortunate enough to be caught and suspended from school on both occasions, would appropriately be diagnosed with cannabis abuse. At the other end of the continuum, a high school student who had actually been using cannabis every day for three years and met the criteria for dependence, who was also caught and suspended from school twice but denied symptoms of dependence, would incorrectly be diagnosed with cannabis abuse.

The difference between people with cannabis abuse and those with cannabis dependence is that the people with dependence have been using more regularly (one or more times per day) and for a longer duration (one or more years), and the acute problems associated with abuse have turned into the chronic problems associated with dependence. For example, what started as failure to fulfill obligations at work or school has resulted in dropping out of school or working at jobs with extremely low expectations. Multiple car accidents or arrests have led to chronic injuries (often associated with obtaining SSDI), loss of licenses, probation and even periods of time in prison. Social or interpersonal problems have resulted in isolation or at least separation from people who are not regular cannabis users. If there is a committed relationship where the partner is typically cannabis dependent, and if children are involved, chronic neglect is present if caring for children while intoxicated with cannabis represents neglect.

Cannabis Intoxication

There are four criteria necessary to make this diagnosis (see DSM-IV criteria for intoxication). The first is that recent use of cannabis must be established. This cannot be done with toxicology screening because the result may be negative after a single episode of smoking or, alternatively, may be positive even if the individual has not used the drug for a time much longer than the period of intoxication (see section on Cannabis botany and pharmacology). Thus, the recent use of cannabis must be reported by the patient or another person who witnessed the patient's use. In addition, the symptoms resulting from cannabis use must produce "clinically significant maladaptive behavioral or psychological changes". Thirdly, the patient must exhibit some physical signs of cannabis use. DSM-IV-TR requires the patient to have at least two of four signs – conjunctival injection, increased appetite, dry mouth and tachycardia – within 2 hours of cannabis use. Fourthly, symptoms cannot be accounted for by a general medical condition or another mental disorder. There is a specifier, "with perceptual disturbances", that can be used if the patient is experiencing illusions or hallucinations while not delirious and while maintaining intact reality testing.

Table 37.2   Physiological Effects of Cannabis Intoxication
Common and Transient
Tachycardia
Hypertension
Thirst
Increased appetite
Constipation
Decreased intraocular pressure
Mydriasis
Mild bronchoconstriction followed by bronchodilation
Increased reaction time
Impaired coordination
Distorted time perception
Decreased libido
Mild analgesia
Mild anti-emetic effects
Uncommon and Transient
Ataxia
Ptosis
Miosis
Drowsiness
Bradycardia
Hypotension
Peripheral vasoconstriction
Hypothermia

There has been extensive research on the effects of acute cannabis intoxication. In addition to the symptoms and signs required for a DSM-IV-TR diagnosis, many psychological and physiological effects have been reported. Awareness of these may enhance the psychiatrist's ability to recognize cannabis intoxication. Physiological effects are listed in Table 37.2, and are divided into commonly observed effects and rare effects that have been described only after the use of very high doses of cannabis (Hall and Solowij, 1998; Ameri, 1999; Perez-Reyes, 1999). Cannabis has low toxicity, and to our knowledge, no deaths from cannabis overdose have been reported (Hall and Solowij, 1998). Similarly, psychological effects are listed in Table 37.3, divided into commonly observed effects and uncommon effects. Most people find the commonly experienced psychological effects enjoyable. However, some individuals, especially women (Thomas, 1996)

Table 37.3   Psychological Effects of Cannabis Intoxication
Common and Transient
Euphoria
Distortions in perception, including time perception
Enhancement of sensations
Uncommon and Transient
Dysphoria
Anxiety, and less commonly panic reactions
Restlessness
Depersonalization
Derealization
Paranoid ideation

and inexperienced users in an unfamiliar environment, find them frightening and experience anxiety and even have panic reactions (Hall and Solowij, 1998; Johns, 2001; Thomas, 1996). Although all of these effects typically persist only for the period of acute intoxication, some reports have described individuals who report "flashbacks" of cannabis intoxication long after use, and depersonalization persisting long after acute intoxication (Keeler et al., 1968, 1971; Levi and Miller, 1990; Annis and Smart, 1973; Stanton and Bardoni, 1972). At this time there is insufficient evidence to ascertain whether these reports are attributable to cannabis itself, to confounding factors such as the concomitant use of other drugs, or the presence of other Axis I disorders (Johns, 2001).

In addition, cannabis use produces deficits in a number of neuropsychological functions, both during acute intoxication and after up to a week or more of abstinence in chronic, long-term users. These tasks include short-term memory, sustained or divided attention, and complex decision-making (Ehrenreich et al., 1999; Pope et al., 1995, 1997, 2001a; Pope and Yurgelun-Todd, 1996; Schwartz et al., 1989; Solowij et al., 1991, 1995; Solowij, 1995, 1998). A study of chronic, long-term users found that these deficits were reversible after 28 days of abstinence (Pope et al., 2001a). However, a few studies have found that subtle electrophysiologic changes, of uncertain clinical significance, may persist even after years of abstinence (Solowij, 1995, 1998; Struve et al., 1998).

Cannabis Intoxication Delirium

We have not located any original reports of this entity, although it is mentioned in various reviews and is included in DSM-IV. Thus, if cannabis intoxication delirium does occur in neurologically intact individuals, it is probably a rare complication. If the delirium does not resolve within 24 to 48 hours, it is almost certainly a result of an underlying neurological or medical condition. Therefore, in a patient with delirium, even if recent cannabis use has been reported, a full diagnostic work-up should be performed to rule out a concomitant, treatable neurological condition (Halikas, 1974; Johns, 2001).

The following two substance-induced conditions are not generally diagnosed unless the symptoms are in excess of those usually associated with the intoxication or withdrawal state and are sufficiently severe to warrant independent clinical attention.

Cannabis-induced Psychotic Disorder

There are two subtypes of cannabis-induced psychotic disorder: one featuring delusions, the other hallucinations. The diagnosis of this disorder is readily made in individuals who have psychotic symptoms that appear immediately after ingestion of cannabis. However, a careful history is required to establish whether the individual has a preexisting psychotic disorder (as is often the case in such situations) or whether the symptoms arose de novo after cannabis consumption. There is little evidence that cannabis-induced psychotic disorders can arise in previously asymptomatic individuals (Gruber and Pope, 1994). Therefore, if psychotic symptoms persist for 24 to 48 hours after the period of acute intoxication, they are likely due to an underlying psychiatric disorder which must be diagnosed and treated (Hall and Degenhardt, 2000; Johns, 2001, Gruber and Pope, 1994).

Cannabis-induced Anxiety Disorder

This disorder may be further described by the following specifiers: with generalized anxiety, with panic attacks, with

obsessive–compulsive symptoms and with phobic symptoms. The literature contains papers that report individuals who have anxiety, panic reactions and paranoid ideation during the period of acute intoxication, but we are unaware of any papers that report obsessive–compulsive or phobic symptoms. People who experience anxiety after using cannabis are typically inexperienced users who react to the novel experiences of perceptual distortions and intensified sensations with anxiety and even panic reactions, rather than enjoyment (Thomas, 1996; Johns, 2001; Szuster et al., 1988). Women are more likely than men to experience cannabis-induced anxiety (Thomas, 1996). As with cannabis-induced psychotic disorders, we have been unable to find clear cases of cannabis-induced anxiety disorders in individuals without a preexisting Axis I disorder. Again, if symptoms of severe anxiety or panic persist for 24 to 48 hours after the period of acute intoxication, they are likely due to an underlying psychiatric disorder that must be diagnosed and treated (Johns, 2001).

A diagnostic decision tree for cannabis use disorders is presented in Figure 37.1.

Epidemiology and Comorbidity

Cannabis Use Disorders

Cannabis is probably the most commonly used illicit substance in the world, with an estimated 200 to 300 million regular users (Johnson, 1990). In the USA, cannabis is generally thought to be the most widely used illicit drug, with more than 50% of Americans reporting at least one episode of use (Johnson, 1990; Mueser et al., 1992; Chen and Kandel, 1998; Hubbard et al., 1999). As with most other illicit drugs cannabis use occurs more often in men though the difference between the sexes is decreasing (Greenfield and O'Leary, 1999). Also, like other illicit drugs cannabis use typically begins in adolescence and is most prevalent in people between the ages of 18 to 30 years (Chen and Kandel, 1995, 1998; Johnston et al., 2001; Kandel and Chen, 2000). The age of first cannabis use in America has been decreasing; in 1997 the average age of first use was reported to be 14 by the National Household Survey on Drug Abuse (NHSDA) (SAMHSA, 1997). The annual, monitoring the future study of high school students, reported that in 2000, 15.6% of 8th graders, 32.2% of 10th graders and 36.5% of 12th graders reported using cannabis in the past year. Approximately 20% of 12th grade cannabis users reported daily use (Johnston et al., 2001).

Adolescents appear more vulnerable to developing cannabis dependence than adults, becoming dependent after using cannabis at a lower dose and frequency of use (Chen et al., 1997). Although earlier onset of use during adolescence is a predictor for continued use and the development of dependency, frequency of use is a stronger predictor (Chen and Kandel, 1998; Kandel and Chen, 2000; DeWit et al., 2000; SAMHSA, 2000). Of those adolescents who use cannabis more than once, about a third will subsequently use cannabis regularly for some period of time, with 20% using daily, and an additional 10 to 20% using near daily (Hall and Solowij, 1998; Johnston et al., 2001; Zoccollilo et al., 1999). It is estimated that a third of those who use cannabis daily meet the criteria for cannabis dependence, and that of all adolescents who use cannabis at least once, approximately 9% will develop dependence (Anthony et al., 1994; Chen et al., 1997). However, most adolescents who use cannabis regularly will have stopped use by the time they are 30 (Chen and Kandel, 1995, 1998).

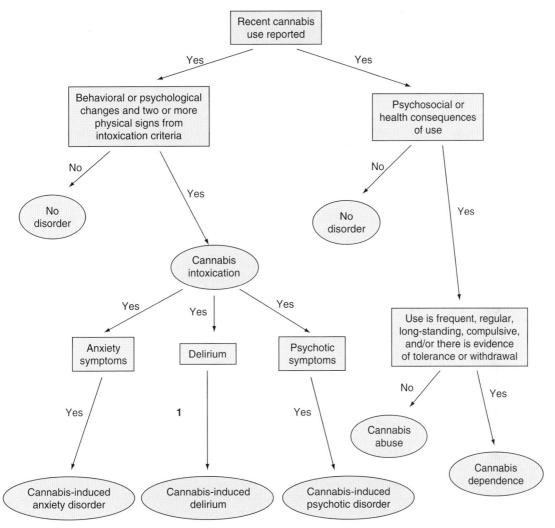

Figure 37.1   *Diagnostic decision tree for cannabis use disorders.*

Studies have reported that individuals with cannabis use disorders have high rates of other substance abuse disorders (Miller *et al.*, 1990) as well as other types of Axis I disorders (Regier *et al.*, 1990; Troisi *et al.*, 1998). It is possible, however, that these findings reflect "spurious comorbidity" (Smoller *et al.*, 2000) because individuals with cannabis dependence and other Axis I disorders are probably more likely to present for treatment or research studies than those with cannabis dependence alone.

Conversely, studies of several psychiatric populations (Brady *et al.*, 1991; Alterman *et al.*, 1982; Miller *et al.*, 1989; Cantwell *et al.*, 1999; Menezes *et al.*, 1996; Johns, 2001) with a number of different Axis I diagnoses other than panic disorder (Szuster *et al.*, 1988) have found high rates of cannabis use. The course of the Axis I illnesses is often adversely affected by cannabis use; cannabis may exacerbate psychotic symptoms in patients with schizophrenia, possibly precipitate schizophrenia in predisposed individuals (Andreasson *et al.*, 1987, 1989), precipitate hypomanic or manic episodes in bipolar patients (Gruber and Pope, 1994) and trigger panic reactions in patients with panic disorder (Szuster *et al.*, 1988). Cannabis use, abuse and dependence are also commonly comorbid with conduct disorder in children and adolescents and with antisocial personality disorder in adults (Weller and Halikas, 1985; Henry *et al.*, 1993; True *et al.*, 1999; Crowley *et al.*, 1998). Despite these findings of

comorbidity, cannabis use has not been shown to induce any psychiatric disorders *de novo* in nonpredisposed individuals (Hall and Degenhardt, 2000; Johns, 2001).

Cannabis-induced Disorders

The prevalence of cannabis intoxication should be approximately the same as the prevalence of cannabis use described at the beginning of this section. No formal epidemiological data exist regarding the prevalence of cannabis intoxication delirium, cannabis-induced psychotic disorder, or cannabis-induced anxiety disorder. In fact, it is not entirely certain that any of these three entities actually occurs in individuals free of preexisting DSM-IV-TR Axis I disorders (Hall and Degenhardt, 2000; Johns, 2001).

For example, no original reports of cannabis-induced delirium in the literature were found except for comments about it in review articles. Whereas cannabis use occasionally causes anxiety, or even panic reactions, especially among inexperienced users, there is again no known published study exhibiting a cohort of previously asymptomatic subjects who developed clinically significant cannabis-induced anxiety disorder. One investigator (Pillard, 1970) observed that there were five to seven cases of cannabis-associated anxiety reactions reported to a university health service per year; he hypothesized that more cases occurred but were not reported. However, he noted that reassurance was all the treatment necessary, suggesting that these patients had not developed clinically significant anxiety disorders. Finally, although anecdotal reports and even case series of cannabis-induced psychotic disorder have appeared, many of these have been collected outside the USA and most provide insufficient evidence to assess whether the subjects studied were suffering from preexisting psychotic disorders before their ingestion of cannabis (Gruber and Pope, 1994). In one US study, the investigators reviewed approximately 10 000 discharges from two psychiatric units. All cases of possible cannabis-induced mental disorders were investigated by chart review. No cases of clear-cut cannabis-induced psychotic disorder or cannabis-induced anxiety disorder were found. Thus, it appears that these disorders, at least of sufficient magnitude to prompt a psychiatric admission, are rare or do not exist at all (Gruber and Pope, 1994; Hall and Degenhardt, 2000; Johns, 2001).

Course

Cannabis Use Disorders

As discussed in the epidemiology section, about a third of those adolescents who try cannabis will use it regularly for some period of time, whereas only about 10% will go on to develop long-term dependence lasting into adulthood (Hall and Solowij, 1998). Even among these persistent users, the majority will stop use by age 30 years. Thus, it is possible to extrapolate from these figures that less than 2% of adults will exhibit cannabis dependence during their twenties and probably less than 1% of adults will continue use into their thirties, suggesting a good prognosis for the majority of cannabis-dependent patients under age 30 years. However, for the small minority who continue to suffer from cannabis dependence into their thirties, most follow a chronic or relapsing course similar to those who suffer from dependence on other substances (Miller *et al.*, 1989; Hall and Solowij, 1998; Johnston *et al.*, 2001; Zoccolillo *et al.*, 1999; Anthony *et al.*, 1994; Chen and Kandel, 1995, 1998; Chen *et al.*, 1997; Kandel and Chen, 2000, Stephens *et al.*, 1993a, 1993b, 1994, 2000; Baer *et al.*, 1998; Hser *et al.* 2001; Hubbard *et al.*, 1985).

Cannabis abuse and dependence appear to pursue a benign course in many individuals; many studies have suggested that individuals suffering from these disorders do not differ in ability to function in society from matched control subjects who are not users (Kouri *et al.*, 1995; Simon *et al.*, 1974; Pope *et al.*, 1990, 2001b; Zinberg and Weil, 1970; Comitas, 1976; Hochman and Brill, 1973; Boulougouris *et al.*, 1976; Robins *et al.*, 1970; Mendelson *et al.*, 1976; Brill and Christie, 1974; Pope and Yurgelun-Todd, 1996). However, a few studies have described an "amotivational syndrome" associated with chronic cannabis use, characterized by subjective reports of lack of direction, motivation and ambition (Mellinger *et al.*, 1976; Lessin and Thomas, 1976; Kupfer *et al.*, 1973; Burdsal *et al.*, 1973; Campbell, 1976; Hendin and Haas, 1985; Musty and Kaback, 1995; Gruber *et al.*, in press). This "amotivational syndrome" appears to result from the effects of continuous intoxication and resolves when cannabis is discontinued (Johns, 2001). In the context of a recent study involving 108 chronic, long-term cannabis users (Pope *et al.*, 2001a; Gruber *et al.*, in press), the authors encountered a number of chronic long-term cannabis users who reported lack of direction, motivation and ambition while using cannabis heavily, but then reported increased productivity and success in their work and social lives after discontinuing use.

Cannabis-induced Disorders

Cannabis intoxication is a self-limiting state that remits as cannabis is metabolized and eliminated from the body. If symptoms suggestive of cannabis intoxication persist, other diagnoses should be considered. Similarly, although there are few data regarding the course of the other cannabis-induced disorders, it appears that cannabis-induced psychotic and anxiety disorders, as well as cannabis intoxication delirium, rarely persist beyond the period of acute intoxication with the drug. For example, although there have been reports of cannabis-induced psychoses persisting for days or even weeks beyond the time of acute intoxication, a review of the literature (as discussed earlier) was unable to exhibit a series of unequivocal cases in which such symptoms persisted in the absence of an underlying Axis I disorder. Therefore, symptoms of delirium, psychosis, or anxiety persisting more than 24 to 48 hours after acute cannabis intoxication suggest that another Axis I disorder, rather than cannabis itself, is responsible for the symptoms (Gruber and Pope, 1994; Hall and Degenhardt, 2000; Johns, 2001).

Treatment

Cannabis Use Disorders

Standard Approaches to Treatment

Up until the last few years, the prevailing opinion was that cannabis use did not produce addiction and dependence and that cannabis users could discontinue use without the help of treatment programs. In fact, this was the prevailing attitude even amongst users, many of whom had tried unsuccessfully to discontinue use (Weiner *et al.*, 1999). Although it is undeniably true that the majority of cannabis users are able to stop without assistance, it is also becoming apparent that many cannabis-dependent individuals cannot stop without help. The generally held opinion among cannabis users is that there are few substance abuse programs that will accept them if their primary substance is cannabis and that those programs that do exist are not effective for cannabis users (Weiner *et al.*, 1999).

However, mounting evidence documents the existence of a population of cannabis-dependent individuals who desire treatment (Roffman and Barnhart, 1987; Budney *et al.*, 1999; Stephens *et al.*, 1993a, 1993b, 1994, 2000; Weiner *et al.*, 1999). For example, a survey of 335 adolescent cannabis users reported that 80% had considered quitting, 52% had tried unsuccessfully to quit, and only 24% believed that they would never quit (Weiner *et al.*, 1999). In one investigation, a public service announcement directed at chronic marijuana users resulted in interviews of 225 people who responded. It was found that 74% reported negative consequences of their marijuana use and 92% wanted to be treated (Roffman and Barnhart, 1987). In 1998, 48% of adolescent admissions to state-funded substance abuse programs were for primary cannabis dependence, indicating a significant need for treatment programs for cannabis dependence (SAMHSA, 1999).

With the recognition that cannabis use produces dependence and withdrawal, and that cannabis-dependent individuals may benefit from treatment, many substance abuse programs have started offering treatment to people whose primary drug of abuse or dependence is marijuana. Unfortunately, these programs are not generally designed specifically for cannabis dependence and they have not achieved high success rates (Baer et al., 1998; Hser et al., 2001; Hubbard et al., 1985; SAMHSA, 2000). Similarly, many nonprofessional organizations that offer support groups, such as Alcoholics Anonymous (AA), Narcotics Anonymous (NA) and Self-Management and Recovery Training (SMART), have also begun to welcome people whose primary drug is cannabis. In addition, there is now a nonprofessional support organization, Marijuana Anonymous (MA), started by and run for cannabis-dependent individuals.

We are aware of only four controlled studies of treatment of cannabis-dependent individuals. In three of the studies, the subjects were seeking treatment specifically for cannabis dependence, whereas the fourth study involved schizophrenic patients undergoing treatment for marijuana dependence. The first study found no difference in the outcome between a cognitive–behavioral relapse prevention group and a support group – overall, 16% of subjects had decreased use and 15% were abstinent when assessed 12 months after treatment (Stephens et al., 1994). Higher quantity and frequency of marijuana use prior to treatment were strongly correlated with poorer outcome (Stephens et al., 1993b). A second study compared a motivational enhancement group, a motivational enhancement plus cognitive–behavioral therapy group, and a motivational enhancement plus cognitive–behavioral therapy group combined with a voucher-based incentive program that rewarded bi-weekly urine screens that were negative with vouchers for retail items. The group that received the voucher-based incentive program achieved a higher rate of abstinence during the study period and at the end of the study than either of the other two treatment groups (Budney et al., 2000). Similar success using monetary rewards for negative urines was also reported in a small trial of schizophrenic patients undergoing treatment for marijuana dependence (Sigmon et al., 2000). The last study compared brief motivational therapy with a cognitive–behavioral relapse prevention support group and a control group consisting of subjects put on a waiting list. Although no difference was found between the two active-treatment groups, subjects in both treatment groups were using significantly less marijuana and reported significantly fewer symptoms of dependence and fewer marijuana-related problems than subjects in the control group. Nevertheless, only 22% of the subjects in the active-treatment groups remained abstinent throughout a 16-month follow-up period (Stephens et al., 2000).

The strongest predictor of successful outcome is longer retention in treatment programs (Simpson, 1981). Predictors of dropping out of an outpatient treatment program and presumably continuing use, were found to be young age, financial difficulties and psychological stress (Crits-Christoph and Siqueland, 1996; Grella et al., 1999; Hser et al., 2001; Simpson et al., 1997; Roffman et al., 1993). More research is clearly required to discover effective ways to retain cannabis-dependent patients in treatment.

Currently, there are few substance abuse programs specifically designed to treat cannabis dependence. Most programs are designed to treat all types of substance abuse, so that cannabis-dependent patients typically receive the same treatment as patients with other types of substance abuse. Since many cannabis-dependent patients are also dependent on other substances, this is often a satisfactory treatment strategy. Also, a number of basic principles of treatment of substance use disorders are equally applicable to cannabis dependence and other types of substance dependence.

One of these principles, critical for selecting the most appropriate intervention, is the importance of assessing an individual's stage in the recovery process (Prochaska and Velicer, 1997). Individuals in early stages, such as "precontemplation" and "contemplation", benefit most from strategies aimed at using reliable sources to convey accurate information about cannabis that will help individuals identify personal reasons for discontinuing use. Individuals in later stages, such as "action" and "maintenance", benefit most from cognitive–behavioral relapse-prevention strategies (Botvin, 2000; Prochaska and Velicer, 1997).

As with all other drugs of abuse, the ultimate goal in the treatment of cannabis dependence is abstinence. In a phenomenon similar to that seen in alcohol-dependent people, many cannabis-dependent people have exposure to others who are able to use cannabis in a nonproblematic manner, and will often insist that their goal is to moderate their use, rather than cease use altogether. Unfortunately, if a person is susceptible to cannabis dependence, the most frequent outcome of trying to use moderately after a period of abstinence is that within a few weeks or months they have returned to their preabstinence pattern of use. Although physicians can tell cannabis-dependent people that this is the likely outcome, only after going through this process one or more times do people whose goal is moderation rather than abstinence recognize that like alcoholics, moderation is not an option for them. The process of treatment begins with detoxification followed by maintenance. As discussed in the section on etiology and pathophysiology, chronic users usually experience a withdrawal syndrome during detoxification. Since the cannabis withdrawal syndrome is not life-threatening, detoxification generally does not require hospitalization unless it is complicated by detoxification from other drugs or by comorbid Axis I disorders that do require hospitalization for safe treatment. The intensity of the cannabis withdrawal syndrome varies widely, with some individuals reporting very mild symptoms and others reporting more severe symptoms (Budney et al., 1999; Haney et al., 1999; Kouri and Pope, 2000; Kaymakcalan, 1973, 1981; Tennant, 1986; Compton et al., 1990; Jones et al., 1976, 1981; Jones, 1983; Wiesbeck et al., 1996).

To help a patient tolerate the 7- to 10-day withdrawal period, practitioners should provide psychological support (e.g., reassurance that the symptoms will resolve in a little over a week) and in some cases, provide pharmacological support (Miller et al., 1989; Haney et al., 2001a, 2001b). Research into possible pharmacological interventions is just getting underway. One author suggested the use of long-acting benzodiazepines if the level of discomfort is high or there are abnormal vital signs (Miller et al., 1989). A small placebo-controlled, crossover study of 10 subjects showed that the antidepressant bupropion (Wellbutrin, Zyban) worsened irritability, restlessness, depression and insomnia associated with marijuana withdrawal (Haney et al., 2001a). A second small placebo-controlled, crossover study of seven subjects showed that the antidepressant nefazodone (Serzone) decreased anxiety, muscle aches and restlessness associated with marijuana withdrawal, but not irritability or insomnia (Haney et al., 2001b).

The foundation of maintenance treatment, as with other types of substance use disorders, is regular attendance at groups that provide education and support. It is hypothesized that such groups are effective because fellow group members are best able to confront each other's denial and minimization of the substance abuse problem and the rationalizations put forth by the substance abuser for continued use despite negative consequences. Also, substance users typically report that they are most likely to believe information if it is provided by former users (Weiner *et al.*, 1999). Since cannabis dependence, like other types of substance abuse, is characterized by a chronic, relapsing course, these groups provide an important function by addressing issues around relapse prevention and provide support for dealing with relapses when they do occur.

Special Features Influencing Treatment

Several approaches that are more important to the treatment of cannabis dependence should be employed in addition to the basic, general substance abuse program. Recent studies examining reasons for cannabis use have provided information to guide treatment strategies. For example, both adolescent and adult cannabis users frequently report that they use cannabis to relax, or as a stress reduction or coping mechanism. This observation suggests that treatment programs should teach healthier and more effective coping mechanisms and cognitive–behavioral strategies for relaxation and stress reduction (Botvin, 2000; Hendin and Haas, 1985; Weiner *et al.*, 1999).

The most salient feature of cannabis abuse or dependence is that it is often comorbid with other Axis I disorders as discussed earlier. Toxicology screening for other drugs of abuse is imperative because the most common comorbid Axis I disorders are other types of substance abuse. Even in the absence of an obvious Axis I diagnosis, psychological reasons for cannabis use should be investigated. For example, use of cannabis for relaxation or improving mood may be indicative of efforts to "self-medicate" underlying anxiety or mood disorders (Chen and Kandel, 1998; Latimer *et al.*, 2000). Thus, treatment programs for cannabis dependence should include a dual-diagnosis component. Because of the high frequency of comorbidity among cannabis-dependent individuals, diagnosing and treating the underlying disorder or symptomatology may be a necessary condition for the individual to stop using marijuana (Brady *et al.*, 1991; Cantwell *et al.*, 1999; Crits-Christoph and Siqueland, 1996; Johns, 2001; Menezes *et al.*, 1996; Regier *et al.*, 1990; Rounds-Bryant *et al.*, 1999; Simpson, 1981; Simpson *et al.*, 1997; Troisi *et al.*, 1998).

Another treatment situation frequently encountered is that of an individual with a known Axis I disorder that is being exacerbated by cannabis use. Some studies, performed in popu-

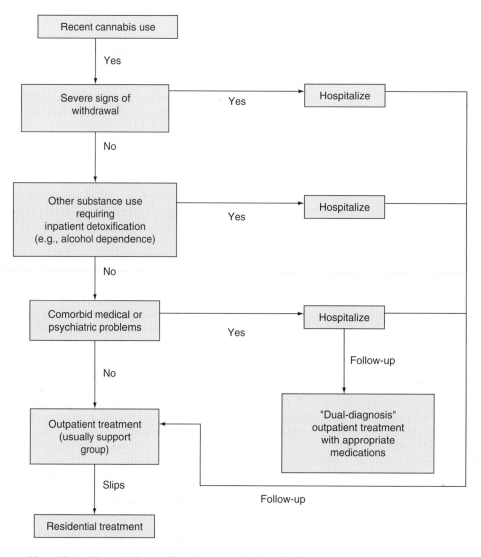

Note: Most of these patients will not be commitable and will have to voluntarily seek treatment

Figure 37.2 *Treatment decision tree for cannabis use disorders.*

lations of patients with schizophrenia, have found that cannabis use worsens the course of the illness, whereas others have found that it does not affect the course (Negrete *et al.*, 1986; Treffert, 1978; Cuffel *et al.*, 1993; Linszen *et al.*, 1994). It is a reasonable assumption that at least some patients with Axis I disorders are adversely affected by cannabis use even if they use the drug only occasionally. In such cases, the role of cannabis as an exacerbating factor must be assessed and discussed with the patient. These patients may or may not be suitable for support groups directed primarily at substance abuse because cannabis may represent a relatively minor portion of the patient's overall clinical picture.

Refractory Patients and Nonresponse to Initial Treatment

Like alcohol, the most common problem in managing cannabis use disorders is the high rate of relapse due to the wide availability of the drug and the large number of people who are users. Users are therefore tempted to resume use soon after a period of treatment when they find themselves in situations where they are surrounded by people using the substance. It is often useful for families and other people important in the patient's life to get involved in treatment to understand the role that they play in the patient's substance abuse. Some treaters advocate periodic random urine testing, which is an inexpensive and reliable method of monitoring abstinence, because THC remains present for such a long time and can be detected with infrequent testing (Miller *et al.*, 1989).

A difficult treatment situation arises when it is hypothesized that the patient is using cannabis to self-medicate a primary Axis I disorder such as depression or an anxiety disorder. In these individuals, abstinence is difficult to achieve because the patient believes that cannabis will alleviate his or her symptoms. Relapse may occur repeatedly until the underlying Axis I disorder is effectively treated (Peralta and Cuesta, 1992; Dixon *et al.*, 1991; Estroff and Gold, 1986; Warner *et al.*, 1994).

Cannabis-induced Disorders

Uncomplicated cannabis intoxication rarely comes to clinical attention and, if it does, it does not require treatment other than reassurance, as it is a self-limiting condition. Similarly, as suggested in the previous sections, symptoms of delirium, psychosis, or anxiety associated with cannabis use typically resolve promptly after the period of acute intoxication is past. Again, no treatment is necessary other than keeping the patient safe and providing reassurance that symptoms caused by the drug will stop, as these are also self-limiting conditions. If the symptoms continue after more than 24 to 48 hours of abstinence from the drug, the possibility of another Axis I diagnosis must be considered. In such cases, treatment should then be directed at the primary Axis I disorder.

In the given treatment decision tree a diagnosis of cannabis use disorders is presented Figure 37.2.

Comparison of DSM-IV/ICD-10 Diagnostic Criteria

The ICD-10 criteria and DSM-IV-TR criteria for Cannabis Intoxication are equivalent.

References

Alterman AI, Erdlen DL, LaPorte DJ *et al.* (1982) Effects of illicit drug use in an inpatient psychiatric population. *Addict Behav* 7, 231–242.

Ameri A (1999) The effects of cannabinoids on the brain. *Prog Neurobiol* 58(4), 315–348.

Andreasson S, Allebeck P, Engstrom A *et al.* (1987) Cannabis and schizophrenia: A longitudinal study of Swedish conscripts. *Lancet ii* (8574), 1483–1486.

Andreasson S, Allebeck P and Rydberg U (1989) Schizophrenia in users and nonusers of cannabis. A longitudinal study in Stockholm County. *Acta Psychiatr Scand* 79(5), 505–510.

Annis HM and Smart RG (1973) Adverse reactions and recurrences from marijuana use. *Br J Addict* 68, 315–319.

Anthony JC, Warner LA and Kessler RC (1994) Comparative epidemiology of dependence on tobacco, alcohol, controlled substances and inhabitants: Basic findings from the National Comorbidity Study. *Clin Exp Psychopharmacol* 2, 244–268.

Ashton CH (2001) Pharmacology and effects of cannabis: A brief review. *Br J Psychiatr* 178, 101–106.

Baer JS, MacLean MG and Marlatt GA (1998) Linking etiology and treatment for adolescent substance abuse: Toward a better match, in *New Perspectives on Adolescent Risk Behavior* (ed Jessor R). Cambridge University Press, New York, pp. 182–220.

Baigent M, Holme G and Hafner RJ (1995) Self-reports of the interaction between substance abuse and schizophrenia. *Aust NZ J Psychiatr* 29, 69–74.

Botvin GJ (2000) Preventing drug abuse in schools: Social and competence enhancement approaches targeting individual-level etiologic factors. *Addict Behav* 25(6), 887–897.

Boulougouris JC, Liakos A and Stefanis C (1976) Social traits of heavy hashish users and matched controls. *Ann NY Acad Sci* 282, 17–23.

Brady K, Casto S, Lydiard RB *et al.* (1991) Substance abuse in an inpatient psychiatric sample. *Am J Drug Alcohol Abuse* 17, 389–397.

Brill NQ and Christie RL (1974) Marijuana use and psychosocial adaptation. *Arch Gen Psychiatr* 31, 713–719.

Budney AJ, Novy PL and Hughes JR (1999) Marijuana withdrawal among adults seeking treatment for marijuana dependence. *Addiction* 94(9), 1311–1322.

Budney AJ, Higgins ST, Radonovich KJ *et al.* (2000) Voucher-based incentives to coping skills and motivational enhancement improves outcomes during treatment for marijuana dependence. *J Consult Clin Psychol* 68(6), 1051–1061.

Burdsal C, Greenberg G and Timpe R (1973) The relationship of marijuana usage to personality and motivational factors. *J Psychol* 85, 45–51.

Campbell I (1976) The amotivational syndrome and cannabis use with emphasis on the Canadian scene. *Ann NY Acad Sci* 282, 33–36.

Cantwell R, Brewin J Glazebrook C *et al.* (1999) Prevalence of substance misuse in first-episode psychosis. *Br J Psychiatr* 174, 150–153.

Chait LD and Burke KA (1994) Preference for high versus low-potency marijuana. *Pharmacol Biochem Behav* 49(3), 643–647.

Chen K and Kandel DB (1995) The natural history of drug use from adolescence to the mid-thirties in a general population sample. *Am J Pub Health* 85(1), 41–47.

Chen K and Kandel DB (1998) Predictors of cessation of marijuana use: An event history analysis. *Drug Alcohol Depend* 50, 109–121.

Chen K, Kandel DB and Davies M (1997) Relationships between frequency and quantity of marijuana use and last year proxy dependence among adolescents and adults in the United States. *Drug Alcohol Depend* 46(1–2), 53–67.

Comitas L (1976) Cannabis and work in Jamaica: A refutation of the amotivational syndrome. *Ann NY Acad Sci* 282, 24–35.

Compton DR, Dewey WL and Martin BR (1990) Cannabis dependence and tolerance production. *Adv Alcohol Subst Abuse* 9, 129–147.

Crits-Christoph P and Siqueland L (1996) Psychosocial treatment for drug abuse. Selected review and recommendations for national health care. *Arch Gen Psychiatr* 53(8), 749–756.

Crowley TJ, Macdonald MJ and Whitmore EA *et al.* (1998) Cannabis dependence, withdrawal, and reinforcing effects among adolescents with conduct symptoms and substance use disorders. *Drug Alcohol Depend* 50(1), 27–37.

Cuffel BJ, Heithoff KA and Lawson W (1993) Correlates of patterns of substance abuse among patients with schizophrenia. *Hosp Comm Psychiatr* 44, 247–251.

DeWit DJ, Hance J, Offord DR *et al.* (2000) The influence of early and frequent use of marijuana on the risk of desistance and of progression to marijuana-related harm. *Prev Med* 31(5), 455–464.

Diana M, Melis M and Gessa GL (1998a) Increase in meso-prefrontal dopaminergic activity after stimulation of CB1 receptors by cannabinoids. *Eur J Neurosci* 10(9), 2825–2830.

Diana M, Melis M, Muntoni AL *et al.* (1998b) Mesolimbic dopaminergic decline after cannabinoid withdrawal. *Proc Natl Acad Sci USA* 95(17), 10269–10273.

Dixon L, Haas G, Weiden PJ *et al.* (1991) Drug abuse in schizophrenic patients: Clinical correlates and reasons for use. *Am J Psychiatr* 148, 224–230.

Ehrenreich H, Rinn T, Kunert HJ *et al.* (1999) Specific attentional dysfunction in adults following early start of cannabis use. *Psychopharmacology* 142(3), 295–301.

Estroff TW and Gold MS (1986) Psychiatric presentations for marijuana abuse. *Psychiatr Ann* 16, 221–224.

Gardner EL (1999) Cannabinoid interaction with brain reward systems, in *Marijuana and Medicine* (eds Nahas GG, Sutin KM, Harvey DJ *et al.*). Humana Press, Totowa, NJ, pp. 187–205.

Green BE and Ritter C (2000) Marijuana use and depression. *J Health Soc Behav* 41(1), 40–49.

Greenfield SF and O'Leary G (1999) Sex differences in marijuana use in the United States. *Harv Rev Psychiatr* 6(6), 297–303.

Grella CE, Hser YI, Joshi V *et al.* (1999) Patient histories, retention, and outcome models for younger and older adults in DATOS. *Drug Alcohol Depend* 57(2), 151–166.

Gruber AJ and Pope HG Jr (1994) Cannabis psychotic disorder: Does it exist? *Am J Addict* 3, 72–83.

Gruber AJ, Pope HG Jr, and Brown ME (1996) Do patients use marijuana as an antidepressant? *Depression* 4(2), 77–80.

Gruber AJ, Pope HG Jr, Hudson JI, and Yurgelun-Todd, D. Attributes of long-term heavy cannabis users: A case–control study. *Psychological Medicine* 33, 1415–1422, 2003.

Halikas JA (1974) Marijuana use and psychiatric illness, in *Marijuana: Effects on Human Behavior* (ed Miller LL). Academic Press, New York, pp. 265–302.

Hall W and Degenhardt L (2000) Cannabis use and psychosis: A review of clinical and epidemiological evidence. *Aust NZ J Psychiatr* 34(1), 26–34.

Hall W and Solowij N (1998) Adverse effects of cannabis. *Lancet* 352 (9140), 1611–1616.

Haney M, Ward AS, Comer SD *et al.* (1999) Abstinence symptoms following smoked marijuana in humans. *Psychopharmacologia* 141(4), 395–404.

Haney M, Ward AS, Comer SD *et al.* (2001a) Bupropion SR worsens mood during marijuana withdrawal in humans. *Psychopharmacologia* 155, 171–179.

Haney M, Ward AS, Hart CL *et al.* (2001b) Effects of nefazodone on marijuana withdrawal in humans. College on Problems of Drug Dependence, 63rd Annual Scientific meeting, Scottsdale, AZ, June 16–21, appears as abstract #241. *Drug Alcohol Depend* 63(Suppl 1), S62.

Harder S and Reitbrock S (1997) Concentration–effect relationship of delta-9-tetrahydrocannabinol and prediction of psychotropic effects after smoking marijuana. *Int J Clin Pharmacol Ther* 35(4), 155–159.

Hendin H and Haas AP (1985) The adaptive significance of chronic marijuana use for adolescents and adults. *Adv Alcohol Subst Abuse* 4(3–4), 99–115.

Henry B, Feehan M, McGee R *et al.* (1993) The importance of conduct problems and depressive symptoms in predicting adolescent substance use. *J Abnorm Child Psychol* 21, 469–480.

Hochman JS and Brill NQ (1973) Chronic marijuana use and psychosocial adaptation. *Am J Psychiatr* 130, 132–140.

Hser Y-I, Grella CE, Hubbard RL *et al.* (2001) An evaluation of drug treatments for adolescents in 4 US cities. *Arch Gen Psychiatr* 58, 689–695.

Hubbard RL, Cavanaugh ER and Craddock SG (1985) Characteristics, behaviors, and outcomes for youth in the TOPS, in *Treatment Services for Adolescent Substance Abusers* (eds Friedman AS and Beschner G). National Institute on Drug Abuse, Rockville, MD, pp. 49–65.

Hubbard JR, Franco SE and Onaivi ES (1999) Marijuana: Medical implications. *Am Fam Physician* 60(9), 2583–2588, 2593.

Johns A (2001) Psychiatric effects of cannabis. *Br J Psychiatr* 178, 116–122.

Johnson BA (1990) Psychopharmacological effects of cannabis. *Br J Hosp Med* 43, 114–122.

Johnston LD, O'Malley PM and Bachman JG (2001) Monitoring the Future National Results on Adolescent Drug Use: Overview of key findings, 2000. (NIH Publication No. 01-4923) National Institute on Drug Abuse, Bethesda, MD.

Jones RT (1983) Cannabis tolerance and dependence, in *Cannabis and Health Hazards* (eds Fehr KO and Kalant H). *Addiction* Research Foundation, Toronto, pp. 617–689.

Jones RT, Benowitz N and Bachman J (1976) Clinical studies of cannabis tolerance and dependence. *Ann NY Acad Sci* 282, 221–239.

Jones RT, Benowitz NL and Herning RI (1981) Clinical relevance of cannabis tolerance and dependence. *J Clin Pharmacol* 21, 143S–152S.

Kandel DB and Chen K (2000) Types of marijuana users by longitudinal course. *J Stud Alcohol* 61(3), 367–378.

Kaymakcalan S (1973) Tolerance to and dependence on cannabis. *Bull Narc* 25, 39–47.

Kaymakcalan S (1981) The addictive potential of cannabis. *Bull Narc* 33, 21–31.

Keeler MH, Reifler CB and Liptzin MB (1968) Spontaneous recurrence of marijuana effect. *Am J Psychiatr* 125, 384–386.

Keeler MH, Ewing JA and Rouse BA (1971) Hallucinogenic effects of marijuana as currently used. *Am J Psychiatr* 128, 213–216.

Kendler KS and Prescott CA (1998) Cannabis use, abuse, and dependence in a population-based sample of female twins. *Am J Psychiatr* 155(8), 1016–1022.

Kouri EM and Pope HG Jr (2000) Abstinence symptoms during withdrawal from chronic marijuana use. *Exp Clin Psychopharmacol* 8(4), 483–492.

Kouri E, Pope HG Jr Todd D *et al.* (1995) Attributes of heavy versus occasional marijuana smokers in a college population. *Biol Psychiatr* 38, 475–481.

Kouri EM, Pope HG Jr and Lukas SE (1999) Changes in aggressive behavior during withdrawal from long-term cannabis use. *Psychopharmacology* 143, 302–308.

Kupfer DJ, Detre T, Koral J *et al.* (1973) A comment on the "amotivational syndrome" in marijuana smokers. *Am J Psychiatr* 130, 1319–1321.

Latimer WW, Winters KC, Stinchfield R *et al.* (2000) Demographic, individual, and interpersonal predictors of adolescent alcohol and marijuana use following treatment. *Psychol Addict Behav* 14(2), 162–173.

Lessin PJ and Thomas SA (1976) Assessment of the chronic effect of marijuana on motivation and achievement: A preliminary report, in *The Pharmacology of Marijuana* (eds Braude MC and Szara S). Raven Press, New York, pp. 681–690.

Levi L and Miller NR (1990) Visual illusions associated with previous drug abuse. *J Clin Neuroophthalmol* 10, 103–110.

Lex BW, Griffin ML, Mello NK *et al.* (1989) Alcohol, marijuana, and mood states in young women. *Int J Addict* 24, 405–424.

Linszen DH, Dingemans PM and Lenior ME (1994) Cannabis abuse and the course of recent-onset schizophrenic disorder. *Arch Gen Psychiatr* 51, 273–279.

Mellinger GD, Somers RH, Davidson ST *et al.* (1976) The amotivational syndrome and the college student. *Ann NY Acad Sci* 282, 37–55.

Mendelson JH, Kuehnle JC, Greenberg I *et al.* (1976) The effects of marijuana use on human operant behavior: Individual data, in *The Pharmacology of Marijuana* (eds Braude MC and Szara S). Raven Press, New York, pp. 643–653.

Menezes PR, Johnson S, Thornicroft G *et al.* (1996) Drug and alcohol problems among individuals with severe mental illness in south London. *Br J Psychiatr* 168, 612–619.

Miller FT, Busch F and Tanenbaum JG (1989) Drug abuse in schizophrenia and bipolar disorder. *Am J Drug Alcohol Abuse* 15, 291–295.

Miller NS, Gold MS and Pottash AC (1989) A 12-step treatment approach for marijuana dependence. *J Subst Abuse Treat* 6, 241–250.

Miller NS, Klahr AL, Gold MS et al. (1990) Cannabis diagnosis of patients receiving treatment for cocaine dependence. *J Subst Abuse* 2(1), 107–111.

Mirin SM, Shapiro LM, Meyer RE et al. (1971) Casual versus heavy use of marijuana: A redefinition of the marijuana problem. *Am J Psychiatr* 127(9), 1134–1140.

Mueser KT, Yarnold PR and Bellak AS (1992) Diagnostic and demographic correlates of substance abuse in schizophrenia and major affective disorder. *Acta Psychiatr Scand* 85, 48–55.

Musty RE and Kaback L (1995) Relationships between motivation and depression in chronic marijuana users. *Life Sci* 56(23–24), 2151–2158.

Negrete JC, Knapp WP, Douglas DE et al. (1986) Cannabis affects the severity of schizophrenic symptoms: Results of a clinical survey. *Psychol Med* 16, 515–520.

Newcombe MD and Bentler P (1988) *Consequences of Adolescent Drug Use: Impact on the Lives of Young Adults.* Sage Publications, Newbury Park, CA.

Peralta V and Cuesta MJ (1992) Influence of cannabis abuse on schizophrenic psychopathology. *Acta Psychiatr Scand* 85, 127–130.

Perez-Reyes M (1999) The psychologic and physiologic effects of active cannabinoids, in *Marijuana and Medicine* (eds Nahas GG, Sutin KM, Harvey DJ et al.). Humana Press, Totowa, NJ, pp. 245–252.

Pillard RC (1970) Marijuana. *New Engl J Med* 283, 294–303.

Pope HG and Yurgelun-Todd D (1996) The residual cognitive effects of heavy marijuana use. *JAMA* 275, 521–527.

Pope HG Jr, Ionescu-Piogga M, Aizley HG et al. (1990) Drug use and lifestyle among college undergraduates in 1989: A comparison with 1969 and 1978. *Am J Psychiatr* 147, 998–1001.

Pope HG Jr, Gruber AJ and Yurgelun-Todd D (1995) The residual neuropsychological effects of cannabis: The current status of research. *Drug Alcohol Depend* 38(1), 25–34.

Pope HG, Jacobs A, Mialet JP et al. (1997) Evidence for a sex-specific residual effect of cannabis on visuospatial memory. *Psychother Psychosom* 66(4), 179–184.

Pope HG Jr, Gruber AJ, Hudson JI et al. (2001a) Neuropsychological performance in long-term cannabis users. *Arch Gen Psychiatr* 58, 909–915.

Pope HG Jr, Ionescu-Pioggia M and Pope KW (2001b) Drug use and life style among college undergraduates: A 30-year longitudinal study. *Am J Psychiatr* 158(9), 1519–1521.

Prochaska JO and Velicer WF (1997) The transtheoretical model of health behavior change. *Am J Health Promot* 12(1), 38–48.

Regier DA, Farmer ME, Rae DS et al. (1990) Comorbidity of mental disorders with alcohol and other drug abuse. Results from the epidemiologic catchment area (ECA) study. *JAMA* 264(19), 2511–2518.

Robins LN, Darvish HS and Murphy GE (1970) The long-term outcome for adolescent drug users: A follow-up study of 76 users and 146 nonusers, in *The Psychopathology of Adolescence* (eds Zubin J and Freedman AM). Grune & Stratton, New York, pp. 159–180.

Rodriguez de Fonseca F, Carrera MRA, Navarro M et al. (1997) Activation of corticotropin-releasing factor in the limbic system during cannabinoid withdrawal. *Science* 276, 2050–2054.

Roffman RA and Barnhart R (1987) Assessing need for marijuana dependence treatment through an anonymous telephone interview. *Int J Addict* 22(7), 639–651.

Roffman RA, Klepsch R, Wertz JS et al. (1993) Predictors of attrition from an outpatient marijuana-dependence counseling program. *Addict Behav* 18, 553–566.

Rounds-Bryant JL, Kristiansen PL and Hubbard RL (1999) Drug abuse treatment outcome study of adolescents: A comparison of client characteristics and pretreatment behaviors in three treatment modalities. *Am J Drug Alcohol Abuse* 25(4), 573–591.

Schwartz RH, Gruenewald PJ, Klitzner M et al. (1989) Short-term memory impairment in cannabis-dependent adolescents. *Am J Dis Child* 143(10), 1214–1219.

Sigmon SC, Steingard S, Badger GJ et al. (2000) Contingent reinforcement of marijuana abstinence among individuals with serious mental illness: A feasibility study. *Exp Clin Psychopharmacol* 8(4), 509–517.

Simon WE, Primavera LH, Simon MG et al. (1974) A comparison of marijuana users and nonusers on a number of personality variables. *J Consult Clin Psychol* 42, 917–918.

Simpson DD (1981) The relation of time spent in drug abuse treatment to posttreatment outcome. *Am J Psychiatr* 136, 1449–1453.

Simpson DD, Joe GW and Brown BS (1997) Treatment retention and follow-up outcomes in the drug abuse treatment outcome study (DATOS). *Psychol Addict Behav* 11(4), 294–307.

Smoller JW, Lunetta KL and Robins J (2000) Implications of comorbidity and ascertainment bias for identifying disease genes. *Am J Med Genet* 96, 817–822.

Solomons K and Neppe VM (1989) Cannabis – its clinical effects. *S Afr Med J* 76, 102–104.

Solowij N (1995) Do cognitive impairments recover following cessation of cannabis use? *Life Sci* 56(23–24), 2119–2126.

Solowij N (1998) *Cannabis and Cognitive Functioning.* Cambridge University Press, Cambridge, UK.

Solowij N, Michie PT and Fox AM (1991) Effects of long-term cannabis use on selective attention: An event-related potential study. *Pharmacol Biochem Behav* 40(3), 683–688.

Solowij N, Michie PT and Fox AM (1995) Differential impairments of selective attention due to frequency and duration of cannabis use. *Biol Psychiatr* 37(10), 731–739.

Stanton MD and Bardoni A (1972) Drug flashbacks: Reported frequency in a military population. *Am J Psychiatr* 129, 751–755.

Stephens RS, Roffman RA and Simpson EE (1993a) Adult marijuana users seeking treatment. *J Consult Clin Psychol* 61(6), 1100–1104.

Stephens RS, Wertz JS and Roffman RA (1993b) Predictors of marijuana treatment outcomes: The role of self-efficacy. *J Subst Abuse* 5(4), 341–353.

Stephens RS, Roffman RA and Simpson EE (1994) Treating adult marijuana dependence: A test of the relapse prevention model. *J Consult Clin Psychol* 62(1), 92–99.

Stephens RS, Roffman RA and Curtin L (2000) Comparison of extended versus brief treatments for marijuana use. *J Consult Clin Psychol* 68(5), 898–908.

Struve FA, Patrick G, Straumanis JJ et al. (1998) Possible EEG sequelae of very long duration marijuana use: Pilot findings from topographic quantitative EEG analysis of subjects with 15 to 24 years of cumulative daily exposure to THC. *Clin Electroencephalogr* 29, 31–36.

Substance Abuse and Mental Health Services Administration. Office of Applied Studies (1997) Preliminary Results From the 1996 National Household Survey on Drug Abuse. SAMHSA, Rockvile, MD.

Substance Abuse and Mental Health Services Association. Office of Applied Studies (1999) National admissions to substance abuse treatment services: The treatment episode data set (TEDS) 1992–1997. US Government Printing Office, Washington DC.

Substance Abuse and Mental Health Services Administration. Office of Applied Studies (2000) Summary of Findings from the 1999 National Household Survey on Drug Abuse. SAMHSA, Rockville, MD.

Szuster RR, Pontuis EB and Campos PE (1988) Marijuana sensitivity and panic anxiety. *J Clin Psychiatr* 49, 427–429.

Tanda G, Pontieri FE and Di Chiara G (1997) Cannabinoid and heroin activation of mesolimbic dopamine transmission by a common microl opioid receptor mechanism. *Science* 276(5321), 2048–2050.

Tennant FS (1986) The clinical syndrome of marijuana dependence. *Psychiatr Ann* 16, 225–234.

Thomas H (1996) A community survey of adverse effects of cannabis use. *Drug Alcohol Depend* 42, 201–207.

Treffert DA (1978) Marijuana use in schizophrenia: A clear hazard. *Am J Psychiatr* 135, 1213–1215.

Troisi A, Pasini A, Saracco M *et al.* (1998) Psychiatric symptoms in male cannabis users not using other illicit drugs. *Addiction* 93(4), 487–492.

True WR, Heath AC, Scherrer JF *et al.* (1999) Interrelationship of genetic and environmental influences on conduct disorder and alcohol and marijuana dependence symptoms. *Am J Med Genet* 88(4), 391–397.

Tsuang MT, Lyons MJ, Harley RM *et al.* (1999) Genetic and environmental influences on transitions in drug use. *Behav Genet* 29(6), 473–479.

Warner R, Taylor D, Wright J *et al.* (1994) Substance use among the mentally ill: Prevalence, reasons for use, and effects on illness. *Am J Orthopsychiatr* 64, 30–39.

Weiner MD, Sussman S, McCuller WJ *et al.* (1999) Factors in marijuana cessation among high-risk youth. *J Drug Educ* 29(4), 337–357.

Weller RA and Halikas JA (1985) Marijuana use and psychiatric illness: A follow-up study. *Am J Psychiatr* 142, 848–850.

Wiesbeck GA, Schuckit MA, Kalmijn JA *et al.* (1996) An evaluation of the history of a marijuana withdrawal syndrome in a large population. *Addiction* 91(10), 1469–1478.

Zinberg NE and Weil AT (1970) A comparison of marijuana users and nonusers. *Nature* 226, 119–123.

Zoccollilo M, Vitaro F and Tremblay RE (1999) Problem drug and alcohol use in a community sample of adolescents. *J Am Acad Child Adolesc Psychiatr* 38(7), 900–907.

Substance Abuse: Cocaine Use Disorders

Definition

Cocaine, a central nervous system stimulant produced by the coca plant, is consumed in several preparations. Cocaine hydrochloride powder is usually snorted through the nostrils, or it may be mixed in water and injected intravenously. Cocaine hydrochloride powder is also commonly heated ("cooked up") with ammonia or baking soda and water to remove the hydrochloride, thus forming a gel-like substance that can be smoked ("freebasing"). "Crack" cocaine is a precooked form of cocaine alkaloid that is sold on the street as small "rocks". Abundant supplies and falling prices for cocaine (the equivalent of 1 gram of cocaine can be purchased for as little as $25 to $50 and a vial of crack [two or three small "rocks"] can be had for about $10) have contributed greatly to the prevalence of cocaine abuse and dependence as well as other related cocaine use disorders.

Cocaine intoxication produces a state of intense euphoria that is a powerful reinforcer and can lead to the development of cocaine use disorders in many individuals, although only 10 to 16% of those who try the drug go on to develop these disorders (Van Etten and Anthony, 1999). Some experience the stimulant effects of cocaine as anxiogenic; others discontinue use because of lack of easy drug availability, fear of loss of control over use, or apprehension regarding possible legal consequences of cocaine abuse. The route of administration is strongly correlated with the development of cocaine use disorders, in that the intravenous and smoked routes of administration allow rapid transport of the drug to the brain, producing intense effects that are short-lived. Rapid tolerance to euphoria occurs and plasma concentrations are not correlated with peak euphoria, producing a need for frequent dosing to regain euphoric effects (binge use) that can place the cocaine abuser at risk for medical and psychiatric complications of cocaine abuse.

Cocaine abuse is characterized by a maladaptive pattern of substance use demonstrated by recurrent and significant adverse consequences related to repeated drug use. Such consequences include family discord, legal and employment problems and interpersonal problems. The person diagnosed with cocaine abuse may have significant periods during which no cocaine-related problems are experienced, but the initiation of cocaine abuse usually heralds the onset of psychosocial difficulties. Cocaine dependence is characterized by a more pervasive pattern of frequent cocaine use and a chronic cycle of psychosocial problems. In addition, medical and psychiatric adverse events associated with cocaine use can result in serious morbidity and, in some cases, mortality.

While the question of whether cocaine is physiologically addictive is not completely clear, the psychological addiction alone is powerful and can completely dominate the life of the cocaine abuser. Binge use of cocaine may be followed by what has been described as a mild withdrawal syndrome characterized by dysphoria and anhedonia. Cocaine withdrawal may resemble a depressive disorder, in some cases requiring emergent psychiatric treatment. Some combination of these consequences of cocaine abuse are usually responsible for the identification and diagnosis of individuals with cocaine use disorders and referral to substance abuse treatment.

Epidemiology

The National Household Survey on Drug Abuse (NHSDA) reported that in 2000, 1.2 million Americans were current cocaine users representing 0.5% of the population over the age of 12 (SAMHSA, 2001a). Since 1975, the monitoring the future (MTF) study has annually examined the extent of drug abuse among 8th to 12th graders. Use of cocaine decreased significantly among 12th graders, from 6.2% in 1999 to 5.0% in 2000; crack cocaine use in the year 2000 decreased from 2.7 to 2.2% for 12th graders. While cocaine use has shown a downward trend, several statistics indicate that cocaine abuse is still a serious threat to the public. For example, cocaine-related emergency department visits constituted 29% of all drug related visits in 2000, more than for any other illicit substance (SAMHSA, 2001b).

Gender Differences in Cocaine Use Disorders

While men continue to have a higher rate of current cocaine use than women, the gap is narrowing (Van Etten and Anthony, 1999; SAMHSA, 1996). Some studies have reported that women cocaine abusers differ from men in several respects, including responses to the direct administration of cocaine.

Much of the research on substance abuse treatment efficacy is based predominantly on male samples. Cocaine dependence in women is as severe as that in men, however women often receive less treatment for their substance abuse (McCance-Katz et al., 1999). Studies have also suggested that cocaine dependence can develop more rapidly in women than in men. Cocaine is one of the most frequently abused illicit drugs during pregnancy (SAMHSA, 1999). It has been estimated that 0.1% of pregnant women are cocaine users (SAMHSA, 1999). The risks of cocaine

Essentials of Psychiatry   Jerald Kay and Allan Tasman
© 2006 John Wiley & Sons, Ltd.

and other substance abuse during pregnancy are significant not only for women but also for their unborn children who may be at increased risk of vascular injury to the central nervous system. Abuse of cocaine has been linked to placental abruption, preterm labor, and low birth weight. Abuse and neglect of children are also common consequences of parental addiction Recent studies have suggested that children exposed to cocaine *in utero* do not appear to have permanent sequelae attributable to maternal cocaine abuse.

Relationship of Psychiatric Disorders to Cocaine Abuse and Dependence

Several studies have documented the high rate of comorbid psychiatric disorders in cocaine abusers entering treatment. These disorders include mood disorders (major depressive disorder, bipolar disorders), schizophrenia, post traumatic stress disorder, attention-deficit hyperactivity disorder, anxiety disorders and antisocial personality disorder. Mood disorders often temporally follow the onset of cocaine abuse in patients presenting for treatment, while attention-deficit hyperactivity disorder and antisocial personality disorder precede the onset of cocaine abuse (McMahon *et al.*, 1999; Clure *et al.*, 1999). However, while high levels of depressive symptoms during treatment were associated with greater craving for cocaine, alcohol and other substances, only limited evidence exists regarding the influence of depression on treatment course and outcome (Carroll *et al.*, 1995; Brown *et al.*, 1998; Simpson *et al.*, 1999).

It is important to note that comorbid psychiatric illnesses are common among cocaine users. Furthermore, the diagnosis of a comorbid primary psychiatric disorder can be challenging to make in cocaine abusers because psychiatric symptoms may be the result of cocaine abuse or acute abstinence. When psychiatric disorders cooccur with cocaine use disorders, it is important to provide treatment for both disorders. Cocaine use disorders will not generally resolve with treatment of the psychiatric disorder alone, nor will substance abuse treatment resolve a comorbid psychiatric disorder.

Course and Natural History

Cocaine produces a sense of intensified pleasure in most activities and a heightened sense of alertness and well-being. Anxiety and social inhibition are decreased. Energy, self-esteem and self-perception of ability are increased. There is enhancement of emotion and sexual feeling. Pleasurable experiences, although heightened, are not distorted and hallucinations are usually absent. The person engaging in low-dose cocaine use often receives positive feedback from others responding to the user's increased energy and enthusiasm. This, in combination with the euphoria experienced by the user, can be reinforcing, and cocaine use is perceived as free of any adverse consequences. The duration of cocaine's euphoric effects depends on the route of administration. Cocaine and alcohol are often consumed together. In addition to the synergistic effects of cocaine and alcohol in humans, an active metabolite, cocaethylene, with cocaine-like pharmacological properties is formed and users of both drugs simultaneously report enhanced euphoria.

Cocaine users quickly learn that higher doses are associated with intensified and prolonged euphoria, resulting in increasing use of the drug and progression to cocaine dependence. The abuser is focused on the cocaine-induced euphoria and begins compulsively to pursue this effect. These behaviors become

pivotal in the lives of cocaine abusers who continue drug abuse despite the presence of increasing personal and social consequences. Uncontrolled use of cocaine often begins with either increased access and resultant escalating dosages and frequency of administration or a change from intranasal use to a route of administration with more rapid onset of effects (i.e., intravenous or smoked). Such binges produce extreme euphoria and vivid memories. These memories are later contrasted with current dysphoria to produce intense craving, which perpetuates the binge use pattern Addicts report that during binge use, thoughts are focused exclusively on the cocaine-induced effects. Normal daily needs, including sleep and nourishment, are neglected. Responsibilities to family and employer and social obligations are given up. This continues until the supply of cocaine is exhausted.

Binges are often separated by several days of abstinence; cocaine-dependent individuals average one to three binges per week. This is in contrast to use patterns for opiate and alcohol dependence which often produce physiological dependence necessitating daily consumption to prevent withdrawal symptoms. This differentiation is crucial to an understanding of the syndrome of cocaine dependence. Newly abstinent cocaine abusers may experience a triphasic abstinence pattern, although this varies by individual, that includes a period of acute abstinence, sometimes referred to as the "crash", lasting several hours to several days consisting of dysphoria, fatigue, insomnia or hypersomnia, increased appetite, and either psychomotor agitation or retardation, subsequent to the more intensive "crash" phase. A more chronic withdrawal period sometimes occurs characterized by minor depressive symptoms and cocaine craving lasting 2 to 10 weeks. This may then be followed by an extinction phase characterized by intermittent drug craving that becomes increasingly manageable with continued abstinence.

Like other drug and alcohol use disorders, cocaine use disorders are chronic relapsing illnesses that present substantial challenges in the treatment process. Cocaine abusers are at high risk for relapse, particularly in the first few months of treatment related to acute craving often in the context of ongoing psychosocial stressors that result from or have been exacerbated by cocaine abuse. Newly abstinent cocaine abusers often lack adequate coping skills necessary to avoid cocaine use, which take time to acquire in the treatment process. Although the ability to cope with cocaine craving improves with continued abstinence, relapse to cocaine abuse or other drug and alcohol abuse will continue to be a risk for those with a history of a cocaine use disorder who relapse to cocaine abuse. Repeated treatments may be required for those with cocaine use disorders. Treatment modalities include inpatient hospitalization for medical or psychiatric complications of cocaine abuse, partial hospital programs, self-help groups, psychotherapy (usually group or family therapy for patients with primary cocaine use disorders), or some combination of these treatments according to the clinical presentation of the patient

Neurobiological Changes Related to Cocaine Use

Cocaine has effects on multiple neurotransmitters, including release and reuptake blockade of dopamine, serotonin (5-hydroxytryptamine [5-HT]) and norepinephrine. The most widely accepted explanation of cocaine-induced euphoria is that dopamine reuptake inhibition results in increased extracellular dopamine concentration in the mesolimbic and mesocortical reward pathways in the brain. Another important phenomenon related to acute cocaine administration is that of "acute tolerance". A single dose of cocaine has been shown experimentally to reduce the response to a second identical dose given 100 minutes later as measured by extracellular dopamine levels and motor activity (Bradberry, 2000). The finding of "acute tolerance" is consistent with the binge pattern of cocaine use in which abusers consume escalating doses of cocaine in an attempt to recapture the intense euphoria of the initial cocaine dose (Bradberry, 2000). A growing body of evidence indicates that chronic cocaine administration can result in sustained neurophysiological changes in brain systems that regulate psychological processes, specifically pleasure and hedonic responsivity. This has been postulated to underlie a physiological addiction to cocaine with associated withdrawal phenomena that are manifested clinically as a psychological syndrome (Koob and Nestler, 1997).

Diagnosis of Cocaine Use Disorders

The initial evaluation period should include the collection of a complete history of all substance abuse, which is essential to accurate diagnosis and appropriate treatment. The history includes the circumstances under which each drug was used, the psychoactive effects sought and obtained, the route of administration, and the frequency and amount of each drug used. Cocaine abusers frequently abuse other drugs and alcohol to enhance euphoria or to alleviate dysphoric effects associated with cocaine abuse (agitation, paranoia). A thorough history with diagnosis of other substance use disorders is important to treatment planning. Patients may need detoxification from other substances prior to initiation of cocaine abuse treatment. It is also important to monitor clinically for relapses to any substance abuse during treatment for cocaine use disorders because the use of other drugs and alcohol often leads to resumption of cocaine abuse. In addition, a thorough history of current and previous substance abuse is important so that treatment can be individualized and patients can be helped to develop coping skills that will assist them in specific situations that they identify as placing them at high risk for relapse.

A complete physical examination is necessary to determine whether medical complications of substance abuse are present. Common medical problems seen in those with cocaine use disorders include poor nutrition, vitamin deficiencies, anemia, human immunodeficiency virus (HIV) infection and sexually-transmitted diseases. In those who self-administer the drug by injection or who abuse other drugs in addition to cocaine by the intravenous route, endocarditis, abscesses, cellulitis, and Hepatitis B and C occur with regularity. The clinical evaluation should include blood studies to determine the presence of abnormalities and urine toxicology screen to determine recent drug use.

Cocaine Dependence

Cocaine has a short half-life requiring frequent dosing to maintain the "high" (binge use). Persons with cocaine dependence often spend large amounts of money for the drug and may be involved in illegal activities to obtain cocaine. Binges may be separated by several days while the individual recovers or attempts to obtain more money for drug purchase. Illegal activities such as theft and prostitution are often engaged in to obtain cash for cocaine. Obligations such as employment and childcare are often neglected. Tolerance to cocaine effects develops quickly, resulting in larger amounts of drug use with time. This is often associated with mental or physical complications of use including

paranoia, aggressive behavior, anxiety and agitation, depression and weight loss. Withdrawal symptoms, most prominently dysphoric mood, may be seen but are usually short-lived and clear within several days of abstinence. The criteria of cocaine dependence is identical to that of substance dependence and may be found on p. 411.

Cocaine Abuse

Substance abuse is described by DSM-IV-TR as a maladaptive pattern of substance use demonstrated by recurrent and significant adverse consequences related to repeated use (see p. 409). For example, there may be neglect of obligations to family or employer, repeated use in hazardous situations, legal problems and recurrent social or interpersonal problems. These problems must recur within the same 12-month period. The intensity and frequency of use are less in cocaine abuse than in cocaine dependence. Episodes of abuse may occur around paydays or special occasions and may be characterized by brief periods (hours to days) of high-dose binge use followed by longer periods of abstinence or nonproblem use.

Cocaine Intoxication

The clinical effects of cocaine intoxication are characterized initially by euphoria (referred to as "high") and also include agitation, anxiety, irritability or affective lability, grandiosity, impaired judgment, increased psychomotor activity, hypervigilance or paranoia, and sometimes hallucinations (visual, auditory, or tactile) may occur. Physical symptoms that can accompany cocaine intoxication include hypertension, tachycardia, hyperthermia, pupillary dilatation, nausea, vomiting, tremor, diaphoresis, chest pain, arrhythmia, confusion, seizures, dyskinetic movements, dystonia and, in severe cases, coma. These effects are more frequently seen in high-dose binge users of cocaine. Cardiovascular effects are probably a result of sympathomimetic properties of cocaine (i.e., release of norepinephrine and blockade of norepinephrine reuptake). The DSM-IV criteria of cocaine intoxication are based on the general criteria for substance intoxication (see p. 410).

Cocaine Withdrawal

The principal feature of substance withdrawal is development of a substance-specific maladaptive behavioral change, which may have associated physiological and cognitive components, resulting from the cessation of or reduction in heavy and prolonged substance use. Depression and suicidal ideation are the most serious complications and require individualized assessment and treatment. The syndrome may last up to several days but generally resolves without treatment. The diagnosis of cocaine withdrawal is predicated on the general DSM-IV criteria for substance abuse withdrawal (see p. 410). Specifically it requires the presence of dysphoria and two of the following symptoms developing as short as a few hours after discontinuation of the drug: insomnia, fatigue, increased appetite, psychomotor agitation or retardation, and vivid, unpleasant dreams.

Medical Complications of Cocaine Abuse

Cardiac toxicity is one of the leading causes of morbidity and mortality associated with cocaine use. The risk of myocardial infarct is well established in cocaine use and is not related to dose, route, or frequency of administration. The risk of acute myocardial infarction is increased 24-fold in 1 hour immediately following cocaine use in persons who are otherwise at relatively low risk for such events (Mittleman *et al.*, 1999). Detection of recent cocaine use by urine toxicology screen has been observed in 25% of those reporting to urban emergency departments and 7% of those evaluated at suburban hospitals and found to have evidence of myocardial infarct (Hollander *et al.*, 1995). About half of the patients with cocaine-related myocardial infarction have no evidence of atherosclerotic coronary artery disease (Hollander *et al.*, 1997a, 1997b). Identifying and diagnosing cocaine-related myocardial infarction can be difficult. The hallmarks of myocardial infarct are a constellation of physical symptoms including chest pain, electrocardiogram (ECG) abnormalities and elevated creatine kinase. Cocaine abusers with chest pain may have ECG abnormalities that are not specific for myocardial infarct (Weber *et al.*, 2000). Cocaine abusers are also often found to have nonspecific elevations in creatine kinase without myocardial infarction. Therefore, the diagnosis of cocaine-related myocardial infarction is often based on the physician's clinical judgment. Evaluation of serum troponin I, a cardiac marker that is not affected by recent cocaine use, can be helpful in determination of whether a myocardial infarct has occurred.

The pathophysiology of cocaine-related myocardial infarction is probably multifactorial. The sympathomimetic effects of cocaine increase myocardial oxygen demand by increasing heart rate, systemic blood pressure and left ventricular contractility while reducing oxygen supply through its coronary artery vasoconstriction effects (Baumann *et al.*, 2000). According to new treatment guidelines for emergency cardiovascular care, nitroglycerine and benzodiazepines are first line agents and phentolamine is a second line agent for patients with cocaine-related myocardial ischemia or infarction. Propranolol is contraindicated as it exacerbates cocaine-induced vasoconstriction of coronary arteries. Thrombolysis is not recommended unless evidence of evolving myocardial infarction persists despite medical therapy and an occluded coronary artery is shown to be present on angiography.

Cocaine use is associated with a wide range of cardiac dysrhythmias including sinus tachycardia, sinus bradycardia, supraventricular and ventricular tachycardia, ventricular premature contractions, ventricular tachycardia and fibrillation, torsades de pointes and asystole. Life-threatening dysrhythmia caused by cocaine in the absence of myocardial ischemia is rare. In many instances, cardiac dysrhythmias have occurred in the context of profound hemodynamic or metabolic disturbances (Wang, 1999). Intranasal abuse of cocaine has been associated with a number of medical complications including chronic sinusitis, septal perforation, subperiosteal abscess, pneumomediastinum, pneumothorax and pulmonary edema (Gendeh *et al.*, 1998). The presence of pulmonary edema in a young, otherwise healthy patient, without predisposing risk factors, should alert the physician to the possibility of cocaine abuse.

Cerebrovascular accidents related to cocaine use have been well documented in the medical literature. Cerebral infarct, subarachnoid hemorrhage, intraparenchymal hemorrhage and intraventricular hemorrhage have been observed as acute complications of cocaine use. Seizures were one of the earliest known complications of cocaine abuse. While anticonvulsants have not been helpful in preventing cocaine-related seizures, intravenous diazepam has been effective in acute management.

Clinical Vignette 1

Mr B is a 34-year-old divorced man with a 10-year history of freebase cocaine abuse characterized by weekly binge use of up to 6 g of cocaine and alcohol use reported as five beers several times per week with cocaine, but no other illicit drug use. He was admitted to the hospital emergency department with a chief complaint of visual hallucinations and paranoid ideation that developed during the course of several hours of binge cocaine use. On physical examination, he was noted to be agitated with mild tachycardia and hypertension, but there were no other concurrent medical illnesses.

Haloperidol 5 mg and lorazepam 2 mg were administered by intramuscular injection for treatment of psychosis and agitation, with rapid abatement in symptoms. The patient was transferred to a dual-diagnosis inpatient unit for further evaluation. Resolution of visual hallucinations and paranoia occurred within 24 hours. After 2 days of hypersomnia, intermittent anxiety and mild depressive symptoms, he reported feeling better and began to engage in substance abuse treatment. He was discharged to an outpatient clinic for further treatment of cocaine and alcohol use disorders.

Final DSM-IV Diagnoses
Axis I: Cocaine dependence, alcohol abuse, cocaine intoxication, cocaine withdrawal
Axis II: Deferred
Axis III: None

Assessment and Treatment Overview

The two primary goals of cocaine treatment are: 1) the initiation of abstinence through disruption of binge cycles and 2) the prevention of relapse. Treatment planning to achieve these goals must be considered in the context of the individual clinical presentation of the patient. Initial assessment to determine immediate needs is necessary to determine the most appropriate level of care (inpatient or outpatient treatment) as well as other psychiatric and medical considerations important to the development of the treatment plan.

The majority of those with cocaine use disorders are most appropriately treated in an outpatient setting. Outpatient treatment may vary by provider but generally includes multiple weekly contacts for the initial months of treatment because less frequent contact is not effective in the initiation or maintenance of abstinence these sessions consist of some combination of individual drug counseling, peer support groups, family or couples therapy, urine toxicology monitoring, education sessions, psychotherapy and psychiatric treatment that may include pharmacotherapy for cocaine addiction or comorbid psychiatric disorders. Inpatient treatment is reserved for those who have been refractory to outpatient treatment, whose compulsive use of cocaine represents an imminent danger (e.g., suicidality associated with cocaine toxicity or acute abstinence), who have other comorbid psychiatric or medical disorders, or who are dependent on more than one substance and require monitored detoxification.

Cocaine Use Disorders: Clinical Course

Cocaine use is characterized by binge use that can occur over extended periods of time and is limited only by the supply of drug or money to purchase the drug. Cocaine toxicity may occur with repeated use of the drug over the course of a binge. Symptoms can include hypervigilance, psychomotor agitation, hyperawareness and psychosis. While these symptoms generally resolve within 24 hours of cessation of cocaine use, prolonged symptoms may be indicative of an underlying bipolar disorder that will need further assessment. Another facet of cocaine toxicity that may be manifested as psychiatric symptoms is that of a syndrome of hyperthermia and agitation resembling neuroleptic malignant syndrome. An additional serious complication of cocaine intoxication is that of stimulant delirium characterized by confusion, disorientation and agitation. This should be treated as a medical emergency since such symptoms may be indicative of cocaine overdose. Cocaine abstinence symptoms occur with the cessation of binge use (Margolin *et al.*, 1996; Foltin and Fischman, 1998; Milby *et al.*, 2000). The abstinence syndrome is characterized by extreme exhaustion after a binge. Initial depression, agitation and anxiety are a common experience, followed by craving for sleep. Prolonged hypersomnolence and hyperphagia are usually followed by a return to normal mood, although some dysphoria may remain.

Cocaine abusers may present to urgent care settings in the context of cocaine toxicity or severe psychiatric symptoms associated with acute abstinence including anxiety, depression, or psychosis. Symptoms may be of a severity that require emergent use of benzodiazepines or antipsychotics. Lorazepam is a good choice for treatment of anxiety, agitation, or psychosis because it can be administered orally; it is also well-absorbed by the intramuscular route. The use of benzodiazepines in the severely agitated patient may decrease the need to employ the use of restraints. Antipsychotics should be used sparingly because, like cocaine, these drugs may lower the seizure threshold. In considering the choice of an antipsychotic, low-potency antipsychotics may be more likely than high-potency neuroleptics to lower seizure threshold and therefore should be avoided. Psychiatric management must also include clinical observation because suicidal ideation is not uncommon. Symptoms resembling those of a major depressive episode occur frequently in newly abstinent cocaine abusers. The occurrence of major depressive disorder must be excluded by observation over several days following the initiation of abstinence.

Individuals with cocaine use disorders will experience a withdrawal syndrome upon cessation of binge cocaine abuse that can last for as long as 10 weeks. Cocaine withdrawal is marked by decreased energy, lack of interest and anhedonia. These symptoms fluctuate and are usually not severe enough to meet diagnostic criteria for a major depressive episode. However, this subjective state experienced by the cocaine abuser is contrasted with vivid memories of cocaine-induced euphoria and constitutes a strong inducement to resume cocaine use. It is during this time that relapse is most likely. Withdrawal symptoms generally diminish over several weeks if abstinence is maintained.

The withdrawal phase is followed by what has been termed "extinction", an indefinite period during which evoked craving can occur, placing the individual at increased risk for relapse. Craving is evoked by moods, people, locations, or objects associated with cocaine use (money, white powder, pipes, mirrors, syringes) that act as cues to conditioned associations with drug use and drug-induced euphoria.

Treatment of Cocaine Use Disorders

One of the greatest challenges in the early stages of cocaine treatment is to prevent early drop out. It has been estimated that up to 80% of patients drop out of treatment programs (Higgins *et al.*, 1994). Frequent clinical contacts, especially in the early weeks of treatment, can help to establish a therapeutic alliance that will assist in engaging the patient in the treatment process. Many programs offer 3 to 6 days per week of substance abuse treatment sessions within outpatient partial hospital programs or intensive outpatient chemical dependency programs. Assessments by the program physician and counseling staff can identify other areas requiring specific interventions (comorbid medical or psychiatric disorders) and can expedite the initiation of appropriate pharmacotherapies. These interventions will increase treatment retention. Often patients must be helped to realize that their drug use is having a significant and adverse impact on their lives. Many patients come to treatment because of family, legal, or social pressures. They can be ambivalent about the need for treatment and require education about their addiction and assistance in reviewing the consequences of cocaine use in their lives. This inventory should occur in the initial visits to the substance abuse treatment program.

Initial treatment should include the encouragement of abstinence from all drug and alcohol use. Patients who abuse alcohol and marijuana often do not perceive these drugs as problems. Education regarding the use of such drugs as conditioned stimuli to the use of cocaine should be emphasized. The "disease model" of chemical dependency may be used to assist in the initiation of abstinence. Emphasis is placed on the patients recognizing chemical dependency as a disease needing treatment to control, but one for which there is no cure. Comprehensive drug education should also be provided in the initial treatment phase. Frequent contact with a drug counselor is an important part of treatment. Individual, group and (where clinically indicated) family or marital therapy should be available. Attendance at 12-step or other self-help groups is often a useful adjunct to treatment and can be particularly helpful during the early stages of treatment when support for sobriety is essential.

The early recovery phase of treatment varies in duration from 3 to 12 months and is characterized by multiple weekly contacts and participation in therapeutic modalities with the goal of initiation and maintenance of abstinence. The focus during early recovery should be on relapse prevention and development of new and adaptive coping skills, healthy relationships and lifestyle changes that will facilitate abstinence.

Relapses are common during early recovery. Patients often feel pleased about their progress in treatment, become overly confident about their ability to control use, and test themselves by deliberately encountering what they know to be a high-risk situation for their drug use. Experimentation with cocaine to prove that drug use can be controlled often results in relapse and is associated with guilt. Patients should be informed about the potential for relapse from the start of the treatment process. Relapse should be reviewed with the patient in a supportive way with an emphasis on helping the patient to gain an understanding of the events leading to relapse. Relapse should, however, also trigger a review of the treatment plan and consideration of the need for additional interventions or whether a higher level of care is needed to assist the patient in the recovery process.

Success with initiating and maintaining abstinence over several months is followed by a reduced frequency of contact (e.g., a decrease to weekly group or individual therapy sessions). The focus should be on maintaining a commitment to abstinence, addressing renewed denial and continued improvement of interpersonal skills. Participation in self-help groups should continue to be encouraged. Self-help groups based on 12-step principles

Table 38.1   Psychotherapies: The Mainstay of Treatment for Cocaine Use Disorders

Interpersonal therapy
Supportive expressive therapy
Cognitive–behavioral therapy/Relapse prevention therapy
Voucher based treatment alternative reinforcement behavioral
  therapy
Individual and group drug counseling
Systematic cue exposure
Self-help groups (e.g., Cocaine Anonymous)

encourage patients to continue to view themselves as addicts in recovery – a cognitive structuring that many recovering drug abusers find helpful in maintaining sobriety.

Psychotherapies for Cocaine Use Disorders

A variety of psychotherapeutic strategies for the treatment of cocaine use disorders have been adopted (Table 38.1). In contrast to opiate addiction, for which psychotherapies alone are insufficient, there appear to be at least some subpopulations of cocaine abusers for whom psychotherapy alone may be adequate (Crits-Christoph *et al.*, 1997, 1998, 1999). Behavioral therapies, in particular cognitive–behavioral therapy and contingency management approaches, have been demonstrated to be effective treatments for some cocaine-dependent patients.

The lack of a medically dangerous withdrawal syndrome from cocaine also suggests that some cocaine abusers may respond to psychotherapy alone in an outpatient treatment setting, compared with opiate- or alcohol-dependent persons for whom hospitalization may be required for detoxification. Another important reason for the development of psychotherapies for the

treatment of cocaine use disorders is that no medication is currently approved for the treatment of these disorders. Psychotherapies are also important platforms on which any pharmacological treatment may be supported.

Physician–Patient Relationship Considerations

The treatment of cocaine use disorders should be undertaken in the context of a thorough understanding of the disease (Table 38.2). The physician should develop individual treatment plans for patients based on the presenting complaints and symptoms related to cocaine abuse and any abstinence syndrome. Treatment plans include assessment for psychiatric and medical illnesses, pharmacological interventions, psychotherapy and other psychosocial interventions.

The physician is the provider who will make decisions regarding pharmacotherapy for cocaine dependence. This is an important consideration because there are currently no medications for cocaine use disorders that are approved by the US Food and Drug Administration. Therefore, any decision to provide medication to assist with the maintenance of abstinence from cocaine abuse must be carefully considered with documentation of the rationale for medication choice, risks and benefits of treatment and informed consent from the patient.

Pharmacotherapies for Cocaine Use Disorders

The development of pharmacological treatments for cocaine abuse has been based on the premise that an altered neurochemical substrate underlies the chronic, high-intensity (binge) use and acute abstinence/withdrawal that follows binge use. This neuroadaptation model has also served as a basis for a number of studies that have evaluated the clinical utility of psychotropic

Table 38.2   Cocaine Use Disorders: Recovery and Treatment

Parameter	Acute Abstinence	Withdrawal Phase	Extinction Phase
Duration	Several hours to 4 d	2–10 wk	3–12 mo
Treatment	Symptomatic May need hospitalization for medical or psychiatric care and assessment	Initiate psychotherapy Individual/group therapy Self-help groups, other therapies, e.g., family, marital, individual, as needed	Continue psychotherapy, decrease intensity with continued abstinence; self-help groups and additional interventions developed for individual patients as needed
Pharmacotherapy	Benzodiazepines for anxiety, agitation, paranoia. Antipsychotics (sparingly) for severe psychosis or agitation	None approved specific for cocaine use disorders Consider disulfiram for cocaine- or alcohol abuse previously refractory to treatment; psychotropics for cormorbid psychiatric disorders or cocaine-related disorders; pharmacotherapies for other substance use disorders	Unusual to initiate in this phase Taper and discontinue pharmacotherapy for cocaine abuse and monitor clinically

agents that, based on their pharmacological profile, might possess anticraving properties, block euphoria, or decrease cocaine abstinence symptoms. To date, no medication has emerged as an accepted effective pharmacotherapy.

Common Problems in Management

Several common problems are encountered in the treatment of patients with cocaine use disorders. These include: 1) relapse to cocaine use, 2) comorbid psychiatric disorders, 3) comorbid substance use disorders, 4) premature treatment termination and 5) treatment refractoriness.

Comparison of DSM-IV/ICD-10 Diagnostic Criteria

The ICD-10 and DSM-IV-TR Criteria sets for Cocaine Intoxication and Withdrawal are almost the same except that ICD-10 criteria set for Withdrawal includes drug-craving as an additional item.

References

Bradberry CW (2000) Acute and chronic dopamine dynamics in a non-human primate model of recreational cocaine use. *J Neurosci* 20, 7109–7115.

Brown RA, Monti PM, Myers MG *et al.* (1998) Depression among cocaine abusers in treatment: Relation to cocaine and alcohol use and treatment outcome. *Am J Psychiatr* 155, 220–225.

Carroll KM, Nich C and Rounsaville BJ (1995) Differential symptom reduction in depressed cocaine abusers treated with psychotherapy and pharmacotherapy. *J Nerv Ment Dis* 183, 251–259.

Clure C, Brady KT, Saladin ME *et al.* (1999) Attention-deficit/hyperactivity disorder and substance use: Symptom pattern and drug choice. *Am J Drug Alcohol Abuse* 25, 441–448.

Crits-Christoph P, Siqueland L, Blaine J *et al.* (1997) The National Institute on Drug Abuse Collaborative Cocaine Treatment Study. Rationale and methods. *Arch Gen Psychiatr* 54, 721–726.

Crits-Christoph P, Siqueland L, Chittams J *et al.* (1998) Training in cognitive, supportive-expressive, and drug counseling therapies for cocaine dependence. *J Consult Clin Psychol* 66, 484–492.

Crits-Christoph P, Siqueland L, Blaine J *et al.* (1999) Psychosocial treatments for cocaine dependence: National Institute on Drug Abuse Collaborative Cocaine Treatment Study. *Arch Gen Psychiatr* 56, 493–502.

Foltin RW and Fischman MW (1998) Effects of "binge" use of intravenous cocaine in methadone-maintained individuals. *Addiction* 93, 825–836.

Gendeh BS, Ferguson BJ, Johnson JT *et al.* (1998) Progressive septal and palatal perforation secondary to intranasal cocaine abuse. *Med J Mal* 53, 435–438.

Higgins ST, Budney AJ, Bickel WK *et al.* (1994) Incentives improve outcome in outpatient behavioral treatment of cocaine dependence. *Arch Gen Psychiatr* 51, 568–576.

Hollander JE, Shih RD, Hoffman RS, *et al.* (1997a) Predicts of coronary artery desease in patients with cacaine-associated myocardial infarction. Cocain-Associated Myocardial Infraction (CAMI) Study Group. *Am J Med.* 102, 158–163.

Hollander JE, Vignona L, and Burnstein J (1997b) Predictors of underlying coronary artery disease in cocaine associated myocardial infarction: A meta-analysis of case reports. *Vet Hum Toxicol* 39, 276–280.

Hollander JE, Todd KH, Green G *et al.* (1995) Chest pain associated with cocaine: An assessment of prevalence in suburban and urban emergency departments. *Am Emerg Med* 26, 671–676.

Koob GF and Nestler EJ (1997) The neurobiology of drug addiction. *J Neuropsychiatr Clin Neurosci* 9, 482–497.

Margolin A, Avants SK and Kosten TR (1996) Abstinence symptomatology associated with cessation of chronic cocaine abuse among methadone-maintained patients. *Am J Drug Alcohol Abuse* 22, 377–388.

McCance-Katz EF, Carroll KM and Rounsaville BJ (1999) Gender differences in treatment-seeking cocaine abusers – implications for treatment and prognosis. *Am J Addict* 8, 300–311.

McMahon RC, Malow R and Loewinger L (1999) Substance abuse history predicts depression and relapse status among cocaine abusers. *Am J Addict* 8, 1–8.

Milby JB, Schumacher JE, McNamara C *et al.* (2000) Initiating abstinence in cocaine abusing dually diagnosed homeless persons. *Drug Alcohol Depend* 60, 55–67.

Mittleman MA, Mintzer D, Maclure M *et al.* (1999) Triggering of myocardial infarction by cocaine. *Circulation* 99, 2737–2741.

Simpson DD, Joe GW, Fletcher BW *et al.* (1999) A national evaluation of treatment outcomes for cocaine dependence. *Arch Gen Psychiatr* 56, 507–514.

Substance Abuse and Mental Health Services Administration (1996) *Trends in the Incidence of Drug Use in the United States.* Rockville, MD.

Substance Abuse and Mental Health Service Administration (1999) *The 1999 National Household Survey on Drug Abuse.* Rockville, MD.

Substance Abuse and Mental Health Administration (2001a) *DASIS Report: Women in Treatment for Smoked Cocaine.* The Office of Applied Studies, Arlington, VA.

Substance Abuse and Mental Health Service Administration (2001b) *Mid-Year 2000 Preliminary Emergency Department Data from the Drug Abuse Warning Network.* Rockville, MD.

Van Etten ML and Anthony JC (1999) Comparative epidemiology of initial drug opportunities and transitions to first use: Marijuana, cocaine, hallucinogens and heroin. *Drug Alcohol Depend* 54, 117–125.

Wang RY (1999) pH-dependent cocaine-induced cardiotoxicity. *Am J Emerg Med* 17, 364–369.

Weber JE, Chudnofsky CR, Boczar M *et al.* (2000) Cocaine-associated chest pain: How common is myocardial infarction? *Acad Emerg Med* 7, 873–877.

Substance Abuse: Phencycline Use Disorders

Phencyclidine (PCP) failed its development as a potential general anesthetic agent during the 1950s because of its propensity to cause psychotic episodes during emergence that were sometimes severe and violent, and lasted from hours to days. PCP psychosis closely resembles schizophrenia in terms of symptoms, signs and thought disorder. A single very small dose of PCP given to a normal subject induces a psychotic state lasting for several hours, while in a person with schizophernia, the psychosis can be exacerbated for several weeks by the fact that it is easy to synthesize. Many users consumed PCP on a daily or near-daily basis for weeks or months at a time. There were numerous instances of severe medical toxicity, a number of deaths from overdoses, and many cases of prolonged (up to six weeks) psychoses in users without preexisting psychotic disorders. In addition to CNS effects, PCP overdose involves sympathomimetic, neuromuscular and renal effects that can result in tissue damage and death. These problems are compounded by PCP's lipophilicity, long half-life and still longer duration of action. The incidence and prevalence of PCP abuse have declined markedly since the late 1970s to early 1980s; however, PCP abuse continues and remains relatively high in certain areas of the USA. PCP exerts its characteristic effects by noncompetitive blockade of the N-methyl D-aspartate class of glutamate receptors. Ketmine is a PCP derivative that shares PCP's mechanism of action and is approved for general effects are less frequent and severe owing to the lower potency and shorter duration of ketamine action compared with PCP.

Epidemiology

As of the year 2000, the highest rates of PCP use during the previous year were observed among 18- to 20-year-olds, followed by 12- to 17-, 21- to 25-, and 26- to 34-year-olds. In 2000, among Americans aged 12 or older, it was estimated that 54 000 had used PCP within the previous month, 264 000 within the previous year and 5 693 000 (2% of the population) within their lifetimes (Substance Abuse and Mental Health Services Administration, 2001). In the same year, PCP ranked 31st among the top 50 drugs mentioned most frequently in drug-related emergency department episodes nationwide showing a 48% increase in ER mentions compared with 1999 (Substance Abuse and Mental Health Services Administration, 2002).

In 1983, more than 66% of PCP-related deaths reported to the Drug Abuse Warning Network involved at least another one drug. Many of the PCP-related deaths were not the result of overdose or drug interaction or reaction, but the direct result of some external event facilitated by intoxication (e.g., homicides, accidents). The various manners of death (such as drowning and being shot by police) reported are consistent with the disorientation and violent aggressive behavior that can be stimulated by PCP (Crider, 1986).

Etiology and Pathophysiology

The effects of low-dose PCP administration have been extensively studied in volunteers. In normal subjects single intravenous doses of 0.05 to 0.1 mg/kg induced withdrawal, negativism and in some cases catatonic posturing; thinking processes became concrete, idiosyncratic and bizarre in the absence of significant physical or neurological findings; and drug effects persisted for 4 to 6 hours In contrast to lysergic acid diethylamide (LSD) or amphetamine PCP was noted to induce disturbances in symbolic thinking perception and attention strikingly similar to those observed in schizophrenia. Administration of PCP to schizophrenic subjects caused exacerbation of illness-specific symptoms persisting up to several weeks, suggesting that schizophrenic or preschizophrenic individuals may be at significantly increased risk of behavioral effects from PCP abuse.

Phenomenology and Variations in Presentation

Physicians must be alert to the wide spectrum of PCP effects on multiple organ systems. Because fluctuations in serum levels may occur unpredictably, a patient being treated for apparently selective psychiatric or behavioral complications of PCP abuse may suddenly undergo radical alterations in medical status; emergency medical intervention may become necessary to avoid permanent organ damage or death. Any patient manifesting significant cardiovascular, respiratory, neurological, or metabolic derangement subsequent to PCP use should be evaluated and treated in a medical service; the psychiatrist plays a secondary role in diagnosis and treatment until physiological stability has been reached and sustained.

PCP-intoxicated patients may come to medical attention on the basis of alterations in mental status; bizarre or violent behavior; injuries sustained while intoxicated; or medical complications, such as rhabdomyolysis, hyperthermia, or seizures (Baldridge and Bessen, 1990). As illicit ketamine use has increased significantly as part of the "club drug" phenomenon, it is important to remember that ketamine can induce the same spectrum of effects and complications, the chief difference from PCP being the much shorter duration of action of ketamine.

Essentials of Psychiatry   Jerald Kay and Allan Tasman
© 2006 John Wiley & Sons, Ltd.

Phencyclidine Intoxication

A. Recent use of phencyclidine (or a related substance).

B. Clinically significant maladaptive behavioral changes (e.g., belligerence, assaultiveness, impulsiveness, unpredictability, psychomotor agitation, impaired judgment, or impaired social or occupational functioning) that developed during, or shortly after, phencyclidine use.

C. Within an hour (less when smoked, "snorted," or used intravenously), two (or more) of the following signs:
   (1) Vertical or horizontal nystagmus
   (2) Hypertension or tachycardia
   (3) Numbness or diminished responsiveness to pain
   (4) Ataxia
   (5) Dysarthria
   (6) Muscle rigidity
   (7) Seizures or coma
   (8) Hyperacusis

D. The symptoms are not due to a general medical condition and are not better accounted for by another mental disorder.

Specify if:
With perceptual disturbances

Reprinted with permission from the Diagnostic and Statistical Manual of Mental Disorders, Fourth Edition, Text Revision. Copyright 2000 American Psychiatric Association.

Studies of normal volunteers suggested that the acute psychosis induced by a single low dose of PCP usually lasts for 4 to 6 hours (Javitt and Zukin, 1991). However, in some PCP users psychotic symptoms including hallucinations, delusions, paranoia, thought disorder and catatonia, with intact consciousness, have been reported to persist from days to weeks after single doses. Sudden and impulsive violent and assaultive behaviors have been reported in PCP-intoxicated patients without previous histories of such conduct.

In PCP intoxication, the central nervous, cardiovascular, respiratory and peripheral autonomic systems are affected to degrees ranging from mild to catastrophic (Table 39.1). The level of consciousness may vary from full alertness to coma. Coma of variable duration may occur spontaneously or after an episode of bizarre or violent behavior.

Table 39.1 Nonpsychiatric Findings in Phencyclidine Intoxication

Altered level of consciousness
Central nervous system changes including nystagmus, hyperreflexia, and motor abnormalities
Hypertension
Cholinergic or anticholinergic signs
Hypothermia or hyperthermia
Myoglobinuria

Nystagmus (which may be horizontal, vertical, or rotatory) has been described in 57% of a series of 1000 patients (McCarron *et al.*, 1981). Consequences of PCP-induced central nervous system hyperexcitability may range from mildly increased deep tendon reflexes to grand mal seizures (observed in 31 of a series of 1000 PCP-intoxicated patients) or status epilepticus (McCarron *et al.*, 1981; Kessler *et al.*, 1974). Seizures are usually generalized, but focal seizures or neurological deficits have been reported, probably on the basis of focal cerebral vasoconstriction (Crosley and Binet, 1979). Other motor signs have been observed, such as generalized rigidity, localized dystonias, facial grimacing and athetosis.

Hypertension, one of the most frequent physical findings, was described in 57% of 1000 patients evaluated, and it was found to be usually mild and self-limiting, but 4% had severe hypertension, and some remained hypertensive for days (McCarron *et al.*, 1981). Tachycardia occurs in 30% of patients. PCP-induced tachypnea can progress to periodic breathing and respiratory arrest (Hurlbut, 1991). Autonomic signs seen in PCP intoxication may be cholinergic (diaphoresis, bronchospasm, miosis, salivation, bronchorrhea) or anticholinergic (mydriasis, urinary retention). Hypothermia and hyperthermia have been observed (McCarron *et al.*, 1981). Hyperthermia may reach malignant proportions (Thompson, 1979). Rhabdomyolysis frequently results from a combination of PCP-induced muscle contractions and trauma occurring in relation to injuries sustained as a result of behavioral effects. Acute renal failure can result from myoglobinuria.

Assessment

Special Issues in Psychiatric Examination and History

The disruption of normal cognitive and memory function by PCP frequently renders patients unable to give an accurate history. Therefore, assay of urine or blood for drugs may be the only way to establish the diagnosis. PCP is frequently taken in forms in which it has been used to adulterate other drugs, such as marijuana and cocaine, often without the user's knowledge. One of the most recent and alarming manifestations of this phenomenon is a preparation known variously as "illy", "hydro", "wet", or "fry", consisting of a marijuana cigarette or blunt containing formaldehyde/formalin (which is advertised) and PCP (which often is not). By disrupting sensory pathways, PCP frequently renders users hypersensitive to environmental stimuli to the extent that physical examination or psychiatric interview may cause severe agitation. If PCP intoxication is suspected, measures should be taken from the outset to minimize sensory input. The patient should be evaluated in a quiet, darkened room with the minimal necessary number of medical staff present. Assessments may need to be interrupted periodically.

Relevant Physical Examination and Laboratory Findings

Vital signs should be obtained immediately on presentation. Temperature, blood pressure and respiratory rate are dose-dependently increased by PCP and may be of a magnitude requiring emergency medical treatment to avoid the potentially fatal complications of malignant hyperthermia, hypertensive crisis and respiratory arrest. In all cases, monitoring of vital signs should continue at 2- to 4-hour intervals throughout treatment, because serum PCP levels may increase spontaneously as a result of mobilization of drug from lipid stores or enterohepatic recirculation. Analgesic and behavioral changes induced by PCP not only predispose patients to physical injury but also mask these injuries, which may be found only with careful physical examination.

Because PCP is usually supplied in combination with other drugs and is often misrepresented, toxicological analysis of urine or blood is essential. However there may be circumstances in which PCP may not be detected in urine even if it is present in the body, for example, when the urine is alkaline. On the other hand, in chronic PCP users, drug may be detected in urine up to 30 days after last use (Simpson *et al.*, 1982–1983). It must be kept in mind that false-positive PCP results can be caused by the presence of venlafaxine and *O*-desmethylvenlafaxine (Sena *et al.*, 2002), or dextromethorphan (Shier, 2000). Urine should be tested for heme because of the possible complication of myoglobinuria.

Differential Diagnosis

The presence of nystagmus and hypertension with mental status changes should raise the possibility of PCP intoxication. Because of the close resemblance of both the acute and the prolonged forms of PCP psychosis to schizophrenia, and the increased sensitivity of patients with schizophrenia to the psychotomimetic effects of the drug, an underlying schizophrenia spectrum disorder should be considered, particularly if paranoia or thought disorder persists beyond 4 to 6 weeks after last use of PCP. PCP psychosis may also resemble mania or other mood disorders. Robust response of psychotic symptoms to treatment with neuroleptics would favor a diagnosis other than simple PCP psychosis.

PCP psychosis is readily distinguishable from LSD psychosis in normal as well as in individuals with schizophrenia by the lack of typical LSD effects, such as synesthesia. In cases involving prominent PCP-induced neurological, cardiovascular, or metabolic derangement, encephalitis, head injury, postictal state and primary metabolic disorders must be ruled out. Either intoxication with or withdrawal from sedative–hypnotics may be associated with nystagmus. Neuroleptic malignan at syndrome should be ruled out in the differential diagnosis of PCP-induced hyperthermia and muscle rigidity.

Course and Natural History

As drug levels decline, the clinical picture recedes in five to 21 days through periods of moderating neurological, autonomic and metabolic impairments to a stage at which only psychiatric impairments are apparent. Once the physical symptoms and signs have cleared the period of simple PCP psychosis may last 1 day to 6 weeks, whether or not neuroleptics are administered, during which the psychiatric symptoms and signs abate gradually and progressively. Even after complete recovery flashbacks may occur if PCP sequestered in lipid stores is mobilized. Any underlying psychiatric disorders can be detected and evaluated only after complete resolution of the drug-induced psychosis.

Overall Goals of Treatment

The hierarchy of treatment goals begins with detection and treatment of physical manifestations of PCP intoxication. Equally important are measures to anticipate PCP-induced impulsive, violent behaviors and provide appropriate protection for the patient and others. The patient must then be closely observed during the period of PCP-induced psychosis, which may persist for weeks after resolution of physical symptoms and signs. Finally, the possibly dramatic medical and psychiatric presentation and its resolution must not divert the attention of the psychiatrist from full assessment and treatment of the patient's drug-seeking behavior.

Physician–Patient Relationship in Psychiatric Management

In contrast to psychotic states induced by drugs such as LSD, in which "talking the patient down" (by actively distracting the patient from his LSD-induced sensory distortions and convincing the patient that his or her distress stems from nothing more than the temporary effects of a drug that soon will wear off) may be highly effective, no such effort should be made in the case of PCP psychosis, particularly during the period of acute intoxication, because of the risk of sensory overload that can lead to dramatically increased agitation. The risk of sudden and unpredictable impulsive, violent behavior can also be increased by sensory stimulation.

Pharmacotherapy and Somatic Treatments

There is no pharmacological competitive antagonist for PCP. Oral or intramuscular benzodiazepines are recommended for agitation. Neuroleptics usually have little or no effect on acute or chronic PCP-induced psychosis or thought disorder. Because they lower the seizure threshold, neuroleptics should be used with caution. Physical restraint may be lifesaving if the patient's behavior poses an imminent threat to his or her safety or that of others; however, such restraint risks triggering or worsening rhabodomyolysis.

Comparison of DSM-IV/ICD-10 Diagnostic Criteria

Unlike DSM-IV-TR, ICD-10 does not have a separate class for Phencyclidine-Related Disorders and instead includes PCP in the Hallucinogen class.

References

Baldridge BE and Bessen HA (1990) *Phencyclidine. Emerg Med Clin N Am* 8, 541–550.

Crider R (1986) Phencyclidine: Changing abuse patterns. *NIDA Res Monogr* 64, 163–173.

Crosley CJ and Binet EF (1979) Cerebrovascular complications in phencyclidine intoxication. *J Pediatr* 94, 316–318.

Hurlbut KM (1991) Drug-induced psychosis. *Emerg Med Clin N Am* 9, 31–53.

Javitt DC and Zukin SR (1991) Recent advances in the phencyclidine model of schizophrenia. *Am J Psychiatr* 148, 1301–1308.

Kessler GF, Demers LM and Berlin C (1974) Phencyclidine and fatal status epilepticus (letter). *New Engl J Med* 291, 979.

McCarron MM, Schulze BW, Thompson GA *et al.* (1981) Acute phencyclidine intoxication: Incidence of clinical findings in 1,000 cases. *Ann Emerg Med* 10, 237–242.

Sena SF, Kazimi S and Wu AH (2002) False-positive phencyclidine immunoassay results caused by venlafaxine and O-desmethylvenlafaxine. *Clin Chem* 48(4), 676–677.

Shier J (2000) Avoid unfavorable consequences: Dextromethorphan can bring about a false-positive phencyclidine urine drug screen. *J Emerg Med* 18(3) (Apr), 379–381.

Simpson JM, Khajawallam AM and Alatorre E (1982–1983) Urinary phencyclidine exceretion in chronic abusers. *J Toxicol Clin Toxicol* 19, 1051–1059.

Substance Abuse and Mental Health Services Administration (2001) Summary of Findings from the 2000 National Household Survey on Drug Abuse. Office of Applied Studies, NHSDA Series H-13, DHHS Publication No. (SMA) 01-3549, Rockville, MD.

Substance Abuse and Mental Health Services Administration (2002) Office of Applied Studies. Emergency Department Trends from the Drug Abuse Warning Network, Preliminary Estimates January–June 2001 with Revised Estimates 1994–2000, DAWN Series D-20, DHHS Publication No. (SMA) 02-3634, Rockville, MD.

Thompson TN (1979) Malignant hyperthermia from PCP (letter). *J Clin Psychiatr* 40, 327.

40 Substance Abuse: Hallucinogen- and MDMA-Related Disorders

Hallucinogens alter perception, cognition and mood as their primary psychobiological action in the presence of an otherwise clear sensorium. LSD is the most common hallucinogen and is readily and cheaply available in the USA. Unlike the chronic use of stimulants amphetamine and cocaine, chronic use of hallucinogen does not lead to physiological dependence. On the other hand tolerance to LSD builds in 4 to 7 days. There is no withdrawal or documented fatalities from overdose of LSD. The 3,4-methylenedioxymethamphetamine (MDMA or Ecstasy) is a synthetic amphetamine analogue that is used to enhance affiliative emotional responses. Its use appears to be increasing, particularly among young adults. Dependence and escalation of dosage are uncommon. All these agents are neurotoxic with deleterious effects on serotonergic neurons, memory and mood. Common naturally occurring compounds include mescaline (and peyote), psilocybin and dimethyltryptamine (DMT). The dawn of modernity for synthetic hallucinogenic drugs can be placed tothe moment in 1943 when Albert Hofmann, a Swiss chemist, discovered the potent psychological effects of LSD. The definition of an hallucinogenic drug has been a matter of controversy. To address the problem of classification, one may define as hallucinogenic "any agent which has alterations in perception, cognition, or mood as its primary psychobiological actions in the presence of an otherwise clear sensorium".

Epidemiology of Hallucinogen Abuse

Among hallucinogens, LSD remains the most popular in its class among American high school students. An annual drug survey of 45 000 students by the Monitoring the Future Program of the University of Michigan has been performed since 1975. There is a stable long-term trend of LSD lifetime use among one in 10 seniors.

Etiology and Pathophysiology

The acute effects of "tripping" on LSD-like (i.e, with similar psychic effects, such as psilocybin or mescaline) hallucinogens are variable and profound. Table 40.1 illustrates a typical time course for the psychiatric effects of LSD.

The effective hallucinogenic doses vary widely between drugs in this class, and between individuals. The conventional explanation of this variability of response is instructional set, anticipation of drug effects due to previous experience, and

Table 40.1	Time Course for the Psychiatric Effects of LSD-like Hallucinogens
Time	Psychiatric Effects
0–30 min	Dizziness, nausea, weakness, anxiety
30–60 min	Blurred vision, visual pseudohallucinations and hallucinations, afterimagery, geometric and imagistic imagery with eyes closed, decreased concentration, dissociation, depersonalization, out of body sensations, reduced coordination
60–240 min	Intensified afterimagery, false perceptions of movement (walls appearing to breathe or melt), loss of rectilinearity of perceptions, a rapid flood of emotions including anxiety, euphoria, and oceanic unity, loss of the sense of time
4–12 hr	Gradual return to previous mental state, but with continued arousal, headache, fatigue, contemplative frame of reference, sense of profundity

Modified from Hollister L (1984) Effects of hallucinogens in humans, in *Hallucinogens: Neurochemical, Behavioral, and Clinical Perspectives* (ed Jacobs B). Raven Press, New York. Copyright, Lippincott, Williams & Wilkins.

environmental setting affect outcome. Additionally, personality, preexisting mental illness and genetic vulnerability are also likely to be important. Unlike the chronic use of stimulants like amphetamine and cocaine, chronic use of hallucinogens does not lead to physiological dependence. On the other hand, tolerance to LSD rapidly builds in 4 to 7 days, and lasts 3 days. Titeler and colleagues (1988) have shown that hallucinogenic potency of LSD and selected phenylisopropylamines correlates with the drug's ability to bind at the postsynaptic 5-HT$_2$ receptor.

Hallucinogens simultaneously decrease spontaneous activity in the locus coeruleus, considered a novelty detector in the midbrain, while enhancing sensory responses of the locus coeruleus by activating N-methyl-D-aspartate receptors. In the cerebral cortex, the drugs both inhibit and induce activity by exciting GABAergic and glutamatergic neurons respectively.

Essentials of Psychiatry Jerald Kay and Allan Tasman
© 2006 John Wiley & Sons, Ltd.

The presence of selective serotonin reuptake inhibitors blunts hallucinogenic effects, possibly through the activation of 5-HT$_1$ receptors (Aghajanian and Marek, 1999). GABA-$_A$ antianxiety agents (e.g., benzodiazepines) promptly bring a bad trip to an end, presumably by inhibition of the locus coeruleus. Opiates are likely to have a similar outcome by reducing glutamatergic excitation of cortical systems. This may explain why hallucinogen abuse appears to be so uncommon among active opioid abusers.

Differential Diagnosis and Treatment of Acute Intoxication

Criteria for the diagnosis of acute hallucinogen intoxication are set forth in the following *Diagnostic and Statistical Manual of Mental Disorders*, Fourth Edition, Text Revision (DSM-IV-TR) (American Psychiatric Association, 2000).

Chemical identification of hallucinogens in emergency specimens with methods such as gas chromatography–mass spectrometry remain costly and time consuming. Thus, clinicians in emergency settings must rely on a careful drug history, the information from the less drug-affected friends of the patient, the mental status examination and signs Pparent from the physical examination. The high potency of this class of drugs permits their distribution in venues of single drops of solution. Thus, blotter paper (often marked with stamps of cartoon characters or New Age symbols) or a single sugar cube can easily carry more than the 50 to 100 μg

---

DSM-IV-TR Criteria 292.89

Hallucinogen Intoxication

A. Recent use of a hallucinogen.

B. Clinically significant maladaptive behavioral or psychological changes (e.g., marked anxiety or depression, ideas of reference, fear of losing one's mind, paranoid ideation, impaired judgment, or impaired social or occupational function) that developed during, or shortly after, hallucinogen use.

C. Perceptual changes occurring in a state of full wakefulness and alertness (e.g., subjective intensification of perceptions, depersonalization, derealization, illusions, hallucinations, synesthesias) that developed during, or shortly after, hallucinogen use.

D. Two (or more) of the following signs, developing during, or shortly after, hallucinogen use:
   (1) pupillary dilation
   (2) tachycardia
   (3) sweating
   (4) palpitations
   (5) blurring of vision
   (6) tremors
   (7) incoordination

E. The symptoms are not due to a general medical condition and are not better accounted for by another mental disorder.

---

of LSD necessary for the user to trip for 6 to 12 hours. Routes of administration other than by ingestion are rare. Autonomic arousal is the rule, with tachycardia, increased deep tendon reflexes, and dilated pupils present regardless of whether euphoria or panic is present. Hypersensitivity to visual and auditory stimuli is common, with atypical affective responses as the result. Motor function is reduced, so that such patients are not likely to act out aggressively.

The differential diagnosis of an acute hallucinogenic intoxication includes intoxication by other agents, (such as phencyclidine [PCP], cocaine, amphetamines, anticholinergics and inhalants, among others). It also includes acute schizophrenia or affective disorder, panic disorder, head injury, sedative, hypnotic, anxiolytic, or alcohol withdrawal (including gamma-hydroxybutyrate [GHB]), metabolic disorders such as hypoglycemia and hyperthyroidism, epilepsy, acute vascular events, release hallucinations of ophthalmologic disease and the complications of central nervous system (CNS) tumors. Age, along with prior clinical history, the history of the current event, physical examination and toxicology screen for suspected nonhallucinogenic agents usually reveal the diagnosis.

A patient presenting with a history of taking LSD is only correct approximately 50% of the time, judging from analysis of street samples analyzed by the Massachusetts Department of Public Health in the last decade. The street practice of adulteration or mislabeling of the drug is common. Psychosis following a smoked agent suggests phencyclidine. Differentiating between PCP and LSD is clinically important, since LSD-induced panic responds well to oral benzodiazepines, while PCP delirium requires high potency antipsychotic medications such as haloperidol. A "palm test" can be employed to differentiate PCP from LSD toxicity (Abraham and Aldridge, 1993). This is performed by the examiner holding an open palm in front of the patient, and asking "the names of all the colors you see in my palm". The LSD patient often ticks off a series of vivid colors and occasional images. The dissociated, aggressive PCP patient attempts to attack the hand. Treatment of hallucinogen intoxication with panic is easily managed with oral benzodiazepines (diazepam 20 mg or lorazepam 2 mg) which bring the terror, as well as the trip, to an end within 30 minutes.

LSD-Related Psychotic Disorders

Criteria for substance-induced psychotic disorders are listed below in the DSM-IV-TR Criteria.

Among the hallucinogens, LSD has been associated with the majority of, but not all, prolonged psychotic reactions following acute drug use. Psychoses are apparently rare with the abuse of botanical preparations, in all likelihood because such agents are of low potency, not widely abused, and often controlled by religious sanctions. By comparison, psychoses have been seen following the administration of LSD to patients and experimental subjects. In addition to exhibiting positive signs of schizophrenia, patients with post-LSD psychoses show affective lability and the novel addition of visual hallucinations uncommon in non-drug-related psychoses. The uniqueness of post-LSD psychosis remains controversial. One comparison of post-LSD psychosis and nondrug-related schizophrenia found no essential clinical differences between the two (Vardy and Kay, 1983).

Differential Diagnosis and Treatment

The differential diagnosis of posthallucinogen psychosis is that for any acute psychotic disorder. This includes protracted psychoses

DSM-IV-TR Criteria

Substance-induced Psychotic Disorder

A. Prominent hallucinations or delusions, **Note:** Do not include hallucinations if the person has insight that they are substance induced.

B. There is evidence from the history, physical examination, or laboratory findings of either (1) or (2):
   (1) the symptoms in Criterion A developed during, or within a month of, substance intoxication or withdrawal
   (2) medication use is etiologically related to the disturbance

C. The disturbance is not better accounted for by a psychotic disorder that is not substance induced. Evidence that the symptoms are better accounted for by a psychotic disorder that is not substance induced might include the following: the symptoms precede the onset of the substance use (or medication use); the symptoms persist for a substantial period of time (e.g., about a month) after the cessation of acute withdrawal or severe intoxication or are substantially in excess of what would be expected given the type or amount of the substance used or the duration of use; or there is other evidence that suggests the existence of an independent nonsubstance-induced psychotic disorder (e.g., a history of recurrent nonsubstance-related episodes).

D. The disturbance does not occur exclusively during the course of a delirium.

Note: This diagnosis should be made instead of a diagnosis of substance intoxication or substance withdrawal only when the symptoms are in excess of those usually associated with the intoxication or withdrawal syndrome and when the symptoms are sufficiently severe to warrant independent clinical attention.

Code specific substance-induced psychotic disorder: 292.11 amphetamine (or amphetamine-like substance), with delusions; 292.12 amphetamine (or amphetamine-like substance), with hallucinations; 292.11 hallucinogen, with delusions; 292.12 hallucinogen, with hallucinations.

Specify:
With onset during intoxication: if criteria are met for intoxication with the substance and the symptoms develop during the intoxication syndrome.

With onset during withdrawal: if criteria are met for withdrawal from the substance and the symptoms develop during, or shortly after, a withdrawal syndrome.

following the use of the dissociative anesthetics phencyclidine and ketamine, amphetamines, and cocaine; schizophrenia and affective disorders, migraine, deliria from CNS infections, closed head injuries, tumors, vascular events, and the toxic effects of

Clinical Vignette

A 19-year-old man used LSD for the fourth time. In the past, his trip on LSD ran an 8-hour course. Now, however, auditory and visual hallucinations persisted over the next week. At the same time his behavior became increasingly agitated and bizarre. His speech became rapid and incoherent. He was unable to sleep. His energy was increased though he talked of committing suicide. He expressed the delusion that he had sexual relations with a pet, and that he was androgynous. He was admitted to a psychiatric hospital where he showered with his clothes on and pulled a towel rack off the wall. Four-point restraints were required. His past history was negative for prior psychosis. There was no history of drug dependency. His family history was positive for depression. The patient was treated at the outset with neuroleptics which were supplemented with lithium carbonate in the fourth week. He remained disoriented, delusional and hallucinatory until the illness remitted 2 months after his last use of LSD.

Comment

This case illustrates the continuum between LSD use and an acute psychotic reaction. Salient are signs consistent with the positive symptoms of schizophrenia, including multimodal hallucinations, bizarre delusions and behavior, and thought disorder. Like other patients in this class, without predisposing factors, this man had a relatively healthy premorbid adjustment and good outcome. The patient has avoided mind-altering drugs since discharge. There has been no relapse in a 16-year follow-up.

bromine, heavy metals and anticholinergic drugs. Central to diagnosis is a careful premorbid history, complemented by data from friends and family on the patient's recent medical history and behavior. Neurological examination, an acute urine for toxicological screening, and computed tomography or magnetic resonance imaging of the brain are helpful in ruling out treatable nonLSD-related psychotic disorders.

Treatment for post-LSD psychoses includes neuroleptics, electroconvulsive therapy (ECT), and lithium.

Hallucinogen Persisting Perception Disorder (HPPD)

The definition of hallucinogen persisting perception disorder is shown in the following DSM-IV-TR Criteria.

Differential Diagnosis and Treatment

It is not uncommon for a patient suffering from HPPD to consult multiple clinicians before a diagnosis is made. Because the symptoms are primarily perceptual, an HPPD subject may consult an ophthalmologist, neurologist, or psychologist before seeing a psychiatrist. Often patients come for help having made their own diagnoses using the DSM-IV or internet chat groups devoted to HPPD. Despite a patient's certainty about their diagnosis, the clinician is obligated to rule out other sources of chronic organic hallucinosis, including other drug toxicities, strokes, CNS tumors, infections and head trauma. Magnetic resonance images of the brain are usually negative. Quantitative electroencephalography shows accelerated alpha and visual evoked potentials, especially in the posterior cerebrum.

DSM-IV-TR Criteria 292.89

Hallucinogen Persisting Perception Disorder (Flashbacks)

A. The reexperiencing, following cessation of use of a hallucinogen, of one or more of the perceptual symptoms that were experienced while intoxicated with the hallucinogen (e.g., geometric hallucinations, false perception of movement in the peripheral visual fields, flashes of color, intensified colors, trails of images of moving objects, positive afterimages, halos around objects, macropsia, and micropsia).

B. The symptoms in Criterion A cause clinically significant distress or impairment in social, occupational, or other important areas of functioning.

C. The symptoms are not due to a general medical condition (e.g., anatomical lesions and infections of the brain, visual epilepsies) and are not better accounted for by another mental disorder (e.g., delirium, dementia, schizophrenia) or hypnopompic hallucinations.

Reprinted with permission from the Diagnostic and Statistical Manual of Mental Disorders, Fourth Edition, Text Revision. Copyright 2000 American Psychiatric Association.

Treatment at the present time is palliative. Benzodiazepines, olanzepine, sertraline, naltrexone and clonidine have anecdotally been reported to help in selected cases. Risperidone has been reported to exacerbate HPPD symptoms Marijuana can chronically induce an exacerbation of HPPD. Because HPPD is also exacerbated by CNS arousal, affect, stress and stimulants, these are to be reduced or avoided. HPPD is worse with one's eyes closed, or when entering a dark environment. Thus, sunglasses, which serve to reduce the difference between outdoor and indoor luminance, may reduce HPPD symptoms when the patient enters an interior space.

MDMA ("Ecstasy")

3,4-methylenedioxymethamphetamine (MDMA, commonly known as "ecstasy," and chemically N-methyl-1-[3,4- methylenedioxyphenyl]-2-aminopropane) is a synthetic amphetamine analogue that is also similar to mescaline. During the 'psychedelic' 1970s, recreational use of MDMA took root due to its psychological effects and the fact that it was available legally. Recreational use was partially fueled by reports of the use of MDMA as a psychotherapeutic adjunct.

The publicity that followed the scheduling of MDMA only served to increase its popularity, particularly on college campuses. Recently, the use of MDMA has increased and its pattern of use has changed. These factors have heightened public awareness of the drug and paradoxically led to an increase in use and adverse consequences. Emerging evidence supports the hypothesis that MDMA is a neurotoxin in humans with long-lived sequelae on cognition, memory and emotions.

Epidemiology

Despite its existence for nearly 90 years, the recreational use of MDMA appears to have had its origins in the 1960s (Pope et al.,

2001). Initial drug use centered around college campuses (Pope et al., 2001; Peroutka et al., 1988). At that time, use of MDMA was generally in small groups in private places (Peroutka et al., 1988). Accurate epidemiologic data are not available for the 1960s. However, by 1977 about 2.8% of US college students used MDMA (Strote et al., 2002). College is the first time that people are likely to begin use of MDMA (Cuomo et al., 1994; Randell, 1992). Nonetheless, use in high school students has also increased, so that in 1998, 4.4% of 10th graders and 5.6% of high school seniors had tried MDMA (Johnston et al., 1999). In a survey of 14 000 college students at 119 American colleges by the Harvard School of Public Health College Alcohol Study, there was a 69% increase in use between 1997 and 1999 (from 2.8 to 4.7%) (Strote et al., 2002). At 10 high use schools with a 1997 rate of 4.7%, the rate increased to 10.6% by the year 2000 (Strote et al., 2002). Over the same time the use of marijuana did not significantly change (38.5% in 1997 and 37.6% in 2000) (Strote et al., 2002). MDMA is the only illicit drug to see continued increase in use. In surveys of a large New England college performed in 1969, 1978, 1989 and 1999, all drug use peaked in 1978 and dropped thereafter but MDMA use has continued to increase. The increasing popularity of MDMA is not just an American phenomenon, but is seen in both Europe (Cregg and Traqcey, 1993; Christophersen, 2000) and Australia (Topp et al., 1999).

In addition to increased popularity of MDMA, the pattern of use appears to have changed. Initial use was in small groups at doses ranging from 75 to 150 mg with an occasional booster of 50 to 100 mg (Peroutka et al., 1988; Downing, 1986; Siegel, 1986; Liester, 1992). The 1990s saw the onset of the rave phenomenon. These are generally large gatherings in warehouses or dance clubs. Dosage utilized in raves are much more variable ranging from 100 to 750 mg and as high as 1 250 mg/night (Brown et al., 1995; Forsyth, 1996). Concomitant drug use is also more common in raves (Strote et al., 2002; Gervin et al., 2001; Gerhard, 2001). These include alcohol, marijuana and opiates. Furthermore, the term "ecstasy", which was originally used to refer specifically to MDMA, has grown to refer to other related compounds such as 3,4-methylenedioxyamphetamine (MDA) and 3,4-methylenedixoyethylamphetamine (MDE or Eve) (Gerhard, 2001). The combination of these variables increases the risks of adverse consequences associated with MDMA use (see later).

MDMA users generally limit the frequency of use of the drug. Most report limiting use of MDMA to twice per month or less. Fridays and Saturdays are the most common days of use because users say they need 1 day to recover after use (Peroutka et al., 1988; Liester et al., 1992). More frequent use is associated with a loss of the desired effect of the drug (Gerhard et al., 2001).

Prior to its placement on Schedule 1 by the DEA, MDMA was considered as an adjunct to psychotherapy (Shulgin and Nichols, 1978; Greer and Tolbert, 1986, 1998). In this setting, a dosage of 50 to 200 mg (with modal doses ranging from 100 to 150 mg), with a booster of 50 to 75 mg several hours later, was used. There are no controlled studies of the use of MDMA in psychotherapy. However, there is one open study of 29 subjects in which the dosage used was 75 to 150 mg after a 6-hour fast with an offered second dose of 50 to 75 mg. All subjects reported positive attitudinal and emotional changes. Twenty-two felt that their insight into their own psychopathology was enhanced. Twenty-one subjects in couples treatment reported increased closeness and communication with their partner (Greer and Tolbert, 1986). All subjects reported adverse consequences similar to those reported by recreational drug users. While the use of MDMA as a psychotherapeutic adjunct appears to have advocates (Greer and

Tolbert, 1998), the documentation of neurotoxicity in humans (Reneman *et al.*, 2002; McCann *et al.*, 1998; Semple *et al.*, 1999) makes such use dubious.

Pharmacology

MDMA is toxic to serotonergic neurons. Serotonergic loss is evident through several markers which include reduced brain serotonin, 5-hydroxyindoleacetic acid (5-HIAA), and the serotonin transporter. Immunocytochemical studies suggest that serotonergic neurons are damaged, but the cell bodies are preserved. Recovery from MDMA-induced serotonergic damage can occur. In monkeys the damage persists at least 7 years. In humans, serotonergic damage after repeated MDMA use is evident through several different types of studies. CSF 5-HIAA levels are reduced in MDMA users, an effect that is more pronounced in women than in men.

Diagnosis

A typical MDMA user is a college student. In a survey of 14 000 college students in 119 American colleges, MDMA users were more likely to use marijuana, smoke cigarettes and engage in binge alcohol consumption (Strote *et al.*, 2002). They were also more likely to have multiple sex partners (Strote *et al.*, 2002). They considered art and parties important, but they were not academic underachievers.

Acute Positive Psychological Effects

Unlike many drugs of abuse which are frequently used alone, MDMA is almost always used in the company of others. Most MDMA users report positive mood and emotional effects as they relate to others. Experienced MDMA users report a greater capacity for empathy, communication and understanding. Users also report increased self-esteem, high energy, relaxation, sensual awareness, euphoria and dissociation.

Physical Consequences of MDMA Use

Humans exhibit complications that are related to both the sympathomimetic and serotonergic properties of MDMA. These include nausea, vomiting, anorexia, hypertension, palpitations, diaphoresis, headaches, difficulty walking, muscle aches and tension, hot and cold flashes, urinary urgency, nystagmus, blurred vision, insomnia and dry mouth. The common complaints of trismus and bruxism may reflect MDMA enhancement of serotonin activation of the $5HT_{1B}$ receptors of the trigeminal motor nuclei (Tancer and Johanson, 2001).

At least two MDMA-related deaths have been associated with automobiles (Hooft *et al.*, 1994; Cifasi and Long, 1996).

Clinical Manifestations of Long-term of MDMA Neurotoxicity

Former chronic ecstasy users (an average of 527 tablets) have higher self-reported depression. The predictors of developing this depressive syndrome are maximum quantity of pills consumed over a 12-hour period and mild, frequent life stress. Heavy MDMA use has also been associated with higher rates of psychopathology including obsessive and compulsive behaviors, anxiety, somatization and loss of libido. The relationship between MDMA use and these syndromes is unclear, but since these syndromes involve serotonergic mechanisms,

additional investigation into these potential long-term sequelae is warranted. MDMA users have been noted to have problems with memory, attention, reasoning, impulse control and sleep abnormalities.

MDMA Somatic Toxicity

MDMA has been associated with a wide range of somatic toxic events. These include thrombotic or hemorrhagic strokes, leukoencephalopathy, myocardial infarction, arrhythymias and pneumothorax. The wide range of manifestations suggests that most of these cases are either idiosyncratic or related to impurities remaining from the synthetic process. Since much of the MDMA supply is synthesized in small "basement" laboratories, the quality control of the manufacturing process may not be adequate. Cases of severe medical illness or death due to electrolyte and fluid are more likely due to MDMA use. These complications may be related to the specific environment in raves. In raves people are exposed to hot, crowded environments. In association with the increased body temperature caused by MDMA dehydration and its consequences are likely. MDMA may also cause serotonergic hyperstimulation and produce a fatal serotonin syndrome-like (illness).

Treatment

There have been no studies examining the treatment of MDMA use. The issue of how a practitioner may help his/her patient discontinue MDMA use is never addressed in the literature. This may be due to the rarity of presentation of subjects seeking treatment for MDMA addiction. Serotonin reuptake inhibiting antidepressants may offer a possible treatment for subjects who present with an MDMA addiction.

Comparison of DSM-IV/ICD-10

The ICD-10 and DSM-IV-TR criteria sets for Hallucinogen Intoxication are almost the same.

References

Abraham HD and Aldridge A (1993) Adverse consequences of lysergic acid diethylamide. *Addiction* 88, 1327–1334.

Aghajanian GK and Marek GJ (1999) Serotonin and hallucinogens. *Neuropsychopharmacology* 21, 18S–23S.

American Psychiatric Association (2000) *Diagnostic and Statistical Manual of Mental Disorders*, 4th edn., Text Rev. APA, Washington, DC.

Brown ER, Jarvie DR and Simpson D (1995) Use of drugs at 'raves.' *Scot Med J* 40, 168–171.

Christophersen AS (2000) Amphetamine designer drugs-an overview and epidemiology. *Toxicol Lett* 112 and 113, 127–131.

Cifasi J and Long C (1996) Traffic fatality related to the use of methylenedioxymethamphetamine. *J Forens Sci* 41, 1082–1084.

Cregg MT and Traqcey JA (1993) Ecstasy abuse in Ireland. *Irish Med J* 86, 118–120.

Cuomo MJ, Dyment PG and Gammino VM (1994) Increasing use of "ecstasy" (MDMA) and other hallucinogens on a college campus. *J Am Coll Health* 42, 272–274.

Downing J (1986) The psychological and physiological effects of MDMA on normal volunteers. *J Psychoact Drugs* 18, 335–340.

Forsyth AJ (1996) Places and patterns of drug use in the Scottish dance scene. *Addiction* 91, 511–521.

Gerhard H (2001) Party-drugs: Sociocultural and individual background and risks. *Int J Clin Pharmacol Ther* 39, 362–366.

Gervin M, Hughes R, Bamford L *et al.* (2001) Heroin smoking by "chasing the dragon" in young opiate users in Ireland: Stability and associations with use to "come down" of "Ecstasy." *J Subst Abuse Treat* 20, 297–300.

Greer G and Tolbert P (1986) Subjective reports of the effects of MDMA in a clinical setting. *J Psychoact Drugs* 18, 319–327.

Greer GR and Tolbert P (1998) A method of conducting therapeutic sessions with MDMA. *J Psychoact Drugs* 30, 371–379.

Hollister L (1984) Effects of hallucinogens in humans, in *Hallucinogens: Neurochemical, Behavioral, and Clinical Perspectives* (ed Jacobs B). Raven Press, New York.

Hooft PJ and Van der Voorde HP (1994) Reckless behavior related to the use of 3,4-methylenedioxymethamphetamine (ecstasy): Apropos of fatal accident during car surfing. *Int J Legal Med* 106, 328–329.

Johnston LD, O'Malley PM and Bachman JG (1999) *National Survey Results on Drug Use from the Monitoring the Future Study, 1975–1998, Vol. I, Secondary School Students.* US Department of Health and Human Services, NIH Publication No. 99-4660, Washington DC.

Liester MB, Grob CS, Bravo GL *et al.* (1992) Phenomenology and sequelae of 3,4-methylenedioxymethamphetamine use. *J Nerv Ment Dis* 180, 345–352.

McCann UD, Szabo Z, Scheffel U *et al.* (1998) Positron emission tomographic evidence of toxic effect of MDMA ("Ecstasy") on brain serotonin neurons in human beings. *Lancet* 352, 1433–1437.

Peroutka SJ, Newman H and Harris H (1988) Subjective effects of 3,4-methylenedioxymethamphetamine in recreational users. *Neuropsychopharmacology* 1, 273–277.

Pope HG Jr., Ionescu-Pioggia M and Pope KW (2001) Drug use and life style among college undergraduates: A 30-year longitudinal study. *Am J Psychiatr* 158, 1519–1521.

Randell T (1992) Rave scene, ecstasy use, leap Atlantic. *J Am Med Assoc* 268, 1506.

Reneman L, Endert E, de Bruin K *et al.* (2002) The acute and chronic effects of MDMA ("Ecstasy") on cortical 5-HT$_{2A}$ receptors in rat and human brain. *Neuropsychopharmacology* 26, 387–396.

Semple DM, Ebmeier KP, Glabus MF *et al.* (1999) Reduced *in vivo* binding to the serotonin transporter in the cerebral cortex of MDMA ("Ecstasy") users. *Br J Psychiatr* 175, 63–69.

Shulgin AT and Nichols DE (1978) Characterization of three new psychomimetics, in *The Psychopharmacology of Hallucinogens* (eds Stillman R and Willette R). Pergamon Press, New York, pp. 74–83.

Strote J, Lee JE and Wechsler H (2002) Increasing MDMA use among college students: Results of a national survey. *J Adolesc Health* 30, 64–72.

Tancer ME and Johanson CE (2001) The subjective effects of MDMA and mCPP in moderate MDMA users. *Drug Alcohol Depend* 65, 97–101.

Titeler M, Lyon RA and Glennon RA (1988) Radioligand binding evidence implicates the brain 5-HT$_2$ receptor as a site of action for LSD and phenylisopropylamine hallucinogens. *Psychopharmacology* 94, 213–216.

Topp L, Hando J, Dillon P *et al.* (1999) Ecstasy use in Australia: Patterns of use and associated harm. *Drug Alcohol Depend* 55, 105–115.

Vardy MM and Kay SR (1983) LSD psychosis or LSD-induced schizophrenia? A multimethod inquiry. *Arch Gen Psychiatr* 40, 877–883.

Substance Abuse: Inhalant-related Disorders

This chapter reviews the disorders of deliberately inhaling large quantities of volatile solvents and gases for minutes to hours, most often repeatedly over days, months and frequently for many years. This is reffered to as inhalant disorders in DSM-IV. The most frequently chemicals now present in the products that are abused include toluene, butane, nitrous oxide, gasoline mixtures (including hexane and benzene), different chlorocarbons such as trichloroethylene, fluorocarbons and organic nitrites. Acute symptoms include: dizziness, headache, disorientation, ataxia foul breath, with conditions proceeding to nausea, slurred speech, belligerence, irritability and delirium. Chronic conditions are characterized by a strong psychological, but weaker physical dependence, without any known dually diagnosed mental disorder. Known associated physical disorders include cognitive dysfunction, limb dysmetria, hearing loss, arrhythmia, metabolic acidosis, peripheral neuropathies, hematologic abnormalities, significant embryopathic changes, and some liver and lung changes.

Several subcategories of inhalants can be established based on chemical classes of products and primary abuse groups as follows: 1) industrial or household cleaning and paint-type solvents including paint thinners or solvents, degreasers or dry cleaning solvents, solvents in glues, art or office supply solvents such as correction fluids, and solvents in magic markers (gasoline is similar to these products); 2) propellant gases used in household or commercial products, such as butane in lighters, or fluorocarbons in electronic (personal computer, office equipment) cleaners or refrigerant gases; 3) household aerosol sprays such as paint, hair and fabric protector sprays; 4) medical anesthetic gases such as ether, chloroform, halothane and nitrous oxide; and 5) aliphatic nitrites. Nitrous oxide is also available in whipped cream dispensers (e.g., whippets) and for octane boosters in car racing, and is used outside the medical theater by nonprofessionals. Most of the foregoing compounds affect the central nervous system (CNS) directly, whereas nitrites act on cardiovascular smooth muscle rather than as an anesthetic in the CNS. The nitrites are also used primarily as sexual enhancers rather than as mood alterants. Therefore, when discussing "inhalant abuse," we will be referring primarily to substances other than nitrites. One item worthy of note: the exclusion of anesthetics from the inhalant-related disorders section in the *Diagnostic and Statistical Manual of Mental Disorders*, Fourth Edition (DSM-IV-TR) is not medically correct, as almost all of the inhalants act physiologically as would any anesthetic and some, particularly the anesthetics nitrous oxide and trichloroethylene (TCE), are abused by the primary inhalant abuser discussed herein.

Many anesthetics have a potential for abuse, mostly by medical personnel. That these substances are abused by middle-class professionals not only demonstrates the diversity of the groups that abuse inhalants but also focuses on the basic nature of the physical properties of most of these volatile agents. That is, many anesthetics produce a light-headedness that relates to euphoria. Almost all solvents would produce anesthesia if sufficient amounts are inhaled with the proper amounts of oxygen present. As with any anesthetic, death is possible and too often occurs with these substances.

Inhalant Use Disorders

Inhalant Dependence

Dependence on inhalants is primarily psychological, with a less dramatic associated physical dependence occurring in some heavy users. There is at least a psychological dependence and often a weak physical dependence on these substances. A mild withdrawal syndrome occurs in 10 to 24 hours after cessation of use (only in those who have excessively abused inhalants) and lasts for several days. Symptoms include general disorientation, sleep disturbances, headaches, muscle spasms, irritability, nausea and fleeting illusions. However, this is not an easily identified or a characteristic withdrawal syndrome that is useful for many practitioners in a clinical setting. The need to continue use is undeniably strong in many individuals; specific treatments for inhalant dependence, other than the drug therapy and/or psychotherapy used for other drug dependence, need to be developed.

Inhalant Abuse

Abuse of inhalants may lead to harm to individuals (e.g., accidents involving automobiles, falling from buildings when in an impaired or intoxicated state [illusionary feelings], or self-inflicted harm such as attempted or successful suicide). Frozen lips caused by rapidly expanding gases or serious burns may also occur. Chronic inhalant use is often associated with familial conflict and school problems.

Inhalant-induced Disorders

The primary disorder is inhalant intoxication, which is characterized by the presence of clinically significant maladaptive behavioral or psychological changes (e.g., belligerence, assaultiveness, apathy, impaired judgment, impaired social or occupational functioning) that develop during the intentional

Essentials of Psychiatry   Jerald Kay and Allan Tasman
© 2006 John Wiley & Sons, Ltd.

hort-term, high-dose exposure to volatile inhalants (diagnostic riteria A and B in DSM-IV-TR). The maladaptive changes oc- urring after intentional and nonintentional exposure include isinhibition, excitedness, light-headedness, visual distur- ances (blurred vision, nystagmus), incoordination, dysarthria, n unsteady gait and euphoria. Higher doses of inhalants may ead to depressed reflexes, stupor, coma and death, sometimes aused by cardiac arrhythmia. Lethargy, generalized muscle veakness, and headaches may occur some hours later depend- ng on the dose.

Epidemiology

Prevalence

nhalant abuse is a worldwide problem. Countries are increas- ngly evaluating the abuse of solvents.

Current estimates of sniffing volatile substances to "get igh" rank inhalants high in the "ever use" category of substance buse, especially for the younger population. Some surveys of eenage use showed that one in six had tried an inhalant and that ver 220000 persons of the US population had done so in the ast month during the year 2000 (Substance Abuse and Mental Iealth Services Administration, 2001). As many as 20000 to 0000 youth got high on inhalants several times a month. Some

---

DSM-IV-TR Criteria 292.89

Inhalant Intoxication

A. Recent intentional use or short-term, high-dose exposure to volatile inhalants (excluding anesthetic gases and short-acting vasodilators).

B. Clinically significant maladaptive behavioral or psychological changes (e.g., belligerence, assaultiveness, apathy, impaired judgment, impaired social or occupational functioning) that developed during, or shortly after, use of or exposure to volatile inhalants.

C. Two (or more) of the following signs developing during, or shortly after, inhalant use or exposure:
  (1) dizziness
  (2) nystagmus
  (3) incoordination
  (4) slurred speech
  (5) unsteady gait
  (6) lethargy
  (7) depressed reflexes
  (8) psychomotor retardation
  (9) tremor
  (10) generalized muscle weakness
  (11) blurred vision or diplopia
  (12) stupor or coma
  (13) euphoria

D. The symptoms are not due to a general medical condition and are not better accounted for by another mental disorder.

Reprinted with permission from the Diagnostic and Statistical Manual f Mental Disorders, Fourth Edition, Text Revision. Copyright 2000 american Psychiatric Association.

---

of the highest rates were noted for 8th graders. The practice of "sniffing", "snorting", "huffing", "bagging", or inhaling to get high describes various methods of inhalation. These terms refer to the inhalation of volatile substances from 1) filled balloons, 2) bags and 3) soaked rags and/or sprayed directly into oral orifices. Abusers can be identified by various telltale clues such as organic odors in the breath or clothes, stains on the clothes or around the mouth, empty spray paint or solvent containers, and other unusual paraphernalia. These clues may enable one to identify a serious problem of solvent abuse before it causes serious health problems or death.

Toxicology of Inhalant Abuse

The majority of inhalant abusers are never seen in a hospital or outpatient facility. Although many do not need medical attention for their inhalant habit, of those who do, many often die before reaching the hospital as a result of asphyxia, cardiac arrhythmia, or related overdose effects after inhaling fluorocarbons, low-mo- lecular-weight hydrocarbon gases (butane, propane), nitrous ox- ide, or other solvents including toluene during either the first or a subsequent episode. Death may also occur after inhalation of toluene-containing substances as a result of metabolic acidosis or related kidney failure if left untreated.

Clinical Manifestations After Chronic Inhalant Abuse

Chronic high-level exposure to organic solvents occurs in the in- halant abuse setting at levels several thousand times higher than in the occupational setting and results in numerous irreversible disease states. Table 41.1 describes several well-characterized disorders and identifies the solvent when corroborated by animal studies. Some substances have been strongly correlated with the development of a disorder through numerous case studies.

Treatment

Individuals need different treatments based on the severity of the dependence and any medical complications. Primary care physi- cians should address the medical issues identified earlier as well as other medical concerns before dealing with the dependence on solvents and other drugs. During this period, sedatives, neu- roleptics and other forms of pharmacotherapy are not useful in the treatment of inhalant abusers and should be avoided in most cases as they are likely to exacerbate the depressed state. Once it is determined that the individual is detoxified, that is, has low levels of solvent or other depressant drug, then therapy with other drugs, such as antianxiety drugs, may be useful. The determina- tion of detoxification, even in the absence of drug (solvent) ad- ministration, is not well defined or systematic. It may take several days for the major "reversible" intoxication state to be reduced to a level at which coherent cognition can occur. The use of various psychological assessment tools can assist not only in evaluating the intoxication but also in following the progress of the treat- ment. Little can be done during this period other than to facili- tate improvement of the basic health of these individuals, provide supportive care and build the individual's self-esteem.

There is no accepted treatment approach for inhalant abuse. Many drug treatment facilities refuse treatment of the inhalant abuser because many feel that inhalant abusers are resistant to treatment) or that there is no standard or accepted treatment. One

Table 41.1   Diseases Observed in Humans After Chronic Inhalant Abuse

Conditiont	Syndrome	Substance	Animal Studies*
Slowly Reversible and/or Irreversible Syndromes			
Encephalopathy	Cognitive dysfunction	"Toluene,"† other solvents	—
Cerebellar syndrome	Limb dysmetria	"Toluene"	Rat
	Dysarthria		—
Sensorineural otic Sensorineural	High-frequency hearing loss	TCE, toluene	Rat, mouse
Optic nerve	Visual loss	"Toluene"	—
Oculomotor	Oculomotor disturbances (nystagmus)	Xylene, TCE	Rabbits
Myeloneuropathy	Sensory loss Spasticity	Nitrous oxide	Rat, mouse
Axonal neuropathy	Distal sensory loss, limb weakness	Hexane, methyl butyl ketone	Rat, monkey
Cardiotoxicity	Arrhythmia	Chlorofluorocarbons, butanes, propanes	Mouse, rat, dog
Leukemia	Myelocytic	Benzene	Rat, mouse
Mostly Reversible Syndromes			
Trigeminal neuropathy	Numbness, paresthesia	TCE and/or dichloroacetylene	Rat
Renal acidosis	Metabolic acidosis	"Toluene"	Rat
	Hypokalemia		—
Carboxyhemoglobin	Hypoxia	Methylene chloride, tobacco	Human, rat
Methemoglobinemia	Syncope, blue	Nitrites, organic	Rat
Neonatal syndrome	Retarded growth, development	"Toluene"	Rat
Hepatotoxicity	Fatty vacuoles, plasma liver enzymes	Chlorohydrocarbons	Rat
Immunomodulatory	Loss of immune cell function	Nitrites, organic	Rat

*Symptoms observed in animal studies with these solvents.
†Quotation marks around substance indicates uncertainty about this solvent (alone) producing these symptoms.

facility that focuses solely on the comprehensive treatment of inhalant abusers, the International Institute on Inhalant Abuse based in Colorado (www.allaboutinhalants.com), uses a three-phase model that allows longer periods of treatment.

The inhalant abuser typically does not respond to usual drug rehabilitation treatment modalities. Several factors may be involved, particularly for the chronic abuser who may have significant psychosocial problems as well as irreversible brain injury. Treatment becomes slower and progressively more difficult when the severity of brain injury worsens as abuse progresses through transient social use (experimenting in groups) to chronic use in isolation. For these and other reasons, longer therapies are necessary than are utilized in most drug treatment facilities. Also, neurological impairment, the breadth of which still needs to be established, may be a major complication slowing the progress of rehabilitation. This is not as significant a problem with other forms of drug abuse.

Drug screening would be useful in monitoring inhalant abusers. Routine urine screening for hippuric acid (the major metabolite of toluene metabolism) performed two or three times weekly can detect the high level of exposure to toluene commonly seen in inhalant abusers. More frequently performed expired breath analysis for toluene or other abused compounds is also available. As alcohol is a common secondary drug of abuse among inhalant abusers, alcohol abuse should be monitored and considered in the approach to treatment.

Comparison of DSM-IV/ICD-10 Diagnostic Criteria

The ICD-10 and DSM-IV-TR criteria sets for Inhalant Intoxication are nearly equivalent (except that DSM-IV-TR lists additional symptoms).

References

Substance Abuse and Mental Health Services Administration (2001) *National Household Survey on Drug Abuse: Population Estimates 2000.* US Government Printing Office, Washington DC.

Substance Abuse: Nicotine Dependence

Nicotine dependence is the most common substance use disorder in the USA and increases morbidity and mortality more than any other substance use disorders. In the USA about 25% of the population is addicted to tobacco. Tobacco use has serious health consequences for the user, family members and others who inhale secondhand environmental tobacco smoke or are exposed during pregnancy. Treatment can be effective. There are six FDA-approved medications for use in tobacco addiction treatment, including bupropion and five nicotine replacement medications (patch, gum, spray, inhaler and lozenge). Behavioral psychosocial therapies are also as effective as medications, however, treatment providers do not often this approach. Integrated medication and behavioral therapy is effective in helping smokers quit in about 45% of cases. About 44% of all cigarettes consumed in the USA are by individuals with mental illness or addiction, and specialized treatments can help this heavy smoker population. The diagnosis of Nicotine Dependence follows the DSM-IV TR criteria for substance dependence found on p. 476.

Definition

The DSM-IV nicotine withdrawal syndrome describes a characteristic set of symptoms that develops after abrupt cessation or a reduction in the use of nicotine products after at least several weeks of daily use and is accompanied by four of the following signs and symptoms: 1) dysphoria or depressed mood; 2) insomnia; 3) irritability, frustration, or anger; 4) anxiety; 5) difficulty concentrating; 6) restlessness or impatience; 7) decreased heart rate; and 8) increased appetite or weight gain (American Psychiatric Association, 1994). The withdrawal symptoms must also cause clinically significant distress or impairment in social, occupational, or other important areas of functioning and must not be secondary to a general medical condition or be accounted for by another mental disorder.

Other symptoms that may be associated with nicotine withdrawal include craving for nicotine, a factor thought to be significant in relapse; a desire for sweets; and impaired performance on tasks requiring vigilance. To some extent, the degree of physiological dependence predicts severity of the withdrawal syndrome and difficulty stopping smoking.

The prevalence of cigarette smoking is higher at lower socioeconomic levels. Slightly more males than females smoke, although more males than females are successful in stopping smoking. There is evidence that the number of cigarettes per smoker is increasing, leaving a more hard-core and potentially more dependent group of smokers. There has also been a recent increase in the rate of smoking among adolescents, particularly in the number of teenage girls smoking. This increased smoking rate amongst adolescents is particularly alarming, as smokers typically start smoking at an early age, with more than 60% of smokers beginning by age 14 years and nearly all by age 18 years.

Cooccurring Psychiatric or Substance Use Disorders

Nicotine dependence and smoking are two to three times more common in individuals with psychiatric and other substance use disorders than in the general population. Smoking-related illnesses are the primary cause of death among those in recovery from other substances. It is estimated that 55 to 90% of individuals with psychiatric disorders smoke versus the 23% of the general population. The prevalence of smoking is especially high in patients with schizophrenia (70–90%), affective disorders (42–70%) and alcohol dependence (60–90%) or other substance use disorders (70–95%).

There is no simple reason why so many psychiatric patients smoke.

Etiology and Pathophysiology

Nicotine dependence has been called a "pediatric disease" since most smokers started during adolescence. By the age of 18, 90% of those who will ever try a cigarette have done so, and age 18 years is the average age at which individuals become daily smokers. As with other substance use disorders, the etiology of nicotine dependence is multifactorial and includes biological, psychological and social factors, including genetic factors.

Nicotine is the primary psychoactive agent in tobacco smoke and smokeless tobacco and has powerful addictive properties. As an indication of the addictive potential of this substance, one-third to one half of all children and adolescents who smoke one cigarette progress to become habitual users. Nicotine is considered to be the "gateway drug" to the use of other substances.

Nicotine has a multitude of effects. Some are acute, while others appear only after chronic usage. It acts in two primary areas of the brain: the mesolimbic dopaminergic system (the brain reward pathway), which is related to the euphoriant effects of the drug, and the locus coeruleus, which mediates stress reactions and vigilance and relates to the higher mental and cognitive functions. There are specific nicotine receptor sites (the nicotinic cholinergic receptors) throughout the central nervous system in

Essentials of Psychiatry   Jerald Kay and Allan Tasman
© 2006 John Wiley & Sons, Ltd.

the hypothalamus, hippocampus, thalamus, midbrain, brain stem and cerebral cortex. In addition, nicotine affects nearly all aspects of the endocrine–neuroendocrine system, including the catecholamine, serotonin, corticosteroid and pituitary hormones. Its endocrine effects are mediated via the hypothalamic–pituitary axis and the adrenal medullary cortex. Centrally it causes release of acetylcholine, norepinephrine, serotonin, dopamine, vasopressin, growth hormone, corticotropin, cortisol, prolactin and endorphins.

Nicotine has stimulant and depressive effects on both the central and the peripheral nervous systems. It also affects the cardiovascular system, the gastrointestinal system and the skeletal motor system. Nicotine stimulates the cholinergic nervous system (sympathetic and parasympathetic). Through this variety of central and peripheral actions, nicotine improves mood and decreases anxiety; decreases distress in response to stressful stimuli and decreases aggression; improves overall cognitive function and performance (improves reaction time, concentration, vigilance and stimulus-processing capacity, increases attention, memory and learning, improves the ability to disregard irrelevant stimuli); and decreases the appetite for simple carbohydrates, decreases stress-induced eating and increases resting metabolic rate. Many individuals soon become tolerant to these effects so that they smoke not to achieve them, but rather to avoid withdrawal symptoms.

Course and Natural History

The National Health Interview Survey found that 70% of smokers interviewed reported they wanted to quit smoking at some point in their lifetime, and about 33% of smokers try to quit each year. Only about 3% of quit attempts without formal treatment are successful, and in recent years about 30% of smokers who want to quit are seeking treatment. Outcomes for nicotine dependence treatment vary by the type of treatment and the intensity of treatment with specific reports ranging from about 15 to 45% 1-year abstinence rates following treatment. Cessation attempts result in high relapse rates, with the relapse curve for smoking cessation paralleling that for opiates. Most individuals relapse during the first 3 days of withdrawal and most others will relapse within the first 3 months. Withdrawal symptoms are most severe within the first 1 to 3 days of abstinence, often continue for 3 to 4 weeks, and in some persons last for up to 6 months or longer. Current depressive symptoms and a history of depression are predictors of relapse. Weight gain may also contribute to relapse, particularly in women. In contrast, several factors have been found to predict worse outcomes at smoking cessation. Predictors include individual factors, manifestations of the addiction such as severity of withdrawal, and social and environmental circumstances.

Nicotine dependence, like other substance use disorders, can be thought of as a chronic relapsing illness with a course of intermittent episodes alternating with periods of remission for most smokers. About 65% of those who stop smoking relapse in 3 months and another 10% relapse in 3 to 6 months, and with treatment the overall relapse rate is still about 75 to 80% by 1 year. However, these reported lower outcome rates do not consider the additive effects over time related to multiple quit attempts, since about 40 to 50% of smokers in the USA have been able to quit smoking in their lifetime. Less than 25% of the individuals who have quit smoking are successful on their first attempt. Repeated failures are common before successful abstinence, with the average smoker attempting to quit five or six times before success.

Table 42.1	Assessing Nicotine Use and Nicotine Dependence

Current and past patterns of tobacco use (include multiple sources of nicotine)
Current motivation to quit
Objective measures: breath co level or cotinine level (saliva, blood, urine)
Assess prior quit attempts (number and what happened in each attempt)
Why quit? How long abstinent? Why relapsed?
What treatment was used (how used and for how long)
Assess withdrawal symptoms and dependence criteria
Psychiatric and other substance use history
Medical conditions
Their common triggers (car, people, moods, home, phone calls, meals, etc.)
Perceived barriers against and supports for treatment success
Preference for treatment strategy

Recent prior attempts at quitting do increase the odds that individuals will be able to quit smoking on a future attempt. Relapse can occur even after a long time of abstinence, with about 33% of former smokers who are abstinent for 1 year eventually relapsing 5 to 10 years after cessation.

Evaluation and Assessment

Before formal intervention is undertaken, it is beneficial and important to perform a comprehensive evaluation to determine the biological, psychological and social factors that are most significant in the initiation and maintenance of nicotine use and dependence. Comprehensive evaluation of the patient is outlined in Table 42.1.

Assessment of the psychiatric history is also important. Numerous studies have shown the significance of current and past depression in relation to smoking, as well as the increased prevalence rates of cigarette smoking in patients with a variety of psychiatric disorders, such as MDD, schizophrenia, and alcohol and substance abuse (see section on comorbidity). The presence of these comorbid disorders may also make successful smoking cessation less likely (see section on special features influencing treatment), especially if undiagnosed and untreated.

Assessing the patient for a history of current alcohol or other substance abuse is also important, as the prevalence of smoking in persons with alcohol dependence as well as in other substance abusers is much higher than in the general population. A careful medical history should also be obtained. The presence of significant tobacco-related medical illness can sometimes serve as crucial leverage to help motivate the individual to attempt cessation. Current medications and medical conditions may also be important considerations in determining the approach to cessation, especially with regard to pharmacotherapy. For example, a history of seizures or an eating disorder is usually a contraindication to the use of bupropion/Zyban (nonnicotine pill medication). The individual should be assessed for pulmonary symptoms and signs (cough), and if there is a long history of significant nicotine use, pulmonary function tests should be considered. The presence of significant cardiovascular disease, especially a history of recent myocardial infarction, is especially relevant to planning psychopharmacological interventions. If the individual is already taking a psychiatric medication, consider it important to realize that quitting smoking may result in an increase in medication blood levels and side effects.

Overall Approach to Treatment

Nicotine dependence treatment targets severity of the problem, co-occurring disorders and the different motivational levels to change. Treatment is provided in a range of levels of intensity of care (self-help, brief treatment and once or twice per week out-patient treatment) and may include different modalities (self-help guides, internet resources, medications and individual or group therapy). Formal treatment options have expanded rapidly in the past 25 years to include six FDA-approved medications, a range of effective psychosocial interventions including internet and phone-line services. Unfortunately, most insurance plans do not cover nicotine dependence treatment, and only some prescription plans will cover the medications. Few individuals receive combined medications and therapy treatment. Most receiving treatment get medication treatments, and only about 3% of the individuals receiving medication treatments will also receive psychosocial treatment despite the fact that this combination improves outcomes by 50%. Primary care treatment providers tend to offer brief counseling treatment services with follow-up visits. In addition, many individuals receive minimal formal treatment and either purchase over-the-counter nicotine replacement patch or gum, or go to Nicotine Anonymous or other self-help groups in attempting to quit on their own.

Phases of Treatment

The general approach to the treatment of nicotine dependence considers three phases of treatment (engagement, quitting, and relapse prevention) (Table 42.2).

The importance of each of the biopsychosocial factors in initiating and maintaining smoking can vary considerably in different individuals. As a result, smoking cessation interventions should be tailored to the individual and his or her particular circumstances. This may be one reason why "one size fits all" generic treatment interventions have had such a low success rate. It must also be kept in mind that nicotine dependence is as complex in its components and determinants as other addictions and that more comprehensive multicomponent treatments may be required. When a smoker is ready for a cessation attempt, a "quit date" should be selected. After cessation, close monitoring should occur during the early period of abstinence. Before the quit date, the person should be encouraged to explore and organize social support for the self-attempt. Plans to minimize cues associated with smoking (e.g., avoiding circumstances likely to contribute to relapse) are important, as is considering alternative coping behaviors for situations with a higher potential for relapse. A telephone or face-to-face follow-up during the first few days after cessation is critical because this is the time that withdrawal symptoms are most severe, with 65% of patients relapsing by 1 week. A follow-up face-to-face meeting within 1 to 2 weeks allows a discussion of problems that have occurred (e.g., difficulties managing craving) and serves as an opportunity to provide reinforcement for ongoing abstinence. Even after the early period of abstinence, periodic telephone or face-to-face contacts can provide continued encouragement to maintain abstinence, allow problems with maintaining abstinence to be addressed, and provide feedback regarding the health benefits of abstinence.

If an initial attempt at cessation using only information and brief advice from the physician has been unsuccessful, pharmacotherapy may be used unless contraindications are present or unless the person has had few or no significant withdrawal symptoms. The most common pharmacotherapy approaches are nicotine replacement therapies (NRTs: patch, gum, spray, or inhaler) or bupropion for nicotine dependence. Combining different types of NRT and bupropion is becoming more common in clinical practice, including using these medications for at least several months and in some cases 1 year or longer. Maintenance medications are being considered in an effort of harm reduction in a more select group of patients. If a detoxification/quit attempt with pharmacotherapy alone fails, psychosocial treatments and the use of higher NRT dosages/multiple medications are possible clinical next steps. Psychosocial treatments are often available through organizations such as the American Cancer Society, American Lung Association, the American Heart Association, or through local hospitals that provide health prevention and public education programs (American Cancer Society/National Cancer Institute, 1989). If pharmacotherapy is unacceptable or contraindicated, behavioral therapy (BT) alone should be provided. Failure with pharmacotherapy or BT alone suggests the need for more detailed in-depth assessment and more intensive and multimodal interventions.

Self-help

Many smokers have successfully quit smoking without participating in formal treatment and the success rate improves with multiple attempts and probable self-learning through trial and error and learning from others. Eventually about 50% of smokers are able to quit and more than 90% of successful quitters have been able to do so without the assistance of professionals or formal programs. These numbers reflect multiple factors including the limitations on access to treatment (nonexistent health insurance coverage and limited number of providers with expertise to help), the cumulative process of multiple attempts and learning from others and from self-help materials, and the severity of the nicotine dependence. The advantage of quitting without professional intervention is the decreased expense and time commitment; however, professional treatment may be necessary for higher severity cases that are often complicated by other behavioral health problems. The primary unassisted method of detoxification from nicotine dependence is precipitous cessation (cold turkey), which is used by more than 80% of smokers. This is followed by spontaneous strategies to handle cravings and triggers. Some smokers attempt to limit intake, taper the number of cigarettes smoked, or switch to a reduced tar or nicotine brand. Special filters and holders are also available to decrease the amount of smoke that is available from a cigarette. These methods are usually less successful because smokers have been shown to alter smoking behavior by increasing the frequency, volume, or duration of the inhalation to ensure maintenance of blood levels of nicotine adequate to prevent withdrawal symptoms. Some smokers use nonprescription pills that are analogues of nicotine, such as lobeline, to help manage or prevent withdrawal symptoms. These agents have not been shown to be effective in controlled studies.

Some geographical areas have Nicotine Anonymous groups that are structured similarly to Alcoholics Anonymous or Narcotics Anonymous groups. These groups are based on the 12-Step approach to recovery from addictions. Nicotine Anonymous is a relatively new organization (founded in 1985)

Table 42.2   Three Phases of Nicotine Dependence Treatment

Engagement Phase
- Do a comprehensive evaluation of nicotine use and dependence
- Provide MET personalized feedback from the assessment
- Assess motivational level to quit and attempt to set a target quit date
- Explore previous quit attempts – what worked? What did not work? What triggered the return to tobacco use?
- Assess patient preference for treatment (medications, psychosocial treatments, group vs. individual, self-help, etc.) and provide education on treatment
- Create a treatment plan
- Strengthen and renew patient's motivation to quit smoking (MET orientation)
- Identify cues and triggers for usage
- Self-monitoring of smoking behavior (write down when use)
- Help patients gain understanding of their own tobacco use patterns
- Help increase knowledge about triggers and cues
- Help patients understand environmental influences on their smoking
- Begin education about nicotine, tobacco addiction, withdrawal symptoms, etc.
- Begin disconnecting smoking behavior and linked behaviors (no smoking while driving car, talking on phone, during meal time, etc.)
- Help them get medication evaluation and medications for the quitting phase

Quitting Phase
- Start medications on quit date (NRT) or before quit date (bupropion), sometimes begin NRT (gum, spray, inhaler, not patch) in small amounts and reduce tobacco usage in an equivalent or greater amount
- Teach specific coping techniques for handling withdrawal symptoms, cues/triggers and how to enhance social support
- Help patient prepare emotionally, behaviorally and physically for the quit date and the early abstinence period
- Help identify support systems, anticipate challenges and address ways to handle people, places, things, and mood challenges
- Address nutrition and exercise components
- Address role of family/friends in supporting or sabotaging treatment
- Continue to strengthen client's resolve to quit
- Continue relapse prevention therapy approaches
- Assess triggers to craving and use and high-risk situations
- Coping with cravings, thoughts and urges
- Problem solving
- Smoke refusal skills
- Planning for emergencies
- Seemingly irrelevant decisions
- Relapse analysis for slips

Relapse Prevention Phase
- Continue relapse prevention strategies for long-term abstinence
- Reinforce specific coping skills, including mood management and patient specific triggers
- Teach positive coping skills for dealing with frustration and anxiety
- Compliment success and provide encouragement
- Continue focus on maintaining motivation and commitment for abstinence
- Monitor progress
- Provide treatment within your discipline and make referrals when appropriate
- Encourage the use of peer support such as Nicotine Anonymous help the client gain personal insight and keep growing in their recovery
- Manage any relapses/slips to continue the course
- Continue medications as needed

and does not have the extensive network that other 12-Step programs like Alcoholics Anonymous or Narcotics Anonymous have developed. No formal controlled studies of the benefits of this intervention have been carried out. In addition, self-help written materials can play an important role in educating patients about the negative health effects of nicotine, the benefits of quitting and the nature of the addiction. Self-help literature, internet resources and Nicotine Anonymous can be effectively integrated into formal treatments of brief interventions, individual and group treatments. Even smokers with major health conditions, such as chronic obstructive pulmonary disease or cardiovascular disease, often have a difficult time attaining and maintaining abstinence. Numerous psychological and pharmacological treatments have been developed to assist with smoking cessation.

Even a brief face-to-face intervention by a physician or other medical staff can increase the likelihood of cessation two- to tenfold (Klesges *et al.*, 1990). The impact of physician's brief advice to quit has received the most study relative to other disciplines such as nursing; however, clearly all disciplines have an opportunity to make an impact. Physicians can inquire about a patient's smoking status, urge the patient to stop smoking, and spend a brief time counseling the patient about cessation strategies. Multiple follow-up interventions, even telephone contacts by other medical staff, can further improve the cessation rate. Resources are available to assist physicians in providing effective antismoking interventions, which can even be used by those not highly skilled in counseling. Physicians' advice appears to be most successful with patients with a serious medical problem or specific medical reason for quitting (e.g., pregnancy or congestive heart disease). In addition, because an estimated 70% of smokers in the USA visit their physicians at least once a year, an important opportunity exists for providing this type of smoking cessation intervention.

Specific Medication and Psychosocial Treatment Interventions

It should be noted that even brief face-to-face intervention by a physician or other medical staff increase the likelihood of cessation two- to tenfold. There are now numerous effective psychosocial and pharmacological approaches that can be used in nicotine dependence treatment. Psychosocial intervention alone, pharmacotherapy alone, or combined approaches may be used. Given patients' preferences and current concerns with cost-effectiveness, less costly single-modality interventions are often used initially, whereas more costly multimodal interventions are often reserved for persons for whom cessation attempts have failed. This may not be the wisest strategy, but it is the most common.

Pharmacological interventions have become an important component of treating nicotine dependence. Approaches used parallel other addictions in treating acute withdrawal (detoxification), protracted withdrawal and even maintenance for harm reduction. The primary medications are NRT and bupropion. All six of these modalities are FDA approved and have demonstrated efficacy.

Nicotine replacement therapy (NRT) is the most widely used medication option and is available over-the-counter (patch and gum) or by prescription (patch, gum, spray and inhaler). The principle behind nicotine replacement is that nicotine is the dependence producing constituent of cigarette smoking, and that smoking cessation and abstinence can be achieved by replacing nicotine without the harmful impurities in cigarette smoke. The abuse liability of nicotine replacement appears to be minimal. The substituted nicotine initially prevents significant withdrawal symptoms that may lead to relapse during the early period of smoking cessation. The substituted nicotine is then gradually tapered and discontinued.

Nicotine gum was the first NRT approved and it slowly releases nicotine from an ion exchange resin when chewed. The nicotine released is absorbed through the buccal mucous membranes. The NRT gum is available in doses of 2 and 4 mg, and the recommended dosing is in the range of nine to 16 pieces per day. Nicotine gum is more effective when used in conjunction with some type of psychosocial intervention, particularly BT. Outcome is more positive when a definite schedule for gum use is prescribed – for example, one piece of gum per hour while awake – than when used on an as-needed basis. (Tapering may be necessary after 4 to 6 months of use, especially for individuals using higher total daily doses of gum. Nicotine gum is often not effectively utilized in patients with temporomandibular joint problems, dental problems and dentures. Nicotine gum requires

a highly motivated patient and a good deal of time in instructing the patient in proper use of the gum. Many individuals find the gum difficult to learn to use properly. Patients must be instructed that nicotine gum is not like bubble gum and that the gum is crunched a few times and "parked" between the gum and cheek. It should not be used soon after drinking acidic substances such as coffee, soda, or orange juice because the acidic environment in the mouth interferes with its release and absorption.

The *nicotine patch* transdermal delivery system provides continual sustained release of nicotine, which is absorbed through the skin. This form of nicotine replacement more than doubles the 1-year cessation rate (Hughes, 1994). There is a dose–response relationship, with patients receiving higher doses attaining higher cessation rates. The nicotine patch eliminates the conditioning of repeated nicotine use, which remains present with the use of other NRT products. Compliance rates are higher because it involves once-daily dosing and its administration is simple and discreet. The typical starting dose of NRT patch is 21 or 15 mg patch, however, in some cases multiple patches are used. Lower dose patches available at 7 and 14 mg are used to taper after smoking cessation. The patch delivers approximately 0.9 mg of nicotine/hour. Steady-state nicotine levels are 13 to 25 ng/mL and the highest levels are seen soon after patch application. The nicotine patch is often used for a total of 6 to 12 weeks but can be used for much longer (American Psychiatric Association, 1996). The transdermal patch does not allow for self-titrated dosing, craving and nicotine withdrawal symptoms like the other NRT routes (gum, spray, inhaler); however, the nicotine blood levels are significantly less than with smoking. The patch can be used more discreetly and can be used despite dental or temporomandibular joint problems.

Although the nicotine patch is well tolerated, about 25% of patients have significant local skin irritation or erythema and 10% discontinue the patch because of intolerable side effects. Other side effects include sleep problems with the 24-hour patches.

Some experts suggest using nicotine gum concurrently with transdermal nicotine on an as-needed basis to cover emergent withdrawal symptoms or craving not controlled by replacement from the transdermal patch, whereas others suggest simply increasing the dose of the transdermal patch or using gum initially and then switching to the patch (Gourley, 1994; Fagerstrom et al., 1993). Combining transdermal nicotine and nicotine gum increases the potential for significant side effects.

The **nicotine nasal spray** is rapidly absorbed and produces a higher nicotine blood level than does transdermal nicotine or gum. A single dose of the spray delivers 0.5 mg to each nostril and it can be used one to three times/hour. It has been suggested that the effective daily dose in nicotine dependent smokers is 15 to 20 sprays (8–10 mg).

The **nicotine inhaler** provides nicotine through a cartridge that must be "puffed". It mimics the upper airway stimulation experienced with smoking; however, absorption is primarily through the oropharyngeal mucosa. Although the blood level of nicotine is lower than with other forms of nicotine replacement (8–10 ng/mL), the inhaler has been shown to be effective. Side effects of the inhaler and spray include local irritation, cough, headache, nausea, dyspepsia, the need for multiple dosing and the impossibility of discreet use.

Bupropion, the non-nicotine pill FDA-approved medication option, is a heterocyclic, atypical antidepressant that blocks the re-uptake of both dopamine and norepinephrine. Its efficacy as an aid to smoking cessation was first demonstrated in three double-blind placebo-controlled trials. Smoking cessation rates appear to improve further when bupropion is combined with the nicotine patch (Nides, 1997).

Combined NRTs/bupropion or serial pharmacotherapeutic approaches may also be beneficial, especially in more difficult to treat cases of nicotine dependence. For example, combining the patch with other nicotine replacement medications like nicotine gum or the spray allows for both more rapid onset of action and reduction of withdrawal symptoms through steady levels of nicotine released by the patch. Combining nicotine replacement with non-nicotine replacement strategies (e.g., bupropion and nicotine patch) has been beneficial in further improving outcomes in some

---

Clinical Vignette 1

A 50-year-old divorced woman, Ms D, had been smoking about 30 cigarettes per day for more than 30 years. She reported only one prior attempt to quit, which resulted in significant depressive symptoms that resolved after she returned to smoking. However, the symptoms had been so disabling that she never again seriously considered another quit attempt. She reported a period of significant depressive symptoms of several months' duration after her divorce 2 years previously, with some lingering symptoms that met the criteria for dysthymic disorder. She had not previously received treatment for her depressive symptoms. She lived alone and had limited social support. With regard to her dysthymia, she complained of low energy, excessive sleeping and poor concentration. Treatment for both the depression and nicotine dependence were reviewed. Ms D was interested to try the bupropion since it may help her with both her mood and the nicotine dependence. The plan was to first stabilize her depression and then select a quit date. She started bupropion SR 150 mg in the morning and after 7 days increased the dosage to 300 mg (second dose at about 5 PM). After approximately 1 month there was substantial improvement in her depressive symptoms. During this time she had been provided with educational materials about nicotine dependence, tobacco and nicotine dependence treatment. She was willing to begin an 8-week behaviorally-oriented group for smoking cessation at the local community hospital clinic. She selected a quit date that would coincide with the projected quit date within the group treatment, and she desired to have an NRT option available in case she continued to have intensive cravings even while on the bupropion and participating in the group treatment. She was prescribed nicotine gum 4 mg and instructed in its use. She reported having persistent cravings on the quit day and began taking about 6 to 10 pieces of the 4 mg dose per day. She successfully completed the Nicotine Dependence Treatment Group and continued both nicotine gum and the bupropion for the next 4 months with monthly monitoring. At that time, she gradually tapered and discontinued the nicotine gum during a period of 2 months. She continued her antidepressant medication, bupropion SR, with monthly monitoring for the next 3 months. At that time, she was free of depressive symptoms, had become more socially active and had remained abstinent from cigarettes. The antidepressant was discontinued after 9 months, and she remained free of depression and abstinent from nicotine 2 years later.

---

studies and is common in clinical practice. The combination approach offers the advantage of multiple neurobiological mechanisms of action.

Psychosocial Treatments

In contrast with the treatment of other substance use disorders, psychosocial treatment is underutilized and has not evolved to be the cornerstone of treatment. This limited utilization of psychosocial treatments does not match the very positive outcomes from either psychosocial treatments alone (25% 1-year abstinence with BT) or when combined with NRT or bupropion (50% improvement compared with NRT or bupropion alone), however, it does match the lack of health care coverage for this service.

As in treating other substance use disorders, the core psychotherapy approaches are motivational enhancement therapy (MET), cognitive–behavioral therapy (CBT) (relapse prevention), and 12-Step facilitation. Psychosocial interventions, particularly BT, have been shown to increase abstinence rates significantly. However, only 7% of smokers attempting to quit smoking are willing to participate in BT (Ferry et al., 1992). In addition, it is more expensive than pharmacotherapy and more labor-intensive.

Combined Psychosocial and Psychopharmacological Therapies

All nicotine dependence treatment practice guidelines recommend the integration of nicotine dependence treatment medications (NRT and bupropion) with behavioral and supportive psychosocial treatment approaches. Empirical evidence supports the finding that medications double the quit rate compared with placebo, and face-to-face BT can double the quit rate compared with minimal psychosocial intervention. BT also can increase medication compliance. Integrated treatment further increases the quit rate by another 50% and triples the outcome rate compared with a control group (Fiore et al., 1990).

Comparison of DSM-IV/ICD-10 Diagnostic Criteria

The DSM-IV-TR and ICD-10 symptom lists for nicotine withdrawal include some different items: the ICD-10 list has craving, malaise, increased cough and mouth ulceration and does not include the DSM-IV-TR decreased heart rate item.

References

American Cancer Society/National Cancer Institute (1989) *Quit for Good: A Practitioners' Stop-Smoking Guide.* National Institutes of Health, Publication 89–1825, Bethesda, MD.

American Psychiatric Association (1994) *Diagnostic and Statistical Manual of Mental Disorders,* 4th edn. APA, Washington, DC.

American Psychiatric Association (1996) *Practice Guideline for the Treatment of Patients with Nicotine Dependence.* APA, Washington, DC.

Fagerstrom KO, Schneider NG and Lunell E (1993) Effectiveness of nicotine patch and nicotine gum in individual versus combined treatments for tobacco withdrawal symptoms. *Psychopharmacology (Berl)* 11, 271–277.

Ferry LH, Robbins AS, Scariati AM et al. (1992) Enhancement of smoking cessation using the antidepressant bupropion (abstract). *Circulation* 86(Suppl), 1–167.

Fiore MC, Novonty TE, Pierce JP *et al.* (1990) Methods used to quit smoking in the United States. Do cessation programs help? *JAMA* 263, 2760–2765.

Gourley S (1994) The pros and cons of transdermal nicotine therapy. *Med J Austral* 160, 152–159.

Hughes JR (1994) Pharmacotherapy of nicotine dependence, in *Pharmacological Aspects of Drug Dependence: Towards an Intergrative Neurobehavioral Approach. Handbook of Experimental Pharmacology* (eds Schuster CR, Sust SW, and Huhar MJ). Springer-Verlag, Forcheim, Germany.

Klesges RC, Klesges LM, Myers AW *et al.* (1990) The effects of phenylpropanolamine on dietary intake, physical activity, and body weight after smoking cessation. *Clin Pharmacol Ther* 47, 747–754.

Nides M (1997) Oral Presentation to the Society for Research on Nicotine and Tobacco (SRNT) (June 13). Nashville, TN.

43

CHAPTER

Substance Abuse: Opioid Use Disorders

Introduction

The term **opioids** describes a class of substances that act on opioid receptors. Numerous opioid receptors have been identified, but the physiologic and pharmacologic responses in man are best understood for the mu (μ) and kappa (κ) receptors. The μ receptor, for which morphine is a prototypical agonist, appears to be the one most closely related to opioid analgesic and euphorigenic effects. Opioids can be naturally-occuring substances such as morphine, semi-synthetics such as heroin, and synthetics with morphine-like effects such as meperidine. These drugs are prescribed as analgesics, anesthetics, antidiarrheal agents, or cough suppressants. In addition to morphine and heroin, the opioids include codeine, hydromorphone, methadone, oxycodone and fentanyl among others. Drugs such as buprenorphine, a partial agonist at the μ receptor, and pentazocine, an agonist-antagonist, are also included in this class because their physiologic and behavioral effects are mediated through opioid receptors (Table 43.1).

Opioids are the most effective medications for relief of severe pain and are widely used for that purpose. Their euphoric properties can also result in inappropriate use, abuse and dependence (i.e., "addiction"), which is why they have been placed under the Controlled Substances Act. The more potent opioids approved for medical use are under schedule II: examples are fentanyl, hydromorphone, methadone, morphine; others are under schedules III and IV.

Epidemiology of Opioid Abuse and Dependence

Heroin is the most commonly abused drug of this class. The 2000 National Household Survey obtained information on nonmedical use of analgesics and heroin separately. For heroin, the survey showed that 1.3% of the population had used in their lifetime; in the adolescent groups, 0.6% of 16- to 17-year-olds had used in their lifetime, but by age 18 to 20 the percentage was the same as in the adult population, 1.3%. When the data for nonmedical use of opioid pain relievers are examined, particularly in adolescent populations, the numbers are more alarming, with 12.4% of 16- to 17-year-olds having used these agents and 15.8% of 18- to 20-year-olds. It is unclear what proportion of the users met criteria for dependence or abuse since diagnoses were not part of the Household Survey (National Household Survey, 2000).

Heroin addiction has traditionally been associated with large urban areas, especially those in the northeast and mid-Atlantic states.

In spite of significant increases in resources that are committed to stop the supply, the purity, and availability of heroin for sale to addicts "on the street" have increased markedly during the last several years. This increase in purity and availability is probably a significant contributor to the increase that has recently occurred in opioid-related emergency room visits and applications for methadone treatment. There also appears to have been an increase in the abuse of prescription opioids, mainly in nonurban areas. Oxycodone and hydrocodone containing products have traditionally been the main prescription opioids of abuse. Attention has recently focused on oxycontin, a long-acting formulation of oxycodone that contains doses up to 80 mg/tablet. Though the slow absorption of this medication is unlikely to result in abuse when taken as prescribed, addicts have discovered that the tablets can be crushed, freeing much of the oxycodone which can then be inhaled or injected to produce a potent euphoria.

Etiology and Pathophysiology of Opioid-related Disorders

Opioid-related disorders are felt to arise from a variety of social, psychological and biological factors that interact to produce a "case". Among those identified as especially important are opioid use within the individual's immediate social environment and peer group; availability of opioids; a history of childhood conduct disorder or adult antisocial personality disorder; and a family history of one or more substance use disorders. The families of persons with opioid dependence are likely to have higher levels of psychopathology, especially an increased incidence of alcohol and drug use disorders, and antisocial personality. The exact mechanism or mix of factors that produce opioid dependence or abuse are unknown, as are the factors that contribute to the chronic relapsing pattern that is typically seen in many of these patients.

Clinical Picture of Opioid-related Disorders

Heroin is usually taken by injection, though it can be smoked, inhaled ("snorted"), or taken orally. Smoking and inhalation are commonly seen only when very pure heroin is available and is currently on the rise in the northeastern US; tar heroin is also commonly smoked in the Pacific Northwest. Hydromorphone (Dilaudid®), morphine and meperidine (Demerol®) are also usually injected though they can be taken orally; fentanyl is always injected. Codeine and other analgesics made for oral ingestion (such as Percodan® or Percocet®) are usually taken orally. All of these drugs can cause intoxication, withdrawal, dependence and abuse.

Essentials of Psychiatry Jerald Kay and Allan Tasman
© 2006 John Wiley & Sons, Ltd.

Table 43.1 Opioids*

Drug	Active Metabolite	Route of Administration	Relative Potency	Medical Use	Plasma Half-Life (Hours)	Duration of Action (Hours)
Morphine		IM	1	Analgesia	2	4–6
Heroin	Morphine	IM	1–2	None	0.5	3–5
Codeine		PO	0.05	Analgesia, antitussive	2–4	4–6
Fentanyl		IM	40–100	Analgesia	3–4	1–2
Hydromorphone		IM	13	Analgesia	2–3	4–6
Oxycodone		PO	0.5–1	Analgesia		4–6
Methadone		PO	0.50	Analgesia, opioid substitution	15–40	18–30
l-α-acetylmethadol (LAAM)		PO	0.40	Opioid substitution	14–104†	48–80
	Nor-LAAM				13–130†	
	Dinor-LAAM				97–430†	
Buprenorphine		SL	N/A (partial agonist)	Analgesia (opioid substitution, investigational)	6–12	4–6 (foranalgesia) 12–48‡

*IM, intramuscular; PO, by mouth; SL, sublingual; N/A, not applicable.
†At steady state.
‡Appears to be dose dependent.

Intoxication

Opioid intoxication is characterized by maladaptive and clinically significant behavioral changes developing within minutes to a few hours after opioid use (see DSM-IV-TR for substance intoxication on p. 410 on general approaches to substance abuse disorder. Symptoms include an initial euphoria sometimes followed by dysphoria or apathy. Psychomotor retardation or agitation, impaired judgment, and impaired social or occupational functioning are commonly seen. Intoxication is accompanied by pupillary constriction unless there has been a severe overdose with consequent anoxia and pupillary dilatation. Persons with intoxication are often drowsy (described as being "on the nod") or even obtunded, have slurred speech, impaired memory and demonstrate inattention to the environment to the point of ignoring potentially harmful events. Dryness of secretions in the mouth and nose, slowing of gastrointestinal activity and constipation are associated with both acute and chronic opioid use. Visual acuity may be impaired as a result of pupillary constriction. The magnitude of the behavioral and physiologic changes depends on the dose as well as individual characteristics of the user such as rate of absorption, chronicity of use and tolerance. Symptoms of opioid intoxication usually last for several hours, but are dependent on the half-life of the particular opioid that has been used. Severe intoxication following an opioid overdose can lead to coma, respiratory depression, pupillary dilatation, unconsciousness and death.

Withdrawal

Opioid withdrawal is a clinically significant, maladaptive behavioral and physiological syndrome associated with cessation or reduction of opioid use that has been heavy and prolonged (see DSM-IV-TR criteria for substance withdrawal from general approaches to substance abuse disorders p. 410. It can also be precipitated by administration of an opioid antagonist such as naloxone or naltrexone. Patients in opioid withdrawal typically demonstrate a pattern of signs and symptoms that are opposite the acute agonist effects. The first of these are subjective and consist of complaints of anxiety, restlessness and an "achy feeling" that is often located in the back and legs. These symptoms are accompanied by a wish to obtain opioids (sometimes called "craving") and drug-seeking behavior, along with irritability and increased sensitivity to pain. Additionally, patients typically demonstrate three or more of the following: dysphoric or depressed mood; nausea or vomiting; diarrhea; muscle aches; lacrimation or rhinorrhea; increased sweating; yawning; fever; insomnia; pupillary dilatation; fever; and piloerection. Piloerection and withdrawal-related fever are rarely seen in clinical settings (other than prison) as they are signs of advanced withdrawal in persons with a very significant degree of physiologic dependence; opioid-dependent persons with "habits" of that magnitude usually manage to obtain drugs before withdrawal becomes so faradvanced. For short acting drugs such as heroin, withdrawal symptoms occur within 6 to 24 hours after the last dose in most dependent persons, peak within 1 to 3 days and gradually subside over a period of 5 to 7 days. Symptoms may take 2 to 4 days to emerge in the case of longer acting drugs such as methadone or levo-alpha-acetylmethadol (LAAM). Less acute withdrawal symptoms are sometimes present and can last for weeks to months. These more persistent symptoms can include anxiety, dysphoria, anhedonia, insomnia and drug craving.

Dependence

Opioid dependence is diagnosed by the signs and symptoms associated with compulsive, prolonged self-administration of opioids which are used for no legitimate medical purpose, or if a medical condition exists that requires opioid treatment, are used in doses that greatly exceed the amount needed for pain relief. Persons with opioid dependence typically demonstrate continued use in spite of adverse physical, behavioral and psychological consequences. Almost all persons meeting criteria for opioid dependence have significant levels of tolerance and will experience withdrawal upon abrupt discontinuation of opioid drugs. Persons with opioid dependence tend to develop such regular patterns of compulsive use that daily activities are typically planned around obtaining and administering drugs.

Opioids are usually purchased on the illicit market, but they can also be obtained by forging prescriptions, faking or exaggerating medical problems, or by receiving simultaneous prescriptions from several physicians. Physicians and other health care professionals who are dependent will often obtain opioids by writing prescriptions or by diverting opioids that have been prescribed for their own patients.

Abuse

Opioid abuse is a maladaptive pattern of intermittent use in hazardous situations (driving under the influence, being intoxicated while using heavy machinery, working in dangerous places, etc.), or periodic use resulting in adverse social, legal, or interpersonal problems (see DSM-IV-TR criteria on p. 409). All of these signs and symptoms can also be seen in persons who are dependent; abuse is characterized by less regular use than dependence (i.e., compulsive use not present) and by the absence of significant tolerance or withdrawal. As with other substance use disorders, opioid abuse and dependence are hierarchical and thus persons diagnosed as having opioid abuse must never have met criteria for opioid dependence.

Assessment and Clinical Picture

Opioid use disorders can occur at any age, including adolescence and the geriatric years, but most affected persons are between 20 and 45 years. Neonates whose mothers are addicted can experience opioid withdrawal. Rarely, young children are affected with some cases of dependence having been reported in persons who are 8 to 10 years of age. Males are more commonly affected, with the male : female ratio typically being 3 or 4 to 1.

A nonjudgmental and supportive yet firm approach to these patients is especially important. They typically have engaged in antisocial or other forms of problematic behavior. They are often embarrassed or afraid to describe the extent of their behavior, and have extremely low self-esteem. At the same time, they are prone to be impulsive, manipulative and to act-out when frustrated. Communicating a feeling of nonjudgmental support in the context of setting limits, along with a clear and informed effort to provide appropriate help will encourage optimum therapeutic opportunities.

Physical Examination

Sclerosed veins ("tracks") and puncture marks on the lower portions of the upper extremities are common in intravenous users. When these veins become unusable or otherwise unavailable, persons will usually switch to veins in the legs, neck or groin. Veins sometimes become so badly sclerosed that peripheral edema develops. When intravenous access is no longer possible, persons will often inject directly into their subcutaneous tissue ("skin-popping") resulting in cellulitis abscesses, and circular-appearing scars from healed skin lesions. Tetanus is a relatively rare but extremely serious consequence of injecting into the subcutaneous tissues. Infections also occur in other organ systems, including bacterial endocarditis, hepatitis B and C, and HIV infection.

Persons who "snort" heroin or other opioids often develop irritation of the nasal mucosa. Difficulties in sexual function are common, as are a variety of sexually transmitted diseases. Males often experience premature ejaculation associated with opioid withdrawal, and impotence during intoxication or chronic use. Females commonly have disturbances of reproductive function and irregular menses.

Laboratory Findings

During dependence, routine urine toxicology tests are often positive for opioid drugs and remain positive for most opioids for 12 to 36 hours. Methadone and LAAM, because they are longer acting, can be identified for several days. Fentanyl is not detected by standard urine tests but can be identified by more specialized procedures. Oxycodone, hydrocodone and hydromorphone are often not routinely included on urine toxicology tests though they can be identified by gas chromatography/mass spectrometry. Testing for fentanyl is not necessary in most programs, but needs to be performed in assessing and treating health care professionals such as anesthesiologists who have access to this drug. Concomitant laboratory evidence of other abuseable substances such as cocaine, marijuana, alcohol, amphetamines and benzodiazepines is common.

Hepatitis screening tests are often positive, either for hepatitis B antigen (signifying active infection) or hepatitis B and/or C antibody (signifying past infection). Mild to moderate elevations of liver function tests are common, usually as a result of chronic infection with hepatitis C but also from toxic injury to the liver due to contaminants that have been mixed with injected opioids, or from heavy use of other hepatotoxic drugs such as alcohol. Low platelet count, anemia, or neutropenia, as well as positive HIV tests or low CD-4 cell counts are often signs of HIV infection. HIV is commonly acquired via the practice of sharing injection equipment, or by unprotected sexual activity that may be related to the substance use disorder, for example, exchanging sex for drugs or money to buy drugs.

Differential Diagnosis

Individuals who are dependent on "street" opioids are usually easy to diagnose due to the physical signs of intravenous use, drug-seeking behavior, reports from independent observers, the lack of medical justification for opioid use, urine test results, and the signs and symptoms of intoxication or withdrawal.

The signs and symptoms of opioid withdrawal are fairly specific, especially lacrimation and rhinorrhea, which are not associated with withdrawal from any other abuseable substances. Other psychoactive substances with sedative properties such as alcohol, hypnotics, or anxiolytics can cause a clinical picture that resembles opioid intoxication. A diagnosis can usually be made by the absence of pupillary constriction, or by the lack of response to a naloxone challenge. In some cases, intoxication is due to opioids along with alcohol or other sedatives. In these cases the naloxone challenge will not reverse all of the sedative drug effects.

Difficult diagnostic situations are seen among persons who fabricate or exaggerate the signs and symptoms of a painful illness (such as kidney stones, migraine headache, back pain, etc.). Because pain is subjective and difficult to measure, and because some of these individuals can be very skillful and deceptive, diagnosis can be difficult and time-consuming. Drugs that are obtained in such deceptions may be used by the individual in the service of his/her dependence or abuse, or may be sold on the illicit drug market for profit. These individuals cause problems not only for physicians, but also for patients with disorders that need opioids for pain relief.

Persons with opioid dependence will often present with psychiatric signs and symptoms such as depression or anxiety. Such subjective distress often serves to motivate the patient to seek treatment, and thus can be therapeutically useful. These symptoms can be the result of opioid intoxication or withdrawal, or they might result from the pharmacological effects of other substances that are also being abused such as cocaine, alcohol, or benzodiazepines. They may also represent independent, non-substance-induced psychiatric disorders that require long-term treatment. The correct attribution of psychiatric symptoms that are seen in the context of opioid dependence and abuse follows the principles that are outlined in the substance-related section and other relevant parts of DSM-IV-TR.

Course and Natural History of Opioid Dependence

Opioid dependence can begin at any age, but problems associated with opioid use are most commonly first observed in the late teens or early twenties. Once dependence occurs it is usually continuous over a period of many years even though periods of abstinence are frequent. Reoccurrence is common even after many years of forced abstinence, such as occurs during incarceration. Increasing age appears to be associated with a decrease in prevalence. This tendency for dependence to remit generally begins after age 40 and has been called "maturing out". However, many persons have remained opioid dependent for 50 years or longer. Thus, though spontaneous remission can and does occur, most cases of untreated opioid dependence follow a chronic, relapsing course for many years.

Treatment

There are currently a number of effective pharmacological and behavioral therapies for the treatment of opioid dependence, with these two approaches often combined to optimize outcome. There are also some newer treatment options, which may take various forms. For example, methadone maintenance is an established treatment, while the use of buprenorphine/naloxone in an office-based setting represents a new variation on that theme. Clonidine has been used extensively to treat opioid withdrawal while lofexidine is a structural analog that appears to have less hypotensive and sedating effects. The depot dosage form of naltrexone, currently under development, may increase compliance with a medication that has been an effective opioid antagonist but which has been underutilized due to poor acceptance by patients. In almost every treatment episode using pharmacotherapy, it is combined with some type of psychosocial or behavioral treatment. Recent research has documented the value of these additional treatments and provided insight into the ones that are the most effective.

Detoxification: Long-term, Short-term, Rapid and Ultra-rapid

Detoxification from opioids, for most patients, is only the first phase of a longer treatment process. Most patients seeking treatment have been addicted to heroin or other opioids for 2 to 3 years, and some for 30 years or more. Thus, treatment usually involves changes in individuals' lifestyles. Though generally ineffective in achieving sustained remission unless combined with long-term pharmacological, psychosocial, or behavioral therapies, detoxification alone continues to be widely used. It is sometimes the only option available for individuals who do not meet the Food and Drug Administration (FDA) criteria for, do not desire, or do not have access to agonist medications such as methadone or methadyl acetate (LAAM).

Pharmacologic detoxification is generally ineffective in achieving sustained remission unless combined with long-term pharmacologic, psychosocial, or behavioral therapies.

The detoxification process may include use of opioid agonists (e.g., methadone); partial agonists (e.g., buprenorphine); antagonists (e.g., naloxone, naltrexone); or nonopioid alternatives such as clonidine, benzodiazepines, or nonsteroidal anti-inflammatory agents. In many cases, one or more medications are combined, such as naloxone with clonidine and a benzodiazepine. The choice of detoxification medication and the duration of the process depend on numerous factors including patient preference, clinician expertise and experience, type of treatment facility, licensing and available resources. Ultimately, however, the goal of detoxification is the achievement (and maintenance) of a drug-free state while minimizing withdrawal. Unfortunately detoxification for some individuals appears to be used in a punitive manner or as an expedient means to achieve a drug-free state rapidly with no follow-up pharmacological or behavioral therapy.

Opioid detoxification paradigms are frequently categorized according to their duration: long-term (typically 180 days), short-term (up to 30 days), rapid (typically 3–10 days) and ultra-rapid (1–2 days). These temporal modifiers provide only a coarse description of the paradigm; they do not provide other important information such as the medications used or whether postdetoxification pharmacological, psychosocial, or behavioral therapy is provided. However, some general guidelines typically apply.

The most common detoxification protocols, and those for which the most data are available, are the long-term (typically 180 days) and short-term (up to 30 days) paradigms involving the use of methadone. Unfortunately, these strategies have not generally been associated with acceptable treatment response using relapse to opioid use as an outcome criterion. Results from more rapid detoxification evaluations using short- or even intermediate term (up to 70 days) medication-tapering protocols are even less encouraging and have an unfortunately low success rate. It should be noted, however, that provision of additional services such as counseling, behavioral therapy, treatment of underlying psychopathologies, job skills training and family therapy to address concomitant treatment needs can improve outcome though success rates remain low, even with these services.

Rapid detoxification involves the use of an opioid antagonist, typically naltrexone or naloxone, in combination with other medications (such as clonidine and benzodiazepines) to mitigate the precipitated withdrawal syndrome. The procedure is intended to expedite and compress withdrawal in order to minimize discomfort and decrease treatment time. Ultra-rapid detoxification also utilizes other medications, along with an opioid antagonist, to moderate withdrawal effects. However, rather than individuals being awake as they are during the rapid detoxification process, they are placed under general anesthesia or, alternatively, deeply sedated. A recently published study (Hensel and Kox, 2000) in which ultra-rapid detoxification was followed by naltrexone maintenance and supportive psychotherapy, indicated that 49 of

72 patients were opioid abstinent 12 months following detoxification. However this study and other studies involved self-selected individuals thus making it impossible to know the overall effectiveness of this type of intervention.

A major concern regarding ultra-rapid detoxification is the occurrence of potentially serious adverse effects, such as respiratory distress or other pulmonary and renal complications during or immediately following the procedure. A high frequency of vomiting has also been reported. The degree to which serious adverse events occur has not yet been determined. In spite of the emerging evidence about serious adverse events, ultra-rapid detoxification may be appropriate for highly selected individuals based on considerations of previous treatment history, economic factors and patient choice. However, patients seeking this treatment must be thoroughly informed that serious adverse events, including sudden unexpected deaths, have occurred in association with this procedure and its use should probably be limited to inpatient settings where monitoring by anesthesiologists and other highly trained staff is available.

Buprenorphine, a μ-opioid partial agonist, has also been used as a detoxification agent. Results from inpatient studies have shown that it is safe, well tolerated and mitigates opioid withdrawal signs and symptoms over a range of doses and detoxification schedules. Clonidine, an alpha-2-adrenergic agonist, has been shown to suppress many of the autonomic signs and symptoms of opioid withdrawal. It can cause sedation and hypotension but has been used with few problems when appropriate monitoring is available. It does not suppress the subjective discomfort of withdrawal and, probably for that reason, is not well accepted by most patients.

Other alpha-2-adrenergic agonists have also been evaluated in order to find agents that are as or more effective, but less sedating and hypotensive than clonidine. Lofexidine, a medication that was originally promoted as an antihypertensive but was shown to lack clinically significant hypotensive effects, has been the most studied. When compared with clonidine, it has been found equally to suppress autonomic signs and symptoms of opioid withdrawal but with less sedation and hypotension. When compared with methadone dose tapering, lofexidine detoxification was associated with opioid withdrawal effects that peaked sooner, but resolved to negligible levels more rapidly. Data regarding the potential effectiveness of guanabenz and guanfacine have also been reported, but further studies are required to assess the potential utility of these medications. In summary, recent studies have shown that lofexidine is likely to be a useful opioid detoxification agent whose efficacy approximates that of clonidine but with fewer side effects.

Opioid Agonist Pharmacotherapy

Methadone maintenance has become the most commonly used pharmacotherapy for opioid dependence. Methadone acts at the μ-opioid receptor and its ability to suppress opioid withdrawal for 24 to 36 hours following a single oral dose makes it an ideal medication for this purpose. Another μ-opioid agonist, LAAM, received FDA approval for maintenance treatment in 1993. LAAM is a long-acting congener of methadone that suppresses withdrawal for 48 to 72 hours and thus has the advantage of requiring less frequent clinic visits than methadone, which must be taken daily. A third medication, buprenorphine, has received FDA approval. It has been mentioned above as a detoxification agent and will be discussed later and in more detail as it has unique properties that are likely to result in it being used with fewer regulatory controls than methadone and LAAM.

Both methadone and LAAM are Schedule II controlled substances and can only be used for maintenance and detoxification in programs that are licensed and regulated by the FDA and the Drug Enforcement Administration (DEA). The regulations specify who is eligible for treatment, procedures that are required for its administration, the number of take-home doses permitted, and the type of medication storage security needed. Treatment programs have been inspected approximately every 3 years for the past 30 years and violations have resulted in sanctions ranging from administrative citations to criminal prosecution.

A combination of regulations has resulted in a treatment system that is separated from the mainstream of other medical care and that consists almost entirely of specially licensed and inspected clinics. Clinics are often located in old buildings that have been converted to comply with regulations but that were never intended for medical use. At the present time, it is estimated that approximately 179 000 patients are being maintained on methadone or LAAM at 940 or more sites, and that this number represents only about 20% of all persons with opioid dependence in the USA (Addiction Treatment Forum, 2000). This situation is very unlike that of some other western countries such as Spain and Switzerland where 50% or more of persons with opioid dependence are reported to be on agonist therapy, with substantial numbers of others in residential treatment.

The appropriate dose of agonist medication has been a subject of both federal and state regulations, although there has been a gradual shift toward allowing more clinical judgment in its determination. A number of studies have been done during the last 25 years to determine the optimal dose and, although it is clear that some patients do well on low doses of methadone or LAAM (about 20–50 mg), studies have consistently shown that most individuals need higher doses if they are to achieve maximum benefit from agonist treatment. The results of these comparison studies are generally supportive of the guidelines originally proposed by Dole and Nyswander, who recommended doses in the 80 to 120 mg/day range (Dole and Nyswander, 1968)

Physicians who choose to treat persons with opioid dependence under new regulations will need to notify the Secretary of Health and Human Services in writing of their intent and show that they are qualified to provide addiction treatment by virtue of certification or experience. No physician will be allowed to treat more than 30 patients at one time without special approval according to the proposed legislation. This change in the regulations will be especially important for buprenorphine and the buprenorphine/naloxone combination as it will provide better access to treatment for persons who are unwilling or unable to be treated in the current methadone or LAAM system. The overall intent of the proposed regulatory reform is better to integrate maintenance treatment into the mainstream of medical care, and to make it more available and improve its quality. These changes are likely to influence the ways that buprenorphine is used in opioid addiction treatment.

The greatest advantage of buprenorphine compared with full agonists such as methadone and LAAM is the plateau effect of μ-agonist activity. A number of large trials have confirmed the utility of buprenorphine for agonist maintenance therapy. Buprenorphine has the potential to be abused and can produce addiction; however, most persons who abuse buprenorphine initiated opioid use with other drugs.

Buprenorphine, in combination with naloxone, has less potential for abuse than buprenorphine alone. The therapeutic utility of combining naloxone with buprenorphine derives from the low sublingual bioavailability of naloxone as compared with buprenorphine. Parenteral misuse of the combination by persons addicted to opioids would be expected to produce antagonist like effects; thus, most persons with opioid dependence would be unlikely to inject the combination more than once. The use of the buprenorphine/naloxone combination in an office-based setting represents an innovative alternative to the restrictive methadone or LAAM maintenance paradigm and should expand the availability of agonist maintenance treatment with a relatively low risk for abuse or diversion. In addition, the partial agonist activity of buprenorphine results in a much lower risk for overdose death than is the case with methadone or LAAM.

Antagonist Maintenance

Naltrexone is the prototypical opioid antagonist used in abstinence therapy, blocking the effects of heroin and other opioids through competitive receptor inhibition. Naltrexone has no opioid agonist effects and is a competitive opioid antagonist. It is orally effective and can block opioid effects for 24 hours when administered as a single daily dose of 50 mg; doses of 100 to 150 mg can block opioid effects for 48 to 72 hours. Despite a favorable adverse event profile (nausea is typically the most common side effect), naltrexone is generally not favored by opioid addicts because, unlike opioid agonists and partial agonists, it produces no positive, reinforcing effects. Furthermore, it may be associated with the precipitation of an opioid withdrawal syndrome if used too soon after opioid use stops, an effect that can be minimized by administering a naloxone challenge prior to giving the first dose of naltrexone.

Psychosocial/Behavioral Treatments

In addition to challenges related to ambivalence about stopping opioid use, patients often have serious problems with nonopioid substance abuse and/or with medical, psychiatric, legal, employment and family/social issues that preexist or result from the addiction. Research has found that addressing these additional problems can be helpful, but is complex and requires coordination between agonist pharmacotherapy staff, and other medical and psychosocial services.

Individual Drug Counseling

The most common type of psychosocial treatment in opioid agonist maintenance is individual drug counseling. Counselors are typically persons at the masters level or below who deliver a behaviorally focused treatment aimed to identify specific problems, help the patient access services that may not be provided in the clinic (e.g., medical, psychiatric, legal, family/social), stop substance use and improve overall adjustment. Functions that counselors perform include monitoring methadone and LAAM doses and requesting changes when needed, reviewing urine test results, responding to requests for take-homes doses, assisting with family problems, responding to crises, writing letters for court or social welfare agencies, recommending inpatient treatment when necessary, and providing support and encouragement for a drug-free lifestyle.

Counseling usually addresses both opioid and nonopioid use. Although nicotine (tobacco) use is not always included, the increased emphasis on adverse health effects of smoking has resulted in more attention to stop smoking at all levels, including drug counseling. Counselors and patients typically have weekly, 30- to 60-minute sessions during the first weeks or months of treatment with reductions in frequency to biweekly or monthly depending on progress. The frequency of counseling can vary widely depending on the severity of the patient's problems, clinic requirements and counselor workload.

The importance of regular counseling was clearly demonstrated in a study by McLellan and coworkers (1993) in which patients were randomly assigned to minimal counseling (one 5- to 10-minute session per month), standard counseling (one 45-minute session per week), or enhanced counseling (standard plus on-site referral to psychiatric, medical and family/social services). Results showed a dose–response relationship with the minimal condition doing significantly worse than standard, and enhanced counseling doing the best overall; however, about 30% of patients did well in the minimal counseling condition. This study clearly demonstrated the positive benefits achieved by drug counseling and showed that, for most patients, counseling is necessary to bring out the maximum benefits from agonist maintenance.

Though most counseling is individual, some programs use group therapy exclusively and others do not use it at all. Most agonist programs that use groups have them only for patients with focal problems such as HIV disease, PTSD, homelessness, or loss of close personal relationships. Many programs encourage patients to participate in self-help groups, but ask them to select a group that accepts persons who are on agonist maintenance treatment. Some programs have self-help groups that meet on site. Counselors, like psychotherapists, can vary widely in the results they achieve. This variability seems more related to the ability to form a positive, helping relationship than to specific techniques.

Contingency management techniques are always included in drug counseling, if only to fulfill regulations about requiring progress in treatment as a condition of providing take-home doses; studies have shown that such contingencies can be helpful. For example, an opportunity to receive take-home medications in return for drug-free urine tests is a powerful and practical motivator for many patients. More flexibility in dispensing take-home doses as contingencies for positive behaviors could be an additionally useful result of the regulatory reforms that were described earlier. Another contingency that is easily applicable and which some programs have used with positive results is requiring a negative alcohol breath test prior to dispensing the daily dose of methadone or LAAM.

Though counseling and other services are effective enhancements of agonist treatment, compliance is often an issue and clinics vary in the way they respond to this problem. Some remind patients of appointments, others do not permit patients to be medicated unless they keep appointments, and others suspend patients who miss appointments. For noncompliant patients, a powerful contingency is requiring certain behaviors for patients to remain on the program, a procedure that is often formalized in a "treatment contract". Here, the patient is given the option of stopping heroin and other drug use, keeping regular counseling appointments, looking for work, or correcting other behaviors that need improvement as a condition for remaining in treatment. Patients who fail are administratively detoxified, suspended for months to years, and referred to another program, although the referrals are not always successful. The long-term effects of this form of contingency management have not been well studied.

Therapeutic Communities (TCs)

These programs are another approach that has been shown to be useful for treating opioid dependence, especially patients with a long history of addiction and a strong motivation to become drug-free, either as a result of internal processes or from external pressures such as being given the choice of entering prison for a drug-related crime, or getting treatment in a TC. These programs are very selective, self-governing and long-term (6–18 months). They occur in residential settings where patients share responsibilities for maintaining the treatment milieu (cleaning, cooking and leading group therapy). Confrontation of denial and behaviors such as lying and "conning", combined with group support for healthy, positive change are used to restructure character and the addictive lifestyle. Medications such as methadone, LAAM, or naltrexone are rarely used; however, medications for specific psychiatric or medical conditions are usually available after careful screening and evaluation. Many TCs have large numbers of individuals who have been referred by the criminal justice system including some who have tried but not responded to agonist maintenance on repeated occasions. Though dropout rates are high, studies have shown that over 80% of individuals who complete TCs have a sustained remission and demonstrate significant improvement in psychiatric symptoms, employment and criminal behavior (Inciardi *et al.*, 1997; DeLeon, 1999).

Addressing Comorbidity

Patients seeking treatment for opioid dependence are typically using one or more other substances (cocaine, alcohol, benzodiazepines, amphetamines, marijuana, nicotine), and have additional problems in the psychiatric, medical, family/social, employment, or legal areas. In fact, it is rare to find a person with only opioid dependence and no other substance use, or without a psychiatric, medical, or family/social problem. The presence of these problems, perhaps with the exception of nicotine dependence, tends to magnify the severity of the opioid dependence and makes the patient even more difficult to treat. An example of a successful treatment of a difficult patient is given in the following clinical vignette.

Clinical Vignette

A 42-year-old male presented for treatment of opioid dependence; this was his sixth episode of methadone maintenance. The patient had a long history of alcoholism that interfered with treatment in the past and had begun using cocaine regularly. Historically, the patient had done fairly well on methadone as far as illicit opioid use was concerned, but clinic attendance and his ability to comply with clinic rules, especially regarding take-home doses, had been severely compromised by alcohol use. In the past, the patient would remain in treatment for about a year, then become angry over his inability to obtain take-home doses (due to ongoing positive Breathalyzer readings) and drop out of treatment; relapse to opioid use always immediately followed. During previous treatment episodes, the patient had frequently been offered inpatient detoxification for alcoholism but always refused because 1) "alcohol was not his problem, heroin was the problem" and 2) he could not take time off work (as a stockperson in a liquor store).

When the patient presented for treatment this time, he had severe social stressors; was unemployed (secondary to his alcohol problems) and living with his parents, who were threatening to put him out because of drug use.

The patient was told that, this time, methadone would not be offered unless he first entered the hospital. After some discussion, he agreed that as part of his treatment plan he would first enter the hospital for 21 to 28 days of treatment including alcohol detoxification and stabilization on methadone; he would then be discharged to maintenance therapy. This approach worked. After inpatient discharge, the patient kept regular counseling appointments, continued to attend self-help meetings to which he had been introduced while on the inpatient unit, "requested" daily Breathalyzer testing, and turned down an offer to return to his job in the liquor store. Over the past 3 years, his liver function tests returned to normal levels, he was stable on 65 mg of methadone/day with urine tests negative for opioids, although occasionally his urine was positive for cocaine. He was able to comply fully with a treatment regimen for a back injury sustained 2 years ago and currently enrolled in school.

Psychiatric

Among the psychiatric disorders seen in persons with opioid dependence, antisocial personality disorder is one of the most common. Diagnostic studies of persons with opioid dependence have typically found rates of antisocial personality disorder ranging from 20 to 50%, as compared with less than 5% in the general population. PTSD is also seen with increased frequency.

Opioid dependent persons are especially at risk for the development of brief depressive symptoms, and for episodes of mild to moderate depression that meet symptomatic and duration criteria for major depressive disorder or dysthymia. These syndromes represent both substance-induced mood disorders as well as independent depressive illnesses. Brief periods of depression are especially common during chronic intoxication or withdrawal, or in association with psychosocial stressors that are related to the dependence. Insomnia is common, especially during withdrawal; sexual dysfunction, especially impotence, is common during intoxication. Delirium or brief, psychotic-like symptoms are occasionally seen during opioid intoxication.

The data on psychiatric comorbidity among opioid addicts and its negative effect on outcome have stimulated research on the effect of combining psychiatric and substance abuse treatment. Studies have shown that tricyclic antidepressants can be useful for chronically depressed opioid dependent persons who are treated with methadone maintenance and that professional psychotherapy can be useful for psychiatrically impaired, methadone-maintained opioid addicts. The main result in most pharmacotherapy and psychotherapy studies with methadone-maintained addicts has usually been a reduction in psychiatric symptoms such as depression, although some have shown reductions in substance use as well.

Less than 5% of persons with opioid dependence have psychotic disorders such as bipolar illness or schizophrenia; however, these patients can present special problems since programs typically have few psychiatric staff. As a result, these patients are sometimes excluded from methadone treatment because they cannot be effectively managed within the constraints of the available resources. Others are treated with methadone, counseling and the same medications used for nonaddicted patients with similar disorders. Women with opioid dependence can present special challenges because many have been sexually abused as children, have other psychiatric disorders, and are involved in difficult family/social situations. Abusive relationships with addicted males are common, sometimes characterized by situations in which the male exerts control by providing drugs. These complex psychiatric and relationship issues have emphasized the need for comprehensive psychosocial services that include psychiatric assessment and treatment, and access to other medical, family and social services.

Medical

Medical comorbidity is a major problem among persons with opioid dependence; HIV infection, AIDS, and hepatitis B and C have become some of the most common problems. Sharing injection equipment including "cookers" and rinse water, or engaging in high-risk sexual behaviors are the main routes of infection. Sexual transmission appears to be a more common route of HIV transmission among females than males because the HIV virus is spread more readily from males to females than from females to males. Females who are intravenous drug users and also engage in prostitution or other forms of high-risk sex are at extremely high risk for HIV infection Cocaine use has been found to be a significant risk factor as a single drug of abuse or when used in combination with heroin or other opioids (Booth *et al.*, 2000).

Recent studies have identified several important interactions between methadone and drugs to treat HIV. One important interaction is that methadone increases plasma levels of zidovudine; the associated symptoms resemble methadone withdrawal. There have been instances in which methadone doses have been increased in response to complaints of withdrawal with increasing doses compounding the problem. Another important interaction involves decreased methadone blood levels secondary to nevirapine that may result in mild to moderate withdrawal. This interaction can be important if the patient is taken off either of these two drugs while on methadone, since the result may be a sudden rise in methadone blood levels with signs and symptoms of over medication.

As mentioned earlier, mortality is high and studies have found annual death rates of approximately 10 per 1000 or greater, which is substantially higher than demographically matched samples in the general population (Gronbladh *et al.*, 1990). Common causes of death are overdose, accidents, injuries, and medical complications such as cellulitis, hepatitis, AIDS, tuberculosis and endocarditis. The cocaine and alcohol dependence that is often seen among opioid-dependent persons contributes to cirrhosis, cardiomyopathy, myocardial infarction and cardiac arrhythmias. Tuberculosis has become a particularly serious problem among intravenous drug users, especially heroin addicts. In most cases, infection is asymptomatic and evident only by the presence of a positive tuberculin skin test. However, many cases of active tuberculosis have been found, especially among those who are infected with HIV.

Other medical complications of heroin dependence are seen in children born to opioid-dependent women. Perhaps the most serious is premature delivery and low birthweight, a problem that can be reduced if the mother is on methadone maintenance and receiving prenatal care. Another is physiological dependence on opioids, seen in about half the infants born to women maintained

on methadone or dependent on heroin or other opioids. Effective treatments for neonatal withdrawal are available and long-term adverse effects of opioid withdrawal have not been demonstrated. A recent study found that methadone is present in the breast milk of women maintained on doses as high as 180 mg but that the concentration is very low and no adverse effects were observed in the infants (McCarthy and Posey, 2000). HIV infection is seen in about one-third of infants born to HIV-positive mothers, but can be reduced to about 10% if HIV-positive pregnant women are given zidovudine prior to delivery. HIV can also be transmitted by breast-feeding, and thus formula is recommended for HIV-positive mothers with the exception of countries where it is unavailable or unaffordable. Thorough washing of infants born to HIV-infected mothers immediately after delivery also appears to reduce the incidence of HIV infection.

Integrated Treatment

The comorbidity data have led to research that has demonstrated the positive effects of integrating psychiatric and medical care within agonist and other substance abuse treatment programs. Clinical experience and National Institute on Drug Abuse demonstration projects have shown that integration of these services can be done, and with very positive results since patients are seen frequently and treatment retention is high (Umbricht-Schneiter *et al.*, 1994). Related to this line of research are studies that have shown improved compliance with directly observed antituberculosis pharmacotherapy. These findings have important implications for tuberculosis control policies in methadone programs since intravenous drug users are at very high risk for tuberculosis infection and because maintenance programs provide settings in which directly observed therapy can be easily applied. Similar principles apply to administration of psychotropic medication in noncompliant patients with schizophrenia or other major Axis I disorders.

Harm Reduction

Harm reduction is concerned with minimizing various negative consequences of addiction. As such, the focus is shifted away from drug use to the consequences of use and its attendant behaviors. Examples of harm reduction include needle exchange programs, efforts directed at reducing drug-use-associated behaviors that may result in the transmission of HIV, and making changes in policies (including increasing treatment availability) that reduce heroin use and the criminal behavior associated with drug procurement. Harm reduction refers not only to reducing harm to the individual addict, but also to family, friends and to society generally. A number of authors have identified the limitations of harm reduction when it is used as a sole strategy to combat the adverse effects of addiction.

With regard to opioids, much of the health-related harm from their improper or illicit use is secondary to elements other than the substances themselves. Sequelae from unhygienic methods of administration and poor injection technique are typically more serious than the constipation or other side effects of the drugs themselves, acute overdoses notwithstanding. At current levels of use, greater harm is expected to result from the use of alcohol and tobacco than from opioids. With regard to opioid addiction treatment, medications such as methadone, LAAM and buprenorphine, among others (including supervised heroin substitution) used for maintenance agonist treatment, may be considered harm-reduction measures.

Comparison of DSM-IV/ICD-10 Diagnostic Criteria

The DSM-IV-TR and ICD-10 criteria sets for opioid intoxication are almost the same. The DSM-IV-TR and ICD-10 symptom lists for opioid withdrawal include some different items: the ICD-10 list has craving, abdominal cramps and tachycardia and does not include the fever and dysphoric mood items from the DSM-IV-TR criteria set.

References

Addiction Treatment Forum (2000) *The Quarterly Newsletter of Addiction Treatment for Clinical Health Care Professionals* IX (2), 2.

Booth RE, Kwiatkowski CF, and Chitwood DD (2000) Sex related HIV risk behaviors: Differential risks among injection drug users, crack smokers, and injection drug users who smoke crack. *Drug Alcohol Depend* 58, 219–226.

DeLeon G (1999) Therapeutic communities, in *Textbook of Substance Abuse Treatment* (eds Galanter M and Kleber HD). American Psychiatric Association Press, Washington DC, pp. 447–462.

Dole VP and Nyswander M (1968) Successful treatment of 750 criminal addicts. *J Am Med Assoc* 26, 2708–2710.

Gronbladh L, Ohlund LS and Gunne LM (1990) Mortality in heroin addiction: Impact of methadone treatment. *Acta Psychiatr Scand* 82, 223–227.

Hensel M and Kox WJ (2000) Safety, efficacy, and long-term results of a modified version of rapid opiate detoxification under general anesthesia: A prospective study in methadone, heroin, codeine, and morphine addicts. *Acta Anaesthesiol Scand* 44, 3226–3233.

Inciardi JA, Martin SS, Butzin CA *et al.* (1997) An effective model of prison-based treatment for drug-involved offenders. *J Drug Issues* 27, 261–278.

McCarthy JJ and Posey BL (2000) Methadone levels in human milk. *J Human Lac* 16, 115–120.

McLellan AT, Arndt IO, Metzger DS *et al.* (1993) The effects of psychosocial services on substance abuse treatment. *J Am Med Assoc* 269, 1953–1959.

National Household Survey on Drug Abuse (2000) *Population Estimates*, 2nd Rev. US Department of Health and Human Services, Public Health Service, Alcohol, Drug Abuse and Mental Health Administration, DHHS Publication No. (ADM) 92–1887.

Umbricht-Schneiter A, Ginn DH, Pabst KM *et al.* (1994) Providing medical care to methadone clinic patients: Referral vs. on-site care. *Am J Pub Health* 84, 207–210.

44

Substance Abuse:
Sedative, Hypnotic,
or Anxiolytic Use Disorders

Sedative–hypnotics and anxiolytics include prescription sleeping medications and most medications used for the treatment of anxiety. Pharmacologically alcohol is appropriately included among sedative–hypnotics; however, it is generally considered separately as it is in DSM-IV-TR (American Psychiatric Association, 2000). The medications usually included in the category of sedative–hypnotics are listed in Table 44.1.

Sedative–hypnotics are among the most commonly prescribed medications. They are also often misused and abused and can produce severe, life-threatening dependence. With the exception of the benzodiazepines and newer hypnotics (e.g., eszopiclone, zaleplon, zopiclone and zolpidem), overdose with sedative–hypnotics can be lethal. Benzodiazepines and the newer hypnotics are rarely lethal if taken alone; in combination with alcohol or other drugs, however, they can be lethal.

When the benzodiazepines were introduced into clinical medicine in the early 1960s, their lack of lethality in overdose led physicians to believe that they were without harmful effects. Over time, it was recognized that the benzodiazepines could produce severe physiological dependence and could be drugs of abuse. Nonetheless, their medical utility in treatment of disabling anxiety, episodic sleep disturbances and seizures has made them indispensable to medical practice.

Considerations of sedative–hypnotic use disorders should reflect a sensible balance between their medical utility, side effects, and abuse and dependence. Some abuse and dependence that inevitably occur must be accepted to keep them available in clinical practice.

Substance-related Disorders of Sedative–Hypnotics

The term "misuse" is commonly applied to prescription sedative–hypnotics, but the DSM-IV-TR does not provide explicit criteria for misuse as it does for abuse and dependence. When medications are taken in higher doses or more frequently than prescribed, or by someone other than the person for whom the medication was prescribed, or for reasons other than what would normally be considered medical use, the behavior is generally considered misuse of the medication.

DSM-IV-TR defines abuse and dependence in terms of behavioral and physiological consequences to the person taking the medication. The criteria for abuse and dependence are intended to apply as uniformly as possible across classes of drugs, and the criteria do not distinguish the source of the medication or the intended purpose for which it was taken. Further, when most people, including physicians speak of drug dependence, they are referring to physical dependence. DSM-IV-TR uses the term dependence to denote a more severe form of substance use disorder than abuse, and it uses the specifier "with or without physiological dependence" to indicate whether the patient has significant physical dependence. Physiological dependence is not necessarily required for a diagnosis of drug dependence. A diagnosis of substance dependence is made only when a patient has dysfunctional behaviors that are a result of the drug use.

The qualification that the dysfunctional behavior is the "result" of drug use is extremely important, and observation of the patient over time in a medication-free state may be necessary to determine which is driving which. The patient, the patient's family members and the treating psychiatrist may disagree about what is causing symptoms or behavioral dysfunction. Likewise, the underlying motivation for "drug-seeking" behavior may vary. For example, a patient whose panic attacks are ameliorated by a medication may exhibit what may be interpreted as drug-seeking behavior if access to the medication is threatened. The terms **anxiolytic** and **minor tranquilizer** are also frequently sources of confusion. In classic pharmacology sedative–hypnotics are drugs or medications that produce a dose-related depression of consciousness. Drug classes are formed by combining drugs or medications that have similar pharmacological profiles.

Etiology and Pathophysiology

Sedative–Hypnotics and GABA Receptors

Many neurons in the central nervous system (CNS) have receptors for the neurotransmitter gamma-aminobutyric acid (GABA). Benzodiazepines attach to receptors that are allosteric to the $GABA_A$ receptor, that is, occupancy of the benzodiazepine receptor potentiates GABA at the $GABA_A$ receptor. The molecular pharmacology of the receptor is exceedingly complex. Chronic exposure to benzodiazepines may uncouple the benzodiazepine receptor from the $GABA_A$ receptor. The uncoupling may explain in part why over time benzodiazepines appear to become less

Essentials of Psychiatry   Jerald Kay and Allan Tasman

Table 44.1   Medications Usually Included in the Category of Sedative–Hypnotics

Generic Name	Trade Names	Common Therapeutic Use	Therapeutic Dose Range (mg/d)
Barbiturates			
Amobarbital	Amytal	Sedative	50–150
Butabarbital	Butisol	Sedative	45–120
Butalbital	Fiorinal, Sedapap	Sedative/analgesic	100–300
Pentobarbital	Nembutal	Hypnotic	50–100
Secobarbital	Seconal	Hypnotic	50–100
Benzodiazepines			
Alprazolam	Xanax	Antianxiety	0.75–6
Chlordiazepoxide	Librium	Antianxiety	15–100
Clonazepam	Klonopin	Anticonvulsant	0.5–4
Clorazepate	Tranxene	Antianxiety	15–60
Diazepam	Valium	Antianxiety	5–40
Estazolam	ProSom	Hypnotic	1–2
Flunitrazepam	Rohypnol*	Hypnotic	1–2
Flurazepam	Dalmane	Hypnotic	15–30
Halazepam	Paxipam	Antianxiety	60–160
Lorazepam	Ativan	Antianxiety	1–16
Midazolam	Versed	Anesthesia	–
Oxazepam	Serax	Antianxiety	10–120
Prazepam	Centrax	Antianxiety	20–60
Quazepam	Doral	Hypnotic	15
Temazepam	Restoril	Hypnotic	7.5–30
Triazolam	Halcion	Hypnotic	0.125–0.5
Others			
Chloral hydrate	Noctec, Somnos	Hypnotic	250–1000
Eszopiclone	Lunesta	Hypnotic	1-3
Ethchlorvynol	Placidyl	Hypnotic	200–1000
Glutethimide	Doriden	Hypnotic	250–500
Meprobamate	Miltown, Equanil, Equagesic	Antianxiety	1200–1600
Methyprylon	Noludar	Hypnotic	200–400
Zaleplon	Sonata, (Stilnox, other countries)	Hypnotic	5–20
Zolpidem	Ambien	Hypnotic	5–10

*Rohypnol is not marketed in the USA.

effective in controlling symptoms in some patients, which give them an impetus to increase dosage.

Epidemiology

The prevalence of sedative–hypnotic disorders is not known with precision. Unlike most drugs of abuse (e.g., cocaine or heroin) that are manufactured in clandestine laboratories and distributed through the street-drug black markets, sedative–hypnotics are exclusively manufactured by pharmaceutical companies. Sedative–hypnotics that are used and abused by addicts are obtained either from the black market, where they have been diverted from medical channels, or from physicians and pharmacies under treatment subterfuge. Drug dependence may arise as an inadvertent consequence of medical treatment or through patient's self-administration of sedative–hypnotics obtained from illicit sources or sequential visits to different physicians. By some indicators, tranquilizer and sedative–hypnotic use is increasing.

Insomnia and anxiety disorders are common and sedative–hypnotics are among the most commonly prescribed medications worldwide. Sedative–hypnotic abuse and dependence disorders are common, but involve only a small percentage of the people who use these medications. Most people do not find the subjective effects of sedative–hypnotics pleasant or appealing beyond their therapeutic effects (e.g., relief of anxiety or facilitation of sleep). Many addicts, on the other hand, have a subjectively different response to sedative–hypnotics and like the subjective effects of sedative–hypnotics. The qualitative difference in subjective response to medications by addicts is one extremely important factor in understanding why medications that are safe and efficacious for nonaddicts cannot be safely prescribed for addicts. In addition, addicts may take doses of medications far in excess of recommended dosage, take them by injection or means other than prescribed (e.g., dissolving tablets and injecting them, crushing tablets and snorting them), or take them in combination with other prescription medications or street drugs such as heroin or cocaine that are extremely likely to produce adverse consequences.

Patterns of Abuse

Some sedative–hypnotics, such as the short-acting barbiturates, are primary drugs of abuse, that is, they are injected for the "rush" or are taken orally to produce a state of disinhibition similar to that achieved with alcohol. Sedative hypnotics may also be taken in combination with other primary intoxicants, such as alcohol or heroin, to intensify the desired subjective effects.

Drug addicts may also use sedative–hypnotics to self-medicate withdrawal of drugs such as heroin. When the avowed intent is to stop the use of drugs such as heroin, physicians may be lured into thinking that addicts' self-administration of sedative–hypnotics is not "abuse" but rather a reasonable approximation of medical use. While on occasion this may be the case, often it is not. Addicts' episodic attempts to stop using heroin by self-medicating opiate withdrawal symptoms with sedative–hypnotics without entering drug abuse treatment is rarely successful, and may result in the secondary development of sedative–hypnotic dependence.

Addicts may also use sedative–hypnotics to reduce un-pleasant side effects of stimulants, particularly cocaine or meth-amphetamine. Impairment of judgment and memory produced by the sedative–hypnotic in combination with wakefulness of a stimulant may result in unpredictable behavior.

Barbiturates

Injection of a barbiturate is associated with the usual infectious risk of injecting street drugs, but the barbiturates are particularly pernicious if inadvertently injected into an artery or if the solution is injected or leaked from a vein or artery into tissue sur-rounding the vessel. Barbiturates are irritating to tissue, and the affected tissue becomes indurated and may abscess. In addition, barbiturate solution injected into an artery produces intense va-soconstriction and blockage of the arterioles, resulting in gan-grene of areas supplied by the artery.

Methaqualone

Methaqualone (Quaalude) was removed from the US market in 1984 because of its abuse. Subsequently, it has continued to be sold on the street-drug black market. Some tablets sold on the black market as Quaalude contain methaqualone, apparently diverted from countries where methaqualone is still available; others con-tain diazepam, phenobarbital, or another sedative–hypnotic.

Benzodiazepines

Benzodiazepines are often used or misused by addicts to self-medicate opiate withdrawal, to intensify the CNS effects of methadone, or to ameliorate the adverse effects of cocaine or methamphetamine.

The benzodiazepine, flunitrazepam (Rohypnol, Narcozep), is singled out for additional discussion in this chapter on benzo-diazepine abuse because of the media and legislative attention it received during the 1990s, and because it is still widely abused in Europe and other areas of the world. Flunitrazepam, a potent benzodiazepine hypnotic, was never marketed in the USA but is widely available by prescription in many other countries in 1- or 2-mg oral dosage forms and for injection.

Flunitrazepam has many street names, including rophies, ropies, roopies, roofies, ruffes, rofinol, loops and wheels. Tablets of Rohypnol have the name of the manufacturer Roche engraved on them and a number indicating the milligram strength (either 1 or 2). Drug abusers usually prefer the 2-mg tablets, which are often called "Roche dos" or just "Roche" (usually pronounced "row-shay"). Although flunitrazepam is similar in many respects to other benzodiazepines in abuse potential flunitrazepam is among the benzodiazepines with highest abuse potential and has considerable appeal among heroin addicts.

In the mid-1990s Rohypnol achieved notoriety as the "date-rape drug". Because of the media attention, considerable public debate ensued and the US Congress was prompted to pass legislation increasing penalties for rape when Rohypnol or other drugs were used to facilitate it. Subsequently, GHB (gamma-hydroxybutyric acid), which has some properties of a sedative–hypnotic, was also called a "date-rape drug."

Flunitrazepam and other benzodiazepines have also been associated with deaths among opiate addicts taking buprenor-phine. Although buprenorphine alone or benzodiazepines alone are rarely fatal, the combination appears to increase the risk of overdose. Benzodiazepines and buprenorphine may have syner-gistic action in suppressing respiration.

Zolpidem

Zolpidem (Ambien) is an imidazopyridine hypnotic, chemically unrelated to the benzodiazepines. However, it binds to a subu-nit of the same GABA–benzodiazepine complex as the benzo-diazepines and its sedative effects are reversed by the benzodi-azepine antagonist flumazenil.

A few case reports of abuse suggest that some patients in-crease the dosage many times above what is prescribed and that zolpidem produces a withdrawal syndrome similar to that of other sedative–hypnotics (Aragona, 2000). The case histories also de-scribe significant tolerance to the sedative effects of zolpidem.

Zolpidem is rapidly absorbed and has a short half-life (2.2 hours). Its sedative effects are additive with alcohol. Like triazolam, zolpidem decreases brain metabolism of glucose. In addition to dependence, zolpidem has produced idiosyncratic psychotic reactions.

Zaleplon

Like zolpidem, this drug is chemically unrelated to the benzodi-azepines and binds to the omega-1 receptor, which is a subunit of the GABA-benzodiazepine receptor. Studies in volunteers with a history of drug abuse suggest abuse potential similar to tria-zolam. Peak plasma concentration occurs about 1 hour following oral ingestion. It is rapidly metabolized with a half-life of about 1 hour. Impairment of short-term memory may occur at dosages of 10 to 20 mg.

Acute Intoxication with Sedative–Hypnotics

The acute toxicity of sedative–hypnotics consists of slurred speech, incoordination, ataxia, sustained nystagmus, impaired judgment and mood lability. When taken in large amounts sedative–hypnotics produce progressive respiratory depression and coma. The amount of respiratory depression produced by the benzodiazepines is much less than that produced by the barbiturates and other sedative–hypnotics. Consistent with its general approach, the DSM-IV-TR diagnosis of intoxication requires "clinically significant maladaptive behavioral or psychological changes" developing after drug use in addition to the signs and symptoms of acute toxicity.

Dependence

Sedative–hypnotics can produce tolerance and physiological dependence. Physiological dependence can be induced within several days with continuous infusion of anesthetic doses. Pa-tients who are taking barbiturates daily, for example, for a month or more above the upper therapeutic range listed in Table 44.1 should be presumed to be physically dependent and in need of medically managed detoxification.

Withdrawal Syndrome

The withdrawal syndrome arising from the discontinuation of short-acting sedative–hypnotics is similar to that from stopping or cutting down on the use of alcohol. Signs and symptoms of sedative–hypnotic withdrawal include anxiety, tremors, nightmares, insomnia, anorexia, nausea, vomiting, postural hypotension, seizures, delirium and hyperpyrexia. The syndrome is qualitatively similar for all sedative–hypnotics; however, the time course of symptoms depends on the particular drug. With short-acting sedative–hypnotics (e.g., pentobarbital, secobarbital, meprobamate, oxazepam, alprazolam and triazolam), withdrawal symptoms typically begin 12 to 24 hours after the last dose and peak in intensity between 24 and 72 hours (symptoms may develop more slowly in patients with liver disease or in the elderly because of decreased drug metabolism). With long-acting drugs (e.g., phenobarbital, diazepam and chlordiazepoxide), withdrawal symptoms peak on the fifth to eighth day. The withdrawal delirium may include confusion, visual and auditory hallucinations. The delirium generally follows a period of insomnia. Some patients may have only delirium; others only seizures; and some may have both delirium and convulsions.

Iatrogenic Dependence

Patients treated for months to years with benzodiazepines and other sedative–hypnotics may become physically dependent on sedative–hypnotics. The possibility of physical dependence should be discussed with the patient and, in some cases, the patient's family. The distinction between physical dependence as a process of neuroadaptation and physical dependence as a component of a substance-use disorder should be explained in detail. Patients need to be advised against abruptly stopping the medication because of the possibility of developing severe withdrawal symptoms, including seizures.

Diagnosis and Differential Diagnosis

The diagnosis of sedative–hypnotic abuse and dependence is based primarily on drug-use history and the DSM-IV-TR criteria of continuing behavior dysfunction caused by the drug. With dependence developing from prescribed use, the practical difficulty is determining when the dysfunction is a result of the drug use rather than the disorder for which the medication was prescribed.

Phenomenology and Variations in Presentations

Long-term use of benzodiazepines can result in physical dependence in nondrug-dependent medical patients. Withdrawal symptoms "or" return of symptoms suppressed by the benzodiazepines may make discontinuation difficult.

Some patients who are physically dependent on or unable to discontinue a medication do not necessarily have a substance-use disorder. Physical dependence results from neuroadaptive changes resulting from long-term exposure to a medication. Inability to discontinue the medication may simply mean that patients are unwilling to tolerate the severity of postwithdrawal symptoms that develop. In the absence of medication-produced dysfunction, the continuation of the medication may be an appropriate choice. Patients who do not have a substance-use disorder take medications in the quantity prescribed. They follow their physicians' recommendations, and they do not mix them with drugs of abuse.

Abusers of alcohol and other drugs rarely present for primary treatment of sedative–hypnotic dependency. From the drug-abusing patient's point of view, sedative–hypnotic use is an effort to self-medicate anxiety or insomnia, which is often the result of alcohol or stimulant abuse.

Assessment

Drug Use History

The patient's drug use history is usually the first source of information that is used in assessing sedative–hypnotic abuse or dependence. If the sedative–hypnotics were being used for treatment of insomnia or anxiety, the history is often best obtained as part of the history of the primary disorder and its response to treatment. A detailed history of use of all sedative–hypnotics, including alcohol, should be elicited from the patient. When framed in terms of the presenting disorder, patients are generally more candid about their drug use and their relationship with past treating physicians.

For many reasons, patients may minimize or exaggerate their drug use and not accurately report the behavioral consequences of their use. High doses of benzodiazepines or therapeutic doses of benzodiazepines in combination with alcohol may disrupt memory. Patients are likely to attribute impairment of function to the underlying disorder rather than to the medication use. Observations of patients' behavior by family members can be a source of valuable information. Whenever possible, the patient's history should be supplemented by medical and pharmacy records to help piece together as accurate a picture of drug use as possible. Pharmacy records may be helpful in establishing and verifying patient's drug use history, and urine testing can be useful in verifying recent drug use history.

Patients who are obtaining some or all of their medication from street sources may not know what they have been taking, as deception in the street-drug marketplace is common. For example, tablets sold as methaqualone have been found to contain phenobarbital or diazepam.

Physical Findings

Sustained horizontal nystagmus is a reliable indicator of sedative–hypnotic intoxication. Onset of tremor, abnormal sweating and blood pressure or pulse increase may be produced by sedative–hypnotic withdrawal.

Laboratory Tests

Urine toxicology can be useful in monitoring patients' use of drugs and in confirming a history of drug or medication use. The detection time varies widely for benzodiazepines. Diazepam or chlordiazepoxide may be detected for weeks following chronic or high-dose use, whereas others, such as alprazolam or clonazepam, may not be detectable in routine toxicology urinalysis. Because of the variability in laboratory cutoffs and detection time and different drugs included in the screening panel, the analytical laboratory should be asked about what they routinely screen for and the detection limits.

Course and Natural History

Once a diagnosis of sedative–hypnotic dependence is manifested it is unlikely that a patient will be able to return to controlled, therapeutic use of sedative–hypnotics. All sedative–hypnotics, including alcohol, are cross-tolerant, and physical dependence and tolerance are quickly re-established if a patient resumes use of sedative–hypnotics.

If after sedative–hypnotic withdrawal the patient has another primarily psychiatric disorder, such as generalized anxiety disorder (GAD), panic attacks, or insomnia, alternate treatment strategies other than sedative–hypnotics should be used if possible. Definitive diagnosis of a psychiatric disorder during early abstinence is often not possible because protracted withdrawal symptoms may mimic anxiety disorders, and disruption of sleep architecture for days to months after drug withdrawal is extremely common.

If the sedative–hypnotic dependence has developed secondary to stimulant or alcohol use, primary treatment of the chemical dependence should be a priority. Often the symptom that was driving the sedative–hypnotic use disappears after the patient is drug abstinent.

Detoxification

Three general strategies are used for withdrawing patients from sedative–hypnotics, including benzodiazepines. The first is to use decreasing doses of the agent of dependence. The second is to substitute phenobarbital or some other long-acting barbiturate for the addicting agent, and gradually withdraw the substitute medication. The third, used for patients with a dependence on both alcohol and a benzodiazepine, is to substitute a long-acting benzodiazepine, such as chlordiazepoxide, and taper it during 1 to 2 weeks.

The pharmacological rationale for phenobarbital substitution is that phenobarbital is long-acting and little change in blood levels of phenobarbital occurs between doses. This allows the safe use of a progressively smaller daily dose. Phenobarbital is safer than the shorter-acting barbiturates; lethal doses of phenobarbital are many times higher than toxic doses, and the signs of toxicity (e.g., sustained nystagmus, slurred speech and ataxia) are easy to observe. Finally, phenobarbital intoxication usually does not produce euphoria or behavioral disinhibition, so most patients view it as a medication, not as a drug of abuse.

The withdrawal strategy selected depends on the particular benzodiazepine, the involvement of other drugs of dependence, and the clinical setting in which the detoxification program takes place. The gradual reduction of the benzodiazepine of dependence is used primarily in medical settings for dependence arising from treatment of an underlying condition. The patient must be cooperative, must be able to adhere to dosing regimens, and must not be abusing alcohol or other drugs.

Substitution of phenobarbital can also be used to withdraw patients who have lost control of their benzodiazepine use or who are polydrug-dependent. Phenobarbital substitution has the broadest use for all sedative–hypnotic drug dependencies and is widely used in drug treatment programs.

Stabilization Phase

The patient's history of drug use during the month before treatment is used to compute the stabilization dose of phenobarbital. Although many addicts exaggerate the number of pills they are taking, the patient's history is the best guide to initiating pharmacotherapy for withdrawal. Patients who have overstated the amount of drug that they have taken will become intoxicated during the first day or two of treatment. Intoxication is easily managed by omitting one or more doses of phenobarbital and reducing the daily dose.

To compute the initial daily starting dose of phenobarbital, the patient's average daily use of each sedative–hypnotic is estimated. Next, the patient's average daily sedative–hypnotic dose for each drug is converted to its phenobarbital withdrawal equivalent by multiplying the average daily dose by the drug's phenobarbital conversion constant shown in either Table 44.2 or 44.3. Finally, the phenobarbital withdrawal equivalences for each drug are added together. In any case, the maximum daily phenobarbital dose is limited to 500 mg/day. The total daily amount of phenobarbital is divided into three doses per day.

Before receiving each dose of phenobarbital, the patient is checked for signs of phenobarbital toxicity: sustained nystagmus, slurred speech, or ataxia. Of these, sustained nystagmus is

Table 44.2	Phenobarbital Withdrawal Equivalents of Nonbenzodiazepines		
Generic Name	Trade Name	Dose Equal to 30 mg of Phenobarbital for Withdrawal* (mg)	Phenobarbital Conversion Constant
Barbiturates			
Amobarbital	Amytal	100	0.33
Butabarbital	Butisol	100	0.33
Butalbital†	Fiorinal	100	0.33
Pentobarbital	Nembutal	100	0.33
Secobarbital	Seconal	100	0.33
Others			
Chloral hydrate	Noctec, Somnos	500	0.06
Ethchlorvynol	Placidyl	500	0.06
Glutethimide	Doriden	250	0.12
Meprobamate	Miltown	1200	0.025
Methyprylon	Noludar	200	0.15
Zaleplon	Sonata	10	3
Zolpidem	Ambien	5	6

*Phenobarbital withdrawal conversion equivalence is not the same as therapeutic dose equivalence.
†Butalbital is in combination with opiate or nonopiate analgesics.

Table 44.3 Phenobarbital Withdrawal Equivalents of Benzodiazepines

Generic Name	Trade Name	Dose Equal to 30 mg of Phenobarbital for Withdrawal* (mg)	Phenobarbital Conversion Constant
Alprazolam	Xanax	1	30
Chlordiazepoxide	Librium	25	1.2
Clonazepam	Klonopin	2	15
Clorazepate	Tranxene	7.5	4
Diazepam	Valium	10	3
Estazolam	ProSom	1	30
Flurazepam	Dalmane	15	2
Halazepam	Paxipam	40	0.75
Lorazepam	Ativan	2	15
Oxazepam	Serax	10	3
Prazepam	Centrax	10	3
Quazepam	Doral	15	2
Temazepam	Restoril	15	2
Triazolam	Halcion	0.25	120

*Phenobarbital withdrawal conversion equivalence is not the same as therapeutic dose equivalence.

the most reliable. If nystagmus is present, the scheduled dose of phenobarbital is withheld. If all three signs are present the next two doses of phenobarbital are withheld, and the daily dosage of phenobarbital for the next day is halved.

If the patient is in acute withdrawal and has had, or is in danger of having withdrawal seizures, the initial dose of phenobarbital is administered by intramuscular injection. If nystagmus and other signs of intoxication develop after 1 to 2 hours after the intramuscular dose, the patient is in no immediate danger from barbiturate withdrawal. Patients are maintained with the initial dosing schedule of phenobarbital for 2 days. If the patient has neither signs of withdrawal nor phenobarbital toxicity (slurred speech, nystagmus, unsteady gait) phenobarbital withdrawal is begun.

Withdrawal Phase

Unless the patient develops signs and symptoms of phenobarbital toxicity or sedative–hypnotic withdrawal, phenobarbital is decreased by 30 mg/day. Should signs of phenobarbital toxicity develop during withdrawal, the daily phenobarbital dose is decreased by 50% and the 30 mg/day withdrawal is continued from the reduced phenobarbital dose. Should the patient have objective signs of sedative–hypnotic withdrawal, the daily dose is increased by 50% and the patient is restabilized before continuing the withdrawal.

Psychotherapy

The self-medication model, even if accurate in a particular case, is not a good one because once drug abuse or dependence becomes established the drug use takes on a life of its own regardless of the underlying reason for initiation. Rarely is treatment with insight-oriented psychotherapy successful in stopping the drug use. During early recovery, most patients are coping with subtle withdrawal symptoms, repairing relationships and learning to function without reliance on psychoactive drugs. Patients with underlying psychiatric disorders may have the additional burden of emergence of symptoms that had been ameliorated by their drug use. Psychotherapy during early recovery should be supportive and focused on coping with current life difficulties. Psychotherapists should remain vigilant for symptoms of panic

attacks, generalized anxiety, depression, or sleep disturbances that interfere with current function and should initiate appropriate psychopharmacological or somatic treatments when appropriate.

Psychotherapy can, however, have an important role in motivating a patient for primary treatment of drug dependency. Therapists can help break down patients' denial of their drug dependence by helping them see how drug use is interfering with relationships and undermining their ability to function. In some instances, it is desirable to continue the psychotherapeutic relationship while the patient is undergoing treatment for chemical dependence. With drug abusers, it is often desirable to separate the medication management from psychotherapy to prevent the psychotherapy from becoming bogged down in discussions of medications and medication side effects.

Twelve-step Recovery

Alcoholics Anonymous, Narcotics Anonymous and Cocaine Anonymous groups are important treatment adjuncts for many people recovering from alcohol and other forms of drug dependence. Although many groups are becoming more tolerant of appropriate use of pharmacotherapies, many individuals who attend 12-step recovery meetings are adamantly opposed to any form of psychotropic medication use and counsel fellow members to stop their use. Strong opposition to medications is usually based on their own or friends' bad experience with medications. Some individuals recover without medications and believe that recovery is of better quality if not supported by a pharmacological crutch.

Patients with underlying psychiatric disorders and the need for treatment with psychopharmacotherapeutic medications often require ongoing support from their psychotherapist if they must have medication.

Additional Treatment Considerations

Psychiatric Comorbidity

Most patients who are being prescribed long-term benzodiazepine therapy have underlying major depressive disorder, panic disorder,

Clinical Vignette

A 33-year-old woman was referred by her internist for treatment of alcohol dependence after an overdose of alprazolam (Xanax) and alcohol. The patient had ingested about 30 tablets of alprazolam (2 mg) and a bottle of wine after an argument with her husband. The patient and her husband were in the process of an acrimonious separation, and during the 3 months before her hospitalization, the patient had increased her alcohol consumption to 1.5 bottles of wine each night. The patient stated that she had wanted to die and that she had heard that the combination of alprazolam and alcohol was lethal. She had not previously made a suicide attempt; however, she was under the ongoing care of a psychiatrist because of panic attacks. A previous psychiatrist had started the patient with alprazolam about 6 years before the overdose. Before she had started alprazolam, the panic attacks had become disabling. While she was taking 4 mg/day of alprazolam, the panic attacks became infrequent, and when they occurred were much attenuated. She had resumed employment as a travel agent. Her usual alcohol consumption consisted of one or, at the most, two glasses of wine with the evening meal. Until the overdose, she took alprazolam exactly as prescribed, 2 mg twice a day at the same time each day. Her psychiatrist verified that her refills were consistent with her history. The patient was frightened by having overdosed and acknowledged that her alcohol use was excessive and that she needed treatment; however, she did not want to discontinue alprazolam because she feared return of the panic attacks.

Discussion

This patient presents a challenging clinical situation, often referred to in the chemical dependence treatment field as dual diagnosis: a major psychiatric disorder and chemical dependence. Alcohol and drug treatment programs generally want patients to discontinue all psychoactive medications when they enter treatment. Chemical dependence treatment staffs often observe that alcohol-abusing patients increase their use of prescription medication when they stop drinking.

Because the patient's panic attacks had been disabling, and because the alcohol abuse seemed a response to an acute situational stress, the patient began outpatient (4 nights/week) chemical dependence treatment, she and her husband began couples therapy, and the patient increased the frequency of visits with her psychiatrist. With the increased support, the patient completed the separation from her husband, remained abstinent from alcohol, and remained on a carefully monitored dose of alprazolam.

or GAD. The clinical dilemma is deciding which patients are receiving appropriate maintenance therapy for a chronic psychiatric condition. Physical dependence on benzodiazepines may be acceptable if the patient's disabling anxiety symptoms are ameliorated. The reason for the patient's request for benzodiazepine withdrawal from long-term, stable dosing should be carefully explored. Valid reasons to discontinue benzodiazepine treatment include: 1) breakthrough of symptoms that were previously well controlled; 2) impairment of memory or other neurocognitive functions; and 3) abuse of alcohol, cocaine, or other medications.

Patients with severe underlying psychiatric disorders may have unrealistic hopes of becoming medication-free. Often the origin of request for benzodiazepine withdrawal comes from concerned friends or relatives.

Abuse Potential of Benzodiazepines

Most people do not like the subjective effects of benzodiazepines, especially in high doses. Even among drug addicts, the benzodiazepines alone are not common intoxicants. They are, however, widely used by drug addicts to self-medicate opiate withdrawal and to alleviate the side effects of cocaine and amphetamines. Patients receiving methadone maintenance use benzodiazepines to boost (enhance) the effects of methadone. Some alcoholic patients use benzodiazepines either in combination with alcohol or as a second-choice intoxicant, if alcohol is unavailable. Fat-soluble benzodiazepines that enter the CNS quickly are usually the benzodiazepines preferred by addicts.

Addicts whose urine is being monitored for benzodiazepines prefer benzodiazepines with high milligram potency, such as alprazolam or clonazepam. These benzodiazepines are excreted in urine in such small amounts that they are often not detected in drug screens, particularly with thin-layer chromatography.

Treatment of High-dose Benzodiazepine Dependence

For high-dose benzodiazepine dependence, the pharmacological treatment strategy is the same as that for barbiturates. The phenobarbital conversion equivalents are shown in Table 44.3. The dose conversions computed using Table 44.3 prevent the emergence of severe withdrawal of the classic sedative–hypnotic types. Some patients who take high doses of benzodiazepines, or even therapeutic doses for months to years, may have prolonged withdrawal symptoms.

Low-dose Benzodiazepine Withdrawal Syndromes

Many people who have taken benzodiazepines in therapeutic doses for months to years can abruptly discontinue the drug without developing withdrawal symptoms. But other patients, taking similar amounts of a benzodiazepine develop symptoms ranging from mild to severe when the benzodiapine is stopped or when the dosage is substantially reduced. Characteristically, patients tolerate a gradual tapering of the benzodiazepine until they are at 10 to 20% of their peak dose. Further reductions in benzodiazepine dose then cause patients to become increasingly symptomatic. In addition medicine literature, the low-dose withdrawal may be called therapeutic-dose withdrawal, normal-dose withdrawal, or benzodiazepine discontinuation syndrome. The symptoms can ultimately be categorized as symptom reemergence, symptom rebound, or a prolonged withdrawal syndrome.

Many patients experience a transient increase in symptoms for 1 to 2 weeks after benzodiazepine withdrawal. The symptoms are an intensified return of the symptoms for which the benzodiazepine was prescribed. This transient form of symptoms intensification is called **symptom rebound**. The term comes from sleep research in which rebound insomnia is commonly observed after sedative–hypnotic use. Symptom rebound lasts a few days to weeks after discontinuation Symptom rebound is the most common withdrawal consequence of prolonged benzodiazepine use.

The symptoms for which the benzodiazepine has been taken may return to the same level as before benzodiazepine therapy. This is called symptom reemergence (or recrudescence). In other words, the patient's symptoms, such as anxiety, insomnia, or muscle tension, that had abated during benzodiazepine treatment return.

The reason for making a distinction between symptom rebound and symptom reemergence is that symptom reemergence suggests that the original symptoms are still present and must be treated. Symptom rebound is a transient withdrawal syndrome that will disappear over time.

A few patients experience a severe, protracted withdrawal syndrome that includes symptoms (e.g., paresthesia and psychosis) that were not present before. This withdrawal syndrome has generated much of the concern about the long-term safety of the benzodiazepines.

Risk Factors for Low-dose Benzodiazepine Withdrawal

Some drugs or medications may facilitate neuroadaptation by increasing the affinity of benzodiazepines for their receptors. Phenobarbital, for example, increases the affinity of diazepam to benzodiazepine receptors and prior treatment with phenobarbital has been found to increase the intensity of chlordiazepoxide (45 mg/day) withdrawal symptoms. Patients at increased risk for development of the low-dose withdrawal syndrome are those with a family or personal history of alcoholism, those who use alcohol daily and those who concomitantly use other sedatives. Case–control studies suggest that patients with a history of addiction, particularly to other sedative–hypnotics, are at high risk for low-dose benzodiazepine dependence. The short-acting, high-milligram-potency benzodiazepines appear to produce a more intense low-dose withdrawal syndrome.

Treatment of Protracted Benzodiazepine Withdraw

Phenobarbital conversions based on Table 44.3 are not adequate to suppress symptoms. For example, someone discontinuing 20 mg of diazepam would have a computed phenobarbital conversion of 60 mg. In managing low-dose withdrawal, an approach is to begin with about 200 mg/day of phenobarbital and then taper the phenobarbital slowly as tolerated. If palpitations or other symptoms of autonomic hyperactivity are bothersome, beta-adrenergic blockers, such as propranolol or 2-adrenergic agonists, such as clonidine, may be useful adjuncts. Reports on the use of clonidine to reduce benzodiazepine withdrawal severity have yielded mixed results.

Comparison of DSM-IV/ICD-10 Diagnostic Criteria

The DSM-IV-TR and ICD-10 Criteria sets for Sedative, Hypnotic, or Anxiolytic Intoxication are almost equivalent (except that ICD-10 also includes "erythematous skin lesions or blisters". The DSM-IV-TR and ICD-10 symptom lists for Sedative, Hypnotic, or Anxiolytic Withdrawal include some different items: the ICD-10 list has craving, postural hypotension, headache, malaise or weakness and paranoid ideation and do not include the DSM-IV-TR anxiety item.

References

American Psychiatric Association (2000) *Diagnostic and Statistical Manual of Mental Disorders*, 4th edn., Text Rev. (DSM-IV-TR). APA, Washington DC.

Aragona M (2000) Abuse, dependence, and epileptic seizures after zolpidem withdrawal: Review and case report. *Clin Neuropharmacol* 23(5), 281–283.

45 Schizophrenia and Other Psychoses

Diagnosis

In DSM-IV, criterion A of schizophrenia includes delusions, hallucinations, disorganized speech, disorganized or catatonic behavior and negative symptoms. Two or more of these symptoms are required during the active phase of the illness. However, if the patient describes bizarre delusions or auditory hallucinations consisting of a voice commenting on the patient's behavior or voices conversing, only one of these symptoms is required to reach the diagnosis. It is important to distinguish negative symptoms, which are often difficult to appreciate, from the myriad factors that may contribute to the severity and serious morbidity associated with schizophrenia. Patients who are not motivated to attend to their personal hygiene or suffer from alogia and a flattened affect are sadly at a disadvantage in society. The addition of negative symptoms as a separate criterion in DSM-IV recognizes the prominence of these symptoms in patients with schizophrenia.

DSM-IV-TR Criteria 295.xx

Schizophrenia

A. Characteristic symptoms: Two (or more) of the following, each present for a significant portion of time during a 1-month period (or less if successfully treated):

   (1) delusions
   (2) hallucinations
   (3) disorganized speech (e.g., frequent derailment or incoherence)
   (4) grossly disorganized or catatonic behavior
   (5) negative symptoms, i.e., affective flattening, alogia, or avolition

Note: Only one criterion A symptom is required if delusions are bizarre or hallucinations consist of a voice keeping up a running commentary on the person's behavior or thoughts, or two or more voices conversing with each other.

B. Social/occupational dysfunction: For a significant portion of the time since the onset of the disturbance, one or more major areas of functioning such as work, interpersonal relations, or self-care are markedly below the level achieved prior to the onset (or when the onset is in childhood or adolescence, failure to achieve expected level of interpersonal, academic, or occupational achievement).

C. Duration: Continuous signs of the disturbance persist for at least 6 months. This 6-month period must include at least 1 month of symptoms (or less if successfully treated) that meet criterion A (i.e., active-phase symptoms) and may include periods of prodromal or residual symptoms. During these prodromal or residual periods, the signs of the disturbance may be manifested by only negative symptoms or two or more symptoms listed in criterion A present in an attenuated form (e.g., odd beliefs, unusual perceptual experiences).

D. Schizoaffective and mood disorder exclusion: Schizoaffective disorder and mood disorder with psychotic features have been ruled out because either (1) no major depressive, manic, or mixed episodes have occurred concurrently with the active-phase symptoms; or (2) if mood episodes have occurred during active-phase symptoms, their total duration has been brief relative to the duration of the active and residual periods.

E. Substance/general medical condition exclusion: The disturbance is not due to the direct physiological effects of a substance (e.g., a drug of abuse, a medication) or a general medical condition.

F. Relationship to a pervasive developmental disorder: If there is a history of autistic disorder or another pervasive developmental disorder, the additional diagnosis of schizophrenia is made only if prominent delusions or hallucinations are also present for at least a month (or less if successfully treated).

Reprinted with permission from the Diagnostic and Statistical Manual of Mental Disorders, Fourth Edition, Text Revision. Copyright 2000 American Psychiatric Association.

DSM-IV Subtypes of Schizophrenia

In DSM-IV, schizophrenia has been divided into clinical subtypes, based on field trials of the reliability of symptom clusters. The subtypes are divided by the most prominent symptoms, although it is acknowledged that the specific subtype may exist simultaneously with or change over the course of the illness. DSM-IV also initiates an optional dimensional descriptor, which allows the condition to be characterized by the presence or absence of a psychotic, disorganized, or negative symptom dimension over the entire course of the illness.

Essentials of Psychiatry   Jerald Kay and Allan Tasman
© 2006 John Wiley & Sons, Ltd.

Paranoid Type

In DSM-IV, paranoid-type schizophrenia is marked by hallucinations or delusions in the presence of a clear sensorium and unchanged cognition. Disorganized speech, disorganized behavior and flat or inappropriate affect are not present to any significant degree. The delusions (usually of a persecutory or grandiose nature) and the hallucinations most often revolve around a particular theme or themes. Because of their delusions, these patients may attempt to keep the interviewer at bay, and thus they may appear hostile or angry during an interview. This type of schizophrenia may have a later age of onset and a better prognosis than the other subtypes.

DSM-IV-TR Criteria 295.30

Paranoid Type

A type of schizophrenia in which the following criteria are met:

A. Preoccupation with one or more delusions or frequent auditory hallucinations.

B. None of the following is prominent: disorganized speech, disorganized or catatonic behavior, or flat or inappropriate affect.

Reprinted with permission from the *Diagnostic and Statistical Manual of Mental Disorders*, Fourth Edition, Text Revision. Copyright 2000 American Psychiatric Association.

Disorganized Type

Disorganized schizophrenia, historically referred to as hebephrenic schizophrenia, presents with the hallmark symptoms of disorganized speech and/or behavior, along with flat or inappropriate (incongruent) affect. Any delusions or hallucinations, if present, also tend to be disorganized and are not related to a single theme. Furthermore, these patients would not be classified as having catatonic schizophrenia. These patients in general have more severe deficits on neuropsychological tests. According to DSM-IV, these patients tend to have an earlier age at onset, an unremitting course, and a poor prognosis.

DSM-IV-TR Criteria 295.10

Disorganized Type

A type of schizophrenia in which the following criteria are met:

A. All of the following are prominent:

(1) disorganized speech
(2) disorganized behavior
(3) flat or inappropriate affect

B. The criteria are not met for catatonic type.

Reprinted with permission from the *Diagnostic and Statistical Manual of Mental Disorders*, Fourth Edition, Text Revision. Copyright 2000 American Psychiatric Association.

DSM-IV-TR Criteria 295.20

Catatonic Type

A type of schizophrenia in which the clinical picture is dominated by at least two of the following:

(1) motoric immobility as evidenced by catalepsy (including waxy flexibility) or stupor

(2) excessive motor activity (that is apparently purposeless and not influenced by external stimuli)

(3) extreme negativism (an apparently motiveless resistance to all instructions or maintenance of a rigid posture against attempts to be moved) or mutism

(4) peculiarities of voluntary movement as evidenced by posturing (voluntary assumption of inappropriate or bizarre postures), stereotyped movements, prominent mannerisms, or prominent grimacing

(5) echolalia or echopraxia

Reprinted with permission from the *Diagnostic and Statistical Manual of Mental Disorders*, Fourth Edition, Text Revision. Copyright 2000 American Psychiatric Association.

Catatonic Type

Catatonic schizophrenia has unique features that distinguish it from other subtypes of schizophrenia in DSM-IV for Catatonic Schizophrenia. During the acute phase of this illness, patients may demonstrate marked negativism or mutism, profound psychomotor retardation or severe psychomotor agitation, echolalia (repetition of words or phrases in a nonsensical manner), echopraxia (mimicking the behaviors of others), or bizarreness of voluntary movements and mannerisms. Some patients demonstrate a waxy flexibility, which is seen when a limb is repositioned on examination and remains in that position as if the patient were made of wax. Patients with catatonic stupor must be protected against bodily harm resulting from the profound psychomotor retardation. They may remain in the same position for weeks at a time. Because of extreme mutism or agitation, patients may not be able to report any difficulties. Some patients may experience extreme psychomotor agitation, with grimacing and bizarre postures. These patients may require careful monitoring to safeguard them from injury or deterioration in nutritional status or fluid balance.

Undifferentiated Type

There is no hallmark symptom of undifferentiated schizophrenia; thus, it is the subtype that meets the criterion A for schizophrenia

DSM-IV-TR Criteria 295.90

Undifferentiated Type

A type of schizophrenia in which symptoms that meet criterion A are present, but the criteria are not met for the paranoid, disorganized, or catatonictype.

Reprinted with permission from the *Diagnostic and Statistical Manual of Mental Disorders*, Fourth Edition, Text Revision. Copyright 2000 American Psychiatric Association.

out does not fit the profile for paranoid, disorganized, or catatonic schizophrenia.

Residual Type

The diagnosis of residual schizophrenia, according to DSM-IV, is appropriately used when there is a past history of an acute episode of schizophrenia but at the time of presentation the patient does not manifest any of the associated psychotic or positive symptoms. However, there is continued evidence of schizophrenia manifested in either negative symptoms or low-grade symptoms of criterion A. These may include odd behavior, some abnormalities of thought processes, or delusions or hallucinations that exist in a minimal form. This type of schizophrenia has an unpredictable, variable course.

DSM-IV-TR Criteria 295.60

Residual Type

A type of schizophrenia in which the following criteria are met:

A. Absence of prominent delusions, hallucinations, disorganized speech, and grossly disorganized or catatonic behavior.

B. There is continuing evidence of the disturbance, as indicated by the presence of negative symptoms or two or more symptoms listed in criterion A for schizophrenia, present in an attenuated form (e.g., odd beliefs, unusual perceptual experiences).

Reprinted with permission from the *Diagnostic and Statistical Manual of Mental Disorders*, Fourth Edition, Text Revision. Copyright 2000 American Psychiatric Association.

One must avoid imposing Western definitions of psychosis on nonWestern societies. Psychosis and delusions, by definition, must be beliefs or experiences that are incongruent with those of the patient's social or cultural background. To determine where culture-bound beliefs end and delusions or inappropriate behaviors begin in a multicultural world is clearly not possible using only a written algorithm such as DSM-IV. A critical step toward sound cross-cultural clinical care is developing an awareness of and a respect for diversity. Utilizing the expertise of persons familiar with a specific culture allows appropriate diagnosis and treatment of schizophrenia worldwide.

Epidemiological Findings: Incidence and Prevalence

The incidence of schizophrenia is defined as the number of new cases in a given population, usually per 1000 persons, during a specific period of time (1 year by convention). In an illness with an insidious onset, such as schizophrenia, accurate incidence rates can be difficult to determine. The incidence varies depending on the methods and the diagnostic criteria used. For example, the US–UK study is often cited as an example of epidemiological variation based on different diagnostic criteria (Kramer, 1969). This study, conducted in the 1960s, found a lower incidence of schizophrenia in the UK than in the USA. It is now widely accepted that this difference was found because a broader definition

of schizophrenia was being used in the USA, and it did not reflect true differences in the incidence of schizophrenia in each country.

The data obtained from World Health Organization (WHO) studies are important in part because the same diagnostic criteria were used in all countries studied. According to the results of the International Pilot Study of Schizophrenia, schizophrenia is found in all cultures and the incidence rates per 1000 people annually ranged from 0.15 in Denmark to 0.42 in India (WHO, 1973).

Because schizophrenia is a chronic illness, the incidence rates must, by definition, be much lower than the prevalence rates. Prevalence is defined as the number of cases present in a specified population at a given time or time interval (e.g., at a specific point in time, during a time period, or over a lifetime). Lifetime prevalence represents the proportion of persons who have ever had the illness at a given time. Lifetime prevalence rates of schizophrenia, based on the Epidemiology Catchment Area (ECA) data, were approximately 1% (range across three sites, 1–1.9%) (Robins *et al.*, 1984). Point prevalence rates based on International Pilot Study of Schizophrenia data showed no significant differences across study centers: schizophrenia was found universally with relatively equal frequencies in a wide variety of cultures.

Sociodemographical Characteristics

Age

An investigation of late-onset schizophrenia found that 28% of patients had the onset of illness after age 44 years and 12% after age 63 years, based on 470 chart reviews of patients who had sought psychiatric help during a period of 20 years (Castle and Murray, 1993). Although the majority of patients have an early age at onset, a certain subgroup of patients may have a disturbance that meets all the criteria of schizophrenia with onset in their forties or later.

The phenomenology of late-onset compared with early-onset schizophrenia may be distinct, with later-onset cases having a higher level of premorbid social functioning and exhibiting paranoid delusions and hallucinations more often than formal thought disorder, disorganization and negative symptoms. Studies have also shown a high comorbid risk of sensory deficits, such as loss of hearing or vision, in patients with late-onset schizophrenia. Specifically, late-onset patients are more likely to report visual, tactile and olfactory hallucinations and are less likely to display affective flattening or blunting. One of the most robust finding among the late-onset cases is the higher prevalence seen in women. This does not appear to be due to sex differences in seeking care, societal role expectations or delay between emergence of symptoms and service contact.

Gender

A large body of data suggests that although men and women have an equivalent lifetime risk; the age at onset varies with sex. Strong evidence that onset of schizophrenia is on average 3.5 to 6 years earlier in men than in women.

There is undoubtedly a subgroup of patients who have a later onset of illness (after age 45 years), and this subgroup is made up predominantly of women Among these female schizophrenia patients, there is a higher incidence of comorbid affective symptoms. When the effects of gender, premorbid personality, marital status and family history of psychosis on the age at onset were removed in a reanalysis of the WHO 10-country study data, there was a significant attenuation of the gender differences (Jablensky and Cole, 1997).

Race

The ECA data have shown that there is no significant difference in the prevalence of schizophrenia between black and white persons when corrected for age, sex, socioeconomic status and marital status (Robins and Regier, 1991). This finding is significant because it refutes prior studies that have shown the prevalence of schizophrenia to be much greater in the black population than in the white population.

Marital Status and Fertility

A study of marriage and fertility rates of individuals with schizophrenia compared with the general population showed that, on average, by the age of 45 years, three times as many of those with schizophrenia as of the general population are still unmarried (40% of men and 30% of women with schizophrenia are still single by age 45). Studies have also shown that fertility rates are lower in patients with schizophrenia compared with the general population. These observations may be related, and further investigation of the role of premorbid function, negative symptoms and fertility rates, including rates among unmarried patients, is warranted. With the advent of the newer and more effective antipsychotic medications, and their increased use in first episode patients, it is possible that we may witness improved fertility and marriage rates in patients with schizophrenia.

Socioeconomic Status

For many years, epidemiological studies revealed a higher incidence and prevalence of schizophrenia in groups with lower socioeconomic status. In the past half century, studies have found that the actual incidence of schizophrenia does not vary with social class, based on first admission rates, adoption studies and a series of studies examining the social class of the fathers of people with schizophrenia. When these findings did not validate the original theory, it became clear that lower socioeconomic status was more a result than a cause of schizophrenia. This led to the acceptance of the downward drift hypothesis, which stated that because of the nature of schizophrenic symptoms, people who develop schizophrenia are unable to attain employment and positions in society that would allow them to achieve a higher social status. Thus, these patients drift down the socioeconomic ladder, and because of the illness itself they may become dependent on society for their well-being.

Season of Birth and Onset

That season of birth differs between individuals with schizophrenia and the general population has by now gained wide acceptance. This factor has been studied in the 20th century, with the predominant view that the birth rate of people with schizophrenia is highest in late winter. Torrey and colleagues (1997) confirmed this, reviewing approximately 250 studies and concluding that there is an excess of schizophrenia births during winter. In fact, there is approximately a 5 to 8% greater likelihood for individuals with schizophrenia to be born during winter months compared with the general population. This higher incidence of winter births has been found in both hemispheres, offering further evidence that this phenomenon is related to the colder months rather than specific calendar months.

Morbidity and Mortality

The economic costs of schizophrenia have been estimated to be six times the costs of myocardial infarction. The WHO has estimated that mental illness accounts for as much as two-fifths of all disability funding in the USA. In the USA, the cost of schizophrenia in 1994 was $44.9 billion and rising. Much of the cost of schizophrenia is due to the high morbidity of this chronic illness. Premorbid deficits, cognitive deficits and negative symptoms account for much of the disability. Also, schizophrenia patients with more severe courses may require repeated hospitalizations and may not be capable of maintaining independent living or stable employment.

The mortality rate of schizophrenia is estimated to be twice that of the general population. Approximately 10% of the mortality is secondary to suicide Young male patients with schizophrenia are most likely to complete suicide attempts, especially early in their illness. Degree of social isolation, agitation, depression, a sense of hopelessness, a history of prior suicide attempts and recent loss may be associated with increased risk of suicide among schizophrenia patients. There is also some evidence that an increased number of relapses, rehospitalizations and discharges lead to an increased risk of suicide. There have been observations that suicide rates of schizophrenia patients may be increasing in the era of shorter hospital stays and community treatment. However, with the advent of the novel antipsychotic medication and especially with clozapine use, it is possible that this risk of suicide may even out or decrease due to their possible protective effects against suicide. Other factors leading to increased mortality rates in schizophrenia patients include an increased incidence of accidents as well as a more frequent association with other medical illnesses (including cardiovascular disease), comorbid substance abuse, a general neglect of health, an increased rate of damaging behaviors such as smoking and poor diet, decreased access to health services and depression.

Comorbidity with Other Illnesses

Schizophrenia is associated with an increased frequency of tuberculosis (not accounted for by institutionalization), celiac disease, myxedema and arteriosclerotic heart disease. Patients who present with atypical psychoses have been noted to have an increased risk of ankylosing spondylitis and uroarthritis, which may indicate a relationship between the histocompatibility complex and schizophrenia. Along these lines, there is a strikingly decreased risk for rheumatoid arthritis among patients with schizophrenia.

Etiology

The cause of schizophrenia is currently not known. A leading view is that schizophrenia may be heterogeneous with respect to etiology. Thus, multiple causative mechanisms may give rise to distinct disease subtypes. If this is true, it is important for psychiatric researchers to differentiate the homogeneous subtypes of this illness. Moreover, it has been proposed that more than one causative mechanism might interact (the so-called double-hit hypothesis) to cause the illness in some individuals. In this section, the main etiological theories of schizophrenia are examined.

Genetics

Schizophrenia represents a daunting challenge for genetic researchers for several reasons: the paucity of extended multigenerational family histories containing large numbers of affected individuals; the possibility of genetic heterogeneity, such as more than one phenotype or more than one genetic variant; and a lack of agreement on the mode of transmission. The focus of research has shifted to multiple genes of small to moderate effects which may compound their effects through interactions with each other and with other nongenetic risk factors.

Family Prevalence Studies

Wide agreement now exists that the rate of schizophrenia among first-degree family members of persons with schizophrenia is higher than in control families. The chance of occurrence is approximately 10 times greater among these individuals than in individuals with no first-degree relatives with schizophrenia. There is approximately six times and two times greater chance of developing schizophrenia in second- and third-degree relatives of individuals with schizophrenia respectively. In addition, the higher prevalence of schizophrenia spectrum disorders among family members of individuals with schizophrenia, such as schizoaffective disorder and schizoid and schizotypal personality disorders, provides support for a common genetic basis for this family of schizophrenia-like illnesses.

Adoption Studies

Adoption studies constitute a powerful experimental strategy for examining the role of genetic versus environmental factors. In these studies, the rates of schizophrenia are compared in relatives of adoptees with and without schizophrenia. Danish adoption studies conducted in the 1960s and 1970s provided compelling evidence that adoptees with schizophrenia had higher rates of schizophrenia in their first-degree relatives than control adoptees. A reanalysis of these data in the late 1980s confirmed the original finding that biological relatives of schizophrenia adoptees had significantly higher rates of schizophrenia (4.1%) than biological relatives of nonschizophrenia (control) adoptees (0.5%). Several methodological issues are important in interpreting the data from adoption studies, including the diagnostic status of biological fathers and levels of psychopathology in adoptive families. Additional factors to consider are the intrauterine environment, birth complications and length of time from birth to adoptive placement.

Twin Studies

Another approach to examining genetic contributions to schizophrenia involves concordance studies of dizygotic (nonidentical) and monozygotic (identical) twin pairs. Available data indicate that the concordance of schizophrenia among dizygotic twins is approximately 8 to 12%. This is much greater than the 1% rate found in the general population and comparable to the rate of concordance of schizophrenia among first-degree siblings. The concordance of schizophrenia among monozygotic twins is approximately 50%. Even though the high rate of concordance among monozygotic twin pairs is compelling evidence for genetic contributions, the fact that it is not higher than 50% suggests a role for additional, perhaps nongenetic, factors in the etiology of schizophrenia. The number of sets of adopted-away, monozygotic twin pairs affected with schizophrenia is relatively small. However, data available on the limited number of pairs meeting these criteria support the strong concordance of schizophrenia in monozygotic twins.

Linkage and Association Studies

The Human Genome Project with its 3 billion base pairs and approximately 35 000 genes has ushered us into the "Genomic Era". However, systematic genome scans done recently have not resulted in strong evidence for linkage to any chromosomal region. At the time of this writing, no genetic linkage or association related to schizophrenia has been discovered. There have been reports of suggestive linkages but there has been a failure to replicate these findings. It has become painfully clear that the replication studies are, in many ways, more important to establishing linkage than the initial report. Genes that have been found not to be associated with schizophrenia include the dopamine D_2 and D_4 genes.

The initial enthusiasm for these strategies has waned as no gene has yet been isolated for schizophrenia or bipolar disorder. Impediments that have limited the success of linkage and association studies are etiologic and phenotypic heterogeneity of schizophrenia, lack of power and high false positive rates. Thus, newer approaches such as multi-investigator collaborative studies to increase the power have already been implemented.

Meanwhile, modern functional genomic approaches such as DNA microarrays, based on the principles of nucleic acid hybridization, can check a tissue sample for presence of thousands of genes simultaneously. For example, Mirnics and colleagues (2000) employed cDNA microarrays and compared transcriptomes in schizophrenia and matched control subjects and found that only a few gene groups consistently differed between subjects and controls. In all subjects with schizophrenia, the most changed gene group was related to **presynaptic group secretory function** (PSYN) gene group and in particular the "mechanics" of neurotransmitter release.

Weinberger and colleagues (2001) suggest that the gene that encodes the postsynaptic enzyme catechol-*o*-methyl transferase (COMT) is preferentially involved in the metabolism of dopamine in frontal lobe. Dopamine is hypothesized to underlie aspects of cognition in frontal lobe such as information processing. Based on animal studies, family-based association studies and fMRI studies in schizophrenia patients and general population, Weinberger and colleagues propose an interesting hypothesis that the COMT genotype with valenine allele (val/val type) may increase the risk of developing schizophrenia due to its effect on dopamine-mediated prefrontal information processing.

Researchers are urgently searching for schizophrenia phenotypes for subgroups or dimensions that may define etiologically or genetically distinct subtypes. Similarly, the field is yearning for **endophenotypes** with simpler architecture than schizophrenia possibly to guide to newer leads in research. Latent genetically influenced traits, which may be related only indirectly to the classic disease symptoms defined in major classification systems, are known as "endophenotypes". They reflect an underlying susceptibility to the disease phenotype (or some form of it). In schizophrenia we are interested in endophenotypes that are measurable by neurophysiological or neuropsychological means. Crucial characteristics of any endophenotype include the fact that it can be measured before the explicit onset of the illness, and that it represents the genetic liability of nonaffected relatives of probands with the disorder.

Viral Hypotheses

Two lines of evidence that have provoked the most interest in the possibility that viral infections are causative of schizophrenia are an increase in birth during influenza epidemics of individuals who subsequently develop schizophrenia and an increase in winter births among patients with schizophrenia because of the higher rate of viral infections in winter months. However, negative results from multiple studies have raised serious questions about this theory. Several studies have demonstrated an excess of winter births among patients with schizophrenia. Although statistically significant, the association between winter births and schizophrenia appears relatively small, occurring in less than 10% of cases. Thus, season of birth remains an interesting (and unresolved) research issue but has little use as a risk factor for the illness from a clinical perspective. Exposure to influenza *in utero* and excess winter births are interesting although indirect lines of evidence for a viral cause of schizophrenia. To date, there has been no direct confirmation for any viral agent causing this illness, such as viral isolates or consistent findings of specific viral antibodies. Advances in neurovirology, however, are providing new insights into the role of viruses in brain diseases, leading to new hypotheses about schizophrenia. One area involves the search for neurotropic retroviruses.

Immune Dysfunction

Several research groups are exploring the possibility that schizophrenia may be associated with impaired immune function including alterations in autoimmunity. Anticardiolipin antibody and antinuclear antibody, two autoantibodies that are used as markers of autoimmune vulnerability, have been shown to be increased in patients with schizophrenia in some but not all studies of this illness. Two other markers relevant to autoimmune function, impaired T lymphocyte proliferative response to the mitogen phytohemagglutinin and impaired interleukin-2 production, have shown more consistent alterations in patients with schizophrenia than in control populations. Some of the most intriguing work in this area is focused on finding autoantibodies to brain tissue.

Birth Complications

Numerous studies have reported a higher rate of pregnancy and birth complications in patients with schizophrenia than in control populations. The complication rates vary widely among studies, probably because of the inherent difficulties in obtaining reliable and valid retrospective data in this area. In one study, two-thirds of schizophrenia patients and less than one-third of control subjects had histories of obstetrical complications. Hypoxia is one possible result of pregnancy and birth complications that has been shown to disrupt brain development. The hippocampus and some neocortical regions are particularly sensitive to shortfalls in oxygen. Thus, one proposed mechanism for a role of pregnancy and birth complications in the cause of schizophrenia involves hypoxia-mediated damage to these areas. Interestingly, some studies suggest that the rate of obstetric complications are higher in early-onset schizophrenia, occur more often in males, in people with prominent negative symptoms, and no family history of schizophrenia.

Pathophysiology

Whereas **etiology** refers to the cause of an illness, **pathophysiology** refers to the abnormal processes that mediate the clinical manifestation of the illness. As was the case with etiology, the brain processes that give rise to schizophrenia are currently not known. However, rapidly converging bodies of neuroanatomical and neurochemical data appear to be closing in on defining the pathophysiology of this illness.

Neuroanatomical Theories

Enlarged Ventricles

The ventricles are the fluid-filled spaces in the center of the brain. The most consistent morphological finding in the literature of schizophrenia is enlarged ventricles which has been confirmed by a large number of CT and MRI studies. The effect size of ventriculomegaly has been reported to be 0.7 (Raz and Raz, 1990). Seventy-nine percent of the well designed studies report enlargement of lateral ventricles. Lawrie and Abukmeil (1998) report approximately 40% difference in volume between schizophrenia patients and controls across all volumetric MRI studies. It should be noted that although the ventricular increases are statistically significant, the ventricles are not grossly enlarged in most cases. In fact, radiologists most often read CT and MRI scans of patients with schizophrenia as normal. In addition, most studies of ventricular size demonstrate overlap between patients and normal control subjects, indicating that many patients have ventricles in the normal range. Nonetheless, enlargement of the ventricles is the first consistently reported finding confirming a brain abnormality in schizophrenia.

The pathophysiological significance of larger than normal ventricles is unclear. Enlarged ventricles are most likely a secondary manifestation of brain atrophy or some other process resulting in either focal or generalized reductions in brain mass. Indeed, there have been many reports of brain atrophy and reduced mass in the illness (Figure 45.1). Enlarged ventricles have also been reported in first-degree relatives of subjects with schizophrenia (Cannon *et al.*, 1998; Seidman *et al.*, 1997) and in persons suffering from schizotypal personality disorder (Buchsbaum *et al.*, 1997) raising interesting speculations of whether ventriculomegaly may be an indicator of neurodevelopmental risk for schizophrenia (Lencz *et al.*, 2001).

Limbic System

The limbic structures that have been implicated in schizophrenia are the hippocampus, entorhinal cortex, anterior cingulate and amygdala. These structures have important functions for memory (hippocampus), attention (anterior cingulate), and emotional expression and social affiliation (amygdala). The entorhinal cortex serves as a "way station" between hippocampus and neocortex in that neurotransmissions between these regions synapse in the entorhinal cortex. The entorhinal cortex, hippocampus and other components of the parahippocampal gyrus are often considered "mesiotemporal" structures because of their close anatomical and functional relationship.

There are more reports of abnormalities in hippocampal and related mesiotemporal structures than other limbic structures in schizophrenia. In fact, mesiotemporal pathology is consistently found in studies of schizophrenia and mesiotemporal structures are leading candidates for the neuroanatomical site of this condition. This region has been implicated by converging brain imaging and postmortem lines of evidence. One of the most consistent MRI morphological findings is reduction in size of the hippocampus. In addition, more than 25 postmortem studies have reported morphological and cytoarchitectural abnormalities in this structure. The findings have included reduced size and

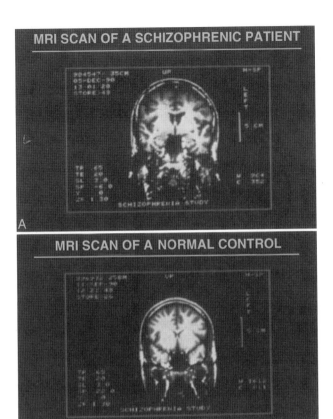

Figure 45.1 *CT scans of a schizophrenic patient* (A) *and a healthy volunteer* (B). *Note enlarged ventricular spaces and brain atrophy in the scan of the patient with schizophrenia.*

cellular number (white matter reductions, and abnormal cell arrangement. There is a bilateral reduction of approximately 4% hippocampal volume in schizophrenia. However, reduced hippocampal volume is not reported by all studies.

The anterior cingulate has been implicated in schizophrenia largely because of postmortem findings of reduced gamma-aminobutyric acid (GABA) interneurons. In addition, functional imaging studies have demonstrated altered metabolic activity both at rest and during selective attention tasks in the anterior cingulate in patients with schizophrenia. Thirty-one studies evaluated one or more of the medial temporal lobe structures – hippocampus, amygdala, parahippocampal gyrus, entorhinal cortex – with 77% reporting positive findings; this is one of the higher percentages of abnormalities reported in all regions of interest throughout the brain.

Prefrontal Cortex

The prefrontal cortex is the most anterior portion of the neocortex, sitting behind the forehead. It has evolved through lower species to become one of the largest regions of the human brain, constituting approximately one-third of the cortex. It is responsible for some of the most sophisticated human functions. It contains a heteromodal association area that is responsible for integrating information from all other cortical areas as well as from several subcortical regions for the execution of purposeful behavior. Among its specific functions are working memory, which involves the temporary storage (seconds to minutes) of information, attention and suppression of interference from internal and external sources. The most inferior portion of the

prefrontal cortex, termed the orbital frontal cortex, is involved in emotional expression. Given its unique role, it is not surprising that the prefrontal cortex has been considered in the etiology of schizophrenia.

Indeed, several lines of evidence have implicated the prefrontal cortex in schizophrenia. CT studies have provided evidence for prefrontal atrophy, and some, although not all, MRI studies have found evidence for decreased volume of this structure. One of the earliest observations from functional imaging studies of schizophrenia was reduced perfusion of the frontal lobes. This finding was subsequently replicated by several PET studies suggesting decreased frontal glucose utilization and blood flow, which came to be known as **hypofrontality**. Subsequent functional imaging studies provided further support for hypofrontality by demonstrating that patients with schizophrenia failed to activate their frontal lobes to the same degree as normal control subjects when performing frontal cognitive tasks. This finding has been questioned because patients with schizophrenia typically perform poorly in many cognitive paradigms, so it is unclear whether their lack of frontal activation is a primary frontal deficit or secondary to poor cognitive task performance related to factors such as lack of motivation, inattention, or cognitive impairment stemming from nonfrontal regions. Auditory hallucinations were found to be associated with increases in Broca's area, a portion of the frontal cortex responsible for language production. This finding was of interest because it supported a hypothesis that auditory hallucinations were a form of abnormal "inner speech".

MRI studies employing diffusion tensor imaging have reported changes suggestive of an abnormality in white matter connectivity possibly due to reduced myelination of fiber tracts in patients with schizophrenia (Buchsbaum *et al.*, 1998). Magnetic resonance spectroscopy (MRS) studies have reported reduced levels of neuronal membrane constituents (phosphomonoesters) and/or increased levels of their breakdown products (phosphodiesters) in patients with schizophrenia, primarily in the frontal cortex. Such abnormalities have been observed in treatment-naive first episode patients and have been correlated with trait-like negative symptoms and neurocognitive performance.

Though sometimes contradictory, the neuroimaging studies consistently report abnormalities in the orbitofrontal region; often, these abnormalities tend to correlate with severity of schizophrenia symptomatology, show gender differences in relation to spatial localization and the gray matter deficits may be more widespread in chronic, as compared with medication-naive first episode patients. Additional support for prefrontal cortical involvement in schizophrenia comes from postmortem studies with a range of findings. There have been reports of reduced cortical thickness, loss of pyramidal cells, malformed cellular architecture, loss of GABA interneurons and evidence of failed neuronal migration. A majority of the abnormalities represented a decline in function suggesting a widespread failure of gene expression. Specifically, abnormalities involving the glycoprotein *Reelin* were observed in schizophrenia, a finding reported previously by other postmortem studies. *Reelin*, an extracellular matrix glycoprotein secreted from different GABAergic interneurons during development and adult life, may be important for the transcription of specific genes necessary for synaptic plasticity and morphological changes associated with learning.

Temporal Lobe

The superior temporal gyrus is involved in auditory processing and, with parts of the inferior parietal cortex, is a heteromodal association area that includes Wernicke's area, a language center. Because of the important role it plays in audition, it was hypothesized to be involved in auditory hallucinations. Indeed, MRI studies have found the superior temporal gyrus to be reduced in size in schizophrenia and have found a significant relationship between these reductions and the presence of auditory hallucinations. Similarly, Wernicke's area, which is involved in the conception and organization of speech, has been hypothesized to mediate the thought disorder of schizophrenia, particularly conceptual disorganization. Support for this hypothesis comes from a report of a patient with vascular and other lesions of this region that produce Wernicke's aphasia, a disruption in the organization of speech that resembles the thought disorder of schizophrenia. MRI studies have found a relationship between morphological abnormalities in this region and conceptual disorganization in schizophrenia. McCarley and colleagues (1999) reviewed 118 MRI studies published from 1988 to 1998; 62% of the 37 studies of whole temporal lobe showed volume reduction and/or abnormal asymmetry especially in the superior temporal gyrus, the highest percentage of any cortical region of interest.

Striatum

The striatum, consisting of the caudate, putamen, globus pallidus, substantia nigra and accumbens, is an output center for the cortex and has been traditionally thought to have a primary role in the execution of motor programs. Subsequent studies have demonstrated an important cognitive role for this structure as well. Moreover, in primary diseases of the striatum, such as Parkinson's and Huntington's diseases, clinical manifestations include psychosis and other schizophrenia type behavior, which has contributed to interest in this region in the pathophysiology of schizophrenia.

Two related bodies of data are most frequently cited regarding the role of the striatum in schizophrenia; these concern the mechanism of antipsychotic drugs and postmortem studies of altered dopamine D_2 receptor numbers. The dorsal striatum (caudate and putamen) is the site of the vast majority of D_2 receptors in the brain. All effective antipsychotic drugs antagonize this receptor and thus, by extrapolation, it was reasoned that this region might be central to the pathophysiology of schizophrenia. Moreover, the most consistent postmortem finding in the schizophrenia literature is an increased density of striatal D_2 receptors. However, neuroleptic exposure causes up-regulation of D_2 receptors, which may account for this postmortem finding. A current view of the antipsychotic mechanism is that the dorsal striatum is involved in mediating the extrapyramidal side effects of antipsychotic medications and, based on rodent studies of antipsychotic drug mechanisms, the ventral striatum (nucleus accumbens) may be involved in antipsychotic efficacy. Thus, attention has shifted toward the possible role of the accumbens in mediating the psychosis of schizophrenia.

Thalamus

The thalamus is a nucleus that receives subcortical input and outputs it to the cortex. One theory posits that the thalamus provides a filtering function for sensory input to the cortex. A deficit in thalamic filtering was proposed to account in part for the experiential phenomena of being overwhelmed by sensory stimuli reported by many patients with schizophrenia. Preclinical studies have demonstrated that antipsychotic drugs modulate thalamic input to the cortex, which has been offered as a model for antipsychotic drug action. Several MRI studies have reported reduced

volume, and functional abnormalities of the thalamus in patients with schizophrenia. Postmortem studies have also found cell loss and reductions in tissue volume in thalamic nuclei. This thalamic tissue reduction is considered as a possible evidence of abnormal circuitry linking the cortex, thalamus and cerebellum.

Neural Circuits

Because of the large number of different neuroanatomical findings in studies of schizophrenia and the appreciation that brain function involves integration of several brain regions, current thinking about the neuroanatomy of this illness is centered on neural circuits. It is conceivable that an isolated lesion anywhere in a neural circuit could result in dysfunction of the entire network, and therefore spurious conclusions could be drawn by investigating only one component of a neural network. Evidence suggests that schizophrenia may be associated with a decrease in synaptic connectivity of the dorsal prefrontal cortex though this is not reported by all studies. McGlashan and Hoffman (2000) have proposed the Developmentally Reduced Synaptic Connectivity (DRSC) model which proposes that cortical gray matter deficits may arise from either reduced baseline synaptic density due to genetic and/or perinatal factors, or excessive pruning of synapses during adolescence and early adulthood or both. There is regionally specific decreased neuronal size in cortical layer III with cytoplasmic atrophy and generally reduced neuropil. The reduced size and increased density of neurons or glia and decreased cortical thickness suggest that cell processes and synaptic connections are reduced in schizophrenia. This is consistent with reports of decreased concentrations of synaptic proteins (e.g., synaptophysin). These cell processes and synapses could be lost as a consequence of a neurochemically mediated (through dopamine and or glutamate) synaptic apoptosis that would compromise cell function and alter brain morphology without, however, producing serious cell injury (and thus inducing glial reactions). However, McCarley and colleagues (1999) suggest that the main neural abnormality in schizophrenia involves neural connectivity (dendrite/neuropil/gray matter changes) rather than the number of neurons or network size. They suggest that a "failure of inhibition" on the cellular level is present in schizophrenia and may be linked to a "failure of inhibition" at the cognitive level. According to Lafargue and Brasic (2000) abnormalities involving the temporolimbic–prefrontal cerebral circuitry is postulated to underlie the organizational and memory deficits commonly observed in schizophrenia patients. Furthermore, as reviewed by these authors, a possible insult or injury to the mechanism of GABAergic and glutamatergic influence during early corticogenesis may largely contribute to the later manifestation of clinical schizophrenia. Malfunction of the cooperating sensory systems of excitation and inhibition during the early stages of development of the brain could result in the failure of "pioneer neurons" properly to differentiate and migrate to their appropriate cerebral locations. Consequently the later migrating projection neurons may fail to reach or invade their preselected area-specific brain sites. A disturbance of the proper GABAergic and glutamatergic influences would upset NMDA mechanisms and normal cortical development. If such disturbance is actively occurring from the onset of cerebral ontogeny, the affected individual may suffer from the signs and symptoms observed in schizophrenia. A challenge for the future is developing new approaches to examining the brain as an integrated and highly interactive system. An unanswered question is whether the morphological differences reflect hypoplasia (failure to develop) or atrophy (shrinkage).

Electrophysiology

Electroencephalogram (EEG) records the electrical activity of brain, which may reflect the mental functions carried out by the neurons possibly in "real time". However, the precise localization of this event in the specific brain region is poor. When EEG activity from repeated presentations of a specific stimulus is summed across trials, some potentials related to the specific processing of the target stimulus can be extracted from the EEG and are referred as **event-related potentials** (ERPs).

The P300 ERP, a positive deflection occurring approximately 300 milliseconds after the introduction of a stimulus, is regarded as a putative biological marker of risk for schizophrenia. The P300 amplitudes are smaller in patients with schizophrenia and is one of the most replicated electrophysiological findings.

Neurochemical Theories

Dopamine

Dopamine is the most extensively investigated neurotransmitter system in schizophrenia. In 1973 it was proposed that schizophrenia is related to hyperactivity of dopamine. This proposition became the dominant pathophysiological hypothesis for the next 15 years. Its strongest support came from the fact that all commercially available antipsychotic agents have antagonistic effects on the dopamine D_2 receptor in relation to their clinical potencies (Creese et al., 1975). In addition, dopamine agonists, such as amphetamine and methylphenidate, exacerbate psychotic symptoms in a subgroup of patients with schizophrenia. Moreover, as noted earlier, the most consistently reported postmortem finding in the literature of schizophrenia is elevated D_2 receptors in the striatum.

The dopamine hyperactivity hypothesis and the primacy of D_2 antagonism for antipsychotic drug action were seriously questioned largely because of the advent of clozapine, an atypical antipsychotic drug. Clozapine has proved to be the most efficacious treatment for chronic schizophrenia and yet it has one of the lowest levels of D_2 occupancy of all antipsychotic drugs. This started an extensive search for explanations underlying the extraordinary efficacy of clozapine. However, new information from PET studies has once again highlighted the central role that the dopaminergic system plays in treatment of psychosis. The typical and atypical antipsychotics are effective only when their D_2 receptor occupancy exceeds 65%, reinforcing the importance of D_2 antagonism in producing antipsychotic effects. However, an important difference between typical and atypical antipsychotics is in their affinity for the D_2 receptors. Medications like clozapine attach loosely to and dissociate rapidly from the dopamine D_2 receptors compared with typical antipsychotic agents (like haloperidol) which have strong affinity for and bind tightly to these receptors.

Five subtypes of dopamine receptor have now been discovered, D_1, D_2, D_3, D_4 and D_5, and interest in dopamine receptors other than the D_2 receptor has arisen. Reduced levels of D_1-like dopamine receptors in the prefrontal cortex of patients with schizophrenia including in those never exposed to antipsychotic agents have been reported. The D_1 receptors are expressed predominantly by pyramidal neurons on their dendritic spines, where they possibly modulate glutamate-mediated inputs to these neurons – inputs that mainly come from other pyramidal and thalamic neurons. Thus the reduced D_1-like receptors seen in the prefrontal cortex of schizophrenia patients may underlie aspects of cognitive dysfunction and severity of negative symptoms (Nestler, 1997).

Clinical trials of dopamine agonists have resulted in improvements in the negative symptoms of schizophrenia. A new model of dopamine dysfunction was proposed which stated that deficits in dopamine, perhaps in the prefrontal cortex, may result in negative symptoms and that concomitant dopamine dysregulation in the striatum, perhaps related to faulty presynaptic control of dopamine release, may be involved in positive symptoms. This bidirectional model is under investigation.

The DA hypothesis of schizophrenia has been critical in guiding schizophrenia research for several decades. Until recently, a main shortcoming of this hypothesis was absence of direct evidence linking DA dysfunction to schizophrenia. Sophisticated in vivo techniques have provided fascinating data directly implicating dopamine in developing psychosis. It is also becoming clear that dopamine works closely with serotonin, glutamate and other systems such that changes in one system affects the balance of the other systems too.

Serotonin

Clozapine has a relatively high affinity for specific serotonin (5-hydroxytryptamine [5-HT]) receptors (5-HT_{2A} and 5-HT_{2C}) and risperidone, has even greater serotonin antagonistic properties. Clozapine, risperidone, olanzapine, quetiapine and ziprasidone, the novel antipsychotic agents, have a greater ratio of serotonin 5-HT_{2A} to dopamine D_2 binding affinity. This has led to the hypothesis that the balance between serotonin and dopamine may be altered in schizophrenia. Serotonin 5-HT_{2A} (and other serotonin) receptor occupancy by the antipsychotic drugs, depending on the areas of the brain involved, could be associated with improvement in cognition, depression and D_2 receptor mediated EPS.

There has been an explosion of new information about the structure and function of 5-HT receptors. To date, 15 serotonin receptor subtypes have been identified. Two receptors, 5-HT_6 and 5-HT_7, have been proposed as candidates for atypical drug action and are therefore reasonable targets for pathophysiological studies of schizophrenia. It is clear that the field is in the early stages of understanding the possible involvement of serotonin in schizophrenia.

Glutamate and *N*-Methyl-ᴅ-aspartate Receptor

Glutamate is a major brain excitatory amino acid neurotransmitter and is critically involved in learning, memory and brain development. Interest in glutamate and the NMDA receptor in schizophrenia arose because of the similarity between phencyclidine (PCP) psychosis and the psychosis of schizophrenia. PCP is a noncompetitive antagonist of the NMDA receptor and produces a psychotic state that includes conceptual disorganization, auditory hallucinations, delusions and negative symptoms. PCP produces more symptoms that are similar to those of schizophrenia than most other pharmacological agents.

PCP and other highly potent NMDA receptor antagonists cause neuronal damage and therefore are not used as research tools in clinical populations. However, ketamine, a widely used dissociative anesthetic, is another noncompetitive NMDA antagonist and, at subanesthetic doses, produces a PCP-like psychosis resembling schizophrenia. The glutamate hypothesis of schizophrenia is one of the most active areas of research currently. The NMDA receptor is reported to play a critical role in guiding axons to their final destination during neurodevelopment. Also, abnormalities with glutamate transmission is reported in many areas of the brain such as frontal cortex, hippocampus, limbic cortex, striatum and thalamus. Moreover, there are changes reported in the gene expression in these areas, Hypoglutamatergia in schizophrenia may have very important downstream modulatory effects on catecholaminergic neurotransmission and play a critical role during neurodevelopment. It also plays an important role in synaptic pruning and underlies important aspects of neurocognition.

GABA

GABA is the major inhibitory neurotransmitter in brain. Support for GABA's involvement in schizophrenia comes from two lines of investigation. First, clinical trials have demonstrated that benzodiazepines, administered both in conjunction with antipsychotic drugs and as the sole treatment, are effective at reducing symptoms in subgroups of schizophrenia patients. Benzodiazepines are agonists at $GABA_A$ receptors. Secondly, postmortem studies have found a deficit in GABA interneurons in the anterior cingulum and prefrontal cortex and decreased GABA uptake sites in the hippocampus. GABAergic neurons are especially vulnerable to glucocorticoid hormones and also to glutamatergic excitotoxicity.

Peptides

Several peptides have been hypothesized to play a pathophysiological role in schizophrenia. Interest in neurotensin arose because of the discovery that it is colocalized in some dopaminergic neurons and acts as a neuromodulator of this and other neurotransmitters. In preclinical studies, neurotensin was found to have effects that resembled those of antipsychotic drugs (Kasckow and Nemeroff, 1991. In addition, schizophrenia patients were found to have lower cerebrospinal fluid neurotensin levels than healthy control subjects and other patients with neuropsychiatric disorders. Other peptides that are under consideration for a pathophysiological role in schizophrenia are somatostatin, dynorphin, substance P and neuropeptide Y.

Norepinephrine

Heightened noradrenergic function has been implicated in psychotic relapse in subgroups of schizophrenia patients (van Kammen *et al.*, 1990). In addition, clozapine, but not other neuroleptic drugs, consistently produces increases in central and peripheral indices of noradrenergic function, and one study found a significant relationship between increases in plasma norepinephrine and improvement in positive symptoms.

The Biochemical Theory

Carlsson and colleagues (2001) provide a multineurotransmitter theory of schizophrenia which improves upon previous biochemical theories of schizophrenia. Accumulating evidence suggests that hyperdopaminergia in schizophrenia is probably secondary to some other phenomena. The data involving glutamatergic system suggests that NMDA receptor antagonism enhances the spontaneous and amphetamine-induced release of dopamine and thus raises the possibility that **hypoglutamatergia** could be related to the **hyperdopaminergia**. Carlsson and colleagues propose that psychotogenesis depends on an interaction between dopamine and glutamate pathways projecting to the striatum from the lower brain stem and cortex respectively. These neurotransmitters are predominantly antagonistic to each other, the former being inhibitory and the latter stimulatory when acting on striatal GABAergic projection neurons. These GABAergic

neurons belong to striatothalamic pathways, which exert an inhibitory action on thalamocortical glutamatergic neurons, thereby filtering off part of the sensory input to the thalamus to protect the cortex from a sensory overload and hyperarousal. Hyperactivity of dopamine or hypofunction of the corticostriatal glutamate pathway should reduce this protective influence and could thus lead to confusion or psychosis. As a result, the indirect striatothalamic pathways have an inhibitory influence on the thalamus with the corresponding direct pathways exerting an opposite and excitatory influence. Both pathways are controlled by glutamatergic corticostriatal pathways enabling the cortex to regulate the thalamic gating in opposite directions. Thus, according to Carlsson and colleagues they appear to serve as **brakes** and **accelerators**.

It has been suggested that the activity of the direct pathways is predominantly phasic and of the indirect pathways is mainly tonic. This difference could have important consequences for a different responsiveness of the direct and indirect pathways to drugs. Thus the NMDA receptor antagonists are behavioral stimulants. AMPA receptor antagonists act in the same direction as NMDA antagonists in some and opposite direction in other experiments. The relationship between glutamate and serotonin is very important and interesting. Serotonin appears to play a more important role than dopamine in the behavioral stimulation induced by hypoglutamatergia. Serotonin may play a more prominent role than dopamine in the behavioral stimulation induced by hypoglutamatergia. Schizophrenia is a syndrome of heterogeneous etiology and pathology. If one neurotransmitter is disturbed, it will inevitably have an impact on other neurotransmitters (Carlsson *et al.*, 2001).

Neurodevelopmental Versus Neurodegenerative Disease Processes

Neurodevelopmental hypotheses of schizophrenia posit that a disruption in normal development causes the illness (Weinberger, 1987). Thus, the "lesion" occurs well before the onset of the illness and interacts with maturation events such as neuronal precursor, glial proliferation and migration; axonal and dendritic proliferation; myelination of axons; programmed cell death and synaptic pruning and is in all likelihood a nonprogressive disease process. Support for the neurodevelopment hypothesis includes the fact that the majority of patients with schizophrenia do not have a course of illness marked by progressive deterioration such as found in dementias. In addition, brain morphological abnormalities commonly found in this illness, such as enlarged ventricles and reduced mesolimbic structures, do not appear to be progressive and, in fact, are present at the onset of the illness. Moreover, gliosis, which occurs during active pathological processes as part of the cellular reparative process in mature brains, is not commonly found in postmortem studies of schizophrenia.

That illness onset typically occurs in the teenage years and early twenties, as opposed to earlier in life when the proposed pathogenic insult occurs, has been explained by the fact that brain regions implicated in this illness, such as prefrontal cortex, are still undergoing myelination during the adolescent years and are therefore not fully functional until that time. Thus, an early lesion involving this region could remain silent until adolescence, when its normal functional capacity is expected to be realized. However, these assumptions have proven to be controversial.

Clinical Manifestations and Phenomenology

Positive and Negative Symptoms

There has been an emphasis on positive and negative symptom clusters in some schizophrenia patients. In the psychiatric literature, positive symptoms have come to mean those that are actively expressed, such as hallucinations, thought disorder, delusions and bizarre behavior, whereas negative symptoms reflect deficit states such as avolition, flattened affect and alogia. How these distinct symptom patterns are related in schizophrenia remains unresolved.

That schizophrenia could be divided into a two-syndrome concept was put forth by Crow (1980). According to his theory, type I schizophrenia patients are those who present, often more acutely, with a predominantly positive symptom profile and who have a good response to neuroleptics. In contrast, type II schizophrenia patients are those who have a more chronic illness, more frequent evidence of intellectual impairment and enlarged ventricular size and cortical atrophy as seen on CT or MRI scans, a poorer response to neuroleptics and predominantly negative symptoms. Crow further postulated that type I schizophrenia may be secondary to a hyperdopaminergic state, whereas type II disease may be due to structural abnormality of the brain.

The idea that positive and negative symptoms may be overlapping end points along a single continuum of biological and clinical manifestations has been described by Andreasen and colleagues (1982). In their study of 52 schizophrenia patients, they found that negative symptoms correlated with the presence of ventricular enlargement and that patients with small ventricles were more likely to manifest positive symptoms. In a separate report, Andreasen and Olsen (1982) posited that negative and positive symptoms reflect opposite extremes of a spectrum and that a mixed symptom pattern can exist and may be present 30% of the time. Others have suggested that although the positive and negative characteristics may be part of a continuum, they may not be related to the presence or absence of structural brain abnormalities; rather, there may be a relationship between the symptom pattern and outcome, depending on the clinical course.

A categorical scheme for differentiation of so-called primary and secondary negative symptoms was developed by Carpenter and colleagues (1985). This distinction is based in part on the fact that negative symptoms are not pathognomonic of schizophrenia. The negative symptoms that can be seen in a number of other illnesses, including depression and medical illness, and as a result of positive symptoms themselves or the side effects of medication, particularly extrapyramidal symptoms, are considered "secondary". The negative symptoms that are a core element of schizophrenia are deemed "primary" or "deficit" symptoms. This distinction enables further exploration of outcome variables and the heterogeneity of this illness and in many ways aids treatment decisions.

Because positive and negative symptoms may be seen differently by individual psychiatrists, valid psychometric scales have become important clinical and research tools. The Brief Psychiatric Rating Scale (BPRS) (Overall and Gorham, 1961), for example, includes subscales for positive and negative symptoms, as does the Positive and Negative Syndrome Scale (PANSS) for schizophrenia (Kay et al., 1988). Others have more broadly defined negative symptoms. Crow (1985) proposed the use of a narrow definition, that is, flattened affect and poverty of speech, for negative symptoms, and Andreasen (1981) supported a broader definition in the widely used Scale for the Assessment of Negative Symptoms (SANS). This psychometric scale includes categories of alogia and flattened affect as well as items such as anhedonia, asociality, avolition, apathy and deficits in attention.

Symptom Cluster Analysis

Although the dichotomous positive–negative distinction has gained clinical and research recognition, several reports suggest that this division is incomplete. Much of the current interest in understanding the heterogeneity of schizophrenia has involved a more detailed look at the symptoms of schizophrenia. Sophisticated statistical techniques utilize factor analysis to reduce data to elucidate clusters of symptoms that are most likely to group together or be found independently.

An application of this approach found that there are three, rather than two, symptom dimensions that better subdivide schizophrenia. Correlational relationships between symptoms reveal that positive symptoms can be divided into two distinct groups. The first includes psychotic symptoms such as hallucinations and delusions, and the second includes symptoms of disorganization, consisting of thought disorder, bizarre behavior and inappropriate affect. A third group is that of negative symptoms. Although these patterns of symptoms may be seen in different proportions in individuals and may change over time, they can be shown to have distinct clinical courses and may be related to independent neuropsychological deficits in a given individual (Andreasen et al., 1995).

Cognitive Impairment

Now it is widely accepted that schizophrenia patients experience neuropsychological deficits that can be characterized by difficulties with attention, information processing, executive function, learning and memory, which leads to a generalized performance deficit. Typically, there is a wide variance with some aspects of performance being more impaired then others. Interestingly, a small subgroup of the patients have cognitive functioning within the normal range Most patients with schizophrenia have only modest reductions in their IQs with an average of 90 and about 0.67 standard deviation below that of the general population. In contrast, their performance is usually worse even in first episode patients. Usually patients with schizophrenia underperform relative to estimates of their premorbid functioning. Cognitive impairments involving verbal learning, verbal delayed recall, working memory, vigilance and executive functioning have a significant negative impact on social and occupational functioning. Two meta-analysis of 24 and nine studies respectively suggest that treatment with novel antipsychotic agents improve cognitive function compared with typical antipsychotic agents (Keefe et al., 1999; Harvey, 2001).

The degree of cognitive deficit appears to be more strongly associated with severity of negative symptoms, symptoms of disorganization and adaptive dysfunction than with positive symptoms. Verbal fluency is severely impaired in patients with psychotic disorders and the use of atypical antipsychotic medications results in significant improvement. Motor functions (e.g., reaction time, motor and graphomotor speed) improve with clozapine, olanzapine and risperidone. Olanzapine improves motor functions more than either haloperidol or risperidone. Furthermore, motor functions are related to outcome, underscoring the importance of this domain. The symbol–digit and digit–symbol tests have been among the most responsive tests to atypical antipsychotic treatment. Though the novel antipsychotic agents appear to have beneficial effects on cognition, much work still remains to eliminate biases; also, effect sizes of these improvements are modest (Harvey and Keefe, 2001).

Information Processing and Attention

The term **information processing** is used to describe the process of taking information and encoding it in such a way that it can be understood and recalled when appropriately cued. This construct is related to neural circuits and a stepwise logical spread of neurochemical messages, which may be impaired in schizophrenia. **Attention**, simply defined, is the ability to focus on a stimulus, either through conscious effort or passively. These two constructs are interrelated, and our understanding of their composite parts has increased in complexity in the past few decades.

Measures of attention were developed from the idea that patients with schizophrenia cannot block out unimportant stimuli in the way that those without schizophrenia can. This phenomenon has come to be called **gating**. Gating is usually seen, for example, when a weak stimulus is delivered before a real stimulus. Normally, the first stimulus would dampen or eliminate the response to the second.

In general, patients with schizophrenia have impairments in information processing, especially when they are exposed to increasing demands on their attentional capabilities, such as under timed conditions or in stressful situations. Therefore, these deficits not only are viewed as trait linked (i.e., a manifestation of the illness itself) but may be compounded when state linked (i.e., when there are increases in symptoms). The trait-linked disturbances in neuropsychological parameters are seen in those at high risk for developing schizophrenia, those who have schizophrenia, and relatives who appear clinically unaffected, which may indicate a genetic vulnerability.

Many of these tests of attention and information processing have been associated with specific symptoms and neuropsychological impairment in schizophrenia. For example, one study showed that impaired prepulse inhibition was related to increased perseveration on neuropsychological tests of higher executive function (Butler et al., 1991). Others have shown that deficits in attention and information processing may be associated with positive and/or negative symptoms (Strauss, 1993). Specifically, deficits in visual processing and motor function (as seen with continuous performance tasks) have been linked to negative symptoms (Nuechterlein et al., 1986), whereas positive symptoms seem to be related to auditory-processing dysfunction (Green and Walker, 1986).

Learning and Memory

Although there are generally no consistent gross deficits of memory in schizophrenia patients, close examination of certain aspects of learning and memory has revealed striking abnormalities. Schizophrenia patients have been shown to be poorer in recall of word lists if the words are not grouped into categories. Furthermore, unlike normal control subjects, schizophrenia patients do not seem to show an improvement in memory when asked to recall words with latent positive emotional meaning. These findings have been attributed to poor cognitive organization in schizophrenia patients.

Others have reported that patients with chronic schizophrenia had impairment in new learning and short-term memory but not remote memory possibly indicating temporal–hippocampal dysfunction. These may be more likely in patients with a poor premorbid course and ventricular enlargement.

Working memory is a cognitive system that stores and processes information needed for planning and reasoning for a brief duration. Some cognitive scientists refer to short-term memory as working memory. Working memory consists of verbal and visual memory subsystems with a central principle that manipulates and coordinates information stored in the two systems for problem solving, planning and organizing activities. Separate areas of the prefrontal cortex may underlie different aspects of the working memory. The workspace used for such memory is capacity-limited. Patients with schizophrenia have significant dysfunction in this area and are unable to change an ineffective strategy (i.e., shift sets) even when feedback is provided. This dysfunction occurs (albeit at a lower level) even in subjects with higher intelligence. Conventional antipsychotics do not appear to impair or improve working memory in patients with schizophrenia. Studies involving evaluation of working memory using neuroimaging, pharmacological models of schizophrenia and neurochemical function should further our understanding of this manifestation of schizophrenia.

Differential Diagnosis

Making an accurate diagnosis of schizophrenia requires high levels of clinical acumen, extensive knowledge of schizophrenia and sophisticated application of the principles of differential diagnosis. It is unfortunately common for patients with psychotic disorders to be misdiagnosed and consequently treated inappropriately. The importance of accurate diagnosis is underlined by an emerging database indicating that early detection and prompt pharmacological intervention may improve the long-term prognosis of the illness.

Mental Status Examination

There is no specific laboratory test, neuroimaging study, or clinical presentation of a patient that yields a definitive diagnosis of schizophrenia. Schizophrenia can present with a wide variety of symptoms, and a longitudinal history of symptoms and comorbid clinical variables such as medical illness and a history of substance abuse are necessary before a diagnosis can be considered. The Mental Status Examination, much like the physical examination, is an additional clinical tool that aids the psychiatrist in generating a differential diagnosis and appropriate treatment recommendations.

Appearance

Although a disheveled look is not pathognomonic for schizophrenia, patients with this disorder often present, especially acutely, with a disordered appearance. The description of a patient's appearance is an objective verbal sketch, much like the description of a heart murmur, that can uniquely identify a particular patient.

A person with schizophrenia often has difficulty attending to activities of daily living, either because of negative symptoms (apathy, social withdrawal, or motor retardation) or because of the presence of positive symptoms, such as psychosis, disorganization, or catatonia, that interfere with the ability to maintain personal hygiene. Also, schizophrenia patients often present with odd or inappropriate attire, such as a coat and hat worn during the summer or dark sunglasses worn during an interview. It is generally thought that the inappropriate dress is a manifestation of symptoms such as disorganization or paranoid ideation. It should be noted that some patients present quite neatly groomed. Thus appearance is noted but is not diagnostic.

Attitude

Individuals with schizophrenia may be friendly and cooperative, or they may be hostile, annoyed and defensive during an interview. The latter may be secondary to paranoid symptoms, which can make patients quite cautious and guarded in their responses to questions.

Behavior

Schizophrenic patients can have bizarre mannerisms or stereotyped movements that can make them look unusual. Patients with catatonia can stay in one position for weeks, even to the point of causing serious physical damage to their body; for example, a patient who stands in one place for days may develop stress fractures, peripheral edema and even pulmonary emboli. Patients with catatonia may have waxy flexibility, maintaining a position after someone else has moved them into it. Patients with catatonic excitement exhibit odd posturing or purposeless, repetitive, and often strange movements.

Behaviors seen in schizophrenia patients include choreoathetoid movements, which may be related to neuroleptic exposure but have been reported in patients even before neuroleptic use. Other behaviors or movement disorders may be seen as parkinsonian features, such as a shuffling gait or a pill-rolling tremor.

Psychomotor retardation may be present and may be a manifestation of catatonia or negative symptoms. On close observation, it is usually characterized, in this group of patients, as a lack of motor movements rather than slowed movements.

Patients may present with agitation, ranging from minimal to extreme. This agitation is often seen in the acute state and may require immediate pharmacotherapy. However, agitation may be secondary to neuroleptic medications, as in akathisia, which is felt as an internal restlessness making it difficult for the person to sit still. Akathisia can manifest itself in limb shaking, pacing, or frequent shifting of position. Severely agitated patients may be unresponsive to verbal limits and may require measures to ensure their safety and the safety of others around them.

Eye Contact

Paranoid patients may look hypervigilant, scanning a room or glancing suspiciously at an interviewer. Psychotic patients may make poor eye contact, looking away, or appear to stare vacuously at the interviewer, making a conversational connection seem distant. Characteristic responding to internal stimuli is seen when a patient appears to look toward a voice or an auditory hallucination, which the patient may hear. A nystagmus may also be observed. This clinical finding has a large differential diagnosis, including Wernicke-Korsakoff syndrome; alcohol, barbiturate, or phenytoin intoxication; viral labyrinthitis; or brain stem syndromes including infarctions or multiple sclerosis.

Speech

In a Mental Status Examination, one usually comments on the rate, tone and volume of a patient's speech, as well as any distinct dysarthrias that may be present. Pressured speech is usually thought of in conjunction with mania; however, it can be seen in schizophrenia patients, particularly on acute presentation. This is often difficult to assess, as it may be a normal variant or a cultural phenomenon, because some languages are spoken faster than others.

Tone refers to prosody, or the natural singsong quality of speech. Negative symptoms may include a lack of prosody, resulting in monotonous speech. Furthermore, odd tones may be consistent with neurological disorders or bizarre behavior.

Speech volume is important for a number of reasons. Loud speech can be a measure of agitation; it can occur in conjunction with psychosis, or it could even be an indication of hearing loss. Speech that is soft may be an indication of guardedness or anxiety.

Dysarthrias are notable because they can be idiopathic and longstanding, or they can be an indication of neurological disturbance. In patients who have been exposed to neuroleptics, orobuccal tardive dyskinesia should be considered when there is evidence of slurred speech.

Mood and Affect

Affect, which is the observer's objective view of the patient's emotional state, is often constricted or flat in patients with schizophrenia. In fact, this is one of the hallmark negative symptoms. Flattened affect may also be a manifestation of pseudoparkinsonism, an extrapyramidal side effect of typical neuroleptics.

Inappropriate affect is commonly seen in patients with more predominant positive symptoms. A smile or a laugh while relating a sad tale is an example. Patients with catatonic excitement or hebephrenia may have bizarre presentations or affective lability, laughing and crying out of context with the situation. Emotional reactivity must alert the clinician to the possibility of neurological impairment as well, as in the case of pseudobulbar palsy.

Mood is based on a patient's subjective report of how he or she feels, emotionally, at the time of the interview. It is not uncommon for patients with schizophrenia to be depressed (especially patients with history of higher premorbid functioning who may have some insight into the losses they are facing) or to be indifferent, with seemingly no emotional awareness of their situation.

Thought Process

Because actual thoughts cannot be measured, thought processes are assessed by extrapolation from the organization of speech. Thought disorders can be more or less obvious, and a trained listener is one who appreciates the normal logical pattern of flow of words and ideas in speech and can thus sense abnormalities.

There are many different versions of thought disorders: lack of logical connections of ideas (looseness of associations); shift of the original theme because of weak connections of ideas (tangentiality); overinclusiveness to the point of loss of the theme (circumstantiality); use of words and phrases with no relation to grammatical rules (word salad); repetition of words spoken by others (echolalia); use of sounds of other words, such as "yellow bellow, who is this fellow?" (clang associations); use of made-up words (neologisms); and repetition of a particular word or phrase, such as "this and that, this and that" (perseveration).

Other thought disorders are part of a constellation of negative symptoms. Examples would be thoughts that appear to stop abruptly, either because of interruption by an auditory hallucination or because the thought is lost (thought blocking);

absence of thoughts (paucity of thought content); and a delayed response to questions (increased latency of response).

Thought Content

Although not necessarily present in every patient, characteristic symptoms of schizophrenia include the belief that outside forces control a person's thought or actions. A patient might report that others can insert thoughts into her or his head (thought insertion), broadcast them to others (thought broadcasting), or take thoughts away (thought withdrawal). Other delusions, or fixed false beliefs, may also be prominent. Patients may describe ideas of reference, which is the phenomenon of feeling that some external event or report relates to oneself specifically; for example, a patient may infer special meaning from an image seen on television or a broadcast heard on the radio.

Paranoid ideation may be manifested as general suspiciousness or frank, well-systematized delusions. The themes may be considered bizarre, such as feeling convinced that aliens are sending signals through wires in the patient's ear, or nonbizarre, such as being watched by the Central Intelligence Agency or believing that one's spouse is having an affair. These symptoms can be quite debilitating and lead to a great deal of personal loss, which patients may not understand because the ideas are so real to them.

Patients with schizophrenia commonly express an abundance of vague somatic concerns, and a particular patient might develop a delusion around a real physiological abnormality. Therefore, somatic symptoms should be evaluated appropriately in their clinical context without automatically dismissing them as psychotic. Preoccupations and obsessions are also seen commonly in this population, and certain patients have comorbid obsessive–compulsive disorder.

The mortality rate for suicide in schizophrenia is approximately 10%. It is therefore imperative to evaluate a patient for both suicidal and homicidal ideation. Patients of all diagnoses, and particularly schizophrenia, may not spontaneously articulate suicidal or homicidal ideation and must therefore be asked directly about such feelings. Moreover, psychotic patients may feel compelled by an auditory hallucination telling them to hurt themselves.

Perceptions

Perceptual disturbances involve illusions and hallucinations. Hallucinations may be olfactory, tactile, gustatory, visual, or auditory, although hallucinations of the auditory type are more typical of schizophrenia. Hallucinations in the other sensory modalities are more commonly seen in other medical or substance-induced conditions. Auditory hallucinations can resemble sounds, background noise, or human voices. Auditory hallucinations that consist of a running dialogue between two or more voices or a commentary on the patient's behavior are typical of schizophrenia. These hallucinations are distinct from verbalized thoughts that most humans experience. They are often described as originating from outside the patient's head, as if they were emanating from the walls or the radiators in the room. Less commonly, a patient with schizophrenia describes illusions or misperceptions of a real stimulus, such as seeing demons in a shadow.

Consciousness and Orientation

Patients with schizophrenia most likely have a clear sensorium unless there is some comorbid medical illness or substance-related phenomenon. A schizophrenia patient may be disoriented, but this could be a result of inattentiveness to details or distraction secondary to psychotic preoccupation.

Attention and Concentration

Studies utilizing continuous performance task paradigms have demonstrated repeatedly that schizophrenia patients have pervasive deficits in attention in both acute and residual phases. On a Mental Status Examination, these deficits may present themselves as the inability to perform mental exercises, such as spelling the word "earth" backward or serial subtractions.

Memory

Careful assessment of memory in patients with schizophrenia may yield some deficits. Acquisition of new information, immediate recall, and recent and remote memory may be impaired in some individuals. Furthermore, answers to questions regarding memory may lead to idiosyncratic responses related to delusions, thought disorder, or other overriding symptoms of the illness. In general, schizophrenia patients do not show gross deficits of memory such as may be seen in patients with dementia or head trauma.

Fund of Knowledge

Schizophrenia is not the equivalent of mental retardation, although these syndromes can coexist in some patients. Patients with schizophrenia generally experience a slight shift in intellectual functioning after the onset of their illness, yet they typically demonstrate a fund of knowledge consistent with their premorbid level. Schizophrenia patients manifest a characteristic discrepancy on standardized tests of intelligence, with the nonverbal scores being lower than the verbal scores.

Abstraction

A classical aberration of mental function in a patient with schizophrenia involves the inability to utilize abstract reasoning, which is similar to metaphorical thinking, or the ability to conceptualize ideas beyond their literal meaning. For example, when the patient is asked what brought him or her to the hospital, a typical answer might be "an ambulance". On a Mental Status Examination, this concrete thinking is best elicited by asking a patient to interpret a proverb or state the similarities between two objects. For example, "a rolling stone gathers no moss" may mean, to the patient with schizophrenia, that "if a stone just stays in one place, the moss won't be able to collect". More profound difficulties in abstraction and executive function, often seen in schizophrenia, such as inability to shift cognitive focus or set, may be assessed by neuropsychological tests.

Judgment and Insight

Individuals suffering from schizophrenia often display a lack of insight regarding their illness. Whether it is a reflection of a negative symptom, such as apathy, or a constricted display of emotion, patients often appear to be emotionally disconnected from their illness and may even deny that anything is wrong. Poor judgment, which is also characteristic and may be related to lack of insight, may lead to potentially dangerous behavior. For example, a patient walking barefoot in the snow because of the feeling that her or his shoes could be traced by surveillance cameras would be displaying both poor judgment and poor insight. On a formal Mental Status Examination, judgment is commonly assessed by asking patients what they would do if they saw a fire in a movie theater or if they saw a stamped, addressed envelope on the street. Insight can be ascertained by asking patients about their understanding of why they are being evaluated by a psychiatrist or why they are receiving a certain medication.

Physical Examination

Although there are no pathognomonic physical signs of schizophrenia, some patients have neurological "soft" signs on physical examination. The neurological deficits include nonspecific abnormalities in reflexes, coordination (as seen in gait and finger-to-nose tests), graphesthesia (recognition of patterns marked out on the palm) and stereognosis (recognition of three-dimensional pictures). Other neurological findings include odd or awkward movements (possibly correlated with thought disorder), alterations in muscle tone, an increased blink rate, a slower habituation of the blink response to repetitive glabellar tap and an abnormal pupillary response.

   The exact etiology of these abnormalities is unknown, but they have historically been associated with minimal brain dysfunction and may be more likely in patients with poor premorbid functioning. These neurological abnormalities have been seen in neuroleptic-naive patients as well as those with exposure to traditional antipsychotic medication. Overall, the literature suggests that these findings may be associated with the disease itself.

   Neuroophthalmological investigations have shown that patients with schizophrenia have abnormalities in voluntary saccadic eye movements (rapid eye movement toward a stationary object) as well as in smooth pursuit eye movements. The influence of attention and distraction, neuroleptic exposure and the specificity of smooth pursuit eye movements for schizophrenia have raised criticisms of this area of study, and further investigation is necessary to determine its potential as a putative genetic marker for schizophrenia.

Other Conditions that Resemble Schizophrenia

Schizoaffective Disorder

Possibly the most difficult diagnostic dilemma in cases in which a patient has both psychotic symptoms and affective symptoms is in the differentiation between schizophrenia and schizoaffective disorder. There has been some controversy regarding this diagnostic entity. It has been included in studies of both affective disorder and schizophrenia and has at times been considered part of a continuum between the two, which has contributed to some of the diagnostic confusion.

   In DSM-IV, schizoaffective disorder is treated as a unique clinical syndrome. A patient with schizoaffective disorder must have an uninterrupted period of illness during which, at some time, they have symptoms that meet the diagnostic criteria for a major depressive episode, manic episode, or a mixed episode concurrently with the diagnostic criteria for the active phase of schizophrenia (criteria A for schizophrenia). Additionally, the patient must have had delusions or hallucinations for at least 2 weeks in the absence of prominent mood disorder symptoms

during the same period of illness. The mood disorder symptoms must be present for a substantial part of the active and residual psychotic period. The essential features of schizoaffective disorder must occur within a single uninterrupted period of illness where the "period of illness" refers to the period of active or residual symptoms of psychotic illness and this can last for years and decades. The total duration of psychotic symptoms must be at least 1 month to meet criteria A for schizophrenia and thus the minimum duration of a schizoaffective episode is also 1 month.

DSM-IV-TR Criteria 295.70

Schizoaffective Disorder

An uninterrupted period of

A. illness during which, at some time, there is either a major depressive episode, a manic episode, or a mixed episode concurrent with symptoms that meet criterion A for schizophrenia.

Note: The major depressive episode must include criterion A1: depressed mood.

B. During the same period of illness, there have been delusions or hallucinations for at least 2 weeks in the absence of prominent mood symptoms.

C. Symptoms that meet criteria for a mood episode are present for a substantial portion of the total duration of the active and residual periods of the illness.

D. The disturbance is not due to the direct physiological effects of a substance (e.g., a drug of abuse, a medication) or a general medical condition.

Specify type:

Bipolar type: if the disturbance includes a manic or a mixed episode (or a manic or a mixed episode and major depressive episodes)

Depressive type: if the disturbance only includes major depressive episodes

---

Reprinted with permission from the *Diagnostic and Statistical Manual of Mental Disorders*, Fourth Edition, Text Revision. Copyright 2000 American Psychiatric Association.

   The criteria for a major depressive episode requires a minimum duration of 2 weeks of either depressed mood or markedly diminished interest or pleasure. As the symptoms of loss of pleasure or interest commonly occur in nonaffective psychotic disorders, to meet the criteria for schizoaffective disorder criteria A, the major depressive episode must include pervasive depressed mood. Presence of markedly diminished interest or pleasure is not sufficient to make a diagnosis as it is possible that these symptoms may also occur with other conditions.

Brief Psychotic Disorder and Schizophreniform Disorder

The distinctions among brief psychotic disorder, schizophreniform disorder and schizophrenia are based on duration of active symptoms. DSM-IV has established the requirement of 6 months of active, prodromal, and/or residual symptoms for a diagnosis of schizophrenia. Brief psychotic disorder is a transient psychotic state, not caused by medical conditions or substance use, that lasts for at least 1 day and up to 1 month. Schizophreniform disorder falls in between and requires symptoms for at least 1 month and not exceeding 6 months, with no requirement for loss of functioning.

DSM-IV-TR Criteria 298.8

Brief Psychotic Disorder

A. Presence of one (or more) of the following symptoms:

   (1) delusions
   (2) hallucinations
   (3) disorganized speech (e.g., frequent derailment or incoherence)
   (4) grossly disorganized or catatonic behavior

Note: Do not include a symptom if it is a culturally sanctioned response pattern.

B. Duration of an episode of the disturbance is at least 1 day but less than 1 month, with eventual full return to premorbid level of functioning.

C. The disturbance is not better accounted for by a mood disorder with psychotic features, schizoaffective disorder, or schizophrenia and is not due to the direct physiological effects of a substance (e.g., a drug of abuse, a medication) or a general medical condition.

Specify if:

With marked stressor(s) (brief reactive psychosis): if symptoms occur shortly after and apparently in response to events that, singly or together, would be markedly stressful to almost anyone in similar circumstances in the person's culture

Without marked stressor(s): if psychotic symptoms do not occur shortly after, or are not apparently in response to events that, singly or together, would be markedly stressful to almost anyone in similar circumstances in the person's culture

With postpartum onset: if onset within 4 weeks postpartum

Reprinted with permission from the *Diagnostic and Statistical Manual of Mental Disorders*, Fourth Edition, Text Revision. Copyright 2000 American Psychiatric Association.

DSM-IV-TR Criteria 295.40

Schizophreniform Disorder

A. Criteria A, D, and E of schizophrenia are met.

B. An episode of the disorder (including prodromal, active, and residual phases) lasts at least 1 month but less than 6 months. (When the diagnosis must be made without waiting for recovery, it should be qualified as "provisional.")

Specify if:

Without good prognostic features

With good prognostic features: as evidenced by two (or more) of the following:

   (1) onset of prominent psychotic symptoms within 4 weeks of the first noticeable change in usual behavior or functioning
   (2) confusion or perplexity at the height of the psychotic episode
   (3) good premorbid social and occupational functioning
   (4) absence of blunted or flat affect

Reprinted with permission from the *Diagnostic and Statistical Manual of Mental Disorders*, Fourth Edition, Text Revision. Copyright 2000 American Psychiatric Association.

Delusional Disorder

If the delusions that a patient describes are not bizarre (e.g., examples of bizarre delusions include the belief that an outside force or person has taken over one's body or that radio signals are being sent through the caps in one's teeth), it is wise to consider delusional disorder in the differential diagnosis. Delusional disorder is usually characterized by specific types of false fixed beliefs such as erotomanic, grandiose, jealous, persecutory, or somatic types. Delusional disorder, unlike schizophrenia, is not associated with a marked social impairment or odd behavior. Moreover, patients with delusional disorder do not experience hallucinations or typically have negative symptoms.

DSM-IV-TR Criteria 297.1

Delusional Disorder

Nonbizarre delusions (i.e., A. involving situations that occur in real life, such as being followed, poisoned, infected, loved at a distance, or deceived by spouse or lover, or having a disease) of at least 1 month's duration.

B. Criterion A for schizophrenia has never been met.
Note: Tactile and olfactory hallucinations may be present in delusional disorder if they are related to the delusional theme.

C. Apart from the impact of the delusion(s) or its ramifications, functioning is not markedly impaired and behavior is not obviously odd or bizarre.

D. If mood episodes have occurred concurrently with delusions, their total duration has been brief relative to the duration of the delusional periods.

E. The disturbance is not due to the direct physiological effects of a substance (e.g., a drug of abuse, a medication) or a general medical condition.

Specify type (the following types are assigned based on the predominant delusional theme):

Erotomanic type: delusions that another person, usually of higher status, is in love with the individual

Grandiose type: delusions of inflated worth, power, knowledge, identity, or special relationship to a deity or famous person

Jealous type: delusions that the individual's sexual partner is unfaithful

Persecutory type: delusions that the person (or someone to whom the person is close) is being malevolently treated in some way

Somatic type: delusions that the person has some physical defect or general medical condition

Mixed type: delusions characteristic of more than one of the above types but no one theme predominates

Unspecified type

Reprinted with permission from the *Diagnostic and Statistical Manual of Mental Disorders*, Fourth Edition, Text Revision. Copyright 2000 American Psychiatric Association.

Affective Disorder with Psychotic Features

If the patient experiences psychotic symptoms solely during times when affective symptoms are present, the diagnosis is more likely to be mood disorder with psychotic features. If the mood disturbance involves both manic and depressive episodes, the diagnosis is bipolar disorder. According to DSM-IV, affective disorders that are seen in patients with schizophrenia may fall in the category depressive disorder not otherwise specified or bipolar disorder not otherwise specified.

Substance-related Conditions

Psychotic disorders, delirium and dementia that are caused by substance use, in DSM-IV, are distinguished from schizophrenia by virtue of the fact that there is clear-cut evidence of substance use leading to symptoms. Examples of psychotomimetic properties of substances include a PCP psychosis that can resemble schizophrenia clinically, chronic alcohol intoxication (Korsakoff's psychosis) and chronic amphetamine administration, which can lead to paranoid states. Therefore, patients who have symptoms that meet criterion A of schizophrenia in the presence of substance use must be reevaluated after a significant period away from the suspected substance, and proper toxicology screens must be performed to rule out recent substance abuse.

General Medical Conditions

General medical conditions ranging from vitamin B_{12} deficiency to Cushing's syndrome have been associated with a clinical presentation resembling that of schizophrenia. Because the prognosis for the associated medical condition is better than that for schizophrenia and the stigma attached to schizophrenia is significant, it is imperative to provide patients with a thorough medical work-up before giving a diagnosis of schizophrenia. This includes a physical examination; laboratory analyses including thyroid function tests, syphilis screening, and folate and vitamin B_{12} levels; a CT or MRI scan; and a lumbar puncture when indicated in new-onset cases.

Course of Illness

In long-term follow-up studies of 20 years or more, surprisingly favorable outcomes were observed: between 40 and 66% of patients had either recovered or were only mildly impaired at follow-up (Table 45.1). In the Vermont Longitudinal Study of Schizophrenia (Harding *et al.*, 1987a, 1987b), 269 backward patients who were chronically institutionalized in the 1950s were followed up an average of 32 years later. The patients who met rigorously applied retrospective DSM-III diagnostic criteria for schizophrenia disorder ($N = 118$) during their index admission in the 1950s were found on follow-up to have outcomes that varied widely; 82% were not hospitalized in the year of the follow-up, 68% displayed slight or no symptoms, 81% were able to meet their own basic needs, and more than 60% had good social functioning. Thus, these data indicate that the long-term outcome of schizophrenia is heterogeneous, with substantially larger numbers of patients having better outcomes than would have been predicted by the Kraepelinian model that postulated this illness was a dementia and worsened over time.

Based on current epidemiological data, a new model of the natural course of schizophrenia has been proposed (Breier *et al.*, 1991). This model has three phases: an early phase marked by deterioration from premorbid levels of functioning; a middle phase characterized by a prolonged period of little change termed the stabilization phase; and the last period, which incorporates the long-term outcome data just cited, which is called the improving phase (Figure 45.2).

First Episode Schizophrenia

An enormous clinical and research effort is directed internationally towards patients in very early stages of their illness and especially during their first psychotic break with a focus on early and effective intervention. First episode provides a unique opportunity to intervene early and effectively and possibly change the course of illness. It is well known that there is a delay of 1

Table 45.1	Long-term Follow-up Studies of Schizophrenia			
Study	Location	Length of Follow-up (mean, year)	Sample Size (*N*)	Recovered or Significantly Improved (%)
DeSisto *et al.* (1992)	Maine	36	117	45
Harding *et al.* (1987)	Vermont	32	82	67
Tsuang *et al.* (1979)	Iowa	35	186	46
Huber *et al.* (1982)	Bonn	22	502	57
Ciompi *et al.* (1982)	Lausanne	37	289	53
Bleuler (1987)	Zurich	23	208	53

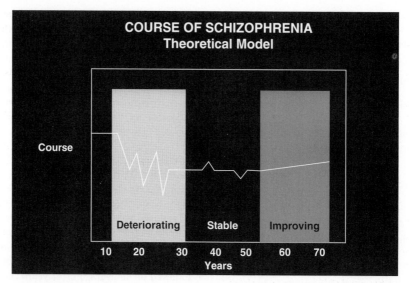

Figure 45.2   *Model of the lifelong course of illness for schizophrenia. Reprinted with permission from Breier A, Schreiber JL, Dyer J, et al. [1991] National Institute of Mental Health longitudinal study of chronic schizophrenia: Prognosis and prediction of outcome. Arch Gen Psychiatr 48, 239–246. Copyright 1991, American Medical Association.*

to 2 years on an average between onset of psychosis and starting of treatment. This duration of untreated psychosis (DUP) is recognized by many though not all as an important indicator of subsequent clinical outcome. Larsen and colleagues (2000) examined 1-year outcome in 43 first episode patients and at 1-year follow-up 56% were in remission, 26% were still psychotic and 18% suffered multiple relapses. Both longer DUP and poor premorbid functioning predicted more negative symptoms and poor global functioning. DUP remained a strong predictor of outcome even after controlling for premorbid functioning. Clinical deterioration appears to be correlated with the duration of psychosis and number of episodes of psychosis. The deterioration usually occurs during the first 5 years after onset and then stabilize at a level where they have persistent symptoms and are impaired in their social and vocational function. After that point additional exacerbation may occur but they are not usually associated with further deterioration.

Long-term studies of schizophrenia suggest that negative symptoms tend to be less common and less severe in the early stages of the illness but increase in prevalence and severity in the later stages. Positive symptoms such as delusions and hallucinations are more common earlier on while thought disorganization, inappropriate affect and motor symptoms occur more commonly in the later stages of illness. A possible decline in the prevalence of the hebephrenic and catatonic subtypes of schizophrenia may be attributed to effective treatment and possible arrest of the progression of illness. Thus with effective treatment, and with long-term compliance it is possible to produce favorable outcomes.

Following onset of the illness, patients experience substantial decline in cognitive functions from their premorbid levels. However, it is unclear whether, after the first episode, there is further cognitive decline due to the illness. Some studies even suggest a slight and gradual improvement. Increased number of episodes and the longer duration of untreated psychosis are associated with greater cognitive dysfunction.

Patients with first episode psychosis usually have excellent clinical response to antipsychotic treatment early in their course of illness when compared with chronic multi-episode patients. Effective and early intervention does help achieve clinical

remission and good outcome (Lieberman et al., 1993). Some suggest that atypical antipsychotic medication should be used preferentially in the treatment of first episode patients with psychotic disorders (Lieberman, 1996) as they are a highly treatment responsive group, and may be best able to optimize the outcome. In addition, first episode patients are sensitive to side effects, especially extrapyramidal and weight gain side effects. They require lower doses of medication to achieve therapeutic responses. The issue of treatment adherence is of critical importance in first episode patients. Although these patients respond very well with 1 year remission rates of greater than >80%, the 1-year attrition rates are as high as 60%. This important issue undermines management of first episode patients during this critical period of their illness.

Treatment

It could be argued that the successful treatment of schizophrenia requires a greater level of clinical knowledge and sophistication than the treatment of most other psychiatric and medical illnesses. It begins with the formation of a therapeutic psychiatrist–patient relationship and must combine the latest developments in pharmacological and psychosocial therapeutics and interventions.

Psychiatrist–Patient Relationship

The psychiatrist–patient relationship is the foundation for treating patients with schizophrenia. Because of the clinical manifestations of the illness, the formation of this relationship is often difficult. Paranoid delusions may lead to mistrust of the psychiatrist. Conceptual disorganization and cognitive impairment make it difficult for patients to attend to what the psychiatrist is saying and to follow even the simplest directions. Negative symptoms result in lack of emotional expression and social withdrawal, which can be demoralizing for the psychiatrist who is attempting to "connect" with the patient.

It is important for the psychiatrist to understand the ways in which the psychopathology of the illness affects the therapeutic relationship. The psychiatrist should provide constancy to the patient, which helps "anchor" patients in their turbulent world.

The qualities of the relationship should include consistency, acceptance, appropriate levels of warmth that respect the patient's needs for titrating emotional intensity, nonintrusiveness and, most important, caring. "Old-fashioned" family doctors who know their patients well, are easily approachable, have a matter-of-fact style, attend to a broad range of needs, and are available and willing to reach out during crises provide a useful model for the psychiatrist–patient relationship in the treatment of schizophrenia.

Psychopharmacological Treatment

Background

The seminal work of Delay and Deniker (1952) provided a pharmacological strategy that would forever change the face of schizophrenia. The implementation of chlorpromazine became the turning point for psychopharmacology. Patients who had been institutionalized for years were able to receive treatment as outpatients and live in community settings. The road was paved for the deinstitutionalization movement, and scientific understanding of the pathophysiology of schizophrenia burgeoned. The introduction of clozapine started the era of antipsychotic agents being referred to as either "typical" (**conventional** or **traditional**) or "atypical" (or **novel**) antipsychotic drugs. If chlorpromazine started the first revolution in the psychopharmacological treatment of schizophrenia, then clozapine ushered in the second and more profound revolution whose impact is felt beyond schizophrenia and its full extent is yet to be realized. Moreover, clozapine has invigorated the psychopharmacology of schizophrenia and rekindled one of the most ambitious searches for new antipsychotic compounds by the pharmaceutical industry. There are now five novel antipsychotics in the USA: risperidone, olanzapine, quetiapine, ziprasidone and aripiprazole.

Clozapine and the Novel Antipsychotic Agents

Double–blind, controlled studies demonstrated the superior clinical efficacy of clozapine compared with standard neuroleptics, without the associated extrapyramidal symptoms. It is clearly superior to traditional neuroleptics for psychosis. Approximately 50% of patients with chronic and treatment-resistant schizophrenia derive a better response from clozapine than from traditional neuroleptics. Its effect on negative symptoms is somewhat controversial and has started an intense and a passionate debate as to whether the efficacy of the medication is with primary or secondary negative symptoms or both (Meltzer, 1989a). There is substantial evidence that clozapine decreases relapses, improves stability in the community, and diminishes suicidal behavior. There have also been reports that clozapine may cause a gradual reduction in preexisting tardive dyskinesia.

Unfortunately, clozapine is associated with agranulocytosis and, because of this risk, it requires weekly white blood cell testing. Approximately 0.8% of patients taking clozapine and receiving weekly white blood cell monitoring develop agranulocytosis. Women and the elderly are at higher risk than other groups. The period of highest risk is the first 6 months of treatment. These data has led to monitoring of white cell counts less frequently after first 6 months to every other week if a person has a history of white cell counts the within the normal range in the preceding 6 months. Current guidelines state that the medication must be held back if the total white blood cell count is 3000/mm³ or less or if the absolute polymorphonuclear cell count is 1500/mm³ or less. Patients who stop clozapine treatment continue to require blood

monitoring for at least 4 weeks after the last dose according to current guidelines. Other side effects of clozapine include orthostatic hypotension, tachycardia, sialorrhea, sedation, elevated temperature and weight gain. Furthermore, clozapine can lower the seizure threshold in a dose-dependent fashion, with a higher risk of seizures seen particularly at doses greater than 600 mg/day.

Clozapine has an affinity for dopamine receptors (D_1, D_2, D_3, D_4 and D_5), serotonin receptors (5-HT_{2A}, 5-HT_{2C}, 5-HT_6 and 5-HT_7), alpha-1- and alpha-2-adrenergic receptors, nicotinic and muscarinic cholinergic receptors and H_1 histaminergic receptors. As clozapine has a relatively shorter half-life, it is usually administered twice a day.

The superior antipsychotic efficacy of clozapine has inspired an abundance of research in the field of modern psychopharmacology for the treatment of schizophrenia. Clozapine and the other novel compounds have an array of biochemical profiles, with affinities to dopaminergic, serotoninergic and noradrenergic receptors. Research on the atypical antipsychotic compounds has led to a greater understanding of the biochemical effects of antipsychotic agents, leaving the basic dopamine hypothesis of schizophrenia insufficient to explain schizophrenic symptoms. Clozapine shows selectivity for mesolimbic neurons and does not increase the prolactin level. Binding studies have shown it to be a relatively weak D_1 and D_2 antagonist, compared with traditional neuroleptics (Farde et al., 1989). Clozapine shares the property of higher serotonin 5-HT_{2A} to dopamine D_2 blockade ratio reported to impart atypicality. The noradrenergic system may also have a role in the mechanism of action of clozapine (Breier, 1994). Clozapine, but not traditional neuroleptics, causes up to fivefold increases in plasma norepinephrine. Moreover, these increases in norepinephrine correlated with clinical response.

Risperidone is a benzisoxazol compound with a high affinity for 5-HT_{2A} and D_2 receptors and has a high serotonin dopamine receptor antagonism ratio. It has high affinity for alpha-1-adrenergic and H_1 histaminergic receptors and moderate affinity for alpha-2-adrenergic receptors. Risperidone is devoid of significant activity against the cholinergic system and the D_1 receptors. The efficacy of this medication is equal to that of other first-line atypical antipsychotic agents and is well tolerated and can be given once or twice a day. It is available in a liquid form as well. The most common side effects reported are drowsiness, orthostatic hypotension, lightheadedness, anxiety, akathisia, constipation, nausea, nasal congestion, prolactin elevation and weight gain. At doses above 6 mg/day EPS can become a significant issue. The risk of tardive dyskinesia at the regular therapeutic doses is low.

Olanzapine, a thienobenzodiazepine compound, has antagonistic effects at dopamine D_1 through D_5 receptors and serotonin 5-HT_{2A}, 5-HT_{2C} and 5-HT_6 receptors. The antiserotonergic activity is more potent than the antidopaminergic one. It also has affinity for alpha-1-adrenergic, M_1 muscarinic acetylcholinergic and H_1 histaminergic receptors. It differs from clozapine by not having high affinity for the 5-HT_7, alpha-2-adrenergic and other cholinergic receptors. It has significant efficacy against positive and negative symptoms and also improves cognitive functions. EPS is minimal when used in the therapeutic range with the exception of mild akathisia. As the compound has a long half-life, it is used once a day and as it is well tolerated, it can be started at a higher dose or rapidly titrated to the most effective dose. It is available as a rapidly disintegrating wafer form, which dissolves immediately in the mouth, and as an intramuscular form. The major side effects of olanzapine include significant weight gain, sedation, dry mouth, nausea, lightheadedness, orthostatic hypotension, dizziness, constipation, headache, akathisia and transient elevation of hepatic transaminases. The risk of tardive dyskinesia and NMS is low. Though used as a once-a-day medication, it is often administered twice a day with the average dose of 15 to 20 mg/day. However, doses higher than 20 mg/day are often used clinically and are thus being evaluated in clinical trials.

Quetiapine, a dibenzothiazepine compound has a greater affinity for serotonin 5-HT$_2$ receptors than for dopamine D$_2$ receptors; it has considerable activity at dopamine D$_1$, D$_5$, D$_3$, D$_4$, serotonin 5-HT$_{1A}$, and alpha-1-, and alpha-2-adrenergic receptors. Unlike clozapine, it lacks affinity for the muscarinic cholinergic receptors. It is usually administered twice a day due to a short half-life. Quetiapine is as effective as typical agents and also appears to improve cognitive function. Among 2035 patients enrolled in seven controlled studies, quetiapine at all doses used did not have an EPS rate greater than placebo. This is in contrast to olanzapine, risperidone and ziprasidone, where there were dose related effects on EPS levels. The rate of treatment emergent EPS was very low even in high at-risk populations such as adolescent, parkinsonian patients with psychosis and geriatric patients. Major side effects include somnolence, postural hypotension, dizziness, agitation, dry mouth and weight gain. Akathisia occurs on rare occasions. The package insert warns about developing lenticular opacity or cataracts and advises periodic eye examination based on data from animal studies. However, recent data suggest that this risk may be minimal.

Ziprasidone has the strongest 5-HT$_{2A}$ receptor binding relative to D$_2$ binding amongst the atypical agents currently in use. Interestingly, ziprasidone has 5-HT$_{1A}$ agonist and 5-HT$_{1D}$ antagonist properties with a high affinity for 5-HT$_{1A}$, 5-HT$_{2C}$ and 5-HT$_{1D}$ receptors. As it does not interact with many other neurotransmitter systems, it does not cause anticholinergic side effects and produces little orthostatic hypotension and relatively little sedation. Just like some antidepressants, ziprasidone blocks presynaptic reuptake of serotonin and norepinephrine. Ziprasidone has a relatively short half-life and thus it should be administered twice a day and along with food for best absorption. Ziprasidone is not completely dependent on CYP3A4 system for metabolism, thus inhibitors of the cytochrome system do not significantly change the blood levels. Ziprasidone at doses between 80 and 160 mg/day is probably the most effective agent for treating symptoms of schizophrenia. To assess the cardiac risk of ziprasidone and other antipsychotic agents a landmark study was designed to evaluate the cardiac safety of the antipsychotic agents, given at high doses alone and with a known metabolic inhibitor in a randomized study involving patients with schizophrenia. This was done to replicate the possible worst-case scenario (overdose or dangerous combination treatment) in the real world. All antipsychotic agents studied caused some degree of QTc prolongation, with the oral form of haloperidol associated with the least and thioridazine with the greatest degree. Major side effects reported with the use of ziprasidone are somnolence, nausea, insomnia, dyspepsia and prolongation of QTc interval. Dizziness, weakness, nasal discharge, orthostatic hypotension and tachycardia occur less commonly.

Ziprasidone should not be used in combination with other drugs that cause **significant** prolongation of the QTc interval. It is also contraindicated for patients with a known history of significant QTc prolongation, recent myocardial infarction, or symptomatic heart failure. Ziprasidone has low EPS potential, does not elevate prolactin levels and causes approximately 1 lb weight gain in short-term studies.

At present, with respect to efficacy, it does not appear that any one of the novel antipsychotic agents (except clozapine) is better than another one in treating schizophrenia. The randomized controlled trials suggest that, on average, these antipsychotic agents are each associated with 20% improvement in symptoms. However, clozapine is the only new antipsychotic agent that is more effective than haloperidol in managing treatment resistant schizophrenia. Unfortunately, its potential for treatment-emergent agranulocytosis, seizures and the new warning of myocarditis, precludes its use as a first line agent for schizophrenia. A major difference amongst the newer antipsychotic agents is the side effect profile and its effect on the overall quality of life of the patient.

Acute Treatment

In last few years, the use of novel antipsychotics has surpassed the use of typical ones in the management of acute phase symptoms of schizophrenia, except for the use of parenteral and liquid forms of antipsychotics where typical antipsychotic agents still hold an upper hand. However, this trend will most likely change once the injectable preparations of the novel antipsychotics enter the market. The primary goal of acute treatment is the amelioration of any behavioral disturbances that would put the patient or others at risk of harm. Acute symptom presentation or relapses are heralded by the recurrence of positive symptoms, including delusions, hallucinations, disorganized speech or behavior, severe negative symptoms or catatonia. Quite frequently, a relapse is a result of antipsychotic discontinuation, and resumption of antipsychotic treatment aids in the resolution of symptoms. There is a high degree of variability in response rates among individuals. When treatment is initiated, improvement in clinical symptoms can be seen over hours, days, or weeks of treatment.

Studies have shown that although typical neuroleptics are undoubtedly effective, a significant percentage (between 20 and 40%) of patients show only a poor or partial response to traditional agents. Furthermore, there is no convincing evidence that one typical antipsychotic is more efficacious as an antipsychotic than any other, although a given individual may respond better to a specific drug. Once an informed choice has been made between using a novel or typical antipsychotic medication by the patient and the clinician, selection of a specific antipsychotic agent should be based on efficacy, side-effect profile, history of prior response (or nonresponse) to a specific agent, or history of response of a family member to a certain antipsychotic agent. (For a pharmacotherapy decision tree based on Texas Medication Algorithm Project, see Figure 45.3.) Amongst the typical antipsychotic medications, low-potency, more sedating agents, such as chlorpromazine, were long thought to be more effective for agitated patients, yet there are no consistent data proving that high-potency agents are not equally useful in this context. The low-potency antipsychotics, however, are more associated with orthostatic hypotension and lowered seizure threshold and are often not as well tolerated at higher doses. Higher potency neuroleptics, such as haloperidol and fluphenazine, are safely used at higher doses and are effective in reducing psychotic agitation and psychosis itself. However, they are more likely to cause EPS than the low potency agents.

The efficacy of novel antipsychotic drugs on positive and negative symptoms is comparable to or even better than the typical antipsychotic. The significantly low potential to cause EPS or dystonic reaction and thus the decreased long-term consequences of TD has made the novel agents more tolerable and acceptable in acute treatment of schizophrenia. Other significant advantages adding to the popularity of novel antipsychotics include their beneficial impact on mood symptoms, suicidal risk and cognition. The selection of the first line treatment with novel antipsychotic

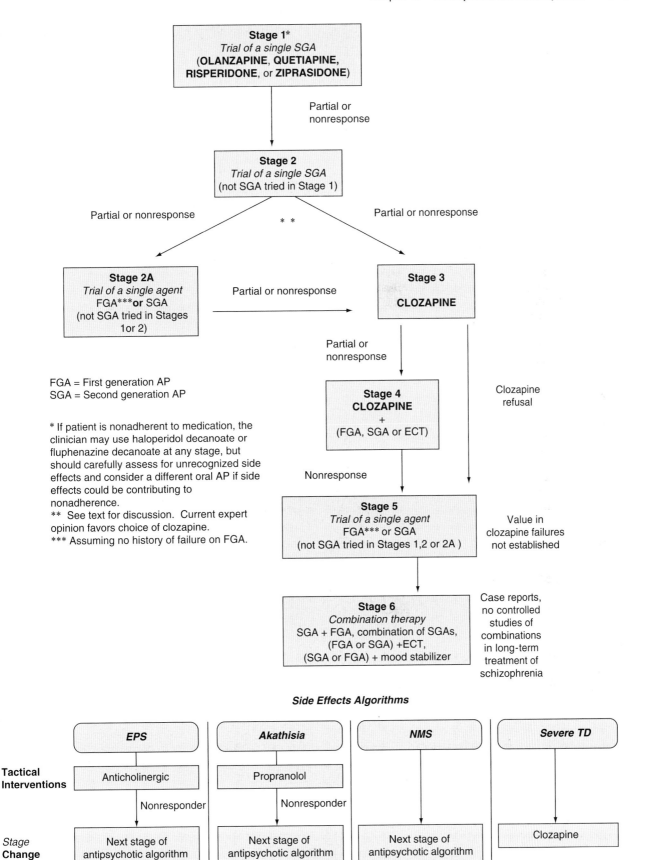

FGA = First generation AP
SGA = Second generation AP

* If patient is nonadherent to medication, the clinician may use haloperidol decanoate or fluphenazine decanoate at any stage, but should carefully assess for unrecognized side effects and consider a different oral AP if side effects could be contributing to nonadherence.

** See text for discussion. Current expert opinion favors choice of clozapine.

*** Assuming no history of failure on FGA.

Side Effects Algorithms

Continues

Coexisting Symptoms Algorithms

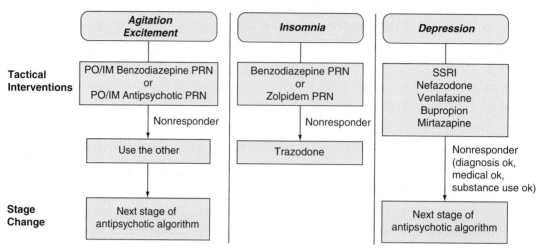

Figure 45.3 *Selecting antipsychotic treatment using Texas Medication Algorithm for Schizophrenia. Choice of antipsychotic (AP) should be guided by considering the clinical characteristics of the patient and the efficacy and side effect profiles of the medication. Any stage(s) can be skipped depending on the clinical picture or history of antipsychotic failures. Texas Medication Algorithm Project for choosing antipsychotic treatment, managing side-effects and coexisting symptoms. This project is a public–academic collaborative effort to develop, implement, and evaluate medication treatment algorithms for public sector patients. For more information or to view the most current version of the algorithm visit www.mhmr.state. tx.us/centraloffice/medicaldirector/tmaptoc.html)*

(and occasionally typical antipsychotic agent) also depends on the circumstances under which the medications are started, for example, extremely agitated or catatonic patients would require intramuscular preparation of the antipsychotic agents which would limit the choice. Except for clozapine, which is not considered first line treatment because of substantial and potentially life threatening side effects, there is no convincing data supporting the preference of one atypical over the other. However, if the patient does not respond to one, a trial with another atypical antipsychotic is reasonable and may produce response.

Once the decision is made to use an antipsychotic agent, an appropriate dose must be selected. Initially, higher doses or repeated dosing may be helpful in preventing grossly psychotic and agitated patients from doing harm. In general, there is no clear evidence that higher doses of neuroleptics (more than 2000 mg chlorpromazine equivalents per day) have any advantage over standard doses (400–600 chlorpromazine equivalents per day).

Some patients who are extremely agitated or aggressive may benefit from concomitant administration of high-potency benzodiazepines such as lorazepam, at 1 to 2 mg, until they are stable. Benzodiazepines rapidly decrease anxiety, calm the person, and help with sedation to break the cycle of agitation. They also help decrease agitation due to akathisia. The use of these medications should be limited to the acute stages of the illness to prevent tachyphylaxis and dependency. Benzodiazepines are quite beneficial in treatment of catatonic or mute patients but the results are only temporary though of enough duration to help with body functions and nutrition.

Maintenance Treatment

There is by now a great deal of evidence from long-term follow-up studies that patients have a higher risk of relapse and exacerbations if not maintained with adequate antipsychotic regimens. Noncompliance with medication, possibly because of intolerable neuroleptic side effects, may contribute to increased relapse rates. In

a double-blind, placebo-controlled study of relapse rates, 50% of patients in a research ward demonstrated clinically significant exacerbation of their symptoms within 3 weeks of stopping neuroleptic treatment. It is estimated that two-thirds of patients relapse after 9 to 12 months without neuroleptic medication, compared with 10 to 30% who relapse when typical neuroleptics are maintained. Long-term outcome studies showed that persistent symptoms that do not respond to standard neuroleptic therapy are associated with a greater risk of rehospitalization. Nonpharmacological interventions may help decrease relapse rates (discussed later).

Long-term treatment of schizophrenia is a complex issue. It is clear that the majority of patients require maintenance medication. Some patients do well with stable doses of neuroleptics for years without any exacerbations. However, many patients who are maintained with a stable neuroleptic dose have episodic breakthroughs of their psychotic symptoms. The difficulty in tolerating neuroleptic side effects often results in noncompliance with medication. It is therefore prudent to assess patients for medication compliance when signs of relapse are suspected. Prodromal cues may be present before an exacerbation of psychotic symptoms. For example, any recent change in sleep, attention to activities of daily living, or disorganization may be a warning sign of an impending increase in psychosis.

For patients for whom compliance is a problem, long-acting, depot neuroleptics are available in the USA for both traditional and novel antipsychotics. This form of medication delivery guarantees that the medication is in the system of the person taking it and eliminates the need to monitor daily compliance. This alternative should be considered if noncompliance with oral agents has led to relapses and rehospitalization. With these patients, maintenance treatment using long-acting preparations should begin as early as possible. Depot antipsychotic drugs are effective maintenance therapy for patients with schizophrenia.

Many studies have investigated appropriate maintenance doses of standard antipsychotics. Effective maintenance treatment s defined as that which prevents or minimizes the risks of symp-tom exacerbation and subsequent morbidity. A series of interest-ing dose-finding studies were performed by Kane and colleagues 1983, 1985) to determine the minimal dosage required to prevent relapse and to reduce the risk of extrapyramidal symptoms and tardive dyskinesia. This group found that the relapse rate (56%) of patients treated with lower doses of fluphenazine decanoate (1.25–mg every 2 weeks) was significantly greater than the relapse rate 14%) of patients receiving standard doses (12.5–50 mg every 2 weeks). Other investigators have found that this low dosage range may appear to prevent relapse for a certain period (Marder *et al.*, 984) but fails to do so if patients are followed up for more than year (Marder *et al.*, 1987). Unfortunately, no specific dosage reliably prevents relapse, and there is no way to predict future relapse. This is true for the novel antipsychotic agents as well.

Depression and Schizophrenia

Symptoms of depression occur in a substantial percentage of schizophrenia patients with a wide range of 7 to 75% and a modal rate of 25% and is associated with poor outcome, impaired func-tioning, suffering, higher rates of relapse or rehospitalization, and suicide. It is important to distinguish depression as a symptom or as a syndrome when it occurs. There is an important overlap of symptoms of depression with the negative symptoms. Differen-tiating these states can sometimes be difficult especially in pa-tients who lack the interpersonal communication skills to articu-late their internal subjective states well. A link between typical antipsychotic use and depression has been suggested with some considering depression to be a form of medication induced aki-nesia. Many patients have a reaction of disappointment, a sense of loss or powerlessness, or awareness of psychotic symptoms or psychological deficits that contributes to depression. Depression in schizophrenia is heterogeneous and requires careful diagnostic clarification. DSM-IV suggests that the term "postpsychotic de-pression" be used to describe depression that occurs at any time after a psychotic episode of schizophrenia, even after a prolonged interval. The atypical antipsychotic medications, with less po-tential to cause motor side effects and different mechanisms of action at receptor levels, themselves may contribute substantially towards a decrease in the rate of depression. Moreover, the atypi-cal antipsychotic medications appear to be superior to standard neuroleptics in treatment of negative symptoms. The clear advan-tage of atypical antipsychotic medications over the typical ones in treatment of psychosis itself can possibly further decrease the rate of depression. The impact of clozapine on the rate of suicide is significantly superior compared with the conventional agents. However, a large number of patients still end up with a depression that will require treatment with an antidepressant.

Risks and Side Effects of Typical Neuroleptics

Extrapyramidal symptoms are side effects of typical antipsy-chotic medications that include dystonias, oculogyric crisis, pseudoparkinsonism, akinesia and akathisia. They are referred to collectively as extrapyramidal symptoms or EPS because they are mediated at least in part by dopaminergic transmission in the extrapyramidal system. Prevalence rates vary among the differ-ent types of extrapyramidal symptoms. When present, they can be uncomfortable for the patient and a reason for noncompliance.

Dystonias are involuntary muscular spasms that can be brief or sustained, involving any muscle group. They can occur with even a single dose of medication. When they develop sud-denly, these spasms can be quite frightening to the patient and potentially dangerous, as in the case of laryngeal dystonias. They are more likely to be seen in young patients. Pseudoparkinsonism and akinesia are characterized by muscular rigidity, tremor and bradykinesia, much as in Parkinson's disease. On examination patients typically have masked facies, cogwheel rigidity, slowing and decreased arm swing with a shuffling gait. This condition is reported to be more prevalent than the dystonias, presenting with a frequency ranging from 15%.

Akathisia is more common, affecting more than 20% of patients taking neuroleptic medications (Ayd, 1961; Marsden *et al.*, 1986). This clinical entity presents as motor restlessness or an internal sense of restlessness. Often patients experiencing akathisia are unable to sit still during an interview. Akathisia is difficult to differentiate from agitation. The tendency to treat agi-tation with neuroleptics may exacerbate akathisia, making treat-ment decisions challenging.

Treatment of EPS can be difficult but usually involves administration of anticholinergic medications. Some advocate the use of prophylactic anticholinergic agents when beginning typical neuroleptic treatment to decrease the incidence of EPS. This option may be appropriate, but it should be used with cau-tion, considering the side effects associated with anticholinergic agents and their potential for abuse. Treatment of acute dystonic reactions usually involves acute intramuscular administration of either an anticholinergic or diphenhydramine. Akathisia may not respond to anticholinergic medications. Both neuroleptic dosage reduction and the use of beta-blocking agents such as propranolol have been found to be efficacious in the treatment of akathisia.

Nonextrapyramidal side effects of the typical antipsy-chotic agents include those that are secondary to blockade of muscarinic, histaminic and alpha-adrenergic receptors. These side effects, which are more commonly seen with the low-po-tency neuroleptics, include sedation, tachycardia and anticholin-ergic side effects such as urinary hesitancy or retention, blurred vision, or constipation. Other nonextrapyramidal side effects include some cardiac conduction disturbances, retinal changes, sexual dysfunction, weight gain, lowered seizure threshold and a risk of agranulocytosis.

Neuroleptic malignant syndrome (NMS) is a relatively rare but serious phenomenon seen in approximately 1% of patients taking neuroleptics. It can be fatal in 15% of cases if not prop-erly recognized and treated. Because the symptoms of NMS may reflect multiple etiologies, making diagnosis difficult, Levenson (1985) has proposed clinical guidelines. According to Levenson, three major or two major and four minor manifestations are in-dicative of a high probability of NMS. Major manifestations of NMS comprise fever, rigidity, and increased creatine kinase levels, and minor manifestations include tachycardia, abnormal blood pressure, tachypnea, altered consciousness, diaphoresis and leukocytosis. Others do not subscribe to the major–minor manifestation distinctions. In general, NMS is considered to be a constellation of symptoms that usually develops during 1 to 3 days. Although its pathogenesis is poorly understood, it has been associated with all antidopaminergic neuroleptic agents and presents at any time during treatment. It must be distinguished from other clinical entities, including lethal catatonia and malig-nant hyperthermia.

The mainstay of treatment is cessation of neuroleptic treat-ment and supportive care, including intravenous hydration, re-versal of fever with antipyretics and cooling blankets, and care-ful monitoring of vital signs because of the risk of cardiac and respiratory disturbance. Rhabdomyolysis is one of the most serious sequelae of NMS; it can lead to renal failure unless patients are well hydrated. In some cases, dantrolene and bromocriptine have been reported to be effective pharmacological treatments. Though quite rare, NMS has been reported even with the use of novel antipsychotic agents. The decision to rechallenge the patient with neuroleptics after an episode of NMS must be made with caution.

One of the major risks of neuroleptic treatment with the traditional antipsychotic agents is that of tardive dyskinesia, a potentially irreversible syndrome of involuntary choreoathetoid movements and chronic dystonias associated with long-term neuroleptic exposure. These buccal, orofacial, truncal, or limb movements can be exacerbated by anxiety and disappear during sleep. They can present with a range of severity, from subtle tongue movements to truncal twisting and pelvic thrusting movements and even possible respiratory dyskinesias. The prevalence rates for this syndrome range from less than 10 to more than 50%), but it is generally accepted that the risk increases 3 to 5% per year for each year the patient is treated with typical neuroleptics. Older age is a considerable risk factor for tardive dyskinesia, and there is some evidence that women are at increased risk for the development of this condition. Of note, a withdrawal dyskinesia that resembles tardive dyskinesia may appear on cessation of the neuroleptic. The specific mechanism involved in tardive dyskinesia remains unclear, although supersensitivity of dopaminergic receptors has been implicated.

All patients receiving traditional neuroleptic treatment should be monitored regularly for any signs of a movement disorder. DSM-IV now includes a diagnosis of neuroleptic-induced tardive dyskinesia. If tardive dyskinesia is suspected, the benefits of antipsychotic treatment must be carefully weighed against the risk of tardive dyskinesia. This should be discussed with the patient, and the antipsychotic should be removed if clinically feasible or at least maintained at the lowest possible dose that provides antipsychotic effect. This would also be an indication to switch to the novel antipsychotic agents with significantly reduced risk of TD or in the case of clozapine no risk of TD. In many instances, clozapine (and possibly quetiapine or olanzapine) may be the best treatment that can be offered for the TD itself. Unfortunately, there is no specific treatment of tardive dyskinesia, although some investigators have proposed the use of adrenergic agents such as clonidine, calcium channel blockers, vitamin E, benzodiazepines, valproic acid, or reserpine to reduce the spontaneous movements.

Sudden death in psychiatric patients treated with typical antipsychotic drugs has been reported for a long time. Sudden cardiac deaths probably occur from prolongation of the ventricular action potential duration represented as the QT interval (or QTc when corrected for heart rate) on the electrocardiogram resulting in a polymorphic ventricular tachycardia termed ***torsades de pointes*** that can degenerate into ventricular fibrillation. The incidence of *torsades de pointes* is unknown and the specific duration of the QTc interval at which the risk of an adverse cardiac event is greatest has not been established. QTc prolongation alone does not appear to explain *torsades de pointes*; several other risk factors must be present simultaneously with QT prolongation before *torsades de pointes* occur. These risk factors may include hypokalemia, hypomagnesemia, hypocalcemia, bradycardia, preexisting cardiac diseases (life-threatening arrhythmias, cardiac hypertrophy, heart failure and congenital QT syndrome), female gender, advancing age, baseline QTc interval of more than 460 m/sec and a long list of medications. In some instances, *torsades de pointes* may be associated with an increase in drug plasma concentrations (e.g., combination with drugs that inhibit the cytochrome P450 systems). Thus, the increase in polypharmacy in psychiatry is especially of concern. The frequency of ECG abnormalities in patients treated with antipsychotic drugs is unclear QTc prolongation has been reported with virtually all antipsychotic drugs. QTc prolongation by more than two standard deviations was reported in 8% of psychiatric patients treated with antipsychotics and especially in those receiving thioridazine (Riley *et al.*, 2000; 2001). Of the typical antipsychotic drugs, haloperidol, chlorpromazine, trifluoperazine, mesoridazine, prochlorperazine, droperidol and fluphenazine have all been reported to cause QTc prolongation and *torsades de pointes*, but thioridazine may be the worst offender. Pimozide, another typical antipsychotic, has also been associated with QTc prolongation, *torsades de pointes* and deaths. A reevaluation by the FDA of the cardiac safety parameters of thioridazine, mesoridazine and droperidol resulted in a black box warning due to significant QTc prolongation. Thus, it is important to monitor QTc interval in the high-risk population to prevent this rare, but potentially fatal side effect.

Side Effects of Novel Antipsychotic Agents

One of the most significant advantages of the newer antipsychotic agent is the relatively less risk of developing EPS and TD. However, treatment emergent substantial weight gain is a harbinger for long-term health consequences and frequently an important reason for noncompliance with medication. According to a meta-analysis done by Allison and colleagues (1999), clozapine and olanzapine are associated with a weight gain of about 10 lb over 10 weeks and ziprasidone was among the agents with the lowest weight gain at an average of 1 lb over the same period. Risperidone and quetiapine are intermediate with approximately 5 lb. Patients with schizophrenia, independent of the use of antipsychotic agents, are at higher risk of developing diabetes mellitus relative to the general. The data from Patient Outcome Research Team (PORT) suggest that the rate of diabetes mellitus and obesity amongst patients with major mental illness was substantially higher even before the advent of the novel antipsychotic drugs. This was more so in women and nonwhite populations. Thakore and colleagues (2002) investigated visceral fat distribution in drug-naïve and drug-free patients with schizophrenia. Compared with controls, patients with schizophrenia had central obesity and signficantly higher levels of plasma cortisol. Thus patients with schizophrenia are at a higher risk to develop major medical problems even before they are exposed to antipsychotic medications. However, this risk has been exacerbated with the introduction of the novel antipsychotic agents as seen by the dramatic rise in number of published cases and reports of significant hyperglycemia associated with the use of these medications, particularly olanzapine and clozapine and to a lesser extent with quetiapine and risperidone. The risk of antipsychotic-induced weight gain and secondary diabetes with clozapine and olanzapine may result from changes in glucose metabolism and insulin resistance induced by these agents. In approximately 40% of the cases of hyperglycemia, insulin resistance appears to occur even in absence of significant weight gain raising some interesting questions about how these medications may interact with the insulin-glycemic control. Unfortunately, in the case of clozapine the risk of developing abnormal glucose and diabetes mellitus appears to be cumulative over the years as reported by Henderson and colleagues (2000). There are no effective countermeasures available to help with weight gain and hyperglycemia. The substantial increased risk to the health of patients with schizophrenia due to these effects is worrisome and an important shortcoming of these efficacious and important medications.

Amongst the novel agents, risperidone, due to its potent dopamine D_2 blockade, remove the inhibitory dopaminergic tone in the tuberoinfundibular neurons resulting in significant increase in prolactin levels. This increase in prolactin is significantly more than usually seen with the typical antipsychotic agents. It is likely that the serotonin system is also involved along with dopamine in raising the prolactin levels. Clozapine and quetiapine on the other hand, are less potent at the D_2 receptors and thus are unlikely to cause prolactin elevations. In some individuals, these elevations of prolactin lead to amenorrhea, galactorrhea, gynecomastia and may possibly decrease bone mineral density. Ziprasidone and olanzapine, within the therapeutic dose range, do not cause significant increases in prolactin levels.

Cases of sudden death while receiving clozapine therapy (in physically healthy young adults with schizophrenia) from myocarditis and cardiomyopathy led to a black box warning from FDA.

Treatment Resistance and Negative Symptoms

The concept of treatment resistance has undergone significant modification in recent years. The original concept of treatment refractory applied to the use of typical antipsychotic agents. With the advent of the novel agents, which are generally more effective than the traditional ones, the patient should fail at least one novel antipsychotic agent before initiating a trial of clozapine mainly to avoid its side effects. The definition of the duration of a drug trial has also evolved over the years. It is increasingly appreciated that a 4 to 6 weeks duration of treatment with an antipsychotic agent at therapeutic doses can be considered an adequate trial. The recommended dosing has also undergone changes. The original recommendation considered a trial of 1000 mg equivalent of chlorpromazine as a necessary minimum requirement but this threshold is now reduced to 400 to 600 mg/day equivalent based on the knowledge that these doses block enough dopamine D_2 receptors with higher doses providing no additional benefit. Thus, a 4 to 6 week trial of 400 to 600 mg of chlorpromazine equivalent is accepted as an adequate antipsychotic trial.

In treatment refractory patients, typical antipsychotic use results in less than 5% response rate. Clozapine is the only antipsychotic drug proven more efficacious in rigorously defined treatment refractory groups. However, monitoring of blood counts and fear of its side effects makes it one of most underused effective treatment for schizophrenia.

Risperidone clearly appears to be superior to typical antipsychotics in treatment refractory patients but does not appear to be as efficacious as clozapine Olanzapine has been reported to have better outcome than haloperidol in the treatment-resistant schizophrenia group. However, when olanzapine was compared with chlorpromazine in a treatment refractory group using a double-blind study design, the outcome with olanzapine was not comparable to what is typically seen with the use of clozapine.

Negative symptoms, such as apathy, amotivational syndrome, flattened affect and alogia, are often the most problematic for patients with schizophrenia, accounting for much of the morbidity associated with this illness. In addition, these symptoms are often the most difficult to treat and do not respond well to traditional neuroleptics. The atypical antipsychotic agents are more effective against the negative symptoms than are the typical agents. However, the magnitude of the effect of these compounds on primary negative symptoms is not clear. Clearly, one of the goals of psychopharmacological research is to develop new antipsychotic agents with low associated risk, a more effective treatment for negative and cognitive symptoms, a further reduction in positive symptoms, and an improvement in long-term relapse rate for patients with chronic schizophrenia.

Augmentation of Typical Neuroleptics

When a patient has shown an inadequate response to traditional neuroleptic agents from different classes and there is a good reason for not switching to a novel antipsychotic drug, other strategies may be necessary to ameliorate residual symptoms. Adding a different type of psychotropic medication may augment the neuroleptic response in some individuals. Several neuroleptic augmentation strategies have been studied, including the addition of beta-blockers, thyrotropin-releasing hormone, clonidine and valproic acid, with mixed results. Lithium has been evaluated extensively for its efficacy as an additional treatment of schizophrenia. In one study, lithium seemed to improve psychotic symptoms of patients who had not adequately responded to neuroleptics alone (Small *et al.*, 1975). Although lithium does not seem to affect positive or negative symptoms specifically, it may be beneficial for patients who present at the depressed end of the spectrum (Meltzer, 1992). Similarly, carbamazepine has had mixed results as an augmentation agent although there is evidence that it can improve anxiety, withdrawal and depression. The use of benzodiazepines as augmenting agents in the treatment of schizophrenia has also been extensively studied. There may be some patients who show improvement in psychotic symptoms, and others who show improvement in negative symptoms. Interestingly, there has been a suggestion that the triazolobenzodiazepines may be more effective than other types of benzodiazepines in augmenting the neuroleptic response.

Antidepressant medications have also been considered in the treatment of depression associated with schizophrenia. Although there is some evidence that typical neuroleptics themselves cause depression there undoubtedly are schizophrenic patients who have primary depressive symptoms. Negative symptoms are often difficult to distinguish from depression (both have features of amotivation, apathy and social withdrawal), but those that are secondary to depression may respond to the addition of an antidepressant to the patient's medication regimen.

With electroconvulsive therapy as an adjuvant treatment, it appears the patient may improve initially, but relapse is likely. However, patients with comorbid affective symptoms may have some increased benefit. In general, however, this option should be considered only if the patient is not a candidate for a trial with an atypical antipsychotic agent and only if the patient has severe persistent symptoms.

When agonists of the glycine site of the NMDA receptor were added to typical antipsychotic agents in a placebo-controlled study, significant improvement were reported in negative symptoms and aspects of cognitive functioning (Heresco-Levy *et al.*, 1999). D-cycloserine, a partial agonist at the glycine site produced a selective improvement of negative symptoms at 6 weeks (Goff *et al.*, 1999). Augmentation with another endogenous full agonist, D-serine was associated with significant improvement in negative, positive, and cognitive symptoms when added to conventional agents in an 8-week trial (Tsai *et al.*, 1998).

Mechanism of Action of the Atypical Antipsychotic Agents

A higher ratio of the serotonin 5-HT_{2A} receptor to dopamine D_2 receptor blockade is reported to predict **atypicality**. This, along with other data, formed the basis of the **serotonin–dopamine hypothesis** that explains the possible mechanism of action underlying the efficacy of the atypical antipsychotics. However, studies using PET paradigm failed to detect differences in the serotonin receptor affinities between typical and atypical antipsychotics. Moreover, atypical antipsychotic agents produce high 5-HT_{2A} receptor occupancy at doses that are not sufficient to produce antipsychotic effects. This has raised some questions about the importance of 5-HT_{2A} blockade for a drug to be either atypical or have antipsychotic efficacy. Though the typical antipsychotics, compared with the atypical ones, show a much higher affinity for the D_2 receptors, both are effective only when their D_2 receptor occupancy exceeds 65%, suggesting that D_2 antagonism is important in producing antipsychotic effects. Thus, some suggest that the major difference between typical and atypical antipsychotic medications may lie in their affinity for the D_2 receptor. **Affinity** is the ratio of the rate at which the drug moves **off** of and **on** to the receptor. Interestingly, Seeman and colleagues found that 99% of the difference in affinity of the antipsychotic was driven by differences in their K_{off} at the D_2 receptor. Difference in the K_{on} did not account for any significant differences in affinity. Thus, PET studies suggest that all antipsychotics (typical as well as atypical) attach to the D_2 receptor with a similar rate constant but differ in how fast they come off the receptor. Thus, Kapur and Seeman (2001) propose that this relationship between fast K_{off} and low receptor affinity of the antipsychotic drug for dopamine D_2 receptor may explain atypicality. Furthermore, *in vivo*, antipsychotic agents modulate dopaminergic transmission and compete with endogenous dopamine. Thus, drugs with fast K_{off} (e.g., clozapine, quetiapine, etc.) modulate dopamine transmission differently from drugs with a slow K_{off} (e.g., haloperidol). For example, clozapine reaches equilibrium and goes on to and off the receptors significantly faster than haloperidol. When the concentration of endogenous dopamine rises physiologically, drugs like clozapine decrease their D_2 occupancy much faster and accommodate to natural surges of dopamine more readily then haloperidol.

Clinically, a significant difference between the typical and the atypical antipsychotic medications is the extent to which EPS occurs during treatment with therapeutic doses of antipsychotic drugs. PET studies suggest that the threshold for clinical antipsychotic response is lower than that of developing EPS and can be separated based on D_2 receptor occupancy. Specifically, D_2 occupancy of 65% or more significantly predicted clinical response, while D_2 occupancy of 78% or above significantly predicted EPS. Similarly, D_2 occupancy of 72% or higher resulted in prolactin elevation (Kapur *et al.*, 1996, 2000). Risperidone and olanzapine achieve strong antipsychotic activity only at doses that occupy 65% or more D_2 receptors, which is similar to haloperidol (Nordstrom and Farde, 1998). On the other hand, although clozapine and quetiapine show less than 60% D_2 occupancy 12 hours after drug administration (Seeman and Tallerico, 1999) these differences partly reflect a fast decline in D_2 occupancy. For example, quetiapine showed 60 and 20% D_2 occupancy 2 and 12 hours after receiving the medication. Similarly, clozapine showed 71% D_2 occupancy 1 to 2 hours after dose administration with a decline to 55% at 12 hours and 26% at 24 hours. It appears that both typical and atypical antipsychotics block sufficient number of D_2 receptors to achieve antipsychotic effect but differ in the kinetics of receptor occupancy.

It has been proposed that 5-HT_{2A} occupancy exerts an attenuating effect on the D_2 related EPS. Antipsychotic agents, both typical and atypical, give rise to EPS only when they exceed 78 to 80% D_2 occupancy; and when they do so, concomitant 5-HT_{2A} blockade does not appear to offer protection from these. Since clozapine and quetiapine never exceed this threshold of D_2 occupancy, they do not give rise to EPS. Since olanzapine and risperidone exceed this threshold in a dose-dependent fashion, they give rise to EPS also in a dose-dependent fashion.

New Directions

Psychopharmacological research has focused on developing compounds with unique combinations of effects at these different neurotransmitter sites. Future strategies for the treatment of schizophrenia are based on novel constructs of its pathophysiology.

One area of interest involves the glutamatergic system. Glutamate, the major excitatory neurotransmitter in the brain, is implicated in information processing and memory, functions that are impaired in schizophrenia. PCP, an NMDA antagonist, causes a syndrome with symptoms clinically similar to those of schizophrenia. These observations have led to the hypothesis that the glutamatergic NMDA receptor is involved in the pathophysiology of schizophrenia. Investigation of compounds that alter NMDA receptor activity is under way to learn more about the clinical significance of this neurotransmitter system.

In another area of drug development, researchers are studying G proteins, ubiquitous proteins found on cell membranes, where they play a critical role in second-messenger systems. These proteins have been found to be related to dopamine receptors in schizophrenic patients and to be involved in the mechanism of action of lithium in the treatment of bipolar disorder. Advanced genetic technology using techniques that could lead to altered receptor function "upstream" is also being explored. Given the enhanced understanding of influential biochemical, genetic and neurodevelopmental interactions, there is promise of developing treatment strategies that would provide a more effective, safe means of amelioriating both the positive and negative symptoms of schizophrenia.

Nonpharmacological Treatment of Schizophrenia

Background

Although psychopharmacological intervention has proved to be the foundation on which the treatment of schizophrenia depends, other approaches to the management of these patients serve a critical function. Studies have shown repeatedly that symptoms of schizophrenia have not only a genetic component but also an environmental aspect, and interactions with family and within the community can alter the course of the illness.

For many years, a dichotomous view of treatment options was tenaciously debated as dynamic psychiatry was challenged by developments in the neurosciences. A more unified view is now accepted, as it has become clear that psychopharmacological treatment strategies are most efficacious if combined with some type of psychosocial intervention and vice versa. It can be said that because of the chronic nature of schizophrenia, one or more treatments may be required throughout the illness and they are likely to have to be modified as symptoms change over time.

Psychosocial Rehabilitation

Bachrach has defined psychosocial rehabilitation as "a therapeutic approach that encourages a mentally ill person to develop his or her fullest capacities through learning and environmental supports" (Bachrach, 2000). According to the author, the rehabilitation process should appreciate the unique life circumstances of each person and respond to the individual's special needs while promoting both the treatment of the illness and the reduction of its attendant disabilities. The treatment should be provided in the context of the individual's unique environment taking into account social support network, access to transportation, housing, work opportunities and so on. Rehabilitation should exploit the patient's strengths and improve his/her competencies. Ultimately, rehabilitation should focus on the positive concept of restoring hope to those who have suffered major setbacks in functional capacity and their self-esteem due to major mental illness. To have this hope grounded in reality, it requires promoting acceptance of one's illness and the limitations that come with it. While work offers the ultimate in sense of achievement and mastery, it must be defined more broadly for the mentally ill and should include prevocational and nonvocational activities along with independent employment. It is extremely important that work is individualized to the talents, skills, and abilities of the individual concerned. However, psychosocial rehabilitation has to transcend work to encompass medical, social and recreational themes. Psychosocial treatment's basic principle is to provide comprehensive care through active involvement of the patient in his or her own treatment. Thus, it is important that a holding environment be created where patients can safely express their wishes, aspirations, frustrations and reservations such that they ultimately mold the rehabilitation plan. Clearly, to achieve these goals, the intervention has to be ongoing.

Given the chronicity of the illness, the process of rehabilitation must be enduring to encounter future stresses and challenges. These goals cannot be achieved without a stable relationship between the patient and rehabilitation counselor, which is central to an effective treatment and positive outcome. Thus, psychosocial rehabilitation is intimately connected to the biological intervention and forms a core component of the biopsychosocial approach to the treatment of schizophrenia. In the real world, programs often deviate from the aforementioned principles and end up putting excessive and unrealistic expectations on patients, thus achieving exactly the opposite of the intended values of the program (see Bachrach, 2000 for more details).

Individual Psychotherapy

Individual therapy in a nontraditional sense can begin on meeting a patient. Even the briefest of normalizing contacts with an agitated, acutely psychotic patient can have therapeutic value. Psychodynamic interpretations are not helpful during the acute stages of the illness and may actually agitate the patient further. The psychiatrist using individual psychotherapy should focus on forming and maintaining a therapeutic alliance (which is also a necessary part of psychopharmacological treatment) and providing a safe environment in which the patient is able to discuss symptoms openly. A sound psychotherapist provides clear structure about the therapeutic relationship and helps the patient to focus on personal goals.

Often, a patient is not aware of or does not have insight into the fact that some beliefs are part of a specific symptom. A psychotherapist helps a patient to check whether his or her reality coincides with that of the therapist. The therapeutic intervention then becomes a frank discussion of what schizophrenia is and how symptoms may feel to the patient. This objectifying of psychotic or negative symptoms can prove of enormous value in allowing the patient to feel more in control of the illness. A good analogy is to diabetic patients, who know they have a medical illness and are educated about the symptoms associated with exacerbation. Just as these patients can check blood glucose levels, schizophrenia patients can discuss with a therapist their sleep patterns, their interpersonal relationships and their internal thoughts, which may lead to earlier detection of relapses.

Schizophrenia often strikes just as a person is leaving adolescence and entering young adulthood. The higher the premorbid level of social adjustment and functioning, the more devastating and confusing the onset of symptoms becomes. Young male patients with a high level of premorbid function are at increased risk of suicide, presumably in part because of the tremendous loss they face. These feelings can continue for years, with schizophrenia patients feeling isolated and robbed of a normal life. Therefore, a component of individual work (which can also be achieved to some degree in a group setting) with these patients is a focus on the impact schizophrenia has had on their lives. Helping patients to grieve for these losses is an important process that may ultimately help them achieve a better quality of life.

Group Psychotherapy

Acutely psychotic patients do not benefit from group interaction. As their condition improves, inpatient group therapy prepares patients for interpersonal interactions in a controlled setting. After discharge, patients may benefit from day treatment programs and outpatient groups, which provide ongoing care for patients living in the community.

Because one of the most difficult challenges of schizophrenia is the inherent deficits in relatedness, group therapy is an important means of gathering patients together and providing them with a forum for mutual support. Insight-oriented groups may be disorganizing for patients with schizophrenia, but task-oriented, supportive groups provide structure and a decreased sense of isolation for this population of patients. Keeping group focus on structured topics, such as daily needs or getting the most out of community services, is useful for these patients. In the era of community treatment and brief hospitalizations, many patients are being seen in medication groups, which they attend regularly to discuss any side effects or problems and to obtain prescriptions.

Psychoeducational Treatment

One of the inherent deficits from which schizophrenia patients suffer is an inability to engage appropriately in social or occupational activities. This debilitating effect is often a lasting feature of the illness, despite adequate psychopharmacological intervention. This disability often isolates patients and makes it difficult for them to advocate appropriate social support or community services. Furthermore, studies have found that there is a correlation between poor social functioning and incidence of relapse One of the challenges of this area of study is the great deal of variability in individual patients. However, standardized measures have been developed to ascertain objective ratings of social deficits. These assessments have become important tools in the determination of effective nonpharmacological treatment strategies.

The literature suggests that schizophrenia patients can benefit from social skills training. This model is based on the idea that the course of schizophrenia is, in part, a product of the environment, which is inherently stressful because of the social deficits from which these patients suffer. The hypothesis is that if patients are able to monitor and reduce their stress, they could potentially decrease their risk of relapse. For this intervention to be successful, patients must be aware of and set their own goals. Goals such as medication management, activities of daily living and dealing with a roommate are achievable examples. Social skills and deficits can be assessed by patients' self-report, observation of behavioral patterns by trained professionals, or a measurement of physiological responses to specific situations (e.g., increased pulse when asking someone to dinner). Patients can then begin behavioral training in which appropriate social responses are shaped with the help of instructors.

One example of such a program, discussed by Liberman and colleagues (1985), is a highly structured curriculum that includes a training manual, audiovisual aids and role-playing exercises. Behaviors are broken down into small bits, such as learning how to maintain eye contact, monitor vocal volume, or ameliorate body language. The modules are learned one at a time, with role-playing, homework and feedback provided to the participants. In several studies, Liberman and coworkers (1986) have shown that patients who were treated with social skills training and medication spent less time hospitalized, with fewer relapses than those treated with holistic health measures (e.g., yoga, stress management) on 2-year follow-up. Research such as this in the field of social skills training is growing as the inherent deficits in information processing, executive function and interpersonal skills are further elucidated.

Social Skills Training

In large number of patients, deficits in social competence persist despite antipsychotic treatment. These deficits can lead to social distress whereas social competence can alleviate distress related to social discomfort. Paradigms using instruction, modeling, role-playing and positive reinforcement are helpful. Controlled studies suggest that schizophrenia patients are able to acquire lasting social skills after attending such programs and apply these skills to everyday life. Besides reducing anxiety, social skills training also improve level of social activity and foster new social contacts. This in turn improves the quality of life and significantly shortens duration of inpatient care. However, their impact on symptom resolution and relapse rates is unclear.

Cognitive Remediation

Patients with schizophrenia generally demonstrate poor performance in various aspects of information processing. Cognitive dysfunction can be a rate-limiting factor in learning and social functioning. Additionally, impaired information processing can lead to increased susceptibility to stress and thus to an increase risk of relapse. Practice appears to improve some of the cognitive dysfunction. Remediation of cognitive dysfunctions with social skills training has been reported to have positive impact. Various types of cognitive behavioral therapies were particularly effective. Social skills training program, cognitive training program to improve neurocognitive functioning and cognitive behavioral therapy approaches are oriented towards coping with symptoms, the disorder and everyday problems.

Cognitive Adaptation Training

Cognitive adaptation training (CAT) is a novel approach to improve adaptive functioning and compensate for the cognitive impairments associated with schizophrenia. A thorough functional needs assessment is done to measure current adaptive functioning. Besides measuring adaptive functioning and quantifying apathy and disinhibition, a neurocognitive assessment using tests to measure executive function, attention, verbal and visual memory, and visual organization is also completed. Treatment plans are adapted to the patient's level of functioning, which includes patient's level of apathy. Interventions include removal of distracting stimuli, use of reminders such as checklists, signs and labels.

Family Therapy

A large body of literature explores the role of familial interactions and the clinical course of schizophrenia. Many of these studies have examined the outcome of schizophrenia in relation to the degree of expressed emotion (EE) in family members. EE is generally defined as excessive criticism and over involvement of relatives. Schizophrenia patients have been found to have a higher risk of relapse if their relatives have high EE levels. Clearly, a patient's disturbing symptoms at the time of relapse may affect the level of criticism and over involvement of family members, but evidence suggests that preexisting increased EE levels in relatives predict increased risk of schizophrenic relapse and that interventions that decrease EE levels can decrease relapse rates.

Hogarty and colleagues (1986) examined the effectiveness of neuroleptics alone, neuroleptics plus psychoeducational family treatment (based on addressing EE levels), social skills training for neuroleptic-treated patients with schizophrenia, and the combination of all three. Perhaps not surprisingly, they found a decreased relapse rate in the patients treated with medication and family therapy as well as in the group treated with neuroleptic and social skills training. The combination of the treatments had an additive effect and was far superior to medication treatment alone.

Though family intervention studies suffer from methodological limitations, the efficacy of family intervention on relapse rate is fairly well supported. This efficacy was particularly evident when contrasted with low quality or uncontrolled individual treatments. The addition of family intervention to standard treatment of schizophrenia has a positive impact on outcome to a moderate extent. Family intervention effectively reduces the short-term risk of clinical relapse after remission from an acute episode. There is evidence of effect on patient's mental state and social functioning, or on any family-related variables. The elements common to most effective interventions are inclusion of the patient in at least some phases of the treatment, long duration, and information and education about the illness provided within a supportive framework. There is sufficient data only for male chronic patients living with high EE parents. Evidence is limited for recent onset patients, women, and people in different family arrangements and families with low EE. Research in family intervention is still a growing field. Thus, at present it is unclear if the effect seen with family therapy is due to family treatment or more intensive care.

Leff (2000) concluded from his review that family interventions reduced relapse rates by one -half over the first year of combined treatment with medications and family therapy. Medications and family therapy augment each other. Psychoeducation by itself is not enough. It also seems that multiple family groups are more efficacious then single family sessions. Attempts are being made to generalize training of mental health workers in effectively implementing these strategies.

Based on these findings, it is clear that there is a significant interaction between the level of emotional involvement and criticism of relatives of probands with schizophrenia and the outcome of their illness. Identifying the causative factors in familial stressors and educating involved family members about schizophrenia lead to long-term benefits for patients. Future work in this field must examine these interactions with an understanding of modern sociological and biological advances in genetics, looking at trait carriers, social skills assessments, positive and negative symptoms, and medication management with the novel antipsychotic agents.

Case Management

Assertive Community Treatment (ACT) is a community care model with a caseload per worker of 15 patients or less in contrast to standard case management (SCM) with a caseload of 30 to 35 patients. Intensive clinical case management (ICCM) differs from ACT by the case manager not sharing the caseload. In the ACT model, most services are provided in the community rather than in the office; the caseloads are shared across clinicians rather than individual separate caseloads. These are time unlimited services provided directly by the ACT team and not brokered out and 24-hour coverage is provided. Research on the ACT model confirms that it is successful in making patients comply with treatment and leads to less inpatient admissions. ACT also improves housing conditions (fewer homeless patients, more patients in stable housing), employment, quality of life and patient satisfaction. No clear differences between ACT and standard or intensive clinical case management are reported with mental condition, social functioning, self-esteem, or number of deaths.

Combining Pharmacological and Psychosocial Treatments

The combination of pharmacological and psychosocial interventions in schizophrenia can have complex interactions. For example, psychotherapies improve medication compliance on one hand but are more effective in the presence of antipsychotic treatment. Family psychoeducation has been reported to decrease the level of expressed emotion in the family resulting in better social adjustment and a need for lower dose of antipsychotic medications. Marder and colleagues (1996) found in their study that pharmacological and psychosocial treatments affect different outcome dimensions. Medications affect relapse risk whereas skills training affect social adjustment. The VA cooperative study by Rosenheck and colleagues (1998) found that patients who received clozapine were more likely to participate in these treatments and led to improved quality of life. The qualitative differences in the interactions between the newer antipsychotic agents and psychotherapy suggest a hopeful trend of better utilization of psychosocial treatments.

Self-directed Treatment

Groups such as the National Alliance for Mentally Ill (NAMI) and the Manic–Depressive Association offer tremendous resources to psychiatric patients and their relatives. They provide newsletters, neighborhood meetings and support groups to interested persons. These nonprofessional self-help measures may feel less threatening to patients and their families and provide an important adjunct to professional settings.

Structured self-help clubs have also been effective means of bolstering patients' social, occupational and living skills. The Fountain House was the first such club aimed at social rehabilitation (Beard *et al.*, 1982). Patients who are involved are called members of the club, giving them a sense of belonging to a group. They are always made to feel welcome, useful, and productive members of the club community.

The clubhouse model has expanded to provide services such as transitional employment programs, apartment programs, outreach programs, and medication management and consultation services, to name a few. A self-supportive rehabilitation program for mentally ill patients is an important option for many schizophrenic patients who might otherwise feel isolated and out of reach.

Stigma

Though tremendous progress has occurred in understanding and treatment of schizophrenia, stigmatizing attitudes still prevail (Crisp *et al.*, 2000); in a survey, schizophrenia elicited the most negative opinions and over 70% of those questioned thought that schizophrenia patients were dangerous and unpredictable. Thus, stigma surrounding schizophrenia can cause people suffering from the illness to develop low self-esteem, disrupt personal relationships and decrease employment opportunities. The World Psychiatric Association (WPA) has initiated an international program aimed at developing tools to fight stigma and discrimination (Sharma, 2001).

Clinical Vignette 1

Mr A first sought psychiatric help at the age of 19 years. During his first year of college he had a difficult adjustment. He had never had close friends, but at school he felt isolated from his family. Although he had always been a good student, averaging As and Bs in high school, he was unable to achieve the same level of academic performance. He became increasingly distressed by his sense of isolation and his inability to maintain an adequate grade point average. Around the middle of his first year of college he saw a psychiatrist, who thought he was having an adjustment reaction to his new surroundings. He was not given medication at the time but was referred for supportive psychotherapy. After two appointments with his therapist, he decided it was not helpful.

Shortly thereafter, he began to feel that the other students were staring at him and laughing at him behind his back. Then he began to feel as if they were playing tricks on him, sending secret messages to him over the radio to torment him. This experience lasted over 6 months. He also began hearing two voices, which he did not recognize. These voices would comment on his behavior and criticize his actions. They began to tell him to stay out of his dormitory room at night. The voices also warned him that the dormitory food was poisoned. One night, he was picked up by police for loitering and was brought to an emergency department.

The emergency department psychiatrist saw him as a disheveled, unshaven man who was agitated during the interview, pacing across the examining room. He was wearing dark sunglasses, although it was the middle of the night, and he said he did not want the examiner to read his mind by looking into his eyes, so he kept the sunglasses on throughout the interview. His speech was of normal rate and prosody, although there were long pauses in some of his responses. He was able to respond to questions clearly, and his thought processes were logical, although he repeatedly spoke angrily as if responding to voices. He did say that the voices had been telling him to kill himself for the past two nights, although he said he was trying not to listen to them. The patient showed only some difficulty

Clinical Vignette 1 *continued*

in concentration on a cognitive examination. His judgment was fair in that he recognized his need
for some help, but he showed no insight into his symptoms.

The psychiatrist felt that the patient was potentially dangerous to himself because of the command auditory hallucinations and required hospitalization. Mr A did not agree to come into the hospital, and the psychiatrist sought involuntary hospitalization through appropriate procedures. In the hospital, the patient was initially quite agitated, requiring intramuscular haloperidol and lorazepam. Almost immediately his behavior calmed, and he was able to agree to hospitalization and treatment. He was treated with risperidone, and the dose was titrated up to 3 mg/day by mouth at bedtime. After 1 week with this medication regimen, he began to experience a decrease in his auditory hallucinations and paranoid ideation. He was sleeping better and was no longer concerned about the foods he was eating.

Other Psychoses

Schizoaffective Disorder

Over the decades, these patients were often classified as having atypical schizophrenia, good prognosis schizophrenia, remitting schizophrenia, or cycloid psychosis. Inherent within these diagnoses was the implication that they shared similarities to schizophrenia and also appeared to have a relatively better course of illness. With the advent of effective treatment of bipolar disorder with lithium salts, some of these patients started responding to lithium, and the term schizoaffective disorder gained further momentum and evolved in the direction of bipolar disorder. Unfortunately, this lack of diagnostic clarity has plagued the diagnosis of schizoaffective disorder such that there is much that is unknown about the illness.

Epidemiology

The diagnosis of schizoaffective disorder has undergone numerous changes through the decades making it difficult to get reliable epidemiology information. When data was pooled together from various clinical studies, approximately 2 to 29% of those patients diagnosed to have mental illness at the time of the study were suffering from schizoaffective disorder with women having a higher prevalence (Keck *et al.*, 2001). This could possibly be explained by a higher rate of depression in women. Relatives of women suffering from schizoaffective disorder have a higher rate of schizophrenia and depressive disorders compared with relatives of male schizoaffective subjects. The estimated lifetime prevalence of schizoaffective disorder is possibly in the range of 0.5 to 0.8%. In the inpatient settings of New York State psychiatric hospitals, approximately 19% of 6000 patients had a diagnosis of schizoaffective disorder (Levinson *et al.*, 1999).

Gender and Age

The depressive type of schizoaffective disorder appears to be more common in older people while the bipolar type probably occurs more commonly in younger adults. The higher prevalence of the disorder in women appears to occur particularly amongst those who are married. As in schizophrenia, the age of onset for women is later than that for men. Depression tends to occur more commonly in women.

Etiology

The etiology of schizoaffective disorder is unknown. There is a dearth of data relating to this illness. Studies involving families of schizoaffective probands suggest that they have significantly higher rates of relatives with mood disorder than families of schizophrenia probands. It is possible that some of the same environmental theories that apply to schizophrenia and bipolar disorder may also apply to schizoaffective disorder. It is most likely that schizoaffective disorder is a heterogeneous condition. Thus, depending on the type of schizoaffective disorder studied an increased prevalence of either schizophrenia or mood disorders may be found in their relatives. As a group, patients with schizoaffective disorder have a prognosis intermediate between mood disorders and schizophrenia. Thus, on an average they have a better course than those suffering from schizophrenia, respond to mood stabilizers more often and tend to have a relatively nondeteriorating course.

Diagnosis

Schizoaffective disorder criteria have evolved over the years and undergone major changes. According to the DSM-IV, a patient with schizoaffective disorder must have an uninterrupted period of illness during which, at some time, they meet the diagnostic criteria for a major depressive episode, manic episode, or a mixed episode concurrently with the diagnostic criteria for the active phase of schizophrenia (criteria A for schizophrenia). Additionally, "the patient must have had delusions or hallucinations for at least 2 weeks in the absence of prominent mood disorder symptoms" during the same period of illness. The mood disorder symptoms must be present for a substantial part of the active and residual psychotic period. The essential features of schizoaffective disorder must occur within a single uninterrupted period of illness where the "period of illness" refers to the period of active or residual symptoms of psychotic illness and this can last for years and decades. The total duration of psychotic symptoms must be at least 1 month to meet the criteria A for schizophrenia and thus, the minimum duration of a schizoaffective episode is also 1 month.

The criteria for major depressive episode requires a minimum duration of 2 weeks of either depressed mood or markedly diminished interest or pleasure. As the symptoms of loss of pleasure or interest commonly occur in nonaffective psychotic disorders, to meet the criteria for schizoaffective disorder criteria A, the major depressive episode must include pervasive depressed mood. Presence of markedly diminished interest or pleasure is not sufficient to make a diagnosis as it is possible that these symptoms may occur with other conditions too.

The DSM-IV diagnosis of schizoaffective disorder can be further classified as schizoaffective disorder **bipolar type** or schizoaffective disorder **depressive type**. For a person to be classified as having the bipolar subtype he/she must have a disorder that includes a manic or mixed episode with or without a history of major depressive episodes. Otherwise the person is classified as having depressive subtype having had symptoms that meet the criteria for a major depressive episode with no history of having had mania or mixed state.

Clinical Features

The clinical signs and symptoms of schizoaffective disorder include all the signs and symptoms of schizophrenia, and a manic episode and/or a major depressive episode. The schizophrenia and mood symptoms may occur together or in an alternate sequence. The clinical course can vary from one of exacerbations and remissions to that of a long-term deterioration. Presence of mood-incongruent psychotic features – where the psychotic content of hallucinations or delusions is not consistent with the prevailing mood – more likely indicate a poor prognosis.

Differential Diagnosis

The possible differential diagnosis consists of bipolar disorder with psychotic features, major depressive disorder with psychotic features and schizophrenia. Clearly, substance induced states and symptoms caused by coexisting medical conditions should be carefully ruled out. All conditions listed in differential diagnosis of schizophrenia, bipolar disorder and major depressive disorder should be considered including but not limited to those patients undergoing treatment with steroids, those abusing substances such as PCP and medical conditions such as temporal lobe epilepsy. In circumstances where there is ambiguity, it may be prudent to delay making a final diagnosis until the most acute symptoms of psychosis have subsided and time is allowed to establish a course of illness and collect collateral information.

Course and Prognosis

Due to the evolving nature of the diagnosis and limited studies done thus far much remains unknown. However, to the extent that this illness has symptoms from both a major mood disorder and schizophrenia, theoretically one can confer a relatively better prognosis then schizophrenia and a relatively poorer prognosis then bipolar disorder, The following variables are harbingers of a poor prognosis:

1. a poor premorbid history;
2. an insidious onset;
3. absence of precipitating factors;
4. a predominance of psychotic symptoms, especially deficit or negative ones;
5. an early age of onset;
6. an unremitting course, and;
7. a family history of schizophrenia.

The corollary would be that the opposite of each of these characteristics would suggest a better prognosis. Interestingly, the presence or the absence of Schneiderian first-rank symptoms does not seem to predict the course of illness. The incidence of suicide in patients with schizoaffective disorder is at least 10%. Some data indicate that the suicidal behavior may be more common in women then men.

In one study, 82% of those patients who were suffering from a first episode of schizoaffective disorder, and had recovered, experienced psychotic relapse within 5 years. These patients had high rates of second and third relapses despite careful monitoring. Medication discontinuations in first episode patients who are stable for 1 year substantially increase relapse risks. Aside from medication status, premorbid social adjustment was the only predictor of relapse in their study. Poor adaptation to school and premorbid social isolation predicted initial relapse independent of medication status. Thus, like schizophrenia, the risk of relapse is diminished by antipsychotic maintenance treatment (Robinson et al., 1999).

Treatment

With the shifting definitions of schizoaffective disorder, evaluating the treatment of schizoaffective disorder is not easy. Mood stabilizers, antidepressants and antipsychotic medications clearly have a role in management of these patients. The presenting symptoms, their duration and intensity, and patient choices need to be incorporated into deciding what treatment(s) to choose.

Antipsychotic Medications

Atypical antipsychotic medications are reported to be more effective than the typical ones in the treatment of schizoaffective disorder. They appear to have a more broad-spectrum effects then the typical agents. Optimizing antipsychotic treatment, especially with the novel agents, is more likely to be effective than the routine use of adjunctive antidepressants or mood stabilizers. However, when indicated, the use of antidepressants is well supported in schizoaffective patients who present with a full depressive syndrome after stabilization of psychosis.

Olanzapine, ziprasidone and risperidone appear to be effective against symptoms of psychosis, mania and depression. Clozapine use may be beneficial in the treatment of refractory schizoaffective disorder as it has both mood stabilizing and antipsychotic properties, a substantial advantage.

Mood Stabilizers

A small number of studies suggest that valproic acid, lithium and lamotrigine are effective in treating the manic symptoms associated with schizoaffective disorder, bipolar type.

Antidepressants The novel antipsychotic agents are often efficacious against depression in patients who suffer from both depression and psychosis negating the need for routine use of antidepressants. However, there are patients who remain depressed even with optimal antipsychotic and mood stabilizer treatment. SSRIs are widely used in patients who present with schizoaffective disorder with depression. If the SSRIs and newer antidepressants do not show efficacy, tricyclic antidepressants do have a role. Interestingly, chlorpromazine in combination with amitriptyline was reported to be as effective as chlorpromazine alone. Many studies suggest that addition of antidepressants helps in effective treatment of depression in schizoaffective disorder. Occasionally, antidepressants may worsen the course. For patients suffering from depression where they are not responding adequately and are at risk for suicide, ECT is an effective alternative.

Psychosocial Treatment To the extent that schizoaffective disorder shares symptoms with schizophrenia, most of the psychosocial treatments used in the treatment of schizophrenia are likely to be useful in the treatment of schizoaffective disorder. Specifically, patients benefit from individual supportive therapy, family therapy, group therapy, cognitive–behavioral therapy and social skills training. Many patients would be suitable candidates for assertive community therapy (ACT). Depending on the level of recovery, some of the patients may need rehabilitation services to assist them with either developing skills for some form of employment or assistance to maintain a job. Family members benefit from support groups such as NAMI or MDA groups.

Brief Psychotic Disorder

Brief psychotic disorder is defined by DSM-IV-TR as a psychotic disorder that lasts more than 1 day and less than a month.

Moreover, the disorder may develop in response to severe psychosocial stressors or group of stressors European and Scandinavian countries have traditionally diagnosed this type of psychosis as **psychogenic psychoses**, **reactive psychosis**, or **brief reactive psychosis**.

Epidemiology

This illness is not uncommon, but, unfortunately, reliable estimates of the incidence, prevalence, sex ratio and average age of onset are not available. It is believed that this disorder is more common among young people with occasional cases involving older people. This disorder may be seen more commonly in patients from low socioeconomic classes and in those with personality disorders such as histrionic, paranoid, schizotypal, narcissistic and borderline. Though immigrants and people who have experienced major disasters are reported to be at a higher risk, well-controlled studies have failed to show this.

Diagnosis

The DSM-IV diagnostic criteria specify the presence of at least one clear psychotic symptom lasting a minimum of 1 day to a maximum of 1 month. Furthermore, DSM-IV allows the specification of two additional features: the presence or the absence of one or more marked stressors and a postpartum onset. DSM-IV describes a continuum of diagnosis for psychotic disorder based primarily on duration of the symptoms. Once the duration criteria are met, other conditions such as etiological medical illnesses and substance-induced psychosis need to be excluded. In those cases where the duration of psychosis lasts more than 1 month, appropriate diagnosis to be considered are other psychotic conditions based on reevaluation of the clinical features, duration of psychosis and presence of mood symptoms.

Clinical Features

People suffering from this disorder usually present with an acute onset, manifest at least one major symptom of psychosis, and do not always include the entire symptom constellation seen in schizophrenia. Affective symptoms, confusion and impaired attention may be more common in brief psychotic disorders than in chronic psychotic conditions. Some of the characteristic symptoms include emotional lability, outlandish behavior, screaming or muteness and impaired memory for recent events. Some of the symptoms suggest a diagnosis of **delirium** and may warrant a more complete medical workup. The symptom patterns include acute paranoid reactions, reactive confusions, excitations and depressions.

Precipitating Stressors

The precipitating stressors most commonly encountered are major life events that would cause any person significant emotional turmoil. Such events include the death of a close family member or severe accidents. Rarely, it could be accumulation of many smaller stresses.

Differential Diagnosis

Although the classical presentation may be short in duration and associated with stressors, a thorough and careful evaluation is necessary. Additional information is critical to rule out other major psychotic conditions as temporal association of stressors to the acute manifestation of symptoms may be coincidental and thus misleading. Other conditions to be ruled out include psychotic disorder due to a general medical condition, substance-induced psychosis, factitious disorder with predominantly psychological

signs and symptoms, and malingering. Patients with epilepsy and delirium may also present with similar symptoms. Additional conditions to be considered are dissociative identity disorder and psychotic episodes associated with borderline and schizotypal personality disorder that may last for less than a day.

Course and Prognosis

As defined by DSM-IV, the duration of the disorder is less than 1 month. Nonetheless, the development of such a significant psychiatric disorder may indicate a patient's mental vulnerability. An unknown percentage of patients who are first classified as having brief psychotic disorder later display chronic psychiatric syndromes such as schizophrenia and bipolar disorder. Patients with brief psychotic disorders generally have good prognosis, and European studies indicate that 50 to 80% of all patients have no further major psychiatric problems.

The length of the acute and residual symptoms is often just a few days. Occasionally, depressive symptoms follow the resolution of the psychosis. Suicide is a concern during both the psychotic phase and the postpsychotic depressive phase. Indicators of good prognosis are good premorbid adjustment, few premorbid schizoid traits, severe precipitating stressors, sudden onset of symptoms, confusion and perplexity during psychosis, little affective blunting, short duration of symptoms and absence of family history of schizophrenia.

Treatment

These patients may require short-term hospitalizations for a comprehensive evaluation and safety. Antipsychotic drugs are often most useful along with benzodiazepines. Long-term use of medication is often not necessary and should be avoided. If maintenance medications are necessary, the diagnoses may need to be revised. Clearly, the newer antipsychotic agents have a better neurological side effect profile and would be preferred over the typical agents.

Psychotherapy is necessary to help the person reintegrate the experience of psychosis and possibly the precipitating trauma. Individual, family and group therapies may be necessary in some individuals. Many patients need help to cope with the loss of self-esteem and confidence.

Schizophreniform Disorder

Gabriel Langfeldt (1939) suggested the term **Schizophreniform Disorder** in 1937 for a heterogeneous group of patients characterized by the similarity of their symptoms to those of schizophrenia albeit with a good clinical outcome. Langfeldt observed that those patients whose diagnosis was questionable as schizophrenia had a much better outcome than those whose diagnosis was confirmed as schizophrenia; these patients were thus classified as having schizophreniform psychosis. Langfeldt also noted that these patients often had good premorbid adjustment, an abrupt onset of symptoms, frequent presence of psychosocial stressor(s) and a good prognosis.

Family History

Several studies suggest that the relatives of patients with schizophreniform psychosis are at a high risk of having psychiatric disorders. The relatives of patients with schizophreniform psychosis are more likely to have mood disorders than are the relatives of patients with schizophrenia. In addition, the relatives of patients with schizophreniform disorder are more likely to have a diagnosis of a psychotic mood disorder than are the relatives of patients with bipolar disorders.

Biological Measures

Although brain-imaging studies suggest a similarity between schizophreniform disorder and schizophrenia, one study of electrodermal activity has indicated a difference. Patients with schizophrenia born during the winter and spring months had hyporesponsive skin conductances, but this association was absent in patients with schizophreniform disorder. Though the significance of this one study would be difficult to interpret, the results do suggest caution in assuming similarity between patients with schizophrenia and those with schizophreniform disorder. Data from a study of eye tracking in the two groups also indicate that there are differences on some biological measures between schizophrenia and schizophreniform psychosis.

Diagnosis

Schizophreniform disorder shares a majority of the DSM-IV-TR diagnostic features with schizophrenia (see diagnostic criteria above) except the following two criteria: 1) the total duration of the illness which includes the prodrome, active, and residual phases is at least 1 month but less than 6 months in duration; and 2) though impairment in social and occupational functioning may occur during the illness, it is not required or necessary. Thus, the duration of more than 1 month eliminates brief psychotic disorder as a possible diagnosis; if the illness lasts or has lasted for more than 6 months, the diagnosis has to be reevaluated for other possible conditions including schizophrenia. Therefore, the diagnosis of schizophreniform disorder is intermediate between brief psychotic disorder and schizophrenia. Hence, those patients whose duration of episode lasted more than a month and less than 6 months, and have recovered, would be diagnosed as having schizophreniform disorder. On the other hand those patients who have not recovered from an episode, which is less than 6 months but more than one month in duration, and are likely to have schizophrenia would be diagnosed as having schizophreniform disorder until the 6 months criteria is met for schizophrenia. The diagnosis of 'provisional' schizophreniform disorder is made while the clinician monitors the evolving course of the illness, waits for the symptoms to resolve, or when the clinician cannot obtain a reliable history from a patient about the duration of the symptoms.

Specifiers for Prognostic Features

The DSM-IV has specifiers for the presence or absence of good prognostic features. These features include a rapid onset (within 4 weeks) of prominent psychotic symptoms, presence of (psychogenic) confusion or perplexity at the height of the psychotic episode, good premorbid adjustment as evidenced by social and occupational functioning, and the absence of deficit symptoms such as blunted or flat affect.

Clinical Features

The clinical signs and symptoms and the Mental Status Examination of the patient with schizophreniform disorder are often similar to those with schizophrenia, but the presence of affective symptoms usually predict a favorable course. Alternatively, a flat or blunted affect may predict an unfavorable course.

Differential Diagnosis

This is similar to schizophrenia. Psychotic disorder caused by a general medical condition and substance-induced psychotic disorder must be ruled out. General medical conditions to be considered are HIV infection, temporal lobe epilepsy, CNS tumors and cerebrovascular disease, all of which can also be associated with relatively short-lived psychotic episodes. The increasing number of reports of psychosis associated with the use of anabolic steroids by young men who are attempting to build up their muscles to perform better in athletic activities require careful history. Factitious disorder with predominantly psychological signs and symptoms and malingering may need to be ruled out in some instances.

Course and Prognosis

This is, as anticipated, variable. The DSM IV specifiers "with good prognostic features" and "without good prognostic features" though helpful in guiding the clinician, require further validation. However, confusion or perplexity at the height of the psychotic episode is the feature best correlated with good outcome. Also, the shorter the period of illness, the better the prognosis is likely to be. There is a significant risk of suicide in these patients. Postpsychotic depression is quite likely and should be addressed in psychotherapy. Psychotherapy may help speed the recovery and improve the prognosis. By definition, schizophreniform disorder resolves within 6 months with a return to baseline mental functioning.

Treatment

Hospitalization is often necessary and allows for effective assessment, treatment and supervision of a patient's behavior. The psychotic symptoms, usually treated with a 3- to 6-month course of antipsychotic drugs, respond more rapidly than in patients with schizophrenia. One study found that 75% of the patients with schizophreniform psychosis compared with 20% of those with schizophrenia responded to antipsychotic agents within 8 days. ECT may be indicated for some patients, especially those with marked catatonic features or depression. If a patient has recurrent episodes, trials of lithium carbonate, valproic acid, or carbamazepine may be warranted for prophylaxis. Psychotherapy is usually necessary to help patients integrate the psychotic experience into their understanding of their minds, brains and lives.

Delusional Disorder

Delusional disorder refers to a group of disorders, the chief feature of which is the presence of **nonbizarre** delusions. People suffering from this illness do not regard themselves as mentally ill and actively oppose psychiatric referral. Because they may experience little impairment, they generally remain outside hospital settings, appearing reclusive, eccentric, or odd, rather than ill. They are more likely to have contacts with professionals such as lawyers and other medical specialists for health concerns. The current shift in diagnosis from **paranoid** to **delusional** helps avoid the ambiguity around the term "paranoid". This also emphasizes that other delusions besides the paranoid ones are included in this diagnosis. It is important to understand the definition of nonbizarre delusion so as to reach an unambiguous diagnosis. Nonbizarre delusions typically involve situations or circumstances that can occur in real life (e.g., being followed, infected, or deceived by a lover) and are believable.

Diagnostic Criteria

According to DSM-IV-TR, the diagnosis of delusional disorder can be made when a person exhibits nonbizarre delusions of at least 1 month's duration that cannot be attributed to other psychiatric disorders. Nonbizarre delusions must be about phenomena that, although not real, are within the realm of being possible. In general, the patient's delusions are well systematized and have been logically developed. If the person experiences auditory or visual hallucinations, they are not prominent except for tactile or olfactory hallucinations where they are tied in to the delusion (e.g., a person who believes that he emits a foul odor might experience an olfactory hallucination of that odor). The person's behavioral and emotional responses to the delusions appear to be appropriate. Usually the person's functioning and personality are well preserved and show minimal deterioration if at all.

Epidemiology

Though the existence of delusional disorder has been known for a long time, relatively little is known about the demographics, incidence and prevalence. Unfortunately, people suffering from this illness function reasonably well in the community and lack insight resulting in minimal or no contact with the mental health system. However, the crude incidence is roughly 0.7 to 3.0 per 100 000 with a more frequent occurrence in females.

Etiology

Etiology of the delusional disorder is unknown. Risk factors associated with the disorder include advanced age, sensory impairment/isolation, family history, social isolation, personality features (e.g. unusual interpersonal sensitivity) and recent immigration. Some have reported higher association of delusional disorder with widowhood, celibacy and history of substance abuse. Age of onset is later than schizophrenia and earlier in men compared with women.

Subtypes

Persecutory Type

This is the most common form of delusional disorder. Here the person affected believes that he or she is being followed, spied on, poisoned or drugged, harassed, or conspired against. The person affected may become preoccupied by small slights that can become incorporated into the delusional system. These individuals may resort to legal actions to remedy perceived injustice. Individuals suffering from these delusions often become resentful and angry with a potential to become violent against those believed to be against them.

Jealous Type

Individuals with this subtype have the delusional belief that their spouses/lovers are unfaithful. This is often wrongly inferred from small bits of benign evidence which is used to justify the delusion. Delusions of infidelity have also been called **conjugal paranoia**. The term **Othello syndrome** has been used to describe morbid jealousy. This delusion usually affects men, with no history of prior psychiatric problems. The condition is difficult to treat and may diminish only on separation, divorce or death of the spouse. Marked jealousy (pathological jealousy or morbid jealousy) is a symptom of many disorders including schizophrenia and not unique to delusional disorder. Jealousy is a powerful emotion and when it occurs in delusional disorder or as part of another condition, it can be potentially dangerous and has been associated with violence including suicidal and homicidal behavior.

Erotomanic Type

These patients have delusions of secret lovers. Most frequently, the patient is a woman, though men are also susceptible to these delusions. The patient believes that a suitor, usually more socially prominent than herself, is in love with her. This can become central focus of the patient's existence and the onset can be sudden. Erotomania is also referred to as **de Clerambault's syndrome**. Again, these delusions can occur as part of other disorders too. Generally women (but not exclusively so), unattractive in appearance, working at a lower-level jobs, who lead withdrawn, lonely single lives with few sexual contacts are reported to be more prone to develop this condition. They select lovers who are substantially different from them. They exhibit what has been called paradoxical conduct, the delusional phenomenon of interpreting all denials of love no matter how clear as secret affirmations of love. Separation from the love object may be the only satisfactory means of intervention. When it affects men, it can manifest with more aggressive and possibly violent pursuit of love. Thus, such people are often in the forensic system. The object of aggression is often companions or protectors of the love object who are viewed as trying to come between the lovers. However, resentment and rage in response to an absence of reaction from all forms of love communication may escalate to a point that the love object may be in danger too.

Approximately 10% of stalkers have a primary diagnosis of erotomania. Menezies and colleagues (1995) conducted the first predictive study of violence among erotomanic males and found that serious antisocial behavior (a criminal history) unrelated to the delusion and concurrent multiple objects of fixations discriminated between the dangerous and the nondangerous men. In a review by Meloy (1996), if violence occurred the object of love was target at least 80% of the time. The next most likely target was a third party perceived as impeding access to the object. He referred to this latter behavior as **triangulation**. Triangulation when present in jealousy, whether delusional or not, is motivated by a perceived competition for the love object.

Somatic Type

Delusional disorder with somatic delusions has been called **monosymptomatic hypochondriacal psychosis**. This disorder differs from other conditions with hypochondriacal symptoms in degree of reality impairment Munro (1991) has described the largest series of cases and has used content of delusions to define three main types.

Delusions of Infestations (Including Parasitosis) Delusional parasitosis is one of the most common presentations of monohypochondriacal psychosis, which occurs in absence of other psychiatric illness. The onset is insidious and chronic.

Matchbox sign describes the common phenomenon that occurred not so long ago in patients suffering from this condition. During their clinic visit, the patient would present with peeled skin, and other substances connected to delusional thinking in an empty old-fashioned matchbox as evidence that they were infested with insects. Delusional parasitosis has been described in association with many physical illnesses such as vitamin B12 deficiency, pellagra, neurosyphilis, multiple sclerosis, thalamic dysfunction, hypophyseal tumors, diabetes mellitus, severe renal disease, hepatitis, hypothyroidism, mediastinal lymphoma and leprosy. Use of cocaine and presence of dementia has also been reported.

Psychogenic parasitosis was also known as Ekbom's syndrome before being referred to as **delusional parasitosis**. Females experienced this disorder twice as often as males. Entomologists, pest control specialists and dermatologists had often seen the patient before seen by a psychiatrist. All investigators have been impressed by the concurrent medical illnesses associated with this condition. Others have attempted to distinguish between delusional and nondelusional aspects of presentation to establish clearer diagnosis and thus management.

Delusions of Dymorphophobia   This condition includes delusions such as of misshapenness, personal ugliness, or exaggerated size of body parts.

Delusions of Foul Body Odors or Halitosis   This is also called **olfactory reference syndrome**.

    The frequency of these conditions is low, but they may be under diagnosed because patients present to dermatologists, plastic surgeons and infectious disease specialists more often than to psychiatrists. Patients with these conditions do respond to pimozide, a typical antipsychotic medication and also to SSRIs. Usually prognosis is poor without treatment. It affects both sexes equally. Suicide apparently motivated by anguish is not uncommon.

Grandiose Type

This is also referred to as **megalomania**. In this subtype, the central theme of the delusion is the grandiosity of having made some important discovery or having great talent. Sometimes there may be a religious theme to the delusional thinking such that the person believes that he or she has a special message from god.

Mixed Type

This subtype is reserved for those with two or more delusional themes. However, it should be used only where it is difficult to clearly discern one theme of delusion.

Unspecified Type

This subtype is used for cases in which the predominant delusion cannot be subtyped within the above mentioned categories. A possible example is certain delusions of misidentification, for example, **Capgras's syndrome**, named after the French psychiatrist who described the 'illusions of doubles'. The delusion here is the belief that a familiar person has been replaced by an imposter. A variant of this is **Fregoli's syndrome** where the delusion is that the persecutors or familiar persons can assume the guise of strangers and the very rare delusion that familiar persons could change themselves into other persons at will (intermetamorphosis). Each disorder is not only a rare delusion but is highly associated with other conditions such as schizophrenia and dementia.

Course and Prognosis

Though the onset can occur in adolescence, generally it begins from middle to late adulthood with variable patterns of course, including lifelong disorder in some cases. Delusional disorder does not lead to severe impairment or change in personality, but rather to a gradual, progressive involvement with the delusional concern. Suicide has often been associated with this disorder. The base rate of spontaneous recovery may not be as low as previously thought, especially because only the more severely afflicted are referred for psychiatric treatment. The more chronic forms of the illness tend to have their onset early in the fifth decade. Onset is acute in nearly two-thirds of the cases and gradual in the remainder. In almost half of the cases the delusion disappears at follow-up, improves in 10%, and is unchanged in 31%. In the more acute forms of the illness, the age of onset is in the fourth decade, a lasting remission occurs in over half of the patients and a pattern of chronicity develops in only 10%; a relapsing course has been observed in 37%. Thus, the more acute and earlier the onset of the illness, the more favorable the prognosis.

The presence of precipitating factors, married status and female gender are associated with better outcome. The persistence of delusional thinking is most favorable for cases with persecutory delusions and somewhat less favorable for delusions of grandeur and jealousy. However, the outcome in terms of overall functioning appears somewhat more favorable for the jealous subtype.

Comorbidity

Depression occurs frequently and is often an independent disorder in these patients.

Treatment

Though generally considered resistant to treatment and interventions, the management is focused on managing the morbidity of the disorder by reducing the impact of the delusion on the patient's (and family's) life. However, in recent years the outlook has become less pessimistic or restricted in planning effective treatment for these conditions. An effective and therapeutic clinician–patient relationship is important but difficult to establish.

Somatic Treatment

Overall, treatment results suggest that 80.8% of cases recover either fully or partially. Pimozide, the most frequently reported treatment produced full remission in 68.5% and partial recovery in 22.4% ($N = 143$). There are reports of treatment with other typical antipsychotic agents with variable success in small number of subjects. SSRIs have been used and reported to be helpful. The newer atypical antipsychotic agents have been used in small number of cases with success but the data is anecdotal. Bhatia and colleagues (2000) report that pimozide, fluoxetine and amitriptyline were used in their study with pimozide showing good response.

Psychosocial Treatment

As mentioned earlier, developing a therapeutic relationship is very important and yet significantly difficult, and requires a frank and supportive attitude. Supportive therapy is very helpful in dealing with emotions of anxiety and dysphoria generated because of delusional thinking. Cognitive therapy, when accepted and implemented, is helpful. Confrontation of the delusional thinking usually does not work and can further alienate the patient.

Shared Psychotic Disorder

Shared psychotic disorder is a rare disorder, which is also referred to as **shared paranoid disorder, induced psychotic disorder, folie a deux** and **double insanity**. In this disorder, the transfer of delusions takes place from one person to another. Both persons are closely associated for a long time and typically live together in relative social isolation. In its more common form, **folie imposee**, the individual who first has the delusion is often chronically ill and typically is the influential member of the close relationship with another individual, who is more suggestible and who develops the delusion too. The second individual is frequently less intelligent, more gullible, more passive, or more lacking in self-esteem than the primary case. If the two people involved are separated, the second individual may abandon the delusion. However, this is not seen consistently. Other forms of shared psychotic disorder reported are **folie simultanee**, where similar delusional systems develop independently in two closely associated people. The most common dyadic relationships who develop this disorder are sister–sister, husband–wife and mother–child. Almost all cases involve members of a single family.

Epidemiology

More than 95% of all cases of shared psychotic disorder involve two members of the same family. About a third of the cases involve two sisters, another one-third involve husband and wife or a mother and her child. The dominant person is usually affected by schizophrenia or a similar psychotic disorder. In 25% of all cases, the submissive person is usually affected with physical disabilities such as deafness, cerebrovascular diseases, or other disability that increases the submissive person's dependence on the dominant person. This condition is more common in people from low socioeconomic groups and in women.

Etiology

There is some data that suggest that people suffering from shared psychotic disorder may have a family history of schizophrenia. The dominant person suffering from this illness often has schizophrenia or a related psychotic illness. The dominant person is usually older, more intelligent, better educated and has stronger personality traits than the submissive person, who is usually dependent on the dominant person. The affected individuals usually live together or have an extremely close personal relationship, associated with shared life experiences, common needs and hopes, and, often, a deep emotional rapport with each other. The relationship between the people involved is usually somewhat or completely isolated from external societal cultural inputs. The submissive person may be predisposed to a mental disorder and may have a history of a personality disorder with dependent or suggestible qualities as well as a history of depression, suspiciousness and social isolation. The dominant person's psychotic symptoms may develop in the submissive person through the process of identification. By adopting the psychotic symptoms of the dominant person, the submissive person gains acceptance by the other.

Diagnosis

An important feature in the diagnosis is that the person with shared psychotic disorder does not have a preexisting psychotic disorder. The delusions arise in the context of a close relationship with a person who suffers from delusional thinking and resolve on separation from that person.

Clinical Features

The key symptom of shared psychosis is the unquestioning acceptance of another person's delusions. The delusions themselves are often in the realm of possibility and usually not as bizarre as those seen in patients with schizophrenia. The content of the delusion is often persecutory or hypochondriacal. Symptoms of a coexisting personality disorder may be present, but signs and symptoms that meet criteria for schizophrenia, mood disorders and delusional disorder are absent. The patient may have ideation about suicide or pacts about homicide; clinicians must elicit this information during the interview.

Differential Diagnosis

Malingering, factitious disorder with predominantly psychological sign and symptoms, psychotic disorder due to a general medical condition and substance-induced psychotic disorder must be considered.

Course and Prognosis

Though separation of submissive person from the dominant person should resolve the psychosis, this probably occurs only in 10 to 40% of the cases. Unfortunately, when these individuals are discharged from hospital, they usually move back together.

Treatment

The initial step in treatment is to separate the affected person from the source of the delusions, the dominant individual. Antipsychotic agents may be used if the symptoms have not abated in a week after separation. Psychotherapy with the nondelusional members of the patient's family should be undertaken, and psychotherapy with both the patient and the person sharing the delusion may be indicated later in the course of treatment. To prevent redevelopment of the syndrome the family may need family therapy and social support to modify the family dynamics and to prevent redevelopment of the syndrome. Steps to decrease the social isolation may also help prevent the syndrome from reemerging.

Comparison of DSM-IV/ICD-10 Diagnostic Criteria

The ICD-10 and DSM-IV-TR criteria sets for schizophrenia are similar in many important ways although not identical. The ICD-10 Diagnostic Criteria for Research provide two ways to satisfy the criteria for schizophrenia: having one Schneiderian first-rank symptom or having at least two of the other characteristic symptoms (hallucinations accompanied by delusions, thought disorder, catatonic symptoms and negative symptoms). In contrast to DSM-IV-TR which requires 6 months of symptoms (including prodromal, active and residual phases), the ICD-10 definition of schizophrenia requires only a 1-month duration thereby encompassing the DSM-IV-TR diagnostic categories of both schizophrenia and schizophreniform disorder. Thus, cases of DSM-IV-TR schizophreniform disorder are diagnosed in ICD-10 as schizophrenia.

The DSM-IV-TR and ICD-10 definitions of schizoaffective disorder differ with regard to the relationship of the schizoaffective disorder category with the category mood disorder with psychotic features. In DSM-IV-TR, the differentiation depends on the temporal relationship between the mood and psychotic symptoms (i.e., mood disorder with psychotic features is diagnosed whenever the psychotic symptoms occur only in the presence of a mood episode, regardless of the characteristics of the psychotic symptoms). In contrast, the ICD-10 definition of schizoaffective disorder is much broader. It includes situations in which certain specified psychotic symptoms (i.e., thought echo, insertion, withdrawal, or broadcasting; delusions of control or passivity; voices giving a running commentary; disorganized speech, catatonic behavior) occur even if they are confined to a mood episode. Therefore, many cases of DSM-IV-TR mood disorder with mood-incongruent psychotic features would be considered to be schizoaffective disorder in ICD-10. Furthermore, the ICD-10 definition suggests that there should be an "approximate balance between the number, severity, and duration of the schizophrenic and affective symptoms". For delusional disorder, the ICD-10 Diagnostic Criteria for Research specify a minimum 3-month duration in contrast to the 1-month minimum duration in DSM-IV-TR.

In contrast to the single DSM-IV-TR category brief psychotic disorder, ICD-10 has a much more complex way of handling brief psychotic disorders. It includes criteria sets for four specific brief psychotic disorders that differ based on types of symptoms (i.e., with or without symptoms of schizophrenia) and course (i.e., whether they change rapidly or not). Further-more, the maximum duration of these brief psychotic episodes varies depending on the type of symptoms (i.e., 1 month for schizophrenia-like symptoms and 3 months for predominantly delusional). In contrast, DSM-IV-TR has a single criteria set and a maximum 1-month duration.

Finally, the ICD-10 and DSM-IV-TR definitions of shared psychotic disorder are almost identical.

References

Allison DB, Mentore JL, Heo M *et al.* (1999) Antipsychotic-induced weight gain: A comprehensive research synthesis. *Am J Psychiatr* 156, 1686–1696.

American Psychiatric Association (2000) *Diagnostic and Statistical Manual of Mental Disorders*, 4th edn. Text Revision. APA, Washington DC.

Andreasen NC (1981) *Scale for the Assessment of Negative Symptoms (SANS)*. University of Iowa, Iowa City, IA.

Andreasen NC and Olsen SA (1982) Negative vs. positive schizophrenia: Definition and validation. *Arch Gen Psychiatr* 39, 789–794.

Andreasen NC, Olsen SA. Dennert JW *et al.* (1982) Ventricular enlargement in schizophrenia: Relationship to positive and negative symptoms. *Am J Psychiatr* 139, 297–302.

Andreasen NC, Arndt S, Alliger R *et al.* (1995) Symptoms of schizophrenia: Methods, meanings and mechanisms. *Arch Gen Psychiatr* 52, 341–351.

Ayd FJ (1961) A survey of drug induced extrapyramidal reactions. *JAMA* 175, 1054–1061.

Bachrach LL (2000) Psychosocial rehabilitation and psychiatry in the treatment of schizophrenia: What are the boundaries? *Acta Psychiatr Scand* 102(Suppl 407), 6–10.

Beard JH, Propst RN and Malamud TJ (1982) The Fountain House model of psychiatric rehabilitation. *Psychosoc Rehabil J* 5, 47–53.

Bhatia MS, Jagawat T and Choudhary S (2000) Delusional Parasitosis: A clinical profile. *Int J Psychiatr Med* 30, 83–91.

Breier A (1994) Clozapine and noradrenergic function: Support for a novel hypothesis for superior efficacy. *J Clin Psychiatr* 55, 122–125.

Breier A, Schreiber JL, Dyer J *et al.* (1991) National Institute of Mental Health longitudinal study of chronic schizophrenia: Prognosis and prediction of outcome. *Arch Gen Psychiatr* 48, 239–246.

Buchsbaum MS and Hazlett E (1998) Positron emission tomography studies of abnormal glucose metabolism in schizophrenia. *Schizophr Bull* 24, 343–364.

Buchsbaum MS, Yang S, Hazlett E *et al.* (1997) Ventricular volume and asymmetry in schizotypal personality disorder and schizophrenia assessed with magnetic resonance imaging. *Schizophr Res* 27, 45–53.

Butler RW, Jenkins MA, Geyer MA *et al.* (1991) Wisconsin Card Sorting deficits and diminished sensorimotor gating in a discrete subgroup of pharmacology, in *Schizophrenia Research*, Vol. 1 (eds Tamminga CA and Schulz SC).

Cannon TD, van Erp TG, Huttunen M *et al.* (1998) Regional gray matter, white matter, and cerebrospinal fluid distributions in schizophrenic patients, their siblings, and controls. *Arch Gen Psychiatr* 55, 1084–1091.

Carlsson A, Waters N, Holm-Waters S *et al.* (2001) Interactions between monoamines glutamate, and GABA in schizophrenia: New evidence. *Annu Rev Pharmacol Toxicol* 41, 237–260.

Castle DJ and Murray RM (1993) The epidemiology of late-onset schizophrenia. *Schizophr Bull* 19, 691–700.

Carpenter WT, Heinrichs DS and Alphs LD (1985) Treatment of negative symptoms. *Schizophr Bull* 11, 440–452.

Creese I, Burt DR and Snyder SH (1975) Dopamine receptor binding predicts clinical and pharmacological potencies of antischizophrenic drugs. *Science* 192, 481–483.

Crisp A, Gelder M, Rix S *et al.* (2000) Stigmatization of people with mental illness. *Br J Psychiatr* 177, 4–7.

Crow TJ (1980) Molecular pathology of schizophrenia: More than one disease process? *Br Med J* 280, 66–68.

Crow TJ (1985) The two-syndrome concept: Origins and current status. *Schizophr Bull* 11, 471–486.

Delay J and Deniker P (1952) Trente-huit cas de psychoses traités par la cure prolongée et continué de 4560 RP. LeCongres des AI et Neurol. de Langue Fr, in *Comptes Rendu du Congrès*. Masson et Cie, Paris.

Goff DC, Tsai G, Levitt J *et al.* (1999) A placebo-controlled crossover trial of D-cycloserine added to conventional neuroleptics in patients with schizophrenia. *Arch Gen Psychiatr* 56, 21–27.

Green M and Walker E (1986) Attentional performance in positive and negative-symptom schizophrenia. *J Nerv Ment Dis* 174, 203–213.

Harding CM, Brooks GW, Ashikaga T *et al.* (1987a) The Vermont longitudinal study of persons with severe mental illness. I. Methodology, study sample, and overall status 32 years later. *Am J Psychiatr* 144, 718–726.

Harding CM, Brooks GW, Ashikaga T *et al.* (1987b) The Vermont longitudinal study of persons with severe mental illness II. Long-term outcome of subjects who retrospectively met DSM-III criteria for schizophrenia. *Am J Psychiatr* 144, 727–735.

Harvey PD (2001) Abbreviated cognitive assessment in schizophrenia: Recent data on feasibility. *J Adv Schizophr Brain Res* 3, 73–78.

Harvey PD and Keefe RSE (2001) Studies of cognitive change in patients with schizophrenia following novel antipsychotic treatment. *Am J Psychiatr* 158, 176–184.

Henderson DC, Cagliero E, Gray C *et al.* (2000) Clozapine, diabetes mellitus, weight gain and lipid abnormalities: A five-year naturalistic study. *Am J Psychiatr* 157, 975–981.

Heresco-Levy U, Javitt DC, Ermilov M *et al.* (1999) Efficacy of high-dose glycine in the treatment of enduring negative symptoms of schizophrenia. *Arch Gen Psychiatr* 56, 29–36.

Hogarty GE, Anderson CM, Reiss DH *et al.* (1986) Family psychoeducation, social skills training, and maintenance chemotherapy in the aftercare treatment of schizophrenia. I. One-year effects of a controlled study on relapse and expressed emotion. *Arch Gen Psychiatr* 43, 633–642.

Jablensky A and Cole SW (1997) Is the earlier age at onset of schizophrenia in males a confounded finding? Results from a cross-cultural investigation. *Br J Psychiatr* 170, 234–240.

Kane JM, Rifkin A, Woerner MG *et al.* (1983) Low-dose neuroleptic treatment of outpatient schizophrenics. *Arch Gen Psychiatr* 40, 893–896.

Kane JM, Rifkin A, Woerner MG *et al.* (1985) High-dose versus low-dose strategies in the treatment of schizophrenia. *Psychopharmacol Bull* 21, 533–537.

Kapur S and Seeman P (2001) Does fast dissociation from the dopamine D_2 receptor explain the action of atypical antipsychotics? A new hypothesis. *Am J Psychiatr* 158, 360–369.

Kapur S, Remington G, Jones C *et al.* (1996) The D_2 occupancy with low-dose haloperidol treatment: A PET study. *Am J Psychiatr* 153, 948–950.

Kapur S, Zipursky R, Jones C *et al.* (2000) Relationship between D_2 occupancy, clinical response, and side effects: A double-blind PET study of first-episode schizophrenia. *Am J Psychiatr* 157, 514–520.

Kasckow J and Nemeroff C (1991) The neurobiology of neurotensin: Focus on neurotensin–dopamine interactions. *Regul Peptides* 36, 153–164.

Kay SR, Opler LA and Lindemayer JP (1988) Reliability and validity of the positive and negative syndrome scale for schizophrenics. *Psychiatr Res* 23, 99–110.

Keck PE Jr., Reeves K, Harrigan E *et al.* (2001) Ziprasidone in the short-term treatment of patients with schizoaffective disorder: Results from two double-blind, placebo-controlled, multicenter studies. *J Clin Psychopharmacol* 21, 27–35.

Keefe RS, Perkins D, Silva SG *et al.* (1999) The effects of atypical antipsychotic drugs on neurocognitive impairment in schizophrenia. *Schizophr Bull* 25, 201–222.

Kramer M (1969) Cross-national study of diagnosis of the mental disorders: Origin of the problem. *Am J Psychiatr* 10(Suppl), 1–11.

Lafargue T and Brasic J (2000) Neurodevelopmental hypothesis of schizophrenia: A central sensory disturbance. *Med Hypotheses* 55, 314–318.

Langfeldt G (1939) *The Schizophreniform States.* Oxford University Press, London.

Larsen TR, Moe LC, Vibe-Hansen L *et al.* (2000) Premorbid functioning versus duration of untreated psychosis in 1-year outcome in first-episode psychosis. *Schizophr Res* 45, 1–9.

Lawrie SM and Abukmeil SS (1998) Brain abnormality in schizophrenia: A systematic and quantitive review of volumetric magnetic resonance imaging studies. *Br J Psychiatr* 172, 110–120.

Leff J (2000) Family work for schizophrenia: Practical application. *Acta Psychiatr Scand* 102(Suppl 407), 78–82.

Lencz T, Bilder RM and Cornblatt B (2001) The timing of neurodevelopmental abnormality in schizophrenia: An integrative review of the neuroimaging literature. *CNS Spectrums* 6, 233–255.

Levenson JL (1985) Neuroleptic malignant syndrome. *Am J Psychiatr* 142, 1137–1145.

Levinson DF, Umapathy C and Musthaq M (1999) Treatment of schizoaffective disorder and schizophrenia with mood symptoms. *Am J Psychiatr* 156, 1138–1148.

Lieberman JA (1996) Atypical antipsychotic drugs as a first-line treatment of schizophrenia: A rationale and hypothesis. *J Clin Psychiatr* 57(Suppl 11), 68–71.

Lieberman JA, Jody D, Geisler S *et al.* (1993) Time course and biologic correlates of treatment response in first-episode schizophrenia. *Arch Gen Psychiatr* 50, 369–376.

Liberman RP, Massel HK, Mosk MD *et al.* (1985) Social skills training for chronic mental patients. *Hosp Comm Psychiatr* 36, 396–403.

Liberman RP, Mueser KT and Wallace CJ (1986) Social skills training for schizophrenic individuals at risk for relapse. *Am J Psychiatr* 143, 523–526.

Marder SR, Van Patten T, Mintz J *et al.* (1984) Costs and benefits of two doses of fluphenazine. *Arch Gen Psychiatr* 41, 1025–1029.

Marder SR, Van Patten T, Mintz J *et al.* (1987) Low- and conventional-dose maintenance therapy with fluphenazine decanoate: Two-year outcome. *Arch Gen Psychiatr* 44, 518–521.

Marder SR, Wirshing W, Mintz J *et al.* (1996) Two-year outcome of social skills training and group psychotherapy for outpatients with schizophrenia. *Am J Psychiatr* 153, 1585–1592.

Marsden CD, Mindham RHS and Mackay AVP (1986) Extrapyramidal movement disorders produced by antipsychotic drugs, in *The Psychopharmacology and Treatment of Schizophrenia* (eds Bradley PB and Hirsch SR). Oxford University Press, Oxford.

McCarley RW, Wible CG, Frumin M *et al.* (1999) MRI anatomy of schizophrenia. *Biol Psychiatr* 45, 1099–1119.

McGlashan TH and Hoffman RE (2000) Schizophrenia as a disorder of developmentally reduced synaptic connectivity. *Arch Gen Psychiatr* 57, 637–648.

Meloy JR (1996) Stalking (obsessional following): A review of some preliminary studies. *Aggr Viol Behav* 1, 147–162.

Meltzer HY (1989) Duration of a clozapine trial in neuroleptic-resistant schizophrenia. *Arch Gen Psychiatr* 46, 672.

Meltzer HY (1992) Treatment of the neuroleptic–nonresponsive schizophrenic patient. *Schizophr Bull* 18, 515–542.

Menzies R, Federoff J, Green C *et al.* (1995) Prediction of dangerous behavior in male erotomania. *Br J Psychiatr* 166, 529–536.

Mirnics K, Middleton FA, Marquez A *et al.* (2000) Molecular characterization of schizophrenia viewed by microarray analysis of gene expression in prefrontal cortex. *Neuron* 28, 53–67.

Munro A (1991) Phenomenologic aspects of monodelusional disorders. *Br J Psychiatr* 159(suppl 14), 62–64.

Nestler EJ (1997) Schizophrenia: An emerging pathophysiology. *Nature* 385, 578–579.

Nordstrom AL and Farde L (1998) Plasma prolactin and central D_2 receptor occupancy in antipsychotic drug-treated patients. *J Clin Psychopharmacol* 18, 305–310.

Nuechterlein KH, Edell WS, Norris M *et al.* (1986) Attentional vulnerability indicators, thought disorder and negative symptoms. *Schizophr Bull* 12, 408–426.

Overall JE and Gorham DE (1961) The Brief Psychiatric Rating Scale. *Psychol Rep* 10, 799–812.

Ray WA, Meredith S, Thapa PB *et al.* (2001) Antipsychotics and the risk of sudden cardiac death. *Arch Gen Psychiatr* 58, 1161–1167.

Raz S and Raz N (1990) Structural brain abnormalities in the major psychoses: A quantitative review of the evidence from computerized imaging. *Psychol Bull* 108, 93–108.

Riley JG, Ayis SA, Ferrier IN *et al.* (2000) QTc-interval abnormalities and psychotropic drug therapy in psychiatric patients. *Lancet* 355, 1048–1052.

Robins LN and Regier DA (eds) (1991) *Psychiatric Disorders in America: The Epidemiologic Catchment Area Study.* Free Press, New York.

Robins LN, Helzer JE, Weissman MM *et al.* (1984) Lifetime prevalence of specific psychiatric disorders in 3 sites. *Arch Gen Psychiatr* 41, 949–958.

Robinson D, Woerner MG, Alvir JMJ *et al.* (1999) Predictors of relapse following response from a first episode of schizophrenia or schizoaffective disorder. *Arch Gen Psychiatr* 56, 241–247.

Rosenheck R, Teckett J, Peters J *et al.* (1998) Does participation in psychosocial treatment augment the benefit of clozapine? *Arch Gen Psychiatr* 55, 618–625.

Seeman P and Tallerico T (1999) Rapid release of antipsychotic drugs from dopamine D_2 receptors: An explanation for low receptors occupancy and early clinical relapse upon withdrawl of clozapine or quetiapine. *Am J Psychiatr* 156, 876–884.

Seidman LJ, Faraone SV, Goldstein JM *et al.* (1997) Reduced subcortical brain volumes in nonpsychotic siblings of schizophrenic patients: A pilot magnetic resonance imaging study. *Am J Med Genet* 74, 507–514.

Sharma T (2001) Schizophrenia in the UK – A mark of shame? *J Adv Schizophr Brain Res* 3, 70–73.

Strauss ME (1993) Relations of symptoms to cognitive deficits in schizophrenia. *Schizophr Bull* 19, 215–231.

Thakore JH, Mann JN, Vlahos I *et al.* (2002) Increased visceral fat distribution in drug-naïve and drug-free patients with schizophrenia. *Int J Obstet Rel Metab Disord* 26, 137–141.

Torrey EF, Bowler AE and Clark K (1997) Urban birth and residence as risk factors for psychoses: An analysis of 1880 data. *Schizophr Res* 25, 169–176.

Tsai GE, Yang P, Chung LC *et al.* (1998) D-Serine added to antipsychotics for the treatment of schizophrenia. *Biol Psychiatr* 44, 1081–1089.

van Kammen DP, Peters J, Yao J *et al.* (1990) Norepinephrine in acute exacerbations of chronic schizophrenia. *Arch Gen Psychiatr* 47, 161–168.

Weinberger DR (1987) Implications of normal brain development for the pathogenesis of schizophrenia. *Arch Gen Psychiatr* 44, 660–669.

Weinberger DR, Egan MF, Bertolino A *et al.* (2001) Prefrontal neurons and the genetics of schizophrenia. *Biol Psychiatr* 50, 825–844.

World Health Organization (1973) *Report of the International Pilot Study of Schizophrenia*, Vol. 1. World Health Organization, Geneva.

Mood Disorders: Depression

Definition

The depressive disorders are characterized by lifelong vulnerability to episodes of disease, involving depressed mood or loss of interest and pleasure in activities. Individuals may demonstrate ongoing potential for cycling of mood from euthymia to depression to recovery and sometimes to hypomania or mania. When individuals cycle to hypomania or mania, then a diagnosis of bipolar II (in the case of hypomania) or bipolar I (in the case of mania) is made. When the mood disorder is severe, assessment for psychosis is essential.

In most definitions of depression, a distinction is drawn between a feeling state of dejection, sadness, or unhappiness, which may be brief in duration, and a clinical syndrome characterized by persistent sadness, profound discouragement, or despair which persists two weeks or more and is associated with a change from previous functioning. This clinical syndrome invariably involves alterations in mood experienced by an individual as a feeling of sadness, irritability, dejection, despair, or loss of interest or pleasure. Associated neurovegetative or biological signs of depression include impairment in sleep, appetite, energy level, libido and psychomotor activity. Cognitive manifestations of the depressive syndrome include distortions about oneself, one's experience in the world and the future, accompanied by self-blame and indecision. These core symptoms of depression are evident in children or adolescents with MDD although the depressed mood may be manifested by irritability or social withdrawal. Older adults may show a preponderance of somatic preoccupation and memory impairment in association with the signs of MDD. The current DSM-IV-TR criteria (A) for MDD are noted below.

The use of the term melancholia to refer to the depressive syndrome became less common as depression and manic–depressive disease were used more frequently in the early 20th century. Currently, the specifier with melancholic features is applied to the diagnosis of MDD if it is associated with a profound loss of interest and lack of reactivity to favorable external events. Other symptoms characteristic of melancholia include a distinct quality to the depressive mood characterized by marked worsening in the morning, early morning awakening, psychomotor retardation or agitation, significant anorexia and excessive guilt. These melancholic features are noted as a modifier of MDD in III-R, and in DSM-IV (American Psychiatric Association, 1994).

Suicidal Phenomena

Our current definitions of MDD emphasize suicidal ideation, thoughts of death and suicide attempts as a cardinal criterion symptom of the disorder. Suicidality is the feature of depressive disorder that poses substantial risk of mortality in the disease. Prevention of suicide, more than any other treatment goal, requires immediate intervention and may require hospitalization. The risk for subsequent completed suicide for an individual hospitalized for an episode of severe MDD is estimated to be 15%.

Epidemiology

Prevalence and Incidence

Across epidemiologic studies, MDD is found to be a common psychiatric disorder. The lifetime risk for MDD in community samples vary from 10 to 25% for women and 5 to 12% for men (American Psychiatric Association, 2000). The point prevalence of MDD for adults in community samples has varied from 5 to 9% for women and from 2 to 3% for men (American Psychiatric Association, 2000). While the incidence rates of MDD in prepubertal boys and girls are equal, women over the course of their lifetime are two to three times more likely to have MDD after puberty. Whereas a strong relationship exists between low social class and schizophrenia, a weaker but nevertheless meaningful relationship may exist between low income status and the occurrence of MDD. Analyses of the Epidemiological Catchment Area (ECA) data indicated that the lowest income group manifested twice the risk of MDD than the highest income group while the National Comorbidity Survey (NCS) concluded that individuals with low socioeconomic status demonstrate higher risk for MDD than individuals who are economically well-off. The rates of MDD may also be influenced by childhood adversity including severe physical abuse, sexual abuse, neglect and poor care (Harkness and Monroe, 2002). The NCS identified the risk factors associated with having MDD comorbid with another mental disorder as opposed to MDD alone. These risk factors include younger age, lower level of education and lower income.

Lifetime Risk and Lifetime Prevalence

Lifetime risk refers to the proportion of individuals being studied who would go on to develop the disorder during their lifetime. Estimates of lifetime risk of MDD in community samples vary from 20 to 25% for women and 7 to 12% for men (Depression Guideline Panel, 1993). Lifetime prevalence refers to those individuals who, up to the time of assessment, have had symptoms that met diagnostic criteria at some point in their lives. The NCS estimated overall lifetime prevalence of MDD as 17.1%. The estimated prevalence was twice as high in females than males. The ECA study and NCS identified higher lifetime prevalence in younger age groups consistent with the birth cohort effect and possible recall bias. In the survey replication of the NCS (NCS-R) (Kessler *et al.*, 2005), the lifetime prevalence estimate of major depression was 16.6%. Lifetime prevalence for all mood disorders was 20.8%. Both of these estimates were considered to be conservative.

Essentials of Psychiatry   Jerald Kay and Allan Tasman
© 2006 John Wiley & Sons, Ltd.

DSM-IV-TR Criteria 296.xx

Major Depressive Episode

Five (or more) of the following symptoms have A. been present during the same 2-week period and represent a change from previous functioning; at least one of the symptoms is either (1) depressed mood or (2) loss of interest or pleasure. **Note:** Do not include symptoms that are clearly due to a general medical condition, or mood-incongruent delusions or hallucinations.

    (1) Depressed mood most of the day, as indicated by either subjective report (e.g., feels sad or empty) or observation made by others (e.g., appears tearful). **Note:** In children and adolescents, can be irritable mood.

    (2) Markedly diminished interest or pleasure in all, or almost all, activities most of the day, nearly every day (as indicated by either subjective account or observation made by others).

    (3) Significant weight loss when not dieting or weight gain (e.g., a change of more than 5% of body weight in a month), or decrease or increase in appetite nearly every day. **Note:** In children, consider failure to make expected weight gains.

    (4) Insomnia or hypersomnia nearly every day.

    (5) Psychomotor agitation or retardation nearly every day (observable by others, not merely subjective feelings of restlessness or being slowed down).

    (6) Fatigue or loss of energy nearly every day.

    (7) Feelings of worthlessness or excessive or inappropriate guilt (which may be delusional) nearly every day (not merely self-reproach or guilt about being sick).

    (8) Diminished ability to think or concentrate, or indecisiveness, nearly every day (either by subjective account or as observed by others).

    (9) Recurrent thoughts of death (not just fear of dying), recurrent suicidal ideation without a specific plan, or a suicide attempt or a specific plan for committing suicide.

B. The symptoms do not meet criteria for a mixed episode.

C. The symptoms cause clinically significant distress or impairment in social, occupational, or other important areas of functioning.

D. The symptoms are not due to the direct physiological effects of a substance (e.g., a drug of abuse, a medication) or a general medical condition (e.g., hypothyroidism).

The symptoms are not better accounted for by E. bereavement, i.e., after the loss of a loved one, the symptoms persist for longer than 2 months or are characterized by marked functional impairment, morbid preoccupation with worthlessness, suicidal ideation, psychotic symptoms, or psychomotor retardation.

Reprinted with permission from the *Diagnostic and Statistical Manual of Mental Disorders*, Fourth Edition, Text Revision. Copyright 2000 American Psychiatric Association.

Point Prevalence

Point prevalence or current prevalence refers to the proportion of the individuals that have the disorder being studied at a designated time. The specific point prevalence of MDD in community samples has ranged from 5 to 9% for women and 2 to 3% for men. The current point prevalence estimates in the NCS were 4.9%. Of the more prevalent 12 month disorders, the NCS-R found that major depressive disorder was the third most common disorder (6.7%). Although more than one third of cases were found to be mild, the prevalence of moderate and serious cases was 14% of this population and mood disorders was considered the second most common disorder of those serious cases. The point prevalence of MDD in primary care outpatient settings ranges from 4.8 to 8.6% (Depression Guideline Panel, 1993a). In hospitalized patients for all medical conditions, more than 14% had MDD.

Children and Adolescents

For preschool children, the point prevalence is thought to be of 0.8% (Depression Guideline Panel, 1993). Point prevalences of major and minor depressive disorder of 1.8 and 2.5%, respectively, were found in a sample of 9-year-old children from the general population, based upon the use of a semistructured diagnostic instrument (Kashani *et al.*, 1983). A semistructured diagnostic instrument was used to find a 4.7% point prevalence

rate of major depression in a community sample of 150 adolescents. Those adolescents diagnosed with MDD had symptoms that met criteria for dysthymia as well. A point prevalence rate of 3.3% was found for dysthymia. Weller and Weller (1990) have shown the prevalence of MDD in clinical samples of children and adolescents to be 58% in educational clinics, 28% in outpatient psychiatric clinics and 40 to 60% in psychiatric hospitals. By comparison, a prevalence of 7% is found in hospitalized pediatric patients. Emslie *et al.*, (1990) assessed depressive symptoms by self-report in a large sample of high school students of mixed ethnic background in an urban school district. They found that hispanic females reported more severe depression whereas white males reported the least severe scores of depression. For males and females, African-Americans and hispanics reported significantly more depression than whites. Female gender, being behind in school and nonwhite ethnicity predicted higher self-report scores of depressive symptoms.

Older Adult

Weissman and colleagues (1991) found a 1% prevalence of MDD in adults 65 years and older who lived in the community. The data indicate that a lower lifetime prevalence of MDD was found in the oldest age group ($\geq$ age 65) in comparison to younger age groups. Women manifest an increased prevalence of MDD in comparison to men and no significant differences were found across racial or ethnic groups. However, other community samples of older adults were found to have a high prevalence (8–15%) of clinically significant depressive symptoms (but not a formal diagnosis of MDD). In a recent Stockholm group, the frequency of MDD was 5.9% and the rate of DD was 8.3% (Forsell *et al.*, 1994).

In comparison to community settings, higher prevalence rates for MDD are found in treatment settings for older adults: 11% in hospitals, 5% in outpatient nonpsychiatric clinics and 12% in long-term care settings. There is also a higher prevalence rate in treatment settings of clinically significant depression that is not severe enough to warrant a formal diagnosis of MDD: 25% prevalence in hospitals and 30.5% in long-term care facilities.

Birth Cohort

Klerman and Weissman (1989) as well as The Cross-National Collaborative Group (1992) called attention to a changing rate of MDD for recent birth cohorts found in: North America, Puerto Rico, Western Europe, Middle East, Asia and the Pacific Rim. Specifically, earlier age of onset and increased rate of depression occur in individuals born in more recent decades. This finding was supported in NCS-R as well. Historical, social, economic, or biological events most likely account for the variability in rate of depression noted in different countries included in the study. However, an overall increase in the rate of depression was noted across many of the geographic locations.

Older adults continue to manifest a higher suicide rate than in younger age groups. However, suicide rates have increased in younger age groups as the changing rate of MDD is observed in younger cohorts. In keeping with the birth cohort effect, recurrences of MDD in late life may become a significant health concern as the population ages.

Risk Factors

Familiarity with risk factors for MDD may help the clinician recognize or diagnose this common and serious psychiatric illness. Accordingly, The Depression Guideline Panel (1993) enumerated 10 primary risk factors for depression:

1. History of prior episodes of depression;
2. Family history of depressive disorder especially in first-degree relatives;
3. History of suicide attempts;
4. Female gender;
5. Age of onset before age 40;
6. Postpartum period;
7. Comorbid medical illness;
8. Absence of social support;
9. Negative, stressful life events;
10. Active alcohol or substance abuse.

In the NCS, 4.9% of subjects were diagnosed as having a current episode of MDD. Of the subjects with depression, 43.7% had noncomorbid depression while 56.3% had comorbid conditions. This distribution of comorbid versus noncomorbid conditions is consistent with other reports of community and clinical samples examining the extent of cooccurrence. In the NCS, certain risk factors, including: 1) younger age, 2) lower level of education, and 3) lower income, were more associated with comorbid depression than noncomorbid depression.

Comorbidity Patterns: General Medical Conditions

Whereas a 4 to 5% current prevalence rate of MDD exists in community samples, symptoms of depression are found in 12 to 36% of patients with a general medical condition (Depression Guideline Panel, 1993). The rate of depression may be higher in patients with a specific medical condition. MDD is identified as an independent condition and calls for specific treatment when it occurs in the presence of a general medical condition.

The Depression Guideline Panel includes four possible relationships between depression and a general medical condition: 1) depression is biologically caused by the general medical condition; 2) an individual who carries a genetic vulnerability to MDD manifests the onset of depression triggered by the general medical condition; 3) depression is psychologically caused by the general medical condition; and 4) no causal relationship exists between the general medical condition and mood disorder. The first two cases warrant initial treatment directed at the general medical disorder. Treatment is advocated for persistent depression upon stabilization of the general medical condition. When the general medical condition causes depression, specific treatment for the former condition is optimized, while psychiatric management, education and antidepressant medication are administered to treat the depression. In cases where the two conditions are not etiologically related, appropriate treatment is indicated for each disorder.

Stroke

Some poststroke patients manifest depression due to cerebrovascular disease related to cerebral infarction in left frontal and left subcortical brain regions. Mood disorder due to cerebrovascular disease is diagnosed when an individual manifests a recent stroke and has significant symptoms of depression. A point prevalence of mood disorder due to cerebrovascular disease in poststroke patients between 10 and 27% has been documented, with an average duration of depression lasting approximately 1 year. Case reports of mood disorder due to cerebrovascular disease in poststroke patients suggest poor treatment compliance, irritability and personality change (Ross and Rush, 1981).

Dementia

According to DSM-IV-TR, when symptoms of clinically significant depressed mood accompany dementia of the Alzheimer's Type and, in the clinician's judgment, the depression is due to the direct physiological effects of the Alzheimer's disease, mood disorder due to Alzheimer's disease is diagnosed. When dementia consistent with cerebrovascular disease leads to prominent cognitive deficits, focal neurological signs and symptoms, significant impairment in functioning as well as predominant depressed mood, vascular dementia with depressed mood is diagnosed. The distinction between depressive disorders and dementing disorders is often complicated because depression and dementia commonly cooccur. Treatment of cooccurring depressive features may relieve symptoms and improve overall quality of life.

Parkinson's Disease

Fifty percent of patients with Parkinson's disease experience a MDD during the course of the illness. When depression occurs in this context, one diagnoses mood disorder due to Parkinson's disease. Active treatment of the depressive disorder may result in improvement in the signs and symptoms of depression without alleviation of the involuntary movement disorder or cognitive changes associated with subcortical brain disease. The underlying etiology of associated dementia and depressive disorder in Parkinson's disease appears to involve physiologic changes in subcortical brain regions.

Diabetes

It is estimated that the prevalence of depression in treated patients with diabetes is three times as frequent as in the general population. Further, there is no difference in the prevalence rate of depression in patients with insulin-dependent diabetes mellitus (Type I) in comparison to patients with noninsulin-dependent mellitus (Type II). The symptomatic presentation of MDD in patients with diabetes is similar to patients without diabetes. Consequently, full assessment of and treatment for MDD is recommended in patients who become depressed during the course of diabetes. The relatively high point prevalence rate may be due to higher detection rate in this treated population, having a chronic illness, as well as metabolic and endocrine factors.

Coronary Artery Disease

When MDD is present, increased morbidity and mortality is reported in postmyocardial infarction patients as well as in patients having coronary artery disease without myocardial infarction (MI). Therefore, treatment of MDD in patients with coronary artery disease is indicated. Prevalence estimates of MDD in postmyocardial infarction range from 40 to 65%. Over a 15-month period, patients 55 years or older who had mood disorder evidenced a mortality rate four times higher than expected, and coronary heart disease or stroke accounted for 63% of the deaths. Depression may promote poor adherence to cardiac rehabilitation and worse outcome. During the first year following MI, depression is considered to be associated with a three- to fourfold increase in subsequent cardiovascular morbidity and mortality. Depression in patients with coronary artery disease is associated with more social problems, functional impairment and increased health care utilization. Recent studies of erectile dysfunction, cardiovascular disease and depression demonstrate that all three conditions share many of the same risk factors.

Cancer

MDD occurs in 25% of patients with cancer at some time during the illness. MDD should be assessed and treated as an independent disorder. The intense reaction in patients diagnosed with cancer may lead to dysphoria and sadness without evolving a full syndrome of MDD. The consulting psychiatrist must evaluate the patient's response to chemotherapy, side effects of the treatment, and medication interactions in the overall assessment of the patient. Among patients with cancer, MDD is typically characterized by heightened distress, impaired functioning and decreased capacity to adhere to treatment. Treating comorbid MDD with psychotherapy or pharmacotherapy may improve the overall outcome in patients with cancer and mitigate complications of MDD.

Chronic Fatigue Syndrome

Lifetime rates of MDD in patients with chronic fatigue syndrome range from 46 to 75%. Comorbid anxiety and somatization disorders are also common in patients with chronic fatigue. According to the Centers for Disease Control (CDC) criteria, the diagnosis of chronic fatigue syndrome is excluded in patients whose symptoms meet criteria for a formal psychiatric disorder, such as MDD or DD. Patients whose symptoms meet criteria for both a mood disorder and chronic fatigue syndrome should be maximally treated for the mood disorder with appropriate pharmacotherapy and cognitive–behavioral psychotherapy. The etiological relationship between mood disorder and chronic fatigue syndrome is unclear.

Depression Due to Medications

If MDD is judged to be a direct physiologic effect of a medication, then substance induced mood disorder is diagnosed. Medications reported to cause depression involve several drugs from the associated groups listed in Table 46.1.

Among antihypertensive treatment, beta-adrenergic blockers have been studied regarding the risk of depression. No significant differences are found between individuals treated with beta-blockers and those treated with other antihypertensives regarding the propensity to develop depressive symptoms. Lethargy is the most common side effect reported. No significant depressive complications are reported with calcium channel blockers or angiotensin converting enzyme (ACE) inhibitors.

Hormonal treatments, such as corticosteroids and anabolic steroids, can elicit depression, mania, or psychosis. Oral contraceptives require monitoring regarding the possible precipitation of depressive symptoms. Because patients with seizure disorders and Parkinson's disease are at high risk for concomitant MDD, it is difficult to establish a link between anticonvulsant or antiParkinsonian treatment and the precipitation of depression. Nevertheless, patients require close monitoring and evaluation for evolution of depressive symptomatology.

Table 46.1   Medications Associated with Depression

Cardiovascular Drugs	Hormones	Psychotropics
Methyldopa	Oral contraceptives	Benzodiazepines
Reserpine	Corticotropin and glucocorticoids	Neuroleptics
Propranolol	Anabolic steroids	
Guanethidine		
Clonidine		
Thiazide diuretics		
Digitalis		
Anticancer Agents	Anti-inflammatory and Anti-infective Agents	Others
Cycloserine	Nonsteroidal antiinflammatory agents	Cocaine (withdrawal)
	Ethambutol	Amphetamines (withdrawal)
	Disulfiram	Levodopa
	Sulfonamides	Cimetidine
	Baclofen	Ranitidine
	Metoclopramide	

Comorbidity Patterns: Other Clinical Psychiatric Disorders

The presence of a comorbid psychiatric disorder may alter the course of major mood disorder in a dramatic fashion and is identified as a primary risk factor for poor treatment response. More than 40% of patients with MDD have additional symptoms that meet criteria during their lifetime for one or more additional psychiatric disorders. In a sample, assessing both pure and comorbid MDD based upon findings from the NCS, the current prevalence of major depression was 4.9% (Blazer *et al.*, 1994). Of the sample with current MDD, 56.3% also had another psychiatric disorder. Among respondents to the NCS-R, the 12 month prevalence of disorders were considered to be serious in 22%, moderate in 37.3% and mild in 40.4%. Twenty–two percent of those with disorders carried two diagnoses, and 23% carried three more diagnoses. The most common comorbid conditions were with major depression and included:

- bipolar disorder (major depression with either hypomania or mania;
- double depression (major depression with dysthymia);
- anxious depression (major depression with generalized anxiety disorder).

Alcohol/Drug Dependence

Results of family and twin studies in a population-based female sample are consistent with a modest correlation of the liability between alcohol dependence and MDD (Kendler *et al.*, 1993). It is common for individuals with alcohol dependence to evidence signs of depression or MDD, but alcoholism is not thought to be a common consequence of mood disorder. Between 10 and 30% of patients with alcoholism manifest depression (Petty, 1992), whereas alcoholism is thought to occur in under 5% of depressed patients (Depression Guideline Panel, 1993).

Depressed women are more likely to self-medicate their mood disorder with alcohol than are depressed men. The effect of comorbid alcoholism on the course of major mood disorder is unclear. Some evidence suggests that remission of depression occurs within the first month of sobriety. The effect of comorbid depression requires further attention in relation to the course of drug dependence. Drug dependence is often associated with major mood disorder and the presence of associated comorbid personality disorder.

Anxiety Disorders

The cooccurrence of symptoms of anxiety and depression is very common. Kendler *et al.* (1986) found very high genetic correlations between MDD and generalized anxiety disorder in contrast to a modest overlap between phobic disorders and MDD. Anxiety symptoms commonly appear in depressive syndromes and MDD is frequently comorbid with anxiety disorders. From a longitudinal perspective, either symptom constellation can be a precursor to the development of the other disorder. The combination of anxiety and depression predicts greater severity and impairment than the presence of each syndrome in isolation. The association of severe panic and MDD is one of the predictors of suicidal risk. The clinician is advised to assess for symptoms of each disorder and to obtain a thorough family history. Patients with anxiety disorders often experience prior episodes of MDD or have relatives who suffer from mood disorder.

Ten to 20% of outpatients with MDD evidence comorbid panic disorder while 30 to 40% of depressed outpatients have had symptoms that met criteria for generalized anxiety disorder during the course of the mood disorder. In both cases, the anxiety disorder has preceded the major mood disorder about 50% of the time. An increased incidence of MDD is noted in patients with anxiety disorders who are followed over time.

The clinician is advised to evaluate three factors in order to determine treatment approaches when MDD cooccurs with panic disorder or social phobia: 1) the patient's family history; 2) the constellation of symptoms that were first evident in the current episode; and 3) the symptoms that cause the patient the most distress.

Recovery is less likely and symptomatology more severe in patients with comorbid MDD and panic disorder than in cases with a single diagnosis. Lifetime suicide rate is twice as high for patients with comorbid panic disorder and MDD than in panic disorder alone. It is imperative to assess for the presence of mood disorder and suicidality in patients who present with symptoms of anxiety.

Obsessive–Compulsive Disorder

The occurrence of symptoms of depression is very common in patients with obsessive–compulsive disorder (OCD), although full symptom criteria may not be reached to warrant a formal diagnosis of MDD. Ten to 30% of patients with OCD have mood symptoms that meet full criteria for MDD. The relationship between OCD and schizophrenia is less clear. Patients with OCD are at increased risk to develop MDD but not schizophrenia. It is important to distinguish between obsessive–compulsive personality features which can accompany and are exacerbated during an episode of depression and OCD itself. Symptoms of depression often diminish with successful initial treatment of OCD, since biological treatments typically involve use of selective serotonergic antidepressant medications such as clomipramine, fluoxetine, or fluvoxamine.

Post Traumatic Stress Disorder

Individuals with PTSD often experience cooccurring depressive disorders, anxiety disorders and substance use disorders. The range of reported rates of concurrent depressive disorder in patients with PTSD is 30 to 50%. Many of the symptoms of PTSD overlap with signs and symptoms of depression such that both PTSD and MDD can be considered to be the result of traumatic events. In addition, depressive disorder may be associated with worse outcome in individuals with cooccurring PTSD.

Somatization Disorder

It is common for patients with MDD to experience somatic symptoms including pain, although the intensity and frequency of the somatic complaints and the range of body systems affected do not usually meet criteria for somatization disorder. Patients who have mood symptoms that meet criteria for MDD evidence more complaints of pain, experience more physical, interpersonal and occupational limitations, and perceive their overall health as worse than patients with chronic medical illness. The clinician should carefully evaluate for the presence of MDD in cases where the patient reports unexplained pain. Typically, pain complaints are relieved upon successful treatment of the MDD. However, somatoform disorders, as outlined in DSM-IV, may be associated with demoralization and depression.

Eating Disorders

There are little data available regarding prevalence of eating disorders in patients with MDD. However, 33 to 50% of patients with anorexia nervosa or bulimia nervosa experience a comorbid mood disorder. Between 50 and 75% of patients with an eating disorder have a history of a MDD over a lifetime. Initial treatment is aimed at the eating disorder. If depression continues after proper nourishment has been re-established in anorexia nervosa, treatment is directed at the primary mood disorder.

Personality Disorders

High rates of personality disorders are found in depressed inpatients and outpatients. Most studies report a rate of cooccurrence between 30 and 40% in outpatients and 50 to 60% in inpatient samples. Sixty-three percent of our sample of acutely ill patients (mostly inpatients) with a MDD were assigned at least one Axis II diagnosis on the basis of a semistructured diagnostic instrument (Gruenberg *et al.*, 1993). Several studies have found that patients with comorbid MDD and personality disorder evidence an earlier age of onset for the first episode of depression, increased severity of depressive symptoms, more episodes, longer duration of episodes, poorer response to both pharmacotherapy and psychotherapy, and increased risk for self-injury.

A particular relationship is noted for comorbid MDD and borderline personality disorder (BPD). In a general psychiatric population, depressed patients show an estimated rate of 6% for cooccurring BPD. The link between BPD and MDD remains controversial. Anecdotally, there appear to be significant levels of depression accompanying PTSD in those women who have been sexually abused. Herman (1997) has made a cogent argument for conceptualizing these women as suffering from complex PTSD rather than BPD.

Grief and Bereavement

Depressive symptoms associated with normal grieving usually begin within 2 to 3 weeks of the loss and resolve spontaneously over 6 to 8 weeks. If full symptom criteria for MDD persist for more than 2 months beyond the death of a loved one, then an episode of MDD can be diagnosed. Specific treatment for a major depressive episode such as short-term psychotherapy focusing on unresolved grief or pharmacotherapy is indicated.

Etiology and Pathophysiology

Depressive disorders are common and recurrent, and associated with substantial psychosocial dysfunction as well as excess morbidity and mortality. Greater understanding of the underlying etiology and pathophysiology of MDD is the focus of genetic, neurobiologic and psychosocial investigation.

Integration of Genetic and Environmental Theories

Unipolar or nonbipolar MDD has been demonstrated to cluster in the first-degree relatives of patients with depression. The observation that MDD is familial, however, does not address whether the familial aggregation may be due to genetic or familial environmental factors. All attempts to develop integrated etiologic models of depression have identified multiple psychosocial risk factors. In particular, female gender, limited social support, dependent, self-critical and neurotic personality traits, and stressful life events appear to influence the vulnerability to MDD. Whether specific life events are as important later in the course of MDD as in the precipitation of initial episodes is the subject of ongoing investigation. Post (1992) argued that negative, stressful life events are associated with the initial or second episode of recurrent MDD whereas neurobiological factors are most relevant with subsequent recurrent episodes. Post asserted that sensitization to stressors and episodes may become encoded at the level of gene expression, underscoring the role of neurobiological factors in the progression of the illness.

Since genetic factors are operative in the etiology of MDD and prior depressive episodes place an individual at risk for future depression, indirect genetic factors operate in the vulnerability to lifetime risk. In summary, clinical and genetic epidemiologic studies suggest that MDD is a multifactorial disorder influenced by several genetic and environmental risk factors. The effectiveness of the individual's social support network in association with successful treatment may protect the individual from the vulnerability to recurrent MDD.

Neurobiological Theories

The complex interrelation and interdependence of neurochemical systems involving critical neurotransmitters, synaptic regulation, nerve cell mediation and modulation, neuropeptides and neuroendocrine systems are poorly understood. In the past four decades, explorations of these mechanisms have focused on simpler hypotheses derived from clinical observations of drug effects. The interaction of these multiple systems has been difficult to investigate in the laboratory.

Recent studies challenging the simpler paradigm of catecholamine deficit or excess in depression have focused upon neurotransmitter modulation of nerve cell regulation as well as effects of neurotransmitter systems on receptor sensitivity. Additional studies show that patients with depression as well as those who have died by suicide are reported to have lower levels of the serotonin transporter (SERT) than in control subjects (Owens and Nemeroff, 1998). As the pharmacology of the neurotransmitters and receptors is further explicated, receptor changes leading to effects on second messenger systems and the generation of new proteins affecting gene expression will become the focus of the neurobiology of MDD.

Sleep Studies and Biological Rhythm Disturbances

Specific abnormalities in sleep and circadian rhythms are among the most consistent findings in biological psychiatry. Clinical observations of insomnia and hypersomnia are commonly noted as a central feature of depressive disorder. Polysomnography (PSG) demonstrates that the progression of sleep from nonrapid eye movement (nonREM) stages 1 to 4 to rapid eye movement (REM) sleep is disrupted in MDD. EEG recordings demonstrate a shorter than normal onset of REM sleep termed reduced or shortened REM latency. The frequency of eye movements during REM sleep is greater, termed increased REM density. During the sleep laboratory evaluation, increased awakening during sleep leads to the reduction in total sleep time in MDD. NonREM abnormalities include prolonged sleep latency, increased wakefulness, decreased arousal threshold and early morning awakening. Giles and colleagues (1989) have suggested that sleep EEG parameters are more trait-like and that some sleep EEG alterations may precede the onset of clinical depression.

Biological rhythm abnormalities include advances in the timing of daily rhythms such as REM sleep, cortisol and body temperature. Endogenous processes within a day (approximately 25 hours) are **circadian rhythms**. Episodic recurrences of the illness over days, months, or years are called **infradian rhythms** (a period of more than a day). **Ultradian rhythms** are oscillations that occur more than once daily and occur at the cellular and neurohormonal level. Mechanisms which explain the alterations in oscillation of biological rhythms in depression are not well delineated. Clearly, homeostatic regulation of cellular, biochemical and psychological phenomenon is necessary to maintain euthymia. Seasonal variation in mood disorders represents the effect of change in light and temperature on the individual's biological vulnerability to depression. Treatments involving light manipulation have begun to address the impact of seasonal change on those individuals vulnerable to depression with seasonal pattern.

Neurohormonal Theories

The contribution of endocrine system alterations in depression has been examined extensively in biological studies. Both hypothyroidism and hypercortisolism may result in depression.

Hypothalamic–Pituitary–Thyroid Axis

Hypothalamic–pituitary–thyroid (HPT) axis abnormalities are commonly seen in patients with bipolar disorder. Thyroid hormone has been used in antidepressant augmentation as well as in the modulation of rapid cycling bipolar disorder. Neurotransmitters regulate hypothalamic functioning and initiate release of thyrotropin-releasing hormone (TRH) into the portal circulation. TRH is transported to the pituitary causing release of thyroid-stimulating hormone (TSH). TSH modulates synthesis and release of T_3 and T_4.

Thyroid studies in depression are not conclusive. There are more reports of slightly increased peripheral T_4 in major depression than low T_4. Some patients have mild or "sub-clinical" hypothyroidism as reflected in slight TSH abnormalities and associated antithyroid antibodies. The TRH stimulation test has provided suggestive findings: 1) blunted TSH response to TRH occurs in approximately 30% of depressed patients; 2) a possible bipolar/unipolar difference has been reported with bipolar depression showing an augmented TSH response while unipolar depression shows a blunted response; and 3) CSF TRH is found to be raised in some patients with depression, possibly responsible for the blunted response of TSH to TRH, and lower levels of circulating T_3 and T_4. One implication of the suggested bipolar–unipolar distinction is that bipolar depressed patients may demonstrate a false hypothyroidism, when their TSH response is consistent with the underlying bipolar disorder. Effective treatment of the bipolar disorder may reverse the TSH abnormality.

Hypothalamic–Pituitary–Adrenal Axis

The hypothalamic–pituitary–adrenal axis (HPA) has been the subject of intensive investigation as well. The observation of elevated cortisol secretion from the adrenal glands has been replicated consistently in patients with major depression. Corticotropin-releasing factor (CRF) is the hypothalamic hormone that regulates pituitary secretion of corticotropin (ACTH). CRF activity is influenced by multiple neurotransmitters such as 5HT, NE, ACh and GABA. ACTH binds to cells in the adrenal cortex producing release of glucocorticoids, particularly cortisol. Cortisol inhibits secretion of ACTH at the anterior pituitary and CRF at the hypothalamus. Measurements of 24-hour urinary cortisol, cortisol in the CSF and cortisol following dexamethasone suppression suggested increased cortisol secretion in MDD. The dexamethasone suppression test (DST) performed by offering dexamethasone at 11PM followed by serum cortisol at 8AM, 4PM and 11PM is a neuroendocrine probe that demonstrated adrenocortical hyperactivity in depression. DST nonsuppression normalizes with recovery from depression. Persistent nonsuppression is associated with early relapse of MDD. Increased CRF secretion may explain the hypercortisolemia and HPA overactivity. Hypercortisolemia is one of the most consistent findings in biological studies of MDD.

Intracellular Abnormalities

A number of intracellular changes, which involve alteratations in cellular second messenger systems and ion channels, are postulated to occur in depression. The may involve changes in guanine triphosphate binding proteins, G-proteins on the receptor, cyclic adenosine monophosphate (cAMP) regulation, reduced protein kinase activity and brain derived neurotrophic factor (BDNF). Stress itself has been associated with lowered levels of BDNF, which leaves vulnerable to neurotoxic effects of stress. Antidepressants as well as ECT increase BDNF and BDNF has been found to increase functioning of serotonin.

Psychosocial Theories

Psychoanalytic theory as postulated by both Freud and Abraham emphasized the connection between mourning and melancholia. wherein the melancholic patient experiences a loss of self-esteem with associated helplessness, prominent guilt and self-denigration. According to the theory, this results from internally directed anger which or aggression turned against the self, leading to a depressive experience. Self-psychologists have described the effects of loss and trauma on the development of a coherent sense of self. Bowlby's work on attachment elucidates the impact of very early loss and trauma with a resultant predisposition to depression among other things.

Behavioral theory holds that depression is an overgeneralized response to loss of social support. Indeed, the lack of social support appears to be one of the strongest factors in promoting vulnerability to depression. The experience of depression may also elicit negative responses from others which reinforces negatively held personal beliefs.

The cognitive-behavioral perspective emphasizes a set of dysfunctional attitudes, cognitions and images associated with depressive symptomatology. This theory is the most empirically examined psychosocial theory in relation to the management and treatment of the depressed patient, and emphasizes how cognitive distortions and negative self-image cause depression and are associated with maintenance of the disorder.

The cognitive perspective as well as contributions from the helplessness–hopelessness models formed an empirical basis for CBT. In CBT, education, behavioral assignments and cognitive retraining form the active components of the psychotherapy.

This cognitive therapy has been demonstrated to be an effective short-term psychotherapy for depression. Another current therapy called interpersonal therapy derives from a focus on difficulties in current interpersonal functioning. The relationship between psychological health and one's interpersonal environment has received substantial attention.

The current iteration of the interpersonal approach is reflected in the development of a specific treatment for depression termed interpersonal psychotherapy of depression (IPT). IPT involves a formal diagnostic assessment, inventory of important current and past relationships, and definition of the current problem area. In IPT, four areas of focus that could relate to depressive symptoms are: 1) grief, 2) interpersonal role disputes, 3) role transitions, and 4) interpersonal deficits.

The loss of "social zeitgebers" has been proposed as a link between biological and psychosocial formulations. The social zeitgebers theory suggests that social relationships, interpersonal continuity and work tasks entrain biological rhythms. Disruptions of social rhythms due to loss of relationships interfere with biological rhythms that maintain homeostasis. This disruption leads to changes in neurobiological processes including alterations in neurotransmitter functions, neuroendocrine regulation, and neurophysiologic control of sleep/wake cycle and other normal circadian oscillations.

Diagnosis and Differential Diagnosis

The detection of depression in both primary care settings and mental health settings requires the presence of mood disturbance or loss of interest and pleasure in activities for 2 weeks or more accompanied by at least four other symptoms of depression. There are problems in differential diagnosis because depressive experiences vary from individual to individual. MDD is sometimes called unipolar depression or recurrent unipolar depression because the depressive episodes tend to recur in a lifetime. Dysthymic disorder (DD) is characterized by at least 2 years of depressed mood accompanied by two or three depressive symptoms which falls short of threshold criteria for a major depressive episode. Depressive disorder not otherwise specified (DDNOS) includes a set of conditions which do not meet criteria for MDD, DD, or adjustment disorder with depressed mood. These syndromes include premenstrual dysphoric disorder, minor depressive disorder, recurrent brief depressive disorder and postpsychotic depressive disorder occurring during the residual phase of schizophrenia. In DSM-IV, two other depressive disorders are diagnosed based upon etiology and include mood disorder due to a general medical condition and substance-induced mood disorder.

The core symptoms comprising a major depressive episode are illustrated in the DSM-IV criteria. Each symptom is critical to evaluate in a patient with depressive symptomatology since each represents one of the essential features of a major depressive episode. Their persistence for much of the day, nearly every day for at least 2 weeks, is the criterion for diagnosis. The clinical syndrome is associated with significant psychological distress or impairment in psychosocial or work functioning.

The clinical observation of mood reveals variations in presentation. An individual may have depressed symptomatology and experience typical sadness. Another individual may deny sadness and experience internal agitation and dysphoria. Another individual with depression may experience no feelings at all, and the depressed mood is inferred from the degree of psychological pain that is exhibited. Some individuals experience irritability, frustration, somatic preoccupation and the sensation of being numb.

An equally important aspect of the depressive experience involves loss of interest or pleasure, when an individual feels no sense of enjoyment in activities which were previously considered pleasurable. There is associated reduction in all drives including energy and alteration in sleep, interest in food and interest in sexual activity.

A common experience of insomnia or hypersomnia is noted in individuals with persistent depression. Observations of psychomotor activity include profound psychomotor retardation leading to stupor in more severe cases or alternatively significant agitation leading to inability to sit still and profound pacing in agitated forms of depression.

The complaint of guilt or guilty preoccupation is a common aspect of the depressive syndrome. Delusional forms of guilt are a common presentation of depressive disorder with psychotic features.

The loss of ability to concentrate, to focus attention and to make decisions is a particularly distressing symptom for individuals. One may experience a loss of memory which simulates dementia. Loss of concentration is reflected in an inability to perform both complicated and more simple tasks. The loss of ability to perform in school may be a symptom of MDD in children, and memory difficulties in the older adult may be mistaken for a primary dementia. In some older adults, a depressive episode with memory difficulties occurs in the early phase of an evolving dementia.

The most common psychiatric syndrome associated with thoughts of death, suicidal ideation, or completed suicide is MDD. The experience of hopelessness is commonly associated with suicidal ideation. The preoccupation with suicide in MDD requires that the assessment always includes careful monitoring of suicidality.

Subtyping of MDD

The current subtyping of MDD is based on severity, cross-sectional features and course features.

Severity

The rating of severity is based on a clinical judgment of the number of criteria present, the severity of the symptomatology, and the degree of functional distress. The ratings of current severity are classified as mild, moderate, severe without psychotic features, severe with psychotic features, in partial remission, or in full remission. The definition of "mild" refers to a episode results in only mild impairment in occupational or psychosocial functioning or mild disability. "Moderate" implies a level of severity which is intermediate between mild and severe and is associated with moderate impairment in psychosocial functioning. The definition of "severe" describes an episode which meets several symptoms in excess of those required to make a diagnosis of major depressive episode and is associated with marked impairment in occupational or psychosocial functioning and definite disability characterized by inability to work or perform basic social functions. Severe with psychotic features indicates the presence of delusions or hallucinations which occur in the context of the major depressive episode. The categories of mood-congruent versus mood-incongruent psychotic features are made in the context of a psychotic depressive disorder. When the content of delusions or hallucinations is consistent with depressive themes, a mood-congruent psychotic diagnosis is made. When the psychotic features are not related to depressive themes or include symptoms such as thought insertion, broadcast, or withdrawal, the modifier of mood-incongruent psychotic features is used. A recent review has suggested that mood-incongruent psychosis in MDD is associated with a poorer prognosis. For depression with psychotic features, whether they are mood-congruent or mood-incongruent, antipsychotic medication in combination with antidepressant medication or electroconvulsive therapy (ECT) is required to treat the disorder.

Partial remission indicates that the episode no longer meets full criteria for major depressive episode but that some symptoms are still present or the period of remission has been less than 2 months. In full remission, the individual has no significant symptoms of depression for a period of at least 2 months.

Cross-sectional Features

The assessment of cross-sectional features involves the presence or absence of catatonic, melancholic, or atypical features during an episode of depression. The specifier with catatonic features is used when profound psychomotor retardation, prominent mutism, echolalia, echopraxia, or stupor dominate the clinical picture. The presentation of catatonia requires a differential diagnosis which includes schizophrenia, catatonic type, bipolar I disorder, catatonic disorder due to a general medical condition, medication-induced movement disorder leading to catatonic features, or neuroleptic malignant syndrome.

The specifier with melancholic features is applied when the depressive episode is characterized by profound loss of interest or pleasure in activities and lack of reactivity to external events as well as usual pleasurable stimuli. In addition, at least three of the following melancholic features must be present: depression is typically worse in the morning, early morning awakening, psychomotor change with marked retardation or agitation, significant weight loss, or profound and excessive guilt. MDD with melancholic features is particularly important to diagnose because of the prediction that it is more likely to respond to somatic treatment including electroconvulsive therapy. Individuals with melancholic features experience more recurrence of MDD. The findings of hypercortisolism following dexamethasone as well as reduced REM latency is associated with the melancholic subtype of MDD.

Finally, the category of MDD with atypical features was previously called "atypical depression". This syndrome is characterized by prominent mood reactivity in which there is excessive responsiveness of mood to external events and at least two of the following associated features: increased appetite or weight gain, hypersomnia, leaden paralysis (a feeling of profound anergia or heavy feeling) and interpersonal hypersensitivity (rejection sensitivity). Depressive episodes with atypical features are also common in individuals with bipolar I or II disorder as well as seasonal affective disorder.

Course Features

MDD is diagnosed with certain course features such as postpartum onset, seasonal pattern, recurrent, chronic, and with or without full interepisode recovery. Depression with onset in the postpartum period has been the subject of increasing attention in psychiatric consultation to obstetrics and gynecology. The presence of a MDD may occur from 2 weeks to 12 months after delivery, beyond the usual duration of postpartum "blues" (3–7 days). Postpartum blues are brief episodes of labile mood and tearfulness which occur in 50 to 80% of women within 5 days of delivery. However, depression is seen in 10 to 20% of women after childbirth (Miller, 2002), which is higher than rates of depression found in matched controls. There is greater vulnerability in women with prior episodes of major mood disorder particularly bipolar disorder, and there is a high risk of recurrence with subsequent deliveries after an MDD with postpartum onset. The postpartum onset episodes can present either with or without psychosis. Postpartum psychotic episodes occur in 0.1 to 0.2% of deliveries. Depression in postpartum psychosis is associated with prominent guilt and may involve individuals with a prior history of bipolar I disorder. If an episode of postpartum psychosis occurs, there is a high risk of recurrence with subsequent deliveries. Heightened attention to identification of postpartum episodes is required because of potential risk of morbidity and mortality to mother and newborn child.

The specifier with seasonal pattern is diagnosed when episodes of MDD occur regularly in fall and winter seasons and subsequently remit during spring and summer. When the pattern of onset and remission occurs for the last 2 years, one diagnoses an MDD with seasonal pattern. Often, this pattern is characterized by atypical features including low energy, hypersomnia, weight gain and carbohydrate craving. Although the predominant pattern is fall–winter depression, a minority of individuals show the reverse seasonal pattern with spring–summer depression. Specific forms of light therapy with 2500 lux exposure has been shown to be effective in MDD with seasonal pattern. Because seasonal depression has clinical features which are similar to atypical features, the risk of a possible bipolar II disorder must be considered since atypical features are more common in depressive episodes occurring as part of bipolar II. These individuals when exposed to antidepressant medication or bright light therapy may evolve a switch into hypomanic or manic episode.

Clinical and scientific attention to the course of MDD focuses upon the depiction of longitudinal course. Life charting of MDD involves the use of several course specifiers. Each episode is denoted with or without full recovery. MDD manifests either a single or recurrent pattern of episodes. Remission of depression requires a 2-month interval in which the criteria are not met for a major depressive episode. The specifier chronic MDD involves the persistence of a major depressive episode continually, satisfying full MDD criteria for at least 2 years.

Depression in Children and Adolescents

In prepubertal children, MDD occurs equally among boys and girls (Depression Guideline Panel, 1993). MDD in childhood is considered to have high recurrence rates with up to 70% recurrence in 5 years. After puberty, girls experience an increased rate of depression as compared with boys. There is increased risk of depressive disorder in children and adolescence when one or more of the parents are depressed. The earlier the age of onset of depression, the higher the familiar loading. In addition, a number of childhood psychosocial risk factors have been identified to be associated with juvenile-onset MDD. These risk factors include: more perinatal insults, motor skill abnormalities, instability in caregivers and psychopathology in the first-degree relatives. Adolescent-onset depression often takes on a more chronic course associated with dysthymic symptoms. In adolescence, MDD appears to be associated with greater fatigue, worthlessness and more prominent vegetative signs while DD has more prominent changes in mood, irritability, anger and hopelessness. The signs and symptoms used for diagnosis in children and adolescents are identical to those used for diagnosis in adults. The sequelae of depression in children and adolescents is often characterized by disruption in school performance, social withdrawal, increased behavioral disruption and substance abuse. Differential diagnosis among children and adolescents with MDD include behavioral disorders such as conduct disorder, attention deficit hyperactivity disorder and bipolar disorder.

Later-onset MDD in adolescents is also associated with decline in school performance, social withdrawal, or disruptive behavior. The critical differential diagnostic consideration in adolescents with MDD is the misdiagnosis of depression when the clinical presentation will evolve into a diagnosis of bipolar disorder. When depression occurs during adolescence, it often heralds a severe disorder with recurrent course and a family history of MDD is often noted. An additional psychosocial risk factor in later-onset depression in adolescence is childhood sexual abuse.

In a community sample of adolescents, ages 14 to 18 years, onset of MDD was associated with female gender and suicidal ideation. The mean age of onset for the first episode of MDD was 14.9 years. Episodes of MDD were relatively longer in adolescents who had onset before the age of 15.

Major Depressive Disorder in the Older Adult

Older adults with depression often experience cognitive impairment as part of the clinical syndrome. Symptoms of depression may simulate dementia with concentration difficulties, memory loss and distractibility. Commonly, MDD and dementia cooccur. It is less frequent that findings of dementia are fully explained on the basis of depression (pseudodementia). The prevalence of MDD in older adults residing in nursing homes is estimated to be approximately 30%. MDD in the elderly often cooccurs in the presence of medical conditions which complicates the treatment for both the depression and the primary medical condition. Careful evaluation of medications may also reveal explanations for associated symptoms of depression. Older adults with first onset of depression must be carefully evaluated for cooccurring medical conditions. Among the common disorders to be considered are silent cerebral ischemic events, undiagnosed cancer, or complications of metabolic conditions such as adult-onset diabetes mellitus and thyroid dysfunction.

Depression in Ethnic Groups

In working with individuals of different ethnic groups, the language which expresses depressive symptomatology varies. Nonwestern cultural expressions emphasize somatic complaints more prominently than psychological complaints. Depending on the particular ethnic group understanding the specific "language of depression" is important, because the prevalence estimates cross-culturally do not appear to differ significantly from those reported in the USA.

Assessment

The assessment of MDD involves the specific identification of five of nine criterion symptoms which would constitute a diagnosis of MDD. A careful general medical assessment to ascertain the presence of an etiologic general medical condition is required. After the assessment for general medical conditions, one examines the individual for the presence of alcohol or drug dependence. Then the clinician is required to assess retrospectively the occurrence of prior episodes of mood disorder, either depression or mania. It is necessary to examine for other comorbid psychiatric disorders as well. Depressive illnesses are very common and recurrent, but an individual with MDD may or may not recall prior episodes. It is therefore essential to interview a significant other in addition to the patient to identify prior manic, hypomanic, or prior depressive episodes. Family inquiry allows one to elicit the family history of addiction, anxiety, depressive disorder, mania, psychosis, trauma, or neurologic disorders in first-degree relatives.

To assess risk for suicide, one inquires about the presence of active suicidal ideation in relation to the current episode of depression and a history of prior suicide attempts. The occurrence of significant life events such as separation, divorce and death of significant others may precipitate the episode. It is also necessary to review onsets of other medical conditions which may precipitate a new episode of depression. When alcohol or other drug use cooccurs with such significant life events, the risk of suicidal behavior during an episode of depression increases. The presence of a recent suicide attempt may suggest the need for immediate hospitalization and treatment.

General Medical Assessment

The individual who presents for outpatient or hospital treatment for a primary depressive disorder will require general medical examination including a physical examination and laboratory testing to rule out an associated medical condition. Clinical assessment, including the cognitive mental status examination, will direct the extent of the general medical examination.

Laboratory studies in the management of the individual with MDD includes complete blood count with differential, electrolytes, chemical screening for renal and liver function, as well as thyroid function studies. More detailed evaluation will depend upon the nature of the clinical presentation as well as neuropsychological examination. These studies may identify cerebral vulnerability factors that would complicate the treatment for MDD.

When clinical signs suggest cognitive disruption or cognitive impairment, the clinician may also consider administering neuropsychological tests or conducting more focused neurologic examination to explore cognitive, behavioral and neurologic correlates of brain function. Neuropsychological assessment may help to clarify the relative contribution of depression or another disease process to the patient's clinical presentation. Further, neuropsychological assessment will provide a functional analysis of the patient's cognitive and behavioral strengths and limitations. Neurological examination may reveal minor neurological abnormalities suggesting early neurodevelopmental vulnerability.

Psychodiagnostic Assessment

Traditional psychological testing may complement structured diagnostic instruments developed to ascertain the presence or absence of depressive disorders according to DSM-IV criteria. Psychological testing such as the Rorschach Inkblot Test are sensitive to the degree of affective lability, intensity of suicidality and impulse control in individuals with depression. In addition, inventories are commonly used in outpatient and inpatient settings to establish scores of clinical severity of depressive symptoms. Self-administered scales include the Beck Depression Inventory, the Zung Self-Rating Depression Scale and the Inventory for Depressive Symptomatology (self-report). Psychiatrist-administered scales used for assessment of depressive symptoms include the Hamilton Rating Scale for Depression, the Montgomery Asberg Depression Rating Scale and the Inventory for Depressive Symptomatology (psychiatrist rated). Structured diagnostic interviews that have been developed to confirm major psychiatric syndromes include the present state examination, the schedule for affective disorders and schizophrenia (SADS) and structured clinical interview for DSM-IV Axis I disorders (SCID-I). The use of these structured diagnostic interviews reliably predicts the presence of an MDD. It is essential to recognize that a cross-sectional assessment is only one component of the total assessment. Corroborative family data and longitudinal assessment and reassessment of mood disorder symptoms are crucial in following the natural history and course of MDD.

Course and Natural History

Clinical Course and Age of Onset

In order to document onset of depressive phases as well as periods of remission, psychiatrists must pay careful attention to clinical course. Improvements in assessment procedures, including structured interview guides for the assessment of depression as well as rating scales for depression, will promote better attention to course and natural history of MDD. Long-term studies of depression must incorporate information on recovery, recurrence and chronicity. The mean age of onset of major depression is 27 years of age, although an individual can experience the onset of MDD at any age.

Natural History of Episodes

New symptoms of MDD often develop over several to several weeks. Early manifestations of an episode of MDD include anxiety, sleeplessness, worry and rumination prior to the experience of overt depression. Over a lifetime, the presence of one major depressive episode is associated with a 50% chance of a recurrent episode. A history of two episodes is associated with a 70 to 80% risk of a future episode. Three or more episodes are associated with extremely high rates of recurrence. Because the majority of cases of MDD recur, continuation treatment and ongoing education regarding warning signs of relapse or recurrence are essential in ongoing clinical care. In an MDD when single episode recurs, a change in diagnosis to MDD recurrent is necessitated.

In comparison to individuals who develop a single episode (many of whom return to premorbid functioning), individuals with recurrent episodes of depression are at greater risk to manifest bipolar disorder. Individuals who experience several recurrent episodes of depression may develop a hypomanic or manic episode requiring rediagnosis to bipolar disorder. In children and adolescents, the transformation of a diagnosis of depression to a diagnosis of bipolar disorder is higher. Approximately 40% of adolescents who are depressed, evolve a bipolar course. Because bipolar disorder is initiated with a depressive episode in four of five cases, it is important to identify those patients who are most likely to develop a bipolar disorder. Therefore, the clinician is confronted with significant diagnostic and treatment challenges when called upon to evaluate a patient, particularly an adolescent, who presents with depression and has no previous history of mania. Several risk factors have been identified, which predict when a first episode of MDD will evolve into bipolar disorder: 1) the first episode of depression emerges during adolescence; 2) the depression is severe and includes psychotic features; 3) psychomotor retardation and hypersomnia are present; 4) a family history of bipolar disorder exists, particularly across two to three generations; and 5) the patient experiences hypomania induced by antidepressant medication.

Recurrent MDD requires longitudinal observation because of its highly variable course. Generally, complete remission of an episode of MDD heralds a return to premorbid levels of social, occupational and interpersonal functioning. Therefore, the goal of treatment is a focus on achieving full remission of depressive symptoms and recovery. Untreated episodes of depression last 6 to 24 months. Symptom remission and a return to premorbid level of functioning characterize approximately 66% of depressed patients. By comparison, roughly 5 to 10% of patients continue to experience a full episode of depression for greater than 2 years and approximately 20 to 25% of patients experience partial recovery between episodes. Furthermore, 25% of patients manifest "double depression", characterized by the development of MDD superimposed upon a mild, chronic depression (DD). Patients with double depression often demonstrate poor interepisode recovery. Four characteristics are seen in a partial remission of an episode: 1) increased likelihood of a subsequent episode; 2) partial interepisode recovery following subsequent episodes; 3) longer-term treatment may be required; and 4) treatment with a combination of pharmacotherapy and psychotherapy may be indicated.

Follow-up naturalistic studies have indicated that 40.3% of individuals with MDD carry the same diagnosis 1 year later, 2.6% evidence DD, 16.7% manifest incomplete recovery and 40.5% do not meet criteria for MDD. Keller and colleagues (1992) highlight the potential for chronicity in MDD. A 5-year follow-up study indicated that 50% of 431 patients showed recovery by 6 months but 12% of the sample continued to be depressed for the entire 5-year period. The authors noted that inadequate treatment may have contributed to chronicity.

Definitions of Remission, Relapse, Recovery and Recurrence

The precise nature of severity and duration of phases during the natural course of MDD has not been empirically demonstrated in longitudinal, prospective studies. Definitions of remission, recovery, relapse and recurrence proposed by Frank and colleagues are illustrated in Table 46.2.

Factors Affecting Recurrence and Outcome

Poor outcome and likelihood of recurrent episodes is associated with comorbid conditions such as personality disorder, active substance or alcohol abuse, organicity, or medical illness. Recurrence and outcome may be affected by the rapidity of clinical intervention. Inadequate treatment (e.g., insufficient dosing or duration of pharmacotherapy) contributes to poor outcome, including chronic MDD. Several authors have asserted that early treatment intervention in an episode of MDD is considered to be somewhat more effective than later intervention in an episode.

Prognosis and Morbidity

MDD must be viewed as a serious medical illness. Although depression is treatable, the prognosis for an individual diagnosed with MDD involves important implications regarding morbidity, social functioning and mortality Patients with MDD report

Table 46.2	Proposed Definitions of Remission, Recovery, Relapse and Recurrence
Remission	A period in which the individual is asymptomatic. Does not meet syndromal criteria for MDD, and has no more than minimal symptoms; in clinical practice, this remission extends from 2 to 9 mo.
Recovery	A remission that lasts more than 9 mo without relapse after appropriate treatment.
Relapse	A return of symptoms meeting criteria for a full syndrome of an episode of MDD that occurs during a period of remission but before recovery.
Recurrence	A manifestation of a new episode of MDD that occurs during recovery.

health difficulties and actively use health services. Studies have indicated that as many as 23% of depressed patients report health difficulties severe enough to keep them bedridden. A community sample of patients with MDD demonstrated increased health care utilization in comparison to patients in the general medical setting (Regier *et al.*, 1988). The Medical Outcomes Study (Wells *et al.*, 1989) examined role functioning, social functioning and number of days in bed secondary to poor health, and compared the degree of impact of depression and other chronic medical conditions. Depression was associated with more impairment in occupational and interpersonal functioning, and more days in bed, in comparison to several common medical illnesses.

Patients with MDD were shown to be as functionally impaired as patients with serious, chronic medical conditions as well (Katon *et al.*, 1990). Patients with MDD evidence severely impaired occupational functioning, such as loss of work time. Further, long-term diminished activity has been shown to characterize depressed patients.

Mortality

A significant relationship exists between MDD and mortality, characterized by suicide and accidents. Therefore, an accurate diagnosis of MDD, early appropriate intervention and specific assessment of suicidality is essential. Fifteen percent of patients with MDD who require hospitalization due to severe depression will die by committing suicide. Approximately 10% of patients with MDD who attempt suicide will eventually succeed in killing themselves. Roughly 50% of individuals who have successfully committed suicide carried a primary depressive diagnosis.

Factors associated with suicide 1 year after assessment included severe anhedonia, insomnia, concentration difficulties and comorbid panic attacks or substance abuse. Factors associated with suicide at 1 to 5 years after the assessment included prior suicide attempts, suicidal ideation and hopelessness.

Patients with MDD who were admitted to nursing homes were found to have a 59% greater likelihood of death within the first year of admission in comparison with nondepressed admissions. The ECA study indicated that patients with MDD 55 years of age and older evidence a mortality rate over the next 15 months four times higher than nondepressed controls matched for age.

The occurrence of MDD in patients who previously have been hospitalized following MI is demonstrated as an independent risk factor for mortality at 6 months. The consequences of MDD were at the very least commensurate with that of left ventricular dysfunction and history of past MI.

Goals of Treatment

The goals of treatment in MDD are full remission of symptoms of depression with restoration of optimal work and social functioning. During the course of treatment ongoing education of the individual and family regarding remission, relapse and recurrence is critical. This education alerts both those affected by the illness and their families to the early signs of relapse and can assist in prevention of recurrence. Improved social and work functioning following an episode of depression is an important associated goal of treatment. Many studies have demonstrated the benefit of depression-specific psychotherapy as an important aspect of maintaining remission and improving work and social functioning. The establishment of a collaborative working relationship among the patient, family and psychiatrist is an essential aspect of recovery. The data which demonstrate efficacy in psychiatric management and treatment infers that a collaborative relationship is present.

Phases of Treatment

All psychiatric treatment whether pharmacotherapy or psychotherapy or the integration of pharmacotherapy and psychotherapy, first requires a well-established diagnostic formulation in order to achieve optimal response to treatment. As the diagnostic process is undertaken an ongoing therapeutic alliance must be established. In the treatment of MDD an understanding of the clinical history of each individual's distress is necessary. As the clinical history is elicited the appropriate target signs and symptoms of MDD are obtained and the patient is educated as to the nature of the symptom patterns which represent his or her unique form of depressive disorder.

The phases of treatment include:

1. An acute phase directed at reduction and elimination of depressive signs and symptoms, and active restoration of psychosocial and work functioning.
2. A continuation phase directed at prevention of relapse and reduction of recurrence through ongoing education, pharmacotherapy and depression-specific psychotherapy.
3. A maintenance phase of treatment directed at prevention of future episodes of depression based upon the patient's personal history of relapse and recurrence.

Acute phase treatment may involve all interventions that are directed toward decreasing signs and symptoms of depression and maintaining the individual's capacity to work and interact with others in a manner consistent with premorbid levels of social and work functioning. The acute phase treatments may include supportive psychotherapy focusing on resolution of current disputes. A form of supportive therapy may be combined with recommendations for pharmacotherapy. The standard pharmacotherapies which are available for treatment of depression have increased dramatically in the past two decades. In mild to moderate depressive disorder, more depression-specific forms of psychotherapy have been established including cognitive–behavioral psychotherapy, interpersonal psychotherapy, or short-term dynamic psychotherapy. In these forms of psychotherapy, which have been studied to address mild to moderate nonbipolar depressive disorder, the focus of the psychotherapy is very clearly explicated to the patient before the initiation of the psychotherapy. For severe depressive disorder with melancholic or psychotic features, these specific forms of short-term psychotherapy may not be as effective as focused pharmacotherapy. Pharmacotherapy in these conditions is associated with more rapid treatment response than is psychotherapy. During the acute phase of treatment for depressive disorder the optimal treatment should result in resolution of depressive signs and symptoms anytime between week 8 and week 16 of treatment. If resolution of depressive signs and symptoms does not occur during the first 2 to 4 months then the initial diagnostic formulation must be reviewed and alternative treatment strategies must be introduced. Some of the factors associated with lack of complete treatment response include the presence of cooccurring personality disorders, concurrent alcohol or substance abuse, a poor therapeutic alliance leading to lack of adherence to treatment recommendations, and persistent or unfavorable side effects of treatment.

When acute phase treatment does lead to remission of signs and symptoms, then the next phase of treatment begins. This phase of treatment is termed continuation treatment and its goal is prevention of relapse. It is often necessary to maintain ongoing pharmacotherapy for 6 to 12 months after an acute episode of depression during this continuation phase, because there is substantial vulnerability to relapse if medication treatment is prematurely interrupted. During the continuation phase ongoing psychotherapy may be particularly important to address residual symptoms of depression, and to alert the individual to a depressive response to subsequent traumatic circumstances, as well as ongoing clinical interaction with significant others is required in order to address persisting interpersonal conflicts, and may promote even more complete recovery from the depressive episode. The continuation phase of treatment typically lasts 9 to 12 months to minimize the risk of recurrent episode. If this represents the initial episode of depression, then medication treatment may be carefully withdrawn at the end of the continuation phase. However, if this represents a history of recurrence of depression (particularly two or more episodes in the preceding 3 years), maintenance treatment may well be recommended. In addition, maintenance treatment is recommended if two prior episodes have occurred within one's lifetime.

Maintenance treatment of MDD is focused on prevention of future episodes of depression, after a recent recurrence of MDD and a prior history of two or more episodes of MDD. Often the maintenance phase of treatment involves ongoing treatment with antidepressants or alternatively mood-stabilizing treatment (particularly lithium carbonate), or a combination to sustain recovery from depression. When there is early onset (adolescent onset) of depressive symptoms with associated psychosocial impairment, then ongoing maintenance treatment along with rehabilitative psychotherapy may be most critical. During maintenance treatment, continuing education of the patient and family, identification of prodromal symptoms, and continuing efforts at work and psychosocial rehabilitation are indicated. Often the trials of maintenance pharmacotherapy in depression demonstrate the preventive benefit of maintenance medication. In the most often quoted study, recurrence rates of 20 to 25% were found in individuals maintained with full dose of imipramine, while the recurrence rate was 80 to 100% in those patients treated with placebo. The advantage of ongoing maintenance medicine has also been demonstrated at 5 to 10 years. With tricyclic antidepressants, maintenance medication is likely more effective at full dose rather

than lower doses. Limited data exists as to the dosing of SSRIs or other types of antidepressants in maintenance treatment.

Site of Treatment

The site of treatment for MDD is based upon the severity of the acute episode and the psychiatrist's judgment of the individual's potential for suicide. Individuals with mild to moderate depression are often treated in primary care or psychiatry office settings. Acute phase pharmacotherapy involving antidepressant medication is often initiated by a primary care physician. However, the overall longitudinal care of MDD in primary care is the subject of increasing attention. Typically, individuals do not receive treatment for long enough periods and there is limited attention to the domains of social or work functioning. The referral to a psychiatrist may include a request for more expertise regarding medication as well as the need for depression-specific psychotherapy. In addition, there has been a lack of focused attention to the role of integrated psychotherapy and pharmacotherapy in primary care. Inpatient treatment for depression is recommended when there is an immediate risk for suicide or recent suicide attempt. In these settings safety of the individual is the primary concern and often more intensive treatments including electroconvulsive therapy may be initiated. When there are comorbid general medical conditions and psychiatric disorders, inpatient psychiatric hospitalization may be useful to stabilize both the general medical condition as well as the associated psychiatric disorder.

General Approaches to Treatment

Initiation of treatment follows a careful psychiatric diagnostic interview. Assessment of the longitudinal clinical history must rule out bipolar disorder, comorbid PTSD, other anxiety disorders, and personality disorder. A completed mental status examination is used to rule out associated psychosis or marked cognitive disruption. When these procedures are conducted empathically, the beginning of a favorable therapeutic alliance is established. In all circumstances an effective therapeutic alliance facilitates recovery from MDD.

Pharmacotherapy and Other Somatic Treatment

Treatment during the acute phase with medication is highly efficacious in reducing signs and symptoms of MDD. Antidepressant medication has the most specific effect on reduction of symptoms and is often associated with improved psychosocial functioning. When symptoms of depression are mild to moderate, a course of depression-specific psychotherapy without medicine may also be effective. If symptoms of depression are moderate to severe, acute phase treatment with medications is often indicated. A wide variety of antidepressant medications have been documented as effective in moderate to severe MDD.

The range of treatments available in the USA has included the tricyclic antidepressants, monoamine oxidase inhibitors (MAOIs), heterocyclic antidepressants and SSRIs. In addition, antidepressants with both serotonergic and noradrenergic activity or noradrenergic activity alone have become available. Clearly, clinical trials comparing the efficacy of newer treatments with standard tricyclic antidepressants have shown equal efficacy with improvement in overall tolerance to side effects with newer treatments.

Antidepressant medications which are currently available for acute treatment of MDD are listed in the associated table (Table 46.3).

Table 46.3   Antidepressant Medications Category

	Category			Side Effects		
Trade Name	Compound	Usual Therapeutic Dose (mg)	Sedation	Hypotension (Decreased Blood Pressure)	Anticholinergic (i.e., Dry Mouth Constipation)	Cardiac (Slowed Heart Rate)
Tricyclics						
Tertiary Amines						
Anafranil	Clomipramine	150–300	High	High	High	Yes
Elavil	Amitriptyline	150–300	High	High	High	Yes
Sinequan	Doxepin	150–300	High	Moderate	Moderate	Yes
Surmontil	Trimipramine	150–300	High	Moderate	Moderate	Yes
Tofranil	Imipramine	150–300	Moderate	High	Moderate	Yes
Norpramine	Desipramine	100–300	Low	High	Low	Yes
Pamelor	Nortriptyline	50–150	Moderate	Low	Low	Yes
Vivactil	Protriptyline	20–60	Low	Low	High	Yes
Monoamine						
Oxidase Inhibitors						
Marplan	Isocarboxazid	30–60	Low	Moderate	Low	Low
Nardil	Phenelzine	45–90	Low	Moderate	Low	Low
Parnate	Tranylcypromine	30–90	Low	Moderate	Low	Low
Atypical Agents						
Ascendin	Amoxapine	200–300	Low	Moderate	Low	Yes
Desyrel	Trazodone	300–600	High	High	Minimal	Low
Ludiomil	Maprotiline	150–200	Moderate	Moderate	Low	Low
Wellbutrin	Bupropion	150–450	Minimal	Low	Minimal	Yes
Selective Serotonin						
Reuptake Inhibitors						
Paxil	Paroxetine	20–50	Low	Minimal	Minimal	Low
Prozac	Fluoxetine	20–100	Minimal	Minimal	Minimal	Low
Zoloft	Sertraline	50–300	Minimal	Minimal	Minimal	Low
Luvox	Fluvoxamine	150–400	Low	Low	Low	Low
Celexa	Citalopram	20–50	Minimal	None	None	Minimal
Lexapro	Escitalopram	10–30	Minimal	None	None	Minimal
Serotonin/ Norepinephrine						
Reuptake Inhibitors						
Effexor	Venlafaxine	75–450	Low	None	None	Minimal
Serotonin Transport						
Blocker and Antagonist						
Serzone	Nefazadone	200–600	Minimal	Low	Minimal	Minimal
Alpha-2- Adrenergic Antagonist						
Remeron	Mirtazapine	30–60	Moderate	Low	Minimal	Minimal

Choice of treatment with a specific antidepressant treatment in a given clinical situation is based on prior treatment response to medication, consideration of potential side effects, history of response in first-degree relatives to medicines, and the associated presence of cooccurring psychiatric disorders that may lead to a more specific choice of antidepressant treatment. Table 46.4 illustrates an algorithm developed for pharmacotherapy of MDD which includes a staged trial of newer medications (because of their superior side-effect profiles) followed by treatments with older medicines available for the treatment of MDD. The ultimate goal of pharmacotherapy is complete remission of symptoms during a standard 6- to 12-week course of treatment.

Selective Serotonin Reuptake Inhibitors

The most commonly prescribed antidepressant medicines in the past 10 years are SSRIs. They are selectively active at serotonergic neurochemical pathways and are effective in mild to moderate nonbipolar depression. They may also be particularly effective in MDD with atypical features as well as DD. Often these treatments are well tolerated and involve single daily dosing for MDD. Because of selective serotonergic activity, these treatments have also been demonstrated to be effective with cooccurring OCD, panic disorder, generalized anxiety disorder, PTSD, premenstrual dysphoric disorder, bulimia nervosa, social anxiety disorder, as well as MDD. They tend to be reasonably well tolerated in individuals with comorbid medical conditions. There are particular medication-specific interactions based on inhibition of cytochrome P-450 liver enzyme systems which require attention if an individual is taking other medications for primary medical conditions or associated psychiatric conditions. The currently available SSRIs in the USA include fluoxetine, paroxetine, sertraline, fluvoxamine, citalopram and escitalopram.

Other Newer Antidepressants

In addition to SSRIs, greater attention has been brought to medicines with dual noradrenergic and serotonergic pathways including venlafaxine which has become available in both immediate release (IR) and extended release formulations. In addition, an alpha-2-adrenergic agonist, mirtazapine has become available, as well as a serotonin transport blocker and antagonist nefazodone. Recent concerns about hepatic complications associated with nefazodone has required liver function monitoring. A predominantly noradrenergic and dopaminergic agonist, bupropion is also available in an immediate release and sustained release (SR) preparation. The newest dual acting antidepressant marketed in the USA is duloxetine.

Table 46.4 Pharmacotherapy Algorithm in Major Depressive Disorder
Major Depressive Disorder, Single or Recurrent Episode, without Psychotic Features
Begin effective monotherapy with bupropion SR, citalopram, escitalopram, fluoxetine, nefazodone, paroxetine, sertraline, or venlafaxine XR (augment with lithium carbonate 600–900 mg).
or
Begin effective monotherapy with alternative antidepressant from list above (augment with bupropion SR, mirtazepine, or tricyclic antidepressant, either nortriptyline or desipramine, recognizing important drug interactions).
If ineffective, consider tranylcypromine, augmented with lithium carbonate, if necessary, for anergic features.
or
Consider phenelzine, augmented with lithium carbonate, if necessary, for anxious, dependent and phobic features.
Augment with atypical antipsychotics for agitation, rumination, or suspicion.
or
Offer electroconvulsive therapy to remission (ECT).
Major Depressive Disorder, Single or Recurrent Episode, with Psychotic Features
Begin typical or atypical antipsychotic to adequate doses in order to interrupt delusional features, augmented with SSRI, venlafaxine XR, or tricyclic antidepressants, either nortriptyline or desipramine, recognizing important drug interactions.
or
Begin amoxapine as alternative.
or
Begin electroconvulsive therapy as alternative, in context of immediate suicide risk, physical deterioration, or prior response to electroconvulsive therapy.
Major Depressive Disorder with Atypical Features
Begin SSRI starting at low dose to minimize early side effects.
or
Begin MAOI, either phenelzine or tranylcypromine, to therapeutic doses.
Major Depressive Disorder with Catatonic Features
Begin lorazepam 1–3 mg/d, to interrupt catatonic symptoms; evaluate for presence of psychotic features or longitudinal history of bipolar disorder.
Add antipsychotic medication to therapeutic doses or lithium carbonate to therapeutic doses, if bipolar or schizoaffective disorder emerges from the longitudinal history.

Tricyclic Antidepressants in Individuals with Severe MDD Including Melancholic Features

Tricyclic antidepressants have been best studied in individuals with MDD with melancholic features and with psychotic features. The combination of typical antipsychotic pharmacotherapy in association with tricyclic antidepressants has been recommended. The side-effect profile of tricyclic antidepressants has included moderate to severe sedation, anticholinergic effects including constipation and cardiac effects which has made these medicines less popular in typical primary care or psychiatric practice. Nevertheless, the secondary amines which are metabolites of imipramine and amitriptyline, specifically desipramine and nortriptyline, have continued to be useful agents in more refractory depression.

Monoamine Oxidase Inhibitors

There continues to be a role for the use of MAOIs in patients with MDD with atypical features. These agents particularly may be useful in intervention in depressive episodes with atypical features, characterized by prominent mood reactivity, reverse neurovegetative symptom patterns (i.e., overeating and oversleeping) and marked interpersonal rejection sensitivity. MAOIs continue to have a significant role in treatment of comorbid panic disorder, social phobia and agoraphobia if individuals are not responsive to SSRIs. The ongoing prescription of phenelzine or tranylcypromine requires continued education of the patient regarding standard food interactions involving tyramine as well as specific drug–drug interactions involving sympathomimetic medications. These cautions regarding diet and drug interaction makes MAO inhibitors less attractive to primary care physicians and most psychiatrists. However, they continue to be effective treatments which may be useful in depression with atypical features as well as anergic bipolar depression.

Therapeutic Blood Levels

Although therapeutic blood level monitoring in the treatment of MDD may have a role in future treatments, the only group of medicines where there has been reliable assessment of blood levels are the tricyclic antidepressants. Because tricyclic antidepressants have significant drug–drug interactions with certain SSRIs there continues to be a need for therapeutic blood monitoring particularly with nortriptyline and desipramine.

General Pharmacotherapy Recommendations

Increasingly, a trial of one class of antidepressants may be associated with incomplete response leading to a question of augmenting a treatment with another medicine versus switching from one medicine to another within the same class or to a different class altogether. Augmentation strategies with other medications, including adding lithium carbonate and other antidepressants, particularly those with a different mechanism of action, atypical antipsychotics, thyroid and stimulants, have been the focus of a number of reviews of treatment resistance. A staging system for treatment resistant depression (TRD) has been proposed and ranges from failure to respond to a single agent (Stage 1) to failure of multiple treatments and electroconvulsive therapy (Stage 5) as shown in Table 46.5.

Clinical Management

All of the antidepressant medications used in the treatment of MDD must be prescribed in the context of an overall clinical

Table 46.5	Staging Criteria for Treatment Resistant Depression
Stage	**Description**
1. Failure of at least one adequate trial of an antidepressant	
2. Stage 1 resistance plus failure of adequate trial of an antidepressant from a distinctly different class than in Stage 1	
3. Stage 2 resistance plus failure of an adequate trial of a tricyclic antidepressant (TCA)	
4. Stage 3 resistance plus failure of an adequate trial of a monoamine oxidase inhibitor (MAOI)	
5. Stage 4 resistance plus failure of a course of bilateral electroconvulsive therapy (ECT).	

psychiatric relationship characterized by supportive interaction with the patient and family and ongoing education about the nature of the disorder and its treatment. Clinical management optimally involves careful monitoring of symptoms using standardized instruments and careful attention to side effects of medication in order to promote treatment adherence. Outpatient visits, which may be scheduled weekly at the outset of treatment, and subsequently biweekly encouragement and sustain collaborative treatment relationships. These office consultations allow the psychiatrist to make dosage adjustments as indicated, monitor side effects and measure clinical response to treatment.

For the majority of individuals with MDD, a course of 6 to 8 weeks of acute treatment with weekly outpatient visits is indicated. Subsequent office visits may be scheduled every 2 to 4 weeks during the continuation phase of treatment. Appropriate adjustments of dose are determined by the psychiatrist as indicated by best clinical judgments of medication effect. The dose of an SSRI may be adjusted every 3 days on the basis of telephone contact and follow-up visits may be scheduled every 7 to 10 days. Similarly, the adjustment of dosing of tricyclic antidepressants and MAOIs must be attended to carefully in the first 2 to 3 weeks of treatment. Optimal dosing ranges of SSRIs, tricyclics and MAOIs are noted in Table 46.3. Because of the early anxiety, agitation and occasional insomnia associated with SSRIs, somewhat lower doses may be initiated early in the course before achieving the typical standard therapeutic dose.

Incomplete response, which entails the failure to respond to acute treatment with an antidepressant medication at 6 to 8 weeks, requires reassessment of diagnosis and determination of adequacy of dosing. Ongoing substance abuse, associated general medical condition or concurrent psychiatric disorder may partially explain a lack of complete response. If substance dependence is present, a full substance-free interval (preferably

4 weeks or longer) with appropriate detoxification and rehabilitation may be indicated. If a reassessment discloses an associated psychiatric disorder, then more specific treatment of that associated disorder, whether it be bipolar disorder or concurrent post traumatic disorder, is necessary. If the reassessment suggests an associated comorbid personality disorder, then appropriate and more specialized psychotherapy may be necessary in order to achieve a complete response to treatment. As indicated before, if the MDD has psychotic features, then antipsychotic pharmacotherapy to adequate doses must be initiated prior to initiating a course of standard tricyclic antidepressants or a combined serotonin norepinephrine uptake inhibitor such as venlafaxine. If MDD is associated with severe personality disorder (e.g., borderline personality disorder), then adjunctive psychotherapy and low dose antipsychotic medications may be necessary. If the patient has severe melancholic, delusional, or catatonic features, a course of electroconvulsive therapy may be necessary to achieve remission of symptoms.

There is also evidence that continuation of treatment beyond 6 to 12 weeks may convert some partial responders to responders if drug treatment is increased to full doses. This time allows for evaluation of the role of focused psychotherapy to address residual interpersonal disputes, loss or grief, or ongoing social deficits. The associated augmentation strategies to standard treatments include lithium carbonate augmentation, tricyclic antidepressant augmentation of SSRIs, thyroid hormone augmentation and bupropion augmentation of SSRIs.

Electroconvulsive Therapy

Electroconvulsive therapy (ECT) remains an effective treatment in patients with severe MDD and those individuals with psychotic MDD. Many patients who have responded to electroconvulsive therapy do not respond to pharmacotherapy. There is increased need for understanding the role of maintenance electroconvulsive therapy in those individuals who respond to electroconvulsive therapy because ongoing pharmacotherapy does not always prevent recurrence of depression after ECT is successful. ECT can be particularly useful in interrupting acute suicidality for those patients who may require rapid resolution of symptoms. ECT may be indicated in older adults when lack of self-care and weight loss may represent a greater risk. The most common side effect associated with electroconvulsive therapy is amnesia for the period of treatment. There is no consistent evidence to suggest chronic cognitive or memory impairment as a result of ECT.

Other Somatic Treatments

Light therapy investigators have continued to demonstrate benefit in individuals with seasonal MDD by providing greater than 2500 lux light therapy for 1 to 2 hours/day. Many of these patients experience recurrent winter depression in the context of a recurrent MDD or bipolar II disorder. Bright light exposure has been associated with favorable response within 4 to 7 days. As with electroconvulsive therapy, light therapy is best prescribed by specialists who have experience in its use and can appropriately evaluate the indication for light therapy and monitor carefully the response to treatment.

Ongoing investigation of alternative brain stimulation techniques have been the subject of recent investigation. The use of a powerful magnet to provide transcranial magnetic stimulation has been the subject of several open trials. It is not yet determined whether the repetitive transcranial magnetic stimulation demonstrates its effectiveness through reduction of inhibitory neurotransmission or other mechanisms.

In addition, open clinical trials of vagus nerve stimulation (VNS) which has been found to be effective in epilepsy has been the subject of attention in refractory MDD. Several sites of investigation have begun to reveal positive effects at 9 months using VNS implantation. This procedure requires the implantation of a stimulating device in the chest with the capacity to stimulate the vagus nerve at regular intervals through the course of the day.

Psychosocial Treatment

The past decade has also led to the development of more specific depression-based treatment for MDD. These treatments have included supportive psychiatric management techniques during pharmacotherapy, interpersonal psychotherapy, cognitive–behavioral therapy, brief dynamic psychotherapy, and marital and family therapy.

Psychiatric Management and Supportive Psychotherapy

Psychiatric management and supportive psychotherapy is the standard in psychiatric office practice. The psychiatrist focuses on establishing a positive therapeutic relationship in the course of diagnosis and initiation of treatment of depression. The psychiatrist is attentive to all signs and symptoms of the disorder with particular attention to suicidality. The psychiatrist provides ongoing education, collaboration with the patient, and supportive feedback to the patient regarding ongoing response and prognosis. The supportive psychotherapeutic management of depression facilitates the ongoing pharmacologic response. Brief supportive psychotherapy in individuals with mild to moderate depression is indicated to improve medication compliance, to facilitate reduction of active depressive signs and symptoms, and to provide education regarding relapse and recurrence.

Interpersonal Psychotherapy

Interpersonal psychotherapy in outpatients with nonbipolar MDD has been demonstrated to be effective in acute treatment trials. Interpersonal psychotherapy of depression addresses four areas of current interpersonal difficulties:

1. Interpersonal loss or grieving;
2. Role transitions;
3. Interpersonal disputes;
4. Social deficits.

This type of treatment, like other psychotherapies for depression, also involves education about the nature of MDD and the relationship between symptoms of depressive disorder and current interpersonal difficulties. Prior studies demonstrated efficacy of interpersonal psychotherapy for outpatients with depression. Interpersonal psychotherapy, cognitive–behavioral psychotherapy and medication treatment were comparable on several outcome measures and superior to placebo. Medication treatment was associated with the most rapid response and was superior to both interpersonal psychotherapy and cognitive–behavioral therapy in more severely depressed patients. Continuation studies with interpersonal psychotherapy offered monthly, as well as during maintenance treatment, have demonstrated response in prevention of recurrence, and was superior to placebo treatment. Those patients who received ongoing interpersonal psychotherapy and medication had the longest intervals without recurrence of depressive symptoms.

Cognitive–Behavioral Therapy

Cognitive–behavioral therapy for depression is a form of treatment aimed at symptom reduction through the identification and correction of cognitive distortions. These involve negative views of the self, one's current world and the future. Several controlled studies have demonstrated the efficacy of cognitive therapy in resolution of MDD in adults. Cognitive–behavioral therapy as well as interpersonal psychotherapy are somewhat less effective than medication treatment in moderate to severe MDD although some have suggested a relatively equal response to cognitive–behavioral therapy and medication in more severely depressed outpatients.

Brief Dynamic Psychotherapy

Brief dynamic psychotherapy addresses current conflicts as manifestations of difficulty in early attachment and disruption of early object relationships. Brief dynamic psychotherapy was not specifically designed for treatment of MDD and is currently the subject of ongoing studies as well as controlled clinical trials in comparison with medication treatment. The results of these trials will allow us to address the appropriate role of brief dynamic psychotherapy in outpatients with mild to moderate depression. In addition, it will be important to understand whether dynamic psychotherapy may address demoralization or response to traumatic circumstances.

Marital and Family Therapy

It has been difficult to assess the specific efficacy of marital or family therapy in individuals with MDD based on current studies to date. There is substantial evidence that marital distress is a major event associated with the development of a depressive episode. Marital discord will often persist after the remission of depression and subsequent relapses are frequently associated with disruptions of marital relationships. There has been no controlled clinical trial of marital therapy in relation to other treatments for promoting the resolution of depressive signs and symptoms. Both acute and continuation phase treatment of MDD will require ongoing attention to marital and family issues to prevent recurrence of depression.

Factors Influencing Treatment Response

There are a number of factors which influence ultimate treatment response in MDD including patient characteristics, diagnostic issues, comorbidity, treatment-related complications including side effects and demographic factors. Reevaluation of diagnosis, comorbidity and the physician–patient relationship itself is often critical.

Suicide Risk

Patients with MDD are often at increased risk for suicide. Suicidal risk assessment is especially indicated as patients begin to recover from depression with increased energy and simultaneous continued despair. Persistent suicidal ideation coupled with increased energy can often lead to impulsive suicidal acts. The careful attention to the physician–patient relationship can mediate suicidal urges through availability and accessibility. Outpatients and inpatients with MDD and melancholic features will often require antidepressant therapy addressing multiple neurotransmitter systems, or ECT as well.

Psychotic Features

MDD with psychotic features requires careful assessment to rule out comorbid psychiatric conditions. The combined treatment with antipsychotic as well as antidepressant medication is indicated. In addition, electroconvulsive therapy is an effective intervention in psychotic depression and may be considered as a first line alternative.

Catatonic Features

MDD with catatonic features can be associated with significant morbidity due to the individual's refusal to eat or drink. Active treatment with a benzodiazepine such as lorazepam 1 to 3 mg daily may offer short-term treatment response. Subsequent treatment with lithium alone or in association with antidepressants may be indicated given the possible link between catatonic features and bipolar vulnerability. If psychosis is associated with catatonia, then atypical antipsychotic medication or a course of electroconvulsive therapy may be indicated as well.

Atypical Features

Atypical features are associated with significant comorbid anxiety disorders, reverse neurovegetative symptoms such as hypersomnia, increased appetite and weight gain, as well as fatigue and leaden paralysis. SSRIs are likely to be effective in individuals with MDD with atypical features as well as MAOIs. Conversely, tricyclic antidepressants, in particular, are unlikely to be effective in such individuals.

Severity

Individuals with mild to moderate depression may be effectively treated with psychotherapy, pharmacotherapy, or the combination. Individuals with severe MDD often require somatic intervention with antidepressant medication or electroconvulsive therapy.

Recurrence

Because MDD is a recurrent disorder, current treatment guidelines (Hirschfeld, 1994) suggest maintenance antidepressant treatment at full therapeutic doses if there is a history of more than two prior episodes of MDD.

History of Hypomania or Mania

Any of the antidepressant treatments including medication, electroconvulsive therapy, light therapy, or newer somatic interventions may induce hypomania or mania in individuals who are vulnerable to bipolar disorder. Individuals who may have a family history of bipolar disorder should be carefully evaluated for treatment with lithium carbonate or other anticonvulsant mood stabilizers before antidepressant treatment because they are at particular risk for antidepressant-induced mania. Attention to this history of prior hypomania or mania as well as family history may promote treatment response if such individuals have mood stabilizing treatment offered initially.

Comorbid Psychiatric Disorders with Major Depressive Disorder

Alcohol or Substance Dependence

The comorbidity of MDD and alcohol or other substance dependence requires careful attention to both diagnoses. The first priority in treatment is abstinence from alcohol or substance use. Cooccurring addiction will complicate depressive disorders and increases risk for suicide. If detoxification from alcohol or other substance abuse is required, this should be undertaken before initiation of any somatic antidepressant therapy. Individuals who have a family history of depression or bipolar disorder are likely to require early initiation of appropriate mood disorder treatment following detoxification.

Obsessive–Compulsive Disorder

In individuals with OCD, lifetime risk of MDD approaches 70%. The use of higher dose SSRI treatment is often indicated to treat both conditions. Alternatively, the tricyclic antidepressant, clomipramine (Anafranil), may be effective for those individuals with both OCD and MDD who do not respond to SSRIs.

Panic Disorder

Lifetime risk of MDD approaches 50% in individuals with panic disorder. Because many of the SSRI and other antidepressants are effective treatments to treat panic as well as depression, these treatments have gained increasing popularity. One may continue to prescribe short-term courses of benzodiazepines, including lorazepam or clonazepam to alleviate acute symptoms of panic as low doses of antidepressant treatments are introduced into the treatment for comorbid panic and MDD. In addition, MAOIs continue to be effective treatments for both panic and MDD.

Generalized Anxiety Disorder

Lifetime risk of MDD in individuals with generalized anxiety disorder (GAD) approaches 40%. New studies demonstrating efficacy of venlafaxine as well as paroxetine make these effective interventions in situations in which an individual has both MDD and GAD.

Post traumatic Stress Disorder

An essential feature of PTSD is the vulnerability to the development of MDD. Recent studies (Friedman, 1998) demonstrate effectiveness in treating the core symptoms of PTSD as well as MDD. In addition, specific psychotherapy which addresses the core aspects of PTSD may be appropriate in individuals with comorbid PTSD and MDD in order to minimize the vulnerability to depression because of persistent PTSD symptomatology.

Cognitive Impairment

When cognitive impairment is due to depressive disorder (as in "pseudodementia"), active treatment of depression may minimize associated cognitive difficulties. Many seniors evolve mild cognitive impairment and depression as early signs of dementia. Nevertheless, when MDD is mild it requires specific antidepressant treatment, or when severe or psychotic, electroconvulsive therapy.

Dysthymic Disorder

The exacerbation of a persistent or chronic DD into a more severe depressive episode is termed "double depression". Many treatments for MDD are also useful in DD. It is likely that SSRIs, newer antidepressants as well as tricyclic antidepressants are effective for both DD and MDD. Specific forms of psychotherapy which are cognitive–behavioral have been investigated as effective in addressing poor inter-episode recovery from MDD associated with DD.

Personality Disorder

Increasing evidence of the cooccurrence of MDD with personality disorder with rates up to 40 to 50% in outpatient clinics suggests incomplete response to antidepressants alone. Specific psychotherapy treatments which focus on maladaptive personality traits may facilitate the ongoing response to antidepressant pharmacotherapy.

General Medical Conditions Cooccurring with Major Depressive Disorder

Asthma

Ongoing attention to pharmacotherapy of individuals with asthma relates to the use of bronchodilators and steroid inhalers for asthma. These may complicate associated anxiety and depression and must be addressed carefully in consideration of appropriate antidepressant therapy. Generally, SSRIs and newer antidepressants appear to be well tolerated with typical asthma treatments.

Cardiac History

SSRIs, newer mixed noradrenergic and serotonergic reuptake inhibitors, bupropion and ECT are likely to be safe treatments for patients with cardiac disease (Glassman *et al.*, 2002).

Epilepsy

In individuals with epilepsy and MDD, adjunctive antidepressant medications, particularly SSRIs and bupropion are well tolerated in combination with most anticonvulsant treatments.

Glaucoma

Previously, tricyclic antidepressants with anticholinergic properties were known to precipitate acute angle closure glaucoma in vulnerable patients. The effect on intraocular pressure is benign with newer antidepressant treatments.

Hypertension

Many older antihypertensive treatments including reserpine and alpha methyldopa were reported to precipitate depression. Fatigue, lethargy and possible depression were associated with beta-adrenergic blockers. Newer antihypertensive drugs including angiotensin converting enzyme inhibitors (ACEI) and calcium channel blockers have fewer side effects and are tolerated well in combination with standard antidepressant treatments.

Parkinson's Disease

There is prominent cooccurrence of MDD with Parkinson's disease. The prescription of low dose SSRIs, bupropion and mixed noradrenergic serotonergic reuptake inhibitors may be helpful in the management of comorbid MDD and Parkinson's disease without risk of worsening the underlying movement disorder or promoting psychosis.

Demographic and Sociocultural Factors in Treatment

Children

It is increasingly important to identify children at risk for MDD. There have been insufficient controlled studies of pharmacotherapy or psychotherapy in children with MDD. However, early studies of SSRIs appear promising in terms of overall treatment efficacy in children with MDD.

Adolescents

Adolescent-onset depression with psychotic features may be an early predictor of bipolar course. Adolescent-onset depression, therefore, must be carefully diagnosed, ruling out a bipolar history in the family and assessing evidence for mixed hypomanic or manic states in the prepubertal or pubertal period. The appropriate prescription of lithium carbonate in those individuals with bipolar vulnerability must precede antidepressant pharmacotherapy. Alternatively, early studies suggest the role for standard SSRIs in adolescents with nonbipolar depression.

Older Adults

MDD in older adults is often characterized by more prominent somatic signs and cognitive impairment. It is important to diagnose and treat depression to minimize associated morbidity and mortality. Standard SSRI pharmacotherapy is likely to be associated with demonstrated efficacy as is depression-specific psychotherapy assuming the level of depression is mild to moderate.

Gender

Because of substantial hormonal changes associated with the onset of menses, pregnancy and delivery, and menopause, hormonal effects must be part of the standard assessment of depression. Woman may be at somewhat higher risk for depression at these critical intervals of hormonal change. Standard antidepressant pharmacotherapy as well as depression-specific psychotherapy appear to be equally effective in both men and women. Both men and women require careful attention to sexual side effects of antidepressant pharmacotherapy in the course of the longitudinal management.

Refractory Major Depressive Disorder

A staging system for treatment-resistant depression (TRD) has been proposed and ranges from failure to respond to a single agent (Stage 1) to failure of multiple treatments and electroconvulsive therapy (Stage 5; Thase and Rush, 1995), and is presented in Table 46.5. The term refractory depression has been proposed to describe patients who have Stage 5 treatment-resistant depression.

Refractory MDD or Stage 5 in Table 46.5 is estimated to occur in up to 20% of patients. A larger percentage of patients with MDD, up to 30%, may show only partial improvement. The concept of treatment-resistant depression or refractory depression describes this lack of response to a number of clinical trials using optimal dosing and duration of antidepressant medication. One must typically offer the patient a rational series of treatment trials using optimal dosing and duration of each antidepressant. Many individuals consider a patient refractory if a course of three, four, or five treatments is offered without substantial clinical response. The standard approach to the management of refractory depression includes increasing the antidepressant dose and monitoring for a full 8 to 12 week course augmenting the treatment with several augmentation strategies using an adequate combination of antidepressant drug treatment and psychotherapy and switching to alternative somatic treatments including ECT when indicated.

Refractory MDD is ameliorated in the context of a caring and collaborative treatment relationship based on a favorable ther-

apeutic alliance. Patients sometimes will undermine treatment through their own persistent use of substances such as alcohol or lack of adherence to specific pharmacotherapy recommendations. In this context the attention to the therapeutic alliance is particularly critical. In assessing an individual with refractory symptoms, pharmacologic factors including pharmacokinetic considerations, drug–drug interactions and extreme sensitivity to antidepressant drugs must be considered.

Despite many alternative strategies, substantial morbidity and occasional mortality are associated with refractory MDD. In addition, careful attention to psychosocial factors associated with refractoriness is critical. These psychosocial factors include early childhood adversity and abuse, early family dysfunction, increased neuroticism and marked disruption in the development of a stable sense of self.

Dysthymic Disorder

Definition

Dysthymic disorder is defined by the presence of chronic depressive symptoms most of the day, more days than not, for at least 2 years. While chronic depressive conditions were traditionally conceptualized as characterological and amenable to psychotherapy and resistant to pharmacotherapy, recent pharmacologic trials of antidepressants as well as depression-specific psychotherapy have demonstrated effectiveness in the overall treatment of DD. Both focused interpersonal and variations of cognitive–behavioral psychotherapy have demonstrated response in dysthymia. Individuals with DD have a substantial risk for the development of MDD. This highlights the importance of early assessment and treatment to minimize subsequent long-term complications.

If signs and symptoms of DD follow a MDD, then a diagnosis of MDD, in partial remission, is made. A diagnosis of DD can be made if the individual develops full remission of MDD for 6 months and subsequently develops signs and symptoms of DD which then last a minimum of 2 years. In contrast, the diagnosis of chronic MDD is made when an episode of MDD meets full criteria for MDD continuously for at least 2 years. If DD has been present for at least 2 years in adults (or 1 year in children and adolescents) and is subsequently followed by a superimposed MDD, then both DD and MDD are diagnosed, which is often referred to as "double depression". The following specifiers apply to DD as noted in DSM-IV:

1. Early onset – if the onset of dysthymic symptomsoccurs before age 21.
2. Late onset – if the onset of dysthymic symptoms occurs at age 21 or older, and with atypical features.

Atypical features refer to a pattern of symptoms which include mood reactivity and two of the additional atypical symptoms (i.e., weight gain or increased appetite, hypersomnia, leaden paralysis, or interpersonal rejection sensitivity). Early-onset DD is usually associated with subsequent episodes of MDD. DD with atypical features may herald a bipolar I or II course.

Ongoing studies have not completely clarified the distinction between DD and depressive personality disorder. Depressive temperaments may predispose an individual to a condition within the spectrum of Axis I mood disorders. However, it may not be

DSM-IV-TR Criteria 300.4

Dysthymic Disorder

A. Depressed mood for most of the day, for more days than not, as indicated either by subjective account or by observation by others, for at least 2 years. **Note:** In children and adolescents, mood can be irritable and duration must be at least 1 year.

B. Presence, while depressed, of two (or more) of the following:
   (1) poor appetite or overeating
   (2) insomnia or hypersomnia
   (3) low energy or fatigue
   (4) low self-esteem
   (5) poor concentration or difficulty making decisions
   (6) feelings of hopelessness

C. During the 2-year period (1 year for children or adolescents) of the disturbance, the person has never been without the symptoms in criteria A and B for more than 2 months at a time.

D. No major depressive episode has been present during the first 2 years of the disturbance (1 year for children and adolescents); i.e., the disturbance is not better accounted for by chronic major depressive disorder or major depressive disorder, in partial remission.

Note: There may have been a previous major depressive episode provided there was a full remission(no significant signs or symptoms for 2 months) before development of the dysthymic disorder. In addition, after the initial 2 years (1 year in children or adolescents) of dysthymic disorder, there may be superimposed episodes of major depressive disorder, in which case both diagnoses may be given when the criteria are met for a major depressive episode.

E. There has never been a manic episode, a mixed episode, or a hypomanic episode, and criteria have never been met for cyclothymic disorder.

F. The disturbance does not occur exclusively during the course of a chronic psychotic disorder, such as schizophrenia or delusional disorder.

G. The symptoms are not due to the direct physiological effects of a substance (e.g., a drug of abuse, a medication) or a general medical condition (e.g., hypothyroidism).

H. The symptoms cause clinically significant distress or impairment in social, occupational, or other important areas of functioning.

Specify if:

Early onset: if onset is before age 21 years
Late onset: if onset is age 21 years or older *Specify* (for most recent 2 years of dysthymic disorder):

With atypical features

specifically associated with MDD. This depressive temperament may also be associated with vulnerability to bipolar disorder.

Epidemiology

A lifetime prevalence of 4.1% for women and 2.2% for men was reported for DD (Weissman *et al.*, 1988). In adults, DD is more common in women than in men. In children DD occurs equally in both sexes. Across both women and men, DD has a 2.5% 12-month prevalence (Kessler *et al.*, 1994, 2005).

Comorbidity Patterns

Individuals with early-onset DD are at substantial risk for development of other psychiatric conditions including alcohol or substance dependence, MDD and personality disorders. Up to 15% of patients with DD may also have a substance use pattern that meets criteria for comorbid alcohol or substance dependence diagnosis. The most common associated personality disorders include mixed, dependent and borderline. Childhood and adolescent-onset DD is associated with a substantial risk for later occurrence of both MDD and bipolar disorder.

Etiology and Pathophysiology

Biological Findings

Sleep abnormalities demonstrate reduced REM latency, increased REM density, reduced slow wave sleep and impaired sleep continuity in 25 to 50% of individuals with DD. There are minimal data on cortisol or thyroid abnormalities in individuals with DD. Other neurobiological studies have not yielded consistent results.

Diagnosis and Differential Diagnosis

The diagnosis of DD cannot be made, if depressive symptoms occur during the course of a nonaffective psychosis such as schizophrenia, schizoaffective disorder, or delusional disorder. Diagnosis of depressive disorder NOS is made if there are symptoms which meet criteria for MDD during the residual phase of a psychotic disorder. If DD is determined to be etiologically related to a chronic medical condition, then one diagnoses secondary mood disorder due to a general medical condition. If substance dependence is judged to be the etiologic factor, then a substance-induced mood disorder is diagnosed. Individuals with DD often have cooccurring personality disorders and in these situations separate diagnoses on Axis I and II are made.

Course and Natural History

Dysthymic disorder often begins in late childhood or early adolescence and by definition takes a chronic course. The risk for development of MDD among children who have DD is significant because childhood onset of DD is an early marker for recurrent mood disorder, both recurrent MDD and bipolar disorder.

The course of DD suggests impairment in functional status including social and occupational, and physical functioning. Patients who have both DD and MDD have more severe functional impairment. Untreated DD contributes to significant occupational and financial burden. There is substantial reduction in activity, more days spent in bed, more complaints of poor general medical health, and more disability days than reported in the general population.

The treatment goals in DD are similar to those in MDD. They include full remission of symptoms and full psychosocial recovery.

Depressive Disorder not Otherwise Specified

Depressive disorder NOS refers to a variety of conditions listed in DSM-IV that are distinguished from MDD, DD, adjustment disorder with depressed mood, or adjustment disorder with mixed anxiety and depressed mood. These conditions involve a large number of depressed individuals who do not meet formal criteria for MDD or DD. In the ECA study, 11% of subjects had DD NOS. In a primary care outpatient sample, the prevalence of DD NOS was 8.4 to 9.7%. DD NOS is associated with impairment in overall functioning and general health. Among the conditions listed as occurring within this category are premenstrual dysphoric disorder, minor depressive disorder, recurrent brief depressive disorder, postpsychotic depressive disorder of schizophrenia and depressive episode superimposed on delusional disorder or other psychotic disorder.

Premenstrual Dysphoric Disorder

Premenstrual DD is characterized by depressed mood, marked anxiety, affective lability and decreased interest in activities, experienced during the last week of the luteal phase which remits during the follicular phase of the menstrual cycle. This pattern occurs for most months of the year. The severity of symptoms is comparable to MDD, but the duration is briefer by definition. The symptoms disappear with the onset of menses. Current criteria emphasize the disturbance in mood as well as impairment in social functioning associated with premenstrual DD. Current assessments require that the typical cyclical patterns be confirmed by at least 2 months of prospective daily ratings. Premenstrual DD often worsens with increasing age, but then diminishes at menopause. Premenstrual DD appears to respond to standard SSRI treatments including fluoxetine as well as sertraline and dual acting agents but may not respond to other types of antidepressants, such as bupropion. This responsiveness to SSRIs suggests a premenstrual serotonergic hypoactivity which may account for the premenstrual dysphoric symptomatology.

Minor Depressive Disorder

Minor depressive disorder is characterized by episodes lasting 2 weeks and characterized by at least two but fewer than five depressive symptoms. Minor depressive disorder is also associated with less psychosocial impairment than MDD. The prevalence of minor depressive disorder reported in primary care settings ranges from 3.4 to 4.7%. A number of general medical conditions have been associated with minor depressive disorder including stroke, cancer and diabetes. Maier and colleagues report increased symptoms of minor depressive disorder in families in which a proband with MDD is present. In the differential diagnosis of minor depressive disorder, one must consider adjustment disorder with depressed mood and other experiences of sadness that may be part of grieving. Because of frequent cooccurrence with general medical condition, one must rule out a secondary mood disorder due to a general medical condition.

Minor depressive disorder tends to begin in late adolescence and probably affects men and women equally. Minor depressive disorder is often associated with greater impairment of routine activities in older adults. Consultation psychiatrists should pay careful attention to depressive symptoms in association with medical illness in order to establish the impact of depressive disorder on the overall course and recovery from general medical conditions (Cassem, 1990).

Recurrent Brief Depressive Disorder

Recurrent brief depressive disorder refers to brief episodes of recurrent depressive symptoms that last for at least 2 days but less than 2 weeks and meet full criteria (except duration) for MDD. These episodes typically occur monthly for 12 months, but are not specifically related to menstrual cycles. These depressive episodes typically cause clinically significant distress and impairment in social and occupational functioning. In some individuals, RBDD is associated with a high degree of suicidality.

Associated clinical features may include comorbid substance dependence or anxiety disorders. By definition, recurrent brief depressive episodes are not associated with menstrual cycles and are equally common among men as women.

Up to 12 to 20% of first-degree relatives of patients with recurrent brief depressive disorder have MDD. Ongoing research focusing on familial aggregation and associated comorbid conditions is important. It will be particularly important to address its association with personality characteristics and the overlap between personality disorder and the syndrome of RBDD.

Mixed Anxiety–Depressive Disorder

The syndrome of mixed anxiety–depressive disorder is commonly diagnosed in outpatient medical practices internationally and it is included as a disorder in ICD-10. It is typically associated with dysphoric mood lasting at least 1 month and at least four associated clinical symptoms which are derived from both symptoms associated with MDD, DD, panic disorder and generalized anxiety disorder. These symptom characteristics include: difficulty concentrating or mind going blank; sleep disturbance characterized by difficulty falling or staying asleep or restless; unsatisfying sleep; fatigue or low energy; irritability; worry; being easily moved to tears; hypervigilance; anticipating the worst; hopelessness and pessimism about the future; and low self-esteem or feelings of worthlessness. The symptoms cause significant impairment in social and occupational functioning or other aspects of functioning. These symptoms must not be due to the direct physiologic effects of a substance or a general medical condition. Finally, the symptoms are present in the absence of criteria being met for MDD, DD, panic disorder, or generalized anxiety disorder. The presence of these common mixed anxious and depressive symptoms is estimated to range from 1 to 2% in primary care settings.

Post-psychotic Depressive Disorder of Schizophrenia

The diagnosis of postpsychotic depressive disorder of schizophrenia is intended to cover depressive episodes occurring during the residual phase of schizophrenia. In the residual phase there may be associated negative symptoms which can be difficult to differentiate from mood symptoms. The diagnosis should be made only if the full criteria are met for a major depressive episode and if the symptoms are not due to substance abuse, akinesia, or other antipsychotic medication effects.

Features associated with the development of a postpsychotic depressive episode include limited social support, the impact of prior hospitalization, or the trauma of having a major mental illness. It is estimated that up to 25% of individuals with schizophrenia experience postpsychotic depressive disorder. There is no significant age of onset difference between men and women. Individuals who have a family history of MDD may be at higher risk for postpsychotic depression. Treatment studies have demonstrated the efficacy of standard antidepressant medication in the postpsychotic depressive disorder of schizophrenia.

References

American Psychiatric Association (1994) *Diagnostic and Statistical Manual of Mental Disorders*, 4th edn. APA, Washington DC.

American Psychiatric Association (2000) *Diagnostic and Statistical Manual of Mental Disorders*, 4th edn. Text Rev. APA, Washington DC.

Blazer DG (1994) Epidemiology of late-life depression. in *Diagnosis and Treatment Depression in Late Life: Results of the NIH Consensus Development Conference* (eds Schneider LS, Reynolds CF, Lebowityz BD, *et al.* American Psychiatric Press, Washington DC, pp. 9–19.

Cassem EH (1990) Depression and anxiety secondary to medical illness. *Psychiatr Clin N Am* 13, 597–612.

Cross National Collaborative Group (1992) The changing rate of major depression: Cross-national comparisons. *J Am Med Assoc* 268, 3098–3105.

Depression Guideline Panel (1993) Depression in Primary Care: Vol. 1. Detection and Diagnosis, Clinical Practice Guideline, No. 5. (April) U.S. Department of Health and Human Services, Public Health Agency, Agency for Health Care and Policy Research, AHCPR Publication No. 93-0550.

Emslie GE, Weinberg WA and Rush JA (1990) Depressive symptoms by self-report in adolescent: Phase I of the development of a questionnaire for depression by self-report. *J Child Neurol* 5, 114–121.

Forsell Y, Jorm AF and Wonblad B (1994) Association of age, sex, cognitive dysfunction and disability with major depressive symptoms in an elderly sample. *Am J Psychiatr* 11, 1600–1604.

Giles DE, Jarret RB and Roff HP (1989) Clinical predictors of recurrence in depression. *Am J Psychiatr* 146, 764–767.

Glassman AH, O'Connor CM, Califf RM *et al.* (2002) Sertraline treatment of major depression in patients with acute mi or unstable angina. *J Am Med Assoc* 288, 701–707.

Gruenberg AM, Goldstein RD and Bruss GS (1993) Cooccurrence of major mood disorder and personality disorder. Poster presented at Third International Congress on the Disorders of Personality, Cambridge, Massachusetts.

Harkness KL and Monroe SM (2002) Childhood adversity and the endogenous versus nonendogenous distinction in women with major depression. *Am J Psychiatr* 159, 387–393.

Herman J (1997) *Trauma and Recovery*. Basic Books, New York City.

Hirschfeld RMA (1994) Guidelines for the long-term treatment of depression. *J Clin Psychiatr* 55(Suppl), 61–69.

Kashani JH, McGee RO and Clarkson SE (1983) Depression in a sample of 9-year old children. *Arch Gen Psychiatr* 40, 1217–1223.

Katon W, vonKorff M and Lin E (1990) Distressed high utilizers of medical care: DSM-III-R diagnoses and treatment needs. *Gen Hosp Psychiatr* 12, 355–362.

Keller MB, Lavori PW and Mueller JI (1992) Time to recovery, chronicity and levels of psychopathology in major depression: A 5-year prospective follow-up of 431 subjects. *Arch Gen Psychiatr* 49, 809–816.

Kendler KS, Heath AC, Martin AG *et al.* (1986) Symptoms of anxiety and symptoms of depression: Same genes, different environments? *Arch Gen Psychiatr* 44, 451–457.

Kendler KS, Heath AC and Neale AC (1993) Alcoholism and major depression in women: A twin study of the causes of comorbidity. *Arch Gen Psychiatr* 50, 690–698.

Kessler RC, Berglund P, Demler O *et al.* (2005). Lifetime prevalence and age-of-onset distributions of DSM-IV disorders in the National Comorbidity Survey Replication. *Arch Gen Psychiatr* 62, 593-602.

Kessler RC, McGonagle KA and Zhao S (1994) Lifetime and 12-month prevalence of DSM-III-R psychiatric disorders in United States. *Arch Gen Psychiatr* 51, 8–19.

Klerman GI and Weissman MM (1989) Increasing rates of depression. *J Am Med Assoc* 261, 2229–2235.

Miller LJ (2002) Postpartum depression. *J Am Med Assoc* 287(6), 762–765.

Owens MJ and Nemeroff CB (1998) The serotonin transporter and depression. *Depress Anx* 8(Suppl 1), 5–12.

Petty F (1992) The depressed alcoholic: Clinical features and medical management. *Gen Hosp Psychiatr* 14, 458–464.

Post RM (1992) Transduction of psychosocial stress into the neurobiology of recurrent affective disorder. *Am J Psychiatr* 149, 999–1010.

Regier DA, Boyd JH and Burke JD Jr. (1988) One-month prevalence of mental disorders in the United States: Based on five epidemiologic catchment area sites. *Arch Gen Psychiatr* 145, 1351–1357.

Ross ED and Rush AJ (1981) Diagnosis and neuroanatomical correlates of depression in brain-damaged patients: Implications for a neurology of depression. *Arch Gen Psychiatr* 38, 1344–1354.

Thase ME and Rush AJ (1995) Treatment-resistant depression, in *Psychopharmacology: The Fourth Generation of Progress* (eds Bloom F and Kupfer DJ). Raven Press, New York, pp. 1081–1097.

Weissman MM, Leaf PJ and Bruce ML (1988) The epidemiology of dysthymia in five communities: Rates, risks, comorbidity, and treatment. *Am J Psychiatr* 145, 815–819.

Weissman MM, Bruce ML and Leaf PJ (1991) Affective disorders, in *Psychiatric Disorders in America* (eds Robins LN and Regier DA). Free Press, New York, pp. 53–80.

Weller EB and Weller RA (1990) Depressive disorders in children and adolescents, in *Psychiatric Disorders in Children and Adolescents* (eds Garfinkle BD, Carlson GA, and Weller EB). WB Saunders, Philadelphia, pp. 3–20.

Wells KB, Stewart A and Hays RD (1989) The functioning and well-being of depressed patients: Results from the medical outcomes study. *J Am Med Assoc* 262, 914–919.

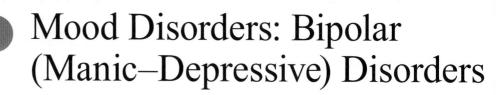

Mood Disorders: Bipolar (Manic–Depressive) Disorders

Until recently, the disorders in this chapter were referred to as "Bipolar Disorders", yet this book includes the older term "manic–depressive disorder". An increasing amount of data indicates that mania and hypomania do not typically take the classic, euphoric, optimistic form that appears to be the polar opposite of depression. Rather, hyperactivation appears to be the core symptom of mania and hypomania while mood itself is quite variable; dysphoria and depression rather than euphoric mood are the rule rather than the exception; and patients rate their quality of life during mania or hypomania as worse than or no better than normal, rather than being enhanced as commonly supposed. Thus the term **manic–depressive** is more accurate and less misleading than **bipolar**, which implies that the two characteristic mood states are somehow polar opposites.

Episodes as the Basis for Diagnosis of Manic–Depressive Disorder

The DSM-based definition of manic–depressive disorder is built on the identification of individual mood **episodes** (Table 47.1). DSM-IV criteria for individual mood episodes are summarized below for manic, mixed and hypomanic episodes. Criteria for these episodes are reviewed in greater detail in the subsequent section on diagnosis. It is important to understand that the diagnosis of manic–depressive disorder derives from the occurrence of individual episodes over time. Persons who experience a manic, hypomanic, or mixed episode, virtually all of whom also have a history of one or more major depressive episodes, are diagnosed with manic–depressive disorder. Those who experience major depressive and manic episodes are diagnosed with **bipolar I** disorder, and those with major depressive and hypomanic (milder manic) episodes are diagnosed with **bipolar II** disorder.

Not surprisingly, most data regarding manic–depressive disorder come from the study of the more severe end of the spectrum, primarily type I disorder. Throughout this chapter, data on manic–depressive disorder derive from studies of type I disorder unless otherwise noted. DSM-IV-TR is the first version of the DSM series to include a specific category for bipolar II disorder. Previously, persons with depressive and hypomanic episodes were grouped under the broad "bipolar disorder not otherwise specified", which included a variety of unusual presentations.

Study of the course over time of type II disorder indicated that persons with hypomania tended to have recurrent hypomanic episodes and did not convert into type I by developing mania. In addition, persons with type II disorder may have more episodes over

time than persons with type I indicating that the course of type II differs from that of type I. However, biological differences between these manic–depressive types have not been reliably demonstrated. However, it should not be construed that manic–depressive disorder type II is in all respects milder than type I, although hypomania is by definition less severe than mania. Specifically, the social and occupational function and quality of life for persons with type II disorder are similar to those for persons with type I disorder.

Persons who experience subsyndromal manic–depressive mood fluctuations over an extended period without major mood episodes are diagnosed with **cyclothymic disorder**. Much less is known about this milder disorder because afflicted persons present for medical attention less frequently than those with full-blown manic–depressive disorder. Cyclothymic disorder has been considered at various times a temperament, a personality disorder and a disorder at the milder end of the manic–depressive. DSM-IV-TR Criteria 301.13

Etiology and Pathophysiology

It is clear from current data that no single paradigm can explain the occurrence, and variability in course and severity of manic–depressive disorder. Rather, a more integrative approach to understanding the causes of manic–depressive disorder is needed, one which recognizes the contributions of varying degrees of importance from several sources.

Further, in trying to understand the source of symptoms at a particular time in a particular person with manic–depressive disorder we must keep in mind that there may be multiple sources that lead to the symptoms that we are trying to treat. It is not likely that biological theories will explain all the pathology seen in manic–depressive disorder. Similarly, the effectiveness of medications such as lithium renders purely psychosocial theories untenable. An integrative **biopsychosocial** mindset will likely be the most successful approach to treatment, as Engel articulated for all illnesses, both medical and psychiatric.

Genetic Hypotheses

Available evidence indicates that familial factors are important determinants of who will develop manic–depressive disorder. Numerous studies have shown that relatives of manic–depressive **probands** (identified cases) have higher rates of manic–depressive disorder than controls or unipolar probands. Overall, rates of manic–depressive disorder in first-degree relatives (parents, siblings, children) of probands with manic–depressive

Table 47.1	Summary of Mood Episodes and Mood Disorders
Episode	**Disorder**
Major depressive episode	Major depressive disorder, single episode
Major depressive episode + major depressive episode	Major depressive disorder, recurrent
Major depressive episode + manic/mixed episode	Manic–depressive disorder, type I
Manic/mixed episode	Manic–depressive disorder, type I
Major depressive episode + hypomanic episode	Manic–depressive disorder, type II
Chronic subsyndromal depression	Dysthymic disorder
Chronic fluctuations between subsyndromal depression and hypomania	Cyclothymic disorder

DSM-IV-TR Criteria

Manic Episode

A. A distinct period of abnormally and persistently elevated, expansive, or irritable mood, lasting at least 1 week (or any duration if hospitalization is necessary).

B. During the period of mood disturbance, three (or more) of the following symptoms have persisted (four if the mood is only irritable) and have been present to a significant degree:
   (1) inflated self-esteem or grandiosity
   (2) decreased need for sleep (e.g., feels rested after only 3 hours of sleep)
   (3) more talkative than usual or pressure to keep talking
   (4) flight of ideas or subjective experience that thoughts are racing
   (5) distractibility (i.e., attention too easily drawn to unimportant or irrelevant external stimuli)
   (6) increase in goal-directed activity (either socially, at work or school, or sexually) or psychomotor agitation
   (7) excessive involvement in pleasurable activities that have a high potential for painful consequences (e.g., engaging in unrestrained buying sprees, sexual indiscretions, or foolish business investments)

C. The symptoms do not meet criteria for a mixed episode.

D. The mood disturbance is sufficiently severe to cause marked impairment in occupational functioning or in usual social activities or relationships with others, or to necessitate hospitalization to prevent harm to self or others, or there are psychotic features.

E. The symptoms are not due to the direct physiological effects of a substance (e.g., a drug of abuse, a medication, or other treatment) or a general medical condition (e.g., hyperthyroidism).

Note: Manic-like episodes that are clearly caused by somatic antidepressant treatment (e.g., medication, electroconvulsive therapy, light therapy) should not count toward a diagnosis of manic–depressive I disorder.

Reprinted with permission from the *Diagnostic and Statistical Manual of Mental Disorders*, Fourth Edition, Text Revision. Copyright 2000 American Psychiatric Association.

DSM-IV-TR Criteria

Mixed Episode

A. The criteria are met both for a manic episode and for a major depressive episode (except for duration) nearly every day during at least a 1-week period.

B. The mood disturbance is sufficiently severe to cause marked impairment in occupational functioning or in usual social activities or relationships with others, or to necessitate hospitalization to prevent harm to self or others, or there are psychotic features.

C. The symptoms are not due to the direct physiological effects of a substance (e.g., a drug of abuse, a medication, or other treatment) or a general medical condition (e.g., hyperthyroidism).

Note: Mixed-like episodes that are clearly caused by somatic antidepressant treatment (e.g., medication, electroconvulsive therapy, light therapy) should not count toward a diagnosis of manic–depressive I disorder.

Reprinted with permission from the *Diagnostic and Statistical Manual of Mental Disorders*, Fourth Edition, Text Revision. Copyright 2000 American Psychiatric Association.

disorder are elevated 5 to 10 times over rates found in the general population. In the latter group, the rates are 0.5 to 1.5%. while in the former group rates are 5 to 15%. Interestingly, rates of unipolar depression in first-degree relatives are about twofold elevated over those in the general population. Because of the rate of depression in the general population (5–20%), this means that a twofold increase is a rate of about 20%. Important for genetic counseling, this in turn means that the probability that a manic–depressive proband will have a unipolar child is greater than the probability that they will have a manic–depressive child (5–15% versus 20%); note that it is most likely that they will have neither (100 minus 25–35%).

Most genetic research has been done on manic–depressive type I disorder. However, manic–depressive type II also appears to have a familial component. Manic–depressive type II probands have more manic–depressive type I disorder and more manic–depressive type II disorder than unipolar depressives and less type I disorder than type I probands. Familial occurrence

DSM-IV-TR Criteria

Hypomanic Episode

A. A distinct period of persistently elevated, expansive, or irritable mood, lasting throughout at least 4 days, that is clearly different from the usual nondepressed mood.

B. During the period of mood disturbance, three (or more) of the following symptoms have persisted (four if the mood is only irritable) and have been present to a significant degree:
   (1) inflated self-esteem or grandiosity
   (2) decreased need for sleep (e.g., feels rested after only 3 hours of sleep)
   (3) more talkative than usual or pressure to keep talking
   (4) flight of ideas or subjective experience that thoughts are racing
   (5) distractibility (i.e., attention too easily drawn to unimportant or irrelevant external stimuli)
   (6) increase in goal-directed activity (either socially, at work or school, or sexually) or psychomotor agitation
   (7) excessive involvement in pleasurable activities that have a high potential for painful consequences (e.g., the person engages in unrestrained buying sprees, sexual indiscretions, or foolish business investments)

C. The episode is associated with an unequivocal change in functioning that is uncharacteristic of the person when not symptomatic.

D. The disturbance in mood and the change in functioning are observable by others.

E. The episode is not severe enough to cause marked impairment in social or occupational functioning, or to necessitate hospitalization, and there are no psychotic features.

F. The symptoms are not due to the direct physiological effects of a substance (e.g., a drug of abuse, a medication, or other treatment) or a general medical condition (e.g., hyperthyroidism).

Note: Hypomanic-like episodes that are clearly caused by somatic antidepressant treatment (e.g., medication, electroconvulsive therapy, light therapy) should not count toward a diagnosis of manic–depressive II disorder.

Reprinted with permission from the *Diagnostic and Statistical Manual of Mental Disorders*, Fourth Edition, Text Revision. Copyright 2000 American Psychiatric Association.

DSM-IV-TR Criteria 301.13

Cyclothymic Disorder

A. For at least 2 years, the presence of numerous periods with hypomanic symptoms and numerous periods with depressive symptoms that do not meet criteria for a major depressive episode.

Note: In children and adolescents, the duration must be at least 1 year.

B. During the above 2-year period (1 year in children and adolescents), the person has not been without the symptoms in criterion A for more than 2 months at a time.

C. No major depressive episode, manic episode, or mixed episode has been present during the first 2 years of the disturbance.

D. The symptoms in criterion A are not better accounted for by schizoaffective disorder and are not superimposed on schizophrenia, schizophreniform disorder, delusional disorder, or psychotic disorder not otherwise specified.

E. The symptoms are not due to the direct physiological effects of a substance (e.g., a drug of abuse, a medication) or a general medical condition (e.g., hyperthyroidism).

F. The symptoms cause clinically significant distress or impairment in social, occupational, or other important areas of functioning.

Reprinted with permission from the *Diagnostic and Statistical Manual of Mental Disorders*, Fourth Edition, Text Revision. Copyright 2000 American Psychiatric Association.

does not differentiate between inborn and environmental factors. Familial aggregation could be due to sharing genetic material, nongenetic congenital factors (e.g., similar inherited or acquired intrauterine factors, or exposure to similar perinatal risk factors), or physiologic or psychological environmental factors.

Data from other types of studies indicate that at least part of this risk is due to biological, and likely genetic factors. Twin studies indicate that **monozygotic** have higher concordance rates for manic–depressive disorder than do **dizygotic** twins 60 to 80% for monozygotic twins versus 20 to 30% for dizygotic twins. Linkage studieshave suggested that in certain families manic–depressive disorder may be linked to specific genes. On

the other hand, studies of monozygotic twins also indicate that only 40 to 70% are concordant for manic–depressive disorder. Thus, although there is clearly a genetic component to this illness, genetics is not destiny.

Several **genetic loci** have been proposed but independent confirmations have been lacking. Overall, the number of families in which a single gene has been associated with manic–depressive disorder is small. Further, no single locus has been replicated in multiple studies. It is likely that genes may confer susceptibility to the disorder without actually determining that the disorder occurs. That is, to have the disorder one must have both the gene and another factor.

A related approach to investigating genetic contributions to manic–depressive disorder is to look for differences in genes that code for components of systems thought to be involved in the pathophysiology of the disorder. Chief among such candidate genes have been those responsible for dopamine and serotonin receptors, transporters and metabolic enzymes. The recent study by Mundo and coworkers (2001) showed that individuals who developed manic symptoms when treated with serotonin-active antidepressants had higher rates of the gene coding for a particular form of the serotonin transporter, compared with those similarly treated who did not develop manic symptoms. In addition, several studies have indicated that the gene coding for the norepinephrine-metabolizing enzyme catechol-*O*-methyl transferase (COMT) may be associated with the rapid cycling form of manic–depressive disorder.

In addition, recent evidence raises the possibility that the expression of a psychiatric illness that is coded genetically may not be due simply to the presence or absence of specific genes, but rather to modifying pieces of DNA in close proximity to important genes. Specifically, small sections of DNA, three base-pairs in length (called **trinucleotide repeats**), appear to be overrepresented in genetic disorders with prominent psychiatric symptoms.

Neurotransmitter Hypotheses

Many theories have something of value to contribute regarding the pathologic basis of manic–depressive disorder. Nonetheless we do not yet have data to indicate whether the disorder is basically a disorder of a particular neurotransmitter, a particular neuroanatomic locus, or a particular physiologic system. Integration of these hypotheses awaits development of new methodologies for clinical neurobiologic investigations.

Second-messenger System Hypotheses

When neurotransmitters bind to postsynaptic neuronal receptors, a series of intracellular events are initiated that are mediated by chemical systems linked to those receptors. So-called G-proteins link the receptors to second-messenger systems, which in turn are linked to protein kinases that control the synthesis and operation of cellular components.

The cyclic AMP and phosphatidyl inositol systems are the most extensively studied of these second-messenger systems. Recent data have generated substantial interest in the phosphatidyl inositol system as a possible mediator of the clinical effects of lithium in manic–depressive disorder, particularly since this second-messenger system is linked to subtypes of adrenergic, serotonergic, dopaminergic and cholinergic neurotransmitter systems. Persons with manic–depressive disorder have alterations in platelet phosphatidyl inositol levels and responsiveness of neutrophil phosphoinositol accumulation.

Neuroendocrine Hypotheses

Typical neuroendocrine studies investigate peripheral or cerebrospinal fluid abnormalities of a particular system in persons with mood disorders and in controls and propose that either the neuroendocrine system itself or the neurotransmitter system that controls the hormone is in some way linked to the pathophysiology of the mood disorder of interest. Taken together, the literature does not identify particular endocrine findings as characteristic of manic–depressive disorder.

The thyroid axis may be of particular relevance to the pathophysiology of mood disorders since it serves not only as a dependent variable that is studied as a function of mood (as most neuroendocrine systems have been), but because the thyroid axis has also been studied as an independent variable of some impact. Several studies have shown that thyroid hormone administration may actually ameliorate mood disorders in certain paradigms. Further, in the rapid cycling variant of manic–depressive disorder, evidence indicates that supplementation with high doses of the thyroid hormone thyroxine (T_4) may induce remission in persons who are refractory to standard. The mechanism for these effects has been the subject of much speculation. Various models posit that the brain is functionally hypothyroid either due to changes in hormone synthesis, transport, or metabolism, or due to increased demand; alternatively, other models propose that the brain has an excess of a thyroid-related substance, which administration of exogenous thyroid hormone diminishes.

Cell Degeneration and Neuroprotective Effects of Medications

One of the most exciting areas of recent research focuses on the possibility that lithium and perhaps certain anticonvulsants such as valproate may actually exert a **neuroprotective** effect in manic–depressive disorder. Evidence indicates that these agents may protect nerve cells by stimulating production of protective proteins or by stimulating nerve growth. Interestingly, there is some clinical evidence from MRI that lithium treatment may actually increase total brain gray matter, although this will of course require replication. Thus, it is possible that cellular degeneration, albeit not as virulent as in Alzheimer's, may play a role in manic–depressive disorder.

Biological Rhythms

Two types of data indicate that biological rhythms may play a role in the pathogenesis of manic–depressive disorder. First, there are a large number of observational studies that have demonstrated seasonal peaks in the onset of affective episodes or hospitalizations for mood disorders. For manic–depressive disorder, the predominant seasons appear to be spring and fall, although other patterns may occur with some consistency across years. Seasonal affective disorder in which persons become depressed and remit at specific, regular times of year, has been codified in DSM-IV by applying the course modifier "seasonal pattern" to recurrent mood disorders. Although the relationship of seasonal affective disorder, particularly the winter depression variant, to manic–depressive disorder is not yet clear, there does appear to be some overlap. For instance, in most studies a large percentage of persons with seasonal affective disorder have manic–depressive disorder. In addition, the clinical picture of winter depression is similar to the hypersomnolent, anergic, hyperphagic depression common in manic–depressive disorder. Further, treatment with bright light has been shown to be efficacious in winter depression, and also appears to be an effective antidepressant in nonseasonal manic–depressives treated in the winter.

The second type of data which may provide a mechanism for seasonal patterns is that persons with manic–depressive disorder often exhibit abnormalities of circadian or daily rhythms. Many rhythmic parameters have been studied in persons with manic–depressive and other mood disorders, with various abnormalities found regarding the **amplitude** (height of the rhythm) and **phase** (timing of the rhythm). Among the most promising findings is that light sensitivity to suppression of the rhythmic hormone melatonin may be altered in persons with manic–depressive disorder and their relatives. Sleep has also been implicated in the pathogenesis of manic–depressive disorders. However, it should be noted that it is not clear whether it is the rhythmic aspects of sleep or its nonrhythmic, restorative components which are most relevant. One of the most striking findings in mania is the lack of need for sleep and there is evidence that sleep deprivation may be both antidepressant and promanic.

An autonomous pattern of affective episodes in manic–depressive disorder may develop from increasing sensitization of an individual to stressors. This process was proposed to be similar to kindling in animals and humans, in which subthreshold convulsant stimuli can decrease the threshold for seizures and eventually lead to spontaneous seizures. There are several attractive aspects to this hypothesis. It is supported by the increased frequency of episodes over the course of manic–depressive disorder, and the response of many persons with manic–depressive disorder to treatment with the anticonvulsants carbamazepine and valproate. However, the clinical data in support of this heuristically powerful conceptual paradigm are at this point quite limited. Thus it is not clear whether the increase in episode frequency sometimes seen is due to accumulating damage from prior episodes, or is simply the unfolding over time of what was destined from the beginning to be a malignant case of the illness.

Stress and Manic–Depressive Disorder

The possible association of stressful life events and the onset of depression has generated substantial interest among researchers from various theoretical backgrounds. Most of the literature regarding analysis of the relationship between stressful life events and manic–depressive disorder has focused on the precipitation of episodes in established manic–depressive disorder rather than the onset of the disorder *de novo*. There are several studies that demonstrate a relationship between stressful life events and the onset of affective episodes in already established manic–depressive disorder. However, several studies failed to find meaningful associations. It is likely that adverse life events are associated with mood episodes, particularly those episodes that are sufficiently severe to warrant hospitalization. In this respect such life events need to be attended to for clinical purposes. However, from a theoretical point of view it is not clear that such events actually play a pathogenic role.

Conclusions: The Biopsychosocial Approach

Numerous family genetic studies indicate that there is a hereditary biological component to manic–depressive disorder, yet the fact that only 40 to 70% of monozygotic twins are concordant for manic–depressive disorder indicates that genetics is not destiny. Most neurotransmitter systems and most neuroendocrine axes studied to date have shown some abnormalities in manic–depressive disorder, yet it is not clear to what degree these are individual in the pathogenesis of symptoms, and to what degree these findings reflect "downstream", or secondary changes. Each of the complex physiologic and psychosocial hypotheses are attractive heuristically, yet they have in most cases little supporting data and are notoriously difficult to test. Clinicians and educators of individuals and families who suffer with manic–depressive disorder are best advised to take a nonreductionistic and biopsychosocial view of this illness.

Assessment and Differential Diagnosis

Mood episodes are discrete periods of altered feeling, thought and behavior. Typically they have a distinct onset and offset, beginning over days or weeks and eventually ending gradually after several weeks or months. Manic–depressive disorder is defined by the occurrence of depressive plus manic, hypomanic, or mixed episodes, or the occurrence of only manic or mixed episodes. The diagnostic decision tree for manic–depressive disorder is given in Figure 47.1.

It is important to note that the phenomenologic differentiation between hypomania and mania is not as cut-and-dried. Of the three characteristics by which one is "promoted" from hypomania to mania, only the presence of psychosis is firmly grounded in the characteristics of the individual. The other two characteristics, marked social or occupational role impairment or hospitalization, clearly have components that are primarily external to the individual. If, for instance, one individual has relatively mild manic symptoms but is living with a family who is unable to tolerate the behavior, she/he is more likely to be hospitalized. Similarly, the comorbid presence of a severe disorder is more likely to result in hospitalization and a "promotion" from type II to type I disorder. Contrarily, limited insurance benefits, or a more tolerant family increase the probability that a manic syndrome of a given severity will be managed without hospitalization and thus be diagnosed as "hypomania" rather than "mania".

A "Bipolar" Disorder?

Classically, mania has been considered to be the opposite of depression: manic individuals were said to be cheery, optimistic and self-confident, hence the name bipolar disorder. However, in most descriptive studies, substantial proportions of hypomanic and manic patients actually exhibit substantial dysphoric symptoms. Mixed episodes, defined as the simultaneous occurrence of full-blown manic and depressive episodes, are the most prominent example of dysphoria during mania.

Additional Features: Psychosis and Rapid Cycling

Psychosis can occur in either pole of the disorder. If psychotic symptoms are limited to the major mood episode, the individual is considered to have manic–depressive disorder with psychotic features. On the other hand, if psychotic symptoms endure significantly into periods of normal mood, the diagnosis of schizoaffective disorder is made. For formal research diagnostic criteria and DSM definitions, 2 weeks of psychotic symptoms during normal mood is sufficient to convert a diagnosis of manic–depressive or major depressive disorder into schizoaffective disorder, because it is thought that such persons have a clinical course midway

---

DSM-IV-TR Criteria

Rapid-Cycling Specifier

Specify if:

With rapid cycling (can be applied to manic–depressive I disorder or manic–depressive II disorder). At least four episodes of a mood disturbance in the previous 12 months that meet criteria for a major depressive, manic, mixed, or hypomanic episode.

Note: Episodes are demarcated by either partial or full remission for at least 2 months or a switch to an episode of opposite polarity (e.g., major depressive episode to manic episode).

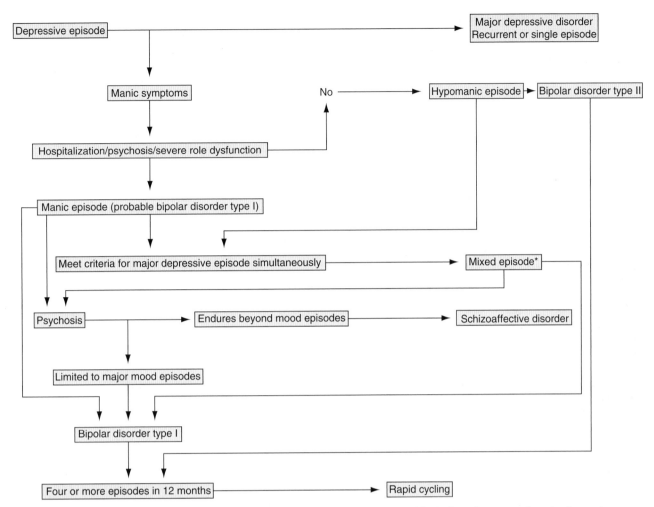

Figure 47.1 *Diagnostic decision tree for manic–depressive disorder. The building blocks for a diagnosis of manic-depressive disorder are individual episodes and their characteristics, as summarized in Table 47.1. This decision tree helps the psychiatrist through the steps that lead to diagnosis of manic-depressive disorder and identification of its subtypes. *Does not apply to hypomanic episode as per DSM-IV. (Source: Bauer M, Whybrow P, Gyulai L, et al. [1994a] Testing definitions of dysphoric mania and hypomania: Prevalence, clinical characteristics, and inter-episode stability. J Affect Disord 32, 201–211; McElroy S, Keck P, Pope H, et al. [1992] Clinical and research implications of the diagnosis of dysphoric or mixed mania or hypomania. Am J Psychiatr 149, 1633–1644.)*

between individuals with mood disorders or schizophrenia. However, this cutoff point is fairly arbitrary, and its validity is not well established. For example, it may be that psychotic symptoms actually represent a separate, comorbid disorder, or they may be integral features of severe manic–depressive disorder that simply take longer to resolve. Identification of pathophysiological and genetic bases of psychosis and of manic–depressive disorder will certainly help to resolve these issues.

Rapid cycling is defined by the occurrence of four or more mood episodes within 12 months. It should be noted that, despite the name, the episodes are not necessarily or even commonly truly cyclical; the diagnosis is based simply on episode counting. This subcategory is of significance because it predicts a relatively poorer outcome and worse response to lithium and other drugs. Although rapid cycling has been considered by some to be an "end stage" of the disorder, empirical evidence indicates that it may have its onset at any time during the disorder and may come and go during the course of illness. Several specific risk factors may be associated with rapid cycling, each of which may give clues to its pathophysiology. These include female gender, antidepressant use and prior or current hypothyroidism.

History, Physical Examination and Laboratory Studies

Although the diagnosis of manic–depressive disorder is made on the basis of phenomenology, there are several reasons to conduct a thorough medical history and physical examination. First, there are several general medical or substance-related causes of manic depression that, if treated, may lead to the resolution of the mood episode. Similarly, mania may be the first sign of a general medical illness that will be progressive and serious in its own right. Secondly, medical evaluation is necessary before starting medications used in the treatment of manic–depressive disorder. Finally, for many patients with psychiatric illnesses, particularly chronic or severe illnesses, their first contact with medical care as an adult is during the psychiatric interview, often under inpatient or even involuntary conditions. Because psychiatric illness is clearly not **protective** against medical illnesses, and since even common general medical illnesses may never have been screened for in the past, a thorough medical history and physical examination are necessary parts of the basic care of patients.

The overall approach to evaluating persons with manic–depressive disorder for medical problems may be generalized as follows: persons with psychiatric disorders, including manic–depressive disorder, should have regular screening for disease detection and health maintenance purposes as recommended for the general population. However, it should also be kept in mind that individuals with manic–depressive disorder, by virtue of having an often severe and disabling behavioral disorder, are less likely than the general population to have had adequate medical screening and treatment. Thus, special care must be made to ensure that health problems are not overlooked and that appropriate treatment or referral is effected. Unfortunately, it is the exception rather than the rule to have well-integrated medical and mental health systems so that the mental health provider can assume that some effort will need to be expended to ensure adequate care is delivered for individuals with manic–depressive disorder.

Which general medical illnesses may cause symptoms of manic–depressive disorder? Most medical illnesses that affect brain function have been described in case reports or small case series to cause one or another psychiatric syndrome. Several general medical illnesses have been associated with the development of manic–depressive disorder (Table 47.2) although none can be considered specific risk factors. Administration of medications has been observed frequently in clinical practice to be associated with the onset of mania, particularly in patients with preexisting depression. Such medications are listed in Table 47.3.

Some controversies have been hotly debated, particularly regarding the role of antidepressants in causing mania and rapid cycling. Of particular importance to psychiatric practice, all efficacious antidepressant treatments have been suspected to cause the induction of mania, with the exception of lithium and the possible exception of psychotherapy. This caveat for antidepressants also includes nonpharmacological antidepressants such as light and electroconvulsive therapy (ECT). The latter effect is paradoxical, as ECT is also used successfully to treat mania.

Age, Gender, and Cultural Issues in Diagnosis and Assessment

It is important to note that manic–depressive disorder is a worldwide problem and is among the top 10 of all diseases in terms of global burden worldwide, and fifth in terms of self-reported disability. There are no major differences in the manifestations of manic–depressive disorder across gender, age, or culture. However, women appear to be at higher risk for rapid cycling dysphoria during mania and comorbid disorders. Note, however, that affective psychoses may be relatively un-

Table 47.2	Medical Disorders Commonly Associated with Mania Neurologic Disorders Endocrine
Stroke	Hyperthyroidism (in those with preexisting manic–depressive disorder)
Head trauma	Postpartum status
Dementia	
Brain tumors	
Infection (including HIV)	
Multiple sclerosis	
Huntington's disease	

Table 47.3	Treatments and Drugs Commonly Associated with Mania	
Antidepressants		**Dopaminergic Agents**
Medications		Levodopa
Bright visible spectrum light treatment		
Electroconvulsant therapy		
Adrenergic Agents		**Drugs of Abuse**
Decongestants		Alcohol
Bronchodilators		Cocaine
Stimulants		Hallucinogens
		Amphetamines
		Caffeine
Other Agents		
Isoniazid		
Corticosteroids		
Anabolic steroids		
Disulfiram		

der-diagnosed and schizophrenia over-diagnosed, in African-Americans compared with Caucasians. Among children and adolescents, the diagnosis of manic–depressive disorder is often complicated by less consistent mood and behavior baseline than occur in adults. Little evidence is available regarding course and outcome in children. Available data indicate that, as with adults, mixed or cycling episodes predict more recurrences; unlike in adults, manic and mixed presentations may be associated with relatively shorter episodes compared with depressive presentations.

Epidemiology

Epidemiological Studies of Manic–Depressive Disorder

Estimates of the lifetime risk for manic–depressive I disorder from epidemiological studies have ranged from 0.2 to 0.9%. The Epidemiological Catchment Area (ECA) study found a lifetime prevalence rate of 1.2% for combined type I and type II variants. These rates are approximately tenfold greater than the prevalence rate for schizophrenia and about one-fifth that for major depressive disorder. Little is known regarding the prevalence of cyclothymic disorder. The National Comorbidity Survey Replication (NCD-R) found a considerably higher lifetime prevalence of bipolar I-II disorders of 3.9% (Kessler *et al.*, 2005). The lifetime prevalence for all mood disorders was 20.8%. Unlike major depressive disorder, manic–depressive disorder has an approximately equal gender distribution. Few consistent data are available regarding differences in prevalence across ethnic, cultural, or rural–urban settings. However, one of the more intriguing puzzles is the tendency of manic–depressive disorder to occur in higher socioeconomic strata than schizophrenia, which tends to aggregate in lower socioeconomic strata. Although many theories have been advanced to explain this phenomenon, no certain mechanism has been identified. However, several issues are clear. First, the finding is most likely not exclusively due to diagnostic bias (i.e., overdiagnosing persons of lower socioeconomic class with schizophrenia more frequently than manic–depressive disorder and the converse in persons of higher socioeconomic class). Secondly, the upward socioeconomic "drift" is not due to highly impaired patients "dragged" upward by higher functioning family members who are normal or who have adaptive subsyndromal manic–depressive spectrum characteristics; rather, patients themselves, at least those with type II disorder, are in many cases highly successful and occupy higher socioeconomic levels. Thirdly, the findings are not limited to the USA but have been replicated in European samples.

Of particular interest in regard to the epidemiology of manic–depressive disorder is that the incidence of manic–depressive disorder (and depressive disorders) appears to have increased since the 1940s. Reasons for this are not clear, although environmental factors, either physiological or psychosocial, may be responsible. For instance, exposure to increasingly severe social stressors, or the breakdown of cultural supports that may buffer stresses, may contribute; increases in exposure to putative environmental toxins might also be considered. In addition, in those families afflicted with manic–depressive disorder across generations, those in later generations tend to have earlier onset. This may be due to changes in genetic loading across generations or to environmental factors either within the family or in the wider environment. Regardless of the cause, the increasing incidence and earlier onset of manic–depressive disorder indicate that this illness is not likely to decrease in importance as a clinical and public health issue.

Comorbidity with Other Psychiatric Disorders

Alcohol and drug abuse and dependence represent the most consistently described and most clinically important psychiatric comorbidities with manic–depressive disorder. Whereas rates of alcohol abuse combined with alcohol dependence are from 3 to 13% in the general population, lifetime rates for alcohol dependence from ECA data indicate that they are greater than 30% in persons with manic–depressive I disorder (Regier et al., 1990). Further, ECA lifetime rates for drug dependence in individuals with manic–depressive I disorder are greater than 25% and rates for any substance abuse or dependence are above 60%. Comparable rates for alcohol, drug, or any substance abuse or dependence in major depressive disorder in ECA data are, respectively, 12%, 11% and 27%. Thus, manic–depressive disorder represents an enriched sample for substance use disorders, with substantially greater rates than for the general population or even those with unipolar depression. The reasons for the co-occurrence of manic–depressive disorder and substance dependence are not clear. In addition to self-medicating for depression, mania and intensifying the manic experience with stimulants, it is possible that some common genetic predisposition for mood instability is associated with both manic–depressive mood phenomenology and increased craving for substances, and the predominant phenotypic expression is then determined by other genetic or environmental factors. According to this hypothesis, some persons possessing the gene develop manic–depressive disorder, some develop substance dependence and some develop both. Regardless of the mechanism, comorbid substance dependence represents an important clinical challenge for clinicians treating persons with manic–depressive disorder.

Lifetime anxiety disorders have been described in as many as 44% of individuals with manic–depressive disorder. Other psychiatric comorbidities have been described in modest proportions of manic–depressive patients. Interestingly, data indicate that comorbidity may be higher in women with manic–depressive disorder than in men which may contribute to the tendency for the female gender to be associated with more complex forms of manic–depressive disorder such as rapid and dysphoric mania.

Clinical Outcome, Functional Outcome and Illness Costs

Clinical Outcome Studies

Manic–depressive disorder has its onset in most persons in adolescence and young adulthood, between the ages of 15 and 30. However, prepubertal mania and first-onset disease in the ninth decade of life are not unheard of. Once developed, multiple episodes are the rule. A review of the literature indicates that the majority of patients have four or more episodes in a lifetime. Among rapid-cycling patients, the basis for the diagnosis is four or more episodes in a year with an average of more than 50 lifetime episodes. There is no typical pattern to episode recurrence, with some patients having isolated manic, hypomanic, or depressive episodes, others switching from one pole to the other in linked episodes, and still others switching continually from one pole to the other in quasi-cyclical fashion. However, even among rapid-cycling patients, episodes are rarely periodic. Rather, the pattern is more accurately described by chaotic dynamics.

Episode length typically ranges from 4 to 13 months, with depressive episodes typically longer than manic or hypomanic episodes. Women appear to have more depressive relapses than manic ones, whereas men have a more even distribution. Also women predominate among rapid-cycling patients, representing 70 to 90% in most studies.

The early optimistic view of outcome, which derived primarily from experience in controlled clinical trials, contrasts with the overall guarded prognosis described by most longitudinal studies in the last three decades, which have been less controlled but more inclusive than formal clinical trials.

Table 47.4	**Classification Schemata for Manic–Depressive Disorder Treatment and Its Goals**

1. Acute versus maintenance
2. Somatic versus psychotherapeutic
3. The intensity-of-care continuum*
  A. Full hospitalization
  B. Partial or day hospitalization
  C. Night hospitalization of respite beds
  D. Ambulatory care
4. Categorization by goal
  A. Improve clinical outcome
  B. Improve functional outcome
  C. Improve host facors
    i. Illness management skills
    ii. Medical and psychiatric comorbidities

*Indications for increased intensity of care: danger to self or others; complicating medical or psychiatric comorbidities; aggressive medication titration; social factors that compromise treatment.

Approximately 20 to 40% of patients with manic–depressive disorder do not respond well to lithium, and that proportion may increase to as much as 80% for certain subgroups such as patients who experience rapid-cycling pattern (Dunner and Fieve, 1974; Maj *et al.*, 1989) or mixed manic and depressive episodes (Keller *et al.*, 1986). When assessed 1.5 years after index hospitalization, between 7 and 32% of manic–depressive patients remain chronically ill, depending on the polarity of index episode (Keller *et al.*, 1986). Only 26% of one sample had good outcome after hospitalization for mania, whereas 40% had moderate and 34% had poor outcome (Harrow *et al.*, 1990). The probability of remaining ill at 1, 2, 3 and 4 years after hospitalization for mania was, respectively, 51%, 44%, 33% and 28% (Tohen *et al.*, 1990). Sixty percent of an ambulatory sample of manic–depressive patients had fair to poor outcome based on a global outcome score after 1-year follow-up (O'Connell *et al.*, 1991).

Relatively little is known regarding clinical outcome in manic–depressive type II patients, although they appear to be at least as impaired in terms of relapse as manic–depressive type I patients. For instance, 70% of manic–depressive II patients followed up for 5 years experienced multiple relapses, whereas only 11% were episode free (Coryell *et al.*, 1989).

Subsyndromal affective symptoms may remain in up to 13 to 34% (Harrow *et al.*, 1990), and substantial interepisode morbidity may remain despite adequate treatment with lithium. It is not clear whether such interepisode pathology represents incompletely resolved major affective episodes, medication side effects, demoralization due to functional impairment, or a combination of these. It should be noted here that side effects are more than a trivial issue, as they may lead to medication discontinuation in 18 to 53%, a figure that is greater in lower socioeconomic classes.

Functional Outcome Studies

Substantial levels of functional impairment are also characteristic of manic–depressive disorder, even when major clinical indices have improved. Tohen and coworkers (1990) found 28% of subjects unemployed after index hospitalization for mania. Bauwens and associates (1991) found that levels of functional disability correlated both with number of prior episodes and with residual interepisode psychopathology. Five-year follow-up data from the NIMH Collaborative Program on the Psychobiology of Depression (Coryell *et al.*, 1989) provide evidence that levels of impairment in manic–depressive type I and type II disorders are similar. This included similarly fair to very poor work (in 30 and 42% of patients with types I and II, respectively), marital (30 and 23%), social (45 and 45%) and recreational (45 and 48%) function; sense of satisfaction or contentment (57 and 62%); and overall social adjustment (68 and 62%). More recent analysis of that data set has revealed enduring deficits in educational and occupational status at 5 years of follow-up in a mixed group of manic–depressive and unipolar patients, even in those who were recovered for 2 years (Coryell *et al.*, 1993). This led the authors to comment succinctly: "Follow-up studies have usually defined recovery as the absence of symptoms. The present findings show that this convention may result in an overly benign portrayal of outcome" (Coryell *et al.*, 1993, pp. 726).

Much less is known about which characteristics predict functional deficits in manic–depressive disorder, an issue of some importance in identifying high-risk groups for particular attention. A recent review (Bauer and Whybrow, 2001) indicates, surprisingly, that baseline demographic and functional outcome do not predict future functional outcome. However ongoing depressive symptoms, even to a mild degree, are strongly associated with ongoing functional deficits. The direction of causability is not clear, however. It is plausible that depressive symptoms render individuals less able to function in work and personal roles. It is equally plausible that unemployment, divorce, social isolation and the like can cause or exacerbate depressive symptoms. In fact, both are likely. In any event, careful attention to functional deficits, depressive symptoms and their interplay is important to optimizing care and hopefully outcome.

Personal and Societal Costs of Manic–Depressive Disorder

Although there are as yet few available data regarding direct and indirect illness costs for manic–depressive disorder, the direct treatment costs of manic–depressive disorder are substantial. Among the major mental disorders, the rate of hospitalization for manic–depressive disorder is exceeded only by that for schizophrenia. It is also clear that substantial loss of productivity, in addition to personal suffering, may occur in manic–depressive disorder. In mental illness in general, functional impairment was responsible for 55% of the costs of nonaddictive mental illness in the USA in 1986 (Rice *et al.*, 1990). It is striking that the functional impairment may be responsible for as much as 75% of the costs of affective illness. Specifically in manic–depressive disorder, evidence indicates that costs from lost productivity are substantial as well. For instance, 19% of persons with manic–depressive disorder attempt suicide at some time in their lives (Klerman *et al.*, 1992), thus placing almost one-fifth of persons with manic–depressive disorder at high risk of loss of life through this one cause alone. Without adequate treatment, a person with manic–depressive disorder from age 25 years can expect to lose 14 years of effective major activity (e.g., work, school, family role function) and 9 years of life. The indirect costs of this disorder are also high, because 15% of persons with manic–depressive disorder are unemployed for at least five consecutive years and more than 25% of those younger than age 65 years receive disability payments (Klerman, 1992). Therefore, it stands to reason that treatments targeted at reducing functional impairment, as well as clinical outcome, can have a substantial impact on the burden of mental illness costs to society and quality of life for the individual and her or his family.

Rating Scales

For clinical usage, clinicians rating scales in general use for depression can also be used for depressive episodes in manic–depressive disorder. Most share in the shortcoming of tending to underrate hypersomnia, hyperphagia and weight gain, "atypical" features that are common in manic–depressive disorder. Among mania scales, the Young Mania Rating Scale (Young *et al.*, 1978) is well validated on outpatients as well as inpatients, and for hypomanic as well as manic episodes. Self-report scales have the advantage of being brief (typically 5 minutes) and amenable to frequent, even daily, usage without undue burden. However, there have been questions about their reliability and validity, particularly in severely ill manic patients, although one instrument, the Internal State Scale (Bauer *et al.*, 1991) has demonstrated reasonable psychometric properties across several replications.

Treatment*

General Considerations

Traditionally, treatment for manic–depressive disorder has been categorized as acute versus prophylaxis, or maintenance; that is, treatment geared toward resolution of a specific episode versus continued treatment to prevent further symptoms. Treatment can also be considered along several other lines. In general, more structured treatment settings, such as full or partial hospitalization, are indicated if patients are likely to endanger self or others, if manic–depressive disorder is complicated by other medical or psychiatric illnesses that make ambulatory management particularly dangerous, or if more aggressive management is desired than is easily available on an ambulatory basis (e.g., intensive psychosocial intervention or rapid dosage titration of psychotropic agents). In addition, social factors play an important role in the decision to hospitalize in the real world of clinical psychiatry. Such reasons may include lack of social support to ensure medication compliance during acute illness, social stresses aggravating symptoms and making treatment compliance difficult (e.g., manipulative or hostile living situation), or lack of transportation to accommodate frequent ambulatory appointments during acute illness. Unfortunately, it is sometimes the case, although less frequent in this era of managed care, that a person's insurance plan covers inpatient but not ambulatory mental health treatment, forcing expensive inpatient care when less costly, time-limited, intensive ambulatory care would suffice.

Finally, treatment can be categorized according to its goals. Treatment can be focused on improving clinical outcome (episodes and symptoms) or functional outcome (social and occupational function and health-related quality of life). Although this categorization appears straightforward, clinical practice reveals many subtleties. For instance, it is erroneous to assume that clinical outcome is the domain of pharmacotherapy and that functional outcome is the domain of psychotherapy. In actuality, most psychotherapies by design focus on improving symptoms. Likewise, pharmacotherapeutic stabilization of symptoms clearly contributes to improved role function. Further, treatments that improve one domain may cause decrements in another. For instance, effective maintenance treatment with lithium may come at the cost of hand tremor, which interfere with work function and causes embarrassment in social situations. Compassionate psychoeducation and alliance building are integral goals of each form of treatment. In analogy to infectious disease treatment, attention to such host factors can often make the difference between success and failure of treatment.

The "Efficacy–Effectiveness Gap"

Great optimism justifiably accompanied the introduction of lithium in the 1960s, with the drug projected to save society millions of dollars in direct and indirect treatment costs. However, there are reasons to be concerned that lithium has made much less of an impact than originally projected, and there is clear evidence that manic–depressive disorder remains a major health concern, even with the addition of anticonvulsants to our armamentarium. For example, readmission rates for manic–depressive disorder may be as high as 90% during 2-year follow-up, with no difference between lithium-treated and nontreated patients (Markar and Mandar, 1989). Overall, the impact of lithium "under ordinary clinical conditions" appears to be much less than would be expected from results of randomized clinical trials.

How can these data be reconciled with early estimates projecting dramatic decreases in treatment costs due to the introduction of lithium? Presumably, the medications themselves do not differ between controlled clinical trials and general clinical practice. If anything, the diffusion over time of the new pharmacological technology into general clinical practice might be expected to lead to further gains in illness management beyond those initially seen. The use of several anticonvulsants such as carbamazepine, valproic acid and lamotrigine in the treatment of manic–depressive disorder holds promise for further improvement in outcome. For instance, these drugs may have **efficacy** in controlled clinical trials, but concerns regarding the **effectiveness** of lithium in clinical practice also apply to the use of these anticonvulsants.

What, then, are the sources of this **efficacy–effectiveness gap** in the treatment of manic–depressive disorder? It is likely that the gap is in part due to the exclusion of "complicated" manic–depressive patients from clinical trials (e.g., those with substance abuse, personality disorders, or medical problems, and those unwilling to risk exposure to placebo. Although such exclusions are appropriate for establishing the efficacy of potential treatments, the exclusivity of structured clinical trials limits their relevance in the general clinical setting. Another likely contributor to the efficacy–effectiveness gap is variation in provider attributes such as attitudes and capabilities. For instance, it is well established that even at academic medical centers, the intensity of medication treatment for mood disorders is much less than that which experts consider optimal. It is possible, then, that supporting providers with specific data regarding treatment options will aid in decreasing the efficacy–effectiveness gap. With this in mind, several organizations have developed clinical practice guideline to assist providers. Finally, the organization and orienttation of care giving systemes may not be optimally supportive.

Somatotherapy

Efficacious Agents for Various Phases of Manic–Depressive Disorder

Over the past 10 years medications have proliferated for the treatment of various phases of the disorder. The clinician must pick through an array of scientific data and marketing claims in order to choose the appropriate treatment. Two conceptual approaches help in this task. First, available scientific data can be reviewed and evaluated according to the techniques of "evidence-based medicine".

The second conceptual approach that we have found useful is to propose an explicit definition for the term "mood stabilizer" and evaluate the role of various medications against this definition. The US Food and Drug Administration (FDA) does not formally define the term, but it stands to reason that an agent would be optimally useful for treatment of manic–depressive disorder if it had efficacy in four roles: 1) treatment of acute manic symptoms; 2) treatment of acute depressive symptoms; 3) prophylaxis of manic symptoms; and 4) prophylaxis of depressive symptoms Table 47.5 summarizes the findings of this approach.

There are additional Class A controlled trials (nonplacebo-controlled) that support efficacy for multiple older, typical neuroleptics as well as the benzodiazepines, lorazepam and clonazepam.

In contrast to evidence regarding acute mania, evidence is scarce concerning efficacy of specific agents for acute

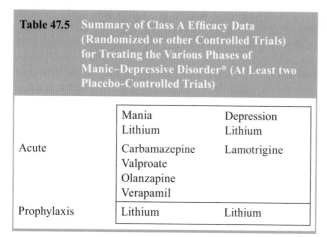

Table 47.5	Summary of Class A Efficacy Data (Randomized or other Controlled Trials) for Treating the Various Phases of Manic–Depressive Disorder* (At Least two Placebo-Controlled Trials)	
	Mania	Depression
Acute	Lithium	Lithium
	Carbamazepine	Lamotrigine
	Valproate	
	Olanzapine	
	Verapamil	
Prophylaxis	Lithium	Lithium

Source: Summarized from Bauer MS and McBride L (2002) *Structured Group Psychotherapy for Manic–depressive Disorder: The Life Goals Program*, 2nd edn. Springer-Verlag, New York.

depressive episodes. Most treatment is undertaken primarily by extension from treatment experience in unipolar depression. In reviewing studies of agents for the prophylaxis of manic or depressive symptoms, most studies report recurrence rates without distinguishing between manic and depressive symptoms. For instance, some studies reported such statistics as time-to-first-episode without specifying whether the first episode was manic or depressed. Other studies reported summary statistics for affective symptoms without separating manic or depressive symptoms. Far and away, the most placebo-controlled support for any prophylactic agent comes from studies of lithium including studies of relapse prevention for depression, with support from controlled trials that are not placebo-controlled for carbamazepine and lamotrigine. The one prophylaxis study of valproate (Bowden *et al.*, 2000) showed no difference from placebo (lithium was also found to be no different from placebo in this study, although the study was under-powered to make definitive conclusions about this comparison).

It may be surprising that, given the paucity of data on treatment of acute depression and prophylaxis of manic–depressive disorder, frequently many other medications are used chronically in this illness, sometimes as first-time agents, for instance, valproate or carbamazepine. Although neuroleptics have acute anti-manic evidence, despite the fact that there is little evidence for prophylactic efficacy, they are often used chronically. This is because these agents are typically started during the course of an acute manic episode and clinicians are reluctant to stop them and switch to a different agent such as lithium. In addition, many individuals have failed or have been intolerant of treatment with lithium and they are therefore treated using the "next best thing". This is not necessarily suboptimal treatment. However, it is important that the clinician recognize that data on long-term prophylactic efficacy is quite scanty for these agents, as it is for many other agents used in psychiatric practice.

Several additional issues in prophylaxis of manic–depressive disorder deserve comment. First, when is lifetime, or at least long-term, prophylaxis warranted? After one manic episode? One hypomanic episode? One depressive episode with a strong family history of manic–depressive disorder? There is insufficient empirical evidence with which to make strong recommendations. In clinical practice without clear guidelines, such decisions need to take into account the capability of the patient and family in

reporting symptoms, rapidity of onset of episodes, episode severity and associated morbidity. Clearly, the risks of a wait-and-see strategy would be different in a person who had a psychotic manic episode than in a person who had mild hypomania.

Secondly, can lithium ever be discontinued? Again, there are no solid data on which to base this decision. However, if lithium discontinuation is contemplated, there is evidence that rapid discontinuation (in less than 2 weeks) is more likely to result in relapse than slow taper (2–4 weeks), with relapse rates higher in type I than in type II patients. In type I patients, relapse rates for rapid discontinuation versus slow taper were, respectively, 96 and 73%, whereas in type II patients they were 91 and 33% (Faedda *et al.*, 1993).

Thirdly, a set sequence of treatment for refractory manic–depressive disorder has yet to be established. In particular, persons with rapid cycling represent a treatment dilemma. Although antidepressants may induce rapid cycling, they often leave the person in a protracted, severe depression. Switching from one antimanic agent to another often results in resumption of cycling. Complex treatment strategies may be required, such as anticonvulsants plus lithium, combinations of anticonvulsants, or adjuvant treatment with high doses of the thyroid hormone thyroxine.

A Simple Treatment Algorithm for Manic–Depressive Disorder

A treatment algorithm for refractory manic–depressive disorder, including strategies to deal with rapid cycling is found in Figure 47.2. It is derived from clinical practice guidelines from the US Veterans Administration and, by design, primarily specifies drug classes rather than individual agents. The entry point for this algorithm is the occurrence of any major mood episode (depression, hypomania, mania, or mixed episode) in an unmedicated patient. Patients with recurrence on medications may enter the algorithm at the appropriate point along the flow diagram. For simplicity of presentation, only depressive and cycling outcomes are illustrated. This is because depressive episodes are more common than manic or hypomanic episodes, and all but the most refractory of the latter episodes are relatively easily treated by the addition (or resumption) of lithium or anticonvulsants or the use of neuroleptics, as summarized above.

Balancing Beneficial and Unwanted Effects of Medications

All psychotropic medications have side effects. Some are actually desirable (e.g., sedation with some antidepressants in persons with prominent insomnia), and specific medications are often chosen on the basis of desired side effects. However, side effects usually represent factors that decrease a patient's quality of life and compromise compliance. Reviews of side effects of antidepressants and neuroleptics can be found in the chapters on depression and schizophrenia, respectively. It should be recalled in regard to antidepressants, however, that all can cause rapid cycling and mixed states in persons with manic–depressive disorder. These effects are not uncommonly encountered in clinical practice and should be watched for, even in persons taking mood-stabilizing agents.

A brief overview of the most frequent or important side effects of lithium, carbamazepine and valproic acid can be found in Table 47.6a–c. Note that some side effects may be encountered at any serum level of the drug, even within the therapeutic range. Some side effects may be dose-related even within that range and

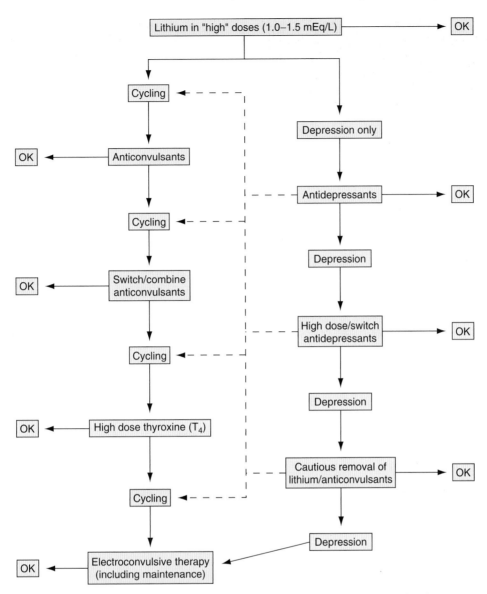

Figure 47.2 *Treatment algorithm for manic–depressive disorder. (Source: Reprinted by permission of Taylor & Francis, from Bauer MS [1994] Rapid cycling, in Anticonvulsants in Mood Disorders [eds], Joffe RT and Calabrese JR. Marcel Dekker, New York, pp. 1–26.) Note: Refractory mania is relatively rare. This general algorithm addresses the more common clinical scenarios of depression and rapid cycling. *For a complete discussion of this topic, see Bauer and McBride (2002); of how to use various psychopharmacologic agents, see Bauer (2003).*

Table 47.6a	Side Effects of Lithium and Commonly Used Anticonvulsants, I: Life-threatening		
	At Therapeutic Levels		At Toxic Levels
	Idiopathic	**Dose-Related**	**Dose-Related**
Lithium			Renal failure
			Encephalopathy
CBZ	Agranulocytosis*		
	Aplastic anemia*		
	Stevens–Johnson*		
VPA	Hepatic necrosis	Thrombocytopenia	Thrombocytopenia
LMT	Stevens–Johnson*		

*Typically during first 1–6 months of treatment.

Table 47.6b	Side Effects of Lithium and Commonly Used Anticonvulsants, II: Clinically Significant Side Effects			
	Lithium	CBZ	VPA	LMT
Neurologic/muscular	Lethargy Memory (anomia) Tremor* Myoclonus	Lethargy Blurred vision Ataxia*	Lethargy Depression Tremor* Ataxia	Lethargy Ataxia Blurred vision Headache
Endocrine/metabolic	Weight gain* Hypothyroidism		Weight gain*	
Cardiopulmonary				
Hematologic			Thrombocytopenia	
Renal	Polyuria			
Hepatic		Jaundice	Jaundice	
Gastrointestinal	Nausea* Diarrhea*	Nausea*	Nausea*	Nausea*
Dermatologic	Maculopapular rash Psoriasis Acne	Maculopapular rash Alopecia	Maculopapular rash	Maculopapular rash
Other			Back pain	

*Most common reasons in our experience for noncompliance.

Table 47.6c	Side Effects of Lithium and Commonly Used Anticonvulsants, III: Subclinical Laboratory Abnormalities			
	Lithium	CBZ	VPA	LMT
Neurologic/muscular				
Endocrine/metabolic	Increased TSH	Decreased FTI		
Cardio-pulmonary	EKG T-wave depression			
Hematologic	Leukocytosis (to 20 000)	Leukopenia	Thrombocytopenia (OK > 20 000)	
Renal	Decreased urine specific gravity, GFR			
Hepatic		Increased LFTs	Increased LFTs	

may respond to dosage reduction. Others are more idiosyncratic and may need other management, as detailed in a subsequent section. Note that not all laboratory findings represent pathological processes that are associated with or presage morbidity for the patient; that is, not all are clinically significant.

Note also that the concept of the "therapeutic level" is not straightforward. The lower limit is usually established by the lowest level necessary for therapeutic effect, whereas the upper limit is set by the lowest level associated with regular, significant toxicity. This range is never established with complete precision. For some medications such as lithium, the therapeutic window is actually quite narrow, with toxic effects developing with some regularity after the upper limit of the therapeutic range is surpassed and with serious toxicity developing at only modestly higher serum levels. As a further complication, for many persons the minimum level of lithium for good response may be substantially above the 0.5 to 0.8 mEq/L that is usually set as the lower therapeutic limit, but this is reached only at the cost of increased incidence of side effects. On the other hand, experience with valproic acid, the upper limit of the therapeutic range for mood stabilization may actually be 125 mg/dL rather than the listed range of 100 mg/dL usually accepted for antiepileptic effect, and this level may be reached without undue side effects. Thus, established therapeutic levels should be used as important guidelines, and therapeutic levels should only be exceeded with careful monitoring. However, one must not be falsely reassured that reaching the lower level of a therapeutic range is equally effective for all patients, while taking with a grain of salt the upper limits of the therapeutic range in drugs with a wider therapeutic window.

Another important issue to consider is drug–drug interactions, which may lead to side effects. Such interactions are often associated with increases in serum levels of the drug of interest. For example, addition of thiazide diuretics, or nonsteroidal antiinflammatory agents, the latter available over the counter, is a common reason for increase in lithium level and development of toxicity. However, at other times the drug–drug interactions may not be reflected in an increased serum level if the main interaction is displacement of protein-bound drug. Because free drug concentrations are usually 1 to 10% of total serum drug, a displacement of even 50% of bound drug may be associated with negligible if any changes in total serum level. However, since both therapeutic and toxic effects are due to free, not bound, drug, unwanted side effects may develop despite total drug levels measured in the therapeutic range.

Guiding Principles of Managing Side Effects

Although some side effects may be desirable, in many cases they are impediments to treatment, frequently of sufficient importance to lead to noncompliance. Clinicians might reframe the noncompliance issue more appropriately as "insufficient provider–patient cost–benefit analysis". Stressing compliance when a person suffers from significant side effects is usually much less effective than working to set appropriate expectations of the patient and to find a regimen of minimal toxicity. Managing side effects is as much psychotherapeutic as medical.

There are several strategies available to improve patients' tolerance of medications. First, dose reduction may be achieved without compromising efficacy in some patients. Some side effects, such as lithium-induced nausea, usually respond well to this, whereas others, such as lithium-induced memory loss, improve less reliably. Secondly, simple changes in preparation may be helpful, such as using enteric-coated lithium. Uncoated valproic acid causes nausea so frequently that only the coated forms are routinely used; however, the pediatric "sprinkle" preparation may be of some benefit in persons with nausea even with enteric-coated valproic acid. Thirdly, changing the administration schedule may ameliorate side effects. Commonsense strategies such as taking nausea-inducing medications after a meal should not be overlooked. Single daily dosing of lithium, carbamazepine, or valproic acid may decrease daytime sedation without compromising efficacy. For more obscure reasons, single daily dosing of lithium appears to decrease polyuria quite effectively.

Fourthly, addition of medications to counteract side effects can sometimes be the only way to continue treatment. Addition of beta-blockers can reduce lithium- or valproic acid-induced tremors. Judicious use of thiazide diuretics, often in conjunction with potassium-sparing diuretics or potassium supplements, can reduce lithium-induced polyuria. Finally, change to another drug may be the only alternative. This is clearly indicated in the case of serious allergic reactions. Polypharmacy should be avoided wherever possible.

Psychotherapies

It is important to note that psychotherapy has been studied almost exclusively in the context of ongoing medication management, rather than as a substitute for, or alternative to, medication treatment. Rather, psychotherapy has been utilized as an adjuvant treatment to optimize outcome in the illness. Psychotherapy has been viewed as having one or more of several roles in the management of the disorder.

Recall that both somatic therapies and psychotherapies to date have been predominantly oriented toward improving clinical outcome. Under this conceptualization psychotherapy has been thought directly to address symptoms, such as cognitive therapy for depressive symptoms. Less frequently has psychotherapy been developed with an explicit component geared toward addressing the functional deficits in manic–depressive disorder. However, functional outcome has often been measured in formal trials of various types of psychotherapy. A third conceptualization has been to use psychotherapy as a predominantly educative method to assist patients in participating more effectively in treatment. In this latter regard, treatment is geared toward improving "host factors", that is, those factors not directly due to the disease but that have an impact on its course or treatment, through education, support and problem solving. Such host factors include illness management skills, which may be improved through psychoeducation and attention to building the therapeutic alliance. Basics of education are summarized in Table 47.7.

An evidence-based review similar to that for somatotherapy has recently been carried out for psychotherapeutic interventions. Bauer and McBride (2002) identified five main types of psychotherapy that have been studied in manic–depressive disorder: couples–partners, group interpersonal or psychoeducative, cognitive–behavioral, family, and interpersonal and social-rhythms. Couples–partners, cognitive–behavioral and family methods all have some Class A data supporting a role in improving clinical outcome or functional outcome or the intermediate outcome variable of improving illness management skills. An additional finding in this review is the degree of convergent validity across interventions regarding agenda for disease management information and skills to be imparted. Specifically, imparting education, focusing on early warning symptoms and triggers of episodes, and developing detailed and patient-specific action plans are found across most of the other interventions as well. For instance, this core agenda is also an important part of such diverse approaches as the cognitive–behavioral interventions of Palmer and Williams (1995) and Lam and coworkers (2000); the psychoeducational interventions of Bauer and coworkers (1998), Perry and coworkers (1999) and Weiss and coworkers (2000); the interpersonal and social rhythms therapy (IPSRT) intervention of Frank and coworkers (1999); and the family intervention of Miklowitz and coworkers (1999). Thus, given the positive results most of these interventions with explicit disease management components (i.e., patient education, collaborative management strategies with the patient, inclusion of as wide a social support system as is available) have produced, it is likely that this basic approach will be critical. It will perhaps be more critical even than the specific type of intervention in which these disease management components are embedded.

Special Features Influencing Treatment

Treatment of Comorbid Disorders

As noted earlier, several reversible "organic" factors may cause mood episodes, either *de novo* or in the course of already established manic–depressive disorder. For instance, removal of pro-manic drugs, both illicit and prescribed, is advisable in the treatment of substance-induced manic episodes. Treatment of

Table 47.7   Basics of Education to Improve Disease Management Skill 1.

1. Principles

A. Gear education to educational, cultural, motivational factors of individuals and their families.

B. Include both knowledge about the disorder in general and exploration of the individual's specific form of illness and how it affects their own life.

C. Pay close attention to opportunities for destigmatization and demystification.

D. Emphasize the role of the person in treatment and his/her family as comanagers of the illness, including judging costs and benefits of specific treatment options according to the individual's priorities

2. Components of Psychoeducation

A. The disorder

  a. Biological basis

    i. Genetic factors (especially for persons of childbearing age)

    ii. Possible brain mechanisms

  b. Environmental components

    i. Psychosocial factors

    ii. Physical environmental factors

  c. Course and outcome

    i. Prevalence

    ii. Episode types and patterns

    iii. Potential triggers for episodes

    iv. Comorbidities and complications

B. Treatment

  a. Somatic therapies: somatic and psychosocial

    i. Goals

    ii. Side effect recognition and management

    iii. Costs and benefits of individual treatment options

  b. Coping skills

    i. Recognition of early warning signs of relapse

    ii. Avoidance/management of triggers for episodes

    iii. Activation of adaptive coping behaviors and avoidance of maladaptive responses

general medical conditions, such as hypothyroidism, that may complicate course or treatment is also important.

Several conceptual approaches, not always explicit, underlie the choice of approach to managing comorbid disorders. Psychiatrists may assume that the comorbid disorder is caused by manic–depressive disorder and consequently that treatment of the manic–depressive disorder will lead to resolution of the comorbidity. For instance, panic attacks might be considered a consequence of mood episodes, or alcohol use a means of self-medication of depressive symptoms or a function of increased appetitive drive due to mania. On the other hand, psychiatrists may assume that the mood instability of manic–depressive disorder is due to the comorbid illness. For instance, mood episodes may be thought to be due to alcohol or drug intoxication or withdrawal or to intrapsychic or psychophysiological effects of prior trauma. There are few data available to support either approach. Even the temporal sequence of onsets (e.g., manic–depressive disorder preceding substance abuse or vice versa) provides little information and in fact may be misleading in planning treatment.

The literature on alcohol dependence comorbidity, which is perhaps the most extensively studied of the comorbidities, provides no data with which to plan treatment strategy.

It stands to reason, however, that some type of **parallel** (simultaneous) treatment is preferable to **sequential** treatment (treating one disorder until resolution and then attending to the other), as the prognosis of manic–depressive disorder is worse when complicated by substance use and the course of alcoholism is worse when complicated by mood disorders. It is also likely that the highly confrontative approaches of some traditional substance dependence treatment programs will not likely serve the needs of often highly impaired depressed or manic persons.

Treatment of Manic–Depressive Disorder Across the Life-cycle

Although the somatotherapeutic and psychotherapeutic mainstays of treatment endure across the life-cycle, several phases of life present particular challenges. There is mounting data on treatment of manic–depressive disorder in childhood. Treatments are chosen by extension from the adult literature, with the one caveat that there have been rare cases of liver failure in conjunction with valproic acid use in children younger than 10 years of age who have been exposed to multiple anticonvulsants (Dreifuss, 1989).

In pregnancy, there is some early evidence that lithium may be teratogenic, associated with increased rates of cardiac abnormalities although more recent data indicate that this risk may be overestimated. Valproic acid and perhaps have been associated with neural tube defects leaving the neuroleptics, antidepressants and ECT as the preferable management strategies during pregnancy, particularly during the first trimester. It should be kept in mind, however, that treatment decisions are based on **risk**, not **certainty**. Risk of fetal malformation, parental attitude toward raising children with birth defects, severity of illness and ease of management with alternative therapies all need to be considered in conjunction with the woman and her partner.

Aging also presents certain treatment concerns. Tricyclic antidepressants may be associated with clinically significant cardiac conduction abnormalities, hypotension, sedation, glaucoma and urinary retention, particularly in the presence of prostatic hypertrophy. These are of even greater concern in the elderly. The risk of sedation due to neuroleptics and benzodiazepines and of hypotension due to low-potency neuroleptics can also particularly complicate treatment of elderly persons with manic–depressive disorder. Such side effects can cause far-reaching and serious complications, such as hip fracture which is not infrequently the initial event in a cascade of complications that can be terminal.

By contrast, lithium, carbamazepine and valproic acid are relatively well tolerated in the elderly once attention is given to the slower clearance of drugs in general in this population group. The risk of clinically significant renal toxicity with appropriately dosed lithium is not great. Although glomerular filtration rate decreases with age in persons treated with lithium, the rate of decline does not appear to be accelerated by lithium treatment. Nonetheless, careful monitoring of renal function is needed in the elderly. In addition, increasing age is clearly a risk factor for hypothyroidism as is lithium use. Thus, elderly persons taking lithium should be followed up carefully for decrements in thyroid function, although hypothyroidism is not an indication for lithium discontinuation but rather simply for thyroid hormone supplementation.

Comparison of DSM-IV/ICD-10 Diagnostic Criteria

The ICD-10 item set for a manic episode contains nine items in contrast to the seven items in the DSM-IV-TR criteria set, the two additional items being marked sexual energy or indiscretions and loss of normal social inhibitions. However, the number of items required by ICD-10 Diagnostic Criteria for Research remains the same as the number in DSM-IV-TR (i.e., three items if mood is euphoric, four items if mood is irritable) which is likely to result in a more inclusive diagnosis of a manic episode in ICD-10. Furthermore, the duration of mixed episodes differ, with DSM-IV-TR requiring a duration of 1 week (as is the case for a manic episode), whereas the ICD-10 Diagnostic Criteria for Research require a duration of at least 2 weeks.

The criteria sets for hypomanic episode differ as well. The ICD-10 Diagnostic Criteria for Research contain several additional items (increased sexual energy and increased sociability) and does not include the DSM-IV-TR items inflated self-esteem and flight of ideas. Furthermore, ICD-10 does not require that the change in mood be observed by others.

Regarding the definition of bipolar I disorder, in addition to differences in the diagnostic criteria for a manic and major depressive episode, the ICD-10 definition of "Bipolar Affective Disorder" (i.e., any combination of hypomanic, manic, mixed and depressive episodes) does not distinguish between bipolar I and bipolar II disorder (i.e., cases of DSM-IV-TR Bipolar II Disorder are diagnosed as Bipolar Affective Disorder in ICD-10). However, ICD-10 Diagnostic Criteria for Research does include diagnostic criteria for bipolar II in its appendix that is identical to the criteria set in DSM-IV-TR.

For cyclothymic disorder, the ICD-10 Diagnostic Criteria for Research provides list of symptoms that must be associated with the periods of depressed mood and hypomania which differ from the ICD-10 item sets for dysthymic disorder and hypomania. In contrast, the DSM-IV-TR definition of cyclothymic disorder.

References

American Psychiatric Association (2000) *Diagnostic and Statistical Manual of Mental Disorders*, 4th edn. Rev. APA, Washington DC.

Bauer MS (1994) Rapid cycling, in *Anticonvulsants in Mood Disorders* (eds Joffe RT and Calabrese JR). Marcel Dekker, New York, pp. 1–26.

Bauer MS (2003) *Field Guide to Psychiatic Assessment and Treatment*. Lippincott, Williams & Wilkins, Philadelphia.

Bauer M and Whybrow PC (2001) Thyroid hormone, neural tissue, and mood modulation. *World J Biol Psychiatr* 2, 59–69.

Bauer MS and McBride L (2002) *Structured Group Psychotherapy for Manic–depressive Disorder: The Life Goals Program*, 2nd edn. Springer-Verlag, New York.

Bauer MS, Crits-Christoph P, Ball W *et al.* (1991) Independent assessment of manic and depressive symptoms by self-rating scale: Characteristics and implications for the study of mania. *Arch Gen Psychiatr* 48, 807–812.

Bauer M, Whybrow P, Gyulai L *et al.* (1994) Testing definitions of dysphoric mania and hypomania: Prevalence, clinical characteristics, and inter-episode stability. *J Affect Disord* 32, 201–211.

Bauer MS, McBride L, Chase C *et al.* (1998) Manual-based group psychotherapy for bipolar disorder: A feasibility study. *J Clin Psychiatr* 59, 449–455.

Bauwens F, Tracy A, Pardoen D *et al.* (1991) Social adjustment of remitted bipolar and unipolar out-patients. A comparison with age- and sex-matched controls. *Br J Psychiatr* 151, 239–244.

Bowden CL, Calabrese JR, McElroy SL *et al.* (2000) A randomized, placebo-controlled 12 month trial of divalproex and lithium in treatment of outpatients with bipolar I disorder. *Arch Gen Psychiatr* 57, 481–489.

Coryell W, Keller M, Endicott J *et al.* (1989) Bipolar II illness: Course and outcome over a five-year period. *Psychol Med* 19, 129–141.

Coryell W, Scheftner W, Keller M *et al.* (1993) The enduring psychosocial consequences of mania and depression. *Am J Psychiatr* 150, 720–727.

Dreifuss FE (1989) Valproate toxicity, in *Antiepileptic Drugs*, 3rd edn (eds Levy R, Mattson RH, Meldrum B *et al.*). Raven Press, New York, pp. 643–651.

Dunner DL and Fieve RR (1974) Clinical factors in lithium prophylaxis failure. *Arch Gen Psychiatr* 30, 229–233.

Faedda GL, Tondo L, Baldessarni RJ *et al.* (1993) Outcome after rapid vs gradual discontinuation of lithium treatment in bipolar disorders. *Arch Gen Psychiatr* 50, 448–455.

Frank E, Swartz H, Mallinger AG *et al.* (1999) Adjunctive psychotherapy for bipolar disorder: Effects of changing treatment modality. *J Abnorm Psychol* 108, 579–587.

Harrow M, Goldberg J, Grossman L *et al.* (1990) Outcome in manic disorders. A naturalistic follow-up study. *Arch Gen Psychiatr* 47, 665–671.

Keller M, Lavori P, Coryell W *et al.* (1986) Differential outcome of episodes of illness in bipolar patients: Pure manic, mixed/cycling, and pure depressive. *JAMA* 255, 3138–3142.

Kessler RC, Berglund MBA, Demler O *et al.* (2005) Lifetime prevalence and age-of-onset distributions of DSM-IV disorders in the National COmorbidity Survey Replication. *Arch Gen Psychiat* 62, 593–602.

Klerman G, Olfson M, Leon A *et al.* (1992) Measuring the need for mental health care. *Health Affairs* 11, 23–33. (Statistics from prepublication draft from Dr. A. Leon).

Lam DH, Bright J, Jones S *et al.* (2000) Cognitive therapy for bipolar illness – a pilot study of relapse prevention. *Cogn Ther Res* 24, 503–520.

Maj M, Pitrozzi R and Starace F (1989) Previous pattern of course of the illness as a predictor of a response to lithium prophylaxis in bipolar illness. *J Affect Disord* 17, 237–241.

Markar H and Mander A (1989) Efficacy of lithium prophylaxis in clinical practice. *Br J Psychiatr* 155, 496–500.

McElroy S, Keck P, Pope H *et al.* (1992) Clinical and research implications of the diagnosis of dysphoric or mixed mania or hypomania. *Am J Psychiatr* 149, 1633–1644.

Miklowitz DJ, Simoneau TL, George EL *et al.* (1999) Family-focused treatment of bipolar disorder: 1-year effects of a psychoeducational program in conjunction with pharmacotherapy. *Biol Psychiatr* 48, 582–592.

Mundo E, Walker M, Cate T *et al.* (2001) The role of serotonin transporter protein gene in antidepressant-induced mania in bipolar disorder: Preliminary findings. *Arch Gen Psychiatr* 58(6), 539–544.

O'Connell R, Mayo J, Flatow L *et al.* (1991) Outcome of bipolar disorder on long-term treatment with lithium. *Br J Psychiatr* 159, 123–129.

Palmer AG and Williams H (1995) CBT in a group format for bipolar affective disorder. *Behav Cogn Psychother* 23, 153–168.

Perry A, Tarrier N, Morriss R *et al.* (1999) Randomised controlled trial of efficacy of teaching patients with bipolar disorder to identify early symptoms of relapse and obtain treatment. *Br Med J* 318, 149–153.

Regier D, Farmer M, Rae D *et al.* (1990) Comorbidity of mental disorders with alcohol and other drugs. Results from the Epidemiological Catchment Area (ECA) Study. *JAMA* 264, 2511–2518.

Rice D, Kelman S, Miller L *et al.* (1990) *The Economic Costs of Alcohol and Drug Abuse and Mental Illness: 1985.* National Institute of Mental Health, DHHS publication (ADM) 90-1694, Rockville, MD.

Tohen M, Waternaux C and Tsuang M (1990) Outcome in mania: A 4-year prospective follow-up of 75 patients utilizing survival analysis. *Arch Gen Psychiatr* 47, 1106–1111.

Weiss RD, Griffin ML, Greenfield SF *et al.* (2000) Group therapy for patients with bipolar disorder and substance dependence: Results of a pilot study. *J Clin Psychiatr* 61, 361–367.

Young RC, Biggs JT, Ziegler VE *et al.* (1978) A rating scale for mania: Reliability, validity, and sensitivity. *Br J Psychiatr* 133, 429–435.

48 Mood Disorders: Premenstrual Dysphoric Disorder

Definition

Premenstrual syndrome (PMS) is a combination of emotional, behavioral and physical symptoms that occur in the premenstrual or luteal phase of the menstrual cycle. The term "premenstrual tension" appeared in the medical literature 70 years ago but widely accepted diagnostic criteria for PMS do not exist. Approximately 80% of women report at least mild premenstrual symptoms, 20 to 50% report moderate to severe premenstrual symptoms, and approximately 5% of women report severe symptoms for several days with impairment of role and social functioning. The 5% of women with the severest form of PMS generally have symptoms that meet the diagnostic criteria for premenstrual dysphoric disorder (PMDD).

The diagnostic criteria for PMDD are listed in the appendix of DSM-IV (American Psychiatric Association, 1994). A clinician can indicate that a woman has symptoms that meet the diagnostic criteria for PMDD by using the DSM-IV diagnosis 311, depressive disorder not otherwise specified. To meet the PMDD criteria, at least five out of 11 possible symptoms must be present in the premenstrual phase; these symptoms should be absent shortly following the onset of menses; and at least one of the five symptoms must be depressed mood, anxiety, lability, or irritability. The PMDD criteria require that role functioning be impaired as a result of the premenstrual symptoms. The functional impairment reported by women with PMDD is similar in severity to the impairment reported in major depressive disorder and dysthymic disorder (Pearlstein et al., 2000). Unlike the functional impairment reported in depressive disorders, women with severe PMS and PMDD report more disruption in their relationships and parenting roles than in their work roles.

The PMDD criteria require that a woman prospectively rate her emotional, behavioral and physical symptoms over two menstrual cycles to confirm the diagnosis. Charting two menstrual cycles is advantageous, since some women have variability of symptom severity from cycle to cycle due to factors such as seasonal worsening, or a woman might have the unusual presence of follicular phase psychological symptoms due to a transient stressor. Recent studies tend to utilize visual analog scales, or Likert scale daily rating forms such as the Daily Record of Severity of Problems (Endicott and Harrison, 1990), with a scoring method that compares the average of symptom scores during the premenstrual days to the average of symptom scores postmenses.

A woman presenting with PMS should ideally bring to her clinician two cycles of an established daily rating form, or alternatively ratings of her most problematic symptoms, rated with anchor points ranging from "not present" to "severe". The clinician should review the daily ratings to confirm that the symptoms are in fact confined largely to the premenstrual phase, with the relative absence of symptoms in the follicular phase, and the clinician should also assess premenstrual functional impairment (Figure 48.1). Ratings that demonstrate follicular symptoms with increased symptom severity in the premenstrual phase suggest "premenstrual exacerbation" of an underlying disorder rather than PMDD. The DSM-IV-TR PMDD criteria state

DSM-IV-TR Criteria

Diagnostic Criteria for PMDD

Research Criteria for Premenstrual Dysphoric Disorder

A. In most menstrual cycles during the past year, five (or more) of the following symptoms were present for most of the time during the last week of the luteal phase, began to remit within a few days after the onset of the follicular phase, and were absent in the week postmenses, with at least one of the symptoms being either (1), (2), (3), or (4):
   (1) markedly depressed mood, feelings of hopelessness, or self-deprecating thoughts
   (2) marked anxiety, tension, feelings of being "keyed up," or "on edge"
   (3) marked affective lability (e.g., feeling suddenly sad or tearful or increased sensitivity to rejection)
   (4) persistent and marked anger or irritability or increased interpersonal conflicts
   (5) decreased interest in usual activities (e.g., work, school, friends, hobbies)
   (6) subjective sense of difficulty in concentrating
   (7) lethargy, easy fatigability, or marked lack of energy
   (8) marked change in appetite, overeating, or specific food cravings
   (9) hypersomnia or insomnia
   (10) a subjective sense of being overwhelmed or out of control
   (11) other physical symptoms, such as breast tenderness or swelling, headaches, joint or muscle pain, a sensation of "bloating," weight gain

Essentials of Psychiatry Jerald Kay and Allan Tasman
© 2006 John Wiley & Sons, Ltd.

B. The disturbance markedly interferes with work or school or with usual social activities and relationships (e.g., avoidance of social activities, decreased productivity and efficiency at work or school).

C. The disturbance is not merely an exacerbation of the symptoms of another disorder such as major depressive disorder, panic disorder, dysthymic disorder, or a personality disorder (although it may be superimposed on any of these disorders).

D. Criteria A, B, and C must be confirmed by prospective daily ratings during at least two consecutive symptomatic cycles. (The diagnosis may be made provisionally prior to this confirmation).

Reprinted with permission from the *Diagnostic and Statistical Manual of Mental Disorders*, Fourth Edition, Text Revision. Copyright 2000 American Psychiatric Association.

that the premenstrual symptoms should not be an exacerbation of an underlying disorder, but that PMDD could be superimposed on another disorder, like panic disorder. No formal guidelines exist for how to apply this criterion clinically.

Differential Diagnosis

Depression and anxiety disorders are the most common Axis I psychiatric disorders that may be concurrent and exacerbated premenstrually, with less clear evidence for bipolar disorder, eating disorders and substance abuse. Since most PMDD symptoms are affective or anxiety-related, "pure PMS" or PMDD is generally not diagnosed when an underlying depression or anxiety disorder is present; these women would be considered to have premenstrual exacerbation of their underlying depression or anxiety disorder. Personality disorders are not elevated in prevalence in women with PMDD, but women with PMDD and a personality disorder may demonstrate premenstrual phase amplification of personality dysfunction. Schizophrenia may be an example of a disorder that does not have premenstrual exacerbation of psychotic symptoms but may have the superimposition of affective and anxiety symptoms of PMDD. The prevalence of premenstrually exacerbated disorders is unknown, but women with these conditions present frequently to their primary care clinician or gynecologist. Since most recent treatment studies have been conducted on women with PMS and PMDD without follicular symptomatology, this literature is not particularly informative on how to treat women with premenstrually exacerbated disorders. The general guideline is to treat the underlying disorder first and see if subsequent daily ratings suggest persistence of premenstrual symptoms that might meet criteria for PMDD.

Several medical conditions should also be considered when evaluating a woman with premenstrual complaints. Symptoms of endometriosis, polycystic ovary disease, thyroid disorders, disorders of the adrenal system, hyperprolactinemia and panhypopituitarism may mimic symptoms of PMS. Several medical disorders may demonstrate a premenstrual increase in

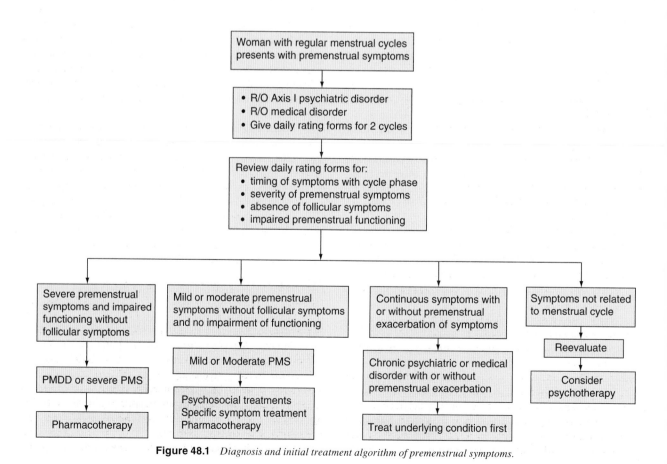

Figure 48.1 *Diagnosis and initial treatment algorithm of premenstrual symptoms.*

symptoms without accompanying emotional symptoms, such as migraines, asthma, epilepsy, irritable bowel syndrome, diabetes, allergies and autoimmune disorders. It is presumed that the menstrual cycle fluctuations of gonadal hormones influence some of the symptoms of these medical conditions.

Epidemiology

Irritability has been identified as the most common premenstrual symptom in USA and European samples. Studies examining age, menstrual cycle characteristics, cognitive attributions, socioeconomic variables, lifestyle variables and number of children have not yielded consistent conclusions. Studies have suggested some genetic liability for PMS, but the overlap with genetic liability for major depression or personality characteristics has received mixed. A polymorphism in the serotonin transporter promoter gene has been suggested in women who have both PMDD and seasonal affective disorder (Praschak-Rieder *et al.*, 2002). Elevated lifetime prevalence of major depressive disorder in women with PMDD has been reported in several studies as well as an elevated lifetime prevalence of postpartum. Even though premenstrual symptoms are described in women from menarche to menopause, it is unclear if symptoms remain stable or increase in severity with age. PMS has been described in several countries and cultures and some have a preponderance of somatic rather than emotional symptoms.

Etiology

Since abnormalities in the hypothalamic-pituitary-gonadal axis (HPG) have not been identified, it is thought that premenstrual symptoms may occur due to a differential sensitivity to mood-perturbing effects of gonadal steroid fluctuations in women with PMS and PMDD. It is probable that the etiology of the "differential sensitivity" is multifactorial. The specific neurotransmitter, neuroendocrine and neurosteroid abnormalities in women with PMS and PMDD are not known, but serotonin, norepinephrine, gamma-aminobutyric acid (GABA), allopregnanolone (an anxiolytic metabolite of progesterone that acts at the $GABA_A$ receptor) and factors involved in calcium homeostasis are all possibly involved.

A large number of studies have reported abnormalities in the serotonin system in women with PMS and PMDD. Several studies have also suggested that women with PMDD have decreased luteal phase levels of GABA, abnormal allopregnanolone levels, and decreased sensitivity of the $GABA_A$ receptor as shown by flumazenil challenge, and the sedative and saccadic eye velocity responses to benzodiazepines. It is possible that the rapid efficacy of selective serotonin reuptake inhibitors (SSRIs) in PMDD may be due in part to their ability to increase allopregnanolone levels in the brain, thus enhancing GABA transmission as well as serotonin transmission.

Several factors that influence calcium and bone homeostasis fluctuate with the menstrual cycle and it is possible that some of these factors are abnormal in women with PMS and PMDD Thys-Jacobs and colleagues (1995) reported that women with PMS had reduced periovulatory calcium levels and elevated parathyroid hormone levels compared with controls, perhaps secondary to elevated preovulatory estrogen levels, and these authors proposed that women with PMS may have a cyclical, transient secondary hyperparathyroidism. It has been reported that when calcium homeostasis is corrected in

primary hyperparathyroidism, cerebrospinal fluid monoamine metabolites normalize and affective symptoms are reduced. It is possible that the administration of supplemental calcium normalizes the peri-ovulatory fluctuations in calcium and parathyroid hormone, thus regulating calcium effects on neurotransmitter synthesis and release leading to symptom relief in women with PMS.

Treatment

Antidepressant Treatment

The treatment studies of SSRIs and venlafaxine in PMDD have suggested a similar efficacy rate to treatment studies of SSRIs in major depressive disorder, with 60 to 70% of women responding to SSRIs compared with approximately 30% of women responding to placebo. In general, the effective doses for all SSRIs are similar to the doses recommended for the treatment of major depressive disorder (Figure 48.2) The efficacy of the continuous versus intermittent dosing is equivalent.

A large RCT has reported that fluoxetine 20 mg/day during the luteal phase only was superior to placebo in reducing premenstrual emotional and physical symptoms in 252 women with PMDD (Cohen *et al.*, 2002). There have not been reports of discontinuation symptoms from these doses of SSRIs when abruptly stopped from the first day of menses. There are no published studies to date of the efficacy of "symptom onset" dosing of SSRIs, that is, administering SSRIs the postovulatory day that premenstrual symptoms appear until menses. The efficacy of intermittent dosing, as well as the findings from most SSRI trials that efficacy is achieved by the first treatment cycle, has suggested a more rapid and different mechanism of action of SSRIs in PMDD compared with its effect in major depressive disorder, which typically takes 2 to 6 weeks. As discussed above, it has been hypothesized that the rapid improvement of premenstrual symptoms by SSRIs may be due to an increase in allopregnanolone levels. The selective superiority of serotonergic antidepressants for PMDD is compatible with the postulated serotonin dysfunction in PMDD.

Most SSRI trials have been 6 months or less in duration, so efficacy-based long-term treatment recommendations do not exist. Clinically, many women note the recurrence of premenstrual symptoms after SSRI discontinuation and many clinicians treat women over a long period of time. As reviewed, a few open studies report maintenance of SSRI efficacy over a couple of years (Yonkers, 1997). Studies are needed to identify whether or not some women develop tolerance to the SSRI and need a higher dose over time and whether or not some women stay in remission for a period of time following SSRI discontinuation.

Ovulation Suppression Treatments

Gonadotropin releasing hormone (GnRH) agonists suppress ovulation by downregulating GnRH receptors in the hypothalamus, leading to decreased follicle-stimulating hormone and luteinizing hormone release from the pituitary, resulting in decreased estrogen and progesterone levels. GnRH agonists are administered parenterally (e.g., subcutaneous monthly injections of goserelin, intramuscular monthly injections of leuprolide, daily intranasal buserelin) (see Figure 48.2). GnRH agonists lead to improvement in most emotional and physical premenstrual symptoms, with possible decreased efficacy for premenstrual dysphoria and severe premenstrual symptoms

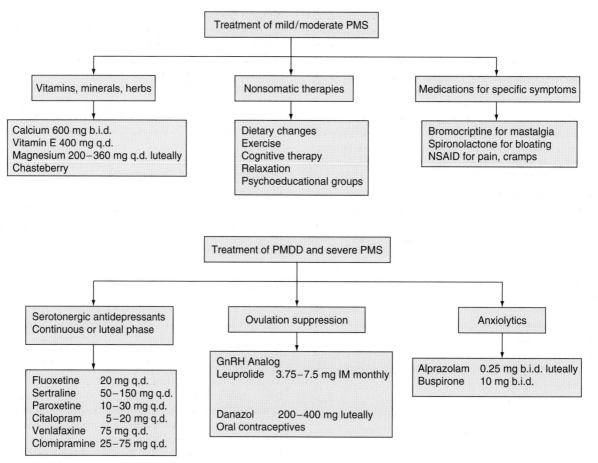

Figure 48.2 *Treatment algorithm of premenstrual symptoms.*

or for the exacerbation of chronic depression. After relief of PMS is achieved with a GnRH agonist, "add-back" hormone strategies have been investigated due to the undesirable medical consequences of the hypoestrogenic state resulting from prolonged anovulation. The addition of estrogen and progesterone to goserelin and leuprolide led to the reappearance of mood and anxiety symptoms. Since women with severe PMS and PMDD have an abnormal response to normal hormonal fluctuations, it is not surprising that women had the induction of mood and anxiety symptoms from the addition of gonadal steroids, reducing the benefit of the replacement strategy.

Oral Contraceptives

Even though oral contraceptives (OCs) are a commonly prescribed treatment for PMS, there is minimal literature endorsing its efficacy. Anecdotally, women report that oral contraceptives may benefit, worsen, or not affect their premenstrual symptoms. The induction of dysphoria may be related to the type and dose of the progestin component, the androgenic properties of the progesterone, or to the estrogen/progestin ratio (Kahn and Halbreich, 2001). A more recent RCT compared an oral contraceptive to placebo in 82 women with PMDD (Freeman *et al.*, 2001). Even though the OC containing ethinyl estradiol 30 µg and drospirenone 3 mg improved most premenstrual symptoms, due in large part to a placebo response rate of 40%, the OC was significantly more efficacious than placebo only in decreasing food cravings, increased appetite and acne. Oral contraceptives have been reported not to alter the response to SSRIs in women with PMDD.

Progesterone

The early assumption that PMS was due to a progesterone deficiency, which has never been substantiated, led to luteal phase progesterone being one of the earliest treatments of PMS in the literature. A recent systematic review of published double-blind placebo-controlled randomized studies of luteal phase progesterone (given as vaginal suppositories or oral micronized tablets) and progestogens reported that there was no clinically meaningful difference between all progesterone forms and placebo, although there was a small statistically significant superiority of progesterone over placebo (Wyatt *et al.*, 2001).

Other Medications

Alprazolam (administered during the luteal phase) has been reported to be superior to placebo in most studies, and although it has a lower efficacy rate than SSRIs, it is effective for premenstrual emotional symptoms. Alprazolam should be tapered over the first few days of menses each cycle. Buspirone at 25 mg/day during the luteal weeks has some efficacy. Spironolactone has been reported to decrease premenstrual emotional and physical symptoms. Bromocriptine has been reported to decrease premenstrual breast.

Herbal Treatments and Dietary Supplementation

Most RCTs have shown little efficacy from herbal treatments and therefore at this time no herbal treatment can be recommended. With respect to dietary supplementation, calcium is reported to have a nearly 50% efficacy rate for reducing the emotional and physical symptoms of the PMDD diagnostic criteria, except for fatigue and insomnia, compared with 30% for placebo. However, women with concurrent psychiatric illness were not clearly excluded, and other treatments except for analgesics were allowed. The efficacy of calcium was somewhat less in women who were also taking oral contraceptives (Thys-Jacobs et al., 1998). The results of this study were notable, and calcium deserves further study. Like herbal preparation, there is a paucity of data to support the efficacy of vitamin supplementation.

Lifestyle Modifications and Psychosocial Treatments

Many lifestyle modifications and psychosocial treatments have been suggested for PMS. Lifestyle modifications are often suggested through self-help materials or in an individual or group psychoeducation format. A recent study reported that a weekly peer support and professional guidance group for four sessions was superior to waitlist control in terms of reducing premenstrual symptoms. The treatment consisted of diet and exercise regimens, self-monitoring and other cognitive techniques and environment modification (Taylor, 1999). Studies have not been conducted on individual lifestyle or psychosocial treatments to identify which components are most efficacious.

Dietary recommendations include decreased caffeine, frequent snacks or meals, reduction of refined sugar and artificial sweeteners, and increase in complex carbohydrates. Premenstrual increased appetite and carbohydrate craving increases the availability of tryptophan in the brain, leading to increased serotonin synthesis. There is little data at this time supporting dietary interventions.

Exercise is likewise a frequently recommended treatment for PMS that has yet to be tested in a sample of women with prospectively-confirmed PMS or PMDD. As reviewed, negative effect and other premenstrual symptoms improve with regular exercise in women in general. Cognitive therapy (CT) is reported to be a promising treatment for PMS. There are limited studies in the use of light therapy, massage therapy, reflexology, chiropractic manipulation, acupuncture and biofeedback.

Conclusion

Women with severe PMS and PMDD comprise a substantial proportion of menstruating women. These women have several symptomatic days each month that lead to disrupted relationships and decreased quality of life. Women presenting with premenstrual complaints need prospectively to rate their symptoms for two menstrual cycles to rule out the presence of a concurrent psychiatric or medical disorder. Once the diagnosis of severe PMS or PMDD is confirmed, SSRI medication is considered the first line treatment. SSRI medication may be administered daily or intermittently (from ovulation to menses) to be effective. Nutritional approaches, exercise and cognitive therapy may be appropriate as first treatments in mild cases, otherwise they should accompany medication treatment. Second line treatment options include changing to a second SSRI, gonadal

hormone therapy (such as GnRH analogs or oral contraceptives), or adding adjunctive anxiolytics, calcium, or other medications targeted to specific symptoms (American College of Obstetrics and Gynecology, 2000; Altshuler et al., 2001). Future studies are still needed for women with severe PMS and PMDD, such as to identify predictors for which women may benefit from hormonal strategies, to determine the optimal duration for medication treatment, and to determine whether or not some women may maintain remission following successful medication treatment.

Comparison of DSM-IV/ICD-10 Diagnostic Criteria

Premenstrual Dysphoric Disorder is not included in ICD-10. A related condition "premenstrual tension syndrome" is included in Chapter 14 for diseases of the genitourinary system.

References

Altshuler LL, Cohen LS, Moline ML et al. (2001) The Expert Consensus Guideline Series. Treatment of depression in women. *Postgrad Med* 1–107.

American College of Obstetrics and Gynecology (2000) *Premenstrual Syndrome*. ACOG Practice Bulletin. American College of Obstetrics and Gynecology, Washington DC.

American Psychiatric Association (1994) *Diagnostic and Statistical Manual of Mental Disorders*, 4th edn. APA, Washington DC.

Cohen LS, Miner C, Brown E et al. (2002) Premenstrual daily fluoxetine for premenstrual dysphoric disorder: A placebo-controlled, clinical trial using computerized diaries. *Obstetr Gynecol* 100(3), 435–444.

Endicott J and Harrison W (1990) *Daily Rating of Severity of Problems Form*. Department of Research Assessment and Training. New York State Psychiatric Institute, New York.

Freeman EW, Kroll R, Rapkin A et al. (2001) Evaluation of a unique oral contraceptive in the treatment of premenstrual dysphoric disorder. *J Women's Health Gender-Based Med* 10, 561–569.

Kahn LS and Halbreich U (2001) Oral contraceptives and mood. *Expert Opin Pharmacother* 2, 1367–1382.

Pearlstein TB, Halbreich U, Batzar ED et al. (2000) Psychosocial functioning in women with premenstrual dysphoric disorder before and after treatment with sertraline or placebo. *J Clin Psychiatr* 61, 101–109.

Praschak-Rieder N, Willeit M, Winkler D et al. (2002) Role of family history and 5-HTTLPR polymorphism in female seasonal affective disorder patients with and without premenstrual dysphoric disorder. *Eur Neuropsychopharmacol* 12, 129–134.

Taylor D (1999) Effectiveness of professional–peer group treatment: Symptom management for women with PMS. *Res Nurs Health* 22, 496–511.

Thys-Jacobs S, Silverton M, Alvir J et al. (1995) Reduced bone mass in women with premenstrual syndrome. *J Women's Health* 4, 161–168.

Thys-Jacobs S, Starkey P, Bernstein D et al. (1998) Calcium carbonate and the premenstrual syndrome: Effects on premenstrual and menstrual symptoms. Premenstrual Syndrome Study Group. *Am J Obstetr Gynecol* 179, 444–452.

Wyatt K, Dimmock P, Jones P et al. (2001) Efficacy of progesterone and progestogens in management of premenstrual syndrome: Systematic review. *Br Med J* 323, 776–780.

Yonkers KA (1997) Antidepressants in the treatment of premenstrual dysphoric disorder. *J Clin Psychiatr* 58, 4–10.

49

Anxiety Disorders: Panic Disorder With and Without Agoraphobia

Definitions and Diagnostic Criteria

According to the *Diagnostic and Statistical Manual of Mental Disorders*, Fourth Edition, Text Revision (DSM-IV-TR) (American Psychiatric Association, 2000), panic disorder is defined by recurrent and unexpected panic attacks. At least one of these attacks must be followed by one month or more of:

1. persistent concern about having more attacks;
2. worry about the implications or consequences of the attack; or
3. changes to typical behavioral patterns (e.g., avoidance of work or school activities) as a result of the attack.

In addition, the panic attacks must not stem solely from the direct effects of illicit substance use, medication, or a general medical condition (e.g., hyperthyroidism, vestibular dysfunction) and are not better explained by another mental disorder (e.g., such as social phobia for attacks that occur only in social situations). A diagnosis of panic disorder with agoraphobia is warranted when the criteria for panic disorder are satisfied and accompanied by agoraphobia.

Although panic attacks are a cardinal feature of panic disorder and in combination with agoraphobia (i.e., anxiety about being in a place or a situation that is not easily escaped or where help is not easily accessible if panic occurs) are essential to a diagnosis of panic disorder with agoraphobia, the criteria sets for panic attacks and for agoraphobia are listed separately as standalone noncodable conditions that are referred to by the diagnostic criteria for panic disorder and agoraphobia without history of panic disorder. Notwithstanding, accurate diagnosis is difficult without a proficient understanding of these features. Tables 49.1 and 49.2 show the DSM-IV-TR criteria for panic attack and agoraphobia, respectively. While the criteria for agoraphobia are generally straightforward, panic attacks can be difficult to understand.

A number of investigations indicate that people report having what they consider to be a panic attack during or in association with actual physical threat (i.e., a true alarm situation). It is, however, important to distinguish between a fear reaction in response to actual threat and a panic attack. In an attempt to do so, the DSM-IV-TR has clarified that panic attacks occur "in the absence of real danger". Such attacks involve a paroxysmal occurrence of intense fear or discomfort accompanied by a minimum of four of the 13 symptoms shown in Table 49.1. The DSM-IV-TR recognizes three characteristic types of panic attacks, including those that are **unexpected** (i.e., not associated with an identifiable internal or external trigger and appear to occur "out of the blue"), **situationally bound**

Table 49.1	Definition and Criteria for Panic Attack

A panic attack is a discrete period of intense fear or discomfort in the absence of real danger that develops abruptly, reaches a peak within 10 min, and is accompanied by four (or more) of the following symptoms:

  (1) palpitations, pounding heart, or accelerated heart rate
  (2) sweating
  (3) trembling or shaking
  (4) sensations of shortness of breath or smothering
  (5) feeling of choking
  (6) chest pain or discomfort
  (7) nausea or abdominal distress
  (8) fee ling dizzy, unsteady, light-headed, or faint
  (9) derealization (feelings of unreality) or depersonalization (being detached from oneself)
(10) fear of losing control or going crazy
(11) fear of dying
(12) paresthesias (numbness or tingling sensations)
(13) chills or hot flushes

Adapted from American Psychiatric Association (2000) *Diagnostic and Statistical Manual of Mental Disorders*, 4th edn., Text Rev. American Psychiatric Association, Washington DC.

(i.e., almost invariably occur when exposed to a situational trigger or when anticipating it) and **situationally predisposed** (i.e., usually, but not necessarily, occur when exposed to a situational trigger or when anticipating it). The term **limited symptom attacks** is used to refer to panic-like episodes comprising fewer than four symptoms.

Although unexpected panic attacks are required for a diagnosis of panic disorder, not all panic attacks that occur in panic disorder are unexpected. The occurrence of unexpected attacks can wax and wane and over the developmental course of the disorder they tend to become situationally bound or predisposed. Moreover, unexpected panic attacks as well as those that are situationally bound or predisposed can occur in the context of other psychiatric disorders, including all of the other anxiety disorders, e.g., a person with social phobia might have an occasional unexpected panic attack without the other feature required to diagnose panic disorder; a dog phobic might panic whenever a large dog is encountered) and some general meda conditions. A clear understanding of the

Table 49.2	Criteria for Agoraphobia

A. Agoraphobia is characterized by anxiety about being in places or situations from which escape might be difficult (or embarrassing) or in which help may not be available in the event of having an unexpected or situationally predisposed panic attack or panic-like symptoms. Agoraphobic fears typically involve characteristic clusters of situations, such as being outside the home alone, being in a crowd, standing in a line, being on a bridge, or traveling in a motor vehicle.

B. The situations are avoided or are endured with marked distress or worry about having a panic attack or panic-like symptoms. Confronting situations is aided by the presence of a companion.

C. The anxiety or avoidance is not better accounted for by another mental disorder.

Adapted from American Psychiatric Association (2000) *Diagnostic and Statistical Manual of Mental Disorders*, 4th edn., Text Rev. American Psychiatric Association, Washington DC.

distinction between types of panic attacks outlined in the DSM-IV-TR provides a foundation for diagnosis and differential diagnosis. However, consideration of other characteristics of panic – including duration of attacks, frequency of attacks, number and intensity of symptoms, nature of catastrophic thinking and mechanism responsible for termination of an attack – can be important in identifying exacerbating and controlling factors.

Historical Overview

Descriptions of cases resembling agoraphobia date back thousands of years, appearing in the writings of Hippocrates and others. The term **agoraphobia** was, however, coined less than 150 years ago to describe patients who seemingly experienced unexpected and situational panic attacks accompanied by anticipatory anxiety and functional incapacitation when walking the streets of their neighborhoods. Freud (1894/1949), whose description of anxiety attacks holds many similarities (but also some notable differences) to contemporary descriptions of panic disorder, was the first to explicate this association. In describing agoraphobia, he specifically mentioned the role of panic, anticipatory anxiety and escape concerns as central to the condition.

The origin of the panic disorder construct as a separate diagnostic entity was influenced by the work of a number of researchers but none so much as Donald Klein in the late 1950s and early 1960s. Klein observed that contrary to expectation a subgroup of patients with anxiety neurosis did not improve on chlorpromazine and in some cases became worse. When he gave this subgroup imipramine, a new compound derived from modifications to chlorpromazine, marked improvements were observed. Prior to taking imipramine these patients unlike those who were responsive to chlorpromazine had been experiencing rapid rushes of terror, racing hearts and other physical sensations, which prompted them to rush to the nurses station with reports that they were about to die. On the basis of this differential drug response, Klein concluded that imipramine was effective against these seemingly spontaneous episodes of panic and, importantly, that these attacks were distinct from other forms of anxiety. He also suggested that agoraphobia was a consequence of spontaneous panic attacks.

Prevalence and Course

The one-year prevalence for any panic attack, whether unexpected or situationally cued, is approximately 28%. Lifetime prevalence rates for unexpected panic attacks and agoraphobia are approximately 4 and 9%, respectively. The National Comorbidity Survey Replication (NCS-R) found lifetime prevalence rates of 4.7% for panic disorder and 1.4% for agoraphobia without panic (Kesseler *et al.*, 2005). Investigations of unexpected panic attacks in college student samples using self-report methodology have revealed similar rates, ranging from approximately 5 to 11%.

The National Comorbidity Study (Eaton *et al.*, 1994) has reported the lifetime prevalence of panic disorder (with or without agoraphobia) in the general population to be 3.5%. However, despite uncertainty as to the reason, this rate is somewhat of an anomaly in the literature. Most epidemiological studies, including those based on Epidemiologic Catchment Area and other data sources, have consistently shown lifetime rates between 1 and 2%. The National Comorbidity Survey Replication (NCS-R) found lifetime prevalence rates of 4.7% for panic disorder and 1.4% for agoraphobia without panic (Kesseler *et al.*, 2005). In

DSM-IV-TR Criteria

Summary of DSM-IV-TR diagnostic criteria for 300.01 Panic Disorder Without Agoraphobia and 300.21 Panic Disorder With Agoraphobia

A. Both (1) and (2):
  (1) recurrent unexpected panic attacks
  (2) at least one of the attacks has been followed by one month (or more) of one (or more) of the following:
     (a) persistent concern about having additional attacks
     (b) worry about the implications of the attack or its consequences (e.g., losing control, having a heart attack, "going crazy")
     (c) a significant change in behavior related to the attacks

B. This criterion differs for Panic Disorder With and Without Agoraphobia as follows:

For 300.21 Panic Disorder With Agoraphobia: the presence of Agoraphobia

For 300.01 Panic Disorder Without Agoraphobia: absence of Agoraphobia

C. The panic attacks are not due to the direct physiological effects of a substance (e.g., a drug of abuse, a medication) or a general medical condition (e.g., hyperthyroidism).

D. The panic attacks are not better accounted for by another mental disorder, such as social phobia (e.g., occurring on exposure to feared social situations), specific phobia (e.g., on exposure to a specific phobic situation), obsessive–compulsive disorder (e.g., on exposure to dirt in someone with an obsession about contamination), posttraumatic stress disorder (e.g., in response to stimuli associated with a severe stressor), or separation anxiety disorder (e.g., in response to being away from home or close relatives).

Reprinted with permission from DSM-IV Guidebook (2004) Frances A, First MB, Pincus HA. American Psychiatric Press Inc, Washington, DC p. 235. Copyright 2004 American Psychiatric Press, Inc

treatment seeking individuals, the prevalence of panic disorder is considerably higher. Approximately 10% of patients in mental health clinics and between 10 and 60% in various medical specialty clinics (e.g., cardiology, respiratory, vestibular) have panic disorder. Panic disorder with agoraphobia is more common than panic disorder without agoraphobia in clinical samples.

Age of onset for panic disorder is distributed bimodally, typically developing between 15 and 19 or 25 and 30 years. The clinical features of panic disorder such as number and severity of symptoms are much the same across the sexes. However, women are diagnosed with panic disorder more than twice as often as men. Recent research indicates that women are more likely to have panic disorder with agoraphobia and that they are more likely to have recurrence of symptoms after remission of their panic attacks than are men (Yonkers *et al.*, 1998). Men, on the other hand, are more likely to have panic disorder without agoraphobia (Yonkers *et al.*, 1998) and are more likely to self-medicate with alcohol than are women. The literature remains unclear as to why these sex differences exist but alludes to the possible role of biological and/or socialization factors.

Panic disorder symptoms may wax and wane but, if left untreated, the typical course is chronic. Data from a sample of patients assessed and treated through the Harvard/Brown Anxiety Disorders Research Program and followed prospectively over a 5-year period indicated remission rates in both men and women to be 39% (Yonkers *et al.*, 1998). In general among those receiving tertiary treatment, approximately 30% of patients have symptoms that are in remission, 40 to 50% are improved but still have significant symptoms, and 20 to 30% are unimproved or worse at 6 to 10 years follow-up.

Costs of Panic Disorder

Panic disorder with or without agoraphobia is associated with impaired occupational and social functioning and poor overall quality of life. People with panic disorder, compared with people in the general population, report poorer physical health. Panic disorder is a leading reason for seeking emergency department consultations and a leading cause for seeking mental health services, surpassing both schizophrenia and mood disorders. Panic disorder exceeds the economic costs associated with many other anxiety disorders such as social phobia, generalized anxiety disorder and obsessive–compulsive disorder. The high medical costs are partly because panic disorder patients quite often present to their primary care physician or hospital emergency departments, thinking they are in imminent danger of dying or "going crazy." In these settings, patients may undergo a series of extensive medical tests before panic disorder is, if ever, finally diagnosed. Ruling out general medical conditions is good clinical practice but the process contributes substantially to the costs that panic disorder places on health care systems.

Comorbidity

Lifetime comorbidity (i.e., the cooccurrence of two or more disorders at any point in a person's life, regardless of whether or not they overlap) in panic disorder is common, with over 90% of community-dwelling and treatment seeking patients having had symptoms meeting diagnostic threshold for at least one other disorder (Robins *et al.*, 1991). Comorbidity can pose considerable challenge to treatment. The most common comorbid diagnoses with panic disorder are other anxiety disorders, major

depression, somatoform, pain-related, substance use and personality disorders.

Other Anxiety Disorders

The rates of lifetime comorbidity between panic disorder and other anxiety disorders, although variable across epidemiological studies, are high. The most common comorbid anxiety disorders are social phobia and generalized anxiety disorder (15–30%) followed by specific phobia (2–20%), obsessive compulsive disorder (10%), and post traumatic stress disorder (2–10%) (American Psychiatric Association, 2000). To date, there are no studies that have reported comorbid panic disorder and acute stress disorder. The most parsimonious explanation of high comorbidity between panic disorder and the other anxiety disorders is that they share a common diathesis.

Major Depressive Disorder

Epidemiological studies indicate that major depressive disorder occurs in up to 65% of patients with panic disorder at some point in their lives. In approximately two-thirds of these cases, the symptoms of depression develop along with, or secondary to, panic disorder. However, since depression precedes panic disorder in the remaining third, depressive symptoms cooccurring with panic disorder cannot be considered simply as a demoralized response to paroxysms of anxiety. While the risk of developing secondary depression appears to be more closely associated with the severity of agoraphobia than with the severity or frequency of panic attacks, this may be a confound of misdiagnosing some behavioral manifestations of depression as agoraphobia. Panic disorder and depression do not appear to be identical disorders and their co-occurrence may be due to a shared diathesis or mutual exacerbation of symptoms.

Somatoform and Pain-related Disorders

Somatoform and pain-related disorders are frequently comorbid with panic disorder. For example, hypochondriasis has been diagnosed in approximately 20% of panic disorder patients attending general medical clinics and in almost 50% of those attending anxiety disorders clinics. Acute and chronic musculoskeletal pain (i.e., pain that persists for six months or longer), respectively, are reported by approximately 85 and 40% of panic disorder patients attending anxiety disorders clinics. Irritable bowel syndrome, a condition characterized persistent abdominal pain and defecation difficulties, cooccurs in 17 to 41% of treatment seeking panic disorder patients. Emerging evidence suggests that comorbidity between panic disorder and both somatoform and pain-related disorders may be best explained by a shared diathesis model.

Substance Use Disorders

Panic disorder can be precipitated by the use of psychotropic drugs and risk is higher with chronic use. Alcohol has been identified as playing a precipitating, maintaining and aggravating role in panic disorder. The 6-month prevalence of alcohol abuse or dependence in panic disorder has been reported to be 40% in men and 13% in women. These rates are higher than those observed in people with other anxiety disorders and those with no anxiety disorder. Although alcohol problems have been reported to precede panic disorder in a majority of cases, most reports indicate that alcohol problems develop secondary to panic disorder, often as a means of self-medication. Those having panic disorder with agoraphobia appear to be at greater risk for comorbid alcohol abuse or dependence than those without agoraphobia.

Personality Disorders

Lack of reliable assessment instruments for personality disorders as well as overlapping diagnostic criteria necessarily limit the degree of confidence in reports of comorbidity with panic disorder. Notwithstanding, 40 to 50% of panic disorder patients have been reported to qualify for one or more personality disorders, a rate which exceeds that of 13% observed in community control samples. The most commonly reported cooccurring personality disorders are avoidant, dependant, and histrionic personality disorders. These disorders do not cooccur uniquely with panic, also being common in patients with depression and other anxiety disorders, and they often persist despite remission of panic symptoms.

Etiology

Cognitive Models – The Vicious Cycle

There are several contemporary cognitive models of panic disorder which, for the most part, are based on variations of the "fear of anxiety" construct. Goldstein and Chambless (1978) proposed that fear of anxiety arises through the association of interoceptive cues with panic attacks. In other words, people with panic disorder are thought to learn to fear the recurrence of aversive panic episodes and thereby develop a fear of panic-related symptoms. Refuting the premise that fear of anxiety develops from the experience of panic attacks, Clark (1986) posited that panic attacks are the product of a tendency **catastrophically misinterpret** to autonomic arousal sensations that occur in the context of nonpathological anxiety (as well as physical illness, exercise and ingestion of certain substances). Reiss and colleagues (Reiss, 1999; Reiss and McNally, 1985), incorporating components of the Goldstein and Chambless and Clark models, proposed that panic attacks arise as a consequence of both:

1. a predispositional tendency to catastrophically misinterpret and respond with fear to the benign arousal sensations, and
2. a learned fear of anxiety that is maintained by the experience of panic episodes.

Most recently, Bouton, Mineka and Barlow (2001) have described a variant of the original fear of anxiety model, suggesting that panic disorder develops when exposure to panic attacks conditions a person to respond with anticipatory anxiety (and sometimes with panic) to internal arousal and contextual cues.

The vicious cycle model makes several assumptions. First, while recognizing that initial panic attacks may be caused by other factors (e.g., drug-related autonomic surges), it assumes that people prone to panic disorder have an enduring tendency catastrophically to misinterpret benign arousal sensations. Secondly, it assumes that misinterpretations can occur at the conscious and unconscious level. Thirdly, the cycle can be entered into at any point. For example, the cycle can be initiated by a contextual trigger or simply by having catastrophic thoughts about bodily sensations. Fourthly, physiological changes are viewed as one of several components in a process, rather than as a pathogenic mechanism.

Cognitive models can also account for agoraphobia. Agoraphobia has long been regarded as a product of operant conditioning. As noted above, it most often develops as a consequence of panic attacks. These attacks typically occur in particular situations (e.g., when in line at a shopping mall, when driving) and motivate the person to avoid or escape these situations. The avoidance and escape behaviors are negatively reinforced by the reduction of aversive autonomic arousal and other anxiety-related sensations. Cognitive factors such as expectations that an attack will be imminent and harmful and that coping will be ineffective play a significant role by influencing and maintaining avoidance behavior.

A growing body of literature supports the vicious cycle model. Thoughts of imminent catastrophe have been identified as triggers of panic attacks. Patients with panic disorder relative to healthy and patient controls have been shown to be:

1. characterized by strategic and automatic information processing (i.e., memory, attention) biases for physical threat cues;
2. more accurate, in some instances, at detecting body sensations;
3. more likely to report fear of somatic sensations and beliefs in their harmful consequences; and
4. more susceptible to the influence of instructional manipulations of control in response to pharmacological panic provocation challenges, panicking less often under the illusion of greater control in some (but not all cases).

Research shows that treatments stemming from the cognitive model (reviewed later in this chapter) are effective.

Biological Models

Evidence suggests that several neurotransmitter systems, involving neurotransmitters or neuromodulators such as serotonin, noradrenalin, adenosine, gamma-aminobutyric acid and cholecystokinin-4, play a role in panic disorder. Various brain structures in the limbic system and associated regions have also been implicated. Contemporary biological models of panic have grown in number and complexity in recent years in an effort to integrate and explain these findings. Recent emphasis has focused on the amygdala, a limbic structure that appears to be involved in coordinating the different neurotransmitters involved in anxiety disorders (Goddard and Charney, 1997). Today, there is no single, leading biological model of panic. However, there are a number of useful models that guide research and clinical practice. Among the most promising is the neuroanatomical hypothesis recently revised by Gorman and colleagues (2000). This hypothesis is useful for several reasons. First, it integrates a wide range of findings, including animal research and studies of humans. Secondly, it provides a unifying framework for understanding why panic disorder is associated with so many biological dysregularities such as abnormalities in neurotransmitter systems and irregularities on various indices of autonomic functioning. Thirdly, the model accounts for treatment-outcome data, which show that both pharmacological and psychological therapies are effective treatments for panic disorder (as reviewed later in this chapter).

Neuroanatomical Hypothesis

Gorman and colleagues (2000) begin with the observation that there is a remarkable similarity between the physiological and behavioral consequences of panic attacks in humans and conditioned fear responses in animals. Similarities include autonomic arousal, fear evoked by specific cues (i.e., contextual fear) and avoidance of these cues. Animal research indicates that conditioned fear responses are mediated by a "fear network" in the brain, consisting of the amygdala and its afferent and efferent projections, particularly its connections with the hippocampus, medial prefrontal cortex, hypothalamus and brainstem. Animal studies also show that activation of this network produces biological and behavioral reactions that are similar to those associated with panic attacks. Thus, Gorman and colleagues (2000) posit that a similar network is involved in panic disorder.

The fear network consists of a complex matrix of interconnections, implicating a number of brain structures and neurotransmitter systems. Sensory input passes through the anterior thalamus to the lateral nucleus of the amygdala. Input is then transferred to the central nucleus of the amygdala, which coordinates autonomic and behavioral responses. Direct sensory input to the amygdala from brainstem structures and the sensory thalamus enables a rapid response to potentially threatening stimuli. The central nucleus of the amygdala projects to the following structures:

1. the parabrachial nucleus, producing an increase in respiratory rate;
2. the lateral nucleus of the hypothalamus, causing autonomic arousal and sympathetic discharge;
3. the locus coeruleus, leading to an increase in norepinephrine and to increases in blood pressure, heart rate and behavioral fear responses (e.g., freezing);
4. the paraventricular nucleus of the hypothalamus, resulting in an increase in the release of adrenocorticoids; and
5. the periaqueductal gray region, leading to avoidance behaviors.

In addition, there are reciprocal connections between the amygdala and the sensory thalamus, prefrontal cortex, insula, and primary somatosensory cortex.

Panic attacks arise from excessive activation of the fear network (Gorman *et al.*, 2000). The fear network becomes sensitized (conditioned) to respond to noxious stimuli such as internal (bodily sensations) and external (contexts or situations) that the person associates with panic. Sensitization of the network may be manifested by the strengthening of various projections from the central nucleus of the amygdala to brainstem sites (such as the locus coeruleus, periaqueductal gray region and hypothalamus). The network could be over-activated if brainstem inputs to the amygdala are dysregulated. However, autonomic activation (e.g., increased respiration and heart rate) and neuroendocrine activation (e.g., increased cortisol secretion) does not occur in all panic attacks. Moreover, a variety of biological agents with diverse physiological properties can trigger panic attacks in people with panic disorder (e.g., sodium lactate, yohimbine, CO_2, caffeine, cholecystokinin-4). It is, therefore, unlikely that a single brainstem dysregulation is responsible for panic or, in turn, that brainstem dysregulation is the only way of producing an over-active fear network.

There may be other ways of activating the fear network. For example, the amygdala receives input from cortical regions involved in the processing and evaluation of sensory information. Therefore, a neurocognitive deficit in these cortico-amygdala pathways could result in the catastrophic misinterpretation of sensory information (i.e., misinterpretation of bodily sensations), leading to an inappropriate activation of the fear network. Notice that this pathway resembles the cognitive model of panic

described earlier in this chapter. Thus, Gorman and colleagues (2000) model integrates the cognitive model and places it in a neuroanatomical context.

In addition to playing a role in panic disorder, the fear network is thought to play a role in other anxiety disorders and in mood disorders. This is consistent with the comorbidity between panic disorder and these disorders. Abnormalities in the fear network may vary from disorder to disorders. For example, the strength of various connections between components of the network may distinguish various disorders.

Medications, particularly selective serotonin reuptake inhibitors (SSRIs), are thought to desensitize the fear network. This may happen in a number of ways. SSRIs increase serotonergic transmission in the brain. Serotonergic neurons originate in the brainstem raphe and project throughout the central nervous system and some of these projections have inhibitory influences. For example, the greater the activity in the raphe, the greater the inhibition of noradrenergic neurons in the locus ceruleus, resulting in a reduction of cardiovascular symptoms associated with panic attacks, such as tachycardia. Similarly, the greater the activity in the raphe, the greater the inhibition in the periaqueductal gray region, resulting in a reduction in avoidance behavior. Increased serotonergic activity also may reduce hypothalamic release of corticotropin-releasing factor, thereby resulting in a reduction of cortisol and a reduction in activity of the locus ceruleus thereby leading to a reduction in fear. SSRIs may also directly inhibit activity of the lateral nucleus of the amygdala. Thus, there appear to be several ways in which SSRIs could desensitize the fear network. Effective psychological therapies are thought to reduce contextual fear and catastrophic misinterpretations at the level of the medial prefrontal cortex and hippocampus.

Environmental and Genetic Factors

The fear network is thought to be influenced by genetic factors and stressful life events, particularly events in early childhood. The search for genetic markers and candidate genes for panic disorder has revealed several possible loci but, to date, none has been replicated across studies. Research with monozygotic and dizygotic twins show that panic disorder is moderately heritable, with 32 to 46% of variance in liability for panic being attributed to genetic factors (Kendler *et al.*, 1993).

Vulnerability to panic disorder appears to result from a combination of disorder-specific and disorder-nonspecific factors. The importance of nonspecific genetic factors is consistent with observation that panic disorder is often comorbid with other disorders. Twin studies suggest that nonspecific factors influence the vulnerability to several disorders, including panic disorder, bulimia nervosa, generalized anxiety disorder and alcohol dependence. Genetic factors specific to panic disorder may be those that influence the tendency catastrophically to misinterpret bodily sensations. This cognitive tendency is a distinguishing feature of panic disorder, as described above. Recent twin research indicates that it is moderately heritable in women but not men (Jang *et al.*, 1999). Thus, some specific genetic factors in panic disorder appear to be sex-linked.

Environmental events occurring during particular developmental phases such as separation from the primary caregiver during early childhood may activate the genes that modulate the fear network, thereby creating a vulnerability to panic disorder. Research suggests that later events, occurring during adolescence or early adulthood, then precipitate panic disorder in vulnerable individuals. These events may stress the individual at a psychological or physiological level. Events commonly associated with the onset of panic disorder include:

1. separation, loss, or illness of a significant other;
2. being the victim of sexual assault or other forms of interpersonal violence;
3. financial or occupational stressors; and
4. intoxication with, or withdrawal from, a psychoactive substance such as marijuana, cocaine, or anesthetic.

Dynamic Models

The most promising psychodynamic models for understanding panic disorder are those that focus specifically on this disorder. Rather than review all the models, we will summarize the model developed by the Cornell Panic-Anxiety Study Group (Milrod *et al.*, 1997; Shear *et al.*, 1993) because it has led to a promising treatment. According to the Cornell group, people at risk for panic disorder have 1) a neurophysiological vulnerability to panic attacks, and/or 2) multiple experiences of developmental trauma. These factors lead the child to become frightened of unfamiliar situations and to become excessively dependent on the primary caregiver to provide a sense of safety. The caregiver is unable to provide support always, so the child develops a fearful dependency. This leads, in turn, to the development of unconscious conflicts about dependency (independence versus reliance on others) and anger (expression versus inhibition). The dependency conflict is said to express itself in a number of ways. Some panic-vulnerable people are sensitive to separation and overly reliant on others, while others are sensitive to suffocation and overly reliant on a sense of independence. These conflicts can activate conscious or unconscious fantasies of catastrophic danger, which can trigger panic attacks. In addition, the conflicts evoke aversive emotions, such as anxiety, anger and guilt. The otherwise benign arousal sensations accompanying these emotions can become the focus of "conscious as well as unconscious cognitive catastrophizing" (Shear *et al.*, 1993, p. 862), thereby leading to panic attacks.

Assessment

The most comprehensive and accurate diagnostic information emerges when the clinician uses open ended questions and empathic listening, combined with structured inquiry about specific events and symptoms. Useful structured interviews include the *Structured Clinical Interview for DSM-IV* (SCID-IV) and the *Anxiety Disorders Interview Schedule for DSM-IV* (ADIS-IV). A complete assessment for panic disorder also includes a general medical evaluation consisting of a medical history, review of organ systems, physical examination and blood tests. A general medical evaluation is important for identifying general medical conditions that mimic or exacerbate panic attacks or panic-like symptoms (e.g., seizure disorders, cardiac conditions, pheochromocytoma). These disorders should be investigated and treated before contemplating a course of panic disorder treatment. It is also important to rule out the other anxiety disorders and major depressive disorder as primary factors in the person's panic attacks and avoidance prior to initiating treatment for panic disorder (Figure 49.1).

Diagnostic information can be usefully supplemented by short self-report questionnaires to assess the severity of symptoms and other variables. The **Beck Depression Inventory** and

Beck Anxiety Inventory (Beck and Steer, 1987, 1993) are quick, reliable and valid measures that can be administered at the start of each treatment session to assess the severity of past-week general anxiety and depression. The **Anxiety Sensitivity Index** (Peterson and Reiss, 1992) is another useful short questionnaire that can be used to gauge the severity of the patient's fear of bodily sensations. Scores on this scale can be used to assess whether treatment is altering the patient's tendency catastrophically to misinterpret bodily sensations. This scale has good reliability and validity, is sensitive to treatment-related effects, and its post treatment scores predict who is likely to relapse after panic treatment.

Another useful questionnaire to monitor treatment progress is the **Panic and Agoraphobia Scale** (Bandelow, 1995). This 13-item scale was designed as a short, sensitive measure for treatment outcome studies. The patient is asked to rate the past-week frequency and/or severity of the following: 1) panic attacks, 2) agoraphobia, 3) anticipatory anxiety (i.e., worry about having an panic attack), 4) panic-related disability in various areas of functioning, and 5) worry about the health-related implications of panic (e.g., worry that panic attacks will lead to a heart attack). The Panic and Agoraphobia Scale has good reliability and validity and is sensitive in detecting treatment-related change. It has the advantage of providing a broad assessment of many features of panic disorder and agoraphobia. A limitation is that it does not distinguish between full and limited symptom panic attacks or among the types of panics (i.e., unexpected, situationally bound, situationally predisposed). When asked to recall their attacks, patients may have difficulty making these distinctions. Prospective (ongoing) monitoring is needed to provide this information.

To gain more detailed information on panic attacks, clinicians and clinical researchers are increasingly including some form of prospective monitoring in their assessment batteries. The most widely used are the **panic attack records**. The patient is provided with a definition of a panic attack and then given a pad of panic attack records that can be readily carried in a purse or pocket. The patient is instructed to carry the records at all times and to complete one record (sheet) for each full-blown or limited symptom attack, soon after the attack occurs. Variants on the panic diaries developed by Barlow and colleagues (Barlow and Craske, 1994) are among the most informative and easy to use. These records are then reviewed during treatment sessions to glean information about the links among beliefs, bodily sensations and safety behaviors, and to assess treatment progress.

Treatment

There are a number of approaches that can be taken in treating panic disorder with and without agoraphobia. Both single and combined treatment modalities are presented in Figure 49.2.

Pharmacotherapies

Controlled studies show that effective anti-panic medications include tricyclic antidepressants (e.g., imipramine), monoamine oxidase inhibitors (MAOIs; e.g., phenelzine), high-potency benzodiazepines (e.g., alprazolam) and SSRIs (e.g., fluvoxamine). These treatments have broadly similar efficacy, although there is some evidence that SSRIs tend to be most effective. The classes of medication differ in their side effects and their contraindications. Anticholinergic effects (e.g., blurred vision, dry mouth) are common problems with tricyclics. They are also contraindicated

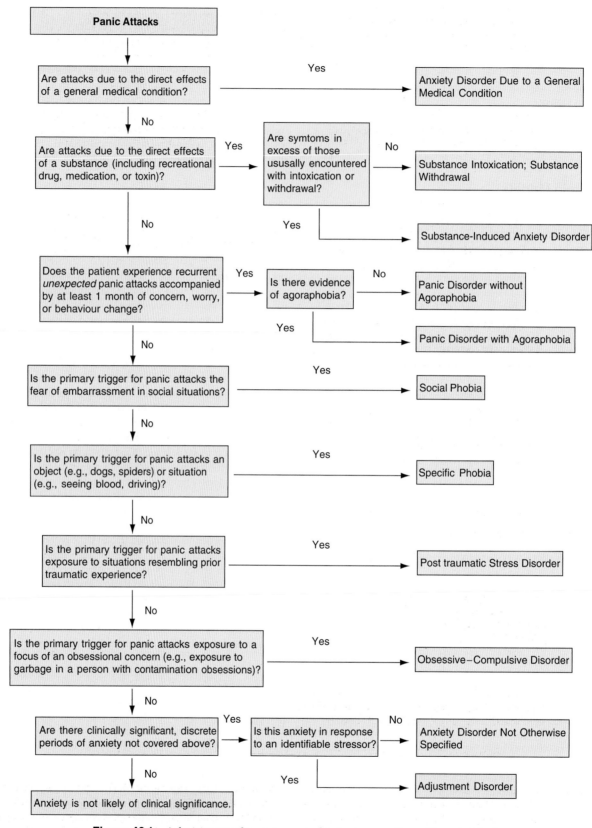

Figure 49.1 *A decision tree for assessment of patients presenting with panic attacks.*

in patients with particular comorbid cardiac disorders. Dietary restrictions (i.e., abstaining from foods containing tyramine) are a limitation of many MAOIs. Sedation, impaired motor coordination and addiction are concerns with benzodiazepines.

When efficacy and side effects are considered together, SSRIs emerge as the most promising drug treatments for panic disorder. However, even SSRIs have side effects, with the most problematic being a short-term increase in arousal-related

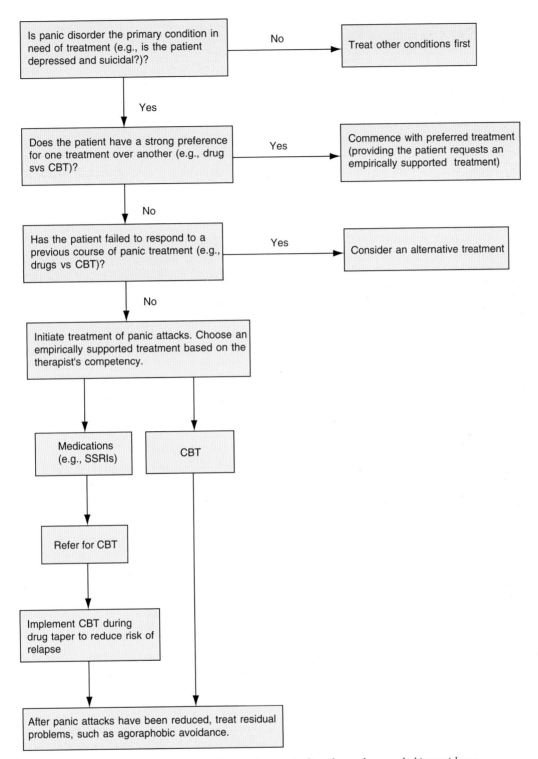

Figure 49.2   *A decision tree for treating panic disorder and agoraphobic avoidance.*

sensations. To overcome this problem, SSRIs can be started at a low dose (e.g., 5–10 mg/d for paroxetine; 12.5–25 mg/d for sertraline) and then increased gradually (e.g., up to 10–50 mg/d for paroxetine; up to 25–200 mg/d for sertraline). The choice of SSRI is determined on the basis of several factors, including side effects, patient preference and the patient's history of responding (or not responding) to particular agents.

For drug refractory patients, or patients who are unable to tolerate SSRI side effects, combination medications are sometimes used. For example, SSRIs can be augmented with benzodiazepines. The latter are used to dampen the side effects of SSRIs. Despite some positive preliminary reports supporting this strategy, its value in the treatment of panic disorder remains to be properly evaluated. An alternative strategy is to change the patient's medication. Some of the newer, nonSSRI antidepressants could be considered, such as venlafaxine, nefazodone, buproprion, duloxetine, or gabapentin. A concern with using these newer medications to treat panic disorder is that there are few data to guide the clinician. Another approach to the drug refractory patient is to use a psychosocial treatment such as cognitive–behavioral therapy (CBT), as an alternative or adjunctive intervention.

Cognitive–Behavioral Therapy

CBT treatment packages include a number of components, such as psychoeducation (e.g., information about the cognitive model of panic), breathing retraining, cognitive restructuring, relaxation exercises, interoceptive exposure and situational exposure. Breathing retraining involves teaching the patient to breathe with the diaphragm rather than with the chest muscles. Cognitive restructuring focuses on challenging patient's beliefs about the dangerousness of bodily sensations (e.g., challenging the belief that palpitations lead to heart attacks). Interoceptive exposure involves inducing feared bodily sensations to further teach patients that the sensations are harmless. Situational exposure involves activities that bring the patient into feared situations such as shopping malls, bridges, or tunnels. Despite the advantages of exposure exercises, they are medically contraindicated in some cases. For example, a hyperventilation exercise would not be used in a patient with severe asthma.

A large body of evidence shows that CBT is effective in reducing panic attacks, agoraphobia and associated symptoms such as depression. However, not all CBT interventions may be necessary. Interoceptive exposure, situational exposure and cognitive restructuring are the most widely used and supported interventions. Several studies suggest that breathing retraining reduces panic frequency. However, recent research casts doubt about the importance of hyperventilation in producing panic attacks. This suggests that breathing retraining may only be useful for a minority of patients, for which chest breathing or hyperventilation plays a role in producing panic symptoms. Breathing retraining may be counterproductive if it prevents patients from learning that their catastrophic beliefs are unfounded. Given these concerns, breathing retraining should be used sparingly in the treatment of panic disorder. If used at all, the clinician should ensure that the patient understands that breathing exercises are used to remove unpleasant but harmless sensations. Interoceptive exposure and cognitive restructuring are important for helping patients learn that the sensations are not dangerous.

How effective is CBT compared with other therapies? A small but growing literature suggests that the efficacy of CBT is equal to or greater than that of alprazolam and imipramine at post treatment. Future research is needed to compare CBT with other pharmacotherapies, such as SSRIs. Preliminary evidence suggests that CBT is effective in treating patients who have failed to respond to pharmacotherapies. Follow-up studies suggest that CBT is effective in the long term and is likely to be more effective than short-term pharmacological treatment. It is not known whether drug treatments would be as effective as CBT if patients remained on their medications. Any conclusions about the long-term efficacy of panic treatments are necessarily tentative because patients sometimes seek additional treatment during the follow-up interval.

Other Psychosocial Interventions

Several other approaches have been used in the treatment of panic disorder, including psychodynamic psychotherapies (Milrod et al., 2000; Wiborg and Dahl, 1996), hypnosis (e.g., Delmonte, 1995), Eye Movement Desensitization and Reprocessing (EMDR)

(Shapiro, 1995), and mindfulness meditation (Miller et al., 1995). Support for these treatments is limited largely to case studies and uncontrolled trials. Controlled studies, although few in number, indicate that hypnosis and EMDR are of limited value in treating panic disorder. and may be no better than placebo. Interventions that look more promising are mindfulness meditation (Miller et al., 1995) and psychodynamic psychotherapies modified specifically to focus on panic symptoms (Milrod et al., 2000; Wiborg and Dahl, 1996). However, none have been extensively evaluated as panic treatments and none has been compared with empirically supported treatments such as CBT or SSRIs.

Combining CBT with Pharmacotherapies

Simultaneous Treatments

Many clinicians believe the optimal treatment consists of drugs combined with some form of psychosocial intervention. This view arose from observations that even the most effective drugs and the most effective psychosocial interventions do not eliminate panic disorder in all cases. It was thought that combination treatments might be a way to improve treatment outcome. The available evidence provides mixed support for this view. Evidence suggests that the efficacy of CBT is not improved when it is combined with either diazepam or alprazolam. In fact, some studies have found that the efficacy of situational exposure is **worsened** when alprazolam is added.

Several studies have compared CBT with CBT combined with imipramine. These results have also been mixed. Adding imipramine in the range of 150–300 mg/day to either situational exposure or CBT sometimes improves treatment outcome in the short term, provided that patients are able to tolerate the dose. Any advantage of combined treatment tends to be lost at follow-up. Similarly, studies of combining CBT with SSRIs (fluvoxamine or paroxetine) have produced mixed results, with some studies finding the combination is no better than CBT.

It remains unclear whether treatment outcome is enhanced by combining CBT with SSRIs. The neuroanatomical model with its dual emphasis on cortical and serotonergic mechanisms suggests that this combined treatment might be superior to CBT alone and to SSRIs alone. On the other hand, pharmacotherapies such as SSRIs might undermine the patient's confidence in implementing CBT, particularly if they attribute their gains to medications rather than to their own efforts at using the skills learned in CBT. Large, well-designed studies are needed to explore these important issues.

Sequential Treatments

A more promising type of combined therapy is a sequential approach, where patients are treated with pharmacotherapy during the acute phase, and then are treated with CBT as the medication is phased out. Several studies have shown that adding CBT during the tapering period for alprazolam and clonazepam reduces the relapse rate associated with these drugs. It remains to be demonstrated that CBT can reduce relapse when patients are tapered off other antipanic drugs such as SSRIs. However, there is no reason to expect that CBT would not be helpful in these cases.

Conclusion

Panic disorder with or without agoraphobia is a common condition with a lifetime prevalence of approximately 2%. Panic disorder is often comorbid with major depressive disorder and also commonly co-occurs with other disorders such as anxiety disorders and substance use disorders. Treatment planning typically begins with a thorough assessment, including a medical history, a structured diagnostic interview and prospective monitoring of symptoms. Based on contemporary biological and cognitive–behavioral models, there are several treatment options that can be considered. These include various pharmacotherapies, particularly SSRIs and psychosocial interventions that have proven effective in controlled trials. While mixed, there is evidence to suggest that treatments that combine SSRIs and CBT may be more effective than either treatment alone, at least in some symptom domains.

Comparison of DSM-IV/ICD-10 Diagnostic Criteria

The ICD-10 Diagnostic Criteria for Research for a panic attack are identical to the DSM-IV-TR criteria set except that ICD-10 includes an additional item (i.e., dry mouth). In contrast to the DSM-IV-TR algorithm which does not give special weight to any particular symptom, the ICD-10 algorithm requires that at least one of the symptoms be palpitations, sweating, trembling, or dry mouth. Like DSM-IV-TR, ICD-10 requires recurrent panic attacks but, in contrast to DSM-IV-TR, it does not include a criterion requiring that the panic attacks be clinically significant.

The ICD-10 Diagnostic Criteria for Research for Agoraphobia differ markedly from the DSM-IV-TR criteria. The ICD-10 Diagnostic Criteria for Research specify that there be fear or avoidance of at least two of the following situations: crowds, public places, traveling alone, or traveling away from home. Furthermore, ICD-10 requires that at least two symptoms of anxiety (i.e., from the list of 14 panic symptoms) be present together on at least one occasion and that these anxiety symptoms be "restricted to, or predominate in, the feared situations or contemplation of the feared situations". In contrast, DSM-IV-TR Agoraphobia is defined in terms of "anxiety about being in places or situations from which escape might be difficult (or embarrassing) or in which help may not be available in the event of having an unexpected or situationally predisposed panic attack". No specific avoided situations or specific types of anxiety symptoms are required for a diagnosis.

References

American Psychiatric Association (2000) *Diagnostic and Statistical Manual of Mental Disorders* 4th edn. Text Rev. American Psychiatric Association, Washington DC.

Bandelow B (1995) Assessing the efficacy of treatments for panic disorder and agoraphobia. II. The panic and agoraphobia scale. *Int Clin Psychopharmacol* 10, 73–81.

Barlow DH and Craske MG (1994) *Mastery of Your Anxiety and Panic II: Client Workbook.* Psychological Corporation, San Antonio, TX.

Beck AT and Steer RA (1987) *Manual for the Revised Beck Depression Inventory.* Psychological Corporation, San Antonio, TX.

Beck AT and Steer RA (1993) *Manual for the Beck Anxiety Inventory.* Psychological Corporation, San Antonio, TX.

Bouton ME, Mineka S and Barlow DH (2001) A modern learning theory perspective on the etiology of panic disorder. *Psychol Rev* 108, 4–32.

Clark DM (1986) A cognitive approach to panic. *Behav Res Ther* 24, 461–470.

Delmonte MM (1995) The use of hypnotic regression with panic disorder: A case report. *Aust J Clin Hypnother Hypnosis* 16, 69–73.

Eaton WW, Kessler RC, Wittchen HU *et al.* (1994) Panic and panic disorder in the United States. *Am J Psychiatr* 151, 413–420.

Freud S (1895/1949) Obsessions and phobias: Their psychical determinants and aetiology, in *Collected Papers of Sigmund Freud*, Vol. I (ed E Jones). Hogarth Press, London, pp. 128–137.

Goddard AW and Charney DS (1997) Toward an integrated neurobiology of panic disorder. *J Clin Psychiatr* 58(Suppl 2), 4–12.

Goldstein AJ and Chambless DL (1978) A reanalysis of agoraphobia. *Behav Ther* 9, 47–59.

Gorman J, Kent JM, Sullivan GM *et al.* (2000) Neuroanatomical hypothesis of panic disorder, *Rev. Am J Psychiatr* 157, 493–505.

Jang KL, Stein MB, Taylor S *et al.* (1999) Gender differences in the etiology of anxiety sensitivity: A twin study. *J Gender Specific Med* 2, 39–44.

Kendler KS, Neale MC, Kessler RC *et al.* (1993) Panic disorder in women: A population-based twin study. *Psychol Med* 23, 397–406.

Kessler RC, Berglund MBA, Demler O *et al.* (2005) Lifetime prevalence and age-of-onset distributions of DSM-IV disorders in the National Comorbidity Survey Replication. *Arch Gen Psychiatr* 62, 593–602

Miller JJ, Fletcher K and Kabat-Zinn J (1995) Three-year follow-up and clinical implications of a mindfulness meditation-based stress reduction intervention in the treatment of anxiety disorders. *Gen Hosp Psychiatr* 17, 192–200.

Milrod BL, Busch FN, Cooper AM *et al.* (1997) *Manual of Panic-focused Psychodynamic Psychotherapy.* American Psychiatric Association, Washington, DC.

Milrod B, Busch F, Leon AC *et al.* (2000) Open trial of psychodynamic psychotherapy for panic disorder: A pilot study. *Am J Psychiatr* 157, 1878–1880.

Peterson RA and Reiss S (1992) *Anxiety Sensitivity Index Manual*, 2nd edn. International Diagnostic Systems, Worthington, OH.

Reiss S (1999) The sensitivity theory of aberrant motivation, in *Anxiety Sensitivity: Theory, Research, and Treatment of the Fear of Anxiety* (ed Taylor S). Lawrence Erlbaum, Mahwah, NJ, pp. 35–58.

Reiss S and McNally RJ (1985) The expectancy model of fear, in *Theoretical Issues in Behavior Therapy* (eds Reiss S and Bootzin RR). Academic Press, New York, pp. 107–121.

Robins LN, Locke BZ and Regier DA (1991) An overview of psychiatric disorders in America, in *Psychiatric Disorders in America: The Epidemiologic Catchment Area Study* (eds Robins LN and Reiger DA). Free Press, New York, p. 328.

Shapiro F (1995) *Eye Movement Desensitization and Reprocessing: Basic Principles, Protocols, and Procedures.* Guilford Press, New York.

Shear MK, Cooper AM, Klerman GL *et al.* (1993) A psychodynamic model of panic disorder. *Am J Psychiatr* 150, 859–866.

Wiborg IM and Dahl AA (1996) Does brief dynamic psychotherapy reduce the relapse rate of panic disorder? *Arch Gen Psychiatr* 53, 689–694.

Yonkers KA, Zlotnick C, Allsworth J *et al.* (1998) Is the course of panic disorder the same in women and men? *Am J Psychiatr* 155, 596–602.

CHAPTER
50

Anxiety Disorders:
Social and Specific Phobias

Definition

The experience of fear and the related emotion of anxiety are universal and familiar to everyone. Fear exists in all cultures and appears to exist across species. Presumably, the purpose of fear is to protect an organism from immediate threat and to mobilize the body for quick action to avoid danger. Emotion theorists consider fear to be an alarm response that fires in the presence of imminent threat or danger. The function of the primarily noradrenergic mediated fear response is to facilitate immediate escape from threat (flight) or attack on the source of threat (fight). Therefore, fear is often referred to as a fight-or-flight response. All the manifestations of fear are consistent with its protective function. For example, heart rate and breathing rate increase to meet the increased oxygen needs of the body, increased perspiration helps to cool the body to facilitate escape, and pupils dilate to enhance visual acuity.

Anxiety, on the other hand, is a future-oriented mood state in which the individual anticipates the possibility of threat and experiences a sense of uncontrollability focused on the upcoming negative event. In the *Diagnostic and Statistical Manual of Mental Disorders*, Fourth Edition, Text Revision (DSM-IV-TR) (American Psychiatric Association, 2000), anxiety is defined as "the apprehensive anticipation of future danger or misfortune accompanied by a feeling of dysphoria or somatic symptoms of tension" (p. 820). If one were to put anxiety into words, one might say, "Something bad might happen soon. I am not sure I can cope with it but I have to be ready to try". Anxiety is primarily mediated by the gamma-aminobutyric acid-benzodiazepine system.

Despite evidence that fear and anxiety are mediated by different brain systems, anxiety and fear are related, which makes sense ethologically. Experiencing anxiety after encountering signals of impending danger seems to lower the threshold for fear which is triggered when danger actually occurs (e.g., being attacked by a mugger or almost being hit by an automobile). Anxiety leads to a shift in attention toward the source of danger so that individuals become more vigilant for relevant threat cues and therefore are more likely to experience fear in the face of perceived immediate threat.

Fear and anxiety are not always adaptive. At times, the responses can occur in the absence of any realistic threat or out of proportion to the actual danger. Almost everyone has situations that arouse anxiety and fear despite the fact that the actual risk is minimal. It is not unusual to become anxious before a job interview or a speech. Many individuals feel fearful when exposed to situations such as dental visits, seeing certain animals, or being at certain heights. For some people, these fears reach extreme levels and

may cause significant distress or impairment in functioning. It is at this point that what we typically refer to as shyness and fearfulness might meet diagnostic criteria for social phobia or specific phobia, respectively (see DSM-IV-TR Criteria 300.23 and 300.29).

As discussed later, phobias are the most common of the anxiety disorders and among the most common of all mental disorders. However, despite the frequency with which phobias occur in the general population, they have tended to be relatively ignored by clinicians and researchers. The introduction of social phobia to the diagnostic nomenclature has led to a slow but steady increase in research on the disorder, so that social phobia has now become a more popular topic of study among researchers on anxiety disorders. In addition to being widespread, social phobia is associated with significant functional impairment. Also, social phobia often presents comorbidly with other mental disorders. Despite the high prevalence rate and significant impairment, generalized social phobia is rarely diagnosed or treated in a primary care setting

With respect to specific phobias, the lack of attention is probably due to several factors. First, many physicians and researchers may view specific phobias to be less severe than other disorders, therefore warranting less attention. In addition, few individuals with specific phobias present for treatment, and the ones who do seek help tend to differ from untreated individuals with phobias with respect to the number and types of specific phobias. As with social phobia, there has been an increase in attention paid to specific phobias, along with increased recognition that these phobias can interfere seriously with an individual's ability to function. It is not unusual for flying phobias to lead individuals to refuse job promotions that involve travel or to avoid visiting distant family members. Likewise, individuals with insect phobias may avoid being outside during the summer.

Psychological Factors

Psychoanalytic Perspectives

Historically, the etiology of phobic disorders was typically explained from a psychoanalytic perspective. Although the defense mechanism of repression is typically used to protect the individual from experiencing the anxiety (and the underlying conflict), when repression is insufficient the ego must use additional defense mechanisms. In the case of individuals with phobias, Freud proposed that displacement of the anxiety to a less relevant object or situation occurs (such as a dog or some other animal), so that the feared object is used to symbolize the primary source of the conflict. Patients with phobias use avoidance further to escape

Essentials of Psychiatry   Jerald Kay and Allan Tasman
© 2006 John Wiley & Sons, Ltd.

DSM-IV-TR Criteria 300.23

Social Phobia (Social Anxiety Disorder)

A. A marked and persistent fear of one or more social or performance situations in which the person is exposed to unfamiliar people or to possible scrutiny by others. The individual fears that he or she will act in a way (or show anxiety symptoms) that will be humiliating or embarrassing. **Note:** In children, there must be evidence of the capacity for age-appropriate social relationships with familiar people and the anxiety must occur in peer settings, not just in interactions with adults.

B. Exposure to the feared social situation almost invariably provokes anxiety, which may take the form of a situationally bound or situationally predisposed panic attack. **Note:** In children, the anxiety may be expressed by crying, tantrums, freezing, or shrinking away from social situations with unfamiliar people.

C. The person recognizes that the fear is excessive or unreasonable. **Note:** In children, this feature may be absent.

D. The feared social or performance situations are avoided or else are endured with intense anxiety or distress.

E. The avoidance, anxious anticipation, or distress in the feared social or performance situation(s).

E. interferes significantly with the person's normal routine, occupational (or academic) functioning, or social activities or relationships, or there is marked distress about having the phobia.

F. In individuals under age 18 years, the duration is at least 6 months.

G. The fear or avoidance is not due to the direct physiological effects of a substance (e.g., a drug of abuse, a medication) or a general medical condition and is not better accounted for by another mental disorder (e.g., panic disorder with or without agoraphobia, separation anxiety disorder, body dysmorphic disorder, a pervasive developmental disorder, or schizoid personality disorder).

H. If a general medical condition or another mental disorder is present, the fear in criterion A is unrelated to it, for example, the fear is not of stuttering, trembling in Parkinson's disease, exhibiting abnormal eating behavior in anorexia nervosa or bulimia nervosa.

Specify if:

Generalized: if the fears include most social situations (also consider the additional diagnosis of avoidant personality disorder)

DSM-IV-TR Criteria 300.29

Specific Phobia

A. Marked and persistent fear that is excessive or unreasonable, cued by the presence or anticipation of a specific object or situation (e.g., flying, heights, animals, receiving an injection, seeing blood).

B. Exposure to the phobic stimulus almost invariably provokes an immediate anxiety response, which may take the form of a situationally bound or situationally predisposed panic attack. **Note:** In children, the anxiety may be expressed by crying, tantrums, freezing, or clinging.

C. The person recognizes that the fear is excessive or unreasonable. **Note:** In children, this feature may be absent.

D. The phobic situation(s) is avoided or else is endured with intense anxiety or distress.

E. The avoidance, anxious anticipation, or distress in the feared situation(s) interferes significantly with the person's normal routine, occupational (or academic) functioning, or social activities or relationships, or there is marked distress about having the phobia.

F. In individuals under age 18 years, the duration is at least 6 months.

G. The anxiety, panic attacks, and phobic avoidance associated with the specific object or situation are not better accounted for by another mental disorder, such as obsessive–compulsive disorder (e.g., fear of dirt in someone with an obsession about contamination), post traumatic stress disorder (e.g., avoidance of stimuli associated with a severe stressor), separation-anxiety disorder (e.g., avoidance of school), social phobia (e.g., avoidance of social situations because of fear of embarrassment), panic disorder with agoraphobia, or agoraphobia without history of panic disorder.

Specify type:

Animal type

Natural environment type (e.g., heights, storms, water)

Blood-injection-injury type

Situational type (e.g., airplanes, elevators, enclosed places)

Other type (e.g., fear of choking, vomiting, or contracting an illness; in children, fear of loud sounds or costumed characters)

the effects of the anxiety. Although Freud's theory was once influential, its impact on current thinking among researchers has waned. Rather, most current research on psychological factors in the development of phobias has tended to focus on conditioning and information-processing theories and their interaction with neurobiological processes.

Learning and Conditioning Perspectives

Emotions are "contagious". That is, we learn to respond to stimuli, in part, by observing other people's responses and also by our own experiences in these situations. In other words, we come to fear dangerous situations easily. This is important from an ethological perspective because our ancestors who could learn to fear threatening objects or situations easily were more likely to survive and pass these genes to their offspring. This inherited tendency to learn to experience fear in particular situations is the basis of conditioning models of phobia development.

Rachman's Pathways to Fear Development Rachman (1977) proposed three pathways to the development of fear. The first of these is **direct conditioning**, which typically involves the experience of being hurt or frightened by the phobic object or situation. Examples include being involved in an automobile accident, being humiliated in front of a group, falling or almost falling from a high place, or fainting at the sight of blood. Rachman's second pathway is called **vicarious acquisition**, which involves witnessing some traumatic event or seeing someone behave fearfully in the presence of a phobic situation. For example, a child might develop a fear of snakes after seeing her father behave fearfully around snakes, or someone might develop a fear of public speaking after seeing another individual heckled by the audience during a presentation. For the third pathway, Rachman proposed that fears can develop through **informational and instructional pathways**. It is not surprising that individuals might develop flying phobias, given the frequency with which plane crashes are reported in the news. Similarly, a child might develop a fear of heights if his parents frequently warned him of the dangers of being near high places.

In addition to these pathways, Rachman acknowledged the role of biological constraints on the development of fear. Of particular relevance is the fact that fears are not randomly distributed. To explain this observation, Seligman (1971) proposed that organisms are predisposed to learn certain associations and not others. Seligman called his theory "preparedness" and hypothesized that individuals are "prepared" to develop some associations that lead to fear and not others. For example, an individual might be more likely to develop a fear of dogs after being bitten than to develop a fear of flowers after being pricked by a thorn. Seligman proposed that these associations evolved through natural selection processes to facilitate survival.

Evidence for the theory of preparedness is mixed. Although some authors have concluded that the studies to date do not support preparedness, it may be argued that these studies have not adequately tested the theory. Most studies examining preparedness have attempted to associate dangerous objects (e.g., snakes) and nondangerous objects (e.g., flowers) with an aversive electrical shock and have found few differences in the subsequent development of fear. However, preparedness predicts that some "associations" are more difficult to establish than others, not that some "objects" are more easily feared than others. The theory does not necessarily predict that shock should be more easily associated with snakes than with flowers. A more appropriate experiment might be to compare the effects of a minor snakebite to the effects of being pricked by a thorny flower on the development of fear of each object. In any event, there is now strong evidence that conditioning processes play an important role in the development of phobic disorders.

Numerous studies have examined the prevalence of Rachman's three pathways to fear development. Most of these studies have focused on the development of specific phobias, although a few studies included social phobia groups. The majority of studies have found support for the model, indicating that both direct and indirect forms of phobia acquisition occur frequently across a wide range of phobias. However, numerous people report onsets that are unrelated to these pathways (e.g., "I have had this fear for

as long as I can remember" or "I have always had this fear"). Overall, it appears that direct and indirect methods of fear development are relatively common, although the frequency of these onsets varies greatly across studies for a variety of reasons.

Despite the prevalence of direct and indirect conditioning events and informational onsets, it appears that they are not the whole story. In fact, studies have begun to include normal comparison groups and have found that these events are equally common in individuals who do not have phobias. Ultimately, to answer the question of how phobias begin, we must discover the variables that lead only certain individuals to develop phobias after experiencing conditioning events or receiving information that leads to fear. For example, several investigators have found that a tendency to feel "disgust" in response to certain stimuli may be important in the development of some animal phobias and blood phobias. In addition, heightened disgust sensitivity in parents has been found to predict fear of disgust-relevant animals (e.g., snakes, mice, slugs and cockroaches) in children. Several other variables have also been suggested as mediating factors in the development of fear. Stress at the time of the event may make individuals more likely to react fearfully. In addition, previous and subsequent exposure to the phobic object may protect an individual from the development of a phobia. For example, someone who grew up around dogs may be less likely to develop a phobia after being bitten than someone who has spent little time around dogs. The context of the event may also influence the reaction. For example, being with another supportive individual at the time of the trauma may protect an individual from developing fear. Finally, a number of individual difference variables such as perceived control, trait anxiety and various personality factors may influence an individual's likelihood of developing a phobia after a conditioning event. In fact, there is evidence that personality factors and parenting styles may be especially relevant to the development of social phobia.

It has been proposed that a fourth nonassociative pathway be added to Rachman's three associative pathways to fear development. Nonassociative fear models propose that a limited number of fears are not acquired by conditioning or other learning processes. Rather, these evolutionary adaptive fears are proposed to be innate or biologically determined. This is similar to preparedness theory, however, it maintains that fears are acquired through a learning or conditioning process and that some fears are more easily learned than others. The nonassociative pathway to fear acquisition helps to explain a number of research findings that run counter to associative models of fear development, including the nonrandom distribution of common fears, and the emergence of some fears without any prior specific associative learning experiences (i.e., direct conditioning, vicarious conditioning, or informational transmission).

Personality Variables It appears that at as early as 18 months of age children differ with respect to their tendency to interact with other individuals, toys and objects. Although about 70% of children are somewhat exploratory in these situations, about 15% of children are extremely exploratory, and the remaining 15% are quite shy and withdrawn. The behavior exhibited by the shy and withdrawn children has been called "behavioral inhibition" and has been proposed to be a predisposing factor in the development of social phobia and other anxiety disorders. One study found that the prevalence of social phobia was significantly greater (17%; $N = 64$) in children with behavioral inhibition than without (5%; $N = 152$) (Biederman et al., 2001). In addition, compared with nonanxious individuals, patients with social phobia describe their parents as having 1) discouraged them from socializing; 2) placed undue importance on the opinions of others; and 3) used shame as a means of discipline. Other predictors of the development of social phobia include a childhood history of separation anxiety, self-consciousness or shyness in childhood and adolescence, and a low frequency of dating in adolescence.

Perfectionism is another personality variable that has been associated with social phobia. Although several other anxiety disorders have also been associated with perfectionism, concern about making mistakes and a perception of having critical parents are highest among individuals with social phobia compared with individuals with other anxiety disorders (e.g., panic disorder, obsessive–compulsive disorder, or specific phobia).

Cognitive Variables Numerous studies have examined the role of cognitive variables in social and specific phobias and have consistently found that individuals with these disorders exhibit attentional and attributional biases regarding the phobic object or situation. In studies of information processing, people with social and specific phobias devote more attention to threat-related information than do nonphobic individuals. They also show perceptual and cognitive distortions consistent with their phobias. For example, individuals with snake or spider phobias tend to overestimate the degree of activity in the feared animal before treatment but not after treatment. Likewise, people with social phobia tend to rate their own performance during public speaking more critically than do nonphobic control subjects. Furthermore, the discrepancy between self-ratings and observer ratings is greater for people with social phobia than control subjects. In addition, individuals with social phobia tend to report more negative self-evaluative thoughts and underestimate their performance when interacting with others relative to nonanxious subjects. More recent research has found that compared with nonanxious individuals, individuals with social phobia are more likely to experience negative imagery and to take an observer's point of view (i.e., see themselves from an external perspective) when exposed to feared social situations. Other research has found that social phobia is associated with impaired thought suppression affecting both social phobia-related stimuli as well as nonsocial phobia-related stimuli. Although it is clear that cognitive biases exist in individuals with phobias and that attentional and attributional biases improve after effective treatment, it is not known whether the cognitive biases exhibited by patients contribute to the development of the fear or whether they are simply a manifestation of the fear.

Genetic and Family Factors

Specific phobias and social phobia tend to run in families. It appears that being a first-degree relative of an individual with a specific phobia puts one at a greater risk for a specific phobia compared with first-degree relatives of never mentally ill controls (31% versus 11%). However, the particular phobia that is transmitted is usually different from that in the relative, although it is often from the same general type (e.g., animal, situational). Furthermore, relatives of people with specific phobias are not at increased risk for other types of anxiety disorders (including social phobia) or subclinical fears. There is no increased risk among relatives of people with social phobia to develop other anxiety disorders. A recent study found that in comparison to probands in a comparison group, the relative risk for generalized social phobia and avoidant personality disorder were tenfold for first-degree relatives of probands with social phobia.

Of course, the existence of a disorder in multiple family members does not necessarily imply genetic transmission. Family members often share learning experiences and other environmental factors. To establish a genetic relationship among family members with a particular disorder, twin studies, adoption studies and molecular genetics studies are typically conducted. Currently, there are no adoption or molecular genetics studies of social or specific phobias, and twin studies have yielded conflicting results.

Although there are conflicting findings on whether there is a general genetic factor (influencing risk for any anxiety disorder) or a specific genetic factor (influencing risk for specific anxiety disorders such as specific and social phobias), some general conclusions can be made. In the case of social phobia, there seems to be a moderate (based on the strength of the correlations from twin studies) disorder-specific genetic influence combined with specific and nonspecific environmental influences. In the case of specific phobia, evidence supports a disorder-specific genetic contribution combined with disorder-specific environmental influences (e.g., traumatic conditioning experiences involving the phobic object or situation).

Although the nature of the genetic contribution has yet to be specified (a low threshold for alarm reactions or vasovagal responses is one possibility), specific and social phobias may be related to personality factors that have been found to be highly heritable. Two traits that may be relevant are neuroticism (or emotionality) and extroversion (or sociability). Average heritability estimates for these traits are about 50% across a wide range of genetic studies. Emotionality probably predisposes individuals to develop a range of anxiety and mood disorders whereas sociability may be most relevant to social phobia. Furthermore, certain phobias may have other specific genetic contributions. Up to 70% of individuals with blood phobia report a history of fainting on exposure to blood. It has been suggested that an inherited overactive baroreflex may contribute to the high rate of familial transmission of blood phobias.

Other Biological Factors

In contrast to the situation with other anxiety disorders, little is known about the physiological correlates of specific and social phobias. However, effective drug treatments have been identified for social phobia, leading to an increased interest in the biological factors underlying this disorder. There has been some evidence to suggest a relationship between dopamine and social phobia. Unlike panic disorder, which responds well to a variety of tricyclic antidepressants and monoamine oxidase inhibitors, social phobia tends to have a positive response to MAOIs and shows little response to tricyclic antidepressants. Whereas tricyclic antidepressants tend to act on noradrenergic and serotonergic systems, MAOIs affect noradrenergic, serotonergic and dopaminergic systems. This finding has led some investigators to suggest that the dopamine system is primarily involved in social phobia, which would explain why biological challenges that appear to affect noradrenergic activity (e.g., sodium lactate infusion, carbon dioxide inhalation) have little effect on patients with social phobia, despite having panicogenic effects in patients with panic disorder. The dopamine hypothesis is consistent with findings that dopamine metabolite levels correlate with measures of extroversion as well as findings that mice bred to be timid have been shown to be deficient in brain dopamine concentration.

With respect to neuroendocrine correlates in social phobia, studies of the hypothalamic–pituitary–thyroid and hypothalamic–pituitary–adrenal axes in social phobia have found few differences between patients with social phobia and control persons. Some recent studies have found evidence of cortisol differences associated with social anxiety.

Recent imaging studies have found a number of differences between social phobia patients and controls. One study using functional magnetic resonance imaging (fMRI) found that conditioned aversive stimuli were associated with increased activation in the amygdala and hippocampus of social phobia patients, whereas decreased activation in these areas was observed in normal controls (Schneider *et al.*, 1999). Another study using single photon emission computer tomography (SPECT) found that after an 8-week trial of citalopram there was significantly decreased activity in the anterior and lateral part of the left temporal cortex, the left cingulum and the anterior, lateral and posterior part of the left midfrontal cortex in a small ($N = 15$) sample of social phobia patients (Van der Linden *et al.*, 2000). Compared with treatment responders, treatment nonresponders had higher activity at baseline in the lateral left temporal cortex and the lateral left midfrontal regions. Further research is necessary to understand the significance of these imaging findings as well as their specificity to social phobia.

A few studies have examined patterns of brain activity associated with shyness. In a study on high and low shyness (anxious self-preoccupation and avoidance of social situations) and sociability (preference to be socially active and seek out social situations) in college students, it was found that shyness was associated with greater relative right frontal EEG activity, whereas sociability was associated with greater relative left frontal EEG.

Finally, there may be good reason to consider different underlying mechanisms in patients with performance-related phobias (e.g., public speaking) than in patients with generalized social phobia (i.e., those who fear most social situations). Individuals with performance-related phobias tend to show more autonomic reactivity (e.g., rapid heart beat) in the phobic situation than do patients with generalized social phobia. In addition, beta-blockers such as atenolol may be useful for decreasing performance anxiety in normal individuals, although they have little effect on patients with generalized social phobia. These facts have led some investigators to suggest that adrenergic hyperactivity may be involved in performance anxiety but not in generalized social phobia. However, it should be noted that despite limited evidence for the use of beta-blockers in normal groups (e.g., musicians with performance anxiety), their utility for treating patients with a diagnosis of social phobia (e.g., performance fears that lead to significant distress or impairment) has not been established.

Assessment

Special Issues in Psychiatric Examination and History

During all parts of the initial evaluation, the psychiatrist should be sensitive to several issues. First, for many patients with phobias, even discussing the phobic object can provoke anxiety. For example, some patients with spider phobias experience panic attacks when they discuss spiders. Some patients with blood phobias faint when they discuss surgical procedures. Therefore, the psychiatrist should ask the patient whether discussing the phobic object or situation will provoke anxiety. If the interview is likely to be a source of stress, the psychiatrist should emphasize the importance of the information that is being collected, as well as

the potential therapeutic value of discussing the feared object. As described in a later section, exposure to the feared stimulus is an essential component of the treatment of most specific phobias. Of course, the interviewer should use his or her judgment when deciding how much to push the patient in the first session. For treatment to be effective, establishing trust in the psychiatrist early in the course of treatment is essential.

With respect to social phobia, the assessment itself may be considered a phobic stimulus. Because individuals with social phobia fear the evaluation of others, a psychiatric interview may be especially frightening. Even completing self-report questionnaires in the waiting room may be difficult for patients who fear writing in front of others. The psychiatrist should be sensitive to this possibility and provide reassurance when appropriate.

Structured and Semistructured Interviews

Although there are numerous structured and semistructured interviews available, two of the most commonly used interviews for diagnosing anxiety disorders are the Anxiety Disorders Interview Schedule for DSM-IV (ADIS-IV) (Brown *et al.*, 1994) and the Structured Clinical Interview for Axis I DSM-IV-TR Disorders-Patient Edition (SCID-I/P for DSM-IV-TR) (First *et al.*, 2001). Current and lifetime diagnoses of specific phobia and social phobia based on the ADIS-IV have been shown to have good to excellent reliability for the specific phobia types and the generalized type of social phobia. Each interview has advantages and disadvantages. Although the SCID-I provides detailed assessment of a broader range of disorders relative to the ADIS-IV (including eating disorders and psychotic disorders), the ADIS-IV provides more detailed information on each of the anxiety disorders and, like the SCID-I, includes sections to provide DSM-IV diagnoses for the mood disorders and other disorders that are typically associated with the anxiety disorders (e.g., substance use and somatoform disorders). In addition, the ADIS-IV includes more questions to help differentiate specific and social phobias from other disorders with which they share features.

Self-report Measures

Numerous self-report measures have been created for the assessment of specific phobias and social anxiety. The main advantage of self-report measures is the time that they save for the psychiatrist. Relevant self-report measures are recommended before the clinical interview if possible. This will allow the interviewer to follow up specific responses during the interview. Measures can be administered again, periodically, to assess progress and outcome. It should be noted that questionnaire measures do not always correlate highly with performance on behavioral measures. Furthermore, there is evidence that men are more likely than women to underestimate their fear on specific phobia measures. The most common questionnaires used to screen for specific phobias are the various versions of the Fear Survey Schedule. In addition, a variety of measures exist to assess fear of specific objects and situations. For example, the Mutilation Questionnaire (Klorman *et al.*, 1974) is among the most common tests for assessing fear of situations involving blood and medical procedures. Self-report measures for assessing both specific phobia and social anxiety are listed in Table 50.1.

Behavioral Tests

Behavioral testing is an important part of any comprehensive evaluation for a phobic disorder. This is particularly the case

Table 50.1	Common Measures for Specific and Social Phobias

Specific Phobia

Fear Survey Schedule (FSS)
Fear Questionnaire (FQ)
Fear of Flying Scale (FFS)
Acrophobia Questionnaire (AQ)
Mutilation Questionnaire (MQ)
Medical Fear Survey (MFS)
Dental Anxiety Inventory (DAI)
Claustrophobia Situations Questionnaire (CSQ)

Social Phobia

Social Phobia Inventory (SPIN)
Mini-Social Phobia Inventory (Mini-SPIN)
Social Phobia and Anxiety Inventory (SPAI)
Social Interaction Anxiety Scale (SIAS)
Social Phobia Scale (SPS)

if behavioral or cognitive–behavioral treatment will be used. Because most individuals with phobias avoid the objects and situations that they fear, patients may find it difficult to describe the subtle cues that affect their fear in the situation. In addition, it is not unusual for patients to misjudge the amount of fear that they typically experience in the phobic situation. A behavioral approach test can be useful for identifying specific fear triggers as well as for assessing the intensity of the patient's fear in the actual situation.

To conduct a behavioral approach test, patients should be instructed to enter the phobic situation for several minutes. For example, an individual with a snake phobia should be instructed to stand as close as possible to a live snake and note the specific cues that affect the fear (e.g., size of snake, color, movement) and the intensity of the fear (perhaps rating it on a 0–100-point scale). Patients should pay special attention to their physical sensations (e.g., palpitations, sweating, blushing), negative thoughts (e.g., "I will fall from this balcony") and anxious coping strategies (e.g., escape, avoidance, distraction).

The behavioral approach test will help in the development of a specific treatment plan. However, before treatment patients will often be reluctant to enter the feared situation. If this is the case, the information collected during the behavioral approach test may be elicited during the early part of behavioral treatment.

Differences in Sex, Cultural and Developmental Presentation

Sex Differences

As mentioned earlier, specific phobias tend to be more common among women than men. This finding seems to be strongest for phobias from the animal type, whereas sex differences are smaller for height phobias and blood-injury-injection phobias. In addition, social phobia tends to be slightly more prevalent among women than men, although these differences are relatively small.

There are several reasons why women may be more likely than men to report specific phobias. First, men tend to underreport their fear. Also, women may be more likely than men to seek treatment for their difficulties, which would account for the fact that sex differences are often larger in treatment samples compared with epidemiological samples. In addition sex ratios for phobias differ across cultures, which may be explained by cultural differences in treatment seeking. Finally, the sex difference in prevalence may reflect actual differences between men and women in susceptibility to develop phobias.

Women and men are taught to deal differently with typical phobic stimuli. Traditionally, boys more than girls are often encouraged to play with spiders and toy snakes and to engage in more adventurous activities (e.g., hiking in high places). In addition, women may have more role models for the development of fear than do men. Images of women standing on chairs when they see a mouse or running away from spiders are common in children's cartoons and other media, but men are rarely depicted as being frightened by these objects. Therefore, it is possible that in Western cultures women learn to fear certain situations more strongly than do men. Of course, it is difficult to know whether culture and the media are responsible for sex differences or simply reflect differences that exist for other reasons (e.g., different predisposing factors). It will be interesting to see whether sex ratios for phobias change as traditional gender roles continue to change.

Cultural Differences

Little is known about cultural differences in specific and social phobias. Nevertheless, a few studies bear on the issue of cultural differences in phobias. For example, there is evidence from epidemiological studies that African-Americans are 1.5 to 3 times as likely as whites to report phobic disorders, even after controlling for education and socioeconomic status. Several explanations for this finding have been provided. For example, some of the fears reported by African-American individuals may reflect realistic concerns that were misdiagnosed as phobias. For example, African-American persons in inner city communities may have more realistic reasons to fear violence. Furthermore, African-Americans experience more negative evaluation from others, and some of their social concerns may be realistic. Another possibility is that African-Americans experience more chronic stress than whites and therefore may be more susceptible to the development of phobias and other problems. Finally, there may be cultural differences in response biases on questionnaire measures of fear and during interviews.

Research has found that specific phobias, but not social phobias, are more common among US-born Mexican-Americans than in US-born whites or immigrant Mexican-Americans, after controlling for sex, age, socioeconomic status and various other variables. A variety of studies have shown that specific phobias, social phobia and related conditions exist across cultures. For example, in Japan, a condition exists called *taijin kyôfu* in which individuals have an "obsession of shame". This condition has much overlap with social phobia in that it is often accompanied by fears of blushing, having improper facial expressions in the presence of others, looking at others, shaking and perspiring in front of others. In addition, studies have identified individuals with social and specific phobias in a variety of other nonWestern countries including Saudi Arabia, India, Japan and other East Asian countries. Interestingly, in some other cultures, the sex ratio for phobias tends to be reversed. For example, in studies from Saudi Arabia and India, up to 80% of individuals reporting for treatment of phobias were male.

Psychiatrists treating patients from different cultures should be aware of cultural differences in presentation and response to treatment, such as cultural differences in verbal communication styles, proxemics (i.e., use of interpersonal space), nonverbal communication and other verbal cues (e.g., tone and loudness). Many cues that a psychiatrist might use to aid in the diagnosis of social phobia in white Americans may not be useful for diagnosing the condition in other cultures. For example, although many psychiatrists interpret a lack of eye contact as indicating shyness or a lack of assertiveness, avoidance of eye contact among Japanese and Mexican-Americans is often viewed as a sign of respect. In contrast to white Americans, Japanese are apparently more likely to view smiling as a sign of embarrassment or discomfort. Furthermore, cultural differences in tone and volume of speech may lead psychiatrists to misinterpret their patients. For example, whereas white Americans are often uncomfortable with silence in a conversation, British and Arab individuals may be more likely to use silence for privacy and other cultures use silence to indicate agreement among the parties or a sign of respect. In addition, Asian individuals have been reported to speak more quietly than white Americans, who in turn speak more quietly than those from Arab countries. Therefore, differences in the volume of speech should not be taken to imply differences in assertiveness or other indicators of social anxiety.

Treatment methods may have to be adapted for different cultures. For example, the direct style of many cognitive and behavioral therapists may be more likely to be perceived as rude or insensitive by individuals with certain cultural backgrounds than those with other backgrounds. It should be noted that individuals within a culture differ on these variables just as individuals across cultures differ. Therefore, although psychiatrists should be aware of cultural differences, these differences should not blind the psychiatrist to relevant factors that are unique to each individual patient.

Developmental Differences

Among children, specific and social fears are common. Because these fears may be transient, DSM-IV-TR has included a provision that social and specific phobias not be assigned in children unless they are present for more than 6 months. In addition, children may be less likely than adults to recognize that their phobia is excessive or unrealistic. The specific objects feared by children are often similar to those feared by adults, although children may be more likely to fear objects and situations that are not easily classified in the four main specific phobia types in DSM-IV-TR (e.g., balloons or costumed characters). In addition, children often report specific and social phobias having to do with school. Children with social phobia tend to avoid changing for gym class in front of others, eating in the cafeteria, or speaking in front of the class. They may stay home sick on days when frightening situations arise or may make frequent trips to the school nurse. Whereas some investigators have found that boys and girls are equally likely to present for treatment of phobias, others have found social phobia to be more common among girls. In one prospective study of childhood anxiety disorders, Last and colleagues (1996) found that almost 70% of children with a specific phobia were recovered over a 3- to 4-year period compared with a recovery rate of 86% for social phobia. Thus, almost a third of the clinical sample with specific phobia had symptoms that still met clinical criteria for specific phobia at the end of the follow-up period. This was the lowest recovery rate among the anxiety disorders that were studied. However, those in the clinical sample with specific phobia had the lowest rate of development of new psychiatric disorders (15%) compared with the other anxiety disorders studied (e.g., the rate of development for new psychiatric disorders was 22% for those in the clinical sample with social phobia).

Diagnosis and Differential Diagnosis

Panic disorder with agoraphobia may easily be misdiagnosed as social phobia or a specific phobia (especially the situational type). For example, many patients with panic disorder avoid a variety of social situations because of anxiety about having others notice their symptoms. In addition, some individuals with panic disorder may avoid circumscribed situations, such as flying, despite reporting no other significant avoidance. Four variables should be considered in making the differential diagnosis: 1) type and number of panic attacks; 2) focus of apprehension; 3) number of situations avoided; and 4) level of intercurrent anxiety.

Patients with panic disorder experience unexpected panic attacks and heightened anxiety outside of the phobic situation, whereas those with specific and social phobias typically do not. In addition, individuals with panic disorder are more likely than those with specific and social phobias to report fear and avoidance of a broad range of situations typically associated with agoraphobia (e.g., flying, enclosed places, crowds, being alone, shopping malls). Finally, patients with panic disorder are typically concerned only about the possibility of panicking in the phobic situation or about the consequences of panicking (e.g., being embarrassed by one's panic symptoms). In contrast, individuals with specific and social phobias are usually concerned about other aspects of the situation as well (e.g., being hit by another driver, saying something foolish).

Consider two examples in which the differential diagnosis with panic disorder might be especially difficult. First, individuals with claustrophobia are typically extremely concerned about being unable to escape from the phobic situation as well as being unable to breathe in the situation. Therefore, like patients with panic disorder and agoraphobia, they usually report heightened anxiety about the possibility of panicking. The main variable to consider in such a case is the presence of panic attacks outside of claustrophobic situations. If panic attacks occur exclusively in enclosed places, a diagnosis of specific phobia might best describe the problem. In contrast, if the patient has unexpected or uncued panic attacks as well, a diagnosis of panic disorder might be more appropriate.

A second example is a patient who avoids a broad range of situations including shopping malls, supermarkets, walking on busy streets, and various social situations including parties, meetings and public speaking. Without more information, this patient's problem might appear to meet criteria for social phobia, panic disorder with agoraphobia, or both diagnoses. As mentioned earlier, patients with panic disorder often avoid social situations because of anxiety about panicking in public. In addition, patients with social phobia might avoid situations that are typically avoided by individuals with agoraphobia for fear of seeing someone that they know or of being observed by strangers. To make the diagnosis in this case, it is necessary to assess the reasons for avoidance.

Other diagnoses that should be considered before a diagnosis of specific phobia is assigned include post traumatic stress disorder (PTSD) (if the fear follows a life-threatening trauma and is accompanied by other PTSD symptoms such as reexperiencing the trauma), obsessive–compulsive disorder (if the fear is related to an obsession, e.g., contamination), hypochondriasis (if the fear is related to a belief that he or she has some serious illness), separation-anxiety disorder (if the fear is of situations that might lead to separation from the family, for example, traveling on an airplane without one's parents), eating disorders (if the fear is of eating certain foods but not related to a fear of choking) and psychotic disorders (if the fear is related to a delusion).

Social phobia should not be diagnosed if the fear is related entirely to another disorder. For example, if an individual with obsessive–compulsive disorder avoids social situations only because of the embarrassment of having others notice her or his excessive hand washing, a diagnosis of social phobia would not be given. Furthermore, individuals with depression, schizoid personality disorder, or a pervasive developmental disorder may avoid social situations because of a lack of interest in spending time with others. To be considered social phobia, an individual must avoid these situations specifically because of anxiety about being evaluated negatively.

In the case of generalized social phobia, the diagnosis of avoidant personality disorder should be considered as well. Individuals with avoidant personality disorder tend to display more interpersonal sensitivity and have poorer social skills than social phobic patients without avoidant personality disorder. Furthermore, most studies suggest that the differences between avoidant personality disorder and social phobia are more quantitative than qualitative and that the former may simply be a more severe form of the latter. Therefore, most patients who meet criteria for avoidant personality disorder will meet criteria for social phobia as well.

Finally, social and specific phobias should be distinguished from normal states of fear and anxiety. Many individuals report mild fears of circumscribed situations or mild shyness in certain social situations. Others may report intense fears of public speaking or heights but insist that these situations rarely arise and that they have no interest in being in these situations. For the criteria for a specific or social phobia to be met, the individual must report significant distress about having the fear or must report significant impairment in functioning.

A variety of factors should be considered in deciding whether a patient's fear exceeds the threshold necessary for a diagnosis of specific or social phobia. To make the differential diagnosis between normal fears and clinical phobias, the psychiatrist should consider the extent of the individual's avoidance, the frequency with which the phobic stimulus is encountered, and the degree to which the individual is bothered by having the fear. For example, an individual who fears seeing snakes in the wild but who lives in the city never encounters snakes, and never even thinks about snakes would probably not be diagnosed with a specific phobia. In contrast, when an individual's fear of snakes leads to avoidance of walking through parks, camping, swimming and watching certain television programs, despite having an interest in doing these things, a diagnosis of specific phobia would be appropriate.

Similar factors should be considered in deciding at what point normal shyness reaches an intensity that warrants a diagnosis of social phobia. An individual who is somewhat quiet in groups or when meeting new people but does not avoid these situations and is not especially distressed by his or her shyness would probably not receive a diagnosis of social phobia. In contrast, an individual who frequently refuses invitations to socialize because of anxiety, quits a job because of anxiety about having to talk to customers, or is distressed about her or his social anxiety would be likely to receive a diagnosis of social phobia.

Diagnostic decision trees for social and specific phobias are presented in Figures 50.1 and 50.2.

Specific Phobia Phenomenology and Subtypes

DSM-IV defines five main types of specific phobia: animal, natural environment, blood-injection-injury, situational and other. These types were introduced on the basis of a series of reports showing that specific phobia types tend to differ on a variety of dimensions including age at onset, sex composition, patterns of covariation among phobias, focus of apprehension, timing and predictability of the phobic response, and type of physiological reaction during exposure to the phobic situation.

Although anxiety about physical sensations and the occurrence of panic is a feature typically associated with panic disorder, several studies have shown that panic-focused and symptom-focused apprehensions are not unique to panic disorder and agoraphobia. Individuals with specific phobias tend to report anxiety about the sensations (e.g., racing heart, breathlessness, dizziness) typically associated with their fear. Also, there is evidence that in addition to fearing danger from the phobic object (e.g., a plane crash, being bitten by a dog) many individuals with specific phobias fear danger as a result of their reaction in the phobic situation (e.g., having a panic attack, losing control, being embarrassed). Also, the few relevant studies that have been conducted suggest that there may be differences in sensation-focused apprehension across specific phobia types.

Data are converging to indicate that individuals with phobias from the situational (e.g., claustrophobia) and blood-injury-injection types may be especially internally focused on their fear. Whereas individuals with situational phobias tend to fear the possible consequences of panic, those with blood-injury-injection phobias seem uniquely concerned about sensations that indicate that fainting is imminent (e.g., lightheadedness, hot flashes). Delayed and unpredictable panic attacks may be more characteristic of situational phobias than of other phobia types, consistent with the argument that situational phobias share more features with agoraphobia than do other specific phobia types.

Perhaps the most consistent difference among specific phobia types is the tendency for individuals with blood-injury-injection phobias to report a history of fainting in the phobic situation. Although all phobia types are associated with panic attacks in the phobic situation, only patients with blood and injection phobias report fainting. The different responses experienced in different phobias have been explained from an evolutionary perspective. As mentioned earlier, the typical phobic responses of fear and panic are adaptive in that the increased arousal facilitates escape. In contrast, the most adaptive response during serious injury may be a drop in blood pressure to prevent excessive bleeding. It has been suggested that this response is mediated by an overactive

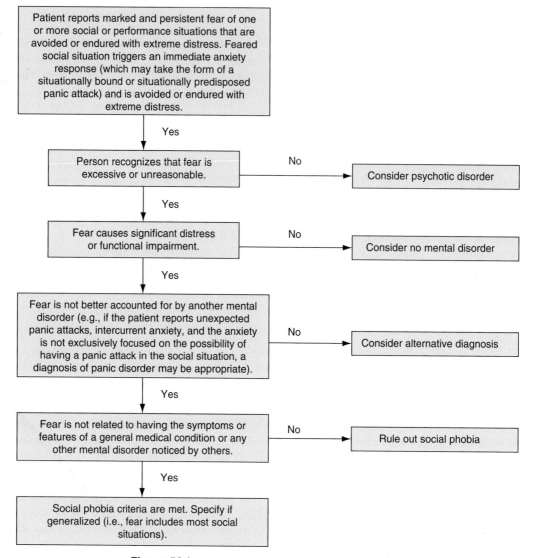

Figure 50.1 *Diagnostic decision tree for social phobia.*

sinoaortic baroreflex that is triggered by heightened arousal in situations involving blood or needles. Of course, in people with blood and injection phobias, the response is excessive and unwarranted, as there is typically no danger of excessive blood loss.

Social Phobia Phenomenology and Subtypes

Many researchers in the area of social phobia tend to classify the disorder into two main subtypes. DSM-IV requires that diagnosticians specify whether a social phobia diagnosis is "generalized", or includes most social situations. In addition, a "discrete or circumscribed" subtype is often used by investigators to describe patients with only one domain of social anxiety, usually involving performance-related situations (e.g., public speaking).

Several studies have examined differences among these subtypes. Specifically, patients with generalized social phobias tend to be younger, less educated and less likely to be employed than are patients with discrete social phobias. In addition, generalized social phobias are associated with more depression, anxiety, general distress and concerns about negative evaluation from others. Discrete social phobias appear to be associated with greater cardiac reactivity.

Epidemiology and Comorbidity

Prevalence and Incidence

Phobias are among the most common psychiatric disorders. Findings based on large community samples from five sites in the Epidemiological Catchment Area (ECA) study (Eaton *et al.*, 1991) yielded lifetime prevalence estimates of 11.25% for specific phobias and 2.73% for social phobia. Estimates from the National Comorbidity Survey (NCS) (Kessler *et al.*, 1994) were consistent with previous findings on specific phobias: a lifetime prevalence of 11.30% in a sample of more than 8000 individuals from across the USA. The recent NCS-Replication study found lifetime prevalence rates of 12.5% and 12.1 respectively for specific phobia and social phobia (Kessler *et al.*, 2005).

Specific phobias are more common in women than in men, although there are differences in sex ratio among phobia types. Specifically, the ratio of females to males is smaller for height phobias than for other specific phobia types. Among social phobia situations, sex differences are less pronounced than for most specific phobia types. In the NCS, relatively small sex differences in social phobia prevalence were confirmed, with lifetime estimates of 11.1% for males and 15.5% for females. In addition,

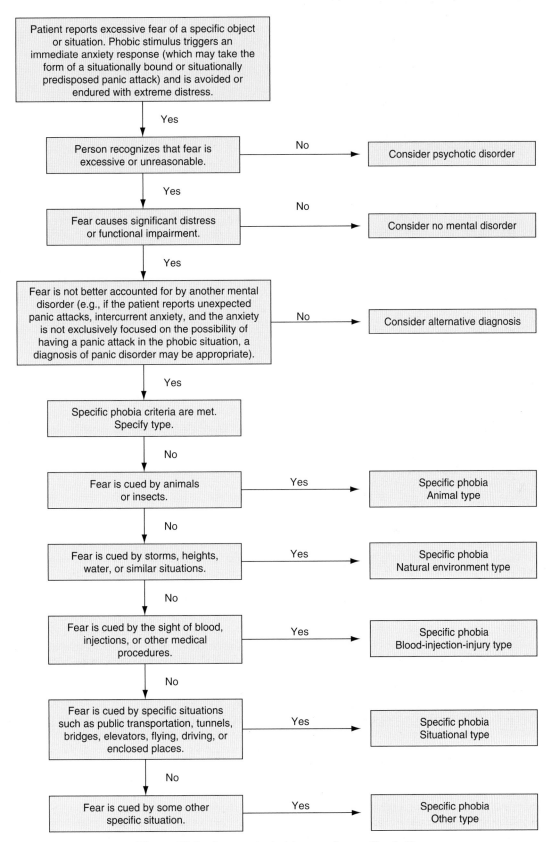

Figure 50.2 *Diagnostic decision tree for specific phobia.*

the relatively equal numbers of men and women with social phobia in epidemiological studies is consistent with findings from samples of individuals presenting for treatment.

Most studies have found the mean age at onset of social phobia to be in the middle to late teens. This is supported by research finding that social phobia is common in children and is diagnosed in a significant percentage of children referred to a specialty anxiety disorders clinic. A history of childhood anxiety has been associated with an earlier age of onset of social phobia as well as greater severity and comorbidity. Mean age at onset for specific phobias appears to differ depending on the type of phobia. Phobias of animals, blood, storms and water tend to begin in early childhood, whereas phobias of heights tend to begin in the teens, and phobias of the situational type (e.g., claustrophobia) begin even later, with mean ages at onset in the late teens to middle twenties.

Comorbidity Patterns

The issue of comorbidity is important for several reasons. First, covariation among disorders provides valuable information about the nature of specific disorders as well as the utility of current diagnostic nomenclature. For example, high rates of cooccurrence between two disorders could reflect overlap in the definitions of two disorders (as may be the case with social phobia and avoidant personality disorder) or shared etiological pathways. In addition, comorbidity may have implications for treatment. For example, an individual with social phobia who abuses alcohol might be less likely to benefit from treatment for social phobia if the alcohol abuse affects compliance with the social phobia treatment.

Specific Phobias

About 70% of individuals with blood phobias tend to have injection phobias as well. In addition, numerous factor analytical studies have found that blood-injection-injury phobias tend to cluster together as do animal phobias, natural environment phobias and situational phobias. In other words, having a phobia of one specific phobia type makes an individual more likely to have additional phobias of the same type than of other types. However, the clustering is not perfect and many studies show exceptions to this pattern. The research on the classification of specific phobia types is inconsistent. For example, in several of these studies, height phobias tend to be associated with situational phobias (e.g., claustrophobia), despite height phobias being listed as an example of the natural environment type in DSM-IV.

Specific phobias tend to cooccur with other specific phobias. A recent methodologically rigorous study found that 15% of patients with a principal diagnosis of specific phobia also met criteria for another type of specific phobia and that 33% of patients presenting with a principal diagnosis of specific phobia had additional symptoms that met criteria for an Axis I anxiety or mood disorder (Brown *et al.*, 2001a). However, compared with individuals who have other anxiety disorders, individuals with principal diagnoses of a specific phobia are less likely to have additional diagnoses. Rather, specific phobias typically occur on their own or as additional diagnoses of lesser severity than the principal diagnosis. Studies confirm that specific phobias are a frequently occurring additional diagnosis, particularly with other anxiety disorders. However, specific phobias tend to occur less frequently in the context of other disorders such as depression (and alcohol use disorders.

Whereas the above mentioned studies reflect "syndrome" comorbidity, one can also discuss comorbidity at the "symptom"

level. In other words, one can examine the frequency with which specific fears are associated with disorders regardless of whether they meet criteria for specific phobia. It appears that specific phobias commonly occur as additional diagnoses, at both clinical and subclinical levels.

Social Phobia

Social anxiety is a feature of many disorders. Individuals with panic disorder, obsessive–compulsive disorder, or eating disorders often avoid social situations because of the possibility of being judged negatively if their symptoms are noticed by others. However, to meet diagnostic criteria for social phobia, one's concerns must not be exclusively related to the symptoms of another disorder. With this criterion in mind, social phobia still tends to be associated with a variety of other DSM-IV disorders. Furthermore, unlike specific phobias, social phobia is frequently associated with additional disorders of lesser severity. One study conducted in two outpatient clinics in a managed care setting found a comorbidity rate of 43.6% in patients with generalized social phobia (Katzelnick *et al.*, 2001). In another study, almost 60% of patients with social phobia had additional symptoms that met criteria for one or more additional diagnoses (Sanderson *et al.*, 1990). The most frequently assigned additional diagnoses in this study were specific phobias (25%), dysthymia (21%) and panic disorder with agoraphobia (17%). The presence of comorbid mood disorders has been associated with a greater duration of social phobia as well as more severe impairment before and after cognitive–behavioral therapy (CBT). Other studies have found that panic disorder with or without agoraphobia, generalized anxiety disorder, major depressive disorder and substance abuse are common additional diagnoses as well. In one prospective study, an estimated relative risk ratio of 2.30 for alcohol abuse or dependence was found in individuals with subclinical social phobia relative to individuals without social phobia or subclinical social fears, suggesting that individuals with subclinical social phobia were more than twice as likely to develop alcohol use disorders than were individuals without social phobia or subclinical social anxiety (Crum and Pratt, 2001).

As an additional diagnosis, social phobia is often assigned in patients with panic disorder with agoraphobia, generalized anxiety disorder, obsessive–compulsive disorder and major depressive disorder. Social phobia is also common among patients with eating disorders and alcohol abuse. When social phobia coexists with a mood disorder, substance abuse disorder, or another anxiety disorder, the social phobia tends to predate the other disorder. Treatment of these disorders should include components that address the social phobia when both disorders occur together.

Course and Natural History

As discussed earlier, the mean age at onset of social phobia is in the middle teens. The age at onset of specific phobias varies depending on the phobia type, with phobias of animals, blood, storms and water tending to begin in early childhood, phobias of heights beginning in the teens, and situational phobias beginning in the late teens to middle twenties. Although childhood fears are often transient (e.g., most children outgrow fear of the dark without treatment), fears that persist into adulthood usually have a chronic course unless treated.

Although many phobias begin after a traumatic event, many patients do not recall the specific onset of their fear, and

Ms K is a 29-year-old student who presented with social phobia. She reported being shy as a child and could remember pretending to be ill to stay home from school. As she got older, she met more children and by high school was quite comfortable with her friends at school. Meeting new people was still difficult, as was public speaking in class. Fortunately, neither situation came up often.

In college, Ms K's problem became worse. Several of her classes required her to make presentations. In addition, because she lived off campus, she found it particularly difficult to meet friends. The few times she tried to talk to people in class, she felt as though she had nothing to say. Before long, she stopped trying. Ms K did not avoid her class presentations at first. Rather, she tended to overprepare for them and tried to use overheads when possible because the dark room helped to decrease her anxiety. Still during presentations she could feel her heart pounding and she tended to have difficulty breathing. Her mouth became dry and she was sure that her classmates could see her shaking and perspiring.

After her first year of college, Ms K began to avoid any class that required presentations. In addition, she found herself avoiding other situations in which people might notice her shaking. Specifically, she avoided writing in front of others, holding drinking glasses and other situations that might focus other people's attention on her hands. She also avoided engaging in conversation with others and when people approached her, she tried to end the conversation as quickly as possible. In addition to fearing that others would notice her anxiety, Ms K felt that others might see her as weak, unattractive, or foolish.

During a diagnostic interview, it was found that Ms K was suffering from social phobia. She seemed bright and motivated, and it was decided that she might benefit from CBGT for social phobia. However, the patient initially rejected this option because of anxiety about participating in a group. Therefore, she started 10 mg of paroxetine and gradually increased the dosage to 50 mg. Because of difficulties due to sexual dysfunction, the dosage was decreased to 40 mg and her sexual symptoms subsided.

During a period of 6 weeks, Ms K felt more comfortable around people and decided that she was willing to participate in a 12-session CBGT program. Treatment included a variety of components, including information about the nature of anxiety and social phobia, cognitive restructuring, role-play exposures to anxiety-provoking situations (e.g., group presentations) and homework assignments to enter feared situations. In addition, Ms K practiced purposely shaking in front of others, until the symptom was no longer frightening to her. Over the course of the CBGT, Ms K's medication was gradually discontinued. By the end of treatment, Ms K was essentially symptom free and criteria for social phobia were no longer met. Furthermore, she had met several new friends and had enrolled in a few classes that required her to make presentations. Although she still became nervous before speaking in public, she looked forward to the presentations. She rarely experienced shaking in front of others and was no longer particularly concerned about shaking.

few empirical data have examined the initial period after the fear onset. Clinically, however, some patients report a sudden onset of fear, whereas others report a more gradual onset. Studies examining the onset of phobias have tended to assess the onset of the **fear** rather than the onset of the **phobia** (i.e., the point at which the fear creates significant distress or functional impairment). A study by Antony and colleagues (1997) suggests that the fear and phobia onset are often not the same. Patients with specific phobias of heights, animals, blood-injection, or driving were asked to estimate the earliest age at which they could recall having their fear and the earliest age at which they could recall experiencing distress or functional impairment due to their fear. Anecdotally, the types of factors leading to the transition from fear to phobia included gradual increases in the intensity of fear, additional traumatic events (e.g., panic attacks, car accidents), increased life stress and changes in living situation (e.g., starting a job that requires exposure to heights). Similarly, it is not unusual for individuals with social phobia to report having been shy as children, although their anxiety may not have reached phobic proportions until later.

Treatment

Goals and Nature of Treatment

The main goal of treatment is to decrease fear and phobic avoidance to a level that no longer causes significant distress or functional impairment. In some cases, treatment includes strategies for improving specific skill deficits as well. For example, individuals with social phobia may lack adequate social skills and can sometimes benefit from social skills training. Likewise, some individuals with specific phobias of driving may have poor driving skills if their fear prevented them from learning how to drive properly. Typically, effective treatment for social phobia lasts several months, although treatment of discrete social phobias (e.g., public speaking) may take less time. Specific phobias can usually be treated relatively quickly. In fact, for certain phobias, the vast majority of individuals are able to achieve clinically significant, long-lasting improvement in as little as one session of behavioral treatment.

Effective treatments fall into one of two main categories: pharmacological treatment and CBT. Pharmacological treatments have been used effectively for treating social phobia, although it is generally accepted that they are of limited utility for treating specific phobias. In contrast, CBT has been used with success for the treatment of specific and social phobias. Despite the existence of effective treatments, fewer than half of those who seek treatment in an anxiety disorders specialty clinic have previously received evidence-based treatments for their social anxiety (Rowa *et al.*, 2000). Tables 50.2 and 50.3 summarize various treatments for social and specific phobias.

Pharmacotherapy

Specific Phobia

Pharmacotherapy is generally thought to be ineffective for specific phobias. However, little research has been conducted to assess the utility of medications for specific phobias, and it is not uncommon for phobic patients occasionally to be prescribed low dosages of benzodiazepines to be taken in the phobic situation (e.g., while flying). The few relevant studies that have been conducted have

Table 50.2   Treatments for Social Phobia

Treatment	Advantages	Disadvantages	Rating
Cognitive–behavioral therapy (CBT) (e.g., exposure, cognitive restructuring, social skills training, education)	Good treatment response Brief course of treatment Treatment gains maintained at follow-up Considered first line	May lead to temporary increases in discomfort or fear.	++++
SSRIs (e.g., paroxetine, fluvoxamine, sertraline)	Good treatment response Early response, relative to CBT Broad spectrum efficacy for comorbid disorders (i.e., depression) Lack of abuse potential Considered first line	Side effects are common. Cost is a factor. May be a risk of relapse after discontinuation.	+++
Moclobemide	Good treatment response in some studies Fewer side effects than phenelzine Considered second line	Side effects common. Does not separate from placebo in some studies. Potential exists for relapse after discontinuation	++
Benzodiazepines (e.g., clonazepam, alprazolam)	Good treatment response Considered adjunctive or second line	Side effects and withdrawal occur. Potential for abuse. Relapse after discontinuation is likely. Does not treat certain comorbid conditions (i.e., depression)	++
MAOIs (e.g., phenelzine)	Good treatment response Early response Considered third line	Relatively high rate of adverse effects. Dietary restrictions must be followed. Numerous drug interactions. Potential exists for relapse after discontinuation.	++
Gabapentin	Possibly beneficial Considered third line	Side effects are common. More research is needed	++
β-blockers (e.g., atenolol)	Appears to be useful for "stage fright" in actors, musicians, and other performers	Drugs are not effective for generalized social phobia. Benefits for discrete social phobias are questionable. Side effects occur. Potential exists for relapse after discontinuation.	+

+++++ First treatment of choice. Helpful for most patients, with few side effects. Good long-term benefits.
+++ Helpful for most patients. Potential for relapse after treatment is discontinued.
++ More controlled research needed, although preliminary studies suggest potential benefit OR research has been mixed.
+ Not especially effective for generalized social phobia.

examined the use of benzodiazepines and beta-blockers alone or in combination with behavioral treatments for specific phobias and in general have found that drugs do not contribute much to the treatment of specific phobias. However, one problem with the research to date is that it has not taken into account differences among specific phobia types. For example, claustrophobia and other phobias of the situational type appear to share more features with panic disorder than with the other specific phobia types. Therefore, medications that are effective for panic disorder (e.g., imipramine, alprazolam) may prove to be effective for situational phobias. Although there are few studies examining this hypothe-

sis, preliminary data suggest that benzodiazepines may be helpful in the short term but lead to greater relapse in the long term and possibly interfere with the therapeutic effects of exposure across sessions. There have been very few controlled studies to date examining the effectiveness of antidepressants for specific phobia.

Social Phobia

In contrast to specific phobias, social phobia has been treated successfully with a variety of pharmacological interventions including SSRIs such as sertraline, fluvoxamine and paroxetine, benzodiazepines such as alprazolam, traditional monoamine

Table 50.3	Treatments for Specific Phobias		
Treatment	Advantages	Disadvantages	Rating
In vivo exposure	Highly effective Early response Treatment gains maintained at follow-up	May lead to temporary increases in discomfort or fear.	++++
Applied tension	Highly effective for patients with blood-injection phobias who faint Early response Treatment gains maintained at follow-up	Treatment is relevant for a small percentage of patients with specific phobias.	+++
Applied relaxation	May be effective for some patients	Treatment has not been extensively researched for specific phobias.	++
Cognitive therapy	May help to reduce anxiety about conducting exposure exercises	Treatment has not been extensively researched for specific phobias. Treatment is probably not effective alone.	++
Benzodiazepines	May reduce anticipatory anxiety before patient enters phobic situation, and may reduce fear, particularly in situational specific phobias	Treatment has not been extensively researched for specific phobias. Treatment is probably not effective alone, in many cases. Side effects (e.g., sedation) occur. Discontinuation of symptoms may undermine benefits of treatment.	
SSRIs	May reduce panic sensations for individuals with situational phobias that are similar to panic disorder (e.g., claustrophobia)	Treatment has not been extensively researched for specific phobias. There are a few studies (primarily case reports) with promising results. Discontinuation of medication may result in a return of fear.	++

++++ Treatment of choice. Effective for almost all patients.
+++ Very effective for a subset of patients.
++ May be helpful for some patients. More research needed.

oxidase inhibitors (MAOIs) such as phenelzine and reversible inhibitors of monoamine oxidase A (RIMA), such as moclobemide and brofaromine.

Numerous controlled trials across a range of SSRIs including sertraline, fluvoxamine and paroxetine have demonstrated their effectiveness in the treatment of social phobia, such that the SSRIs are currently considered the first-line medication treatment. Due to their tolerability and efficacy, the SSRIs have been referred to as "the new gold standard" in pharmacological treatment for social phobia. Uncontrolled open trials and case series studies with citalopram and fluoxetine suggest that these SSRIs may also be beneficial in the treatment of social phobia. Another benefit of SSRIs is their broad spectrum efficacy for common comorbid disorders such as depression and panic disorder.

Research on the use of anxiolytics for the treatment of social phobia have focused on high potency benzodiazepines (e.g., clonazepam, alprazolam) and the nonbenzodiazepine buspirone. Several studies have examined the significant utility of clonazepam for treating social phobia. Alprazolam may also be effective but there are too few studies to establish this. The findings on buspirone are mixed.

Due to the potentially severe side effects of MAOIs as well as the necessity for certain dietary restrictions, they are not recommended as a first-line treatment. The findings from more recent trials involving RIMAs have been less encouraging than initial studies suggested. Discontinuation of MAOIs and RIMAs have been associated with a tendency to relapse.

Research on beta-blockers indicates that they are no better than placebo for most patients with generalized social phobia. Although beta-blockers have been used to treat individuals from nonpatient samples with heightened performance anxiety (e.g., people with public speaking anxiety, musicians with stage fright), their efficacy for treating individuals with discrete social phobia has not been established. Nevertheless, beta-blockers are often prescribed for discrete performance-related social phobias. Preliminary findings suggest that gabapentin, a medication typically used in the treatment of partial seizures, may be effective in the treatment of social phobia, but more research is needed to confirm this finding.

Psychosocial Treatments

Specific Phobias

Numerous studies have shown that exposure-based treatments are effective for helping patients to overcome a variety of specific phobias including fears of blood, injections dentists, spiders, snakes, rats), enclosed places, thunder and lightning, water, flying, heights, choking and balloons. Furthermore, the way in which exposure is conducted may make a difference. Exposure-based treatments can vary on a variety of dimensions including the degree of therapist involvement, duration and intensity of exposure, frequency and number of sessions, and the degree to which the feared situation is confronted in imagination versus in real life. In addition, because individuals with certain specific phobias often report a fear of panicking in the feared situation, investigators have suggested that adding various panic management strategies (e.g., cognitive restructuring, exposure to feared sensations) may help to increase the efficacy of behavioral treatments for specific phobias. It remains to be shown whether the addition of these strategies will improve the efficacy of treatments that include only exposure.

Exposure seems to work best when sessions are spaced close together. Secondly, prolonged exposure seems to be more effective than exposure of shorter duration. Thirdly, during exposure sessions, patients should be discouraged from engaging in subtle avoidance strategies (e.g., distraction) and over-reliance on safety signals (e.g., being accompanied by one's spouse during exposure). Fourth, real-life exposure is more effective than exposure in imagination. Fifthly, exposure with some degree of therapist involvement seems to be more effective than exposure that is exclusively conducted without the therapist present. Exposure may be conducted gradually or quickly. Both approaches seem to work equally well, although patients may be more compliant with a gradual approach. Finally, in the case of blood and injection phobias, the technique called applied muscle tension should be considered as an alternative or addition to exposure therapy. Applied muscle tension involves having patients repeatedly tense their muscles, which leads to a temporary increase in blood pressure and prevents fainting upon exposure to blood or medical procedures.

Cognitive strategies have also been used either alone or in conjunction with exposure for treating specific phobias. The evidence suggests that the addition of cognitive strategies to exposure may provide added benefit for some individuals. For a detailed guide to integrating cognitive strategies with exposure see Antony and Swinson (2000).

Specific phobias are among the most treatable of the anxiety disorders. For example, in as little as one session of guided exposure lasting 2 to 3 hours, the majority of individuals with animal or injection phobias are judged much improved or completely recovered. A recent study demonstrated that one session of exposure treatment was effective in the treatment of children and adolescents with various specific phobias and exposure conducted with a parent present was equally effective as exposure treatment conducted alone. However, despite how straightforward the concept of exposure may seem, many subtle clinical issues can lead to problems in implementing exposure-based treatments. For example, although a patient might be compliant with therapist-assisted exposure practices, he or she may refuse to attempt exposure practices alone between sessions. In such cases, involving a spouse or other family member as a coach during practices at home may help. In addition, gradually increasing the distance between therapist and patient during the therapist-assisted exposures will help the patient to feel comfortable when practicing alone. However, to maintain the patient's trust and to maximize the effectiveness of behavioral interventions, it is important that exposure practices proceed in a predictable way, so that the patient is not surprised by unexpected events. Several

self-help books and manuals for treating a range of specific phobias have been published in the past decade. Whereas some of these manuals were developed to be used with the assistance of a therapist (Bourne, 1998; Antony et al., 1995; Craske et al., 1997), others were developed for self-administration (Brown, 1996).

Recent developments in technology have started to have an impact on the treatment of specific phobias. Videotapes are commonly used to show feared stimuli to patients during exposure. Computer administered treatments have also been used. More recent is the use of virtual reality to expose patients to simulated situations that are more difficult to replicate *in vivo* such as flying (Kahan et al., 2000) and heights (Rothbaum et al., 1995). Emerging data on the effectiveness of virtual reality is encouraging. However, other preliminary studies indicate that *in vivo* exposure is still superior (Dewis et al., 2001).

Social Phobia

Empirically validated psychosocial interventions for social phobia have primarily come from a cognitive–behavioral perspective and include four main types of treatment: 1) exposure-based strategies; 2) cognitive therapy; 3) social skills training; and 4) applied relaxation. Exposure-based treatments involve repeatedly approaching fear-provoking situations until they no longer elicit fear. Through repeated exposure, patients learn that their fearful predictions do not come true despite their having confronted the situation. Table 50.4 illustrates an example of an exposure hierarchy that might be used to structure a patient's exposure practices. An exposure hierarchy is a list of feared situations that are rank ordered by difficulty and used to guide exposure practices for phobic disorders including social phobia and specific phobia. The patient and therapist generate a list of situations that the patient finds anxiety provoking. Items are placed in descending order from most anxiety provoking to least anxiety provoking, and each item is rated with respect to how anxious the patient might be to practice the item. Exposure practices are designed to help the patient become more comfortable engaging in the activities from the hierarchy. Cognitive therapy helps patients identify and change anxious thoughts (e.g., "Others will think I am stupid

Table 50.4	Exposure Hierarchy for Generalized Social Phobia	
Item	Fear Rating (0–100)
Have a party and invite everyone from work.	99
Go to work Christmas party for 1 h without drinking	90
Invite Cindy to have dinner and see a movie.	85
Go for a job interview	80
Ask boss for a day off from work	65
Ask questions in a meeting at work	65
Eat lunch with coworkers	60
Talk to a stranger on the bus	50
Talk to cousin on the telephone for 10 min	40
Ask for directions at the gas station.	35

if I participate in a conversation at work") by teaching them to consider alternative ways of interpreting situations and to examine the evidence for their anxious beliefs. Social skills training is designed to help patients to become more socially competent when they interact with others. Treatment strategies may include modeling, behavioral rehearsal, corrective feedback, social reinforcement and homework assignments. Finally, applied relaxation involves learning to relax one's muscles during rest, during movement and eventually in anxiety-provoking social situations.

Although these methods are presented as four distinct treatment approaches, there is often overlap among the various treatments. Social skills training typically requires exposure to the phobic situation so that new skills may be practiced (e.g., behavioral rehearsal). The same may be said of applied relaxation, which includes learning to conduct relaxation exercises in the phobic situation. In fact, most treatments for social phobia involve some type of exposure to anxiety-provoking social interactions and performance-related tasks. Furthermore, many cognitive–behavioral therapists treat patients using several different strategies delivered in a comprehensive package.

Studies demonstrating the efficacy of CBT for social phobia are too numerous to describe in detail. Several studies have compared various cognitive–behavioral strategies and their combinations for treating social phobia. For example, Wlazlo and colleagues (1990) compared social skills training to exposure therapy conducted either individually or in groups. All three treatments led to significant improvements and there were no differences between treatments. However, exposure therapy conducted in groups tended to be more effective for the subset of patients with social skills deficits, most likely by enabling those individuals with deficits to develop their skills through exposure to social situations and interactions in the group. There is conflicting evidence that guided exposure is more effective when cognitive therapy is included than when exposure is conducted without cognitive therapy.

Heimberg and colleagues (1990) compared supportive psychotherapy with a comprehensive CBGT package that included exposure to simulated and real social situations as well as cognitive restructuring for the treatment of social phobia. Although both groups improved on most measures, patients receiving CBGT were significantly more improved immediately after treatment and at 3- and 6-month follow-up. CBGT was more effective despite that patient ratings of treatment credibility and expectations for improvement were equal for both treatments. Patients receiving CBGT continued to be more improved at 5-year follow-up, although only 41% of the original sample participated in the follow-up study, which limited the validity of these findings.

Four treatments for social phobia have been compared: 1) CBGT, 2) phenelzine, 3) supportive psychotherapy, and 4) placebo. Overall, both phenelzine and CBGT were equally effective after 12 weeks of treatment and were significantly more effective than placebo or supportive psychotherapy. Phenelzine tended to work more quickly than CBGT and appeared to be more effective on a few measures. However, preliminary analyses of long-term outcome showed that after discontinuing treatment, patients receiving CBGT were more likely than patients who received phenelzine to maintain their gains, with approximately half of patients taking phenelzine relapsing, compared with none of the patients who responded to CBGT.

In a randomized clinical trial comparing cognitive therapy to moclobemide for social phobia, Oosterbaan and colleagues (2001) found that cognitive therapy was significantly better than moclobemide, but not placebo, after 15 weeks of active treatment. After a 2-month follow-up period, cognitive therapy was significantly better than both moclobemide and placebo. In addition, treatment gains in the cognitive therapy group were maintained over a 15-month follow-up period.

Exposure therapy alone or in combination with sertraline for generalized social phobia in a primary care setting has been studied. Family physicians (FPs) were trained for 30 hours in assessment of social phobia and in the application of exposure therapy. FPs reported satisfaction with the training program and found that the exposure treatment was also useful for treating patients with other conditions. Although exposure therapy and sertraline were effective alone, the combination of exposure therapy and sertraline appeared to confer added benefit.

According to cognitive models of social phobia, one of the mechanisms by which CBT works is by causing a positive shift in an individual's self-representation (e.g., decreased negative self-focused thoughts and increased task-focused thoughts and positive self-focused thoughts). Indeed, there is evidence that following CBT, individuals report significantly fewer negative self-focused thoughts. Similarly, cognitive biases are reduced following successful pharmacotherapy treatment as well and are related to the degree of symptomatic improvement in both psychological and pharmacological treatments.

In summary, it seems clear that effective psychosocial treatments and medications for social phobia exist. Although both types of treatments appear to be equally effective, each has advantages and disadvantages. Medication treatments may work more quickly and are less time-consuming for the patient and therapist. In contrast, improvement after CBT appears to last longer. Due to medication side effects, CBT may be more appropriate for some individuals. More studies are needed to examine the efficacy of combined medication and psychosocial treatments for social phobia. A meta-analysis of 24 studies examining cognitive–behavioral and medication treatments for social phobia found that both treatments were more effective than control conditions (Gould et al., 1997). In this study, the SSRIs and benzodiazepines tended to have the largest effect sizes among medications and treatments involving exposure either alone or with cognitive therapy had the largest effect sizes among CBT. Another meta-analytic study of 108 psychological and pharmacological treatment-outcome trials found that the pharmacotherapies (SSRIs, benzodiazepines, MAO inhibitors) were the most consistently effective treatments, with both SSRIs and benzodiazepine treatments equally effective and more effective than control groups (Fedoroff and Taylor, 2001). Further, maintenance of treatment gains for CBT was moderate and continued during follow-up intervals. In comparison, it is not known the extent to which treatment gains for medication treatments are maintained following discontinuation. Treatment decision trees for social and specific phobias are presented in Figures 50.3 and 50.4.

Predictors of Treatment Outcome

Few studies have examined predictors of outcome for treatment of specific and social phobias. However, the few studies that do exist fall into two main categories. First, several investigators have attempted to match treatment strategies to specific characteristics of patients. Secondly, several studies have examined the relationship between individual differences (e.g., duration and severity of illness, personality factors) and response to treatment.

Much more research is needed to identify predictors of outcome with CBT and especially with pharmacological treatment. For example, little is known about the effectiveness of treatments for specific and social phobias in special populations (e.g., elderly persons, culturally diverse groups). There has also been a lack of research on the impact of comorbidity on success of treatment with specific phobias.

Relapse and Return of Fear

With respect to specific phobia, it is common for some return of fear to occur in the presence of the phobic stimulus Relapse following treatment of a specific phobia is believed to be rare. A number of variables have been identified that predict return of fear including distraction during exposure, a relatively quick reduction in fear during exposure, a relatively slow reduction in fear during exposure, higher initial heart rate, spacing of exposure sessions and the degree to which the exposure stimuli are varied, the tendency to over associate fear-relevant stimuli with aversive.

Refractory Patients and Nonresponse to Initial Treatment

Several variables may lead to an initially poor treatment response. Anticipating potential difficulties will help increase treatment efficacy. Possible reasons for a worse outcome include poor compliance, poor motivation and poor understanding of the treatment procedures. In addition, interpersonal issues and other possible conflicts may interfere with the successful treatment of specific and social phobias.

Patients fail to comply with treatment procedures for a variety of reasons. In the case of pharmacological treatments, patients may avoid taking medications because of side effects, lack of confidence in efficacy, or preference for an alternative type of treatment. If patients are not compliant with medications, the physician should attempt to identify the reasons for poor compliance and to suggest methods of increasing compliance or changing to another type of treatment.

In the case of CBT, common reasons for poor compliance are anxiety about conforming to treatment, lack of time and lack of motivation to conduct the treatment properly. Because CBT requires patients to confront the situations they fear most, patients often feel extreme anxiety about participating in the treatment. Patients should be reassured that their anxiety is normal and that they will never be forced to do anything that they are unwilling to try. Furthermore, the difficulty of exposure tasks should be increased gradually to maximize treatment compliance. If patients do not have the time or motivation to conduct treatment as suggested, therapists should be willing to find ways to make the treatment more accessible to the patient. For example, involvement of a friend or relative of the patient as a coach may allow the patient to conduct more practices without the therapist's assistance. The therapist could also explore the possibility that the patient consider beginning treatment later, when more time is available.

Poor motivation can lead to poor compliance with the treatment procedures. If a patient's symptoms are not especially se-

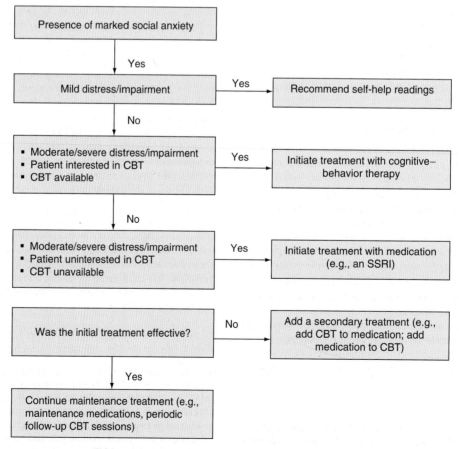

Figure 50.3   *Treatment decision tree for social phobia.*

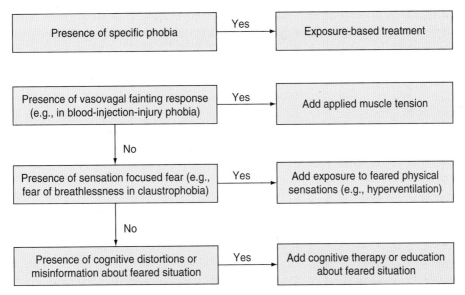

Figure 50.4 *Treatment decision tree for specific phobia.*

vere, the distress and impairment created by the disorder may not be enough to motivate the patient to take medications regularly or to confront the phobic situation in a systematic way. Furthermore, as a patient improves in treatment, she or he may experience a decrease in motivation. Patients should be encouraged to continue with treatment assignments even after improvement. More complete improvements may protect against a return of symptoms.

Finally, treatment procedures may be complicated for some patients. This is especially the case for CBT. Patients may fail to complete homework assignments (e.g., monitoring anxious cognitions) simply because the treatment rationale and the specifics of how to conduct the treatment procedures were not made clear. Therefore, therapists should continually assess the patient's understanding of the treatment procedures.

Comparison of DSM-IV/ICD-10 Diagnostic Criteria

The ICD-10 Diagnostic Criteria for Research for Social Phobia specify that at least two symptoms of anxiety (i.e., from the list of 14 panic symptoms) be present together on at least one occasion along with at least one of the following anxiety symptoms: blushing or shaking, fear of vomiting, and urgency or fear of micturition or defecation. Furthermore, these anxiety symptoms must be "restricted to, or predominated in, the feared situations or contemplation of the feared situations". In contrast, the DSM-IV criteria do not specify any particular types of anxiety symptoms nor is any restriction placed on whether anxiety can occur in situations other than social situations.

For specific phobia, the ICD-10 Diagnostic Criteria for Research also specify that the anxiety symptoms be "restricted to, or predominated in, the feared situations or contemplation of the feared situation". DSM-IV again does not impose any such restriction.

References

American Psychiatric Association (2000) *Diagnostic and Statistical Manual of Mental Disorders*, 4th edn. Text Rev. APA, Washington DC.

Antony MM and Swinson RP (2000) *Phobic Disorders and Panic in Adults: A Guide to Assessment and Treatment.* American Psychological Association, Washington DC.

Antony MM, Craske MG and Barlow DH (1995) *Mastery of Your Specific Phobia.* The Psychological Corporation, San Antonio, TX.

Antony MM, Brown TA and Barlow DH (1997) Heterogeneity among specific phobia types in DSM-IV. *Behav Res Ther* 35, 1089–1100.

Biederman J, Hirshfeld-Becker DR, Rosenbaum JF *et al.* (2001) Further evidence of association between behavioral inhibition and social anxiety in children. *Am J Psychiatr* 158, 1673–1679.

Bourne EJ (1998) *Overcoming Specific Phobia: A hierarchy and exposure-based protocol for the treatment of all specific phobias (therapist protocol).* New Harbinger, Oakland, CA.

Brown D (1996) *Flying Without Fear.* New Harbinger, Oakland, CA.

Brown TA, Di Nardo PA and Barlow DH (1994) *Anxiety Disorders Interview Schedule for DSM-IV (ADIS-IV).* The Psychological Corporation, San Antonio, TX.

Brown TA, Campbell LA, Lehman CL *et al.* (2001) Current and lifetime comorbidity of the DSM-IV anxiety and mood disorders in a large clinical sample. *J Abnorm Psychol* 110, 585–599.

Craske MG and Rowe MK (1997) A comparison of behavioral and cognitive treatments for phobias, in *Phobias: A Handbook of Theory, Research, and Treatment* (ed Davey GCL). John Wiley, New York.

Crum RM and Pratt LA (2001) Risk of heavy drinking and alcohol use disorders in social phobia: A prospective analysis. *Am J Psychiatr* 158, 1693–1700.

Dewis LM, Kirkby KC, Martin F *et al.* (2001) Computer-aided vicarious exposure versus live graded exposure for spider phobia in children. *J Behav Ther Exp Psychiatr* 32, 17–27.

Eaton WW, Dryman A and Weissman MM (1991) Panic and phobia, in *Psychiatric Disorders in America: The Epidemiologic Catchment Area Study* (eds Robins LN and Regier DA). Free Press, New York, pp. 155–179.

Fedoroff IC and Taylor S (2001) Psychological and pharmacological treatments for social phobia: A meta-analysis. *J Clin Psychopharmacol* 21, 311–324.

First MB, Spitzer RL, Gibbon M *et al.* (2001) *Structured Clinical Interview for DSM-IV-TR Axis I Disorders, Research Version, Patient Edition. (SCID-I/P).* New York State Psychiatric Institute, Biometrics Research, New York.

Gould RA, Buckminster S, Pollack MH *et al.* (1997) Cognitive–behavioral and pharmacological treatment for social phobia: A meta-analysis. *Clin Psychol Sci Pract* 4, 291–306.

Heimberg RG, Dodge CS, Hope DA *et al.* (1990) Cognitive–behavioral group treatment for social phobia: Comparison with a credible placebo control. *Cog Ther Res* 14, 1–23.

Kahan M, Tanzer J, Darvin D *et al.* (2000) Virtual reality-assisted cognitive-behavioral treatment for fear of flying: Acute treatment and follow-up. *Cyber Psychol Behav* 3, 387–392.

Katzelnick DJ, Kobak KA, DeLeire T *et al.* (2001) Impact of generalized social anxiety disorder in managed care. *Am J Psychiatr* 158, 1999–2007.

Kessler RC, McGonagle KA, Zhao S *et al.* (1994) Lifetime and 12-month prevalence of DSM-III-R psychiatric disorders in the United States: Results from the National Comorbidity Survey. *Arch Gen Psychiatr* 51, 8–19.

Kessler RC, Berglund MBA, Demler O et al. (2005) Lifetime prevalence and age-of-onset distributions of DSM-IV disorders in the National Comorbidity Survey Replication. *Arch Gen Psychiatr* 62, 593–602.

Klorman R, Hastings J, Weerts T *et al.* (1974) Psychometric description of some specific-fear questionnaires. *Behav Ther* 5, 401–409.

Last CG, Perrin S, Hersen M *et al.* (1996) A prospective study of childhood anxiety disorders. *J Am Acad Child Adolesc Psychiatr* 35, 1502–1510.

Oosterbaan DB, vab Balkom AJLM, Spinoven P, *et al.* (2001) Coginitive therapy versus moclobemide in social phobia: A controlled study. Clin Psychol Psychother 8, 263–273.

Rachman S (1977) The conditioning theory of fear-acquisition: A critical examination. *Behav Res Ther* 15, 375–387.

Rothbaum BO, Hodges LF, Kooper R *et al.* (1995) Effectiveness of computer-generated (virtual reality) graded exposure in the treatment of acrophobia. *Am J Psychiatr* 152, 626–628.

Rowa K, Antony MM, Brar S *et al.* (2000) Treatment histories of patients with three anxiety disorders. *Depress Anx* 12, 92–98.

Sanderson WC, Di Nardo PA, Rapee RM *et al.* (1990) Syndrome comorbidity in patients diagnosed with a DSM-III-R anxiety disorder. *J Abnorm Psychol* 99, 308–312.

Schneider F, Weiss U, Kessler C *et al.* (1999) Subcortical correlates of differential classical conditioning of aversive emotional reactions in social phobia. *Biol Psychiatr* 45, 863–871.

Seligman MEP (1971) Phobias and preparedness. *Behav Ther* 2, 307–320.

Van Der Linden G, Van Heerden B, Warwick J *et al.* (2000) Functional brain imaging and pharmacotherapy in social phobia: Single photon emission computed tomography before and after treatment with the selective serotonin reuptake inhibitor citalopram. *Prog Neuro-Psychopharmacol Biol Psychiatr* 24, 419–438.

Wlazlo Z, Schroeder-Hartwig K, Hand I *et al.* (1990) Exposure in vivo vs. social skills training for social phobia: Long-term outcome and differential effects. *Behav Res Ther* 28, 181–193.

Obsessive–Compulsive Disorder

Definition and Overview

Obsessive–compulsive disorder (OCD) is an intriguing and often debilitating syndrome characterized by the presence of two distinct phenomena: obsessions and compulsions. Obsessions are intrusive, recurrent, unwanted ideas, thoughts, or impulses that are difficult to dismiss despite their disturbing nature. Compulsions are repetitive behaviors, either observable or mental, that are intended to reduce the anxiety engendered by obsessions. Both obsessions and compulsions have been described in a wide variety of psychiatric and neurological disorders. However, obsessions and compulsions that clearly interfere with functioning and/or cause significant distress are the hallmark of OCD.

Although OCD was originally considered rare, findings from the Epidemiologic Catchment Area (ECA) survey in 1984 demonstrated that OCD was 50 to 100 times more common than had been previously believed. With increasing recognition of OCD, both in the mental health field and in the media, many individuals with OCD have pursued treatment for this disorder. This has led to systematic investigation of clinical features such as symptom subtype, course, comorbidity, and the role of insight both descriptively and as mediators of treatment response.

These studies, conducted over the past 15 years, have greatly furthered our understanding of the clinical characteristics of this disorder. OCD is now considered a relatively common disorder that usually has its onset during puberty, although it may begin as early as age 2 years and infrequently begins after age 35 years. Women develop OCD slightly more often than men. Earlier studies found that the course of OCD is usually chronic, with symptom severity waxing and waning over time. However, those studies, which had a number of methodological limitations, were conducted prior to the availability of effective treatments for this disorder. More recent evidence suggests that some individuals have a more episodic and favorable course.

Several large studies have found that the most common obsession is contamination, and the most common compulsion is checking. However, most individuals with this disorder have multiple obsessions and compulsions over time. A number of psychiatric disorders cooccur with OCD, major depressive disorder being most frequent. Comorbidity with tic disorders is well established. That association plus a familial relationship between OCD and tic disorders has led to suggestions that tic-related OCD is a specific phenotype of OCD that is more closely related to tic disorders.

There has been considerable interest in the role of insight, or awareness, in OCD. An ability to recognize the senselessness of

the obsessions and the ability to resist obsessional ideas have been considered fundamental components of OCD. However, research findings during the past decade have demonstrated a continuum of insight in this disorder, which ranges from excellent (i.e., complete awareness of the senselessness of the content of the obsessions), through poor insight, to delusional thinking (i.e., the obsessions are held with delusional conviction). To reflect these findings, the *Diagnostic and Statistical Manual of Mental Disorders*, Fourth Edition (DSM-IV) established a new OCD specifier – with poor insight – and also noted that, in cases of delusional OCD, an additional diagnosis of delusional disorder or psychotic disorder not otherwise specified may be appropriate (American Psychiatric Association, 1994).

Epidemiology

The ECA study found that OCD was the fourth most common psychiatric disorder (after the phobias, substance use disorders and major depressive disorder), with a prevalence of 1.6% over 6 months and a lifetime prevalence of 2.5% (Myers *et al.*, 1984; Robins *et al.*, 1984). Although the ECA survey has been criticized as overestimating OCD's prevalence a subsequent study in the USA and several epidemiological studies in other countries have supported its findings. The National Comorbidity Survey Replication (NCS-R) found the lifetime prevalence for OCD to be 1.6% (Kessler *et al.*, 2005). Using the same instrument as the ECA, studies have been done in diverse cultures, including Puerto Rico, Canada, Germany, Taiwan, New Zealand and Korea, as part of the Cross National Collaborative Group (Weissman *et al.*, 1994). The lifetime (range 1.9–2.5%) and annual (range 1.1–1.8%) prevalence rates of OCD were remarkably consistent across countries with the exception of Taiwan. The rates in Taiwan were substantially lower than in all the other sites, paralleling Taiwan's low rates of other psychiatric disorders.

Demographic Characteristics

Gender Distribution

Women appear to develop OCD slightly more frequently than do men. A pooled sample from two studies with a total of 991 subjects found that 52% of the subjects were women. However, a study that assessed the presence of comorbid disorders characterized by psychosis (schizophrenia, delusional disorder) or psychosis-like features (schizotypal personality disorder) in 475 patients with OCD found a different sex ratio. Fifty-six percent of the patients with OCD who did not have one of these comorbid disorders were women, whereas 85% of those with one

Essentials of Psychiatry   Jerald Kay and Allan Tasman
© 2006 John Wiley & Sons, Ltd.

DSM-IV-TR Criteria 300.3

Definition of Obsessive–Compulsive Disorder

Either obsessions or compulsions:

Obsessions as defined by (1), (2), (3), and (4):

   (1) recurrent and persistent thoughts, impulses, or images that are experienced, at some time during the disturbance, as intrusive and inappropriate and that cause marked anxiety or distress

   (2) the thoughts, impulses, or images are not simply excessive worries about real-life problems

   (3) the person attempts to ignore or suppress such thoughts, impulses, or images, or to neutralize them with some other thought or action

   (4) the person recognizes that the obsessional thoughts, impulses, or images are a product of his or her own mind (not imposed from without as in thought insertion)

Compulsions as defined by (1) and (2):

   (1) repetitive behaviors (e.g., hand washing, ordering, checking) or mental acts (e.g., praying, counting, repeating words silently) that the person feels driven to perform in response to an obsession, or according to rules that must be applied rigidly

   (2) the behaviors or mental acts are aimed at preventing or reducing distress or preventing some dreaded event or situation; however, these behaviors or mental acts either are not connected in a realistic way with what they are designed to neutralize or prevent or are clearly excessive

At some point during the course of the disorder, the person has recognized that the obsessions or compulsions are excessive or unreasonable. Note: This does not apply to children.

The obsessions or compulsions cause marked distress, are time consuming (take more than 1 hour a day), or significantly interfere with the person's normal routine, occupational (or academic) functioning, or usual social activities or relationships.

If another Axis I disorder is present, the content of the obsessions or compulsions is not restricted to it (e.g., preoccupation with food in the presence of an eating disorder; hair pulling in the presence of trichotillomania; concern with appearance in the presence of body dysmorphic disorder; preoccupation with drugs in the presence of a substance use disorder; preoccupation with having a serious illness in the presence of hypochondriasis; preoccupation with sexual urges or fantasies in the presence of a paraphilia; or guilty ruminations in the presence of major depressive disorder).

The disturbance is not due to the direct physiological effects of a substance (e.g., a drug of abuse, a medication) or a general medical condition.

Specify if:

With poor insight: if, for most of the time during the current episode, the person does not recognize that the obsessions and compulsions are excessive or unreasonable

of these comorbid disorders were men. A predominance of males has also been observed in child and adolescent OCD populations. In a study of 70 probands with OCD who were aged 6 to 18 years, 67% were males. This finding may be due to the fact that males develop OCD at a younger age than do females.

Marital Status

Although marital status was not found to be a predictor of course in a number of earlier studies, a recent prospective study of 107 subjects with OCD found that being married significantly increased the probability of partial remission, with married patients more than twice as likely to remit as unmarried ones (Steketee *et al.*, 1999).

Course and Natural History

Age at Onset

Age at onset usually refers to the age when OCD symptoms (obsessions and compulsions) reach a severity level wherein they

lead to impaired functioning or significant distress or are time-consuming (i.e., meet DSM-IV criteria for the disorder). Reported age at onset is usually during late adolescence. In one study drawn from an OCD clinic sample ($N = 560$), the onset for males occurred significantly earlier than for females (19.5 ± 9.2 years versus 22.0 ± 9.8 years). In this study, 83% of patients experienced the onset of significant symptoms between ages 10 and 24 years, whereas less than 15% experienced onset after age 35 years (Rasmussen and Eisen, 1998). People with OCD, however, usually describe the onset of minor symptoms in childhood, well before the onset of symptoms meeting full criteria for the disorder.

   In several studies, earlier age at onset has been associated with an increased rate of OCD in first-degree relatives and suggest that there is a familial type of OCD characterized by early onset. Age at onset of OCD may also be a predictor of course. The vast majority of patients report a gradual worsening of obsessions and compulsions prior to the onset of full-criteria OCD, which is followed by a chronic course (see later). However, Swedo and colleagues (1998) have described a subtype of OCD that begins before puberty and is characterized by an episodic course with intense exacerbations. Exacerbations of OCD symptoms in this subtype have been linked with Group A beta-hemolytic streptococcal infections, which has led to the subtype designation of pediatric autoimmune neuropsychiatric disorders associated with streptococcal infections (PANDAS). In their study of 50 children with PANDAS, the average age of onset was 7.4 years. Whether the course of illness in patients with PANDAS continues to be episodic into adulthood, or, as is the case with postpubertal onset, tends to be chronic, is not known.

In keeping with the older literature, a recent 2-year naturalistic prospective study of 65 adults with OCD, in which the effect of treatment was assessed, supported earlier findings that OCD is usually chronic with fluctuations in symptom intensity but no lasting remission; it is notable that this course was most common even during an era when effective treatments were available. Although 50% of the subjects achieved partial remission in the first year of the study, the probability of subsequent relapse was 48%. Only 12% achieved full and sustained remission (Eisen et al., 1999). In contrast, a better outcome was found in a follow-up study of 144 people with OCD assessed in the 1950s and again in the 1990s (mean length of follow-up from illness onset was 47 years). Most subjects reported a significant decrease in OCD symptom severity, which varied from complete recovery (20%), to recovery with continued subclinical symptoms (28%), to continued OCD but with clear improvement (35%). Better outcome was associated with later age of onset and poorer social functioning at baseline (Skoog and Skoog, 1999).

In a prospective study of children with OCD, the majority (52%) of the 25 patients had moderate to severe OCD in the 2- to 7-year follow-up period (Flament et al., 1990), which is consistent with the data on adults. A more recent prospective study of 54 children with OCD who were treated with clomipramine yielded a more hopeful picture of OCD's course. At 2 to 7 years after initial referral, 43 of these patients still had symptoms that met criteria for OCD, but 73% were considered much or very much improved, and 11% were completely asymptomatic (Leonard et al., 1993). This study suggested that appropriate somatic treatment may improve outcome only while the patient continues to receive this treatment (see later).

Phenomenology

OCD's clinical presentation is characterized by phenomenological subtypes based on the content of the obsessions and corresponding compulsions. The list of subtypes in the Yale-Brown Obsessive–Compulsive Scale (Y-BOCS) (Table 51.1) was generated on

Table 51.1   Yale-Brown Obsessive–Compulsive Scale Symptom Checklist

Aggressive obsessions
  Fear might harm others
  Fear might harm self
  Violent or horrific images
  Fear of blurting out obsessions or insults
  Fear of doing something embarrassing
  Fear of acting on other impulses (e.g., robbing a bank, stealing groceries, overeating)
  Fear of being responsible for things going wrong (e.g., others will lose their job because of patient)
  Fear something terrible might happen (e.g., fire, burglary)
  Other
Contamination obsessions
  Concerns or disgust with bodily waste (e.g., urine, feces, saliva)
  Concern with dirt or germs
  Excessive concern with environmental contaminants (e.g., asbestos, radiation, toxic wastes)
  Excessive concern with household items (e.g., cleansers, solvents, pets)
  Concerned will become ill
  Concerned will become ill (aggressive)
  Other
Sexual obsessions
  Forbidden or perverse sexual thoughts, images, or impulses
  Content involves children
  Content involves animals
  Content involves incest
  Content involves homosexuality
  Sexual behavior toward others (aggressive)
  Other
Hoarding or collecting obsessions
  Religious obsessions

Obsession with need for symmetry or exactness
Miscellaneous obsessions
  Need to know or remember
  Fear of saying certain things
  Fear of not saying things just right
  Intrusive (neutral) images
  Intrusive nonsense sounds, words, or music
  Other
Somatic obsession–compulsion
  Cleaning or washing compulsions
  Excessive or ritualized hand washing
  Excessive or ritualized showering, bathing, brushing the teeth, or grooming
Involves cleaning of household items or inanimate objects
Other measures to prevent contact with contaminants

Counting compulsions
  Checking compulsions
  Checking that did not or will not harm others
  Checking that did not or will not harm self
  Checking that nothing terrible did or will happen
  Checking for contaminants
  Other
Repeating rituals
Ordering or arranging compulsions
Miscellaneous compulsions
  Mental rituals (other than checking or counting)
  Need to tell, ask, or confess
  Need to touch
Measures to prevent
  Harm to self
  Harm to others
  Terrible consequences
  Other

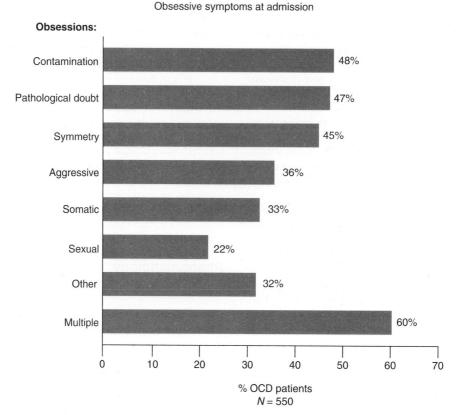

Obsessive symptoms at admission

Figure 51.1   *Obsessive symptoms at the time of initial evaluation in 550 patients with OCD.*

the basis of clinical interviews with OCD patients in the 1980s. These subtypes are remarkably consistent with phenomenological descriptions in the psychiatric literature beginning with scrupulosity in the 15th century.

The basic types of obsessions and compulsions seem to be consistent across cultures. The most common obsession is fear of contamination, followed by pathological doubt, a need for symmetry and aggressive obsessions (Figure 51.1). The most common compulsion is checking, which is followed by washing, symmetry, the need to ask or confess and counting (Figure 51.2). Children with OCD present most commonly with washing compulsions, which are followed by repeating rituals.

Most patients have multiple obsessions and compulsions over time, with a particular fear or concern dominating the clinical picture at any one time. The presence of obsessions without compulsions, or compulsions without obsessions, is unusual. In the DSM-IV OCD field trial of 431 patients, only 2% had predominantly obsessions and 2% had predominantly compulsions; the remaining 96% endorsed both obsessions and compulsions (Foa and Kozak, 1995). Patients who appear to have obsessions without compulsions frequently have unrecognized reassurance rituals or mental compulsions, such as repetitive, ritualized praying, in addition to their obsessions. Pure compulsions are also unusual in adults, although they do occur in children, especially in the young (e.g., 6 to 8 years of age). Most people have both mental and behavioral compulsions; in the DSM-IV field trial 79.5% reported having both mental and behavioral compulsions, 20.3% had behavioral compulsions only and 0.2% had only mental compulsions.

The search for whether specific obsessions and compulsions have predictive value in terms of treatment response,

biologic markers, or genetic transmission has not been particularly fruitful. There has been considerable interest in exploring whether certain clusters of obsessions and compulsions represent specific OCD phenotypes. A number of studies have addressed this question systematically using the Y-BOCS Symptom Checklist to identify groups of obsessions and compulsions that cluster together on factor analysis. Several studies have found between three and five such symptom dimensions: *symmetry/ordering, hoarding, contamination/cleaning, aggressive obsessions/checking* and *sexual/religious obsessions.* The symmetry dimension has been associated with comorbid tic disorder; in one study, patients who scored high on this dimension had a relative risk for chronic tic disorder that was 8.5 times higher than those scoring low on this factor (Leckman *et al.*, 1997). It appears that these symptom dimensions are stable over time, that is, although a patient's specific obsessions and compulsions may change over time, new obsessions and compulsions that develop are often within the same symptom dimension as the previous symptoms. A study using positron emission tomography to evaluate neural correlates of these symptom dimensions suggests that dysfunction in separate regions of the brain (e.g., striatum and prefrontal cortex) may mediate these factors (Rauch *et al.*, 1998).

Data were analyzed from a number of placebo-controlled serotonin reuptake inhibitor (SRI) treatment studies to assess whether symptom factors or dimensions were associated with treatment response. No clear pattern emerged except that patients with hoarding obsession had a significantly poorer response to SRIs. Whether these identified dimensions are associated with response to behavioral treatment, biological markers, or genetic transmission has yet to be investigated.

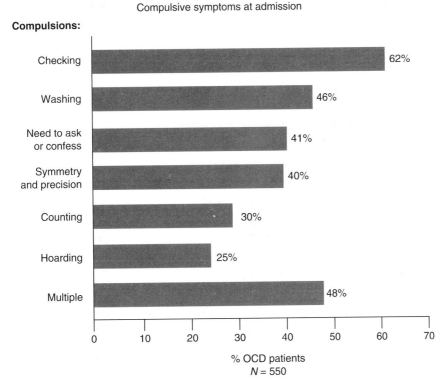

Figure 51.2 *Compulsive symptoms at the time of initial evaluation in 550 patients.*

The following descriptions of some common obsessions and compulsions illustrate the clinical presentation of these symptoms. In some cases a particular symptom may belong to more than one "type" of obsessive or compulsive grouping. Thus it is often up to the clinician to decide which category to place a symptom so that it best describes the patient's symptoms overall; it may even be best to classify it in more than one category. For instance, a patient who has concerns about cancer may have handwashing as a compulsion related to her somatic obsession. If this is the only reason that she washes her hands, to avoid getting cancer, you might simply classify this as a somatic obsession with the accompanying compulsion. However if the patient also washes repeatedly to avoid contamination in general, not just for cancer, she would have both contamination and somatic obsessions and compulsions.

Contamination

Contamination obsessions are the most frequently encountered obsessions in OCD. Such obsessions are usually characterized by a fear of dirt or germs. Contamination fears may also involve toxins or environmental hazards (e.g., asbestos or lead) or bodily waste or secretions. Patients usually describe a feared consequence of contacting a contaminated object, such as spreading a disease or contracting an illness themselves. Occasionally, however, the fear is based not on a fear of disease but on a fear of the sensory experience of not being clean. The content of the contamination obsession and the feared consequence commonly changes over time; for example, a fear of cancer may be replaced by a fear of a sexually transmitted disease.

Many patients with contamination fears use avoidance to prevent contact with contaminants, as is illustrated by a 58-year-old housewife who spent the entire day sitting in a chair to avoid touching anything in the house that might be dirty. In some cases, a specific feared object and associated avoidance become more generalized. For example, a woman with a fear of acquired immunodeficiency syndrome (AIDS) initially avoided anything that looked like dried blood but eventually avoided anything red.

Excessive washing is the compulsion most commonly associated with contamination obsessions. This behavior usually occurs after contact with the feared object; however, proximity to the feared stimulus is often sufficient to engender severe anxiety and washing compulsions, even though the contaminated object has not been touched. Most patients with washing compulsions perform these rituals in response to a fear of contamination, but these behaviors occasionally occur in response to a drive for perfection or a need for symmetry. Some patients, for example, repeatedly wash themselves in the shower until they feel "right" or must wash their right arm and then their left arm the same number of times.

Need for Symmetry

Need for symmetry is a term that describes a drive to order or arrange things perfectly or to perform certain behaviors symmetrically or in a balanced way. Patients describe an urge to repeat motor acts until they achieve a "just right" feeling that the act has been completed perfectly. Patients with a prominent need for symmetry may have little anxiety but rather describe feeling unsettled or uneasy if they cannot repeat actions or order things to their satisfaction. In addition to a need for perfection, the drive to achieve balance or symmetry may be connected with magical thinking. The desire to "even up" or balance movements may be present in patients with tapping or touching rituals. Such a patient may, for example, feel that the right side of the chair must be tapped after the left side has been tapped. Such urges and behaviors are frequently seen in patients with comorbid tic disorders, who may, for example, describe an urge to tic on the right side of their body after experiencing a tic on the left side. Patients with a need for symmetry frequently present with obsessional slowness, taking hours to perform acts such as grooming or brushing their teeth.

Somatic Obsessions

Patients with somatic obsessions are worried about the possibility that they have or will contract an illness or disease. In the past, the most common somatic obsessions consisted of fears of cancer or venereal diseases. However, a fear of developing AIDS has become increasingly common. Checking compulsions consisting of checking and rechecking the body part of concern, as well as reassurance seeking, are commonly associated with this fear. While it may be difficult to distinguish the somatic obsessions of OCD from those of hypochondriasis, there are several distinguishing features, which are discussed later in the chapter. Somatic obsessions are more easily distinguished from somatization disorder in which patients with somatic obsessions usually focus on one illness at a time and are not preoccupied with a diverse, apparently unrelated array of somatic symptoms.

Sexual and Aggressive Obsessions

People with sexual or aggressive obsessions are plagued by fears that they might harm others or commit a sexually unacceptable act such as molestation. Often, they are fearful not only that they will commit a dreadful act in the future but also that they have already committed the act. Patients are usually horrified by the content of their obsessions and are reluctant to divulge them. It is striking that the content of these obsessions tends to consist of ideas that patients find particularly abhorrent. Patients with these highly distressing obsessions frequently have checking and confession or reassurance rituals. They may report themselves to the police or repeatedly seek out priests to confess their imagined crimes

Pathological Doubt

Pathological doubt is a common feature of patients with OCD who have a variety of different obsessions and compulsions. Individuals with pathological doubt are plagued by the concern that, as a result of their carelessness, they will be responsible for a dire event. They may worry, for example, that they will start a fire because they neglected to turn off the stove before leaving the house. Although many patients report being fairly certain that they performed the act in question (e.g., locking the door, unplugging the hairdryer, paying the correct amount on a bill), they cannot dismiss the nagging doubt "What if?" Such patients often describe doubting their own perceptions. A 42-year-old man felt incapable of throwing grocery bags away because he feared he might not have completely emptied them. Immediately after staring into an empty bag, he inevitably thought, "What if I missed something important in there?"

Excessive doubt and associated feelings of excessive responsibility frequently lead to checking rituals. For example, individuals may spend several hours checking their home before they leave. As with contamination obsessions, pathological doubt can lead to marked avoidance behavior. Some patients become housebound to avoid the responsibility of potentially leaving the house unlocked. Pathological doubt is also embedded in the cognitive framework of a number of other obsessions. Patients with aggressive obsessions may be plagued by the doubt that they inadvertently harmed someone without knowing that they did so.

Insight

An awareness of the senselessness or unreasonableness of obsessions (often referred to as insight) and the accompanying struggle against the obsessions (referred to as resistance) have generally been considered fundamental components of OCD and its diagnosis. However, during the past century there have been numerous descriptions of patients with OCD who are completely convinced of the reasonableness of their obsessions and need to perform compulsions. In 1986, Insel and Akiskal described several such patients and presented the hypothesis that patients with OCD have varying degrees of insight and resistance, with obsessive–compulsive psychosis at one extreme of a hypothesized continuum. They also noted a fluidity between neurotic (i.e., associated with insight) and psychotic states in these patients.

Degree of insight in OCD was addressed during the DSM-IV field trial in which patients were asked if they feared consequences other than anxiety if they did not perform their compulsions (Foa and Kozak, 1995). Fifty-eight percent believed that harmful consequences would occur. The degree of certainty that their obsessions were reasonable ranged across the entire spectrum of insight: 30% were uncertain whether they actually needed to perform their compulsions to avoid harm; however, 4% were certain and 26% were mostly certain. Again, this finding supports the notion that patients with OCD do not always maintain good insight but rather have varying degrees of insight. Although patients may be aware that their obsessions are excessive – that is, recognizing that they spend too much time thinking about them – they may have little insight into the fact that the belief underlying their obsession (e.g., that they will get cancer from stepping on a chemically treated lawn) is senseless, unreasonable, or unrealistic.

To reflect these findings, DSM-IV established a new OCD specifier, with poor insight. This specifier applies to "an individual who, for most of the time in the current episode, does not recognize that the obsessions or compulsions are excessive or unreasonable". DSM-IV also acknowledges that the beliefs that underlie OCD obsessions can be delusional and notes that in such cases an additional diagnosis of delusional disorder or psychotic disorder not otherwise specified may be appropriate Most people with OCD are aware that other people think their symptoms are unrealistic and that the obsessions are caused by a psychiatric illness. Whether insight is an important predictor of prognosis and treatment response is an intriguing issue that has received little investigation. More studies are needed to determine the effect of insight on treatment response. For example, to our knowledge no studies have assessed whether adding an antipsychotic to an SRI is more effective in patients with poor insight than in those with good insight. Studies that assess the impact of insight on compliance with and refusal of behavioral therapy are also needed.

Comorbidity

OCD frequently occurs in association with other Axis I disorders. In a study of 100 patients with primary OCD, 67 had a lifetime history of major depressive disorder, and 31 had symptoms that met criteria for current major depressive disorder (Rasmussen and Eisen, 1991). Although it may be difficult to distinguish a primary from a secondary diagnosis, some individuals with OCD view their depressive symptoms as occurring secondary to the demoralization and hopelessness accompanying their OCD and report that they would not be depressed if they did not have OCD. However, others view their major depressive symptoms as occurring independently of their OCD symptoms, which may be less severe when they cycle into an episode of major depression, because they feel too apathetic to be as concerned with their obsessions and too fatigued to perform compulsions. Conversely, OCD symptoms may intensify during depressive episodes.

Although findings have varied, the generally accepted frequency of tic disorders in patients with OCD is far higher than in the general population, with a rate of approximately 5 to 10% for Tourette's disorder and 20% for any tic disorder. Conversely, patients with Tourette's disorder have a high rate of comorbid OCD, with 30 to 40% reporting obsessive–compulsive symptoms. The likelihood of childhood onset of OCD is greater in this group, and the presence of tics is associated with more severe OCD symptoms in children. There is an increased rate of both OCD and tic disorders in the first-degree relatives of OCD probands with a family lifetime history of tics, and an increased frequency of tic disorders in the first-degree relatives of OCD probands compared with controls. There are also phenomenologic observations that link OCD and tic disorders. Individuals with both OCD and tics have several features that distinguish them from individuals with OCD alone. They more frequently have symmetry, ordering and arranging, and hoarding compulsions, and they more frequently try to attain a "just right" feeling. These data strengthen the notion that tic disorders and OCD are highly related. In fact, it has been suggested that tic disorders are an alternative expression or phenotype of the familial OCD subtype.

Anxiety disorders frequently coexist with OCD, with relatively high lifetime rates of specific phobia (22%), social phobia (18%) and panic disorder (12%) in patients with OCD (Rasmussen and Eisen, 1991). In one study, 17 of 100 subjects with OCD had a lifetime history of an eating disorder. Conversely, in 93 subjects with an eating disorder, 37 had symptoms that met criteria for comorbid OCD.

Several studies of OCD and comorbid schizophrenia found that compared with subjects with OCD alone, those with comorbid schizophrenia have a worse prognosis in terms of long-term outcome (social relations, employment, psychopathology and global functioning). Similarly, treatment studies of patients with OCD and comorbid schizotypal personality disorder have shown a poorer prognosis and poorer response to psychotropic medications for the comorbid group. Thus, it appears important to differentiate OCD plus a comorbid psychotic disorder, which may have a relatively poor outcome, from delusional OCD, which may be more similar to OCD with insight and without comorbid psychosis.

Studies of patients with schizophrenia or schizoaffective disorder have found rates of OCD ranging from 8 to 46%. This strikingly large range is most likely due to the OCD criteria used (i.e., subclinical OCD symptoms versus OCD symptoms severe enough to cause significant impairment or distress). Regardless, it is clear that a significant number of people with schizophrenia have OCD symptoms which require assessment and may benefit from treatment.

The relationship between OCD and personality disorders, particularly obsessive–compulsive personality disorder (OCPD), has received considerable attention. Early observations noted the presence of OCPD traits in patients with OCD. Systematic studies have yielded inconsistent findings however. Although personality disorders are considered to be stable over time, one study found that of 17 OCD patients with a personality disorder, nine of the 10 treatment responders no longer met criteria for either avoidant or dependent personality disorder after successful pharmacotherapy, raising the question of whether these personality disorders actually represented a coping style in response to OCD (Ricciardi *et al.*, 1992).

Differential Diagnosis

OCD is sometimes difficult to distinguish from certain other disorders. Obsessions and compulsions may appear in the context of other syndromes, which can raise the question whether the obsessions and compulsions are a symptom of another disorder or whether both OCD and another disorder are present (see section on Comorbidity). A general guideline is that if the content of the obsessions is not limited to the focus of concern of another disorder (e.g., an appearance concern, as in body dysmorphic disorder, or food concerns, as in an eating disorder) and if the obsessions or compulsions are preoccupying as well as distressing or impairing, OCD should generally be diagnosed.

Diagnostic dilemmas may also arise when it is unclear whether certain thoughts are obsessions or whether, instead, they are ordinary worries, ruminations, overvalued ideas, or delusions. In a similar vein, questions may develop about whether certain behaviors constitute true compulsions or whether they should instead be conceptualized as impulses, tics, or addictive behaviors.

Obsessive–Compulsive Disorder Versus Other Anxiety Disorders

Both OCD and the other anxiety disorders are characterized by the use of avoidance to manage anxiety. However, OCD is distinguished from these disorders by the presence of compulsions. For OCD patients with preoccupying fears or worries but no rituals, several other features may be useful in establishing the diagnosis of OCD. In social phobia and specific phobia, fears are circumscribed and related to specific triggers (in specific phobia) or social situations (in social phobia). Although circumscribed situations may initially trigger obsessions and compulsions in OCD, triggers in OCD become more generalized over time, unlike the triggers in social and specific phobias, in which the evoking situations remain circumscribed.

As many as 60% of people with OCD experience full-blown panic symptoms. However, unlike panic disorder, in which panic attacks occur spontaneously, panic symptoms occur in OCD only during exposure to specific feared triggers such as contaminated objects. The worries that are present in generalized anxiety disorder (GAD) are more ego syntonic and involve an exaggeration of ordinary concerns, whereas the obsessional thinking of OCD is more intrusive, is limited to a specific set of concerns (e.g., contamination, blasphemy), and usually has an irrational, senseless, or unreasonable quality. Also, whereas the worry of GAD is considered primarily thoughtlike in nature, obsessional symptoms may consist of thoughts, impulses, or images.

Obsessive–Compulsive Disorder Versus Psychotic Disorders

One question is how to differentiate OCD from psychotic disorders such as schizophrenia and delusional disorder. Another question is how to distinguish OCD with insight from OCD without insight (delusional OCD). One distinguishing feature between OCD and the psychotic disorders is that the latter are not characterized by prominent ritualistic behaviors. If compulsions are present in a patient with prominent psychotic symptoms, the possibility of a comorbid OCD diagnosis should be considered. Furthermore, although schizophrenia may be characterized by obsessional thinking, other characteristic features of the disorder, such as prominent hallucinations or thought disorder, are also present. With regard to delusional disorder, paranoid and grandiose concerns are generally not considered to fall under the OCD rubric. However, some other types of delusional disorder, such as the somatic and jealous types, seem to bear a close resemblance to OCD and are not always easily distinguished from it. It will be interesting to see whether future research indicates that certain types of somatic delusional disorder (e.g., the delusional variant of hypochondriasis) and the jealous type of delusional disorder (also referred to as pathological jealousy) are actually variants of OCD.

The second issue noted above – how to distinguish OCD with insight from OCD without insight – is complex. As previously discussed, insight in OCD is increasingly being recognized as spanning a spectrum from good to poor to absent. Both clinical observations and research findings indicate that some individuals hold their obsessional concerns with delusional intensity and believe that their concerns are reasonable. In DSM-IV, delusional OCD may be double-coded as both OCD and delusional disorder or as both OCD and psychotic disorder not otherwise specified, in other words, patients with delusional OCD would receive both diagnoses. This double coding reflects the fact that it is unclear whether OCD with insight and OCD without insight constitute the same or different disorders. Further research using validated scales to assess insight in OCD is needed to shed light on this question.

Obsessive–Compulsive Disorder Versus Impulse Control Disorders

Differential diagnosis questions have been raised with regard to kleptomania, trichotillomania, pathological gambling and other disorders involving impulsive behaviors. Several features have been said to distinguish these disorders from OCD. For example, compulsions – unlike behaviors of the impulse control disorders – generally have no gratifying element, although they do diminish anxiety. In addition, the affective state that drives the behaviors associated with these disorders may differ. In OCD, fear is frequently the underlying drive that leads to compulsions, which, in turn, decrease anxiety. In the impulse control disorders, patients frequently describe heightened tension, but not fear, preceding an impulsive behavior. However, OCD and the impulse control disorders have some features in common. Research is ongoing to explore the relationship between OCD and the impulse control disorders by examining similarities and differences in treatment response, biological markers and familial transmission.

Obsessive–Compulsive Disorder Versus Tourette's Disorder

Complex motor tics of Tourette's disorder may be difficult to distinguish from OCD compulsions. Both tics and compulsions are preceded by an intrusive urge and are followed by feelings of relief. However, OCD compulsions are usually preceded by both anxiety and obsessional concerns, whereas, in Tourette's disorder, the urge to perform a tic is not preceded by an obsessional fear. This distinction breaks down to some extent when considering the "just right" perceptions of some patients with OCD. The "just right" perception refers to the need to perform a certain motor action, such as touching, tapping, checking, ordering, arranging, or counting, until it feels right. Determining when an action has been performed enough or perfectly may depend on tactile, visual, or auditory perceptions. In a study of patients with Tourette's disorder and OCD symptoms, most patients could distinguish between the mental urge to do something repeatedly until it felt right and a physical urge to perform a motor tic. However, it is sometimes difficult for psychiatrists to distinguish between complex tics and compulsions, especially when a patient has both disorders.

Obsessive–Compulsive Disorder Versus Hypochondriasis

Fears of illness that occur in OCD, referred to as somatic obsessions, may be difficult to distinguish from hypochondriasis. Usually, however, patients with somatic obsessions have other current or past classic OCD obsessions unrelated to illness concerns. Patients with OCD also often engage in classic OCD rituals, such as checking or reassurance seeking, in an attempt to diminish their illness concerns. Unlike patients with OCD, patients with hypochondriasis experience somatic and visceral sensations. Although insight and resistance have been used to distinguish OCD from hypochondriasis, with the concern in hypochondriasis being said to be egosyntonic (realistic and totally justified) and that of OCD to be egodystonic (unacceptable and undesirable thoughts, actions, or both), studies have demonstrated a range of insight in OCD. Attempting to differentiate these disorders by degree of insight or egosyntonicity may therefore be of limited usefulness.

Obsessive–Compulsive Disorder Versus Body Dysmorphic Disorder

Body dysmorphic disorder (BDD), a preoccupation with an imagined or slight defect in appearance (e.g., thinning hair, facial scarring, or a large nose), has many similarities to OCD (Phillips, 1991). Patients with BDD experience obsessional thinking about the supposed defect and usually engage in associated repetitive ritualistic behaviors, such as mirror checking and reassurance seeking. Preliminary evidence suggests that BDD also appears similar to OCD in terms of age of onset, course of illness and other variables. Nonetheless, emerging data suggest that there are some important differences between the two disorders, and they are currently classified separately in DSM-IV. Insight, for example, is more frequently impaired in BDD than in OCD. If the content of a patient's obsessions involves a concern about a supposed defect in appearance, BDD, rather than OCD, is the diagnosis that should be given.

Obsessive–Compulsive Disorder Versus Obsessive–Compulsive Personality Disorder

Obsessive–compulsive personality disorder is a lifelong maladaptive personality style characterized by perfectionism, excessive attention to detail, indecisiveness, rigidity, excessive devotion to work, restricted affect, lack of generosity and hoarding. OCD and OCPD have historically been considered variants of the same disorder on a continuum of severity, with OCD viewed as the more severe manifestation of illness. Contrary to this notion, studies using structured interviews to establish diagnosis have found that not all patients with OCD also have OCPD. One reason for the perception that these disorders are linked lies in the frequency of several OCPD traits in patients with OCD. In one study, the majority of 114 patients with OCD had perfectionism and indecisiveness (82 and 70, respectively). In contrast, other OCPD traits, such as restricted affect, excessive devotion to work and rigidity, were seen infrequently.

Although perfectionism and indecisiveness are relatively common traits in patients with OCD, the distinction between OCD and OCPD is important, and several guidelines may be useful in distinguishing them. Unlike OCPD, OCD is characterized by distressing, time-consuming egodystonic obsessions and repetitive rituals aimed at diminishing the distress engendered by obsessional thinking. One of the hallmarks that traditionally has been used to distinguish OCD from OCPD is that, in contrast, OCPD features are considered egosyntonic. In addition, as previously noted, the traits of restricted affect, excessive devotion to work and rigidity are generally characteristic of OCPD but not OCD. Although useful, these guidelines are not absolute, and some patients defy easy categorization. Some patients, for example, spend hours each day engaged in egosyntonic behaviors such as excessive cleaning; such patients may seek treatment not because they are disturbed by their behaviors but because the behaviors cause problems in functioning or family friction. It is unclear whether some of these patients should be diagnosed with OCPD or subthreshold OCD.

Obsessive–Compulsive Spectrum Disorders

Certain disorders other than OCD, such as BDD, hypochondriasis, and eating disorders, are characterized by obsessional thinking and/or ritualistic behaviors. On the basis of these apparent similarities with OCD, the concept of OCD spectrum disorders has been developed. They have been defined as disorders that share features with OCD (Hollander, 1993) and are posited to have "spectrum membership" on the basis of their similarities with OCD across multiple domains. These domains include not only symptoms but also treatment response, comorbidity, joint familial loading, sex ratio, age at onset, course, premorbid personality characteristics and presumed cause. Cause is inferred from characteristics such as neurological deficits, response to biological challenges, biochemical indices, brain imaging patterns (functional and anatomical) and epidemiological risk factors. It is worth noting that there are currently no operational criteria for what constitutes an OCD spectrum disorder; for example, in which of the preceding domains must similarities be documented, and how similar in each domain must the disorder be to OCD?

Disorders postulated to be OCD spectrum disorders include BDD, hypochondriasis, eating disorders, "grooming" disorders such as nail biting and trichotillomania, and the impulse

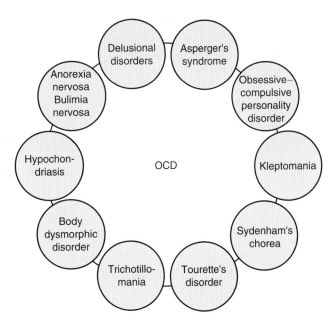

Figure 51.3 *OCD spectrum disorders.*

disorders (see Figure 51.3). Of interest is a recent study investigating the frequency of these disorders in first-degree relatives of people with OCD. BDD, hypochondriasis, any eating disorder (although not anorexia or bulimia individually) and grooming disorders (but not the impulse control disorders) were found more frequently in probands with OCD than in general population controls. In addition, BDD and grooming disorders (although not the other disorders) were significantly more common in the first-degree relatives of OCD probands than in relatives of controls (Bienvenu *et al.*, 2000). This finding suggests that certain of the proposed OCD spectrum disorders may have a familial link to OCD. The relationship of these disorders with OCD is an area in which exciting research will be conducted in coming years.

Etiology and Pathophysiology

A number of intriguing avenues have been investigated to determine the etiology and pathophysiology of OCD. Although our understanding of what causes this disorder has continued to grow, there is still much to learn. It is likely that OCD is caused by a complex interaction of factors rather than a single defect. However, for the purpose of clarity, these factors are described separately.

Genetic Factors

A number of approaches have been used to evaluate the role of heredity in OCD. Twin studies have examined rates of concordant monozygotic twins versus discordant monozygotic twins with OCD. A review of this literature reveals a concordance rate of 63% in monozygotic twins and supports the notion that genetic factors are implicated in the expression of OCD. Given the concordance rate of less than 100% in monozygotic twins, it is clear that environment also plays a role in OCD's phenotypic expression.

A second approach to examining the role of genetics in OCD has been to investigate the rate of OCD in family members of OCD probands. Evidence supporting familial transmission of OCD has been obtained by studying the frequency of OCD in relatives of patients with Gilles de la Tourette's Syndrome (TS). Available data support familial transmission in some cases of OCD and suggest that genetic factors play an important role in its etiology, particularly in patients with comorbid tic disorder. Thus, in recent years a molecular genetics approach has begun to be applied to OCD, although there have been not significant findings to date.

Neurobiological Factors

Neuroanatomical Aspects

Brain imaging techniques have advanced the search for abnormalities in brain functioning and/or structure in patients with OCD. Numerous studies have now been done with both structural imaging – CT (computed tomography) and MRI (magnetic resonance imaging) – and functional imaging – PET (positron emission tomography), SPECT (single photon emission computed tomography), fMRI (functional magnetic resonance imaging) and MRS (magnetic resonance spectroscopy). These techniques have demonstrated abnormalities in OCD patients. These abnormalities occur at rest and with symptom provocation and they are "normalized" with effective treatment.

While not all results are in agreement, a majority of these studies have implicated abnormalities in the orbitofrontal cortex, anterior cingulate cortex, and structures of the basal ganglia and thalamus. These structures are proposed to be linked in neuroanatomical circuits. One well-articulated model by Saxena and colleagues (1998) proposes that OCD symptoms are mediated by hyperactivity in orbitofrontal–subcortical circuits, which might be due to an imbalance in tone between direct and indirect striato–pallidal pathways. Some studies have implicated a preferential role for right anterolateral orbitofrontal cortex in both OCD symptoms and symptom response. This view has neurocognitive implications because studies of executive function in OCD patients have shown that patients have difficulty with alternation tasks and tasks that involve making choices. A number of treatment studies (see later) with clomipramine, fluoxetine, paroxetine and cognitive–behavioral therapy (CBT) have shown a decrease in caudate glucose metabolism with successful treatment.

Further indirect evidence implicating a role for basal ganglia dysfunction in OCD lies in the clinical relationship between neurological insults to the basal ganglia and the subsequent development of obsessions and compulsions. There is an association between OCD and Tourette's disorder, Sydenham's chorea, bilateral necrosis of the globus pallidus and postencephalitic parkinsonian symptoms.

Neurochemical Aspects

The hypothesis that OCD involves an abnormality in the serotonin neurotransmitter system has been called the serotonin hypothesis. Several different lines of investigation support this hypothesis: 1) therapeutic response of patients to chronic administration of medication; 2) measurements of central and peripheral neurotransmitter or metabolite concentration; and 3) pharmacologic challenge paradigms which measure behavioral and neuroendocrine effects produced by acute administration of selective pharmacologic agents.

All the evidence from treatment studies points to a role for serotonin and speaks of a need for prolonged administration to see a positive effect. All of the antidepressants that effectively treat OCD affect serotonin. These antidepressants are potent inhibitors of the presynaptic reuptake of serotonin (i.e., SRIs). Those antidepressants that primarily affect the noradrenergic system have not been found to have antiobsessional properties. Exactly how the SRIs improve OCD symptoms remains unclear; while the immediate action of these agents may be to increase serotonin in the synapse, they undoubtably cause a cascade of changes, both presynaptically and postsynaptically.

The role of the dopamine system in OCD's pathophysiology has also been investigated. When added to the SRIs, dopamine antagonists (neuroleptic agents) decrease symptoms of OCD in patients with OCD and comorbid tics, as well as in patients with OCD and comorbid schizotypal personality disorder. It has been hypothesized that some forms of OCD, particularly OCD plus Tourette's disorder, may involve an imbalance in activity between serotonergic and dopaminergic systems.

Given the complex interactions and overlap among monoaminergic and other receptors in the brain, it is likely that a number of neurotransmitters are involved in OCD's pathophysiology and etiology. The effect of long-term treatment with SRIs is probably several: to change the ratio of dopamine to serotonin turnover, alter the gene expression of target neurons to stress-related neuropeptides, and decrease the sensitivity of subtypes of presynaptic serotonin auto- and heteroceptors belonging to the $5-HT_1$ receptor family. Ongoing research is expected to elucidate further the likely role of serotonin and the possible role of other neurotransmitters in OCD.

Animal Models

Animal models may provide an important window on treatment efficacy and the influence of environmental and genetic factors in OCD. Because of the inherent difficulties in studying cognitive aspects of OCD (such as guilt, over-responsibility and doubt) in animals, attention has focused on repetitive motor actions that are similar to compulsions. Ethologists have observed that when specific, goal-directed actions are thwarted, animals may substitute unrelated behaviors, known as displacement behaviors, which frequently involve digging, pecking, or grooming. These motor actions have several elements: they are triggered by conflict over territory or by frustration, they continue in a stereotyped fashion, and they are excessive and/or inappropriate to the context in which they are performed. Thus, they are similar to the compulsive behaviors of OCD. Another animal model for OCD is acral lick disorder, in which dogs and cats groom themselves excessively, causing cutaneous lesions. As in OCD, stress increases these excessive grooming behaviors. Of interest is the positive responsive of acral lick disorder to clomipramine, fluoxetine and sertraline but not to placebo, which lends support to the hypothesis that this behavior represents an animal model of OCD.

A number of models implicate excessive dopaminergic activity in repetitive behaviors. For example, dopamine antagonists such as haloperidol decrease stereotyped behaviors in animals induced by amphetamine administration, stimulation, or stress. Animal models offer the advantage of accessibility and ease of manipulation for controlled trials and as such can play a valuable role in understanding OCD's etiology.

Learning Theory

A model based on the psychological concept of conditioning has also been used to understand the development of obsessions and

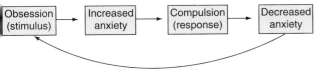

Figure 51.4 *Learning theory of OCD.*

compulsions. Compulsions, whether mental or observable, usually decrease the anxiety engendered by obsessional thoughts. Thus, if a person is preoccupied with fears of contamination from germs, repetitive handwashing usually decreases the anxiety caused by these fears. The compulsion becomes a conditioned response to anxiety. Because of the tension-reducing aspect of the compulsion, this learned behavior becomes reinforced and eventually fixed. Compulsions, in turn, actually reinforce anxiety because they prevent habituation from occurring; that is, by performing a compulsion, contact with the fear-evoking stimulus (e.g., dirt) is not maintained, and habituation (a decrease in fear associated with the stimulus) does not occur. Thus, the vicious circle linking obsessions and compulsions is maintained (Figure 51.4). This learning theory model of OCD has had a major influence on the way behavioral therapy is used in its treatment.

Psychoanalytic Theory

Much of the psychoanalytic literature on OCD does not distinguish between the phenomena observed in OCD (obsessions and compulsions) and the traits of OCPD. This distinction has relevance because of treatment implications. Although the clinical observations of earlier psychoanalysts, such as Freud's famous Ratman case (Freud, 1963), reflect current clinical presentations of Axis I OCD, understanding symptoms from the psychoanalytic perspective have not yielded improvement in this disorder's symptoms. Conversely, characterologic problems such as perfectionism, indecisiveness and rigidity, seen in OCPD, may benefit from a psychoanalytic orientation that focuses on the meaning of these symptoms or traits; such traits have typically not responded well to medications alone, although further investigation of this question is needed.

Recent theory has attempted to integrate the biology of OCD with psychological models by proposing a phylogenetic model based on systems theory. In this model, behavioral inhibition and harm-assessment systems, which develop early in human phylogeny, are disrupted. This disruption can occur at a hierarchically primary level of biological organization, resulting in neurobiologic disturbance, or at a hierarchically higher level of organization, leading to psychological disturbances. Such a model can help to explain the diversity of symptoms seen in OCD, from the more primitive biologically based behaviors based on fight/flight and risk to more psychologically sophisticated behaviors involving morality and guilt. This model might also explain why neither biological or psychological treatments alone always lead to complete remission of symptoms (Cohen *et al.*, 1997).

Treatment

General Considerations

Both pharmacologic and behavioral therapies have proved effective for OCD. The majority of controlled treatment trials have been performed with adults age 18 to 65 years. However, these therapies have been shown effective for patients of all ages. In general, children and the elderly tolerate most of these medications well. For children, lower doses are indicated because of lower body mass. For instance, the recommended dose for clomipramine in children is up to 150 mg/day (3 mg/kg/day) versus 250 mg/day in adults. Use of lower doses should also be considered in the elderly because their decreased ability to metabolize medications can increase the risk of side effects and toxicity. Behavioral therapy has also been used successfully in all age groups, although when treating children with this modality it is usually advisable to use a parent as a cotherapist. A flowchart that outlines treatment options for OCD is shown in Figure 51.5.

In general, the goals of treatment are to reduce the frequency and intensity of symptoms as much as possible and to minimize the amount of interference the symptoms cause. It should be noted that few patients experience a cure or complete remission of symptoms. Instead, OCD should be viewed as a chronic illness with a waxing and waning course. Symptoms are often worse during times of psychosocial stress. Even when on medication, individuals with OCD are often upset when they experience even a mild symptom exacerbation, anticipating that their symptoms will revert to their worst, which is rarely the case. Anticipating with the patient that stress may make the symptoms worse can often be helpful in long-term treatment. Expert consensus guidelines, based on completion of a survey by 79 experts in the field, provide a reasonable approach to clinical practice in treating patients with OCD. However like any consensus report, based on clinical practice, not all of the recommendations are supported by empirical data (March *et al.*, 1997). Further work in neurosurgical techniques, particularly less invasive approaches like gamma knife and possibly transmagnetic stimulation, may offer other options in the future for treating OCD.

Pharmacological Treatments

The most extensively studied agents for OCD are medications that affect the serotonin system. Many studies implicate the serotonin system in OCD's pathophysiology, although comparative studies also seem to implicate other neurotransmitter systems, including the dopaminergic system, in treatment response. The principal pharmacologic agents used to treat OCD are the SRIs, which include clomipramine, fluoxetine, fluvoxamine, sertraline, paroxetine and citalopram.

Outcome measures in OCD treatment trials generally include the Yale-Brown Obsessive–Compulsive Scale (Y-BOCS; Goodman *et al.*, 1989), a reliable and valid 10-item, 40-point semi-structured instrument that assesses the severity of obsessions and rituals during the preceding week. Studies conducted since 1989 have generally used the Y-BOCS as one of the major outcome measures. Most studies have used Y-BOCS scores of 16 to 20 as a study entry criterion, although it has been argued that higher scores (e.g., 20–21) might reduce the increasing placebo response rates being obtained in OCD studies. Treatment response is generally considered to constitute at least a 25 to 35% reduction in OCD symptoms as measured by the Y-BOCS. Another frequently used global outcome measure is the National Institute of Mental Health Global Obsessive–Compulsive Scale (NIMH-OC) (Pato *et al.*, 1994).

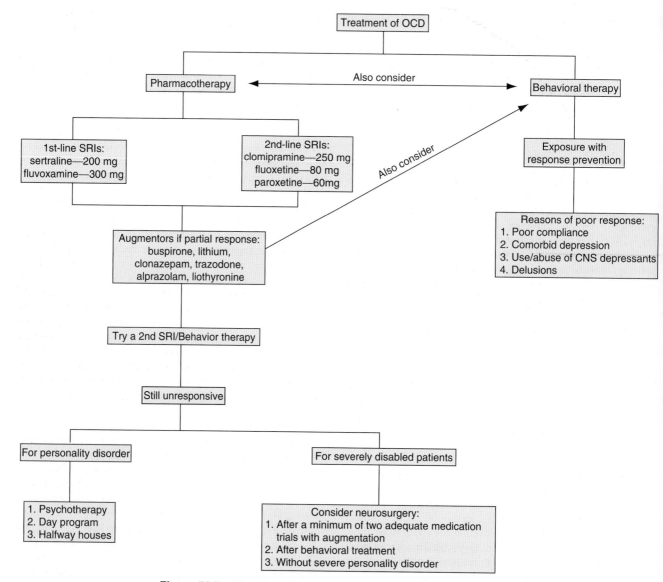

Figure 51.5   *Flowchart of treatment options for OCD.*

Clomipramine

The tricyclic antidepressant clomipramine is among the most extensively studied pharmacological agents in OCD. This drug is unique among the antiobsessional agents in which in addition to its potency as an SRI, it has significant affinity for noradrenergic, dopaminergic, muscarinic and histaminic receptors. The most common side effects are those typical of the tricyclic antidepressants, including dry mouth, dizziness, tremor, fatigue, somnolence, constipation, nausea, increased sweating, headache, mental cloudiness and sexual dysfunction. Previous data have indicated that at doses of 300 mg/day or more, the risk of seizures is 2.1% but at doses of 250 mg/day or less, the risk of seizures is low (0.48%) and comparable to that of other tricyclic antidepressants. It is therefore recommended that doses of 250 mg/day or less be used. Elderly patients may be more prone to tricyclic side effects, such as orthostatic hypotension, constipation (which may lead to fecal impaction), forgetfulness and mental cloudiness, which might be confused with dementia. Most of these side effects can be treated by simply lowering the dose, although the cardiac conduction effects of tricyclic anti-

depressants may preclude the use of clomipramine in patients with preexisting cardiac conduction problems, especially atrioventricular block.

Recent studies of IV clomipramine have been particularly promising because it seems to have a quicker onset of action and fewer side effects than the oral form, and it may be effective even in patients who do not respond to oral clomipramine. Oral clomipramine, like other SRIs, usually takes a minimum of 4 to 6 weeks to produce a clinically significant clinical response, but in at least one study using IV pulse doses patients showed a response within 4.5 days. The reasons for this unique response are not fully understood, but it is postulated that the IV preparation avoids first-pass hepatoenteric metabolism, leading to increased bioavailability of the parent compound clomipramine. This in turn may play a role in rapidly desensitizing serotonergic receptors or initiating changes in postsynaptic serotonergic neurons. This preparation is still not FDA-approved for clinical use in the USA. Cardiac monitoring is recommended during the use of IV clomipramine.

Fluoxetine

Despite their different chemical structures, all of the SSRIs appear to have similar efficacy in treating OCD. Fluoxetine has not been shown to be more effective than clomipramine. The fixed-dose trials of fluoxetine are particularly noteworthy because there are few published fixed-dose trials with any of the antiobsessional agents in OCD. Although these studies indicated that doses of 20, 40 and 60 mg/day were all effective when compared with placebo, there was a trend toward 60 mg/day being more effective. Some patients who did not respond at lower doses responded at higher doses, and others who responded at lower doses showed increased improvement at a higher dose. In addition, patients maintained their improvement or experienced increased improvement during the 5- to 6-month follow-up period.

Fluoxetine has fewer side effects than clomipramine, reflecting its more selective mechanism of action. The most common side effects are headache, nausea, insomnia, anorexia, dry mouth, somnolence, nervousness, tremor and diarrhea. Side effects occur more frequently at higher doses. Fluoxetine's long half-life, which is unique among the SRIs, is 2 to 4 days for the parent compound and 4 to 16 days for its active metabolite. This long half-life can be beneficial for patients who do not comply with treatment, because relatively high steady-state levels are maintained even when several doses are missed. However, the long half-life can present problems when switching or discontinuing fluoxetine, because 5 weeks or more may be required for the medication to be completely cleared from the body. Hence the added delay, 5 weeks rather than 2 weeks for the other SRIs, is required when switching from fluoxetine to an MAOI.

Fluvoxamine

Fluvoxamine is a unicyclic agent which differs from the other SSRIs in that it does not have an active metabolite. A number of systematic blinded clinical trials, most of which were placebo-controlled, have demonstrated fluvoxamine's effectiveness in treating OCD. As has been demonstrated for the other SSRIs, relatively long treatment trials are indicated before concluding that an SSRI is ineffective in OCD.

The largest and most recent fluvoxamine study was a 10-week multicenter double-blind placebo-controlled study of 320 patients. The mean dose of fluvoxamine was 249 mg/day. As in the other studies, the fluvoxamine-treated patients had a significant reduction in OCD symptoms; however, unlike most of the earlier medication trials there was a relatively high placebo response rate of 11%. One of the important conclusions from this study was that prior failure to respond to another SSRI was associated with a lower likelihood of responding to fluvoxamine. All of the fluvoxamine studies show a similar side-effect profile, which included insomnia, nervousness, fatigue, somnolence, nausea, headache and sexual dysfunction. Insomnia and nervousness tended to occur early in treatment, whereas fatigue and somnolence occurred later. Overall, the medication is well tolerated, with only 10 to 15% of patients dropping out of treatment because of side effects.

Sertraline

As is true of other studies, higher doses of sertraline 200 mg/day being is more effective than 50 mg/day or 100 mg/day. Typical side effects included nausea, headache, diarrhea, insomnia and dry mouth. A recent study compared sertraline with the non-SRI antidepressant desipramine for patients with OCD and comorbid depression. Although these medications were similarly efficacious for depression, sertraline was more effective for OCD symptoms, supporting the use of an SRI-like sertraline rather than a norepinephrine reuptake inhibitor like desipramine in such patients. In addition, even though desipramine did improve depressive symptoms, a significantly greater number of patients treated with sertraline achieved remission from depression (Hoehn-Saric et al., 2000).

Paroxetine

Paroxetine is another SSRI that differs in structure from those previously discussed. It is a phenylpiperidine compound that is marketed as an antidepressant and, like sertraline, shows promise in the treatment of OCD. Results of a fixed-dose multicenter trial of 348 patients indicated that paroxetine is effective for OCD. As was suggested in the sertraline study, higher doses (40 or 60 mg/day) may be needed because 20 mg/day was no more effective than placebo (Wheadon et al., 1993). Paroxetine's efficacy is comparable to that of other SRIs, and side effects are similar to those of other SSRIs and include lethargy, dry mouth, nausea, insomnia, somnolence, tremor, sexual dysfunction and decreased appetite. Reports of an acute discontinuation syndrome, which can include general malaise, asthenia, dizziness, vertigo, headache, myalgia, loss of appetite, nausea, diarrhea and abdominal cramps, warrant a gradual reduction in dose if this medication is to be discontinued. Occasional patients may experience some of these symptoms even if their dose is delayed by only a few hours.

Citalopram

Citalopram is the newest SSRI available for the treatment of OCD and is unique in its selectivity for serotonin reuptake compared with the other SRIs. It has few significant secondary binding properties, and its minimal effect on hepatic metabolism probably makes it safer to combine with other medications. A multicenter fixed-dose-placebo-controlled trial with 401 patients showed that 52 to 65% of patients responded in the three dosage groups compared with a 37% response rate in the placebo group. While there was a trend for a higher dose to lead to a higher response rate, as with other SRIs, there was no statistical difference between the three doses used (20, 40 and 60 mg/day). Typical side effects included fatigue, sweating, dry mouth, ejaculation failure, nausea and insomnia, although many patients habituated to these side effects in 4 to 6 weeks. Thus, citalopram is a good choice for OCD treatment because of its side-effect profile and low probability of causing drug–drug interactions (Montgomery et al., 2001).

Other Agents

Most studies of other medications (venlafaxine, buspirone, trazoadone, clonazepam and MAOIs for OCD have consisted of only case reports or small samples. However, few of these agents have been promising enough to warrant large blinded efficacy trials.

Which SRI to Choose?

The efficacy of each SRI – clomipramine, fluoxetine, fluvoxamine, sertraline, paroxetine, and citalopram – is supported by existing data. During the last 12 years at least seven head-to-head SRI comparison studies have been done, six of which compared clomipramine with fluoxetine, fluvoxamine, paroxetine and sertraline. All of the studies found that the agents studied were equally efficacious, although they may have been underpowered to detect differences among medications. However, several meta-analyses of OCD trials, which compared SRIs across large placebo-controlled multicenter trials, lend some support to the notion that clomipramine might be more effective than the more selective agents. These meta-analyses support a trial of clomipramine in all patients who do not respond to SRIs, even though clomipiramine tends to cause more side effects.

A number of studies have assessed predictors of medication response. Predictors of poor response include failure to respond to a previous SRI, early age of OCD onset, presence of schizotypal personality disorder and presence of hoarding. However, not all studies have had consistent findings, and more investigation of this issues is needed using larger and more narrowly defined samples.

It is worth noting that the SSRIs, via their effect on the liver cytochrome system, can inhibit the metabolism of certain other drugs. Fluoxetine can elevate blood levels of a variety of coadministered drugs, including tricyclic antidepressants (such as clomipramine), carbamazepine, phenytoin and trazodone. However, the other SSRIs (with the exception of citalopram) can theoretically cause similar elevations, although fewer reports on such interactions are currently available. Some clinicians have taken advantage of these interactions by carefully combining fluvoxamine with clomipramine in order to block clomipramine's metabolism to desmethylclomipramine; this in turn favors serotonin reuptake inhibition provided by the parent compound rather than the norepinephrine reuptake inhibition provided by the metabolite. However, caution should be used with this approach since the elevation in clomipramine levels, and perhaps other compounds, can be nonlinear and quickly lead to dangerous toxicity; at the very least, clomipramine levels should be carefully monitored.

All of the SSRIs are generally well tolerated, with a relatively low percentage of patients experiencing notable side effects or discontinuing them because of side effects. In addition, these compounds are unlikely to be lethal in overdose, except for clomipramine, which can lead to cardiac arrhythmias and death. All these agents can cause sexual side effects, ranging from anorgasmia to difficulty with ejaculatory function. However, such symptoms are not readily volunteered by the patient, thus it is important to ask. Should such symptoms be experienced, conservative measures may include dosage reduction, transient drug holidays for a special weekend or occasion, or switching to another SRI since patients may not have the same degree of dysfunction with a different agent. However if the clinician feels that it is critical to continue with same agent, various treatments have been reported in the literature. Usually taken within a few hours of sexual activity, no one agent has been shown to work consistently. Among those that have been tried are yohimbine, buspirone, cyproheptadine, buproprion, dextroamphetamine, methylphenidate, amantidine, nefazodone, to name but a few.

Assessing Treatment Resistance

Before concluding that a patient is treatment-resistant, the adequacy of previous treatment trials must be assessed (see Table 51.2). In particular, it is critical to know both the duration and dose of every medication that has been used. Typically, patients who appear treatment-resistant have received an inadequate duration of treatment, which should be a minimum of 10 to 12 weeks, or an inadequate medication dose, which should be the maximum dose for any particular agent. Some psychiatrists consider patients truly treatment-resistant only if they have failed

Table 51.2	Things to Consider in Patients with Obsessive–Compulsive Disorder in Whom Initial Treatment Fails

Was the diagnosis correct?
Is there an Axis II disorder, especially schizotypal or obsessive–compulsive personality disorder?
Are there comorbid diagnoses that could interfere with treatment response?
Is there a major depressive disorder?
Are there obsessive thoughts, overvalued ideas, or delusions?

Was the pharmacotherapy trial adequate?
Was a known effective agent used?
Was the dose adequate?
Was the duration of treatment long enough?

Was behavioral therapy performed?
Were an adequate number of sessions attended?
Did the patient comply with homework assignment?
Was there cognitive impairment inhibiting the ability to implement treatment?
Was there concurrent use of central nervous system depressants that affect ability to attend to evoked anxiety?

several adequate pharmacologic trials, including one with clomipramine, and several augmentation strategies including behavioral therapy. With this kind of aggressive treatment, 80 to 90% of patients usually experience some improvement, although few patients become symptom-free.

When inadequate treatment is not the reason for poor treatment response, it is important to assess the accuracy of the diagnosis. Schizotypal personality disorder, borderline personality disorder, avoidant personality disorder and OCPD seem to be associated with poorer response to pharmacotherapy, particularly if the personality disorder is the primary diagnosis. Behavioral therapy seems less effective in patients with comorbid major depressive disorder. Comorbid depression may inhibit the ability to learn and to habituate to anxiety. Initial pharmacotherapy sometimes improves depression, as well as OCD symptoms, and may increase the likelihood of success with behavioral treatment.

Augmentation Strategies

If a patient has had only a partial response to an antiobsessional agent of adequate dose and duration, the next question is whether to change the SRI or add an augmenting agent. Current clinical practice suggests that if there is no response at all to an SRI, it may be best to change to another SRI. However, if there has been some response to treatment, an augmentation trial of at least 2 to 8 weeks may be warranted. No augmentation agent has been firmly established as efficacious. Many questions about augmentation remain unanswered, including the optimal duration of augmentation, comparative efficacy of different agents, predictors of response and mechanism of action. Nonetheless, these agents do help some patients significantly, and thus their systematic use should be considered (see Table 51.3).

In patients with severe symptoms or comorbid psychosis or tic disorder, pimozide 1 to 3 mg/day, haldol 2 to 10 mg/day, and other neuroleptic agents (risperdone 2–8 mg/day and olanzapine 2.5–10 mg/day) have been used with some success.

Table 51.3   Potential Augmenting Agents for Treatment-Resistant Obsessive–Compulsive Disorder

Augmenting Agent	Suggested Dosage Range*†
Lithium	300–600 mg/d†
Clonazepam	1–3 mg/d
Tryptophan	2–10 g/d‡
Trazodone	100–200 mg/d
Buspirone	15–60 mg/d
Alprazolam	0.5–2 mg/d
Methylphenidate	10–30 mg/d
Haloperidol	2–10 mg/d
Pimozide	2–10 mg/d
Nifedipine	10 mg t.i.d
Liothyronine sodium	10–25 mg/d
Clonidine	0.1–0.6 mg/d
Fenfluramine	Up to 60 mg/d

*Add these to an ongoing trial of antidepressant medication. It should be noted that most of these dosages have not been tested with rigorous clinical trials but simply represent some of the reported doses tried in the current literature. Some would not recommend augmentation unless the initial treatment showed some response.

†*Use with caution* – there have been some reports of elevated lithium levels with ongoing fluoxetine treatment.

‡Because the use of l-tryptophan has been implicated in an increased incidence of eosinophilia, the authors advise against the prescribing and use of this agent until the issue is resolved.

Reprinted with permission from Management of patients with treatment-resistant obsessive–compulsive disorder, Jenike MA (1991). In Current Treatments of Obsessive–Compulsive Disorder, p. 146. Copyright 1991, American Psychiatric Press.

However, the use of a neuroleptic agent should be considered carefully in light of the risk of extrpyramidal symptoms and side effects such as weight gain, lethargy and tardive dyskinesia. Thus, when a neuroleptic drug is used, target symptoms should be established before beginning treatment, and the medication discontinued within several months if target symptoms do not improve.

The use of lithium (300–600 mg/day) and buspirone (up to 60 mg/day) as augmentation agents has also been explored. Both agents looked promising in open trials but failed to be effective in more systematic trials. Augmentation with fenfluramine (up to 60 mg/day), clonazepam (up to 5 mg/day), clonidine (0.1–0.6 mg/day) and trazodone (100–200 mg/day), as well as the combination of clomipramine with any of the SSRIs, has had anecdotal success but has not been evaluated in methodologically rigorous studies. Some potential augmenting agents and their dosage ranges are presented in Table 51.3.

Behavioral Therapy

Behavioral therapy is effective for OCD both as a primary treatment and as an augmentation agent. This form of therapy is based on the principle of exposure and response prevention. The patient is asked to endure, in a graduated manner, the anxiety that a specific obsessional fear provokes while refraining from compulsions that allay that anxiety. The principles behind the efficacy of treatment are explained to the patient in the following way. Although compulsions, either covert or overt, usually immediately relieve anxiety, this is only a short-term solution; the

anxiety will ultimately return, requiring the performance of another compulsion. However, if the patient resists the anxiety and urge to ritualize, the anxiety will eventually decrease on its own (i.e., habituation will occur), and the need to perform the ritual will eventually disappear. Thus, behavioral therapy helps the patient habituate to the anxiety and extinguish the compulsions.

Compulsions, especially overt behaviors like washing rituals, are more successfully treated by behavioral therapy than are obsessions alone or covert rituals like mental checking. This is because covert rituals are physically harder to resist than are rituals like handwashing and checking a door. In fact washing rituals are the most amenable to behavioral treatment, followed by checking rituals and then mental rituals.

For rituals that do not constitute overt behaviors, techniques other than exposure and response prevention have been used in conjunction with exposure and response prevention. These approaches include imaginal flooding and thought stopping. In imaginal flooding, the anxiety provoked by the obsessions is evoked by continually repeating the thought, often with the help of a continuous-loop tape or the reading of a "script" composed by the patient and therapist, until the thought no longer provokes anxiety. In thought stopping, an compulsive mental ritual (e.g., continually repeating a short prayer in one's head) is stopped by simply shouting, making a loud noise, or snapping a rubber band on the wrist in an attempt to interrupt the thought.

In the early stages of treatment, a behavioral assessment is performed. During this assessment, the content, frequency, duration, amount of interference and distress, and attempts to resist or ignore the obsessions and compulsions are catalogued. An attempt is made to clarify the types of symptoms, any triggers that bring on the obsessions and compulsions, and the amount and type of avoidance used to deal with the symptoms. For instance, in the clinical vignette described later, the fact that Ms Z stopped preparing meals to deal with her obsessional concerns about contamination was carefully documented. The patient, usually with the help of a therapist, then develops a hierarchy of situations according to the amount of anxiety they provoke. During treatment, patients gradually engage in the anxiety-provoking situations included in their hierarchy without performing anxiety-reducing rituals.

Behavioral therapy can be used with patients of any age and has been used in young children, often with the help of a parent as a cotherapist. However, systematic trials of behavioral treatment in children have not been performed. More recently, behavioral therapy in a group setting has been explored and found as effective as, and perhaps even more effective than, individual behavioral treatment. The group seems to act as a catalyst for change by promoting group cohesion, support and encouragement. Groups can include patients with different symptoms, though each has a personalized hierarchy, so that one patient can encourage another. Van Noppen and associates (1991) included family members in groups because families are often affected by the patient's rituals and often function as unwilling participants in rituals. As members of the group, family members not only gain knowledge and understanding about OCD but can be cotherapists at home for homework assignments.

Despite its efficacy, behavioral therapy has limitations. To begin with, about 15 to 25% of patients refuse to engage in behavioral treatment initially or drop out early in treatment because it is so anxiety-provoking. Behavioral treatment fails in another 25% of patients for a variety of other reasons, including concomitant depression; the use of central nervous system depressants, which

Clinical Vignette 1 *Pharmacology*

Ms M was a 38-year-old married teacher who had experienced OCD symptoms since age 10 years. At that time, she had a need to reread sentences, as well as a need to check things like doors and faucets to guard against something bad happening. Her symptoms subsided somewhat during her teenage years but resurfaced during her early twenties. She sought treatment from a hypnotherapist in her late twenties and subsequently did relatively well, with only minimal symptoms, for the next 10 years. She noted, however, that during that time she continued to be a nervous person who worried about everything.

At the time of her initial visit, she reported a significant worsening of her OCD symptoms during the previous weeks. In particular, she began to have trouble driving her car. She often found herself retracing her route to ascertain that she had not hit something or to pick up road debris that she was worried might get in her way. This behavior greatly lengthened her driving time and, as a result, Ms M began to drive less and to avoid unnecessary trips like driving to stores to shop. As her symptoms worsened, she began to avoid driving at night because she worried that she would not see debris and other objects in the road. In addition, much to her chagrin, she began to involve her husband in her rituals by asking him to drive back with her to make sure that nothing was wrong. She also experienced increased checking behavior, for example, rechecking how she had written a check or retracing her steps at school to ascertain that she had not kicked something down the stairs. Overall, she estimated that her symptoms were moderately severe and taking about 3 hours per day. Ms M had also begun to experience prominent neurovegetative symptoms of depression, including early morning awakening, decreased energy and initiative, psychomotor slowing and a 10-pound weight loss.

Ms M was entered in a 10-week placebo-controlled blinded clomipramine trial and received clomipramine 250 mg/day. Within 3 weeks of starting treatment, she began to show some signs of improvement. She reported less frequent episodes of driving back and less avoidance of driving to go shopping; however, she did not experience much change in other checking behaviors. After 5 to 6 weeks at 250 mg/day of clomipramine, Ms M noted marked improvement (approximately 85%) in her symptoms. She had only transient episodes of needing to drive back, which lasted less than 5 minutes, and no avoidance of driving; her checking had also improved. She began to have some symptom-free days. Ms M also had no depressive symptoms and experienced a general sense of well-being that was a significant improvement from her baseline. However, she began to complain of significant drowsiness and fatigue, despite adequate sleep, as well as dry mouth and tremor.

Within 10 weeks of beginning treatment, Ms M was virtually free of OCD symptoms, experiencing only a few mild and transient episodes. Because she was at the end of the blinded medication period, her clomipramine dose was decreased from 250 to 150 mg/day. Within 1 week, she reported that she had started retracing her route while driving and had other symptoms of OCD that occupied about 1 hour per day. Her dose was increased to 200 mg/day, but in 1 week she called her physician to say that she was distressed because her OCD symptoms had interfered with her ability to pick up her child and that her symptoms had increased to 3 hours per day. Her clomipramine was increased to 250 mg/day. Within 8 weeks, Ms M had returned to her previous level of good health. She was driving normally, was not checking or engaging in avoidance behavior, and had no obsessional fear of harm coming to others. Although on some days she experienced about 45 minutes of fleeting symptoms, on other days she was totally symptom-free. However, she was experiencing some side effects, such as dry mouth, tremor, weight gain and fatigue. Her fatigue became marked to the point that she came home from her job as a school teacher exhausted and slept 16 hours a day on the weekend.

After 1 year at 250 mg/day of clomipramine, a taper was again attempted, and the medication was discontinued within a month. Before the taper, Ms M's Y-BOCS score was 4 (out of a possible total score of 40), but after 2 weeks without medication it rose to 6, indicating an increased effort on her part to resist her obsessions and compulsions. After 7 weeks of not taking medication, her Y-BOCS score rose to 10, and after 15 weeks it rose to 16, indicating moderate symptom severity. She noted that she had 1 to 3 hours of obsessions and 1 hour of compulsions per day, with increasing effort needed to resist symptoms. In addition, she noted the return of her nervousness and tendency to worry. However, Ms M also had a lessening of her fatigue and lost five of the 10 pounds she had gained on the medication.

The return of symptoms was distressing to Ms M, and she decided to try another medication. Sertraline was begun, and after only 6 to 8 weeks of treatment, at 200 mg/day, she had a remission of all OCD symptoms and the return of a sense of well-being. She had no side effects. At 5 months of follow-up she remained symptom-free, and her Y-BOCS score had decreased to 1, with only 15 minutes of symptoms per week.

may inhibit the ability to habituate to anxiety; lack of insight; poor compliance with homework, resulting in inadequate exposure; and poor compliance on the part of the therapist in enforcing the behavioral paradigm. Thus, overall, 50 to 70% of patients are helped by this form of therapy.

One of the issues that has emerged in treating OCD with CBT is the lack of trained therapists and the cost of repeated individual exposure sessions. Thus, in addition to developing group treatments which allow therapists to treat a number of patients simultaneously, researchers have begun to develop computer-guided behavior therapy. Several recent reports have shown that while this modality is not as effective as individual behavior therapy, it does allow for significant improvement in symptoms over a control condition like relaxation therapy.

Behavior therapy can be used as the sole treatment of OCD, particularly with patients whose contamination fears or somatic obsessions make them resistant to taking medications. Behavioral treatment is also a powerful adjunct to pharmacotherapy. Some research appears to indicate that combined treatment may be more effective than pharmacotherapy or behavioral therapy alone, although these findings are still preliminary. Some studies have even suggested that adding pharmacotherapy to behavior therapy may be particularly helpful in reducing obsessions while compulsions respond to behavior therapy. From a clinical perspective, it may be useful to have patients begin treatment with medication to reduce the intensity of their symptoms or comorbid depressive symptoms if present; patients may then be more amenable to experiencing the anxiety that will be evoked by the behavioral challenges they perform.

Work by Baxter and colleagues (1992) has illustrated some interesting correlations between treatment response and changes in neuroanatomy and neurophysiology. Positron emission tomography scans with ^{18}F-fluorodeoxyglucose were performed on all patients before and after treatment. Compared with nonresponders and control subjects, responders in both the medication and the behavioral treatment groups showed a decrease in activity in the right head of the caudate nucleus. This finding seems to support the notion that both forms of treatment bring about similar changes in neurophysiology which lead to improvement in symptoms. These results also provide important theoretical links with the serotonin hypothesis described earlier in this chapter, as basal ganglion structures like the caudate nucleus have been postulated to mediate serotonin function.

Psychotherapy

The use of psychotherapeutic techniques of either a psychoanalytic or a supportive nature has not been proved successful in treating the specific obsessions and compulsions that are a hallmark of OCD. However, the more characterological aspects that are part of obsessive–compulsive personality disorder may be helped by a more psychoanalytically oriented approach. As noted earlier, the defense mechanisms of reaction formation, isolation and undoing, as well as a pervasive sense of doubt and need to be in control, are hallmarks of the obsessive–compulsive character. Salzman (1983) and MacKinnon and Michels (1971) have written elegantly on how to approach the maladaptive aspects of this character style in therapy. In essence, the patient must be encouraged to take risks and learn to feel comfortable with, or at least less anxious about, making mistakes and to accept anxiety as a natural and normal part of human experience. Techniques for meeting such goals in treatment may include the psychiatrist's being relatively active in therapy to ensure that the patient focuses on the present rather than getting lost in perfectly recounting the past, as well as the psychiatrist's being willing to take risks and present herself or himself as less than perfect.

Neurosurgery

Occasionally, even after receiving adequate pharmacotherapy (including augmentation), adequate behavioral therapy, and a combination of behavioral therapy and pharmacotherapy, patients may still experience intractable OCD symptoms. Such patients may be candidates for neurosurgery. Although criteria for who should receive neurosurgery vary, it has been suggested that failure to respond to at least 5 years of systematic treatment is a reasonable criterion. Frequently used criteria are the following: a minimum of two adequate medication trials with augmentation plus adequate behavioral therapy in the absence of severe personality disorder.

The procedures that have been most successful interrupt tracts involved in the serotonin system. The surgical procedures used – anterior capsulotomy, cingulotomy and limbic leukotomy – all aim to interrupt the connection between the cortex and the basal ganglia and related structures. Current stereotactic surgical techniques involve the creation of precise lesions, which are often only 10 to 20 mm, to specific tracts. These procedures have often been done with radiofrequency heated electrodes and,

more recently, with gamma knife techniques. Postsurgical risks have been minimized, and in some cases cognitive function and personality traits improve along with symptoms of OCD.

Data compiled from a number of small studies have yielded success rates of 25 to 84% with treatment. However, most samples are small, and the procedures have often differed in both lesion location and size, making it difficult to compare them. However, in a recent prospective long-term follow-up study, all 44 patients received the same procedure (cingulotomy), although some had single procedures and others multiple procedures (Dougherty *et al.*, 2002). This study had several important findings. Clinical improvement occurred in 32 to 45% of patients, depending on the criteria used to rate full or partial response, and the average effect size was 1.27, comparable to that seen in pharmacologic trials (1.09–1.53). However, these changes were not immediately apparent postoperatively, and most patients were encouraged to engage in pharmacotherapy and/or behavior therapy postoperatively. The longitudinal follow-up component of the study, which was a mean duration of 32 months, allowed the researchers to assess the longer-term impact of the procedure in ways other studies could not. Of particular note, patients continued to show improvement for up to 29 months after surgery without receiving further procedures. As a result, the authors noted that the typical 6-month wait before deciding whether to repeat and extend the lesion may be too brief. In conclusion, neurosurgical treatments offer hope to some of the most severely ill and treatment-resistant patients and should therefore be considered. However, which surgical lesions are most effective in which patients still needs much more study.

Issues in the Physician–Patient Relationship

Treatment for OCD is often effective, leading to at least some response in a majority of patients. However, treatment adherence is difficult for some patients, which may interfere with treatment efficacy. Short- and long-term compliance with treatment can be greatly facilitated by considering how the nature of the illness affects the treatment modalities used.

At the core of OCD are the concepts of obsessional doubt, risk aversion and a need to feel in control of one's environment. These three concepts affect behavioral and pharmacological treatment. In the initial phases of behavioral treatment, it may be difficult to engage the patient in treatment because of his or her doubt that the treatment will be effective and an unwillingness to experience the anxiety that results from exposure to feared stimuli. Extra time must often be spent convincing patients of the potential efficacy of treatment and lack of serious side effects from behavioral treatment. Unlike pharmacological treatment, in which the side effects can be quantified in medical terms, the side effects that patients fear from behavioral treatment are related to their cognitive distortions. For instance, those with contamination fears may be thoroughly convinced that simply walking by an AIDS clinic will put them at risk of contracting AIDS or that simply using a public bathroom will give them a communicable disease. Thus, reassurance that this is not the case and that it is safe to engage in behavioral treatment may first involve playing out the catastrophic consequences in their mind or role-playing and discussing the irrational nature of the fear to the fullest extent possible.

When behavioral treatment is started, it is customary to develop a hierarchy of subjective units of distress, which rate particular events according to how much anxiety they produce. For some patients, the ability to develop this hierarchy and thereby obtain a sense of control over their fears, and the ability to begin with the least stressful challenges, can allow them to engage in behavioral treatment.

Similar concerns related to doubt, risk aversion and control must also be addressed when pharmacological treatment is undertaken. In the initial treatment phases, the major task is getting the patient to engage in treatment. Patients with OCD, particularly those with contamination and somatic obsessions, often have numerous questions about medication safety and may be hesitant to take them. Patients with contamination and somatic obsessions may be more likely to engage in behavioral treatment initially.

Although it is important that patients have a thorough understanding of side effects, the psychiatrist should not be thorough to an obsessional degree. Many patients with OCD want a detailed understanding of every side effect and have difficulty differentiating which side effects are of concern and which are not. Thus, it is critical when discussing side effects to present an objective assessment of the relative frequency and severity of various side effects. It is important to emphasize that even though some of the rare side effects are more serious than the more common side effects, they are unlikely to occur. It is also worth keeping in mind that the patient's concerns about a particular side effect may be different from the psychiatrist's. Again, it may help to elicit the catastrophic fears that the patient has and address the irrational obsessional qualities of those fears.

The initial phase of treatment is often the most difficult. This has to do with both risk aversion and a need to be in control. With pharmacologic treatment, patients may occasionally experience an initial worsening of symptoms in addition to side effects. This can be terrifying to the patient and can lead to an abrupt discontinuation of the medication. Warning the patient before treatment that this might occur increases the patient's sense of control. Similarly, the antiobsessional effects of treatment often take 6 to 10 weeks to be seen and are often gradual in onset. This gradual response is usually delayed until after the patient experiences side effects. Thus, the early phase of treatment may need to focus on encouraging the patient to stay on medication despite side effects and no improvement. Side effects can often be framed as a good sign that the medication is being actively absorbed by the body. Again, preparing patients in advance helps them feel in control and able to continue treatment. The gradual onset of improvement, although in some cases frustrating, is also reassuring to patients who might feel out of control if improvement occurred too rapidly.

Unlike many patients with mood disorders, most patients with OCD do not have full recovery from their symptoms. Although the majority of patients, perhaps as many as 85%, experience some improvement, most tend to remain symptomatic to some degree. Nonetheless, symptom improvement of even 10 to 15% can have a dramatic effect on their lives.

Duration and Discontinuation of Treatment

Little systematic research has been performed to guide decisions about continuation, maintenance and discontinuation of treatment. The largest study of extended pharmacologic treatment involved fluoxetine (Tollefson et al., 1994b). In this study, 70 patients who had responded to fluoxetine and 198 patients who had not responded during an acute 13-week trial were given the

opportunity to continue on medication for another 6 months. At the end of the 6 months, 74.3% of those who had responded initially experienced further improvement. In the nonresponder group, 91.7% experienced a decrease in symptoms when the medication dose was increased from the previous unsuccessful dose. Only 19% of patients ($N - 13$) experienced a significant worsening of symptoms during the follow-up period. Similar to previous reports on fluoxetine, this study suggested that symptom improvement was maintained over time. Even more important, further improvement occurred in responders with longer treatment and in nonresponders with continued treatment at higher doses.

In another study, 85 patients who had been treated with a variety of antiobsessional medications were followed up 1 to 3.5 years after initial treatment (Orloff et al., 1994). Ninety-four percent of the patients were still taking medication, and 87% had maintained previous gains or achieved further improvement. Thus, from a clinical point of view, it seems wise to continue medication for an extended period, perhaps for 6 months to a year after initiating treatment, because during this period improvement is maintained and some patients experience further improvement. Overall, this extended duration of treatment did not result in worsening side effects; in fact, in most cases patients habituated to side effects. In general, the most bothersome side effects that persist with SRI treatment appear to be fatigue, weight gain and sexual dysfunction.

In recent years a number of studies of long-term efficacy have emerged. One study that included a follow-up period of 2 years for 38 OCD patients on sertraline showed continued efficacy with fewer side effects with longer-term treatment. Another study assessed a larger group of patients and attempted to answer important clinical questions not only about long-term efficacy but about the effects of medication discontinuation after 1 year of treatment. The latter is an important question because few studies of systematic discontinuation have been carried out and in those that have been done relapse rates were quite high, above 90%. This sertraline study (Koran et al., 2002) involved 223 patients who had been successfully treated with single-blind sertraline for 52 weeks who were then randomized in a double-blind manner to continue treatment for another 6 months or placebo. One-third of the patients in the placebo group relapsed; this was surprisingly lower than the percentage found in earlier studies. The authors offered several plausible explanations for this, which included the possibility that 1 year of effective treatment may provide sustained benefit for patients, and that patients may have engaged in self-directed behavior therapy, something that was not readily available at the time of the previous discontinuation studies. They also noted that while OCD symptom ratings did not worsen in the placebo-treated group as a whole, quality of life did significantly deteriorate. This finding points to the need for more sensitive measures of patient improvement and for further studies of long-term treatment efficacy.

Some preliminary data have suggested that in treatment responders it may be possible to decrease the dose of clomipramine over the longer term without subsequent relapse, although this important issue needs further investigation.

The data on discontinuation of behavioral therapy are also encouraging and overall, about 75% of patients continue to do well at follow-up. However, most studies also noted that few patients were symptom-free.

Conclusion

For many patients with OCD the illness is life long, starting in early childhood and extending into adulthood. It is often familial and accompanied by comorbid conditions including depression, other anxiety disorders, Tourette's syndrome and even psychosis. However, with a combination of pharmacologic and behavioral treatment, at adequate dose and duration, patients can often have significant improvement in symptoms and overall function.

Comparison of DSM-IV/ICD-10 Diagnostic Criteria

The ICD-10 Diagnostic Criteria for Research for Obsessive–Compulsive Disorder differentiate between obsessions and compulsions based on whether they are thoughts, ideas, or images (obsessions) or acts (compulsions). In contrast, DSM-IV-TR distinguishes between obsessions and compulsions based on whether the thought, idea, or image causes anxiety or distress or prevents or reduces it. Thus, in DSM-IV-TR, there can be cognitive compulsions which would be considered obsessions in ICD-10. In addition, ICD-10 sets a minimum duration of at least 2 weeks whereas DSM-IV-TR has no minimum duration.

References

American Psychiatric Association (1994) *Diagnostic and Statistical Manual of Mental Disorders*, 4th edn. American Psychiatric Association, Washington DC.

Baxter LR, Schwartz JM, Bergman KS *et al.* (1992) Caudate glucose metabolic rate changes with both drug and behavior therapy for obsessive–compulsive disorder. *Arch Gen Psychiatr* 49, 681–689.

Bienvenu OJ, Samuels JF, Riddle MA *et al.* (2000) The relationship of obsessive–compulsive disorder to possible spectrum disorders: Results from a family study. *Biol Psychiatr* 48(4), 287–293.

Cohen LJ, Stein D and Galykner I (1997) Towards an intergration of psychological and biological models of obsessive–compulsive disorder: Phylogenetics considerations. *CNS Spect* 2(10), 26–44.

Dougherty DD, Laer L, Cosgrove GR *et al.* (2002) Prospective long-term follow-up of 44 patients who received cingulotomy for treatment refractory obsessive–compulsive disorder. *Am J Psychiatr* 159, 269–275.

Eisen JL, Goodman W, Keller MB *et al.* (1999) Patterns of remission and relapse in OCD: A 2-year prospective study, *J Clin Psychiatr* 60, 346–351.

Flament MF, Koby E, Rapoport JL, *et al.* (1990) Childhood obsessive–compulsive disorder: A prospective follow-up study. *J Child Psychol Psychiatr* 31, 363–380.

Foa EB and Kozak MJ (1995) DSM-IV field trial: Obsessive–compulsive disorder. *Am J Psychiatr* 152, 90–96.

Freud S (1963) An infantile neurosis, in *The Standard Edition of the Complete Psychologic Works of Sigmund Freud*, Vol. 17. (trans-ed Strachey J). Hogarth Press, London. Originally published in 1955.

Goodman WK, Price LH, Rasmussen SA *et al.* (1989) The Yale-Brown Obsessive–Compulsive Scale. Development, use, and reliability. *Arch Gen Psychiatr* 46, 1006–1011.

Hoehn-Saric R, Ninan P, Black DW *et al.* (2000) Multicenter double-blind comparison of sertraline and desipramine for concurrent obsessive–compulsive and major depressive disorders. *Arch Gen Psychiatr* 57, 76–82.

Hollander E (1993) Introduction. In Obsessive–Compulsive Related Disorders, Hollander E (ed). American Psychiatric Press, Washington DC, pp. 1–16.

Jenike MA (1991) Management of patients with treatment-resistant obsessive–compulsive disorder, in *Current Treatments of Obsessive–Compulsive Disorder* (eds Pato MT and Zohar J). American Psychiatric Press, Washington DC, p. 146.

Kessler RC, Berglund MBA, Demler O *et al.* (2005) Lifetime prevalence and age-of-onset distributions of DSM-IV disorders in the National Comorbidity Survey Replication. *Arch Gen Psychiatr* 62, 593–602.

Koran LM, Hackett E, Rubin A *et al.* (2002) Efficacy of sertraline in the long term treatment of obsessive–compulsive disorder. *Am J Psychiatr* 159, 88–95.

Leckman JF, Boardman J, Grice DE *et al.* (1997) Symptoms of obsessive–compulsive disorder. *Am J Psychiatr* 154, 911–917.

Leonard HL, Swedo SE, Lenane MC *et al.* (1993) A 2- to 7-year follow-up study of 54 obsessive–compulsive children and adolescents. *Arch Gen Psychiatr* 50, 429–439.

MacKinnon RA and Michels R (1971) The obsessive patient, in *The Psychiatric Interview in Clinical Practice* (eds MacKinnon RA and Michels R). WB Saunders, Philadelphia, pp. 89–109.

March JS, Frances A, Carpenter D *et al.* (1997) The expert consensus guildine series: Treatment of obsessive–compulsive disorder. *J Clin Psychiatr* 58(suppl 4).

Montgomery SA, Kasper S, Stein DL *et al.* (2001 March) Citalopram 20 mg, 40 mg and 60 mg are all effective and well tolerated compared with placebo in obsessive–compulsive disorder. *Int Clin Psychopharmacol* 16(2), 75–86.

Myers JK, Weissman MM, Tischler GL *et al.* (1984) Six-month prevalence of psychiatric disorders in three communities, 1980 to 1982. *Arch Gen Psychiatr* 41, 949–958.

Orloff LM, Battle MA, Baer L *et al.* (1994) Long-term follow-up of 85 patients with obsessive–compulsive disorder. *Am J Psychiatr* 151, 441–442.

Pato MT, Eisen JL and Pato CN (1994) Rating scales for obsessive–compulsive disorder, in *Current Insights in Obsessive–Compulsive Disorder* (eds Hollander E, Zohar J, Marazziti D *et al.*). John Wiley, West Sussex, UK, pp. 77–92.

Phillips KA (1991) Body dysmorphic disorder: The distress of imagined ugliness. *Am J Psychiatr* 148, 1138–1149.

Rasmussen SA and Eisen JL (1991) Phenomenology of obsessive–compulsive disorder, in *Psychobiology of Obsessive–Compulsive Disorder* (eds Insel J and Rasmussen S). Springer-Verlag, New York, pp. 743–758.

Rasmussen SA and Eisen JL (1998) The epidemiology and clinical features of obsessive–compulsive disorder, in *Obsessive–Compulsive Disorders: Practical Management* (eds Jenike M, Baer L and Minichiello W). Mosby, St Louis, Missouri.

Rauch SL, Dougherty DD, Shin LM *et al.* (1998) Neural correlates of factor-analyzed OCD symptom dimensions: A PET Study CNS Spectrums 1998; 3(7), 37–43.

Ricciardi JN, Baer L, Jenike MA *et al.* (1992) Changes in DSM-III-R axis II diagnoses following treatment of obsessive–compulsive disorder. *Am J Psychiatr* 149, 829–831.

Robins LN, Helzer JE, Weissman MM *et al.* (1984) Lifetime prevalence of specific psychiatric disorders in three sites. Arch Gen Psychiatr 41, 958–967.

Salzman L (1983) Psychoanalytic therapy of the obsessional patient. *Curr Psychiatr Ther* 9, 53–59.

Saxena S, Brody AL, Schwartz JM *et al.* (1998) Neuroimaging and frontal–subcortical circuitry in obsessive–compulsive disorder. *Br J Psychiatr* 173(Suppl 35), 26–37.

Skoog G and Skoog I (1999) A 40-year follow-up of patients with obsessive–compulsive disorder. *Arch Gen Psychiatr* 56, 121–127.

Steketee G, Eisen JL, Dyke I *et al.* (1999) Predictors of Course in Obsessive–Compulsive Disorder. *Psychiatr Res* 89, 229–238.

Swedo SE, Leonard HL, Garvey M *et al.* (1998) Pediatric autoimmune neuropsychiatric disorders associated with streptococcal infection: Clinical description of the first 50 cases. *Am J Psychiatr* 155, 264–271.

Tollefson GD, Rampey AH, Potvin JH, *et al.* (1994b) A multicenter investigation of fixed dose fluoxetine in the treatment of obsesssive–compulsive disorder. *Arch Gen Psychiatr* 51, 559–567.

Van Noppen BL, Rasmussen SA, McCartney L *et al.* (1991) A multifamily group approach as an adjunct to treatment of obsessive–compulsive disorders, in *Current Treatments of Obsessive–Compulsive Disorder* (eds Pato MT and Zohar J). American Psychiatric Press, Washington DC, pp. 115–134.

Weissman MM, Bland RC, Canino GL, *et al.* (1994) The cross-national epidemiology of obsessive–compulsive disorder. *J Clin Psychiatr* 55, 5–10.

Wheadon D, Bushnell W and Steiner M (1993) A fixed-dose comparison of 20, 40, or 60 mg paroxetine to placebo in the treatment of obsessive–compulsive disorder. Presented at the Annual Meeting of the American College of Neuropsychopharmacology Honolulu, Hawaii.

52 Anxiety Disorders: Traumatic Stress Disorders

Post Traumatic Stress Disorder

Definition

PTSD is defined in the *Diagnostic and Statistical Manual of Mental Disorders*, Fourth Edition (DSM-IV) by six different criteria (American Psychiatric Association, 1994, see pp. 427–429). First, the disorder arises in a person who has been exposed to a traumatic event in which he or she experienced, witnessed, or was confronted with actual or threatened death or serious injury or a threat to the physical integrity of self or others. Furthermore, the response must have involved intense fear, helplessness, or horror. In children, it is allowed that the response may take the form of disorganized or agitated behavior.

Secondly, there must have been at least one of five possible intrusive symptoms occurring as a result of exposure to the trauma, as exhibited in either dream activity or waking life. These include recollections, images, thoughts, or perceptions of the event, recurrent distressing dreams, acting as if the trauma were recurring, and intense psychological or physical distress on exposure to internal or external cues resembling the trauma. Allowance is made for a different set of reactions in children, in whom intrusive symptoms may take the form of repetitive play, frightening dreams without recognizable content, or reenactment of the trauma.

Thirdly, persistent avoidance of stimuli associated with the trauma and numbing of general responsiveness must occur as exhibited by at least three of seven symptoms. Although grouped together as one criterion, it is likely that phobic avoidance, numbing and withdrawal do not reflect the same underlying phenomenon.

Fourthly, there must be at least two symptoms indicating the presence of increased arousal (i.e., difficulty sleeping, irritability or anger, difficulty concentrating, hypervigilance, or exaggerated startle response). Symptoms of PTSD should last at least 1 month, and it is necessary that the disturbances cause clinically significant distress or impairment in social, occupational, or other areas of functioning.

PTSD is considered to be "acute" if the duration of symptoms is between 1 and 3 months or "chronic" if it is 3 months or greater. If symptoms do not occur until at least 6 months have passed since the stressor, the delayed-onset subtype is given.

Epidemiology

Community-based studies conducted in the USA have documented a lifetime prevalence rate for PTSD of approximately 8% of the adult population (Kessler *et al.*, 1995). In the National Comorbidity

---

DSM-IV-TR Criteria 309.81

Post Traumatic Stress Disorder

A. The person has been exposed to a traumatic event in which both of the following were present:

    (1) the person experienced, witnessed, or was confronted with an event or events that involved actual or threatened death or serious injury, or a threat to the physical integrity of self or others

    (2) the person's response involved intense fear, helplessness, or horror. **Note:** In children, this may be expressed instead by disorganized or agitated behavior

B. The traumatic event is persistently reexperienced in one (or more) of the following ways:

    (1) recurrent and intrusive distressing recollections of the event, including images, thoughts, or perceptions. **Note:** In young children, repetitive play may occur in which themes or aspects of the trauma are expressed

    (2) recurrent distressing dreams of the event. **Note:** In children, there may be frightening dreams without recognizable content

    (3) acting or feeling as if the traumatic event were recurring (includes a sense of reliving the experience, illusions, hallucinations, and dissociative flashback episodes, including those that occur on awakening or when intoxicated). **Note:** In young children, trauma-specific reenactment may occur

    (4) intense psychological distress at exposure to internal or external cues that symbolize or resemble an aspect of the traumatic event

    (5) physiological reactivity on exposure to internal or external cues that symbolize or resemble an aspect of the traumatic event

C. Persistent avoidance of stimuli associated with the trauma and numbing of general responsiveness (not

---

Essentials of Psychiatry Jerald Kay and Allan Tasman
© 2006 John Wiley & Sons, Ltd.

present before the trauma), as indicated by three (or more) of the following:

   (1) efforts to avoid thoughts, feelings, or conversations associated with the trauma

   (2) efforts to avoid activities, places, or people that arouse recollections of the trauma

   (3) inability to recall an important aspect of the trauma

   (4) markedly diminished interest or participation in significant activities

   (5) feeling of detachment or estrangement from others

   (6) restricted range of affect (e.g., unable to have loving feelings)

   (7) sense of a foreshortened future (e.g., does not expect to have a career, marriage, children, or a normal life span)

D. Persistent symptoms of increased arousal (not present before the trauma), as indicated by two (or more) of the following:

   (1) difficulty falling or staying asleep

   (2) irritability or outbursts of anger

   (3) difficulty concentrating

   (4) hypervigilance

   (5) exaggerated startle response

E. Duration of the disturbance (symptoms in criteria B, C, and D) is more than 1 month.

F. The disturbance causes clinically significant distress or impairment in social, occupational, or other important areas of functioning.

Specify if:

Acute: if duration of symptoms is less than 3 months

Chronic: if duration of symptoms is 3 months or more

Specify if:

With delayed onset: if onset of symptoms is at least 6 months after the stressor

Reprinted with permission from the *Diagnostic and Statistical Manual of Mental Disorders*, Fourth Edition, Text Revision. Copyright 2000, American Psychiatric Association.

Survey replication this figure was 6.8% (Kessler *et al.*, 2005). The highest rates of PTSD occurrence for particular traumatic exposures (occurring in one-third to three-fourths of those exposed) are among survivors of rape, military combat and captivity, graves registration (i.e., registering dead bodies through the morgue), and ethnically or politically motivated internment and genocide.

    Epidemiological studies show that PTSD often remains chronic, with a significant number of people remaining symptomatic several years after the initial event. In support of this view are epidemiological data that show that recovery frequently

does not occur. For example, the National Vietnam Veterans Readjustment study (Kulka *et al.*, 1990) found lifetime and current prevalence rates of PTSD to be, respectively, 30.9% and 15.2% in men and 26.9% and 8.5% in women. In a population of rape victims, Kilpatrick and colleagues (1987) found a lifetime prevalence rate of 75.8% and a current prevalence rate of 39.4%. In children, studies by Pynoos and associates (1993) revealed prevalence rates of 58.4% in children exposed to sniper attacks in the USA and 70.2% in those exposed to an earthquake in Armenia. Kessler and colleagues (1995) documented that one-third of those diagnosed with PTSD fail to recover even after many years. Therefore, chronicity of PTSD is not limited to the more severe treatment-seeking samples.

Etiology and Pathophysiology

The Event

PTSD is defined in terms of etiology as much as phenomenology. The disorder cannot exist unless the individual has been exposed to a traumatic event with a particular set of properties. Community-based epidemiological studies suggest that 70% of individuals will experience at least one traumatic event meeting criterion A(1) over the course of their lifetime. The relative severity of the traumatic event, predisposing factors and peritraumatic environmental factors must all be considered in understanding the etiology of PTSD. In most instances, occurrence of the disorder represents the outcome of an interaction among these three groups of factors. The likelihood of developing PTSD with regard to the nature of the event has shown consistent relationship occurred between magnitude of stress exposure and risk of developing PTSD. This association held up in many different trauma populations in adults and children.

    Cognitive and affective responses to the stressor are also important in determining the likelihood that PTSD will develop. A traumatic event is defined as an event that involves experiencing or witnessing actual or threatened death or serious injury or learning about an unexpected or violent death and having a response that involves intense fear, helplessness, or horror.

Biological Factors

Patients with chronic PTSD have increased circulating levels of norepinephrine and increased reactivity of the alpha-2-adrenergic receptors. These changes have been hypothesized possibly to account for some of the somatic symptoms that occur in individuals with PTSD. Neuroanatomical studies have implicated alterations in the amygdala and hippocampus in patients with PTSD. Functional magnetic resonance imaging and positron-emission tomography have demonstrated increased reactivity of the amygdala and anterior paralimbic region to trauma-related stimuli. Furthermore, in response to trauma-related stimuli, there is decreased reactivity of the anterior cingulate and orbitofrontal areas. These biological alterations suggest that there may be a neuroanatomical substrate for symptoms (intrusive recollections and other cognitive problems) that characterize PTSD. However, it is unknown whether these changes are preexisting, a result of traumatic exposure, or a result of having PTSD.

Sympathetic Nervous System Alterations

There is a positive association between the diagnosis of PTSD and basal cardiovascular activity. Particularly, individuals with a current PTSD diagnosis have a higher resting heart rate relative to both trauma-exposed individuals without a PTSD diagnosis and nontrauma-exposed controls and this appears to be greatest in studies with the most chronic PTSD samples. Along with increased 24-hour urinary catecholamines, results suggest an increase in sympathetic tone. There has been repeated demonstration that there is heightened sympathetic arousal in PTSD patients when reexposed to the original trauma in controlled settings.

Although a conditioning model provides a viable explanation of the process through which trauma-related cues may generate the heightened physiological responses characteristic of PTSD, it does not explain why some individuals develop PTSD when exposed to traumatic events, while others do not. It has been hypothesized that differential susceptibility to developing PTSD might be attributable in part to individual differences in conditionability, such that some individuals more readily acquire and maintain a conditioned response compared with others, and thus may be more likely to develop PTSD after a traumatic event.

There is evidence of brain dysfunction in individuals with PTSD as evidenced by abnormalities in evoked potentials. These ERP findings suggest that PTSD patients have increased cortical inhibition to high-intensity stimuli, impairments in memory and concentration, auditory gating deficits and heightened selective attention to trauma-related stimuli. However, whether these processing abnormalities are a precursor or a result of PTSD awaits further study.

Psychophysiological response to acute trauma exposure may predict the development of PTSD. Shalev and colleagues (1990) demonstrated that on arrival to the emergency department, regardless of whether PTSD ultimately developed, survivors of traumatic events showed elevated heart rates upon arrival to the emergency department, which at later assessment occasions were normal. However, those who subsequently developed PTSD showed higher emergency department and 1-week heart rates than those who did not.

Neuroendocrine Factors

The hypothalamic–pituitary–adrenal (HPA) axis has been the most extensively studied neuroendocrine system in PTSD. The principal findings are as follows: reduced 24-hour urinary cortisol excretion, supersuppression of cortisol after low-dose dexamethasone administration, blunting of corticotropin in response to corticotropin-releasing hormone and increased numbers of glucocorticoid receptors. This suggests that chronic PTSD is accompanied by supersuppression of the emergency HPA response to acute stress. This may result from the organism's attempt to protect itself from the potentially toxic effect of high levels of corticosteroids that might occur with repeated exposure to stress or from reminders of the trauma. In further support of the importance of HPA axis alteration in PTSD is the finding that glucocorticoid receptor changes also correlate with the severity of PTSD symptoms, but not with the less specific anxiety and depressive symptoms measured on other rating scales. More recently, in a large sample of Vietnam veterans, combat-exposed veterans with current PTSD had lower cortisol compared with noncombat-exposed veterans without PTSD or combat-exposed veterans with lifetime PTSD but without current PTSD (Boscarino, 1996).

Further evidence for abnormalities in neurotransmitter regulation comes from provocation studies conducted with Vietnam veterans. Administration of yohimbine, an alpha-$_2$-adrenergic antagonist, provoked symptoms of PTSD in combat veterans who had PTSD as did the serotoninergic challenge with m-chlorophenylpiperazine. Of considerable interest is that there was no overlap between these two groups, suggesting some selectivity in the way in which neurotransmitter systems can be affected between individuals (Southwick *et al.*, 1993; Krystal *et al.*, 1989). Finally, evidence to support alteration of noradrenergic and serotoninergic pathways in PTSD comes from the clinical effects of medications that are selective for these neurotransmitter systems, as discussed later. The opioid system has also been investigated, but less extensively and without any consensus being obtained.

Sleep Studies

Studies support that there are two distinct, but possibly interrelated types of sleep complaints in individuals with PTSD: nightmares that replicate traumatic events and impairment in initiating and maintaining sleep. Data further suggest that sleep problems in PTSD can also include excessive motor activity and awakenings with somatic anxiety symptoms. There is support for these complaints using polysomnography (PSG) studies, particularly in reduced sleep time or efficiency, and increased awakenings in the PTSD patients. There has also been documentation of PTSD subgroups that evidence breathing-related sleep disorders. PTSD is associated with a more fragmented rapid eye movement sleep as well.

Psychological Factors

Behavioral Models

Conditioning theory has been helpful in explaining the process through which stimuli that are associated with a traumatic event can alone elicit intense emotional responses in individuals who have PTSD. Cues (i.e., conditioned stimuli) that are present at the time of the trauma (the unconditioned stimulus) become associated with the unconditioned emotional response (fear, helplessness, or horror). Following the traumatic event, these cues alone can then repeatedly elicit the strong emotional response. For example, a woman who has been raped (unconditioned stimulus) in a dark alley (conditioned stimulus) by a man (conditioned stimulus) and has an intense fear response (unconditioned response) may demonstrate a fear response (now the conditioned response) when she sees a dark alley (conditioned stimulus) or is in the presence of a man (conditioned stimulus). Avoidance behaviors develop to decrease anxiety associated with the conditioned stimuli. For example, the woman who has been raped may avoid going outside when it is dark and also avoid being in the company of men. Behavioral treatments using exposure principles require confrontation with the feared situation and may ultimately lead to reduction of anxiety.

Cognitive and Information Processing

Exposure to a severe or unexpected event may result in an inability to process and assimilate the experience adequately or to deal effectively with its impact. A period of prolonged, difficult and often incomplete assimilation occurs. The experience is kept alive in active memory, intruding itself into awareness either during the day or at night. The pain of the unbidden experience is followed by active attempts to avoid reminders of the trauma. These intrusive and avoidance phases often alternate (Horowitz, 1973).

Fear can be considered a cognitive structure with three elements: stimulus, response and meaning. To reduce fear, the fear memory must first be activated and then new information provided to modify the fear structure. Cognitive interventions can be used to recognize and change maladaptive cognitions and to replace interpretations of danger by realistic or safer interpretations, with the ultimate hope that the patient will integrate the new information into the fear structure, leading to a more realistic appraisal of the degree of danger.

Genetic–Familial Factors

From the available literature, which is based on male combat veterans, general population surveys and rape-trauma-related PTSD, there is evidence to suggest that anxiety and depression in families is a risk factor for PTSD. A twin study of Vietnam veterans concordant and discordant for combat exposure has shown that a significant part of the variance is explained on the basis of genetic factors with respect to all three symptom clusters (i.e., intrusive, avoidant and hyperarousal symptoms) (True et al., 1993). McLeod and colleagues (2001) examined the role of genetic and environmental influences on the relationship between combat exposure, post traumatic stress disorder symptoms and alcohol use in 4072 male–male twin pairs; the authors found that alcohol problems occur together because of a shared vulnerability that increases risk for both disorders. These findings are most consistent with the shared vulnerability hypothesis in which combat exposure, PTSD symptoms and alcohol use are associated because some portion of the genes that influence vulnerability to combat also influence vulnerability to PTSD symptoms and alcohol consumption. It is important to note, however, that specific unique environmental factors the twins did not share were more important than genetic factors for combat exposure and PTSD symptoms, whereas environmental influences appeared about equally important as genetic influences on alcohol use. Overall, the evidence suggests that psychiatric history, both personal or in family members, increases the likelihood of being exposed to a trauma and of developing PTSD once exposed.

Other Factors

Although systematic research is scant, it may be that individuals exposed to repeated or continuous trauma, particularly of an interpersonal nature, may be more likely to develop PTSD. Trauma involving loss of community or support structures is likely to be particularly damaging. Because social support has been held to produce a buffering effect, lack of support might be considered an additional vulnerability factor. Women are at more risk than men for PTSD.

Diagnosis

Assessment and Diagnostic Features

The diagnosis of PTSD is based on a history of exposure to a traumatic stressor, the simultaneous appearance of three different symptom clusters, a minimal duration and the existence of functional disturbance. To qualify as traumatic the event must have involved actual or threatened death or serious injury or a threat to the patient or others, and exposure to this event must arouse an intense affective response characterized by fear, helplessness, or horror. In children, disorganized or agitated behavior can be seen in lieu of an intense affective response. Symptomatically, there must be at least one of five possible intrusive-reexperiencing symptoms. These have the quality of obsessive, recurring, intrusive and distressing recollections either in the form of imagery or thoughts, or in the form of recurrent distressing dreams. Intense psychological distress or physiological reactivity on exposure to either an external reminder or an internal reminder of the trauma

can also occur. The flashback experience, or reliving of the event, is less common.

Symptom cluster C in the DSM-IV-TR criteria in actuality embodies two somewhat different psychopathologies, namely, phobic avoidance and numbing or withdrawal. The phobic avoidance is expressed either in 1) efforts to avoid thoughts and feelings, and conversations associated with the trauma or 2) in efforts to avoid activities places or people that arouse recollections of the trauma; 3) psychogenic amnesia, a more dissociative symptom, is also in this symptom grouping, followed by 4) markedly diminished interest; 5) feeling detached or estranged; 6) having a restricted range of affect; and 7) having a sense of a foreshortened future. At least three of these seven symptoms must be present.

Hyperarousal symptoms, somewhat similar to those of generalized anxiety disorder, are also present in PTSD and at least one of five of the following symptoms is required: difficulty sleeping, irritability or anger, poor concentration, hypervigilance and exaggerated startle response.

With regard to the symptoms as a whole, it is evident that they embody features of different psychiatric disorders, including obsessive–compulsive processes, generalized anxiety disorder, panic attacks, phobic avoidance, dissociation and depression. Finally, it is necessary for symptoms to have lasted at least 1 month and for the disturbance to have caused clinically significant distress or impairment.

Assessment and Differential Diagnosis

PTSD symptoms may overlap with symptoms of a number of other disorders in the DSM-IV. Both PTSD and adjustment disorder are etiologically related to stress exposure. PTSD may be distinguished from adjustment disorder by assessing whether the traumatic stress meets the severity criteria described earlier. Also, if there are an insufficient number of symptoms to qualify for the diagnosis, this might merit a diagnosis of adjustment disorder.

Specific phobia may arise after traumatic exposure. For example, after an automobile accident, victims may develop phobic avoidance of traveling, but without the intrusive or hyperarousal symptoms. In such cases, a diagnosis of specific phobia should be given instead of a diagnosis of PTSD.

The criteria set for generalized anxiety disorder include a list of six symptoms of hyperarousal, of which four are common to PTSD: being on edge, poor concentration, irritability and sleep disturbance. PTSD requires the additional symptoms as described earlier, and the worry in PTSD is focused on concerns about reexperiencing the trauma. In contrast, the worry in generalized anxiety disorder is about a number of different situations and concerns. However, it is possible for the two conditions to coexist.

In obsessive–compulsive disorder, recurring and intrusive thoughts occur, but the patient recognizes these to be inappropriate and unrelated to any particular life experience. Obsessive–compulsive disorder is a common comorbid condition in PTSD and may develop with generalization (e.g., compulsive washing for months after a rape to reduce contamination feelings). It may also develop by activation of an underlying obsessive–compulsive disorder diathesis.

Autonomic hyperarousal is a cardinal part of panic attack, which may indicate a diagnosis of panic disorder. To distinguish between panic disorder and PTSD, the therapist needs to assess whether panic attacks are related to the trauma or reminders of the same (in which case they would be subsumed under a diagnosis of

PTSD) or whether they occur unexpectedly and spontaneously (in which case a diagnosis of panic disorder would be justified).

Depression and PTSD share a significant overlap, including four of the criterion C cluster symptoms and three of the criterion D cluster symptoms. Thus, an individual who presents with reduced interest, estrangement, numbing, impaired concentration, insomnia, irritability and sense of a foreshortened future may manifest either disorder. PTSD may give rise to depression as well, and it is possible for the two conditions to coexist. In a few instances, a patient with prior depression may be more vulnerable to developing PTSD. Reexperiencing symptoms are present only in PTSD.

Dissociative disorders also overlap with PTSD. In the early aftermath of serious trauma, the clinical picture may be predominantly one of the dissociative states (see the section on acute stress disorder [ASD]). ASD differs from PTSD in that the symptom pattern occurs within the first few days after exposure to the trauma, lasts no longer than 4 weeks, and is typically accompanied by prominent dissociative symptoms.

More rarely, PTSD must be distinguished from other disorders producing perceptual alterations, such as schizophrenia and other psychotic disorders, delirium, substance use disorders and general medical conditions producing psychosis (e.g., brain tumors).

The differential diagnosis is important but, notwithstanding, PTSD is unlikely to occur in isolation. Psychiatric comorbidity is the rule rather than the exception, and a number of studies have demonstrated that, in both clinical and epidemiological populations, a wide range of disorders is likely to occur at an increased probability. These include major depressive disorder, all of the anxiety disorders, alcohol and substance use disorders, somatization disorder, and schizophrenia and schizophreniform disorder. A few studies have documented the course of comorbid conditions. Major depressive disorder cooccurs with PTSD, but can take a separate course. Comorbid substance abuse tends to be a consequence rather than a precursor of PTSD.

Assessment

The comprehensive evaluation of PTSD should include information from the individual, collaterals, psychometric indices (such as self-reported questionnaires) and a clinical interview. The standard for diagnosis in clinical research studies is always to use a structured clinical interview. The use of self-report instruments can be used to corroborate information obtained in the clinical interview, or can be used as a screening assessment for a clinical interview. All information would then be integrated on the basis of clinical judgment, especially if discrepancies existed. A number of structured interviews exist, along with other self-rating scales. The "gold standard" of clinical interviewing is the Clinician-Administered PTSD scale (Blake *et al.*, 1990). Other instruments that have been used to evaluate PTSD are the Structured Clinical Interview for DSM-IV, the Diagnostic Interview Schedule and the Structured Interview for PTSD. Self-rated measures that can be used include self-rating psychometric assessments, such as the Davidson Trauma Scale, the Short PTSD Rating Instrument (SPRINT), the PTSD Checklist, the PK scale on the Minnesota Multiphasic Personality Inventory, the Mississippi Scale for Combat-Related PTSD, the Impact of Events Scale and the PTSD Scale.

Structured interview and psychometric measures are also available for children with PTSD but are less well developed with regard to validity and reliability. A version of the Clinician-Administered PTSD Scale for children and adolescents allows for current and lifetime diagnoses as well as the dimensional assessment of PTSD symptoms and related psychopathology. It has also been suggested that the use of additional measures (such as the Conners Parent Rating Scale and Conners Teacher Rating Scale) are important adjuncts to assess externalizing collateral symptoms, whereas the Children's Depression Inventory can be used to assess internalizing symptoms found in PTSD.

Course and Natural History

Immediately following traumatic exposure, a high percentage of individuals develop a mixed symptom picture, which includes disorganized behavior, dissociative symptoms, psychomotor change and, sometimes, paranoia. The diagnosis of ASD (described later) accounts for many of these reactions. These reactions are generally short-lived, although by 1 month the symptom picture often settles into a more classic PTSD presentation, such that after rape, for example, as many as 90% of individuals may qualify for the diagnosis of PTSD. Approximately 50% of people with PTSD recover, and approximately 50% develop a persistent, chronic form of the illness still present 1 year following the traumatic event.

The longitudinal course of PTSD is variable and permanent recovery occurs in some people, whereas others show a relatively unchanging course with only mild fluctuation. Still others show a more obvious fluctuation with intermittent periods of well-being and recurrences of major symptoms. In a limited number of cases, the passage of time does not bring a resolution of symptoms, and the patient's condition tends to deteriorate with age. Particular symptoms that have been noted to increase with time in many people include startle response, nightmares, irritability and depression. Clinicians during World War II also observed that the existence of marked startle response and hypervigilance in the acute aftermath of exposure to combat often represented a comparatively poor prognostic sign. In children, PTSD can be, and often is, chronic and debilitating.

General medical conditions may occur as a direct consequence of the trauma (e.g., head injury, burns). In addition, chronic PTSD may be associated with increased rates of adverse physical outcomes, including musculoskeletal problems and cardiovascular morbidity.

Overall Goals of Treatment

General principles of treating PTSD involve explanation and destigmatization, which can be provided both to the patient and to family members. This often includes a description of the symptoms of PTSD and the way in which it can affect behaviors and relationships. Information can be given about general treatment principles, pointing out that sometimes cure is attainable but that at other times symptom containment is a more realistic treatment goal, particularly in chronic and severe PTSD. Regaining self-esteem and attaining greater control over impulses and affect are also desired in many instances. Information can be provided as to appropriate literature, local support groups and resources, and names and addresses of national advocacy organizations. If the therapist attends to these important issues early in treatment, the patient is able more readily to build trust and also to appreciate that the therapist shows a good understanding both of the condition and of the patient.

PTSD is sometimes comparatively straightforward to treat and at other times it is more complicated. However, treatment by a mental health provider (rather than a primary care provider) is almost always indicated. The initial history taking can evoke strong affect to a greater degree than is customarily found in other disorders. In fact, it may take several interviews for the details to emerge. A sensitive yet persistent approach is needed on the part of the interviewer. During treatment, although the mental health care provider will clearly want to impart a sense of optimism to the patient, it is also a reflection of reality to point out early that recovery may be a slow process and that some symptoms (e.g., phobic avoidance, startle response) may persist. It is important for the mental health care provider to be comfortable in hearing and tolerating unpleasant affect and often horrifying stories. All these must take place in a noncritical and accepting manner.

Pharmacotherapy

PTSD may be accompanied by enduring neurochemical and psychophysiological changes and can lead to substantial impairment and distress. Sometimes the intensity of symptoms is severe enough to preclude the effective use of trauma-focused psychotherapy. In these situations, the use of medication should not be delayed unnecessarily. Initial studies showed benefit for the tricyclic antidepressant and monoamine oxidase inhibitor medications, however, the selective serotonin reuptake inhibitors (SSRIs) have now replaced these as first-line agents, based upon evidence from several placebo-controlled trials. A suggested sequencing of treatment is outlined in Table 52.1.

Two double-blind clinical trials in more than 100 patients support the efficacy of amitriptyline and imipramine in combat veterans with PTSD (Frank et al., 1988; Davidson et al., 1990). In both studies, the medication was effective on intrusive PTSD symptoms and, to a weaker extent, on avoidant symptoms (Table 52.2). Of importance was that clinical efficacy occurred in patients who did not suffer from depressive illness, suggesting that the effect of tricyclic agents in PTSD is independent of

Table 52.2	**Factors Associated with Good Response to Tricyclic Drug Therapy and Direct Therapeutic Exposure in Combat Veterans with Post traumatic Stress Disorder**	
	Pharmacotherapy	Psychotherapy
Older age	No effect	Yes
Lower level of trauma intensity	Yes	Yes
Fewer comorbid disorders	Yes	Yes
Low depression score	Yes	Yes
Low PTSD symptom severity score	Yes	Yes
Low anxiety symptom score	Yes	Yes
Low avoidance of trauma cues	Yes	Unknown
Low autonomic arousal	Yes	Unknown
Low neuroticism	Yes	Unknown
Good social adjustment	Unknown	Yes

Table 52.1	**Pharmacotherapy Steps for Post Traumatic Stress Disorder**
Step 1	

Selective serotonin reuptake inhibitor (SSRI)
Adjunctive medications:
  If prominent hyperarousal: benzodiazepine or buspirone
  If prominent mood liability or explosiveness:
    anticonvulsant or lithium
  If prominent dissociation: valproic acid
  If persistent insomnia: trazodone
  If psychotic: atypical antipsychotic

Step 2

If no response or intolerance to SSRI:
  Dual action antidepressant, e.g., mirtazapine, venlafaxine
  Adjunctive medications as above

Step 3

If no response to Step 1 or 2:
  Monoamine oxidase inhibitor
  Adjunctive medications as above

Step 4

Other useful drugs:
  Propranolol – hyperarousal
  Clonidine – startle response
  Neuroleptics – psychosis, poor impulse control

antidepressant properties. In fact response was inversely correlated with baseline depression level.

Phenelzine has been found to be effective in symptom reduction and that avoidant symptoms improve to a much greater degree with phenelzine than with the tricyclic agents. However, the side effects of phenelzine limit its use to a third- or fourth-line drug to be used only when other, safer medications have failed to work. Several placebo-controlled trials have shown positive effects for the SSRI medications, including fluoxetine, sertraline and paroxetine. Long-term use of sertraline is associated with a substantial reduction in relapse over a 15-month period. Data support positive effects for SSRI in men and women and in adults who have survived all major classes of trauma (e.g., combat, sexual violence, nonsexual violence and accident). Each of these medications has broad-spectrum properties across the full symptom range of the disorder as well as improving function and, perhaps, resilience or stress-coping. They also support the benefit of SSRI in those with and without comorbid major.

At this point, the indications for antipsychotic and mood-stabilizing drugs are poorly defined, but clinical experience suggests that they continue to have a role in the pharmacologic treatment of PTSD. Antipsychotic medications can be useful in patients with poor impulse control or in those who manifest features of borderline personality disorder. Lithium and carbamazepine can also be useful in such patients but might benefit individuals who are subject to mood swings and angry or explosive outbursts. The appropriate role for the use of benzodiazepines is not well-defined. The antiphobic and antiarousal effects of the benzodiazepines should, in theory, be helpful in PTSD. However, withdrawal from short-acting benzodiazepines may also introduce an additional set of problems with intense symptom rebound. In patients who have a propensity to abuse alcohol and other substances, benzodiazepines are not recommended.

Overall, the antidepressants, mood stabilizers and anticonvulsants are the medication groups that are generally considered primary for treating PTSD; beta-blockers, alpha-$_2$-agonists and anxiolytics have a less clearly defined place. Often, patients need a combination of drugs but polypharmacy should be utilized in a carefully planned fashion. Also, since the time course of response may be slow, it is advisable to persist with a particular course of action for at least 8 weeks before deciding that it has been unhelpful. It is possible that avoidance and numbing symptoms respond more effectively to SSRI drugs.

Cognitive, Cognitive–Behavioral and Behavioral Therapies

Despite theoretical differences, most schools of psychotherapy recognize that cognitively oriented approaches to the treatment of anxiety must include an element of exposure. Because PTSD involves aberrant and voluntary programs for the avoidance of danger that are conditioned by real experience, correction of these "fear structures" requires exposure to ensure habituation. Although a range of possible PTSD interventions has recently been reviewed (Foa *et al.*, 2000) including group therapy, cognitive–behavioral therapy, eye movement desensitization and reprocessing, and psychodynamic therapy, the preponderance of current evidence suggests that the primary effective component of PTSD treatment is prolonged exposure (Rothbaum *et al.*, 2000). Prolonged exposure depends on the fact that anxiety will be extinguished in the absence of real threat, given a sufficient duration of exposure *in vivo* or in imagination to traumatic stimuli. In PTSD, the patient retells the traumatic experience as if it were happening again, until doing so becomes a pedestrian exercise and anxiety decreases. Between sessions, patients perform exposure homework, including listening to tapes of the flooding sessions and limited exposure *in vivo*. A review of 12 studies suggests that prolonged exposure is a component of the most well-controlled study designs and is associated with positive results (Rothbaum *et al.*, 2000). However, not every patient may be a candidate for exposure. Due to the high anxiety and temporarily increased symptoms associated with prolonged exposure, there are patients who will be reluctant to confront traumatic reminders. Patients in whom guilt or anger are primary emotional responses to the traumatic event (as opposed to anxiety) may not profit from prolonged exposure. More empirical research is needed to evaluate how this efficacious treatment can be most effectively implemented in nonacademic settings. In addition, additional research is needed to identify methods to increase patient tolerability of the treatment.

Anxiety management techniques are designed to reduce anxiety by providing patients with better skills for controlling worry and fear. Among such techniques are muscle relaxation, thought stopping, control of breathing and diaphragmatic breathing, communication skills, guided self-dialogue and stress inoculation training (SIT). Although these interventions have less empirical evidence regarding treatment efficacy for PTSD, generally the results are positive and further controlled evaluation across trauma population samples is needed.

Further, cognitive approaches to the treatment of PTSD have also gained empirical support. A cognitive approach to treatment includes training patients in challenging problematic cognitions such as self-blame. In a recent comparison of cognitive therapy to imaginal exposure in the treatment of chronic PTSD, both treatments were associated with positive improvements at post treatment and follow-up, with no differences in outcome between treatments. However, patients who received imaginal exposure were more likely to experience an increase in PTSD symptoms during the treatment course, and those who did were more likely to miss treatment sessions, rate the therapy as less credible and be rated as less motivated by the therapist.

In contrast to the treatment-efficacy literature for adults with PTSD, the child-focused PTSD literature is limited to open trials and case reports. Treatment practices for childhood PTSD have recently been surveyed (Cohen *et al.*, 2001). Clearly, adult treatment approaches need to be empirically evaluated for use in children with PTSD. As no single treatment for PTSD has been shown to be curative, patient characteristics, characterization of the nature and range of stress responses of trauma victims, partial response, treatment combinations, sequencing of treatment approaches and further well-controlled investigations of current approaches are all important empirical topics to be addressed.

Psychodynamic Therapy

Psychodynamically based approaches emphasize the interpretation of the traumatic event as being a critical determinant of symptoms. Treatment is geared to alter attributions, usually by means of slow exposure and through confrontation and awareness of the negative affect that have been generated by the trauma. Conflictual meanings begin to appear, and it is the task of treatment to reinterpret the experience in a more realistic and adaptive fashion. During such treatment, it is important to ensure that the affect intensity is not overwhelming or disorganizing. Obviously, support needs to be provided throughout, and sometimes other treatment approaches are used adjunctively. Excessive and maladaptive behaviors such as avoidance, use of alcohol or work, or risk taking may occur as a means of coping with the experience and these need to be identified and addressed.

Using psychodynamic concepts, Horowitz (1973) developed a trauma-focused, time-limited, psychotherapeutic approach. Periods of intrusion are considered an attempt at mastery rather than a failure in defenses, whereas emotional numbness is seen as a result of defensive overcontrol. Overwhelmingly intrusive symptoms are counteracted by means of structuring, and avoidance and numbing are met with procedures to minimize such behavior. With this approach, as with any psychotherapeutic approach, the establishment of a safe therapeutic alliance is essential and medications are used sparingly. The goal of such trauma-focused therapy is to achieve an end point in which the trauma is meaningfully integrated into the survivor's life schema, with reduction of intensity and frequency of the intrusive and avoidant phases of PTSD. Although this approach awaits controlled testing, it aspires to reduce all aspects of PTSD symptoms.

Roth and Newman (1991) presented a conceptual framework for understanding the emotional impact of sexual trauma. The survivor must come to understand the affective impact of the event so that she or he is no longer preoccupied or driven by negative feelings or self-defeating behaviors. It is also important for the survivor to grapple with the meaning of the trauma so as to reach adaptive resolution. Preliminary studies utilizing this approach show promise of efficacy.

Special Features Influencing Treatment

Psychiatric Features

Several important issues of comorbidity need to be considered in the treatment of PTSD. These may suggest either a contraindication to a particular treatment or the need first to treat the comorbid state before embarking energetically on the PTSD problems. Thus, comorbid depression needs to be treated, as it is likely to interfere with the benefits of behavioral therapy or other psychotherapies. In fact, as mentioned earlier, in some instances guilt-bound issues may worsen with exposure. A suicidally depressive individual with PTSD needs to be adequately treated before dealing with issues of PTSD, which may in fact worsen suicidality in some instances.

Occasionally, severe depression comorbid with PTSD may need to be treated with electroconvulsive therapy. Although this form of treatment has no proven place as a major intervention for PTSD per se, in comorbid cases it has been noted that PTSD symptoms may also abate when they are tied to the presence of depression. Amitriptyline is less likely to help combat veterans with PTSD if they have been exposed to more severe forms of combat trauma, and also if they have more severe symptoms of depression, anxiety and PTSD. Antisocial and severe borderline personality disorder may be contraindications to various forms of psychotherapy and are unlikely to respond well to pharmacotherapy.

General Medical Comorbidity

PTSD patients have been shown to have an increased risk of physical conditions, with particular conditions perhaps being more prevalent (gastrointestinal disease and cardiovascular disease). There is also evidence that chronic pain and PTSD are commonly associated, even when PTSD has not followed serious physical injury.

Demographical Features

It is not known to what extent sex or age is likely to determine treatment outcome. However, it is generally believed that lack of psychosocial supports can interfere with successful adaptation to trauma and response to treatment.

Nonresponse to Treatment

A stepwise sequence of approaches may be used in the treatment of PTSD but it must be said that there are no definitive guidelines currently in place. As a result, the particular order in which treatments are considered varies based on individual circumstances. Also, no uniform definition exists as to what constitutes a good or poor response to treatment. In general, some symptoms of chronic PTSD persist, albeit at a considerably reduced level, in people who have undergone treatment. A summary of the limited information available for predicting response to pharmacotherapy and behavioral therapy in PTSD arising from combat trauma is given elsewhere (Davidson and Fairbank, 1993).

Management problems are likely to occur as a result of both therapist-related factors and factors related to the patient. With regard to the therapist, it must be recognized that much of the material offered by the patient is charged with affect and, at times, may strain credibility and lead to high levels of doubt. The therapist may fall into the error of being unable to accept such an emotionally charged experience and thus rejecting or denying its validity. Equally, the therapist may fall into the error of overidentification with the patient such that impartiality is lost. It is important for therapists not to become overinvolved with rescue or to break down customary therapist–patient boundaries.

Although not unique to PTSD, powerful violent urges may arise in the patient during treatment, which may challenge the therapist's feeling of safety. Simple strategies, such as where the patient and therapist sit with respect to proximity of escape, merit attention. For example, a female therapist dealing with a highly hostile and threatening male patient would do well to be sure that she can exit the room quickly if necessary and not be trapped behind a desk with the patient having control of the exit. Another simple yet important issue calling for attention is whether there is an available alarm if the therapist is dealing regularly with violent or threatening patients.

With respect to the patient, there are times when decompensation occurs to such an extent that the provider will have to judge whether hospitalization is indicated. Denial of particularly painful issues can lead to avoidance of therapy and missed appointments. Similarly, the emergence of unpleasant or troubling side effects with medication may also lead to treatment discontinuation. At all times, it is advisable for the therapist to remind the patient that difficult issues will arise periodically and that, rather than the patient taking unilateral action to drop out of treatment, these issues are best discussed with the therapist, with the hope that they can be resolved and further treatment progress can be made.

At times, it is helpful to engage the spouse or significant family member in treatment because of the difficulties and stresses to which they may be subjected. Furthermore, they can provide information that might help the therapist to acquire a better grasp of the severity of symptoms as well as their effects on the lives of others. For example, sleeping partners can give a more graphic account of the nocturnal disturbances that may occur in symptomatic patients with PTSD. They may also provide important supplementary information as to the effects of poor impulse regulation or impaired memory or concentration on daytime behaviors in an individual.

Given that many patients with PTSD are receiving more than one treatment, coordination of effort between providers is important. At times, different philosophical persuasions may result in one provider being somewhat less supportive of another's efforts, a situation in which everybody loses. Mutual respect for each other's efforts is essential if optimal progress is to be made by the patient.

Summary of Treatment

Whatever the type of treatment administered, a number of goals are common to all and can be summarized as follows: 1) to reduce intrusive symptoms; 2) to reduce avoidance symptoms; 3) to reduce numbing and withdrawal; 4) to dampen hyperarousal; 5) to reduce psychotic symptoms when present; and 6) to improve impulse control when this is a problem.

By reducing troublesome symptoms, a number of other important goals can also be accomplished as follows: 1) to develop the capacity to interpret events more realistically with respect to their threat content; 2) to improve interpersonal work and leisure functioning; 3) to promote self-esteem, trust and feelings of safety; 4) to explore and clarify meanings attributed to the event; 5) to promote access to memories that have been dissociated or repressed when judged to be clinically appropriate; 6) to strengthen social support systems; and 7) to move from identification as a victim to that of a survivor.

The three major treatment approaches, pharmacotherapeutic, cognitive–behavioral and psychodynamic, all emphasize different aspects of the problem. Pharmacotherapy targets the underlying neurobiological alterations found in PTSD and attempts to control symptoms so that the above treatment goals can be more effectively accomplished. Cognitive–behavioral treatments emphasize the phobic avoidance and counterproductive reenactments that often occur, along with the identification of faulty beliefs that arise owing to the trauma, and replace them with more adaptive beliefs, usually in association with direct therapeutic exposure. The psychodynamic approach emphasizes the associations that arise from the trauma experience and that lead to unconscious and conscious representations. Defense mechanisms that lead to lack of memory, and the contributions from early development, are also brought into play in psychodynamic therapy.

Acute Stress Disorder

Definition

It has long been recognized that clinically significant dissociative states are seen in the immediate aftermath of overwhelming trauma. In addition, many individuals may experience less clinically severe dissociative symptoms or alterations of attention and time sense. Because such syndromes, even when short-lasting, can produce major disruption of everyday activities, they may require clinical attention. During triage situations after a disaster, it can be important to recognize this clinical picture, which may require treatment intervention and which may also be predictive of later PTSD. As a result of these considerations, a decision was made to include in DSM-IV a new entity, acute stress disorder (ASD), grouped together with PTSD in the anxiety disorders section. Essentially, it represents the clinical features of PTSD along with conspicuous dissociative symptoms, of which at least three must be present. The possible dissociative symptoms in ASD are a subjective sense of numbing; detachment or absence of emotional response; reduced awareness of one's surroundings; derealization; depersonalization; and dissociative amnesia.

However, there is a lack of empirical evidence for some of the assumptions inherent in the conceptualization of ASD, and there has been a call for empirical evidence of acutely traumatized individuals to address these assumptions. The current emphasis placed on acute dissociative responses may be flawed in that there are multiple pathways to PTSD, and most trauma survivors who display severe acute stress reactions without dissociation can develop PTSD.

Epidemiology

Little is known about the epidemiology of ASD as defined in DSM-IV, but after events such as rape and criminal assault, the clinical picture of acute PTSD is found in between 70 and 90% of individuals, although frequency of the particular dissociative symptoms is unknown. One problem of most postdisaster surveys is that they evaluate subjects at points several months or years after the event. This makes any meaningful assessment of acute stress syndromes difficult. One exception was the self-report-based assessment of morbidity 2 months after an earthquake in Ecuador, which found a 45% rate of caseness (being a clinical case), with most prominent symptoms being fear, nervousness, tenseness, worry, insomnia and fatigue (Lima *et al.*, 1989).

Retrospective reports of acute stress symptoms should be interpreted cautiously because of the influence of current

---

DSM-IV-TR Criteria 308.3

Acute Stress Disorder

A. The person has been exposed to a traumatic event in which both of the following were present:

   (1) the person experienced, witnessed, or was confronted with an event or events that involved actual or threatened death or serious injury, or a threat to the physical integrity of self or others

   (2) the person's response involved intense fear, helplessness, or horror

B. Either while experiencing or after experiencing the distressing event, the individual has three (or more) of the following dissociative symptoms:

   (1) a subjective sense of numbing, detachment, or absence of emotional responsiveness

   (2) a reduction in awareness of his or her surroundings (e.g., "being in a daze")

   (3) derealization

   (4) depersonalization

   (5) dissociative amnesia (i.e., inability to recall an important aspect of the trauma)

C. The traumatic event is persistently reexperienced in at least one of the following ways: recurrent images, thoughts, dreams, illusions, flashback episodes, or a sense of reliving the experience; or distress on exposure to reminders of the traumatic event.

D. Marked avoidance of stimuli that arouse recollections of the trauma (e.g., thoughts, feelings, conversations, activities, places, people).

E. Marked symptoms of anxiety or increased arousal (e.g., difficulty sleeping, irritability, poor concentration, hypervigilance, exaggerated startle response, motor restlessness).

F. The disturbance causes clinically significant distress or impairment in social, occupational, or other important areas of functioning or impairs the individual's ability to pursue some necessary task, such as obtaining necessary assistance or mobilizing personal resources by telling family members about the traumatic experience.

G. The disturbance lasts for a minimum of 2 days and a maximum of 4 weeks and occurs within 4 weeks of the traumatic event.

H. The disturbance is not due to the direct physiological effects of a substance (e.g., a drug of abuse, a medication) or a general medical condition is not better accounted for by brief psychotic disorder, and is not merely an exacerbation of a preexisting Axis I or Axis II disorder.

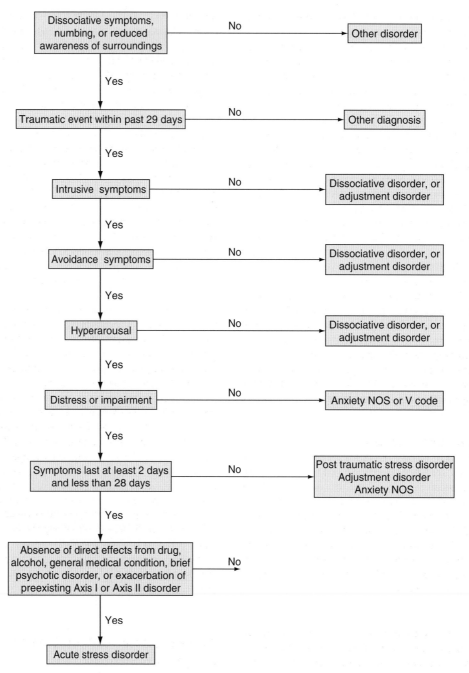

Figure 52.1 *Diagnostic decision tree for acute stress disorder.*

symptoms on recall of acute symptoms. In a longitudinal study evaluating report of acute stress symptoms at 1 month and 2 years post trauma, at least one of the four ASD diagnostic clusters was recalled inaccurately by 75% of patients (Harvey and Bryant, 2000).

Etiology

Little is known about the etiology of ASD specifically, but it is likely that many of the same factors that apply to PTSD are relevant for ASD that is, trauma intensity, preexisting psychopathology, family and genetic vulnerability, abnormal personality, lack of social supports at the time of the trauma and physical injury are all likely to increase vulnerability for ASD.

The role of acute arousal in the development of PTSD has been evaluated in one study (Bryant *et al.*, 2000). Resting heart rate (HR) and ASD symptoms together were found to account for 36% of the variance in PTSD prediction. Further, a formula using resting HR following the trauma exposure (HR > 90 beats/minute) and the diagnosis of ASD to predict PTSD development possessed strong sensitivity (88%) and specificity (85%).

Diagnosis and Differential Diagnosis

ASD may need to be distinguished from several related disorders (Figure 52.1). Brief psychotic disorder may be a more appropriate diagnosis if the predominant symptoms are psychotic. It is possible that major depressive disorder can develop post traumatically and that there may be some overlap with ASD, in which case both disorders are appropriately diagnosed.

When ASD-like symptoms are caused by direct physiological perturbation, the symptoms may be more appropriately diagnosed with reference to the etiological agent. Thus, an ASD-like picture that develops secondary to head injury is more appropriately diagnosed as mental disorder due to a general medical condition, whereas a clinical picture related to substance use (e.g., alcohol intoxication) is appropriately diagnosed as substance-induced disorder. Substance-related ASD is confined to the period of intoxication or withdrawal. Head injury-induced ASD needs substantiating by evidence from the history, physical examination and laboratory testing that the symptoms are a direct physiological consequence of head trauma. Recently, a self-report scale of ASD has been developed, the Acute Stress Disorder Scale (ASDS). The scale has demonstrated good test–retest reliability ($r = 0.94$), and in one sample (bushfire survivors), the ASDS predicted 91% of survivors who developed PTSD and 93% of those who did not (Bryant *et al.*, 2000).

Because ASD by definition cannot last longer than 1 month, if the clinical picture persists, a diagnosis of PTSD is appropriate. Some increased symptoms are expected in the great majority of subjects after exposure to major stress. These remit in most cases and only reach the level of clinical diagnosis if they are prolonged, exceed a tolerable quality, or interfere with everyday function. Resolution may be more difficult if there has been previous psychiatric morbidity, subsequent stress and lack of social support.

Course and Natural History

Although data do not exist on the course and natural history of ASD as now defined, studies by Kooopman and coworkers (1994) indicated that dissociative and cognitive symptoms, which are so common in the immediate wake of trauma, improve spontaneously with time. However, they also found that the likelihood of developing PTSD symptoms at 7-month follow-up was more strongly related to the occurrence of dissociative symptoms than to anxiety symptoms immediately after exposure to the trauma. However, other studies have questioned the dissociative criteria as critical for the prediction of later PTSD.

Treatment

There are six general principles involved in administering any treatment immediately after trauma. These include principles of brevity, immediacy, centrality, expectancy, proximity and simplicity. That is, treatment of acute trauma is generally aimed at being brief, provided immediately after the trauma whenever possible, administered in a centralized and coordinated fashion with the expectation of the person's return to normal function and as proximately as possible to the scene of the trauma, and not directed at any uncovering or explorative procedures but rather at maintaining a superficial, reintegrating approach.

People most highly at risk, and therefore perhaps most in need of treatment, are as follows: survivors with psychiatric disorders; traumatically bereaved people; children, especially when separated from their parents; individuals who are particularly dependent on psychosocial supports, such as the elderly, handicapped and mentally retarded individuals; and traumatized survivors and body handlers.

Different components of treatment include providing information, psychological support, crisis intervention and emotional first aid. Providing information about the trauma is important as it can enable the survivor fully to recognize and accept all the details of what happened. Information needs to be given in a way that conveys hope and the possibility that psychological pain and threat of loss may be coped with. Unrealistic hope needs to be balanced by the provision of realistic explanations as to what happened. Psychological support helps to strengthen coping mechanisms and promotes adaptive defenses. The survivor benefits if he or she recognizes the need to take responsibility for a successful outcome and is as actively involved with this as possible. Crisis intervention is often used after disasters and acts of violence or other serious traumas. It has been described by a number of investigators. Emotional first aid has been described by Caplan (1984) using the six principles presented earlier and is used to achieve any of the following: acceptance of feelings, symptoms, reality and the need for help; recognition of psychologically distressing issues; identification of available resources; acceptance of responsibility and absence of blame; cultivation of an optimistic attitude; and efforts to resume activities of daily life as much as possible.

Civilian trauma survivors with ASD were found to engage in the cognitive strategies of punishment and worry more than survivors without ASD (Warda and Bryant, 1998), and cognitive–behavioral therapy has been shown to reduce these strategies and increase the use of reappraisal and social control strategies. However, the relation of these findings to the development of PTSD has not yet been determined.

There is little investigation as to whether early recognition and effective treatment of acute stress reactions prevent the development of PTSD, although it is safe to assume that they are likely to have beneficial effects in this regard. Nonetheless, as was recognized during World War II, rapid and effective treatment of acute combat stress did not always prevent veterans from developing subsequent chronicity. More recently, an intervention designed to prevent the development of PTSD and administered in the acute phase, critical incident stress debriefing, has been found to be ineffective in preventing the development of PTSD. However, there has been an initial study with motor vehicle accident survivors that suggested exposure therapy and exposure therapy with anxiety management training may be effective in preventing PTSD (Bryant *et al.*, 1999).

Comparison of DSM-IV/ICD-10 Diagnostic Criteria

The ICD-10 Diagnostic Criteria for Research for Post traumatic Stress Disorder provides a different stressor criterion: a situation or event "of exceptionally threatening or catastrophic nature, which would be likely to cause pervasive distress in almost everyone" which is similar to the DSM-III-R definition of a traumatic stressor. DSM-IV-TR instead defines a traumatic stressor as "an event or events that involved actual or threatened death or serious injury, or a threat to the physical integrity of self or others". Furthermore, the ICD-10 diagnostic algorithm differs from that specified in DSM-IV-TR in that the DSM-IV criterion D (i.e., symptoms of increased arousal) is not required. In contrast to DSM-IV-TR which requires that the symptoms persist for more than one month, the ICD-10 Diagnostic Criteria for Research do not specify a minimum duration.

For acute stress disorder, the ICD-10 Diagnostic Criteria for Research differs in several ways from the DSM-IV-TR criteria: 1) primarily anxiety symptoms are included; 2) it is required that the onset of the symptoms be within 1 hour of the stressor; and 3) the symptoms must begin to diminish after not more than 8 hours (for transient stressors) or 48 hours (for extended stressors). In contrast to DSM-IV-TR, the ICD-10 Diagnostic Criteria for Research does not require dissociative symptoms or that the event be persistently reexperienced.

References

American Psychiatric Association (1994) *Diagnostic and Statistical Manual of Mental Disorders*, 4th edn. APA, Washington DC.

Blake DD, Weathers FW, Nagy LM *et al.* (1990) A clinician rating scale for assessing current and lifetime PTSD: The CAPS-1. *Behav Ther* 13, 187–188.

Boscarino JA (1996) Posttraumatic stress disorder, exposure to combat, and lower plasma cortisol among Vietnam veterans: Findings and clinical implications. *J Consult Clin Psychol* 64, 191–201.

Bryant RA, Sackville T, Dang ST *et al.* (1999) Treating acute stress disorder: An evaluation of cognitive behavior therapy and supportive counseling techniques. *Am J Psychiatr* 156, 1780–1786.

Bryant RA, Harvey AG, Guthrie R *et al.* (2000) A prospective study of psychophysiological arousal, acute stress disorder, and posttraumatic stress disorder. *J Abnorm Psychol* 109, 341–344.

Caplan G (1984) *Principles of Preventive Psychiatry*. Basic Books, New York.

Cohen JA, Mannarino AP and Rogal S (2001) Treatment practices for childhood posttraumatic stress disorder. *Child Abuse Neglect* 25, 123–135.

Davidson JRT and Fairbank JA (1993) The epidemiology of posttraumatic stress disorder, in *Posttraumatic Stress Disorder: DSM-IV and Beyond* (ed Foa EB). American Psychiatric Press, Washington DC, pp. 147–172.

Davidson JRT, Kudler HS, Smith BD *et al.* (1990) Treatment of posttraumatic stress disorder with amitriptyline and placebo. *Arch Gen Psychiatr* 47, 259–266.

Foa EB, Keane TM and Friedman MJ (2000) *Effective Treatments for PTSD: Practice Guidelines from the International Society for Traumatic Stress Studies*. Guilford Press, New York.

Frank JB, Giller ELJ, Kosten TB *et al.* (1988) A randomized clinical trial of phenelzine and imipramine for posttraumatic stress disorder. *Am J Psychiatr* 145, 1289–1291.

Harvey AG and Bryant RA (2000) Memory for acute stress disorder symptoms: A two year prospective study. *J Nerv Ment Dis* 188, 602–607.

Horowitz MJ (1973) Phase-oriented treatment of stress response syndromes. *Am J Psychother* 27, 506–515.

Kessler RC, Sonnega A, Bromet E *et al.* (1995) Posttraumatic stress disorder in the National Comorbidity Survey. *Arch Gen Psychiatr* 52, 1048–1060.

Kessler RC, Berglund MBA, Demler O *et al.* (2005) Lifetime prevalence and age-of-onset distributions of DSM-IV disorders in the National Comorbidity Survey Replication. *Arch Gen Psychiatr* 62, 593–602.

Kilpatrick DB, Saunders BE, Veronen LJ *et al.* (1987) Criminal victimization: Lifetime prevalence, reporting to police, and psychological impact. *Crime Delinquency* 33, 479–489.

Koopman C, Classen C and Spiegel D (1994) Predictors of posttraumatic stress symptoms among survivors of the Oakland/Berkeley, California firestorm. *Am J Psychiatr* 151, 888–894.

Krystal JH, Kosten TB, Perry BD *et al.* (1989) Neurobiological aspects of PTSD: Review of clinical and preclinical studies. *Behav Ther* 20, 177–198.

Kulka RA, Schlenger WE, Fairbank JA, *et al.* (1990) Trauma and the Vietnam War generation: Report of Findings from the National Vietnam Veterans Readjustment Study. Brunner/Mazel, New York.

Lima BR, Chavez H, Samniego N *et al.* (1989) Disaster severity and emotional disturbance: Implications for primary mental health care in developing countries. *Acta Psychiatr Scand* 79, 74–82.

McLeod DS, Koenen KC, Meyer JM *et al.* (2001) Genetic and environmental influences on the relationship among combat exposure, posttraumatic stress disorder symptoms, and alcohol use. *J Traum Stress* 14, 259–275.

Pynoos RS, Goenjian A, Tashjian M, *et al.* (1993) Posttraumatic stress reactions in children after the 1988 American earthquake. *Br J Med Psychol* 163, 239–247.

Pynoos RS, Frederick CJ, Nader K *et al.* (1987) Life threat and posttraumatic stress in school-age children. *Arch Gen Psychiatr* 44, 1057–1063.

Roth S and Newman E (1991) The process of coping with sexual trauma. *J Traum Stress* 4, 279–297.

Rothbaum BO, Meadows EA, Resick PA *et al.* (2000) Cognitive–behavioral therapy, in *Effective Treatments for PTSD: Practice Guidelines from the International Society for Traumatic Stress Studies* (eds Friedman MJ). Guilford Press, New York, pp. 320–325.

Shalev A, Bleich A and Ursano RJ (1990) Posttraumatic stress disorder: Somatic comorbidity and effort tolerance. *Psychosom* 31, 197–203.

Southwick SM, Krystal JH, Morgan CA *et al.* (1993) Abnormal noradrenergic function in posttraumatic stress disorder. *Arch Gen Psychiatr* 50, 266–274.

True WR, Rice J, Eisen SA *et al.* (1993) A twin study of genetic and environmental contributions to liability for posttraumatic stress symptoms. *Arch Gen Psychiatr* 50, 257–265.

Warda G and Bryant RA (1998) Thought control strategies in acute stress disorder. *Behav Res Ther* 36, 1171–1175.

CHAPTER

53

Anxiety Disorders: Generalized Anxiety Disorder

Definition

In the *Diagnostic and Statistical Manual of Mental Disorders*, Fourth Edition (DSM-IV) (American Psychiatric Association, 1994) GAD is currently defined as excessive anxiety and worry (apprehensive expectation) occurring for a majority of days during at least a 6-month period, about a number of events or activities (such as work or school performance; see DSM-IV). In individuals with GAD, the anxiety and worry are accompanied by at least three of six somatic symptoms (only one accompanying symptom is required in children), which include restlessness or feeling keyed up or on edge, being easily fatigued, difficulty concentrating or mind going blank, irritability, muscle tension and sleep disturbance. In addition, the affected individual has difficulty controlling his/her worry, and the anxiety, worry, or somatic symptoms cause clinically significant distress or impairment in social, occupational, and/or other important areas of functioning. Further, the GAD symptoms should not be due to the direct physiological effects of a substance such as drugs or alcohol or a general medical condition, and should not occur exclusively during a mood disorder, psychotic disorder, or pervasive developmental disorder.

Worry and anxiety are part of normal human behavior and it may be difficult to define a cutoff point distinguishing normal or trait anxiety (i.e., a relatively stable tendency to perceive various situations as threatening) from GAD. However, as described in the DSM-IV definition of GAD, individuals suffering from a "disorder" exhibit significant distress and impairment in functioning as a result of their anxiety symptoms.

Etiology and Pathophysiology

Family Studies

Family studies suggest a familial (and probably a genetic) basis for certain anxiety disorders such as panic disorder. Genetic transmission of a disorder suggests that certain gene-encoded changes in proteins and the resulting biological abnormalities may play a role in the pathophysiology of specific disorders. Skre and collaborators (1993) examined 20 monozygotic and 29 dizygotic twins with DSM-III-R-defined GAD. They found GAD to be diagnosed in 22% of first-degree relatives of 33 probands with anxiety disorders. In the largest twin study to date which included 1033 female twin pairs, Kendler and associates (1992) found that genetic factors play a significant, but not overwhelming role in the etiology of GAD, with the heritability of GAD estimated at

---

DSM-IV-TR Criteria 300.02

Generalized Anxiety Disorder

A. Excessive anxiety and worry (apprehensive expectation), occurring more days than not for at least 6 months, about a number of events or activities (such as work or school performance).

B. The person finds it difficult to control the worry.

C. The anxiety and worry are associated with three (or more) of the following six symptoms (with at least some symptoms present for more days than not for the past 6 months).

   Note: Only one item is required in children.
   (1) restlessness or feeling keyed up or on edge
   (2) being easily fatigued
   (3) difficulty concentrating or mind going blank
   (4) irritability
   (5) muscle tension
   (6) sleep disturbance (difficulty falling or staying asleep, or restless unsatisfying sleep)

D. The focus of anxiety and worry is not confined to features of an Axis I disorder, e.g., the anxiety or worry is not about having a panic attack (as in panic disorder), being embarrassed in public (as in social phobia), being contaminated (as in obsessive–compulsive disorder), being away from home or close relatives (as in separation anxiety disorder), gaining weight (as in anorexia nervosa), having multiple physical complaints (as in somatization disorder), or having a serious illness (as in hypochondriasis), and the anxiety and worry do not occur exclusively during posttraumatic stress disorder.

E. The anxiety, worry, or physical symptoms cause clinically significant distress or impairment in social, occupational, or other important areas of functioning.

F. The disturbance is not due to the direct physiological effects of a substance (e.g., a drug of abuse, a medication) or a general medical condition (e.g., hyperthyroidism) and does not occur exclusively during a mood disorder, a psychotic disorder, or a pervasive developmental disorder.

Essentials of Psychiatry   Jerald Kay and Allan Tasman
© 2006 John Wiley & Sons, Ltd.

around 30% in comparison to 70% heritability in major depression. In addition, the authors found that the vulnerability to GAD and major depression is influenced by the same genetic factors. In short, the available data suggest at most a modest genetic contribution to the etiology of GAD.

Biological Studies

Relatively few studies have addressed issues regarding the biological aspects of GAD. Existing studies have focused on the evaluation of catecholamine and autonomic responses, neuroendocrine measures, sleep, neuroanatomical/neuroimaging studies, infusion studies and evaluation of other neurotransmitter systems. There is not strong evidence for abnormalities in catecholamine or thyroid function in GAD patients. Some studies have shown a higher prevalence of an "escape" (nonsuppression) response in following dexamethasone administration (that was not attributable to the presence of depression) in GAD patients when compared with normal comparison subject. These data indicate that there may be dysregulation of the HPA axis in these patients, as observed following dexamethasone.

Although restless and decreased sleep are common complaints in GAD patients, there have been only a few polysomnographic studies in this patient population. There is some evidence suggesting that patients with GAD have a longer rapid eye movement (REM) latency, shorter REM duration, increased sleep onset latency and less total sleep time compared with control subjects (Papadimitriou et al., 1988). These findings may differentiate patients with GAD from patients with depression, who show shorter REM latencies.

Alterations in different neurotransmitter systems have been implicated in the pathophysiology of various anxiety disorders. It is generally accepted that anxiety disorders are not associated with abnormalities in only one neurotransmitter system; rather dynamic interactions among several different neurotransmitter systems are believed likely to underlie different anxiety states. Presently, there are data suggesting that the catecholamine serotonin and GABA-benzodiazepine systems may be involved in the pathophysiology of anxiety disorders.

GABA-benzodiazepines

Benzodiazepines have been the treatment of choice for many patients with GAD. They act at specific recognition sites in the brain, the benzodiazepine receptors, which are located in a subu-nit of a receptor for gamma-aminobutyric acid (GABA), the major inhibitory neurotransmitter in the brain. Several lines of evidence suggest that the GABA-benzodiazepine receptor complex may be involved in the mediation of anxiety responses. Studies with animals suggest a relationship between benzodiazepine receptors, fear and anxiety. Models using gamma-2 knockout mice have shown a reduction in $GABA_A$ receptor clustering in the hippocampus and cerebral cortex along with behavioral inhibition to aversive stimuli and increased responsiveness in trace fear conditioning (Lesch, 2001).

Serotonin

Alterations in serotonergic (5-HT) neurotransmission have been implicated in the mediation of fear and anxiety responses in animal models and in humans. Specifically, researchers hypothesize that anxiety may represent dysregulated serotonergic activity in critical brain areas. Given the available data, whether overactivity or underactivity of the 5-HT system is the mechanism for GAD development remains unclear.

Neuropeptides

Cholecystokinin (CCK), a highly abundant neurotransmitter in the brain, has also been implicated in anxiety in humans. CCK may be possibly involved in the pathophysiology of panic disorder and may also play a role in the biology of GAD. Corticotropin-releasing factor (CRF), a major physiological regulator of adreno corticotropic hormone (ACTH), appears to be involved in stress and anxiety responses. Administration of CRF to various parts of animal brains has elicited anxiety and fear responses, e.g., suppression of exploratory behavior, shock-induced freezing. Interestingly, both these peptides are functionally antagonized by benzodiazepines. Neuropeptide Y, glutamate and tachykinins may also play a role in anxiety.

Neuroanatomic Sites of Anxiety

Several potential neuroanatomic anxiogenic sites in the central nervous system (CNS) have been proposed based on brain imaging and neuroanatomic studies. The areas potentially involved in anxiety are the parts of the limbic system involving the hippocampus, prefrontal cortex, occipital lobes, basal ganglia and brain stem structures, specifically the locus coeruleus, nucleus paragigantocellularis and periaqueductal gray (Gray, 1988). These structures are rich in noradrenergic, GABAergic and serotonergic receptors which are believed to be involved in the pathophysiology of different anxiety states such as GAD.

Cerebral Blood Flow and Metabolism Studies

Only a few imaging studies in GAD have appeared in the literature. In one study, patients with GAD displayed decreases in cortical blood flow compared with control subjects. Significant negative correlations between state anxiety and cerebral blood flow in most brain regions were observed. Wu and colleagues (1991) evaluated 18 patients who met DSM-III criteria for GAD using positron emission tomography (PET) measurements of cerebral glucose at "baseline" (during a passive viewing task), following a cognitive vigilance task designed to stimulate anxiety, and following treatment with benzodiazepines. They found a higher relative metabolic rate for GAD patients in parts of the occipital, temporal, frontal lobes and cerebellum relative to normal control subjects during a passive viewing task. The authors also found a decrease in absolute basal ganglia metabolic activity in GAD patients. During the vigilance task, GAD patients showed a significant increase in relative basal ganglia metabolism. The authors did not find a global decrease in cortical metabolism, as had been predicted by blood flow studies. Finally, benzodiazepine treatment resulted in a significant decrease in glucose metabolism in cortical surface (especially in the occipital cortex), the limbic system and basal ganglia compared with patients receiving placebo.

MRI and SPET studies have found that those with GAD have decreased benzodiazepine receptor binding in the left temporal pole as compared with matched healthy controls. In a study using functional MRI in GAD patients, Lorberbaum and colleagues (2001) found greater activity in the right cingulate, right medial prefrontal and orbitofrontal cortex, right temporal poles and right dorsomedial thalamus, during periods of anticipatory anxiety, compared with rest periods, than matched control subjects. Further, only matched control subjects displayed increased activity in the medial prefrontal cortex.

Psychological Mechanisms

Cognitive–Behavioral Model

Psychological models, which emphasize the cognitive–behavioral processes involved in the onset and maintenance of GAD, have emerged in recent years. Individuals' thoughts, cognitive style and behaviors are thought to instigate and maintain episodes of anxiety. In support of cognitive theories of GAD, anxious individuals with GAD are more likely to perceive ambiguous information as threatening and/or negative, and to perceive that they are more likely than others to experience threatening situations. Patients with GAD also pay more attention to the detection of potentially threatening information and incorporate this information into highly elaborate cognitive schemas, thus lowering their threshold for activation of an anxiety response. The threatening information then elicits anxious affect and the individual begins to worry in an attempt further to define the problem.

Patients with GAD are likely to be characterized by a perception of lack of control over threatening. In addition, these patients are likely to believe that they have little control over their emotions, especially their worrying, leading to further distress. It has been suggested that the interaction between perceived uncontrollability and a cognitive focus on negative/threatening stimuli may amplify the general worry to pathological.

Psychodynamic Theories

Freud's concept of signal anxiety followed the development of Freud's structural model of the mind, which proposes three interacting psychological functions: ego (which mediates between the demands of primitive drives, the social and parental prohibitions, and reality), superego (representing the internalized parental and social prohibitions) and id (representing the primitive drives and urges). Freud believed that anxiety serves as a signal to the ego of a threat (in the form of an unconscious drive or wish arising from the id), which, if enacted, may be dangerous to the ego, signaling the potential punishment by the superego or the external world. According to this model, the ego can activate defense mechanisms, such as repression, and prevent the actualization of the forbidden urge either by preventing the expression of the wish or by avoiding the life situations in which the wish might be potentially expressed. Ideally, repression into the unconscious (i.e., out of subject's awareness) should successfully contain the drives. However, if the defenses fail, one may experience symptomatic anxiety and other distressing psychological symptoms. Implicit in this model is the concept that the individuals themselves are not consciously aware of these processes. Therefore, the promotion of subjects' insight into unconscious conflicts and the uncovering of the unconscious origins of anxiety through interpretation and other techniques is the primary goal (and method) of the psychoanalytic treatment approach.

Sullivan developed a theory of anxiety based on the importance of interpersonal relationships. He viewed affects (such as anxiety) as forms of interpersonal communication. According to this model, anxiety communicates the sense of insecurity in interpersonal relationships. For example, a mother who is insecure in her role may communicate her insecurity to the infant when she is anxious in her child's presence. The child in turn identifies her anxiety and expresses anxious affect himself. Another approach to the understanding of the origins of anxiety was offered by object relations theorists such as Klein and Bowlby. They believed that anxiety reflects a fear of the loss of the nurturing object or fear of being hurt by the antagonistic object.

Finally, self-psychology theorists, such as Kohut, believed that the individual strives to achieve and maintain an integrated, cohesive sense of self. Beginning in early age, the individual develops this sense of self through idealization of important others, such as important caregivers (called self-objects), and through a process of positive interaction with caregivers (called mirroring). He believed that inadequate provision of these experiences can lead to anxiety (fear of disintegration) and the loss of the cohesive self.

Assessment and Differential Diagnosis

GAD patients frequently report that they have been anxious all their lives. Typically, they were moderately anxious during childhood, later developing full-blown GAD when their stress levels increased through activities such as attending college or starting to work. Patients with early onset of symptoms report experiencing significant anxiety and fears, social isolation, obsessionality, more academic difficulties and disturbed home environment during their childhood. The social maladjustment and emotional overreactivity persist into adulthood. Epidemiological studies and clinical studies suggest that the onset of GAD typically begins between the late teens and late twenties. However, not all GAD patients have a lifelong history of excessive anxiety. Some patients develop their disorder at a later age, that is, in one's thirties or later. These patients frequently report identifiable, precipitating stressful events, specifically unexpected, negative, important events in the year preceding development of GAD.

Patients with GAD experience chronic anxiety and tension. They find the worry as being uncontrollable. However, some patients intentionally initiate and maintain worry with an almost superstitious assumption that, by doing so, they can avert a negative event. Patients tend to worry predominantly about family, personal finances, work and illness. They are also likely to report worrying over minor matters, such as making a slight social faux pas. The majority report being anxious for at least 50% of the time during an average day. In children and adolescents, the worries often revolve around quality of performance in school/competitive areas; catastrophic events; and physical/mental inadequacies. They typically require excessive reassurance and often appear shy, overcompliant and perfectionistic. Frequent multiple physical complaints are common. They may have an unusually mature and serious manner and appear older than their actual age. These children are often the eldest in small, competitive, achievement-oriented families.

Individuals with GAD commonly complain of feeling tense, jumpy and irritable. They have difficulty falling or staying asleep, and tire easily during the day. Particularly distressing to patients is the difficulty in concentrating and collecting their thoughts. Cognitions appear to play a central role in GAD, as well as other anxiety disorders. Patterns of cognitions, however, appear to be disorder-specific. Cognitions about interpersonal conflict or acceptance by others are quite common.

Patients may present complaining of muscular tension, especially in their neck and shoulders and headaches which frequently are described as frontal and occipital pressure or tension. Patients commonly experience sweaty palms, feel shaky and tremulous, complain of dryness of the mouth, and experience palpitations and difficulty breathing. They may also experience gastrointestinal symptoms such as heartburn and epigastric fullness and approximately 30% of patients experience severe gastrointestinal symptoms of irritable bowel syndrome. Physical complaints frequently lead patients to seek medical attention,

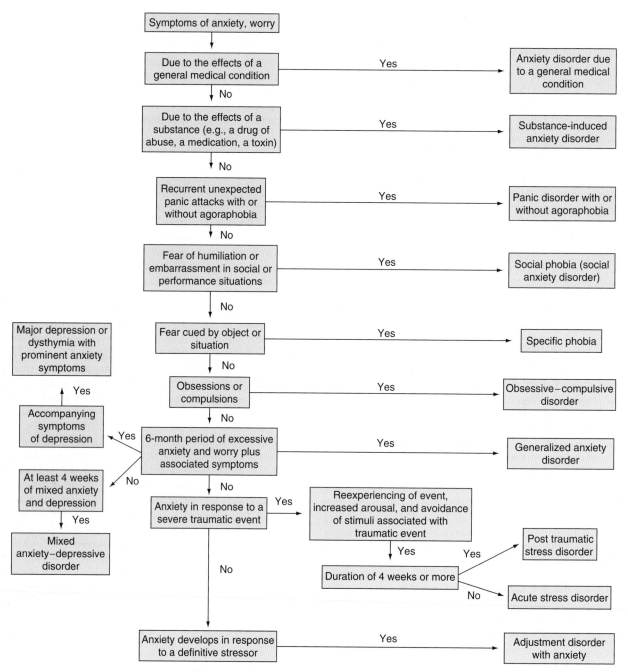

Figure 53.1   *Diagnostic decision tree for GAD.*

and most will initially consult a primary care physician. Although chest pain is more frequently reported by patients with panic disorder, Carter and Maddock (1992) observed that 34% of patients with GAD without panic attacks experienced chest pain. They also found that these patients were predominantly males and many had undergone extensive cardiac evaluations that revealed no demonstrable cardiac pathology.

Differential Diagnosis

Psychiatric Conditions

Anxiety can be a prominent feature of many psychiatric disorders. In addition, the substantial overlap of symptoms between GAD and other psychiatric disorders such as major depressive disorder, often creates diagnostic and treatment dilemmas for the clinician and may complicate the difficult task of differential diagnosis and treatment planning. This section will highlight the major disorders that should be considered in the differential diagnosis of GAD (Figure 53.1).

Major Depressive Disorder and Dysthymic Disorder

Several symptom profiles discriminate between major depressive disorder or dysthymic disorder and GAD. Patients with major depressive disorder exhibit higher rates of dysphoric mood, psychomotor retardation, suicidal ideation, guilt, hopelessness and helplessness, as well as more work impairment than patients with GAD. In contrast, patients with GAD show higher rates of somatic symptoms, specifically, muscle tension and autonomic symptoms (e.g., respiratory or cardiac complaints) than depressed patients.

Panic Disorder With/Without Agoraphobia

Some researchers have suggested that GAD is attributable to panic disorder. However, clear differences exist between GAD and panic disorder. For example, panic disorder is characterized by the presence of panic attacks; that is, recurrent, discrete episodes of intense anxiety or fear associated with a cluster of somatic symptoms reflecting autonomic hyperactivity such as rapid heartbeat, dizziness, numbness or tingling, trouble breathing or choking, and nausea or vomiting. In contrast, patients with GAD experience predominantly symptoms of muscle tension and vigilance such as fatigue, muscle soreness, insomnia, difficulty concentrating, restlessness and irritability. Patients with panic disorder tend to seek treatment earlier in life than patients with GAD. Additionally, reports of types of worry differ between those diagnosed with GAD and those with panic disorder. For example, panic patients worry about having additional panic attacks, whereas GAD patients worry unrealistically about a number of everyday issues.

Obsessive–Compulsive Disorder

Anxiety is part of the clinical picture of obsessive–compulsive disorder (OCD) and may be a central factor in initiating and maintaining obsessions and compulsions. Interestingly there are also some data suggesting that OCD and GAD may be related. For example, Black and associates (1992) found an increased prevalence of GAD among relatives of patients with OCD. However, several features distinguish the excessive worry that accompanies GAD from the obsessional thoughts of OCD. Obsessive thoughts are described as ego-dystonic intrusions that often take the form of urges, impulses, or images. They are often senseless and are frequently accompanied by time-consuming compulsions designed to reduce mounting anxiety. In contrast, the worries in GAD are about realistic concerns, such as health and finances.

Other Anxiety Disorders

In phobic disorders, the anxiety is characteristically associated with a specific phobic object or situation that is frequently avoided by the patient. Such is the case with social anxiety disorder as well, in which the individual is afraid of or avoids situations in which he or she may be the focus of potential scrutiny by others. Anxiety is also a characteristic part of the presentation of post traumatic stress disorder (PTSD) and acute stress disorder. However, unlike in GAD, the principal symptoms experienced in PTSD and acute stress disorder follow exposure to a traumatic event and are characterized by avoidance of reminders of the event and persistent reexperiencing of the traumatic event. In addition, in contrast to GAD which must last at least 6 months, acute stress disorder does not persist for more than 4 weeks. Finally, in adjustment disorders anxiety when present occurs in response to a specific life stressor or stressors and generally does not persist for more than 6 months (American Psychiatric Association, 1994).

Normal Anxiety

Worry and anxiety are part of normal human behavior, and it may be difficult to define a cutoff point distinguishing normal or trait anxiety (i.e., a relatively stable tendency to perceive various situations as threatening) from GAD. However, individuals suffering from a "disorder" exhibit significant distress and impairment in functioning as a result of their anxiety symptoms.

Anxiety Disorder due to a General Medical Condition

Many general medical conditions may present with prominent anxiety symptoms. If not identified and properly addressed, these conditions may adversely affect the treatment outcome of the anxious patient. In this section we will highlight important medical conditions in the differential diagnosis of generalized anxiety (see Table 53.2).

Cardiovascular Disorders

Patients with GAD may complain of palpitations, skipped heartbeats and chest pain. In addition, many GAD patients, especially males, fear having an acute myocardial infarction and often present to the emergency room for evaluation. However, most patients with GAD without a concomitant cardiovascular disease do not experience severe chest pain. Following the controversial evidence suggesting an association between mitral valve prolapse (MVP) and panic disorder, researchers evaluated the prevalence of MVP in patients with GAD and found no evidence of increased prevalence in patients with GAD. Nevertheless, patients with anxiety symptoms associated with unexplained chest pain should be evaluated for possible cardiovascular disease.

Hyperthyroidism

Anxiety is a prominent feature of hyperthyroidism with some overlap in the symptomatology of thyrotoxicosis and GAD. Symptoms such as tachycardia, tremulousness, irritability, weakness and fatigue are common to both disorders. In GAD, however, the peripheral manifestations of excessive concentrations of circulating thyroid hormones are absent, including symptoms such as weight loss, increased appetite, warm and moist skin, heat intolerance and dyspnea on effort. Presence of goiter makes the diagnosis of hyperthyroidism likely; however, the absence of thyroid enlargement does not exclude it. Thus, confirmatory laboratory tests (free T_4, T_3 and TSH) assume significant diagnostic importance. In mild cases, laboratory tests may be within the upper limit of the normal range, in which case a thyroid releasing hormone stimulation test is indicated.

Pheochromocytomas

Pheochromocytomas, also known as chromaffin tumors, produce, store and secrete catecholamines. They are derived most often from the adrenal medulla, as well as the sympathetic ganglia and occasionally from other sites. The clinical features of these tumors, most commonly hypertension and hypertensive paroxysms, are predominantly due to the release of catecholamines. Patients may also experience diaphoresis, tachycardia, chest pain, flushing, nausea and vomiting, headache and significant apprehension. Although the clinical presentation frequently mimics spontaneous panic attacks, pheochromocytomas should also be considered in the differential diagnosis of GAD. The diagnosis of pheochromocytoma can be confirmed by increased levels of catecholamines (epinephrine and norepinephrine) or catecholamine metabolites (metanephrines and vanillylmandelic acid) in a 24-hour urine collection.

Other Medical Conditions

Menopause is commonly referred to as the period that encompasses the transition between the reproductive years and beyond the last episode of menstrual bleeding. Frequently associated with significant anxiety, menopause should be considered in the differential diagnosis of GAD. However, other associated symptoms such as vasomotor instability, atrophy of urogenital epithelium and skin, and osteoporosis make the diagnosis of menopause probable. Another endocrinologic disorder, hyperparathyroidism, can present with anxiety symptoms, and the initial evaluation of serum calcium levels may be indicated. Finally, certain neurologic conditions such as complex partial seizures, intracranial tumors and strokes, and cerebral ischemic attacks may be associated with symptoms typically observed in anxiety disorders and may require appropriate evaluation.

Substance-induced Anxiety Disorder

Anxiety disorders can occur frequently in association with intoxication and withdrawal from several classes of substances (see Table 53.1). Excessive use of caffeine, especially in children and adolescents, may cause significant anxiety. Cocaine intoxication may be associated with anxiety, agitation and hypervigilance. During cocaine withdrawal, patients may also present with prominent anxiety, irritability, insomnia, fatigue, depression and cocaine craving. Adverse reaction to marijuana includes extreme anxiety that usually lasts less than 24 hours. Mild opioid withdrawal presents with symptoms of anxiety and dysphoria. However, accompanying symptoms such as elevated blood pressure, tachycardia, pupilary dilatation, rhinorrhea, piloerection and lacrimation are rare in patients with GAD.

The clinical phenomenology observed both in alcohol and sedative–hypnotic drug withdrawal and in GAD, although variable, may be highly similar. In both conditions, nervousness, tachycardia, tremulousness, sweating, nausea and hyperventilation occur prominently. Additionally, the same drugs (i.e., benzodiazepines) can be used to treat anxiety symptoms, and some patients may use alcohol in an attempt to alleviate anxiety. Thus, the symptoms of an underlying anxiety disorder may be difficult to differentiate from the withdrawal symptoms associated with the use of benzodiazepines or alcohol.

The use of many commonly prescribed medications may produce side effects manifesting as anxiety (see Table 53.1). Such medications include sympathomimetics or other bronchodilators such as theophilline, anticholinergics, antiparkinsonian preparations, corticosteroids, thyroid supplements, oral contraceptives, antihypertensive, and cardiovascular medications such as digitalis, insulin (secondary to hypoglycemia), and antipsychotic and antidepressant medications. Finally, heavy metals and toxins such as organophosphates, paint and insecticides may also cause anxiety symptoms.

Epidemiology and Comorbidity

Current data indicate that GAD is probably one of the more common psychiatric disorders. The National Comorbidity Survey (NCS) of psychiatric disorders (Kessler *et al.*, 1994) found prevalence rates of 1.6% for current GAD (defined as the most recent 6-month period of anxiety), 3.1% for 12-month GAD, and 5.1% for lifetime GAD, with lifetime prevalence higher in females (6.6%) than males (3.6%). The more recent National Comorbidity Survey replication (NCS-R) found a lifetime prevalence of 5.7% (Kessler *et al.*, 2005).

Table 53.1 **Medical Conditions and Drugs That May Cause Anxiety**

Endocrine Disorders	Cardiovascular and Circulatory Disorders
Addison's disease	Anemia
Cushing's syndrome	Congestive heart failure
Hyperparathyroidism	Coronary insufficiency
Hyperthyroidism	Dysrhythmia
Hypothyroidism	Hypovolemia
Carcinoid	Myocardial infarction
Pheochromocytoma	

Drug Intoxication	Respiratory Disorders
Anticonvulsants	Asthma
Antidepressants	Chronic obstructive pulmonary disease
Antihistamines	Pulmonary embolism
Antihypertensive agents	Pulmonary edema
Antiinflammatory agents	
Antiparkinsonian agents	
Caffeine	
Digitalis	
Sympathomimetics	
Thyroid supplements	

Substance Use Related	Immunological, Collagen and Vascular Disorders
Cocaine	Systemic lupus erythematosus
Hallucinogens	Temporal arteritis
Amphetamines	

Withdrawal Syndromes	Metabolic Conditions
Alcohol	Acidosis
Narcotics	Acute intermittent porphyria
Sedatives–hypnotics	Electrolyte abnormalities
	Hypoglycemia

Gastrointestinal Disorders	Neurological Disorders
Peptic ulcer disease	Brain tumors
	Cerebral syphilis
	Cerebrovascular disorders
	Encephalopathies
	Epilepsy (especially temporal lobe epilepsy)
	Postconcussive syndrome
	Vertigo
	Akathisia

Infectious Diseases
Miscellaneous viral and bacterial infections

GAD appears at even higher rates in clinical settings, particularly in primary care settings. For example, Shear and colleagues (1994) found prevalence rates of GAD, using DSM-III-R criteria, reported by patients at four primary care centers, to be twice as high as those reported in community samples (i.e., 10 versus 5.1%). Similarly, a collaborative study by the World Health Organization (WHO) across 15 international sites reported prevalence rates of GAD at approximately 8% in primary care settings (Maier *et al.*, 2000).

Those with anxiety symptoms meeting criteria for GAD in the Epideiological Catchment Area (ECA) study reported receiving more outpatient mental services during the previous year than those diagnosed with other psychiatric disorders (Blazer *et al.*, 1991). Many of those with GAD in the National Comorbidity Survey sought professional help for GAD (66% of participants) and used medications to reduce their symptoms of GAD (44% of participants). Over 80% of the GAD group in the Harvard/Brown Anxiety Disorders Research Program (HARP) data indicated that they received psychotherapy and/or pharmacotherapy (Yonkers *et al.*, 1996).

Rates of GAD appear similar in special populations such as children and the elderly. GAD appears to be less prevalent in children than in adults. Data from the NCS indicate that for both lifetime and 12-month prevalence rates, GAD occurs at the lowest rate in younger ages and at the highest rate in older adults Epidemiological data on prevalence of GAD in childhood using DSM-IV criteria are currently lacking. In the elderly, GAD appears to account for the majority of anxiety disorders, with prevalence rates ranging from 0.7 to 7.3%.

Although it is unclear whether childhood GAD predisposes to the development of adult GAD or represents an early manifestation of adult GAD, these studies further suggest that generalized anxiety is highly prevalent both in the community and in the clinical population.

GAD: Comorbidity with Other Disorders

Despite different methodological approaches in early studies, the available studies report a high prevalence of psychiatric comorbidity in patients with GAD. For example, in some studies more than 90% of GAD patients had additional symptoms that fulfilled criteria for at least one or more concurrent disorders (range of 45–91%). An examination of the relative frequencies of various comorbid diagnoses in patients with GAD obtained from the available studies reveals that other anxiety and mood disorders frequently complicate the course of GAD (see diagnostic decision tree for GAD: Figure 53.1).

The National Comorbidity Survey showed 90% of respondents with lifetime GAD had at least one other lifetime disorder and of those with current GAD, 66% had at least one other current disorder. The most common comorbidities (specifically that criteria for both disorders were met) were found for mood disorders (major depression and dysthymia), panic disorder and (for current comorbidity only) agoraphobia. High 12 month rates for comorbidity for GAD and major depression were reaffirmed in the NCS-R (Kessler *et al.*, 2005). Other studies have also found that the highest comorbidities were with depressive disorders and panic disorders. GAD usually has an earlier onset than other anxiety and depressive disorders when comorbid disorders are present. Brawman-Mintzer and associates (1993) found that GAD had an onset before dysthymia and panic disorder, and after simple and social phobia. Further, onset of major depression

seemed to follow the onset of anxiety. Similar findings have been reported by other investigators.

As in adult GAD, childhood GAD (or overanxious anxiety disorder as it was earlier labeled) is also characterized by an unusual degree of comorbidity. Kashani and coworkers (1990) observed that over 50% of children with overanxious disorder had symptoms that met criteria for at least one additional psychiatric diagnosis. Among the most prevalent current comorbid diagnoses are social phobia (16–59%), simple phobia (21–55%), panic disorder (3–27%) and depression (8–39%). Furthermore, Masi and coworkers (1999) found, in those children and adolescents they sampled, that 87% had a comorbid disorder. In particular, high rates of separation anxiety, social anxiety and depressive disorders were found.

Alcoholism also complicates the clinical course of GAD for some patients; however, the available literature suggests that the diagnosis of alcohol abuse is not as prevalent in GAD as in other anxiety disorders, and the pattern of abuse is often a brief and nonpersistent one. GAD onset is usually later than that of the alcohol use disorder. Personality disorders have been observed to co-occur in approximately 50% of patients with GAD. For example, rates of GAD and personality disorders in clinical populations have ranged from 31 to 46%. Cluster C personality disorders, specifically avoidant personality disorder, dependent personality disorder and obsessive–compulsive personality disorder are common. Interestingly, Cluster A personality traits, in particular suspiciousness and mistrust, may be prominent in GAD as well.

Comorbid GAD is associated with increased severity of comorbid disorders (Kessler, 2000; Kessler *et al.*, 2005). Additionally, the presence of comorbid disorders in GAD patients is related to increased rates of negative outcomes such as disability, impairment and cost of care. Rates of relapse for GAD patients with comorbid depression appear higher than in noncomorbid GAD patients. Further, comorbidity is also associated with greater treatment seeking. Unsurprisingly, data indicate that patients with comorbid GAD and depression may have poorer response to treatment than patients with either disorder only.

Course

Retrospective and prospective reports indicate that the typical course of GAD is chronic, nonremitting, and that it often persists for a decade or longer. Rickels and colleagues (1986) reported that two-thirds of patients treated initially with diazepam relapsed within 1 year of discontinuation of treatment. Other studies utilizing criteria prior to the DSM-III-R for GAD found comparable levels of chronicity, with almost half the patients reporting moderate symptoms at follow-up (Yonkers *et al.*, 2000).

HARP, a prospective, naturalistic study of 711 adults with DSM-III-R anxiety disorders, recruited initially from psychiatric clinics and hospitals in the Boston Metropolitan area, indicated that only 15% of those with GAD at baseline experienced a full remission for 2 months or longer at any time during the first year after baseline, and only 25% had a full remission in the 2 years after baseline (Yonkers *et al.*, 1996). Further, among patients who experienced full or partial remission, 27 and 39% respectively, experienced a full relapse during a 3-year follow-up period (Yonkers *et al.*, 2000). Chronicity of GAD was also associated with cluster B and C personality disorders or a concurrent Axis I comorbidity. Wittchen and coworkers (1994) found that approximately 80% of subjects with GAD reported substantial interference with their life, a high degree of professional help-seeking, and a high prevalence of taking medications because of

Clinical Vignette 1

RJ is a 27-year-old graduate student who presented to his primary care physician with complaints of recurrent frontal headaches. He asked his physician to order a CT scan or an MRI because he feared that this may be a sign of a serious and a life-threatening illness. However, the headaches appeared to worsen during times of stress, and abated when the patient was on vacation with a friend. During the interview the patient admitted that he is very worried about the quality of his research at the university, even though he had received consistently positive evaluations. He attributed the perceived academic difficulties to his forgetfulness and diminished ability to concentrate during the last 6 months. He also described feeling fatigued, as well as significant indigestion, abdominal pain associated with bouts of changes in bowel movements (alternating diarrhea and constipation).

For the past 6 months he had few social contacts because of his symptoms and his girlfriend demanded that he seek professional help. Following complete physical evaluation, including consultation with a gastroenterologist, a diagnosis of generalized anxiety disorder and irritable bowel syndrome was made.

their GAD symptoms. The disability associated with GAD was found to be similar to that found in individuals with panic disorder or major depression.

Treatment Approaches

GAD is a chronic, relapsing illness, which means that most treatments do not cure the patient. Furthermore, it also suggests that when treatments are discontinued, symptoms may return. It follows that a thorough understanding of the long-term benefits and risks associated with the different treatments available is important. Thus, each case must be considered individually according to the severity and chronicity of the disorder, the severity of somatic symptoms, the presence of stressors, and the presence of specific personality traits. The clinician may also need to work with the patient to determine how much improvement is sufficient. For example, a reduction in disability may occur without a marked change in symptoms. Symptoms may persist but occur less frequently, or their intensity may be reduced. All these variations have important treatment implications, including decisions regarding the need for long-term treatment. Patients with milder forms of GAD may respond well to simple psychological interventions, and require no medication treatment. In more severe forms of GAD, it may become necessary to see the patient regularly and to provide both more specific psychological and pharmacological interventions. Figure 53.2 can be used as a guide to the treatment of GAD.

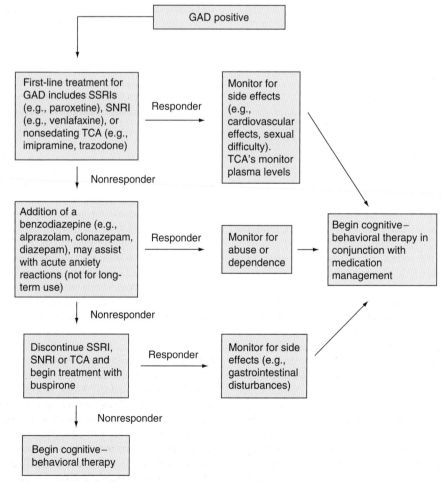

Figure 53.2   *Generalized anxiety disorder treatment flowchart.*

During the early (acute) phase of treatment, an attempt should be made to control the patient's symptomatology. It may take 3 to 6 months for an optimal response to be achieved. However, there may be a considerable variation in the length of the initial treatment phase. For example, clinical response to benzodiazepines occurs early in treatment. Response to other anxiolytic medications or to cognitive–behavioral treatment generally requires longer periods of time. During the maintenance phase, treatment gains are consolidated. Unfortunately, studies suggesting how long treatment should be continued are limited. Routinely, pharmacological treatment is continued for a total of 6 to 12 months before attempting to discontinue medications. Recent data indicate that "maintenance" psychotherapeutic treatments such as cognitive–behavioral therapy may be helpful in maintaining treatment gains in patients with anxiety disorders following the discontinuation of pharmacotherapy. It is clear that many patients may experience chronic and continuous symptoms that require years of long-term treatment.

Doctor–Patient Relationship

The vast majority of patients with GAD who present for treatment have been ill for many years and frequently have received a variety of treatments. Some patients have been sent to psychiatrists for treatment as a "last resort" in order to learn how to cope with their various ill-defined somatic and emotional complaints. Patients may feel shame and guilt over their inability to control symptoms. They are often demoralized and angry, and feel that their symptoms are not taken seriously. Thus, it is important to help the patient understand their illness and to conceptualize it as a health problem rather than a "personal weakness". Once the burden of perceived responsibility is lifted from the patient, and they believe that effective treatment of their illness is possible, a working alliance with the treating physician can begin. The treatment plan should be outlined clearly, and the patient cautioned that recovery may have a gradual, variable course. Finally, during the critical early stages of treatment, the clinician should make a special effort to be available in person or by phone to answer questions and provide support.

Pharmacotherapy

Below, we will discuss the use of various anxiolytic agents in the treatment of GAD. Table 53.2 provides a summarization of this information.

Benzodiazepines

Benzodiazepines are commonly used for the treatment of GAD and are still considered by some clinicians to be the first-line treatment for GAD. Several controlled studies have demonstrated the efficacy of different benzodiazepines such as diazepam, chlordiazepoxide and alprazolam in the treatment of GAD. The available placebo-controlled studies found that diazepam, alprazolam and lorazepam were effective in the treatment of GAD. The benzodiazepines have a broad spectrum of effects including sedation, muscle relaxation, anxiety reduction and decreased physiologic arousal (e.g. palpitations, tremulousness, etc.). Interestingly, available studies indicate that benzodiazepines have the most pronounced effect on hypervigilance and somatic symptoms of GAD, but exhibited fewer effects on psychic symptoms such as dysphoria, interpersonal sensitivity and obsessionality (Hoehn-Saric et al., 1988).

The main difference between individual benzodiazepines is potency and elimination half-life. These differences may have important treatment implications. For example, benzodiazepines with relatively short elimination half-lives such as alprazolam (range of 10–14 hours) may require dosing at least three to four times a day in order to avoid interdose symptom rebound. Conversely, the use of longer-acting compounds such as clonazepam (range of 20–50 hours) may minimize the risk of interdose symptom recurrence. In comparative studies of different benzodiazepines, alprazolam appeared to perform somewhat better than lorazepam. Data from the HARP study indicate that the most frequently reported medication used by GAD patients was alprazolam (31%), followed by clonazepam (23%) (Yonkers et al., 1996).

Benzodiazepines exert their therapeutic effects quickly, often after a single dose. However, concern has emerged over the use of benzodiazepines, particularly long-term benzodiazepine use. Side effects of benzodiazepines, such as sedation, psychomotor impairment and memory disruption, were noted by treating clinicians, and confirmed in research studies. Further, although it was suggested that the use pattern of benzodiazepines by patients with anxiety disorders may not represent abuse, addiction, or drug dependence as typically understood, the chronic use of benzodiazepines in the treatment of GAD has been increasingly discouraged in recent years.

When initiating treatment with benzodiazepines, it is helpful for patients to take an initial dose at home in the evening to see how it affects them. Gradual titration to an effective dose allows for limiting unwanted adverse effects. A final daily dosage of alprazolam between 2 and 4 mg/day, 1 and 2 mg/day for clonazepam, or 15 and 20 mg/day of diazepam is usually sufficient for the majority of patients. Upon treatment discontinuation, it is important to consider appropriate taper in order to avoid withdrawal symptoms. Possible factors that may contribute to the severity of withdrawal and the ultimate outcome of benzodiazepine taper include the dosage, duration of treatment, the benzodiazepine elimination half-life and potency, and the rate of benzodiazepine taper (gradual versus abrupt). Additionally, patient factors such as premorbid personality features have been implicated. It appears that a taper rate of 25% per week is probably too rapid for many patients. We, therefore, recommend a slow benzodiazepine taper of at least 4 to 8 weeks, with the final 50% of the taper conducted even more gradually, with the patient decreasing by the lowest possible daily dose of the benzodiazepines during this period. We also recommend continuing to use divided doses of short to intermediate half-life benzodiazepines (alprazolam, lorazepam) during taper to minimize fluctuations in benzodiazepine levels over a 24-hour period, or using longer half-life benzodiazepines (such as clonazepam) which have the advantage of maintaining a once- or twice-daily dosing schedule.

Tricyclic Antidepressants

Clinical trials conducted in the early 1990s have confirmed that tricyclic antidepressants (TCAs) may also be effective in the treatment of GAD. These studies, as well as other trials, suggest that TCAs may be especially effective in the treatment of psychic symptoms of GAD (Brawman-Mintzer and Lydiard, 1994). The relationship between plasma levels of TCAs and their anxiolytic efficacy in patients with GAD has not been studied. Until this relationship is clarified, decisions regarding the total daily doses and the monitoring of plasma levels should be based on

Drug	Daily Dosage Range (mg)	Advantages	Disadvantages
Table 53.2 Anxiolytic Agents			
Selective serotonin reuptake inhibitors			
Paroxetine	20–40	Efficacy with GAD	Gastrointestinal side effects
Fluoxetine	20–60	Efficacy with comorbid depression	Delayed onset
Sertraline	50–200		Sexual side effects
Citalopram	20–40	Favorable side effects profile compared with TCAs	
Fluvoxamine	100–300	Easy dosing schedule	
Serotonergic and noradrenergic reuptake inhibitors			
Venlafaxine extended release (XR)	75–225	Efficacy with GAD Efficacy with comorbid depression	Gastrointestinal side effects Sexual side effects Potential for increased blood pressure
Benzodiazepines			
Alprazolam	2–6	Rapid onset of action	Sedation
Clonazepam	1–3	Favorable side-effects profile	Multiple doses for shorter acting agents
Lorazepam	4–10		Physical dependence
Diazepam	15–20		Limited antidepressant effects Sexual side effects
Tricyclic antidepressants			
Imipramine	75–300	Once-daily dosage Efficacy with comorbid depression	Delayed onset Need for titration Activation Anticholinergic effects Orthostatic hypotension Weight gain Toxicity in overdose Sexual side effects
Atypical antidepressants			
Trazodone	150–600	Once-daily dosage Efficacy with comorbid depression Low anticholinergic effects	Delayed onset Orthostatic hypotension Weight gain Sexual side effects Priapism (rare) Sedation
Azapirones			
Buspirone	30–60	No withdrawal symptoms No physical dependence Favorable side-effects profile	Multiple doses

the patient's treatment response and side-effects profile. Further, due to potential jitteriness, restlessness and agitation during the initial stages of treatment, we suggest that the initial dose of the TCAs in patients with GAD may need to be low (for example 10 mg/day of imipramine), and increased gradually.

Adverse effects commonly associated with the use of TCAs include anticholinergic effects (dry mouth, blurred vision,

constipation), cardiovascular effects (orthostatic hypotension, slightly increased heart rate), sexual side effects and weight gain. As mentioned, patients may also experience significant jitteriness, restlessness and agitation during the initial stages of treatment. These side-effects often limit the acceptability of TCAs by many patients. Potential toxicity in overdose has been of concern to clinicians as well. Due, in part, to the side-effect profile, need for dose titration and importantly the emergence of new and effective agents (as described below), the use of TCAs in the treatment of GAD has been reserved for those resistant to these newer agents.

Serotonin Reuptake Inhibitors

Selective serotonin reuptake inhibitors (SSRIs) are rapidly becoming a key tool in the treatment of GAD. SSRIs are generally well tolerated. The most problematic side effect associated with SSRI use is interference with sexual function (e.g., delayed orgasm or abnormal ejaculation) in women and men. A variety of treatment strategies have been suggested for the management of SSRI-induced sexual dysfunction. Such strategies include waiting for tolerance to develop, dosage reduction, drug holidays and various augmentation strategies with 5-hydroxytryptamine-2 (5-HT_2), 5-HT_3 and alpha-2-adrenergic receptor antagonists, 5-HT_{1A} and dopamine receptor agonists, and phosphodiesterase (PDE5) enzyme inhibitors.

Serotonergic and Noradrenergic Reuptake Inhibitors

The antidepressant venlafaxine extended release (XR) is an inhibitor of both 5-HT and NE reuptake (SNRI). Several large, placebo-controlled trials have evaluated it in the treatment of patients with DSM-IV-diagnosed GAD. As a result, venlafaxine XR was the first antidepressant approved by the FDA for the treatment of GAD. Results from two short-term studies indicate that venlafaxine XR (75, 150 and 225 mg/day) was significantly more effective than placebo and superior to buspirone on certain anxiety measures and in the prevention of relapse (Sheehan, 2001). The adverse events for GAD patients treated with venlafaxine XR resembled those in depression trials. The most common adverse events included nausea, somnolence, dry mouth, dizziness, sweating, constipation and anorexia.

Other Antidepressants

Both trazodone and imipramine have comparable efficacy to diazepam. In addition, trazodone and imipramine exhibit higher efficacy in the treatment of psychic symptoms such as tension, apprehension and worry. The alpha-2-adrenoreceptor antagonist mitrazapine, which is also a 5-HT_2, 5-HT_3 and H(1) receptors antagonist, has been evaluated as a potential anxiolytic in the treatment of patients with major depressive disorder and comorbid GAD in an 8-week, open-label study (Goodnick *et al.*, 1999). Results suggest that this antidepressant may be useful in the treatment of anxiety symptoms.

Azapirones

Buspirone hydrochloride, the only currently marketed azapirone, was the first nonbenzodiazepine anxiolytic agent approved for the treatment of persistent anxiety by FDA. Results have been mixed about the efficacy of buspirone over placebo. For example, in four placebo-controlled studies that compared buspirone with a standard benzodiazepine, two showed no benefit for diazepam and buspirone over placebo, and two showed no benefit for buspirone over placebo. Benzodiazepines may also be slightly more effective than buspirone in the treatment of somatic symptoms of anxiety but no significant differences appear to exist between buspirone and benzodiazepines in measures of psychic anxiety (Rickels *et al.*,

1997). Side effects most frequently associated with buspirone use included gastrointestinal system-related side effects, such as appetite disturbances and abdominal complaints, and dizziness. Prior use of benzodiazepines may adversely affect the therapeutic response to buspirone. DeMartinis and colleagues (2000) found that buspirone treatment was less effective for patients who had been taking benzodiazepines within 30 days of initiating buspirone treatment. Delle Chiaie and colleagues (1995) reported that a gradual 2-week taper of lorazepam with a simultaneous addition of buspirone for 6 weeks prevents the development of clinically significant rebound anxiety or benzodiazepine withdrawal. This approach was shown to provide clinically significant relief of anxiety symptoms in GAD patients previously treated with benzodiazepines for 8 to 14 weeks.

Perhaps the most significant problem with the use of buspirone has been that experts have advocated too low a dose to produce symptom reduction. In order to achieve optimal response, buspirone dosing in the range of at least 30 to 60 mg/day is currently recommended.

Other Agents

Hydroxyzine is a histamine-1 receptor blocker and a muscarinic receptor blocker. Recent controlled trials with the antihistamine have suggested that this compound may be effective in the acute treatment of GAD symptoms. Finally, the potential use of the anticonvulsant gabapentin in the treatment of anxiety symptoms has also been suggested.

Nonpharmacological Treatments

Numerous studies have shown that psychological interventions are beneficial in the comprehensive management of anxiety disorders. However, data suggesting that specific psychotherapeutic techniques yield better results in the treatment of patients with GAD are inconclusive and more evidence is needed on the comparative efficacy and long-term effects of different psychological treatments.

Cognitive–Behavioral Therapy

In recent years specific cognitive–behavioral therapy (CBT) interventions for the treatment of patients with anxiety disorders have been developed. Components of CBT include teaching patients to identify and label irrational thoughts and to replace them with positive self-statements or modify them by challenging their veracity. The cognitive modification approaches are combined with behavioral treatments such as exposure or relaxation training. There is currently evidence suggesting that CBT may be more effective in the treatment of GAD than other psychotherapeutic interventions, such as behavioral therapy alone or nonspecific supportive therapy (Chambless and Gillis, 1993). Six additional studies confirmed the efficacy of CBT compared with waiting list or pill placebo and patients tend to maintain improvement following CBT over 6 to 12 months of follow-up.

CBT targeting intolerance of uncertainty, erroneous beliefs about worry, poor problem orientation and cognitive avoidance demonstrated effectiveness at post treatment (no change in the delayed treatment control group) 6- and 12-month follow-up, with 77% of the treatment group no longer having symptoms meeting criteria for a GAD diagnosis (Ladouceur *et al.*, 2000).

Cognitive therapy was also compared with analytic psychotherapy, and was found to be significantly more effective (Borkovec and Costello, 1993). Overall, two-thirds in the cognitive therapy group achieved clinically significant improvements and cognitive therapy was associated with significant reductions in medication usage.

A meta-analytic review of controlled trials examining CBT and pharmacotherapy for GAD, which included 35 studies, demonstrated the robustness of CBT in the treatment of GAD (Gould *et al.*, 1997). Overall, both modalities offered clear efficacy to patients, with the effect size for CBT not being statistically different from psychopharmacological approaches. CBT demonstrated greater effects in reducing depression and was associated with clear maintenance of treatment gains, whereas long-term efficacy of pharmacologic treatment was attenuated following medication discontinuation.

Barlow and colleagues (1986) developed a CBT approach to GAD which concentrates on the behavioral element of direct exposure to the contents of patients' worry and apprehension (i.e., a deconditioning strategy) in addition to relaxation techniques (progressive muscle relaxation) and cognitive restructuring. The authors found that this technique is effective in reducing anxiety symptoms in patients with GAD.

Supportive Psychotherapy

Many patients with milder forms of GAD will benefit from simple psychological interventions such as supportive psychotherapy. They may experience lessening of anxiety when given the opportunity to discuss their difficulties with a supportive clinician and to become better informed about their illness. Thus, basic supportive techniques such as reassurance, clarification of patient concerns, direct suggestions and advice are often effective in reducing anxiety symptoms.

Relaxation and Biofeedback

Relaxation techniques such as progressive muscle relaxation and biofeedback have also been utilized in the treatment of patients with anxiety symptoms. Few controlled studies have examined their effectiveness. In a recent controlled study, Borkovec and Costello (1993) compared a comprehensive relaxation treatment and cognitive–behavioral therapy in the treatment of patients with DSM-III-R-defined GAD. The authors found that both treatments were equally effective and superior to a nonspecific supportive treatment intervention.

Psychodynamic Psychotherapy

Although there are no controlled studies evaluating the efficacy of psychodynamic psychotherapies in the treatment of patients with GAD, some of its important principles in understanding patients may be helpful. First, it is important to note that the psychoanalytic theories view anxiety as an indicator of certain unconscious conflicts, rather than as a primary target symptom to be alleviated. It is, therefore, the clinician's task to use various techniques to help the patient uncover these unconscious conflicts. It is believed that the newly gained understanding of the underlying reasons for symptoms will have a therapeutic effect, thereby reducing anxiety. Through interpretation of previously unconscious conflicts and unconscious origins of anxiety, the patient will be able to utilize new insights and find more adaptive outlets or solutions to problems. In Harry Stack Sullivan's theory, anxiety reflects the failure to develop secure interpersonal interactions, such as an emphatic and secure mother–infant relationship. He believed that the child learns to identify anxiety states in himself and significant others and develops protective defensive strategies which enable him to avoid experiencing anxiety. However, the defenses employed (termed security operations) are generally restrictive and may result in limiting the subject's interpersonal interactions. Therefore, the task of the therapist, according to Sullivan's model, is to trace the patterns of interpersonal interactions throughout the patient's developmental stages (rather than to uncover the unconscious drives), thereby promoting a more accurate perception of self and others and subsequently better social adaptation.

Another therapeutic approach to the treatment of anxiety symptoms was offered by object relation and self-psychology theorists. They view anxiety as a result of the loss of or inadequate emotional relationships with significant others. Therefore, the primary focus of therapy shifts to emphasize the importance of the relationship to the therapist, who functions as an empathic object providing emotionally corrective experiences. For example, the patient may learn that an important person may be imperfect but still be trusted and nurturing.

Finally, most psychodynamically oriented therapists agree that the outcome of psychodynamic psychotherapy is determined by factors reflecting a patient's maturity and strength. Specifically factors such as the patient's capacity for introspection, intelligence, ability to relate to the therapist, and ability to bear painful feelings should be carefully evaluated.

Long-term Management of Generalized Anxiety Disorder

As mentioned, GAD is a chronic, continuous condition in the majority of patients. Frequently beginning in adolescence or early adulthood, the course of GAD can persist for decades, with relatively low remission rates. The HARP data indicate that among the 164 GAD patients followed, only 15% had a full remission for 2 months or longer at any time during the first follow-up year, 25% had a full remission during the 2-year follow-up, and only 35% had a full remission after 5 years (Yonkers *et al.*, 1996). In a 5-year follow-up study of 64 GAD patients, only 18% of GAD subjects achieved a full remission compared with 45% of panic disorder subjects (Woodman *et al.*, 1999).

Despite these findings, less research has been conducted to assess the efficacy of chronic long-term anxiolytic therapy. To our knowledge, only three double-blind, controlled studies evaluating the long-term pharmacological treatment of GAD have been conducted. The first, a 1-year follow-up of patients who participated in a 6-month diazepam maintenance study, found that two-thirds of all patients relapsed within a 1-year period after diazepam discontinuation. In the second study, GAD patients were treated for 6 months with buspirone or clorazepate, and reevaluated them after discontinuation at 6 and 40 months. The authors found that the improvement achieved in both treatment groups was sustained during the 6-month maintenance phase, with no need for an increase in medication intake, and no evidence of tolerance or abuse. At follow-up, approximately 60% of patients treated initially with clorazepate compared with 30% of patients treated initially with buspirone were experiencing at least moderate anxiety symptoms. Finally, in a recent study, Stocchi and colleagues (2001) found that many patients with GAD are not able to remain symptom-free for long periods without treatment. Therefore, a long-term therapy may be needed in many patients.

Generally, the current recommendation for GAD treatment suggests a treatment period of approximately 1 year after response has been established prior to considering treatment discontinuation. Stress management and problem-solving techniques, along with specific psychotherapeutic approaches such as cognitive–behavioral therapy, should be attempted in addition to medication treatment.

Comorbidity and the Treatment of GAD

GAD is often accompanied by other concurrent psychiatric disorders, specifically anxiety and mood disorders. The presence of these comorbid conditions may reflect more severe loading for psychopathology, and may have important implications on the course and treatment response of the primary disorder. In the National Comorbidity Survey, more patients with comorbidity experienced interference with daily activities than did patients with pure GAD (Wittchen *et al.*, 1994). The presence of a comorbid anxiety disorder and major depressive disorder is frequently associated with a poorer overall outcome than for patients with a single psychiatric disorder (Kessler *et al.*, 1999). Currently, there are treatment options that can target both GAD and major depressive disorder simultaneously. The use of SSRIs and the SNRI venlafaxine is recommended as the first-line treatment for comorbid GAD and depression.

Social anxiety disorder frequently complicates the course GAD takes. With the recent data indicating that the SSRIs such as sertraline and paroxetine are effective in the treatment of social anxiety, these agents may be useful in the treatment of comorbid social anxiety disorder and GAD. The benzodiazepines that have been established as effective in the treatment of patients with GAD also appear to be effective in the treatment of patients with social anxiety disorder. Thus, these agents (considering the caveats associated with their use described earlier) may have a therapeutic role in patients with GAD and coexisting social phobia. Finally, patients with GAD and concurrent panic disorder or panic attacks may be effectively treated with SSRIs, TCAs and benzodiazepines. However, buspirone is probably ineffective in the treatment of panic disorder.

Concurrent alcohol and substance abuse tend to confuse the clinical picture of GAD and can interfere with the therapeutic efforts. Additionally, symptoms associated with alcohol withdrawal or other sedative–hypnotics may mimic the underlying anxiety disorder. If a substance abuse problem exists, the clinician and the patient should take the necessary steps to discontinue the use of the abused substance. This may well include specific substance abuse treatment. Specifically, the need for detoxification should be assessed and discussed with the patient. Following cessation of substance abuse the patient's symptomatology should be reevaluated. The use of benzodiazepines in these patients may be contraindicated, and alternative treatments with SSRIs, SNRIs, TCAs, buspirone, or gabapentin may be needed.

Treatment of GAD in the Elderly

Epidemiological data suggests that GAD is highly prevalent in the geriatric population (prevalence rates ranging from 0.7 to 7.1%), accounting for the majority of anxiety disorder cases in this group. GAD is the most common of the pervasive late-life anxiety disorders. In the elderly, anxiety symptoms are often associated with depression, medical conditions and cognitive

dysfunction. Thus, a careful differential diagnosis to eliminate exogenous causes of anxiety and identification of other coexisting conditions is necessary. For example, treatment of medical illness, depression, or underlying dementia may reduce anxiety symptoms. Dose reductions or elimination of anxiety-inducing medications as well as reducing stressful life circumstances may also reduce anxiety symptoms. However, if these interventions are not effective in reducing anxiety, pharmacotherapy may be necessary. Several factors influencing pharmacologic treatment in the elderly should be considered. These factors include alterations in pharmacokinetics and pharmacodynamics of psychotropic drugs, primarily because of reduced hepatic clearing efficiency, alterations in the response of the central nervous system to drugs, such as changes in receptor sensitivity, and concurrent medical conditions that may alter drug effect, side-effect profile, and toxicity.

Benzodiazepines can be effective in the treatment of anxiety symptoms. However, older patients are often sensitive to their effects. Adverse effects may include increased sedation, tendency to fall, psychomotor discoordination and cognitive impairment. Older patients may become disinhibited by benzodiazepines and experience agitation and aggression. The administration of long-acting benzodiazepines such as diazepam and chlorazepate may result in increased accumulation of the drug predisposing the patient to these side effects. Conversely, the use of short half-life high potency benzodiazepines such as alprazolam may be associated with more severe withdrawal symptoms following rapid discontinuation. Because of these factors, benzodiazepines should be prescribed for the briefest period of time, at the lowest therapeutic dose, giving preference for the short half-life, low-potency benzodiazepines such as oxazepam. We recommend initiating treatment with oxazepam at low doses (10 mg t.i.d.), to be increased gradually, while carefully monitoring for the emergence of side effects.

Buspirone has been extensively used in the treatment of GAD symptoms. The lack of associated sedation, discoordination and dependence with the use of buspirone makes its use in the elderly less problematic. However, additional research is needed to determine its long-term efficacy in the GAD elderly population. The average therapeutic doses of buspirone for elderly patients range from 5 to 20 mg/day.

The use of TCAs in the anxious elderly patient should be viewed in light of the side-effect profile of TCAs. Side effects commonly associated with the use of TCAs, such as the anticholinergic effects and orthostatic hypotension, may be especially troublesome in these patients. We therefore recommend the use of TCAs with low anticholinergic and hypotensive effects such as desipramine and nortryptiline, starting at low doses (10 mg/day) that are raised slowly and gradually.

Finally, despite the widespread use of the newer antidepressant agents, specifically the SSRIs and the SNRIs, in the treatment of adult GAD patients, very limited data exist regarding their use in the anxious elderly population. However, preliminary evidence suggests that they can decrease symptoms, improve quality of life and potentially promote healthier outcomes in geriatric patients who have comorbid anxiety and depression and/or comorbid mental and physical illness. A potential drawback of venlafaxine in this population is the need to monitor for drug-induced blood pressure elevation in those taking the medication.

Most controlled studies examining CBT in older adults have focused on the treatment of GAD. This literature suggests that CBT is effective in the treatment of GAD in this population.

For example, group-administered CBT was found to be effective in reducing GAD and coexistent symptoms in older adults. In conclusion, several agents may play an important role in the treatment of anxiety in the elderly. However, until more studies in the elderly GAD population are available, treatment choices should be guided by clinical judgment and specific factors relevant to this patient population, such as medical comorbidity and age-associated changes in the drug metabolism.

Treatment of GAD in Adolescents and Children

The treatment of GAD in adolescents and children should be multifaceted, including psychotherapy for the patient, psychoeducation for the parents, and pharmacotherapy when other psychotherapeutic interventions have not produced satisfactory outcome. CBT is successful in treating GAD in children. The addition of family anxiety management skills taught to parents appears to increase treatment success.

Pharmacotherapy in children and adolescents differs from that of the adult population primarily because of the difference in the hepatic biotransformation and elimination of many psychotropic drugs that may require some adjustments in treatment regimen. Hepatic metabolic rate is faster in children and adolescents than in adults, reaching adult values around 15 years of age. Thus a particular milligram per kilogram (mg/kg) dose will yield a lower blood level in a child than in an adult, and higher mg/kg doses than based on those for adults may be necessary. This applies for all liver-metabolized drugs, such as antidepressants, anxiolytics, anticonvulsants and neuroleptics. In addition, the higher clearance of these drugs requires more frequent administration of medications (i.e., small divided doses rather than one large dose).

Over the years, a number of medications have been used in the treatment of childhood GAD (previously classified as overanxious anxiety disorder). Unfortunately, only a few studies have been conducted in children with overanxious anxiety disorder. Given these limited findings and the reported occurrence of significant behavioral activation, other side effects, and their addictive potential, the use of benzodazepines to treat children with GAD is suspect.

The use of SSRIs in the treatment of GAD in children and adolescents appears promising; however, no controlled trials with large samples have been conducted. Buspirone may also be effective in the treatment of GAD in children and adolescents. No controlled studies have been completed for the treatment of GAD with buspirone in children to date. TCAs have not been studied in overanxious anxiety disorder. It should be noted that cardiovascular side effects may occur more frequently in children and adolescents than in adults, and preexisting conduction abnormalities may be associated with significant TCA effect on cardiac conduction. However, the clinical significance of TCA-induced changes in cardiac conduction is not clear. Given this lack of efficacy data for GAD and the concern of significant cardiovascular side effects in children, TCAs should not be a first-line treatment in children and adolescents with GAD.

Treatment Resistance

The clinician is frequently faced with a patient whose anxiety symptomatology is not responding satisfactorily to the standard treatment. Different factors, such as inadequate length of treatment, low dose and noncompliance, may contribute to treatment failure in the management of patients with GAD. Pharmacologic treatment is often complicated by the occurrence of side effects, which may impair quality of life, deter clinicians from prescribing adequate doses and contribute to noncompliance. For example, some antidepressants, including SSRIs, TCAs and venlafaxine, are associated with activation, overstimulation, or "jitters" primarily during the initial stage of treatment. When evaluating noncompliance, clinicians should also assess for akathisia and worsening of anxiety and hypomania or mania. Further, the presence of comorbid general medical and psychiatric conditions in GAD patients may be associated with nonresponse or lower response rates and should be carefully assessed during patient evaluation. Finally, the use of concurrent medications that can precipitate anxiety symptoms may affect the response to treatment.

The clinician should always evaluate whether an adequate treatment trial was complete. We believe that an attempt should be made to maintain the patient on medication for at least 6 weeks. Although there are no data suggesting that certain doses may be particularly effective in the treatment of GAD, it is advisable to titrate the medication up to maximally tolerated doses prior to discontinuing the medication for nonresponse. It is important to inquire about the presence of side effects such as sedation, anticholinergic effects, or sexual side effects, which may limit the attainment of a therapeutic dosage and reduce compliance. Additionally, many patients with GAD fear that they may become "drug-dependent" and thus avoid dose increases. Some estimate of the patient's compliance may be helpful in determining whether a treatment was adequate, as indicated by blood plasma levels or pill counts. Drug plasma levels may also be useful to identify patients who are rapid metabolizers. A careful evaluation for the presence of psychiatric comorbid conditions that may contribute to treatment refractoriness should follow. As mentioned, comorbidity which may reflect more severe loading for psychopathology is often associated with increased severity of illness and poorer response to treatment in comparison to patients with an uncomplicated (i.e., single) disorder. Thus, treatment strategies in GAD patients with a concurrent disorder may differ from those in an uncomplicated disorder, often requiring multiple drug therapy. The clinician should also be alert to the presence of underlying general medical conditions such as hyperthyroidism which may present with refractory anxiety, or conditions/medications which may alter the effects of treatment such as hepatic disease or medications (e.g., steroids) that affect hepatic clearance.

The use of psychotherapy, such as cognitive–behavioral therapy, in conjunction with pharmacotherapy may also enhance response in the treatment-resistant patient. Finally, education and psychological support for patients and their families may help them better to understand and deal with their illness, especially during periods of increased stress, and consequently improve treatment outcome.

Summary

In conclusion, GAD appears to be a chronic, frequently comorbid condition, often requiring long-term management. Benzodiazepines were, at one time, the first-line treatment choice for GAD. However, newer medication may offer more hope for those with GAD. SSRIs and SNRIs are promising new pharmocotherapies for GAD. Additionally, these treatments may be especially effective for patients presenting with depressive symptomatology. Further, buspirone and TCAs have been shown to be an important treatment alternative to benzodiazepines, and the TCAs may be especially effective in patients presenting with depressive symptomatology. Finally psychotherapy, specifically cognitive–behavioral therapy, is an additional treatment strategy, potentially effective in maintaining treatment gains. Further information is needed on long-term treatment, medication discontinuation and comparative efficacy of pharmacotherapies, psychotherapies and combination in the treatment of uncomplicated and comorbid GAD.

Comparison of DSM-IV/ICD-10 Diagnostic Criteria

The ICD-10 Diagnostic Criteria for Research specify that four symptoms from a list of 22 be present. In contrast, DSM-IV-TR requires three out of a list of six (of which five are included among the ICD-10 list of 22).

References

American Psychiatric Association (1994) *Diagnostic and Statistical Manual of Mental Disorders*, 4th edn. APA, Washington DC.

Barlow DH, Blanchard RB, Vermilyea JB et al. (1986) Generalized anxiety and generalized anxiety disorder: Description and reconceptualization. *Am J Psychiatr* 143, 40–44.

Black DW, Noyes R, Goldstein RB et al. (1992) A family study of obsessive–compulsive disorder. *Arch Gen Psychiatr* 49, 362–368.

Blazer DG, Hughes D, George LK et al. (1991) Generalized anxiety disorder, in *Psychiatric Disorders in America: The Epidemiologic Catchment Area Study* (eds Robins LN and Regier DA). Free Press, New York, pp. 180–203.

Borkovec TD and Costello E (1993) Efficacy of applied relaxation and cognitive–behavioral therapy in the treatment of generalized anxiety disorder. *J Consult Clin Psychol* 61(4), 611–619.

Brawman-Mintzer O, Lydiard RB, Emmanuel N et al. (1993) Psychiatric comorbidity in patients with generalized anxiety disorder. *Am J Psychiatr* 150, 1216–1218.

Brawman-Mintzer O, Lydiard RB (1994) Psychopharmacology of anxiety disorders. *Psychiatr Clin N AM* 1, 51–79.

Carter CS and Maddock RJ (1992) Chest pain in generalized anxiety disorder. *Int J Psychiatr Med* 22(3), 291–298.

Chambless DL and Gillis MM (1993) Cognitive therapy of anxiety disorders. *J Clin Consult Psychol* 61(2), 248–260.

Delle Chiaie R, Pancheri P, Casacchia M et al. (1995) Assessment of the efficacy of buspirone in patients affected by generalized anxiety disorder, shifting buspirone from prior treatment with lorazepam: A placebo-controlled, double-blind study. *J Clin Psychopharmacol* 15(1), 12–19.

DeMartinis N, Rynn M, Rickels K et al. (2000) Prior benzodiazepine use and buspirone response in the treatment of generalized anxiety disorder. *J Clin Psychiatr* 61(2), 91–94.

Goodnick PJ, Puig A, DeVane CL et al. (1999) Mirtazapine in major depression with comorbid generalized anxiety disorder. *J Clin Psychiatr* 60, 446–448.

Gould RA, Otto MA, Pollack MH, et al. (1997) Cognitive–behavioral and pharmacological treatment of generalized anxiety disorder: A preliminary meta-analysis. *Behav Ther* 28(2), 285–305.

Gray JA (1988) The neuropsychological basis of anxiety. In Handbook of Anxiety Disorders, Last CG and Hersen M (eds). Pergamon Press, New York, pp. 10–37.

Hoehn-Saric R, McLeod DR and Zimmerli WD (1988) Differential effects of alprazolam and imipramine in generalized anxiety disorder: Somatic versus psychic symptoms. *J Clin Psychiatr* 49, 293–301.

Kashani JH, Vaidya AF and Soltys SM (1990) Correlates of anxiety in psychiatrically hospitalized children and their parents. *Am J Psychiatr* 147, 319–323.

Kendler KS, Neale MC, Kessler RC et al. (1992) Generalized anxiety disorder in women. *Arch Gen Psychiatr* 49, 267–272.

Kessler RC (2000) The epidemiology of pure and comorbid generalized anxiety disorder: A review and evaluation of recent research. *Acta Psychiatr Scand* 406(Suppl), 7–13.

Kessler RC, McGonagle KA, Zhao S et al. (1994) Lifetime and 12-month prevalence of DSM-III-R psychiatric disorders in the United States: Results from the National Comorbidity Survey. *Arch Gen Psychiatr* 51, 8–19.

Kessler RC, DuPont RL, Berglund P et al. (1999) Impairment in pure and comorbid generalized anxiety disorder and major depression at 12 months in two national surveys. *Am J Psychiatr* 156, 1915–1923.

Kessler RC, Berglund MBA, Demler O et al. (2005) Lifetime prevalence and age-of-onset distributions of DSM-IV disorders in the National Comorbidity Survey Replication. *Arch Gen Psychiatr* 62, 593–602.

Ladouceur R, Dugas MJ, Freeston MH et al. (2000) Efficacy of a cognitive–behavioral treatment for generalized anxiety disorder: Evaluation in a controlled clinical trial. *J Clin Consult Psychol* 68(6), 957–964.

Lesch KP (2001) Genetic dissection of anxiety and related disorders, in *Anxiety Disorders* (eds Nutt D and Ballenger J). Blackwell Science, Oxford.

Lorberbaum JP, Varon D, Brawman-Minzter O et al. (2001) The functional neuroanatomy of anticipatory anxiety in healthy adults and patients with generalized anxiety disorder. Presented at the 21st National Conference of Anxiety Disorders Association of America, Atlanta.

Maier W, Gaeniscke M, Freyberger HJ et al. (2000) Generalized anxiety disorder (ICD-10) in primary care from a cross-cultural perspective: A valid diagnostic entity? *Acta Psychiatr Scand* 101, 29–36.

Masi G, Mucci M, Favilla L et al. (1999) Symptomatology and comorbidity of generalized anxiety disorder in children and adolescents. *Compr Psychiatr* 40, 210–215.

Papadimitriou GN, Kerkhofs M, Kempenaers C et al. (1988) EEG sleep studies in patients with generalized anxiety disorder. *Psychiatr Res* 26, 183–190.

Rickels K, Case WG, Downing RW et al. (1986) One-year follow-up of anxious patients treated with diazepam. *J Clin Psychopharmacol* 6, 32–36.

Rickels K, Schweizer E, DeMartinis N et al. (1997) Gepirone and diazepam in generalized anxiety disorder: A placebo-controlled trial. *J Clin Psychopharmacol* 17(4), 272–277.

Shear MK, Schulberg HC and Madonia M (1994) Panic and generalized anxiety disorder in primary care. Paper presented at a meeting of the Association for Primary Care, Washington DC.

Sheehan DV (2001) Attaining remission in generalized anxiety disorder: Venlafaxine extended release comparative data. *J Clin Psychiatr* 62(9S), 26–31.

Skre I, Torgersen S, Lygren S et al. (1993) A twin study of DSM-III-R anxiety disorders. *Acta Psychiatr Scand* 88, 85–92.

Stocchi F, Jokinen R and Lepola U (2001) Efficacy and tolerability of paroxetine for long-term treatment of generalized anxiety disorder. Presented at 2001 Annual Meeting of the American Psychiatric Association (May 5–10), New Orleans.

Wittchen HU, Zhao S, Kessler RC et al. (1994) DSM-III-R generalized anxiety disorder in the National Comorbidity Survey. *Arch Gen Psychiatr* 51, 355–364.

Woodman CL, Noyes R, Black DW et al. (1999) A 5-year follow-up study of generalized anxiety disorder and panic disorder. *J Nerv Ment Disord* 187, 3–9.

Wu JC, Buchsbaum MS, Hershey TG et al. (1991) PET in generalized anxiety disorder. *Biol Psychiatr* 29, 1181–1199.

Yonkers KA, Dyck IR, Warshaw M et al. (2000) Factors predicting the clinical course of generalized anxiety disorder. *Br J Psychiatr* 176, 544–549.

Yonkers KA, Massion A, Warshaw M et al. (1996) Phenomenology and course of generalized anxiety disorder. *Br J Psychiatr* 168, 308–313.

54 Somatoform Disorders

Definition

The somatoform disorders are a major diagnostic class in the *Diagnostic and Statistical Manual of Mental Disorders*, Fourth Edition, Text Revision (DSM-IV-TR) (American Psychiatric Association, 2000) that groups together conditions characterized by physical symptoms suggestive of but not fully explained by a general medical condition or the direct effects of a substance. In this class, symptoms are not intentionally produced and are not attributable to another mental disorder. To warrant a diagnosis, symptoms must be clinically significant in terms of causing distress or impairment in important areas of functioning. As summarized in Table 54.1, the disorders included in this class are somatization disorder, undifferentiated somatoform disorder, conversion disorder, pain disorder, hypochondriasis, body dysmorphic disorder and somatoform disorder not otherwise specified (NOS).

The somatoform disorders class was created for clinical utility, not on the basis of an assumed common etiology or mechanism. In DSM-IV-TR terms, it was designed to facilitate the differential diagnosis of conditions in which the first diagnostic concern is the need to "exclude occult general medical conditions or substance-induced etiologies for the bodily symptoms". As shown in Figure 54.1, only after such explanations are reasonably excluded should somatoform disorders be considered.

Many criticisms of the somatoform disorder category have been raised and they include contentions that because the category is delineated on the basis of presenting symptoms, it is "superficial"; that the individual disorders are not qualitatively distinct from one another or from "normality" and hence would be better described dimensionally rather than differentiated categorically; that the disorders are derived from hospital rather than community- or primary care-based populations; and, perhaps the most serious challenge, that the grouping "gives the spurious impression of understanding". On the other hand, proponents maintain that the somatoform grouping represents a major advance over previous systems and that segregation of such disorders into a class has helped clarify the conceptualization of the "mind–body" distinction, promoted greater consistency in terminology, and led to better descriptive distinctions between specific disorders. Supporters contend that maintaining this diagnostic class will foster more generalizable and thereby more clinically applicable research.

The somatoform disorder concept should be distinguished from traditional concepts of "psychosomatic illness" and "somatization". The psychosomatic illnesses involved structural or physiological changes hypothesized as deriving from psychological factors. In the DSM-IV somatoform disorders, such objective changes are generally not evident. The "classic" psychosomatic illnesses of Alexander (1950) included bronchial asthma, ulcerative colitis, thyrotoxicosis, essential hypertension, rheumatoid arthritis, neurodermatitis and peptic ulcer. In DSM-IV, most of these illnesses would be diagnosed as a general medical condition on Axis III, and in some cases with an additional designation of psychological factors affecting medical condition on Axis I. By definition, the diagnosis of "psychological factors affecting medical condition" is not a psychiatric disorder, but it is included in DSM-IV in the section for other conditions that may be a focus of clinical attention; it involves the presence of one or more specific psychological or behavioral factors that adversely affect a general medical condition.

The descriptive use of the term "somatization" in somatization disorder is not to be confused with theories that generally postulate a somatic expression of psychological distress. Empirical studies suggest that there is no single theory that can adequately explain somatization, which is not only multifactorially determined but is an exceedingly complex phenomenon. Furthermore, treatment strategies derived from somatization theories have not proven effective. For example, the postulation that patients with somatoform disorders are alexithymic, that is, are unable to process emotions and psychological conflicts verbally and therefore do so somatically, suggested that teaching such patients to "appreciate" and "verbalize" their emotions would circumvent the need to "somatize" them. Such treatment approaches have been ineffective.

Diagnosis and Differential Diagnosis

As shown in Figure 54.1, after it is determined that physical symptoms are not fully explained by a general medical condition or the direct effect of a substance, somatoform disorders must be differentiated from other mental conditions with physical symptoms.

In contrast to malingering and factitious disorder, symptoms in somatoform disorders are not under voluntary control, that is, they are not intentionally produced or feigned. Determination of intentionality may be difficult and must be inferred from the context in which symptoms present. Somatic symptoms may also be involved in disorders in other diagnostic classes. However, in such instances, the overriding focus is on the primary symptom complex (i.e., anxiety, mood, or psychotic symptoms) rather than the physical symptoms. In panic disorder and in generalized anxiety disorder, physical symptoms such as chest pain, shortness of breath, palpitations, sweating and tremulousness may occur. However, such somatic symptoms occur only in the context of fear or anxious foreboding. In general, there is a lack of a consistent physical focus. In mood disorders (particularly major depressive disorder) and in schizophrenia and other psychotic disorders, somatic preoccupations, fears, and even

Essentials of Psychiatry   Jerald Kay and Allan Tasman
© 2006 John Wiley & Sons, Ltd.

Table 54.1   DSM-IV Somatoform Disorders Criteria Indicating Changes from DSM-III-R*

DSM-IV Disorder	General Description	Temporal Requirements	Threshold for Diagnosis†	Exclusion Criteria‡
Somatization disorder	"A history of many physical complaints" ***Symptoms required: 4 pain, 2 nonpain gastrointestinal, 1 nonpain sexual or reproductive, and 1 pseudoneurological (conversion or dissociative)*** *No exclusive list of symptoms*	Onset "…before age 30 years" "…occur for a period of several years"	"…result in treatment being sought or significant impairment in social, occupational, or other important areas of functioning"	"…cannot be fully explained by a known GMC or the DES" or "…when there is a related GMC… complaints or… impairment is in excess of …expected" ***"…not intentionally produced or feigned"*** *No exclusion based on other mental disorder*
Undifferentiated somatoform disorder	"One or more physical complaints (e.g., fatigue, loss of appetite, gastrointestinal or urinary complaints)"	"…duration…at least 6 months"	***"…clinically significant distress or impairment in social, occupational, or other important areas of functioning"***	"…cannot be fully explained by a known GMC or the DES" or "… when there is a related GMC…complaints or…impairment is in excess of…expected" ***"…not intentionally produced or feigned"*** "…not better accounted for by another mental disorder"
Conversion disorder	***"One or more symptoms or deficits affecting voluntary motor or sensory function that suggest a neurological or other GMC"*** "Psychological factors judged…associated with the symptom…symptom is preceded by conflicts or other stressors" *Specify: "with motor symptom or deficit," "with sensory symptom or deficit," "with seizures or convulsions," or "with mixed presentation"*	No temporal requirements	***"…clinically significant distress or impairment in social, occupational, or other important areas of functioning or warrants medical evaluation"***	"…cannot be…fully explained by a GMC, or by the DES, or as a culturally sanctioned behavior or experience" "…not intentionally produced or feigned" "…not limited to pain or sexual dysfunction *… not exclusively… during the course of somatization disorder… not better accounted for by another mental disorder"*
Pain disorder	***"Pain in one or more anatomical sites is the predominant focus of the clinical presentation"*** *"Psychological factors …judged… important role in onset, severity, exacerbation, or maintenance of the pain"* *Code: "…with psychological factors," "…with both psychological factors and a GMC" ("…with a GMC" not a mental disorder)*	*"Specify if: acute: duration of less than 6 months"* or *"chronic: duration of 6 months or longer"*	***"…sufficient severity to warrant clinical attention"*** "… clinically significant distress or impairment in social, occupational, or other important areas of functioning"	"… not intentionally produced or feigned" ***"…not better accounted for by a mood, anxiety, or psychotic disorder …not… dyspareunia"***

Continues

Table 54.1   **DSM-IV Somatoform Disorders Criteria Indicating Changes from DSM-III-R*** *Continued*

DSM-IV Disorder	General Description	Temporal Requirements	Threshold for Diagnosis†	Exclusion Criteria‡
Hypochondriasis	"Preoccupation…fears of having, or…idea…one has, a serious disease based on…misinterpretation of bodily symptoms" "…persists despite appropriate medical evaluation and reassurance" **"Specify if: with poor insight"**	"…duration…at least 6 months"	**"…clinically significant distress or impairment in social, occupational, or other important areas of functioning"**	"…not of delusional intensity…***not restricted to a circumscribed concern about appearance***" "***…not better accounted for by generalized anxiety disorder, obsessive–compulsive disorder, panic disorder, a major depressive episode, separation anxiety, or another somatoform disorder***"
Body dysmorphic disorder	"Preoccupation with an imagined defect in appearance. If a slight physical anomaly… concern is markedly excessive"	No temporal requirements	**"…clinically significant distress or impairment in social, occupational, or other important areas of functioning"**	***No exclusion for delusional disorder, somatic type*** "…not better accounted for by another mental disorder (e.g.,…anorexia nervosa)"
Somatoform disorder not otherwise specified	"Disorders…somatoform symptoms…not meet criteria for any specific somatoform disorder" Examples: ***pseudocyesis***, nonpsychotic hypochondriacal symptoms, unexplained physical complaints	Less than 6 months in duration (except for ***pseudocyesis***)		"…not meet criteria for any specific somatoform disorder"

*Actual DSM-IV criteria wording is in quotation marks. Criteria substantively changed from DSM-III-R are in boldface and italicized. GMC, General medical condition, DES, direct effects of a substance. Although not specified in the criteria for each the DSM-IV text specifies that for all somatoform disorders:

†"the symptoms must cause clinically significant distress or impairment in social, occupational, or other areas of functioning;"

‡"the physical symptoms are not intentional (i.e., under voluntary control)," and "there is no diagnosable GMC to fully account for the physical symptoms."

Source: Reprinted from Martin RL (1995) DSM-IV changes for the somatoform disorders. Psychiatr Ann 25, 29–39, copyright 1995 Slack Publications.

delusions and false perceptions may be evident. In the mood disorders, these are generally mood congruent (e.g., "I'm so worthless not even my organs work anymore"), whereas in the psychoses, bizarre and mood-incongruent beliefs are typical (e.g., "Half of my brain was removed by psychic neurosurgery").

Differentiation Among the Various Somatoform Disorders

Whereas it is assumed that the specific disorders in the somatoform grouping are heterogeneous in terms of pathogenesis and pathophysiology, they are also phenomenologically diverse. In somatization disorder, undifferentiated somatoform disorder, conversion disorder and pain disorder, the focus is on the physical complaints themselves, and thus on perceptions. In hypochondriasis and body dysmorphic disorder, emphasis is on physically related preoccupations or fears, and thus on cognitions. Somatization disorder and, to a lesser extent, undifferentiated somatoform disorder are characterized by multiple symptoms of different types; conversion disorder, pain disorder, hypochondriasis and body dysmorphic disorder are defined on the basis of a single symptom or a few symptoms of a certain type (see Figure 54.1). Whereas somatization disorder, undifferentiated somatoform disorder and hypochondriasis are, by definition, at least 6 months in duration, conversion disorder, pain disorder, body dysmorphic disorder and somatoform disorder NOS may be of short duration as long as they are associated with clinically significant distress or impairment.

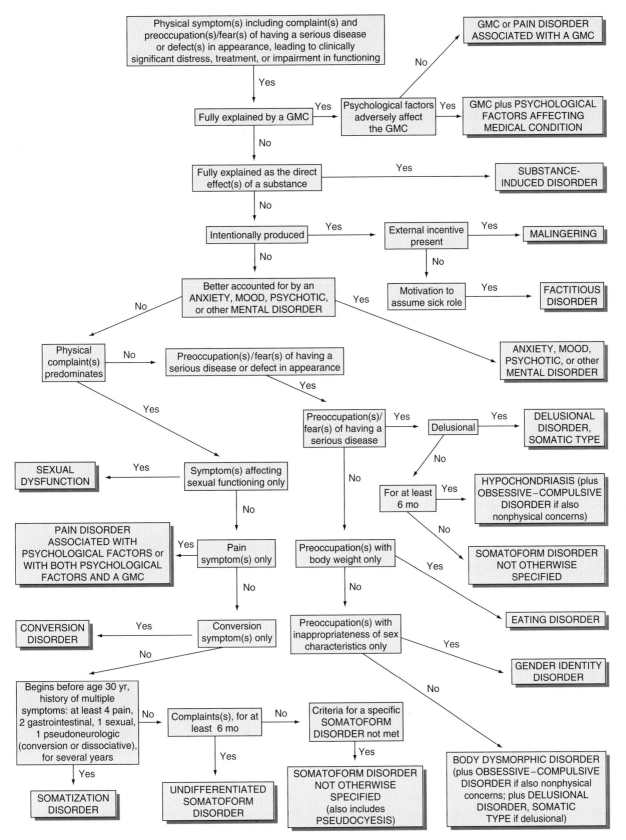

Figure 54.1 *Somatic symptom diagnostic exploration and treatment algorithm. Differential diagnosis of clinically significant physical symptoms. Shadowed boxes represent diagnostic categories; GMC, General medical condition.*

Epidemiology

In view of the vicissitudes of diagnostic approaches and the recency of the current somatoform disorder grouping, it is not surprising that estimates of the frequency of this group of disorders in the general population as well as in clinical settings are inconsistent if not nonexistent. Yet, existing data seem to indicate that such problems are indeed common and account for a major proportion of clinical services, especially in primary care settings.

Table 54.2 summarizes what is known about the epidemiology of these disorders.

In consideration of the substantial frequency of somatoform disorders in nonpsychiatric settings, instruments have been designed to aid primary care physicians in diagnosing psychiatric conditions. The Primary Care Evaluation of Mental Disorders (PRIME-MD) (Spitzer *et al.*, 1994) includes somatoform items in its screening questionnaire and in its physician education guide. The DSM-IV Primary Care Edition (DSM-IV-PC) includes an "unexplained physical symptoms" algorithm among the nine it included to address the most common psychiatric symptom groups presenting in primary care settings (American Psychiatric Association, 1995).

Table 54.2   Epidemiology and Natural History of the Somatoform Disorders

Somatoform Disorder	Prevalence and Incidence	Age at Onset	Course and Progress
Somatization disorder	US women 0.2–2%; women/men = 10:1	First symptoms by adolescence, full criteria met by mid-20s, not after 30 yr by definition	Chronic with fluctuations in severity Most active in early adulthood Full remissions rare
Undifferentiated somatoform disorder	"Abridged somatization disorder" type estimated as 11–15% of US adults, 20% in Puerto Rico Preponderance of women in US but not Puerto Rico	Variable	Variable conversion disorder
Conversion disorder	Conversion symptoms common, as high as 25% Treated conversion symptoms: 11–500 per 100 000 5–14% of general hospital admissions 5–24% of psychiatric outpatients 1–3% of psychiatric outpatient referrals 4% of neurological outpatient referrals 1% of neurological admissions	Late childhood to early adulthood, most before age 35 yr medical neurological or general If onset in middle or late life, condition more likely	Individual conversion symptoms generally remit within days to weeks Relapse within 1 yr in 20–25%
Pain disorder	10–15% of US adults with work disability owing to back pain yearly more A predominant symptom in hospital admissions than half of general psychiatric Present in as many as 38% of psychiatric outpatients admissions, 18%	Any age	Good if less than 6 mo in duration disorder Unemployment, personality drugs habituation to addictive compensation, and potential for prognosis associated with poorer
Hypochondriasis	Perhaps 4–9% in general medical settings, but unclear whether full syndrome criteria are met Equal in both sexes	Early adulthood typical	10% recovery, two-thirds a chronic but fluctuating course, 25% do poorly absence Better prognosis if acute onset, secondary gain disorder, absence of personality
Body dysmorphic disorder	Not routinely screened for in psychiatric or general population studies corrective Perhaps 2% of patients seeking cosmetic surgery	Adolescence or early adulthood Perhaps in women at menopause	Generally chronic, fluctuating severity perceived In a lifetime, multiple defects Incapacitating: one-third housebound
Somatoform disorder NOS	Unknown	Variable	Variable

The epidemiology of the specific somatoform disorders is discussed individually in following sections.

Treatment

Whereas specific somatoform disorders indicate specific treatment approaches, some general guidelines apply to the somatoform disorders as a whole (Figure 54.2 and Table 54.2). Therapeutic goals include 1) as an overriding goal, prevention of the adoption of the sick role and chronic invalidism; 2) minimization of unnecessary costs and complications by avoiding unwarranted hospitalizations, diagnostic and treatment procedures, and medications (especially those of an addictive potential); and 3) effective treatment of comorbid psychiatric disorders, such as depressive and anxiety syndromes. The three general treatment strategies include 1) consistent treatment, generally by the same physician, with careful coordination if multiple physicians are involved; 2) supportive office visits, scheduled at regular intervals rather than in response to symptoms; and 3) a gradual shift in focus from symptoms to an emphasis on personal and interpersonal problems.

Somatization Disorder

Definition

As defined in DSM-IV, somatization disorder is a polysymptomatic somatoform disorder characterized by multiple recurring pains and gastrointestinal, sexual and pseudoneurological symptoms occurring for a period of years with onset before age 30 years. The physical complaints are not intentionally produced and are not fully explained by a general medical condition or the direct effects of a substance. To warrant diagnosis, they must result in medical attention or significant impairment in social, occupational, or other important areas of functioning. Table 54.1 summarizes the criteria for this disorder.

Despite efforts to simplify it, the somatization disorder construct has remained somewhat cumbersome.

It remains to be seen whether the DSM-IV diagnosis of somatization disorder will be used broadly and appropriately. Unresolved problems include that the term somatization disorder has acquired a pejorative connotation; a tendency to diagnose more readily treatable symptoms such as anxiety and depressive syndromes without considering the underlying illness; and that authorization and reimbursement for treatment of this chronic condition are often challenged or denied. It is relatively easier to obtain approval for an intervention on the basis of major depressive disorder, for example, than on the basis of a disorder that is much more likely to be poorly understood by case reviewers.

Epidemiology

In the USA, somatization disorder is found predominantly in women, with a female/male ratio of approximately 10:1 (see Table 54.1). This ratio is not as large in some other cultures (e.g., in Greeks and Puerto Ricans). Thus, gender- and culture-specific rates are more meaningful than generalized figures. The lifetime prevalence of somatization disorder in US women has been estimated to be between 0.2 and 2%. The magnitude of this discrepancy is attributable, at least in part, to methodological differences. The Epidemiological Catchment Area study (Robins *et al.*, 1984), the most recent large-scale general population study in the USA to include an assessment for somatization disorder, found a lifetime risk of somatization disorder of only 0.2 to 0.3% in US women. However, this study may have underestimated the prevalence of somatization disorder because nonphysician interviewers were used. It is argued that it is difficult for lay interviewers critically to assess whether somatic symptoms are fully explained by physical conditions. As a result, they may more readily accept patients' general medical explanations of symptoms, resulting in fewer diagnoses of somatization disorder. With age and method of assessment taken into account, the lifetime risk for somatization disorder was estimated to be 2% in US women.

Etiology and Pathophysiology

Many theories on the cause of somatization disorder have been proposed, however, the etiology remains unknown. Psychodynamic hypotheses regarding the physical expression of unconscious conflict by conversion or somatization have been influential. Even Freud assumed a "constitutional diathesis", as had Charcot before him. Evidence exists for both biological and psychosocial contributions.

Somatization disorder has been shown to be familial. It is observed that in 10 to 20% of female relatives of patients affected by somatization disorder there is a lifetime risk in US women 10 to 20 times greater than that of the general population. Yet, aggregation in families may be attributable to both genetic and environmental factors. A cross-fostering study of a Swedish population demonstrated that genetic background and postnatal influences contribute to the risk of somatization disorder independently (Bohman *et al.*, 1984). Of additional interest are observations that male relatives of patients with somatization disorder show increased rates of antisocial personality and alcoholism, suggesting an etiological link.

Certain promising theories have focused on learning principles with possible organic underpinnings. Some have postulated a social communication model based on learning theory to explain somatization disorder. This theory hypothesizes that individuals learn to somatize as a means of expressing their wants and needs and evoking care, nurturance and support from family and caregivers. That different sex ratios may exist in different cultures suggests that such learning differs from culture to culture.

In the 1970s, impaired information-processing problems involving attention and memory were identified in experimental neuropsychological testing. Such deficits may result in vague, nonspecific and impressionistic description for experience. These may underlie a tendency for excessive somatic complaints and, together with tendencies for impulsiveness and monotony intolerance, may contribute to the often associated multiple personal and social problems. Early studies also reported that the pattern of neuropsychological defects found in subjects with somatization disorder differed from that in normal control, schizophrenic and psychotic depression comparison groups. Subjects with somatization disorder had greater bilateral, symmetrical patterns of frontal lobe dysfunction in comparison with normal control subjects and greater dominant hemisphere impairment than control and depressive subjects. Nondominant hemisphere dysfunction was also identified, with greater impairment in the anterior as opposed to posterior regions. However, subjects with somatization disorder had less nondominant hemisphere disorganization than schizophrenic subjects. Of interest, these findings were similar to findings in male patients with antisocial personality disorder, giving further support to an etiological link with this disorder.

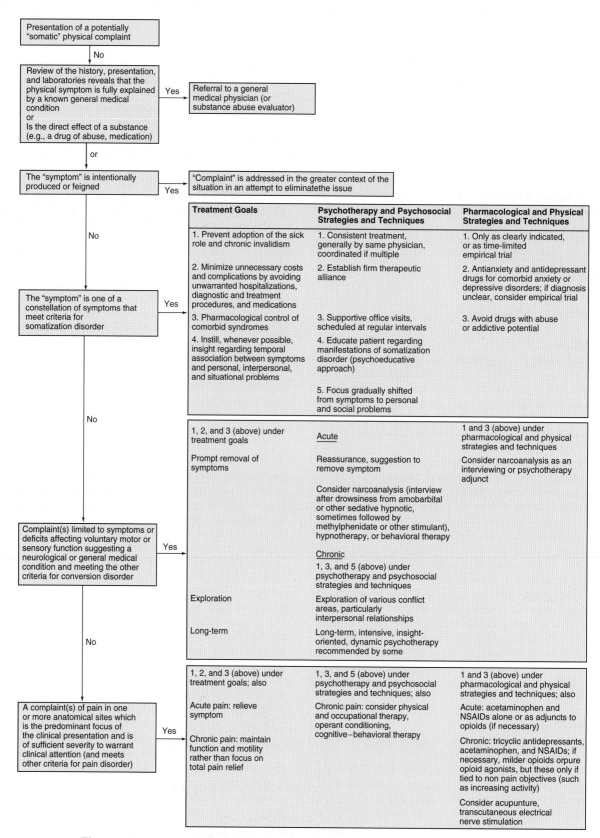

Figure 54.2   *Diagnostic decision tree and treatment algorithm for Somatoform Disorders.*

Diagnosis and Differential Diagnosis

As defined in DSM-IV, somatization disorder is characterized by multiple recurring physical symptoms and, as will be described, often multiple psychiatric complaints. Thus, it is not surprising that somatization disorder may present in a manner suggestive of multiple general medical and, although too often forgotten, psychiatric disorders (Table 54.3). Indeed, it can be said that an essential aspect of somatization disorder is its simulation of other syndromes. As described by Preskorn (1995), "Somatization disorder is fundamentally a syndrome of apparent syndromes" (see Table 54.4). Thus, the first task in the diagnosis of somatization disorder is the exclusion of other suggested medical and psychiatric conditions.

To help in this, Cloninger (1986) identified three features that generally characterize somatization disorder but rarely general medical disorders and these are described in Table 54.5. Another way of characterizing the distinction is the "reverse funnel effect". With most general medical conditions, the process of investigation "funnels down" to fewer and fewer specific diagnostic possibilities; in somatization disorder, the more extensive the investigation, the greater the number of suggested disorders.

Several general medical disorders may also fit this pattern and may be confused with somatization disorder. These include multiple sclerosis, other neuropathies, systemic lupus erythematosus, acute intermittent porphyria, other hepatic and hematopoietic porphyrias, hypercalcemia, certain chronic systemic

Table 54.3	Treatment of DSM-IV-TR Somatoform Disorders		
Somatoform Disorder	Treatment Goals	Psychotherapy and Psychosocial Strategies and Techniques	Pharmacological and Physical Strategies and Techniques*
Somatoform disorders, as a group	1. Prevent adoption of the sick role and chronic invalidism 2. Minimize unnecessary costs and complications by avoiding unwarranted hospitalizations, diagnostic and treatment procedures, and medications 3. Pharmacological control of comorbid syndromes	1. Consistent treatment, generally by same physician, coordinated if multiple 2. Supportive office visits, scheduled at regular intervals 3. Focus gradually shifted from symptoms to personal and social problems	1. Only as clearly indicated, or as time-limited empirical trial 2. Avoid drugs with abuse or addictive potential
Somatization disorder	1, 2 and 3; also • Instill, whenever possible, insight regarding temporal association between symptoms and personal, interpersonal, and situational problems	1, 2 and 3; also • Establish firm therapeutic alliance • Educate patient regarding manifestations of somatization disorder (psychoeducative approach) • Consistent reassurance	1 and 2, also • Antianxiety and antidepressant drugs for comorbid anxiety or depressive disorders; if diagnosis unclear, consider empirical trial
Undifferentiated somatoform disorder	1, 2 and 3	1, 2 and 3	1 and 2
Conversion disorder	1, 2 and 3; also • Prompt removal of symptoms	Acute: • Reassurance, suggestion to remove symptom • Consider narcoanalysis (interview after drowsiness from amobarbital or other sedative–hypnotic, sometimes followed by methylphenidate or other stimulant), hypnotherapy, or behavioral therapy Chronic: 1, 2 and 3 • Exploration of various conflict areas, particularly interpersonal relationships • Long-term, intensive, insight-oriented dynamic psychotherapy recommended by some	1 and 2; also • Consider narcoanalysis as an interviewing or psychotherapy adjunct

Continues

Table 54.3   Treatment of DSM-IV-TR Somatoform Disorders *Continued*

Somatoform Disorder	Treatment Goals	Psychotherapy and Psychosocial Strategies and Techniques	Pharmacological and Physical Strategies and Techniques*
Pain disorder	1, 2 and 3; also • Acute pain: Relieve symptom • Chronic pain: Maintain function and motility rather than focus on total pain relief	1, 2 and 3; also • Chronic pain: Consider physical and occupational therapy, operant conditioning, cognitive–behavioral therapy	1 and 2; also • Acute: Acetaminophen and NSAIDs alone or as adjuncts to opioids (if necessary) • Chronic: Tricyclic antidepressants, acetaminophen, and NSAIDs; if necessary, milder opioids or pure opioid agonists, but these only if tied to nonpain objectives (such as increasing activity) • Consider acupuncture, transcutaneous electrical nerve stimulation
Hypochondriasis	1, 2 and 3; also • Pharmacological control of central syndrome itself	1, 2 and 3; also • Cognitive–behavioral therapy involving prevention of checking rituals and reassurance seeking	2; also • Attempt to decrease hypochondriacal symptoms with SSRIs at higher than antidepressant doses or clomipramine
Body dysmorphic disorder	1, 2 and 3, especially avoiding corrective surgery; also • Pharmacological control of central syndrome itself	1, 2 and 3; also • Cognitive–behavioral therapy involving prevention of checking rituals and reassurance seeking	2; also • Attempt to decrease hypochondriacal symptoms with SSRIs at higher than antidepressant doses or clomipramine
Somatoform disorder NOS	1, 2 and 3; also • Evaluate carefully for alternative general medical or other psychiatric disorder to which the symptoms can be attributed	1, 2 and 3	1 and 2

*NSAIDs, Nonsteroidal antiinflammatory drugs; SSRIs, selective serotonin reuptake inhibitors.

infections such as brucellosis and trypanosomiasis, myopathies and vasculitides. In general, such conditions begin with disseminated, nonspecific subjective symptoms and transient or equivocal physical signs or laboratory abnormalities.

Somatization disorder is characterized by excessive psychiatric as well as physical complaints. Thus, other psychiatric disorders, including anxiety and mood disorders and schizophrenia, may be suggested. Although no specific exclusion criteria regarding other psychiatric disorders are given, one must be careful in accepting "comorbidity" and critically evaluate whether suggested syndromes are truly additional syndromes or simply manifestations of somatization disorder.

The overlap between somatization disorder and anxiety disorders may be a particular problem. Patients with somatization disorder frequently complain of many of the same somatic symptoms as patients with anxiety disorders, such as increased muscle tension, features of autonomic hyperactivity and even discrete panic attacks. Likewise, anxiety disorder patients may

report irrational disease concerns and such somatic complaints as those involving gastrointestinal function that are commonly seen in somatization disorder. However, patients with anxiety disorders neither typically report sexual and menstrual complaints or conversion or dissociative symptoms as in somatization disorder, nor do they have the associated histrionic presentation and personal, marital and social maladjustment common in patients with somatization disorder.

It must be remembered that an anxiety disorder may be comorbid with somatization disorder. Here, objective observation of the patient rather than reliance on the patient's report may facilitate an additional diagnosis. For example, patients with somatization disorder may report that they are presently overwhelmed by anxiety while speaking calmly or even cheerfully about their symptoms, or they may be redirectable while in the midst of a reported panic attack.

Mood disorders (in particular depression) frequently present with multiple somatic complaints, especially in cer-

Table 54.4   Somatoform Disorders: A Syndrome of Simulated Syndromes

Symptom Examples	Examples of Simulated Neurological Conditions	Examples of Simulated Nonneurological General Medical Conditions	Examples of Simulated Psychiatric Conditions
Symptoms* of somatization disorder			
Pain			
Headache	Migraine	Temporal arteritis	Pain disorder
Abdomen	"Abdominal epilepsy"	Peptic ulcer disease	Pain disorder
Back	Lumbosacral radiculopathy	Ruptured disk	Pain disorder
Joints or extremities		Fibromyalgia	Pain disorder
Chest		Angina	Panic disorder
Menstruation, intercourse		Endometriosis	Dyspareunia, vaginismus
Urination	Neurogenic bladder	Urinary tract infection	
Gastrointestinal (nonpain)			
Difficulty swallowing	Myasthenia gravis	Esophageal motility disorder	Eating disorder
Nausea	Raised intracranial pressure	Meniere's disease	Eating disorder
Bloating		Galactase deficiency	Eating disorder
Vomiting (nonpregnancy)	Raised intracranial pressure		Eating disorder
Diarrhea		Irritable bowel syndrome	Eating disorder
Intolerance to several foods		Food allergy	Eating disorder
Sexual (nonpain)			
Loss of interest			Major depressive episode
Erectile–ejaculatory dysfunction	Diabetic neuropathy	Antihypertensive drug effect	
Menorrhagia		Leiomyofibroma	
Vomiting throughout pregnancy		Preeclampsia, eclampsia	
Pseudoneurological			
Conversion			
Sensory	Stroke (hemianesthesia)		Schizophrenia/(hallucinations)
Motor	Huntington's disease	Myopathy	Catatonia
Seizures	Epilepsy	Electrolyte imbalance	Catatonia
Mixed	Multiple sclerosis	Electrolyte imbalance	Catatonia
Dissociative			
Amnesia	Amnestic disorder	Anticholinergic drug effects	Dissociative identity disorder
Loss of consciousness (nonfainting)	Coma	Metabolic encephalopathy	Catatonia
Symptoms* often associated with somatization disorder			
Anxiety, panic		Pheochromocytoma	Generalized anxiety and panic disorders
Dysphoria, affective lability	Frontal lobe syndrome	Endocrinopathy	Major mood disorders
Cluster B personality features	Frontal lobe syndrome	Acute intermittent porphyria	Brief psychotic disorder

*All of these symptoms may be reported by patients with somatization disorder, without the clinical consistency and pathological findings to support the diagnosis of neurological, general medical, or psychiatric conditions separate from somatization disorder.

Developed in conjunction with Sheldon H. Preskorn.

tain cultures such as in India, where somatic but not mental complaints are acceptable. A longitudinal history identifying age at onset and course of illness may facilitate discrimination of a mood disorder from somatization disorder. In mood disorders, the age at onset of the somatic symptoms is generally later than in somatization disorder; their first appearance generally correlates discretely with the onset of mood symptoms, and a lengthy pattern of multiple recurring somatic complaints is not seen. Also, resolution of the underlying mood disorder will generally result in disappearance of the somatic complaints.

From the other perspective, patients with somatization disorder often present with depressive complaints. In somatization disorder, a thorough investigation will reveal a multitude of somatic as well as "depressive" symptoms. Interestingly, somatization disorder patients complaining of depression have been found to proffer greater depressive symptoms than individuals with major depression. As in anxiety disorders, major depressive

Table 54.5 *Discrimination of Somatization Disorder from General Medical Conditions*

Features Suggesting Somatization Disorder	Features Suggesting a General Medical Condition
Involvement of multiple organ systems	Involvement of single or few organ systems
Early onset and chronic course without development of physical signs or structural abnormalities	If early onset and chronic course, development of physical signs and structural abnormalities
Absence of laboratory abnormalities characteristic of the suggested general medical condition	Laboratory abnormalities evident

Reprinted with permission from The American Psychiatric Press Textbook of Psychiatry, 2nd ed., Hales RE, Yudofsky SC, and Talbott JA (eds), p. 600. Copyright 1994, American Psychiatric Press, Washington DC.

episodes may occur in patients with somatization disorder and must be differentiated from the tendency to have multiple complaints, which is characteristic of somatization disorder. As with anxiety disorders, in considering comorbidity with a depressive disorder, the patient's reports should be corroborated by collateral information or by direct observation. Thus, the veracity of the self-report of overwhelming depression and suicidal ideation should be doubted if the patient appears cheerful and charming, at least at times, when interviewed, or if the patient is reported to be actively involved in social activities on an inpatient psychiatric service.

Schizophrenia may present with generally single but occasionally multiple unexplained somatic complaints. Interview usually uncovers psychotic symptoms such as delusions, hallucinations, or disorganized thought. In some cases, the underlying psychosis cannot be identified initially but, in time, schizophrenia will become manifest. Hallucinations are included as examples of conversion symptoms in DSM-IV. As discussed in the conversion disorder section, careful analysis of this symptom is warranted so that a misdiagnosis is not made, relegating a patient to long-term neuroleptic treatment on the basis of conversion hallucinations.

Patients with histrionic, borderline and antisocial personality disorders frequently have an excess of somatic complaints, at times presenting with somatization disorder. Antisocial personality disorder and somatization disorder cluster in individuals and within families and may share common causes. Dissociative phenomena, in particular dissociative identity disorder, are commonly associated with somatization disorder. Because dissociative symptoms are included in the diagnostic criteria for somatization, a separate diagnosis of a dissociative disorder is not made if such symptoms occur only in the course of somatization disorder.

Unlike in hypochondriasis and body dysmorphic disorder, in which preoccupations and fears concerning the interpretation of symptoms predominate, the focus in somatization disorder is on the physical complaints themselves. Unlike in pain disorder and conversion disorder, multiple complaints of different types are reported; by definition in DSM-IV, the history is of pain in at least four sites or functions (e.g., pain with intercourse, pain in swallowing), at least two nonpain gastrointestinal symptoms, at least one nonpain sexual or reproductive symptom, and at least one conversion or dissociative (i.e., pseudoneurological) symptom.

Whereas criteria require the onset of symptoms before the age of 30 years, most patients will have had some symptoms at least by adolescence or early adulthood. Symptoms are often described in a dramatic yet imprecise way and may be reported inconsistently from interview to interview. The medical history is usually complicated with multiple medical investigations, procedures and medication trials. If there have been symptoms for at least 6 months but the onset is later than at age 30 years, or if the required number and distribution of symptoms are not evident, undifferentiated somatoform disorder is diagnosed. If the duration has been less than 6 months, somatoform disorder NOS applies. In general, the greater the number and diversity of symptoms, and the longer they have been present without development of signs of an underlying general medical condition, the greater can be the confidence that a diagnosis of somatization disorder is correct.

Course, Natural History and Prognosis

Somatization disorder is rare in children younger than 9 years of age. Characteristic symptoms of somatization disorder usually begin during adolescence, and the criteria are met by the mid-twenties. Somatization disorder is a chronic illness characterized by fluctuations in the frequency and diversity of symptoms. Full remissions occur rarely, if ever. Whereas the most active symptomatic phase is in early adulthood, aging does not appear to lead to total remission. Pribor and colleagues (1994) found that women with somatization disorder older than 55 years did not differ from younger somatization patients in the number of somatic symptoms. Longitudinal follow-up studies have confirmed that 80 to 90% of patients initially diagnosed with somatization disorder will maintain a consistent clinical picture and be rediagnosed similarly after 6 to 8 years. Women with somatization disorder seen in psychiatric settings are at increased risk for attempted suicide, although such attempts are usually unsuccessful and may reflect manipulative gestures more than intent to die. It is not clear whether such risk is true for patients with somatization disorder seen only in general medical settings.

Treatment

First, a "management" rather than a "curative" strategy is recommended for somatization disorder. With the current absence of an identified definitive treatment, a modest, practical, empirical approach should be taken. This should include efforts to minimize distress and functional impairments associated with the multiple somatic complaints; to avoid unwarranted diagnostic and therapeutic procedures and medications; and to prevent potential complications including chronic invalidism and drug dependence.

In such regard, the general recommendations outlined for somatoform disorders should be followed (see Table 54.3). The patient should be encouraged to see a single physician with an understanding of and, preferably, experience in treating somatization disorder. This helps limit the number of unnecessary evaluations and treatments. Most clinicians advocate routine, brief, supportive office visits scheduled at regular intervals to provide reassurance and prevent patients from "needing to develop" symptoms to obtain care and attention. This "medical" management can well be provided by a primary care physician, perhaps with consultation with a psychiatrist. The study by Smith and colleagues (1986) demonstrated that such a regimen led to markedly decreased health care costs, with no apparent decrements in health or satisfaction of patients.

The foundations of treatment for this disorder are: 1) establishment of a strong physician–patient relationship or bond; 2) education of the patient regarding the nature of the psychiatric condition; and 3) provision of support and reassurance.

The first component, establishing a strong therapeutic bond, is important in the treatment of somatization disorder. Without it, it will be difficult for the patient to overcome skepticism deriving from past experience with many physicians and other therapists who "never seemed to help". In addition, trust must be strong enough to withstand the stress of withholding unwarranted diagnostic and therapeutic procedures that the patient may feel are indicated. The cornerstone of establishing a therapeutic relationship is laid when the psychiatrist indicates an understanding of the patient's pain and suffering, legitimizing the symptoms as real. This demonstrates a willingness to provide direct compassionate assistance. A full investigation of the medical and psychosocial histories, including extensive record review, will illustrate to patients the willingness of the psychiatrist to gain the fullest understanding of them and their plight. This also provides another opportunity to evaluate for the presence of an underlying medical disorder and to obtain a fuller picture of psychosocial difficulties that may relate temporally to somatic symptoms.

Only after the diagnosis has been clearly established and the therapeutic alliance is firmly in place can the psychiatrist confidently limit diagnostic evaluations and therapies to those performed on the basis of objective findings as opposed to merely subjective complaints. Of course, the psychiatrist should remain aware that patients with somatization disorder are still at risk for development of general medical illnesses so that a vigilant perspective should always be maintained.

The second component is education. This involves advising patients that they suffer from a "medically sanctioned illness", that is, a condition recognized by the medical community and one about which a good deal is known. Ultimately, it may be possible to introduce the concept of somatization disorder, which can be described in a positive light (i.e., the patient does not have a progressive, deteriorating, or potentially fatal medical disorder, and the patient is not "going crazy" but has a condition by which many symptoms will be experienced). A realistic discussion of prognosis and treatment options can then follow.

The third component is reassurance. Patients with somatization disorder often have control and insecurity issues, which often come to the forefront when they perceive that a particular physical complaint is not being adequately addressed. Explicit reassurance should be given that the appropriate inquiries and investigations are being performed and that the possibility of an underlying physical disorder as the explanation for symptoms is being reasonably considered.

In time, it may be appropriate gradually to shift emphasis away from somatic symptoms to consideration of personal and interpersonal issues. In some patients, it may be appropriate to posit a causal theory between somatic symptoms and "stress", that is, that there may be a temporal association between symptoms and personal, interpersonal and even occupational problems. In patients for whom such "insight" is difficult, behavioral techniques may be useful.

Even following such therapeutic guidelines, patients with somatization disorder are often difficult to treat. Attention-seeking behavior, demands and manipulation are common, necessitating firm limits and careful attention to boundary issues. This, again, is a management rather than a curative approach. Thus, such behaviors should generally be dealt with directively rather than interpreted to the patient.

Pharmacological and Other Somatic Treatments

No effective somatic treatments for somatization disorder itself have been identified.

Patients with somatization disorder may complain of anxiety and depression, suggesting readily treatable comorbid psychiatric disorders. As previously discussed, it is often difficult to distinguish actual comorbid conditions from aspects of somatoform disorder itself. Pharmacological interventions are likely to be helpful in the former but not in the latter. At times, such discrimination will be impossible, and an empirical trial of such treatments may be indicated. Patients with somatization disorder are often inconsistent and erratic in their use of medications. They will often report unusual side effects that may not be explained pharmacologically. This makes evaluation of treatment response difficult. In addition, drug dependence and suicide gestures and attempts are not uncommon.

Undifferentiated Somatoform Disorder

Definition

As defined in DSM-IV, this category includes disturbances of at least 6 months' duration, with one or more unintentional, clinically significant, medically unexplained physical complaints (see Table 54.1). In a sense, it is a residual category, subsuming syndromes with somatic complaints that do not meet criteria for any of the "differentiated" somatoform disorders yet are not better accounted for by any other mental disorder. On the other hand, it is a less residual category than somatoform disorder NOS, in that the disturbance must last at least 6 months (see Figure 54.1). Virtually any unintentional, medically unexplained physical symptoms causing clinically significant distress or impairment can be considered. In effect, this category serves to capture syndromes that resemble somatization disorder but do not meet full criteria.

Epidemiology

Some have argued that undifferentiated somatoform disorder is the most common somatoform disorder. Escobar and coworkers (1991), using an abridged somatization disorder construct requiring six somatic symptoms for women and four for men, reported that 11% of nonHispanic US whites and Hispanics, 15% of US blacks and 20% of Puerto Ricans in Puerto Rico fulfilled criteria. A preponderance of women was evident in all groups except the Puerto Rican sample (see Table 54.1). According to Escobar, such an abridged somatoform syndrome is 100 times more prevalent than a full somatoform syndrome.

Diagnosis and Differential Diagnosis

In comparison to when the full criteria for the well-validated somatization disorder are met, exclusion of an as yet undiscovered general medical or substance-induced explanation for physical symptoms is far less certain when the less stringent criteria for undifferentiated somatoform disorder are met. Thus, the diagnosis of undifferentiated somatoform disorder should remain tentative, and new symptoms should be carefully investigated.

Because undifferentiated somatoform disorder represents somewhat of a residual category, the major diagnostic process, once occult general medical conditions and substance-induced explanations have been considered, is one of exclusion. As shown in Figure 54.1, whether the somatic symptoms are intentionally produced as in malingering and factitious disorder must be addressed. Here, motivation for external rewards (for malingering) and a pervasive intent to assume the sick role (for factitious disorder) must be assessed. The next consideration is whether the somatic symptoms are the manifestation of another psychiatric disorder. Anxiety and mood disorders commonly present with somatic symptoms; high rates of anxiety and major depressive disorders are reported in patients with somatic complaints attending family medicine clinics. Of course, undifferentiated somatoform disorder could be diagnosed in addition to one of these disorders, so long as the symptoms are not accounted for by the other psychiatric disorder. Crucial in this determination is whether the symptoms are present during periods in which the anxiety or mood disorders are not actively present.

Next, other somatoform disorders must be considered. In general, undifferentiated somatoform disorders are characterized by unexplained somatic complaints; the most common according to Escobar and coworkers (Escobar *et al.*, 1989) are female reproductive symptoms, excessive gas, abdominal pain, chest pain, joint pain, palpitations and fainting, rather than preoccupations or fears as in hypochondriasis or body dysmorphic disorder. However, a patient with some manifestations of these two disorders but not meeting full criteria could conceivably receive a diagnosis of undifferentiated somatoform disorder. An example is a patient with recurrent yet shifting hypochondriacal concerns that do respond to medical reassurance. If symptoms are restricted to those affecting the domains of sexual dysfunction, pain, or pseudoneurological symptoms, and the specific criteria for a sexual dysfunction, pain disorder and/or conversion disorder are met, the specific disorder or disorders should be diagnosed. If other types of symptoms or symptoms of more than one of these disorders have been present for at least 6 months, yet criteria for somatization disorder are not met, undifferentiated somatoform disorder should be diagnosed. By definition, undifferentiated somatoform disorder requires a duration of 6 months. If this criterion is not met, a diagnosis of somatoform disorder NOS should be considered.

Patients with an apparent undifferentiated somatoform disorder should be carefully evaluated for somatization disorder. Typically, patients with somatization disorder are inconsistent historians, at one evaluation reporting a large number of symptoms fulfilling criteria for the full syndrome, at another time endorsing fewer symptoms. In addition, with follow-up, additional symptoms may become evident, and criteria for somatization disorder will be satisfied. Patients with multiple somatic complaints not diagnosed with somatization disorder because of a reported onset later than 30 years of age may be inaccurately reporting a later age at onset. If the late age at onset is accurate, the patient should be carefully scrutinized for an occult general medical disorder.

In addition to the range of symptoms specified in the other somatoform disorders, patients complaining primarily of fatigue (chronic fatigue syndrome), bowel problems (irritable bowel syndrome), or multiple muscle aches/weakness (fibromyalgia) can be considered for undifferentiated somatoform disorder. Substantial controversy exists regarding the etiology of such syndromes. Even if an explanation on the basis of a known pathophysiological mechanism cannot be established, many argue that the syndromes should be considered general medical conditions. However, for the time being, these syndromes could be considered in a highly tentative manner under the undifferentiated somatoform disorder rubric. Careful reconsideration of the psychiatric label should be undertaken at regular intervals if the symptoms persist. The psychiatrist should remain ever vigilant to the emergence of another general medical or psychiatric condition. When patients are diagnosed with chronic fatigue syndrome, careful evaluation procedures are recommended.

Course, Natural History and Prognosis

As shown in Table 54.1, it appears that the course and prognosis of undifferentiated somatoform disorder are highly variable. This is not surprising, because the definition of this disorder allows a great deal of heterogeneity.

Treatment

In view of the broad inclusion and minimal exclusion criteria for undifferentiated somatoform disorder, it is difficult to make treatment recommendations beyond the generic guidelines outlined for the somatoform disorders in general. More definitive recommendations await a more extensive empirical database. A substantial proportion of patients with undifferentiated somatoform disorders improve or recover with no formal therapy. However, appropriate psychotherapy and pharmacological intervention may accelerate the process.

Some recommendations for patients with symptoms of headache, fibromyalgia, and chronic fatigue syndrome, conditions that some would include under undifferentiated somatoform disorder. Generally recommended are brief psychotherapy of a supportive and educative nature. As with somatization disorder, the physician–patient relationship is of great importance. Judicious use of pharmacotherapy may also be of benefit, particularly if the somatoform syndrome is intertwined with an anxiety or depressive syndrome. Here, usual antianxiety and antidepressant medications are recommended. Patients with unexplained pains may benefit from pain management strategies as outlined in the pain disorder section.

Conversion Disorder

Definition

As defined in DSM-IV, conversion disorders are characterized by symptoms or deficits affecting voluntary motor or sensory function that suggest yet are not fully explained by a neurological or other general medical condition or the direct effects of a substance (see Table 54.1). The diagnosis is not made if the presentation is explained as a culturally sanctioned behavior or experience, such as bizarre behaviors resembling a seizure during a religious ceremony. Symptoms are not intentionally produced or feigned, that is, the person does not consciously contrive a symptom for external rewards, as in malingering, or for the intrapsychic rewards of assuming the sick role, as in factitious disorder.

Four subtypes with specific examples of symptoms are defined: with motor symptom or deficit (e.g., impaired coordination or balance, paralysis or localized weakness, difficulty swallowing or lump in throat, aphonia and urinary retention); with sensory symptom or deficit (e.g., loss of touch or pain sensation, double vision, blindness, deafness and hallucinations); with seizures or convulsions; and with mixed presentation (i.e., has symptoms of more than one of the other subtypes). The list of examples is also contained among the pseudoneurological symptoms listed in the diagnostic criteria for somatization disorder. Although determination is highly subjective and of questionable reliability and validity, association with psychological factors is required.

Whereas conversion symptoms are among the most dramatic symptoms, somatization disorder is characterized by multiple unexplained symptoms in many organ systems; in conversion disorder, even a single symptom affecting voluntary motor or sensory function may suffice. Such nosological inconsistencies have resulted in a great deal of confusion, both in research and in clinical practice.

The relationship of conversion disorder to the dissociative disorders warrants comment. Long recognized as related, they were subsumed as subtypes of hysterical neurosis in DSM-II: conversion involving voluntary motor and sensory functioning, and dissociation affecting memory and identity. DSM-IV-TR text acknowledges the symptomatic, epidemiological and probable pathogenetic similarities between conversion and dissociative symptoms. Such symptoms have been attributed to similar psychological mechanisms, and they often occur in the same individual, sometimes during the same episode of illness. DSM-IV-TR does suggest that patients with conversion disorder be carefully scrutinized for dissociative symptoms.

Hallucinations are included among the sensory nervous symptoms in DSM-IV. The concept of conversion hallucinations has a long tradition and its inclusion as a conversion symptom was supported by the somatization disorder field trial, in which one-third of a large sample of nonpsychotic women with evidence of unexplained somatic complaints reported a history of hallucinations. Among the 40% who had symptoms that met criteria for somatization disorder, more than half reported hallucinations. Women with other conversion symptoms were more likely to report hallucinations than were those with no other conversion symptoms.

In general, conversion hallucinations (referred to by some as pseudohallucinations) differ in several ways from those in psychotic conditions. Conversion hallucinations typically occur in the absence of other psychotic symptoms, insight that the hallucinations are not real may be retained, and they often involve more than one sensory modality, whereas hallucinations in psychoses generally involve a single sensory modality, usually auditory. Conversion hallucinations also often have a naive, fantastic, or childish content, as if they are part of a fairy tale, and are described eagerly, sometimes even provocatively, as an interesting story (e.g., "I was driving downtown and a flying saucer flew over my car and I saw you [the psychiatrist] in a window and I heard your voice calling to me"). They often bear some understandable psychological purpose, although the patient may not be aware of intent. In the example given, the "sighting" was reported at the time that no further sessions were scheduled.

Epidemiology

Vastly different estimates of the incidence and prevalence of conversion disorder have been reported. Much of this difference may be attributable to methodological differences from study to study, including the changing definition of conversion disorder, ascertainment procedures and populations studied. General population estimates have generally been derived indirectly, extrapolating from clinic or hospital samples.

Conversion symptoms themselves may be common; it was reported that 25% of normal postpartum and medically ill women had a history of conversion symptoms at some time during their life (Cloninger, 1993), yet in some instances, there may have been no resulting clinically significant distress or impairment. Lifetime prevalence rates of treated conversion symptoms in general populations are much more modest, ranging from 11 to 500 per 100 000 (see Table 54.1). About 5 to 24% of psychiatric outpatients, 5 to 14% of general hospital patients and 1 to 3% of outpatient psychiatric referrals reported a history of conversion symptoms, although their current treatment was not necessarily for conversion symptoms. A rate of nearly 4% of outpatient neurological referrals and 1% of neurological admissions (Ziegler and Paul, 1954) involved conversion disorder. In virtually all studies, an excess (to the extent of 2:1 to 10:1) of women reported conversion symptoms relative to men. In part, this may relate to the simple fact that women seek medical evaluation more often than men do, but it is unlikely that this fully accounts for the sex difference. There is a predilection for lower socioeconomic status; less educated, less psychologically sophisticated and rural populations are overrepresented. Consistent with this, higher rates (nearly 10%) of outpatient psychiatric referrals are for conversion symptoms in "developing" countries. As countries develop, there may be a declining incidence in time, which may relate to increasing levels of education, and medical and psychological sophistication.

Etiology and Pathophysiology

The term conversion implies etiology because it is derived from a hypothesized mechanism of converting psychological conflicts into somatic symptoms, often symbolically (e.g., repressed rage is converted into paralysis of an arm that could be used to strike). A number of psychological factors have been promoted as part of such an etiological process, but evidence for their essential involvement is scanty at best. Theoretically, anxiety is reduced by keeping an internal conflict or need out of awareness by symbolic expression of an unconscious wish as a conversion symptom (primary gain). However, individuals with active conversion symptoms often continue to show marked anxiety, especially on psychological tests. Symbolism is infrequently evident, and its evaluation involves highly inferential and unreliable judgments. Overinterpretation of symbolism in persons with occult medical disorder may contribute to misdiagnosis. Secondary gain, whereby conversion symptoms allow avoidance of noxious activities or the procurement of otherwise unavailable support, may also occur in persons with medical conditions, who may take advantage of such benefits.

Individuals with conversion disorder may show a lack of concern out of keeping with the nature or implications of the symptom (the so-called **la belle indifférence**). However, indifference to symptoms is not invariably present in conversion disorder and is also seen in individuals with general medical conditions, on the basis of denial or stoicism. Conversion symptoms may present in a dramatic or histrionic fashion and may be highly suggestible. A dramatic presentation is also seen in distressed individuals with medical conditions. Even symptoms based on an underlying medical condition may respond to suggestion, at least temporarily. In many instances, preexisting personality disorders (in particular histrionic personality disorder) are evident and may predispose to conversion disorder. Persons with conversion disorder may often have a history of disturbed sexuality many (one-third) report a history of sexual abuse, especially incestuous.

If not directly etiological, many psychosocial factors have been suggested as predisposing to conversion disorder. At a minimum, many persons with conversion disorder are in chaotic domestic and occupational situations. As previously mentioned, individuals from rural backgrounds and those who are psychologically and medically unsophisticated appear to be predisposed, as are those with existing neurological disorders. In the last case, a tendency to conversion symptoms has been attributed to "modeling", that is, patients with neurological disorders are likely to have observed in others, as well as in themselves, various neurological symptoms, which they then may simulate as conversion symptoms.

Available data suggest a genetic contribution. Conversion symptoms are more frequent in relatives of individuals with conversion disorder. In a nonblinded study, rates of conversion disorder were found to be elevated tenfold in female (fivefold in male) relatives of patients with conversion disorder. Nongenetic familial factors, particularly incestuous childhood sexual abuse, may also be involved in some. Nearly one-third of individuals with medically unexplained seizures reported childhood sexual abuse, compared with less than 10% of those with complex partial epilepsy.

Diagnosis and Differential Diagnosis

As shown in Figure 54.1, the first consideration is whether the conversion symptoms are explained on the basis of a general medical condition. Because conversion symptoms by definition affect voluntary motor or sensory function (thus pseudoneurological), neurological conditions are usually suggested, but other general medical conditions may be implicated as well. Neurologists are generally first consulted by primary care physicians for conversion symptoms; psychiatrists become involved only after neurological or general medical conditions have been reasonably excluded. Nonetheless, psychiatrists should have a good appreciation of the process of making such exclusions. More than 13% of actual neurological cases are diagnosed as functional before the elucidation of a neurological illness (Perkin, 1989). Even after referral, vigilance for an emerging general medical condition should continue. A significant percentage – 21 to 50% – of patients diagnosed with conversion symptoms are found to have neurological illness on follow-up.

Apparent conversion symptoms mandate a thorough evaluation for possible underlying physical explanation. This evaluation must include a thorough medical history; physical (especially neurological) examination; and radiographical, blood, urine and other tests as clinically indicated. Reliance should not be placed on determination of whether psychological factors explain the symptom. Such determinations are unreliable except, perhaps, in cases in which there is a clear and immediate temporal relationship between a psychosocial stressor and the symptom, or in cases in which similar situations led to conversion symptoms in the past. A history of previous conversion or other unexplained symptoms, particularly if somatization disorder is diagnosable, lessens the probability that an occult medical condition will be identified. Although conversion symptoms may occur at any age, symptoms are most often first manifested in late adolescence or early adulthood. Conversion symptoms first occurring in middle age or later should increase suspicion of an occult physical illness.

Symptoms of many neurological illnesses may appear inconsistent with known neurophysiological or neuropathological processes, suggesting conversion and posing diagnostic problems. These illnesses include multiple sclerosis, in which blindness due to optic neuritis may initially present with normal fundi; myasthenia gravis, periodic paralysis, myoglobinuric myopathy, polymyositis and other acquired myopathies, in which marked weakness in the presence of normal deep tendon reflexes may occur; and Guillain–Barré syndrome, in which early extremity weakness may be inconsistent.

Complicating diagnosis is the fact that physical illness and conversion or other apparent psychiatric overlay are not mutually exclusive. Patients with physical illnesses that are incapacitating and frightening may appear to be exaggerating symptoms. Also, patients with actual neurological illness will also have "pseudo" symptoms. For example, patients with actual seizures may have pseudoseizures as well. Considering these observations, psychiatrists should avoid a rash and hasty diagnosis of conversion disorder when faced with symptoms that are difficult to interpret.

As with the other somatoform disorders, symptoms of conversion disorder are not intentionally produced, in distinction to malingering or factitious disorder. To a large part, this determination is based on assessment of the motivation for external rewards (as in malingering) or for the assumption of the sick role (as in factitious disorder). The setting is often an important consideration. For example, conversion-like symptoms are frequent in military or forensic settings, in which obvious potential rewards make malingering a serious consideration.

A diagnosis of conversion disorder should not be made if a conversion symptom is fully accounted for by a mood disorder or by schizophrenia (e.g., disordered motility as part of a catatonic syndrome of a psychotic mood disorder or schizophrenia). If the symptom is a hallucination, it must be remembered that the descriptors differentiating conversion from psychotic hallucinations should be seen only as rules of thumb. Differentiation should be based on a comprehensive assessment of the illness. In the case of hallucinations, post traumatic stress disorder and dissociative identity disorder (multiple personality disorder) must also be excluded. If the conversion symptom cannot be fully accounted for by the other psychiatric illness, conversion disorder should be diagnosed in addition to the other disorder if it meets criteria (e.g., an episode of unexplained blindness in a patient with a major depressive episode). In hypochondriasis, neurological illness may be feared ("I have strange feelings in my head; it must be a brain tumor"), but the focus here is on preoccupation with fear of having the illness rather than on the symptom itself as in conversion disorder.

By definition, if symptoms are limited to sexual dysfunction or pain, conversion disorder is not diagnosed. Criteria for somatization disorder require multiple symptoms in multiple organ systems and functions, including symptoms affecting motor or sensory function (conversion symptoms) or memory or identity (dissociative symptoms). Thus, it would be superfluous to make an additional diagnosis of conversion disorder in the context of a somatization disorder.

A last consideration is whether the symptom is a culturally sanctioned behavior or experience. Conversion disorder should not be diagnosed if symptoms are clearly sanctioned or even expected, are appropriate to the sociocultural context, and are not associated with distress or impairment. Seizure-like episodes, such as those that occur in conjunction with certain religious ceremonies, and culturally expected responses, such as women "swooning" in response to excitement in Victorian times, qualify as examples of these symptoms.

Course, Natural History and Prognosis

Age at onset is typically from late childhood to early adulthood. Onset is rare before the age of 10 years and after 35 years, but cases with an onset as late as the ninth decade have been reported. The likelihood of a neurological or other medical condition is increased when the age at onset is in middle or late life. Development is generally acute, but symptoms may develop gradually as well. The course of individual conversion symptoms is generally short; half to nearly all symptoms remit by the time of hospital discharge. However, symptoms relapse within 1 year in one-fifth to one-fourth of patients. Typically, one symptom is present in a single episode, but multiple symptoms are generally involved longitudinally. Factors associated with good prognosis include acute onset, clearly identifiable precipitants, a short interval between onset and institution of treatment, and good intelligence. Conversion blindness, aphonia and paralysis are associated with relatively good prognosis, whereas patients with seizures and tremor do more poorly. Some patients diagnosed initially with conversion disorder will have a presentation that meets criteria for somatization disorder when they are observed longitudinally.

Individual conversion symptoms are generally self-limited and do not lead to physical changes or disabilities. Rarely, physical sequelae such as atrophy may occur. Marital and occupational problems are not as frequent in patients with conversion disorder as they are in those with somatization disorder.

Treatment

Reports of the treatment of conversion disorder date from those of Charcot, which generally involved symptom removal by suggestion or hypnosis. Breuer and Freud, using such psychoanalytic techniques as free association and abreaction of repressed affects, had more ambitious objectives in their treatment of Anna O, including the resolution of unconscious conflicts. To date, whereas some recommend long-term, intensive, insight-oriented psychodynamic psychotherapy in pursuit of such goals, most psychiatrists advocate a more pragmatic approach, especially for acute cases.

Therapeutic approaches vary according to whether the conversion symptom is acute or chronic. Whichever the case, direct confrontation is not recommended. Such a communication may cause a patient to feel even more isolated. An undiscovered physical illness may also underlie the presentation.

In acute cases, the most frequent initial aim is removal of the symptom. The pressure behind accomplishing this depends on the distress and disability associated with the symptom (Ford, 1995). If the patient is not in great distress and the need to regain function is not immediate, a conservative approach of reassurance, relaxation and suggestion is recommended. With this technique, the patient is reassured that on the basis of evaluation the symptom will disappear completely and, in fact, is already beginning to do so. The patient can then be encouraged to ventilate about recent events and feelings, without any causal relationships being suggested. This is in contrast to attempts at abreaction, by which repressed material, particularly regarding a painful experience or a conflict, is brought back to consciousness.

If symptoms do not resolve with such conservative approaches, a number of other techniques for symptom resolution may be instituted. It does appear that prompt resolution of conversion symptoms is important because the duration of conversion symptoms is associated with a greater risk of recurrence and chronic disability. The other techniques include narcoanalysis (e.g., amobarbital interview), hypnosis and behavioral therapy. In narcoanalysis, amobarbital or another sedative–hypnotic medication such as lorazepam is given intravenously to the point of drowsiness. Sometimes this is followed by administration of a stimulant medication, such as methamphetamine. The patient is then encouraged to discuss stressors and conflicts. This technique may be effective acutely, leading to at least temporary symptom relief as well as expansion of the information known about the patient. This technique has not been shown to be especially effective with more chronic conversion symptoms. In hypnotherapy, symptoms may be removed with the suggestion that the symptoms will gradually improve posthypnotically. Information regarding stressors and conflicts may be explored as well. Formal behavioral therapy, including relaxation training and even aversive therapy, has been proposed and reported by some to be effective. In addition, simply manipulating the environment to interrupt reinforcement of the conversion symptom is recommended.

Anecdotally, somatic treatments including phenothiazines, lithium and electroconvulsive therapy have been reported effective. However, in many cases, this may be attributable to simple suggestion. In other cases, resolution of another psychiatric disorder, such as a psychotic disorder or a mood disorder, may have led to the symptom's removal. It should be evident from the preceding discussion that in acute conversion disorders, it may be not the particular technique but the influence of suggestion that is specifically associated with symptom relief. It is likely that in various rituals, such as exorcism and other religious ceremonies, immediate "cures" are based on suggestion. Suggestion seems to play a major role in the resolution of "mass hysteria", in which a group of individuals who believe that they have been exposed to some noxious influence such as a "toxin" or even a "spell" experience similar symptoms that do not appear to have any organic basis. Often, the epidemic can be contained if affected individuals are segregated. Simple announcements that no such factor has been identified and that symptoms experienced by the group have been linked to mass hysteria have been effective.

Thus far, this discussion has centered on acute treatment primarily for symptom removal. Longer-term approaches include strategies previously discussed for somatization disorder – a pragmatic, conservative approach involving support and exploration of various conflict areas, particularly of interpersonal relationships. A certain degree of insight may be attained, at least in terms of appreciating relationships between various conflicts and stressors and the development of symptoms. Others advocate long-term, intensive, insight-oriented dynamic psychotherapy.

Pain Disorder

Definition

As defined in DSM-IV, the essential feature of pain disorder is pain with which psychological factors "have an important role in the onset, severity, exacerbation, or maintenance" (see Table 54.1). Pain disorder is subtyped as pain disorder associated with psychological factors and pain disorder associated with both psychological factors and a general medical condition. The third possibility, pain disorder associated with a general medical condition, is not considered to be a mental disorder, because the requirement is not met that psychological factors play an important role. Thus, the DSM-IV concept of pain disorder allows the psychiatrist greater specificity in considering etiological factors and a more useful schema for differential diagnosis. The focus is placed on the presence of psychological factors rather than the exasperating determination of whether the pain is attributable to organic disease.

In addition, DSM-IV requires that pain be the predominant focus of the clinical presentation and that it cause clinically significant distress or impairment. Specifiers of acute (duration of less than 6 months) and chronic (duration of 6 months or longer) are provided.

Epidemiology

As to pain itself, some empirical studies suggest that it is common. Perhaps as indirect evidence of this is the proliferation of pain clinics nationally. Of course, many patients attending these clinics fall into the category of pain disorder associated with a general medical condition, but undoubtedly, some also have involvement of psychological factors as required for a diagnosis of pain disorder as a mental disorder. The same would apply to the 10 to 15% of adults in the USA in any given year who have work disability because of back pain. Pain has been found to be a predominant symptom in 75% of consecutive general medical patients, with 75% of these (thus 50% overall) judged as having no identifiable physical cause. No apparent physical basis is found in 40 to 50% of patients presenting with nonspecific abdominal pain. At least half of such patients show major personality problems in addition, with such aberrations associated with poor outcome. Whereas primary care and other nonpsychiatric physicians probably see most pain patients, 38% of psychiatric inpatient admissions and 18% attending a psychiatric outpatient clinic report pain as a significant problem.

Etiology and Pathophysiology

In considering the etiology of pain disorder, possible mechanisms of pain itself must be considered. The definition of pain sanctioned by the International Association for the Study of Pain Subcommittee on Taxonomy is "an unpleasant sensory and emotional experience associated with actual or potential tissue damage". It goes on to acknowledge that pain is not simply "activity induced in the nociceptor and nociceptive pathways by a noxious stimulus" but "is always a psychological state…". Thus, it accepts the hypothesis that pain involves psychological as well as physical factors.

Many theories of the etiology and pathophysiology of pain involving both biological and psychological factors have been proposed. It is known that a neuropathway descends from the cerebral cortex and medulla, which inhibits the firing of pain transmission neurons when it is activated. This system is apparently mediated by the endogenous opiate-like compounds, endorphins and by serotonin. Indeed, metabolites of both of these neurotransmitters may be reduced in the cerebrospinal fluid of chronic pain patients.

The gate control theory links biological and psychological factors. It hypothesizes a gate-like mechanism involving the dorsal horn of the spinal cord by which large A-beta fibers as well as small A-delta and C fibers carry impulses from the periphery to the substantia gelatinosa and T-cells in the spinal cord. Activation of the large fibers inhibits, whereas activation of the small fibers facilitates transmission to the T-cells. In addition, impulses descending from the brain, influenced by cognitive processes, may either inhibit or facilitate transmission of pain impulses. Such a

mechanism may explain how psychological processes affect pain perception.

By definition, both pain disorder associated with psychological factors and pain disorder associated with both psychological factors and a general medical condition involve psychological factors. In the case of the former, it is presumed that there is little contribution from general medical conditions; in the latter, both physical and psychological factors contribute. A plethora of not necessarily mutually exclusive theories has been proposed to explain how this takes place.

Psychological constructs involving learning theories, both operant and classical conditioning, may apply. In operant paradigms, pain-related complaints are reinforced by increased attention, relief from obligations, monetary compensation and the pleasurable effects of analgesics. In classical conditioning, originally neutral settings such as a workplace or bedroom where pain was experienced come to evoke pain-related behavior. Social and cultural attitudes may also have effects. Patients with unexplained pain are more likely than others to have close relatives with chronic pain. Although findings have differed from study to study, ethnic differences may also have effects, such as greater pain tolerance in Irish and Anglo-Saxon groups in comparison to southern Mediterranean groups.

Diagnosis and Differential Diagnosis

As shown in Figure 54.1, the diagnostic approach begins with assessment of whether the presentation is fully explained by a general medical condition. If not, it may be assumed that psychological factors play a major role. If it is judged that psychological factors do not play a major role, a diagnosis of pain disorder associated with a general medical condition may apply. As previously mentioned, this does not have a mental disorder code.

If psychological factors are involved, the first consideration is whether the pain is feigned. If so, either malingering or factitious disorder is diagnosed, depending on whether external incentives or assumption of the sick role is the motivation. Evidence of malingering includes consideration of external rewards relative to the chronology of the development and maintenance of the pain. In factitious disorder, a pattern of successive hospitalizations and medical evaluations is evident. Inconsistency in presentation, lack of correspondence to known anatomical pathways or disease patterns, and lack of associated sensory or motor function changes suggest malingering or factitious disorder, but pain disorder associated with psychological factors may show this pattern as well. The key question is whether the patient is experiencing rather than feigning the pain.

Determination of the relative contributions of psychological and general medical factors is difficult. Of course, careful assessment of the nature and severity of the potential underlying medical condition and the nature and degree of pain that would be expected should be made. Traditionally, the so-called conversion V or neurotic triad (consisting of elevation of the hypochondriasis and hysteria scales with a lower score on the depression scale) on the Minnesota Multiphasic Personality Inventory has been purported to indicate emotional indifference to the somatic concerns as might be expected if the symptom is attributable to psychological factors rather than organic disease. However, evidence indicates that this configuration may also occur as an adjustment to chronic illness.

A diagnosis of pain disorder requires that the pain be of sufficient severity to warrant clinical attention, that is, it causes clinically significant distress or impairment. A number of instruments have been developed to assess the degree of distress associated with the pain. Such measures include the numerical rating scale and visual analog scale as described by Scott and Huskisson (1976), the McGill Pain Questionnaire and the West Haven-Yale Multidimensional Pain Inventory (Osterweis *et al.*, 1987).

DSM-IV includes a number of exclusionary conventions. By definition, if pain is restricted to pain with sexual intercourse, the sexual disorder, dyspareunia, not pain disorder, is diagnosed. If pain occurs in the context of a mood, anxiety, or psychotic disorder, pain disorder is diagnosed only if it is an independent focus of clinical attention and is not better accounted for by the other disorder, a highly subjective judgment.

If pain occurs exclusively during the course of somatization disorder, pain disorder is not diagnosed because pain symptoms are part of the criteria for somatization disorder and are thereby subsumed under the more comprehensive diagnosis. Because somatization disorder is virtually a lifelong condition, this exclusion generally applies in someone with somatization disorder by history. Important here is that, in addition to pain, somatization disorder involves multiple symptoms of the gastrointestinal system, the reproductive system, and the central and peripheral nervous systems; whereas in pain disorder, the focus is on pain symptoms only.

Specification of acute versus chronic pain disorder on the basis of whether the duration is less than or greater than 6 months is an important distinction. Whereas acute pain, in most cases, will be linked with physical disorders, when pain remains unexplained after 6 months, psychological factors are often involved (Cloninger, 1993). However, the psychiatrist must remember that a significant minority (in one study 19%) of patients with chronic pain of no apparent physical origin will ultimately be found to have occult organic disease (Cloninger, 1993).

In patients with unexplained pelvic pain, psychiatrists should be warned about cavalier conclusions regarding the absence of physical disease. With laparoscopy, a high frequency of occult organic disease has been identified in several studies. Thus, laparoscopy may be indicated in patients with pelvic pain. Electromyography may be helpful in distinguishing muscle contraction headaches. Failure to show coronary artery spasm with provocative procedures and failure to respond to nitroglycerin may be useful in distinguishing patients with pain disorder from those in whom the pain is attributable to coronary artery disease.

Course, Natural History and Prognosis

Given the heterogeneity of conditions subsumed under the pain disorder rubric, course and prognosis vary widely. The subtyping at 6 months is of significance. The prognosis for total remission is good for pain disorders of less than 6 months' duration. However, for syndromes of greater than 6 months' duration, chronicity is common. The site of the pain may be another factor. Certain anatomically differentiated pain syndromes can be distinguished, and each has its own characteristic pattern. These include syndromes characterized primarily by headache, facial pain, chest pain, abdominal pain and pelvic pain. In such syndromes, symptoms tend to be recurrent, with relapses occurring in association with stress. A high rate of depression has been observed among patients with unexplained facial pain. Facial pain is often alleviated by antidepressant medication. This effect has been observed in both patients with depressive symptoms and those without.

Other factors affecting course and prognosis include associated psychiatric illness and external reinforcement. Employment at the outset of treatment predicts improvement. Chronicity is more likely in the presence of certain personality diagnoses or traits, such as pronounced passivity and dependency. External reinforcement includes litigation involving potential financial compensation or disability. Continuation of the pain disorder may prove more lucrative than its resolution and return to work. Level of activity, which is generally associated with improvement, is discouraged by fears of losing compensation. Thus, although outright malingering may be rare pain behaviors are often reinforced and maintained. Habituation with addictive drugs is associated with greater chronicity.

Treatment

An overriding guideline is that the psychiatrist does not do anything that will actually perpetuate and even promote "pain-related behavior". Thus, a major goal is to encourage activity. Other guidelines include avoidance of sedative–antianxiety drugs, judicious use of analgesics on a fixed interval schedule so as not to reinforce pain-related behaviors, avoidance of opioids and consideration of alternative treatment approaches such as relaxation therapy. Depression should be treated with appropriate antidepressant drugs, not sedative–antianxiety medications. The difficulties in managing pain disorder patients have resulted in the establishment of many clinics and programs especially designed for pain. Referral to such a service may be indicated. Intervention should best be provided early in the course of the syndrome, before pain-related behaviors become entrenched. Once continuing disability compensation is established, therapeutic efforts become much more difficult.

The preceding general guidelines apply whether or not a general medical basis for the pain is involved. Of course, if only pain disorder associated with psychological factors is involved, psychological management will be the mainstay. For patients with pain associated with general medical factors (not a mental disorder) in which psychological factors do not play a major role, efforts should be made to prevent the development of psychological problems in response to the resulting distress, isolation and loss of function, and iatrogenic effects such as exposure to potentially addicting drugs.

In acute pain, the major goal is to relieve the pain. Thus, pharmacological agents generally play a more significant role than in chronic syndromes. Whereas the risk of developing opioid dependence appears to be surprisingly low (four per 12 000) among patients without a prior history of dependence, nonopioid agents should be used whenever they can be expected to be effective. As discussed for chronic pain, these include particularly acetaminophen and the nonsteroidal antiinflammatory drugs (NSAIDs), of which aspirin is considered a member. Even if an opioid analgesic is employed, these drugs should be continued as adjuncts; often, they lessen the required dose of the opioid.

It is with the chronic syndromes that proper management is crucial to ease distress and prevent the development of additional problems. As advised by King (1994), the overriding goal is to maintain function, because total relief of the pain may not be possible. Physical and occupational therapy may play a major role. There may be resistance to the involvement of a psychiatrist as an indication that the pain is not seen as real. Such issues must first be resolved. An attempt should be made to ascertain the roles that psychological and general medical factors play in the maintenance of the pain.

A large variety of psychotherapies including individual, group and family strategies have been employed. Two techniques that warrant special attention are operant conditioning and cognitive–behavioral therapy. In operant conditioning, the pattern of reinforcement of pain behavior by medication, attention and excuse from responsibilities is to be interrupted and reinforcement shifted to usual daily activities. To assess the role of operant conditioning, it may be necessary to have patients keep a diary and to interview family members to identify any conditioning patterns. In cognitive–behavioral therapies, the goal is the identification and correction of attitudes, beliefs and expectations. Biofeedback and relaxation techniques may be used to minimize muscle tension that may aggravate if not cause pain. Hypnosis may also be used to achieve muscle relaxation and to help the patient "dissociate" from the pain.

Pharmacological intervention may also be useful in chronic syndromes. Effort should be made to avoid opioids if possible. Agents to be tried first include antidepressants, acetaminophen, NSAIDs (including aspirin) and anticonvulsants such as carbamazepine. Antidepressants seem particularly useful for neuropathic pain, headache, facial pain, fibrositis and arthritis (including rheumatoid arthritis). Analgesic action seems to be independent of antidepressant effects. Most work has been done with the tricyclic antidepressants; other classes, such as the monoamine oxidase inhibitors (MAOIs) and the selective serotonin reuptake inhibitors (SSRIs), may be effective as well. Although it was thought that the action is mediated by serotoninergic effects, agents such as desipramine with predominantly noradrenergic activity seem to be effective as well. NSAIDs, of which aspirin, ibuprofen, naproxen and piroxicam are commonly used examples, may alleviate pain through inhibition of prostaglandin synthesis. Unfortunately, this effect may also contribute to side effects, such as aggravation of peptic or duodenal ulcers and interference with renal function. For patients unable to tolerate NSAIDs, acetaminophen should be tried.

If opioid analgesics are used, it is recommended that use be tied to objectives such as increasing level of activity rather than simply pain alleviation. Milder opioids, such as codeine, oxycodone and hydrocodone, should be implemented first. The once widely used propoxyphene has less analgesic effect than these drugs; it is not devoid of abuse potential as once thought and is not recommended. Pure opioid agonists such as morphine, methadone and hydromorphone should be tried next. Meperidine, also in this class, is contraindicated for prolonged use because accumulation of the toxic metabolite, normeperidine, a cerebral irritant, may result in anxiety, psychosis, or seizures. Meperidine may also have a lethal interaction with MAOIs. There are no advantages to mixed opioid agonist–antagonists. The commonly used pentazocine should be avoided because it has abuse potential and psychotomimetic effects in some patients. It remains to be seen whether newer agents (buprenorphine, butonphanol and nalbuphine) have lower abuse potential as claimed. Above all, psychiatrists should be judicious in the use of opioid analgesics, considering not only their abuse potential but their large number of side effects including constipation, nausea and vomiting, excessive sedation and, in higher doses, respiratory depression that may be fatal.

In addition to pharmacotherapy, a number of other "physical" techniques have been used, such as acupuncture and transcutaneous electrical nerve stimulation. These carry little risk of adverse effects or aggravation of the pain disorder. Other procedures such as trigger point injections, nerve blocks and surgical ablation may be recommended if specifically indicated by an underlying general medical disorder.

As can be seen in the preceding discussion, the management of pain disorders is not monomodal. A great number of psychological and physical factors and interventions may be considered.

Hypochondriasis

Definition

The essential feature in hypochondriasis is preoccupation with fears or the idea of having a serious disease based on the "misinterpretation of bodily symptoms". (see Table 54.1). This is in contrast to somatization disorder, conversion disorder and pain disorder, in which the symptoms themselves are the predominant focus. There was some debate in the development of DSM-IV as to whether it was necessary that a body complaint be present. On the basis of empirical data, however, it was determined that this requirement was a valid one and helped to distinguish the "disease conviction" of hypochondriasis from "disease fear" as in phobic disorder. Bodily symptoms may be interpreted broadly to include misinterpretation of normal body functions. In hypochondriasis, the preoccupation persists despite reassurance from physicians and the accumulation of evidence to the contrary. As in the other somatoform disorders, symptoms must result in clinically significant distress or impairment in important areas of functioning. The duration must be at least 6 months. Hypochondriasis is not diagnosed if the hypochondriacal concerns are better accounted for by another psychiatric disorder, such as major depressive episodes or various psychotic disorders with somatic delusions.

Throughout the modern period, there has been controversy as to whether hypochondriasis represented an independent, discrete disease entity. Some maintain that hypochondriasis is virtually always secondary to another psychiatric disorder, usually depression. A number of studies suggested that of the many patients with hypochondriacal complaints, few meet criteria for the full diagnosis. Moreover, the lack of bimodality to the complaints suggests a continuum rather than a discrete entity.

In the development of DSM-IV, owing to observations that the disease conviction resembled disease phobia or the incorrigible ideas of obsessive–compulsive disorder, placement of hypochondriasis with the anxiety disorders was considered. Similarly, a case can be made that disease conviction is on a continuum with somatic delusions of disease, suggesting inclusion with the delusional disorders. In the end, such considerations were resolved by keeping hypochondriasis with the somatoform disorders, defining it in terms of an idea that one already has a particular illness rather than fears of acquiring one to distinguish it from a disease phobia, and by excluding cases in which the idea was of delusional proportions to differentiate hypochondriasis from delusional disorder, somatic type.

Epidemiology

Some degree of preoccupation with disease is apparently common. As reviewed by Kellner (1991), 10 to 20% of "normal" and 45% of "neurotic" persons have intermittent unfounded worries about illness, with 9% of patients doubting reassurances given by physicians. Kellner also estimated that 50% of all patients attending physicians' offices "suffer either primary hypochondriacal symptoms or have minor somatic disorders with hypochondriacal overlay". How these relate to hypochondriasis as a disorder is difficult to assess because these estimates do not appear to distinguish between a focus on the symptoms themselves (as in somatization disorder) and preoccupation with the implications of the symptoms (as in hypochondriasis). The Epidemiological Catchment Area study (Robins *et al.*, 1984) did not consider hypochondriasis. A 1965 study reported prevalence figures ranging from 3 to 13% in different cultures, but it is not clear whether this represents a syndrome comparable to the current definition or just hypochondriacal symptoms. As already noted, many patients manifest some hypochondriacal symptoms as part of other psychiatric disorders, and others have transient hypochondriacal symptoms in response to stresses such as serious physical illness yet never fulfill the inclusion criteria for DSM-IV hypochondriasis. Assessment of the incidence and prevalence of hypochondriasis undoubtedly requires study of general or primary care rather than psychiatric populations, because patients with hypochondriasis are convinced that they suffer from some physical illness. To date, study of such populations suggests that 4 to 9% of patients in general medical settings suffer from hypochondriasis.

It does appear that hypochondriasis is equally common in males and females.

Etiology and Pathophysiology

Until recently, psychoanalytic hypotheses of etiology predominated. Freud hypothesized that hypochondriasis represented "the return of object libido onto the ego with cathexis of the body" (Viederman, 1985). Subsequently, the cathexis to the body hypothesis was elaborated on to include interpretations involving disturbed object relations – displacement of repressed hostility to the body to communicate anger indirectly to others. Dynamic mechanisms involving masochism, guilt, conflicted dependency needs and a need to suffer and be loved at the same time have also been suggested (Stoudemire, 1988). The presence of such "narcissistic" mechanisms has been suggested as the reason that patients with hypochondriasis were "unanalyzable". Other psychological theories involve defense against feelings of low self-esteem and inadequacy, perceptual and cognitive abnormalities, and operant conditioning involving reinforcement for assumption of the sick role.

Biological theories have been suggested as well. Hypochondriacal ideas have been attributed to a hypervigilance to insult, including overperception of physical problems. This has been posited in particular in reference to hypochondriasis as an aspect of depression or anxiety disorders. Hypochondriasis has been included by some in the posited obsessive–compulsive spectrum disorders along with obsessive–compulsive and body dysmorphic disorders, anorexia nervosa, Tourette's disorder, trichotillomania, pathological gambling and other impulsive disorders. All these disorders involve repetitive thoughts or behaviors that patients are unable to delay or inhibit without great difficulty. Evidence for this clustering includes observations of clinical improvement with SSRIs such as fluoxetine even in nondepressed patients with hypochondriasis, body dysmorphic disorder, obsessive–compulsive disorder and anorexia nervosa. Because such a response is not evident with nonSSRI antidepressants, some type of common serotonin dysregulation is suggested for these disorders.

Diagnosis and Differential Diagnosis

As shown in Figure 54.1, the first step in approaching patients with distressing or impairing preoccupation with or fears of having a serious disease is to exclude the possibility of explanation on the basis of a general medical condition. Fears that may seem excessive may also occur in patients with general medical conditions with vague and subjective symptoms early in their disease course. These include neurological diseases, such as myasthenia gravis and multiple sclerosis; endocrine diseases; systemic diseases that affect several organ systems, such as systemic lupus erythematosus; and occult malignant neoplasms. The disease conviction of hypochondriasis may actually be less amenable to medical reassurance than the fears of patients, with general medical illnesses, who may at least temporally accept such encouragement. Hypochondriacal complaints are not often intentionally produced such that differentiation from malingering and factitious disorder is seldom a problem.

Exclusion is made if the preoccupation is better accounted for by another psychiatric disorder. DSM-IV lists generalized anxiety disorder, obsessive–compulsive disorder, panic disorder, a major depressive episode, separation anxiety, or another somatoform disorder as candidates. Chronology will be of utmost importance in such discriminations. Hypochondriacal concerns occurring exclusively during episodes of another disturbance, such as an anxiety or depressive disorder, do not warrant an additional diagnosis of hypochondriasis. The presence of other psychiatric symptoms will also be helpful. For example, a patient with hypochondriacal complaints as part of a major depressive episode will show other symptoms of depression, such as sleep and appetite disturbance, feelings of worthlessness and self-reproach, although depressed elderly patients may deny sadness or other expressions of depressed mood. A confounding factor is that patients with hypochondriasis often have comorbid anxiety or depressive syndromes. Again, characterizing the symptoms by chronology will be useful. Treatment trials may also have diagnostic significance. Depressed patients who are hypochondriacal may respond to nonSSRI antidepressant medications or electroconvulsive therapy (often necessary to reverse a depressive state of sufficient severity to lead to such profound symptoms), with resolution of the hypochondriacal as well as the depressive symptoms.

Hypochondriasis is differentiated from other somatoform disorders such as pain, conversion and somatization disorders by its predominant feature of preoccupation with and fears of having an underlying illness based on the misinterpretation of body symptoms, rather than the physical symptoms themselves. Patients with these other somatoform disorders at times are concerned with the possibility of underlying illness, but this will generally be overshadowed by a focus on the symptoms themselves.

The next consideration is whether the belief is of delusional proportions. Patients with hypochondriasis, although preoccupied, generally acknowledge the possibility that their concerns are unfounded. Delusional patients do not. Somatic delusions of serious illness are seen in some cases of schizophrenia and in delusional disorder, somatic type. In general, patients with schizophrenia that have such delusions also show other signs of schizophrenia, such as disorganized speech, peculiarities of thought and behavior, hallucinations and other delusions. Belief that an underlying illness is being caused by some bizarre process may also be seen (e.g., "I'm trying not to defecate because it will cause my brain to turn to jelly"). Schizophrenic patients may also show improvement with neuroleptic treatment, at least in the "active" symptoms of their illness, under which somatic delusions are included.

Differentiation from delusional disorder, somatic type, may be more difficult. It is often a thin line between preoccupation and fear that is a conviction and that which is a delusion. Often, the distinction is made on the basis of whether the patient can consider the possibility that the conviction is erroneous. Yet, patients with hypochondriasis vary in the extent to which they can do this. DSM-IV acknowledges this by its inclusion of the specifier with poor insight. In the past, some argued that differentiation could be made on the basis of response to neuroleptics, especially pimozide; patients with delusional disorder, but not hypochondriasis, respond.

If it is concluded that the preoccupations are not delusional, the next consideration is whether the duration requirement of 6 months has been met (see Figure 54.1). Syndromes of less than 6 months' duration are diagnosed under either somatoform disorder NOS or adjustment disorder if the symptoms are an abnormal response to a stressful life event. The reason to make such a distinction is to distinguish hypochondriasis from transient syndromes, the longitudinal course of which have been shown to be more variable, suggesting heterogeneity.

Other diagnostic considerations include whether the preoccupations or fears are restricted to preoccupations with being overweight, as in anorexia nervosa; with the inappropriateness of one's sex characteristics, as in a gender identity disorder; or with defects in appearance, as in body dysmorphic disorder. The preoccupations of hypochondriasis resemble the obsessions, and the health checking and efforts to obtain reassurance resemble the compulsions of obsessive–compulsive disorder. However, if such manifestations are health centered only, obsessive–compulsive disorder is not diagnosed. If, on the other hand, nonhealth related obsessions and compulsions are present, obsessive–compulsive disorder may be diagnosed in addition to hypochondriasis.

Course, Natural History and Prognosis

Data are conflicting, but it appears that the most common age at onset is in early adulthood. Available data suggest that approximately 25% of patients with a diagnosis of hypochondriasis do poorly, 65% show a chronic but fluctuating course and 10% recover. This pertains to the full syndrome. A much more variable course is seen in patients with just some hypochondriacal concerns. It appears that acute onset, absence of a personality disorder and absence of secondary gain are favorable prognostically.

Treatment

Until recently, it appeared that patients with hypochondriasis as a primary condition benefited, but only modestly, from psychiatric intervention. Patients referred early for psychiatric evaluation and treatment showed a slightly better prognosis than those continuing with only medical evaluations and treatments. Of course, the first step in treatment is getting the patient to a psychiatrist. Patients with hypochondriasis generally present initially to nonpsychiatric physicians and are often reluctant to see a psychiatrist. Referral should be done sensitively, with the referring physician stressing to the patient that his or her distress is real and that psychiatric evaluation will be a supplement to, not a replacement for, continued medical care.

Initially, the generic techniques outlined for the somatoform disorders in general should be followed. However, it has not been demonstrated that a specific psychotherapy for hypochondriasis is available. Dynamic psychotherapy is of minimal effectiveness; supportive–educative psychotherapy is only somewhat helpful, and primarily for those with syndromes of less than 3 years' duration; and cognitive–behavioral therapy, especially response prevention of checking rituals and reassurance seeking,

is of only moderate effectiveness at best. All of these techniques seem to lack definitive effects on hypochondriasis itself.

Until recently, this could also be said of pharmacological approaches. Pharmacotherapy of comorbid depressive or anxiety syndromes was often effective, and control of such syndromes aided in general management, yet hypochondriasis itself was not ameliorated. Although controlled trials are lacking, anecdotal and open-label studies suggest that serotoninergic agents such as clomipramine and the SSRI fluoxetine may be effective in ameliorating hypochondriasis. Similar effects are expected from the other SSRIs. Response to fluoxetine has been reported with doses recommended for obsessive–compulsive disorder, rather than usual antidepressant doses (i.e., 60–80 mg rather than 20–40 mg/day). Such pharmacotherapy is best combined with the generic psychotherapy recommendations for somatoform disorders, as well as with cognitive–behavioral techniques to disrupt the counterproductive checking and reassurance-seeking behaviors.

Body Dysmorphic Disorder

Definition

The essential feature of this disorder is preoccupation with an imagined defect in appearance or a markedly excessive concern with a minor anomaly (see Table 54.1). In body dysmorphic disorder, a person could be preoccupied with an imagined defect while she or he actually had some other anomaly and was not normal appearing. To exclude conditions with trivial or minor symptoms, the preoccupation must cause clinically significant distress or impairment. By definition, body dysmorphic disorder is not diagnosed if symptoms are limited to preoccupation with body weight, as in anorexia nervosa or bulimia nervosa, or to perceived inappropriateness of sex characteristics, as in gender identity disorder.

Preoccupations most often involve the nose, ears, face, or sexual organs. Common complaints include a diversity of imagined flaws of the face or head, including defects in the hair (e.g., too much or too little), skin (e.g., blemishes), and shape or symmetry of the face or facial features (e.g., nose is too large and deformed). However, any body part may be the focus, including genitals, breasts, buttocks, extremities, shoulders and even overall body size.

Body dysmorphic disorder has been well described in the European and Japanese literature, generally designated dysmorphophobia, often under the rubric of the monosymptomatic hypochondriacal psychoses. Until recently, it had been virtually ignored in the US literature as well as clinically.

The definition of the disorder was reexamined for DSM-IV on several counts, but especially as to its relationship to other psychiatric disorders (Phillips and Hollander, 1996). After much deliberation, it was determined that body dysmorphic disorder, although often comorbid with anxiety and mood disorders, was sufficiently discrete to be maintained as a separate disorder. As discussed in the differential diagnosis section, it can be distinguished from depressive disorders and from most anxiety disorders, although it resembles obsessive–compulsive disorder in phenomenology, course and even response to treatment. It was also decided to keep it with the somatoform disorders grouping, although it does not share much with the other disorders in this grouping (with the exception of hypochondriasis), beyond the fact that affected patients are generally referred to psychiatrists from other physicians and that they also present with medically unexplained physical complaints (defects in appearance in body dysmorphic disorder).

As De Leon and colleagues (1989) pointed out, it is extremely difficult to determine whether a dysmorphic concern is delusional as in that with body dysmorphic disorder, for a continuum exists from clearly nondelusional preoccupations to unequivocal delusions such that defining a discrete boundary between the two ends of the spectrum would be artificial. Furthermore, individual patients seem to move back and forth along this continuum. Support for rejecting the exclusion is preliminary evidence that dysmorphic preoccupations may respond to the same pharmacotherapy (SSRIs), regardless of whether the concerns are delusional. Perhaps as a reflection of the state of knowledge at this point, both body dysmorphic disorder and delusional disorder, somatic type, can be diagnosed on the basis of the same symptoms, in the same individual, at the same time. Thus, the definition of body dysmorphic disorder differs from hypochondriasis, which is not diagnosed if hypochondriacal concerns are determined to be delusional.

Epidemiology

Knowledge of such parameters is still incomplete. In general, patients with body dysmorphic disorder first present to nonpsychiatrists such as plastic surgeons, dermatologists and internists because of the nature of their complaints and are not seen psychiatrically until they are referred (De Leon *et al.*, 1989). Many resist or refuse referral because they do not see their problem as psychiatric; thus, study of psychiatric clinic populations may underestimate the prevalence of the disorder. It has been estimated that 2% of patients seeking corrective cosmetic surgery suffer from this disorder. Although women outnumber men in this population, it is not known whether this sex distribution holds true in the general population.

Etiology and Pathophysiology

A number of sociological, psychological and neurobiological theories have been proposed. Body dysmorphic disorder has been explained, at least in part, as an exaggerated incorporation of societal ideals of physical perfection and acceptance of cosmetic plastic surgery to attain such goals. A high frequency of insecure, sensitive, obsessional, schizoid, anxious, narcissistic, introverted and hypochondriacal personality traits in body dysmorphic patients have been described (Phillips, 1991). Various psychodynamic mechanisms and symbolic meanings of dysmorphic symptoms have been suggested (Phillips, 1991), going back to Freud's case of the Wolfman who had dysmorphic preoccupations regarding his nose.

Some interesting neurobiological possibilities have emerged, particularly concerning observations that hypochondriasis, body dysmorphic disorder and a number of other conditions involving compelling repetitive thoughts or behaviors may respond preferentially to SSRIs, not to other antidepressant drugs. An obsessive–compulsive spectrum disorders grouping, the pathological process of which is mediated by serotoninergic dysregulation, has been suggested. As further evidence, symptoms of body dysmorphic disorder as well as those of obsessive–compulsive disorder may be aggravated by the partial serotonin agonist *m*-chlorophenylpiperazine.

Diagnosis and Differential Diagnosis

The preoccupations of body dysmorphic disorder must first be differentiated from usual concerns with grooming and appearance. Attention to appearance and grooming is universal and socially sanctioned. However, diagnosis of body dysmorphic disorder requires that the preoccupation cause clinically significant distress or impairment. In addition, in body dysmorphic disorder, concerns focus on an imaginary or exaggerated defect, often of something, such as a small blemish, that would warrant scant attention even if it were present. Persons with histrionic personality disorder may be vain and excessively concerned with appearance. However, the focus in this disorder is on maintaining a good or even exceptional appearance, rather than preoccupation with a defect. Such concerns are probably unrelated to body dysmorphic disorder. In addition, by nature, the preoccupations in body dysmorphic disorder are essentially unamenable to reassurance from friends or family or consultation with physicians, cosmetologists, or other professionals.

Next, the possibility of an explanation by a general medical condition must be considered (see Figure 54.1). As mentioned, patients with this disorder often first present to plastic surgeons, oral surgeons and others, seeking correction of defects. By the time a mental health professional is consulted, it has generally been ascertained that there is no physical basis for the degree of concern. As with other syndromes involving somatic preoccupations (or delusions), such as olfactory reference syndrome and delusional parasitosis (both included under delusional disorder, somatic type), occult medical disorders, such as an endocrine disturbance or a brain tumor, must be excluded.

In terms of explanation on the basis of another psychiatric disorder, there is little likelihood that symptoms of body dysmorphic disorder will be intentionally produced as in malingering or factitious disorder. Unlike in other somatoform disorders, such as pain, conversion and somatization disorders, preoccupation with appearance predominates. Somatic preoccupations may occur as part of an anxiety or mood disorder. However, these preoccupations are generally not the predominant focus and lack the specificity of dysmorphic symptoms. Because patients with body dysmorphic disorder often become isolative, social phobia may be suspected. However, in social phobia, the person may feel self-conscious generally but will not focus on a specific imagined defect. Indeed, the two conditions may coexist, warranting both diagnoses. Diagnostic problems may present with the mood-congruent ruminations of major depression, which sometimes involve concern with an unattractive appearance in association with poor self-esteem. Such preoccupations generally lack the focus on a particular body part that is seen in body dysmorphic disorder. On the other hand, patients with body dysmorphic disorder commonly have dysphoric affects described by them variously as anxiety or depression. In some cases, these affects can be subsumed under body dysmorphic disorder; but in other instances, comorbid diagnoses of anxiety or mood disorders are warranted.

Differentiation from schizophrenia must also be made. At times, a dysmorphic concern will seem so unusual that such a psychosis may be considered. Furthermore, patients with this disorder may show ideas of reference in regard to defects in their appearance, which may lead to the consideration of schizophrenia. However, other bizarre delusions, particularly of persecution or grandiosity, and prominent hallucinations are not seen in body dysmorphic disorder. From the other perspective, schizophrenia with somatic delusions generally lacks the focus on a particular body part and defect. Also in schizophrenia, bizarre interpretations and explanations for symptoms are often present, such as "this blemish was a sign from Jesus that I am to protect the world from Satan". Other signs of schizophrenia, such as hallucinations and disorganization of thought, are also absent in body dysmorphic disorder. As previously mentioned, the preoccupations in body dysmorphic disorder appear to be on a continuum from full insight to delusional intensity whereby the patient cannot even consider the possibility that the preoccupation is groundless. In such instances, both body dysmorphic disorder and delusional disorder, somatic type, are to be diagnosed.

Body dysmorphic disorder is not to be diagnosed if the concern with appearance is better accounted for by another psychiatric disorder. Anorexia nervosa, in which there is dissatisfaction with body shape and size, is specifically mentioned in the criteria as an example of such an exclusion. Although not specifically mentioned in DSM-IV, if a preoccupation is limited to discomfort or a sense of inappropriateness of one's primary and secondary sex characteristics, coupled with a strong and persistent cross-gender identification, body dysmorphic disorder is not diagnosed.

The preoccupations of body dysmorphic disorder may resemble obsessions and ruminations as seen in obsessive–compulsive disorder. Unlike the obsessions of obsessive–compulsive disorder, the preoccupations of body dysmorphic disorder focus on concerns with appearance. Compulsions are limited to checking and investigating the perceived physical defect and attempting to obtain reassurance from others regarding it. Still, the phenomenology is similar, and the two disorders are often comorbid. If additional obsessions and compulsions not related to the defect are present, obsessive–compulsive disorder can be diagnosed in addition to body dysmorphic disorder.

Course, Natural History and Prognosis

Age at onset appears to peak in adolescence or early adulthood. Body dysmorphic disorder is generally a chronic condition, with a waxing and waning of intensity but rarely full remission. In a lifetime, multiple preoccupations are typical; in one study, the average was four (Phillips *et al.*, 1993). In some, the same preoccupation remains unchanged. In others, new perceived defects are added to the original ones. In others still, symptoms remit, only to be replaced by others. The disorder is often highly incapacitating, with many patients showing marked impairment in social and occupational activities. Perhaps a third becomes housebound. Most attribute their limitations to embarrassment concerning their perceived defect, but the attention and time-consuming nature of the preoccupations and attempts to investigate and rectify defects also contribute. The extent to which patients with body dysmorphic disorder receive surgery or medical treatments is unknown. Superimposed depressive episodes are common, as are suicidal ideation and suicide attempts. Actual suicide risk is unknown.

In view of the nature of the defects with which patients are preoccupied, it is not surprising that they are found most commonly among patients seeking cosmetic surgery. Preoccupations persist despite reassurance that there is no defect to correct surgically. Surgery or other corrective procedures rarely if ever lead to satisfaction and may even lead to greater distress with the perception of new defects attributed to the surgery.

Treatment

First, the generic goals and treatments as outlined for the somatoform disorders overall should be instituted. These are beneficial in interrupting an unending procession of repeated evaluations and the possibility of needless surgery, which may lead to additional perceptions that surgery has resulted in further disfigurement.

Traditional insight-oriented therapies have not generally proved to be effective. Results with traditional behavioral techniques, such as systematic desensitization and exposure therapy, have been mixed. At least without amelioration with effective pharmacotherapy, the preoccupations do not extinguish as would be expected with phobias. A cognitive–behavioral approach similar to what was recommended for hypochondriasis may be more effective. This includes response prevention techniques whereby the patient is not permitted repetitively to check the perceived defect in mirrors. In addition, patients are advised not to seek reassurance from family and friends, and these persons are instructed not to respond to such inquiries. Some patients adopt such behaviors spontaneously, avoiding mirrors and other reflecting surfaces, refusing even to allude to their perceived defects to others. Such "self-techniques" may be encouraged and refined.

Biological treatments have long been used but until recently were of limited benefit to patients with body dysmorphic disorder. Approaches have included electroconvulsive therapy, tricyclic and MAOI antidepressants, and neuroleptics, particularly pimozide. In most reports of positive response to tricyclic or MAOI antidepressant drugs, it is unclear whether response was truly in terms of the dysmorphic syndrome or simply represented improvement in comorbid depressive or anxiety syndromes. Response to neuroleptic treatment has been suggested as a diagnostic test to distinguish body dysmorphic disorder from delusional disorder, somatic type. The delusional syndromes often respond to neuroleptics; body dysmorphic disorders, even when the body preoccupations are psychotic, generally do not. Pimozide has been singled out as a neuroleptic with specific effectiveness for somatic delusions, but this specificity does not appear to apply to body dysmorphic disorder.

An exception to this uninspiring picture is the observation of a possible preferential response to antidepressant drugs with serotonin reuptake blocking effects, such as clomipramine, or SSRIs, such as fluoxetine and fluvoxamine (Hollander *et al.*, 1992). Phillips and coworkers (1993) reported that more than 50% of patients with body dysmorphic disorder showed a partial or complete remission with either clomipramine or fluoxetine, a response not predicted on the basis of coexisting major depressive or obsessive–compulsive disorder. As with hypochondriasis, effectiveness is generally achieved at levels recommended for obsessive–compulsive disorder rather than for depression (e.g., 60–80 mg rather than 20–40 mg/day of fluoxetine). The SSRIs appear to ameliorate delusional as well as nondelusional dysmorphic preoccupations. Successful augmentation of clomipramine or SSRI therapy has been suggested with buspirone, another drug with serotoninergic effects. Neuroleptics, particularly pimozide, may also be helpful adjuncts, particularly if delusions of reference are present. Little seems to be gained with the addition of anticonvulsants, or benzodiazepines to the SSRI therapy.

As yet, rigorous studies have not been conducted, but anecdotal observations and open-label studies show promise for effective treatment with SSRIs and other serotoninergic agents for this, until now, therapeutically exasperating disorder. If such approaches fulfill their initial promise, integrated approaches using pharmacotherapy and other modalities such as cognitive–behavioral therapy may provide effective treatment options.

Somatoform Disorder not Otherwise Specified

Definition

Somatoform disorder NOS is the true residual category (see Table 54.1). Disorders considered under this category are characterized by somatic symptoms, but criteria for any of the specific somatoform disorders are not met. Several examples are given, but syndromes potentially included under this category are not limited to these. Unlike for undifferentiated somatoform disorder, no minimal duration is required. DSM-IV lists as examples pseudocyesis, disorders involving hypochondriacal complaints but of less than 6 months' duration, and disorders involving unexplained physical complaints such as fatigue or body weakness not due to another mental disorder and again of less than 6 months' duration. This last syndrome would seem to resemble neurasthenia of short duration, a syndrome with a long historical tradition.

Inclusion of pseudocyesis deserves special mention. With the restriction of conversion in DSM-IV to include only symptoms affecting voluntary motor and sensory function, pseudocyesis was excluded from the conversion disorder definition. In a sense, it is placed in the somatoform disorder NOS category for lack of a more appropriate place. Pseudocyesis is a reasonably discrete syndrome for which specific criteria as listed in DSM-IV can be delineated. However, given its rarity, it is not listed as a specified somatoform disorder.

Diagnosis and Differential Diagnosis

As a residual category, somatoform disorder NOS is to be diagnosed after all other possibilities are excluded (see Figure 54.1). After it is determined that a syndrome with somatoform symptoms is not attributable to a nonsomatoform psychiatric disorder and does not meet criteria for any of the specific somatoform disorders (including, on the symptom-focused side, pain, conversion and somatization disorders and, on the preoccupation-focused side, hypochondriasis or body dysmorphic disorder), the two diagnostic possibilities that remain are undifferentiated somatoform disorder and somatoform disorder NOS. Except in the case of pseudocyesis, these two are differentiated on the basis of whether the disturbance is of 6 months' duration. If symptoms last more than 6 months, undifferentiated somatoform disorder is diagnosed; if less than 6 months, somatoform disorder NOS.

Conclusion

As a group, the syndromes now subsumed under the rubric of somatoform disorders are relatively common and are associated with great direct and indirect costs to society. Yet, they have remained a "stepchild" of psychiatry, underdiagnosed and underresearched. Therapeutic direction is emerging, with some general guidelines for all of these disorders; some specific ways of managing patients with somatization disorder, undifferentiated somatoform disorder and conversion disorder; and a more utilitarian approach to management of patients with pain disorders.

It appears that pharmacological inroads are being made in the treatment of hypochondriasis and body dysmorphic disorder in terms of the possible efficacy of SSRIs. This pharmacological "probe" suggests that these disorders may be more closely linked with the so-called obsessive–compulsive spectrum disorders than with the other somatoform disorders, a linkage that may be reflected in future diagnostic systems. Even if this turns out to be the case, the somatoform disorder concept will have served its purpose in stimulating and making possible research leading to a better understanding and ultimately more effective treatments for these complex conditions.

Much work remains to be done before the knowledge concerning the somatoform disorders and their treatment catch up with the understanding of other groupings of psychiatric disorders.

Comparison of DSM-IV/ICD-10 Diagnostic Criteria

The ICD-10 Diagnostic Criteria for Research for Somatization Disorder has both a different item set and algorithm. Six symptoms are required out of a list of 14 symptoms which are broken down into the following groups: six gastrointestinal symptoms, two cardiovascular symptoms, three genitourinary symptoms, and three "skin and pain" symptoms. It is specified that the symptoms occur in at least two groups. In contrast, DSM-IV-TR requires four pain symptoms, two gastrointestinal symptoms, one sexual symptom and one pseudoneurological symptom. Furthermore, the ICD-10 Diagnostic Criteria for Research specify that there must be "persistent refusal to accept medical reassurance that there is no adequate physical cause for the physical symptoms". DSM-IV-TR only requires that the symptoms result in treatment being sought or significant impairment in social, occupational, or other important areas of functioning and that the symptoms cannot be fully explained by a known general medical condition or substance. For Undifferentiated Somatoform Disorder, the ICD-10 Diagnostic Criteria for Research and the DSM-IV-TR criteria are almost identical.

Regarding conversion disorder, ICD-10 considers conversion a type of dissociative disorder and includes separate criteria sets for dissociative motor disorders, dissociative convulsions and dissociative anesthesia and sensory loss in a section that also includes dissociative amnesia and dissociative fugue.

For pain disorder, the ICD-10 Diagnostic Criteria for Research require that the pain last at least 6 months and that it not be "explained adequately by evidence of a physiological process or a physical disorder". In contrast, DSM-IV-TR does not force the clinician to make this inherently impossible judgment and instead requires the contribution of psychological factors. Furthermore, DSM-IV-TR includes both acute (duration less than 6 months) and chronic pain (more than 6 months). This disorder is referred to in ICD-10 as "Persistent Somatoform Pain Disorder".

ICD-10 provides a single criteria set that applies to both the DSM-IV-TR categories of hypochondriasis and body dysmorphic disorder. The ICD-10 Diagnostic Criteria for Research for Hypochondriasis specifies that the belief is of a "maximum of two serious physical diseases" and requires that at least one be specifically named by the individual with the disorder. The DSM-IV-TR has no such requirement.

References

Alexander F (1950) *Psychosomatic Medicine.* WW Norton, New York.

American Psychiatric Association (1995) *Diagnostic and Statistical Manual of Mental Disorders,* 4th edn. Primary Care ed. APA, Washington DC.

American Psychiatric Association (2000) *Diagnostic and Statistical Manual of Mental Disorders,* 4th edn. Text Rev. APA, Washington DC.

Bohman M, Cloninger CR, von Knorring A-L *et al.* (1984) An adoption study of somatoform disorders. III. Cross-fostering analysis and genetic relationship to alcoholism and criminality. *Arch Gen Psychiatr* 41, 872–878.

Cloninger CR (1986) Somatoform and dissociative disorders, in *Medical Basis of Psychiatry* (eds Winokur G and Clayton PJ). WB Saunders, Philadelphia, pp. 123–151.

Cloninger CR (1993) Somatoform and dissociative disorders, in *Medical Basis of Psychiatry,* 2nd edn. (eds Winokur G and Clayton PJ). WB Saunders, Philadelphia, pp. 169–192.

De Leon J, Bott A and Simpson G (1989) Dysmorphophobia: Body dysmorphic disorder or delusional disorder, somatic subtype? *Compr Psychiatr* 30, 457–472.

Escobar JI, Rubio-Stipec, Canino G *et al.* (1989) Somatic Symptom Index (SSI): A new and abridged somatization construct: Prevalence and epidemiological correlates in two large community samples. *J Nerv Ment Dis* 177, 140–146.

Escobar JI, Swartz M, Rubio-Stipec M *et al.* (1991) Medically unexplained symptoms: Distribution, risk factors, and comorbidity, in *Current Concepts of Somatization: Research and Clinical Perspectives* (eds Kirmayer LJ and Robbins JM). American Psychiatric Press, Washington DC, pp. 63–68.

Ford CV (1995) Conversion disorder and somatoform disorder not otherwise specified. In Treatments of Psychiatric Disorders, Vol. 2, 2nd edn., (ed Gabbard GO). American Psychiatric Association, Washington DC, pp. 1735–1753.

Hollander E, DeCaria CM, Nitescu A *et al.* (1992) Serotonergic function in obsessive–compulsive disorder. Behavioral and neuroendocrine responses to oral *m*-chlorophenylpiperazine and fenfluramine in patients and healthy volunteers. *Arch Gen Psychiatr* 49, 21–28.

Kellner R (1991) *Psychosomatic Syndromes and Somatic Symptoms.* American Psychiatric Press, Washington DC.

King SA (1994) Pain disorders, in *The American Psychiatric Press Textbook of Psychiatry,* 2nd edn. (eds Hales RE, Yudofsky SC, and Talbott JA). American Psychiatric Press, Washington DC, pp. 591–622.

Martin RL and Yutzy SH (1994) Somatoform disorders, in *The American Psychiatric Press Textbook of Psychiatry,* 2nd edn. (eds Hales RE, Yudofsky SC, and Talbott JA). American Psychiatric Press, Washington DC, pp. 591–622.

Osterweis M, Kleinman A and Mechanic D (eds). (1987) *Pain and Disability.* National Academy Press, Washington DC.

Perkin GD (1989) An analysis of 7836 successive new outpatient referrals. *J Neurol Neurosurg Psychiatr* 52, 447–448.

Phillips KA (1991) Body dysmorphic disorder: The distress of imagined ugliness. *Am J Psychiatr* 148, 1138–1149.

Phillips KA and Hollander E (1996) Body dysmorphic disorder, in *DSM-IV Sourcebook,* Vol. 2 (eds Widiger TA, Frances AJ, Pincus HA *et al*). American Psychiatric Association, Washington DC, 949–960.

Phillips KA, McElroy S, Keck PE *et al.* (1993) Body dysmorphic disorder: 30 cases of imagined ugliness. *Am J Psychiatr* 150, 302–308.

Preskorn SH (1995) Beyond DSM-IV: What is the cart and what is the horse? *Psychiatr Ann* 25, 53–62.

Pribor EF, Smith DS and Yutzy SH (1994) Somatization disorder in elderly patients. *Am J Geriatr Psychiatr* 2, 109–117.

Robins LN, Helzer JE, Weissman MM *et al.* (1984) Lifetime prevalence of specific psychiatric disorders in three sites. *Arch Gen Psychiatr* 41, 949–958.

Scott J and Huskisson EC (1976) Graphic representation of pain. *Pain* 2, 175–184.

Smith GR Jr, Monson RA and Ray DC (1986) Psychiatric consultation in somatization disorder. A randomized controlled study. *N Engl J Med* 314, 1407–1413.

Spitzer RL, Williams JBW, Kroenke K, *et al.* (1994) Utility of a new procedure for diagnosing mental disorders in primary care: The PRIMEMD 100 Study. *JAMA* 272, 1749–1756.

Stoudemire GA (1988) Somatoform disorders, factitious disorders, and malingering, in *Textbook of Psychiatry* (eds Talbott JA, Hales RE, and Yudofsky SC). American Psychiatric Press, Washington DC, pp. 533–556.

Viederman M (1985) Somatoform and factitious disorders, in *Psychiatry,* Vol. 1 (ed Cavenar JO). JB Lippincott, Philadelphia, pp. 1–20.

Ziegler DK and Paul N (1954) On the natural history of hysteria in women. *Dis Nerv Syst* 15, 3–8.

55 Factitious Disorders

Introduction

A patient with factitious disorder consciously induces or feigns illness in order to obtain a psychological benefit by being in the sick role. It is the conscious awareness of the production of symptoms that differentiates factitious disorder from the somatoform disorders in which the patient unconsciously produces symptoms for an unconscious psychological benefit. It is the underlying motivation to produce symptoms that separates factitious disorders from malingering. Patients who malinger consciously feign or induce illness in order to obtain some external benefit such as money, narcotics, or excuse from duties. While the distinctions among these disorders appear satisfyingly clear, in practice, patients often blur the boundaries. Patients with somatoform disorders will sometimes consciously exaggerate symptoms which they have unconsciously produced, and it is a rare patient who consciously creates illness and yet receives no external gain at all, be it disability benefits, excuse from work, or even food and shelter.

Talcott Parsons described the "sick role" in 1951 and noted that in our society there are four aspects of this role. First, the patient is not able to will himself or herself back to health but instead must "be taken care of". Secondly, the patient in the sick role must regard the sickness as undesirable and want to get better. Thirdly, the sick patient is obliged to seek medical care and cooperate with his or her medical treatment. Finally, the sick patient is exempted from the normal responsibilities of his or her social role (Parsons, 1951).

Patients with factitious disorder seek, often desperately, the sick role. They usually have little insight into the motivations of their behaviors but are still powerfully driven to appear ill to others. In many cases, they endanger their own health and life in search of this role. Patients with this disorder will often induce serious illness or undergo numerous unnecessary, invasive procedures. As most people avoid sickness, the actions of these patients appear to run counter to human nature. Also, since entry into the "sick role" requires that the sick person should try to get better, patients with factitious disorder must conceal the voluntary origin of their symptoms. The inexplicability of their actions combined with their deceptive behavior stir up both intense interest and intense (usually negative) countertransference in health care providers.

Patients have been known to create or feign numerous illnesses, both acute and chronic, in all of the medical specialties. These illnesses can be either physical or psychological. It appears that the only limit is the creativity and knowledge of a given patient. In fact, there is at least one case report of a patient who feigned factitious disorder itself (Gurwith and Langston, 1980). The patient claimed to have Munchausen's syndrome, to have

DSM-IV-TR Criteria

Factitious Disorder

A. Intentional production or feigning of physical or psychological signs or symptoms.

B. The motivation for the behavior is to assume the sick role.

C. External incentives for the behavior (such as economic gain, avoiding legal responsibility, or improving physical well-being, as in malingering) are absent.

Code based on type

300.16 With Predominantly Psychological Signs and Symptoms: if psychological signs and symptoms predominate in the clinical presentation 300.19 With Predominantly Physical Signs and Symptoms: if physical signs and symptoms predominate in the clinical presentation 300.19 With Combined Psychological and Physical Signs and Symptoms: if both psychological and physical signs and symptoms are present and neither predominates in the clinical presentation

Reprinted with permission from the *Diagnostic and Statistical Manual of Mental Disorders*, Fourth Edition, Text Revision. Copyright 2000 American Psychiatric Association.

undergone numerous unnecessary procedures and operations and, as a result, to need immediate hospitalization. He displayed his abdomen, which appeared to have numerous surgical scars and hinted that searches of his hospital room would be fruitful. However, collateral information revealed that the physicians and hospitals he had reported had never treated the patient, and his "scars" washed off with soap and water. Patients with factitious disorder are often quite medically sophisticated. Even though acquired immune deficiency syndrome was not described until the early 1980s, the first factitious cases followed shortly thereafter, at least as early as 1986.

Definition

For a diagnosis of factitious disorder (see DSM-IV-TR criteria for factitious disorder) to be justified, a person must be intentionally producing illness; his or her motivation is to occupy the sick role, and there must not be external incentives for the behavior. The diagnosis is further subclassified, depending on whether the factitious symptoms are predominantly physical, psychological, or a combination. The DSM also includes a category (see DSM-IV-TR criteria for factitious disorder not otherwise specified) for patients with factitious symptoms who do not meet the listed criteria. The most common example of factitious disorder not otherwise specified is factitious disorder by proxy, in which the individual creates symptoms in another person, usually a dependent, in order to occupy the sick role. Patients who readily admit to inducing symptoms, such as self-mutilating patients, are not diagnosed with factitious disorder as they are not using their symptoms to occupy the sick role.

Factitious Disorder with Predominantly Physical Signs and Symptoms

Patients with this subtype of factitious disorder present with physical signs and symptoms. The three main methods patients use to create illness are: 1) giving a false history, 2) faking clinical and laboratory findings, and 3) inducing illness (e.g., by surreptitious medication use, inducing infection, or preventing wound healing). There are reports of factitious illnesses in all of the medical specialties. Particularly common presentations include fever, self-induced infection, gastrointestinal symptoms, impaired wound healing, cancer, renal disease (especially hematuria and nephrolithiasis), endocrine diseases, anemia, bleeding disorders and epilepsy (Wise and Ford, 1999). True Munchausen's syndrome fits within this subclass and is the most severe form of the illness. According to the DSM-IV, patients with Munchausen's syndrome have chronic factitious disorder with physical signs and symptoms, and in addition, have a history of recurrent hospitalization, peregrination, and **pseudologia fantastica** – dramatic, untrue, and extremely improbable tales of their past experiences (American Psychiatric Association, 2000).

Factitious Disorder with Predominantly Psychological Signs and Symptoms

Another subtype of factitious disorder includes patients who present feigning psychological illness. They both report and mimic psychiatric symptoms. These patients can be particularly difficult to diagnose as psychiatric diagnosis depends greatly on the patient's report. There are reports of factitious psychosis, post traumatic stress disorder and bereavement. In addition, there are reports of psychological distress due to false claims of being a victim of stalking, rape, or sexual harassment, and these cases are often diagnosed with a factitious psychological disorder such as post traumatic stress disorder. While patients with factitious psychological symptoms feign psychiatric illness, they also often suffer from true comorbid psychiatric disorders, particularly Axis II disorders and substance abuse. Case reports suggest that patients with psychological factitious disorder have a high rate of suicide and a poor prognosis. While Munchausen's syndrome is considered a subset of physical factitious disorder, there are case reports of patients presenting with psychological symptoms who also have some of the key features of Munchausen's (pathological lying, wandering and recurrent hospitalizations).

Factitious Disorder with Combined Psychological and Physical Signs and Symptoms

DSM-III separated factitious disorder into two disorders, based on whether the symptoms were physical or psychological.

Clinical Vignette 1

Factitious Disorder with Psychological Features
A 46-year-old man presented complaining of symptoms of post traumatic stress disorder (PTSD). He reported intense flashbacks, numbing and avoidance, and irritability resulting from his experience as a combat veteran. He began intensive treatment for PTSD including support groups, individual therapy and medication management. He was an extremely active participant in the support groups and would recount detailed horrors of his time in combat. A staff member verifying the patient's history learned the patient had served in the military but was not a combat veteran. The patient was confronted in a supportive manner, and he admitted that he had fabricated his history. It was recommended that the patient continue in psychiatric treatment, and he agreed to do so.

However, case reports clarified that this distinction was often artificial (Merrin *et al.*, 1986; Parker, 1993). Some patients present with simultaneous psychological and physical factitious symptoms, and some patients move between physical and psychological presentations over time. For example, a patient who presented with factitious post traumatic stress disorder was confronted about the nature of his symptoms and then began complaining of physical symptoms. DSM-IV was revised to account for patients who present with both psychological signs and symptoms, though this category of patients is the least well-studied.

Factitious Disorder not Otherwise Specified (Factitious Disorder by Proxy)

Some individuals pursue the sick role not by feigning illness in themselves, but instead by creating it in another person, usually someone dependent on the perpetrator. They seek the role of caring for an ill individual (the sick role by proxy). While the victim is usually a child, there are reports of victimization of elders and developmentally delayed adults. The veterinary literature even reports cases of factitious disorder by proxy in which the victim is a pet. Due to the unique characteristics of this disorder, it will be discussed in a separate section at the end of the chapter.

Clinical Findings

Due to the inherently deceptive nature of patients with factitious disorder, the literature is largely confined to case reports and case series. It is likely that many patients with less severe forms of the disease escape detection and their clinical characteristics might be quite different. In addition, the literature on factitious disorder with physical symptoms is much more extensive than the literature on the other subtypes. As a result, we will discuss the features of the factitious disorders as a whole, referring to specific characteristics of patients with psychological symptoms (either alone or accompanying physical symptoms) when they are known.

Numerous reports in the literature describe two different subclasses of factitious patients. The first type fits with the classic Munchausen's syndrome diagnosis: they have chronic factitious symptoms associated with antisocial traits, pathological lying, minimal social supports, wandering from hospital to hospital, and very poor work and relationship functioning. They are often very familiar with hospital procedure and use this knowledge to present dramatically during off-hours or at house officer transition times when the factitious nature of their symptoms is least likely to be discovered. Male patients compromise the majority of these cases. Patients with Munchausen's syndrome appear to have an extremely poor prognosis. Fortunately, this most severe class of patients makes up the minority of factitious patients, probably fewer than 10%.

The second, and more typical, type of patient does not display pathological lying or wandering. Their recurrent presentations are usually within the same community, and they become well known within the local health care system. They often have stable social supports and employment, and a history of a medically related job. This larger class of factitious patients is mostly made up of women, and is more likely to accept psychiatric treatment and to show improvement. Plassmann (1994a) reviewed 1070 cases of patients with factitious, but not Munchausen's disorder. He found that 78% of the patients were women and 58% had a medically related job. Finally, there are individuals who may have an episode of factitious disorder in reaction to a life stressor, but may return to premorbid functioning after the stressor is resolved.

All types of factitious disease show a strong association with substance abuse as well as borderline and narcissistic personality disorders. In a case series by Ehlers and Plassman (1994), nine of 18 patients had personality features that met criteria for borderline personality disorder, and another six of 18 had personality features that met criteria for narcissistic personality disorder. Factitious patients span a broad age range. Reports in the literature show patients ranging from four to 85 years. Of note, a 4-year-old patient with factitious disorder reported that he had been coached by his mother and may be better diagnosed as a victim of factitious disorder by proxy. The next youngest case found was 8 years old. Ethnicity is frequently not reported in case studies and series, so it is difficult to determine if there are any ethnic differences in the prevalence or presentation of factitious disorder.

Diagnosis and Differential Diagnosis

The diagnosis of factitious disorder is made in several ways. Factitious disorder is occasionally diagnosed accidentally when the patient is discovered in the act of creating symptoms. A history of inconsistent or unexplainable signs and symptoms or failure to respond to appropriate treatment can prompt health care providers to probe for evidence of the disorder, as can evidence of peregrination or pathological lying. In some cases, it is a diagnosis of exclusion in an otherwise inexplicable case. The differential diagnosis of factitious disorder includes rare or complex physical illness, somatoform disorders, malingering, other psychiatric disorders and substance abuse. It is especially important to rule out genuine physical illness since patients with factitious disorder often induce real physical illness. Furthermore, it is always important to remember the patients with factitious disorder are certainly not immune to the physical illnesses that plague the general population.

If there is suspicion of factitious disorder, confirmation can be difficult. Laboratory examination can confirm some factitious diagnoses such as exogenous insulin or thyroid hormone administration. Collateral information from family members or previous health care providers can also be extremely helpful. Factitious disorder with psychological signs and symptoms can

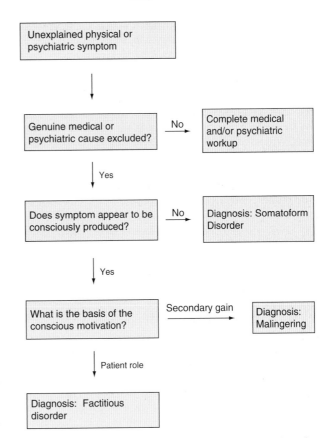

Figure 55.1 *Diagnostic decision tree for factitious disorder.*

be particularly difficult to diagnose, as so much of psychiatric diagnosis relies on the patient's report. However, there is some evidence that neuropsychological testing may be helpful in making the diagnosis. There are conflicting reports about the ability to detect over 90% of cases of factitious post traumatic stress disorder using the MMPI. In addition, there is a report of MMPI test results being used to support a diagnosis of factitious disorder with psychological features in a woman thought to be feigning symptoms of multiple personality disorder (see Figure 55.1).

Epidemiology

The nature of factitious disorder makes it difficult to determine how common it is within the population. Patients attempt to conceal themselves, thereby artificially lowering the prevalence. The tendency of patients to present several times at different facilities, however, may artificially raise the prevalence. Most estimates of the prevalence of the disease, therefore, rely on the number of factitious patients within a given inpatient population. Such attempts have generated estimates that 0.5 to 3% of medical and psychiatric inpatients suffer from factitious disorder. Of 1288 patients referred for psychiatric consultation at a Toronto general hospital, 10 (0.8%) were diagnosed with factitious disorder. A prospective examination of all 1538 patients hospitalized in a Berlin neurology department over 5 years found five (0.3%) cases of factitious disorder. An examination of 506 patients with fever of unknown origin (FUO) revealed that 2.2% of the fevers were of factitious origin, and a review of 199 Belgian patients with FUO found seven of 199 (3.5%) to be factitious. A similar study of patients with FUO at the National

Institutes of Health (NIH) revealed that 9.3% of the fevers were factitious. The increased prevalence found at the NIH may be due to the fact that the study was undertaken in a more tertiary setting, and it is a reminder that the prevalence of factitious disorder likely varies widely depending on the population and the setting. Gault and colleagues (1988) examined 3300 renal stones brought in by patients and found that 2.6% of these stones were mineral and felt to be submitted by factitious or malingering patients. There is much less data on the prevalence of factitious disorder with psychological features. A study of psychiatric inpatients showed a prevalence of 0.5% of admissions determined to be a result of a factitious psychological condition. There are few data about the prevalence of factitious disorder in an outpatient population. Because factitious patients do not readily identify themselves in large community surveys, it is not currently possible to determine the prevalence of the disorder in the general population.

Etiology

Both psychological and biological factors have been postulated to play a role in the etiology of factitious disorder. Although numerous case reports have generated speculation that factitious disorder may run in families, this could be explained by environmental factors, genetic factors, or both. The presence of central nervous system (CNS) abnormalities in some patients with factitious disorders have led some to hypothesize that underlying brain dysfunction contributes to factitious disorder. One review of factitious patients with pseudologia fantastica found CNS abnormalities (such as EEG abnormality, head injury, imaging abnormalities, or neurological findings) in 40% of the patients (King and Ford, 1988). There have been case reports of MRI and SPECT abnormalities, but it is unknown if these abnormalities were related to the disorder.

In addition, childhood developmental disturbances are thought to contribute to factitious disorder. Predisposing factors are thought to include 1) serious childhood illness or illness in a family member during childhood, especially if the illness was associated with attention and nurturing in an otherwise distant family, 2) past anger with the medical profession, 3) past significant relationship with a health care provider, and 4) factitious disorder in a parent (McKane and Anderson, 1997).

Patients with factitious disorder create illness in pursuit of the sick role. For these patients, being in the sick role allows them to compensate for an underlying psychological deficit. Most authors identify several common psychodynamic motivations for factitious disorder. First, patients with little sense of self may seek the sick role in order to provide a well-defined identity around which to structure themselves. Others may seek the sick role in order to meet dependency needs which have gone unmet elsewhere. As a patient, they receive the attention, caring and nurturing of the health care environment and are relieved of many of their responsibilities. In addition, some patients may engage in factitious behaviors for masochistic reasons. They feel they deserve punishment for some forbidden feelings and thus they should suffer at the hands of their physicians. Other patients may be motivated by anger at physicians and dupe them in retaliation. Patients with a history of childhood illness or abuse may attempt to master past traumas by creating a situation over which they have control. Finally, some authors have speculated that some patients may be enacting suicidal wishes through their factitious behavior.

Treatment and Prognosis

The goals in treating patients with factitious disorder are twofold; first to minimize the damage done by the disorder to both the patient's own health and the health care system. The second goal is to help patients recover, at least partially, from the disorder. These goals are furthered by treating comorbid medical illnesses, avoiding unnecessary procedures, encouraging patients to seek psychiatric treatment and providing support for health care clinicians. Because the literature is based exclusively on case reports and series, determining treatment effectiveness is difficult. As mentioned before, patients with true Munchausen's syndrome (including antisocial traits, pathological lying, wandering and poor social support) are felt to be refractory to treatment. While factitious disorder is extremely difficult to cure, effective techniques exist to minimize morbidity, and some patients are able to benefit greatly from psychiatric intervention.

The course of untreated factitious disorder is variable. While patients with factitious disorder commonly suffer a great deal of morbidity, fatal cases appear to be less common. One survey of 41 cases noted only one fatality, though many of the other cases were life-threatening (Reich and Gottfried, 1983). However, patients with psychological signs and symptoms are reported to have a high rate of suicide and a poor prognosis.

Soon after the widely noted publication of the first article on factitious disorders (Asher, 1951) many patients with factitious disorder were vigorously confronted once the nature of their illness was discovered. Unfortunately, most patients would deny their involvement and seek another provider who was unaware of their diagnosis (Eisendrath, 2001). In addition, the idea of "blacklists" was proposed in order to aid detection of these patients. However, issues regarding patient confidentiality as well as concerns about cursory medical evaluations that might miss genuine physical illness prevented this idea from being adopted. Although aggressive confrontation is usually unsuccessful, supportive, nonpunitive confrontation may be helpful for some. In one case series, 33 patients were confronted with the factitious nature of their illness. While only 13 admitted feigning illness, most of the patients' illnesses subsequently improved, at least in the short term (Reich and Gottfried, 1983).

Eisendrath suggested three alternatives to confrontation that he found effective. First is inexact interpretation, in which the psychiatrist interprets the psychodynamics thought to be underlying the patient's behavior without explicitly identifying the factitious behavior. He gave the example of a patient suspected of having factitious disorder who developed septicemia after her boyfriend proposed marriage. The consultant suggested that the patient might feel a need to punish herself when good things happened to her. She agreed and, soon after, admitted that she had injected a contaminant intravenously (Eisendrath, 2001). The second technique is the therapeutic double-blind. The physician presents the patient with a new medical intervention to treat his or her illness. The patient is told that one possibility is that the patient's illness has a factitious origin, and that, if so, the treatment would not be expected to work while, if the illness is biological, the treatment will work and the patient will improve. The patient must decide to give up the factitious illness or admit it. A third technique is to provide the patient with a face-saving way, such as hypnosis or biofeedback, of giving up his or her symptoms without admitting that they are not genuine. Eisendrath (2001) points out that in emergent situations, there may not be time for nonconfrontational techniques, and more directly confrontational means may be necessary.

Another important component in the treatment of patients with factitious disorder is the coordination of health care among all providers. This allows for fewer unnecessary interventions, minimizes splitting among the health care team, and allows the health care team to vent and process the strong emotions that arise when caring for factitious patients. This decreases both the negative impact on the providers and the chance that anger will be acted out on the patient.

There are no clear data supporting the effectiveness of medications in treating factitious disorder. There is a case report of effective pimozide treatment in a patient thought to have delusional symptoms (Prior and Gordon, 1997), as well as a case report of a factitious patient with comorbid depression improving when treated with an antidepressant in addition to intensive psychotherapy.

While many patients with factitious disorder are hesitant to pursue psychiatric treatment, there are numerous case reports of successful treatment of the disorder with long-term psychotherapy. In many of these cases, the therapy lasted several years, including one patient who received treatment while imprisoned for over 10 years. Plassman reports a case series of 24 factitious patients. Twelve of these patients accepted psychotherapy and 10 continued with long-term treatment, lasting up to 4½ years. He reports "significant, or at least marked, improvement" in those 10 patients (Plassmann, 1994b). These case reports support the idea that treatment of patients with factitious disorder is not impossible, and these patients can improve. However, expectations must be realistic as improvement in the disorder itself can take several years. Techniques that target short-term reduction in the production of factitious symptoms can be effective more quickly. See Figure 55.2 for a treatment flowchart for factitious disorder.

Ethical Considerations

Treating patients with factitious disorder often raises ethical questions including those regarding confidentiality, privacy and medical decision-making, and it is important to be alert to these issues. Often, patients with factious disorder will want to keep their diagnosis confidential, even when to do so may harm the patient or others. For example, although a consulting physician may diagnose a patient with factitious disorder, the patient may refuse consent to reveal this information to the referring physician. If the consultant does inform the referring physician, she has violated the patient's confidentiality, but if she does not, the referring physician is likely to continue to treat the patient for the incorrect diagnosis. Dilemmas regarding patient privacy also arise with factitious patients. For example, hospital room searches could often help clarify the diagnosis or remove materials the patient is using to harm himself, but these searches also violate the patient's privacy. Dilemmas surrounding medical decision-making can arise when a patient with factitious disorder refuses treatment or requests potentially harmful treatments. It can often be difficult to resolve these ethical dilemmas. In general, even though the factitious patient is deceptive within the doctor–patient relationship, the physician is not released from his or her responsibilities within that relationship, and the patient retains his or her rights of confidentiality, privacy and autonomy. As with all patients, emergency situations require different ethical guidelines. Often, an ethics consultation can be very helpful in sorting through the difficult issues of patient care in the setting of factitious disorder.

Factitious Disorder by Proxy

In factitious disorder by proxy, one person creates or feigns illness in another person, usually a child, though occasionally the victim is an elder or developmentally delayed adult. Factitious

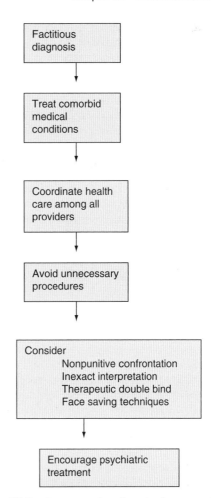

Figure 55.2 *Treatment flowchart for factitious disorder.*

disorder by proxy is not defined as a specific disorder in DSM-IV but instead is listed under the "not otherwise specified" heading with research criteria included. While rare instances of fathers perpetrating factitious disorder by proxy have been reported, the perpetrator is usually the mother. Usually the victim is a preverbal child. While numerous symptoms have been reported, common presentations include apnea, seizures and gastrointestinal problems. The mothers appear extremely caring and attentive

---

DSM-IV-TR Criteria

Factitious Disorder by Proxy

A. Intentional production of or feigning of physical or psychological signs or symptoms in another person who is under the individual's care.

B. The motivation for the perpetrator's behavior is to assume the sick role by proxy.

C. External incentives for the behavior (such as economic gain) are absent.

D. The behavior is no better accounted for by another mental disorder.

Reprinted with permission from the *Diagnostic and Statistical Manual of Mental Disorders*, Fourth Edition, Text Revision. Copyright 2000 American Psychiatric Association.

when observed, but appear indifferent to the child when they are not aware of being observed (Eisendrath, 2001).

As in factitious disorder, the exact prevalence of factitious disorder by proxy is unknown. There have been studies of the annual incidence of factitious disorder by proxy in the general population in both the UK and New Zealand. In the former, the annual incidence of factitious disorder by proxy in children less than 16 years was found to be 2.0/100 000 (18 total cases) and in the latter, the annual incidence in children under 16 was 0.5/100 000 (128 total cases). As for the incidence within clinical populations, an Argentinean survey of 113 children with FUO found four (3.5%) cases of factitious fever. A survey of 20 090 children brought in with apnea found 54 (0.27%) to be victims of factitious disorder by proxy (Kravitz and Willmott, 1990). Finally, a review of children brought in for treatment of acute, life threatening episodes of diverse etiologies ranging from seizure disorders to electrolyte abnormalities found 1.5% to be factitious (Rahilly, 1991). Factitious disorder by proxy appears to have a much higher mortality rate than self-inflicted factitious disorder. In Rosenberg's survey of 117 victims, there was a 9% mortality rate (Rosenberg, 1987), and of the 54 victims of the disorder in the apnea survey, three index cases and five siblings were dead at follow-up (Kravitz and Wilmott, 1990). More recently, McClure found that eight of 128 index cases in the UK were fatal (6.25%) (McClure *et al.*, 1996) while Denny reported no fatalities in 18 index cases (Denny *et al.*, 2001).

The diagnosis of factitious disorder by proxy is usually made by having an index of suspicion in a child with unexplained illnesses. The diagnosis is supported if symptoms occur only in the parent's presence and resolve with separation. Covert video surveillance has been used to diagnose this condition, though it raises questions of invasion of privacy. In general, it has been felt that the welfare of the child overrides the parent's right to privacy.

As counterintuitive as it is to comprehend why anyone would induce illness in oneself, it can be even more difficult to understand inducing illness in one's own child. The perpetrator in factitious disorder by proxy appears to seek not the "sick role" but the "parent to the sick child" role. This role is similar to the sick role in that it provides structure, attention from others, caring and relief from usual responsibilities. The parent also receives some psychological benefit from inducing illness in his or her child. Based on case reports, the parent often has a comorbid personality disorder and a history of family dysfunction.

Treatment

Due to the high morbidity and mortality, treatment requires at least temporary separation from the parent and notification of local child protective agencies. The perpetrators often face criminal charges of child abuse. There is high psychiatric morbidity in the children: many go on to develop factitious disorder or other psychiatric illnesses themselves. Psychiatric intervention is necessary to ameliorate this morbidity as much as possible in these children. There are some case reports of successful psychotherapeutic treatments of the parents in this disorder.

Summary

Patients with factitious disorder seek, often desperately, the sick role. Due to the nature of the disorder, the literature on factitious disorder is largely confined to case reports and case series, limiting the information available. Patients with factitious disorder present

with a broad spectrum of signs and symptoms, and effective diagnosis often requires a high index of suspicion. The differential diagnosis of factitious disorder includes physical illness, somatoform disorders, malingering, psychiatric illness and substance abuse. While factitious disorder is extremely difficult to cure, effective techniques exist to minimize morbidity, and some patients are able to benefit greatly from psychiatric intervention.

Comparison of DSM-IV/ICD-10 Diagnostic Criteria

The ICD-10 Diagnostic Criteria for Research and the DSM-IV criteria sets are almost identical.

References

American Psychiatric Association (2000) *Diagnostic and Statistical Manual of Mental Disorders*, 4th edn., Text Rev. APA, Washington DC.

Asher R (1951) Munchausen's syndrome. *Lancet* i, 339–341.

Denny SJ, Grant CC and Pinnock R (2001) Epidemiology of Munchausen syndrome by proxy in New Zealand. *J Paediatr Child Health* 37(3) (June), 240–243.

Ehlers W and Plassmann R (1994) Diagnosis of narcissistic self-esteem regulation in patients with factitious illness (Munchausen syndrome). *Psychother Psychosom* 62(1–2), 69–77.

Eisendrath SJ (2001) Factitious disorders and malingering, in *Treatment of Psychiatric Disorders*, 3rd edn., (ed Gabbard GO). American Psychiatric Publishing, Washington DC, pp. 1825–1844.

Gault MH, Campbell NR and Aksu AE (1988) Spurious stones. *Nephron* 48(4), 274–279.

Gurwith M and Langston C (1980) Factitious Munchausen's syndrome. *New Engl J Med* 302(26) (June), 1483–1484.

King BH and Ford CV (1988) Pseudologia fantastica. *Acta Psychiatr Scand* 77(1) (Jan), 1–6.

Kravitz RM and Wilmott RW (1990) Munchausen syndrome by proxy presenting as factitious apnea. *Clin Pediatr (Phila)* 29(10) (Oct), 587–592.

McClure RJ, Davis PM, Meadow SR *et al.* (1996) Epidemiology of Munchausen syndrome by proxy, nonaccidental poisoning, and nonaccidental suffocation. *Arch Dis Child* 75(1) (July), 57–61.

McKane JP and Anderson J (1997) Munchausen's syndrome: Rule breakers and risk takers. *Br J Hosp Med* 58(4) (Aug 207–Sep 2), 150–153.

Merrin EL, Van Dyke C, Cohen S *et al.* (1986) Dual factitious disorder. *Gen Hosp Psychiatry* 8(4) (July), 246–250.

Parker PE (1993) A case report of Munchausen syndrome with mixed psychological features. *Psychosomatics* 34(4) (July–Aug), 360–364.

Parsons T (1951) *The Social Structure*. Free Press, Glencoe, Illinois, pp. 436–439.

Plassmann R (1994a) Munchausen's syndrome and factitious diseases. *Psychother Psychosom* 62(1–2), 7–26.

Plassmann R (1994b) Inpatient and outpatient long-term psychotherapy of patients suffering from factitious disorders. *Psychother Psychosom* 62(1–2), 96–107.

Prior TI and Gordon A (1997) Treatment of factitious disorder with pimozide. *Can J Psychiatr* 42(5) (June), 532.

Rahilly PM (1991) The pneumographic and medical investigation of infants suffering apparent life threatening episodes. *J Paediatr Child Health* 27(6) (Dec), 349–353.

Reich P and Gottfried LA (1983) Factitious disorders in a teaching hospital. *Ann Int Med* 99(2) (Aug), 240–247.

Rosenberg DA (1987) Web of deceit: A literature review of Munchausen syndrome by proxy. *Child Abuse Neglect* 11(4), 547–563.

Wise MG and Ford CV (1999) Factitious disorders. *Prim Care* 26(2) (June), 315–326.

56 Dissociative Disorders

Dissociative phenomena are best understood through the term *désagrégation* (disaggregation) originally given by Janet (1920). Events normally experienced as connected to one another on a smooth continuum are isolated from the other mental processes with which they would ordinarily be associated. The dissociative disorders are a disturbance in the organization of identity, memory, perception, or consciousness. When memories are separated from access to consciousness, the disorder is dissociative amnesia. Fragmentation of identity results in dissociative fugue or dissociative identity disorder (DID; formerly multiple personality disorder). Disintegrated perception is characteristic of depersonalization disorder. Dissociation of aspects of consciousness produces acute stress disorder and various dissociative trance and possession states. Numbing and amnesia are diagnostic components of post traumatic stress disorder (PTSD). These dissociative and related disorders are more a disturbance in the organization or structure of mental contents than in the contents themselves. Memories in dissociative amnesia are not so much distorted or bizarre as they are segregated from one another. The identities lost in dissociative fugue or fragmented in DID are two-dimensional aspects of an overall personality structure. In this sense, patients with DID suffer not from having more than one personality but rather from having less than one personality. The problem involves information processing: the failure of integration of elements rather than the contents of the fragments.

The dissociative disorders have a long history in classical psychopathology, being the foundation on which Freud began his explorations of the unconscious and Janet developed dissociation theory. Although much attention in psychiatry has shifted to diagnosis and treatment of mood, anxiety and thought disorders, dissociative phenomena are sufficiently persistent and interesting that they have elicited growing attention from both professionals and the public. There are at least four reasons for this:

1. They are fascinating phenomena in and of themselves, involving the loss of or change in identity, or memory, or a feeling of detachment from extreme and traumatic physical events.
2. Dissociative disorders seem to arise in response to traumatic stress.
3. Dissociative disorders remain an area of psychopathology for which the best treatment is psychotherapy, although adjunctive pharmacological interventions can be helpful.
4. Dissociation as a phenomenon has much to teach us about information processing in the brain.

Development of the Concept
The dissociative disorders might have been studied more intensively during the 20th century had not Janet's and Charcot's work

been so thoroughly eclipsed by Freud's psychoanalytic theory, emphasizing as it did repression rather than dissociation.

Hilgard (1977) developed a neodissociation theory that revived interest in Janetian psychology and dissociative psychopathology. He postulated divisions in mental structure that were horizontal rather than vertical, as was the case in Freud's archeological model. This model allowed for immediate access to consciousness of any of a variety of warded-off memories, which is not the case in Freud's system. In the dynamic unconscious model, repressed memories must first go through a process of transformation as they are accessed and lifted from the depths of the unconscious, for example, through the interpretation of dreams or slips of the tongue. In Hilgard's model, amnesia is a crucial mediating mechanism that creates barriers dividing one set of mental contents from another. Thus, flexible use of amnesia is conceptualized as a key defensive strategy. Therefore, reversal of amnesia is an important therapeutic tool.

Repression as a general model for keeping information out of conscious awareness differs from dissociation in four important ways:

1. In repression, information is disguised as well as hidden. Dissociated information is stored in a discrete and untransformed manner, for example, as a memory of some element of a traumatic experience, whereas repressed information is usually disguised and fragmented. Even when repressed information becomes available to consciousness, its meaning is hidden, for example, in dreams or slips of the tongue.
2. Retrieval of repressed information requires translation. Retrieval of dissociated information can often be direct. Techniques such as hypnosis can be used to access warded-off memories. By contrast, uncovering of repressed information often requires repeated recall trials through intense questioning, psychotherapy, or psychoanalysis with subsequent interpretation (i.e., of dreams).
3. Repressed information is not discretely organized temporally. The information kept out of awareness in dissociation is often for a discrete and sharply delimited time, whereas repressed information may be for a type of encounter or experience scattered across times.
4. Repression is less specifically tied to trauma. Dissociation seems to be elicited as a defense most commonly after episodes of physical trauma, whereas repression is in response to warded-off fears, wishes and other dynamic conflicts.

Whether dissociation is a subtype of repression or vice versa, both are important methods for managing complex and affectively charged information. Given the complexity of human information processing, the synthesis of perception, cognition and

Essentials of Psychiatry   Jerald Kay and Allan Tasman
© 2006 John Wiley & Sons, Ltd.

Table 56.1	Models of Mental Experience	
Mental Function	Dissociation	Repression
Organization	Horizontal	Vertical
Barriers	Amnesia	Dynamic conflict
Etiology	Trauma	Developmental conflict over unacceptable wishes
Nature of contents	Untransformed: traumatic memories	Disguised, primary process: dreams, slips
Means of access	Hypnosis	Interpretation
Treatment	Psychotherapy emphasizing access, control, and working through traumatic memories	Psychotherapy emphasizing interpretation, transference

DSM-IV-TR Criteria 308.12

Dissociative

A. The predominant disturbance is one or more episodes of inability to recall important personal information, usually of a traumatic or stressful nature, that is too extensive to be explained by ordinary forgetfulness.

B. The disturbance does not occur exclusively during the course of dissociative identity disorder, dissociative fugue, posttraumatic stress disorder, acute stress disorder, or somatization disorder and is not due to the direct physiological effects of a substance (e.g., a drug of abuse, a medication) or a neurological or other general medical condition (e.g., amnestic disorder due to head trauma).

C. The symptoms cause clinically significant distress or impairment in social, occupational, or other important areas of functioning.

Reprinted with permission from the *Diagnostic and Statistical Manual of Mental Disorders*, Fourth Edition, Text Revision. Copyright 2000 American Psychiatric Association.

affect is a major task. Mental function is composed of a variety of reasonably autonomous subsystems involving a perception, memory storage and retrieval, intention and action. Indeed, the accomplishment of a sense of mental unity is an achievement, not a given. It is remarkable not that dissociative disorders occur at all, but rather that they do not occur more often. Models of mental experience are presented in Table 56.1.

Epidemiology

Dissociative disorders are not among the more common psychiatric illnesses but are not rare. Few good epidemiological studies have been performed. Some estimate the prevalence at only 1 per 10 000 in the population, but far higher proportions are reported among psychiatric populations. In fact, the prevalence of the disorder seems to be associated to the specific population under study. For example, data from the general population suggest that the numbers are as high as 1%. On the other hand, the data seem to indicate that the numbers are even higher in specialized inpatient populations, as high as 3%.

There has been a rise in reported cases, which may be attributed to greater awareness of the diagnosis among mental health professionals, to the availability of specific criteria, and to previous misdiagnosis of DID as schizophrenia or borderline personality disorder. Some experts attribute possible underdiagnosis to family disavowal of sexual and physical abuse. However, there is also controversy about possible overdiagnosis of the syndrome, while others propose that the increase is the result of hypnotic suggestion and inadequate handling by therapists. Individuals who most commonly have the disorder are highly hypnotizable and therefore especially sensitive to suggestion or cultural influences. Although psychiatrists' expectations amplified with hypnosis may account for some cases, they cannot account for many patients diagnosed without benefit of hypnosis or by "skeptical" psychiatrists.

Women make-up the majority of cases, accounting for 90% of the cases or more, in some studies. Strangely, the most common dissociative disorder diagnosis falls into the "not otherwise specified" category, both in the USA and in nonWestern countries, where dissociative trance and possession trance are the most common dissociative disorder diagnoses. Dissociative disorders are ubiquitous around the world, although the structure of the symptoms varies across cultures. Indeed, the symptomatology reflects cultural biases. In Western cultures, which emphasize the importance of the individual, dissociation often takes the form of dissociated elements of individual personality, while in Eastern cultures, which are more sociocentric, possession trance, in which patients feel themselves to be taken over by an outside entity or entities, is more common.

Diagnostic Criteria and Treatment

Dissociative Amnesia

This is the classical functional disorder of episodic memory. It does not involve procedural memory or problems in memory storage, as in Wernicke–Korsakoff syndrome. Furthermore, unlike dementing illnesses, dissociative amnesia is reversible for example, by using hypnosis or narcoanalysis. It has three primary characteristics:

1. Type of memory lost: The memory loss is episodic. The first-person recollection of certain events, rather than knowledge of procedures, is lost.
2. Temporal structure: The memory loss is for one or more discrete time periods, ranging from minutes to years. It is not vagueness or inefficient retrieval of memories but rather a dense unavailability of memories that were encoded and stored. Unlike the situation in amnestic disorders, for example, resulting from damage to the medial temporal lobe in surgery (the case of H.M. [Milner, 1959]), in Wernicke–Korsakoff syndrome, or in Alzheimer's dementia, there is usually no difficulty in learning new episodic information. Thus, the amnesia

of dissociative disorders is typically retrograde rather than anterograde. However, a dissociative syndrome of continuous difficulty in incorporating new information that mimics organic amnestic syndromes has been observed.

3. Type of events forgotten: The memory loss is usually for events of a traumatic or stressful nature. This fact has been noted in the language of the DSM-IV diagnostic criteria. In one study (Coons and Milstein, 1986), the majority of cases involved child abuse (60%) but disavowed behaviors such as marital problems, sexual activity, suicide attempts, criminal activity, and the death of a relative have also been reported as precipitants.

Dissociative amnesia most frequently occurs after an episode of trauma, and its onset may be gradual or sudden.

Dissociative amnesia occurs most often in the third and fourth decades of life. It usually involves one episode, but multiple periods of lost memory are not uncommon. Comorbidity with conversion disorder, bulimia nervosa, alcohol abuse and depression are common, and Axis II diagnoses of histrionic, dependent, or borderline personality disorders occur in a substantial minority of such patients.

Such individuals typically demonstrate not vagueness or spotty memory but rather a loss of any episodic memory for a finite period. They may not initially be aware of the memory loss; that is, they do not remember that they do not remember. They often report being told that they have done or said things that they cannot remember.

Some individuals do suffer from episodes of selective amnesia, usually for specific traumatic incidents, which may be interwoven with periods of intact memory. In these cases, the amnesia is for a type of material remembered rather than for a discrete time period.

Implicit Effects of Dissociated Memories

Although information is kept out of consciousness in dissociative amnesia, it may well exert an influence on consciousness: out of sight does not mean out of mind. For example, a rape victim with no conscious recollection of an assault nonetheless behaves like someone who has been sexually victimized. Such individuals often suffer detachment and demoralization, are unable to enjoy intimate relationships, and show hyperarousal to stimuli reminiscent of the trauma. This loss of explicit memory with retention of implicit knowledge is similar to priming in memory research. Individuals who have read a word in a list complete a word stem (a partial word such as "pre" for "present") more quickly if they have seen that word minutes or even hours earlier. This priming effect occurs despite the fact that they cannot consciously recall having read the word, or even the list in which it occurred. When asked in a free recall format to list the word they have seen, they cannot name it, yet they act as though they have seen it and do remember it. Similarly, individuals instructed in hypnosis to forget having seen a list of words nonetheless demonstrate priming effects of the hypnotically suppressed list. It is the essence of dissociative amnesia that material kept out of conscious awareness is nonetheless active and may influence consciousness indirectly.

Individuals with dissociative amnesia generally do not suffer disturbances of identity, except to the extent that their identity is influenced by the warded-off memory. It is not uncommon for such individuals to develop depressive symptoms as well, especially when the amnesia occurs in the wake of a traumatic stressor.

Treatment

Psychotherapy
Often, patients suffering from dissociative amnesia experience spontaneous recovery when they are removed from the stressful or threatening situation, when they feel safe, and/or when exposed to personal cues from their past (i.e., home, pets, family members). In cases where exposure to a safe environment is not enough to restore normal memory functioning, pharmacologically-facilitated interviews may prove useful.

Hypnosis
Most patients with dissociative disorder are highly hypnotizable on formal testing and are therefore easily able to make use of hypnotic techniques such as age regression. Hypnosis can enable such patients to reorient temporally and therefore achieve access to otherwise dissociated and unavailable memories.

Abreaction
If there is traumatic content to the warded-off memory, patients may abreact, that is, express strong emotion as these memories are elicited. Such abreactions are rarely damaging in themselves but are not intrinsically therapeutic either. They may be experienced by the patient as a reinflicting of the traumatic stressor. Such patients need psychotherapeutic help in integrating these warded-off memories and the associated affect into consciousness, thereby gaining a sense of mastery over them.

Screen Technique
One technique that can help bring such memories into consciousness while modulating the affective response to them is a projective technique known as "the screen technique" (Spiegel, 1981). While using hypnosis, such patients are taught to recall the traumatic event as if they were watching it on an imaginary movie or television screen. This technique is often helpful for individuals who are unable to remember the event as if it were occurring in the present, either because for some highly hypnotizable individuals that approach is too emotionally taxing or because others are not sufficiently hypnotizable to be able to engage in such hypnotic age regression. The screen can be employed to facilitate cognitive restructuring of the traumatic memory, for example, by picturing on the left side of the screen some component of the traumatic experience, and on the right side something they did to protect themselves or someone else during it. This makes the memory both more complex and more bearable.

A particularly useful feature of this technique is that it allows for the recollection of traumatic events without triggering an uncontrolled reliving of the trauma, as is the case of traumatic flashbacks. The screen technique provides a "controlled dissociation" between the psychological and somatic aspects of memory retrieval. Individuals can be put into self-hypnosis and instructed to get their body into a state of floating comfort and safety. They can do this by imagining that they are somewhere safe and comfortable: "Imagine that you are floating in a bath, a lake, a hot tub, or just floating in space". They are reminded that no matter what they see on the screen their bodies are safe and comfortable: "Do the work on your imaginary screen, not in your body". In this way the tendency for physiological arousal to accompany and intensify the working through of traumatic memories can be controlled, facilitating the psychotherapeutic work.

The psychotherapy of dissociative amnesia involves accessing the dissociated memories, working through affectively loaded aspects of these memories, and supporting the patient through the process of integrating these memories into consciousness.

Dissociative Fugue

Dissociative fugue combines failure of integration of certain aspects of personal memory with loss of customary identity and automatisms of motor behavior. It involves one or more episodes of sudden, unexpected, purposeful travel away from home, coupled with an inability to recall portions or all of one's past, and a loss of identity or the assumption of a new identity. The onset is usually sudden, and it frequently occurs after a traumatic experience or bereavement. A single episode is not uncommon, and spontaneous remission of symptoms can occur without treatment. Dissociative fugue has the identical DSM-IV TR criteria as that of dissociative amnesia with the exception that it involves travel.

It was originally thought that the assumption of a new identity, as in the classical case of the Reverend Ansel Bourne (James, 1984), was typical of dissociative fugue. However, a review of the literature shows that in the majority of cases there is loss of personal identity but no clear assumption of a new identity.

Many cases of dissociative fugue remit spontaneously. Again, hypnosis can be useful in accessing dissociated material. Not infrequently, fugue episodes represent dissociated but purposeful activity.

Hypnosis can be helpful in treating dissociative fugue by accessing otherwise unavailable components of memory and identity. The approach used is similar to that for dissociative amnesia. Hypnotic age regression can be used as the framework for accessing information available at a previous time. Demonstrating to patients that such information can be made available to consciousness enhances their sense of control over this material and facilitates therapeutic working through of emotionally laden aspects of it.

Once reorientation is established and the overt identity and memory loss of the fugue have been resolved, it is important to work through interpersonal or intrapsychic issues that underlie the dissociative defenses. Such individuals are often relatively unaware of their reactions to stress because they can so effectively dissociate them. Thus, effective psychotherapy is anticipatory, helping patients to recognize and modify their tendency to set aside their own feelings in favor of those of others.

Patients with dissociative fugue may be helped with a psychotherapeutic approach that facilitates conscious integration of dissociated memories and motivations for behavior previously experienced as automatic and unwilled. It is often helpful to address current psychosocial stressors, such as marital conflict, with the involved individuals, as in the case of the woman found on the army base. To the extent that current psychosocial stress triggers fugue, resolution of that stress can help resolve it and reduce the likelihood of recurrence. Highly hypnotizable individuals prone to these extreme dissociative symptoms often have great difficulty in asserting their own point of view in a personal relationship. Rather, they interact with others as though they were undergoing a spontaneous trance experience. One such individual described herself as a "disciple in search of a teacher". Psychotherapy can help such individuals recognize and modify

their tendency to unthinking compliance with others and extreme sensitivity to rejection and disapproval.

In the past, medication facilitated interviews were used to reverse dissociative amnesia or fugue. However, such techniques offer no advantage over hypnosis and are not especially effective. Not infrequently, the ceremony of injecting the drug elicits spontaneous hypnotic phenomena before the pharmacological effect is felt, and sedation, respiratory depression and other side effects can be troublesome. It also promotes dependency on the therapist. On the contrary, when hypnosis is used, patients are trained on self-hypnotic techniques, promoting the use of hypnosis instead of spontaneous dissociation. This enhances the patients' level of control while enhancing a sense of mastery and self-control.

Clinical Vignette 1

A woman who appeared dazed but physically unharmed was brought into an army hospital emergency department by the base guards because she had been found wandering nearby. She said that she did not know who she was, where she lived, or how she happened to be there. Initially, plans were made to admit her to the hospital for a full neurological and psychiatric evaluation. She proved to be highly hypnotizable, and hypnosis age regression was used to take her back to an earlier year. She then reported her name and that she lived some 500 miles away. The time was changed again to a period just before this apparent fugue episode. She reported having received unsigned letters from someone at that army base, where, it turned out, her husband was stationed. These letters suggested that her husband was having an affair. This had deeply upset her. She and her husband were reunited and reconciled, and the fugue episode ended.

Depersonalization Disorder

This dissociative disorder involves lack of integration of one or more components of perception. The essential feature of depersonalization disorder is the occurrence of persistent feelings of unreality, detachment, or estrangement from oneself or one's body, usually with the feeling that one is an outside observer of one's own mental processes (American Psychiatric Association, 2000). Individuals suffering depersonalization are distressed by it. They are aware of some distortion in their perceptual experience and therefore are not hallucinating or delusional. Affected individuals often fear that they are "going crazy". The symptom is not infrequently transient.

Derealization, in which affected individuals notice an altered perception of their surroundings, resulting in the world seeming unreal or dream-like, frequently occurs as well. Such individuals often ruminate anxiously about this symptom and are preoccupied with their own somatic and mental functioning.

Depersonalization frequently cooccurs with a variety of other symptoms, especially anxiety, panic, or phobic symptoms. It is often a symptom of PTSD and also occurs as a symptom of alcohol and drug abuse, as a side effect of the use of prescription medication, and during stress and sensory deprivation. The symptom of depersonalization is also commonly seen in the course of a number of other neurological and psychiatric disorders. It is considered a disorder when it is a persistent and predominant symptom. The phenomenology of the disorder involves both the initial symptoms themselves and the reactive anxiety caused by them.

Treatment

Depersonalization is most often transient and may remit without formal treatment. Recurrent or persistent depersonalization should be thought of both as a symptom in itself and as a component of other syndromes requiring treatment, such as anxiety disorders and schizophrenia.

DSM-IV-TR Criteria 300.6

Depersonalization Disorder

A. Persistent or recurrent experiences of feeling detached from, and as if one is an outside observer of, one's mental processes or body (e.g., feeling like one is in a dream).

B. During the depersonalization experience, reality testing remains intact.

C. The depersonalization causes clinically significant distress or impairment in social, occupational, or other important areas of functioning.

D. The depersonalization experience does not occur exclusively during the course of another mental disorder, such as schizophrenia, panic disorder, acute stress disorder, or another dissociative disorder, and is not due to the direct physiological effects of a substance (e.g., a drug of abuse, a medication) or a general medical condition (e.g., temporal lobe epilepsy).

Reprinted with permission from the *Diagnostic and Statistical Manual of Mental Disorders*, Fourth Edition, Text Revision. Copyright 2000 American Psychiatric Association.

The symptom itself may respond to training in self-hypnosis. Paradoxically, induction or deliberate worsening of symptoms may provide relief by teaching a method of controlling them. For example, a hypnotic induction may induce transient depersonalization symptoms, such as a sense of detachment from part of the body, in such individuals. This is a useful exercise, in that by having a structure for inducing the symptoms, one provides the patient with a context for understanding and controlling them. They are presented as a spontaneous form of hypnotic dissociation that can be modified. Such individuals can be taught to induce a pleasant sense of floating lightness or heaviness in place of the anxiety-related somatic detachment. The use of an imaginary screen to picture problems in a way that detaches them from the typical somatic response is also helpful. Other relaxation techniques such as systematic desensitization, progressive muscle relaxation and biofeedback may also be of help. Psychotherapy aimed at working through emotional responses to any traumatic or other stressors that tend to elicit the depersonalization is also helpful.

Pharmacological approaches involve balancing therapeutic benefit and risk. Antianxiety medications are most commonly used and may be helpful in reducing the amplification of depersonalization caused by anxiety. However, depersonalization and derealization are also side effects of antianxiety drugs, so their use should be carefully monitored. Increasing dosage, a standard technique when there is lack of therapeutic response, may also increase symptoms, leading to a spiral of increasing symptoms and drug dosage but without therapeutic benefit.

However, appropriate pharmacological treatment for comorbid disorders is an important part of treatment. Use of antianxiety medications for generalized anxiety or phobic disorders or of antipsychotic medications for psychotic disorders is often beneficial in conditions in which there is contributory comorbidity.

Dissociative Identity Disorder (Multiple Personality Disorder)

Dissociative identity disorder is a rare but real disorder that is the most widely discussed of the dissociative disorders. It involves the "presence of two or more distinct identities or personality states (each with its own relatively enduring pattern of perceiving, relating to, and thinking about the environment and self)" (American Psychiatric Association, 2000). The diagnostic criteria also require that "At least two of these identities or personality states recurrently take control of the person's behavior" (American Psychiatric Association, 2000), and that there be amnesia: "Inability to recall important personal information that is too extensive to be explained by ordinary forgetfulness" (American Psychiatric Association, 2000). It is a failure of integration of various aspects of identity and personality structure. Often different relationship styles (dependent versus assertive/aggressive) and mood states (depressed versus hostile) segregate with different identities and personal memories. Such patients may be mystified by events that occurred in another "state", or by responses of others to them for behavior that occurred in a different "state". This fragmentation of personality often occurs in response to trauma in childhood, and is perceived by the patient as protective, allowing him or her to tolerate and partially evade chronic abuse. These patients thus view treatment ambivalently as an attempt to deprive them of a defense against attack. They also tend to see others as irrational

---

DSM-IV-TR Criteria 308.14

Dessociative Identity Disorder

A. The presence of two or more distinct identities or personality states (each with its own relatively enduring pattern of perceiving, relating to, and thinking about the environment and self).

B. At least two of these identities or personality states recurrently take control of the person's behavior.

C. Inability to recall important personal information that is too extensive to be explained by ordinary forgetfulness.

D. The disturbance is not due to the direct physiological effects of a substance (e.g., blackouts or chaotic behavior during alcohol intoxication) or a general medical condition (e.g., complex partial seizures). **Note:** In children, the symptoms are not attributable to imaginary playmates or other fantasy play.

Reprinted with permission from the *Diagnostic and Statistical Manual of Mental Disorders*, Fourth Edition, Text Revision. Copyright 2000 American Psychiatric Association.

and unfair, since response to one aspect of their personality frequently reflects experience with other aspects. One DID patient (prior to diagnosis) reported puzzlement about accusations by friends and acquaintances that she had made hostile comments for which she had no memory. She would find people angry at her for no reason. Thus their personality fragmentation renders them vulnerable to interpersonal problems yet gives them the belief that they are relatively protected from them.

Prevalence

There are no convincing studies of the absolute prevalence of DID, although there is widespread agreement that the number of diagnosed cases has increased considerably in the USA and some European countries in the past two decades. Two studies have estimated the prevalence as approximately 1% of psychiatric inpatients (Saxe *et al.*, 1993; Ross *et al.*, 1991). Factors that may account for the increase in the number of true reported cases include 1) more general awareness of the diagnosis among mental health professionals, 2) the availability of specific diagnostic criteria starting with DSM-III and 3) reduced misdiagnosis of DID as schizophrenia or borderline personality disorder.

Other authors attribute the increase in reported cases to social contagion, hypnotic suggestion and misdiagnosis Proponents of this point of view argue that these individuals are highly hypnotizable and therefore quite suggestible. They would therefore be especially vulnerable to direct or implicit hypnotic suggestion. They note that not infrequently a few specialist psychiatrists make the vast majority of diagnoses. However, it has been observed that the symptoms of patients diagnosed by specialists in dissociation do not differ from those of patients diagnosed by psychiatrists, psychologists and physicians in more general practice who diagnose one or two cases a year. Furthermore, such patients have been noted to persist in presenting symptoms for an average of 6.5 years before attaining the diagnosis. They encounter many psychiatrists who are convinced that they do not have DID and that they have some other disorder, such as schizophrenia. Were they so easily suggestible, it seems likely that they would accept a suggestion that they have other disorders as well, such as schizophrenia or borderline personality disorder.

Nonetheless, because these patients are indeed highly hypnotizable and therefore suggestible, care must be taken in the manner in which the illness is presented to them. However, it is unlikely that the increased number of cases currently reported is accounted for by suggestion alone. Reduction in previous misdiagnosis and increased recognition of the prevalence and sequelae of physical and sexual abuse in childhood are also reasonable explanations.

Course

The disorder is more frequently recognized during childhood but typically emerges between adolescence and the third decade of life; it rarely presents as a new disorder after age 40 years, but there is often considerable delay between initial symptom presentation and diagnosis.

Untreated, it is a chronic and recurrent disorder. It rarely remits spontaneously, but the symptoms may not be evident for certain time periods. DID has been called "a disease of hiddenness" (Schacter, 1995). The dissociation itself hampers self-monitoring and accurate reporting of symptoms and history. Many patients with the disorder are not fully aware of the extent of their dissociative symptoms. They may be reluctant to bring up symptoms because of confusion or shame about the illness

or because they encountered previous skepticism. Furthermore, because the majority of patients report histories of sexual and physical abuse, the shame associated with that and fear of retribution may inhibit reporting of symptoms as well.

Comorbidity

The major comorbid psychiatric illnesses are the depressive disorders, substance use disorders and borderline personality disorder. Sexual, eating, and sleep disorders cooccur less commonly. Such patients frequently display self-mutilative behavior, impulsiveness, and overvaluing and devaluing of relationships. Indeed, approximately a third of patients with DID have symptoms that fit criteria for borderline personality disorder as well. Such individuals are also more frequently depressed. Conversely, research shows dissociative symptoms in many patients with borderline personality disorder, especially those who report histories of physical and sexual abuse. Indeed, the impulsiveness, splitting, hostility and fear of abandonment, frequently seen in certain personality states, are similar to the presentation of many patients with borderline personality disorder. Many such patients also have symptoms that meet criteria for PTSD, with intrusive flashbacks, recurrent dreams of physical and sexual abuse, avoidance of and loss of pleasure in usually pleasurable activities, and symptoms of hyperarousal, especially when exposed to reminders of childhood trauma.

Thus, comorbidity is a complex issue. In addition, these patients are not infrequently misdiagnosed as having schizophrenia (Kluft, 1987). This diagnostic confusion is understandable in that they have an apparent delusion that their bodies are occupied by more than one person. In addition, they frequently have auditory hallucinations when one personality state speaks to or comments on the activities of another. When misdiagnosed as schizophrenic, patients with DID are frequently given neuroleptics, which results in a poor therapeutic response and a flattening of affect, which tends to confirm the misdiagnosis (since flat affect is characteristic of schizophrenia).

Individuals with DID commonly report somatic or conversion symptoms and other psychosomatic symptoms, such as migraine headaches. Studies have shown that approximately a third of these patients have complex partial seizures (Schenk and Bear, 1981), although later studies did not show seizure rates that high. Furthermore, the studies did not show substantial elevations in scores on Dissociative Experiences Scale in patients with complex partial seizures as compared with those of other neurological patients (Loewenstein and Putnam, 1988). However, there is sufficient comorbidity that patients recently diagnosed with DID should be evaluated for the possibility of a seizure disorder.

Psychological Testing

The diagnosis can be facilitated by psychological testing. Scales of trait dissociation have been developed (Bernstein and Putnam, 1986; Ross, 1989; Carlson *et al.*, 1993), and patients with DID score extremely high on these scales, in contrast to normal populations and other groups of patients. Those with DID score far higher than normal individuals on standard measures of hypnotizability, whereas schizophrenic patients tend to have lower than normal scores or the absence of high hypnotizability. Thus, there is comparatively little overlap in the hypnotizability scores of patients with schizophrenia and those with DID. Form level on the Rorschach test is usually within the normal range, but there are frequent emotionally dramatic responses, often involving mutilation (especially with the color cards) of a type that is often seen in histrionic personality disorder as well. Form level is an assessment of the match between the percept (what the subject reports seeing) and the inkblot structure. Good form level involves relatively little distortion of the image to match percept to inkblot. Good form level is useful in distinguishing patients with DID from those with schizophrenia, who have poor form level.

Treatment

Psychotherapy

Therapeutic Direction

It is possible to help patients with DID gain control over the dissociative process underlying their symptoms in several ways. The fundamental psychotherapeutic stance should involve meeting patients halfway, a form of structured empathy in which their experience of themselves as fragmented is acknowledged while the reality that the fundamental problem is a failure of integration of disparate memories and aspects of the self is kept in view. In this sense, such individuals suffer from having less than one personality rather than more than one. Therefore, the goal in therapy is to facilitate integration of disparate elements. This can be done in a variety of ways.

Secrets are frequently a problem with such patients, who attempt to use the psychiatrist to reinforce a dissociative strategy of withholding relevant information from certain personality states. Such patients often like to confide in the psychiatrist with the idea that the information is to be kept from other parts of the self, for example, traumatic memories or plans for self-destructive activities.

Clear limit setting and commitment on the part of the psychiatrist to helping all portions of the patient's personality structure learn about warded-off information are important. It is wise to clarify explicitly that the psychiatrist will not become involved in secret collusion. Furthermore, when important agreements are negotiated, such as commitments on the part of patients to seek medical help before acting on a thought to harm themselves or others, it is useful to discuss with the patients that this is an "all-points bulletin", requiring attention from all the relevant personality states. The excuse that certain personality states were "not aware" of the agreement should not be accepted.

Hypnosis

Hypnosis can be helpful in facilitating psychotherapy as well as establishing the diagnosis. First of all, the simple structure of hypnotic induction may elicit dissociative phenomena. Hypnosis can be helpful in facilitating access to dissociated personalities. They may simply occur spontaneously during hypnotic induction. An alternative strategy is to hypnotize the patient and use age regression to reorient to a time when a different personality state was manifest. An instruction later to change times back to the present usually elicits a return to the other personality state. This then becomes a means of teaching such an individual how to control the dissociative process.

Alternatively, entering the state of hypnosis may make it possible simply to address and elicit different identities or personality states. Patients can be taught a simple self-hypnosis exercise for this purpose. For example, the patient can be told to count to herself or himself from one to three. After some formal exercises such as this, it is often possible to ask the patient to speak with a given alter personality, without the formal use of hypnosis. Merely asking to talk with a given identity usually suffices after a while.

Memory Retrieval

Because the loss of memory in DID is complex and chronic, its retrieval is likewise a more extended and integral part of the psychotherapeutic process. The therapy becomes an integrating experience of information sharing among disparate personality elements. Conceptualizing DID as a chronic PTSD, the psychotherapeutic strategy involves a focus on working through traumatic memories in addition to controlling the dissociation.

Controlled access to memories greatly facilitates psychotherapy. As with dissociative amnesia, a variety of strategies can be employed to help patients with DID break down amnesic barriers. Eliciting various identities or personality states can facilitate access to memories previously unavailable to consciousness. While so-called "pseudomemories" can occur, previously dissociated traumatic memories are often accurate.

Once these memories of earlier traumatic experience have been brought into consciousness, it is crucial to help the patient work through the painful affect, inappropriate self-blame and other reactions to these memories. It may be useful to have patients visualize the memories rather than relive them as a means of making their intensity more manageable. It can also be useful to have patients divide the memories, for example, picturing on one side of an imaginary screen something an abuser did to them and on the other side how they tried to protect themselves from the abuse.

Such techniques can help make the traumatic memories more bearable by placing them in a broader perspective, one in which trauma victims can also identify adaptive aspects of their response to the trauma.

This and similar approaches can help these individuals work through traumatic memories, enabling them to bear them in consciousness and therefore reducing the need for dissociation as a means of keeping such memories and associated painful affect out of consciousness. Although these techniques can be helpful and often result in reduced fragmentation and integration, a number of complications can occur in the psychotherapy of these patients.

The therapeutic process can be thought of as a kind of grief work in which information retrieved from memory is reviewed, traumatic memories are put into perspective, and emotional expression is encouraged and worked through, thereby making it more possible to endure and disseminate the information as widely as possible among various parts of the patient's personality structure. Instructions to other alter personalities to "listen" while a given one is talking and reviewing previously dissociated material can be helpful.

The Rule of Thirds

The psychotherapy of DID can be a time-consuming and emotionally taxing process. The rule of thirds (Kluft, 1991; Schacter, 1995) is a helpful guideline. Spend the first third of the psychotherapy session assessing the patient's current mental state and life problems and defining a problem area that might benefit from retrieval into conscious memory and working through. Spend the second third of the session accessing and working through this memory. Allow a final third for helping the patient assimilate the information, regulate and modulate emotional responses, and discuss any responses to the psychiatrist and plans for the immediate future. The psychiatrist may resist doing this because the intense abreactive materials are often so compelling and interesting. The patient may also resist sharing information across personalities. Nonetheless, the psychiatrist can be helpful in imposing structure on often chaotic memories and identity states.

Given the intensity of the material that often emerges involving memories of sexual and physical abuse and sudden shifts in mental state accompanied by amnesia, the psychiatrist is called on to take a clear and structured role in managing the psychotherapy. Appropriate limits must be set concerning self-destructive or threatening behavior, agreements must be made regarding physical safety and treatment compliance, and other matters must be presented to the patient in such a way that dissociative ignorance is not an acceptable explanation for failure to live up to the agreements.

Traumatic Transference

Transference applies with special meaning to patients who have been physically and sexually abused, especially in childhood. They have experienced individuals who are presumed to be caretakers acting instead in an exploitative and sometimes sadistic fashion. They thus expect similar betrayal from psychiatrists. Although their reality testing is good enough that they can perceive genuine caring, they often unconsciously expect psychiatrists to exploit them. They may experience working through of traumatic memories as a reinflicting of the trauma, with the psychiatrist taking sadistic pleasure in their suffering. They may expect excessive passivity on the part of the psychiatrist, identifying the psychiatrist with some uncaring family figure who knew that abuse was occurring but did little or nothing to stop it. It is important in managing the therapy to keep these issues in mind and make them frequent topics of discussion. This can diffuse, if not eliminate, such traumatic transference distortions of the therapeutic relationship.

Integration

The ultimate goal of psychotherapy is integration of these multiple ego states. It is often the case that one or more of the personality states may exert considerable resistance to the process of integration, particularly early in the process of therapy. Also patients may experience efforts of integration as an attempt on the part of the therapist to "kill" personalities. These fears must be worked through and the patient needs to understand that the goal is to learn how to control the episodes of dissociation. This gives patients a sense of gradually being able to control their dissociative processes in order to work through the traumatic memories. In order to enhance mastery and control, the process of the psychotherapy must help patients minimize rather than reinforce the content of traumatic memories, which often involves reexperiencing a sense of helplessness in a symbolic reenactment of the trauma.

At the same time, the dissociative defense represents an internalization of the abusive people in the patient's past, a kind of identification with the aggressor, which makes the patient feel powerful rather than helpless. Setting aside the defense also means acknowledging and bearing the helplessness of having been victimized and working through the irrational self-blame that gave such individuals a fantasy of control over events during which they were helpless. Yet, difficult as it is, ultimately the goal of psychotherapy is mastery over the dissociative process, controlled access to dissociative states, integration of warded-off painful memories and material, and a more integrated continuum of identity, memory and consciousness. Although there have been no controlled trials of the outcome of psychotherapy

| Table 56.2 Stages of Therapy ||
Stage	Technique
Establishing treatment	Education, atmosphere of safety, instill confidence
Preliminary interventions	Confirm diagnosis, set limits, access dissociation with hypnosis
History gathering	Explore components of dissociative structure
Working through trauma	Grief work
Move toward integration	Enhance communication across dissociative states
Integration–resolution	Encourage development of integrated self
Learning coping skills	Help with life decisions and relationships
Solidification of gains	Transference examination
Follow-up	Maintenance

Source: Kluft RP (1991) Multiple personality disorder. Reprinted with permission from the American Psychiatric Press Review of Psychiatry, Vol. 10, Tasman A and Goldfinger SM (eds). Copyright 1991, American Psychiatric Press, Washington DC.

for this disorder, case series reports indicate a positive outcome in a majority of cases (Kluft, 1984, 1986, 1991).

The stages of therapy are presented in Table 56.2.

Psychopharmacology

As with other dissociative disorders, there is little evidence that psychoactive drugs are of great help in reversing dissociative symptoms (Maldonado *et al.*, 2000). In the past, short-acting barbiturates such as sodium amobarbital were used intravenously to reverse functional amnesia, but this technique is no longer employed, largely because of poor results. Research data provide no evidence suggesting that any medication regimen has any significant therapeutic effect on the dissociative process manifested by DID patients. To date, pharmacological treatment has been limited to symptom control or the management of comorbid conditions (e.g., depression).

Of all available classes of psychotropic agents, antidepressants are the most useful class for the treatment of patients with DID. That is because patients suffering from dissociation frequently experience comorbid dysthymic or major depressive disorder. The newer agents – selective serotonin reuptake inhibitors (SSRIs) – are particularly useful, given their high level of effectiveness, low side-effect profile, and even lower danger in overdose, compared with tricyclic antidepressants and monoamine oxidase inhibitors. Nevertheless, medication compliance may be a problem with dissociative patients because dissociated personality states may interfere with medication taking or may take the medication in an overdose attempt.

Benzodiazepines have mostly been used to facilitate recall by controlling secondary anxiety associated with retrieval of traumatic memories (i.e., medication facilitated interviews). Nevertheless, despite their short-term usefulness, CNS-depressant agents may cause sudden mental state transitions, which may in turn increase rather than decrease amnesic barriers. Therefore, as useful as they could be on short-term basis (i.e., acute management of a panic attack), the long term of these agents may, in fact, contribute rather than treat dissociative episodes.

There are several uses for anticonvulsant agents. We know that seizures disorders have a high rate of comorbidity with DID. Thus, anticonvulsant agents may help control the dissociation associated with epileptogenic activity. On the other hand, anticonvulsant agents have proven to be effective in the management of mood disorders, as well as the impulsiveness associated with personality disorders and brain injury. Also despite their effectiveness, these agents produce less amnestic side effects than the benzodiazepines and thus may be preferred. On the other hand, the need for closer monitoring due to potential toxicity, particularly in overdoses, makes their use less desirable than the newer SSRIs.

Of all pharmacological agents available, antipsychotics may be the less desirable. First, they are rarely useful in reducing dissociative symptoms. In fact, there have been reports of increased levels of dissociation and an increased incidence of side effects when used in patients suffering from dissociative disorders.

Dissociative Trance Disorder

Dissociative Trance

Dissociative trance disorder has been divided into two broad categories, dissociative trance and possession trance (American Psychiatric Association, 2000). Dissociative trance phenomena are characterized by a sudden alteration in consciousness, not accompanied by distinct alternative identities. In this form the dissociative symptom involves an alteration in consciousness rather than identity. Also, in dissociative trance, the activities performed are rather simple, usually involving sudden collapse, immobilization, dizziness, shrieking, screaming, or crying. Memory is rarely affected, and if there is amnesia, it is fragmented.

Dissociative trance phenomena frequently involve sudden, extreme changes in sensory and motor control. A classic example is the *ataque de nervios*, prevalent in Latin American countries. For example, this phenomenon is estimated to have a 12% lifetime prevalence rate in Puerto Rico (Lewis-Fernandez, 1994). A typical episode involves a sudden feeling of anxiety, followed by total body shakes, which may mimic convulsions. This is then followed by hyperventilation, unintelligible screaming, agitation and often violent bodily movements. Often, this is followed by collapse and probably transient loss of consciousness. After the episode is over, subjects complain of fatigue and having been confused, although this behavior is dramatically different from classic postictal states. Some subjects may experience amnesia at least to some aspects of the event (Lewis-Fernandez, 1994).

Other examples include **lata** and "falling out". Lata represents the Malay version of trance disorder. In these episodes, afflicted individuals usually experience a sudden vision, mostly of a threatening spirit. The observable behavior includes screaming or crying and physical manifestation of overtly violent behavior which often requires the sufferer to be physically restrained. Patients often report episodes of amnesia, but there is no clear possession by the offending spirit. On the other hand, "falling out" more commonly occurs among African-Americans in the southern USA. Similarly to other trance episodes, the affected individual may enter a trance state, followed by bodily collapse, the

---

inability to see or speak, despite the fact that they are fully conscious. Temporary confusion may be observed, although subjects are not usually amnesic to what occurred during the episode.

Possession Trance

In contrast to dissociative trance episodes, possession trance involves the assumption of a distinct alternative identity. The new identity is presumed to be that of a deity, ancestor, or spirit who has transiently taken possession of the subject's mind and body. Different from dissociative trance episodes, which are characterized by rather crude, simplistic, regressive-like behaviors, possession trance victims often exhibit rather complex behavior. During these episodes, subjects may, for example, express otherwise forbidden thoughts or needs, engage in unusually and uncharacteristic aggressive behavior (e.g., verbal or physical expressions of aggression), or may attempt to negotiate for change in family or social status. Also, in contrast to dissociative trance episodes, possession trance episodes often are followed by dense amnesia for a large portion of the episode during which the spirit identity was in control of the subject's behavior.

Cultural Context

Dissociative-like phenomena have been described in virtually every culture. Yet they appear to be more prevalent in the less heavily industrialized Second and Third World countries. Studies on the prevalence of dissociative disorders in India have suggested that the 1-year prevalence of dissociative trance disorder is approximately 3.5%; of all psychiatric hospitalizations, making it a highly frequent mental disorder. Trance and possession syndromes are by far the most common type of dissociative disorders seen around the world. On the other hand, DID, which is relatively more common in the USA, is virtually never diagnosed in underdeveloped countries. This difference in prevalence and distribution of dissociative disorder across different populations may be mediated by cultural as well as biological factors. For example, Eastern culture is far more sociocentric than Western culture. Thus, being "possessed" by an outside entity would be more culturally comprehensible and acceptable in the East. On the other hand, an apparent proliferation of individual identities would fit better with the Western preoccupation with individualism. Nonetheless, the underlying dissociative mechanism inhibiting integration of perception, memory and identity may suggest a common underlying mechanism amongst these dissociative syndromes.

Trance and possession episodes are usually understood as an idiom of distress and yet they are not viewed as normal. That is, they are not a generally accepted part of cultural and religious practice, which often does involve normal trance phenomena, such as trance dancing in the Balinese Hindu culture. Trance dancers enjoy the remarkable privilege of being the only portion of this socially rigid society able to elevate their social status. The way they are able to do that is by developing the ability to enter trance states. During these altered states of consciousness, which usually occur within the context of a socially acceptable ceremony setting, they dance over hot coals, hold a sword at their throat, or in other ways exhibit supernormal powers of concentration and physical prowess. The mechanism mediating these phenomena is not fully understood, but there is evidence of elevations in plasma noradrenaline, dopamine and beta-endorphin among Balinese trance dancers during trance states. This form of trance is considered socially normal and even exalted.

By contrast, disordered trance and possession trance are viewed by the local community as an aberrant form of behavior that requires intervention. Such symptoms often arise in the context of family or social distress, for example, discomfort in a new family environment. Thus, cultural informants make it clear that people with dissociative trance disorder are abnormal.

Treatment

Dissociation and Trauma

One of the important developments in the modern understanding of dissociative disorders is the establishment of a clearer link between trauma and dissociation. Trauma can be understood as the experience of being made into an object, a thing, the victim of someone else's rage or of nature's indifference. Trauma represents the ultimate experience of helplessness: loss of control over one's own body. There is growing clinical evidence that dissociation occurs as a defense during traumatic experiences, constituting

an attempt to maintain mental control at the moment when physical control has been lost. Assault victims report floating above their body, feeling sorry for the person being assaulted beneath them. Patients, victims of childhood abuse, have reported "taking themselves elsewhere" where they could "safely play" by themselves or with imaginary friends, while their bodies were brutally abused by a perpetrator. In fact, there is evidence (Terr, 1991) that children exposed to multiple traumas as opposed to single-blow traumas are more likely to use dissociative defense mechanisms, which include spontaneous trance episodes and amnesia.

As noted in the section on DID, there is an accumulating literature suggesting a connection between a history of childhood physical and sexual abuse and the development of dissociative symptoms. Similarly, dissociative symptoms have been found to be more prevalent in patients with Axis II disorders, such as borderline personality disorder, when there has been a history of childhood abuse. Another means of examining the putative connection between dissociation and trauma is to look at the prevalence of dissociative symptoms after recent trauma. If it is indeed the case that trauma seems to elicit dissociative symptoms, they should be observable in the immediate aftermath of trauma. In the early literature examining responses to trauma, Lindemann (1944), studying the aftermath of the Coconut Grove fire, observed that the individuals who acted as though little or nothing had happened had an extremely poor long-term prognosis. These were individuals who had been injured or had lost loved ones. Indeed, it was the absence of post traumatic symptoms in this group, compared with the agitation, dysphoria, and restlessness that typified the majority of survivors, that led him to formulate the normal process of acute grief. Several subsequent researchers have observed that psychic numbing is a predictor of later PTSD symptoms.

Research on survivors of other life-threatening events, including hostage taking, indicated that more than half have experienced a sense of detachment, feelings of unreality (i.e., depersonalization), lack of emotions, hyperalertness, and automatic movements. Although these dissociative responses to traumatic stressors have been conceptualized as adaptive defenses to overwhelming situations, the thrust of the literature indicates that the presence of dissociative symptoms in the immediate aftermath of trauma is a strong predictor of the development of later PTSD. Physical trauma seems to elicit dissociation, perhaps in individuals who are prone to the use of this defense by virtue of either previous traumatic experience or a constitutional tendency to dissociate. This dissociative reaction may, in some cases, resolve quickly. However, in others it may become the matrix for later post traumatic symptoms, such as dissociative amnesia for the traumatic episode. Indeed, more extreme dissociative disorders, such as DID, have been conceptualized as chronic PTSDs (Kluft, 1984, 1991; Speigel, 1985, 1986b). Recollection of trauma tends to have an off–on quality involving either intrusion or avoidance (Horowitz, 1976), in which victims either intensively relive the trauma as though it were recurring or have difficulty remembering it. Thus, physical trauma seems to elicit dissociative responses, which, in turn, predispose to the development of later PTSD, perhaps by reducing the likelihood of working through the traumatic experiences afterward.

Acute Stress Disorder

Although acute stress disorder is classified among the anxiety disorders in DSM-IV-TR (American Psychiatric Association, 2000) (see acute stress disorder criteria on p. 635) mention is made of it in this chapter because half of the symptoms of this disorder are dissociative in nature. These diagnostic criteria would designate approximately a third of individuals exposed to serious trauma as symptomatic. As noted, dissociative symptoms occurring at the time of the trauma are strongly predictive of later development of PTSD and are associated with higher cortisol levels during exposure to uncontrollable stress. Similarly, the occurrence of PTSD is predicted by intrusion, avoidance and hyperarousal symptoms in the immediate aftermath of rape and combat trauma. Although most individuals experiencing serious trauma are initially symptomatic, the majority recover without developing PTSD. Most studies demonstrate that 25% or less of those who experience serious trauma later become symptomatic.

This diagnostic category is useful not only for research on the normal and abnormal processes of adjusting to trauma, but also as a means of providing an important opportunity for early intervention and thus prevention of later psychopathology. Even though dissociation has a role at the time of trauma, if the defense persists too long it may interfere with the working through of traumatic material. Lindemann (1944) described the term **grief work**, referring to process needed to put traumatic experience into perspective and reduce the likelihood of later symptoms. In this context, psychotherapy, aimed at helping individuals acknowledge, bear and put into perspective a traumatic experience shortly after the trauma, should be helpful in reducing the incidence of later PTSD.

Theoretical and Research Issues: Models and Mechanisms of Dissociation

Dissociation and Information Processing

Dissociation may seem like a historical aberration, a throwback to earlier and more primitive models of the mind. Yet these disorders are surprisingly congruent with information processing–based theories of mental function. For example, connectionist and parallel distributed processing models (Rumelhart and McClelland, 1986) take a bottom-up rather than a top-down approach to cognitive organization. Traditional models emphasize a supraordinate structure in which broad categories of information structure the processing of specific examples of those categories, that is, the category "sweet" must exist to make sense of "sugar", "candy" and "jelly". In the parallel distributed processing models, subunits or neural nets process information through patterns of cooccurrence of input stimuli that lead to activation patterns in these neural nets, which produce pattern recognition. The output of one neuronal system becomes the input to another, thereby gradually building up integrated and complex patterns of activation and inhibition. A bottom-up processing model system has the advantage of accounting for the processing of vast amounts of information and the ability to recognize patterns with approximate information. Nevertheless, such models make the classification and integration of information problematical.

Information seems to be processed on the basis of the cooccurrence of patterns of activation rather than its appearance in a predefined category. Therefore, in parallel distributed processing system models, failures in integration of mental contents are theoretically likely to occur. Inappropriate but apparent similarities may appear when activation patterns are similar and, conversely, no two pieces of information are necessarily connected. There have been models created to explain psychotic, dissociative and mood disorders, based on abnormal or defective neuronal association network patterns. These neural models assumed that when there are problems with the processing of input information (a model for traumatic input), the brain is more likely to have difficulty achieving a coherent and balanced output. This could then lead to the development of dissociation of information and data manifested in the subject's inability to process smoothly all of the incoming information.

Dissociation and Memory Systems

There are two broad categories of memory known as explicit and implicit, declarative and procedural, or episodic and semantic. These two basic memory systems serve different functions. Explicit or episodic memory involves recall of personal experience identified with the self, for example, "I went dancing last night". The second type is known as implicit or procedural memory. This involves the execution of routine operations, such as driving a car, or typing on a keyboard. Most of these rather automatic operations could be carried out with little conscious awareness, but yet with a high degree of proficiency. These two types of memory seem to reside in different cerebral anatomical localizations. Episodic memory seems to be primarily associated with limbic system function, primarily involving the hippocampal formation and mamillary bodies. On the other hand, procedural memory appears to be a function of basal ganglia and cortical functioning.

The fact that there are separate memory systems may account for certain types of dissociative phenomena. For example, the automaticity observed in certain types of dissociative disorders reflect the separation of self-identification associated with explicit memory from routine activity in implicit or procedural memory. It is thus not at all foreign to our mental processing to act in an automatic way devoid of explicit self-identification. Future research on the neurobiology of memory may well provide insights into the functional disintegration of memory, perception, identity and consciousness seen in dissociative disorders.

Comparison of DSM-IV/ICD-10 Diagnostic Criteria

The ICD-10 Diagnostic Criteria for Research for dissociative amnesia specify that there be a "convincing association in time between the onset of symptoms of the disorder and stressful events, problems, or needs". In DSM-IV-TR, the criteria set notes that the forgotten information is usually of a stressful or traumatic nature.

For dissociative fugue, in contrast to DSM-IV-TR, the ICD-10 Diagnostic Criteria for Research specify "amnesia for the journey". Furthermore, in contrast to DSM-IV-TR, the ICD-10 Diagnostic Criteria for Research do not indicate that there is an inability to recall one's past during the fugue or that there be confusion about personal identity.

Dissociative identity disorder is included in ICD-10 as an example of an "other dissociative (conversion) disorder" under the rubric "multiple personality disorder". The ICD-10 Diagnostic Criteria for Research and the DSM-IV-TR criteria are almost identical.

Finally, ICD-10 has a single category "depersonalization–derealization syndrome" for presentations characterized by either depersonalization or derealization. In contrast, the DSM-IV-TR category includes only depersonalization and mentions derealization as an associated feature. Furthermore, unlike DSM-IV-TR which includes this category in the dissociative disorders section, ICD-10 includes the category within the "other neurotic disorders" grouping.

Conclusion

The dissociative disorders constitute a challenging and fascinating spectrum of psychiatric illnesses. The failure of integration of memory, identity, perception and consciousness seen in these disorders results in symptoms that illustrate fundamental problems in the organization of mental processes. Dissociative phenomena often occur during and after physical trauma but may also represent transient or chronic defensive patterns. Dissociative disorders are generally treatable and are a domain in which psychotherapy is a primary modality, although pharmacological treatment of comorbid conditions such as depression can be quite helpful. The dissociative disorders are ubiquitous around the world, although they take a variety of forms. They represent a fascinating diagnostic, therapeutic and investigative challenge.

References

American Psychiatric Association (2000) *Diagnostic and Statistical Manual of Mental Disorders*, 4th edn., Text Rev. APA, Washington DC.

Bernstein EM and Putnam FW (1986) Development, reliability, and validity of a dissociation scale. *J Nerv Ment Dis* 174, 727–735.

Carlson EB, Putnam FW, Ross CA *et al.* (1993) Validity of the Dissociative Experiences Scale in screening for multiple personality disorder: A multicenter study. *Am J Psychiatr* 150, 1030–1036.

Coons PM and Milstein V (1986) Psychosexual disturbances in multiple personality: Characteristics, etiology, treatment. *J Clin Psychiatr* 47, 106–110.

Hilgard ER (1977) *Divided Consciousness: Multiple Controls in Human Thought and Action*. Wiley-Interscience, New York.

Horowitz MJ (1976) Stress Response Syndromes. Jason Aronson, New York.

James W (1984) *William James on Exceptional Mental States. The 1896 Lowell Lectures* (ed Taylor E). The University of Massachusetts Press, Amherst, MA.

Janet P (1920) The Major Symptoms of Hysteria. Macmillan, New York, p. 332.

Kluft RP (1984) Treatment of multiple personality disorder: A study of 33 cases. *Psychiatr Clin N Am* 7, 9–29.

Kluft RP (1986) Personality unification in multiple personality disorder: A follow-up study, in *Treatment of Multiple Personality Disorder* (ed Braun BG). American Psychiatric Press, Washington DC, pp. 29–60.

Kluft RP (1987) First rank symptoms as diagnostic indicators of multiple personality disorder. *Am J Psychiatr* 144, 293–298.

Kluft RP (1991) Multiple personality disorder, in *American Psychiatric Press Review of Psychiatry*, Vol. 10 (eds Tasman A and Goldfinger SM). American Psychiatric Press, Washington DC, pp. 161–188.

Lewis-Fernandez (1994) Culture and dissociation: A comparison of ataque de nervios among Puerto Ricans and "possession syndrome" in India, in *Dissociation: Culture, Mind and Body* (ed Spiegel D). American Psychiatric Press, Washington DC, pp. 123–167.

Lindemann E (1944) Symptomatology and management of acute grief. *Am J Psychiatr* 101, 141–148.

Loewenstein RJ and Putnam FW (1988) A comparative study of dissociative symptoms in patients with complex partial seizures, multiple personality disorder, and posttraumatic stress disorder. *Dissociation* 1, 17–23.

Maldonado JR, Butler LD and Spiegel D (2000) Treatment of dissociative disorders, in *Treatments That Work* (eds Nathan P and Gorman JM). Oxford University Press, New York, pp. 463–496.

Milner B (1959) The memory defect in bilateral hippocampal lesions. *Psychiatr Res Rep* 11, 42–52.

Ross CA (1989) *Multiple Personality Disorder: Diagnosis, Clinical Features, and Treatment*. John Wiley, New York.

Ross CA, Anderson G, Fleisher WP *et al.* (1991) The frequency of multiple personality disorder among psychiatry inpatients. *Am J Psychiatr* 148, 1717–1720.

Rumelhart DE and McClelland JL (1986) *Parallel Distributed Processing: Explorations in the Microstructure of Cognition*. The MIT Press, Cambridge, MA.

Saxe GN, van der Kolk BA, Berkowitz R *et al.* (1993) Dissociative disorders in psychiatric patients. *Am J Psychiatr* 150, 1037–1042.

Schacter DL (1995) Memory distortion: History and current status, in *Memory Distortion: How Minds, Brains, and Societies Reconstruct the Past* (ed Schacter DL). Harvard University Press, Cambridge, MA, pp. 1–42.

Schenk L and Bear D (1981) Multiple personality and related dissociative phenomena in patients with temporal lobe epilepsy. *Am J Psychiatr* 138, 1311–1316.

Spiegel D (1981) Vietnam grief work using hypnosis. *Am J Clin Hypn* 24, 33–40.

Spiegel D (1986b) Dissociation, double binds, and posttraumatic stress in multiple personality disorder. In *Treatment of Multiple Personality Disorder*, Braun B (ed). American Psychiatric Press, Washington DC, pp. 61–77.

Terr LC (1991) Childhood traumas: An outline and overivew. Am J Psychiatr 148, 10–20.

57 Sexual Disorders

A wide array of sexuality topics impact psychiatry. These topics range from those constituting a major social burden, such as teenage pregnancy, sex crimes and sexually transmitted diseases, to those involving ethical and moral values, such as abortion, extramarital affairs, commercial sex industries and crossing sexual boundaries with patients. They include those with a developmental or medical focus, such as sexual dysfunction or sexual dysfunction due to substance abuse or medical conditions, and those involving lifestyles, such as sexual minority status and drugs for sexual enhancement. There are also those that center on psychiatry's undisputed responsibility, such as psychotropic medication-induced sexual dysfunction and the sexual consequences of psychiatric illness. No discipline, no ideology, no religion and certainly no textbook chapter is sufficient fully to understand and encompass the myriad expressions of human sexuality.

Psychiatry has known for almost a century that child development lays the foundation for a wide variety of adult sexual outcomes (Freud, 1905). These are reflected in the variations of gender, orientation, intention and ease of sexual expression with chosen partners. Psychiatry has also been long aware that the conduct of adolescent and adult sexual life is laden with concern, and sometimes anguish, in every person. In the last generation, we have acquired greater convictions about the profound public health implications of several sexual patterns. First came awareness of the high incidence of childhood sexual abuse and its long-term consequences. Then came the data showing that some psychiatrists and other trusted professionals engaged in genital intimacies with patients. Psychiatry responded by unambiguously clarifying our ethical standards. At about the same time the AIDS epidemic led to a greater awareness of the lives of homosexual and bisexual men. In the 1990s when the Internet usage grew without regulation, addictions to at-home pornography appeared. As the use of SSRIs became widespread, psychiatrists learned about their negative sexual impact. In 1998 an effective pill for erectile dysfunction created an explosion of media interest across the world. The Viagra story reminded us that sexual function is really important to people.

Psychiatry prides itself about being the only field that can comprehend the biopsychosocial aspects of illness. We understand that all sexual expression is simultaneously constituted by biological, psychological and social forces. We also know that sexual disorders are a high prevalence, high incidence source of personal suffering, affecting almost every person at some time in the life-cycle. Sexual disorders often play a subtle role in the genesis of other psychiatric disorders as presented in Figure 57.1.

Patients assume their psychiatrists know about sexuality. Therapists can be helpful to many individuals and couples with these problems if they have an interest in the area, a comfort with the subject and a modest fund of knowledge. Sometimes the help can be given quite efficiently. The assistance is often based on knowledge of the diverse origins of these problems. To be able to treat a broad range of sexual disorders the psychiatrist needs to be diagnostically competent, skillful with medications and willing to engage in psychotherapeutic processes. This chapter provides background information for these three goals.

The Components of Sexuality

An adult's sexuality has seven components – gender identity, orientation, intention (what one wants to do with a partner's body and have done with one's body during sexual behavior), desire, arousal, orgasm and emotional satisfaction. The first three components constitute our sexual identity. The second three comprise our sexual function. The seventh, emotional satisfaction, is based on our personal reflections on the first six (Table 57.1). The DSM-IV-TR designates impairments of five of these components as pathologies. Variations in orientation and the failure to find ordinary sexual experience emotionally satisfying, although problems for some, are not designated as "disorders".

Sexual Development Through the Life-cycle

While the psychological foundations for a healthy sexual life are laid down during childhood through parent–child relationships, each subsequent phase of life – adolescence, young adulthood, middle-life, and older age – has inherent developmental challenges and potentials. The normal tasks of sexual development at each phase provide the clinician with an understanding of age-related etiologies of sexual disorders. Adolescent sexual troubles often reflect difficulties consolidating a personally acceptable sexual identity. Young adult dysfunctions often indicate the presence of psychological obstacles to growing comfortable as a sexual pleasure-seeking, pleasure-giving person while integrating sex into the larger context of human attachment. Middle-life disorders often represent failures to maintain psychological intimacy and diplomatically to negotiate tensions within an increasingly complex interpersonal relationship. The dysfunctions of older persons often represent failures to preserve sexual function in the face of biological assaults of menopause, aging, illness, medications, radiation and surgery. Most etiologic factors can operate in another epoch as well. For instance, a young person's new indifference to sexual behavior may be due to an

Essentials of Psychiatry   Jerald Kay and Allan Tasman
© 2006 John Wiley & Sons, Ltd.

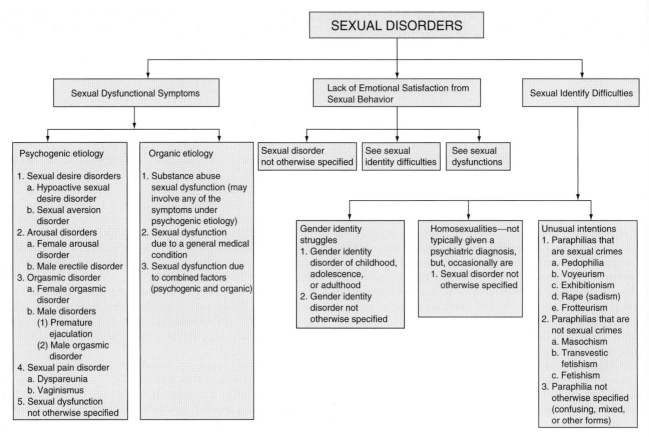

Figure 57.1   *Diagnostic decision tree for sexual disorders.*

SSRI or an older person's new marriage may expose previously avoided personal discomfort with receiving and giving sexual pleasure.

Table 57.1	Mechanisms of Sexual Equilibrium

Interplay I. of Each Person's Seven Sexual Components

Person A		*Person B*
Gender identity	⇆	Gender identity
Orientation	⇆	Orientation
Intention	⇆	Intention
Desire	⇆	Desire
Arousal	⇆	Arousal
Orgasm	⇆	Orgasm
Emotional satisfaction	⇆	Emotional satisfaction

Regard II. That Each Person Has for the Partner's Component Characteristics

Positive regard leads to:
   Increased sensual abandon,
   Positive attitudes toward self and partner, and
   Frequent sexual behavior
Negative regard leads to:
   Increased personal inhibition,
   Hostile critical attitudes toward self and partner, and
   Limited motivation to engage in partner sexual behavior

The Sexual Dysfunctions

Significance of Sexual Dysfunction

While sex is widely thought of as recreation, psychiatrists recognize it as an important means of establishing and reaffirming emotional attachments. Sexual competence – the ability to desire a partner, become aroused and attain orgasm in a cooperative manner when together – is a valuable developmental accomplishment because it enables a person to experience the physical expressions and emotional complexities of love. Mutually pleasurable sexual behavior tends to recur far more often in couples than unilaterally satisfying behavior. Mutually pleasurable sexual behavior allows both partners to be comforted and stabilized by loving and feeling loved. The dysfunctions are symptomatic deficits in the quest for these widespread ideals: sexual competence, fun and stabilization of the self.

DSM-IV Diagnoses

DSM-IV specifies three criteria for each sexual dysfunction (American Psychiatric Association, 1994). The first criterion describes the psychophysiologic impairment – for example, absence of sexual desire, arousal, or orgasm. The second and third criteria are the same for each impairment: the dysfunction causes marked distress or interpersonal difficulty and the dysfunction is not better accounted for by another Axis I diagnosis or not due exclusively to the direct physiological effects of a substance (e.g., a drug of abuse, a medication) or a general medical condition. Table 57.2 lists the first criterion of each of the 12 sexual dysfunction diagnoses. DSM-IV gives the clinician additional latitude

Table 57.2   Delineating Criteria of 12 Sexual Dysfunction Diagnoses

Sexual Desire Disorders	Sexual Arousal Disorders	Orgasmic Disorders	Sexual Pain Disorders
Hypoactive sexual desire disorder: persistently or recurrently deficient (or absent) sexual fantasies and desire for sexual activity	Female sexual arousal disorder: persistent or recurrent inability to attain, or to maintain until completion of the sexual activity, an adequate lubrication-swelling response of sexual excitement	Female orgasmic disorder: persistent or recurrent delay in, or absence of, orgasm after a normal sexual excitement phase	Dyspareunia: recurrent or persistent genital pain associated with sexual intercourse in either a male or a female
Sexual aversion disorder: persistent or recurrent extreme aversion to, and avoidance of, all (or almost all) genital sexual contact with a sexual partner	Male erectile disorder: persistent or recurrent inability to attain, or to maintain until completion of the sexual activity, an adequate erection	Male orgasmic disorder: persistent or recurrent delay in, or absence of, orgasm after a normal sexual excitement phase during sexual activity	Vaginismus: recurrent or persistent involuntary spasm of the musculature of the outer third of the vagina that interferes with sexual intercourse
		Premature ejaculation: persistent or recurrent ejaculation with a minimal sexual stimulation before, on, or shortly after penetration and before the person wishes it	
Sexual Dysfunction Due to a General Medical Condition	**Substance-Induced Sexual Dysfunction**	**Sexual Dysfunction Not Otherwise Specified**	
any of the above-mentioned diagnoses must be judged to be exclusively due to the direct physiological effects of a medical condition	a sexual dysfunction that is fully explained by substance use in that it develops within a month of substance intoxication	for problems that do not meet the categories just described	

for deciding when a person who meets the first criterion qualifies for a disorder. The doctor is asked to consider the effects of the individual's age, experience, ethnicity and cultural background, the degree of subjective distress, adequacy of sexual stimulation and symptom frequency. No instructions are provided about how to exercise this judgment. In this way DSM-IV makes it clear that understanding sexual life requires more than counting symptoms; it requires judgment.

Epidemiology

Numerous attempts to describe the prevalence of sexual dysfunction have been made in the previous 25 years. These range from attempts to define the frequency of a particular dysfunction, for instance male erectile disorder, to attempts to estimate the prevalence of a series of separate dysfunction, for example, desire, arousal and orgasmic disorders of women. All such efforts quickly confront methodological influences of sampling, means of obtaining the information, definition of each dysfunction, purpose of the study and perspective of its authors. These data not surprisingly, therefore, demonstrate a range of prevalence depending on the problem studied. Gender identity disorders are relatively rare (<1–2%). Lifelong sexual desire disorders among women may involve 15% but are less

frequent among men. Acquired desire disorders among older individuals are probably three times as common. Perhaps more than half of women at age 55 years have recognized a deterioration in their sexual function. Perhaps 25% of women in their twenties have difficulty having orgasm and 33% of men less than age 40 claim to ejaculate too rapidly. The majority of men by age 70 years are likely to be having erection problems. The recent careful epidemiologic study, designed by sociologists, successfully generated a representative sample of the USA (Laumann *et al.*, 1994a). They interviewed men and women between age 18 and 59 years and found that sexual dysfunction is common, particularly among young women and older men. This is noteworthy for psychiatrists because our studies of sexual dysfunction caused by medications or acquired psychiatric disorders tend to assume that patients are generally functionally intact prior to becoming ill or taking medications. This assumption is not tenable based on a generation of epidemiologic studies.

Sexual Equilibrium

Etiologic ideas about sexual dysfunction are a relatively simple conceptual challenge involving notions about the individual's psychology and his or her cultural expectations. In contrast, for couples, they involve two individual psychologies, their interpersonal impact on one another and their cultures. The clinician must be wary when one coupled person is presented as having a sexual dysfunction and the partner is presented as "normal". Sexual dysfunction in a couple is a two-person problem in terms of immediate effects and often in terms of cause as well (Table 57.1). How a partner regards the sexual characteristics of the other is a subtle ingredient of sexual comfort, competence and dysfunction. For instance, a young woman's new inability to attain orgasm with her husband may be traced to her embarrassment at sharing her excitation with him because she perceives him to be generally critical of her. Similarly, the origin of a husband's erectile dysfunction may be traced to the emergence of his wife's negative regard for him, which stemmed from something other than his sexual behavior. This **ordinary** connectivity of a couple's sexual function is referred to as the couple's sexual equilibrium (Levine, 1998). The sexual equilibrium explains five observations:

1. Improvement and deterioration of sexual function can rapidly occur;
2. When a couple's nonsexual relationship is good, their sexual life may not be;
3. Individual psychotherapy is often insufficient to help coupled patients improve their sexual life;
4. A negative attitude from the partner can block improvement in a couple's sexual life regardless of the therapy format and therapist skill;
5. A conversation with a therapist who is attuned to the emotional meanings of a couple's interaction can shift a dysfunctional equilibrium back to mutually satisfying sexual behavior.

The Problems of Sexual Desire

Sexual desire manifestations are diverse: erotic fantasies, sexual dreams, initiation of sexual behavior, receptivity to partner-initiated sexual behavior, masturbation, genital sensations, heightened responsivity to erotic environmental cues and sincere statements about wanting to behave sexually. For most of the 20th century, these have been referred to as manifestations of libido. Psychiatrists spoke of libido as if it was a homogeneous instinctive force. Clinicians will find it far more useful to conceptualize that the diverse and changeable desire manifestations are produced by the intersection of three mental forces: drive (biology), motive (psychology) and wish (culture).

Drive

By only partially understood psychoneuroendocrine mechanisms, the preoptic area of the anterior-medial hypothalamus and the limbic system periodically produce sexual drive. **Drive** is recognized by genital tingling, heightened responsivity to erotic environmental cues, plans for self or partner sexual behavior, nocturnal orgasm and increased erotic preoccupations. These are often spontaneous. Although people can become aroused and attain orgasm without evident drive, it propels the entire sexual psychophysiological process. Without drive, the sexual response system is far less efficient and capable. While men as a group seem to have significant more drive than women as a group, in both sexes, drive requires the presence of a modest amount of testosterone. Drive is frequently dampened by medications that act within the central nervous system, substances of abuse, psychiatric illness, systemic physical illness, despair and aging. It is heightened by low doses of a few often-abused substances such

as alcohol or amphetamine, manic mechanisms, falling in love, joy, and some dopaminergic compounds such as those used to treat Parkinson's disease.

Motive

The psychological aspect of desire is referred to as **motive** and is recognized by willingness to bring one's body to the partner for sexual behavior either through initiation or receptivity. Motive often directly stems from the person's perception of the context of the nonsexual and sexual relationship. Sexual desire diagnoses are often made in persons who have adequate drive manifestations. Most sexual desire problems in physically healthy adults are simply generated by one partner's unwillingness to engage in sexual behavior. This is often a secret, however. Sexual motives are originally programmed by social and cultural experiences. Children and adolescents acquire values, beliefs, expectations and rules for sexual expression. Young people have to find a way to negotiate their way through the fact that their early motives to behave sexually frequently coexist with their motives **not** to engage in sexual behavior. Conflicted motives often persist throughout life but the reasons for the conflict evolve. A teenager possessed of considerable drive and motive to make love may inhibit all sexual activities because of moral considerations emanating from religious education or the sense that he or she is just not developmentally ready yet.

Wish

An 80-year-old man who had no drive manifestations and had avoided all sexual contact with his wife for a decade because he could not get an erection, passionately answered a doctor's query about his sexual desire, "Of course, I have sexual desire! I am a red-blooded American male! Why do you think I am here?" In fact, he was only speaking about his wish to be sexually capable now that an effective treatment for erectile problems existed. The doctor asked an imprecise question. The doctor should have separately explored his drive manifestations, his sexual motivation to exchange sexual pleasure with his wife in recent years and his wish for sexual rejuvenation.

The appearance and disappearance of sexual desire is often enigmatic to a patient, but its ebb and flow result from the ever-changing intensities of its components, biological **drive**, psychological **motive** and socially acquired concepts, **wish** (Table 57.3) (Levine, 2002). In women, this interplay is generally more difficult to delineate because drive and motive are sometimes inseparable.

Sexual Desire Diagnoses

Two official diagnoses are given to men and women whose desires for partner sexual behavior are deficient: hypoactive sexual desire disorder (HSDD) and sexual aversion disorder (SAD). The differences between the two revolve around the emotional intensity with which the patient avoids sexual behavior. When visceral anxiety, fear, or disgust is routinely felt as sexual behavior becomes a possibility, sexual aversion is diagnosed. HSDD is far more frequently encountered. It is present in at least twice as many women than men; female to male ratio for aversion is far higher. Like all sexual dysfunctions, the desire diagnoses may be lifelong or may have been acquired after a period of ordinary fluctuations of sexual desire. Acquired disorders may be partner specific ("situational") or may occur with all subsequent partners ("generalized").

Table 57.3	Three Interactive Components of Sexual Desire

Sexual Drive = Biological Component

Evolves over time, decreasing with increasing age

Diminished by many psychotropic and antihypertensive medications

Manifested by the internally stimulated genital sensations and thoughts of sexual behavior that occur within a person's privacy

Sexual Motivation = Psychological Component

Highly contextual in terms of relationship status

The most socially and psychologically responsive of the three components

Evolves over time but not predictably

Manifested by a person's willingness to bring his or her body to a specific person for sexual behavior

Sexual Wish = Social Component

Expectations for sexual behavior based on membership in various subcultural groups such as family, religion, gender, region and nation

These expectations begin as cognitions of what is right and wrong and what a person is entitled to sexually and are influenced by what people think others in their cohort are experiencing

Often clinically difficult to distinguish from motivation, which wishes influence

When the psychiatrist concludes that the patient's acquired generalized HSDD is either due to a medical condition, a medication, or a substance of abuse, the diagnosis is further elaborated to sexual dysfunction due to general medical condition (for instance, HSDD due to multiple sclerosis). The frequency of the specific etiologies are heavily dependent on the clinical setting. In oncology settings, medical causes occur in high frequency; in drug rehabilitation programs, methadone maintenance will be a common cause. In marital therapy clinics, anger and loss of respect for the partner, hidden incompatibility of sexual identity between the self and the partner because of covert homosexuality or paraphilia, an affair, or childhood sexual abuse will commonly be the basis. In general psychiatry settings, medication side effects will often be the top layer of several causes. When a major depression disorder is diagnosed, for instance, the desire disorder is often assumed to be a symptom of the depression. This usually is incorrect. The desire disorder often preceded the decompensation into depression.

From a Desire Diagnosis to Dynamics

Those with **lifelong** deficiencies of sexual desire are often perceived to be struggling with either: 1) sexual identity issues involving gender identity, orientation, or a paraphilia; 2) having failed to grow comfortable as a sexual person due to extremely conservative cultural backgrounds, developmental misfortunes, or abuses. Occasionally the etiology is enigmatic, raising the important question whether it is possible to never have any sexual drive manifestations on a biological basis. (Theoretically, the answer is yes.) Both acquired and lifelong desire disorders are

often associated with past or chronic mood disorders. Disorders of desire are often listed as "of unknown etiology", but clinicians should be skeptical of this idea because:

1. The patient may not tell the doctor the truth early in the relationship;
2. The patient may have strong defenses against knowing the truth;
3. The patient may not be able to speak freely in front of the partner;
4. The patient may not know what is occurring in the partner's life, despite being influenced negatively by it;
5. The doctor may not realize the usual causes of the problem;
6. The doctor may not believe in developmental influences on the organization of adult sexual function.

Sexual aversion should strongly suggest three possibilities to the clinician:

1. that a remote traumatic experience is being relived by the partner's expression of interest in sexual behavior;
2. that without the symptom the patient feels powerless to say "no" to sexual advances;
3. the patient feels guilty about her own sexual behavior with another person.

The doctor's attention should focus on the patient's sexual development as a child, adolescent and young adult when the aversion is lifelong, whereas when it is **acquired**, the focus of the history should be on the period immediately prior to the onset of the symptom.

Desire disorders require the clinician to think both in terms of development and personal meanings of sex to their individual patients (Table 57.4). Because all explanations are speculative, they should at least make compelling sense of the patients' life experiences. Some explanations are based on the influence

Table 57.4	Obstacles to Discovering the Psychological Contributants to a Sexual Desire Disorder

Obstacles That Reside in the Patient

The patient may not tell the psychiatrist the truth about life circumstances

The patient may have strong defenses against knowing the truth

The patient may be unable to tell the truth in front of the partner

The patient may not actually know what is occurring in the partner's life, although she or he is reactive to it

Obstacles That Reside in the Psychiatrist

The psychiatrist may not realize the psychological factors that usually cause these problems

The psychiatrist may not believe that developmental influences can organize an adult sexual function such as sexual motivation

The psychiatrist may not like to deal with the murky complexity of nonbiological developmental and interpersonal issues when thinking about etiology of remote developmental processes. The term **madonna–whore complex** misleads us into thinking this is only a male pattern. The syndrome is manifested by normal sexual capacity with anyone but the fiancé or spouse. Freud interpreted this as a sign of incomplete resolution of the oedipal complex. The man was thought to be unable sexually to desire his beloved because he had unconsciously made her into his mother. He withdrew his sexual interest from her to protect himself from symbolic incest. Some women are comparably unable sexually to enjoy their partners because they unconsciously confuse their beloved with their father. Another form can be seen among patients whose parents were grossly inadequate caregivers. When these men and women find a reliable, kind, supportive person to marry, they quickly discover a strong motive to avoid sexual behavior with their fiancé. The patient makes the partner into a good-enough parent, experiences anxiety as an unconscious threat of incest associated with the possibility of sex, and becomes skillful at avoiding sexual opportunities.

Most sexual desire disorders are difficult to overcome quickly. Brief treatment generally should not be undertaken. Serious individual or couple issues frequently underlie these diagnoses. They have to be afforded time to emerge and to be worked through. However, clinicians need not be pessimistic about all of these conditions. For example, helping a couple resolve a marital dispute may return them to their usual normal sexual desire manifestations. For many individuals and couples, therapy assists the couple to accept more calmly the profound implications of continuing marital discord, infidelity, homosexuality, or other contributing factors. Some treatment failures lead to divorce and the creation of a relationship with a new partner. There is then no further sign of the desire problem. Problems rooted in early developmental experiences are particularly difficult to overcome. While DSM-IV asks the clinician to make many distinctions among the desire disorders, no follow-up study has been published in which either the subtypes (lifelong, acquired, situational, generalized) or etiologic organizers (relationship deterioration with and without extramarital affairs, sexual identity incompatibilities, parental, and medical) are separated into good and poor prognosis categories.

Developmental and identity matters are typically approached in long-term individual psychotherapy. In these sessions women often discuss the development of their femininity from adolescence to young womanhood, focusing on issues of body image, beauty, social worth to others, moral sensibilities, social awkwardness and whether they consider themselves deserving of personal physical pleasure. Men often discuss similar issues in terms of masculinity.

Anger, loss of respect, marital discord and extramarital affairs may be approached in either individual or conjoint formats. In either setting, patients often formulate the etiology as having fallen out of love with the partner. Those whose cultural backgrounds limit their ease in being a sexual person are often encouraged in educational and cultural experiences that might help them outgrow their earliest notions about what is proper sexual behavior.

The Problems of Sexual Arousal

The emotion interchangeably referred to as sexual arousal or sexual excitement generates changes in respiration, pulse and muscular tension as well as an increased blood flow to the genitals. Genital vasocongestion creates vaginal lubrication, clitoral tumescence, labial color changes, and penile erection, testicular elevation and penile color changes. How arousal is centrally coordinated in either sex remains mysterious. During lovemaking, men and women do not necessarily maintain or progressively increase their arousal; rather often there is a fluctuating intensity of arousal which is reflected in variations in vaginal wetness and penile turgidity and nongenital signs of arousal.

Female Sexual Arousal Disorder

The specificity and validity of this disorder is unclear. In women it is far more difficult to separate arousal and desire problems than in men. The perimenopausal period is now recognized as generating complaints about decreased drive, motivation, lubrication and arousal in at least 35 to 50% of women. However, it is unclear whether to label the problem as primarily of desire or arousal. It is assumed to be endocrine in origin even though estrogen, progesterone and testosterone replacement do not reliably reverse the pattern. Even in younger regularly menstruating women, however, diminished motivation and dampened drive makes it difficult to sustain arousal. Many have called into question the accepted notions that desire necessarily precedes arousal and that they are separate physiological processes. Female arousal disorder implies that drive and motivation are relatively intact although arousal is difficult. The disorder is usually an **acquired** diagnosis. Premenopausal women who have it focus on the lack of moisture in the vagina or their failure to be excited by the behaviors that previously reliably brought pleasure. They have drive and motive and wish, but enigmatically are unable to sustain arousal. Some mental factor arises to distract them from their excitement during lovemaking. Therapy is focused, therefore, on the meaning of what preoccupies them. This often involves the dynamics of their current individual or partnered life or the influence of their past relationships on their present. With therapy the diagnosis often is changed to a HSDD.

In peri- and postmenopausal women, arousal problems are more often focused on the body as a whole rather than just genital moisture deficiencies. Skin insensitivity, often a euphemism for decreased pleasure in response to oral and manual nipple, breast and vulvar stimulation, is often initially treated as a symptom of "estrogen" deficiency. Early in the menopause, a small minority of women have an increase in drive due to changing testosterone–estrogen ratios. Yet, they may still subjectively experience arousal as different than it used to be. Therapy often focuses on the women's concerns about estrogen replacement and the consequences of menopause in terms of body image, attractiveness, fears of partner infidelity, loss of health and vigor, and aging.

Aging of the female arousal mechanisms, whether simply due to shifts in ovarian endocrine production or systemic aging mechanisms, occurs earlier than deterioration of orgasmic physiology. Women with decreasing arousal are often, therefore, still reliably orgasmic with the use of vaginal lubricants well into old age. Women who have been treated with chemotherapy for breast cancer are a particularly problematic group to offer assistance to for their new arousal problems. Fear of stimulating remaining cancerous cells makes systemic estrogen replacement contraindicated.

In 1999 a renewed interest in female arousal disorder, sometimes casually called female sexual dysfunction surfaced in response to the efficacy of Viagra for men's arousal problems. It was reasoned that since the penis and clitoris are embryologic homologues with comparable adult histology, the drug would improve women's arousal. Placebo-controlled trials concluded that the drug did not improve arousal any more than placebo (Basson *et al.*, 2002).

Male Erectile Disorder

The mechanisms of erection – the sequestering and maintaining arterial blood within the corpora cavernosa – are being elucidated by urological research. Their research has led to a diminishing emphasis on "psychogenic impotence" diagnosis. Urologists may refer to male erectile disorders (ED) of a psychogenic origin as "adrenergic" ED, a reference to the preponderance of sympathetic tone on the corporal mechanisms that maintain flaccidity. Adrenergic dominance of the penile arterial tone is created by a mind that perceives the sexual context as a dangerous, frightening, or as unwanted.

The prevalence of ED rises dramatically in the sixth decade of life from less than 10 to 30%; it increases further during the seventh decade. Aging, medical conditions such as diabetes, prostatic cancer, hypertension and cardiovascular risk factors predict the most common pattern of ED due to a medical condition in this age group. While medication-induced, neurological, endocrine, metabolic, radiation and surgical causes of erectile dysfunction also exist, in population studies diabetes, hypertension, smoking, lipid abnormalities, obesity and lack of exercise are correlated with the progressive deterioration of erectile functioning in the sixth and seventh decades. These factors are thought to create a relative penile anoxemia which stimulates the conversion of corporal smooth muscle cells into fibrocytes. The gradual loss of elasticity of the corpora interferes with filling and sequestering of arterial blood. Erections at first become unreliable and finally impossible to obtain or sustain.

At every age, **selectivity** of erectile failure is the single most important diagnostic feature of primary erectile dysfunction. Clinicians should inquire about the relative firmness and duration of erections under each of these circumstances: masturbation, sex other than intercourse, sex with other female or male partners, upon stimulation with explicit media materials, in the middle of the night and upon awakening. If under some circumstances the erection is firm and lasting, the clinician can usually assume that the man's neural, endocrine and vascular physiology is sufficiently normal and that the problem is psychogenic in origin. This is true even for men in their fifties and older. Clinicians often feel more certain about this diagnosis when no diseases thought to lead to erectile dysfunction are present.

Lifelong male ED typically is psychogenic and involves either a sexual identity dilemma: such as transvestism, gender identity disorder, a homoerotic orientation, a paraphilia, or another diagnosis that expresses the patient's fear of being sexually close to a partner. Sexual identity problems are often initially denied unless the clinician is nonjudgmental and thorough during the inquiry. However, obsessive–compulsive disorder, schizoid personality, a psychotic disorder, or severe character disorders may be present. Occasionally, a reasonably normal young man with an unusually persistent fear of sexual intercourse seeks attention. These good prognosis cases are sometimes informally referred to as anxious beginners (Table 57.5). With that exception, men with lifelong male arousal disorder (MAD), when taken into individual therapy are usually perceived as having a strong motive to avoid sexual behavior and while dysfunctional with a partner during much of their therapy might equally be diagnosed as having HSDD with normal drive but a motive to avoid partner sex. The prognosis with older men with lifelong erectile dysfunction is poor even with modern erectogenic agents. Long-term therapy, even if it does not enable regular intercourse, may enable more emotional and sexual closeness to a partner. Some reasonably masculine appearing men with mild gender identity problems

Table 57.5	What the Psychiatrist Should Expect to Encounter Among Men Who Have Never Been Able to Have Intercourse with a Woman

Unconventional Sexual Identity

Gender identity problem
  Wish to be a woman
  A history of cross-dressing in women's clothing in public or private and/
  Suspected by psychiatrist but information initially withheld
Homoeroticism
  Without sexual behavior with men partner
  With sexual behavior with men but not known to the female
  With sexual behavior with men and known to the female partner
Paraphilia
  One or more of a wide range of paraphilic patterns
  Preference for prepubertal or young adolescents often initially denied unless thoroughly, systematically and nonjudgmentally questioned
  Compulsivity with or without obvious paraphilia confined to masturbation with the help of pornographic images for stimulation

Serious Character Disorders (Men Have Strong Fear of Closeness to Women)

Obsessive–compulsive
Schizotypal
Schizoid
Avoidant
Past history of psychotic decompensation

Anxious Beginners

Psychiatrically normal young men with inordinate anxiety and shyness that quickly respond to psychiatrist's encouragement and optimism and partner warmth and patience

can quickly become potent if they can reveal their need during sexual relationship to cross-dress (use a fetish article of clothing) to a partner who calmly accepts his requirement. However, most of these men have inordinate fears of sexually bonding to any woman and, in therapy, become preoccupied with basic developmental issues. Some of them marry and form companionate relationships that are rarely or never consummated.

In dramatic contrast, men with long-established good potency who have recently lost their erectile capacities with their partner – acquired psychogenic ED – have a far better prognosis (Table 57.6). They may be treated in individual or couples format, depending on the precipitants of the sexual problem and the status of their relationship with their partner. Many of these therapies become focused on resentments that have not been identified, discussed and worked through by the couple. Such distressed couples are most efficiently helped in a conjoint format. When extramarital affairs are part of the relationship deterioration and cannot be discussed, most clinicians simply work with one spouse. Potency is frequently lost following a separation or divorce. Impaired potency after a spouse's death is either about unresolved grief or problems that exist prior to the wife's terminal illness. Men are also often worried about their potency when their financial or

Table 57.6	Apparent Precipitants of Recently Acquired Psychogenic Erectile Disorder and Their Associated Private Emotions*

Deterioration of marital relationship: anger, guilt, disdain, sadness

Divorce: abandonment, anger, guilt, sadness, shame

Deterioration of personal or spousal health: sadness, anxiety, anger, shame

Death of spouse ("widower's impotence"): sadness, longing, guilt

Threat of or actual unemployment: anxiety, worthlessness, guilt, anger, shame

Financial reversal: shame, guilt, anxiety

Surreptitious extramarital affair: guilt

Reunited marriage after extramarital affair: shame, anxiety

*These short lists of simple emotions are a mere introduction to what transpires within the man's mind as a result of the meanings that the sexual behavior has for him. Although incomplete and oversimplified, they are listed to remind the psychiatrist that what the man feels about his life competes with sexual arousal during sexual behavior to generate the psychogenic erectile dysfunction.

Table 57.7	Pathogenesis Model for Acquired Erectile Dysfunction

Functional cognitive predispositions
  A normal (or real, adequate, or competent) man is able to have intercourse with anyone under any circumstances
  Feelings are a womanly intrusion on my reason; I am disinterested and relatively unaware of them.
Precipitating events (see Table 57.6)
  ↓
One episode of erectile failure
  ↓
Performance anxiety
  ↓
Another episode of erectile failure
  ↓
More performance anxiety
  ↓
Decreased frequency of sexual initiation
  ↓
Changes in the sexual equilibrium
  ↓
Established pattern of impotence with partner

vocational lives crumble, when they have a serious new physical illness such as a myocardial infarction or stroke, or when their wives become seriously ill. The esthetics of lovemaking require a context of reasonable physical health; when one spouse becomes chronically ill or disfigured by illness or surgery, either one of the couple may lose their willingness to be sexual. This may be reflected in impaired erections or sexual avoidance.

Regardless of the precipitating factors, men with arousal disorders have performance anxiety. They anticipate erectile failure before sex begins and vigilantly monitor their state of tumescence during sex (Masters and Johnson, 1970). Performance anxiety is present in almost all impotent men. Performance anxiety is efficiently therapeutically addressed by identifying it to the patient and asking him to make love without trying intercourse on several occasions to demonstrate to himself how different lovemaking can feel for him when he is not risking failure. This enables many to relax, concentrate on sensation and return to previous states of sensual abandon during lovemaking. This technique is known as **sensate focus**.

The psychological treatment of acquired arousal disorders is often highly satisfying for the professional because many of the men are anxious for help. Motivation to behave sexually is often present, fear can be allayed and men can learn to appreciate the emotional complexity of their lives. They can be shown how their minds prevented intercourse until they could acknowledge what has been transpiring within and around them. Many recently separated men, for example, are grieving, angry, guilty, uncertain and worried about their finances. Yet, they may propel themselves into a new relationship. Two characteristics seem to predispose to erectile problems at key life transitions: 1) The pursuit of the masculine standard that men ought to be able to perform intercourse with anyone, anywhere, under any circumstances; 2) The inability to readily grasp the nature and significance of his inner experiences. "Yes, my schizophrenic daughter became homeless in another city, my wife was depressed and began drinking to excess in response, and I had a financially costly affair with my secretary. What do these have to do with my loss of potency?" (Table 57.7).

Sildenafil revolutionized the treatment of erectile dysfunction in 1998. This phosphodiesterase type 5 inhibitor maintains corporal vasodilatation by preventing the degradation of cGMP. Sexual arousal leads to the corporal secretion of nitric oxide which is converted by an enzyme into cGMP. Sildenafil is increasingly effective as the dose is increased from 25 to 50 up to 100 mg. The drug must not be used when any organic nitrate is being taken because it dangerously potentiates the hypotensive effect of the nitrates risking brain and myocardial infarction. Sildenafil is dramatically underutilized by psychiatrists.

Prior to sildenafil, urologists argued that most erectile dysfunction was organic in origin, but since the drug works at about the same rate regardless of the pretreatment etiology, most erectile dysfunction is now recognized to be of mixed – organic and psychosocial – origin. Three conditions have unique response profiles: after prostatectomy the response rate is approximately 34%, among diabetics it is approximately 43%, and among the spinal cord injured it is approximately 80%; the same rate seems to improve psychogenic ED. Other medical interventions are also effective in varying degrees for largely organic erectile dysfunction: vacuum pump, the intracavernosal injection of vasodilating substances, intraurethral aprostadil, the surgical implantation of a penile prostheses and, outside the USA, sublingual apomorphine. Because sildenafil's rate of improving erections is significantly higher than the restoration of a mutually satisfactory sexual equilibrium (approximately 44%), psychological ED that persists after medication should be treated by a mental health professional.

Problems with Orgasm

Female Orgasmic Disorder

The attainment of reasonably regular orgasms with a partner is a crucial personal developmental step for young women. This task of adult sexual development rests upon a subtle interplay of physiology, individual psychology and culture. Reliable orgasmic attainment is usually highly valued by the woman and is often reflected in enhanced self-esteem, confidence in her femininity, relationship satisfaction and the motive to continue to behave sexually.

Orgasm is the reflexive culmination of arousal. It is manifested by rhythmic vaginal wall contractions and the release of muscular tension and pelvic vasocongestion, accompanied by varying degrees of pleasurable body sensations. Its accomplishment requires: 1) the physiologic apparatus to augment and sustain arousal; 2) the psychological willingness to be swept away by excitement; and 3) tenacious focus on the required physical work of augmenting arousal. The diagnosis of female orgasmic disorder (FOD) is made when the woman's psychology persistently interferes with her body's natural progression through arousal.

Estimates of prevalence of both lifelong and acquired psychological FOD range from 10 to 30% (Laumann *et al.*, 1994b). Some of this variability is due to the different definitions of anorgasmia. It remains a difficult scientific judgment, however, where to draw the line between dysfunction and normality, for example, is it normal to attain orgasms during one-third of partner sexual experiences? (Tiefer, 1998). Few women are always orgasmic.

During most of the 20th century, psychoanalysts thought that almost 90% of women were orgasmically dysfunctional. Prior to 1970, the accepted concept of normality required a woman to be brought to orgasm by penile thrusting. Orgasmic fulfillment through solitary masturbation or partner manual or oral stimulation was viewed as signifying the presence of a neurotic obstacle to mature femininity. This paternalistic idea has weakened considerably in the last generation.

The biologic potential for orgasmic attainment is an inborn endowment of nearly all physically healthy women. The cultural and psychological factors that influence orgasmic attainment are usually fundamental to the etiology of FOD. Centuries-old beliefs that sexual knowledge, behavior and sexual pleasure were not the prerogative of "good girls" powerfully affects some women's sexual adjustment. These beliefs cause young women to be uninformed about the location and role of their clitoris and ashamed of their erotic desires and sexual sensations. For women with FOD, modern concepts of equality of sexual expression are insufficient to overcome these traditional beliefs. These emotionally powerful beliefs often lay behind their classic dysfunctional pattern: the women can become aroused to a personal plateau beyond which they cannot progress; thereafter, their excitement dissipates. After numerous repetitions, they begin to lose motivation to participate in sex with their partner. They may eventually meet criteria for HSDD.

Diagnosis

The doctor should know the answers to the following questions. Does the patient have orgasms under any of the following sexual circumstances: solitary masturbation, partner manual genital stimulation, oral–genital stimulation, vibratory stimulation, any other means? Does she have orgasms with a partner different from her significant other? How are they stimulated? Does a particular fantasy make orgasmic attainment easier or possible? Under what conditions has she ever been orgasmic? Has she had an orgasm during her sleep?

Lifelong Varieties

The lifelong **generalized** variety of the disorder is recognized when a woman has never been able to attain orgasm alone or with a partner by any means, although she regularly is aroused. When a woman can only readily attain orgasm during masturbation, she is diagnosed as having a lifelong **situational** type. Women with any form of lifelong FOD more clearly have conflicts about personal sexual expression due to fear, guilt, ignorance, or obedience to tradition than those with the acquired variety. Women who can masturbate to orgasm often feel fear and embarrassment about sharing their private arousal with any other person.

Acquired Varieties

The acquired varieties of this disorder are more common and are characterized by both complete anorgasmia, too-infrequent orgasms and too-difficult orgasmic attainment. The most common cause of this problem are serotonergic compounds. Prospective studies of various antidepressants have demonstrated up to 70% incidence of this disorder among those treated with serotonergic antidepressants. Bupropion and nefazodone do not cause this problem. When medications are not the cause of an acquired FOD, the doctor needs carefully to assess the meaning of the changes in her life prior to the onset of the disorder. Some of these women are in the midst of making a transition to a new partner after many years in another relationship. Some seem to suffer from memories of earlier shame-ridden behaviors such as incest.

Treatment

When a doctor applies a label of disorder to a relatively anorgasmic woman, the woman often privately interprets the diagnosis as meaning that she has a serious and difficult problem to overcome. Physicians need to be careful about this because some of these women are relatively easy to help. It must be realized that many women gradually undo the effects of their culture on their own and grow to be increasingly responsive sexually with time and growing trust of their partners. Clinicians can do many women a great service by offering education and reassurance. Giving an inhibited woman new-to-her information in an encouraging manner can subdue her anxiety and foster her optimism. On the other hand, some women with this disorder are profoundly entrenched in not being too excited and treatments fail. The ideal era to begin treatment is young adulthood.

Four formats are known to be of help. Individual therapy is the most commonly employed. In lifelong varieties of the disorder, therapy focuses on the cultural sources of sexual inhibition and how and when they impacted upon the patient. In the situational varieties, the therapist focuses on the meaning of the life changes that preceded the onset of the disorder. Group therapy is highly effective in helping women reliably to masturbate to orgasm and moderately effective in overcoming partner inhibition. It is typically done with college and graduate students in campus settings, not older women. Couple therapy may be useful to assist the couple with the subtleties of their sexual equilibrium. The personal and interpersonal dimensions of orgasmic attainment can be stressed. Often other issues then come to the fore that initially seemed to have little to do with orgasmic attainment. The most cost-effective treatment is bibliotherapy. Female orgasmic attainment has been widely written about in the popular press since the early 1970s. It is widely believed that these articles and books, which strongly encourage knowledge of her genital anatomy, masturbation and active pursuit of orgasm, have enabled many women to grow more comfortable and competent in sexual expression.

Male Orgasmic Disorder

When a man can readily attain a lasting erection with a partner, yet is consistently unable to attain orgasm in the body of the partner, he is diagnosed with male orgasmic disorder (MOD). The disorder has three levels of severity: 1) the most common form is characterized by the **ability** to attain orgasm with a partner outside of her or his body, either through oral, manual, or personal masturbation; 2) the more severe form is characterized by the man's inability to ejaculate in his partner's presence; and 3) the rarest form is characterized by the inability to ejaculate when awake. The disorder is usually lifelong and not partner specific. These men cannot allow themselves to be swept away in arousal by another person. They are sexually vigilant not to allow themselves to be controlled by the partner's power to convey them to orgasm. This power would provide the partner with personal pleasure and the man with this disorder, while initially appearing to be a sexual superman, ultimately disappoints the partner. Their psychological dysfunction represents a capacity to use a mental mechanism which other men would love to possess in smaller degrees. Both the partners and the therapists of these men tend to describe them as controlling, unemotional, untrusting, hostile, obsessive–compulsive, or paranoid. Some of these men improve with psychotherapy, others improve spontaneously with time and, for others, the dysfunction leads to the cessation of the aspiration for sex with a partner. One controlled study of patients with numerous sexual dysfunctions suggested that bupropion 300 to 450 mg/day may improve the capacity to ejaculate in a minority of patients.

Premature Ejaculation

Premature ejaculation is a high prevalence (25–40% disorder seen primarily in heterosexuals characterized by an untameably low threshold for the reflex sequence of orgasm. The problem, a physiological **efficiency** of sperm delivery, causes social and psychological distress. In failing to develop a sense of control over the timing of his orgasm in the vagina, the man fails to meet his standards of being a satisfying sexual partner. However, if his partner does not explicitly or implicitly object, his rapidity is not likely to cause him to seek medical attention. The range of intravaginal containment times among self-diagnosed patients extends from immediately before or upon vaginal entry (rare), to less than a minute (usual), to less than the man and his partner desire (not infrequent). Time alone is a misleading indicator, however. The essence of the self-diagnosis is an emotionally unsatisfying sexual equilibrium apparently due to the man's inability to temper his arousal. Most men sometimes ejaculate before they wish to, but not persistently.

Clinical Approach

The history should clarify the answers to following questions: Why is he seeking therapy now? Is the patient a sexual beginner or a beginner with a particular partner? Does he have inordinately high expectations for intravaginal containment time for a man his age and experience? Is he desperate about losing the partner because of the rapid ejaculation? Is the relationship in jeopardy for another reason? Does his partner have a sexual dysfunction? Does she have orgasms with him other than through intercourse? Is he requesting help in order to cover his infidelity? Is his partner now blaming the man's sexual inadequacy for her infidelity? Is his new symptom a reflection of his fear about having a serious physical problem during sex such as angina, a stroke, or another myocardial infarction? The answers will enable the doctor to classify the rapid ejaculation into an acquired or lifelong and specific or general pattern, to sense the larger

context in which his sexual behavior is conducted and to plan treatment.

Premature ejaculation reflects to the man's sense that his contribution to the sexual equilibrium is deficient. It implies that he considers that he is far behind most men in his vaginal containment time and that he wants to provide his partner with a better opportunity to be nurtured during lovemaking through prolonged intercourse. Typically, he aspires to "bring" his partner to orgasm during intercourse. If anxiety lowers the ejaculatory threshold and keeps it from its natural evolution to a higher level over time, then premature ejaculation is a self-perpetuating pattern. Premature ejaculation may last a lifetime.

Therapy

There are three efficient approaches to this dysfunction. The first is simply to refuse to confirm the patient's self- diagnosis. Some anxious beginners, men with reasonable intravaginal containment times of two or more minutes, and those with exaggerated notions of sexual performance can be calmed down by a few visits. When they no longer think of themselves as dysfunctional their intravaginal containment times improve. The second is the use of serotonergic medications. In a study of 15 carefully selected stable couples, daily administration of clomipramine 25 and 50 mg increased intravaginal containment times on average of 249% and 517% over baseline observations (Althof *et al.*, 1995). At these dosage levels, there were few side effects. Numerous similar reports testify to the fact that various serotonergic reuptake inhibitors can significantly lengthen the duration of intercourse. Clinicians need to determine with each patient whether the medication can be taken within hours or days of anticipated intercourse. Improvement is not sustained after medication is stopped. Serotonergic medications are the most common treatment of rapid ejaculation because they are so quickly effective in over 90% of men. The third approach is behaviorally-oriented sex therapy that trains the man to focus his attention on his penile sensations during vaginal containment and to signal his partner to cease movement or to apply a firm squeeze of the glans/ shaft area to interrupt the escalation of arousal. This requires an increase in communication and full cooperation of the partner which in themselves can go a long way in improving their sexual equilibrium.

Rapid ejaculation in some men reflects mere inexperience; for others it is stubborn physiological efficiency; for others it reflects fear of personal harm, which is either related to physical illness or to unresolved fears of closeness to a woman; and yet for others it reflects a partnership with a profoundly inhibited blaming partner. If the psychodynamic question is asked of men with persistent rapid ejaculation, "Why does this man want to finish intercourse so quickly?" the answers vary from, "It is not a relevant question!" to "I'm afraid of her!" to "I'm afraid of what will happen to me". For instance, a large percentage of men ejaculate quickly for the first months after a myocardial infarction.

The advantages of costlier couple psychotherapy are to allow the man and his partner to understand their lives better, to address both of their sexual anxieties, and to deal with other important nonsexual issues in their relationship. Effective psychotherapy allows the man to become positioned to continue the usual biological evolution that occurs during the life-cycle from rapid ejaculation, which is true for many young men, to occasional difficulty in ejaculating, which is true for many men in their sixties.

Sexual Pain Disorders

The clinician needs to consider a series of questions when dealing with a woman who reports painful intercourse. Does she have a known gynecologic abnormality which is generally associated with pain? Is there anything about her complaint of pain that indicates a remarkably low pain threshold? Does she now have an aversion to sexual intercourse? At what level of physical discomfort did she develop the aversion? Does her private view of her current relationship affect her willingness to be sexual and her experience of pain? Does her partner's sexual style cause her physical or mental discomfort, for example, is he overly aggressive or does he stimulate memories of former abuse? What has been the partner's response to her pain? What role does her anticipation of pain play in her experience of pain?

These clinical questions are typical biopsychosocial ones. Sex-limiting pain often is the result of the subtle interplay of personal and relational, cognitive and affective, and fundamental biological processes that are inherent in other human sexual struggles that operate to produce these confusing disorders.

The DSM-IV presents dyspareunia and vaginismus as distinct entities. However, they have been viewed as inextricably connected in much of the modern sexuality literature: vaginismus is known to create dyspareunia and dyspareunia has been known to create vaginismus.

Dyspareunia

Terminology

Recurrent uncomfortable or painful intercourse in either gender is known as dyspareunia. Women's dyspareunia varies from discomfort at intromission, to severe unsparing pain during penile thrusting, to vaginal irritation following intercourse. In both sexes, recurring coital pain leads to inhibited arousal and sexual avoidance. "Dyspareunia" is used as both a symptom and a diagnosis. When coital pain is caused solely by defined physical pathology, dyspareunia due to a medical condition is diagnosed. When coital pain is due to vaginismus, insufficient lubrication, or other presumably psychogenic factors, dyspareunia not due to a medical condition diagnosis is made. Psychogenic etiologies may include a CNS pain perception problem raising the question, "What do we mean by psychogenic?" This arena's nomenclature will undoubtably change when a breakthrough in understanding the causes of coital pain occurs.

Psychogenic Sources of Dyspareunia

Pain associated with intercourse may have purely subjective or psychologic origin. Couple dynamics are often relevant, but the pain may be seen as a means of not allowing painful memories of childhood sexual abuse into clear focus. Fear of or helplessness about negotiating interpersonal conflicts may eventually lead to pain becoming a solution for avoiding unwanted sexual behaviors. While physicians tend to assume that pain has unconscious origins, sometimes it is merely faked; more often the patient is quite aware of its developmental origins but is too embarrassed quickly to communicate it to the doctor.

Personal psychological origins of painful intercourse pass through the common denominator of anxiety. Such anxiety may take the forms of dread of physical damage, worry about the psychological dependence that might result from physical union, fear of a first or another pregnancy, or a sexually transmitted disease. Intense anxiety, the psychological source of her pain, may lead to involuntary contraction of vaginal muscles which is the mechanical source of her pain. Thus, dyspareunia and vaginismus reinforce each other. Both situational and acquired dyspareunia may reflect a woman's conscious or unconscious motivation to avoid sex with a particular partner; it may be her only means to express her despair about their nonsexual relationship. Lifelong dyspareunia draws the clinicians attention to developmental experiences.

Differential Diagnosis

Because the **symptom** dyspareunia is produced by numerous organic conditions, the psychiatrist should be certain that the patient has had a pelvic examination by a person equipped to assess a broad range of regional pathology. Vulvovestibulitis is diagnosed by pain in response to cotton swab touching in a normal appearing vulvar vestibule. A fundamental question remains unanswered about this often devastating problem: "Is the disorder of local or central origin?" In these patients and some others, the pain can not be classified with certainty as a **symptom** or a **disorder**. Pain upon penile or digital insertion may be due to an intact hymen or remnants of the hymenal ring, vaginitis, cervicitis, episiotomy scars, endometriosis, fibroids, ovarian cysts, and so on. Postcoital dyspareunia often begins at orgasm when uterine contractions occur. Fibroids, endometriosis and pelvic inflammatory disease should be considered. Postmenopausal pain, particularly if the woman has had many years without intercourse, is often a result of thinning of the vaginal mucosa, loss of elasticity of the labia and vaginal outlet, and decreased lubrication. Normal menopause, however, is often associated with mild pain due to inadequate lubrication (in both partners).

Dyspareunia in men is usually due to a medical condition. Herpes, gonorrhea, prostatitis and Peyronie's disease cause pain during intercourse. Remote trauma to the penis may cause penile chordee or bowing which makes intercourse mechanically difficult and sometimes painful. Pain experienced upon ejaculation can be a side effect of trazodone.

Vaginismus

Vaginismus is an involuntary spasm of the musculature of the outer third layer of the vagina which makes penile penetration difficult or impossible. The diagnosis is not made if an organic cause is known. Although a woman with vaginismus may wish to have intercourse, her symptom prevents the penis from entering her body. It is as though her vagina says, "No!" In lifelong vaginismus, the anticipation of pain at the first intercourse causes muscle spasm. Pain reinforces the fear and, on occasion, the partner's response gives her good reason to dread a second opportunity to have intercourse. Early episodic vaginismus may be common among women, but most of the cases that are brought to medical attention are chronic. Lifelong vaginismus is relatively rare. The clinician needs to focus attention on what may have made the idea of intercourse so overwhelming to her: parental intrusiveness, sexual trauma, childhood genital injury, illnesses whose therapy involved orifice penetration and surgery?

The woman with lifelong vaginismus not only has a history of unsuccessful attempts at penetration but displays an avoidance of finger and tampon penetration. The most dramatic aspect of her history, however, is her inability to endure a speculum examination of her vagina. Vaginismus is a phobia of vaginal entrance.

Treatment of Dyspareunia and Vaginismus

While vaginismus has the reputation of being readily treatable by gynecologists by pairing relaxation techniques with progressively larger vaginal dilators, the mental health professional typically approaches the problem differently. The psychiatric approach to both vaginismus and dyspareunia is attuned to the role that her symptom plays in her life. The therapy, therefore, does not begin with a cavalier, optimistic attempt to remove the symptom, which only frightens some patients. Rather, it begins with a patient exploration of the developmental and interpersonal meanings of the need for the symptom. "I wonder how this problem originally got started? Can you tell me a bit more about your life?" In the course of assisting women with these problems a variety of techniques may be utilized including relaxation techniques, sensate focus, dilatation, marital therapy and medication. Short-term therapies should not be expected to have lasting good results because once the symptom is relieved, other problematic aspects of the patient's sexual equilibrium and nonsexual relationship often come into focus. Clinicians have developed an impression that women with a diagnosis of dyspareunia are particularly difficult to help permanently. However, this is a largely unstudied topic.

Sexual Dysfunction Not Otherwise Specified

This diagnosis is reserved for circumstances that leave the doctor uncertain as to how to diagnose the patient. This may occur when the patient has too many fluctuating dysfunctional symptoms without a clear pattern of prominence of anyone of them. Sometimes the psychiatrist is unable to determine whether the dysfunction is the basic complaint or when the sexual complaints are secondary to marital dysfunction. At other times the etiology is the uncertain: psychogenic, due to a general medical condition, or substance-induced. When the patient does not emphasize the dysfunction as the problem but emphasizes instead the lack of emotional satisfaction from sex, the psychiatrist may temporarily provide this NOS diagnosis. It is usually possible to find a better dysfunction diagnosis after therapy begins.

Gender Identity Disorders

The organization of a stable gender identity is the first component of sexual identity to emerge during childhood. The processes that enable this accomplishment are so subtle that when a daughter consistently acts as though she realizes that "I am a girl and that is all right", or when a son's behavior announces that "I am a boy and that is all right", families rarely even remember their children's confusion and behaviors to the contrary. Adolescent and adult gender problems are not rare. They are however commonly hidden from social view, sometimes long enough to developmentally evolve into other less dramatic forms of sexual identity.

Early Forms

Extremely Feminine Young Boys

Although occasionally the parents of a feminine son have a convincing anecdote about persistent feminine interests dating from early in the second year of life, boyhood femininity is more typically only apparent by the third year. By the fourth year playmate preferences become obvious. Same-sex playmate preference is a typical characteristic of young children. Cross-gender–identified children consistently demonstrate the opposite sex playmate preference. The avoidance of other boys has serious consequences in terms of social rejection and loneliness throughout the school years. The peer problems of feminine boys cause some of their behavioral and emotional problems which are in evidence by middle-to-late childhood. However, psychometric studies support clinical impressions that feminine boys have emotional problems even before peer relationships become a factor, that is, something more basic about being cross-gender-identified creates problems. Young feminine boys have been shown to be depressed and have difficulties with separation anxiety.

Speculations about the origin of boyhood femininity generally suggest converging cumulative forces. Any child's cross-gender identifications are likely to involve a host of factors: constitutional forces, problematic interactions with parents, problematic internal processing of life experiences and family misfortune: financial, reproductive, physical disease, emotional illness, or death of vital persons. These factors are sometimes restated as temperament, disturbed family functioning, separation–individuation problems and trauma.

Temperament is a dual phenomenon being both the child's predisposition to respond to the world in a certain way and the aspects of the child to which others respond. The common temperamental factors of feminine boys have been described as: a sense of body fragility and vulnerability that leads to the avoidance of rough-and-tumble play; timidity and fearfulness in the face of new situations; a vulnerability to separation and loss; an unusual capacity for positive emotional connection to others; an ability to imitate; sensitivities to sound, color, texture, odor, temperature and pain (Coates *et al.*, 1992).

The development of boyhood femininity may occur within the mind of the toddler in response to a loss of emotional availability of the nurturant mother. The child creates a maternal (feminine) self through imitation and fantasy in order to make up for the mother's emotional unavailability. This occurs beyond the family's awareness and is left in place by the family either ignoring what has transpired in the son or valuing it. The problem for the effeminate boy is that reality – the social expectations of other people – is unyielding on gender issues; the adaptive early life solution becomes progressively more maladaptive with time.

The answer to the question whether boyhood femininity is entirely constitutional, an adaptive solution, or due to a combination that includes some other process is not known. A few reports of femininity giving way to psychotherapeutic interventions with young boys and their families are of heuristic value but limited in follow-up duration.

Green prospectively studied a large well-matched group of feminine boys for over a decade and discovered that boyhood effeminacy was a frequent precursor of adolescent homoeroticism and homosexual behavior rather than gender identity disorders. He observed, as had others before, that without therapy feminine gender role behaviors give rise to more masculine behavioral styles as adolescence emerges (Green, 1987).

Masculine Girls: Tomboys

The masculinity of girls may become apparent as early as age 2 years. The number of girls brought to clinical attention for cross-gendered behaviors, self-statements and aspirations is consistently less than boys by a factor of 1:5 at any age of childhood in Western countries (except Poland). It is not known whether this reflects a genuine difference in incidence of childhood gender disorders, cultural perceptions of femininity as a negative in boys versus the neutral-to-positive perception of boy-like behaviors in girls, the broader range of cross-gender expression permitted to girls but not to boys, or an intuitive understanding that cross-gender identity more accurately predicts homosexuality in boys than girls.

The distinction between tomboys and gender-disordered girls is often difficult to make. Tomboys are thought of as not as deeply unhappy about their femaleness, not as impossible occasionally to dress in stereotypic female clothing, and not thought to have a profound aversion to their girlish and future womanly physiologic transformations. Tomboys are able to enjoy some feminine activities along with their obvious pleasures in masculine-identified toys and games and the company of boys. Girls who are diagnosed as gender-disordered generally seem to have a relentless intensity about their masculine preoccupations and an insistence about their future. The onset of their cross-gendered identifications is early in life. Although most lesbians have a history of tomboyish behaviors, most tomboys develop a heterosexual orientation.

The Subjectivity of a Well-developed Gender Disorder

Children, teenagers and adults exist who rue the day they were born to their biological sex and who long for the opportunity simply to live their lives in a manner befitting the other gender. They repudiate the possibility of finding happiness within the broad framework of roles given to members of their sex by their society. Their repudiation is not motivated by an intellectual attack on sexism, homophobia, or any other injustice imbedded in cultural mores. A gender-disordered person literally repudiates his or her body, repudiates the self in that body and rejects performing roles expected of people with that body. It is a subtle, usually self-contained rebellion against the need of others to designate them in terms of their biological sex.

The repudiation and rebellion may first occur as a subjective internal drama of fantasy, as behavioral expression in play, or a preference for the company of others. Regardless of when and how it is displayed, the drama of the gender-disordered involves the relentless feeling that "life would be better – easier, fuller, more enjoyable – if I and others could experience me as a member of the opposite sex".

By mid-adolescence, the extremely gender-disordered have often envisioned the solution for their paralyzing self-consciousness: to live as a member of the opposite gender, to transform their bodies to the extent possible by modern medicine, and to be accepted by all others as the opposite sex. Most people with these cross-gender preoccupations, however, do not go beyond the fantasy or private cross-dressing. Those that do eventually come to psychiatric attention. When a clinician is called in, the family has one set of hopes, the patient another. The clinician has many tasks, one of which is to mediate between the ambitions of the gender-disordered person and society and see what can be done to help the patient. Negative countertransference may steer the clinician to deal with the opportunity expeditiously: "Obviously the patient is sick, maybe psychotic, and needs help. I don't take care of people who do these things. Refer it out!" With a little supervisory encouragement to perform a thorough evaluation, therapists soon find that these patients possess many of the ordinary aspects of life and one unusual ambition: they often want to be the opposite sex so badly that they are willing to make it a priority over family, friends, vocation and material acquisition.

Diagnostic Criteria of Gender Identity Disorder

Adults who permanently change their bodies to deal with their gender dilemmas represent the far end of the spectrum of adaptations to gender problems. Even the lives of those who reject bodily change, however, have considerable pain because the images of a better gendered self may recur throughout life, becoming more powerful whenever life becomes strained or disappointing.

The diagnosis of the extreme end of the gender identity disorder spectrum is clinically obvious. The challenging diagnostic task for clinicians is to suspect a gender problem and inquire about gender identity and its evolution in those whose manner suggest a unisexed or cross-gendered appearance, those with dissociative gender identity disorder (GID), severe forms of character pathology and those who seem unusual in some undefinable manner.

DSM-IV provides the clinician with two Axis I gender diagnoses. To qualify for the first, a patient of any age must meet four criteria:

Criterion 1: Strong, persistent cross-gender identification Because young children may not verbalize enough about their inner experiences for the clinician to be certain that this criterion is met, at least four of five manifestations of cross-gender identification must be present: 1) repeatedly stated desire to be, or insistence that he or she is, the opposite sex; 2) in boys, preference for cross-dressing or simulating female attire; in girls, insistence on wearing stereotypical masculine clothing; 3) strong and persistent preferences for cross-gender roles in fantasy play or persistent fantasies of being the opposite sex; 4) intense desire to participate in the games and pastimes of the opposite sex; 5) strong preference for playmates of the opposite sex.

In adolescence and adulthood, this criterion is fulfilled when the patient states the desire to be the opposite sex, has frequent social forays into appearing as the opposite sex, desires to live or be treated as the opposite sex, or has the conviction that his or her feelings and reactions are those typical of the opposite sex.

Criterion 2: Persistent discomfort with one's gender or the sense of inappropriateness in a gender role This criterion is fulfilled in boys who assert that their penis or testicles are disgusting or will disappear or that it would be better not to have these organs; or who demonstrate an aversion toward rough-and-tumble play and rejection of male stereotypical toys, games and activities. In girls, rejection of urinating in a sitting position or assertion that they do not want to grow breasts or menstruate, or marked aversion towards normative feminine clothing fulfill this criterion.

Among adolescents and adults, this criterion is fulfilled by the patients' exhibiting the following characteristics: preoccupation with getting rid of primary and secondary sex characteristics; preoccupation with thoughts about hormones, surgery, or other alterations of the body to enhance the capacity to pass as a member of the opposite sex such as electrolysis for beard removal, cricoid cartilage shave to minimize the Adam's apple, breast augmentation, or preoccupation with the belief that one was born into the wrong sex.

Criterion 3: Not due to an intersex condition In the vast majority of clinical circumstances the patient possesses normal genital anatomy and sexual physiology. When a patient with a gender identity disorder and an accompanying intersex condition such as congenital adrenal hyperplasia, an anomaly of the genitalia, or a chromosomal abnormality is encountered, the clinician will be uncertain whether the intersex condition is the cause of the GID. The clinician may either diagnose gender identity disorder not otherwise specified (GIDNOS) or classify the patient as having a GID and list the physical factor on Axis III as a comorbid condition. The relationship between GID and intersex conditions is controversial topic that may be clarified with further research being done in Germany.

Criterion 4: Significant distress and impairment   It is likely that many children, adolescents and adults struggle for a while to consolidate their gender identity but eventually find an adaptation that does not impair their capacities to function socially, academically, or vocationally as a member of their sex. These persons do not qualify for GID nor do those who simply are not stereotypic in how they portray their gender roles. Mental health professionals occasionally encounter parents who are disturbed by their adolescent child's gender roles. Parental distress is not the point of criterion 4; this criterion refers to patient distress.

Diagnostic Criteria of Gender Identity Disorder Not Otherwise Specified (GIDNOS)

If an accurate community-based study of the gender-impaired could be conducted, most cases would be diagnosed as GIDNOS. The diagnostician needs to understand that gender identity development is a dynamic evolutionary process and clinicians see people at crisis points in their lives. At any given time, although it is clear that the patient has some form of GID, it may not be that which is described in DSM-IV as GID. Here is one example: an adult female calls herself a "neuter". She wants her breasts removed because she hates to be perceived as a woman. For 2 years she has been exploring "neuterdom" and "I am definitely not interested in being a man!" If in 2 years, she evolves to meet criterion 1, her current GIDNOS diagnosis will change.

GIDNOS is a large category designed to be inclusive of those with unusual genders who do not clearly fit the criteria of GID. There is no implication that if a patient is labeled GIDNOS that his or her label cannot change in the future. GIDNOS would contain the many forms of transvestism: masculine-appearing boys and teenagers with persistent cross-dressing (former fetishistic transvestites) who are evolving toward GID, socially isolated men who want to become a woman shortly after their wives or mothers die (secondary transvestites) but express considerable ambivalence about the very matter they passionately desired at their last visit, extremely feminized homosexuals including those with careers as "drag queens" who seem to want to change their sex when depressed, and so on. GIDNOS would also capture men who want to be rid of their genitals without being feminized, unisexual females who imagine themselves as males but who are terrified of any social expression of their masculine gender identity, hypermasculine lesbians in periodic turmoil over their gender, and those women who strongly identify with both male and female who lately want mastectomies. In using gender identity diagnoses, clinicians need to remember that extremely masculine women or extremely feminine men are not to be dismissed as homosexual. "Lesbian" or "gay" is only a description of orientation. They are more aptly described as also cross-gendered.

The Relationship of Gender Identity Disorders to Orientation

The usual clarity of distinctions between heterosexual, bisexual and homosexual orientations rests upon the assumption that the biological sex and psychological gender of the person and the partner are known. A woman who designates herself as a lesbian is understood to mean she is erotically attracted to other women. "Lesbian" loses its meaning if the woman says she feels she **is** a man and lives as one. She insists, "I am a heterosexual man; men are attracted to women as am I!" The baffled clinician may erroneously think, "You are a female therefore you are a lesbian!" DSM-IV suggests that adults with GIDs should be

subgrouped according to which sex the patient is currently sexually attracted: males, females, both, or neither. This makes sense for most gender patients because it is their gender identity that is most important to them. Some are rigid about the sex of those to whom they are attracted because it supports their idea about their gender, others are bierotic and are not too concerned with their orientation, still others have not had enough experiences to overcome their uncertainty about their orientation. A few gender patients find all partners too complicated and are only interested in themselves.

Treatment Options for the Gender Identity Disorders

The treatment of these conditions, although not as well-based on scientific evidence as some psychiatric disorders, has been carefully scrutinized by multidisciplinary committees of specialists within the Harry Benjamin International Gender Dysphoria Association for over 20 years. For more details in managing an individual patient, please consult its "Standards of Care" (Meyer et al., 2001). The treatment of any GID begins after a careful evaluation, including parents, other family members, spouses, psychometric testing, and occasionally physical and laboratory examination. The details will depend on age of the patient. It is possible, of course, to have a GID as well as mental retardation, a psychosis, dysthymia, severe character pathology, or any other psychiatric diagnosis (Table 57.8).

Individual Psychotherapy

No one knows how to cure an adult's gender problem. People who have lived long with profound cross-gender identifications do not

Table 57.8	Steps in Evaluation of the Profoundly Gender Disordered*

Formal evaluation and diagnosis—gender identity disorder or gender identity disorder NOS. Can the patient be referred to a gender program? Is another treatable psychiatric or physical disorder present?

Individual psychotherapy within the gender program or with yes,interested professional. Do the diagnoses remain the same? Ifan does the patient consistently want to

Discuss his (or her) situation but make no changes?

Increase cross-dressing toward cross-living?

Prepare the family for the real-life test?

Obtain permission to proceed with hormones?

Approval for hormones from a gender committee or on written recommendation from the psychiatrist to an endocrinologist. Individual or group psychotherapy should continue.

Real-life test of living and working full time in the aspired-to gender role for at least 1 year. Does the patient want to continue to surgery?

Gender committee approval for surgery. Many patients have cosmetic surgery other than that listed with only ordinary patient–surgeon consent. This most often involves breast augmentation but may include numerous other attempts to improve ability to pass as opposite sex and be attractive.

Men—genital reconstruction

Women—mastectomy, hysterectomy, genital reconstruction

*Most patients will not complete all of these steps.

get insight – either behaviorally modified or medicated – and find that they subsequently have a conventional gender identity. Psychotherapy is useful, nonetheless. If the patient is able to trust a therapist, there can be much to talk about: family relationships are often painful, barriers to relationship intimacy are profound, work poses many difficult issues, and the patient has to make monumental decisions. The central one is, "How am I going to live my life? Should I go through with cross-gender living, hormone therapy, mastectomy, or genital surgery?" The therapist can help the patient recognize the drawbacks and advantages of the various available options and to respect the initially unrecognized or unstated ambivalence. Completion of the gender transformation process usually takes longer than the patient desires, and the therapist can be an important source of support during and after these changes.

Group Therapy

Group therapy for gender-disordered people has the advantages of allowing patients to know others with gender problems, of decreasing their social isolation, and of being among people who do not experience their cross-gender aspirations and their past behaviors as weird. Group members can provide help with grooming and more convincing public appearances. The success of these groups depends on the therapist's skills in patient selection and using the group process. Groups are generally only available in a few specialized treatment programs.

"Real-life Test"

Living in the aspired-to-gender role – working, relating, conducting the activities of daily living – is a vital process that enables one of three decisions: to abandon the quest, to simply live in this new role, or to proceed with breast or genital surgery (Peterson and Dickey, 1995). Some clinicians use the real-life test as a criterion for recommending hormones but this varies because some patients' abilities to present themselves in a new way is definitely enhanced by prior administration of cross-sex hormones. The reason for the real-life test is to give the patient, who created a transsexual solution in fantasy, an opportunity to experience the solution in social reality. Passing the real-life test is expected to be associated with improved psychological function.

Hormone Therapy

Ideally, hormones should be administered by endocrinologists who have a working relationship with a mental health team dealing with gender problems. The effects of administration of estrogen to a biological male are: breast development, testicular atrophy, decreased sexual drive, decreased semen volume and fertility, softening of skin, fat redistribution in a female pattern and decrease in spontaneous erections. Breast development is often the highest concern to the patient. Because hair growth is not affected by estrogens, electrolysis is often used to remove beard growth. Side effects within recommended doses are minimal but hypertension, hyperglycemia, lipid abnormalities, thrombophlebitis and hepatic dysfunction have been described. The most dramatic effect of hormones is on the sense of well-being. Patients report feeling calmer, happier knowing that their bodies are being demasculinized and feminized. All results derive from open-labeled studies.

The administration of androgen to females results in an increased sexual drive, clitoral tingling and growth, weight gain, and amenorrhea and hoarseness. An increase in muscle mass may be apparent if weight training is undertaken simultaneously. Hair growth depends on the patient's genetic potential. Androgens are administered intramuscularly 200 to 300 mg/month and are generally safe. It is prudent, however, periodically to monitor hepatic, lipid and thyroid functioning. Most patients are delighted with their bodily changes, although some are disappointed that they remain short, wide-hipped, relatively hairless men with breasts that do not significantly regress.

Surgical Therapy

Surgical intervention is the final external step. It should not occur without mental health professional's input, even when the patient provides a heart-felt convincing set of reasons to bypass the real-life test, hormones and therapeutic relationship. Genital surgery is expensive, time-consuming, at times painful, and has frequent anatomic complications and functional disappointments. Surgery can be expected to add further improvements in the lives of patients: more social activities with friends and family, more activity in sports, more partner sexual activity and improved vocational status.

Males Surgery consists of penectomy, orchiectomy, vaginoplasty and fashioning of a labia. The procedures used for the creation of a neovagina have evolved over the years. Postoperatively, the patient must maintain the patency of the neovagina by initially constantly wearing and then periodically using a vaginal dilator. Vaginal stenosis or shortening is a frequent complication. The quest for an unmistakable feminine shape leads many young adult patients to augmentation mammoplasty and the shaving of their cricoid cartilage.

Females The creation of a male-appearing chest through mastectomies and contouring of the chest wall requires only a brief hospital stay. Patients are usually immediately delighted with their new-found freedom, but their fantasies of going shirtless are often not fulfilled due to the presence of two noticeable horizontal chest scars. The creation of a neophallus that can become erect, contain a functional urethra throughout its length (enabling urination while standing), and pass as an unremarkable penis in a locker room has been a significant surgical challenge. It is far from perfected. The surgery is, however, the most time-consuming, technically difficult and expensive of all the sex reassignment procedures. Erection is made possible by a penile prosthesis. Many prudent patients consider themselves reassigned when they have a hysterectomy, oophorectomy and mastectomy. Some just have a mastectomy. They find a partner who understands the situation and supports the idea of living with, and loving with, female genitals.

The Paraphilias

A paraphilia is a disorder of intention, the final component of sexual identity to develop in children and adolescents. Intention refers to what individuals want to do with a sexual partner and what they want the partner to do with them during sexual behavior. Normally, the images and the behaviors of intention fall within ranges of peaceable mutuality. The disorders of intention are recognized by unusual eroticism (images) and often socially destructive behaviors such as sex with children, rape, exhibitionism, voyeurism, masochism, obscene phone calling, or sexual touching of strangers. While 5% of the diagnoses of paraphilia are given to women, etiologic speculations refer to male sexual identity development gone awry. This raises the important question about what happens to girls who have the same developmental misfortunes that are speculated to create male paraphilia. Accounts of paraphilic behaviors have been in the nonmedical literatures for centuries.

Now it is apparent that paraphilias occur among individuals of all orientations and among those with conventional and unconventional gender identities. A homosexual sadist is paraphilic only on the basis of sexual cruelty. A transsexual who desires to be beaten during arousal is paraphilic only on the basis of masochism.

Three General Characteristics of the Paraphilias

A Longstanding, Unusual, Highly-arousing Erotic Preoccupation

Erotic intentions that are not longstanding, unusual, and highly arousing may be problematic in some way but they are not clearly paraphilic. The *sine qua non* of the diagnosis of paraphilia is unusual, often hostile, dehumanized eroticism which has preoccupied the patient for most of his adolescent and adult life. The paraphilic fantasy is often associated with this preoccupying arousal when it occurs in daydreams and masturbation reveries or is encountered in explicit films or magazines. The specific imagery varies from one paraphilic patient to the next, but both the imagined behavior and its implied relationship to the partner are unusual in that they are preoccupied with aggression. Images of rape, obscene phone calling, exhibitionism and touching of strangers, for example, are rehearsals of victimization. In masochistic images, the aggression is directed at the self, for instance, autoerotic strangulation, slavery, torture, spanking. In others, the aggression is well-disguised as **love** of children or teenagers. In some, such as simple clothing fetishism, the aggression may be absent. Aggression is so apparent in most paraphilic content, however, that when none seems to exist, the clinician needs to wonder whether it is actually absent or being hidden from the doctor. Paraphilic fantasies often rely heavily upon the image of a partner who does not possess "personhood". Some imagery in fact has no pretense of a human partner at all; clothing, animals, or excretory products are the focus. Other themes such as preoccupation with feet or hair, combine both human and inanimate interests. Paraphilic images are usually devoid of any pretense of caring or human attachment. The hatred, anger, fear, vengeance, or worthlessness expressed in them require no familiarity with the partner. Paraphilic images are conscious – clearly known to the individual. They should not be confused with speculations about "unconscious" aggression or sadomasochism that some assume are part of all sexual behavior (Kernberg, 1991). Clinicians should expect occasionally to see paraphilic patients whose preoccupations are not hostile to others.

An individual's paraphilic themes often change in intensity or seem to change in content from time to time. The stimuli for these changes often remain unclear. It is a moot point whether changes should be considered a shift to a different disorder, a new paraphilia, or a natural evolution of the basic problem. The shifts from imagining talking "dirty" on the phone in order to scare a woman to imagining raping can be considered an intensification of sadism. Switches between sadism and masochism or voyeurism and exhibitionism are common. Changes from voyeurism to pedophilia or from pedophilia to rape, however, raise the question whether a new disorder has developed. The most socially significant shifts are from erotic imagery to sexual behavior. In most instances, it is reasonable to consider that paraphilia is a basic developmental disorder in which particular erotic

and sexual manifestations are shaped by the individuality of the person's history.

Most paraphilic adults can trace their fantasy themes to puberty and many can remember these images from earlier years. When adolescent rapists or incest offenders are evaluated, they often are able to report prepubertal aggressive erotic preoccupations. Men who report periodic paraphilic imagery interspersed with more usual eroticism have had their paraphilic themes from childhood or early adolescence. To make a diagnosis of paraphilia, the patient must evidence at least 6 months of the unusual erotic preoccupation. Duration is usually not in question, even among adolescents, however (Shaw, 1999).

Pressure to Act Out the Fantasy

To be paraphilic means that the erotic imagery exerts a pressure to play out the often imagined scene. In its milder forms, the pressure results merely in a preoccupation with a behavior. For instance, a man who prefers to be spoken to harshly and dominated by his wife during sex thinks about his masochistic images primarily around their sexual behaviors. He does not spend hours daydreaming of his erotic preferences. In its more intense forms, paraphilias create a **drivenness** to act out the fantasy in sexual behavior – usually in masturbation. Frequent masturbation, often more than once daily, continues long after adolescence. In the most severe situations, the need to attend to the fantasy and masturbate is so overpowering that life's ordinary activities cannot efficiently occur. Masturbation and sometimes partner-seeking behavior – such as finding a woman to shock through exhibiting an erection – is experienced as driven. The patient reports either that he cannot control his behavior or he controls it with such great effort that his work, study, parenting and relationships are disrupted. This pressure to behave sexually often leads the man to believe he has a high sex drive. Some severe paraphilics describe their masturbation-to-orgasm frequencies as 10/day. Even when the patient's estimate of his frequency of orgasm strains credulity less, the return of sexual drive manifestations so soon after orgasm suggests that either something is wrong with the patients' sexual drive generator, their satiety mechanisms, or that their existential anxiety overpowers their other defense mechanisms.

Paraphilic men often report collecting and viewing pornography, visiting sexual book stores to see explicit videos or peep shows, frequenting prostitutes for their special sexual behaviors, downloading explicit images from the Internet, or extensively using telephone sex services or strip clubs. Victimization of others, the public health problem, is the least common form of sexual acting out but it is by no means rare (Abel *et al.*, 1987). When the behavioral diagnosis of exhibitionism, pedophilia, or sadism is made, the clinician should assume that the numbers of victims far exceed the number stated in the criminal charges.

Two other conditions, compulsive sexual behavior and sexual addiction not part of the DSM-IV, are informally and synonymously used to refer to heterosexual and homosexual men and women who display an intense drivenness to behave sexually without paraphilic imagery. The personal, interpersonal and medical consequences of paraphilic and nonparaphilic sexual compulsivity seem indistinguishable as do their usual psychiatric comorbidities: depression, anxiety disorders, substance abuse and attention deficit disorders (Kafka and Prentky, 1998).

Partner Sexual Dysfunction

A severe sexual dysfunction involving desire, arousal, or orgasm with a partner, although not invariably, often is present among paraphilics (Pawlak, 1991). The wives of paraphilics tell stories with these themes: "He is not interested in sex with me". "He never initiates." "He doesn't seem to enjoy our sexual life together except when…." "He is usually not potent." "Even when we do make love, he rarely ejaculates." Some paraphilic men however are able to function well without paraphilic fantasies but others are either able primarily to function when their partners are willing to meet their special requirements for arousal or when they fantasize about their paraphilic script (Abel, 1989).

Speculations About the Underlying Problem

Paraphilia has been considered in 15 somewhat different ways, depending on era, ideology and region: 1) an impairment in the bonding function of sexuality; 2) a courtship disorder; 3) the erotic form of hatred motivated by the need for revenge for childhood trauma; 4) a fixation to childhood misunderstandings that women had penises and that men could lose theirs during sex (castration anxiety); 5) the unsuccessful repair of early life passive, helpless experiences with a terrifying, malignant, malicious preoedipal mother; 6) a strategy to stabilize a conventional masculine or feminine gender identity; 7) a strategy to deny the differences between the sexes and the generations of child and parent; 8) an outcome of childhood sexual abuse; 9) a consequence of far less than ideal parent–child relationships; 10) a soft neurological sign of a neural wiring defect; 11) a released behavior due to cerebral pathology, for example, temporal lobe dysfunction, or substance abuse; 12) the sexual face of an addiction disorder; 13) an unusual manifestation of an affective disorder; 14) an obsessive–compulsive spectrum disorder; 15) a defective self-system requiring a patch – that is, a sexual preoccupation – to shore up the private, carefully-hidden-from-others sense of inadequate subjective masculinity.

Whatever its ultimate etiologies and nature, the paraphilias are sexual identity disorders that generally make normal erotic and sexual loving unattainable. Culture asks us to have some image of attachment, some ability to neutralize anger toward others, some ability to contain the anxiety over closeness, and some psychological motive simultaneously to enhance the self and the partner through sexual contact. Ordinary intentions aim for peaceable mutuality between real people; paraphilic ones aim at aggressive one-sidedness. This sexual identity disorder could be referred to as a disorder of self, specifically of that part of the self that maintains a sense of masculinity. Paraphilics often bear an enigmatic paradox between what they want to be and what they are. They often hunger for a behavior which feels uncontrollable or sick and which robs them of autonomy. This is why the behaviors are often thought of as addictions and are often associated with other forms of substance abuse, obsessive–compulsive phenomena and affective symptoms. Relative to the dynamic fluctuations of sexual dysfunctions, intention disorders are tenacious throughout life.

The Specific Paraphilias

Criminal Sex Offending Behaviors

Exhibitionism

Exhibitionism generally involves teenagers and men displaying their penises so that the witness will be shocked or (in the paraphilic's fantasy) sexually interested. They may or may not masturbate during or immediately following this act of victimization. This diagnosis is not usually made when a man is arrested for "public indecency" and his penile exposures are motivated to arrange homosexual contact in a public place generally unseen by heterosexuals. Penile display in parks is one way to make anonymous contact. The presence or absence of exhibitionistic imagery allows the clinician to make the distinction between paraphilia and homosexual courting.

Pedophilia

Pedophilia is the most widely and intensely socially repudiated of the paraphilias. Pedophiles are men who erotically and romantically prefer children or young adolescents. They are grouped into categories depending upon their erotic preferences for boys or girls and for infant, young, or pubertal children. Some pedophiles have highly age- and sex-specific tastes, others are less discriminating. Since the diagnosis of pedophilia requires that over a period of at least 6 months, recurrent, intense sexually arousing fantasies, sexual urges, or behaviors involving sexual activity with a prepubescent child or children, the disorder should not be expected to be present in every person who is guilty of child molestation. Some intrafamilial child abuse occurs over a shorter time interval and results from combinations of deteriorated marriages, sexual deprivation, sociopathy and substance abuse. Child molestation, whether paraphilic or not, is a crime, however. Child molesters show several patterns of erectile responses to visual stimulation in the laboratory. Some have their largest arousal to children of a specific age and others respond to both children and adults (Barbaree and Marshall, 1989). Others respond with their greatest arousal to aggressive cues.

Voyeurism

Men whose sexual life consist of watching homosexual or heterosexual videos in sexual book stores occasionally come to psychiatric attention after being charged with a crime following a police raid. They may or may not qualify for this diagnosis. The voyeurs who are more problematic for society are those who watch women through windows or break into their dwellings for this purpose. Some of these crimes result in rape or nonsexual violence, but many are motivated by pure voyeuristic intent (which is subtly aggressive).

Sexual Sadism

While rape is an extreme variety of sadism, paraphilic sadism is present only in a minority of rapists. It is defined by the rapist's prior use of erotic scripts that involve a partner's fear, pain, humiliation and suffering. Rapists are highly dangerous men whose antisocial behaviors are generally thought to be unresponsive to ordinary psychiatric methods. Their violence potential often makes psychiatric therapy outside of institutions imprudent. Noncriminal paraphilic sadism, that is, arousal to images of harming another that has not crossed into the behavioral realm, can be treated in outpatient settings.

Frotteurism

Frotteurism, the need to touch and rub against nonconsenting persons, although delineated as a criminal act, is probably better understood as the most socially benign form of paraphilic sadism. Frotteurism often occurs in socially isolated men who become sexually driven to act out. They often are unaware of how frightening they can be.

Stalking

Stalking is the latest erotic preoccupation to be criminalized. Forensic psychiatry has defined various motivations for arrested stalkers, including those who have made the transition from romantic to violent preoccupation with the victim. Stalking is particularly frightening because murder occasionally results. It is likely that stalking as a behavior is the product of further deterioration of an already compromised mind, although not necessarily a paraphilic one.

Noncriminal Forms of Paraphilia

Because the individual manifestations of paraphilia depend on the particular individual life history of the affected, over 40 paraphilic categories have been identified although only a few are listed in the DSM-IV. Most of these are unusual means of attaining arousal during masturbation or consenting partner behaviors. Each of the themes identified below demonstrate a wide range of manifestations from the bizarre to the more "reasonable" and from the common to the unique. They often subtly combine elements of more than one paraphilia.

Fetishism

Fetishism, the pairing of arousal with wearing or holding an article of clothing or inanimate object such as an inflatable doll, has a range of manifestations from infantilism in which a person dresses up in diapers to pretend he is a baby to the far more common use of a female undergarment for arousal purposes. Fetishism when confined to one garment for decades is classified as a paraphilia, but many cases involve more complex varieties of cross-dressing and overlap with gender identity disorders, usually GIDNOS. Fetishistic transvestism is the diagnosis used when it is apparent that the urges to use the clothing of the opposite sex is part of a larger mental preoccupation with that sex.

Sexual Masochism

Sexual masochism is diagnosed over a range of behaviors from the sometimes fatal need to nearly asphyxiate oneself to the request to be spanked by the partner in order to be excited. Masochism may be the most commonly reported or acknowledged form of female paraphilia, although it is more common among men. Sadists and masochists sometimes find one another and work out arrangement to act out their fantasies and occasionally reverse roles.

Paraphilia Not Otherwise Specified

Paraphilia not otherwise specified is a DSM-IV category for other endpoints of abnormal sexual development that lead to preoccupations with amputated body parts, feces, urine, sexualized enemas and sex with animals.

Treatment

Four general approaches are employed to treat the paraphilias. The treatments are not mutually exclusive, rather they are often multimodal in application.

Evaluation Only

Evaluation only is often selected when the evaluator concludes that the paraphilia is benign in terms of society, the patient will be resistant to the other approaches, and does not suffer greatly in terms of social and vocational functioning in ways that might be improved. Often these are isolated men with private paraphilic sexual pleasures, such as telephone sex with a masochistic scenario.

Psychotherapy

What constitutes psychotherapy for paraphilia heavily depends on the therapist training rather than strident declarations of treatment of choice. Little optimism exists that any form of therapy can permanently change the nature of a long established paraphilic erotic script, even among teenage sex offenders. Individual psychodynamic psychotherapy can be highly useful in diminishing paraphilic intensifications and gradually teaching the patient better management techniques of the situations that have triggered acting out. Well-described cognitive–behavioral interventions exist for interrupting paraphilic arousal via pairing masturbatory excitement with either aversive imagery or aversive stimuli. Comprehensive behavioral treatment involves social skills training, assertiveness training and confrontation with the rationalizations that are used to minimize awareness of the victims of sexual crimes, and marital therapy (Abel and Osborn, 1995). The self-help movement has created 12-step programs for sexual addictions to which many individuals now belong. Group psychotherapy is offered by trained therapists as well. When the lives of paraphilics are illuminated in various therapies, it becomes apparent that the emotional pain of the patients is thought to be great; the sexual acting out is often perceived as a defense against recurrent unpleasant emotions from any source. These often, however, involve self-esteem and primitive anxiety.

Medications

In the early 1980s, depo-medroxy-progesterone (Provera) was first used to treat those who were constantly masturbating, seeking out personally dangerous sexual outlets, or committing sex crimes. The weekly 400 to 600 mg injections often led to the men being able to work, study, or participate in activities that were previously beyond them because of concentration or attention difficulties. In the late 1980s, the use of oral Provera, 20 to 120 mg/day led to similar results: the drug enabled these men to leave their former state in which their sexual needs took priority over other life demands, and they did not have depo-Provera's side-effect profile: weight gain, hypertension, muscle cramps and gynecomastia. Today, gonadotrophin-releasing blockers are occasionally used for this. The possible side effects are similar to oral Provera. Despite the fact that the clinical results are among the most powerful effected by any psychopharmacologic treatment, many psychiatrists cannot overcome their disinclination about giving a "female" hormone to a man or working with patients who victimize others sexually. Serotonergic agents are now more commonly used as a first line of treatment and their administration, of course, creates fewer countertransference obstacles. While these studies are not as methodologically sophisticated as they need to be, the SSRIs are in widespread use for compulsive sexual behaviors and sexual obsessions. Their efficacy is the source of the speculation that some of the paraphilias may be an obsessive–compulsive spectrum disorder.

External Controls

Sexual advantage-taking, whether it be by a paraphilic physician with his patients, by a pedophilic mentally retarded man in the neighborhood, or of a grandfather who has abused several generations of his offspring, can often be stopped by making it **impossible** for these behaviors to be **un**known to most people in his life. The doctor's staff can be told, the neighbors can know, the family can meet to discuss the current crisis and review who has been abused over the years and plan to never allow grandfather alone with any child in or outside the family. The concept of external control is taken over by the judicial system when sex crimes are highly repugnant or heinous. The offender is removed from society for punishment and the protection of the public. Increasing pressure exists to criminalize sexual advantage-taking by physicians who are even more susceptible to losing their medical licenses at least for several years.

Psychiatrists need to be realistic about the limitations of various therapeutic ventures. Sexual acting out may readily continue during therapy beyond the awareness of the therapist. The more violent and destructive the paraphilic behavior to others, the less the therapist should risk ambulatory treatment. Since paraphilia occurs in patients with other psychiatric conditions, the psychiatrist needs to remain vigilant that the treatment program is comprehensive and does not lose sight of the paraphilia just because the depressive or compulsive symptoms are improved. Paraphilia may be improved by medications and psychotherapy but the clinician should expect that the intention disorder is the patient's lasting vulnerability.

Sexual Disorder Not Otherwise Specified

If the clinician is uncertain about how to categorize a person's problem, it is more reasonable to use this diagnosis than one that does not encompass the range of the patient's suffering. Sexual disorder not otherwise specified can be used when the therapist perceives a dramatic interplay between issues of sexual identity and sexual dysfunction, or when "everything" seems to be amiss. DSM-IV-TR, however, encourages the clinician to make multiple sexual diagnoses involving, for instance, a gender identity disorder, a desire disorder, erectile and orgasmic disorder.

DSM-IV-TR provides two examples when it would be appropriate to use the diagnosis sexual disorder NOS: 1) nonparaphilic compulsive sexual behaviors, that is, relentless pursuit of masturbatory or heterosexual or homosexual partner experiences without evidence of paraphilic imagery; and 2) complicated or exaggerated struggles to manage homosexual urges. Despite the removal of homosexuality from the DSM in 1974 men (particularly) and women still generate symptoms in their struggle to balance the demands of their homoeroticism with their ambitions to participate in conventional family life. This ongoing struggle can generate a variety of anxiety, depressive, compulsive, substance abusing and suicidal states.

Final Thoughts

A specific diagnosis like vaginismus or GIDNOS does not, per se, dictate the type and course of therapy. The clinician is called upon to weigh many factors in planning treatment. Accurate diagnosis is a vital first step but it quickly gives way to other, more artful considerations. "What factors set up this problem and what forces maintain it? What is the essence of this situation? What does this diagnosis mean in ordinary human terms? Can medication play a useful role? How am I to help? What am I to say? When and how should I say it?" These are essentially psychotherapy considerations. The sexual disorders challenge the doctor to integrate the advances of modern psychiatry with the traditions of less biologically-oriented psychiatry and the knowledge accumulating in forensic settings for the purpose of seeing if the patient's distress can be lastingly altered. In this challenge, clinical science inevitably gives way to clinical art. The art involves enabling the patient's distress to make sense so that the

underlying struggle – the developmental task – can be successfully negotiated.

For gender identity disorder, ICD-10 defines three separate disorders: "Gender Identity Disorder of Childhood", "Dual-role Transvestism" and "Transsexualism", all of which are included under the single DSM-IV-TR category Gender Identity Disorder.

Comparison of DSM-IV/ICD-10 Diagnostic Criteria

For hypoactive sexual desire disorder, the ICD-10 Diagnostic Criteria for Research and the DSM-IV-TR criteria are essentially identical except that ICD-10 specifies a minimum duration of at least 6 months (DSM-IV-TR has no minimum duration).

The ICD-10 Diagnostic Criteria for Research for Sexual Aversion Disorder differs from the DSM-IV-TR criteria in several ways. In contrast to DSM-IV-TR which restricts the condition to the aversion to, and avoidance of, sexual genital contact, ICD-10 also includes presentations characterized by sexual activity resulting in "strong negative feelings and an inability to experience any pleasure". Furthermore, ICD-10 excludes cases in which the aversion is due to performance anxiety. Finally, ICD-10 specifies a minimum duration of at least 6 month whereas DSM-IV-TR does not specify any minimum duration.

For female sexual arousal disorder and male erectile disorder, the ICD-10 Diagnostic Criteria for Research and the DSM-IV-TR criteria are essentially equivalent except that ICD-10 specifies a minimum duration of at least 6 months. ICD-10 includes a single category ("Failure of Genital Response") with two separate criteria sets by gender. In contrast, DSM-IV-TR includes two separate categories.

For female and male orgasmic disorders, the ICD-10 Diagnostic Criteria for Research and the DSM-IV-TR criteria are essentially equivalent except that ICD-10 specifies a minimum duration of at least 6 months. In contrast to DSM-IV-TR which has male and female versions defined separately, ICD-10 has a single category that applies to both genders.

For premature ejaculation, the ICD-10 Diagnostic Criteria for Research and the DSM-IV-TR criteria are essentially equivalent except that ICD-10 specifies a minimum duration of at least 6 months. Similarly, the ICD-10 Diagnostic Criteria for Research and the DSM-IV-TR criteria for Dyspareunia and Vaginismus are essentially equivalent except that ICD-10 specifies a minimum duration of at least 6 months. Furthermore, these conditions are referred to in ICD-10 as "Nonorganic Dyspareunia" and "Nonorganic Vaginismus".

The definition of a paraphillia is essentially the same in DSM-IV-TR and ICD-10. However, ICD-10 does not include a separate category for Frotteurism and has a combined "Sado-masochism" category.

For gender identity disorder, ICD-10 defines three separate disorders: "Gender Identity Disorder of Childhood", "Dual-role Transvestism" and "Transsexualism", all of which are included under the single DSM-IV-TR category Gender Identity Disorder.

References

Abel GG and Osborn CA (1995) Behavioral therapy treatment for sex offenders, in *Sexual Deviation*, 3rd edn. (ed Rosen I). Oxford University Press, London.

Abel GG, Becker JV, Mittelman MS *et al.* (1987) Self-reported sex crimes of nonincarcerated paraphiliacs. *J Interpers Viol* 2, 3.

Abel GG (1989) Paraphilias. In Comprehensive Textbook of Psychiatry, Vol. V, Kaplan and Sadock (eds). Williams & Wilkins, Baltimore, pp. 1069–1085.

Althof SE, Levine SB, Corty E, *et al.* (1995) Double-blind crossover study of clomipramine for rapid ejaculation in 15 couples. *J Clin Psychiatr* 56(9), 402–407.

American Psychiatric Association (1994) *Diagnostic and Statistical Manual*, 4th edn. APA, Washington DC.

Barbaree HE and Marshall WL (1995) Erectile responses amongst heterosexual child molesters. *Can J Behav Sci.*

Barbaree, H.E., & Marshall, W.L. (1989) Erectile resposees amongst heterosexual child molesters, father-daughter incest offenders and matched nonoffenders: five distint age preference profilses. Canadian Journal of Behavioral Science, 21, 70–82.

Basson R, McInnes R, Smith MD *et al.* (2002) Efficacy and safety of sildenafil citrate in women with sexual dysfunction associated with female sexual arousal disorder. *J Women's Health Gender-Based Stud* 11(4), 367–377.

Coates S, Friedman RC and Wolfe S (1992) The etiology of boyhood gender identity disorder: A model for integrating psychodynamics, temperament, and development. *Psychoanal Dialogues* 1, 481–523.

Freud S (1905) Three essays on the theory of sexuality, in *The Standard Edition of the Complete Works of Sigmund Freud* (ed Strachy J) (1953) Hogarth Press, London, pp. 125–243.

Green R (1987) *"Sissy Boy Syndrome" and the Development of Male Homosexuality.* Yale University Press, New Haven.

Kafka MP and Prentky RA (1998) Attention-deficit/hyperactivity disorder in males with paraphilia and paraphilia-related disorder: A comorbidity study. *J Clin Psychiatr* 59(7), 388–396.

Kernberg OF (1991) Aggression and love in the relationship of a couple. In Perversions and Near-Perversions in Clinical Practice: New Psychoanalytic Perspectives, Fogel GI and Myers WA (eds). Yale University Press, New Haven.

Laumann EO, Gagnon J and Michael RT (1994a) *Sex In America.* University of Chicago Press, Chicago.

Laumann EO, Gagnon JH, Michael RT *et al.* (1994b) *The Social Organization of Sexuality.* University of Chicago Press, Chicago.

Levine SB (1998a) The Nature of Love in Sexuality in Mid-Life. Kluwer Academic/Plenum Publishers, New York, pp. 1–22.

Levine SB (2002) Re-exploring the concept of sexual desire. *J Sex Marit Ther* 28(1), 39–51.

Masters WH and Johnson V (1970) *Human Sexual Inadequacy.* Little, Brown & Co, Boston.

Meyer W (Chairman), Bockting WO, Cohen-Kettenis P *et al.,* (2001) *Harry Benjamin International Gender Dysphoria Association's The Standard of Care for Gender Identity Disorders*, Sixth Version, 6th Rev. Symposion Publishing, Dusseldorf.

Pawlak AE, Boulet JR and Bradford JMW (1991) Discriminant analysis of a sexual-function inventory with intrafamilial and extrafamilial child molesters. *Arch Sex Behav* 20(1), 27–34.

Petersen ME and Dickey R (1995) Surgical sex reasssignment: A comparative survey of international centes. *Arch Sex Bahav* 24(2), 135–156.

Shaw J (ed) (1999) *Sexual Aggression.* American Psychiatric Press, Washington DC.

Tiefer L (1998) A feminist critique of the sexual dysfunction nomenclature. *Women Ther* 7, 3–21.

58   Eating Disorders

In the current psychiatric nomenclature of the *Diagnostic and Statistical Manual of Mental Disorders*, Fourth Edition (DSM-IV-TR), the eating disorders consist of two clearly defined syndromes: anorexia nervosa and bulimia nervosa. Many individuals presenting for treatment of an eating disorder (Figure 58.1) fail to meet formal criteria for either anorexia nervosa or bulimia nervosa, which raises an important theoretical and practical question: What is an eating disorder? Although this topic has received surprisingly little attention, it has been suggested that a working definition of an eating disorder might be "a persistent disturbance of eating behavior or behavior intended to control weight, which significantly impairs physical health or psychosocial functioning" (Fairburn and Walsh, 2002). This definition clearly encompasses the recognized disorders, anorexia nervosa and bulimia nervosa. In addition, it provides a basis for viewing eating disorders as clinically significant problems that do not meet criteria for anorexia nervosa or bulimia nervosa. The term atypical eating disorder is often applied to such problems, even though the number of individuals suffering from them may well outnumber those with "typical" eating disorders. One example of an atypical eating disorder is that of women who are overly concerned about their weight, have dieted to a below-normal weight, but have not ceased menstruating and, therefore, do not meet full criteria for anorexia nervosa. Another is that of individuals who binge and vomit regularly, but at less than the twice-a-week frequency required for bulimia nervosa.

An additional example of a clinically important atypical eating disorder is the occurrence of frequent binge-eating that is not followed by the self-induced vomiting or other inappropriate attempts to compensate that are characteristic of bulimia nervosa. This disturbance, for which the name binge-eating disorder has been proposed (DSM-IV appendix B) is a common behavioral pattern among obese individuals who present for treatment at weight loss clinics.

At present, obesity is not considered an eating disorder. Obesity refers to an excess of body fat and is viewed as a general medical, not a psychiatric, condition. At this stage of our knowledge, obesity is conceived as an etiologically heterogeneous condition. Obese individuals are at increased risk for a number of serious medical problems and are subject to significant social stigmatization and its psychological sequelae. However, the widely held assumption that obesity is the result of a psychiatric disorder in which eating is used as a coping mechanism for depression or anxiety has not been substantiated by empirical research. Studies of obese and normal-weight subjects from the general (nonpatient) population have found no more psychiatric disturbance in those who are overweight than in those who are of normal weight.. Therefore, it seems appropriate at present to describe as having an eating disorder only those obese individuals who manifest a clear behavioral abnormality that impairs health or psychosocial functioning.

Anorexia Nervosa

Definition

The DSM-IV-TR criteria require the individual to be significantly underweight for age and height. Although it is not possible to set a single weight loss standard that applies equally to all individuals, DSM-IV-TR provides a benchmark of 85% of the weight considered normal for age and height as a guideline. Despite being of an abnormally low body weight, individuals with anorexia nervosa are intensely afraid of gaining weight and becoming fat, and remarkably, this fear typically intensifies as the weight falls.

DSM-IV-TR criterion C requires a disturbance in the person's judgment about his or her weight or shape. For example, despite being underweight, individuals with anorexia nervosa often view themselves or a part of their body as being too heavy. Typically, they deny the grave medical risks engendered by their semistarvation and place enormous psychological importance on whether they have gained or lost weight. For example, someone with anorexia nervosa may feel intensely distressed if her or his weight increases by half a pound. Finally, criterion D requires that women with anorexia nervosa be amenorrheic.

The DSM-IV-TR criteria for anorexia nervosa are generally consistent with recent definitions and descriptions of this illness. In addition, in DSM-IV-TR, a new subtyping scheme was introduced. DSM-IV-TR suggests that individuals with anorexia nervosa be classed as having one of two variants, either the binge-eating/purging type or the restricting type. Individuals with the restricting type of anorexia nervosa do not engage regularly in either binge-eating or purging and, compared with individuals with the binge-eating/purging form of the disorder, are not as likely to abuse alcohol and other drugs, exhibit less mood lability and are less active sexually. There are also indications that the two subtypes may differ in their response to pharmacological intervention.

Epidemiology

Anorexia nervosa is a relatively rare illness. Even among high-risk groups, such as adolescent girls and young women, the prevalence of strictly defined anorexia nervosa is only about 0.5%. The prevalence rates of partial syndromes are substantially higher. Despite the infrequent occurrence of anorexia nervosa, most studies suggest that its incidence has increased significantly during the last 50 years, a phenomenon usually attributed to changes in cultural norms regarding desirable body shape and weight.

Essentials of Psychiatry Jerald Kay and Allan Tasman
© 2006 John Wiley & Sons, Ltd.

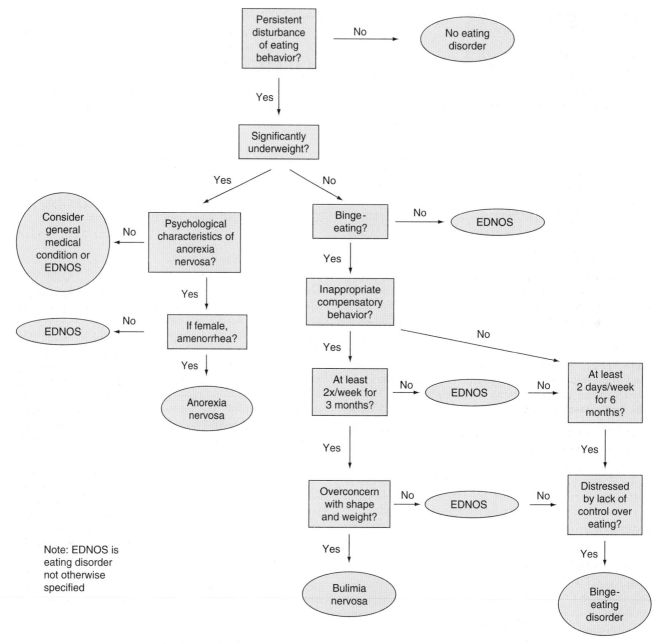

Figure 58.1   *Algorithm for diagnosis of eating disorders.*

Anorexia nervosa usually affects women; the ratio of men to women is approximately 1:10 to 1:20. Anorexia nervosa occurs primarily in industrialized and affluent countries and some data suggest that even within those countries, anorexia nervosa is more common among the higher socioeconomic classes. Some occupations, such as ballet dancing and fashion modeling, appear to confer a particularly high risk for the development of anorexia nervosa. Thus, anorexia nervosa appears more likely to develop in an environment in which food is readily available but in which, for women, being thin is somehow equated with higher or special achievement.

Etiology

At present, the etiology of anorexia nervosa is fundamentally unknown. However, from several sources, such as the epidemiological data just reviewed, it is possible to identify risk factors whose presence increases the likelihood of anorexia nervosa. It is also possible to describe the course and complications of the syndrome and to suggest interactions between features of the disorder, for example, between malnutrition and psychiatric illness. Thus, as indicated in Figure 58.2, the difficulties that lead to the development of anorexia nervosa may be distinct from the forces that intensify the symptoms and perpetuate the illness once it has begun.

Genetic and Twin Studies

Anorexia nervosa occurs more frequently in biological relatives of patients who present with the disorder. The prevalence rate of anorexia nervosa among sisters of patients is estimated to be approximately 6%; the morbid risk among other relatives ranges from 2 to 4%. Some evidence for a genetic component in the etiology of anorexia nervosa comes from twin studies, which reported

Anorexia Nervosa

A. weight at or above a minimally normal weight Refusal to maintain body for age and height (e.g., weight loss leading to maintenance of body weight less than 85% of that expected; or failure to make expected weight gain during period of growth, leading to body weight less than 85% of that expected).

B. or becoming fat, Intense fear of gaining weight even though underweight.

C. one's body Disturbance in the way in which weight or shape is experienced, undue influence of body weight or shape on self-evaluation, or denial of the seriousness of the current low body weight.

D. In postmenarcheal females, amenorrhea, i.e., the absence of at least three consecutive menstrual cycles. (A woman is considered to have amenorrhea if her periods occur only following hormone, e.g., estrogen, administration.)

Specify type:

Restricting type: during the current episode of anorexia nervosa, the person has not regularly engaged in binge-eating or purging behavior (i.e., self-induced vomiting or the misuse of laxatives, diuretics, or enemas).

Binge-eating/purging type: during the current episode of anorexia nervosa, the person has regularly engaged in binge-eating or purging behavior (i.e., self-induced vomiting or the misuse of laxatives, diuretics, or enemas).

Reprinted with permission from the *Diagnostic and Statistical Manual of Mental Disorders*, Fourth Edition, Text Revision. Copyright 2000 American Psychiatric Association.

substantially higher concordance rates for monozygotic than for dizygotic twin pairs (Klump *et al.*, 2001). However, conclusive data for genetic transmission of the disorder are not yet available.

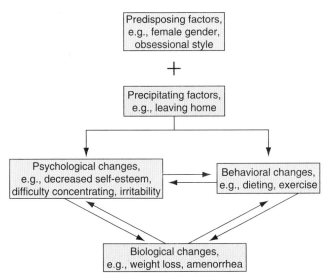

Figure 58.2 *Schematic diagram illustrating how an interplay of factors may lead to the initiation and persistence of anorexia nervosa.*

Family Studies

Individual psychiatric disorders in parents, dysfunctional family relationships and impaired family interaction patterns have been implicated in the etiology of anorexia nervosa. Mothers of individuals with anorexia nervosa are often described as overprotective, intrusive, perfectionistic and fearful of separation; fathers are described as withdrawn, passive, emotionally constricted, obsessional, moody and ineffectual. Family systems theorists have suggested that impaired family interactions such as pathological enmeshment, rigidity, overprotectiveness, and difficulties confronting and resolving conflicts are central features of anorexic pathology. However, few empirical studies have been conducted to date, particularly studies that also examine psychiatrically or medically ill comparison groups. Therefore, the precise role of the family in the development and course of anorexia nervosa, although undoubtedly important, has not been clearly delineated.

Psychosocial Factors

The increased prevalence of anorexia nervosa has been connected to the current emphasis in contemporary Western society on an unrealistically thin appearance in women. There is substantial evidence that a desire to be slim is common among middle- and upper-class white women and that this emphasis on slimness has increased significantly during the past several decades. In the USA, anorexia nervosa develops much more frequently in white adolescents than in adolescents from other racial groups. It has been suggested that a variety of characteristics may protect African-American girls from having eating disorders, including more acceptance of being overweight, more satisfaction with their body image and less social pressure regarding weight.

It has also been suggested that the emphasis of contemporary Western society on achievement and performance in women, which is a shift from the more traditional emphasis on deference, compliance and unassertiveness, has left many young women vulnerable to the development of eating disorders such as anorexia nervosa. These multiple and contradictory role demands are embodied within the modern concept of a superwoman who performs all of the expected roles (e.g., is competent, ambitious and achieving, yet also feminine, nurturing and sexual) and, in addition, devotes considerable attention to her appearance (Gordon, 1990).

Psychodynamic Factors

Various psychoanalytic theories have been postulated (e.g., defense against fantasies of oral impregnation; underlying deficits in the development of object relations; deficits in self-structure), but such hypotheses are difficult to verify. Bruch (1973, 1982) suggested that anorexia nervosa stems from failures in early attachment, attempts to cope with underlying feelings of ineffectiveness and inadequacy, and an inability to meet the demands of adolescence and young adulthood. These ideas, as well as her conceptualization that the single-minded focus on losing weight in anorexia nervosa is the concrete manifestation of a struggle to achieve a sense of identity, purpose, specialness and control, are compelling and clinically useful. Cognitive–behavioral theories emphasize the distortions and dysfunctional thoughts (e.g., dichotomous thinking) that may stem from various causal factors, all of which eventually focus on the belief that it is essential to be thin.

Although the existence of a specific predisposing personality style has not been conclusively documented, certain traits have commonly been reported among women with anorexia nervosa. Women hospitalized for anorexia nervosa have greater self-discipline, conscientiousness and emotional caution than women hospitalized for bulimia nervosa and women with no eating disorders. In addition, even after they have recovered from their illness, women who have had anorexia nervosa tend to avoid risks and to exhibit high levels of caution in emotional expression and strong compliance with rules and moral standards.

Developmental Factors

Because anorexia nervosa typically begins during adolescence, developmental issues are thought to play an important etiological role. Critical challenges at this time of life include the need to establish independence, a well-defined personal identity, fulfilling relationships, and clear values and principles to govern one's life. Family struggles, conflicts regarding sexuality and pressures regarding increased heterosexual contact are also common. However, it is not clear that difficulties over these issues are more salient for individuals who will develop anorexia nervosa than for other adolescents. Depression has been implicated as a nonspecific risk factor, and higher levels of depressive symptoms as well as insecurity, anxiety and self-consciousness have been documented in adolescent girls in comparison with adolescent boys. Similarly, the progression of physical and sexual maturation and the concomitant increase in women's percentage of body fat may have a substantial impact on the self-image of adolescent girls, particularly because the relationship between self-esteem and satisfaction with physical appearance and body characteristics is stronger in women than in men.

Pathophysiology

An impressive array of physical disturbances has been documented in anorexia nervosa and the physiological bases of many are understood (Table 58.1). Most of these physical disturbances appear to be secondary consequences of starvation, and it is not clear whether or how the physiological disturbances described here contribute to the development and maintenance of the psychological and behavioral abnormalities characteristic of anorexia nervosa. The remainder of this section briefly describes the major physical abnormalities of anorexia nervosa and what is understood about their etiology.

The central nervous system is clearly affected. Computed tomography has demonstrated that individuals with anorexia nervosa have enlarged ventricles, an abnormality that improves with weight gain. The cerebrospinal fluid concentrations of a variety of neurotransmitters and their metabolites are altered in underweight patients with anorexia nervosa and tend to normalize as weight is restored. An intriguing exception may be the serotonin metabolite 5-hydroxyindoleacetic acid, which has been reported to be elevated in the cerebrospinal fluid of patients with anorexia nervosa after they have achieved a normal or near-normal weight. Kaye (1997) has suggested that the elevated 5-hydroxyindoleacetic acid levels may reflect a serotoninergic abnormality that is tied to the obsessional traits often observed in anorexia nervosa.

Some of the most striking physiological alterations in anorexia nervosa are those of the hypothalamic–pituitary–gonadal axis. In women, estrogen secretion from the ovaries is markedly reduced, accounting for the occurrence of amenorrhea. In analogous fashion, testosterone production is diminished in men with anorexia nervosa. The decrease in gonadal steroid production is due to a reduction in the pituitary's secretion of the gonadotropins luteinizing hormone and follicle-stimulating hormone, which in turn is secondary to diminished release of gonadotropin-releasing

Table 58.1	Medical Problems Commonly Associated with Anorexia Nervosa

Skin
  Lanugo
Cardiovascular system
  Hypotension
  Bradycardia
  Arrhythmias
Hematopoietic system
  Normochromic, normocytic anemia
  Leukopenia
    Diminished polymorphonuclear leukocytes
Fluid and electrolyte balance
  Elevated blood urea nitrogen and creatinine concentrations
  Hypokalemia
  Hyponatremia
  Hypochloremia
  Alkalosis
Gastrointestinal system
  Elevated serum concentration of liver enzymes
  Delayed gastric emptying
  Constipation
Endocrine system
  Diminished thyroxine with normal thyroid-stimulating level hormone level
  Elevated plasma cortisol level
  Diminished secretion of luteinizing hormone, hormone, estrogen, or testosterone follicle-stimulating
Bone
  Osteoporosis

hormone from the hypothalamus. Therefore, the amenorrhea of anorexia nervosa is properly viewed as a type of hypothalamic amenorrhea. It is of interest that in a significant minority amenorrhea begins before substantial weight loss has occurred, suggesting that factors other than malnutrition, such as psychological distress, contribute significantly to the disruption of the reproductive endocrine system.

In an adult with anorexia nervosa, the status of the hypothalamic–pituitary–gonadal axis resembles that of a pubertal or prepubertal child – the secretion of estrogen or testosterone, of luteinizing hormone and follicle-stimulating hormone and of gonadotropin-releasing hormone is reduced. This endocrinological picture may be contrasted with that of postmenopausal women who have a similar reduction in estrogen secretion but who, unlike women with anorexia nervosa, show increased pituitary gonadotropin secretion. Furthermore, even the circadian patterns of luteinizing hormone and follicle-stimulating hormone secretion in adult women with anorexia nervosa closely resemble the patterns normally seen in pubertal and prepubertal girls. Although similar abnormalities are also seen in other forms of hypothalamic amenorrhea and are therefore not specific to anorexia nervosa, it is nonetheless striking that this syndrome is accompanied by a physiological arrest or regression of the reproductive endocrine system.

The functioning of other hormonal systems is also disrupted in anorexia nervosa, although typically not as profoundly as is the reproductive axis. Presumably as part of the metabolic response to semistarvation, the activity of the thyroid gland is reduced.

Plasma thyroxine levels are somewhat diminished, but the plasma level of the pituitary hormone and thyroid-stimulating hormone is not elevated. The activity of the hypothalamic–pituitary–adrenal axis is increased, as indicated by elevated plasma levels of cortisol and by resistance to dexamethasone suppression. The regulation of vasopressin (antidiuretic hormone) secretion from the posterior pituitary is disturbed, contributing to the development of partial diabetes insipidus in some individuals.

Anorexia nervosa is often associated with the development of leukopenia and of a normochromic, normocytic anemia of mild to moderate severity. Surprisingly, leukopenia does not appear to result in a high vulnerability to infectious illnesses. Serum levels of liver enzymes are sometimes elevated, particularly during the early phases of refeeding, but the synthetic function of the liver is rarely seriously impaired so that the serum albumin concentration and the prothrombin time are usually within normal limits. Serum cholesterol levels are sometimes elevated in anorexia nervosa, although the basis of this abnormality remains obscure. In some patients, self-imposed fluid restriction and excessive exercise produce dehydration and elevations of serum creatinine and blood urea nitrogen. In others, water loading may lead to hyponatremia. The status of serum electrolytes is a reflection of the individual's salt and water intake and the nature and the severity of the purging behavior. A common pattern is hypokalemia, hypochloremia and mild alkalosis resulting from frequent and persistent self-induced vomiting.

It has become clear that individuals with anorexia nervosa have decreased bone density compared with age- and sex-matched peers and, as a result, are at increased risk for fractures. Low levels of estrogen, high levels of cortisol and poor nutrition have been cited as risk factors for the development of reduced bone density in anorexia nervosa. Theoretically, estrogen treatment might reduce the risk of osteoporosis in women who are chronically amenorrheic because of anorexia nervosa, but controlled studies indicate that this intervention is of limited, if any, benefit.

Abnormalities of cardiac function include bradycardia and hypotension, which are rarely symptomatic. The pump function of the heart is compromised, and congestive heart failure occasionally develops in individuals during overly rapid refeeding. The electrocardiogram shows sinus bradycardia and a number of nonspecific abnormalities. Arrhythmias may develop, often in association with fluid and electrolyte disturbances. It has been suggested that significant prolongation of the QT interval may be a harbinger of life-threatening arrhythmias in some individuals with anorexia nervosa, but this has not been conclusively demonstrated.

The motility of the gastrointestinal tract is diminished, leading to delayed gastric emptying and contributing to complaints of bloating and constipation. Rare cases of acute gastric dilatation or gastric rupture, which is often fatal, have been reported in individuals with anorexia nervosa who consumed large amounts of food when binge-eating.

As already noted, virtually all of the physiological abnormalities described in individuals with anorexia nervosa are also seen in other forms of starvation, and most improve or disappear as weight returns to normal. Therefore, weight restoration is essential for physiological recovery. More surprisingly, perhaps, weight restoration is believed to be essential for psychological recovery as well. Accounts of human starvation amply document the profound impact of starvation on mental health. Starving individuals lose their sense of humor, their interest in friends and family fades and mood generally becomes depressed. They may develop peculiar behavior similar to that of patients with anorexia nervosa, such as hoarding food or concocting bizarre food combinations. If starvation disrupts psychological and behavioral functioning in normal individuals, it presumably does so as well in those with anorexia nervosa. Thus, correction of starvation is a prerequisite for the restoration of both physical and psychological health.

Diagnosis and Differential Diagnosis

Phenomenology
Anorexia nervosa often begins innocently. Typically, an adolescent girl or young woman who is of normal weight or, perhaps, a few pounds overweight decides to diet. This decision may be prompted by an important but not extraordinary life event, such as leaving home for camp, attending a new school, or a casual unflattering remark by a friend or family member. Initially, the dieting seems no different from that pursued by many young women, but as weight falls, the dieting intensifies. The restrictions become broader and more rigid; for example, desserts may first be eliminated, then meat, then any food that is thought to contain fat. The person becomes increasingly uncomfortable if she is seen eating and avoids meals with others. Food seems to assume a moral quality so that vegetables are viewed as "good" and anything with fat is "bad". The individual has idiosyncratic rules about how much exercise she must do and when, where and how she can eat.

Food avoidance and weight loss are accompanied by a deep and reassuring sense of accomplishment, and weight gain is viewed as a failure and a sign of weakness. Physical activity, such as running or aerobic exercise, often increases as the dieting and weight loss develop. Inactivity and complaints of weakness usually occur only when emaciation has become extreme. The person becomes more serious and devotes little effort to anything but work, dieting and exercise. She may become depressed and emotionally labile, socially withdrawn and secretive and she may lie about her eating and her weight. Despite the profound disturbances in her view of her weight and of her calorie needs, reality testing in other spheres is intact, and the person may continue to function well in school or at work. Symptoms usually persist for months or years until, typically at the insistence of friends or family, the person reluctantly agrees to see a physician.

In general, anorexia nervosa is not difficult to recognize. Uncertainty surrounding the diagnosis sometimes occurs in young adolescents, who may not clearly describe a drive for thinness and the fear of becoming fat. Rather, they may acknowledge only a vague concern about consuming certain foods and an intense desire to exercise. It can also be difficult to elicit the distorted view of shape and weight (criterion C) from patients who have had anorexia nervosa for many years. Such individuals may state that they realize they are too thin and may make superficial efforts to gain weight, but they do not seem particularly concerned about the physical risks or deeply committed to increasing their calorie consumption.

Assessment

Special Issues in Psychiatric Examination and History
In assessing individuals who may have anorexia nervosa, it is important to obtain a weight history including the individual's highest and lowest weights and the weight he or she would

like to be now. For women, it is useful to know the weight at which menstruation last occurred, because it provides an indication of what weight is normal for that individual. The patient should be asked to describe a typical day's food intake and any food restrictions and dietary practices such as vegetarianism. The psychiatrist should ask whether the patient ever loses control over eating and engages in binge-eating and, if so, the amounts and types of food eaten during such episodes. The use of self-induced vomiting, laxatives, diuretics, enemas, diet pills, and syrup of ipecac to induce vomiting should also be queried.

Probably the greatest problem in the assessment of patients with anorexia nervosa is their denial of the illness and their reluctance to participate in an evaluation. A straightforward but supportive and nonconfrontational style is probably the most useful approach, but it is likely that the patient will not acknowledge significant difficulties in eating or with weight and will rationalize unusual eating or exercise habits. It is therefore helpful to obtain information from other sources such as the patient's family.

Physical Examination and Laboratory Findings

The patient should be weighed, or a current weight should be obtained from the patient's general physician. Blood pressure, pulse and body temperature are often below the lower limit of normal. On physical examination, lanugo, a fine, downy hair normally seen in infants, may be present on the back or the face. The extremities are frequently cold and have a slight red–purple color (acrocyanosis). Edema is rarely observed at the initial presentation but may develop transiently during the initial stages of refeeding.

The basis for laboratory abnormalities is presented in the earlier section on pathophysiology. Common findings are a mild to moderate normochromic, normocytic anemia and leukopenia, with a deficit in polymorphonuclear leukocytes leading to a relative lymphocytosis. Elevations of blood urea nitrogen and serum creatinine concentrations may occur because of dehydration, which can also artificially elevate the hemoglobin and hematocrit. A variety of electrolyte abnormalities may be observed, reflecting the state of hydration and the history of vomiting and diuretic and laxative abuse. Serum levels of liver enzymes are usually normal but may transiently increase during refeeding. Cholesterol levels may be elevated.

The electrocardiogram typically shows sinus bradycardia and, occasionally, low QRS voltage and a prolonged QT interval; a variety of arrhythmias have also been described.

Differences in Presentation

The symptoms of anorexia nervosa are remarkably homogeneous, and differences between patients in clinical manifestations are fewer than in most psychiatric illnesses. As described before, younger patients may not express verbally the characteristic fear of fatness or the overconcern with shape and weight, and some patients with longstanding anorexia nervosa may express a desire to gain weight but be unable to make persistent changes in their behavior. It has been suggested that in other cultures, the rationale given by patients for losing weight differs from the fear of fatness characteristic of cases in North America.

Men have anorexia nervosa far less frequently than women. However, when the syndrome does develop in a man, it is typical. There may be an increased frequency of homosexuality among men with anorexia nervosa.

Differential Diagnosis

Although depression, schizophrenia and obsessive–compulsive disorder may be associated with disturbed eating and weight loss, it is rarely difficult to differentiate these disorders from anorexia nervosa. Individuals with major depression may lose significant amounts of weight but do not exhibit the relentless drive for thinness characteristic of anorexia nervosa. In schizophrenia, starvation may occur because of delusions about food, for example, that it is poisoned. Individuals with obsessive–compulsive disorder may describe irrational concerns about food and develop rituals related to meal preparation and eating but do not describe the intense fear of gaining weight and the pervasive wish to be thin that characterize anorexia nervosa.

A wide variety of medical problems cause serious weight loss in young people and may at times be confused with anorexia nervosa. Examples of such problems include gastric outlet obstruction, Crohn's disease and brain tumors. Individuals whose weight loss is due to a general medical illness generally do not show the drive for thinness, the fear of gaining weight and the increased physical activity characteristic of anorexia nervosa. However, the psychiatrist is well advised to consider any chronic medical illness associated with weight loss, especially when evaluating individuals with unusual clinical presentations such as late age at onset or prominent physical complaints, for example, pain and gastrointestinal cramping while eating.

Course and Natural History

The course of anorexia nervosa is enormously variable. Some individuals have mild and brief illnesses and either never come to medical attention or are seen only briefly by their pediatrician or general medical physician. It is difficult to estimate the frequency of this phenomenon because such individuals are rarely studied.

Most of the literature on course and outcome is based on individuals who have been hospitalized for anorexia nervosa. Although such individuals presumably have a relatively severe illness and adverse outcomes, a substantial fraction, probably between one-third and one-half, make full and complete psychological and physical recoveries. On the other hand, anorexia nervosa is also associated with an impressive long-term mortality. The best data currently available suggest that 10 to 20% of patients who have been hospitalized for anorexia nervosa will, in the next 10 to 30 years, die as a result of their illness. Much of the mortality is due to severe and chronic starvation, which eventually terminates in sudden death. In addition, a significant fraction of patients commit suicide.

Between these two extremes are a large number of individuals whose lives are impaired by persistent difficulties with eating. Some are severely affected maintaining a chronic state of semistarvation, bizarre eating rituals and social isolation; others may gain weight but struggle with bulimia nervosa and strict rules about food and eating; and still others may recover initially but then relapse into another full episode. There is a high frequency of depression among individuals who have had anorexia nervosa and a significant frequency of drug and alcohol abuse, but psychotic disorders develop only rarely. Thus, in general, individuals either recover or continue to struggle with psychological and behavioral problems that are directly related to the eating disorder. It is of note that it is rare for individuals who have had anorexia nervosa to become obese.

It is difficult to specify factors that account for the variability of outcome in anorexia nervosa. A significant body of experience suggests that the illness has a better prognosis when it begins in adolescence, but there are also suggestions that pre-pubertal onset may portend a difficult course. It is likely that the severity of the illness (e.g., the lowest weight reached, the number of hospitalizations) and the presence of associated symptoms, such as binge-eating and purging, also contribute to poor outcome. However, it is impossible to predict course and outcome in an individual with any certainty.

Goals of Treatment

The first goal of treatment is to engage the patient and her or his family. For most patients with anorexia nervosa, this is challenging. Patients usually minimize their symptoms and suggest that the concerns of the family and friends, who have often been instrumental in arranging the consultation, are greatly exaggerated. It is helpful to identify a problem that the patient can acknowledge, such as weakness, irritability, difficulty concentrating, or trouble with binge-eating. The psychiatrist may then attempt to educate the patient regarding the pervasive physical and psychological effects of semistarvation and about the need for weight gain if the acknowledged problem is to be successfully addressed.

A second goal of treatment is to assess and address acute medical problems, such as fluid and electrolyte disturbances and cardiac arrhythmias. Depending on the severity of illness, this may require the involvement of a general medical physician. The additional but most difficult and time-consuming goals are the restoration of normal body weight, the normalization of eating and the resolution of the associated psychological disturbances. The final goal is the prevention of relapse.

Treatment

A common major impediment to the treatment of patients with anorexia nervosa is their disagreement with the goals of treatment; many of the features of their illness are simply not viewed by patients as a problem. In addition, this may be compounded by a variety of concerns of the patient, such as basic mistrust of relationships, feelings of vulnerability and inferiority, and sensitivity to perceived coercion. Such concerns may be expressed through considerable resistance, defiance, or pseudocompliance with the psychiatrist's interventions and contribute to the power struggles that often characterize the treatment process. The psychiatrist must try to avoid colluding with the patient's attempts to minimize problems but at the same time allow the patient enough independence to maintain the alliance. Dealing with such dilemmas is challenging and requires an active approach on the part of the psychiatrist. In most instances, it is possible to preserve the alliance while nonetheless adhering to established limits and the need for change.

The initial stage of treatment should be aimed at reversing the nutritional and behavioral abnormalities (Figure 58.3). The intensity of the treatment required and the need for partial or full hospitalization should be determined by the current weight, the rapidity of weight loss, and the severity of associated medical and behavioral problems and of other symptoms such as depression. In general, patients whose weights are less than 75% of expected should be viewed as medically precarious and require intensive treatment such as hospitalization.

Most inpatient or day treatment units experienced in the care of patients with anorexia nervosa use a structured treatment approach that relies heavily on supervision of calorie intake by the staff. Patients are initially expected to consume sufficient calories to maintain weight, usually requiring 1500 to 2000 kcal/day

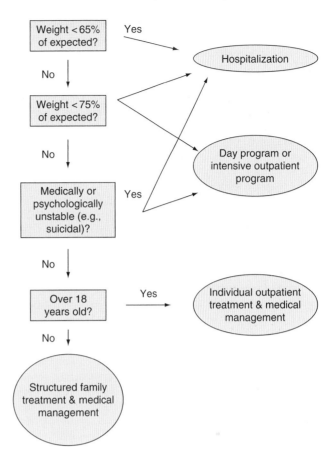

Figure 58.3 *Algorithm for choice of initial treatment of anorexia nervosa.*

in four to six meals. After the initial medical assessment has been completed and weight has stabilized, calorie intake is gradually increased to an amount necessary to gain 2 to 5 lb/week. Because the consumption of approximately 4000 kcal beyond maintenance requirements is needed for each pound of weight gain, the daily calorie requirements become impressive, often in the range of 4000 kcal/day. Some eating disorder units provide only food while others rely on nutritional supplements such as Ensure or Sustacal. During this phase of treatment it is necessary to monitor patients carefully; many will resort to throwing food away or vomiting after meals. Careful supervision is also required to obtain accurate weights; patients may consume large amounts of fluid before being weighed or hide heavy articles under their clothing.

During the weight restoration phase of treatment patients require substantial emotional support. It is probably best to address fears of weight gain with education about the dangers of semistarvation and with the reassurance that patients will not be allowed to gain "too much" weight. Most eating disorders units impose behavioral restrictions, such as limits on physical activity, during the early phase of treatment. Some units use an explicit behavior modification regimen in which weight gain is tied to increased privileges and failure to gain weight results in bed rest.

A consistent and structured treatment approach, with or without an explicit behavior modification program, is generally successful in promoting weight recovery but requires substantial energy and coordination to maintain a supportive and nonpunitive treatment environment. In most experienced treatment units, parenteral methods of nutrition, such as nasogastric feeding or intravenous hyperalimentation, are only rarely needed. Nutritional counseling and behavioral approaches can also be effective in helping patients expand their dietary repertoire to include foods they have been frightened of consuming.

As weight increases, individual, group and family psychotherapy can begin to address other issues in addition to the distress engendered by gaining weight. For example, it is typically important for patients to recognize that they have come to base much of their self-esteem on dieting and weight control and are likely to judge themselves according to harsh and unforgiving standards. Similarly, patients should be helped to see how the eating disorder has interfered with the achievement of personal goals such as education, sports, or making friends.

There is, present, no general agreement about the most useful type of psychotherapy or the specific topics that need to be addressed. Most eating disorders programs employ a variety of psychotherapeutic interventions. A number of psychiatrists recommend the use of individual and group psychotherapy using cognitive–behavioral techniques to modify the irrational overemphasis on weight. Although most authorities see little role for traditional psychoanalytic therapy, individual and group psychodynamic therapy can address such problems as insecure attachment, separation and individuation, sexual relationships and other interpersonal concerns. There is good evidence supporting the involvement of the family in the treatment of younger patients with anorexia nervosa. Family therapy can be helpful in addressing family members' fears about the illness; interventions typically emphasize parental cooperation, mutual support and consistency, and establishing boundaries regarding the patient's symptoms and other aspects of his or her life.

Despite the multiple physiological disturbances associated with anorexia nervosa, there is no clearly established role for medication. The earliest systematic medication trials in anorexia nervosa focused on the use of neuroleptics. Theoretically, such agents might help to promote weight gain, to reduce physical activity and to diminish the distorted thinking about shape and weight, which often reaches nearly delusional proportions. Early work in the late 1950s and 1960s using chlorpromazine led to substantial enthusiasm, but two placebo-controlled trials of the neuroleptics, sulpiride and pimozide, were unable to establish significant benefits. In recent years interest has grown in taking advantage of the impressive weight gain associated with some atypical antipsychotics; however, no controlled data supporting this intervention have yet appeared. Despite the frequency of depression among patients with anorexia nervosa, there is no good evidence supporting the use of antidepressant medication in their treatment.

Unfortunately, although controlled trials have provided some evidence of benefit, the impact of cyproheptadine, an antihistamine, in anorexia nervosa appears limited.

A large percentage of patients with anorexia nervosa remain chronically ill; 30 to 50% of patients successfully treated in the hospital require rehospitalization within 1 year of discharge. Therefore, posthospitalization outpatient treatments are recommended to prevent relapse and improve overall short- and long-term functioning. Several studies have attempted to evaluate the efficacy of various outpatient treatments for anorexia nervosa including behavioral, cognitive–behavioral and supportive psychotherapy, as well as a variety of nutritional counseling interventions. Although most of these treatments seem to be helpful, the clearest findings to date support two interventions. For patients whose anorexia nervosa started before age 18 years and who have had the disorder for less than 3 years, family therapy is effective, and for adult patients, cognitive–behavioral therapy reduces the rate of relapse. Preliminary information suggests that fluoxetine treatment may reduce the risk of relapse among patients with anorexia nervosa who have gained weight, but additional controlled data are required to document the usefulness of this intervention.

Refractory Patients

Some patients with anorexia nervosa refuse to accept treatment and thereby can raise difficult ethical issues. If weight is extremely low or if there are acute medical problems, it may be appropriate to consider involuntary commitment. For patients who are ill but more stable, the psychiatrist must weigh the short-term utility of involuntary treatment against the disruption of a potential alliance with the patient.

The goals of treatment may need to be modified for patients with chronic illness who have failed multiple previous attempts at inpatient and outpatient care. Treatment may be appropriately aimed at preventing further medical, psychological and social deterioration in the hope that the anorexia nervosa may eventually improve with time.

Clinical Vignette 1

When Ms A was first evaluated for admission to an inpatient eating disorders program, she had been restricting her food intake for approximately 5 years and had been amenorrheic for 4 years. At the time of her admission, this 24-year-old, single, white woman weighed 71 lb at a height of 5 feet 1.5 inches. In 12th grade, Ms A menstruated for the first time and also developed "very large" breasts. She had a difficult first year at college, where she gained to her maximum weight of 120 lb. The following year, Ms A transferred to a smaller college, became a vegetarian "for ethical reasons", and began to significantly restrict her food intake. She limited herself to a total of 700 to 800 cal/day, with a maximum of 200 calories per meal and gradually lost weight in the next 5 years. Ms A did not binge, vomit, abuse laxatives, or engage in excessive exercise. She considered herself to be "obsessed with calories" and observed a variety of rituals regarding food and food preparation (e.g., obsessively weighing her food).

Although Ms A excelled academically, she had no close friends and had never been involved in a romantic relationship. She was quite close to her mother and sister and had always been dependent on her parents. After graduating (with honors) from college, Ms A worked at a series of temporary jobs but was unemployed and living at home with her mother at the time of admission. She had been in outpatient psychotherapy with two different therapists during the previous 2 years. The first therapist did not address her eating disorder, and Ms A continued to lose weight, from 90 to 80 lb. Although her second therapist confronted her about her anorexia nervosa and started her on desipramine at 20 mg/day for depressive symptoms, Ms A continued to lose weight.

During her first 5-month hospitalization, Ms A was treated with a multimodal program (behavioral weight gain protocol, individual and family therapy, fluoxetine at 60–80 mg for obsessive–compulsive traits and depressive symptoms) and gained to a weight of 98 lb. At discharge, she was maintaining her weight on food but remained concerned about her weight and was particularly frightened of reaching "the triple digits" (i.e., ≥100 lb). After leaving the hospital, Ms A continued with outpatient psychotherapy and fluoxetine for several months. She was then seriously injured in a car accident and, during a prolonged convalescent period, discontinued treatment for her eating disorder. Ms A remained unemployed, eventually moved in with her sister and her sister's family, and gradually lost weight.

About 3.5 years after discharge, at age 27 years, Ms A again sought inpatient treatment. At admission, she weighed 83 lb but still felt "fat". During hospitalization, she steadily gained weight and was prescribed sertraline at 100 mg/day for feelings of low self-esteem, anxiety and obsessional thinking. When she was discharged 5 months later, at a weight of 108 lb, she noted menstrual bleeding for the first time in more than 7 years. After leaving the hospital, Ms A continued taking medication and began outpatient cognitive–behavioral psychotherapy. For the next year, she continued to struggle with eating and weight issues but managed to maintain her weight and successfully expand other aspects of her life by independently supporting herself with a full-time job, making new friends and becoming involved in her first romantic relationship.

Bulimia Nervosa

Definition

The salient behavioral disturbance of bulimia nervosa is the occurrence of episodes of binge-eating. During these episodes, the individual consumes an amount of food that is unusually large considering the circumstances under which it was eaten. Although this is a useful definition and conceptually reasonably clear, it can be operationally difficult to distinguish normal overeating from a small episode of binge-eating. Indeed, the available data do not suggest that there is a sharp dividing line between the size of binge-eating episodes and the size of other meals. On the other hand, while the border between normal and abnormal eating may not be a sharp one, both patients' reports and laboratory studies of eating behavior clearly indicate that, when binge-eating, patients with bulimia nervosa do indeed consume larger than normal amounts of food.

Episodes of binge-eating are associated, by definition, with a sense of loss of control. Once the eating has begun, the individual feels unable to stop until an excessive amount has been consumed. This loss of control is only subjective, in that most individuals with bulimia nervosa will abruptly stop eating in the midst of a binge episode if interrupted, for example, by the unexpected arrival of a roommate.

After overeating, individuals with bulimia nervosa engage in some form of inappropriate behavior in an attempt to avoid weight gain. Most patients who present to eating disorders clinics with this syndrome report self-induced vomiting or the

---

DSM-IV-TR Criteria 307.51

Bulimia Nervosa

A. binge-eating. An episode Recurrent episodes of of binge-eating is characterized by both of the following:

  (1) eating in a discrete , period of time (e.g., within any 2-hour period), an amount of food that is definitely larger than most people would eat during a similar period of time and under similar circumstances.

  (2) a sense of lack of control over eating during the episode (e.g., a feeling that one cannot stop eating or control what or how much one is eating).

Recurrent

B. compensatory behavior in order to prevent weight gain, inappropriate such as self-induced vomiting; misuse of laxatives, diuretics, enemas, or other medications; fasting; or excessive exercise.

C. inappropriate compensatory The binge-eating and behaviors both occur, on average, at least twice a week for 3 months.

D. influenced by body Self-evaluation is unduly shape and weight.

E. exclusively The disturbance does not occur during episodes of anorexia nervosa.

Specify type:

Purging type: during the current episode of bulimia nervosa, the person has regularly engaged in self-induced vomiting or the misuse of laxatives, diuretics, or enemas.

Nonpurging type: during the current episode of bulimia nervosa, the person has used other inappropriate compensatory behaviors, such as fasting or excessive exercise, but has not regularly engaged in self-induced vomiting or the misuse of laxatives, diuretics, or enemas.

Reprinted with permission from the *Diagnostic and Statistical Manual of Mental Disorders*, Fourth Edition, Text Revision. Copyright 2000 American Psychiatric Association.

---

abuse of laxatives. Other methods include misusing diuretics, fasting for long periods and exercising extensively after eating binges.

The DSM-IV-TR criteria require that the overeating episodes and the compensatory behaviors both occur at least twice a week for 3 months to merit a diagnosis of bulimia nervosa. This criterion, although useful in preventing the diagnostic label from being applied to individuals who only rarely have difficulty with binge-eating, is clearly an arbitrary one.

Criterion D in the DSM-IV-TR definition of bulimia nervosa requires that individuals with bulimia nervosa exhibit an over concern with body shape and weight. That is, they tend to base much of their self-esteem on how much they weigh and how slim they look.

Finally, in the DSM-IV-TR nomenclature, the diagnosis of bulimia nervosa is not given to individuals with anorexia nervosa. Individuals with anorexia nervosa who recurrently engage in binge-eating or purging behavior should be given the diagnosis of anorexia nervosa, binge-eating/purging subtype, rather than an additional diagnosis of bulimia nervosa.

In DSM-IV-TR, a subtyping scheme was introduced for bulimia nervosa in which patients are classed as having either the purging or the nonpurging type of bulimia nervosa. This scheme was introduced for several reasons. First, those individuals who purge are at greater risk for the development of fluid and electrolyte disturbances such as hypokalemia. Secondly, data suggest that individuals with the nonpurging type of bulimia nervosa weigh more and have less psychiatric illness compared with those with the purging type. Finally, most of the published literature on the treatment of bulimia nervosa has been based on studies of individuals with the purging type of this disorder.

Epidemiology

Soon after bulimia nervosa was recognized as a distinct disorder, surveys indicated that many young women reported problems with binge-eating, and it was suggested that the syndrome of bulimia nervosa was occurring in epidemic proportions. Later careful studies have found that although binge-eating is frequent, the full-blown disorder of bulimia nervosa is much less common, probably affecting 1 to 2% of young women in the USA. Although sufficient research data do not exist to pinpoint specific epidemiological trends in the occurrence of bulimia nervosa, research suggests that women born after 1960 have a higher risk for the illness than those born before 1960.

Evidence suggests an important role of sociocultural influences in the development of bulimia nervosa. For example, the frequency of the disorder has been reported to be increasing among immigrants to the USA and UK from nonWestern countries (Hsu, 1990). Although the rate of the disorder appears to be lower among nonwhite and nonWestern cultures, the frequency of bulimia nervosa has been reported to be increasing among these groups, especially among the higher socioeconomic classes. Surprisingly, several epidemiological and clinical studies in the USA found no relationship between bulimia nervosa and social class (Kendler et al., 1991).

Among patients with bulimia nervosa who are seen at eating disorders clinics, there is an increased frequency of anxiety and mood disorders, especially major depressive disorder and dysthymic disorder, of drug and alcohol abuse, and of personality disorders. It is not certain whether this comorbidity is also observed in community samples or whether it is a characteristic of individuals who seek treatment.

Etiology

As in the case of anorexia nervosa, the etiology of bulimia nervosa is uncertain. Several factors clearly predispose individuals to the development of bulimia nervosa, including being an adolescent girl or young adult woman. A personal or family history of obesity and of mood disturbance also appears to increase risk. Twin studies have suggested that inherited factors are related to the risk of developing bulimia nervosa, but what these factors are and how they operate are unclear.

Many of the same psychosocial factors related to the development of anorexia nervosa are also applicable to bulimia nervosa, including the influence of cultural esthetic ideals of thinness and physical fitness. Similarly, bulimia nervosa primarily affects women; the ratio of men to women is approximately 1 : 10. It also

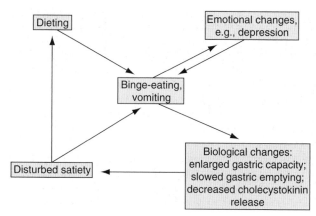

Figure 58.4 *Diagram illustrating factors that may perpetuate bulimia nervosa.*

occurs more frequently in certain occupations (e.g., modeling) and sports (e.g., wrestling, running).

Although not proven, it seems likely that several factors serve to perpetuate the binge-eating once it has begun (Figure 58.4 First, most individuals with bulimia nervosa, because of both their concern regarding weight and their worry about the effect of the binge-eating, attempt to restrict their food intake when they are not binge-eating. The psychological and physiological restraint that is thereby entailed presumably makes additional binge-eating more likely. Secondly, even if mood disturbance is not present at the outset, individuals become distressed about their inability to control their eating, and the resultant lowering of self-esteem contributes to disturbances of mood and to a reduced ability to control impulses to overeat. In addition, cognitive–behavioral theories emphasize the role of rigid rules regarding food and eating, and the distorted and dysfunctional thoughts that are similar to those seen in anorexia nervosa. Interpersonal theories also implicate interpersonal stressors as a primary factor in triggering binge-eating. There is no evidence to suggest that a particular personality structure is characteristic of women with bulimia nervosa.

There are also indications that bulimia nervosa is accompanied by physiological disturbances that disrupt the development of satiety during a meal and therefore increase the likelihood of binge-eating. These disturbances include an enlarged stomach capacity, a delay in stomach emptying and a reduction in the release of cholecystokinin, a peptide hormone secreted by the small intestine during a meal that normally plays a role in terminating eating behavior. All these abnormalities appear to predispose the individual to overeat and therefore to perpetuate the cycle of binge-eating.

It has been suggested that childhood sexual abuse is a specific risk factor for the development of bulimia nervosa. Scientific support for this hypothesis is weak. The best studies to date have found that compared with women without psychiatric illness, women with bulimia nervosa do indeed report increased frequencies of sexual abuse. However, the rates of abuse are similar to those found in other psychiatric disorders and occur in a minority of women with bulimia nervosa. Thus, while early abuse may predispose an individual to psychiatric problems generally, it does not appear to lead specifically to an eating disorder and most patients with bulimia nervosa do not have histories of sexual abuse.

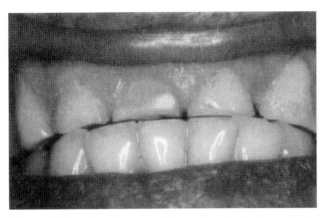

Figure 58.5 *Dental erosion of upper front teeth of a patient with longstanding bulimia nervosa.*

Pathophysiology

In a small fraction of individuals, bulimia nervosa is associated with the development of fluid and electrolyte abnormalities that result from the self-induced vomiting or the misuse of laxatives or diuretics. The most common electrolyte disturbances are hypokalemia, hyponatremia and hypochloremia. Patients who lose substantial amounts of stomach acid through vomiting may become slightly alkalotic; those who abuse laxatives may become slightly acidotic.

There is an increased frequency of menstrual disturbances such as oligomenorrhea among women with bulimia nervosa. Several studies suggest that the hypothalamic–pituitary–gonadal axis is subject to the same type of disruption as is seen in anorexia nervosa but that the abnormalities are much less frequent and severe.

Patients who induce vomiting for many years may develop dental erosion, especially of the upper front teeth (Figure 58.5). The mechanism appears to be that stomach acid softens the enamel, which in time gradually disappears so that the teeth chip more easily and can become reduced in size. Some patients develop painless salivary gland enlargement, which is thought to represent hypertrophy resulting from the repeated episodes of binge-eating and vomiting. The serum level of amylase is sometimes mildly elevated in patients with bulimia nervosa because of increased amounts of salivary amylase.

Most patients with bulimia nervosa have surprisingly few gastrointestinal abnormalities. As indicated earlier, it appears that the disorder is associated with an enlarged gastric capacity and delayed gastric emptying, but these abnormalities are not so severe as to be detectable on routine clinical examination. Potentially life-threatening complications such as an esophageal tear or gastric rupture occur, but fortunately rarely.

The longstanding use of syrup of ipecac to induce vomiting can lead to absorption of some of the alkaloids and to permanent damage to nerve and muscle.

Diagnosis and Differential Diagnosis

Phenomenology

Bulimia nervosa typically begins after a young woman who sees herself as somewhat overweight starts a diet and, after some initial success, begins to overeat. Distressed by her lack of control and by her fear of gaining weight, she decides to compensate for the overeating by inducing vomiting or taking laxatives, methods

she has heard about from friends or seen in media reports about eating disorders. After discovering that she can successfully purge, the individual may, for a time, feel pleased in that she can eat large amounts of food and not gain weight. However, the episodes of binge-eating usually increase in size and in frequency and occur after a variety of stimuli, such as transient depression or anxiety or a sense that she has begun to overeat. Patients often describe themselves as "numb" while they are binge-eating, suggesting that the eating may serve to avoid uncomfortable emotional states. Patients usually feel intensely ashamed of their "disgusting" habit and may become depressed by their lack of control over their eating.

The binge-eating tends to occur in the late afternoon or evening and almost always while the patient is alone. The typical patient presenting to eating disorders clinics has been binge-eating and inducing vomiting five to 10 times weekly for 3 to 10 years. Although there is substantial variation, binges tend to contain 1000 or more calories and to consist of sweet, high-fat foods that are normally consumed as dessert, such as ice cream, cookies and cake. Although patients complain of "carbohydrate craving", they only rarely binge-eat foods that are pure carbohydrates, such as fruits. Patients usually induce vomiting or use their characteristic compensatory behavior immediately after the binge and feel substantial relief that the calories are "gone". In reality, it appears that vomiting is the only purging method capable of disposing of a significant number of ingested calories. The weight loss associated with the misuse of laxatives and diuretics is primarily due to the loss of fluid and electrolytes, not calories.

When not binge-eating, patients with bulimia nervosa tend to restrict their calorie intake and to avoid the foods usually consumed during episodes of binge-eating. Although there is some phenomenological resemblance between binge-eating and substance abuse, there is no evidence that physiological addiction plays any role in bulimia nervosa.

Assessment

Special Issues in Psychiatric Examination and History

The assessment of individuals who may have bulimia nervosa is similar to that described for anorexia nervosa. The patient should be asked to describe a typical day's food intake and a typical binge and the interviewer should assess whether the patient does indeed consume an unusually large amount of food as required by the DSM-IV definition of a binge. The interviewer should explicitly inquire about self-induced vomiting and whether syrup of ipecac is ever used to promote vomiting. The interviewer should ask about the use of laxatives, diuretics, diet pills and enemas. A weight history should be obtained, so the interviewer can determine whether the binge-eating was preceded by obesity or by anorexia nervosa, as is often the case. Because there is substantial comorbidity, the interviewer should ascertain whether there is a history of anxiety or mood disturbance or of substance abuse.

Physical Examination and Laboratory Findings

The patient should be weighed and the presence of dental erosion noted. Routine laboratory testing reveals an abnormality of fluid and electrolyte balance such as those described in the section on pathophysiology in about 10% of patients with bulimia nervosa.

Differences in Presentation

Probably the greatest difference in presentation is between those individuals who purge and those who do not. Individuals with the nonpurging form of bulimia nervosa are more likely to be overweight at the time of presentation and to exhibit less general psychiatric illness compared with individuals who induce vomiting.

Differential Diagnosis

Bulimia nervosa is not difficult to recognize if a full history is available. The binge-eating/purging type of anorexia nervosa has much in common with bulimia nervosa but is distinguished by the characteristic low body weight and, in women, amenorrhea. Some individuals with atypical forms of depression overeat when depressed; if the overeating meets the definition of a binge described previously (i.e., a large amount of food is consumed with a sense of loss of control) and if the binge-eating is followed by inappropriate compensatory behavior, occurs sufficiently frequently and is associated with over concern regarding body shape and weight, an additional diagnosis of bulimia nervosa may be warranted. Some individuals become nauseated and vomit when upset; this and similar problems are probably not closely related to bulimia nervosa and should be viewed as a somatoform disorder.

Many individuals who believe they have bulimia nervosa have a symptom pattern that fails to meet full diagnostic criteria because the frequency of their binge-eating is less than twice a week or because what they view as a binge does not contain an abnormally large amount of food. Individuals with these characteristics fall into the broad and heterogeneous category of atypical eating disorders. Binge-eating disorder (see section on binge-eating disorder), a category currently included in the DSM-IV appendix B for categories that need additional research, is characterized by recurrent binge-eating similar to that seen in bulimia nervosa but without the regular occurrence of inappropriate compensatory behavior.

Course and Natural History

Over time, the symptoms of bulimia nervosa tend to improve although a substantial fraction of individuals continue to engage in binge-eating and purging. On the other hand, some controlled clinical trials have reported that structured forms of psychotherapy have the potential to yield substantial and sustained recovery in a significant fraction of patients who complete treatment. It is not clear what factors are most predictive of good outcome, but those individuals who cease binge-eating and purging completely during treatment are least likely to relapse.

Goals of Treatment

The goals of the treatment of bulimia nervosa are straightforward. The binge-eating and inappropriate compensatory behaviors should cease and self-esteem should become more appropriately based on factors other than shape and weight.

Treatment

The power struggles that often complicate the treatment process in anorexia nervosa occur much less frequently in the treatment of patients with bulimia nervosa. This is largely because the critical behavioral disturbances, binge-eating and purging, are less egosyntonic and are more distressing to these patients. Most bulimia nervosa patients who pursue treatment agree with the primary treatment goals and wish to give up the core behavioral features of their illness.

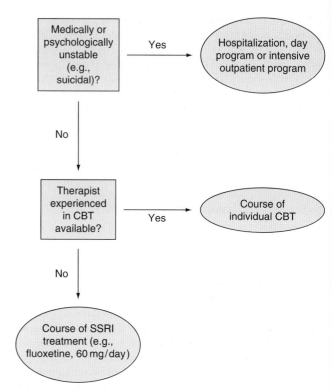

Figure 58.6   *Algorithm for choice of initial treatment of bulimia nervosa.*

The treatment of bulimia nervosa has received considerable attention in recent years and the efficacies of both psychotherapy and medication have been explored in numerous controlled studies (Figure 58.6). The form of psychotherapy that has been examined most intensively is cognitive–behavioral therapy, modeled on the therapy of the same type for depression. Cognitive–behavioral therapy for bulimia nervosa concentrates on the distorted ideas about weight and shape, on the rigid rules regarding food consumption and the pressure to diet and on the events that trigger episodes of binge-eating. The therapy is focused and highly structured and is usually conducted in 3 to 6 months. Approximately 25 to 50% of patients with bulimia nervosa achieve abstinence from binge-eating and purging during a course of cognitive–behavioral therapy and in most, this improvement appears to be sustained. The most common form of cognitive–behavioral therapy is individual treatment, although it can be given in either individual or group format. The effect of cognitive–behavioral therapy is greater than that of supportive psychotherapy and of interpersonal therapy, indicating that cognitive–behavioral therapy should be the treatment of choice for bulimia nervosa.

The other commonly used mode of treatment that has been examined in bulimia nervosa is the use of antidepressant medication. This intervention was initially prompted by the high rates of depression among patients with bulimia nervosa and has now been tested in more than a dozen double-blind, placebo-controlled studies using a wide variety of antidepressant medications. Active medication has been consistently found to be superior to placebo, and although there have been no large "head-to-head" comparisons between different antidepressants, most antidepressants appear to possess roughly similar antibulimic potency. Fluoxetine at a dose of 60 mg/day is favored by many investigators because it has been studied in several large trials and appears to be at least as effective as, and better tolerated than, most other alternatives. It is notable that it has not been possible to link the effectiveness of antidepressant treatment for bulimia nervosa to the pretreatment level of depression. Depressed and nondepressed patients with bulimia nervosa respond equally well in terms of their eating behavior to antidepressant medication.

Although antidepressant medication is clearly superior to placebo in the treatment of bulimia nervosa, several studies suggest that a course of a single antidepressant medication is generally inferior to a course of cognitive–behavioral therapy. However, patients who fail to respond adequately to, or who relapse following a trial of psychotherapy, may still respond to antidepressant medication.

Special Features Influencing Treatment

A major factor influencing the treatment of bulimia nervosa is the presence of other significant psychiatric or medical illness. For example, it can be difficult for individuals who are currently abusing drugs or alcohol to use the treatment methods described, and many psychiatrists suggest that the substance abuse needs to be addressed before the eating disorder can be effectively treated. Other examples include the treatment of individuals with bulimia nervosa and serious personality disturbance and those with insulin-dependent diabetes mellitus who "purge" by omitting insulin doses. In treating such individuals, the psychiatrist must decide which of the multiple problems must be first addressed and may elect to tolerate a significant level of eating disorder to confront more pressing disturbances.

Refractory Patients

Although psychotherapy and antidepressant medication are effective interventions for many patients with bulimia nervosa, some individuals have little or no response. There is no clearly established algorithm for the treatment of such refractory patients. Alternative interventions that may prove useful include other forms of psychotherapy and other medications such as opiate antagonists and the serotonin agonist fenfluramine. Hospitalization should also be considered as a way to normalize eating behavior, at least temporarily, and perhaps to initiate a more effective outpatient treatment.

Binge-eating Disorder

History

As noted earlier, binge-eating disorder is a proposed diagnostic category related to, but quite distinct from, bulimia nervosa. Individuals with binge-eating disorder, like individuals with bulimia nervosa, repeatedly engage in episodes of binge-eating but, unlike patients with bulimia nervosa, do not regularly utilize inappropriate compensatory behaviors. Binge-eating disorder has been the focus of sustained attention only in the last decade. The clinical utility of the information which quickly developed following the recognition of bulimia in the DSM nomenclature was an important source of interest in binge-eating disorder.

Definition

Suggested diagnostic criteria for binge-eating disorder are included in an appendix of DSM-IV-TR which provides criteria sets for further study. These criteria require recurrent episodes of binge-eating, which are defined just as for bulimia nervosa. The major difference from bulimia nervosa is that individuals with binge-eating disorder do not regularly use inappropriate

compensatory behavior, although the precise meaning of "regularly" is not specified. Other differences from the definition of bulimia nervosa relate to the frequency of binge-eating: individuals with bulimia nervosa must binge-eat, on average, at least two times per week over the last 3 months, whereas individuals with binge-eating disorder must binge-eat at least 2 days per week over the last 6 months. A major reason for the difference in the criteria is that the end of a binge episode in bulimia nervosa is usually clearly marked by the occurrence of inappropriate compensatory behavior, like purging, whereas in binge-eating disorder, the end of a binge episode may be more difficult to identify precisely. The criteria attempt to deal with this definitional difficulty by requiring the frequency of binge-eating to be measured in terms of the number of days per week on which episodes occur and, because of the potential difficulty in distinguishing "normal" overeating from binge-eating, to require a 6 month duration, rather than 3 months for bulimia nervosa. In addition, the suggested DSM-IV-TR criteria for binge-eating disorder require that individuals report behavioral evidence of a sense of loss of control over eating, such as eating large amounts of food when not physically hungry. Finally, while there is some evidence that individuals with binge-eating disorder tend to be more concerned about body image than individuals of similar weight, the criteria for binge-eating disorder require only that there is marked distress over the binge-eating. Thus, the criteria for binge-eating disorder do not require that self-evaluation be overly influenced by concerns regarding body weight and shape, as is required for bulimia nervosa.

Epidemiology

The epidemiology of binge-eating disorder is uncertain. Cross-sectional studies suggest that the prevalence of binge-eating disorder among adults is a few percent and that the prevalence is higher among obese individuals in the community and among obese individuals who attend weight loss clinics. Similarly, the frequency of binge-eating disorder increases with the degree of obesity. In contrast to anorexia nervosa and bulimia nervosa, individuals with binge-eating disorder are more likely to be men (the female to male ratio is roughly 1.5 : 1 compared with approximately 10 : 1 for anorexia nervosa and bulimia nervosa), from minority ethnic groups and middle-aged.

Etiology

Very little is known about the etiology of binge-eating disorder. Binge-eating disorder is clearly associated with obesity, but it is uncertain to what degree the binge-eating is a contributor to and to what degree a consequence of, the obesity.

Diagnosis and Differential Diagnosis

Phenomenology

In theory, binge-eating disorder should be easy to recognize on the basis of patient self-report: the individual describes the frequent consumption of large amounts of food in a discrete period of time about which he or she feels distressed and unable to control. Difficulties arise, however, because of uncertainty about what precisely constitutes a "large amount of food", especially for an obese individual and regarding what constitutes a discrete period of time. Many individuals describe eating continuously during the day or evening, thereby consuming a large amount of food, but it is not clear whether such behavior is best viewed as binge-eating. Individuals who meet the proposed definition of binge-eating disorder clearly have increased complaints of depression and anxiety compared with individuals of similar weight without binge-eating disorder.

Assessment

The assessment of individuals who may have binge-eating disorder parallels that of individuals who may have bulimia nervosa. It is important to obtain a clear understanding of daily food intake and of what the individual considers a binge. As in the assessment of bulimia nervosa, the interviewer should inquire about the use of purging and other inappropriate weight control methods. Individuals who describe binge-eating disorder are likely to be obese, and it is important to obtain a history of changes in weight and of efforts to lose weight. The interviewer should also inquire about symptoms of mood disturbance and anxiety.

Physical Examination and Laboratory Findings

The salient general medical issue is that of obesity. Individuals with binge-eating disorder who are obese should be followed by a primary care physician for assessment and treatment of the complications of obesity. There is no evidence suggesting that the behavioral disturbances characteristic of binge-eating disorder add to the physical risks of obesity. Whether the presence of binge-eating disorder affects the natural history of obesity is an intriguing but unanswered question.

Differential Diagnosis

As noted above, the most difficult issue in the diagnostic assessment of binge-eating disorder is determining whether the eating pattern of concern to the individual meets the proposed definition of binge-eating. There are numerous varieties of unhealthy eating, such as the consumption of high fat foods and the nosology of these patterns of eating is poorly worked out.

Some individuals with atypical depression binge-eat when depressed; if the individual meets criteria for both binge-eating disorder and an atypical depression, both diagnoses should be made.

Course and Natural History

As the recognition of binge-eating disorder is quite recent, there is little definitive information about the natural history of this disorder. However, both controlled treatment studies and follow-up studies of community samples indicate that there is substantial fluctuation over time in the frequency and severity of the cardinal symptoms of this disorder.

Goals of Treatment

For most individuals with binge-eating disorder, there are three related goals. One is behavioral, to cease binge eating. A second focuses on improving symptoms of mood and anxiety disturbance which frequently are associated with binge-eating disorder. The third is weight loss for individuals who are also obese.

Treatment

Treatment approaches to binge-eating disorder are currently under active study. There is good evidence that psychological (e.g.,

CBT) and pharmacological (e.g., SSRI) interventions which are effective for bulimia nervosa are also useful in reducing the binge frequency of individuals with binge-eating disorder and in alleviating mood disturbance. However, it is not clear how helpful these approaches are in facilitating weight loss. Standard behavioral weight loss interventions employing caloric restriction appear useful in helping patients to control binge-eating, but the benefits of such treatment have not been compared with those of more psychologically-oriented treatments, such as CBT.

Comparison of DSM-IV/ICD-10 Diagnostic Criteria

The ICD-10 Diagnostic Criteria for Research and the DSM-IV-TR criteria for anorexia nervosa differ in several ways. ICD-10 specifically requires that the weight loss be self-induced by the avoidance of "fattening foods" and that in men there be a loss of sexual interest and potency (corresponding to the amenorrhea requirement in women). Finally, in contrast to DSM-IV-TR which gives anorexia nervosa precedence over bulimia nervosa, ICD-10 excludes a diagnosis of anorexia nervosa if regular binge eating has been present.

For bulimia nervosa, the ICD-10 Diagnostic Criteria for Research and the DSM-IV-TR criteria for bulimia nervosa are similar except that ICD-10 requires a "persistent preoccupation with eating and a strong desire or sense of compulsion to eat". Furthermore, whereas the ICD-10 definition requires a self-perception of being too fat (identical to an item in anorexia nervosa), the DSM-IV-TR criteria set requires instead that "self-evaluation is unduly influenced by body shape and weight".

Both DSM-IV-TR and ICD-10 include categories unique to their systems. DSM-IV-TR has a category for "Binge-Eating Disorder" in its appendix of research categories whereas ICD-10 has categories for "Overeating associated with other psychological disturbances" and "Vomiting associated with other psychological disturbances".

References

Bruch H (1973) *Eating Disorders. Obesity, Anorexia Nervosa, and the Person Within*. Basic Books, New York.

Bruch H (1982) Anorexia nervosa: Therapy and theory. *Am J Psychiatr* 132, 1531.

Fairburn CG and Walsh BT (2002) Atypical eating disorders, in *Eating Disorders and Obesity: A Comprehensive Textbook*, 2nd edn. (eds Brownell KD and Fairburn CG). Guilford Press, New York, p. 171.

Gordon RA (1990) *Anorexia and Bulimia: Anatomy of a Social Epidemic*. Basil Blackwell, Cambridge, MA.

Hsu KL (1990) *Eating Disorders*. Guilford Press, New York.

Kaye WH (1997) Anorexia nervosa, obsessional behavior, and serotonin. *Psychopharmacol Bull* 33, 335.

Kendler KS, Maclean C, Neale M *et al.* (1991) The genetic epidemiology of bulimia nervosa. *Am J Psychiatr* 148, 1627.

Klump KL, Kaye W and Strober M (2001) The evolving genetic foundations of eating disorders. *Psychiatr Clin N Am* 24, 215.

Sleep and Sleep–Wake Disorders

Physiological Regulation of Sleep and Wakefulness

Three physiological processes regulate sleep and wakefulness.

Ultradian Rhythm of Rapid Eye Movement (REM) and Non-rapid Eye Movement (Non-REM) Sleep

Sleep consists of two major REM and non-REM sleep, which alternate throughout the sleep period. Sleep normally begins in the adult with non-REM sleep and is followed after about 70 to 90 minutes by the first REM period. Thereafter, non-REM sleep and REM sleep oscillate with a cycle length (the interval between onset of each non-REM or REM period) of about 80 to 110 minutes. This cycle of REM and non-REM sleep is an example of an ultradian rhythm, a biological rhythm with a cycle length considerably less than 24 hours.

On the basis of electroencephalographical (EEG) characteristics, non-REM sleep in humans is further divided into four stages: stage 1, a brief transitional stage between wakefulness and sleep; stage 2, which occupies the greatest amount of time during sleep; and stages 3 and 4, sometimes called delta sleep because of the characteristic high-amplitude slow EEG waves (delta waves) (Table 59.1). The amount of ocular activity per minute of REM sleep is quantified as REM density; this can be measured by either visual scoring (e.g., on an analogue scale from 0 to 8 per minute) or by computer analysis. Dreaming is commonly reported and is usually vivid when subjects are awakened from REM sleep but also occurs during non-REM sleep, especially at sleep onset during stage 1 sleep.

Circadian (24-Hour) Rhythm of Sleep and Wakefulness

The rest–activity or sleep–wake cycle is an example of a circadian rhythm (Table 59.2). Other examples include the hypothalamic–pituitary–adrenal axis, thyroid-stimulating hormone and core body temperature. [Circadian rhythms can be characterized by three difference measures: 1) cycle length (**tau**) (e.g., the time between two peaks of the ~24 hour temperature curve); 2) amplitude (e.g., the difference between the minimum value of the cycle (**nadir**) and maximum value (**acrophase**), for example, the difference between the lowest and highest points in the 24 hour temperature curve; and 3) phase position of the rhythm (e.g., the time of day when the acrophase occurred).]

The propensity for sleep and wakefulness varies in a circadian fashion, at least after infancy, and is modulated in part by one or more biological clocks. The suprachiasmatic nucleus (SCN) in the anterior hypothalamus plays a decisive role in the regulation of most circadian rhythms in humans and animals. The endogenous activity rhythms of the SCN are synchronized with the environment primarily by ambient light. Information regarding light reaching the retina is conveyed to the SCN directly through the retinohypothalamic tract and indirectly through the intergeniculate leaflet of the lateral geniculate body. Changes in light intensity, especially at dawn and dusk, are particularly important in synchronizing endogenous oscillators controlling rhythms of sleep–wake, cortisol, melatonin and core body temperature with one another and with the outside world.

If humans are allowed to choose their sleep–wake cycles in the absence of time cues such as daily light–dark signals or clocks, they usually show, as most mammalian species do, a sleep–wake cycle longer than 24 hours. The self-selected rest–activity cycle is typically about 24.5 to 25 hours in length, although it may increase, for example, to 36 hours (24 hours awake and 12 hours asleep). These observations imply that neurons within the SCN have an inherent rhythmicity of approximately 24.5 to 25 hours. Subjects in a time-free environment are said to be "free- running" because endogenous processes, such as a circadian oscillator, rather than environmental cues, determine their sleep–wake, endocrine and other rhythms.

The propensity for, character and duration of sleep are closely related to the phase position of the underlying circadian oscillator. If the daily temperature curve is used to index the phase position of the biological clock, sleep in general and REM sleep in particular occur most commonly near the nadir of the temperature rhythm. Thus, in persons who live a conventional sleep schedule (11 PM–7 AM), REM sleep is more common in the last half of the night when core body temperature is lowest than in the first half and more likely in morning naps than in afternoon naps. Furthermore, subjects tend to awaken on the rising phase of the temperature rhythm.

Appropriate exposure to light and darkness can change the phase position of the underlying biological oscillator or, in some circumstances, the amplitude of circadian rhythms. Bright light at the beginning of the subjective evening in conjunction with dark during the subjective morning delays and resets the phase position of the temperature, cortisol, melatonin and sleep–wake rhythms; dark in the subjective evening and bright light in the subjective morning have the opposite effect. The magnitude and direction of the changes induced by bright light or other Zeitgebers ("timegivers") at any particular time form the **phase-response curve**.

Essentials of Psychiatry   Jerald Kay and Allan Tasman
© 2006 John Wiley & Sons, Ltd.

Table 59.1	Commonly Used Terms in Human Sleep Studies
Term	**Definition**
Delta wave	Electroencephalographic pattern conventionally defined as ≤ 75 mV, ≤ 0.5 Hz or cycles per second wave; the amplitude tends to decrease with normal aging
Non-REM sleep	Stages 1, 2, 3, and 4 sleep
Total sleep time	Non-REM and REM sleep time
REM latency	Time from onset of sleep to onset of REM sleep; declines from about 70–100 min in the 20s to 55–70 min in the elderly, short REM latency associated with narcolepsy, depression, and a variety of clinical conditions
REM sleep	Rapid eye movement sleep; characterized by low-voltage, relatively fast frequency EEG, bursts of rapid eye movements, and loss of tone (atonia) in the major antigravity muscles; associated with dreaming
Sleep efficiency	Percentage of time in bed spent in sleep; usually above 90% in the young, falls somewhat with age
Sleep latency	Time from "lights out" to onset of sleep
Stage 1 sleep	A brief transitional state of sleep between wakefulness and sleep, characterized by low-voltage, mixed-frequency EEG and slow eye movements; about 5% of total sleep time
Stage 2 sleep	Characterized by K complexes and sleep spindles (12–14 per cycle rhythms) in the EEG; usually about 45–75% of total sleep time
Stages 3 and 4 sleep	Sometimes referred to as delta sleep, based on amount of sleep delta waves in EEG, 20–50% of an epoch (i.e., 30 or 60 s) for stage 3, more than 50% for stage 4; amount per night declining from about 20–25% of total sleep time in the teens to nearly zero in the elderly
WASO	Wake time sleep onset
REM density	A measure of amount of ocular activity per minute of REM sleep

Table 59.2	Commonly Used Terms in Chronobiology
Term	**Definition**
Acrophase	The time, at which the maximal point of a circadian rhythm occurs, i.e., maximal secretion of cortisol normally occurs at midmorning in humans.
Circadian rhythm	Refers to biological rhythms having a cycle length of about 24 h, derived from Latin *circa dies*, "about 1 d"; examples include the sleep–wake cycle in humans, temperature, cortisol and psychological variation in the 24-h day; characterized by exact cycle length (tau), amplitude and phase position.
Constant routine	An experimental method used to estimate amplitude and phase position of circadian temperature and neuroendocrine rhythms; the subject remains awake for about 36 h under dim light, with head elevated slightly, eating frequent equal-calorie meals, while blood samples are withdrawn unobtrusively every 20–30 min and rectal temperature is measured about once a minute.
Dim light melatonin onset (DLMO)	An experimental method for estimating the phase of melatonin onset; under dim light conditions starting in late afternoon, blood samples are withdrawn every 20–30 min to determine when melatonin secretion begins.
Nadir	Time when the minimal point of a circadian rhythm occurs.
Phase position	Temporal relationship between rhythms or between one rhythm and the environment; e.g., maximal daily temperature peak (acrophase) usually occurs in the late afternoon.
Phase-advanced rhythm	Phase position of biological rhythm occurs earlier than reference, i.e., the patient retires and arises early.
Phase-delayed rhythm	Phase position of biological rhythm occurs later than reference, i.e., the patient retires and arises late.
Phase-response curve	Graph showing the magnitude and direction of change in phase position of circadian rhythm depending upon timing of Zeitgeber with reference to the endogenous oscillator.
Tau	Cycle length, e.g., from one acrophase to the next of temperature.
Zeitgebers	Time cues, such as social activities, meals and bright lights, that influence phase position of rhythm.

The phase position of the circadian oscillator can also be estimated in humans by the 24-hour rhythms of cortisol or melatonin secretion. Because these rhythms can be affected by exercise, meals, light and so forth, the conditions under which they are measured should be controlled. For example, clinical investigators may use a "constant routine" condition in which the subjects are kept awake in bed for 36 hours, under constant low-intensity. An alternative is to determine the onset of melatonin secretion under dark conditions (dim light melatonin onset). As discussed later, various strategies are under experimental development with the hope that appropriate administration of light–dark cycles, melatonin, vitamin B_{12}, or specific medications will "nudge" and "squash" the circadian oscillator correctly better to manage clinical disorders of sleep–wakefulness, such as jet lag, delayed sleep syndrome and shift work. In addition, bright light has been shown to have antidepressant effects in patients with winter depression, some patients with major depressive disorder and patients with premenstrual dysphoric disorder.

If animals suffer lesions of the SCN, they no longer exhibit circadian rhythms of temperature, cortisol secretion, eating, drinking, or sleep–wakefulness. Sleep and wakefulness, for example, are taken in brief bouts throughout the 24-hour day. Total sleep time, however, may increase under these circumstances. No selective lesion of the human SCN has been documented.

Homeostatic Regulation of Sleep–Wakefulness

Common experience suggests that the longer one is awake, the more likely one is to fall asleep. Furthermore, sleep reverses the sleepiness and other consequences of wakefulness. Thus, sleep can be said to perform a homeostatic function; it is a time of rest and restoration that overcomes the "ravages of wakefulness" (Daan *et al.*, 1984). Consistent with the hypothesis, sleep deprivation usually decreases sleep latency and increases sleep efficiency and delta sleep on recovery nights.

The precise regulation of sleep and wakefulness remains an area of intense investigation and theory. Two of the current theories of sleep–wake regulation include the two-process model (Daan *et al.*, 1984) and the opponent process model (Edgar *et al.*, 1993). The first postulates that sleep and wakefulness are regulated by a circadian process (process C), which sets the circadian thresholds for sleep and wakefulness, and a homeostatic process (process S), in which sleep propensity builds up with wakefulness and dissipates during non-REM sleep, especially delta sleep. The opponent process model postulates that the SCN promotes alertness and that duration of wakefulness facilitates sleep.

Normal Age-related Changes in Sleep and Wakefulness

The newborn spends nearly 50% of total sleep time in REM sleep. Because infants may sleep up to 16 hours a day, the infant may spend 8 hours in REM sleep per day. Often to the consternation of the parents, the newborn has a polyphasic sleep–wake pattern, with short bouts of sleep and wakefulness throughout the 24-hour day, until several months of age when the child eventually sleeps through the night. Daytime napping, however, often persists until the age of 4 to 6 years. Stages 3 and 4 sleep increase in the early years. Maximal "depth" of sleep may occur during the prepubertal period, when children are often difficult to awake at night. Adolescents often still need at least 10 hours of sleep. Yet, during adolescence, stages 3 and 4 sleep decline and daytime sleepiness increases, partially in association with the normal Tanner stages of pubertal development. Teenagers are also phase delayed which means that they may not get sleepy until the early morning hours (e.g., 2–3 AM) and do not naturally wake up until the later morning hours. Early school start times and social pressures may produce mild sleep deprivation during weekdays, with some catch-up on weekends.

As adults enter middle age and old age, sleep often becomes more shallow, fragmented, and variable in duration and circadian timing compared with that of young adults. Stages 1 and 2 and wake time after sleep onset tend to increase; REM latency and stages 3 and 4 decline, probably at an earlier age in men than in women and possibly related to changes in brain structure and metabolism. Daytime sleepiness and napping usually increase with age, often as a function of disturbed nocturnal sleep. The elderly frequently choose an "early-to-bed, early-to-rise" pattern reflecting, in part, an apparent phase advance of the circadian clock. Even when they retire at the same time that they did when they were young, they still tend to wake up early, thus sleep-depriving themselves. This can lead to daytime sleepiness and napping. Although average total sleep time actually increases slightly after age 65 years, greater numbers of persons fall into either long-sleeping (>8 hours) or short-sleeping (<7 hours) subgroups. Psychiatrists should always consider the role of chronobiological factors when evaluating patients with sleep disorders, especially the elderly, who have more sleep–wake complaints than younger persons. The sleep–wake patterns of the early bedtimes of the elderly, short REM latency, sleep fragmentation at night and napping during the day may reflect a phase-advance and reduced amplitude of the circadian oscillator.

Factors that could contribute to these age-related patterns include loss of influence from Zeitgebers (light, work schedules, social demands, physical exercise) and a weaker signal from the circadian oscillator to effector systems. Indoor living conditions or loss of hearing and sight may deprive individuals of cues that synchronize the circadian system. In a significant number of totally blind persons, for example, the circadian oscillator free-runs in the normal environment, with resulting regular periods of insomnia and hypersomnia every 3 weeks as the circadian oscillator delays by about 45 minutes each 24 hours while the subject tries to maintain a normal sleep period (11PM–7AM). In a study of normally sighted elderly individuals in San Diego, California, exposure to self-selected bright light averaged 45 minutes and 90 minutes per day for healthy women and men, respectively; 30 minutes per day for patients with Alzheimer's disease living at home; and 2 minutes for chronically ill, institutionalized patients (Jacobs *et al.*, 1989). Perhaps not surprisingly, the elderly in one nursing home study never spent more than an hour in either consolidated sleep or wakefulness throughout a 24-hour period (Jacobs *et al.*, 1989).

Neurophysiology and Neurochemistry of Sleep

The non-REM–REM sleep cycle is regulated within the brain stem. Consistent with the concept that the brain stem regulates REM sleep, an Israeli soldier ceased having REM sleep after suffering a shrapnel wound to the brain stem (Lavie *et al.*, 1984). Some antidepressant medications, notably monoamine oxidase inhibitors (MAOIs), completely eliminate REM sleep when they are taken at high clinical doses for more than 2 weeks. No specific deleterious effects have been attributed to the loss of REM sleep in these patients. These observations underscore the mystery about the fundamental functions of REM sleep in particular and sleep in general.

No specific "sleep neurotransmitter" has been identified that is responsible for the induction or maintenance of sleep, but many different types of neurochemicals (neurotransmitters, neuromodulators, neuropeptides, immune modulators) have been implicated. Adenosine is a potential sleep promoting neurotransmitter; its concentration in basal forebrain increases with prolonged wakefulness. Caffeine probably promotes alertness by blocking the adenosine A_1-receptor. Of particular importance to psychiatry, acetylcholine, released from neurons originating in the dorsal tegmentum, induces REM sleep and cortical activation. Serotonin and norepinephrine, on the other hand, inhibit REM sleep, possibly by inhibition of cholinergic neurons responsible for REM sleep. These physiological mechanisms may be involved in both depression and the sleep disturbances associated with depression and other neuropsychiatric disorders, such as short REM latency (see later). For example, depression may be associated with a functional serotonin deficiency. The suppression of REM sleep during treatment with antidepressants may reflect either enhanced serotoninergic or noradrenergic neurotransmission or anticholinergic effects.

In addition, considerable current research suggests that sleep and immunological processes are intimately related. Several neuroimmunomodulators, such as specific interleukins or tumor necrosis factor, may promote sleep and sleep deprivation may alter immune function, for example, reducing activity of natural killer cells.

Sleep Disorders

Sleep disorders can be divided into four major categories: 1) insomnias, disorders associated with complaints of insufficient, disturbed, or nonrestorative sleep; 2) hypersomnias, disorders of excessive sleepiness; 3) disturbances of the circadian sleep–wake cycle; and 4) parasomnias, abnormal behaviors or abnormal physiological events in sleep (American Psychiatric Association, 1994). By definition, the *Diagnostic and Statistical Manual of Mental Disorders*, Fourth Edition (DSM-IV) limits itself to chronic disorders (at least 1 month in duration). On the other hand, the *International Classification of Sleep Disorders* includes sleep disorders of short-term and intermediate duration, which in fact are more common than chronic disorders (Diagnostic Classification Steering Committee Therapy MJC, 1990).

General Approach to the Patient with a Sleep Disorder

Disorders of sleep and wakefulness are common. Insomnia complaints are reported by about one-third of adult Americans during a 1-year period; clinically significant obstructive sleep apnea may be seen in as many as 10% of working, middle-aged men; and sleepiness is an underrecognized cause of dysphoria, automobile accidents and mismanagement of patients by sleep-deprived physicians. Nearly all physicians will hear complaints of sleep problems. Psychiatrists may be even more likely than other medical specialists to receive these complaints. Of particular importance for mental disorders, prospective epidemiological studies suggest that persistent complaints of either insomnia or hypersomnia are risk factors for the later onset of depression, anxiety disorders and substance abuse.

This chapter attempts to provide a framework for psychiatrists and other mental health specialists to use in understanding the multiple causes of the sleep disorders, their diagnostic evaluation and their treatment. To assist the patient with a sleep

complaint, the psychiatrist needs to have a diagnostic framework with which to obtain the information needed about both the patient as a person and his or her disorder. Two issues are particularly important: 1) How long has the patient had the sleep complaint? Transient insomnia and short-term insomnia, for example, usually occur in persons undergoing acute stress or other disruptions, such as admission to a hospital, jet lag, bereavement, or change in medications. Chronic sleep disorders, on the other hand, are often multidetermined and multifaceted: 2) Does the patient suffer from any preexisting or comorbid disorders? Does another condition cause the sleep complaint, modify a sleep complaint, or affect possible treatments? In general, because common sleep disorders are frequently secondary to underlying causes, treatment should be directed at underlying medical, psychiatric, pharmacological, psychosocial, or other disorders.

A detailed history of the complaint and attendant symptoms must be obtained (Tables 59.3 and 59.4). Special attention should be given to the timing of sleep and wakefulness; qualitative and quantitative subjective measures of sleep and wakefulness; abnormal sleep-related behaviors; respiratory difficulties; medications or other substances affecting sleep, wakefulness, or arousal; expectations, concerns, attitudes about sleep, and efforts used by the patient to control symp-

---

Table 59.3   Office Evaluation of Chronic Sleep Complaints

Detailed history and review of the sleep complaint: predisposing, precipitating and perpetuating factors

Review of difficulties falling asleep, maintaining sleep and awakening early

Timing of sleep and wakefulness in the 24-h day

Evidence of excessive daytime sleepiness and fatigue

Bedtime routines, sleep setting, physical security, preoccupations, anxiety, beliefs about sleep and sleep loss, fears about consequences of sleep loss

Medical and neurological history and examination, routine laboratory examinations: look for obesity, short fat neck, enlarged tonsils, narrow upper oral airway, foreshortened jaw (retrognathia) and hypertension

Psychiatric history and examination

Use of prescription and nonprescription medications, alcohol, stimulants, toxins, insecticides and other substances

Evidence of sleep-related breathing disorders: snoring, orthopnea, dyspnea, headaches, falling out of bed, nocturia

Abnormal movements or behaviors associated with sleep disorders: "jerky legs," leg movements, myoclonus, restless legs, leg cramps, cold feet, nightmares, enuresis, sleepwalking, epilepsy, bruxism, sleep paralysis, hypnagogic hallucinations, cataplexy, night sweats and so on

Social and occupational history, marital status, living conditions, financial and security concerns, physical activity

Sleep–wake diary for 2 wk

Interview with bed partners or persons who observe patient during sleep

Tape recording of respiratory sounds during sleep to screen for sleep apnea

Table 59.4	Selected Disorders and Terms Used in Clinical Sleep Disorders Medicine
Term	**Definition**
Apnea index	Number of apneic events per hour of sleep; usually is considered pathological if ≥5.
Cataplexy	Sudden, brief loss of muscle tone in the waking stage, usually triggered by emotional arousal (laughing, anger, surprise), involving either a few muscle groups (i.e., facial) or most of major antigravity muscles of the body; may be related to muscle atonia normally occurring during REM sleep; is associated with narcolepsy.
Hypopnea	50% or more reduction in respiratory depth for 10 s or more during sleep.
Multiple Sleep Latency Test	An objective method for determining daytime sleepiness; sleep latency and REM latency are determined for four or five naps (i.e., a 20-min opportunity to sleep every 2 h between 10 AM and 6 PM); normal mean values are above 15 min.
Periodic limb movements in sleep index	Number of leg kicks per hour of sleep; usually is considered pathological if ≥5.
Polysomnography	Describes detailed, sleep laboratory-based, clinical evaluation of patient with sleep disorder; may include electroencephalographical measures, eye movements, muscle tone at chin and limbs, respiratory movements of chest and abdomen, oxygen saturation, electrocardiogram, nocturnal penile tumescence, esophageal pH, as indicated.
Respiratory disturbance index	Number of apneas and hypopneas per hour of sleep.
Sleep apnea	Sleep-related breathing disorder characterized by at least five episodes of apnea per hour of sleep, each longer than 10 s in duration.

toms; and the sleep–wake environment. The psychiatrist must be alert to the possibility that sleep complaints are somatic symptoms, which reflect individual ways of experiencing, expressing and coping with psychosocial distress, stress, or psychiatric disorders.

Sleep disorders vary with age and gender and, possibly, with culture and social class. As mentioned previously, the circadian timing of rest–activity, sleep duration at night, and daytime napping and sleepiness vary with age and gender. In addition, parasomnias are most common in boys, Kleine–Levin syndrome in adolescent boys, delayed sleep phase syndrome in adolescents and young adults, insomnia in middle-aged and elderly women, REM sleep behavior disorder and sleep-related breathing disorders in middle-aged men, and advanced sleep phase syndrome in the elderly. Sleep–wake patterns are also influenced by cultural or geographical factors, such as the siesta and late bedtime commonly associated with tropical climates, or the winter hypersomnia and summer hyposomnia said to occur near the Arctic circle. Insomnia is more common in lower than in middle and upper socioeconomic classes, perhaps reflecting the stress of poverty, crowding and lack of privacy, poor medical care, drugs and alcohol, lack of physical security and so forth.

One approach to the differential diagnosis of persistent sleep disorders is suggested in the algorithm in Figure 59.1. First, determine whether the sleep complaint is due to another medical, psychiatric, or substance abuse disorder. Secondly, consider the role of circadian rhythm disturbances and sleep disorders associated with abnormal events predominantly during sleep. Finally, evaluate in greater detail complaints of insomnia (difficulty initiating or maintaining sleep) and excessive sleepiness.

Role of the Sleep Laboratory in Clinical Sleep Disorders

Psychiatrists can usually diagnose most sleep disorders by traditional, simple but systematic clinical methods. Referral to a specialized sleep disorders center, however, should be considered in patients suspected of having severe intractable insomnia, persistent excessive daytime sleepiness and sleep disorders due to a general medical condition (such as narcolepsy, REM sleep behavior disorder, sleep apnea, periodic limb movements in sleep [PLMS], or sleep-related epilepsy). Specialists in sleep disorders medicine will evaluate the patient and, if necessary, arrange for sleep laboratory or ambulatory diagnostic procedures.

One of the most important and common laboratory examinations is all-night polysomnography, which typically records the EEG activity's eye movements with the electrooculogram, and muscle tone with the electromyogram from the chin (submental) muscles. These measures are used to determine sleep stages visually scored as 20- or 30-second epochs by a sleep technician. To evaluate sleep-related respiration and cardiovascular function, measures are made of nasal and oral air flow with a thermistor; of sounds of breathing and snoring with a small microphone near the mouth; of respiratory movements of the chest and abdominal walls; of heart rate with the electrocardiogram; and of blood-oxygen saturation with finger oximetry. To evaluate PLMS, an electromyogram from the shin (anterior tibial) muscles is obtained. Other more specialized tests include intraesophageal pressures, which increase during the upper airway resistance syndrome if respiration is impeded, nocturnal penile tumescence in the evaluation of impotence and core body temperature (usually rectal or tympanic membrane).

Daytime sleepiness can be evaluated in the sleep laboratory with the Multiple Sleep Latency Test, which measures sleep latency during opportunities for napping during the day (see Table 59.4). In addition, subjective sleepiness can be assessed by

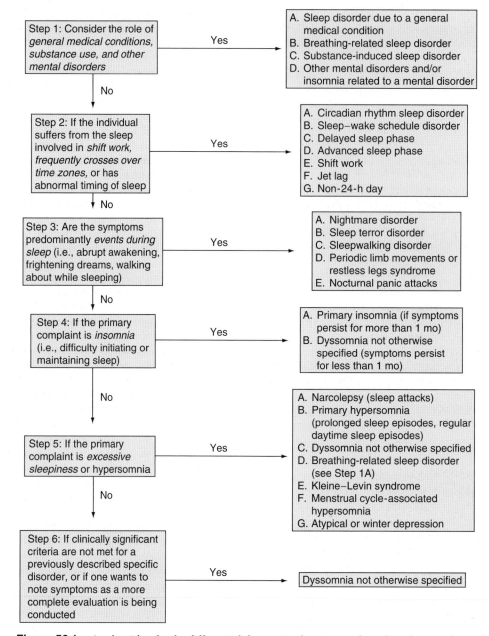

Figure 59.1   *An algorithm for the differential diagnosis of persistent sleep disorder complaints.*

a questionnaire, the Stanford Sleepiness Scale, in which the subject rates sleepiness on a 7-point scale at set intervals throughout the day.

Two research laboratory procedures have been developed for experimental measurement of circadian phase in humans: the constant routine method for temperature and neuroendocrine secretions, and the dim light melatonin onset method for melatonin (see Table 59.2).

According to DSM-IV-TR definitions (American Psychiatric Association, 1994), primary sleep disorders are presumed to arise from endogenous abnormalities in sleep–wake-generating mechanisms, timing mechanisms, sleep hygiene, or conditioning, rather than occurring secondary to medical or psychiatric disorders. Two types of primary sleep disorders are defined: **dyssomnias** (abnormalities in the amount, quality, or timing of sleep) and **parasomnias** (abnormal behaviors associated with sleep, such as

nightmares or sleepwalking). In addition, sleep disorders may be related to other mental disorders, general medical conditions, and substance abuse.

Dyssomnias

Primary Insomnia

According to DSM-IV-TR criteria, primary insomnia is a subjective complaint of poor, insufficient, or nonrestorative sleep lasting more than a month; associated with significant distress or impairment; and without obvious relationships to another sleep, medical, or psychiatric disorder or physiological effects of a substance. Primary insomnia is similar to some insomnia diagnoses in the *International Classification of Sleep Disorders*, including psychophysiological insomnia, which is often ascribed to conditioned arousal factors; sleep state misperception, in which the magnitude of the subjective complaint often exceeds that of the objective abnormality; and idiopathic insomnia, with a childhood onset and lifelong course.

The etiology of primary insomnia is unclear, but it may be dependent more on the factors that perpetuate it than on those that precipitated it. In general surveys of the prevalence of insomnia in the population, about one in three people reported "insomnia" during the previous year, about one in six described it as "serious", and about one in 12 called it "chronic" (Ancoli-Israel and Roth, 1999). The rates of insomnia are higher in women than in men, in the elderly than in the young, and in the lower than in the higher socioeconomic classes. In a survey conducted by the Gallup Poll for the National Sleep Foundation (Ancoli-Israel and Roth, 1999), the most common complaint of insomniacs is waking up feeling drowsy rather than specific complaints about sleep, implying that the sleepiness insomniacs experience could be associated with some morbidity. Compared with transient insomniacs or normal control subjects, chronic insomniacs reported greater difficulty enjoying family and social relationships, greater difficulty concentrating, more problems with memory, greater frequency of falling asleep while visiting friends, and more automobile accidents due to sleepiness. Nevertheless, only about 5% of patients with chronic insomnia ever sought medical attention specifically for insomnia. Only a minority of patients have ever used prescription sleeping pills. On the other hand, most psychiatrists do not routinely inquire about difficulties with sleep and wakefulness. If these patients with chronic or serious insomnia are to be helped, psychiatrists must be proactive and ask specific questions about sleep and its disorders.

DSM-IV-TR Criteria 307.42

Primary Insomnia

A. The predominant complaint is difficulty initiating or maintaining sleep, or nonrestorative sleep, for at least 1 month.

B. The sleep disturbance (or associated daytime fatigue) causes clinically significant distress or impairment in social, occupational, or other important areas of functioning.

C. The sleep disturbance does not occur exclusively during the course of narcolepsy, breathing-related sleep disorder, circadian rhythm sleep disorder, or a parasomnia.

D. The disturbance does not occur exclusively during the course of another mental disorder (e.g., major depressive disorder, generalized anxiety disorder, a delirium).

E. The disturbance is not due to the direct physiological effects of a substance (e.g., a drug of abuse, a medication) or a general medical condition.

Reprinted with permission from the *Diagnostic and Statistical Manual of Mental Disorders*, Fourth Edition, Text Revision. Copyright 2000 American Psychiatric Association.

The prevalence of primary insomnia is not known. Treatment of insomnia should, insofar as possible, be directed at identifiable causes, or those factors that perpetuate the disorders,

such as temperament and lifestyle, ineffective coping and defense mechanisms, inappropriate use of alcohol or other substances, maladaptive sleep–wake schedules and excessive worry about poor sleep. The harder these individuals try to sleep, the worse it is. They keep themselves awake by their apprehensions: "If I don't get to sleep right now, I'll make a bad impression tomorrow". Cognitive–behavioral therapy (CBT) therefore is very effective, as shown by Morin and colleagues (1993). An 8-week group intervention aimed at changing maladaptive sleep habits and altering dysfunctional beliefs and attitudes about sleeplessness was effective in reducing sleep latency, waking up after sleep onset, and early morning awakening, and in increasing sleep efficiency. In a second study, Morin and colleagues (1999) found that CBT and pharmacological approaches were both effective for the short-term management of insomnia but that improvement was better sustained over time with the behavioral treatment.

Diagnosis

Diagnosis and treatment of chronic insomnia are often challenging and difficult. Both the psychiatrist and the patient must be forbearing and realistic as they jointly explore the evolution, causes, manifestations and ramifications of the sleep complaint. In part, the diagnosis of primary insomnia is reached by exclusion after a careful differential diagnosis of other causes. Simple answers and simple solutions are rare. Even if insomnia is initially precipitated by a single event or condition, chronic insomnia is usually maintained by various predisposing and perpetuating factors. For example, a business woman in her early thirties had insomnia during a period of intense stress in her business, but it continued long after the stress had been satisfactorily resolved. Factors that contributed to chronicity included her lifelong somewhat obsessive, anxious personality structure and after the onset of her insomnia, her gradually escalating concerns about her insomnia; these resulted in advanced sleep phase as she tried to spend more time in bed for "rest" and use of wine and sleeping pills at bedtime to sleep. If all these factors can be properly sorted out and dealt with, both the psychiatrist and the patient will be gratified.

Treatment of Chronic Primary Insomnia

Clinical management is often multidimensional, involving psychosocial, behavioral and pharmacological approaches. The relationship with the psychiatrist can often be important since many insomniac patients are skeptical that they can be helped overtly. They are focused on the symptom rather than the underlying causes, and are not psychologically minded. Behavioral treatments, in combination with addressing sleep hygiene, may be helpful in treating psychophysiological and other insomnias. Relaxation training (progressive relaxation, autogenic training, meditation, deep breathing) can all be effective if overtaught to become automatic. Two other behavioral therapies have been shown to be effective for insomnia: stimulus control and sleep restriction therapy (Bootzin and Nicassio, 1978; Spielman *et al.*, 1987; Morin *et al.*, 1994).

The aim of stimulus control therapy is to break the negative associations of being in bed unable to sleep (Table 59.5). It is especially helpful for patients with sleep-onset insomnia and prolonged awakenings. Sleep restriction therapy (Table 59.6) is based on the observation that more time spent in bed leads to more fragmented sleep. Both therapies may take 3 to 4 weeks or longer to be effective.

A wide variety of sedating medications have commonly been used as sleeping pills including benzodiazepines,

Table 59.5	Sleep Hygiene and Stimulus Control Rules

Curtail time spent awake while in bed.
Go to bed only when sleepy.
Do not remain in bed for more than 20–30 min while awake.
Get up at the same time each day.
Avoid looking at the bedroom clock.
Avoid caffeine, alcohol and tobacco near bedtime.
Exercise during the morning or afternoon.
Eat a light snack before bed.
Adjust sleeping environment for optimal temperature, sound and darkness.
Do not worry right before and in bed. Use the bed for sleeping.
Do not nap during the day.

Table 59.6	Sleep Restriction Therapy

Stay in bed for the amount of time you think you sleep each night, plus 15 min.
Get up at the same time each day.
Do not nap during the day.
When sleep efficiency is 85% (i.e., sleeping for 85% of the time in bed), go to bed 15 min earlier.
Repeat this process until you are sleeping for 8 h or the desired amount of time.
Example: if you report sleeping only 5 h a night and you normally get up at 6 AM, you are allowed to be in bed from 12:45 AM until 6 AM.

imidazopyridines (zolpidem), pyrazolopyrimidines (zaleplon), chloral hydrate, antihistamines (diphenhydramine, hydroxyzine, doxylamine), certain antidepressants (amitriptyline, doxepin, trimipramine, and trazodone), barbiturates and over-the-counter medications. However, they do vary in their pharmacokinetic properties and side effects (Table 59.7). The ideal sleeping pill would shorten latency to sleep; maintain normal physiological sleep all night without blocking normal behavioral responses to the crying baby or the alarm clock; leave neither hangover nor withdrawal effects the next day; and be devoid of tolerance and side effects such as impairment of breathing, cognition, ambulation and coordination. Furthermore, sleeping pills should not be habit-forming or addictive. Unfortunately, the ideal sleeping pill has not yet been found. Sleeping pills, if given in appropriate doses, are effective compared with placebo at least from a few days to a few weeks. More recent, developed sleeping pills (such as zaleplon) have demonstrated their superiority after 1 year in double-blind studies with a parallel placebo group. The question, however, is what is the lowest adequate dose for an individual patient, that is, the dose that will promote sleep with the least number of side effects.

The duration of action of these medications is important for several reasons (Table 59.8). Drugs with long half-life metabolites may have next-day hangover effects and tend to accumulate with repeated nightly administration, especially in the elderly, who metabolize and excrete the drugs more slowly than do the young. In addition, long half-life metabolites may act addictively or synergistically the next day with alcohol, with drugs with sedative side effects, or during periods of decreased alertness, such as the afternoon dip in arousal levels. Because the elderly are more sensitive to both the benefits and the side effects at a given dose than are younger patients, a dose for the elderly

Table 59.7	Clinical Characteristics of Sedative–Hypnotics			
Name	Dose (mg)	Absorption	Active Metabolite	Half-life
Chlordiazepoxide (Librium)	5–10	Intermediate	Yes	2–4 d
Diazepam (Valium)	2–10	Fast	Yes	2–4 d
Estazolam (ProSom)*	0.5–2.0	Intermediate	Yes	17 h
Flurazepam (Dalmane)*	7.5–30	Intermediate to fast	Yes	2–4 d
Clorazepate (Tranxene)	7.5–15	Fast	Yes	2–4 d
Clonazepam (Klonopin)	0.5–1.0	Intermediate	Yes	2–3 d
Quazepam (Doral)*	7.5–15	Intermediate	Yes	2–4 d
Oxazepam (Serax)	10–15	Slow	No	8–12 h
Lorazepam (Ativan)	0.5–4.0	Intermediate	No	10–20 h
Temazepam (Restoril)*	7.5–15	Slow	No	10–20 h
Alprazolam (Xanax)	0.25–2	Intermediate	No	14 h
Eszopiclone (Lunesta)*	1-3	Fast	Yes	4–6.5 h
Triazolam (Halcion)*	0.125–0.5	Intermediate	No	2–5 h
Zolpidem (Ambien)*	5–10	Fast	No	2–5 h
Zaleplon (Sonata)*	5–10	Fast	No	1 h

*Marketed as a sleeping pill in the USA.
NB: At publication time the US Food and Drug Administration has approved ramelteon (Rozerem), the first medication to bind melatonin receptors MT_1 and MT_2.

Table 59.8   Comparison of Long and Short Half-life Hypnotics

Measure	Half-life	
	Short	**Long**
Sedative hangover effects	+	++++
Accumulation with consecutive nightly use	0	+++
Tolerance	+++	+
Withdrawal insomnia	+++	+
Anxiolytic effects next day	0	+++
Amnesia	+++	++
Full benefits the first night	+++	++

Note: Although zaleplon is short acting, research suggests that it does not have some of the problems of other short-acting hypnotics, such as tolerance or withdrawal insomnia.

and debilitated patient should normally be about half of that for young and middle-aged patients.

Short half-life hypnotics usually produce less daytime sedation than long half-life drugs, but they often result in more rebound insomnia when they are discontinued. Whereas nearly all hypnotics and sedatives can produce amnesia, the problem may be more common with some short half-life drugs, especially for material that is learned during the periods of peak concentrations of drugs, for example, if the subject is awakened during the middle of the night. Administration of zaleplon 4 hours or more before arising in the morning does not appear to be associated with impairment in motor performance.

Patients should be educated about the anticipated benefits and limitations of sleeping pills, side effects and appropriate use, and should be followed up by office visits or phone calls regularly if prescriptions are renewed. Although hypnotics are usually prescribed for relatively short periods of time (2–6 weeks at most), about 0.5 to 1% of the population uses a hypnotic nearly every night for months or years. Whether this practice is good, useless, or bad remains controversial. Treatment of these patients should focus on the lowest possible effective dose – intermittently if possible – for the treatment of insomnia.

Hypnotics are relatively contraindicated in patients with sleep-disordered breathing; during pregnancy; in substance abusers, particularly alcohol abusers; and in those individuals who may need to be alert during their sleep period (e.g., physicians on call). In addition, caution should be used in prescribing hypnotics to patients who snore loudly; to patients who have renal, hepatic, or pulmonary disease; and to the elderly.

Melatonin

Melatonin is synthesized and released from the pineal gland under dark ambient conditions at a time that is determined by the individual's internal biological clock located within the SCN at the anterior portion of the hypothalamus. For individuals who are synchronized with the local light–dark environment, melatonin is usually secreted at night. The duration of secretion is approximately 8 to 12 hours, depending partially on age, season of the year and lighting conditions. Bright light prevents or terminates secretion of melatonin. For these reasons, melatonin has sometimes been called the "hormone" of the night or of sleep. In addition, nocturnal melatonin secretion appears to be blunted with normal aging, with administration of beta-adrenergic blockers (propranolol, pindolol, metoprolol), and in some populations of patient (including patients with mood disorders, premenstrual depression and panic disorder).

The functions of melatonin in humans are poorly understood, although in animals it has been implicated in seasonal behaviors, breeding, reproductive physiology and timing of adolescence.

The limited database available suggests that melatonin may eventually have a role in the prevention and treatment of circadian and sleep disturbances. Some evidence suggests that it has intrinsic hypnotic effects. Laboratory studies suggest that people are more likely to sleep during the period of endogenous melatonin secretion than during periods of the day without melatonin secretion. Furthermore, some but not all studies suggest that melatonin (0.3–10.0 mg) may induce and maintain sleep when administered to normal subjects or, in a few studies, to individuals with insomnia, jet lag, or other circadian rhythm disturbances. In addition, it is possible that melatonin administration can shift the phase position of the underlying biological clock. The entraining effects of a dose of 0.5 mg melatonin act like a "dark pulse", that is, the phase-response curve is nearly opposite that of light. Melatonin-induced phase-advanced rhythms when administered in the late afternoon or early evening, and it delayed the circadian clock when administered in the early morning. Future research is needed to fulfill the promise that melatonin can be used to prevent or treat some forms of insomnia or other sleep disorders, especially in the elderly, or in cases associated with circadian rhythm disorders (jet lag, shift work, the non-24-hour-day syndrome, phase displacement), neurological disorders, or psychiatric disorders.

The scientific clinical database for the use of melatonin in humans is limited at this time. Few well-designed clinical trials exist to establish clinical benefits or risks in specific disorders or conditions. Little is known about optimal doses, timing of melatonin administration, duration of treatment, drug interactions, or populations at risk, if any. The safety of melatonin, especially melatonin available in health food stores, is unknown. Melatonin is currently treated by the US Food and Drug Administration as a nutritional supplement rather than a medication. Therefore, purity of the product, safety, efficacy, and claims by manufacturers are not carefully regulated in the USA. Physicians are advised to maintain a watchful eye at this time and to be prudently cautious about recommendations to patients and the public about the uses and benefits of melatonin.

Because the timing of melatonin secretion is regulated by the SCN, investigators and clinicians can measure plasma levels of melatonin in dim light conditions to determine the phase position of the circadian clock. A useful revision of this technique is called the dim light melatonin onset (DLMO, pronounced "dil-mo") (Lewy and Sack, 1989). Using repeated measures of DLMO over periods of weeks, Lewy and Sack (1989) demonstrated that the circadian clock was "free-running" in a significant proportion of totally blind individuals, that is, the time of day at which melatonin secretion began completely drifted around the clock in a clockwise direction about every 3 weeks. Since the patients tried to maintain a conventional bedtime (approximately 11PM–7AM), their wake–sleep cycle was in and out of synchrony with their own internal clock, creating significant difficulties in sleep and alertness at times during the month. Furthermore, Lewy and Sack found that appropriately-timed administration of melatonin synchronized the internal clock with the external light–dark cycle.

As footnoted in Table 59.7, the US FDA has very recently approved the first noncontrolled medication to offer a unique mechanism of action that permits extended use for problems with sleep onset in adults. Through the selective binding of melatonin receptors in the SCN, the alerting signal is dampened thereby facilitating sleep onset. The recommended dosage for ramelteon is 8 mg. It is rapidly absorbed from the stomach and and broken down by first-pass metabolism in the liver through the CYP1A2 enzyme. Ramelteon should not be taken with high fat foods which apparently decrease absorption.

Primary Hypersomnia

A specific diagnostic category for primary hypersomnia exists in DSM-IV-TR, defining a disorder characterized by clinically significant excessive sleepiness of at least 1 month's duration, with significant distress or impairment. The hypersomnia is not caused by another primary sleep disorder, a psychiatric disorder, a medical disorder, or a substance. Patients with primary hypersomnia usually present with complaints of long and nonrestorative nocturnal sleep, difficulty awakening ("sleep drunkenness"), and daytime sleepiness and intellectual dysfunction; do not experience the accessory symptoms of narcolepsy such as cataplexy, sleep paralysis and hypnagogic hallucinations; and often report frequent headaches and Raynaud's phenomena.

Differential Diagnosis

Previously called non-REM narcolepsy, this relatively rare disorder is represented by perhaps 5 to 10% of patients presenting to sleep disorders centers for evaluation of hypersomnia. The diagnosis must be made on the basis of polysomnographic confirmation of hypersomnia; subjective complaints of excessive sleepiness are not adequate. A family history of excessive sleepiness may be present.

Although usually seen as a persistent complaint, primary hypersomnia includes recurrent forms, well defined with periods of excessive sleepiness of at least 3 days' duration occurring several times a year for at least 2 years. Among the recurrent or intermittent hypersomnia disorders are Kleine–Levin syndrome, usually seen in adolescent boys, and menstrual cycle-associated hypersomnia syndrome. In addition to hypersomnia (up to 18 hours per day), patients with Kleine–Levin syndrome often demonstrate aggressive or inappropriate sexuality, compulsive overeating and other bizarre behaviors. The rare nature of this syndrome and its unusual behaviors may be mistaken for psychosis, malingering, or a personality disorder.

Another syndrome, idiopathic recurring stupor, has been described and may be confused with hypersomnia. Patients experience attacks of stupor or coma as infrequently as once or twice a year to as often as once a week. The duration of each episode varies from 2 hours to 4 days. Unlike patients with hypersomnia, these patients are in a stuporous coma-like state and cannot be easily aroused or awakened. Furthermore, unlike the EEG of hypersomnia with its sleep spindles and K complexes, the EEG during stupor is characterized by diffuse activity at 13 to 18 Hz. Because the episode can be promptly but temporarily

reversed by administration of flumazenil, a benzodiazepine receptor antagonist, a search was made for an endogenous ligand for the benzodiazepine receptor in plasma and cerebrospinal fluid. The investigators discovered significantly increased levels of "endozepine 4" in blood and cerebrospinal fluid during periods of coma or stupor, suggesting that this syndrome is caused by this endogenous benzodiazepine-like compound. The syndrome occurs predominantly in men; mean age at onset is age 47 years (range, age 22–67 years). The cause is unknown.

Aside from associated medical and psychiatric disorders, the frequency and importance of hypersomnia and daytime sleepiness in otherwise healthy individuals have been increasingly recognized. Sleepiness, for example, as a result of sleep deprivation, disrupted sleep, or circadian dyssynchronization, probably plays a major role in mistakes and accidents in sleepy drivers, interns and medical staff, and industrial workers. Psychiatrists have an obligation to recognize and advise their patients about the dangers inherent in acute or chronic sleepiness.

Treatment

Clinical management is controversial owing to the lack of controlled studies. As in narcolepsy, the stimulant compounds are the most widely used and most often successful of the treatment options available. However, some patients are intolerant of stimulants or report no significant therapeutic effects. For patients intolerant of, or insensitive to, stimulants, some success has been obtained with the use of stimulating antidepressants, both of the MAOI and the selective serotonin reuptake inhibitor (SSRI)

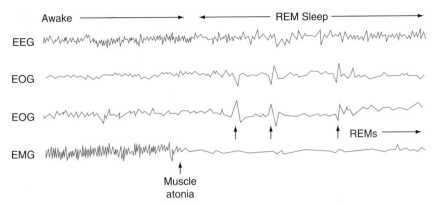

Figure 59.2 *REM-onset sleep in a patient with narcolepsy. EEG, electroencephalogram; EOG, electrooculogram; EMG, electromyogram; REMs, rapid eye movements.*

classes. Methysergide, a serotonin receptor antagonist, may be effective in some treatment-resistant cases but must be used with caution in view of the possibility of pleural and retroperitoneal fibrosis with persistent, uninterrupted use. Careful documentation should be maintained of interruption of drug use at regular intervals and of physical examinations that find the absence of obvious side effects of any sort.

Narcolepsy

Narcolepsy is associated with a pentad of symptoms: 1) excessive daytime sleepiness, characterized by irresistible "attacks" of sleep in inappropriate situations such as driving a car, talking to a supervisor, or social events; 2) cataplexy, which is sudden bilateral loss of muscle tone, usually lasting seconds to minutes, generally precipitated by strong emotions such as laughter, anger, or surprise; 3) poor or disturbed nocturnal sleep; 4) hypnagogic hallucinations, varied dreams at sleep onset; and 5) sleep paralysis, a brief period of paralysis associated with the transitions into, and out of, sleep.

The disorder is lifelong. The first symptom is usually excessive sleepiness, typically developing during the late teens and early twenties. The full syndrome of cataplexy and other symptoms unfolds in several years.

Narcolepsy is now understood as an inherited, physiological disturbance of REM sleep regulation. Narcoleptic patients often enter REM sleep right after sleep onset (the "sleep-onset REM periods"), reflecting an abnormally short or even nonexistent first non-REM sleep period (Figure 59.2). Several of the core symptoms of narcolepsy can be understood as abnormal physiological representations of normal REM sleep. For example, cataplexy can be understood as an abrupt presentation during wakefulness of the paralysis normally seen in REM sleep. Cataplexy is usually triggered by an emotional stimulus. Sleep-onset REM periods may be subjectively appreciated as hypnagogic hallucinations, which may be accompanied by sleep paralysis. Dissociated REM sleep inhibition of the voluntary musculature may lead to complaints of cataplexy and sleep paralysis.

In recent years, a potential biochemical abnormality has been identified in both canine and human narcolepsy. Narcoleptic dogs appear to have a nonfunctional receptor (OX2R) for orexin (hypocretin), a peptide neurotransmitter that has also been associated with feeding and energy metabolism. "Knockout" mice, which no longer make this peptide, appear to have a narcoleptic-like syndrome. Levels of orexin/hypocretin have been reported to be low in both autopsied brains and spinal fluid in human narcoleptics.

Diagnosis

Narcolepsy is not a rare disease; the prevalence rate of 0.03 to 0.16% approximates that of multiple sclerosis. Observers may mistake classic sleepiness in its mild form as withdrawal, poor motivation, negativism and hostility. The hypnagogic imagery and sleep paralysis symptoms, alone and in combination, may resemble bizarre psychiatric illness. Like many medical disorders, narcolepsy presents a wide range of severity, from mild to cases so severe that employment is functionally impossible. Partial remissions and exacerbations occur. Sleep paralysis and hypnagogic imagery may be seen without cataplexy; cataplexy may present in isolation without other REM-associated phenomena. The presence of REM sleep onset at night or during daytime naps, an important sleep laboratory parameter, remains the most valid and reliable method available for diagnosing narcolepsy. Because of the seriousness of the disorder and likelihood that amphetamine or other stimulants will be used to treat the patient at some time, it is important that the diagnosis of narcolepsy be objectively verified as soon as possible. Furthermore, stimulant abusers have been known to feign symptoms of narcolepsy to obtain prescriptions. Narcolepsy is associated with significant social and financial impairment for affected individuals and their families. For example, automobile accidents may result from either sleepiness or cataplexy. Most states prohibit narcoleptic patients from driving, at least as long as they are symptomatic.

Treatment

The major goals of treatment of narcolepsy include: 1) to improve quality of life, 2) to reduce excessive daytime sleepiness (EDS), and 3) to prevent cataplectic attacks.

The major wake-promoting medications are: modafinil, amphetamine, dextraamphetamine and methylphenidate. Modafinil is preferred on grounds of efficacy, safety, availability, and low risk of abuse and diversion. The pharmacological treatment of cataplexy, sleep paralysis and hypnogogic hallucinations includes administration of activating SSRIs such as fluoxetine and tricyclic antidepressants such as protriptyline. Another new drug, sodium oxybate xyrem, appears to be well tolerated and beneficial for the treatment of cataplexy, daytime sleepiness and inadvertent sleep attacks (Littner *et al.*, 2001; US Xyrem Multicenter Study Group, 2002).

Breathing-related Sleep Disorder

The essential feature of this disorder is sleep disruption resulting from sleep apnea or alveolar hypoventilation, leading to complaints of insomnia or, more commonly, excessive sleepiness. The disorder is not accounted for by other medical or psychiatric disorders or by medications or other substances.

Diagnosis

The major diagnostic criterion for sleep apnea is cessation of breathing lasting at least 10 seconds and an apnea index (number of apneic events per hour of sleep) of five or more. Most apneic episodes are terminated by transient arousals. Hypopneas (50% decrease in respiration) may also produce arousal or hypoxia even when complete apneas do not occur. Therefore, rather than just the apnea index, a respiratory disturbance index (number of respiratory events, or number of apneas plus hypopneas per hour of sleep) is used. Whereas the criterion for the respiratory disturbance index has not been fully established, many psychiatrists use a respiratory disturbance index of 10 or greater for purposes of diagnosis. Each time respiration ceases, the individual must awaken to start breathing again. Once the person goes back to sleep, breathing stops again. This pattern continues throughout the night. Clinically, however, it is not unusual to see patients who stop breathing for 60 to 120 seconds with each event and experience hundreds of events per night. Many individuals with BRSD cannot sleep and breathe at the same time and therefore spend most of the night not breathing and not sleeping. In contrast, the central alveolar hypoventilation syndrome is not associated with either apneas or hypopneas, but impaired ventilatory control or hypoventilation results in hypoxemia. It is most common in morbid obesity.

Sleep apnea is characterized by repetitive episodes of upper airway obstruction that occur during sleep, resulting in numerous interruptions of sleep continuity, hypoxemia, hypercapnia, bradytachycardia, and pulmonary and systemic hypertension. It may be associated with snoring, morning headaches, dry mouth on awakening, excessive movements during the night, falling out of bed, enuresis, cognitive decline and personality changes, and complaints of either insomnia or, more frequently, hypersomnia and excessive daytime sleepiness. The typical patient with clinical sleep apnea is a middle-aged man who is overweight or who has anatomical conditions narrowing his upper airway.

DSM-IV-TR Criteria 780.59

Breathing-related Sleep Disorder

A. Sleep disruption, leading to excessive sleepiness or insomnia, that is judged to be due to a sleep-related breathing condition (e.g., obstructive or central sleep apnea syndrome or central alveolar hypoventilation syndrome).

B. The disturbance is not better accounted for by another mental disorder and is not due to the direct physiological effects of a substance (e.g., a drug of abuse, a medication) or another general medical condition (other than a breathing-related disorder).

Coding note: Also code sleep-related breathing disorder on Axis III.

Reprinted with permission from the *Diagnostic and Statistical Manual of Mental Disorders*, Fourth Edition, Text Revision. Copyright 2000 American Psychiatric Association.

There are three types of apnea. The first is obstructive sleep apnea, which involves the collapse of the pharyngeal airway during inspiration, with partial or complete blockage of airflow. The person still attempts to breathe, and one can observe the diaphragm moving, but the airway is blocked and therefore there is no air exchange. It can be caused by bagginess or excessive pharyngeal mucosa and a large uvula, fatty infiltration at the base of the tongue, or collapse of the pharyngeal walls. The resulting decreased air passage compromises alveolar ventilation and causes blood-oxygen desaturation and strenuous attempts at inspiration through the narrowed airway, all of which lighten and disrupt sleep. Hypercapnia, which results either from obstructive sleep apnea or from lung disease, reduces breathing without the presence of disruptive inspiratory efforts.

The second type is central sleep apnea, which results from failure of the respiratory neurons to activate the phrenic and intercostal motor neurons that mediate respiratory movements. There is no attempt to breathe, and although the airway is not collapsed, there is no respiration. This type of apnea is more commonly associated with heart disease. The third type is mixed sleep apnea, which is a combination, generally beginning with a central component and ending with an obstructive component.

The lifetime prevalence of BRSD in adults has been estimated to be 9% in men and 4% in women. The prevalence does increase with age, particularly in postmenopausal women. The prevalence in the elderly has been estimated to be 28% in men and 19% in women.

During apneas and hypopneas, the blood-oxygen level often drops to precarious levels. In addition, one often sees cardiac arrhythmias and nocturnal hypertension in association with the respiratory disturbances. The cardiac arrhythmias include bradycardia during the events and tachycardia after the end of the events. It is not unusual to see premature ventricular contractions, trigeminy and bigeminy, asystole, second-degree atrioventricular block, atrial tachycardia, sinus bradycardia and ventricular tachycardia. However, the electrocardiogram taken during the waking state might be normal. It is only during the respiratory events during sleep that the abnormalities appear.

BRSD, especially central sleep apnea, is commonly seen in patients with congestive heart failure. Cor pulmonale may also be a consequence of longstanding BRSD and is seen in both sleep apnea syndrome and primary hypoventilation. Patients may present with unexplained respiratory failure, polycythemia, right ventricular failure and nocturnal hypertension. About 50% of patients with BRSD have hypertension, and about one-third of all hypertensive patients have BRSD. In the large cross-sectional study, it was found that both systolic and diastolic blood pressure (SDB) as well as the prevalence of hypertension increased significantly with increasing SDB (Nieto *et al.*, 2000). It has also been shown that there is a dose–response association between SDB at baseline and hypertension 4 years later suggesting that SDB may be a risk factor for hypertension and consequent cardiovascular morbidity.

The most common symptoms of BRSD include excessive daytime sleepiness and snoring. The excessive daytime sleepiness probably results from sleep fragmentation caused by the frequent nocturnal arousals occurring at the end of the apneas and possibly from hypoxemia. The excessive daytime sleepiness is associated with lethargy, poor concentration, decreased motivation and performance, and inappropriate and inadvertent attacks of sleep. Sometimes the patients do not realize they have fallen asleep until they awaken.

The second complaint is loud snoring, sometimes noisy enough to be heard throughout or even outside the house. Often the wife has complained for years about the snoring and has threatened to sleep elsewhere if she has not moved out already. Bed partners describe a characteristic pattern of loud snoring interrupted by periods of silence, which are then terminated by snorting sounds. Snoring results from a partial narrowing of the airway caused by multiple factors, such as inadequate muscle tone, large tonsils and adenoids, long soft palate, flaccid tissue, acromegaly, hypothyroidism, or congenital narrowing of the oral pharynx. Snoring has been implicated not only in sleep apnea but also in angina pectoris, stroke, ischemic heart disease and cerebral infarction, even in the absence of complete sleep apneas. Because the prevalence of snoring increases with age, especially in women, and because snoring can have serious medical consequences, the psychiatrist must give serious attention to complaints of loud snoring. Snoring is not always a symptom of BRSD. Approximately 25% of men and 15% of women are habitual snorers.

Patients with BRSD are frequently overweight. In some patients, a weight gain of 20 to 30 lb might bring on episodes of BRSD. The same fatty tissue seen on the outside is also present on the inside, making the airway even more narrow. Because obstructive sleep apnea is always caused by the collapse of the airway, in patients of normal weight, anatomical abnormalities (such as large tonsils, long uvula) must be considered.

Other symptoms of BRSD include unexplained morning headaches, nocturnal confusion, automatic behavior, dysfunction of the autonomic nervous system, or night sweats. The severity of BRSD will depend on the severity of the cardiac arrhythmias, hypertension, excessive daytime sleepiness, respiratory disturbance index, amount of sleep fragmentation and amount of oxygen desaturation.

Mild to moderate sleep-related breathing disturbances increase with age, even in elderly subjects without major complaints about their sleep. The frequency is higher in men than in women, at least until the age of menopause, after which the rate in women increases and may approach that of men. With use of the apnea index of five or more apneic episodes per hour as a cutoff criterion, prevalence rates range from 27 to 75% for older men and from 0 to 32% for older women. In general, the severity of apnea in these older persons is mild (an average apnea index of about 13) compared with that seen in patients with clinical sleep apnea. However, older men and women with mild apnea have been reported to fall asleep at inappropriate times significantly more often than older persons without apnea. Furthermore, the frequency of sleep apnea and other BRSDs is higher in individuals with hypertension, congestive heart failure, obesity, dementia and other medical conditions.

Increased mortality rates have been noted in excessively long sleepers, therefore sleep apnea may account for some of these excess deaths. This is also consistent with evidence that excess deaths from all causes increase between 2 and 8 AM, specifically deaths related to ischemic heart disease in patients older than 65 years. There have been several studies suggesting that untreated sleep apnea in the elderly may lead to shorter survival.

The clinical significance of relatively mild "subclinical" sleep apneas is not fully understood yet. Psychiatrists should be aware, however, that such disturbances might be associated with either insomnia or excessive daytime sleepiness. Furthermore, for some patients with sleep apnea, administration of hypnotics, alcohol, or other sedating medications is relatively contraindicated. The risk is not yet known, but reports indicate that benzodiazepines as well as alcohol may increase the severity of mild sleep apnea. Therefore, psychiatrists should inquire about snoring, gasping, and other signs and symptoms of sleep apnea before administering a sleeping pill. If patients have excessive sleepiness or morning hangover effects while taking benzodiazepines, major tranquilizers, or other sedating medications, the psychiatrist should consider the possibility of an iatrogenic BRSD due to medications.

The diagnosis of BRSD must be differentiated from other disorders of excessive sleepiness such as narcolepsy (Table 59.9). Patients with BRSD will not have cataplexy, sleep-onset paralysis, or sleep-onset hallucination. Narcolepsy is not usually associated with loud snoring or sleep apneas. In laboratory recordings, patients with BRSD do not usually have sleep-onset REM periods either at night or in multiple naps on the Multiple Sleep Latency Test. However, one must be aware that both BRSD and narcolepsy can be found in the same patient. BRSD must also be distinguished from other hypersomnias, such as those related to major depressive disorder or circadian rhythm disturbances.

Table 59.9	Clinical Symptoms of Breathing-related Sleep Disorders	
Daytime Symptoms	**Night-time Symptoms**
Excessive daytime sleepiness	Loud snoring
Memory loss	Hypertension
Decreased mental function	Cardiac arrhythmias
Morning headache	Leg kicks
Automatic behavior	Confusion
Lethargy	Impotence
	Choking–gasping

Treatment of Sleep Apnea

Sleep apnea is sometimes alleviated by weight loss, avoidance of sedatives, use of tongue-retaining devices and breathing air under positive pressure through a face mask (continuous positive airway pressure [CPAP]). Oxygen breathed at night may alleviate insomnia associated with apnea that is not accompanied by impeded inspiration. Surgery may be helpful, for example, to correct enlarged tonsils, a long uvula, a short mandible, or morbid obesity. Pharyngoplasty, which tightens the pharyngeal mucosa and may also reduce the size of the uvula, or the use of a cervical collar to extend the neck, may relieve heavy snoring. Although tricyclic antidepressants are sometimes used in the treatment of clinical sleep apnea in young adults, they may cause considerable toxic effects in older people. The newer shorter-acting nonbenzodiazepine hypnotics seem to be safer in these patients and may be considered in those patients who snore.

Circadian Rhythm Sleep Disorder (Sleep–Wake Schedule Disorders)

Circadian rhythm disturbances result from a mismatch between the internal or endogenous circadian sleep–wake system and the external or exogenous demands on the sleep–wake system. The individual's tendency to sleep–wakefulness does not match that of her or his social circumstances or of the light–dark cycle. Although some individuals do not find this mismatch to be a problem, for others the circadian rhythm disturbance interferes with the ability to function properly at times when alertness or sleepiness is desired or required. For those individuals, insomnia, hypersomnia, sleepiness and fatigue result in significant discomfort and impairment. The circadian rhythm disturbances include delayed sleep phase, advanced sleep phase, shift work, jet lag and non-24-hour-day syndrome.

Diagnosis

The diagnosis is based on a careful review of the history and circadian patterns of sleep–wakefulness, napping, alertness and behavior. According to DSM-IV criteria, the diagnosis of circadian rhythm sleep disorder requires significant social or occupational impairment or marked distress related to the sleep disturbance. It is often useful for patients with chronic complaints to keep a sleep–wake diary covering the entire 24-hour day each day for several weeks. If possible, an ambulatory device that measures rest–activity, such as a wrist actigraph, might supplement the sleep–wake diary. Wrist actigraphs record acceleration of the wrist at frequent intervals, such as every minute, and save it for later display. Because the wrist is mostly at rest during sleep, the record of wrist rest–activity provides a fairly accurate estimate of the timing and duration of sleep–wakefulness. In addition, some commercial wrist activity devices have a built-in photometer, which provides a record of ambient light–darkness against which the rest–activity pattern can be compared.

Delayed and Advanced Sleep Phase Disorders

Delayed sleep phase refers to a delay in the circadian rhythm in the sleep–wake cycle. These individuals are generally not sleepy until several hours after "normal" bedtime (i.e., 2–3 AM). If allowed to sleep undisturbed, they will sleep for 7 or 8 hours, which means they awaken at 10 to 11 AM. People with delayed sleep phase are considered extreme "owls". They may or may

---

Circadian Rhythm Sleep Disorder

A. persistent or recurrent A. pattern of sleep disruption leading to excessive sleepiness or insomnia that is due to a mismatch between the sleep–wake schedule required by a person's environment and his or her circadian sleep–wake pattern.

B. The sleep disturbance causes clinically significant distress or impairment in social, occupational, or other important areas of functioning.

C. The disturbance does not occur exclusively during the course of another sleep disorder or other mental disorder.

D. The disturbance is not due to the direct physiological effects of a substance (e.g., a drug of abuse, a medication) or a general medical condition.

Specify type:

Delayed sleep phase type: a persistent pattern of late sleep onset and late awakening times, with an inability to fall asleep and awaken at a desired earlier time

Jet lag type: sleepiness and alertness that occur at an inappropriate time of day relative to local time, occurring after repeated travel across more than one time zone

Shift work type: insomnia during the major sleep period or excessive sleepiness during the major awake period associated with night shift work or frequently changing shift work

Unspecified type

---

not complain of sleep-onset insomnia. They usually enjoy their alertness in the evening and night and have little desire to sleep beginning at 10 PM or midnight. Their problem is trying to wake up at normal times (i.e., 6–7 AM). In essence, their rhythm is shifted to a later clock time relative to conventional rest–activity patterns.

Individuals with delayed sleep phase often choose careers that allow them to set their own schedules, such as freelance writers. Delayed sleep phase occurs commonly in late adolescence and young adulthood, such as in college students. As many of these individuals age, however, their endogenous sleep–wake rhythm advances and they eventually are able to conform themselves to a normal rest period at night.

For others, however, this phase shift of the endogenous oscillator may lead at a later age to the advanced sleep phase. In this condition, individuals become sleepy earlier in the evening (e.g., 7–8 PM). They will also sleep for 7 to 8 hours, but that means they awaken at 2 to 3 AM. These individuals are" "larks", being most alert in the morning. They complain of sleep maintenance insomnia, that is, they cannot stay asleep all night long. This condition is more prevalent in the elderly than in the young.The etiology of extreme "night owls" and "larks" is probably multifaceted but, in some cases, appears to reflect genetic factors.

Treatment

Clinical management includes chronobiological strategies to shift the phase position of the endogenous circadian oscillator in the appropriate direction. For example, exposure to bright light in the morning advances the delayed sleep phase, that is, individuals will become sleepy earlier in the evening. On the other hand, administration of bright light in the evening acts to delay the circadian rhythm, that is, individuals will become sleepy later in the evening. Light is usually administered in doses of 2500 lux for a period of 2 hours per day, although the ideal intensity and duration are yet to be determined. For some individuals, spending more time outdoors in bright sunlight may be sufficient to treat the sleep phase. For example, individuals with delayed sleep phase should be encouraged to remove blinds and curtains from their windows, which would allow the sunlight to pour into their bedrooms in the morning when they should arise. In addition, gradual adjustments of the timing of the sleep–wake cycle may be used to readjust the phase position of the circadian oscillator. For example, patients with delayed phase disorder can be advised to delay the onset of sleep by 2 to 3 hours each day (i.e., from 4 to 7 to 10 AM, and so on) until the appropriate bedtime. After that, they should maintain regular sleep–wake patterns, with exposure to bright light in the morning.

Shift Work

Shift work problems occur when the circadian sleep–wake rhythm is in conflict with the rest–activity cycle imposed by the externally determined work schedule. Nearly a quarter of all American employees have jobs that require them to work outside the conventional 8 AM to 5 PM schedule. Different patterns include rotating schedules and more or less permanent evening and night schedules. Rotating schedules, particularly rapidly shifting schedules, are difficult because constant readjustment of the endogenous circadian oscillator to the imposed sleep–wake cycle is necessary. In both rotating and shift work schedules, further difficulties are encountered because the worker is usually expected to readjust to a normal sleep–wake cycle on weekends and holidays. Even if the worker can adjust his or her circadian system to the work schedule, he or she is then out of synchrony with the rhythm of family and friends during off-duty hours. These individuals, therefore, are constantly sleep deprived and constantly sleepy. They endure impaired performance and increased risk of accidents, somatic complaints and poor morale; hypnotics, stimulants and alcohol are used excessively in relationship to unusual or shifting work schedules. Shift work schedules may have played a role in human errors that contributed to the Three Mile Island and Chernobyl accidents and the Challenger disaster.

Treatment

No totally satisfactory methods currently exist for managing shift work problems. Because people vary in their ability to adjust to these schedules, self-selection or survival of the fittest may be involved for those who can find other employment or work schedules. Older individuals appear to be less flexible than younger persons in adjusting to shift work. Some experiments suggest that the principles of chronobiology may be useful in reducing the human costs of shift work. For example, because the endogenous pacemaker has a cycle length (tau) longer than 24 hours, rotating shift workers do better when their schedules move in a clockwise direction (i.e., morning to evening to night) rather than in the other direction. Appropriate exposure to bright lights and

darkness may push the circadian pacemaker in the correct direction and help stabilize its phase position, especially in association with the use of dark glasses outside and blackout curtains at home to maintain darkness at the appropriate times for promotion of sleep and shifting of the circadian pacemaker. Naps may also be useful in reducing sleep loss. Modest amounts of coffee may maintain alertness early in the shift but should be avoided near the end of the shift.

Jet Lag

Jet lag occurs when individuals travel across several time zones. Traveling east advances the sleep–wake cycle and is typically more difficult than traveling west (which delays the cycle). Jet lag may be associated with difficulty initiating or maintaining sleep or with daytime sleepiness, impaired performance and gastrointestinal disturbance after rapid transmeridian flights. Individuals older than 50 years appear to be more vulnerable to jet lag than are younger persons.

Management

Considerable research and theorizing are under way better to prevent and manage the problems associated with jet lag. Some efforts before departure may be useful to prevent or ameliorate these problems. For persons who plan to readjust their circadian clock to the new location, it may be possible to move the sleep–wake and light–dark schedules appropriately before departure. In addition, good sleep hygiene principles should be respected before, during and after the trip. For example, many people are sleep deprived or in alcohol withdrawal when they step on the plane because of last-minute preparations or farewell parties. Whereas adequate fluid intake on the plane is necessary to avoid dehydration, alcohol consumption should be avoided or minimized because it causes diuresis and may disrupt sleep maintenance.

On arriving at the destination, it may be preferable to try to maintain a schedule coinciding with actual home time if the trip is going to be short. For example, the individual should try to sleep at times that correspond to the usual bedtime or with the normal midafternoon dip in alertness. If, on the other hand, the trip will be longer and it is desirable to synchronize the biological clock with local time, exposure to appropriate schedules of bright light and darkness may be helpful, at least theoretically. Unfortunately, the exact protocols have not been established in all instances yet and require further research and experimentation. In addition, some of these protocols require avoidance of bright light at certain times, necessitating wearing dark goggles, for example, when traveling.

In addition to synchronizing the clock with the new environment, sleep and rest should be promoted by good sleep hygiene principles, by avoidance of excessive caffeine and alcohol and, possibly, by administration of short-duration hypnotics. Care should be taken, however, to avoid hangover effects or amnesia associated with hypnotics. Because individual responses to sleeping pills vary considerably from person to person, it is often helpful to develop experience with specific compounds and doses before departure.

Non-24-Hour-Day Syndrome

The non-24-hour-day (or "hypernyctohemeral") syndrome is characterized by free-running in the natural environment, that is, the subject goes to bed and arises about 45 minutes later each day. The average duration of the sleep–wake cycle is about 24.5 to 25.0 hours. During the course of about 3 weeks, the subject's sleep–wake cycle "goes around the clock" as the timing of the sleep period gradually delays. The lengthened sleep–wake cycle of these patients in the natural environment is similar to that of normal subjects living in a time-free environment. The disorder appears to be relatively common in patients with total blindness, because they no longer perceive visual Zeitgebers. In many cases, the cause is unknown, but it is sometimes observed in individuals who are socially or linguistically isolated. Management may include bright light therapy in the morning to entrain the endogenous oscillator. Administration of vitamin B$_{12}$ may be helpful, perhaps by enhancing the effectiveness of Zeitgebers.

The prevalence of circadian rhythm disturbances has not been established. Approximately two-thirds of shift workers have difficulty with their schedules. Circadian rhythm disturbances must be differentiated from sleep-onset insomnia due to other causes (such as pain, caffeine consumption), early morning insomnia due to depression or alcohol use, and changes in sleep patterns due to lifestyle or lifestyle changes.

Periodic Limb Movements in Sleep

Periodic limb movements in sleep (PLMS), previously called nocturnal myoclonus, is a disorder in which repetitive, brief and stereotyped limb movements occur during sleep, usually about every 20 to 40 seconds. Dorsiflexions of the big toe, ankle, knee and sometimes the hip are involved (Table 59.10)

Diagnosis

Questioning of the patient or bed partner often yields reports of restlessness, kicking, unusually cold or hot feet, disrupted and torn bedclothes, unrefreshing sleep, insomnia, or excessive daytime sleepiness. Patients may be unaware of these pathological leg movements or arousals, although their bed partners may be all too aware of the kicking, frequent movements and restlessness. If these disorders are strongly suspected, the patient should probably be referred to a sleep disorders laboratory for evaluation and an overnight polysomnogram with tibial electromyograms. These disorders are often associated with transient arousals in the EEG recording. Diagnosis is made when the periodic limb movement index (number of leg jerks per hour of sleep) is five or greater, accompanied by arousals. The jerks occur primarily in the legs but may also appear in less severe forms in the arms. The movements can be bilateral or unilateral and occur in stage 1 and stage 2 sleep. Patients often have reduced deep sleep because the jerks continually awaken them.

A related disturbance, restless legs syndrome, is associated with disagreeable sensations in the lower legs, feet, or thighs that occur in a recumbent or resting position and cause an almost irresistible urge to move the legs. Whereas almost all patients with restless legs syndrome have PLMS, not all patients with PLMS have restless legs syndrome. Restless legs syndrome may be frequent in patients with uremia and rheumatoid arthritis or in pregnant women. Both PLMS and restless legs syndrome usually occur in middle-aged people, but many patients report having had the same sensations as adolescents and even as children. It has been suggested that both conditions are familial, perhaps due to an autosomal dominant gene.

Individuals with PLMS are reported to sleep about an hour less per night than control subjects without PLMS. Interestingly, the prevalence of PLMS is not higher in insomniac patients than in those without insomnia. Complaints of excessive daytime sleepiness increase in individuals with PLMS, probably consequent to the numerous sleep interruptions. The psychiatrist may find it useful to talk with a bed partner, who will often describe kicking and leg twitches during sleep in individuals with PLMS. The myoclonic movements are not related to seizure disorder but should be distinguished from seizures. Because complaints of insomnia and daytime sleepiness are not uncommon, other insomnias, sleep apnea and narcolepsy should be ruled out.

Prevalence of PLMS in young and middle-aged adults has not been fully established. In sleep disorders clinic populations, about 11% of those complaining of insomnia are diagnosed with PLMS. In the elderly, however, this condition is extremely common; more than 45% have at least five leg kicks per hour of sleep.

Treatment

Because the pathogenesis of PLMS is usually unknown, treatment is often symptomatic (Table 59.11). Some studies suggest that the movements arise subcortically from the brain or spinal cord; others suggest subclinical peripheral neuropathy. At the present time, dopaminergic agents such as levodopa (L-dopa), pergolide, or pramipexole generally provide the most effective treatment for both PLMS and restless legs. Opiates, such as oxycodone and propoxyphene, have also been demonstrated to be effective in the treatment of PLMS and restless legs syndrome. Anticonvulsants, such as carbamazepine and gabapentin, have been shown to be effective in treatment of restless legs syndrome. Clonazepam, a benzodiazepine anticonvulsant, is effective in the treatment of PLMS and possibly for restless legs syndrome. Other benzodiazepines have also been used to treat these conditions, as they will decrease some of the awakenings but may have no effect on the number of leg movements.

Parasomnias

The parasomnias are a group of disorders characterized by disturbances of either physiological processes or behavior associated with sleep, but not necessarily causing disturbances of sleep or wakefulness.

Nightmare Disorder

The essential feature of this disorder is the repeated occurrence of frightening dreams that lead to full awakenings from sleep. The dreams or awakenings cause the individual significant distress or dysfunction. By DSM-IV-TR definition, the disorder is excluded if the nightmare occurs in the course of another mental or medical disorder or as a direct result of a medication or

Table 59.10	Features of Periodic Limb Movements in Sleep

Leg kicks every 20–40 s
Duration of 0.5–5 s
  Complaints of:
  Insomnia
  Excessive sleepiness
  Restless legs
  Very cold or hot feet
  Uncomfortable sensations in legs

Table 59.11   Pharmacologic Treatment Options in RLS/PLMS

Medication	Dosage Range	Side Effects	Advantages	Disadvantages
L-dopa/carbidopa	25/100–100/400/D	Dyskinesia Loss of efficacy Nausea Hallucinations	Low cost	Breakthrough restlessness
Pergolide	0.05–1 mg	Dyskinesia Nausea Rhinitis Dizziness	High rate of response	Frequent side effects
Pramipexole	0.25–0.875 mg	Orthostasis Dizziness Sedation	High rate of response Good tolerance	Expense
Anticonvulsants	Variable	Sedation	Low cost Sleep promotion	Variable response
Opiates	Variable	Nausea Constipation	Low cost	Variable response Abuse potential
Clonazepam	0.5–2 mg	Sedation Dizziness	Sleep promotion	Variable response Abuse potential

substance. Many, but not all, nightmares occur during REM sleep; REM nightmares take place most often during the last half of the night when REM sleep is most common (see nightmares in post traumatic stress disorder). Whereas more than half of the adult population probably experiences an occasional nightmare, nightmares start more commonly in children between the ages of 3 and 6 years. The exact prevalence is unknown.

DSM-IV-TR Criteria 307.47

Nightmare Disorder

A. Repeated awakenings from the major sleep period or naps with detailed recall of extended and extremely frightening dreams, usually involving threats to survival, security, or self-esteem. The awakenings generally occur during the second half of the sleep period.

B. On awakening from the frightening dreams, the person rapidly becomes oriented and alert (in contrast to the confusion and disorientation seen in sleep terror disorder and some forms of epilepsy).

C. The dream experience, or the sleep disturbance resulting from the awakening, causes clinically significant distress or impairment in social, occupational, or other important areas of functioning.

D. The nightmares do not occur exclusively during the course of another mental disorder (e.g., a delirium, post traumatic stress disorder) and are not due to the direct physiological effects of a substance (e.g., a drug of abuse, a medication) or a general medical condition.

Reprinted with permission from the *Diagnostic and Statistical Manual of Mental Disorders*, Fourth Edition, Text Revision. Copyright 2000 American Psychiatric Association.

Treatment

The disorder is usually self-limited in children but can be helped sometimes with psychotherapy, desensitization, or rehearsal instructions. Secondary nightmares, as in post traumatic stress disorder (PTSD), can be difficult to treat.

Sleep Terror Disorder

This disorder is defined as repeated abrupt awakenings from sleep characterized by intense fear, panicky screams, autonomic arousal (tachycardia, rapid breathing and sweating), absence of detailed dream recall, amnesia for the episode, and relative unresponsiveness to attempts to comfort the person. Because sleep terrors occur primarily during delta sleep, they usually take place during the first third of the night. These episodes may cause distress or impairment, especially for caretakers who witness the event. Sleep terrors may also be called night terrors, *pavor nocturnus*, or incubus.

The prevalence of the disorder is estimated to be about 1 to 6% in children and less than 1% in adults. In children, it usually begins between the ages of 4 and 12 years and resolves spontaneously during adolescence. It is more common in boys than in girls. It does not appear to be associated with psychiatric illness in children. In adults, it usually begins between 20 and 30 years of age, has a chronic undulating course, is equally common in men and women, and may be associated with psychiatric disorders, such as PTSD, generalized anxiety disorder, borderline personality disorder and others. An increased frequency of enuresis and somnambulism has been reported in the first-degree relatives of patients with night terrors.

Treatment

Nocturnal administration of benzodiazepines has been reported to be beneficial, perhaps because these drugs suppress delta sleep, the stage of sleep during which sleep terrors typically occur.

DSM-IV-TR Criteria 307.46°

Sleep Terror Disorder

A. Recurrent episodes of abrupt awakening from sleep, usually occurring during the first third of the major sleep episode and beginning with a panicky scream.

B. Intense fear and signs of autonomic arousal, such as tachycardia, rapid breathing, and sweating, during each episode.

C. Relative unresponsiveness to efforts of others to comfort the person during the episode.

D. No detailed dream is recalled and there is amnesia for the episode.

E. The episodes cause clinically significant distress or impairment in social, occupational, or other important areas of functioning.

F. The disturbance is not due to the direct physiological effects of a substance (e.g., a drug of abuse, a medication) or a general medical condition.

Reprinted with permission from the *Diagnostic and Statistical Manual of Mental Disorders*, Fourth Edition, Text Revision. Copyright 2000 American Psychiatric Association.

DSM-IV-TR Criteria 307.46

Sleepwalking Disorder

A. Repeated episodes of rising from bed during sleep and walking about, usually occurring during the first third of the major sleep episode.

B. While sleepwalking, the person has a blank, staring face, is relatively unresponsive to the efforts of others to communicate with him or her, and can be awakened only with great difficulty.

C. On awakening (either from the sleepwalking episode or the next morning), the person has amnesia for the episode.

D. Within several minutes after awakening from the sleepwalking episode, there is no impairment of mental activity or behavior (although there may initially be a short period of confusion or disorientation).

E. The sleepwalking causes clinically significant distress or impairment in social, occupational, or other important areas of functioning.

F. The disturbance is not due to the direct physiological effects of a substance (e.g., a drug of abuse, a medication) or a general medical condition.

Reprinted with permission from the *Diagnostic and Statistical Manual of Mental Disorders*, Fourth Edition, Text Revision. Copyright 2000 American Psychiatric Association.

Sleepwalking Disorder

This disorder is characterized by repeated episodes of motor behavior initiated in sleep, usually during delta sleep in the first third of the night. While sleepwalking, the patient has a blank staring face, is relatively unresponsive to others, and may be confused or disoriented initially on being aroused from the episode. Although the person may be alert after several minutes of awakening, complete amnesia for the episode is common the next day. Sleepwalking may cause considerable distress, for example, if a child cannot sleep away from home or go to camp because of it. By DSM-IV definition, pure sleepwalking is excluded if it occurs as a result of a medication or substance or is due to a medical disorder. However, sleepwalking may be an idiosyncratic reaction to specific drugs, including tranquilizers and sleeping pills.

Most behaviors during sleepwalking are routine and of low-level intensity, such as sitting up, picking the sheets, or walking around the bedroom. More complicated behaviors may also occur, however, such as urinating in a closet, leaving the house, running, eating, talking, driving, or even committing murder. A real danger is that the individual will be injured by going through a window or falling from a height.

Whereas about 10 to 30% of children have at least one sleepwalking episode, only about 1 to 5% have repeated episodes. The disorder most commonly begins between the ages of 4 and 8 years and usually resolves spontaneously during adolescence. Genetic factors may be involved, because sleepwalkers are reported to have a higher than expected frequency of first-degree relatives with either sleepwalking or sleep terrors. Sleepwalking may be precipitated in affected patients by gently sitting them up during sleep, by fever, or by sleep deprivation. Adult onset of sleepwalking should prompt the search for possible medical, neurological, psychiatric, pharmacological, or other underlying causes, such as nocturnal epilepsy.

Treatment

No treatment for sleepwalking is established, but some patients respond to administration of benzodiazepines or sedating antidepressants at bedtime. The major concern should be the safety of the sleepwalker, who may injure herself or himself or someone else during an episode.

REM Sleep Behavior Disorder

This disorder, like sleepwalking, is associated with complicated behaviors during sleep such as walking, running, singing and talking. In contrast to sleepwalking, which occurs during the first third of the night during delta sleep, REM sleep behavior disorder usually occurs during the second half of the night during REM sleep. It apparently results from an intermittent loss of the muscle atonia that normally accompanies REM sleep, thus allowing the patient to act out her or his dream. Also, in contrast to sleepwalking, memory for the dream content is usually good. Furthermore, the idiopathic form typically occurs in men during the sixth or seventh decade of life. The cause or causes remain unknown. It has been reported in a variety of neurological disorders and during withdrawal from sedatives or alcohol; during treatment with tricyclic antidepressants or biperiden (Akineton); and in various neurological disorders including dementia, subarachnoid hemorrhage and degenerative neurological disorders.

Treatment

Nocturnal administration of clonazepam, 0.5 to 1 mg, is usually remarkably successful in controlling the symptoms of this disorder. Patients and their families should be educated about the nature of the disorder and warned to take precautions about injuring themselves or others.

Nocturnal Panic Attacks

The typical daytime panic attack, as bizarre and frightening as it may seem to the patient experiencing it, is often fairly obvious to the assessing psychiatrist. Symptoms of anxiety, sweating, tremor, dizziness, chest pain and palpitations occur "out of the blue" with or without specific behavioral or associational stimuli. Once it has been diagnosed, treatment options may include pharmacotherapy with one of several classes of drugs, behavioral therapy, or a combined approach.

When these symptoms occur at night, the task of the assessing psychiatrist is greatly complicated. The patient may assume that the cause is a nightmare or a night terror and may be resistant to the diagnosis of an anxiety disorder, particularly if the symptoms are absent or mild during the daytime. Patients with panic disorder often have not only disturbed subjective sleep but also panic attacks during sleep. Psychiatrists should remember that panic attacks could occur exclusively during sleep, without daytime symptoms, in some patients. Conversely, a report of "awakening in a state of panic" may be associated with a variety of other disorders including obstructive sleep apnea, gastroesophageal reflux, nocturnal angina, orthopnea, nightmares, night terrors and others.

Sleep-related Epilepsy

Some forms of epilepsy occur more commonly during sleep than during wakefulness and may be associated with parasomnia disorders. Nocturnal seizures may at times be confused with sleep terror, REM sleep behavior disorder, paroxysmal hypnogenic dystonia, or nocturnal panic attacks (Culebras, 1992). They may take the form of generalized convulsions or may be partial seizures with complex symptoms. Nocturnal seizures are most common at two times: the first 2 hours of sleep, or around 4 to 6 AM. They are more common in children than in adults. The chief complaint may be only disturbed sleep, torn up bedsheets and blankets, morning drowsiness (a postictal state), and muscle aches. Some patients never realize they suffer from nocturnal epilepsy until they share a bedroom or bed with someone who observes a convulsion.

Sleep Disturbances Related to Other Psychiatric Disorders

Subjective and objective disturbances of sleep are common features of many psychiatric disorders. General abnormalities include dyssomnias (such as insomnia and hypersomnia), parasomnias (such as nightmares, night terrors and nocturnal panic attacks) and circadian rhythm disturbances (early morning awakening). Before assuming that a significant sleep complaint invariably signals a psychiatric diagnosis, mental health specialists should go through a careful differential diagnostic procedure to rule out medical, pharmacological, or other causes. Even if the sleep complaint is primarily related to an underlying psychiatric disorder, sleep disorders in the mentally ill may be exacerbated by many other factors, such as increasing age; comorbid psychiatric, sleep and medical diagnoses; alcohol and substance abuse; effects of psychotropic or other medications; use of caffeinated beverages, nicotine, or other substances; lifestyle; past episodes of psychiatric illness (persisting "scars"); and cognitive, conditioned and coping characteristics such as anticipatory anxiety about sleep as bedtime nears. Some features of these sleep disorders may persist during periods of clinical remission of the psychiatric disorder and may be influenced by genetic factors. Finally, even if the sleep complaint is precipitated by a nonpsychiatric factor, psychiatric and psychosocial skills may be useful in ferreting out predisposing and perpetuating factors involved in chronic sleep complaints.

Although signs and symptoms of sleep disturbance are common in most psychiatric disorders, an additional diagnosis of insomnia or hypersomnia related to another mental disorder is made according to DSM-IV-TR criteria only when the sleep disturbance is a predominant complaint and is sufficiently severe to warrant independent clinical attention. Many of the patients with this type of sleep disorder diagnosis focus on the sleep complaints to the exclusion of other symptoms related to the primary psychiatric disorder. For example, they may seek professional help with complaints of insomnia or oversleeping when they should be at work, excessive fatigue, or desire for sleeping pills, but initially, they minimize or strongly deny signs and symptoms related to poor mood, anxiety, obsessive rumination, alcohol abuse, or a personality disorder.

Sleep Disturbances in Psychiatric Disorders: "Chicken or Egg?"

Whether sleep disturbances "cause" psychiatric disorders can be debated. At one level, this hypothesis seems unlikely because normal subjects vary considerably in their amount and type of sleep. Occasional extreme short sleepers, "needing" and sleeping as little as an hour a day for many years, have been reported, who appeared to be psychologically and medically normal in other respects. Furthermore, prolonged partial or selective sleep deprivation in normal volunteers does not apparently precipitate major psychiatric disorders. Normal control subjects have been kept awake for as long as 11 consecutive days in experiments to test the effect of sleep deprivation. Such experiments may cause dysphoria and dysfunction but not depression or dementia. Moreover, patients with narcolepsy or depression have been deprived of REM sleep for more than a year while being treated with high doses of MAOIs; if anything, they were better because their primary mood disorder improved during the course of treatment. Finally, total or partial sleep deprivation for one night has antidepressant effects in about half of depressed patients, including severely depressed melancholic, endogenous, or delusional patients.

These observations neither prove nor disprove the hypothesis that sleep disturbance does not cause psychiatric disorders. After all, experimental disruption of sleep in normal control subjects is highly artificial, usually conducted in supportive environments in well-screened, self-selected, healthy subjects. Likewise, people may vary in their sleep needs, but as far as we know, everyone needs to sleep; it may just be that individuals vary in the threshold of sleep disturbance beyond which they can go before manifesting psychiatric symptoms. Most important, chronic subjective sleep disturbances may be risk factors for certain vulnerable individuals. Thus, specific sleep characteristics may predispose to, or be a risk factor for, later development of psychiatric or substance abuse disorders. Again, the complaint of chronic insomnia or hypersomnia or normal short sleep cannot always be equated with objective sleep abnormalities, but it should at least alert the psychiatrist to the possibility that the patient deserves careful monitoring for a time.

Sleep disruption may be particularly harmful to some persons, for example, bipolar disorder patients, whether euthymic or depressed, in whom sleep deprivation may precipitate a manic episode. Mania is not uncommon with jet lag or work-related sleep deprivation in bipolar disorder patients. Behavioral and apparent personality changes with sleep deprivation are probably common but more often ignored in everyday life. The irritability of sleep-deprived children is known to most parents; and who of us has not had a "bad day" after a "bad night"?

Whereas insomnia is probably the most common sleep complaint in most psychiatric disorders, hypersomnia is not infrequently reported, especially in association with the following: bipolar mood disorder during depressed periods; major depressive disorder with atypical features (i.e., hypersomniac, hyperphagic patients with "leaden paralysis" and loss of energy); seasonal (winter) depression; stimulant abusers during withdrawal; some patients with personality disorders; and patients who are heavily sedated with anxiolytic, antipsychotic, or antidepressant medications, among other disorders.

Polysomnographic Features of Sleep in Psychiatric Disorders

More studies of sleep and sleep-related phenomenology have been conducted in **depression** than in any other disorder. Despite the common clinical impression that early morning wakefulness is a predominant symptom in depression, most of the objective measures in recent years have implicated abnormalities occurring at sleep onset and during the first non-REM and REM periods: prolonged sleep latency; reduced stages 3 and 4 sleep; increased duration and REM density of the first REM period; and associated neuroendocrine abnormalities, including growth hormone, thyroid-stimulating hormone and melatonin. Furthermore, some studies have suggested that short REM latency or reduced delta sleep ratio (amount of delta waves in first

Table 59.12 **Sleep-related Characteristics Associated with Depression**

Short REM latency (state, possibly trait)

Reduced amounts of stages 3 and 4 sleep (state and trait)

Difficulties initiating and maintaining sleep

Increased amounts of ocular movement during REM sleep (REM density), especially during the first REM period

A redistribution of REM sleep toward the beginning of sleep: increased duration of the first REM period

Low arousal thresholds to auditory stimulation

Elevated core body temperature during sleep

Blunted or reduced levels of plasma growth hormone (state and trait)

Elevated levels of plasma cortisol, increased number of pulses, and earlier onset of the morning rise in cortisol levels

Reduced levels of plasma testosterone

Blunted levels of thyroid-stimulating hormone at sleep onset

Reduced nocturnal levels of plasma melatonin

Longer but flattened periods of prolactin release

Elevated cerebral glucose metabolic rate during the first non-REM period

Faster induction of REM sleep after administration of cholinergic agonists

Antidepressant effect of total and partial sleep deprivation and, possibly, selective REM sleep deprivation

non-REM periods compared with second non-REM periods) may predict relapse in depressed patients. Some of these sleep-related abnormalities appear to persist during periods of clinical remission, such as short REM latency, loss of stages 3 and 4 sleep, and blunted nocturnal growth hormone release. Genetic factors may influence some of these measures, including short REM latency. Preliminary data suggest that short REM latency may be a genetic marker for depression in first-degree relatives of patients with mood disorders.

Even though the polygraphic sleep findings in depression do not appear to be diagnostically specific, they remain among the best documented biological abnormalities of any psychiatric disorder at this time. One challenge is to understand their pathophysiological mechanism. Because of the shallow, fragmented sleep and response to sleep deprivation, the sleep of patients with depression has been described as "overaroused". For instance, the antidepressant response of sleep deprivation may "dampen down" an overly aroused limbic system in a subgroup of patients. Several studies have shown that responders to sleep deprivation differ from nonresponders at baseline assessment before sleep deprivation by having a higher level of metabolic activity in the cingulate gyrus and that this overactivity approaches normality with clinical improvement.

The sleep disturbances of **schizophrenic** patients are often similar to those of depressed patients, including short REM latency and reduced delta sleep, total sleep time and sleep efficiency. Interestingly, while making nightly "sleep checks" on hospitalized patients, nurses are more accurate in judging sleep time in schizophrenic patients than in depressive patients, who often appear to be asleep when they are actually awake.

Although less well studied, the sleep of patients with **anxiety** disorders, such as generalized anxiety disorder, panic disorder, obsessive–compulsive disorder, acute stress disorder and PTSD, is often disturbed. **Panic** attacks, for example, may occur occasionally during sleep itself, usually at the transition between stage 2 and delta sleep. Patients with panic disorders during sleep are also likely to experience panic attacks during wakefulness either with relaxation or after sleep deprivation.

Patients with **obsessive–compulsive** disorder frequently endure difficulties in the initiation and maintenance of sleep. They often have elaborate compulsive rituals before going to bed, for example, concerns about "germs" may necessitate long showers and fresh, clean "sterilized" pajamas and sheets each night. Polysomnographic features are sometimes similar to those described in major depressive disorder, even though the patients do not have symptoms that meet full diagnostic criteria for major depressive disorder.

Classic symptoms of **post traumatic stress** disorder include nightmares, night terrors and violent thrashing about during sleep. These patients are easily aroused. Combat survivors with PTSD sometimes seek a physically "secure" sleeping environment in which to sleep and wake up frequently during the night to "check the perimeter". These sleep problems in Vietnam veterans who suffer from PTSD are often complicated by chronic conditioning, alcohol and substance abuse, depression, anxiety, and significant interpersonal and social problems. Total sleep time is usually reduced with variable and inconsistent disturbances of REM sleep. Successful treatment of the disorder and the sleep complaints has been traditionally difficult. The nightmares of PTSD appear to occur in both non-REM and REM sleep. While SSRIs are often recommended in the treatment of PTSD, some of the activating antidepressants appear to worsen subjective complaints of sleep. Nefazodone, a sedative antidepressant, slowly improved subjective sleep quality, mood, and the number of reported nightmares. Phenelzine and other MAOIs have also been reported to improve sleep and nightmares, but the possibility of serious drug interactions, alcoholism and poor compliance limit their usefulness. More recently, Raskin and colleagues have reported a significant reduction in nightmares and overall improvement in combat veterans with PTSD who were treated with prazosin, an alpha-1-adrenergic receptor antagonist (Taylor and Raskin, 2002).

Changes in sleep patterns may occur in patients with eating disorders. Night bingeing and increased sleep after eating are commonly reported in bulimic patients, who are also reported to eat and shop for food while sleepwalking. The patient frequently does not remember these nocturnal episodes; they often become known from family or friends who have observed the behavior or from physical evidence of shopping or eating behaviors. Patients with anorexia are often hyperactive, needing little sleep. Given the degree of physical and psychic stress associated with eating disorders, it is surprising how limited are the objective sleep disturbances associated with these disorders.

General Approaches to the Clinical Management of Sleep Disorders in Psychiatric Patients

The sleep complaint in the patient with an apparent psychiatric disorder deserves the same careful diagnostic and therapeutic attention that it does in any patient. Just because a patient is depressed does not mean that the complaint of insomnia or hypersomnia can be explained away as a symptom of depression. Too many patients with depression have been found to have a BRSD; too many patients with panic disorder to have insomnia secondary to caffeinism. Chronic sleep complaints are multidetermined and multifaceted, even in many psychiatric patients. Differential diagnosis remains the first obligation of the psychiatrist before definitive treatment, which should be aimed at the underlying cause or causes.

Nonspecific treatments, such as use of sleep hygiene principles, are often helpful for both the sleep complaints and the underlying psychiatric disorders. In particular, bipolar disorder patients and patients whose daily activities are poorly organized (like patients with chronic schizophrenia and patients with certain personality disorders) may benefit from fairly rigid sleep–wake and light–dark schedules to synchronize circadian rhythms and impose structure on their behavior. Physical exercise, meditation, relaxation methods, sleep restriction therapy and cognitive psychotherapy may help patients manage anxiety, rumination and conditioned psychophysiological insomnia that often cause sleeplessness at night and fatigue during the day. Partial or total sleep deprivation may be like "paradoxical intention" therapy in the treatment of major depressive disorder or premenstrual dysphoric disorder but should probably be avoided in bipolar depression.

Medications may either help or hurt. Whether the patient should have drugs with sedating or activating properties should be considered. Timing and dose are important considerations in the context of pharmacokinetic and pharmacodynamic properties of drugs. Night-time administration of sedating drugs may improve sleep and reduce daytime oversedation. Clinically significant drug side effects such as oversedation or activation may

be more likely early in treatment than later, after tolerance has developed. On the other hand, some sedating medications, even short half-life sleeping aids, may have disinhibiting effects, even late into the next day, especially in elderly and cognitively impaired individuals. Doses of sleeping pills and other medications should usually be reduced by about half in the elderly compared with the dose for a young adult.

In general, avoid polypharmacy. Sleeping pills should be prescribed reluctantly to patients who receive adequate doses of antidepressants. Although coadministration of a benzodiazepine may improve sleep during the first week of antidepressant therapy, a low dose of zolpidem, zaleplon, trazodone, or other sedating antidepressant at night in addition to the antidepressant may be less likely to produce tolerance and may have additive antidepressant benefits. Antipsychotic medications should not be administered as sleeping aids unless the patient is psychotic or otherwise unresponsive to other medications.

Sleep Disorders in Other Medical Conditions

A sleep disorder due to a general medical condition is defined in DSM-IV-TR as a prominent disturbance in sleep severe enough to warrant independent clinical attention. Subtypes include insomnia, hypersomnia, parasomnia and mixed types. As a general rule, any disease or disorder that causes pain, discomfort, or a heightened state of arousal in the waking state is capable of disrupting or interfering with sleep. Examples of this phenomenon include pain syndromes of any sort, arthritic and other rheumatological disorders, prostatism and other causes of urinary frequency or urgency, chronic obstructive lung disease and other pulmonary conditions. Many of these conditions increase in prevalence with advancing age, suggesting at least one reason that sleep disorders are more likely to be seen in senior populations. The following include disorders known to cause disturbances in sleep: rheumatoid arthritis, fibromyalgia, chronic obstructive pulmonary conditions, congestive heart failure, peptic ulcer disease, GERD, rectal urgency, Parkinson's disease, Huntington's chorea, advanced Alzheimer's disease and hereditary progressive dystonia.

Sleep in Elderly with Dementia

The sleep of older adults with dementia is extremely disturbed, with severely fragmented sleep, often to the extent that there is not a single hour in a 24-hour day that is spent fully awake or asleep. Patients with mild to moderate dementia have extremely fragmented sleep at night, while those with severe dementia are extremely sleepy during both the day and night. Sleep stages also change with dementia, with significantly lower amounts of stages 3, 4 and REM sleep, and significantly more awakenings, as well as more time spent awake during the night. This results in increased stage 1 sleep and decreased sleep efficiency. It has also been shown that there is a high prevalence of sleep apnea in patients with dementia, with as many as 80% having symptoms that meet the criteria for diagnosis. The sleep changes and disruption seen are likely due to the neuronal degeneration found in Alzheimer's disease. Neuronal structures damaged in patients with dementia include the basal forebrain and the reticular formation of the brain stem, the same structures implicated in sleep regulation.

The nocturnal awakenings seen in dementia patients are often accompanied by agitation, confusion and wandering. These behaviors have been referred to as "sundowning" as it was believed that they typically occurred as the sun set. A recent study (Martin *et al.*, 2000) challenged the idea of sundowning by showing that peak levels of agitation occur during various times of the day, but more often in the afternoon, rather than in the evening or night.

It has been suggested that agitation or sundowning may be a circadian rhythm disorder. Sleep disruption in demented individuals may be amenable to treatment using bright light exposure. Others have tested this theory by exposing patients with dementia to bright light. The results have been mixed, but in general support the theory that increased light exposure, whether during the morning or evening, will improve both sleep and behavior to some extent.

Substance-induced Sleep Disorder

An important aspect of the evaluation of any patient, particularly those with sleep disorders, is the review of medications and other substances (including prescription, over-the-counter and recreational drugs, as well as alcohol, stimulants, narcotics, coffee and caffeine, and nicotine) and exposure to toxins, heavy metals, and so forth. These substances may affect sleep and wakefulness during either ingestion or withdrawal, causing most commonly insomnia, hypersomnia, or, less frequently, parasomnia or mixed types of difficulties. On the basis of DSM-IV-TR criteria, a diagnosis of substance-induced sleep disorder may be made if the disturbance of sleep is sufficiently severe to warrant independent clinical attention and is judged to result from the direct physiological effects of a substance. Substance-induced sleep disorder cannot result from mental disorder or occur during delirium. If appropriate, the context for the development of sleep symptoms may be indicated by specifying with onset during intoxication or with onset during withdrawal.

The recognition of substance-related sleep disturbances usually depends on active searching by the psychiatrist, beginning with a careful history, physical examination, laboratory and toxicological testing, and information (with permission) from former health care providers or friends and relatives. Patients may not know what prescription medications they are taking or the doses, and may forget to mention over-the-counter medications, coffee, occupational or environmental toxins, and so forth. In the case of alcohol and drugs of abuse, they may deny to themselves and others their use, or quantity, or frequency of use. Substance dependence and abuse is often associated with other psychiatric diagnoses or symptoms. When comorbidity does exist, it is important to establish, if possible, whether the sleep disturbance is primary or secondary, that is, whether the sleep disturbance is substance-induced (secondary) or whether the substance use

DSM-IV-TR Criteria

Substance-induced Sleep Disorder

A. prominent disturbance in sleep that is sufficiently severe to warrant independent clinical attention.

B. There is evidence from the history, physical examination, or laboratory findings of either (1) or (2):

    (1) the symptoms in criterion A developed during, or within a month of, substance intoxication or withdrawal

    (2) medication use is etiologically related to the sleep disturbance

C. The disturbance is not better accounted for by a sleep disorder that is not substance induced. Evidence that the symptoms are better accounted for by a sleep disorder that is not substance induced might include the following: the symptoms precede the onset of the substance use (or medication use); the symptoms persist for a substantial period of time (e.g., about a month) after the cessation of acute withdrawal or severe intoxication, or are substantially in excess of what would be expected given the type or amount of the substance used or the duration of use; or there is other evidence that suggests the existence of an independent non-substance-induced sleep disorder (e.g., a history of recurrent non-substance-related episodes).

D. The disturbance does not occur exclusively during the course of a delirium.

E. The sleep disturbance causes clinically significant distress or impairment in social, occupational, or other important areas of functioning.

Note: This diagnosis should be made instead of a diagnosis of substance intoxication or substance withdrawal only when the sleep symptoms are in excess of those usually associated with the intoxication or withdrawal syndrome, and when the symptoms are sufficiently severe to warrant independent clinical attention.

Code

[specific substance]–induced sleep disorder:

(291.8 alcohol; 292.89 amphetamine; 292.89 caffeine; 292.89 cocaine; 292.89 opioid; 292.89 sedative, hypnotic, or anxiolytic; 292.89 other [or unknown] substance)

Specify type:

Insomnia type: if the predominant sleep disturbance is insomnia

Hypersomnia type: if the predominant sleep disturbance is hypersomnia

Parasomnia type: if the predominant sleep disturbance is a parasomnia

Mixed type: if more than one sleep disturbance is present and none predominates

Specify if:

With onset during intoxication: if criteria are met for intoxication with the substance and the symptoms develop during the intoxication syndrome

With onset during withdrawal: if criteria are met for withdrawal from the substance and the symptoms develop during, or shortly after, a withdrawal syndrome

functions as a form of "self-medication" for sleep disturbance, in which the sleep disturbance would be considered primary. Many patients with alcoholism experience secondary depression during the first few weeks of withdrawal from alcohol and exhibit short REM latency and other sleep changes similar to those reported in primary depression. This secondary depression usually remits spontaneously. Likewise, about one-third of patients with unipolar depression and about three-fifths of patients with bipolar disorder, manic type, have a substance use pattern that meets diagnostic criteria for alcoholism or substance abuse at some point. Prognosis and treatment may be altered in comorbid states, depending on whether the sleep disturbance is primary or secondary. In general, treatment should be aimed at the primary diagnosis after management of any acute withdrawal condition that may exist.

Alcohol

Alcohol is probably the most commonly self-administered "sleeping aid". Although it may be sedating, especially in middle-aged or elderly or sleep-deprived persons, its usefulness as a hypnotic is limited by potential disinhibiting and arousing effects, gastric irritation, falling blood-alcohol levels in the early part of the night with mild withdrawal symptoms and sleep fragmentation at the end of the night, morning headaches and hangover effects, tolerance with repeated use, and exacerbation of BRSDs such as apnea.

Virtually any type of sleep disturbance has been attributed to the effects of alcohol or alcohol withdrawal in patients with alcohol abuse or dependence. Insomnia may occur during episodes of drinking and acute and chronic withdrawal. Complaints of insomnia and objective disruption of sleep continuity and stages 3 and 4 sleep have been reported for up to several years in some abstinent patients. Hypersomnia may occur during heavy bouts of drinking, sometimes with peripheral compression neuropathies, or as "terminal hypersomnia" after delirium tremens. Circadian sleep disturbances may also occur during bouts of drinking, including periods of short polyphasic sleep–wake episodes. Parasomnias include sleepwalking and enuresis.

Because alcohol may temporarily improve the poor sleep of the chronic alcoholic individual, sleep disturbance may be a factor in relapse. Treatment of the sleep disturbances of the chronic but abstinent alcoholic individual is difficult. Nonpharmacological approaches include sleep hygiene and sleep restriction, as well as attention to general nutrition, physical health and psychosocial supports. Use of benzodiazepines or other hypnotics is not generally recommended because of cross-tolerance or deliberate or inadvertent overdose.

Nicotine

Aside from medical complications, such as coughing that may interfere with sleep, smoking has been associated with both difficulty in falling asleep and getting up in the morning suggesting that nicotine may phase delay the circadian oscillator. Furthermore, compared with nonsmokers, men who smoked reported more nightmares, women who smoked reported more daytime sleepiness. Furthermore, as blood-nicotine levels fall during the night, smokers go into relative withdrawal and start craving a cigarette. One of the best measures of nicotine dependence is how long the smoker can wait in the morning for the first smoke. Abstinence from smoking is associated with lighter and more fragmented sleep, daytime sleepiness on the Multiple Sleep Latency Test, irritability, craving and other subjective emotional distress.

Amphetamines, Cocaine and Caffeine

Stimulants initially prolong sleep onset and reduce REM sleep, sleep continuity, and sleep duration, but tolerance usually develops. During acute withdrawal, hypersomnia and excessive REM sleep occur for the first week or so but may be followed by a few days of insomnia.

Like the stimulants, caffeine usually promotes arousal and delays sleep, but withdrawal may be associated with hypersomnia. It is probably the most commonly self-administered stimulant, for example, the morning cup of coffee to "get going". Caffeine has some benefits as a mild stimulant to overcome sleepiness.

Opiates

Short-term use of opiates may increase sleep and subjective sleep quality and reduce REM sleep, especially in patients who need an analgesic for relief of pain, but these drugs may also disrupt sleep. Tolerance usually develops with repeated administration. Withdrawal may be associated with hypersomnia or the "nods".

Sedatives, Hypnotics and Anxiolytics

Tolerance usually develops with repeated administration of the sedating effects of barbiturates, chloral hydrate and even benzodiazepines. This is true especially with short half-life agents, with the possible exception of zaleplon. As mentioned earlier, 1 or 2 days of withdrawal insomnia may occur after a few days of administration of short half-life benzodiazepines, such as triazolam, but not with the newer nonbenzodiazepine hypnotics, such as zolpidem and zaleplon.

Potential side effects associated with sedating medications during the sleep period include falls and fractures, difficulty arousing to the telephone or the crying infant, amnesia, impairment of cognitive and motor skills, drug-induced sleepwalking, and possibly, BRSDs.

Other Substances

Many medications produce sleep disturbance, including those with central or autonomic nervous system effects, like adrenergic agonists and antagonists, dopamine agonists and antagonists, cholinergic agonists and antagonists, antihistamines and steroids. Among the prescription drugs associated frequently with sleep disorders are the SSRIs, which have been connected with overarousal and insomnia in some patients and, more commonly, sedation in other patients. Coadministration of trazodone at night has been shown, in a double-blind, placebo-controlled study, to be effective in managing fluoxetine-induced insomnia in depressed patients (Nierenberg *et al.*, 1994). Additional sleep-related disturbances occasionally associated with the SSRIs include sleepwalking, REM sleep behavior disorder and rapid eye movements during non-REM sleep.

Comparison of DSM-IV/ICD-10 Diagnostic Criteria

For primary insomnia, the ICD-10 Diagnostic Criteria for Research and the DSM-IV-TR criteria are almost identical except that ICD-10 requires a frequency of at least three times a week for at least a month, whereas DSM-IV-TR does not specify a required frequency. For primary hypersomnia, the ICD-10 Diagnostic Criteria for Research and the DSM-IV-TR criteria are almost identical except that ICD-10 also counts sleep drunkenness as a presenting symptom. Furthermore, ICD-10 requires that the

Sleep Societies and Associations: Resources for Professional and Patient Information

Name	Address	Phone	Website
American Academy of Sleep Medicine (AASM)	One Westbrook Corporate CenterSuite 920 Westchester, IL 60154	(708) 492–0930	www.apss.org
Academy of Dental Sleep Medicine (ADSM)	10592 Perry Hwy, #220Wexford, PA 15090-9244	(724) 935–0836	www.dentalsleepmed.org
Associated Professional Sleep Societies (APSS)	One Westbrook Corporate CenterSuite 920 Westchester, IL 60154	(708) 492–0930	www.apss.org
American Sleep Apnea Association (ASAA)	1424 K St. NW, Suite 302Washington DC 20005	(202) 293–3650	www.sleepapnea.org
Narcolepsy Network	10921 Reed Hartman Hwy Cincinnati, OH 45242	(513) 891–3522	www.narcolepsynetwork.org
National Sleep Foundation (NSF)	1522 K St. NW, Suite 500 Washington DC 20005	(202) 347–3471	www.sleepfoundation.org
Sleep Medicine Education and Research Foundation (SMERF)	6301 Bandel Rd., Suite 101Rochester, MN 55901	(507) 287–6008	www.aasmnet.org
Sleep Research Society (SRS)	One Westbrook Corporate CenterSuite 920 Westchester, IL 60154	(708) 492–0930	www.sleepresearchsociety.org
Society for Light Treatment and Biological Rhythms (SLTBR)	PO Box 591687San Francisco, CA 94159	(415) 876–0716	www.sltbr.org

problems occur nearly every day for at least 1 month (or recurrently for shorter periods of time).

Since narcolepsy and breathing-related sleep disorder are included in Chapter VI (Diseases of the Nervous System) in ICD-10, there are no diagnostic criteria provided for these conditions.

For circadian rhythm sleep disorder, the ICD-10 Diagnostic Criteria for Research and the DSM-IV-TR criteria are almost identical except that ICD-10 specifies that the problems occur nearly every day for at least 1 month (or recurrently for shorter periods of time) (DSM-IV-TR has no specified duration). This condition is referred to in ICD-10 as "Nonorganic disorder of the sleep–wake cycle".

The ICD-10 Diagnostic Criteria for Research and the DSM-IV-TR criteria for nightmare disorder and sleepwalking disorder are essentially identical. The ICD-10 Diagnostic Criteria for Research and the DSM-IV-TR criteria sets for sleep terror disorder are almost identical except that ICD-10 explicitly limits the duration of the episode to less than 10 minutes.

References

American Psychiatric Association (1994) *Diagnostic and Statistical Manual of Mental Disorders.* APA, Washington DC.

Ancoli-Israel S and Roth T (1999) Characteristics of insomnia in the United States: I. Results of the 1991 National Sleep Foundation Survey. *Sleep* 22, S347–S353.

Bootzin RR and Nicassio PM (1978) Behavioral treatments for insomnia, in *Progress in Behavior Modification* (eds Hersen M, Eisler RM, and Miller PM). Academic Press, New York, pp. 1–45.

Culebras A (1992) Neuroanatomic and neurologic correlates of sleep disturbances. *Neurology* 42(Suppl 6), 19–27.

Daan S, Beersma DGM and Borbely AA (1984) Timing of human sleep: Recovery process gated by a circadian pacemaker. *Am J Physiol* 246, R161–R183.

Diagnostic Classification Steering Committee, Thorpy MJ (Chair) (1990) International Classification of Sleep Disorders: Diagnostic and Coding Manual, Rev. American Academy of Sleep Medicine, Rochester.

Edgar DM, Dement WC, and Fuller CA (1993) Effect of SCN lesions on sleep in squirrel monkeys: Evidence for opponent processes in sleep–wake regulation. *J Neurosci* 13(3), 1065–1079.

Jacobs D, Ancoli-Israel S, Parker L *et al.* (1989) 24-hour sleep/wake patterns in a nursing home population. *Psychol Aging* 4(3), 352–356.

Lavie P, Pratt H, Scharf B *et al.* (1984) Localized pontine lesion: Nearly total absence of REM sleep. *Neurology* 34, 118–120.

Lewy AJ and Sack RL (1989) The dim light melatonin onset as a marker for circadian phase position. *Chronobiol Int* 6, 93–102.

Littner M, Johnson SF, McCall WV *et al.* (2001) Practice parameters for the treatment of narcolepsy: An update for 2000. *Sleep* 24, 451–466.

Martin J, Marler M, Shochat T *et al.* (2000) Circadian rhythms of agitation in institutionalized Alzheimer's disease patients. *Chronobiol Int* 17, 405–418.

Morin CM, Culbert JP and Schwartz SM (1994) Nonpharmacological interventions for insomnia: A meta-analysis of treatment efficacy. *Am J Psychiatr* 151, 1172–1180.

Morin CM, Colecchi C, Stone J *et al.* (1999) Behavioral and pharmacological therapies for late life insomnia. *JAMA* 281, 991–999.

Morin CM, Kowatch RA, Barry T *et al.* (1993) Cognitive–behavior therapy for late-life insomnia. *J Consult Clin Psychol* 61, 137–146.

Nierenberg AA, Adler LA, Peselow E, *et al.* (1994) Trazodone for antidepressant-associated insomnia. *Am J Psychiatr* 151, 1069–1072.

Nieto FJ, Young T, Lind B *et al.* (2000) Sleep-disordered breathing, sleep apnea, and hypertension in a large community-based study. *JAMA* 283, 1829–1836.

Spielman AJ, Saskin P, and Thorpy MJ (1987) Treatment of chronic insomnia by restriction of time in bed. *Sleep* 10, 45–56.

Taylor F and Raskin MA (2002) The alpha-1-adrenergic antagonist prazosin improves sleep and nightmares in civilian trauma posttraumatic stress disorder. *J Clin Psychopharmacol* 1, 82–85.

US Xyrem Multicenter Study Group (2002) A randomized, double-blind, placebo-controlled multicenter trial comparing the effects of three doses of orally administered sodium oxybate with placebo for the treatment of narcolepsy. *Sleep* 25, 42–49.

Impulse Control Disorders

Although dissimilar in behavioral expressions, the disorders in this chapter share the feature of impulse dyscontrol. Individuals who experience such dyscontrol are overwhelmed by the urge to commit certain acts that are often apparently illogical or harmful. The outcome of each of these behaviors is often harmful, either for the afflicted individual (trichotillomania, pathological gambling) or for others (intermittent explosive disorder, pyromania, kleptomania).

The trait of impulsivity has been the subject of increasing interest in psychiatry. New research findings seem to associate various forms of impulsive behavior with biological markers of altered serotonergic function. These include impulsive suicidal behavior, impulsive aggression and impulsive fire-setting. Impulsivity is also a focus of interest in the increasing attention paid to the behavioral phenomenology of borderline personality disorder. In all these circumstances, impulsivity is conceived of as the rapid expression of unplanned behavior, occurring in response to a sudden thought. (This is seen by some as the polar opposite of obsessional behavior, in which deliberation over an act may seem never-ending.) Although the sudden and unplanned aspect of the behavior may be present in the impulse disorders (such as in intermittent explosive disorder and kleptomania), the primary connotation of the word impulsivity, as used to describe these conditions, is the irresistibility of the urge to act.

The National Comorbidity Survey Replication (NCS-R) (Kessler *et al.*, 2005) extended the definition of impulse control disorders described in this chapter to include intermittent explosive disorder, attention deficit hyperactivity disorder (ADHD), conduct disorder (CD) and oppositional defiant disorder (ODD). This decision was based on the fact that ADHD and anger symptoms often persist throughout adulthood. The NCS-R found that the combined lifetime prevalence for these disorders is greater than that of mood (20.8%) or substance abuse disorders (14.6%). Impulse control disorders in the extended definition had a 12 month prevalence of 8.9% and a lifetime prevalence of 24.8%. Moreover, this group was judged to have a greater proportion functioning at the serious level than either anxiety or substance abuse disorders. with approximately half of all lifetime cases receiving no treatment. An important objective in studying the impulse control disorders in this fashion was to highlight how common hostility and aggression are in psychiatric disorders, two dimensions often not receiving sufficient diagnostic consideration but which are significantly present as comorbidities with other disorders.

Trichotillomania, pyromania and pathological gambling may involve episodes in which a sudden desire to commit the act of hair-pulling, fire-setting, or gambling is followed by rapid expression of the behavior. But in these conditions, the individual may spend considerable amounts of time fighting off the urge, trying not to carry out the impulse. The inability to resist the impulse is the common core of these disorders, rather than the rapid transduction of thought to action. A decision tree for the differential diagnosis of impulsive behaviors may be seen in Figure 60.1.

Other than sharing the essential feature of impulse dyscontrol, it is unclear whether the conditions in this chapter bear any relationship to each other. Emerging perspectives on the neurobiology of impulsivity suggest that impulsive behaviors, across diagnostic boundaries, may share an underlying pathophysiological diathesis. As noted earlier, markers of altered serotonergic neurotransmission have been associated with a variety of impulsive behaviors: suicidality, aggressive violence, pyromania and conduct disorder. These observations have led to speculation that decreased serotonergic neurotransmission may result in decreased ability to control urges to act. In accord with this model, these disorders may be varying expressions of a single disturbance – or closely related disturbances – of serotonergic function. Although such markers of altered serotonergic function have been demonstrated among impulsive fire-setters and impulsive violent offenders, there is, as yet, insufficient research on these conditions to accept or dismiss this theory.

It has been noted that these conditions are embedded in similar patterns of comorbidity with other psychiatric disorders. High rates of comorbid mood disorder and anxiety disorder appear typical of these disorders. This contextual similarity, combined with the common feature of impulsivity, may further support the notion that these conditions are – at the level of core diathesis – related to each other.

Although these conditions have historically been considered uncommon, later investigations suggest that some of them may be fairly common. Trichotillomania, for example, was once considered rare. However, surveys indicate that the lifetime prevalence of the condition may exceed 1% of the population. Pathological gambling may be present in up to 3% of the population. Extrapolation from the known incidence of comorbid conditions suggests that kleptomania may have a 0.6% incidence. It would seem reasonable to suspect that individuals with pyromania and kleptomania may seek to avoid detection and may therefore be underrepresented in research and clinical samples.

Treatment protocols for these conditions have not been well studied. Few treatment studies of these specific conditions have been performed. Attempts to treat these conditions are usually formulated by extrapolation from treatments that have been developed for other conditions.

The aggressive quality of kleptomania, pyromania and intermittent explosive disorder and the self-damaging nature of trichotillomania and pathological gambling have presented tempting substrates for the application of traditional analytical concepts. From this perspective, these behaviors have been seen

Essentials of Psychiatry Jerald Kay and Allan Tasman
© 2006 John Wiley & Sons, Ltd.

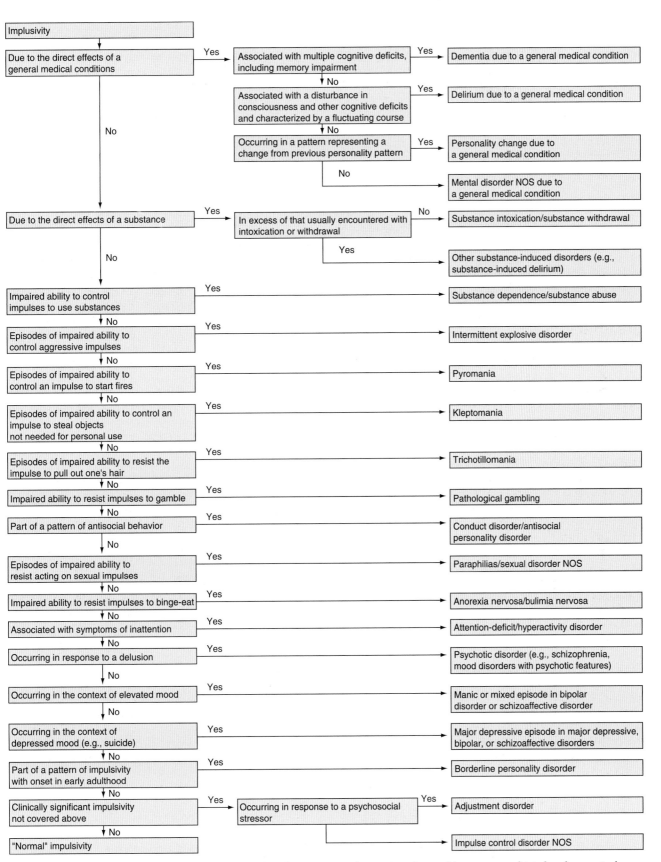

Figure 60.1   *Differential diagnosis of impulsivity. Impulsivity is a tendency to act in a sudden, unpremeditated and excessively spontaneous fashion. Other decision trees that should be considered are those for aggressive behavior, catatonia, delusions, depressed mood, euphoric or irritable mood, disorganized or unusual behavior, distractibility, eating behavior, self-mutilation and suicide ideation or attempt. (NOS, not otherwise specified.)*

as symptomatic expressions of unconscious conflict, often sexual in nature. Other formulations include desires for oral gratification and masochistic wishes to be caught and punished, motivated by a harsh, guilt-inducing superego. The increasing influence of object relations theory was reflected in increasing emphasis on narcissistic psychopathology and histories of disturbed early parenting. As successful behavioral interventions were developed for other conditions, case reports of behavioral treatments for these conditions emerged. Reports of hypnotic treatments are also prominent in the literature.

The contemporary medical and psychological literature reflects, not surprisingly, prevailing general interests in current research and theory. As pharmacological treatments are applied to an increasing range of symptoms, the impulse disorders in this chapter present new opportunities to widen the application of thymoleptic and anxiolytic and, more recently, (atypical) neuroleptic medication. Some are reconceptualizing the idea of mood and obsessional disorders, widening them into affective and obsessional spectrums, encompassing various impulse disorders into these domains.

As part of the ongoing dynamic of evolving theory, the very concept of impulsivity is still in ferment. Attempts further to refine the idea of impulsivity are reflected in a perspective offered by Van Ameringen and associates (1999). In a discussion of preliminary evidence indicating that trichotillomania may be preferentially responsive to neuroleptics, they suggest that individuals with trichotillomania may have features in common with the subgroup of obsessive compulsive disorder (OCD) patients who have comorbid Tourette's syndrome (TS). These authors offer a thoughtful model, applying the idea of an "Impulsion" (Shapiro and Shapiro, 1992), an action performed until a sense of "rightness" is achieved, rather than a compulsion, which is designed to reduce an anxiety brought on by an obsession. They go on to note one formulation of OCD, which divides symptoms into three types: symmetry/hoarding, pure obsessions and contamination/cleaning. The symmetry/hoarding factor – impulsion-driven behavior – was differentially related to OCD with comorbid TS. They point to recent data suggesting that the OCD/TS subgroup is not as responsive to SSRI medication alone as other OCD subtypes, but responds better to SSRI/neuroleptic combinations. These observations, taken together with their report of enhanced response of trichotillomania to neuroleptics, is the basis for their argument that trichotillomania should be seen as more similar to OCD/TS then OCD, more impulsion than compulsion. The idea of anxiously seeking "rightness" is consistent with the clinical experience of many individuals with trichotillomania and is a thoughtful addition to the other attributes associated with impulsivity: anxiety reduction, irresistibility of action and rapidity of its execution.

Trichotillomania provides an example of the convergence of current research techniques and treatment perspectives. The absence of new psychodynamic formulations would seem to reflect not an abandonment of dynamic theory but an acceptance that such models are most useful in understanding individual patients rather than providing universal explanations for the symptom. Dynamic considerations may be useful in trying to understand why particular circumstances may provoke episodes of the problem behavior for a particular individual. But there is no available evidence that dynamic therapy, when employed as a sole mode of treatment, is efficacious in the treatment of trichotillomania or other conditions in this chapter.

Not all these conditions are, as yet, receiving significant attention. Trichotillomania, intermittent explosive disorder and

pathological gambling have become the focus of increasing interest. Kleptomania and pyromania, however, remain stepchildren of research. Perhaps the legal implications of these behaviors and their entanglement with similar, but not impulsively motivated, behaviors complicate the availability of sufficient cases to facilitate research.

Because of the limited body of systematically collected data, the following sections largely reflect accumulated clinical experience. Therefore, the practicing psychiatrist should be particularly careful to consider the exigencies of individual patients in applying treatment recommendations.

Intermittent Explosive Disorder

Definition

Patients with intermittent explosive disorder have a problem with their temper (see DSMIV-TR criteria). This definition highlights the centrality of impulsive aggression in intermittent explosive disorder. Impulsive aggression, however, is not specific to intermittent explosive disorder. It is a key feature of several psychiatric disorders and nonpsychiatric conditions and may emerge during the course of yet other psychiatric disorders. Therefore, the definition of intermittent explosive disorder as formulated in the DSM-IV-TR is essentially a diagnosis of exclusion. As described in criterion C, a diagnosis of intermittent explosive disorder is made only after other mental disorders that might account for episodes of aggressive behavior have been ruled out. The individual may describe the aggressive episodes as "spells" or "attacks". The symptoms appear within minutes to hours and, regardless of the duration of the episode, may remit almost as quickly. As in other impulse control disorders, the explosive behavior may be preceded by a sense of tension or arousal and is followed immediately by a sense of relief or release of tension.

DSM-IV-TR Criteria 312.34

Intermittent Explosive Disorder

A. Several discrete episodes of failure to resist aggressive impulses that result in serious assaultive acts or destruction of property.

B. The degree of aggressiveness expressed during the episodes is grossly out of proportion to any precipitating psychosocial stressors.

C. The aggressive episodes are not better accounted for by another mental disorder (e.g., antisocial personality disorder, borderline personality disorder, a psychotic disorder, a manic episode, conduct disorder, or attention-deficit/hyperactivity disorder) and are not due to the direct physiological effects of a substance (e.g., a drug of abuse, a medication) or a general medical condition (e.g., head trauma, Alzheimer's disease).

Although not explicitly stated in the DSM-IV-TR definition of intermittent explosive disorder, impulsive aggressive behavior may have many motivations that are not meant to be included within this diagnosis. Intermittent explosive disorder should not be diagnosed when the purpose of the aggression is monetary gain, vengeance, self-defense, social dominance, or expressing a political statement or when it occurs as a part of gang behavior. Typically, the aggressive behavior is egodystonic to individuals with intermittent explosive disorder, who feel genuinely upset, remorseful, regretful, bewildered, or embarrassed about their impulsive aggressive acts.

Etiology and Pathophysiology

Since the second half of the 19th century, two main lines of explanation, which are to a large extent complementary, have been developed to account for the existence of individuals with episodic impulsive aggression. One line of explanation viewed the etiology of impulsive aggression as stemming from the effects of early childhood experiences and possibly childhood trauma on the development of self-control, frustration tolerance, planning ability and gratification delay, which are all important for self-prevention of impulsive aggressive outbursts. Early experiences with "good-enough" mothering that fosters phase-appropriate delay of gratification and the development of the potential for imitation and identification with the mother are considered important for normal development. Too much or too little frustration, as well as overgratification or undergratification, may impair the normal development of the ability to anticipate frustration and delay gratification.

A second line of explanation, which has yielded numerous positive findings during the past 15 years, views impulsive aggression as the result of variations in brain mechanisms that mediate behavioral arousal and behavioral inhibition. A rapidly growing body of evidence has shown that impulsive aggression may be related to defects in the brain serotonergic system, which acts as an inhibitor of motor activity. Although the majority of studies involved patients who suffered from impulsive aggression in the context of disorders other than intermittent explosive disorder, their findings may be relevant to the behavioral dimension of impulsive aggression, of which intermittent explosive disorder is a "pure" form. A number of researchers have confirmed a relationship between levels of 5-hydroxyindoleacetic acid (5-HIAA) in the CSF and impulsive or aggressive behaviors. Others have divided aggressive behaviors into impulsive and nonimpulsive forms, and found that reduced CSF 5-HIAA levels were correlated with impulsive aggression only. Pharmacological challenge studies of the serotonergic system have also demonstrated that low serotonergic responsiveness (as measured by the neuroendocrine response to serotonergic agonists) correlates with scores of impulsive aggression. Studies of impulsive aggression among alcoholics have further defined a probable relationship between such behaviors and diminished serotonergic function.

The literature on serotonin and suicide, which may be viewed as an extreme form of self-directed aggression, suggests another link between serotonin and aggression. Postmortem studies found that brain stem levels of serotonin were decreased in suicide victims, and reduced imipramine binding, which is thought to be associated with reduced presynaptic serotonergic binding sites, was found in the brains of suicide completers. Furthermore, an increase in postsynaptic 5-hydroxytryptamine (5-HT$_2$) receptors was found in the brains of suicide completers, and this finding was confirmed in subsequent studies. An increase in 5-HT$_2$ receptors, which are thought to be mostly postsynaptic, may reflect the brain's reaction to a decrease in functional serotonergic neurons, with consequent upregulation of postsynaptic serotonin binding sites.

Another line of neurobiological evidence links impulsive aggression with dysfunction of the prefrontal cortex. Studies of neuropsychiatric patients with localized structural brain lesions have demonstrated that some bilateral lesions in the prefrontal cortex may be specifically associated with a chronic pattern of impulsive aggressive behaviors. Neurological studies suggest that the prefrontal cortical regions associated with impulsive aggression syndromes are involved in the processing of affective information and the inhibition of motor responsiveness, both of which are impaired in patients with impulsive aggression. Interictal episodes of aggression may occur among some individuals with epilepsy. In a quantitative MRI study of such episodes among individuals with temporal lobe epilepsy (TLE) (Woermann et al., 2000) three groups (24 TLE patients with aggressive behavior, 24 TLE patients without such behavior and 35 nonpatient controls) were compared. The researchers concluded that the aggressive behavior was associated with a reduction of frontal neocortical gray matter.

Biological studies implicate the serotonergic system and the prefrontal cortex in the pathogenesis of impulsive aggression. The diagnosis of intermittent explosive disorder is sometimes considered in forensic settings; the biological correlates of impulsive aggression focus attention on, but do not solve, the complicated problem of personal responsibility for impulsive violent acts that are correlated with objective biological findings. Data from a study of visual-evoked potentials and EEGs in a large group of children and adolescents who demonstrated aggressive behavior also suggest that such behavior may be associated with altered innate characteristics of central nervous system function (Bars et al., 2001).

Assessment and Differential Diagnosis

Phenomenology and Variations in Presentation

Episodes of violent behavior appear in several common psychiatric disorders such as antisocial personality disorder, borderline personality disorder and substance use disorders and need to be distinguished from the violent episodes of patients with intermittent explosive disorder, which are apparently rare. The study of Felthous and coworkers (1991), in which 15 men with rigorously diagnosed DSM-III-R intermittent explosive disorder were identified from among a group of 443 men who complained of violence, permitted some systematic observations about the "typical violent episode" as reported by patients with intermittent explosive disorder.

In the vast majority of instances, the subjects with intermittent explosive disorder identified their spouse, lover, or girlfriend or boyfriend as a provocateur of their violent episodes. Only one was provoked by a stranger. For most, the reactions occurred immediately and without a noticeable prodromal period. Only one subject stated that the outburst occurred between 1 and 24 hours after the perceived provocation. All subjects with intermittent explosive disorder denied that they intended the outburst to occur in advance. Most subjects remained well oriented during the outbursts, although two claimed to lose track of where they were. None lost control of urine or bowel function during the episode. Subjects reported various degrees of subjective feelings of behavioral dyscontrol. Only four felt that they completely lost control. Six had good recollection of the event afterward, eight had partial recollection and one lost memory of the event afterward. Most subjects with intermittent explosive disorder attempted to help or comfort the victim afterwards.

Assessment

Special Issues in the Psychiatric Examination and History

The DSM-IV-TR diagnosis of intermittent explosive disorder is essentially a diagnosis of exclusion, and the psychiatrist should evaluate and carefully rule out more common diagnoses that are associated with impulsive violence. The lifelong nonremitting history of impulsive aggression associated with antisocial personality disorder and borderline personality disorder, together with other features of antisocial behavior (in antisocial personality disorder) or impulsive behaviors in other spheres (in borderline personality disorder), may distinguish them from intermittent explosive disorder, in which baseline behavior and functioning are in marked contrast to the violent outbursts. Other features of borderline personality disorder such as unstable and intense interpersonal relationships, frantic efforts to avoid abandonment and identity disturbance may also be elicited by a careful history. More than in most psychiatric diagnoses, collateral information from an independent historian may be extremely helpful. This is especially true in forensic settings. Of note, patients with intermittent explosive disorder are usually genuinely distressed by their impulsive aggressive outbursts and may voluntarily seek psychiatric help to control them. In contrast, patients with antisocial personality disorder do not feel true remorse for their actions and view them as a problem only insofar as they suffer their consequences, such as incarceration and fines. Although patients with borderline personality disorder, like patients with intermittent explosive disorder, are often distressed by their impulsive actions, the rapid development of intense and unstable transference toward the psychiatrist during the evaluation period of patients with borderline personality disorder may be helpful in distinguishing it from intermittent explosive disorder.

Other causes of episodic impulsive aggression are substance use disorders, in particular alcohol abuse and intoxication. When the episodic impulsive aggression is associated only with intoxication, intermittent explosive disorder is ruled out. However, as discussed earlier, intermittent explosive disorder and alcohol abuse may be related, and the diagnosis of one should lead the psychiatrist to search for the other.

Neurological conditions, such as dementias, focal frontal lesions, partial complex seizures and postconcussion syndrome after recent head trauma, may all present as episodic impulsive aggression and need to be differentiated from intermittent explosive disorder. Other neurological causes of impulsive aggression include encephalitis, brain abscess, normal-pressure hydrocephalus, subarachnoid hemorrhage and stroke. In these instances, the diagnosis would be personality change due to a general medical condition, aggressive type, and it may be made with a careful history and the characteristic physical and laboratory findings.

Individuals with intermittent explosive disorder may have comorbid mood disorders. Although the diagnosis of a manic episode excludes intermittent explosive disorder, the evidence for serotonergic abnormalities in both major depressive disorder and impulse control disorders supports the clinical observation that impulsive aggression may be increased in depressed patients, leading ultimately to completed suicide.

Physical Examination and Laboratory Findings

The physical and laboratory findings relevant to the diagnosis of intermittent explosive disorder and the differential diagnosis of impulsive aggression may be divided into two main groups: those associated with episodic impulsive aggression but not diagnostic of a particular disorder and those that suggest the diagnosis of a psychiatric or medical disorder other than intermittent explosive disorder. No laboratory or physical findings are specific for intermittent explosive disorder.

The first group of findings that are associated with impulsive aggression across a spectrum of disorders includes soft neurological signs such as subtle impairments in hand–eye coordination and minor reflex asymmetries. These signs may be elicited by a comprehensive neurological examination and simple pencil-and-paper tests such as parts A and B of the Trail Making Test. Measures of central serotonergic function such as CSF 5-HIAA levels, the fenfluramine neuroendocrine challenge test, and positron emission tomography of prefrontal metabolism also belong to this group. Although these measures advanced our neurobiological understanding of impulsive aggression, their utility in the diagnosis of individual cases of intermittent explosive disorder and other disorders with impulsive aggression is yet to be demonstrated.

The second group of physical and laboratory findings is useful in the diagnosis of causes of impulsive aggression other than intermittent explosive disorder. The smell of alcohol on a patient's breath or a positive alcohol reading with a Breathalyzer may help reveal alcohol intoxication. Blood and urine toxicology screens may reveal the use of other substances, and track marks on the forearms may suggest intravenous drug use. Partial complex seizures and focal brain lesions may be evaluated by use of the EEG and brain imaging. In cases without a grossly abnormal neurological examination, magnetic resonance imaging may be more useful than computed tomography of the head. Magnetic resonance imaging can reveal mesiotemporal scarring, which may be the only evidence for a latent seizure disorder, sometimes in the presence of a normal or inconclusive EEG. Diffuse slowing on the EEG is a nonspecific finding that is probably more common in, but not diagnostic of, patients with impulsive aggression. Hypoglycemia, a rare cause of impulsive aggression, may be detected by blood chemistry screens.

Differential Diagnosis

As discussed earlier, the differential diagnosis of intermittent explosive disorder covers the differential diagnosis of impulsivity and aggressive behavior in general. Aggression and impulsivity are defined as follows:

> Aggression is defined as forceful physical or verbal action, which may be appropriate and self-protective or inappropriate as in hostile or destructive behavior. It may be directed against another person, against the environment, or toward the self. The psychiatric nosology of aggression is still preliminary. Impulsivity is defined as the tendency to act in a sudden, unpremeditated, and excessively spontaneous fashion.

The diagnosis of intermittent explosive disorder should be considered only after all other disorders that are associated with impulsivity and aggression have been ruled out. Chronic impulsivity and aggression may occur as part of a cluster B personality disorder (antisocial and borderline); during the course of substance use disorders and substance intoxication; in the setting of a general medical (usually neurological) condition; and as part of disorders first diagnosed during childhood and adolescence such as conduct disorder, oppositional defiant disorder, attention-deficit/hyperactivity disorder and mental retardation. In addition, impulsive aggression may appear during the course of a mood disorder, especially during a manic episode, which precludes the diagnosis of intermittent explosive disorder, and during the course of an agitated depressive episode. Impulsive aggression may also be an associated feature of schizophrenia, in which it may occur in response to hallucinations or delusions. Impulsive aggression may also appear in variants of OCD, which may present with concurrent impulsive and compulsive symptoms.

A special problem in the differential diagnosis of impulsive aggression, which may arise in forensic settings, is that it may represent purposeful behavior. Purposeful behavior is distinguished from intermittent explosive disorder by the presence of motivation and gain in the aggressive act, such as monetary gain, vengeance, or social dominance. Another diagnostic problem in forensic settings is malingering, in which individuals may claim to have intermittent explosive disorder to avoid legal responsibility for their acts.

Figure 60.2 presents the differential diagnosis of aggression.

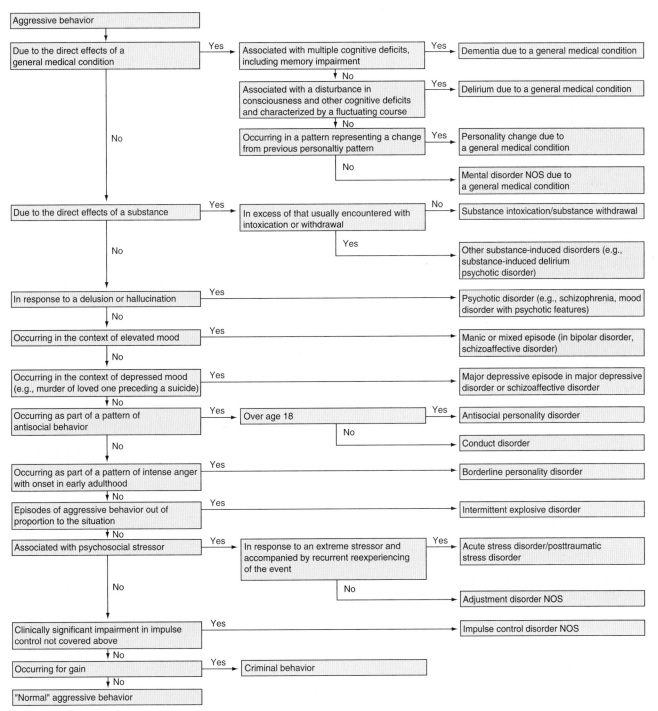

Figure 60.2 *Differential diagnosis of aggression. The psychiatric nosology of aggression has not been well worked out and requires much additional study. This is a particularly unfortunate state of affairs because the attribution (or misattribution) of aggression to a mental disorder is a frequent focus of forensic attention and can mean the difference between a life term in prison or a promotional tour for a bestseller. Because of the inherent difficulties in making these determinations, psychiatric testimony in this regard should be interpreted with caution. Other decision trees that may be of interest include those for catatonia; delusions; euphoria or irritability; disorganized, agitated, or unusual behavior; impulsivity; hallucinations; substance use and general medical condition.*

Epidemiology

Prevalence and Incidence

Intermittent explosive disorder has been subjected to little systematic study. The exclusionary criterion in the DSM-IV-TR definition (criterion C) reflects an ongoing debate over the boundaries of this disorder. In an early study of the prevalence of DSM-III-R intermittent explosive disorder among violent men, Felthous and colleagues (1991) found that of 443 subjects who complained of violence, only 15 (3.4%) met criteria for intermittent explosive disorder. However, the recently completed National Comorbidity Survey Replication (NCS-R) (Kessler *et al.*, 2005) found that intermittent explosive disorder (12 month prevalence 2.6%) was as nearly common as panic disorder (12 month prevalence 2.7%).

Comorbidity

The DSM-IV-TR definition of intermittent explosive disorder allows signs of generalized impulsivity or aggressiveness to be present between episodes. It also allows the psychiatrist to give an additional diagnosis of intermittent explosive disorder in the presence of another disorder if the episodes are not better accounted for by the other disorder. The clinical reality is that most individuals who have intermittent episodes of aggressive behavior also have some impulsivity between episodes and often present with other past or current psychiatric disorders. There is minimal research-based data available regarding comorbidity. But the literature on the comorbidity of impulsive aggressive episodes suggests that it often occurs with three classes of disorders:

1. Personality disorders, especially antisocial personality disorder and borderline personality disorder. By definition, antisocial personality disorder and borderline personality disorder are chronic and include impulsive aggression as an essential feature. Therefore, their diagnosis effectively excludes the diagnosis of intermittent explosive disorder (Figure 60.2).
2. A history of substance use disorders, especially alcohol abuse. A concurrent diagnosis of substance intoxication excludes the diagnosis of intermittent explosive disorder. However, many patients with intermittent explosive disorder report past or family histories of substance abuse, and in particular alcohol abuse. In light of evidence linking personal and family history of alcohol abuse with impulsive aggression and the evidence (reviewed later) linking both with low central serotonergic function, this connection may be clinically relevant. Therefore, when there is evidence suggesting that alcohol abuse may be present, a systematic evaluation of intermittent explosive disorder is warranted, and vice versa.
3. Neurological disorders, especially severe head trauma, partial complex seizures, dementias and inborn errors of metabolism. Intermittent explosive disorder is not diagnosed if the aggressive episodes are a direct physiological consequence of a general medical condition. Such cases would be diagnosed as personality change due to a general medical condition, delirium, or dementia. However, individuals with intermittent explosive disorder often have nonspecific findings on neurological examination, such as reflex asymmetries, mild hand–eye coordination deficits, and childhood histories of head trauma with or without loss of consciousness. Their EEGs may show nonspecific changes. Such isolated findings are compatible with the diagnosis of intermittent explosive disorder and preempt the diagnosis only when they are indicative of a definitely diagnosable general medical or neurological condition. Such "soft" neurological signs may be diagnosed by a full neurological examination and neuropsychological testing.

McElroy and coworkers (McElroy *et al.*, 1998; McElroy, 1999) studied 27 individuals who had symptoms that met criteria for intermittent explosive disorder (IED) and reported: "Twenty-five (93%) subjects had lifetime DSM-IV-TR diagnoses of mood disorders; 13 (48%), substance use disorders; 13 (48%), anxiety disorders; 6 (22%), eating disorders; and 12 (44%), an impulse control disorder other than intermittent explosive disorder. Subjects also displayed high rates of comorbid migraine headaches. First-degree relatives displayed high rates of mood, substance use, and impulse control disorders".

Some children with Tourette's disorder may be prone to rage attacks. The clinical manifestation of these rage attacks are similar to IED and may be more common among children with Tourette's who have comorbid mood disorders. On the basis of these observations, the rage attacks of these children may flow from an underlying dysregulation of brain function (Budman *et al.*, 2000).

Course, Natural History and Prognosis

Little systematic study has been done on the course of intermittent explosive disorder. The onset of the disorder appears to be from late adolescence to the third decade of life, and it may be abrupt and without a prodromal period. Intermittent explosive disorder is apparently chronic and may persist well into middle life unless treated successfully. In some cases, it may decrease in severity or remit completely with old age.

Treatment

Given the rarity of pure intermittent explosive disorder, it is not surprising that few systematic data are available on its response to treatment and that some of the recommended treatment approaches to intermittent explosive disorder are based on treatment studies of impulsivity and aggression in the setting of other mental disorders and general medical conditions. Thus, no standard regimen for the treatment of intermittent explosive disorder can be recommended at this time.

Psychological Treatment

Lion (1992) has described the major psychotherapeutic task of teaching individuals with intermittent explosive disorder how to recognize their own feeling states and especially the affective state of rage. Lack of awareness of their own mounting anger is presumed to lead to the build-up of intolerable rage that is then discharged suddenly and inappropriately in a temper outburst. Patients with intermittent explosive disorder are therefore taught how to first recognize and then verbalize their anger appropriately. In addition, during the course of insight-oriented psychotherapy, they are encouraged to identify and express the fantasies surrounding their rage. Group psychotherapy for temper-prone patients has also been described. The cognitive–behavioral model of psychological treatment may be usefully applied to problems with anger and rage management.

Somatic Treatments

Several classes of medications have been used to treat intermittent explosive disorder. The same medications have also been used to treat impulsive aggression in the context of other disorders. These included beta-blockers (propranolol and metoprolol), anticonvulsants (carbamazepine and valproic acid), lithium, antidepressants (tricyclic antidepressants and serotonin reuptake inhibitors) and antianxiety agents (lorazepam, alprazolam and buspirone). Mattes (1990) compared the effectiveness of two commonly used agents, carbamazepine and propranolol, for the treatment of rage outbursts in a heterogeneous group of patients. He found that although carbamazepine and propranolol were overall equally effective, carbamazepine was more effective in patients with intermittent explosive disorder and propranolol was more effective in patients with attention-deficit/hyperactivity disorder. A substantial body of evidence supports the use of propranolol – often in high doses – for impulsive aggression in patients with chronic psychotic disorders and mental retardation. Lithium has been shown to have antiaggressive properties and may be used to control temper outbursts. In patients with comorbid major depressive disorder, OCD, or cluster B and C personality disorders, SSRIs may be useful. Overall, in the absence of more controlled clinical trials, the best approach may be to tailor the psychopharmacological agent to coexisting psychiatric comorbidity. In the absence of comorbid disorders, carbamazepine, titrated to antiepileptic blood levels, may be used empirically.

Kleptomania

Definition

Kleptomania shares with all other impulse control disorders the recurrent failure to resist impulses. Unfortunately, in the absence of epidemiological studies, little is known about kleptomania. Clinical case series and case reports are limited. Family, neurobiological, and genetic investigations are not available. There are no established treatments of choice. Therefore, in reading this section the reader must keep in mind that much of what is described is based on limited data or on anecdotal information.

DSM-IV-TR Criteria 312.32

Kleptomania

A. Recurrent failure to resist impulses to steal objects that are not needed for personal use or for their monetary value.

B. Increasing sense of tension immediately before committing the theft.

C. Pleasure, gratification, or relief at the time of committing the theft.

D. The stealing is not committed to express anger or vengeance and is not in response to a delusion or a hallucination.

E. The stealing is not better accounted for by conduct disorder, a manic episode, or antisocial personality disorder.

Reprinted with permission from the *Diagnostic and Statistical Manual of Mental Disorders*, Fourth Edition, Text Revision. Copyright 2000 American Psychiatric Association.

Etiology and Pathophysiology

The etiology of kleptomania is essentially unknown, although various models have been proposed in an effort to conceptualize the disorder. The affective spectrum model suggests that kleptomania and other impulse control disorders may share a common underlying biological diathesis with other disorders, such as depression, panic disorder, OCD and bulimia nervosa (McElroy *et al.*, 1992; Hudson and Pope, 1990). In some individuals, kleptomania responds to treatment with thymoleptic agents or electroconvulsive therapy. These observations are cited as support for an affective spectrum model.

Several lines of evidence support kleptomania as belonging to the obsessive-compulsive spectrum disorders. First, there are phenomenological similarities between the classical obsessions and compulsions of OCD and the irresistible impulses and repetitive actions characteristic of kleptomania. In addition, there appears to be a greater than chance occurrence of OCD in probands with kleptomania and in their relatives. In addition, both conditions have significant comorbidity with mood, anxiety, substance use and eating disorders. However, OCD rituals are more clearly associated with relief of anxiety and harm avoidance, whereas kleptomanic acts seem to be associated with gratification or pleasure. In addition, OCD is associated with a clear preferential response to SSRIs as opposed to general thymoleptics. The limited treatment literature does not support a similar response pattern in kleptomania. Unfortunately, the role of the serotonergic or of any other neurotransmitter system has not been investigated in kleptomania. Interestingly, a large study found subjects with mixed anorexia and bulimia nervosa to have a higher lifetime prevalence of kleptomania than those with either anorexia or bulimia nervosa alone (Herzog *et al.*, 1992). This could suggest a relationship between kleptomania and both the obsessive–compulsive (anorexic) and affective (bulimic) spectrum.

Alternatively, kleptomania could be conceptualized as an addictive disorder. The irresistible impulse to steal is reminiscent of the urge and the high associated with drinking or using drugs. Marks (1990) has proposed a constellation of behavioral (i.e., nonchemical) addictions encompassing OCD, compulsive spending, gambling, binging, hypersexuality and kleptomania. This model postulates certain concepts thought to be common in all these disorders, such as craving, mounting tension, "quick fixing", withdrawal, external cuing and habituation. These components have not yet been well investigated in kleptomania.

It should be emphasized that the lack of neurobiological or prospective pharmacological treatment data for kleptomania limits any conclusions that can be drawn with regard to biological models.

A frequent theme, reported by numerous authors is that of kleptomania as an acting-out aimed at alleviating depressive symptoms. From a psychodynamic point of view, kleptomania has been viewed over the decades as a manifestation of a variety of unconscious conflicts, with sexual conflicts figuring prominently in the literature. Case reports have described conscious sexual gratification, sometimes accompanied by frank masturbation or orgasm during kleptomanic acts (Fishbain, 1987). Thus, it has been suggested, kleptomanic behavior serves to discharge a sexual drive that may have forbidden connotations similar to those of masturbation, and the stolen object itself may have unconscious symbolic or overt fetishistic significance. Although no systematic studies exist, there has long been an implication in the literature on kleptomania that those afflicted with kleptomania suffer disproportionately from a variety of sexual dysfunctions. Turnbull (1987) described six patients with a primary diagnosis of kleptomania, all of whom had dysfunctional sexual relationships with their partners, compulsive promiscuity, or anorgasmia.

Other cases of kleptomania have been understood as reflecting conflictual infantile needs and attempts at oral gratification, masochistic wishes to be caught and punished related to a harsh guilt-inducing superego or primitive aggressive strivings, penis envy or castration anxiety with the stolen object representing a penis, a defense against unwelcome passive homosexual longings, restitution of the self in the presence of narcissistic injuries, or the acquisition of transitional objects. One should probably conclude that the psychodynamics associated with kleptomania ought to be carefully tailored to the individual patient. The literature on kleptomania has frequently implicated disturbed childhoods, inadequate parenting and significant character disturbances in kleptomanic patients. From this perspective kleptomania can be more effectively understood in the context of an individual's overall character. Unfortunately, no clinical studies exist that systematically explore Axis II psychopathology in these patients.

Assessment and Differential Diagnosis

Phenomenology and Presentation

At presentation, the typical patient suffering from kleptomania is a 35-year-old woman who has been stealing for about 15 years and may not mention kleptomania as the presenting complaint or in the initial history. The patient may complain instead of anxiety, depression, lability, dysphoria, or manifestations of character pathology. There is often a history of a tumultuous childhood and poor parenting, and in addition acute stressors may be present, such as marital or sexual conflicts. The patient experiences the urge to steal as irresistible, and the thefts are commonly associated with a thrill, a high, a sense of relief, or gratification. Generally, the behavior has been hard to control and has often gone undetected by others. The kleptomania may be restricted to specific settings or types of objects, and the patient may or may not be able to describe rationales for these preferences. Quite often, the objects taken are of inherently little financial value, or have meaningless financial value relative to the income of the person who has taken the object. Additionally, the object may never actually be used. These factors often help distinguish theft from kleptomania. The theft is followed by feelings of guilt or shame and, sometimes, attempts at atonement. The frequency of stealing episodes may greatly fluctuate in concordance with the degree of depression, anxiety, or stress. There may be periods of complete abstinence. The patient may have a past history of psychiatric treatments including hospitalizations or of arrests and convictions, whose impact on future kleptomanic behavior can be variable.

Assessment

Generally, the diagnosis of kleptomania is not a complicated one to make. However, kleptomania may frequently go undetected because the patient may not mention it spontaneously and the psychiatrist may fail to inquire about it as part of the routine history. The index of suspicion should rise in the presence of commonly associated symptoms such as chronic depression, other impulsive or compulsive behaviors, tumultuous backgrounds, or unexplained legal troubles. It could convincingly be argued that a cursory review of compulsivity and impulsivity, citing multiple examples for the patient, should be a part of any thorough and complete psychiatric evaluation. In addition, it is important to make a careful differential diagnosis and pay attention to the

various exclusion criteria before diagnosing theft as kleptomania. Possible diagnoses of sociopathy, mania, or psychosis should be carefully considered. In this regard, the psychiatrist must inquire about the affective state of the patient during the episodes, the presence of delusions or hallucinations associated with the occurrence of the behavior, the motivation behind the stealing, and the fate and subsequent use of the objects.

Although the typical patient may be a 35-year-old woman, it is important to remember that men, children and elderly persons may present with or engage in kleptomania. Interestingly, men may first present for evaluation 15 years later than women. Kleptomania occurs transculturally and has been described in various Western and Eastern cultures. Asian observers have also noted an overlap with eating disorders (Lee, 1994). Atypical presentations should raise a greater suspicion of an organic etiology, and a medical evaluation is then indicated. Medical conditions that have been associated with kleptomania include cortical atrophy, dementia, intracranial mass lesions, encephalitis, normal-pressure hydrocephalus, benzodiazepine withdrawal and temporal lobe epilepsy. A complete evaluation when such suspicions are present includes a physical and neurological examination, general serum chemistry and hematological panels, and an EEG with temporal leads or computed tomography of the brain.

Epidemiology and Comorbidity

Prevalence and Incidence

No epidemiological studies of kleptomania have been conducted, and thus its prevalence can be calculated only grossly and indirectly. Despite the lack of valid epidemiological data, there is general agreement that kleptomania is more common among women than among men. However, women generally seek psychiatric help more frequently than men, whereas men are more likely to become involved with the penal system. Consequently, this may not reflect true gender distribution.

Comorbidity

Among individuals with kleptomania who present for treatment, there is a high incidence of comorbid mood, anxiety and eating disorders, when compared with rates in the general population. Comorbidity patterns among individuals who present for treatment may be greater than among random samples. More reliable comorbidity rates can be found in a prospective investigation of 20 individuals with kleptomania conducted by McElroy and coworkers (1991a). Lifetime DSM-III-R comorbidity rates were 40% major depressive disorder, 50% substance abuse, 40% panic disorder, 40% social phobia, 45% OCD, 30% anorexia nervosa, 60% bulimia nervosa and 40% other impulse control disorders. Dissociative symptoms, significant character pathology and trauma histories are commonly encountered among this group.

Course

In two separate studies, the mean age at onset of kleptomania was reported to be 20 years (Goldman, 1991; McElroy *et al.*, 1991a). The subjects included individuals who had begun stealing as early as 5 to 7 years of age. The disorder appears to be chronic, lasting for decades, albeit with varying intensity. Fifteen or 16 years may elapse before treatment is sought. Onset in and beyond the fifth decade of life appears to be unusual, and in some of these cases remote histories of past kleptomania can be elicited.

At peak frequency, McElroy and colleagues (1991a) found a mean of 27 episodes a month, essentially daily stealing, with one patient reporting four acts daily. The majority of patients may eventually be apprehended for stealing once or more, and a minority may even be imprisoned; more often than not these repercussions do not result in more than a temporary remission of the behavior. Individuals with kleptomania may also have extensive histories of psychiatric treatments, including hospitalization for other conditions, most commonly depression or eating disorders. Because of the unavailability of longitudinal studies, the prognosis is not known. It appears, however, that without treatment the behavior may be likely to persist for decades, sometimes with significant associated morbidity. There may be transient periods of remission.

Treatment

Treatment Goals

The general goal of treatment is the eradication of kleptomanic behavior. Treatment typically occurs in the outpatient setting, unless comorbid conditions such as severe depression, eating disturbances, or more dangerous impulsive behaviors dictate hospitalization. The interview must be conducted in a respectful climate that ensures confidentiality. Patients not only may experience considerable guilt or shame for stealing but also may be unrevealing because of the fear of legal repercussions. In the acute treatment phase, the aim is to decrease significantly or, ideally, eradicate episodes of stealing during a period of weeks to months. Concurrent conditions may compound the problem and require independently targeted treatment. The acute treatment of kleptomania has not been, to date, systematically investigated.

Psychiatrist–Patient Relationship

As with any condition that may be associated with intense guilt or shame, kleptomania must be approached respectfully by the psychiatrist. Patients can be reassured and their negative feelings alleviated to some degree with proper initial psychoeducation. The treatment alliance can be strengthened by consistently maintaining a nonjudgmental and supportive stance. In addition, patients' fears regarding breaks of confidentiality and criminal repercussions must be addressed.

No treatments have been systematically shown to be effective for kleptomania. These treatment recommendations are supported by case reports and retrospective reviews only. In general, it appears that thymoleptic medications and behavioral therapy may be the most efficacious treatments for the short term, whereas long-term psychodynamic psychotherapy may be indicated and have good results for selected patients.

Pharmacological and Somatic Treatments

Mixed results have been reported regarding the pharmacological treatment of kleptomania. In a literature review of 56 cases of kleptomania, McElroy and coworkers (1991b) noted that somatic treatments were described for eight patients. Significant improvement was reported for seven of these. Treatment included antidepressants alone, antidepressants combined with antipsychotics or stimulants, electroconvulsive therapy alone, or electroconvulsive therapy with antidepressants. It is still unclear whether kleptomania responds preferentially to serotonergic antidepressants, and this question awaits further study. Other agents reported to have

treated kleptomania successfully include nortriptyline and amitriptyline. In addition, it remains unclear if the antikleptomanic effect of thymoleptics is dependent on or independent of their antidepressant effect.

A number of other medications have been employed to treat kleptomania. These include antipsychotics, stimulants, valproic acid, carbamazepine, clonazepam and lithium. Lithium augmentation may be of benefit when kleptomania does not respond to an antidepressant alone. Finally, there have been some reports of successful treatment of kleptomania with electroconvulsive therapy, which may have been administered for a concurrent mood disorder.

Although little is known about maintenance pharmacological treatment for kleptomania, there is a suggestion in the literature that symptoms tend to recur with cessation of thymoleptic treatment and again remit when treatment is reinstituted.

Psychosocial Treatments

Formal studies of psychosocial interventions for kleptomania have not been performed. However, a number of clinical reports have supported behavioral therapy for kleptomania. The available clinical literature suggests that for most patients this may be a more efficacious approach than insight-oriented psychotherapy. Different behavioral techniques have been employed with some success, including aversive conditioning, systematic desensitization, covert sensitization and behavior modification. In their review of 56 reported cases of kleptomania, McElroy and colleagues (1991a) noted that the eight patients who were treated with behavioral therapy – mostly aversive conditioning – showed significant improvement. We give here some specific examples of behavioral techniques that have been successfully employed and described. One patient was taught to hold her breath as a negative reinforcer whenever she experienced an impulse to steal. Another patient was taught to use systematic desensitization techniques to control the mounting anxiety associated with the impulse to steal. A patient treated by covert sensitization learned to associate images of nausea and vomiting with the desire to steal. A woman who experienced sexual excitement associated with shoplifting and would masturbate at the site of the act was instructed to practice masturbation at home, while fantasizing kleptomanic acts. There is a suggestion in the literature that these techniques remain effective over the long term.

Finally, it appears that the most effective behavioral treatment of all may be complete abstinence, that is, the patient should no longer visit any of the stores or settings where kleptomanic acts occur. A number of patients who never come to psychiatric attention apparently employ this technique successfully, and it may be an appropriate treatment goal if it does not result in excessive restrictions of activity and lifestyle.

The psychodynamic treatment of kleptomania centers on the exploration and working through of the underlying conflict or conflicts. There are case reports in the literature of successful psychodynamic treatment of kleptomania. Such treatment, possibly in combination with other approaches, may be indicated for patients for whom a clear conflictual basis for the behavior can be formulated, who also have the needed insight and motivation to undertake this type of treatment. In proposing such treatments, which may be long term, the psychiatrist should consider whether there are immediate risks that must be addressed, such as a high risk of legal consequences.

Special Treatment Considerations

Little is known about treating kleptomania and therefore special treatment considerations have not been elucidated. However, it is clear that comorbid conditions, such as depression, bulimia nervosa, OCD, or substance abuse, must be addressed along with the kleptomania. In addition to the inherent suffering and morbidity of these other disorders, their course and severity could compound the kleptomanic behavior. In the rare cases of a precipitating or exacerbating organic etiology, the underlying organic cause must be treated. In addition, the treatment of particular groups such as children or the elderly should take into account special contributing life stage or situational factors. The involvement of family or others on whom the patient is dependent may be indicated.

Pyromania and Fire-setting Behavior

Definition

The primary characteristics of pyromania are recurrent, deliberate fire-setting, the experience of tension or affective arousal before the fire-setting, an attraction or fascination with fire and its contexts, and a feeling of gratification or relief associated with the setting of a fire or its aftermath.

   True pyromania is present in only a small subset of fire-setters. Multiple motivations are cited as causes for fire-setting behavior. These include arson for profit, crime concealment, revenge, vandalism and political expression. In addition, fire-setting may be associated with other psychiatric diagnoses. But true pyromania is rare.

   Fire-setting behavior may be a focus of clinical attention, even when criteria for pyromania are not present. Because the large majority of fire-setting events are not associated with true pyromania, this section also addresses fire-setting behavior in general.

Fire-setting as a Planned, Nonimpulsive Behavior

The following motivations have been suggested for intentional arson: financial reward, to conceal another crime, for political purposes, as a means of revenge, as a symptom of other (nonpyromania) psychiatric conditions (e.g., in response to a delusional belief), as attention-seeking behavior, as a means of deriving sexual satisfaction, and as an act of curiosity when committed by children. Revenge and anger appear to be the most common motivations for fire-setting.

Etiology and Pathophysiology

Arson has been the subject of several investigations of altered neuroamine function. These findings include the observation that platelet monoamine oxidase is negatively correlated with fire-setting behavior of adults who had been diagnosed with attention-deficit disorder in childhood. Investigation of the function of serotonergic neurotransmission in individuals with aggressive and violent behaviors has included studies of CSF concentrations of 5-HIAA in individuals with a history of fire-setting. 5-HIAA is the primary metabolite of serotonin, and its concentration in the CSF is a valid marker of serotonin function in the brain. Virkkunen and colleagues (1994) demonstrated that impulsive fire-setting was associated with low CSF concentrations of 5-HIAA. This finding was consistent with other observations associating impulsive behaviors with low CSF 5-HIAA levels (such as impulsive violence and impulsive suicidal behavior). A history of suicide attempt strongly predicts recidivism of arson.

Assessment and Differential Diagnosis

Presentation

The diagnosis of pyromania emphasizes the affective arousal, thrill, or tension preceding the act, as well as the feeling of tension relief or pleasure in witnessing the outcome. This is useful in distinguishing between pyromania and fire-setting elicited by other motives (i.e., financial gain, concealment of other crimes, political, arson related to other mental illness, revenge, attention seeking, erotic pleasure, part of conduct disorder).

   The onset of pyromania has been reported to occur as early as age 3 years, but the condition may initially present in adulthood. Because of the legal implications of fire-setting, individuals may not admit previous events, which may result in biased perceptions of the common age at onset. Men greatly outnumber women with the disorder. In children and adolescents, the most common elements are excitation caused by fires, enjoyment produced by fires, relief of frustration by fire-setting and expression of anger through fire-setting.

   Fire-setting behavior may be common among more impaired psychiatric patients. In a study of 191 nongeriatric patients in a psychiatric hospital who were admitted for other reasons, 26 had some form of fire-setting behavior (including threats). Of these, 70% had actually set fires. None had a diagnosis of true pyromania (Soltys, 1992).

The Psychiatric Interview

The interviewer must bear in mind that the circumstances of arson, whatever the motive, may pose legal and criminal problems for the individual. This may provide motivation to skew the reporting of events. Individuals who may be at risk for the legal consequences of fire-setting may be motivated to represent themselves as victims of psychiatric illness, hoping that a presumed psychiatric basis of the behavior may attenuate legal penalties. Therefore, the interviewer must maintain a guarded view of the information presented.

Epidemiology and Comorbidity

Prevalence and Incidence

No data are available on the prevalence or incidence of pyromania, but it is apparently uncommon. Although pyromania is a rare event, fire-setting behavior is common in the histories of psychiatric patients. Among children with psychiatric conditions, fire-setting behavior is apparently quite common.

Comorbidity

Limited data are available regarding individuals with pyromania. Reported data of comorbid diagnoses are generally derived from forensic samples and do not distinguish between criminally motivated fire-setters and compulsive fire-setters. Fire-setting behavior may be associated with other mental conditions. These include mental retardation, conduct disorder, alcohol and other substance use disorders personality disorders and schizophrenia.

Course

There are no data regarding the course of and prognosis for pyromania. However, the impulsive nature of the disorder suggests a repetitive pattern. Again, because legal consequences may occur, the individual may be motivated to represent the index episode as a unique event. Fire-setting for nonpsychiatric reasons may be more likely to be a single event.

Treatment

Treatment Goals

Because of the danger inherent in fire-setting behavior, the primary goal is elimination of the behavior. The treatment literature does not distinguish between pyromania and fire-setting behavior of other causes. Much of the literature is focused on controlling fire-setting behavior in children and adolescents.

Psychiatrist–Patient Relationship

Because of the potential legal risks for individuals who acknowledge fire-setting behavior, the psychiatrist must take particular pains to ensure an environment of empathy and confidentiality. A corollary concern involves obligations that may be incumbent on the psychiatrist. Because of the legal implications of these behaviors and the potential for harm to another individual should fire-setting recur, the psychiatrist should be careful to consider both the ethical and the legal constraints that may follow from information learned in the course of treatment.

Pharmacotherapy and Psychosocial Treatments

There are no reports of pharmacological treatment of pyromania. It has been estimated that up to 60% of childhood fire-setting is motivated by curiosity. Such behavior often responds to direct educational efforts. In children and adolescents, focus on interpersonal problems in the family and clarification of events preceding the behavior may help to control the behavior. The treatments described for fire-setting are largely behavioral or focused on intervening in family or intrapersonal stresses that may precipitate episode of fire-setting.

One technique combines overcorrection, satiation and negative practice with corrective consequences. The child is supervised in constructing a controlled, small fire in a safe location. The fire is then extinguished by the child. Throughout the process, the parent verbally instructs the child in safety techniques.

The graphing technique has been used as the basis of several intervention programs with fire-setters. The psychiatrist and the patient agree on a goal of stopping the fire-setting behavior. The psychiatrist and the patient construct a graph that details the events, feelings and behaviors associated with fire-setting episodes. These factors are described on a chronological line graph. The graph is utilized to help the patient see the cause-and-effect relationships between personal events, feelings and subsequent behaviors. The specific intent is to educate patients so that they are able to identify the events that put them at risk for fire-setting. Then patients are equipped to label the feelings as a signal that may allow them to use alternative modes for discharging their feelings. This technique may help the individual curtail other maladaptive behaviors as well. Follow-up reports suggest that individuals who have successfully completed a graphing intervention may be at substantially lower risk for future fire-setting.

Relaxation training may be used (or added to graphing techniques) to assist in the development of alternative modes of dealing with the stress that may precede fire-setting. Principles of cognitive–behavioral therapy have been recently applied to childhood fire-setting.

Pathological Gambling

Definition

Gambling as a behavior is common. Current estimates suggest that approximately 80% of the adult population in the US gamble. The amount of money wagered legally in the USA grew from $17 billion in 1974 to $210 billion in 1988, an increase of more than 1200%, making gambling the fastest growing industry in America. DSM-IV-TR covertly recognized the ubiquity of gambling behavior and the desire to gamble by the careful wording of criterion A for pathological gambling: "Persistent and recurrent maladaptive gambling behavior as indicated by five (or more) of the following". This definition of pathological gambling differs from some other definitions of impulse control disorders not elsewhere classified, which are worded as "Failure to resist an impulse to". This difference implies that neither gambling behavior nor failure to resist an impulse to engage in it is viewed as pathological in and of itself. Rather, the maladaptive nature of the gambling behavior is the essential feature of pathological gambling and defines it as a disorder.

Etiology and Pathophysiology

Pathological gambling has been included as a disorder of impulse control. Pathological gambling can also be viewed as an addictive disorder, an affective spectrum disorder and an obsessive–compulsive spectrum disorder. DSM-IV-TR maintains a close relationship between pathological gambling and addictive disorders in that several of the diagnostic criteria for pathological gambling were intentionally made to resemble criteria for substance dependence.

The parallels between pathological gambling and addictive disorders are manifold. Pathological gambling has been viewed as the "pure" addiction, because it involves several aspects of addictive behavior without the use of a chemical substance. The parallels between substance dependence, in particular alcohol dependence and pathological gambling have led to the successful

Pathological Gambling

A. Persistent and recurrent maladaptive gambling behavior as indicated by five (or more) of the following:

   (1) is preoccupied with gambling (e.g., preoccupied with reliving past gambling experiences, handicapping or planning the next venture, or thinking of ways to get money with which to gamble)

   (2) needs to gamble with increasing amounts of money in order to achieve the desired excitement

   (3) has repeated unsuccessful efforts to control, cut back, or stop gambling

   (4) is restless or irritable when attempting to cut down or stop gambling

   (5) gambles as a way of escaping from problems or of relieving a dysphoric mood (e.g., feelings of helplessness, guilt, anxiety, depression)

   (6) after losing money gambling, often returns another day to get even ("chasing" one's losses)

   (7) lies to family members, therapist, or others to conceal the extent of involvement with gambling

   (8) has committed illegal acts such as forgery, fraud, theft, or embezzlement to finance gambling

   (9) has jeopardized or lost a significant relationship, job, or educational or career opportunity because of gambling

   (10) relies on others to provide money to relieve a desperate financial situation caused by gambling

B. The gambling behavior is not better accounted for by a manic episode.

Reprinted with permission from the *Diagnostic and Statistical Manual of Mental Disorders*, Fourth Edition, Text Revision. Copyright 2000 American Psychiatric Association.

adoption of the self-help group model of Alcoholics Anonymous to Gamblers Anonymous. Patterns of comorbidity also suggest a possible link between pathological gambling and addictions, in particular alcoholism. In addition to the comorbidity of pathological gambling and substance use disorders, family studies have demonstrated a familial clustering of alcoholism and pathological gambling. As high as 50% of patients with pathological gambling have a parent with alcoholism and a family history of substance dependence in patients with pathological gambling. There is also a greater prevalence of pathological gambling in parents of patients with pathological gambling.

The links between pathological gambling and affective disorders are also supported by family studies that demonstrate high rates of affective disorders in first-degree relatives of patients with pathological gambling as well as by high rates of comorbidity of pathological gambling and affective disorders. In addition, as noted by many authors and incorporated in the DSM-IV-TR criteria for pathological gambling, many patients with pathological gambling gamble as a way of relieving dysphoric moods

(criterion A5), and cessation of gambling may be associated with depressive episodes in the majority of recovering gamblers.

The links between pathological gambling and obsessive spectrum disorders are less clear. Although a popular name for pathological gambling is compulsive gambling, the vast majority of patients with pathological gambling do not experience the urge to gamble as egodystonic until late in the course of their illness, after they have suffered some of its consequences. The rates of comorbidity of pathological gambling and OCD and obsessive–compulsive personality disorder are not nearly as high as the rates of comorbidity of pathological gambling and affective and addictive disorders. Nevertheless, pathological gambling shares several characteristics with compulsions: it is repetitive, often has ritualized aspects, and is meant to relieve or reduce distress. Moreover, sporadic reports on the effectiveness of SSRIs in the treatment of pathological gambling suggest a possible link to obsessive spectrum disorders (Hollander *et al.*, 1992).

Neurotransmitter Function in Pathological Gambling

The as sociation between altered function of the serotonin neurotransmitter system and impulsive behaviors has focused attention on a potential role for serotonin function in the neurophysiology of pathological gambling. Several studies have provided data supporting such a link. However, direct measure of cerebrospinal fluid 5-HIAA in pathological gamblers has yielded mixed results. Preliminary data supports potential utility of serotonin reuptake inhibitor medications in the treatment of pathological gambling.

Genetic Contribution

The incidence of pathological gambling among first degree family members of pathological gamblers appears to be approximately 20%. Inherited factors may explain 62% of variance in the diagnosis and some of these genetic factors may also contribute to the risk for conduct disorder, antisocial personality disorder and alcohol abuse (Eisen *et al.*, 2001). At this time, early molecular genetics studies of pathological gamblers point to possible associated polymorphisms in genes that code for both serotonergic and dopaminergic factors (Ibanez *et al.*, 2002).

Psychodynamic Considerations

Psychoanalytic theories of gambling were the first systematic attempts to account for pathological gambling. Erotization of the fear, tension and aggression involved in gambling behavior, as well as themes of grandiosity and exhibitionism, were explored by several authors during the first quarter of the 20th century. Freud (1961), in his influential essay on Dostoyevsky, suggested that the pathological gambler actually gambled to lose, not to win, and traced the roots of the disorder to the ambivalence felt by the young man toward his father. The father, the object of his love, is not only loved but also hated, and this results in unconscious guilt. The gambler then loses to punish himself, in what Freud labeled "moral masochism". Freud also spoke of "feminine masochism" in which losing is a way of gaining love from the father, who will somehow reward the loser for loyalty. To lose is to suffer, and for the feminine masochist, suffering equals love. Interestingly, in the later spirit of DSM-IV-TR, Freud also conceptualized pathological gambling as an addiction and included it in a triad with alcoholism and drug dependence. He saw all three as manifestations of that primary addiction, masturbation, or at least masturbatory fantasies. Like most researchers after him, Freud focused only on male gamblers.

Bergler, a psychoanalyst who actually treated many patients with pathological gambling, expanded on Freud's idea that the pathological gambler gambles to lose. He traced the roots of this desire to lose to the rebellion of gamblers against the authority of their parents and against the parents' intrusive introduction of the reality principle into their lives. The rebellion causes guilt, and the guilt creates the need for self-punishment. Bergler thought that the gambler's characteristic aggression is actually pseudoaggression, a craving for defeat and rejection. He saw the gambler as one who perpetuates an adversarial relationship with the world. The dealer in the casino, the gambler's opponents at the card table, the stock exchange and the roulette wheel are all unconsciously identified with the refusing mother or the rejecting father. Overall, psychoanalytic approaches to pathological gambling (Lesieur and Rosenthal, 1991) generally conceptualized it as either a compulsive neurosis (Freud, Bergler, Rosenthal) or an impulse disorder. Several published case reports documented the successful treatment of pathological gambling by psychoanalysis.

Learning theories of pathological gambling focus on the learned and conditioned aspects of gambling and use the quantifiable nature of the behavior to test specific hypotheses. One hypothesis was that patients with pathological gambling crave the excitement and tension associated with their gambling, as evidenced by the fact that they are much more likely to place last-second wagers than are low-frequency gamblers, to prolong their excitement. Higher wagers placed by patients with pathological gambling also produce greater excitement, and greater amounts of money are required to achieve the same "buzz" over time, an observation incorporated in the diagnostic criteria for pathological gambling (criterion A2).

Assessment and Differential Diagnosis

It is not difficult to diagnose pathological gambling once one has the facts. It is much more of a challenge to elicit the facts, because the vast majority of patients with pathological gambling view their gambling behavior and gambling impulses as egosyntonic and may often lie about the extent of their gambling (criterion A7). Patients with pathological gambling may first seek medical or psychological attention because of comorbid disorders. Given the high prevalence of addictive disorders in pathological gambling and the increased prevalence of pathological gambling in those with alcoholism and other substance abuse, an investigation of gambling patterns and their consequences is warranted for any patient who presents with a substance abuse problem. Likewise, the high rates of comorbidity with mood disorders suggest the utility of investigating gambling patterns of patients presenting with an affective episode.

The spouses and significant others of patients with pathological gambling deserve special attention. Individuals with pathological gambling usually feel entitled to their behavior and often rely on their families to bail them out (criterion A10). As a consequence, it is often the spouse of the patient with pathological gambling who first realizes the need for treatment and who bears the consequences of the disorder. Lorenz (1981) conducted a survey of 103 wives of pathological gamblers who attended Gam-Anon meetings (for family members of patients with pathological gambling). She found that most spouses had to borrow money and were harassed or threatened by bill collectors. Most spouses physically assaulted the gambler, verbally abused their children, and experienced murderous or destructive impulses toward the gambler. Although the gamblers themselves

appeared less violent than the general population norms, their spouses were more violent, possibly because of desperation and anger. Eleven percent of the spouses of patients with pathological gambling admitted to having attempted suicide, and this result was replicated in a later study. These findings have two main implications for the assessment of pathological gambling: first, the spouse may be a valuable and motivated informant who should be questioned about the patient's behavior, and secondly, spouses should be specifically asked about the effects of the patient's illness on their own well-being and functioning and about suicidal ideation and attempts and the control of their own impulsivity.

An important and understudied area is the clinical presentation of pathological gambling in women. Women constitute a third of all patients with pathological gambling in epidemiological studies. However, they are extremely underrepresented in treatment populations, and most psychoanalytic theories of pathological gambling ignore them completely. Part of this bias may be due to the fact that gambling carries a greater social stigma for women, that women gamblers are more likely to live and to gamble alone, and that treatment programs for pathological gambling in the USA were first pioneered in Veterans Hospitals. Compared with men with pathological gambling, women with pathological gambling are more likely to be depressed and to gamble as an escape rather than because of a craving for action and excitement. Pathological gambling begins at a later age in female than in male gamblers, often after adult roles have been established. Big winning is usually less important than the need to impress. Women typically play less competitive forms of gambling in which luck is more important than skill, and they play alone. Their progression into the disorder is often more rapid, and the time between the onset of the disorder and the time they present for treatment is usually much shorter than for men (3 years compared with 20 years). The shorter duration makes for a better prognosis in treatment, but, unfortunately, few of the women with pathological gambling ever come to treatment.

The differential diagnosis of pathological gambling is relatively simple. Pathological gambling should be differentiated from professional gambling, social gambling and a manic episode. Social gambling, engaged in by the vast majority of adult Americans, typically occurs with friends or colleagues, lasts for a specified time, and is limited by predetermined acceptable losses. Professional gambling is practiced by highly skilled and disciplined individuals and involves carefully limited risks. Many individuals with pathological gambling may feel that they are actually professional gamblers. Chasing behavior and unplanned losses distinguish the pathological gamblers. Patients in a manic episode may exhibit a loss of judgment and excessive gambling resulting in financial disasters. A diagnosis of pathological gambling should be given only if a history of maladaptive gambling behavior exists at times other than during a manic episode. Problems with gambling may also occur in individuals with antisocial personality disorder. If criteria are met for both disorders, both can be diagnosed.

Epidemiology and Comorbidity

Prevalence and Incidence

Pathological gambling is considered to be the most common of the impulse control disorders not elsewhere classified. The number of people whose gambling behavior meets criteria for pathological gambling in the USA is estimated to be between 2 million and 6 million. Surveys conducted between 1986 and 1990 in Maryland,

Massachusetts, New York, New Jersey and California estimated the prevalence of "probable pathological gamblers" among the adult population to be between 1.2 and 2.3%. These states have a broad range of legal wagering opportunities and a heterogeneous population. Similar surveys in Minnesota and Iowa, states with limited legal wagering opportunities and more homogeneous populations, yielded prevalence rates of 0.9 and 0.1%, respectively. It thus appears that availability of gambling opportunities as well as demographic make-up may influence the prevalence of pathological gambling. The combined total of "pathological gamblers" and "problem gamblers" is 5.5 million adult Americans. During the past 20 years, many states have turned to lotteries as a way of increasing their revenues without increasing taxes. At this time, some form of gambling is legal in 47 of the 50 states, as well as in more than 90 countries worldwide. From 1975 to 1999 revenues from legal gambling in the USA has risen from $3 to 58 billion. (Given the dramatic increase in the amounts of money wagered in legal gambling activities during the past 20 years, the prevalence and incidence of pathological gambling are expected to increase.)

It is estimated that women make-up to one-third of all Americans with pathological gambling. Nevertheless, they are underrepresented in Gamblers Anonymous, in which only 2 to 4% of the members are women. The reason for this discrepancy was postulated to be the greater social stigma attached to pathological gambling in women and the characteristic pattern of solitary gambling in women. Nonwhites and those with less than a high school education are more highly represented among pathological gamblers than in the general population. The demographic make-up of patients in treatment for pathological gambling differs substantially from the demographics of all patients with pathological gambling. Jewish persons are overrepresented in treatment settings and in Gamblers Anonymous, whereas women, minorities and those younger than age 30 years are underrepresented in Gamblers Anonymous and in treatment.

Comorbidity

Overall, patients with pathological gambling have high rates of comorbidity with several other psychiatric disorders and conditions. Individuals presenting for clinical treatment of pathological gambling apparently have impressive rates of comorbidity. Ibanez and coworkers (2001) reported 62.3% of one group seeking treatment had a comorbid psychiatric disorder. The most frequent diagnosis they found were personality disorders (42%), alcohol abuse or dependence (33.3%) and adjustment disorders (17.4%).

Mood Disorders

There is evidence for extensive comorbidity of pathological gambling with major depressive disorder and with bipolar disorder. In several surveys, between 70 and 80% of all patients with pathological gambling also had mood symptoms that met criteria for a major depressive episode, a manic episode, or a hypomanic episode at some point in their life. More than 50% had recurrent major depressive episodes. A complicating factor is that recovering pathological gamblers may experience depressive episodes after cessation of gambling. In addition, some patients with pathological gambling may gamble to relieve feelings of depression (criterion A5). Despite criterion B for pathological gambling, which essentially precludes the diagnosis of pathological gambling if the behavior occurs exclusively during the course of a manic episode, many patients have a disturbance that meets criteria for both disorders because they gamble both during and between manic and hypomanic episodes. Between 32 and 46% of patients with pathological gambling were reported also to have mood symptoms that meet criteria for bipolar disorder, bipolar II disorder, or cyclothymic disorder.

Suicide

Although data is not yet conclusive, a meaningful association between problem gambling and suicidal behavior and/or ideation appears to exist. Between 12 and 24% of patients with pathological gambling in various settings have had a history of at least one suicide attempt. In one study, 80% of patients with pathological gambling had a history of either suicide attempts or suicidal ideation (Lesieur and Rosenthal, 1991).

Substance Abuse and Dependence

Studies of prevalence of comorbid substance use disorders yield widely varying results; from 9.9% for alcohol and other substance dependence to 44% for alcohol dependence and 40% for illicit drug dependence. Using a structured instrument, between 5 and 25% of substance-abusing patients in several settings were found to meet criteria for pathological gambling and an additional 10 to 15% were considered to have "gambling problems" (Lesieur and Rosenthal, 1991). Among individuals with pathological gambling, individuals with higher socioeconomic status (SES) are more likely to have concurrent problems with alcohol abuse than are gamblers with lower SES.

Other Disorders

Again, current data are inconclusive, but OCD, panic disorder, generalized anxiety disorder and eating disorders have all been reported present in higher rates in patients with pathological gambling than in the general population. The reported prevalence of OCD among pathological gamblers ranges from 0.9 to 16%. Narcissistic and antisocial personality disorders are believed to be overrepresented in patients with pathological gambling, and pathological narcissism is assumed by some psychoanalysts to underlie the entitlement displayed by many patients with pathological gambling. In addition, retrospective studies suggest that many patients with pathological gambling may have had symptoms that met criteria for attention-deficit/hyperactivity disorder as children. In addition to psychiatric disorders, patients with pathological gambling may manifest greater prevalences of stress-related medical conditions, like peptic ulcer disease, hypertension and migraine.

Course

Pathological gambling usually begins in adolescence in men and later in life in women. The onset is usually insidious, although some individuals may be "hooked" by their first bet. There may be years of social gambling with minimal or no impairment followed by an abrupt onset of pathological gambling that may be precipitated by greater exposure to gambling or by a psychosocial stressor. The gambling pattern may be regular or episodic, and the course of the disorder tends to be chronic. Over time, there is usually a progression in the frequency of gambling, the amounts wagered, and the preoccupation with gambling and with obtaining money with which to gamble. The urge to gamble and gambling activity generally increase during periods of stress or depression, as an attempted escape or relief (criterion A5). Rosenthal (1992) described four typical phases in the course of a typical male patient with pathological gambling: winning, losing, desperation and hopelessness.

Typical Phases

Winning Many male gamblers become involved with gambling because they are good at it and receive recognition for their early successes. Women with pathological gambling are less likely to have a winning phase. Traits that foster a winning phase and are typical of male patients with pathological gambling are competitiveness, high energy, ability with numbers and interest in the strategy of games. The early winnings lead to a state in which a large proportion of the gambler's self-esteem derives from gambling, with accompanying fantasies of winning and spectacular success.

Losing A string of bad luck or a feeling that losing is intolerable may be the precipitant of chasing behavior; previous gambling strategies are abandoned as the gambler attempts to win back everything all at once. The gambler experiences a state of urgency, and bets become more frequent and heavy. Debts accumulate, and only the most essential are paid. Covering up and lying about gambling become more frequent. As this is discovered, relationships with family members deteriorate. Losing gamblers use their own and their family's money, go through savings, take out loans and finally exhaust all legitimate sources. Eventually, they cannot borrow any more, and faced with threats from creditors or loss of a job or marriage, they go to their family and finally confess. This results in the "bailout": debts are paid in return for a promise to stop or cut down gambling. Any remission, if achieved at all, is short-lived. After the bailout there is an upsurge of omnipotence; the gambler believes that it is possible to get away with anything, bets more heavily and loses control altogether.

Desperation This stage is reached when the gambler begins to do things that would previously be inconceivable: writing bad checks, stealing from an employer, or other illegal activities. Done once, these behaviors are much more likely to be repeated. The behavior is rationalized as a short-term loan with an intention to pay it back as soon as the winning streak arrives. The gambler feels just one step away from winning and solving all the problems. Attention is increasingly taken up with illegal loans and various scams to make money. The gambler becomes irritable and quick tempered. When reminded of responsibilities or put in touch with guilt feelings, the gambler responds with anger and projective blame. Appetite and sleep deteriorate and life holds little pleasure. A common fantasy at this stage is of starting life over with a new name and identity, the ultimate "clean slate".

Hopelessness For some gamblers, there is a fourth stage in which they suddenly realize that they can never get even, but they no longer care. This is often a revelation, and the precise moment when it occurred is often remembered. From this point on, just playing is all that matters. Gamblers often acknowledge knowing in advance that they will lose and play sloppily so that they lose even if they have the right horse or a winning hand. They seek action or excitement for its own sake and gamble to the point of exhaustion.

Few gamblers seek help in the winning phase. Most seek help only during the later phases and only after a friend, family member, or employer has intervened. Two-thirds of the gamblers have committed illegal activities by then, and the risk of suicide increases as the gambler progresses through the phases of the illness.

Prognosis

Without treatment, the prognosis of pathological gambling is poor. It tends to run a chronic course with increasing morbidity and comorbidity, gradual disruption of family and work roles and relationships, depletion of financial reserves, entanglement with criminals and the criminal justice system and, often, suicide attempts. In the hands of an experienced psychiatrist, it is an "extremely treatable disorder" with a favorable prognosis (Rosenthal, 1992). The difference between a poor and a good prognosis depends on treatment, and treatment depends on a diagnosis. As noted earlier, the diagnosis of pathological gambling is often missed in clinical settings because mental health professionals do not think to ask about it. Because most patients with pathological gambling do not see themselves as having a disorder and many of them do not even consider themselves as having a problem with gambling, collateral information from a family member may be extremely helpful.

Treatment

Overall Goals of Treatment

The goals of treatment of an individual with pathological gambling are the achievement of abstinence from gambling, rehabilitation of the damaged family and work roles and relationships, treatment of comorbid disorders and relapse prevention. This approach echoes the goals of treatment of an individual with substance dependence. Inpatient treatment in specialized programs may be considered if the gambler is unable to stop gambling, lacks significant family or peer support, or is suicidal, acutely depressed, multiply addicted, or contemplating some dangerous activity.

No standard treatment of pathological gambling has emerged. Despite many reports of behavioral and cognitive interventions for pathological gambling, there are minimal data available from well-designed or clearly detailed treatment studies. Pharmacologic treatments offer promise, but research-guided approaches are still insufficient to offer a standardized approach. Therefore, general approaches, based in clinical experience and available resources (such as Gamblers Anonymous or other support groups) should be considered.

The treatment of pathological gambling may consist of participation in Gamblers Anonymous, individual therapy, family therapy, treatment of comorbid disorders and medication treatment. As is the case for substance dependence, the gambler needs to be abstinent to be accessible to any or all of these treatment modalities. For many gamblers, participation in Gamblers Anonymous is sufficient, and it is an essential part of most treatment plans. Gamblers Anonymous is a 12-step group built on the same principles as Alcoholics Anonymous. It utilizes empathic confrontation by peers who struggle with the same impulses and a group approach. Gam-Anon is a peer support group for family members of patients with pathological gambling. Extensive data are lacking, but overall Gamblers Anonymous appears somewhat less effective than Alcoholics Anonymous in achieving and maintaining abstinence.

Individual therapy is often useful as an adjunct to Gamblers Anonymous. Rosenthal (1992) stressed that to maintain abstinence and use Gamblers Anonymous successfully, many gamblers need to understand why they gamble. Therapy involves confronting and teasing out the vicissitudes of the patient's sense of omnipotence and dealing with the various self-deceptions, the defensive aspects of the patient's lying, boundary issues, and problems involving magical thinking and reality. Relapse prevention involves knowledge and avoidance of specific triggers. In addition to psychodynamic therapy, behavioral treatment of pathological gambling has been proposed, with imagined desensitization achieving better rates of remission than aversive conditioning.

The greatest differences between the treatment of pathological gambling and other addictions are in the area of family therapy. Because relapse may be difficult to detect (there is no substance to be smelled on the patient's breath, no dilated or constricted pupils, no slurred speech or staggered gait) and because of a long history of exploitative behavior by the patient, the spouse and other family members tend to be more suspicious of, and angry at, the patient with pathological gambling compared with families of alcoholic patients. Frequent family sessions are often essential to offer the gambler an opportunity to make amends, learn communication skills and deal with preexisting intimacy problems. In addition, the spouse and other family members have often acquired their own psychiatric illnesses during the course of the patient's pathological gambling and need individualized treatment to recover.

Medication

Although research reports of the pharmacological treatment of pathological gambling have begun to emerge, there are still, as yet, insufficient data to come to any conclusions about the utility of medication. Small trials have reported on the use of SSRIs, mood stabilizers and naltrexone with the recommendation of dosing at the high end of usual treatment ranges.

Trichotillomania

Definition

The essential feature of trichotillomania is the recurrent failure to resist impulses to pull out one's own hair. Resulting hair loss may range in severity from mild (hair loss may be negligible) to severe (complete baldness and involving multiple sites on the scalp or body). Individuals with this condition do not want to engage in the behavior, but attempts to resist the urge result in great tension. Thus, hair-pulling is motivated by a desire to reduce this dysphoric state. In some cases, the hair-pulling results in a pleasurable sensation, in addition to the relief of tension. Tension may precede the act or may occur when attempting to stop. Distress over the symptom and the resultant hair loss may be severe.

Etiology and Pathophysiology

The etiology of trichotillomania is unknown. The phenomenological similarities between trichotillomania and OCD have prompted speculations that the pathophysiology of the two conditions may be related. The apparent association between altered serotonergic function and OCD has guided attention toward the possible role of serotonergic function in the underlying cause of trichotillomania. Thus, interest has been spurred in examining serotonergic function in patients with trichotillomania. As yet, however, only limited laboratory investigations have emerged.

In summary, few data are available to support any particular model of the etiological pathophysiology of trichotillomania. Early studies point to some alteration of brain activity. Inconsistent support has been found in these early explorations for a relationship with OCD.

Assessment and Differential Diagnosis

Presentation

Typically, the person complaining of unwanted hair-pulling is a young adult or the parent of a child who has been seen pulling out hair. Hair-pulling tends to occur in small bursts that may last minutes to hours. Such episodes may occur once or many times each day. Hairs are pulled out individually and may be pulled out rapidly and indiscriminately. Often, however, the hand of the individual may roam the afflicted area of scalp or body, searching for a shaft of hair that may feel particularly coarse or thick. Satisfaction with having pulled out a complete hair (shaft and root) is frequently expressed. Occasionally the experience of hair-pulling is described as quite pleasurable. Some individuals experience an itch-like sensation in the scalp that is eased by the act of pulling. The person may then toss away the hair shaft or inspect it. A substantial number of people then chew or consume (trichophagia) the hair. Hair-pulling is most commonly limited to the eyebrows and eyelashes. The scalp is the next most frequently afflicted site. However, hairs in any location of the body may be the focus of hair-pulling urges, including facial, axillary, chest, pubic and even perineal hairs.

Anxiety is almost always associated with the act of hair-pulling. Such anxiety may occur in advance of the hair-pulling behavior. A state of tension may occur spontaneously, driving the person to pull out hair in an attempt to reduce dysphoric feelings. Varying lengths of time must pass before the tension abates. Consequently, the amount of hair that may be extracted in an episode varies from episode to episode and from person to person. Frequently, hair-pulling begins automatically and without conscious awareness. In such circumstances, individuals discover themselves pulling out hairs after some have already been pulled out. In these situations, dysphoric tension is associated with the attempt to stop the behavior.

Circumstances that seem to predispose to episodes of hair-pulling include both states of stress and, paradoxically, moments of particular relaxation. Frequently hair-pulling occurs when at-risk individuals are engaged in a relaxing activity that promotes distraction and ease (e.g., watching television, reading, talking on the phone). It is common for hair-pullers to report that the behavior does not occur in the presence of other people. A frequent exception may be that many pull hair in the presence of members of the nuclear family.

Some individuals have urges to pull hairs from other people and may sometimes try to find opportunities to do so surreptitiously (such as initiating bouts of play fighting). There have been reports of affected individuals pulling hairs from pets, dolls, and other fibrous materials, such as sweaters or carpets.

The distress that usually accompanies trichotillomania varies in severity. Concerns tend to focus on the social and vocational consequences of the behavior. Themes of worry include fear of exposure, a feeling that "something is wrong with me", anxiety about intimate relationships and sometimes inability to pursue a vocation. Because certain kinds of work, such as reading and writing at a desk, seem to precipitate episodes of hair-pulling, some afflicted individuals make career choices based on the avoidance of desk work. Leisure activities that may involve a risk of exposure (ranging from gymnastics class to sexual intimacy) may be avoided.

Patterns of hair-pulling behavior among children are less well described. Usually, the parent observes a child pulling out hair and may note patches of hair loss. Children may sometimes be unaware of the behavior or may, at times, deny it. Childhood trichotillomania has been reported to be frequently associated with thumb-sucking or nail-biting. It has been suggested that trichotillomania with onset in early childhood may occur frequently with spontaneous remissions. Consequently, some have recommended that trichotillomania in early childhood may be considered a benign habit with a self-limited course. However, many individuals who present with chronic trichotillomania in adulthood report onset in early childhood.

Assessment

In general, the diagnosis of trichotillomania is not complicated. The essential symptom – recurrently pulling out hair in response to unwanted urges – is easily described by the patient. When the patient acknowledges the hair-pulling behavior and areas of patchy hair loss are evident, the diagnosis is not usually in doubt. Problems in diagnosis may arise when the diagnosis is suspected but the patient denies it. Such denial may occur in younger individuals and some adults. When the problem is suspected but denied by the patient, a skin biopsy from the affected area may aid in making the diagnosis.

The Psychiatric Interview

The psychiatrist should carefully inquire into the nature of the distress and concerns that may be present in a person with this problem. Although the cosmetic impact may appear slight, distress may be severe. Concerns about disclosure, anticipation of social rejection and concerns about limitations in career choices are frequent and may result in chronic dysphoria. The psychiatrist should be aware of the embarrassment that may accompany inspection of the hair loss, particularly when located in regions of the body that are not usually accessible in the course of a standard psychiatric examination. Because of the apparent frequency of comorbid mood disorders (past or current), the interviewer should pay special attention to the presence of these features.

Physical Examination and Laboratory Findings

Areas of hair loss can be marked by complete alopecia or can appear diffusely thinned or "ratty". Altered scalp appearance can range from small areas of thinned hair to complete baldness. For unclear reasons, several patterns of scalp loss are typical. Frequently, coin-sized areas of alopecia are noted at the vertex or at temporal or occipital regions. Among more severely afflicted people a peculiar pattern, so-called tonsure trichotillomania, may appear: a completely bald head except for a narrow, circular fringe circumscribing the outer boundary of the scalp, producing a look reminiscent of medieval friars.

Despite the hair loss, most individuals with this condition have no overtly unusual appearance on cursory inspection. If the hair loss is not covered by clothing or accessories, artful combing of hair or use of eyeliner and false eyelashes may easily hide it. The ease with which the condition may often be hidden may explain the general underappreciation of its apparent frequency and potential associated distress.

Associated Laboratory Findings

Histological findings are considered characteristic and may aid diagnosis when it is suspected despite denial by the individual. Biopsy samples from involved areas may have the following features. Short and broken hairs are present. The surface of the scalp usually shows no evidence of excoriation. On histological examination, normal and damaged follicles are found in the same area, as well as an increased number of catagen (i.e., nongrowing) hairs. Inflammation is usually minimal or absent. Some hair follicles may show signs of trauma (wrinkling of the outer root sheath). Involved follicles may be empty or contain a deeply pigmented keratinous material. The absence of inflammation distinguishes trichotillomania-induced alopecia from alopecia areata, the principal condition in the differential diagnosis.

Specific Age-, Culture- and Gender-related Features

Secondary avoidance of intimate relationships, which occurs among some individuals with trichotillomania, may be exacerbated for women in cultures in which physical appearance is weighted differently for men and women. Avoidance of sports activities, in which disguised hair loss can be revealed, may also have gender-related effects in cultures in which athletic participation has different social meanings for men and women. Although culture-based expectations regarding appearance may make hair loss a greater burden for women, women may have a greater opportunity to hide hair loss through the use of wigs, hats and scarves. Reliable data regarding sex ratio in the general population are not yet available. For many women hair-pulling may worsen during the premenstrual phase.

Differential Diagnosis

Among individuals presenting with alopecia who complain of hair-pulling urges, the diagnosis is not usually in doubt. When patients deny hair-pulling, other (dermatological) causes of alopecia should be considered. These include alopecia bareata, male pattern hair loss, chronic discoid lupus erythematosus, lichen planopilaris, folliculitis decalvans, pseudopelade and alopecia mucinosa.

Trichotillomania is not diagnosed when hair-pulling occurs in response to a delusion or hallucination. Many people twist and play with their hair. This may be exacerbated in states of heightened anxiety but does not qualify for a diagnosis of trichotillomania.

Some individuals may present with features of trichotillomania but hair damage may be so slight as to be virtually undetectable, even under close examination. In such conditions the disorder should be diagnosed only if it results in significant distress to the individual. Trichotillomania may have a short, self-limited course among children and may be considered a temporary habit. Therefore, among children the diagnosis should be reserved for situations in which the behavior has persisted during several months.

Epidemiology and Comorbidity

Prevalence and Incidence

Trichotillomania was long thought to be an uncommon condition, often accompanied by other psychiatric conditions. Although definitive studies of frequency rates in the general population are still lacking, three surveys of college-age samples support the emerging view that trichotillomania is quite common. In two of these samples, totaling approximately 3000 undergraduate students, a lifetime incidence of self-identified trichotillomania (reaching full symptom criteria as described in DSM-III-R) was present in about 1% of the respondents. Some features of the condition – but not meeting full criteria – were identified in an additional 1 to 2% (Rothbaum *et al.*, 1993).

In addition, because onset may occur later in life than the mean ages of individuals in these groups, the true lifetime incidence would probably be higher. Moreover, these samples consist of a selected population – largely first-year college students – and may not reflect the general population. Nonetheless, these studies indicate that the condition is likely to be far more common than previously assumed. But definitive, controlled studies of the prevalence of the condition have not yet been performed.

Comorbidity

Individuals with trichotillomania have increased risk for mood disorders (major depressive disorder, dysthymic disorder) and anxiety symptoms. The frequency of specific anxiety disorders (such as generalized anxiety disorder and panic).

Course

The age at onset typically ranges from early childhood to young adulthood. Peak ages at presentation may be bimodal, with an earlier peak about age 5 to 8 years among children in whom it has a self-limited course, whereas among patients who present to clinicians in adulthood the mean age at onset is approximately 13 years (Rothbaum *et al.*, 1993). Initial onset after young adulthood is apparently uncommon. There have been reports of onset as early as 14 months of age and as late as 61 years.

Trichotillomania may be one of the earliest occurring conditions in psychiatry. Some parents insist that their child began pulling hair before 1 year of age. When trichotillomania begins before age 6 years it tends to be a milder condition. It often responds to simple interventions and may be self-limited, with a duration of several weeks to several months, even if not treated. It often occurs in association with thumb-sucking. In some cases it remits spontaneously when therapeutic attention is directed at concurrent, severe thumb-sucking. It has been suggested that trichotillomania in childhood may be associated with severe intrapsychic or familial psychiatric conditions. But there is no

reliable evidence that supports such a conclusion. Indeed, some have suggested that because it may be common and frequently self-limiting, it should be considered a normal behavior among young children.

Some individuals have continuous symptoms for decades. For others, the disorder may come and go for weeks, months, or years at a time. Sites of hair-pulling may vary over time. Circumscribed periods of hair-pulling (weeks to months) followed by complete remission are reported among children.

Progression of the condition appears to be unpredictable. Waxing and waning of the severity of hair-pulling and number of hair-pulling sites occur in most individuals. It is not known which factors may predict a protracted and unremitting course.

Prognosis

Because of the unavailability of longitudinal studies of trichotillomania, generalizations about prognosis cannot be made. Patients who present in research clinics typically have histories of many years (up to decades) of hair-pulling. Presentation after age 40 years appears to be far less common than in the previous three decades of life, suggesting that the condition may eventually remit spontaneously, even when untreated. It is likely that the persistent cases seen in research environments reflect the more severe end of the spectrum. As noted earlier, trichotillomania in children may often be a time-limited phenomenon.

Treatment

Treatment Goals

Treatment of trichotillomania typically occurs in an outpatient setting. Eradication of hair-pulling behavior is the general focus of treatment. Distress, avoidant behaviors and cosmetic impairment are secondary to the hair-pulling behavior and would be likely to remit if the hair-pulling behavior is controlled. However, if sufficient control of hair-pulling cannot be attained, treatment goals should emphasize these associated problems as well. Even if hair-pulling persists, therapeutic interventions may be targeted at reducing secondary avoidance and diminishing distress.

Treatment may be considered in three phases:

Initial Contact   The diagnosis is made and the patient and psychiatrist agree on a strategy that may incorporate both pharmacological and psychological interventions. If distress is severe, supportive interventions should be immediately considered in anticipation of incomplete treatment response or of a delay of weeks to months before interventions may be beneficial.

Acute Treatment   Even when treatment of hair-pulling behavior is optimally successful, there may be a delay of several weeks to months before adequate control is attained. Therefore, the acute treatment phase may be prolonged.

Maintenance   It is not known how long patients must maintain active treatment interventions to prevent relapse. It should be anticipated that a substantial number of patients require ongoing treatment for an extended time. Pharmacological treatments may need to be maintained for open-ended periods. Behavioral or hypnotic intervention may require periodic "booster shots" to support continuation of benefits.

Psychiatrist–Patient Relationship

It is important to bear in mind the particular nature of embarrassment that often accompanies this condition. Several factors contribute to feelings of shame for many people with trichotillomania. When hair-pulling has had its onset in childhood or adolescence, there is often a history of the hair-pulling being treated as a family secret. Patients have been frequently castigated by parents or spouses for lack of self-control. In addition, there may be a feeling that the problem is largely cosmetic, causing some individuals to fear they do not have the "right" to utilize health resources for its treatment. This may also be manifest as fears of having their problem minimized or of being derided for seeking help. It is helpful for the psychiatrist to share with patients an understanding that the problem pervades their daily life and may result in meaningful distress and functional inhibition.

A variety of treatment approaches have been advocated for trichotillomania. However, there have, as yet, been few controlled studies of the efficacy of any treatment approach. A number of investigations of the use of antidepressants with specific inhibition of serotonin reuptake (i.e., fluoxetine and clomipramine) have yielded mixed results. A multimodal approach, simultaneously utilizing several complementary treatment options, may turn out to be the most effective approach for most patients. While a number of treatment options can be currently offered to individuals with trichotillomania, the durability of long-term outcomes is unclear.

Stress Management

Before embarking on a course of treatment, the psychiatrist and the patient should first consider the course and severity of the individual's condition. Because early remission may occur in cases of recent onset, mild trichotillomania of short duration does not necessarily require immediate intervention. In particular, if the hair-pulling first occurred during a period of stress, the behavior may spontaneously diminish as the stressful circumstances abate. In such circumstances, therapeutic attention may best be directed toward examining and seeking to diminish the basis for stress. Teaching alternative stress reduction methods may be useful in reducing recent-onset trichotillomania. However, when individuals with trichotillomania present to the psychiatrist, it is often likely to have been a persistent condition and may have been present for many years or decades. Among such patients, stress reduction may also be useful in reducing trichotillomania but complete remission is less likely.

Pharmacotherapy

A variety of medications have been used in the treatment of trichotillomania. Initial reports appeared demonstrating the apparent benefits of fluoxetine and clomipramine. Clomipramine was found to be superior to desipramine (and fluoxetine was reported beneficial in open treatment. Although reports for more than 60 patients have subsequently added support for the use of these medications, the two double-blind studies in which fluoxetine has been compared with placebo did not demonstrate any improvement compared with placebo. Fluvoxamine, citalopram and venlafaxine have been reported to be efficacious in open trials. Although further controlled studies of SSRIs are needed, the use of such medications would be a prudent first step if a pharmacological approach has been agreed upon.

Initial evidence of improvement is usually first reported by the patient as greater awareness of the inclination to pull hair. This is usually followed by an ability to abort hair-pulling episodes more quickly than in the past. The ability to resist the urge follows. In cases with a good outcome, the inclination to pull diminishes and may eventually disappear. Patients who pull from several sites may find that the rate of improvement varies from site to site.

There have been conflicting reports of early relapse of symptoms in some patients treated with clomipramine or fluoxetine. Although good maintenance of benefit has been reported for some patients 6 months and longer after the initiation of treatment, early relapse after several weeks to months has been reported as well. Keuthen and coworkers (2001) have provided long-term data on maintenance of response over time. Following a group of individuals who had varying forms of treatment (pharmacologic and psychological) for several years after an index evaluation, the authors concluded that initial improvement was common, but over time there was an increase in symptom scores and self-esteem scores worsened in the group over time. This problem remains to be further evaluated in long-term treatment studies. If early relapse does turn out to be common, it would distinguish trichotillomania from depression and OCD, in which, once established, medication benefits are often well maintained as long as medication is continued. Optimal duration of treatment for well-treated individuals is also still unknown. In accordance with standards developed for the treatment of other conditions, it would be reasonable to continue medication for at least 6 months before tapering. Reinitiation of treatment may be necessary.

Other Medications

There have been reports of successful treatment with lithium. Adjunctive treatment with pimozide, a neuroleptic agent, has been advocated for some patients who are refractory to other medications. The potential benefits of neuroleptics has been reported and individuals have been described for whom SSRIs provided insufficient benefits. The addition of atypical neuroleptics much improved their outcomes. The greater margin of safety and tolerability associated with atypical neuroleptics have made this a more viable treatment option.

Van Ameringen and colleagues (1999) described the use of haloperidol in nine patients with trichotillomania. Six had previously failed treatment with SSRIs. Eight of nine patients responded to the haloperidol. The possible superiority of neuroleptics prompted these authors to speculate that trichotillomania may be similar to Tourette's syndrome (TS), which responds preferentially to neuroleptics.

Psychosocial Treatments

Behavioral Treatment Various behavioral techniques have been tried. The most successful technique, habit reversal, is based on designing competitive behaviors that should inhibit the behavior of hair-pulling. For example, if hair-pulling requires raising the arm to the scalp and contracting the muscles of the hand to grasp a hair, the behaviorist may design a behavioral program in which the patient is taught to lower the arm and extend the muscles of the hand. As with behavioral techniques in general, these interventions are most successful when the patient is strongly motivated and compliant. In addition, the treating psychiatrist should be experienced in the use of such techniques. If necessary, a referral should be made to such an experienced individual. Modified behavioral approaches have been described for children and adolescents.

Cognitive Behavioral Therapy (CBT) CBT has been developed for, and applied to, individuals with trichotillomania. At this time, the potential for the efficacy of this treatment approach appears good. Ninan and colleagues (2000) compared CBT with clomipramine in the treatment of trichotillomania. The authors reported that CBT had a dramatic effect in reducing symptoms of trichotillomania and was significantly more effective than clomipramine (P 5 0.016) or placebo (P 5 0.026). Clomipramine resulted in symptom reduction greater than that with placebo, but the difference fell short of statistical significance. Placebo response was minimal.

Hypnotherapy There are no formal studies of the use of hypnosis for trichotillomania, but there are many published reports of beneficial treatment. Benefits may be variable. Some patients may have dramatic improvement. For some who improve, the benefits may be short-lived. As with behavioral interventions, the benefits of this approach are sometimes dependent on a highly motivated patient who can regularly carry out self-hypnotic measures as instructed by the psychiatrist. Some patients who have obtained partial benefits from either hypnosis or medication do well when both treatments are combined. Successful use of hypnotherapy for children with trichotillomania has also been reported.

Dynamic Psychotherapy Many psychoanalytically oriented descriptions of individuals with trichotillomania have been published. These reports generally describe the psychodynamic formulations of individual cases and should not be the basis for generalizations about most individuals with trichotillomania. Although patients with trichotillomania may benefit from exploration and attempts to reduce intrapsychic conflict, the literature does not provide persuasive evidence of the efficacy of this approach in reducing hair-pulling.

Self-help and Other Groups Self-help groups for patients with trichotillomania have appeared. Some are based in the structure of other 12-step programs. Some patients appear to experience meaningful reduction in hair-pulling symptoms after beginning participation in such a group. Although the efficacy of such groups in reducing symptoms remains to be established, most patients with trichotillomania can benefit from meeting other individuals with similar symptoms. Because of the lack of general awareness of trichotillomania, these individuals frequently believe that they are "oddball" individuals with a behavior that is unique. Many have experienced parental condemnation for the behavior and have been frequently castigated for a "habit" that may be viewed by others as under their voluntary control. The experience of meeting others with the condition is extremely supportive for such individuals and may help to reduce the attendant stress while supporting self-esteem. Where programs specifically oriented toward trichotillomania may not be generally available, these individuals may benefit from groups oriented toward OCD.

Treatment of Comorbid Conditions

Depression, dysthymic disorder and anxiety symptoms occur frequently in patients with trichotillomania. Successful treatment of depression may not be associated with reduction in trichotillomania. If depression or dysthymic disorder is present and independently provides an indication for medication, one of the antidepressants discussed earlier should be chosen. If fluoxetine is used, the psychiatrist should be aware that a dose that is sufficient for reduction of the depressive symptoms may not be sufficient for reduction of trichotillomania. If panic disorder is present, either medication may still be used, but fluoxetine may initially exacerbate panic attacks in such patients and initiation of treatment at low doses (2.5–5 mg/day) should be considered. With slow titration upward, the patient should generally be able to tolerate usual doses with concomitant amelioration of the

panic disorder. Combined treatment with anxiolytics may be useful for some and may contribute to the reduction in symptoms of trichotillomania. Other conditions that may be present, such as OCD or eating disorders, may require special attention. Although fluoxetine may be useful for patients with eating disorders, medication treatment alone is unlikely to be adequate and the usual multimodal approaches for the treatment of bulimia nervosa or anorexia are appropriate. OCD may respond to treatment directed at trichotillomania, but adjunctive behavioral treatment of symptoms of OCD may be desirable.

Demographical Features

When trichotillomania presents in early childhood, the condition may be likely to be inherently self-limited. Often, all that may be necessary is to draw the child's attention to the behavior in some systematic way and to clarify for the child that the behavior is undesirable. Such methods include daily application of a nonmedicinal ointment to the affected region and reminding the child that the purpose is elimination of the hair-pulling habit. Some suggest that the child be given the responsibility of applying the ointment with parental supervision. Others suggest that parents should monitor the child as much as possible and respond with reminders that the hair should not be pulled and rewards with verbal encouragement for ceasing to pull hair. There have been no systematic studies of the benefits of such interventions, but dermatologists who specialize in the treatment of children have noted that hair-pulling behavior may frequently disappear within a few weeks of initiating such an approach. In circumstances in which childhood trichotillomania is more persistent, the parent and psychiatrist are faced with a dilemma. More elaborate behavioral interventions, such as habit reversal, should be tried. This, however, may be difficult with a child. Hypnosis has been also used in the treatment of habit disorders in children. Medication should be cautiously considered in the treatment of childhood trichotillomania. Although medication may be useful, the absence of data supporting the benefits of such treatments in children indicates a conservative approach. If medication is considered, the use of medication in the treatment of childhood OCD should serve as a guideline.

Should the psychiatrist be presented with trichotillomania in a person of advanced age, special attention should be paid to usual concerns regarding the use of these medications in the elderly. Lower doses of medication should be considered because of potential altered pharmacokinetics in older persons. Medications with anticholinergic side effects (such as clomipramine) may present greater hazards for the older person. Sedative-hypnotic anxiolytics should be used sparingly because of greater vulnerability to cognitive side effects and the increased risk of falling.

Women of childbearing potential (perhaps the majority of individuals who may present for treatment) should be advised regarding the potential risks of these medications to a developing fetus. If the patient is pregnant or considering pregnancy, behavioral treatments may be favored.

The psychiatrist should be sensitive to the interaction between cultural values and trichotillomania. Women of certain cultures may be more prone to distress if trichotillomania is perceived as a hindrance to achieving valued goals, such as marriage. It should also be noted that in some communities, wigs and other hair accessories are generally acceptable and may present a comfortable means of diminishing the cosmetic impact of hair loss. In other communities, such accoutrements may themselves draw undesired attention.

Comparison of DSM-IV/ICD-10 Diagnostic Criteria

The ICD-10 Diagnostic Criteria for Research do not include diagnostic criteria for intermittent explosive disorder. It is included in ICD-10 as an "other habit and Impulse Control Disorder".

The ICD-10 Diagnostic Criteria for Research and the DSM-IV-TR criteria for kleptomania, pyromania and trichotillomania are essentially equivalent.

Finally, the ICD-10 Diagnostic Criteria for Research for pathological gambling are monothetic (i.e., A plus B plus C plus D are required) whereas the DSM-IV-TR criteria set is polythetic (i.e., five out of 10 required) with different items. Furthermore, the ICD-10 criteria specify "two or more episodes of gambling over a period of at least 1 year", whereas DSM-IV-TR does not specify a duration.

References

American Psychiatric Association (2000) *Diagnostic and Statistical Manual of Mental Disorders*, 4th edn. Text Rev. APA, Washington DC.

Bars DR, Heyrend FL, Simpson CD *et al.* (2001) Use of visual evoked-potential studies and EEG data to classify aggressive, explosive behavior of youths. *Psychiatr Serv* 52, 81–86.

Budman CL, Bruun RD, Park KS *et al.* (2000) Explosive outbursts in children with Tourette's disorder. *J Am Acad Child Adolesc Psychiatr* 39, 1270–1276.

Eisen SA, Slutske WS, Lyons MJ *et al.* (2001) The genetics of pathological gambling. *Semin Clin Neuropsychiatr* 6, 195–204.

Felthous AR, Bryant SG, Wingerter CB *et al.* (1991) The diagnosis of intermittent explosive disorder in violent men. *Bull Am Acad Psychiatr Law* 19, 71–79.

Fishbain DA (1987) Kleptomania as risk-taking behavior in response to depression. *Am J Psychother* 41, 598–603.

Freud S (1961) Dostoevsky and parricide. In The Standard Edition of the Complete Psychological Works of Sigmund Freud, Vol. 21, Strachey J (ed). Hogarth Press, London.

Goldman MJ (1991) Kleptomania: Making sense of the nonsensical. *Am J Psychiatr* 148, 986–996.

Herzog DB, Keller MB, Sacks NR *et al.* (1992) Psychiatric comorbidity in treatment-seeking anorexics and bulimics. *J Am Acad Child Adolesc Psychiatr* 31, 810–818.

Hollander E, Frenkel M, Decaria C *et al.* (1992) Treatment of pathological gambling with clomipramine. *Am J Psychiatr* 149, 710–711.

Hudson JI and Pope HG (1990) Affective spectrum disorder: Does antidepressant response identify a family of disorders with a common pathophysiology? *Am J Psychiatr* 147, 552–564.

Ibanez A, Blanco C, Donahue E, *et al.* (2001) Psychiatric comorbidity in pathological gamblers seeking treatment. Am J Psychiar 158, 1733–173.

Ibanez A, Blanco C, and Saiz-Ruiz J (2002) Neurobiology and genetics of pathological gambling. *Psychiatr Ann* 32, 181–185.

Kessler RC, Chiu WT, Demler O *et al.* (2005). Prevalence, severity, and comorbidity of 12 month DSMI-IV disorders in the National Comorbidity Survey. *Arch Gen Psychiatry* 62, 617–627.

Keuthen NJ, Fraim C, Deckersbach T *et al.* (2001) Longitudinal follow-up of naturalistic treatment outcome in patients with trichotillomania. J Clin Psychiatr 62, 101–107.

Lee S (1994) The heterogeneity of stealing behaviors in Chinese patients with anorexia nervosa in Hong Kong. *J Nerv Ment Dis* 182, 304–307.

Lesieur HR and Rosenthal RJ (1991) Pathological gambling: A review of the literature. *J Gambling Stud* 7, 5–39.

Lion JR (1992) The intermittent explosive disorder. *Psychiatr Ann* 2, 64–66.

Lorenz V (1981) Differences found among Catholic, Protestant, and Jewish families of pathological gamblers, in *Fifth National Conference on Gambling and Risk Taking*. Lake Tahoe, CA.

Marks I (1990) Behavioural (non-chemical) addictions. *Br J Addict* 85, 1389–1394.

Mattes JA (1990) Comparative effectiveness of carbamazepine and propranolol for rage outbursts. *J Neuropsychiatr Clin Neurosci* 2, 159–164.

McElroy SL (1999) Recognition and treatment of DSM-IV intermittent explosive disorder. *J Clin Psychiatr* 60, 12–16.

McElroy SL, Hudson JI, Pope HG *et al.* (1991a) Kleptomania: Clinical characteristics and associated psychopathology. *Psychol Med* 21, 93–108.

McElroy SL, Pope HG Jr., Hudson JI *et al.* (1991b) Kleptomania: A report of 20 cases. *Am J Psychiatr* 148, 652–657.

McElroy SL, Hudson JI, Pope HG Jr. *et al.* (1992) The DSM-III-R impulse control disorders not elsewhere classified: Clinical characteristics and relationship to other psychiatric disorders. *Am J Psychiatr* 149, 318–327.

McElroy SL, Soutullo CA, Beckman DA *et al.* (1998) DSM-IV intermittent explosive disorder: A report of 27 cases. *J Clin Psychiatr* 59, 203–210; quiz 211.

Ninan PT, Rothbaum BO, Marsteller FA *et al.* (2000) A placebo-controlled trial of cognitive–behavioral therapy and clomipramine in trichotillomania. *J Clin Psychiatr* 61, 47–50.

Rosenthal RJ (1992) Pathological gambling. *Psychiatr Ann* 22, 72–78.

Rothbaum BO, Shaw L, Morris R *et al.* (1993) Prevalence of trichotillomania in a college freshman population. *J Clin Psychiatr* 54, 72–73.

Shapiro AK and Shapiro E (1992) Evaluation of the reported association of obsessive–compulsive symptoms or disorder with Tourette's disorder. *Compr Psychiatr* 33, 152–165.

Soltys SM (1992) Pyromania and firesetting behaviors. *Psychiatr Ann* 22, 79–83.

Turnbull JM (1987) Sexual relationships of patients with kleptomania. *South Med J* 80, 995–998.

Van Ameringen M, Mancini C, Oakman JM *et al.* (1999) The potential role of haloperidol in the treatment of trichotillomania. *J Affect Disord* 56, 219–226.

Virkkunen M, Rawlings R, Tokola R, *et al.* (1994) CSF biochemistries, glucose metabolism, and diurnal activity rhythms in alcoholic, violent offenders, fire setters, and healthy volunteers. Arch Gen Psychiatr 51, 20–27.

Woermann FG, van Elst LT, Koepp MJ *et al.* (2000) Reduction of frontal neocortical grey matter associated with affective aggression in patients with temporal lobe epilepsy: An objective voxel by voxel analysis of automatically segmented MRI. *J Neurol Neurosurg Psychiatr* 68, 162–169.

61 Adjustment Disorders

Definition

The *Diagnostic and Statistical Manual of Mental Disorders*, Fourth Edition, Text Revision (DSM-IV-TR) states that the essential feature of adjustment disorder (AD) is the development of clinically significant emotional or behavioral symptoms in response to an identifiable psychosocial stressor (American Psychiatric Association, 2000). The symptoms must develop within 3 months after the onset of the stressor (criterion A). The clinical significance of the reaction is indicated either by marked distress that is in excess of what would be expected given the nature of the stressor or by significant impairment in social or occupational (academic) functioning (criterion B). This disorder should not be used if the emotional and cognitive disturbances meet the criteria for another specific Axis I disorder (e.g., a specific anxiety or mood disorder) or are merely an exacerbation of a preexisting Axis I or Axis II disorder (criterion C). AD may be diagnosed if other Axis I or II disorders are present, but do not account for the pattern of symptoms that have occurred in response to the stressor. The diagnosis of AD does not apply when the symptoms represent bereavement (criterion D). By definition, AD must resolve within 6 months of the termination of the stressor or its consequences (criterion E). However, the symptoms may persist for a prolonged period (i.e., longer than 6 months) if they occur in response to a chronic stressor (e.g., a chronic, disabling general medical condition) or to a stressor that has enduring consequences (e.g., the financial and emotional difficulties resulting from a divorce) (American Psychiatric Association, 2000).

Although the above definition provides a certain structure for identifying and describing AD, there is still uncertainty as to when the impairment in functioning or the severity of the psychiatric symptoms that develop in response to a stressor are sufficient to warrant a diagnosis of AD. The DSM-IV-TR describes the boundary issues between conditions that may be a focus of clinical attention (V codes), **subthreshold** disorders (NOS disorders) and the specific mental disorders (American Psychiatric Association, 2000). A compelling literature documents that there is much "physical" in mental disorders and much "mental" in physical disorders. No definition adequately specifies precise boundaries for the concept of a "mental disorder". "The concept...lacks a consistent operational definition that covers all situations. Whatever its original cause, it must currently be considered a manifestation of a behavioral, psychological, or biological dysfunction in the individual". The issue of defining boundaries is especially problematic in the **subthreshold** diagnoses, for example, the AD, in which there are no symptom checklists, algorithms, or guidelines for the "quantification of attributes".

The symptoms of AD are defined in terms of their being a maladaptive response to a psychosocial stressor. There are, in

---

DSM-IV-TR Criteria 309.xx

Adjustment Disorders

A. The development of emotional or behavioral symptoms in response to an identifiable stressor(s) occurring within 3 months of the onset of the stressor(s).

B. These symptoms or behaviors are clinically significant as evidenced by either of the following:

   (1) marked distress that is in excess of what would be expected from exposure to the stressor.

   (2) significant impairment in social or occupational (academic) functioning.

C. The stress-related disturbance does not meet the criteria for another specific Axis I disorder and is not merely an exacerbation of a preexisting Axis I or Axis II disorder.

D. The symptoms do not represent bereavement.

E. Once the stressor (or its consequences) has terminated, the symptoms do not persist for more than an additional 6 months.

Specify if:

Acute: if the disturbance lasts less than 6 months

Chronic: if the disturbance lasts for 6 months or longer

Adjustment disorders are coded based on the subtype, which is selected according to the predominant symptoms. The specific stressor(s) can be specified on Axis IV.

With 309.0 depressed mood

With 309.24 anxiety

With 309.28 mixed anxiety and depressed mood

With 309.3 disturbance of conduct

With 309.4 mixed disturbance of emotions and conduct

Unspecified 309.9

Reprinted with permission from the *Diagnostic and Statistical Manual of Mental Disorders*, Fourth Edition, Text Revision. Copyright 2000 American Psychiatric Association.

---

fact, no specific symptoms of AD; any combination of behavioral or emotional symptoms that occur in association with a stressor may qualify. The lack of specific symptoms or quantifiable

---

Essentials of Psychiatry   Jerald Kay and Allan Tasman
© 2006 John Wiley & Sons, Ltd.

criteria of the AD permits the labeling of early or temporary mental states when the clinical picture does not meet full evidence for a more specific mental disorder, but the morbid state is more than expected in a normal reaction and treatment or intervention may be indicated. AD are an essential "linchpin" in the psychiatric–taxonomic spectrum-hierarchy: 1) disorders with specific diagnostic criteria; 2) disorders not otherwise specified (NOS); 3) adjustment disorders; 4) other conditions that may be a focus of clinical attention (V codes) (American Psychiatric Association, 2000); and 5) normal fluctuations of mental states.

Disorders that do not fulfill the criteria for a specific mental disorder may be accorded a lesser interest by mental health care workers, research institutes and third-party payers, even though they present with serious (or incipient) symptoms that require intervention or treatment. Given this concept, the AD are formulated as a means of classifying psychiatric morbidity that is clinically significant; when the symptom profile is as yet insufficient to meet the more specifically operationalized criteria for another mental disorder; when the symptoms, disturbance of mood, and vocational or interpersonal dysfunction are in excess of a normal reaction to the stressors in question; and for which treatment is indicated. For example, a diagnosis of AD is not given when the clinical picture is a psychosocial problem (V code) requiring clinical attention, such as noncompliance, phase of life problem, bereavement, or occupational (academic) problem. Their etiological and dynamic attributes make the AD a fascinating group of disorders that serve as a fulcrum between normality and more specific mental disorders (Figure 61.1).

Attention to less severe mental symptoms (and psychiatric morbidity) may forestall the evolution to more serious disorders and allow remediation before relationships, work and functioning are so impaired that they are disrupted or permanently sundered.

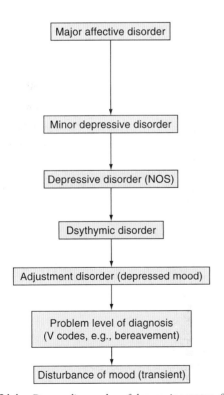

Figure 61.1 *Descending order of depressive states, from most serious to least depressed mood, as a state of being for an occurrence of the moment.*

Yet, in the gray area in which early diagnosis may have enormous value with modest therapeutic investment, guidelines are the most tenuous. It is the professionals at the "front door" – primary care physicians, triage personnel, emergency department staff, walk-in clinic staff – who need assistance in making this difficult call: Is there sufficient psychiatric morbidity to warrant mental health intervention?

Because AD is a nonpejorative psychiatric condition it may have been overdiagnosed in youths to protect them from feared adversities of major psychiatric nomenclature. An early study observed that 25% of a sample of adolescents with AD had attempted suicide and that 17% probably "would have met DSM-III criteria for major depressive disorder" because they had the required symptoms. Nevertheless, in psychological autopsy studies of adolescent suicide completers, approximately 20% do not meet the criteria for any single psychiatric diagnosis, although they present with significant functional impairment and life-threatening behavior.

How to diagnose individuals with suicidal behavior who do not meet criteria for a specific mental is a challenge. Runeson and colleagues (1996) observed from psychological autopsy methods that there was a very short median interval between first suicidal communication and suicide in AD (less than 1 month) compared with major depressive disorder (3 months), borderline personality disorder (30 months), or schizophrenia (47 months).

Recent life events, which would constitute an acute stress, were commonly found to correlate with suicidal behavior in a group that included those with AD (Isometsa *et al.*, 1996). The assessment of suicidal behavior is an important tool in differentiating major depressive disorder, dysthymic disorder and AD. Furthermore, AD patients appear to be among the most common recipients of a deliberate self-harm (DSH) diagnosis, with the majority involving self-poisoning. Thus, DSH with all its variants, e.g., reckless driving, is more common in AD patients, whereas the percentage of completed suicidal behavior *per se* was found to be higher in depressed patients (Spalletta *et al.*, 1996). Of note, biological findings in suicidal patients with AD suggest characteristic patterns of monoamine oxidase (MAO) and noradrenaline turnover. Clearly, what is regarded, as a subthreshold diagnosis – AD – does not necessarily imply the presence of subthreshold symptomatology.

Epidemiology

AD has principally been studied in clinical samples. Epidemiological data in adults are not available. The AD diagnosis was not included in the Epidemiologic Catchment Area Study and there are only a few studies in children and adolescents. Prevalence rates for AD range from 2.3% of walk in clinic patients who had no other Axis I or II disorders to 20% when comorbid axis I and II diagnoses were present. In a Pittsburgh sample, 16% of the children and adolescents younger than 18 years were diagnosed with AD (Fabrega *et al.*, 1986). In adults, women predominated over men by approximately 2 : 1. The sex ratio was more equal in children and adolescents, although there was still a slight excess of female patients.

Prevalence estimates of AD in other clinical populations have been characterized by considerable variability. In general hospital inpatient and psychiatric consultation populations, AD was diagnosed in 21.5 and 11.5%, respectively (Popkin *et al.*, 1988; Snyder and Strain, 1990). Consultation–liaison data from seven university teaching hospitals in the USA, Canada and Australia revealed that AD was diagnosed in 125 patients (12.0%); as the sole diagnosis in 81 (7.8%); and comorbidly with other Axis I and II diagnoses in 44 (4.2%) (Strain *et al.*, 1998). It had been considered as a "rule-out" diagnosis in an additional 110 (10.6%). AD with depressed mood, anxious mood, or mixed emotions were the most common subcategories used. AD was diagnosed comorbidly most frequently with personality disorder and organic mental disorder. Sixty-seven (6.4%) were assigned a V code diagnosis only. Patients with AD compared with other diagnostic categories were referred significantly more often for problems of anxiety, coping and depression; had less past psychiatric illness; and were rated as functioning better – all consistent with the construct of AD as a maladaptation to a psychosocial stressor. Interventions employed for this general hospital inpatient cohort were similar to those for other Axis I and II diagnoses, in particular, the prescription of antidepressant medications. Patients with AD required a similar amount of clinical time and resident supervision.

Oxman and coworkers (1994) observed that 50.7% of elderly patients (aged 55+ years) receiving elective surgery for coronary artery disease developed AD related to the stress of surgery. Thirty percent had symptomatic and functional impairment 6 months following surgery. It is reported that more than 25% of elderly patients examined 5 to 9 days following a cerebral vascular accident had symptoms that fulfilled the criteria for AD. Spiegel (1996) observed that half of all cancer patients have a psychiatric disorder, usually an AD with depression. Since patients treated for their mental states had longer survival time, treatment of depression in cancer patients should be considered integral to their medical treatment. AD is a frequently made diagnosis in patients with head and neck surgery (16.8%), patients with HIV dementia (73%) and cancer patients (27%). AD is seen in dermatology patients and suicide attempters examined in an emergency department. Other studies include diagnosis of AD in more than 60% of inpatients being treated for severe burns, 20% of patients in early stages of multiple sclerosis and 40% of poststroke patients.

There are two published epidemiological studies in populations of children and adolescents that included AD. One determined the prevalence rate of AD was 7.6% if an upper limit of 70 on the Children's Global Assessment Scale (CGAS) is applied. However, if an upper limit of 60 is imposed (corresponding to "moderate" impairment on the CGAS), the prevalence of AD dropped to 4.2%. This indicates that up to 40% of AD diagnosed patients have only mild impairment, more than for any other diagnosis.

The relationship between family functioning and AD was evaluated by administering the Family Assessment Devise (FAD) to families who had a member with one of seven mental disorders: schizophrenia, bipolar disorder, major depression, anxiety disorder, eating disorder, substance abuse and adjustment disorder (Friedmann et al., 1997). Regardless of which specific psychiatric diagnosis was present in the family member, having a family member in an acute phase of any of these psychiatric disorders – even a subthreshold diagnosis such as AD, was a risk factor for poor family functioning. AD in a family member was a significant family stressor.

Etiology

By definition, the ADs are stress-related phenomena in which a psychosocial stressor results in the development of maladaptive states and psychiatric symptoms. The condition is presumed to be time limited, that is, a transitory reaction; symptoms recede when the stressor is removed or a new state of adaptation is defined.

That the relationship between stress and the occurrence of a psychiatric disorder is both complex and uncertain has caused many to question the theoretical basis of AD. The linear model

of stress–disease interaction, which serves as the model for AD, has been questioned as well. The linear model presupposes that a direct and clearly identifiable pathological reaction may follow a stressful event, a scenario that no doubt occurs in some individuals with AD but may not accurately characterize others. For example, there may be multiple stressors, insidious or chronic, as opposed to discrete events. Furthermore, relatively minor precipitating events may generate a disturbance in an individual who has previously been sensitized to stress.

Several authors have criticized the stressor criterion in AD because stressors are difficult to specify and measure, and their clinical implications and impact are uncertain. Questions pertain to whether patients with AD are unusually sensitive to psychosocial events not likely to cause disturbance in others. Are there individuals who have been exposed to high levels of stress, the severity or accumulation of which would probably produce negative consequences in most people?

Diverse variables and modifiers are involved in the presentation of AD after exposure to a stress. Cohen (1981) argued that acute stresses are different from chronic ones in both psychological and physiological terms; that the meaning of the stress is affected by "modifiers" – ego strengths, support systems, prior mastery – and that one must differentiate manifest and latent meaning of the stressors (e.g., loss of a job may be a relief or a catastrophe). An objectively overwhelming stress could have little impact on one individual, whereas another individual could regard a minor one as cataclysmic. A recent minor stress superimposed on a previous underlying (major) stress (which had no observable effect on its own) may have a significant impact, not operating independently but by its additive effect: the concatenation of events (Hamburg, personal communication).

Despite variable findings suggesting a correlation between the acknowledgment of stress and the assignment of an AD diagnosis, stress is not universally related to the development of psychiatric illness, and this has implications for understanding the meaning of stressors in AD. Specific types of stressful events and individual patterns of stress response appear to be preferentially related to the development of psychiatric symptoms in vulnerable individuals.

Diagnosis and Differential Diagnosis

Each of the diagnostic constructs required for the diagnosis of AD is difficult to assess and measure: 1) the stressor, 2) the maladaptive reaction to the stressor, and 3) the time and relationship between the stressor and the psychological response. None of these three components has been operationalized for a diagnostic decision tree, which consequently plagues the AD diagnosis with limited reliability.

In contrast to other DSM-IV-TR disorders, the diagnostic criteria for AD include no clear and specific symptoms (or checklist) that collectively compose a psychiatric (medical) syndrome or disorder.

First, with regard to the maladaptive reaction, it is unclear how this concept can or should be operationalized. The social, vocational and relationship dysfunctions, which are unspecified qualitatively or quantitatively, do not lend themselves to reliable or to valid assessment. The elements of culture (i.e., the expectable reactions within a specific cultural environment), differences in gender responses, developmental level differences and differences in the "meaning" of events and reactions to them by a specific individual further confound it.

The concepts of "average expectable environment" (e.g., the expectation of adequate food in a household in an industrial society) and "patient's explanatory belief model" are examples of an attempt to weigh cultural and subjective differences in the assessment of an individual's mental state and reaction. Such individual cultural–social considerations often require an understanding on the part of the psychiatrist and thereby often render the assessment of whether a reaction is excessive or maladaptive a judgment call.

The criterion and predictive validity of the diagnosis of AD in 92 children who had new onset insulin-dependent diabetes mellitus were examined. DSM-III criteria were employed plus requiring four clinically significant signs or symptoms, and the time frame extended to 6 months (instead of the 3 months specified in the definition) after the diagnosis of diabetes. Thirty-three percent of the cohort developed AD (mean 29 days after the medical diagnosis) and the average episode length was 3 months with a recovery rate of 100%. The five-year cumulative probability of a new psychiatric disorder was 0.48 in comparison to 0.16 for the nonAD subjects. The findings support the criterion validity of the AD diagnosis using the criterion of predicting the future development of psychiatric disorder.

Maladaptation

Although the diagnosis of AD requires evidence of maladaptation, it is notable that no specific requirement for functional impairment has been included (e.g., there is no requirement for a certain decrement in the Global Assessment of Functioning Scale score in order to make the diagnosis). Fabrega and colleagues (1986) stated that both subjective symptoms and decrement in social function can be considered maladaptive and that the severity of either of these is subject to great individual variation. However, they could not conclude that the level of severity of psychiatric illness observed correlates with impaired functioning in three areas: occupational status, family, or other individuals.

The psychiatrist needs to examine the patient's behavior to see whether it is beyond what is expected in a particular situation, and for that patient. In order to do this, the psychiatrist needs to take into account the patient's cultural beliefs and practices, his or her developmental age and the transient nature of the behavior. If the behavior lasts a few moments or is an impulsive outburst, it would not qualify for a maladaptive response to justify the diagnosis of AD. The behavior in question should be maladaptive for that patient, in his/her culture and sufficiently persistent to qualify for the maladaptation attribute of the AD diagnosis.

Stresses

No criteria or guidelines are offered in DSM-IV-TR to quantify the degree of stress required for the diagnosis of AD or assess its effect or meaning for a particular individual at a given time. Many of the statements regarding the problem of assessing maladaptation described above apply equally well to the assessment of stressors. The measurement of the severity of the stressor and its temporal and causal relationship to demonstrable symptoms are often uncertain.

According to DSM-IV-TR, even if a specific and presumably causal stressor is identified, if enough symptoms develop so that diagnostic criteria are met for a specific disorder, then that diagnosis should be made instead of a diagnosis of AD (American Psychiatric Association, 1980, 1987, 2000). Therefore, the presence of stressors does not automatically signify a diagnosis of AD, and conversely, a diagnosis of a specific disorder (e.g., major depressive or anxiety disorder) does not imply the absence of concomitant or concurrent stressful events.

Assessment of the Subtypes of Adjustment Disorder, Comorbidity and Diagnostic Boundaries

The diagnostic criteria for AD define the contextual and temporal characteristics of a subthreshold response to a psychosocial stressor; the specific quality and nature of the resultant psychological morbidity have been used as a means of subtyping.

DSM-IV-TR identifies six AD subtypes; two of the subtypes define discrete disturbances of mood (e.g., depressed, anxious); two describe mixed clinical presentations (e.g., mixed emotional features, mixed disturbance of emotions and conduct); one specifies disturbance of conduct; and the final subtype, unspecified, is a residual category.

Significant occurrence of comorbidity has been reported in studies of AD using structured diagnostic instruments. In a cohort of children, adolescents and adults, approximately 70% of AD patients had at least one additional Axis I diagnosis. In the study of correlates of depressive disorders in children, 45% of those with AD with depressed mood had another disorder. However, comorbidity in AD was less than in dysthymic disorder or major depressive disorder, suggesting a "purer" or more encapsulated disturbance in AD.

Several studies reported an association of suicidal behavior in adolescents and young adults with AD. These studies underscore the seriousness of AD in a subset of individuals and suggest that although the diagnosis may be **subthreshold**, its morbidity can be serious and at times even fatal.

The issue of boundaries between the specific mood and anxiety disorders, depressive disorder or anxiety disorder NOS, and the AD remains problematic. The specific mood and anxiety disorders are often associated with and even precipitated by stress. Therefore, it is not always possible to say one group of diagnoses is accompanied by stress (the AD) and another (e.g., major depressive disorder) is not. Stress may accompany many of the psychiatric diagnoses, but it is not an essential component to make certain diagnoses (e.g., major depressive disorder).

More research is needed carefully to demarcate the boundaries or the meaning of these boundaries among the problem-level, subthreshold and threshold disorders, in particular with regard to the role of stressors as etiological precipitants, concomitants, or factors essentially unrelated to the occurrence of a particular psychiatric diagnosis. In reviewing the diagnosis of AD for DSM-IV, one issue emerges as fundamental. The effect of the imprecision of this diagnosis on reliability and validity, because of the lack of behavioral or operational criteria, must be determined.

Snyder and Strain (1989) observed that in the acute care inpatient hospital setting, many of the psychiatric consultation patients initially thought to have an AD did not maintain that diagnosis at the time of discharge. These same authors also observed that many patients initially diagnosed as having major depressive disorder were reclassified to AD at discharge. It remains to be seen if either the major depressive disorder or the AD diagnosis is significantly altered at a 6-week follow-up and, in particular, when the patient has left the hospital. This evolution of psychiatric morbidity within the acute care general medical setting cautions the psychiatrist to go slowly with treatment until there is a level of certainty to justify an intervention, in particular with a chemotherapeutic modality.

Attempting to diagnose disorders in an early state or before there is a full-blown syndrome or disorder often means that a patient will qualify for the AD criteria or the subsyndromal condition. Just as it is difficult to know when a patient has crossed the diagnostic line (threshold) from normal to disturbed behavior, it is difficult to know how quickly the symptoms will remit with a remission of the stressor, which for the general medical–surgical inpatient include 1) acute hospitalization, 2) uncertain medical diagnosis, 3) pain, 4) medications, 5) separation and 6) lack of ability to function or contain emotions. The AD must be looked at as a **transitory state** for most patients, in that it may subside, respond with treatment, evolve to another diagnosis, or be maintained as the stressor continues.

Furthermore, Monroe and associates (1992) pointed out that "stress does not credit a more favorable treatment course for patients with recurrent depression". For these patients, stress occurring before treatment entry suggests the likelihood of a poorer early treatment response and a longer time to attain relief. Psychiatrists working with recurrent depression should not expect more rapid recovery from patients reporting these types of stress and should not become discouraged if treatment progress is slower or more erratic than usual. The severity of the stressor should be studied as well as its recurrence and its meaning to the patient, all in conjunction with treatment outcome in those with AD.

Clinical Vignette 1

A 35-year-old married woman, mother of three children, was desperate when she learned she had cancer and would need mastectomy followed by chemotherapy and radiation. She was convinced that she would not recover, that her body would be forever distorted and ugly, that her husband would no longer find her attractive, and that her children would be ashamed of her baldness and the fact that she had cancer. She wondered whether anyone would ever want to touch her again. Because her mother and sister had also experienced breast cancer, the patient felt she was fated to an empty future. Despite several sessions dealing with her feelings, the patient's dysphoria remained profound. It was decided to add antidepressant medication (fluoxetine, 20 mg/day) to her psychotherapy to decrease the patient's continuing unpleasant symptoms. Two weeks later, the patient reported that she was feeling less despondent and less concerned about the future and that she had a desire to start resuming her former activities with her family. As the patient came to terms with the overwhelming stressor and, assisted with antidepressant agents, her depressed mood improved, more adequate coping strategies to handle her serious medical illness were mobilized.

Although it is uncommon to use psychotropic medication for the majority of the adjustment disorders, this clinical vignette illustrates the effective use of antidepressant therapy in a patient who was not responding to counseling and psychotherapy; she never had symptoms that met the DSM-IV criteria for a major depressive disorder. It has been found that the addition of a psychotropic medication in adjustment disorder, on the basis of the mood disturbance, may assist those patients who continue to experience disordered mood and adjustment to the stressor despite treatment with verbal therapies. The antidepressant medications have also been found helpful in the terminally ill who exhibit adjustment disorder with depressed mood and who have not responded to counseling alone.

Treatment

There are no reported randomized controlled trials regarding the psychological, social, or pharmacological treatment of AD. In lieu of any substantive randomized controlled trials to guide treatment, the choice of intervention remains a clinical decision.

There are two approaches to treatment. One is based on the understanding that this disorder emanates from a psychological reaction to a stressor. The stressor needs to be identified, described and shared with the patient; plans must be made to mitigate it, if possible. The abnormal response may be attenuated if the stressor can be eliminated or reduced. Popkin and coworkers (1990) have shown that, in the medically ill, the most common stressor is the medical illness itself; and the AD may remit when the medical illness improves or a new level of adaptation is reached. The other approach to treatment is to provide intervention for the symptomatic presentation, despite the fact that it does not reach threshold level for a specific disorder, on the premise that it is associated with impairment and that treatments that are effective for more pronounced presentations of similar pathology are likely to be effective. This may include psychotherapy, pharmacotherapy, or a combination of the two.

Psychotherapy

Psychotherapeutic intervention in AD is intended to reduce the effects of the stressor, enhance coping to the stressor that cannot be reduced or removed, and establish a mental state and support system to maximize adaptation. Psychotherapy can involve any one of several approaches: cognitive–behavioral treatment, interpersonal therapy, psychodynamic efforts, or counseling.

The first goal of these psychotherapies is to analyze the nature of the stressors affecting the patient to see whether they may be avoided or minimized (e.g., assuming excessive responsibility out of keeping with realistic goals; putting oneself at risk, such as dietary indiscretions for a type I diabetic). It is necessary to clarify and interpret the meaning of the stressor for the patient. For example, an amputation of the leg may have devastated a patient's feelings about himself or herself, especially if the individual was a runner. It is necessary to clarify that the patient still has enormous residual capacity; that he or she can engage in much meaningful work, does not have to lose valued relationships, and can still be sexually active; and that it does not necessarily mean that further body parts will be lost. (However, it will also involve redirecting the physical activity to another pastime.) Otherwise, the patient's pernicious fantasies ("all is lost") may take over in response to the stressor (i.e., amputation), make the patient dysfunctional (at work, sex) and precipitate a painful dysphoria or anxiety reaction.

Some stressors may elicit an overreaction (e.g., the patient's attempted suicide or homicide after the abandonment by a lover). In such instances of overreaction with feelings, emotions, or behaviors, the therapist would help the patient put his or her feelings and rage into words rather than into destructive actions and gain some perspective. The role of verbalization and the joining of affects and conflicts cannot be overestimated in an attempt to reduce the pressure of the stressor and enhance coping. Drugs and alcohol are to be discouraged.

Psychotherapy, medical crisis counseling, crisis intervention, family therapy, group treatment, cognitive–behavioral treatment and interpersonal therapy all encourage the patient to express affects, fears, anxiety, rage, helplessness and hopelessness to the stressors imposed. They also assist the patient to reassess reality in the service of adaptation. Following the example given above, the loss of a leg is not the loss of one's life. But it is a major loss. Sifneos (1989) believed that patients with AD could profit most from brief psychotherapy. The psychotherapy should attempt to reframe the meaning of the stress, find ways to minimize it, and diminish the psychological deficit due to its occurrence. The treatment should expose the concerns and conflicts that the patient is experiencing; help the patient gain perspective on the adversity; and encourage the patient to establish relationships and to attend support groups or self-help groups for assistance in the management of the stressor and the self.

Wise (1988), drawing from his experience in military psychiatry, emphasized the variables of **b**revity, **i**mmediacy, **c**entrality, **e**xpectance, **p**roximity and **s**implicity (BICEPS principles). The treatment structure encompasses a simple straightforward approach dealing with the immediate situation at hand which is troubling the patient. The treatment approach is brief, usually no more than 72 hours.

In another sample, interpersonal psychotherapy was applied to depressed outpatients with human immunodeficiency virus, (HIV), infection and found to be useful (Markowitz *et al.*, 1992). Some of the attributes of interpersonal psychotherapy are psychoeducation regarding the sick role; using a here-and-now framework; formulation of the problems from an interpersonal perspective; exploration of options for changing dysfunctional behavior patterns; and identification of focused interpersonal problem areas. Lazarus (1992) described a seven-pronged approach in the treatment of minor depression. The therapy includes assertiveness training, enjoyable events, coping, imagery, time projection, cognitive disputation, role-playing, desensitization, family therapy and biological prophylaxis.

Support groups have been demonstrated to help patients adjust and enhance their coping mechanisms, and they may prolong life as well although the data is conflicting regarding the latter.

Pharmacotherapy

Stewart and colleagues (1992) emphasized the need to consider psychopharmacological interventions as well as psychotherapy for the treatment of minor depression, and this recommendation might be extrapolated to other subthreshold disorders. This group recommends antidepressant therapy if there is no benefit from 3 months of psychotherapy or other supportive measures. Although psychotherapy is the first choice treatment, psychotherapy combined with benzodiazepines may be helpful, especially for patients with severe life stress(es) and a significant anxious component. Tricyclic antidepressants or buspirone are appropriate in place of benzodiazepines for patients with current or past heavy alcohol use because of the greater risk of dependence in these patients.

Psychotropic medication has been used in the medically ill, in the terminally ill and in patients who have been refractory to verbal therapies. Amphetamine derivatives appear helpful in the treatment of these groups of patients. Whether methylphenidate is similarly useful in AD with depressed mood remains

to be examined. Bereavement-related syndromal depression also appears to respond to antidepressant medication. The medication chosen should reflect the nature of the predominant mood that accompanies the AD (e.g., benzodiazepines for AD with anxious mood; antidepressants for AD with depressed mood). The degree to which pharmacotherapy is used for AD has remained elusive.

Some have begun to examine the effect of homeopathic treatments. From a 25-week multicenter randomized placebo-controlled double-blind trial, a special extract from kava-kava was reported to be effective in AD with anxiety and without the adverse side-effect profile associated with tricyclics and benzodiazepines (Volz and Kieser, 1997). Tianeptine, alprazolam and mianserin were found to be equally effective in symptom improvement in patients with AD and anxious mood. In a random double-blind study trazodone was more effective than clorazepate in cancer patients for the relief of anxious and depressed symptoms. Similar findings were observed in HIV positive patients with AD.

Refractory Patients and Nonresponse to Initial Treatment

Those patients who do not respond to counseling or the various modes of psychotherapy that have been outlined and to a trial of antidepressant or anxiolytic medications should be regarded as treatment nonresponders. It is essential to reevaluate the patient to ensure that the diagnostic impression has not altered and, in particular, that the patient has not developed a major mental disorder, which would require a more aggressive treatment, often biological. The psychiatrist must also consider that an Axis II disorder might be interfering with the patient's resolution of the AD. Finally, if the stressor continues and cannot be removed (e.g., the continuation of a seriously impairing chronic illness), additional support and management strategies need to be employed to assist the patient in optimally adapting to the stressor that she or he is confronting (e.g., experiencing the progression of HIV infection).

DSM-IV allows the use of the diagnosis of AD even after 6 months, and then it is described as AD, chronic. With such a contingency (e.g., AD lasting a few years), it is necessary to ensure that the patient is not experiencing dysthymic disorder or an unremitting depressive disorder. However, these diagnoses have a symptom profile that should distinguish them from the AD.

Conclusion

Appropriate and timely treatment is essential for patients with AD so that their symptoms do not worsen; do not further impair their important relationships; and do not compromise their capacity to work, study, or be active in their interpersonal pursuits. Treatment must attempt to forestall further erosion of the patient's capacity to function that could ultimately have grave and untoward consequences. Maladaptation may so impede the patient that irreversible losses in important sectors of his or her life occur. Although this diagnosis lacks rigorous specificity, its treatment is no less challenging or less important. AD's lack of a designated symptom profile results in this diagnosis having insufficient specificity. However, it is this lack of specificity, which permits the psychiatrist to have a "diagnosis" to use when the patient is presenting with early, vague, nonconcrete symptomatology, which should be noted, identified and followed. This is similar to the situation with early fever, or fever of unknown origin, which, by the way, may never go on to a specific medical diagnosis, but be at discharge simply diagnosed as a "fever of unknown origin". Unspecified chest pain is another example where the patient may never have a specific diagnosis even over time. Spitzer has described the ADs as a "wild card" in the psychiatric lexicon that allows a place for an uncertain, early, not completely developed diagnosis to be housed until it disappears, develops into a full blown category, persists in a subsyndromal state, or disappears. As said above, this is not uncommon with physical or mental subsyndromal states.

DSM-III-R has been described as "medical illness and age unfair" (i.e., it does not sufficiently take into account the issues of age and/or medical illness. DSM-IV-TR has tried to take this into account with considerable effort placed on those psychological interface disorders that border between physical and mental phenomena, for example, the somatoform disorders, AD, dissociation and so on. However, in addition to enhancing reliability and validity, the psychiatric taxonomy needs to consider the impact of developmental epochs (e.g., children and youth, adults, young elderly and "old" elderly) and medical illness on symptomatology. With regard to the latter issue, Endicott (1984) has described replacing vegetative with ideational symptoms when evaluating depressed patients with medical illness. Rapp and Vrana (1989) confirmed Endicott's proposed changes in the diagnostic criteria for depression in medically ill elderly persons and observed maintenance of specificity and sensitivity, respectively, when substituting ideational for vegetative symptoms. Recent studies found AD patients to be significantly younger compared with patients who have a major psychiatric diagnosis. Zarb's (1996) study suggests that cognitively impaired elderly, when evaluated using individual items of the Geriatric Depression Scale exhibited AD rather than major depressive disorder. In addition, Despland and colleagues (1995) reported that the patients' group with AD with depressive or mixed symptoms included more women, thus exhibiting a sex ratio resembling that for major depressive disorder or dysthymic disorder. Therefore, future editions of DSM may be able to take into account the differences encountered in symptom profiles for gender, various developmental epochs, and medical and psychiatric comorbidity. Finally, longitudinal observations would describe the outcome of AD over time. Their resolution, evolution to another diagnosis, their response to a variety of treatments would augment our understanding and approach to this important subthreshold diagnosis.

Comparison of DSM-IV/ICD-10 Diagnostic Criteria

In contrast to DSM-IV-TR (which requires the onset of symptoms within 3 months of the stressor), the ICD-10 Diagnostic Criteria for Research specify an onset within 1 month. Furthermore, ICD-10 excludes stressors of "unusual or catastrophic type". In contrast, DSM-IV-TR allows extreme stressors so long as the criteria are not met for post traumatic or acute stress disorder. ICD-10 also provides for several different subtypes, including "brief depressive reaction" (depressive state lasting 1 month or less) and "prolonged depressive reaction" (depressive state lasting up to 2 years).

References

American Psychiatric Association (1980) *Diagnostic and Statistical Manual of Mental Disorders*, 3rd edn. APA, Washington DC.

American Psychiatric Association (1987) *Diagnostic and Statistical Manual of Mental Disorders*, 3rd ed., Rev. APA Washington DC.

American Psychiatric Association (2000) *Diagnostic and Statistical Manual of Mental Disorders*, 4th edn., Text Rev. APA, Washington DC.

Cohen F (1981) Stress and bodily illness. *Psychiatr Clin N Am* 4, 269–286.

Despland JN, Monod L and Ferrero F (1995) Clinical relevance of AD in DSM-III-R and DSM-IV. *Comp Psychiatr* 36, 456–460.

Endicott J (1984) Measurement of depression in patients with cancer. *Cancer* 53, 2243–2249.

Fabrega H Jr, Mezzich J, Mezzich AC *et al.* (1986) Descriptive validity of DSM-I. II. Depressions. *J Nerv Ment Dis* 174, 573–584.

Friedmann MS, McDermut WH, Solomon DA *et al.* (1997) Family functioning and mental illness: A comparison of psychiatric and nonclinical families. *Fam Process* 36, 357–367.

Isometsa E, Heikkinen M, Henriksson M *et al.* (1996) Suicide in nonmajor depressions. *J Affect Disord* 36, 117–127.

Lazarus AA (1992) The multimodal approach to the treatment of minor depression. *Am J Psychother* 46, 50–57.

Markowitz JC, Klerman GL and Perry SW (1992) Interpersonal psychotherapy of depressed HIV-positive outpatients. *Hosp Comm Psychiatr* 43, 885–890.

Monroe SM, Kupfer DJ and Frank E (1992) Life stress and treatment course of recurrent depression. I. Response during index episode. *J Consult Clin Psychol* 60, 718–724.

Oxman TE, Barrett JE, Freeman DH *et al.* (1994) Frequency and correlates of adjustment disorder relates to cardiac surgery in older patients. *Psychosomatics* 35, 557–568.

Popkin MK, Callies AL and Colon EA (1988) *The Treatment and Outcome of Adjustment Disorders in Medically Ill Inpatients*. National Institute of Mental Health Conference, Pittsburgh, PA.

Popkin MK, Callies AL, Colon EA *et al.* (1990) Adjustment disorders in medically ill patients referred for consultation in a university hospital. *Psychosomatics* 31, 410–414.

Rapp SR and Vrana S (1989) Substituting nonsomatic for somatic symptoms in the diagnosis of depression in elderly male medical patients. *Am J Psychiatr* 146, 1197–1200.

Runeson BS, Beskow J and Waern M (1996) The suicidal process in suicides among young people. *Acta Psychiatr Scand* 93, 35–42.

Sifneos PE (1989) Brief dynamic and crisis therapy, in *Comprehensive Textbook of Psychiatry*, Vol. 2, 5th edn. (eds Kaplan HI and Sadock BJ). Williams & Wilkins, Baltimore, pp. 1562–1567.

Snyder S and Strain JJ (1989) Differentiation of major depression and adjustment disorder with depressed mood in the medical setting. *Gen Hosp Psychiatr* 12, 159–165.

Snyder S and Strain JJ (1990) Diagnostic instability in psychiatric consultations. *Hosp Comm Psychiatr* 41, 10–13.

Spalletta G, Troisi A, Saracco M *et al.* (1996) Symptom profile: Axis II comorbidity and suicidal behaviour in young males with DSM-III-R depressive illnesses. *J Affect Disord* 39, 141–148.

Spiegel D (1996) Cancer and depression. *Br J Psychiatr* 168(Suppl 30), 109–116.

Stewart JW, Quitkin FM and Klein DF (1992) The pharmacotherapy of minor depression. *Am J Psychother* 46, 23–36.

Strain JJ, Newcorn JH, Mezzich JE *et al.* (1998) Adjustment disorder: The MacArthur reanalysis, in *DSM-IV Sourcebook*, Vol. 4. American Psychiatric Association, Washington DC, pp. 403–424.

Volz HP and Kieser M (1997) Kava-kava extract WS 1490 versus placebo in anxiety disorders: A randomized placebo-controlled 25-week outpatient trial. *Pharmacopsychiatry* 30, 1–5.

Wise MG (1988) Adjustment disorders and impulse control disorders not otherwise classified. In Textbook of Psychiatry, Talbot JA, Hales R, and Yodofsky SC (eds). American Psychiatric Press, Washington DC, pp. 605–620.

Zarb J (1996) Correlates of depression in cognitively impaired hospitalized elderly referred for neuropsychological assessment. *J Clin Exp Neuropsychol* 18, 713–723.

62 Personality Disorders

Personality traits have long been the focus of considerable research. Their heritability, cross-situational consistency, temporal stability, functional relevance to work, well-being, marital stability and even physical health have been well established across many studies. Everybody has a personality, or a characteristic manner of thinking, feeling, behaving and relating to others. Some persons are typically introverted and withdrawn, others are more extraverted and outgoing. Some persons are invariably conscientious and efficient, whereas other persons might be consistently undependable and negligent. Some persons are characteristically anxious and apprehensive, whereas others are typically relaxed and unconcerned. These personality traits are often felt to be integral to each person's sense of self, as they involve what persons value, what they do, and their innate tendencies and preferences.

It is "when personality traits are inflexible and maladaptive and cause significant functional impairment or subjective distress [that] they constitute Personality Disorders" (American Psychiatric Association, 2000, p. 686). The *Diagnostic and Statistical Manual of Mental Disorders*, Fourth Edition, Text Revision (DSM-IV-TR) (American Psychiatric Association, 2000) provides the diagnostic criteria for 10 personality disorders. Two additional diagnoses are placed within an appendix to DSM-IV for criteria sets provided for further study (passive–aggressive and depressive). This chapter begins with a discussion of the definition, etiology, assessment, epidemiology, course and treatment of personality disorders in general, followed by a discussion of these issues for the 12 individual personality disorders.

Personality Disorder

Definition

A personality disorder is defined in DSM-IV-TR as "an enduring pattern of inner experience and behavior that deviates markedly from the expectations of the individual's culture, is pervasive and inflexible, has an onset in adolescence or early adulthood, is stable over time, and leads to distress or impairment" (American Psychiatric Association, 2000, p. 686). The DSM-IV-TR general diagnostic criteria for a personality disorder are provided below.

Personality disorder is the only class of mental disorders in DSM-IV-TR for which an explicit definition and criterion set are provided. A general definition and criterion set can be useful to psychiatrists because the most common personality disorder diagnosis in clinical practice is often the diagnosis "not otherwise specified" (NOS) (Clark *et al.*, 1995). Psychiatrists provide the NOS diagnosis when they determine that a personality disorder

is present but the symptomatology fails to meet the criterion set for one of the 10 specific personality disorders. A general definition of what is meant by a personality disorder is therefore helpful when determining whether the NOS diagnosis should in fact be provided. Points worth emphasizing with respect to the general criterion set are presented in the following discussion of the assessment, differential diagnosis, epidemiology and course of personality disorders.

DSM-IV-TR Criteria

General Diagnostic Criteria for Personality Disorder

A. An enduring pattern of inner experience and behavior that deviates markedly from the expectations of the individual's culture. This pattern is manifested in two (or more) of the following areas:

1. cognition (i.e., ways of perceiving and interpreting self, other people, and events)

2. affectivity (i.e., the range, intensity, lability, and appropriateness of emotional response)

3. interpersonal functioning

4. impulse control

B. The enduring pattern is inflexible and pervasive across a broad range of personal and social situations.

C. The enduring pattern leads to clinically significant distress or impairment in social, occupational, or other important areas of functioning.

D. The pattern is stable and of long duration and its onset can be traced back at least to adolescence or early adulthood.

E. The enduring pattern is not better accounted for as a manifestation or consequence of another mental disorder.

F. The enduring pattern is not due to the direct physiological effects of a substance (e.g., a drug of abuse, a medication) or a general medical condition (e.g., head trauma).

Reprinted with permission from the *Diagnostic and Statistical Manual of Mental Disorders*, Fourth Edition, Text Revision. Copyright 2000 American Psychiatric Association.

Essentials of Psychiatry   Jerald Kay and Allan Tasman
© 2006 John Wiley & Sons, Ltd.

Etiology and Pathophysiology

A primary purpose of a diagnosis is to lead to scientific knowledge concerning the etiology for a patient's condition and the identification of a specific pathology for which a particular treatment (e.g., medication) would ameliorate the condition. However, many of the mental disorders in DSM-IV-TR, including the personality disorders, may not in fact have single etiologies or even specific pathologies. The DSM-IV-TR personality disorders might be, for the most part, constellations of maladaptive personality traits that are the result of multiple genetic dispositions interacting with a variety of detrimental environmental experiences. The DSM-IV-TR personality disorder diagnoses do provide the clinician with a substantial amount of important information concerning the etiology and pathology for a patient's particular personality syndrome, but there are likely to be alternative pathways to the development of maladaptive personality traits and alternative neurophysiological, cognitive–behavioral, interpersonal and psychodynamic models for their pathology (Livesley, 2001).

Assessment and Differential Diagnosis

Since 1980, the multiaxial system appears to have been successful in encouraging psychiatrists no longer to make arbitrary distinctions between personality disorders and other mental disorders. Ironically, however, the placement of the personality disorders on a separate axis may have also contributed to the development of false assumptions and misleading expectations concerning the distinctions between personality disorders and other mental disorders with respect to etiology, pathology, or treatment. It has been difficult to provide a brief list of specific diagnostic criteria for the broad and complex behavior patterns that constitute a personality disorder. The only personality disorder to be diagnosed reliably in general clinical practice has been antisocial and the validity of this diagnosis has been questioned precisely because of its emphasis on overt and behaviorally specific acts of criminality, irresponsibility and delinquency.

There are assessment instruments, however, that will help psychiatrists obtain more reliable and valid personality disorder diagnoses. Semi-structured interviews will obtain reliable diagnoses of personality disorders and are therefore the preferred method for the assessment of personality disorders in clinical settings. Semi-structured interviews provide a researched set of required and recommended interview queries and observations to assess each of the personality disorder diagnostic criteria. Psychiatrists can find the administration of a semi-structured interview to be constraining but a major strength of semi-structured interviews is their assurance through an explicit structure that each relevant diagnostic criterion has in fact been systematically assessed. Idiosyncratic and subjective interviewing techniques are much more likely to result in gender- and culturally-biased assessments relative to unstructured clinical interviews. The manuals that accompany a semi-structured interview also provide useful information for understanding the rationale of each diagnostic criterion, for interpreting vague or inconsistent symptomatology, and for resolving diagnostic ambiguities. There are currently five semi-structured interviews for the assessment of the DSM-IV-TR (American Psychiatric Association, 2000) personality disorder diagnostic criteria: 1) Diagnostic Interview for Personality Disorders (Zanarini et al., 1995); 2) International Personality Disorder Examination (Loranger, 1999); 3) Personality Disorder Interview-IV (Widiger et al., 1995); 4) Structured Clinical Interview for DSM-IV-TR Axis II Personality

Disorders (First et al., 1997); and 5) Structured Interview for DSM-IV-TR Personality Disorders (Pfohl et al., 1997). The particular advantages and disadvantages of each particular interview have been discussed extensively (Widiger and Coker, 2002).

The administration of an entire personality disorder semi-structured interview can take 2 hours, an amount of time that is impractical for routine clinical practice. However, this time can be reduced substantially by first administering a self-report questionnaire that screens for the presence of the DSM-IV-TR personality disorders (Widiger and Coker, 2002). A psychiatrist can then confine the interview to the few personality disorders that the self-report inventory suggested would be present. Self-report inventories are useful in ensuring that all of the personality disorders were systematically considered and in alerting the clinician to the presence of maladaptive personality traits that might otherwise have been missed. There are a number of alternative self-report inventories that can be used and the advantages and disadvantages of each of them have been discussed extensively (Widiger and Coker, 2002).

Gender and cultural biases are one potential source of inaccurate personality disorder diagnosis that are worth noting in particular. One of the general diagnostic criteria for personality disorder is that the personality trait must deviate markedly from the expectations of a person's culture (see DSM-IV-TR general diagnostic criteria for personality disorders). The purpose of this cultural deviation requirement is to compel clinicians to consider the cultural background of the patient. A behavior pattern that appears to be aberrant from the perspective of one's own culture (e.g., submissiveness or emotionality) could be quite normative and adaptive within another culture. The cultural expectations or norms of the psychiatrist might not be relevant or applicable to a patient from a different cultural background. However, one should not infer from this requirement that a personality disorder is primarily or simply a deviation from a cultural norm. Deviation from the expectations of one's culture is not necessarily maladaptive, nor is conformity to one's culture necessarily healthy. Many of the personality disorders may even represent (in part) extreme or excessive variants of behavior patterns that are valued or encouraged within a particular culture. For example, it is usually adaptive to be confident but not to be arrogant, to be agreeable but not to be submissive, or to be conscientious but not to be perfectionistic. Gender and cultural biases of particular relevance to individual personality disorders will be discussed further in the chapter.

Epidemiology and Comorbidity

Virtually all patients must have had a characteristic manner of thinking, feeling, behaving and relating to others prior to the onset of an Axis I disorder that could have an important impact on the course and treatment of the respective mental disorder and many of these persons would be diagnosed with a DSM-IV-TR personality. Estimates of the prevalence of personality disorder within clinical settings is typically above 50%. As many as 60% of inpatients within some clinical settings would be diagnosed with borderline personality disorder and as many as 50% of inmates within a correctional setting could be diagnosed with antisocial personality disorder. Although the comorbid presence of a personality disorder is likely to have an important impact on the course and treatment of an Axis I disorder the prevalence of personality disorder is generally underestimated in clinical practice due in part to the failure to provide systematic or comprehensive assessments of personality disorder symptomatology and perhaps as well to the lack of funding for the treatment of personality disorders.

Approximately 10 to 15% of the general population would be diagnosed with one of the 10 DSM-IV-TR personality disorders, excluding PDNOS. However the studies of community populations have important limitations that qualify their results. For example, many of the studies sampled persons who would probably have less personality disorder pathology than a randomly selected sample (e.g., some studies have sampled persons without any history of Axis I psychopathology) and the studies have used either the DSM-III (American Psychiatric Association, 1980) or DSM-III-R (American Psychiatric Association, 1987) criterion sets rather than DSM-IV-TR (American Psychiatric Association, 2000). Nevertheless, the prevalence estimates are generally close to those provided in DSM-IV-TR. Prevalence rates for individual personality disorders will be discussed later in this chapter.

There is also considerable personality disorder diagnostic cooccurrence (Table 62.1). Patients who meet the DSM-IV diagnostic criteria for one personality disorder are likely to meet the diagnostic criteria for another DSM-IV instructs psychiatrists that all diagnoses should be recorded because it can be important to consider (for example) the presence of antisocial traits in someone with a borderline personality disorder or the presence of paranoid traits in someone with a dependent personality disorder. However, the extent of diagnostic cooccurrence is at times so extensive that most researchers prefer a more dimensional description of personality. Diagnostic categories provide clear, vivid descriptions of discrete personality types but the personality structure of actual patients might be more accurately described by a constellation of maladaptive personality traits.

Alternative dimensional models of personality disorder are being developed. One such model, based on a theory of temperament and character, consists of seven dimensions. Cloninger (2000) proposes that there are four temperaments (reward dependence, harm avoidance, novelty seeking and persistence), each governed by a particular neurotransmitter system, and three character dimensions (self-directedness, cooperativeness and self-transcendence). The presence of a personality disorder is said to be determined primarily by the four temperaments and the particular form or manner of the personality disorder by the three character dimensions.

Alternative dimensional models of personality disorder are being developed. One such model, based on a theory of temperament and character, consists of seven dimensions. Cloninger (2000) proposes that there are four temperaments (reward dependence, harm avoidance, novelty seeking and persistence), each governed by a particular neurotransmitter system, and three character dimensions (self-directedness, cooperativeness and self-transcendence). The presence of a personality disorder is said to be determined primarily by the four temperaments and the particular form or manner of the personality disorder by the three character dimensions. Another approach has been to apply the predominant model of general personality functioning to the study of personality disorders. Five broad domains of personality functioning have been identified empirically through the study of the languages of a number of different cultures. Language can be understood as a sedimentary deposit of the observations of persons over the thousands of years of the language's development and transformation. The most important domains of personality functioning would be those with the greatest number of terms to describe and differentiate their various manifestations and nuances, and the structure of personality will be evident by the empirical relationship among the trait terms. Such lexical analyses of languages have typically identified five fundamental dimensions of personality: neuroticism (or negative affectivity) versus emotional stability, introversion versus extraversion, conscientiousness versus undependability, antagonism versus agreeableness, and closedness versus openness to experience (Costa and McCrae, 1992). Each of these five broad domains can be differentiated further in terms of underlying facets. For example, the facets of antagonism versus agreeableness include suspiciousness versus trusting gullibility, tough-mindedness versus tender-mindedness, confidence and arrogance versus modesty and meekness, exploitation versus altruism and sacrifice, oppositionalism and aggression versus compliance, and deception and manipulation versus straightforwardness and honesty. Each of the DSM-IV-TR personality disorders can be understood as maladaptive variants of these personality traits that are evident in all persons to varying degrees.

Table 62.1 DSM-III-R Personality Disorder Diagnostic Cooccurrence Aggregated Across Six Research Sites

	PRN	SZD	SZT	ATS	BDL	HST	NCS	AVD	DPD	OCP	PAG
Paranoid (PRN)		8	19	15	41	28	26	44	23	21	30
Schizoid (SZD)	38		39	8	22	8	22	55	11	20	9
Schizotypal (SZT)	43	32		19	4	17	26	68	34	19	18
Antisocial (ATS)	30	8	15		59	39	40	25	19	9	29
Borderline (BDL)	31	6	16	23		30	19	39	36	12	21
Histrionic (HST)	29	2	7	17	41		40	21	28	13	25
Narcissistic (NCS)	41	12	18	25	38	60		32	24	21	38
Avoidant (AVD)	33	15	22	11	39	16	15		43	16	19
Dependent (DPD)	26	3	16	16	48	24	14	57		15	22
Obs-Compulsive (OCP)	31	10	11	4	25	21	19	37	27		23
Pass-Aggressive (PAG)	39	6	12	25	44	36	39	41	34	23	

Sites used DSM-III-R criterion sets. Data obtained for purposes of informing the development of the DSM-IV-TR personality disorder diagnostic criteria.

Widiger TA and Trull TJ (1998) Performance characteristics of the DSM-III-R personality disorder criteria sets. Reprinted with permission from DSM IV Source book Vol. 4. Widiger TA, Francis AJ, Pincus HA et al (Eds.). Copyright 1998, American Psychiatric Association, Washington DC.

Table 62.2   DSM-IV-TR Personality Disorders from the Perspective of the Five-factor Model of General Personality Functioning

	PRN	SZD	SZT	ATS	BDL	HST	NCS	AVD	DPD	OCP
Neuroticism										
Anxiousness			High		High			High	High	
Angry hostility	High			High	High		High			
Depressiveness					High	High		High		
Self-consciousness						High	High	High	High	
Impulsivity					High					
Vulnerability					High			High	High	
Extraversion										
Warmth		Low	Low			High			High	
Gregariousness		Low	Low			HIgh		Low		
Assertiveness								Low	Low	High
Activity										
Excitement-seeking				High		High		Low		
Positive emotionality		Low	Low			High				
Openness										
Fantasy			High			High	High			
Aesthetics										
Feelings		Low				High				
Actions			High							
Ideas			High							
Values										Low
Agreeableness										
Trust	Low		Low		Low	High			High	
Straightforwardness	Low			Low					High	
Altruism				Low			Low		High	
Compliance				Low	Low				High	Low
Modesty							Low		High	
Tender-mindedness				Low			Low			
Conscientiousness										
Competence					Low					High
Order										High
Dutifulness				Low						High
Achievement-striving							High			High
Self-discipline				Low						
Deliberation				Low						

Table 62.2 provides a description of the DSM-IV-TR personality disorders in terms of this five-factor model. For example, the schizoid personality disorder may represent an extreme variant of introversion, avoidant may represent extreme neuroticism and introversion, and antisocial personality disorder an extreme variant of antagonism and undependability. Advantages of understanding personality disorders in terms of this dimensional model are the provision of more specific descriptions of individual patients (including adaptive as well as maladaptive personality functioning) and the avoidance of arbitrary categorical distinctions. An additional factor is the ability to bring to bear on an understanding of personality disorders the extensive amount of research on the heritability, temperament, development and course of general personality functioning.

Course

Personality disorders must be evident since adolescence or young adulthood and have been relatively chronic and stable throughout adult life (see DSM-IV-TR criteria for personality disorders). The World Health Organization's (WHO) *International Classification of Diseases*, 10th Revision (ICD-10, World Health Organization, 1992) does recognize the existence of personality change second-

ary to catastrophic experiences and to brain injury or disease, but only the latter is included within DSM-IV-TR (American Psychiatric Association, 2000). A 75-year-old man can be diagnosed with a DSM-IV-TR dependent personality disorder but the symptoms must have been present throughout the duration of his adulthood (e.g., since the age of 18 years) unless the dependent behavior was a direct, explicit expression of a neurochemical disease or lesion.

The requirement that a personality disorder be evident since late adolescence and be relatively chronic thereafter has been a traditional means with which to distinguish a personality disorder from an Axis I disorder. Mood, anxiety, psychotic, sexual and other mental disorders have traditionally been conceptualized as conditions that arise at some point during a person's life and that are relatively limited or circumscribed in their expression and duration. Personality disorders, in contrast, are conditions that are evident as early as late adolescence (and in some instances prior to that time), are evident in everyday functioning, and are stable throughout adulthood. However, the consistency of this distinction across disorders in the classification has been decreasing with each edition of the DSM, as early-onset and chronic variants of Axis I disorders are being added to the diagnostic manual (e.g., early-onset dysthymia and generalized social phobia). Some researchers have in fact suggested abandoning the concept of personality disorders and replacing them with early-onset and chronic variants of existing Axis I disorders. For example, avoidant personality disorder could become generalized social phobia, obsessive–compulsive personality disorder could become an early-onset variant of obsessive–compulsive anxiety disorder, and borderline personality disorder could become an early-onset and chronic mood dyscontrol.

Treatment

One of the mistaken assumptions or expectations of Axis II is that personality disorders are untreatable. In fact, maladaptive personality traits are often the focus of clinical attention. Personality disorders are among the more difficult of mental disorders to treat as they involve entrenched behavior patterns, some of which will be integral to a patient's self-image. Nevertheless, there is compelling empirical support to indicate that meaningful responsivity to psychosocial and pharmacologic treatment does occur. Treatment of a personality disorder is unlikely to result in the development of a fully healthy or ideal personality structure, but clinically and socially meaningful change to personality structure and functioning does occur. In fact, given the considerable social, occupational, medical and other costs that are engendered by such personality disorders as the antisocial and borderline, even marginal reductions in symptomatology can represent quite significant and meaningful public health care, social and clinical benefits.

DSM-IV-TR includes 10 individual personality disorder diagnoses that are organized into three clusters: 1) paranoid, schizoid and schizotypal (placed within an odd–eccentric cluster); 2) antisocial, borderline, histrionic and narcissistic (dramatic–emotional–erratic cluster); and 3) avoidant, dependent and obsessive–compulsive (anxious–fearful cluster) (American Psychiatric Association, 2000). Each of these personality disorders, along with the two that are included in the appendix to DSM-IV-TR for disorders needing further study (i.e., passive–aggressive and depressive), will be discussed in turn.

Paranoid Personality Disorder

Definition

Paranoid personality disorder (PPD) involves a pervasive and continuous distrust and suspiciousness of the motives of others) but the disorder is more than just suspiciousness. Persons with this disorder are also hypersensitive to criticism, they respond with anger to threats to their autonomy, they incessantly seek out confirmations of their suspicions, and they tend to be quite rigid in their beliefs and perceptions of others. The presence of PPD is indicated by four or more of the seven diagnostic criteria presented in the DSM-IV criteria for PPD.

Etiology and Pathology

Research has indicated a genetic contribution to the development of suspiciousness and mistrust. There is some support for a genetic relationship of PPD with schizophrenia but these findings have not always been replicated and the findings may have been due to the overlap of PPD with the schizotypal personality disorder

---

> ## DSM-IV-TR Criteria 301.0
>
> **Paranoid Personality Disorder**
>
> A. A pervasive distrust and suspiciousness of others such that their motives are interpreted as malevolent, beginning by early adulthood, and present in a variety of contexts, as indicated by four (or more) of the following:
>
> (1) suspects, without sufficient basis, that others are exploiting, harming, or deceiving him or her
>
> (2) is preoccupied with unjustified doubts about the loyalty or trustworthiness of friends or associates
>
> (3) is reluctant to confide in others because of unwarranted fear that the information will be used maliciously against him or her
>
> (4) reads hidden demeaning or threatening meanings into benign remarks or events
>
> (5) persistently bears grudges, i.e. is unforgiving of insults, injuries, or slights
>
> (6) perceives attacks on his or her character or reputation that are not apparent to others and is quick to react angrily or to counterattack
>
> (7) has recurrent suspicions, without justification, regarding fidelity of spouse or sexual partner
>
> B. Does not occur exclusively during the course of schizophrenia, a mood disorder with psychotic features, or another psychotic disorder, and is not due to the direct physiological effects of a general medical condition.
>
> **Note:** if criteria are met prior to the onset of schizophrenia, add "premorbid", e.g., paranoid personality disorder (premorbid).

Reprinted with permission from the *Diagnostic and Statistical Manual of Mental Disorders*, Fourth Edition, Text Revision. Copyright 2000 American Psychiatric Association.

There are no systematic studies on possible psychosocial contributions to the development of PPD. There is some support for the contribution of excessive parental criticism and rejection but there has not yet been adequate prospective longitudinal studies. Paranoid belief systems could develop through parental modeling, a history of discriminatory exploitation or abandonment, or the projection of anger, resentment and bitterness onto a group that is external to, and distinct from, oneself. Mistrust and suspicion is often evident in members of minority groups, immigrants, refugees and other groups for whom such distrust can be a realistic and appropriate response to the social environment. It is conceivable that a comparably sustained experience through childhood and adolescence could contribute to the development of excessive paranoid beliefs that are eventually applied inflexibly and inappropriately to a wide variety of persons, but it can be very difficult to determine what is excessive or unrealistic suspicion and mistrust within a member of an oppressed minority. Paranoid suspiciousness could in fact be more closely associated with prejudicial attitudes, wherein a particular minority group in society becomes the inappropriate target of one's anger, blame and resentment.

There has been little consideration given to the neuro-physiological concomitants of nonpsychotic paranoid personality traits. More attention has been given to cognitive, interpersonal and object-relational models of pathology. Paranoid beliefs do appear to have a self-perpetuating tendency resulting from the narrow and limited focus on signs and evidence for malicious intentions. The pathology of PPD, from this perspective, is inherent to the irrationality of the person's belief systems and is sustained by the biased information processing. There may also be an underlying motivation or need to perceive threats in others and to externalize blame that help to sustain the accusations and distortions.

Differential Diagnosis

PPD paranoid ideation is inconsistent with reality and is resistant to contrary evidence but the ideation is not psychotic, absurd, inconceivable, or bizarre. PPD also lacks other features of psychotic and delusional disorders (e.g., hallucinations) and is evident since early adulthood, whereas a psychotic disorder becomes evident later within a person's life or remits after a much briefer period of time. Persons with PPD can develop psychotic disorders but to diagnose PPD in such cases the paranoid personality traits must be evident prior to and persist after the psychotic episode. If PPD precedes the onset of schizophrenia, then it should be noted that it is premorbid to the schizophrenia (American Psychiatric Association, 2000). However, it may not be meaningful to diagnose a person with both PPD and schizophrenia, as the premorbid paranoid traits may in some cases have simply represented a prodromal phase of the schizophrenic pathology.

Epidemiology and Comorbidity

Trust versus mistrust is a fundamental personality trait along which all persons vary. Thirteen percent of the adult male population and 6% of the adult female population may be characteristically mistrustful of others (Costa and McCrae, 1992). However, only 0.5 to 2.5% of the population are likely to meet the DSM-IV-TR diagnostic criteria for a PPD. It is suggested in DSM-IV-TR that approximately 10 to 30% of persons within inpatient settings and 2 to 10% within outpatient settings have this disorder (American Psychiatric Association, 2000) but the lower end of these rates may represent the more accurate estimate. It does appear that more males than females have the disorder.

Paranoid personality traits are evident in other personality disorders. Persons with avoidant personality disorder are socially withdrawn and apprehensive of others; borderline, antisocial and narcissistic persons may be impatient, irritable and antagonistic; and schizotypal persons may display paranoid ideation. The diagnosis of PPD often cooccurs with these other personality disorder diagnoses. Persons with PPD are prone to develop a variety of Axis I disorders, including substance-related, obsessive–compulsive anxiety, agoraphobia and depressive disorders (American Psychiatric Association, 2000).

Course

Premorbid traits of PPD may be evident prior to adolescence in the form of social isolation, hypersensitivity, hypervigilance, social anxiety, peculiar thoughts, angry hostility and idiosyncratic fantasies (American Psychiatric Association, 2000). As children, they may appear odd and peculiar to their peers and they may not have achieved to their capacity in school. Their adjustment as adults is particularly poor with respect to interpersonal relationships. They may become socially isolated or fanatic members of groups that encourage or at least accept their paranoid ideation. They might maintain a steady employment but are difficult coworkers, as they tend to be rigid, controlling, critical, blaming and prejudicial. They are likely to become involved in lengthy, acrimonious and litigious disputes that are difficult, if not impossible, to resolve.

Treatment

Persons with PPD rarely seek treatment for their feelings of suspiciousness and distrust. They experience these traits as simply accurate perceptions of a malevolent and dangerous world (i.e., egosyntonic). They may not consider the paranoid attributions to be at all problematic, disruptive, or maladaptive. They are not delusional but they also fail to be reflective, insightful, or self-critical. They may recognize only that they have difficulty controlling their anger and getting along with others. They might be in treatment for an anxiety, mood, or substance-related disorder or for various marital, familial, occupational, or social (or legal) conflicts that are secondary to their personality disorder but they also externalize the responsibility for their problems and have substantial difficulty recognizing their own contribution to their internal dysphoria and external conflicts. They consider their problems to be due to what others are doing to them, not to how they perceive, react, or relate to others.

The presence of paranoid personality traits complicate the treatment of an Axis I disorder or a relationship problem. Trust is central to the development of an adequate therapeutic alliance, yet it is precisely the absence of trust that is central to this disorder. It can be tempting to be less than forthright and open in the treatment of excessively suspicious persons because they distort, exaggerate, or escalate minor errors, misunderstandings, or inconsistent statements. However, therapists find that they weave an increasingly tangled web as they walk gingerly around the truth. Also, persons with PPD seize upon any kernel of deception to confirm their suspicion that the therapist is not to be trusted. It is preferable to be especially forthright and precise with paranoid patients. Details that are inconsequential and of no interest to most patients can be important to provide to persons with PPD so that they are ensured that nothing is being withheld or hidden from them.

Clinicians agree on several general principles in the treatment of paranoid personality. It is usually pointless and often harmful to rapport or to confront (or argue with) the paranoid beliefs. Such efforts may only alienate the patient and confirm his or her suspicions. The therapist should maintain a sincere and consistent respect for their autonomy and for their right to make their own decisions. However, one should not attempt to ingratiate oneself by being overly acquiescent and compliant. This can appear to be obviously patronizing, insincere, or manipulative. The goal is to develop, in a nonthreatening way, more self-reflection and self-awareness (e.g., recognition of the contribution of the paranoid traits and behaviors to the difficulties they are experiencing within their lives). A useful approach can be to communicate a sincere and respectful willingness to explore the implications, logic and reality of the suspicions. Whenever one appears to be endangering rapport by moving too quickly, one should retreat to a more neutral and accepting position.

One must also be careful to avoid defensive reactions to the inevitable accusations. Any one of the conflicts they have had with others can develop within the therapeutic relationship and persons with PPD have a tendency to be contentious, rigid, accusatory, suspicious and litigious that can tax the empathy and patience of the therapist. One must attempt to maintain an empathic concern for their feelings of betrayal, and reassure them in an understanding, forthright manner that is neither patronizing nor disrespectful. Termination of treatment may at times be necessary if continuation would only result in further acrimony.

The suspicions, accusations and acrimony often makes the person with PPD a poor candidate for group therapies. There is the potential to learn much about themselves within a group, but it is usually very difficult for them to develop the feelings of trust, respect and security that are necessary for successful group therapy. Their propensity to make unfair hostile accusations alienate them from other group members, and they may quickly become a scapegoat for difficulties and conflicts that develop within the group.

There have been a variety of studies on the pharmacologic treatment of psychotic paranoid ideation and of schizotypal PD (which often includes paranoid personality traits) but little to no research on the pharmacologic responsivity of the nonpsychotic suspiciousness and egosyntonic paranoid ideation of PPD. Persons with PPD may also perceive the use of a medication to represent an effort simply to suppress or control their accusations and suspicions rather than respectfully to consider and address them. However, they may be receptive and responsive to the benefits of a medication to help control feelings of anxiousness or depression that are secondary to their personality disorder.

DSM-IV-TR Criteria 301.20

Schizoid Personality Disorder

A. A pervasive pattern of detachment from social relationships and a restricted range of expression of emotions in interpersonal settings, beginning by early adulthood and present in a variety of contexts, as indicated by four (or more) of the following:

   (1) neither desires nor enjoys close relationships, including being part of a family

   (2) almost always chooses solitary activities

   (3) has little, if any, interest in having sexual experiences with another person

   (4) takes pleasure in few, if any, activities

   (5) lacks close friends or confidants other than first-degree relatives

   (6) appears indifferent to the praise or criticism of others

   (7) emotional coldness, detachment, or flattened affectivity

B. Does not occur exclusively during the course of schizophrenia, a mood disorder with psychotic features, another psychotic disorder, or a pervasive developmental disorder, and is not due to the direct physiological effects of a general medical condition.

Note: if criteria are met prior to the onset of schizophrenia, add "premorbid", e.g., schizoid personality disorder (premorbid).

Reprinted with permission from the *Diagnostic and Statistical Manual of Mental Disorders*, Fourth Edition, Text Revision. Copyright 2000 American Psychiatric Association.

Schizoid Personality Disorder

Definition

The schizoid personality disorder (SZPD) is a pervasive pattern of social detachment and restricted emotional expression. Introversion (versus extraversion) is one of the fundamental dimensions of general personality functioning. Facets of introversion include low warmth (e.g., cold, detached, impersonal), low gregariousness (socially isolated, withdrawn) and low positive emotions (reserved, constricted or flat affect, anhedonic), which define well the central symptoms of SZPD (see Table 62.1). The presence of SZPD is indicated by four or more of the seven diagnostic criteria presented in the DSM-IV criteria for SZPD.

Etiology and Pathology

A fundamental distinction for schizophrenic symptomatology is between positive and negative symptoms. Positive symptoms include hallucinations, delusions, inappropriate affect and loose associations; negative symptoms include flattened affect, alogia, anhedonia and avolition. SZPD has been conceptualized as representing subthreshold negative symptoms, comparable to the subthreshold positive symptoms (cognitive–perceptual aberrations) that predominate schizotypal personality disorder (STPD). However, a genetic link of SZPD to schizophrenia that cannot be accounted for by comorbid STPD symptomatology has not been well established. Research has supported heritability for the personality dimension of introversion–extraversion and for the association of SZPD with introversion. The central pathology of SZPD does appear to be anhedonic deficits, or an excessively low ability to experience positive affect. Psychosocial models for the etiology of SZPD are lacking. It is possible that a sustained history of isolation during infancy and childhood, with an encouragement and modeling by parental figures of interpersonal withdrawal, indifference and detachment could contribute to the development of schizoid personality traits.

Differential Diagnosis

SZPD can be confused with the schizotypal and avoidant personality disorders as both involve social isolation and withdrawal. Schizotypal personality disorder, however, also includes an intense social anxiety and cognitive–perceptual aberrations. The major distinction with avoidant personality disorder is the absence of an intense desire for intimate social relationships. Avoidant persons will also exhibit substantial insecurity and inhibition, whereas the schizoid person is largely indifferent toward the reactions or opinions of others.

The presence of premorbid schizoid traits can have prognostic significance for the course and treatment of schizophrenia but, more importantly, it might not be meaningful to suggest that a person has a schizoid personality disorder that is independent of or unrelated to a comorbid schizophrenia. The negative, prodromal and residual symptoms of schizophrenia resemble closely the features of SZPD. Once a person develops schizophrenia, a diagnosis of SZPD can become rather pointless as all of the schizoid symptoms can then be understood as (prodromal or residual) symptoms of schizophrenia.

Epidemiology and Comorbidity

Approximately half of the general population will exhibit an introversion within the normal range of functioning. However, only a small minority of the population would be diagnosed with a schizoid personality disorder. Estimates of the prevalence of

SZPD within the general population have been less than 1% and SZPD is among the least frequently diagnosed personality disorders within clinical settings. Many of the persons who were diagnosed with SZPD prior to DSM-III are probably now diagnosed with either the avoidant or the schizotypal personality disorders and prototypic (pure) cases of SZPD are likely to be quite rare within the population.

Course

Persons with SZPD are socially isolated and withdrawn as children. They may not have been accepted well by their peers, and may have even borne the brunt of some ostracism (American Psychiatric Association, 2000). As adults, they have few friendships. The friendships that do occur are likely to be initiated by their peers or colleagues. They have few sexual relationships and may never marry. Relationships fail to the extent to which the other person desires or needs emotional support, warmth and intimacy. Persons with SZPD may do well and even excel within an occupation, as long as substantial social interaction is not required. They prefer to work in isolation. They may eventually find employment and a relationship that is relatively comfortable, but they could also drift from one job to another and remain isolated throughout much of their life. If they do eventually become a parent, they have considerable difficulty providing warmth and emotional support, and they may appear neglectful, detached and disinterested.

Treatment

Prototypic cases of SZPD rarely present for treatment, whether it is for their schizoid traits or a concomitant Axis I disorder. They feel little need for treatment, as their isolation is often egosyntonic. Their social isolation is of more concern to their relatives, colleagues, or friends than to themselves. Their disinterest in and withdrawal from intimate or intense interpersonal contact is also a substantial barrier to treatment. They at times appear depressed but one must be careful not to confuse their anhedonic detachment, withdrawal and flat affect with symptoms of depression.

If persons with SZPD are seen for treatment for a concomitant Axis I disorder (e.g., a sexual arousal disorder or a substance dependence) it is advisable to work within the confines and limitations of the schizoid personality traits. Charismatic, engaging, emotional, or intimate therapists can be very uncomfortable, foreign and even threatening to persons with SZPD. A more business-like approach can be more successful.

It is also important not to presume that persons with SZPD are simply inhibited, shy, or insecure. Such persons are more appropriately diagnosed with the avoidant personality disorder. Persons with SZPD are perhaps best treated with a supportive psychotherapy that emphasizes education and feedback concerning interpersonal skills and communication. One may not be able to increase the desire for social involvements but one can increase the ability to relate to, communicate with and get along with others. Persons with SZPD may not want to develop intimate relationships but they will often want to interact and relate more effectively and comfortably with others. The use of role playing and videotaped interactions can at times be useful in this respect. Persons with SZPD can have tremendous difficulty understanding how they are perceived by others or how their behavior is unresponsive to and perceived as rejecting by others.

Group therapy is often useful as a setting in which the patient can gradually develop self-disclosure, experience the interest of others, and practice social interactions with immediate and supportive

feedback. However, persons with SZPD are prone to being rejected by a group due to their detachment, flat affect and indifference to the feelings of others. If the group is patient and accepting, they can benefit from the experience.

There have been many studies on the pharmacologic treatment of the schizotypal PD but no comparable studies on SZPD. The schizotypal and schizoid PDs share many features, but the responsivity of the schizotypal PD to pharmacotherapy will usually reflect schizotypal social anxiety and cognitive–perceptual aberrations that are not seen in prototypic, pure cases of SZPD.

Schizotypal Personality Disorder

Definition

Schizotypal PD (STPD) is a pervasive pattern of interpersonal deficits, cognitive and perceptual aberrations, and eccentricities of behavior (American Psychiatric Association, 2000). The interpersonal deficits are characterized in large part by an acute discomfort with and reduced capacity for close relationships. The symptomatology of STPD has been differentiated further into components of positive (cognitive, perceptual aberrations) and negative (social aversion and withdrawal) symptoms comparable to the distinctions made for schizophrenia. The presence of STPD is indicated by five or more of the nine diagnostic criteria listed in the DSM-IV criteria for STPD.

Etiology and Pathology

There is substantial empirical support for a genetic association of STPD with schizophrenia which is not surprising given that the diagnostic criteria were obtained from the observations of biological relatives of persons with schizophrenia. Research has indicated further that the positive and negative symptoms may even have a distinct genetic relationship with the comparable symptoms of schizophrenia. This suggests that the influence of familial etiological factors determining the expression of these symptom dimensions reaches across the boundary of psychotic illness to phenomena currently classified under the rubric of personality.

A predominant model for the psychopathology of STPD is deficits or defects in the attention and selection processes that organize a person's cognitive–perceptual evaluation of and relatedness to his or her environment. These defects may lead to discomfort within social situations, misperceptions and suspicions, and to a coping strategy of social isolation. Correlates of central nervous system dysfunction seen in persons with schizophrenia have been observed in laboratory tests of persons with STPD, including performance on tests of visual and auditory attention (e.g., backward masking and sensory gating tests) and smooth pursuit eye movement. This dysfunction may be the result of dysregulation along dopaminergic pathways, which could be serving to modulate the expression of an underlying schizotypal genotype.

Differential Diagnosis

Avoidant personality disorder and STPD share the features of social anxiety and introversion, but the social anxiety of STPD does not diminish with familiarity, whereas the anxiety of avoidant PD (AVPD) is concerned primarily with the initiation of a relationship. STPD is also a more severe disorder that includes a variety of cognitive and perceptual aberrations that are not seen in persons with AVPD.

DSM-IV-TR Criteria 301.22

Schizotypal Personality Disorder

A. A pervasive pattern of social and interpersonal deficits marked by acute discomfort with, and reduced capacity for, close relationships as well as by cognitive or perceptual distortions and eccentricities of behavior, beginning by early adulthood, and present in a variety of contexts, as indicated by five (or more) of the following:

   (1) ideas of reference (excluding delusions of reference)

   (2) odd beliefs or magical thinking that influences behavior and is inconsistent with subcultural norms (e.g., superstitiousness, belief in clairvoyance, telepathy, or "sixth sense"; in children and adolescents, bizarre fantasies or preoccupations)

   (3) unusual perceptual experiences, including bodily illusions

   (4) odd thinking and speech (e.g., vague, circumstantial, metaphorical, overelaborate, or stereotyped)

   (5) suspiciousness or paranoid ideation

   (6) inappropriate or constricted affect

   (7) behavior or appearance that is odd, eccentric, or peculiar

   (8) lacks close friends or confidants other than first-degree relatives

   (9) excessive social anxiety that does not diminish with familiarity and tends to be associated with paranoid fears rather than negative judgments about self

B. Does not occur exclusively during the course of schizophrenia, a mood disorder with psychotic features, another psychotic disorder, or a pervasive developmental disorder.

Note: if criteria are met prior to the onset of schizophrenia, add "premorbid", e.g., schizotypal personality disorder (premorbid).

Reprinted with permission from the *Diagnostic and Statistical Manual of Mental Disorders*, Fourth Edition, Text Revision. Copyright 2000 American Psychiatric Association.

An initial concern of many clinicians when confronted with a person with STPD is whether the more appropriate diagnosis is schizophrenia. Persons with STPD closely resemble persons within the prodromal or residual phases of schizophrenia. This differentiation is determined largely by the absence of a deterioration in functioning. It is indicated in DSM-IV that one should note that STPD is "premorbid" if the schizotypal symptoms were present prior to the onset of schizophrenia (American Psychiatric Association, 2000). Premorbid schizotypal traits will have prognostic significance for the course and treatment of schizophrenia and such traits should then be noted. However, as discussed for SZPD, in most of these cases the schizotypal PD symptoms could then be readily understood as prodromal symptoms of schizophrenia.

Epidemiology and Comorbidity

STPD may occur in as much as 3% of the general population although most studies with semistructured interviews have suggested a somewhat lower percentage. STPD might occur somewhat more often in males. STPD cooccurs most often with the schizoid, borderline, avoidant and paranoid personality disorders. Common Axis I disorders are major depressive disorder, brief psychotic disorder and generalized social phobia.

Course

STPD is classified within the same diagnostic grouping as schizophrenia in ICD-10 (World Health Organization, 1992) because of its close relationship in phenomenology, etiology and pathology. However, it is classified as a personality disorder in DSM-IV-TR (American Psychiatric Association, 2000) because its course and phenomenology are more consistent with a disorder of personality (i.e., early onset, evident in everyday functioning, characteristic of long-term functioning and egosyntonic). Persons with STPD are likely to be rather isolated in childhood. They may have appeared peculiar and odd to their peers, and may have been teased or ostracized. Achievement in school is usually impaired, and they may have been heavily involved in esoteric fantasies and peculiar interests, particularly those that do not involve peers. As adults, they may drift toward esoteric–fringe groups that support their magical thinking and aberrant beliefs. These activities can provide structure for some persons with STPD, but they can also contribute to a further loosening and deterioration if there is an encouragement of aberrant experiences. Only a small proportion of persons with STPD develop schizophrenia. The symptomatology of STPD does not appear to remit with age. The course appears to be relatively stable, with some proportion of schizotypal persons remaining marginally employed, withdrawn, and transient throughout their lives.

Treatment

Persons with STPD may seek treatment for their feelings of anxiousness, perceptual disturbances, or depression. Treatment of persons with STPD should be cognitive, behavioral, supportive and/or pharmacologic, as they will often find the intimacy and emotionality of reflective, exploratory psychotherapy to be too stressful and they have the potential for psychotic decompensation.

Persons with STPD will often fail to consider their social isolation and aberrant cognitions and perceptions to be particularly problematic or maladaptive. They may consider themselves to be simply eccentric, creative, or nonconformist. Rapport can be difficult to develop as increasing familiarity and intimacy may only increase their level of discomfort and anxiety. They are unlikely to be responsive to informality or playful humor. The sessions should be well-structured to avoid loose and tangential ideation.

Practical advice is usually helpful and often necessary. The therapist should serve as the patient's counselor, guide, or "auxiliary ego" to more adaptive decisions with respect to everyday problems (e.g., finding an apartment, interviewing for a job and personal appearance). Persons with STPD should also receive social skills training directed at their awkward and odd behavior, mannerisms, dress and speech. Specific, concrete discussions on what to expect and do in various social situations (e.g., formal meetings, casual encounters and dates) should be provided. The rate of progress will tend to be slow, and it is helpful if there remains a continuity in the therapeutic relationship.

Most of the systematic empirical research on the treatment of STPD has been confined to pharmacologic interventions. Low doses of neuroleptic medications (e.g., thiothixene) have shown some effectiveness in the treatment of schizotypal symptoms, particularly the perceptual aberrations and social anxiousness. Group therapy has also been recommended for persons with STPD but only when the group is highly structured and supportive. The emotional intensity and intimacy of unstructured groups will usually be too stressful. Schizotypal patients with predominant paranoid symptoms may even have difficulty in highly structured groups.

Antisocial Personality Disorder

Definition

Antisocial PD (ASPD) is a pervasive pattern of disregard for and violation of the rights of others (American Psychiatric Association, 2000). Persons with ASPD will also be irresponsible and exploitative in their sexual relationships, and irresponsible as employees and parents. They may display a lack of empathy, an inflated or arrogant self-appraisal, a callous, cynical and contemptuous response to the suffering of others, and a glib, superficial charm. This disorder has also been referred to as psychopathy, sociopathy, or dissocial personality disorder. The presence of ASPD is indicated by the occurrence of a conduct disorder prior to age 15 years and by three of the seven adult diagnostic criteria presented in DSM-IV Criteria for ASPD.

Etiology and Pathology

There is considerable support from twin, family and adoption studies for a genetic contribution to the etiology of the criminal, delinquent tendencies of persons with ASPD. The genetic disposition may be somewhat stronger in ASPD females due perhaps to a greater social pressure on females against aggressive, exploitative and criminal behavior. What is inherited by persons with ASPD, however, is unclear; it could be impulsivity, antagonistic callousness, or abnormally low anxiousness.

A predominant theory for the etiology of ASPD is that it results from abnormally low levels of behavioral inhibition and high levels of behavioral activation systems that are important for normal, adaptive functioning. The behavioral inhibition system (BIS) is responsible for inhibiting behavior in response to punishment and acts in opposition to the behavioral activation system (BAS) that activates behavior in response to reward. The BIS has input into the reticular activating system providing experiences of anxiety or arousal. The clinical symptoms of ASPD might be manifestations of a weak or deficient BIS in combination with a normal or strong BAS that reduce normal sensitivity and anxiety in response to threatening and stressful situations. Activities that the average person would find stimulating, antisocial persons would find dull, impelling them to engage in risky, reckless, prohibited and impulsive activities. Low arousal would also help minimize feelings of anxiety, guilt, or remorse and help resist aversive conditioning. Studies have indicated an electrodermal response hyporeactivity in psychopathic persons. This hyporeactivity may be particularly associated with a deficit in anticipatory anxiety and worrying, while not impairing the alarm reactions of flight versus fight. Abnormally low levels of behavioral inhibition may be mediated by the septohippocampal system (and the neurotransmitter serotonin). Deficiencies in response modulation (difficulties suspending a dominant set in

response to negative feedback) are apparent in animals with septohippocampal dysfunction.

There are also substantial data to support the contribution of family, peer, and other environmental factors. No single environmental factor appears to be specific to its development. Modeling by parental figures and peers, excessively harsh, lenient, or erratic discipline, and a tough, harsh environment in which feelings of empathy and warmth are discouraged (if not punished) and tough-mindedness, aggressiveness and exploitation are encouraged (if not rewarded) have all been associated with the development of ASPD. For example, ASPD in some cases could be the result of an interaction of early experiences of physical or sexual abuse, exposure to aggressive parental models and erratic discipline that develop a view of the world as a hostile environment, which is further affirmed over time through selective attention on cues for antagonism, encouragement and modeling of aggression by peers, and the immediate benefits that result from aggressive, exploitative behavior. Persons with ASPD may have had their feelings of anxiety, guilt and remorse extinguished through progressive and cumulative experiences of harsh aggression, violence, abuse and exploitation.

The development of adequate guilt, conscience and shame may also require a degree of distress-proneness (anxiousness or neuroticism) and attentional self-regulation (constraint). Normal levels of neuroticism will promote the internalization of a conscience (the introjection of the family's moral values) by associating distress and anxiety with wrongdoing, and the temperament of self-regulation will help modulate impulses into a socially acceptable manner. Studies have indicated that high levels of arousal at age 15 years serve as a protective factor against criminal activities at age 30 years in persons at high risk for becoming criminals. Additional factors may also help to avoid the development of ASPD, such as high intelligence which may contribute to the availability of alternative life paths, while other factors may exacerbate or escalate its development, such as drug or alcohol dependence. In sum, ASPD appears to be the result of a constellation of factors, including genetic predisposition, experiences within the family and sociological factors, coupled with the absence of preventive factors.

Assessment and Differential Diagnosis

All of the DSM-IV-TR assessment instruments described earlier include the assessment of ASPD. However, an instrument that is focused on the assessment of ASPD is the Psychopathy Checklist – Revised (PCL-R, Hare, 1991). The PCL-R is commonly used within forensic and prison settings and is particularly well suited for the assessment of this disorder within settings that are heavily populated by persons with a criminal history. The PCL-R includes the assessment of psychopathic traits that are relatively more specific to ASPD within prison settings, such as lack of empathy, glib charm and arrogance. However, as suggested by its title, it is perhaps better described as a checklist than as a semistructured interview. Many of its items are scored primarily (if not solely) on the basis of a person's legal, criminal record rather than on the basis of interview questions. The availability of a detailed criminal history within prison settings has contributed to the PCL-R's excellent interrater reliability and predictive validity, but an application of the PCL-R within most other clinical settings will need to rely more heavily on PCL-R interview questions, the administration and scoring of which will be unclear for some PCL-R items.

ASPD will at times be difficult to differentiate from a substance dependence disorder in young adults because many persons with ASPD develop a substance-related disorder and many persons with a substance dependence engage in antisocial acts. The requirement that the ASPD features be evident prior to the age of 15 years will usually assure the onset of ASPD prior to the onset of a substance-related disorder. If both are evident prior to the age of 15 years, then it is likely that both disorders are in fact present and both diagnoses should then be made. ASPD and substance dependence will often interact, exacerbating and escalating each other's development.

Antisocial acts will also be evident in the histrionic and borderline personality disorders, as persons with these disorders will display impulsivity, sensation-seeking, self-centeredness, manipulativeness and a low frustration tolerance. Females with antisocial PD are often misdiagnosed with histrionic personality disorder. Prototypic cases of ASPD might be distinguished from other personality disorders by the presence of the childhood history of conduct disorder and the cold, calculated exploitation, abuse and aggression. Persons with narcissistic personality disorder are also characterized by a lack of empathy and may often exploit and use others. In fact, many of the traits of narcissistic personality disorder are evident in psychopathy, including a lack of empathy, glib and superficial charm and arrogant self-appraisal.

Epidemiology and Comorbidity

The National Institute of Mental Health Epidemiologic Catchment Area (ECA) study indicated that approximately 3% of males and 1% of females have ASPD (Robins *et al.*, 1991). This rate has been replicated in subsequent studies, but it has also been suggested that the ECA finding may have underestimated the prevalence in males due to the failure to consider the full range of ASPD features. Other estimates have been as high as 6% in males (Kessler *et al.*, 1994; Robins *et al.*, 1991). The rate of ASPD within prison and forensic settings has been estimated at 50% but the ASPD criteria may exaggerate the rate within such settings due to the emphasis given to overt acts of criminality, delinquency and irresponsibility that are common to the persons within these settings. More specific criteria for psychopathy provide a more conservative estimate of 20 to 30% of male prisoners with ASPD.

ASPD is much more common in males than in females. A sociobiological explanation for the differential sex prevalence is the presence of a genetic advantage for social irresponsibility, infidelity, superficial charm and deceit in males that contributes to a higher likelihood of developing features of ASPD. It has also been suggested that ASPD and histrionic personality disorder share a biogenetic disposition (perhaps towards impulsivity or sensation-seeking) that is mediated by gender-specific biogenetic and sociological factors toward respective gender variants.

Persons with ASPD are at a high risk for developing substance-related and impulse dyscontrol disorders. They are also likely to display borderline, narcissistic and paranoid personality traits. Females with ASPD will also display histrionic personality traits.

Course

ASPD is evident in childhood in the form of a conduct disorder. Evidence of a conduct disorder prior to the age of 15 years is in fact required for a DSM-IV ASPD diagnosis (American Psychiatric Association, 2000). The continuation into adulthood is particularly likely to occur if multiple delinquent behaviors are evident prior to the age of 10 years. As adults, persons with ASPD are unlikely to maintain steady employment and they may even become impoverished, homeless, or spend years within penal institutions. However, some persons with ASPD characterized by high rather than low levels of conscientiousness may express their psychopathic tendencies within a socially acceptable or at least legitimate profession. They may in fact be quite successful as long as their tendency to bend or violate the norms or rules of their profession and exploit, deceive and manipulate others, contribute to a career advancement. Their success, however, may at some point unravel when their psychopathic behaviors become problematic or evident to others. The same pattern may also occur within sexual and marital relationships. They may at first appear to be charming, engaging and sincere, but most relationships will end due to a lack of empathy, responsibility and fidelity.

There does tend to be a gradual remission of antisocial behaviors, particularly overt criminal acts, as the person ages. Persons with ASPD, however, are more likely than the general population to have died prematurely by violent means (e.g., accidents or homicides) and to engage in quite dangerous, high-risk behavior.

Treatment

The presence of ASPD is important to recognize in the treatment of any Axis I disorder, as their tendency to be manipulative, dishonest, exploitative, aggressive and irresponsible will often disrupt and sabotage treatment. It is also very easy to be seduced by psychopathic charm. Persons with ASPD can be seductive in their engaging friendliness, expressions of remorse, avowed commitment to change, and apparent response to or even fascination with the success, skills, and talents of the therapist, none of which will be sincere or reliable.

The extent to which ASPD is untreatable has at times been overstated and exaggerated. Nevertheless, ASPD is the most difficult personality disorder to treat. Persons with ASPD will often lack a motivation or commitment to change. They might see only the advantages of their antisocial traits and not the costs (e.g., risks of arrest and failure to sustain lasting or meaningful relationships). They are prone to manipulate, abuse, or exploit their fellow patients and the staff. The immediate motivation for treatment is often provided by an external source, such as a court order or the demands of an employer or relative. Motivation may last only as long as an external pressure remains.

The most effective treatment is likely to be prevention through an identification and intervention early in childhood. In adulthood, the most effective treatment may at times be simply some form of sustained incarceration (e.g., imprisonment), as many antisocial behaviors do tend to dissipate (or burnout) with time. The tendency to rationalize irresponsibility, minimize the consequences of acts, and manipulate others needs to be confronted on a daily and immediate basis. Community residential or wilderness programs that provide a firm structure, close supervision and intense confrontation by peers have been recommended. The involvement of family members in the treatment has been shown to be helpful, but there are also data to suggest that interventions with little professional input are less successful and are times counterproductive.

There is some research to suggest that the ability to form a therapeutic alliance is an important indicator of treatment success. Factors to consider are the demographic similarity of the therapist and patient, the quality of the patient's past relationships and the therapist's positive regard for the patient. Many psychiatrists may also experience strong feelings of animosity and distaste for antisocial persons who have a history of abusive and exploitative acts. Rational, utilitarian approaches that help the person consider the long-term consequences of behavior can be useful. This approach does not attempt to develop a sense of conscience, guilt, or even regret for past actions, but focuses instead on the material value and future advantages to be gained by a more prosocial behavior pattern. There are data to suggest the use of pharmacotherapy in the treatment of impulsive aggression but it is unclear whether these findings would generalize to the full spectrum of ASPD psychopathology.

Borderline Personality Disorder

Definition

Borderline personality disorder (BPD) is a pervasive pattern of impulsivity and instability in interpersonal relationships and self-image (American Psychiatric Association, 2000). A broad domain of general personality functioning is neuroticism or emotional instability. characterized by facets of angry hostility, anxiousness, depressiveness, impulsivity and vulnerability; BPD is essentially the most extreme and highly maladaptive variant of emotional instability. This disorder is indicated by the presence of five or more of the nine diagnostic criteria presented in the DSM-IV-TR criteria for BPD.

Etiology and Pathology

There are studies to indicate that BPD may breed true but most research has suggested an association with mood and impulse dyscontrol disorders. There is also consistent empirical support for a childhood history of physical and/or sexual abuse, as well as parental conflict, loss and neglect. It appears that past traumatic events are important in many if not most cases of BPD, contributing to the overlap and association with post traumatic stress and dissociative disorders but the nature and age at which these events have occurred will vary. BPD may involve the interaction of a genetic disposition towards dyscontrol of mood and impulses (i.e., emotionally unstable temperament), with a cumulative and evolving series of intensely pathogenic relationships.

DSM-IV-TR Criteria 301.83

Borderline Personality Disorder

A pervasive pattern of instability of interpersonal relationships, self-image, and affects, and marked impulsivity beginning by early adulthood and present in a variety of contexts, as indicated by five (or more) of the following:

(1) frantic efforts to avoid real or imagined abandonment. **Note:** do not include suicidal or self-mutilating behavior covered in criterion 5

(2) a pattern of unstable and intense interpersonal relationships characterized by alternating between extremes of idealization and devaluation

(3) identity disturbance: markedly and persistently unstable self-image or sense of self

(4) impulsivity in at least two areas that are potentially self-damaging (e.g., spending, sex, substance abuse, reckless driving, binge eating). **Note:** do not include suicidal or self-mutilating behavior covered in criterion 5

(5) recurrent suicidal behavior, gestures, or threats, or self-mutilating behavior

(6) affective instability due to a marked reactivity of mood (e.g., intense episodic dysphoria, irritability, or anxiety usually lasting a few hours and only rarely more than a few days)

(7) chronic feelings of emptiness

(8) inappropriate, intense anger or difficulty controlling anger (e.g., frequent displays of temper, constant anger, recurrent physical fights)

(9) transient, stress-related paranoid ideation or severe dissociative symptoms

---

There are numerous theories regarding the pathogenic mechanisms of BPD, most concern issues regarding abandonment, separation, and/or exploitative abuse, which is one of the reasons that frantic efforts to avoid abandonment is the first item in the DSM-IV-TR diagnostic criterion set. Persons with BPD have quite intense, disturbed, and/or abusive relationships with the significant persons of their past, including their parents, contributing to the development of malevolent perceptions and expectations of others. These expectations, along with an impairment in the ability to regulate affect and impulses may contribute to the perpetuation of intense, angry and unstable relationships. Neurochemical dysregulation is evident in persons with BPD but it is unclear whether this dysregulation is a result, cause, or correlate of prior interpersonal traumas.

Assessment and Differential Diagnosis
All of the DSM-IV assessment instruments described earlier include the assessment of BPD. However, an instrument that is focused on the assessment of BPD is the Diagnostic Interview for Borderlines-Revised (DIB-R; Zanarini et al., 1989). The DIB-R provides a more thorough assessment of components of BPD (e.g., impulsivity, affective dysregulation and cognitive–perceptual aberrations) than is provided by more general DSM-IV-TR personality disorder semi-structured interviews, but psychiatrists might find it impractical to devote up to 2 hours to assess one particular personality disorder, especially when it is likely that other maladaptive personality traits not covered by the DIB-R are also likely to be present.

Most persons with BPD develop mood disorders and it is at times difficult to differentiate BPD from a mood disorder if the assessment is confined to the current symptomatology. A diagnosis of BPD requires that the borderline symptomatology be evident since adolescence, which should differentiate BPD from a mood disorder in all cases other than a chronic mood disorder. If there is a chronic mood disorder, then the additional features of transient, stress-related paranoid ideation, dissociative experiences, impulsivity and anger dyscontrol that are evident in BPD should be emphasized in the diagnosis (Gunderson, 2001).

Epidemiology and Comorbidity
Approximately 1 to 2% of the general population would meet the DSM-IV criteria for BPD. BPD is the most prevalent personality disorder within maximum clinical settings. Approximately 15% of all inpatients (51% of inpatients with a personality disorder) and 8% of all outpatients (27% of outpatients with a personality disorder) have a borderline personality disorder. Approximately 75% of persons with BPD will be female. Persons with BPD meet DSM-IV-TR criteria for at least one Axis I disorder. The range of potential Axis I comorbid psychopathology includes mood (major depressive disorder), anxiety (post traumatic stress disorder), eating (bulimia nervosa), substance (alcohol dependence), dissociative (dissociative identity disorder), and psychotic (brief psychotic) disorders (Gunderson, 2001). Persons with BPD also meet DSM-IV-TR criteria for at least one other personality disorder, particularly histrionic, dependent, antisocial, schizotypal, or passive–aggressive. Researchers and clinicians have at times responded to this extensive cooccurrence by imposing a diagnostic hierarchy whereby other disorders are not diagnosed in the presence of BPD because BPD is generally the most severely dysfunctional disorder (Gunderson et al., 2000). A potential limitation of this approach is that it resolves the complexity of personality by largely ignoring it. This approach may fail to rec-

ognize the presence of maladaptive personality traits that could be important for understanding a patient's dysfunctions and for developing an optimal treatment plan.

Course
As children, persons with BPD are likely to have been emotionally unstable, impulsive and angry or hostile. Their chaotic impulsivity and intense affectivity may contribute to involvement within rebellious groups as a child or adolescent, along with a variety of Axis I disorders, including eating, substance use and mood disorders. BPD is often diagnosed in children and adolescents but considerable caution should be used when doing so as some of the symptoms of BPD (e.g., identity disturbance and unstable relationships) could be confused with a normal adolescent rebellion or identity crisis. As adults, persons with BPD may require numerous hospitalizations due to their affect and impulse dyscontrol, psychotic-like and dissociative symptomatology and risk of suicide. Minor problems quickly become crises as the intensity of affect and impulsivity result in disastrous decisions. They are at a high risk for developing depressive, substance-related, bulimic and post traumatic stress disorders. The potential for suicide increases with a comorbid mood and substance-related disorder. Approximately 3 to 10% commit suicide by the age of 30 years. Relationships tend to be very unstable and explosive and employment history is poor. Affectivity and impulsivity, however, may begin to diminish as the person reaches the age of 30 years, or earlier if the person becomes involved with a supportive and patient sexual partner. Some, however, may obtain stability by abandoning the effort to obtain a relationship, opting instead for a lonelier but less volatile life. The mellowing of the symptomatology, however, can be easily disrupted by the occurrence of a severe stressor (e.g., divorce by or death of a significant other) that results in a brief psychotic, dissociative, or mood disorder episode.

Treatment
Persons with BPD often develop intense, dependent, hostile, unstable and manipulative relationships with their therapists as they do with their peers. At one time they might be very compliant, responsive and even idealizing, but later angry, accusatory and devaluing. Their tendency to be manipulatively as well as impulsively self-destructive is often very stressful and difficult to treat (Stone, 2000).

Persons with BPD are often highly motivated for treatment. Psychotherapeutic approaches tend to be both supportive and exploratory. Therapists should provide a safe, secure environment in which anger can be expressed and actively addressed without destroying the therapeutic relationship. The historical roots of current bitterness, anger and depression within past familial relationships should eventually be explored, but immediate, current issues and conflicts must also be explicitly addressed. Suicidal behavior should be confronted and contained, by hospitalization when necessary. Patients with BPD can be very difficult to treat because the focus of the patient's love and wrath will often be shifted toward the therapist, and the treatment may itself become the patient's latest unstable, intense relationship. Immediate and ongoing consultation with colleagues is often necessary, as it is not unusual for therapists to be unaware of the extent to which they are developing or expressing feelings of anger, attraction, annoyance, or intolerance toward their borderline patient.

A particular form of cognitive–behavioral therapy, dialectical behavior therapy, has been shown empirically to be effective in the treatment of BPD (Linehan, 2000). Part of the strategy entails keeping patients focused initially on the priorities of reducing suicidal threats and gestures, behaviors that can disrupt or resist treatment, and behaviors that affect the immediate quality of life (e.g., bulimia, substance abuse, or unemployment). Once these goals are achieved, the focus can then shift to a mastery of new coping skills, management of reactions to stress and other individualized goals. Individual therapy is augmented by skills-training groups that may be highly structured (e.g., comparable to a classroom format). Patients are taught skills for coping with identity diffusion, tolerating distress, improving interpersonal relationships, controlling emotions and resolving interpersonal crises. Patients are given homework assignments to practice these skills that are further addressed and reinforced within individual sessions. Negative affect is also addressed through a mindful meditation that contributes to an acceptance and tolerance of past abusive experiences and current stress. The dialectical component of the therapy is that "the dialectical therapist helps the patient achieve synthesis of oppositions, rather than focusing on verifying either side of an oppositional argument" (Linehan, 1993, p. 204). An illustrative list of dialectical strategies is presented in Table 62.3.

DBT, however, also includes more general principles of treatment that are important to emphasize in all forms of therapy for BPD (Linehan, 1993; Stone, 1993, 2000), some of which are presented in Table 62.4. For example, exasperated therapists may unjustly experience and even accuse borderline patients of being unmotivated or unwilling to work. It is important to appreciate that they do want to improve and are doing the best that they can. One should not make the therapy personal, but instead identify the sources of the inhibition or interference to their motivation to change. One should take seriously their complaints that their lives are indeed unbearable but not absolve them of their responsibility to solve their own problems. They are unlikely to change simply through a passive reception of insight, nurturance, support and

Table 62.4	Basic Propositions of BPD Treatment from DBT

1. Patients are doing the best they can.
2. Patients want to improve.
3. Patients need to do better, try harder and be more motivated to change.
4. Patients may not have caused all of their own problems, but they have to solve them anyway.
5. The lives of suicidal, borderline individuals are unbearable as they are currently being lived.
6. Patients must learn new behaviors in all relevant contexts.
7. Patients cannot fail in therapy.
8. Therapists treating borderline patients need support.

Reprinted from Cognitive Behavior Treatments of Borderline Personality Disorders. Linehan MM (1993). Guilford Press, New York, p. 106–108.

medication. They will need to work actively on changing their lives. Therapists will often be tempted to rescue their patients, particularly when they are within a crisis. However, it is precisely at such times that there will be the best opportunity to develop and learn new coping strategies. Failures can occur, and it is a failure of the therapy that should be conscientiously and effectively addressed by the therapist. Finally, therapists need honestly to recognize their own limitations. All therapists have their own flaws and limits and patients with BPD invariably strain and overwhelm these limits. Therapists need to be open and receptive to outside support, advice and criticism.

Pharmacologic treatment of patients with BPD is varied, as it depends primarily on the predominant Axis I symptomatology. Persons with BPD can display a wide variety of Axis I symptoms, including anxiety, depression, hallucinations, delusions and dissociations. It is important in their pharmacologic treatment not to be unduly influenced by transient symptoms or by symptoms that are readily addressed through exploratory or supportive techniques. On the other hand, it is equally important to be flexible in the use of medications and not to be unduly resistant to their use. Relying solely upon one's own psychotherapeutic skills can be unnecessary and even irresponsible.

Histrionic Personality Disorder

Definition

Histrionic personality disorder (HPD) is a pervasive pattern of excessive emotionality and attention-seeking (American Psychiatric Association, 2000). Histrionic persons tend to be emotionally manipulative and intolerant of delayed gratification. HPD is indicated by the presence of five or more of the eight diagnostic criteria presented in DSM-IV criteria for HPD.

Etiology and Pathology

There is little research on the etiology of HPD. There is a suggestion that HPD may share a genetic disposition toward impulsivity or sensation-seeking with the antisocial personality. It has also been suggested that HPD is (in part) a severe, maladaptive variant of the personality dimensions of extraversion and neuroticism. Extraversion includes the facets of excitement seeking, gregariousness and positive emotionality, and neuroticism includes the facets of angry hostility, self-consciousness and vulnerability that are all characteristic of persons with HPD

Table 62.3	Dialectical Behavior Therapy Strategies

Alternate between acceptance and change strategies
Balance nurturing with demands for self-help
Balance persistence and stability with flexibility
Balance capabilities with limitations and deficits
Move with speed, keeping the patient slightly off balance
Take positions whole-heartedly
Look for what is not included in patient's own points of view
Provide developmental descriptions of change
Question intransigence of boundary conditions of the problem
Highlight importance of interrelationships in identity
Advocate a middle path
Highlight paradoxical contradictions in patient's own behavior, in the therapeutic process, and in life in general
Speak in metaphors and tell parables and stories
Play the devil's advocate
Extend the seriousness or implications of patient's statements
Add intuitive knowing to emotional experience and logical analysis
Turn problems into assets
Allow natural changes in therapy
Assess the patient, therapist and process dialectically

Reprinted with permission from Cognitive Behavior Treatments of Borderline Personality Disorders. Linehan MM (1993). Guilford Press, New York, p. 206.

Histrionic Personality Disorder

A pervasive pattern of excessive emotionality and attention seeking, beginning by early adulthood and present in a variety of contexts, as indicated by five (or more) of the following:

(1) is uncomfortable in situations in which he or she is not the center of attention

(2) interaction with others is often characterized by inappropriate sexually seductive or provocative behavior

(3) displays rapidly shifting and shallow expression of emotions

(4) consistently uses physical appearance to draw attention to self

(5) has a style of speech that is excessively impressionistic and lacking in detail

(6) shows self-dramatization, theatricality, and exaggerated expression of emotion

(7) is suggestible, i.e. easily influenced by others or circumstances

(8) considers relationships to be more intimate than they actually are

Reprinted with permission from the *Diagnostic and Statistical Manual of Mental Disorders*, Fourth Edition, Text Revision. Copyright 2000, American Psychiatric Association.

and there is considerable empirical support for the heritability of these personality dimensions.

Environmental and social–cultural factors, however, may also play a significant role in the development of HPD. There is some speculation that the fathers of females with HPD combine early sexual seductiveness with subsequent authoritarian puritanical attitudes, while the mother tends to be domineering, controlling and intrusive. Such a history may indeed occur in some cases of HPD but there is unlikely to be a specific, common pattern to all cases. The tendency of a family to emphasize, value, or reinforce attention-seeking in a person with a genetic disposition toward emotionality may represent a more general pathway toward HPD.

Affective instability is an important feature of HPD, which may be associated with a hyperresponsiveness of the noradrenergic system. This instability in the catecholamine functioning may contribute to a pronounced emotional reactivity to rejection and loss. However, the attention-seeking of HPD can be as important to the disorder as the emotionality. The purpose of the exaggerated emotionality is often to evoke the attention and maintain the interest of others. Persons with HPD are intensely insecure regarding the extent to which others appreciate, desire, or want their company. They need to be the center of attention to reassure themselves that they are valued, desired, attractive, or wanted.

Assessment and Differential Diagnosis

HPD involves to some extent maladaptive variants of stereotypically feminine traits. The DSM-IV-TR diagnostic criteria for HPD are sufficiently severe that a normal woman would not

meet these criteria, but studies have indicated that clinicians will at times diagnose HPD in females who in fact have antisocial traits. Both of these disorders can involve impulsivity, sensation-seeking, low frustration tolerance and manipulativeness, and the presence of a female gender may at times contribute to a false presumption of HPD. It is therefore important to adhere closely to the DSM-IV-TR diagnostic criteria when confronted with histrionic and antisocial symptoms in female patients.

Persons with HPD will often have borderline, dependent, or narcissistic personality traits. Prototypic cases of HPD can be distinguished from other personality disorders. For example, the prototypic narcissistic person ultimately desires admiration whereas the histrionic person desires whatever attention, interest, or concern can be obtained. As a result, the histrionic person will at times seek attention through melodramatic helplessness and emotional outbursts that could be experienced as denigrating and humiliating to the narcissistic person. However, most cases will not be prototypic and the most accurate description of a patient's constellation of maladaptive personality traits will be the provision of multiple diagnoses.

Epidemiology and Comorbidity

Approximately 1 to 3% of the general population may be diagnosed with HPD. A controversial issue is its differential sex prevalence. It is stated in DSM-IV-TR that the sex ratio for HPD is "not significantly different than the sex ratio of females within the respective clinical setting" (American Psychiatric Association, 2000, p. 712). However, this should not be interpreted as indicating that the prevalence is the same for males and females. It has typically been found that at least two-thirds of persons with HPD are female, although there have been a few exceptions. Whether or not the rate will be significantly higher than the rate of women within a particular clinical setting depends upon many factors that are independent of the differential sex prevalence for HPD.

Course

Little is known about the premorbid behavior pattern of persons with HPD. During adolescence they are likely to be flamboyant, flirtatious and attention-seeking. As adults, persons with HPD readily form new relationships but have difficulty sustaining them. They may fall in love quite quickly, but just as rapidly become attracted to another person. They are unlikely to be reliable or responsible. Relationships with persons of the same sexual orientation are often be strained due to their competitive sexual flirtatiousness. Employment history is likely to be erratic, and may be complicated by the tendency to become romantically or sexually involved with colleagues, by their affective instability and by their suggestibility. Persons with HPD may become devoted converts to faddish belief systems. They have a tendency to make impulsive decisions that will have a dramatic (or melodramatic) effect on their lives. The severity of the symptomatology may diminish somewhat as the person ages.

Treatment

Persons with HPD readily develop rapport but it is often superficial and unreliable. Therapists may also fail to appreciate the extent of influence they can have on the highly suggestible HPD patient. Persons with HPD can readily become converts to whatever the therapist may suggest or encourage. The transformation to the theoretical model or belief system of the psychiatrist is unlikely to be sustained.

A key task in treating the patient with HPD is countering their global and diffuse cognitive style by insisting on attending to structure and detail within sessions and to the practical, immediate problems encountered in daily life. It is also important to explore within treatment the historical source for their needs for attention and involvement. Persons with HPD are prone to superficial and transient insights but they will benefit from a carefully reasoned and documented exploration of their current and past relationships.

Many clinicians recommend the use of group therapy for persons with HPD. It is quite easy for them to become involved within a group, which may then be very useful in helping them recognize and explore their attention-seeking, suggestibility and manipulation, as well as develop alternative ways to develop more meaningful and sustained relationships. However, it is also important to monitor closely their involvements within the group, as they are prone to dominate and control sessions and they may escalate their attention-seeking to the point of suicidal gestures. The intense affectivity of persons with HPD may also be responsive to antidepressant treatment, particularly those patients with substantial mood reactivity, hypersomnia and rejection sensitivity.

Narcissistic Personality Disorder

Definition

Narcissistic PD (NPD) is a pervasive pattern of grandiosity, need for admiration and lack of empathy (American Psychiatric Association, 2000). Persons with NPD can be very vulnerable to threats to their self-esteem. They may react defensively with rage, disdain, or indifference but are in fact struggling with feelings of shock, humiliation and shame. NPD is indicated by the presence of five or more of the nine diagnostic criteria presented in the DSM-IV-TR Criteria for NPD.

Etiology and Pathology

There are no data on the heritability of the narcissistic PD, although there are data on the heritability of arrogance, modesty and conceit. The etiological theories have been primarily sociological, psychodynamic and interpersonal. For example, it has been suggested that current Western society has become overly self-centered with the decreasing importance of familial bonds, traditional social, religious and political values or ideals, and rising materialism.

Narcissism may also develop through unempathic, neglectful and/or devaluing parental figures (Kernberg, 1991). The child may develop the belief that a sense of worth, value, or meaning is contingent upon accomplishment or achievement. Kohut (1977) has suggested that the parents failed adequately to mirror an infant's natural need for idealization. Benjamin (1993) and Millon and colleagues (1996) suggest that narcissistic persons received excessive idealization by parental figures, which they incorporated into their self-image. The irrationality of this idealization, or its being coupled with inconsistent indications of an actual disinterest and devaluation, may contribute to the eventual difficulties and conflicts surrounding self-image.

Conflicts and deficits with respect to self-esteem have been shown empirically to be central to the pathology of NPD. Narcissistic persons must continually seek and obtain signs and symbols of recognition to compensate for feelings of inadequacy.

DSM-IV-TR Criteria 301.81

Narcissistic Personality Disorder

A pervasive pattern of grandiosity (in fantasy or behavior), need for admiration, and lack of empathy, beginning by early adulthood and present in a variety of contexts, as indicated by five (or more) of the following:

(1) has a grandiose sense of self-importance (e.g. exaggerates achievements and talents, expects to be recognized as superior without commensurate achievements)

(2) is preoccupied with fantasies of unlimited success, power, brilliance, beauty, or ideal love

(3) believes that he or she is "special" and unique and can only be understood by, or should associate with, other special or high-status people (or institutions)

(4) requires excessive admiration

(5) has a sense of entitlement, i.e. unreasonable expectations of especially favorable treatment or automatic compliance with his or her expectations

(6) is interpersonally exploitative, i.e., takes advantage of others to achieve his or her own ends

(7) lacks empathy: is unwilling to recognize or identify with the feelings and needs of others

(8) is often envious of others or believes that others are envious of him or her

(9) shows arrogant, haughty behaviors or attitudes

Reprinted with permission from the *Diagnostic and Statistical Manual of Mental Disorders*, Fourth Edition, Text Revision. Copyright 2000 American Psychiatric Association.

They are not persons who feel valued for their own sake. Value is contingent upon a success, accomplishment, or status. Their feelings of insecurity may be masked by a disdainful indifference towards rebuke and by overt expressions of arrogance, conceit and even grandiosity. However, the psychopathology is still evident in such cases by the excessive reliance and importance that is continually placed upon status and recognition. Some narcissistic persons may in fact envy those who are truly indifferent to success and who can enjoy a modest, simple and unassuming life.

Assessment and Differential Diagnosis

All of the semi-structured interviews and self-report inventories described earlier include scales for the assessment of NPD. There is also a semi-structured interview devoted to the assessment of narcissism (Diagnostic Interview for Narcissism [DIN]; Gunderson *et al.*, 1990), the research with which was highly influential in the development of the DSM-IV-TR diagnostic criteria. There are also a number of self-report inventories devoted to the assessment of narcissistic personality traits, including the Narcissistic Personality Inventory (NPI) that has been used in a number of informative personality and social–psychological studies of narcissism

(Rhodewalt and Morf, 1995). The DIN and NPI have the useful feature of subscales for the assessment of various components of narcissism (e.g., NPI scales for superiority, vanity, leadership, authority, entitlement, exploitativeness and exhibitionism).

Individuals with narcissistic PD may often appear relatively high functioning. Exaggerated self-confidence may in fact contribute to success in a variety of professions and narcissistic traits will at times be seen in highly successful persons. A diagnosis of NPD requires the additional presence of interpersonal exploitation, lack of empathy, a sense of entitlement, and other symptoms beyond simply arrogance and grandiosity.

Both narcissistic and antisocial persons may exploit, deceive and manipulate others for personal gain, and both may demonstrate a lack of empathy or remorse. As indicated above, many of the traits of narcissism, such as arrogance and glib charm, are seen in psychopathic persons. Prototypic cases can be distinguished, as the motivation for the narcissistic person will be for recognition, status and other signs of success, whereas the prototypic antisocial person would be motivated more for material gain or for the subjugation of others. Antisocial persons will also display an impulsivity, recklessness and lax irresponsibility that may not be seen in narcissistic persons.

Epidemiology and Comorbidity

Approximately 18% of males and 6% of females may be characterized as being excessively immodest (i.e., arrogant or conceited; Costa and McCrae 1992) but only a small percent of these persons would be diagnosed with NPD. In fact, the median prevalence rate obtained across 10 community data collections was zero. The absence of any cases within community studies, however, may reflect inadequacies within the diagnostic criteria or limitations of semi-structured interview assessments of narcissism. NPD is observed within clinical settings (approximately 2 to 20% of patients) although it is also among the least frequently diagnosed personality disorders (American Psychiatric Association, 2000). Persons with NPD are considered to be prone to mood disorders, as well as anorexia and substance-related disorders, especially cocaine. Persons with NPD are likely to have comorbid antisocial (psychopathic), histrionic, paranoid and borderline personality traits.

Course

Little is known about the premorbid behavior pattern of NPD, other than through retrospective reports of persons diagnosed when adults. As adolescents, persons with NPD are likely to be self-centered, assertive, gregarious, dominant and perhaps arrogant. They may have achieved well in school or within some other activity. As adults, many persons with NPD will have experienced high levels of achievement. However, their relationships with colleagues, peers and staff will eventually become strained as their exploitative use of others and self-centered egotism become evident. Success may also be impaired by their difficulty in acknowledging or resolving criticism, deficits and setbacks. Interpersonal and sexual relationships are usually easy for them to develop but difficult to sustain due to their low empathy, self-centeredness and need for admiration. Persons who are deferential and obsequious, or who share a mutual need for status and recognition, may help sustain a relationship. As parents, persons with NPD may attempt to live through their children, valuing them as long as they are a source of pride. Their personal sense of adjustment may be fine for as long as

they continue to experience or anticipate success. Some may not recognize the maladaptivity of their narcissism until middle-age, when the emphasis given to achievement and status may begin to wane.

Treatment

Persons with narcissistic personality traits seek treatment for feelings of depression, substance-related disorders and occupational or relational problems that are secondary to their narcissism. Their self-centeredness and lack of empathy are particularly problematic within marital, occupational and other social relationships, and they usually lack an appreciation of the contribution of their conflicts regarding self-esteem, status and recognition. It is difficult for them even to admit that they have a psychological problem or that they need help, as this admission is itself an injury to their self-esteem. In addition, one of the characteristics of NPD is the belief that they can only be understood by persons of a comparably high social status or recognition. They may be unable to accept advice or insight from persons they consider less intelligent, talented, or insightful than themselves, which may eventually effectively eliminate most other persons.

When they are involved in treatment, persons with NPD will often require some indication that their therapist is among the best or at least worth their time. They are prone to idealizing their therapists (to affirm that he or she is indeed of sufficient status or quality) or to devalue them (to affirm that they are of greater intelligence, capacity, or quality than their therapist, to reject the insights that they have failed to identify, and to indicate that they warrant or deserve an even better therapist). How best to respond is often unclear. It may at times be preferable simply to accept the praise or criticism, particularly when exploration will likely be unsuccessful, whereas at other times it is preferable to confront and discuss the motivation for the devaluation (or the idealization).

Psychodynamic approaches to the treatment of NPD vary in the extent to which emphasis is given to an interpretation of underlying anger and bitterness, or to the provision of empathy and a reflection (or mirroring) of a positive regard and self-esteem (Cooper and Ronningstam, 1992; Kernberg, 1991; Kohut, 1977; Gabbard, 2000). It does appear to be important to identify the current extent and historical source of the conflicts and sensitivities regarding self-esteem. Active confrontation may at times be useful, particularly when the therapeutic alliance is strong, but at other times the vulnerability of the patient may require a more unconditional support. Cognitive–behavior approaches to NPD emphasize increasing awareness of the impact of narcissistic behaviors and statements on interpersonal relationships. The idealization and devaluation can be responsive to role playing and rational introspection, an intellectual approach that may itself be valued by some persons with NPD. However, therapists must be careful not to become embroiled within intellectual conflicts (or competitions). This approach may not work well with the narcissistic person who is motivated to defeat or humiliate the therapist.

Group therapy can be useful for increasing awareness of the grandiosity, lack of empathy and devaluation of others. However, these traits not only interfere with the narcissistic person's ability to sustain membership within groups (and within individual therapy), they may also become quite harmful and destructive to the rapport of the entire group. There is no accepted pharmacologic approach to the treatment of narcissism.

RP was a well-regarded clinician with a good publication record and a successful private practice. However, one of his patients filed a complaint with the state board after their sexual relationship ended. He offered in his defense that his behavior was simply the result of marital stress. His license to practice was suspended indefinitely. One of the terms of his probation was to complete successfully 2 years of psychotherapy. RP agreed that treatment would be beneficial but questioned whether any clinician within his local community was sufficiently qualified, as he considered himself to be among the leading clinicians within this community.

Treatment was problematic from the very beginning. RP felt that their discussions should be quid pro quo: if he was going to reveal aspects of himself then the therapist should do likewise. When confronted with the understanding that he was the one in treatment, RP argued that the therapist must be having "narcissistic conflicts" if he is unwilling to accept the insight and guidance that he could offer. Some of the difficulty within the treatment was attributable to the situation (i.e., it would probably be difficult for most therapists to be mandated to receive therapy from a colleague) but as treatment progressed it became apparent that he had similar conflicts with other persons in his life.

RP's wife was threatening divorce in part because of a history of extramarital affairs. RP did not deny the existence of these affairs but argued that his wife was exaggerating their importance: the other women meant little to him, why should they be of concern to her? He said that he did not keep his affairs secret from her prior to marriage (at least those that he was unable to keep secret), and therefore she knew from the beginning that extramarital affairs would occur. In addition, he felt that his affairs were only petty philandering and that his wife should tolerate them because she was "frankly lucky" to have him for a husband. He was good looking, wealthy and professionally successful, and felt that if he had been more patient he might have found someone better than her.

RP was popular with women, at least at the beginning of relationships. He was charming, engaging and verbally facile. However, he acknowledged during the course of therapy that some women eventually became unhappy, dissatisfied and at times even angry with him. It is quite possible that his perception of his past relationships even understated the extent of the dissatisfaction. He attributed their dissatisfaction to "unrealistic and neurotic expectations". He stated that women would flirt with him because he is an "attractive catch" and that he was only fulfilling their fantasies by letting them become involved with him. He would soon lose interest though in the women with whom he became involved, and he acknowledged that it was not always easy to extricate himself from a relationship without any cost to himself.

He evidenced only a marginal insight into the potential harm he had caused the patient with whom he had the sexual relationship. He argued that the proscription against sexual involvements should not have been enforced in this instance because he had been very careful in determining that their relationship was not the intended target of the ethical guidelines: she was herself a "competent" professional who had "freely" entered the relationship and, in any case, no complaint would have been filed if he had been willing to continue the relationship. She was a well-known public figure. She testified to the state board that he repeatedly suggested to her that she accompany him on his business trips, and it was her impression that he wanted to show her off as a "trophy" to his colleagues. She stated that she ended the relationship when she discovered from her colleagues that he was bragging to others about their relationship and revealing details of their sexual activities.

Treatment was terminated by RP after 6 months of treatment upon reading the biannual report by his therapist to the state board regarding his progress. RP felt that he had been making substantial progress that was not being adequately appreciated by his therapist. He noted, for example, that his wife was no longer seeking a divorce and that his ex-patient was engaged to be married. He did indicate that he was dissatisfied with treatment, and felt that progress would be improved by "a more experienced and respected" clinician. He attributed the therapist's negative evaluation of his progress to professional jealousy.

Avoidant Personality Disorder

Definition

Avoidant personality disorder (AVPD) is a pervasive pattern of timidity, inhibition, inadequacy and social hypersensitivity (American Psychiatric Association, 2000). Persons with AVPD may have a strong desire to develop close, personal relationships but feel too insecure to approach others or to express their feelings. AVPD is indicated by the presence of four or more of the seven diagnostic criteria presented in the DSM criteria for AVPD.

Etiology and Pathology

AVPD appears to be an extreme variant of the fundamental personality traits of introversion and neuroticism. Introversion includes such facets as passivity, social withdrawal and inhibition, while neuroticism includes self-consciousness, vulnerability and anxiousness. The personality dimensions of neuroticism and introversion have substantial heritability, as do the more specific traits of social anxiousness and shyness.

In childhood, neuroticism appears as a distress-prone or inhibited temperament. Shyness, timidity and interpersonal insecurity might be exacerbated further in childhood through overprotection and excessive cautiousness. Parental behavior coupled with a distress-prone temperament has been shown to result in social inhibition and timidity. Most children and adolescents will have many experiences of interpersonal embarrassment, rejection, or humiliation, but these will be particularly devastating to the person who is already lacking in self-confidence or is temperamentally passive, inhibited, or introverted.

AVPD may involve elevated peripheral sympathetic activity and adrenocortical responsiveness, resulting in excessive autonomic arousal, fearfulness and inhibition (Siever and Davis, 1991). Just as ASPD may involve deficits in the functioning of

Avoidant Personality Disorder

A pervasive pattern of social inhibition, feelings of inadequacy, and hypersensitivity to negative evaluation, beginning by early adulthood and present in a variety of contexts, as indicated by four (or more) of the following:

(1) avoids occupational activities that involve significant interpersonal contact, because of fears of criticism, disapproval, or rejection

(2) is unwilling to get involved with people unless certain of being liked

(3) shows restraint within intimate relationships because of the fear of being shamed or ridiculed

(4) is preoccupied with thoughts of being criticized or rejected in social situations

(5) is inhibited in new interpersonal situations because of feelings of inadequacy

(6) views self as socially inept, personally unappealing, or inferior to others

(7) is unusually reluctant to take personal risks or to engage in any new activities because they may prove embarrassing

Reprinted with permission from the *Diagnostic and Statistical Manual of Mental Disorders*, Fourth Edition, Text Revision. Copyright 2000 American Psychiatric Association.

a behavioral inhibition system, AVPD may involve excessive functioning of this same. The pathology of AVPD, however, may also be more psychological than neurochemical, with the timidity, shyness and insecurity being a natural result of a cumulative history of denigrating, embarrassing and devaluing experiences. Underlying AVPD may be excessive self-consciousness, feelings of inadequacy or inferiority, and irrational cognitive schemas that perpetuate introverted, avoidant behavior.

Differential Diagnosis

The most difficult differential diagnosis for AVPD is with generalized social phobia. Both involve an avoidance of social situations, social anxiety and timidity, and both may be evident since late childhood or adolescence. Many persons with AVPD in fact seek treatment for a social phobia. To the extent that the behavior pattern pervades the person's everyday functioning and has been evident since childhood, the diagnosis of a personality disorder would be more descriptive. There are arguments to subsume all cases of AVPD into the diagnosis of generalized social phobia (as was done for schizoid disorder of childhood in DSM-IV-TR) but there is considerable empirical support for the existence of the personality dimensions of introversion and neuroticism and for an understanding of AVPD as a maladaptive variant of these personality traits.

Many persons with AVPD may also meet the criteria for dependent personality disorder (DPD). This might at first glance seem unusual, given that AVPD involves social withdrawal whereas DPD involves excessive social attachment. However,

once a person with AVPD is able to obtain a relationship, he or she will often cling to this relationship in a dependent manner. Both disorders include feelings of inadequacy, needs for reassurance and hypersensitivity to criticism and neglect (i.e. abnormally high levels of anxiousness, self-consciousness and vulnerability). A distinction between AVPD and DPD is best made when the person is seeking a relationship. Avoidant persons tend to be very shy, inhibited and timid (and are therefore slow to get involved with someone) whereas dependent persons urgently seek another relationship as soon as one ends (i.e., avoidant persons are high in introversion whereas dependent persons are high in extraversion). Avoidant persons may also be reluctant to express their feelings whereas dependent persons can drive others away by continuous expressions of neediness. The differentiation of AVPD from the schizoid, paranoid and schizotypal personality disorders was discussed in previous sections.

Epidemiology and Comorbidity

Timidity, shyness and social insecurity are not uncommon problems and AVPD is one of the more prevalent personality disorders within clinical settings, occurring in 5 to 25% of all patients (American Psychiatric Association, 2000). However, AVPD may be diagnosed in only 1 to 2% of the general population. It appears to occur equally among males and females, with some studies reporting more males and others reporting more females. Persons with AVPD are likely to have symptoms that meet the DSM-IV criteria for a generalized social phobia, and others may have a mood disorder.

Course

Persons with AVPD are shy, timid and anxious as children. Many are diagnosed with a social phobia during childhood. Adolescence is a particularly difficult developmental period due to the importance at this time of attractiveness, dating and popularity. Occupational success may not be significantly impaired, as long as there is little demand for public performance. Persons with AVPD may in fact find considerable gratification and esteem through a job or career that they are unable to find within their relationships. The job may serve as a distraction from intense feelings of loneliness. Their avoidance of social situations will impair their ability to develop adequate social skills, and this will then further handicap any eventual efforts to develop relationships. As parents, they may be very responsible, empathic and affectionate, but may unwittingly impart feelings of social anxiousness and awkwardness. Severity of the AVPD symptomatology diminishes as the person becomes older.

Treatment

Persons with AVPD seek treatment for their avoidant personality traits, although many initially seek treatment for symptoms of anxiety, particularly social phobia (generalized subtype). It is important in such cases to recognize that the shyness is not due simply to a dysregulation or dyscontrol of anxiousness. There is instead a more pervasive and fundamental psychopathology, involving feelings of interpersonal insecurity, low self-esteem and inadequacy.

Social skills training, systematic desensitization and a graded hierarchy of *in vivo* exposure to feared social situations have been shown to be useful in the treatment of AVPD. However, it is also important to discuss the underlying fears and insecurities regarding attractiveness, desirability, rejection, or intimacy. Persons with AVPD are at times reluctant to discuss such feelings, as they may feel embarrassed, they may fear being ridiculed, or they may not want to "waste the time" of the therapist with such "foolish" insecurities. They may prefer a less revealing or involved form of treatment. It is important to be understanding, patient and accepting, and to proceed at a pace that is comfortable for the patient. Insecurities and fears can at times be addressed through cognitive techniques as the irrationality is usually readily apparent. It remains useful though to identify the historical source of their development as this understanding will help the patient appreciate the irrationality or irrelevance of their expectations and perceptions for their current relationships.

Persons with AVPD often find group therapies to be helpful. Exploratory and supportive groups can provide them with an understanding environment in which to discuss their social insecurities, to explore and practice more assertive behaviors, and to develop an increased self-confidence to approach others and to develop relationships outside of the group. Focused and specialized social skills training groups would be preferable to unstructured groups that might be predominated by much more assertive and extraverted members.

Many persons with AVPD will respond to anxiolytic medications, and at times to antidepressants, particularly such monoamine oxidase inhibitors as phenelzine. Normal and abnormal feelings of anxiousness can be suppressed or diminished through pharmacologic interventions. This approach may in fact be necessary to overcome initial feelings of intense social anxiety that are markedly disruptive to current functioning (e.g., inability to give required presentations at work or to talk to new acquaintances). However, it is also important to monitor closely a reliance on medications. Persons with AVPD could be prone to rely excessively on substances to control their feelings of anxiousness, whereas their more general feelings of insecurity and inadequacy would require a more comprehensive treatment.

Dependent Personality Disorder

Definition

Dependent personality disorder (DPD) involves a pervasive and excessive need to be taken care of that leads to submissiveness, clinging and fears of separation (American Psychiatric Association, 2000). Persons with DPD will also have low self-esteem, and will often be self-critical and self-denigrating. DPD is indicated by the presence of five or more of the eight diagnostic criteria presented in DSM-IV-TR Criteria for DPD.

Etiology and Pathology

Central to the etiology and pathology of DPD is an insecure interpersonal attachment. Insecure attachment and helplessness may be generated through a parent–child relationship, perhaps by a clinging parent or a continued infantilization during a time in which individuation and separation normally occurs., However, DPD may also represent an interaction of an anxious–inhibited temperament with inconsistent or overprotective. Dependent persons may turn to a parental figure to provide a reassurance, security and confidence that they are unable to generate for themselves. They may eventually believe that their self-worth is contingent upon the worth or importance they have to another person.

DSM-IV-TR Criteria 301.6

Dependent Personality Disorder

A pervasive and excessive need to be taken care of that leads to submissive and clinging behavior and fears of separation, beginning by early adulthood and present in a variety of contexts, as indicated by five (or more) of the following:

(1) has difficulty making everyday decisions without an excessive amount of advice and reassurance from others.

(2) needs others to assume responsiblity for most major areas of his or her life.

(3) has difficulty expressing disagreement with others because of fear of loss of support or approval (**Note:** Do not include realistic fears of retribution).

(4) has difficulty initiating projects or doing things on his or her own (because of a lack of self-confidence in judgment or abilities rather than to a lack of motivation or energy).

(5) goes to excessive lengths to obtain nurturance and support from others, to the point of volunteering to do things that are unpleasant.

(6) feels uncomfortable or helpless when alone, because of exaggerated fears of being unable to care for himself or herself.

(7) urgently seeks another relationship as a source of care and support when a close relationship ends.

(8) is unrealistically preoccupied with fears of being left to take care of himself or herself

Reprinted with permission from the *Diagnostic and Statistical Manual of Mental Disorders*, Fourth Edition, Text Revision. Copyright 2000 American Psychiatric Association.

Differential Diagnosis

Excessive dependency will often be seen in persons who have developed debilitating mental and general medical disorders such as agoraphobia, schizophrenia, mental retardation, severe injuries and dementia. However, a diagnosis of DPD requires the presence of the dependent traits since late childhood or adolescence (American Psychiatric Association, 2000). One can diagnose the presence of a personality disorder at any age during a person's lifetime, but if, for example, a DPD diagnosis is given to a person at the age of 75 years, this presumes that the dependent behavior was evident since the age of approximately 18 years (i.e., predates the onset of a comorbid mental or physical disorder).

Deference, politeness and passivity will also vary substantially across cultural groups. It is important not to confuse differences in personality that are due to different cultural norms with the presence of a personality disorder. The diagnosis of DPD requires that the dependent behavior be maladaptive, resulting in clinically significant functional impairment or distress.

Many persons with DPD will also meet the criteria for histrionic and borderline personality disorders. Persons with DPD and HPD may both display strong needs for reassurance, attention and approval. However, persons with DPD tend to be more self-effacing, docile and altruistic, whereas persons with HPD tend to be more flamboyant, assertive and self-centered and persons with BPD will tend to be much more dysfunctional and emotionally dysregulated.

Epidemiology and Comorbidity

DPD is among the most prevalent of the personality disorders (American Psychiatric Association, 2000), occurring in 5 to 30% of patients and 2 to 4% of the general community (Mattia and Zimmerman, 2001). A controversial issue is its differential sex prevalence. DPD is diagnosed more frequently in females but there is some concern that there might be a failure to recognize adequately the extent of dependent personality traits within males. Many studies have indicated that dependent personality traits provide a vulnerability to the development of depression in response to interpersonal loss.

Course

Persons with DPD are likely to have been excessively submissive as children and adolescents, and some may have had a chronic physical illness or a separation anxiety disorder during childhood (American Psychiatric Association, 2000). Persons with DPD fear intensely a loss of concern, care and support from others, particularly the person with whom they have an emotional attachment. They are unable to be by themselves, as their sense of self-worth, value, or meaning is obtained by or through the presence of a relationship. They have few other sources of self-esteem. Along with the need for emotional support are perpetual doubts and insecurities regarding the current source of support. Persons with DPD constantly require reassurance and reaffirmation that any particular relationship will continue, because they anticipate or fear that at some point they may again be alone. Because of their intense fear of being alone they may become quickly attached to persons who are unreliable, unempathic and even exploitative or abusive. More desirable or reliable partners are at times driven away by their excessive clinging and continued demands for reassurance. Occupational functioning is impaired to the extent that independent responsibility and initiative are required. Persons with DPD are prone to mood disorders, particularly major depressive disorder and dysthymic disorder, and to anxiety disorders, particularly agoraphobia, social phobia and perhaps panic disorder. However, the severity of the symptomatology tends to decrease with age, particularly if the person has obtained a reliable, dependable and empathic partner.

Treatment

Persons with DPD are often in treatment for one or more Axis I disorders, particularly a mood (depressive) or an anxiety disorder. They tend to be very agreeable, compliant and grateful patients, at times to excess. An important issue in the treatment of persons with DPD is not letting the relationship with the therapist become an end in itself (Stone, 1993). Many persons with DPD find the therapeutic relationship to satisfy their need for support, concern and involvement. The therapist can be perceived as a nurturing, caring and dependable partner who is always available for as long as the patient desires. Successful treatment can in fact be feared because it suggests the termination of the relationship, an outcome that is at times avoided at all costs. As a result, they may be excessively compliant, submissive, agreeable and cooperative in order to be the patient that the therapist would want to

retain. Therapists need to be careful not unwittingly to encourage or exploit this submissiveness, nor to commit the opposite error of rejecting and abandoning them to be rid of their needy and clinging dependency. Such responses are common in the interpersonal (marital and sexual) history of persons with DPD, and are at times experienced as well within therapeutic relationships. Persons with DPD tend to have unrealistic expectations regarding their therapist. They may attempt to have the therapist take control of their lives, and may make unrealistic requests or demands for their therapist's time, involvement and availability.

Exploration of the breadth and source of the need for care and support is often an important component of treatment. Persons with DPD often have a history of exploitative, rejecting and perhaps even abusive relationships that have contributed to their current feelings of insecurity and inadequacy. Cognitive–behavioral techniques are useful in addressing the feelings of inadequacy, incompetence and helplessness (Beck and Freeman, 1990). Social skills, problem-solving and assertiveness training also makes important contributions.

Persons with DPD may also benefit from group therapy. A supportive group is useful in diffusing the feelings of dependency onto a variety of persons, in providing feedback regarding their manner of relating to others, and in providing practice and role models for more assertive and autonomous interpersonal functioning. There is no known pharmacologic treatment for DPD.

Obsessive–Compulsive Personality Disorder

Definition

Obsessive–compulsive PD (OCPD) includes a preoccupation with orderliness, perfectionism, and mental and interpersonal control (American Psychiatric Association, 2000). OCPD is indicated by the presence of four or more of the eight diagnostic criteria presented in DSM criteria for OCPD.

Etiology and Pathology

A variety of studies have indicated heritability for the trait of obsessionality. OCPD may also relate to the adult personality trait of conscientiousness–constraint and the childhood temperament of attentional self-regulation, both of which have demonstrated substantial heritability.

Early psychoanalytic theories regarding OCPD concerned issues of unconscious guilt or shame (Gunderson and Gabbard, 2000). A variety of underlying conflicts have since been proposed, including a need to maintain an illusion of infallibility to defend against feelings of insecurity, an identification with authoritarian parents, or an excessive, rigid control of feelings and impulses (Gabbard, 2000; Oldham and Frosch, 1991; Stone, 1993). Any one or more of these conflicts might be relevant for a particular person with OCPD but there is quite limited empirical support for these particular models of etiology and pathology. OCPD includes personality traits that are highly valued within most cultures (e.g., conscientiousness) and some instances of OCPD may reflect exaggerated or excessive responses to the expectations of or pressures by parental figures.

Differential Diagnosis

Devotion to work and productivity will vary substantially across cultural groups. One should be careful not to confuse normal cultural variation in conscientiousness with the presence of this personality disorder. A diagnosis of OCPD requires that the

Obsessive–Compulsive Personality Disorder

A pervasive pattern of preoccupation with orderliness, perfectionism, and mental and interpersonal control at the expense of flexibility, openness, and efficiency, beginning by early adulthood and present in a variety of contexts, as indicated by four (or more) of the following:

(1) is preoccupied with details, rules, lists, order, organization, or schedules to the extent that the major point of the activity is lost

(2) shows perfectionism that interferes with task completion (e.g., is unable to complete a project because his or her own overly strict standards are not met)

(3) excessive devotion to work and productivity to the exclusion of leisure activities and friendships (not accounted for by obvious economic necessity)

(4) is overconscientious, scrupulous, and inflexible about matters of morality, ethics, or values (not accounted for by cultural or religious identification)

(5) is unable to discard worn-out or worthless objects even when they have no sentimental value

(6) is reluctant to delegate tasks or to work with others unless they submit to exactly his or her way of doing things

(7) adopts a miserly spending style toward both self and others; money is viewed as something to be hoarded for future catastrophes

(8) shows rigidity and stubbornness

Reprinted with permission from the *Diagnostic and Statistical Manual of Mental Disorders*, Fourth Edition, Text Revision. Copyright 2000 American Psychiatric Association.

devotion to work be maladaptive or to the exclusion of leisure activities and friendships (American Psychiatric Association, 2000).

OCPD resembles to some extent the obsessive–compulsive anxiety disorder (OCAD). However, many persons with OCPD fail to develop OCAD, and vice versa. OCAD involves intrusive obsessions or circumscribed and repetitively performed rituals whose purpose is to reduce or control feelings of anxiety (American Psychiatric Association, 2000). OCPD, in contrast, involves rigid, inhibited and authoritarian behavior patterns that are more egosyntonic. If both behavior patterns are present, both diagnoses should be given as these disorders are sufficiently distinct that it is likely that in such cases two different disorders are in fact present.

OCPD may at times resemble narcissistic PD, as both disorders can involve assertiveness, domination, achievement and a professed perfectionism. However, the emphasis in OCPD will be on work for its own sake whereas narcissistic persons will work only to achieve status and recognition. Persons with OCPD will also be troubled by doubts, worries and self-criticism, whereas the narcissistic person will tend to be overly self-assured.

Epidemiology and Comorbidity

Conscientiousness is one of the fundamental dimensions of personality characterized by the tendency to emphasize duty, order, deliberation, discipline, competence and achievement (Costa and McCrae, 1992). Persons who are excessively organized, ordered, deliberate, dutiful and disciplined would be characterized as having OCPD (Widiger *et al.*, 2002). Only 1 to 2% of the general community may meet the diagnostic criteria for the disorder but this could be an underestimation (Oldham and Frosch, 1991). Up to 10% of the population has been estimated to be maladaptively stubborn, 4% excessively devoted to work, and 8% excessively perfectionistic. OCPD is one of the less frequently diagnosed personality disorders within inpatient settings, occurring in approximately 3 to 10% of patients (American Psychiatric Association, 2000) but its prevalence may be much higher within private practice settings. This disorder does appear to occur more often in males than in females but exceptions to this finding have been reported.

Course

As children, some persons with OCPD may have appeared to be relatively well-behaved, responsible and conscientious. However, they may have also been overly serious, rigid and constrained. As adults, many will obtain good to excellent success within a job or career. They can be excellent workers to the point of excess, sacrificing their social and leisure activities, marriage and family for their job (Oldham and Frosch, 1991; Stone, 1993). Relationships with spouse and children are likely to be strained due to their tendency to be detached and uninvolved, yet authoritarian and domineering with respect to decisions. A spouse may complain of a lack of affection, tenderness and warmth. Relationships with colleagues at work may be equally strained by the excessive perfectionism, domination, indecision, worrying and anger. Jobs that require flexibility, openness, creativity, or diplomacy may be particularly difficult. Persons with OCPD may be prone to various anxiety and physical disorders that are secondary to their worrying, indecision and stress. Those with concomitant traits of angry hostility and competitiveness may be prone to cardiovascular disorders. Mood disorders may not develop until the person recognizes the sacrifices that have been made by their devotion to work and productivity, which may at times not occur until middle-age. However, most will experience early employment or career difficulties or even failures that may result in depression.

Treatment

Persons with OCPD may fail to seek treatment for the OCPD symptomatology. They may seek treatment instead for disorders and problems that are secondary to their OCPD traits, including anxiety disorders, health problems (e.g., cardiovascular disorders), and problems within various relationships (e.g., marital, familial and occupational). Treatment will be complicated by their inability to appreciate the contribution of their personality to these problems and disorders. It is not unusual for persons with OCPD to perceive themselves as being simply conscientious, dutiful, moral and responsible, rather than perfectionistic, stubborn, rigid, domineering and unavailable. Their understanding is complicated further by the contribution of their traits to various achievements and successes (e.g., career advancement) and to the control of negative affect (e.g., ability to control feelings of dysphoria during a crisis). The OCPD traits are not invariably or always maladaptive, and persons with this disorder may not appreciate the disorder's cost to their physical health, psychological well-being and personal relationships.

Cognitive–behavioral techniques that address the irrationality of excessive conscientiousness, moralism, perfectionism, devotion to work and stubborness can be effective in the treatment of OCPD (Beck and Freeman, 1990). Persons with OCPD may in fact appreciate the rational approach to treatment provided by cognitive–behavioral therapy. A common difficulty though is the tendency to drift into lengthy and unproductive ruminations and intellectualized speculations (Beck and Freeman, 1990). Therapeutic techniques that emphasize the acknowledgment, recognition and acceptance of feelings will therefore be useful. Gestalt techniques that focus upon and confront feeling states will often feel threatening to persons with OCPD but precisely for this reason they can also be quite revealing and useful. Persons with OCPD will attempt to control therapeutic sessions, and techniques that encourage uncontrolled, freely expressed associations to explore historical motivations for control, perfectionism and workaholism are often helpful.

Persons with OCPD can be problematic in groups. They will tend to be domineering, constricted and judgmental. There is no accepted pharmacologic treatment for OCPD. Some persons with OCPD will benefit from anxiolytic or antidepressant medications, but this will typically reflect the presence of associated features or comorbid disorders. The core traits of OCPD might not be affected by pharmacologic interventions.

Personality Disorder Not Otherwise Specified

As indicated earlier, DSM-IV includes a diagnostic category, personality disorder not otherwise specified (PDNOS), for persons with a personality disorder who do not meet the diagnostic criteria for any one of the 10 officially recognized diagnoses. PDNOS has in fact been the singly most commonly used personality disorder diagnosis in almost every study in which it has been considered. It would not, of course, be possible to discuss the etiology, pathology, course, or treatment of the PDNOS disorder as the diagnosis refers to a wide variety of personality types. However, one usage of PDNOS is for the two personality disorders presented in the appendix to DSM-IV for criterion sets provided for further study, the passive–aggressive and the depressive (American Psychiatric Association, 2000).

Passive–Aggressive (Negativistic) Personality Disorder

Definition

Passive–aggressive personality disorder (PAPD) is a pervasive pattern of negativistic attitudes and passive resistance to authority, demands, responsibilities, or obligations (American Psychiatric Association, 2000). PAPD would be diagnosed by the presence of four or more of the seven criteria presented in DSM-IV-TR criteria for PAPD.

PAPD is in the appendix of DSM-IV because there has been little research to support its validity. There was concern that the DSM-III-R diagnosis described a situational reaction rather than a pervasive and chronic personality disorder, and the criteria were revised substantially for DSM-IV-TR to describe a more general and pervasive negativism. Compelling objections were

raised in response to the decision to downgrade the recognition of this longstanding diagnosis and the new criteria may eventually prove to have more validity and clinical utility than the DSM-III-R version but this additional research needs to be conducted in order for the diagnosis to be given an official recognition.

DSM-IV-TR Criteria

Passive–Aggressive Personality Disorder

A. A pervasive pattern of negativistic attitudes and passive resistance to demands for adequate performance, beginning by early adulthood and present in a variety of contexts, as indicated by four (or more) of the following:

 (1) passively resists fulfilling routine social and occupational tasks

 (2) complains of being misunderstood and unappreciated by others

 (3) is sullen and argumentative

 (4) unreasonably criticizes and scorns authority

 (5) expresses envy and resentment toward those apparently more fortunate

 (6) voices exaggerated and persistent complaints of personal misfortune

 (7) alternates between hostile defiance and contrition

B. Does not occur exclusively during major depressive episodes and is not better accounted for by dysthymic disorder.

Reprinted with permission from the *Diagnostic and Statistical Manual of Mental Disorders*, Fourth Edition, Text Revision. Copyright 2000 American Psychiatric Association.

Etiology and Pathology

Central to the psychopathology of PAPD appears to be bitter resentment. Passive–aggressive persons have a hostile, angry and bitter attitude towards the world. There are no data on its heritability or psychosocial etiology. It has been suggested that passive–aggressive behavior is due in part to conflicts concerning dependency and resentment, or a history of mistreatment and neglect. One might find a history of being exploited, neglected, mistreated, or abused by persons upon whom the person with PAPD relied. Negativistic traits may also be modeled by parental figures.

Assessment and Differential Diagnosis

Most of the DSM-IV semi-structured interviews include items for the assessment of PAPD. It is particularly important when assessing for PAPD to recognize that passive–aggressive behavior might be confined to settings in which persons have lost freedom, responsibility, or decision-making authority that was previously available to them and overt expressions of assertiveness or opposition are being discouraged. For example, it would not be surprising to observe passive–aggressive behavior within the military, prison, or some inpatient hospitals. It is important in such settings to verify that the negativistic behavior was evident earlier and is currently evident within other situations.

Epidemiology and Comorbidity

Approximately 1 to 2% of the community will meet the DSM-III-R criteria for PAPD. Up to 5% of patients were diagnosed with PAPD earlier. The rate was higher when semi-structured interviews were used but still low compared with most other personality disorders. The prevalence rate with the DSM-IV criteria are likely to be higher, given the expansion of the disorder from simply a passive resistance to demands for adequate performance to a more general negativism. The broader formulation of negativism resembles closely the general trait of oppositionalism (characterized by the tendency to be complaining, discontented, grumbling, whining and argumentative) which does appear to occur more often in males than in females (Costa and McCrae, 1992).

Course

Many persons with PAPD may have met the criteria for an oppositional defiant disorder during childhood, which is also characterized by the tendency to be irritable, complaining, oppositional, argumentative and negativistic (American Psychiatric Association, 1980). As adults, impairment is likely to be most evident with respect to employment. Persons with PAPD are irresponsible, lax and negligent employees, as well as resistant, oppositional and even hostile. Resolution of interpersonal conflicts is difficult due to the tendency of the passive–aggressive person to blame others. They are argumentative, sullen and critical of their peers and friends, who may not tolerate their antagonism.

Treatment

Persons with PAPD rarely enter treatment to make effective changes to their personality or behavior. They are more likely to seek treatment for Axis I disorders (e.g., depression, anxiety, or somatoform disorder), or for marital, family, or occupational problems. The initiation of treatment is often at the insistence of a spouse, relative, or employer. They can be very difficult patients to treat due to their tendency to be blaming, argumentative, pessimistic and passively resistant. It is important for the therapist to remain supportive and empathic; carefully and benignly offering observations, suggestions, and reflections on the patient's tendency to be their own worst enemy. Cognitive treatment can be useful directly to address the false perceptions, assumptions and attributions (Beck and Freeman, 1990) as long as the therapist is not drawn into unproductive disagreements and arguments. It is common for therapists to become frustrated, impatient and defensive in response to the negativism, criticism and complaints. Periodic consultation with colleagues are advisable. Group therapy is often helpful once the patient has developed a commitment to the group, as the various members can provide consistent and confirmatory feedback regarding the negativistic and passive–aggressive behavior. There is no known pharmacologic treatment for PAPD.

Depressive Personality Disorder

Definition

Depressive personality disorder (DPPD) is a pervasive pattern of depressive cognitions and behaviors that have been evident since adolescence and characteristic of everyday functioning (American Psychiatric Association, 2000). These are persons who characteristically display a gloominess, cheerlessness, pessimism, brooding, rumination and dejection. DPPD would be diagnosed by the presence of five or more of the seven criteria presented in the DSM criteria for DPPD.

A field trial by the DSM-IV Mood Disorders Work Group indicated that many persons do meet diagnostic criteria for DPPD rather than early-onset dysthymia (Phillips *et al.*, 1995; Widiger, 1999). In addition, many persons diagnosed with early-onset dysthymia may not be adequately described as having a disorder that is confined to the regulation or control of their mood. However, the DSM-IV diagnostic criteria for DPPD lack sufficient empirical support to warrant full recognition.

DSM-IV-TR Criteria

Depressive Personality Disorder

A. A pervasive pattern of depressive cognitions and behaviors beginning by early adulthood and present in a variety of contexts, as indicated by five (or more) of the following:

  (1) usual mood is dominated by dejection, gloominess, cheerlessness, joylessness, unhappiness

  (2) self-concept centers around beliefs of inadequacy, worthlessness, and low self-esteem

  (3) is critical, blaming, and derogatory toward self

  (4) is brooding and given to worry

  (5) is negativistic, critical, and judgmental toward others

  (6) is pessimistic

  (7) is prone to feeling guilty or remorseful

B. Does not occur exclusively during major depressive episodes and is not better accounted for by dysthymic disorder.

Etiology and Pathology

DPPD may represent a characterologic variant of mood disorder, in the same manner that STPD is perhaps a characterologic variant of schizophrenia. Support for this hypothesis is provided by recent family history and biogenetic studies. Trait depression is also a facet of the personality trait of neuroticism or negative affectivity, which has demonstrated substantial heritability within the general population. A characteristically low self-esteem, self-criticism, pessimism, brooding and guilt may also result from continued, sustained criticism, derogation and discouragement by a significant parental figure that is accepted and incorporated by the child.

Assessment and Differential Diagnosis

Most of the DSM-IV-TR semi-structured interviews include items for the assessment of DPPD (First *et al.*, 1997; Pfohl *et al.*, 1997; Widiger *et al.*, 1995; Zanarini *et al.*, 1995) and there is also available a semi-structured interview that is devoted to its assessment, the Diagnostic Interview for Depressive Personality (Gunderson *et al.*, 1994).

DPPD overlaps substantially with early-onset dysthymia. Early-onset dysthymia was in fact conceptualized previously as depressive personality or a characterologic depression prior to DSM-III-R and the alternative criteria for dysthymia that were placed in the appendix to DSM-IV-TR were developed in part on research on DPPD. It is in fact noted in DSM-IV that there may not be a meaningful distinction between these diagnoses (American Psychiatric Association, 2000). Some may prefer to use the diagnosis of early-onset dysthymia, but a dysregulation in mood may not adequately explain why some persons are characterized by chronic attitudes of pessimism, negativism, hopelessness and dejection.

Epidemiology and Comorbidity

There are not yet published data on the prevalence of DPPD within the general population. DPPD is likely to be comorbid with early onset dysthymia, although not all cases of DPPD will meet the DSM-IV-TR criteria for dysthymia. Many of the persons who meet the DSM-IV-TR criteria for DPPD will also likely meet the DSM-IV-TR criteria for PAPD and BPD.

Course

As children, persons with DPPD are pessimistic, gloomy, passive and withdrawn. Performance in school is often inadequate to poor. This behavior pattern continues essentially unchanged into and through adulthood. Some, however, may eventually become good workers, exhibiting tremendous discipline and devotion to their work. Relationships with peers and sexual partners, however, are invariably problematic. They are gloomy and irritable company, and have difficulty finding pleasure, joy, or satisfaction in leisure activities. They may also be quite withdrawn and lonely, but lack an apparent motivation or energy to seek or maintain relationships.

Treatment

Many persons with DPD are referred or seek treatment for a depressive mood disorder. It is important in such cases to recognize the extent to which the depressed mood reflects their fundamental view of themselves and the world. Their pessimism involves more than simply a dysregulation of mood. Cognitive–behavioral techniques have demonstrated efficacy in the treatment of depressive personality traits (Beck and Freeman, 1990). The depressive individual's pessimistic view of themselves and their future should be systematically challenged. Explorations of the faulty reasoning, arbitrary inferences, selective perceptions and misattributions can be influential in overcoming the pessimistic, gloomy, critical and negativistic attitudes. Audio- or videotaped role playing is useful in helping the person recognize the occurrence and pervasiveness of the depressive cognitions, and in generating, developing and rehearsing more realistic and accurate reasoning. However, exploration of the source for and historical development of self-defeating behaviors may also be helpful, not only to undermine their credibility and validity within current relationships and situations but also to address any motivation for their perpetuation. Persons with DPPD will also be responsive to antidepressant pharmacotherapy, particularly tricyclic antidepressants.

Comparison of DSM-IV/ICD-10 Diagnostic Criteria

The items sets for paranoid, schizoid, schizotypal, antisocial, histrionic, avoidant, dependent and obsessive–compulsive personality disorders in the ICD-10 Diagnostic Criteria for Research and the DSM-IV-TR criteria differ but define essentially the same condition. Furthermore, ICD-10 does not consider schizotypal to be a personality disorder and instead includes this condition in the section containing schizophrenia and other psychotic disorders. ICD-10 also refers to several of the DSM-IV-TR disorders by different names: antisocial is called "dissocial", borderline is called "emotionally unstable personality disorder, borderline type", and obsessive–compulsive is called "anankastic".

ICD-10 includes an "emotionally unstable personality disorder" with two subtypes: impulsive type and borderline type; criteria are provided for each subtype but not for emotionally unstable personality disorder. Neither of these subtypes by themselves correspond to the DSM-IV-TR borderline personality disorder, which includes some items from each of these subtypes. Narcissistic personality disorder in DSM-IV-TR is not included in ICD-10 as a specific personality disorder, although the DSM-IV-TR criteria set is included in Annex I of ICD-10 (i.e., "provisional criteria for selected disorders").

References

American Psychiatric Association (1980) *Diagnostic and Statistical Manual of Mental Disorders*, 3rd edn. APA, Washington DC.

American Psychiatric Association (1987) Diagnostic and Statistical Manual of Mental Disorders, 3rd edn., Rev. APA, Washington DC.

American Psychiatric Association (2000) *Diagnostic and Statistical Manual of Mental Disorders*, 4th edn., Text Rev. APA, Washington DC.

Beck AT and Freeman A (1990) *Cognitive Therapy of Personality Disorders*. Guilford Press, New York.

Benjamin LS (1993) Interpersonal Diagnosis and Treatment of Personality Disorders. Guilford Press, New York.

Clark LA, Watson D and Reynolds S (1995) Diagnosis and classification of psychopathology: Challenges to the current system and future directions. *Annu Rev Psychol* 46, 121–153.

Cloninger CR (2000) A practical way to diagnosis personality disorders: A proposal. *J Pers Disord* 14, 99–108.

Cooper AM and Ronningstam E (1992) Narcissistic personality disorder, in *Review of Psychiatry*, Vol. 11 (eds Tasman A and Riba MB). American Psychiatric Press, Washington DC, pp. 80–97.

Costa PT and McCrae RR (1992) *Revised NEO Personality Inventory (NEO PI-R) and NEO Five-Factor Inventory (NEO-FFI) Professional Manual*. Psychological Assessment Resources, Odessa, FL.

First M, Gibbon M, Spitzer RL *et al.* (1997) *User's Guide for the Structured Clinical Interview for DSM-IV Axis II Personality Disorders*. American Psychiatric Press, Washington DC.

Gabbard GO (2000) *Psychodynamic Psychiatry in Clinical Practice*, 3rd edn. American Psychiatric Press, Washington DC.

Gunderson JG (2001) *Borderline Personality Disorder: A Clinical Guide*. American Psychiatric Press, Washington DC.

Gunderson JG, Ronningstam E and Bodkin A (1990) The diagnostic interview for narcissistic patients. *Arch Gen Psychiatr* 47, 676–680.

Gunderson JG and Gabbard GO (2000) Psychotherapy for Personality Disorders. American Psychiatric Press, Washington DC.

Gunderson JG, Phillips KA, Triebwasser JT, *et al.* (1994) The diagnostic interview for depressive personality. *Am J Psychiatr* 151, 1300–1304.

Gunderson JG, Shea MT, Skodol AE, *et al.* (2000) The Collaborative Longitudinal Personality Disorders Study. I. Development, aims, design, and sample characteristics. *J Pers Disord* 14, 300–315.

Hare RD (1991) The Hare Psychopathy Checklist-Revised Manual. Multi-Healthy Systems, North Tonawanda, New York.

Kernberg OF (1991) Narcissistic personality disorder, in *Psychiatry*, Vol. 1, Ch. 18,(ed Michels R). JB Lippincott, Philadelphia, PA, pp. 1–12.

Kessler K, McGonagle K, Zhao S, *et al.* (1994) Lifetime and 12 month prevalence of DSM-III-R Psychiatric Disorders in the United States. *Arch Gen Psychiatr* 51, 8–19.

Kohut H (1977) *The Restoration of the Self.* International Universities Press, New York.

Linehan MM (1993) *Cognitive–Behavioral Treatment of Borderline Personality Disorder.* Guilford Press, New York.

Linehan MM (2000) The empirical basis of dialectical behavior therapy: Development of new treatments vs. evaluation of existing treatments. *Clin Psychol: Sci Pract* 7, 113–119.

Livesley WJ (ed) (2001) *Handbook of Personality Disorders.* Guilford Press, New York.

Loranger AW (1999) *International Personality Disorder Examination (IPDE).* Psychological Assessment Resources, Odessa, Florida.

Mattia JI and Zimmerman M (2001) Epidemiology. In Handbook of Personality Disorders, (ed Livesley WJ). Guilford Press, New York, pp. 107–123.

Millon T, Davis RD, Millon CM *et al.* (1996) *Disorders of Personality. DSM-IV and Beyond.* John Wiley, New York.

Oldham JM and Frosch WA (1991) Compulsive personality disorder, in *Psychiatry*, Vol. 1, Ch. 22 (ed Michels R). JB Lippincott, Philadelphia, PA, pp. 1–8.

Phillips KA, Hirschfeld RMA, Shea MT, *et al.* (1995) Depressive personality disorder. In the DSM-IV Personality Disorders, (ed Livesley WJ). Guilford Press, New York, pp. 287–302.

Pfohl B, Blum N and Zimmerman M (1997) *Structured Interview for DSM-IV Personality Disorder.* American Psychiatric Press, Washington DC.

Rhodewalt F and Morf CC (1995) Self and interpersonal correlates of the narcissistic personality inventory: A review and new findings. *J Res Pers* 29, 1–23.

Robins LN, Tipp J, and Przybeck T (1991) Antisocial personality, in *Psychiatric Disorders in America*, Robins LN and Regier DA (eds). The Free Press, New York, pp. 258–290.

Siever LJ and Davis KL (1991) A psychobiological perspective on the personality disorders. *Am J Psychiatr* 148, 1647–1658.

Stone MH (1993) *Abnormalities of Personality. Within and Beyond the Realm of Treatment.* WW Norton, New York.

Stone MH (2000) Clinical guidelines for psychotherapy with borderline personality disorder. *Psychiatr Clin N Am* 23, 193–210.

Widiger TA, Mangine S, Corbitt EM *et al.* (1995) *The Personality Disorder Interview – IV: A Semistructured Interview for the Diagnosis of Personality Disorders.* Psychological Assessment Resources, Odessa, Florida.

Widiger TA and Coker LA (2002) Assessing personality disorders, in *Clinical Personality Assessment: Practical Approaches*, 2nd edn, (ed Butcher JN). Oxford University Press, New York, pp. 407–434.

Widiger TA, Verheul R, and van den Brink W (1999) Personality and psychopathology, in *Handbook of Personality*, 2nd edn, Pervin L and John O (eds). Guilford Press, New York, pp. 347–366.

Widiger TA, Trull TJ, Clarkin JF *et al.* (2002) A description of the DSM-IV personality disorders with the five-factor model of personality, in *Personality Disorders and the Five-Factor Model of Personality*, 2nd edn. (eds Costa PT and Widiger TA). American Psychological Association, Washington DC, pp. 89–99.

World Health Organization (1992) *The ICD-10 Classification of Mental and Behavioural Disorders. Clinical Descriptions and Diagnostic Guidelines.* World Health Organization, Geneva.

Zanarini MC, Frankenburg FR, Sickel AE *et al.* (1995) *Diagnostic Interview for DSM-IV Personality Disorders (DIPD-IV).* McLean Hospital, Boston, MA.

Zanarini MC, Gunderson JG, Frankenburg FR *et al.* (1989) The Revised Diagnostic Interview for Borderlines: Discriminating BPD from other Axis II disorders. *J Pers Disord* 3, 10–18.

CHAPTER

63

Psychological Factors Affecting Medical Condition

Definition

This diagnostic category recognizes the variety of ways in which specific psychological or behavioral factors can adversely affect medical illnesses. Such factors may contribute to the initiation or the exacerbation of the illness, interfere with treatment and rehabilitation, or contribute to morbidity and mortality. Psychological factors may themselves constitute risks for medical diseases, or they may magnify the effects of nonpsychological risk factors. The effects may be mediated directly at a pathophysiological level (e.g., psychological stress inducing myocardial ischemia) or through the patient's behavior (e.g., noncompliance).

The criteria in the *Diagnostic and Statistical Manual of Mental Disorders*, Fourth Edition (DSM-IV) includes situations in which psychological factors interfere with medical treatment, pose health risks, or cause stress-related pathophysiological changes. This diagnosis is structured in DSM-IV so that both the psychological factor and the general medical condition are to be specified. The psychological factor can be an Axis I or Axis II mental disorder (e.g., major depressive disorder aggravating coronary artery disease), a psychological symptom (e.g., anxiety exacerbating asthma), a personality trait or coping style (e.g., type A behavior contributing to the development of coronary artery disease), maladaptive health behaviors (e.g., unsafe sex in a person with human immunodeficiency virus [HIV] infection), a stress-related physiological response (e.g., tension headache), or other unspecified psychological factors. The medical condition is noted on Axis III.

The subject of psychological factors affecting medical condition (PFAMC) has become the focus of intense research because of the illumination it may provide of basic disease mechanisms (e.g., psychoneuroimmunology) and because of the deep interest in improving both the outcomes and the efficiency of health care delivery. In epidemiological studies, several psychiatric disorders increase the likelihood of mortality especially depression, bipolar disorder, schizophrenia, and alcohol abuse or dependence. Psychiatric disorders or symptoms in patients with medical illness may increase their use of health care services, particularly the length of costly hospital stays. Interest has been further increased by intervention trials aimed at psychological factors or disorders that have demonstrated improvements in medical outcomes and in quality of life in patients with serious medical disorders.

It should be evident that this diagnosis is not really a discrete diagnostic category but rather a label for the interactive effects of psyche on soma. Mind–body interactions have long been a focus of interest, both in health and in disease. Psychiatric

---

DSM-IV-TR Criteria 361

Psychological Factors Affecting Medical Condition

A. A general medical condition (coded on Axis III) is present.

B. Psychological factors adversely affect the general medical condition in one of the following ways:

(1) the factors have influenced the course of the general medical condition as shown by a close temporal association between the psychological factors and the development or exacerbation of, or delayed recovery from, the general medical condition

(2) the factors interfere with the treatment of the general medical condition

(3) the factors constitute additional health risks for the individual

(4) stress-related physiological responses precipitate or exacerbate symptoms of the general medical condition

Choose name based on the nature of the psycho-logical factors (if more than one factor is present, indicate the most prominent):

Mental disorder affecting... [indicate the general medical condition] (e.g., an Axis I disorder such as major depressive disorder delaying recovery from a myocardial infarction)

Psychological symptoms affecting... [indicate the general medical condition] (e.g., depressive symptoms delaying recovery from surgery; anxiety exacerbating asthma)

Personality traits or coping style affecting... [indicate the general medical condition] (e.g., pathological denial of the need for surgery in a patient with cancer; hostile, pressured behavior contributing to cardiovascular disease)

Maladaptive health behaviors affecting... [indicate the general medical condition] (e.g., overeating; lack of exercise; unsafe sex)

Stress-related physiological response affecting... [indicate the general medical condition] (e.g., stress-related exacerbations of ulcer, hypertension, arrhythmia, or tension headache)

> **Other or unspecified psychological factors affecting...**
> **[indicate the general medical condition]** (e.g.,
> interpersonal, cultural, or religious factors)

Reprinted with permission from the *Diagnostic and Statistical Manual of Mental Disorders*, Fourth Edition, Text Revision. Copyright 2000 American Psychiatric Association.

illness and medical disease frequently coexist. Psychiatrists and investigators of past eras were misled by this frequent comorbidity into premature conclusions that the psychological factors were preeminent in the causation of the medical disorders, and these were designated psychosomatic. A more modern approach has been to recognize that all medical illnesses are potentially affected by many different factors in the biological, psychological and social realms. The earlier designation of certain disorders as psychosomatic (e.g., peptic ulcer disease) overvalued the contribution of psychological factors to those disorders and undervalued their contribution to other medical disorders (e.g., cancer). Furthermore, whereas labeling medical illnesses as psychosomatic drew attention to the importance of mind–body interactions, it unfortunately and falsely implied to many patients and physicians that the illness was basically psychogenic, that the symptoms were not "real", and that the illness was somehow the patient's fault.

The diagnosis of PFAMC focuses attention on one causal direction in the interactions between psyche and soma, that is, the effects of psychological factors on the medical condition (Figure 63.1). This represents a heuristic simplification, highlighting a particular process for further exploration, understanding, and intervention. In most patients, there are effects in the other direction as well (i.e., the effects of general medical illness on psychological function). Furthermore, both mind and body interact with social and environmental factors both dramatic (e.g., poverty, racism, war) and more subtle (e.g., employment status, neighborhood), that affect the incidence and outcome of medical illness. Diagnosing PFAMC may help psychiatrist and patient address an important dimension of care, but the other "arrows" of Figure 63.1 often warrant attention too.

Etiology and Pathophysiology

How do psychological factors affect medical illnesses? Physicians have long recognized that psychological factors seem to affect medical illnesses, and research elucidating the intervening causal mechanisms is now rapidly growing. From their clinical experience, physicians recognize many ways in which psy-

chological factors affect the onset, progression and outcome of their patients' illnesses. First, psychological factors may promote other known risks for medical illness. Smoking is a risk factor for heart disease, cancer and pulmonary and many other diseases, and individuals with schizophrenia or depression are much more likely to smoke than the general population. A wide variety of psychiatric illnesses are associated with an increased likelihood of abuse of other substances. Depression and schizophrenia are also associated with a sedentary lifestyle. Patients with affective disorders often have chronic pain and chronically tend to overuse analgesics. Individuals with schizophrenia, bipolar disorder and some personality disorders are more likely to engage in unsafe sex, which in turn increases the risk of sexually transmitted diseases, including HIV infection and hepatitis B. Depression, eating disorders and other emotional and behavioral factors affect the pattern and content of diet.

In addition to promoting known risk factors for medical illness, psychological factors also have an impact on the course of illness by influencing how patients respond to their symptoms, including whether and how they seek care. For example, the defense mechanism of denial may lead an individual to ignore anginal chest pain, attribute it to indigestion, delay seeking medical attention, or minimize the pain when describing it to a physician. This tends to result in treatment delay after the acute onset of coronary symptoms, with consequently greater morbidity and mortality. Anxiety is also a common cause of avoidance or delay of health care; phobic fears of needles, sight of blood, surgery and other health care phobias are common. Patients may also neglect their symptoms and fail promptly to seek medical care because of depression, psychosis, or personality traits (e.g., procrastination).

Psychological factors also affect the course of illness through their effects on the physician–patient relationship, since they influence both patients' health behaviors and physicians' diagnostic and treatment decisions. A substantial proportion of the excess mortality experienced by individuals with mental disorders is explained by their receiving poorer quality medical care (Druss *et al.*, 2001a). One explanation for the poorer quality and outcomes of medical care in patients with both serious medical and mental illnesses is the lack of integration between their medical and mental health care (Druss *et al.*, 2001b). Psychological factors can also reduce a patient's compliance with diagnostic recommendations, treatment and lifestyle change, and can interfere with rehabilitation through impairment of motivation, understanding, optimism, or tolerance. A recent meta-analysis found that patients with depression are three times as likely to be noncompliant with medical treatment than patients without (DiMatteo *et al.*, 2000). In addition, many of the effects of psychological factors on medical illness appear to be mediated through a wide array of social factors, including social support, job strain, disadvantaged socioeconomic and educational status, and marital stress.

There is an increasing body of scientific evidence that psychological factors, in addition to their impact on classic (nonpsychological) risk factors, patient behaviors and the physician–patient interaction, have direct effects on pathophysiological processes. For example, stress has been experimentally shown to cause myocardial ischemia in patients with coronary disease. Stress and depression are associated with a wide range of immunological effects. Many psychiatric disorders (especially mood disorders) are associated with disruptions in homeostasis including sleep architecture, other circadian rhythms, and

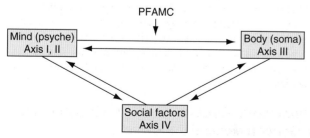

Figure 63.1 *Psychological factors affecting medical condition (PFAMC): Interaction between psyche and soma. Social factors warrant attention as well.*

endocrine secretion and feedback. For example, depression causes increased bone remodeling and decreased bone density (Herran *et al.*, 2000). That such effects occur is well established, but the magnitude of their clinical significance in medical disease is often unclear, and full explanatory causal linkages have for the most part not been demonstrated yet. Nevertheless, investigators have learned a great deal about changes in autonomic, hematologic, endocrine, immunologic and sensory function, as well as gene expression that bring us closer to understanding how psychological factors may affect medical illness. These issues of pathophysiology are discussed later in this chapter for each organ system or specialty category.

Assessment and Diagnosis

The diagnosis of PFAMC differs from most other psychiatric diagnoses in its focus on the interaction between the mental and medical realms. As noted, the criteria require more than that the patient have both a medical illness and contemporaneous psychological factors, because their coexistence does not always include significant interactions between them. To make the diagnosis of PFAMC, either the factors must have influenced the course of the medical condition, interfered with its treatment, contributed to health risks, or physiologically aggravated the medical condition.

Let us consider each of these four ways of making the diagnosis of PFAMC in more detail. The psychological factor's influence on the course of a general medical condition can be inferred from a close temporal relationship between the factor and the development or exacerbation of the medical condition (or delayed recovery). For example, a 45-year-old male executive reports symptoms sounding like typical angina, but occurring only on weekends. Further questioning reveals that he is depressed over deterioration in his marriage. During the week he works late and has limited contact with his family but he spends the weekend at home. The symptoms began after he and his wife started arguing every weekend. The temporal link between onset and recurrence of angina and marital arguments supports a diagnosis of PFAMC.

PFAMC can be diagnosed when the psychological factor interferes with treatment including not seeking medical care, not following up, nonadherence to prescribed drugs or other treatment, or maladaptive modifications in treatment made by the patient or family. The executive with angina rejected his physician's recommendations for further assessment and treatment. He said, "I do get upset at home but I feel just fine at the office, so there couldn't be anything really wrong with me". The patient is able to acknowledge marital discord, but the defense of denial clouds his perception of his physical health and blocks appropriate medical care. This is another form of PFAMC.

PFAMC can also be diagnosed when the psychological factor contributes to health risks, exemplified by the executive increasing his smoking and drinking despite his physician's warnings. ("It's the only way I can cope with my wife.") Finally, PFAMC is an appropriate diagnosis when there are stress-related physiological responses precipitating or exacerbating symptoms of the medical condition. The same man observes that angina is most likely to occur after marital arguments during which he becomes irate, yells, slams doors and throws things.

When a patient's medical illness is faring worse than expected and not responding well to standard treatment, physicians should and often do consider whether a psychological factor may be responsible for the poorer than expected outcome. This is a far from trivial task. To ignore the possibility of PFAMC may miss the crucial barrier to the patient's recovery. On the other hand, premature or facile attribution to psychological factors may lead the physician to overlook medical or social explanations for "treatment-resistant disease" and unfairly blame the patient, with resultant further deterioration in health outcomes and the physician–patient relationship.

To illustrate, a common clinical problem is the brittle diabetic adolescent with labile blood glucose levels and frequent episodes of ketoacidosis and hypoglycemia, despite vigorous attempts by the physician to improve diabetic management and glucose control. The considerable difficulty in controlling such patients' diabetes is often attributed to adolescents' dislike of lifestyle restrictions, their tendency to act out and rebel against authority figures, their denial of vulnerability, their ambivalence about their need for nurturance and their wish to be "normal". There are many adolescent (and some adult) diabetic patients for whom these psychological issues do play an important role in undermining diabetes management through noncompliance regarding medication, diet, visits to the physician, substance use and activity limitations. However, psychological factors do not always account for brittleness and are sometimes incorrectly suspected. It has been demonstrated that much of the difficulty in achieving stable glucose control in adolescent diabetics is the result of the dramatically labile patterns of hormone secretion (cortisol, growth hormone) typical of adolescence, independent of psychological status.

PFAMC has descriptive names for subcategories described as follows.

Mental Disorder Affecting a General Medical Condition

If the patient has a mental disorder meeting criteria for an Axis I or Axis II diagnosis, the diagnostic name is mental disorder affecting medical condition, with the particular medical condition specified. In addition to coding PFAMC, the specific mental disorder is also coded on Axis I or Axis II. Examples include major depressive disorder that reduces energy and compliance in a hemodialysis patient; panic disorder that makes an asthmatic patient hypersensitive to dyspnea; and schizophrenia in a patient with recurrent ventricular tachycardia who refuses placement of an automatic implantable defibrillator because he fears it will control his mind.

Psychological Symptoms Affecting a General Medical Condition

Patients who have psychological symptoms that do not meet the threshold for an Axis I diagnosis may still experience important effects on their medical illness, and the diagnosis would be psychological symptoms affecting a medical condition. Examples include anxiety that aggravates irritable bowel syndrome; depressed mood that hinders recovery from hip replacement surgery; and anger that interferes with rehabilitation after spinal cord injury.

Personality Traits or Coping Style Affecting a General Medical Condition

This may include personality traits or coping styles that do not meet criteria for an Axis II disorder and other patterns of response considered to be maladaptive because they may pose a risk for particular medical illnesses. An example is the competitive hostility component of the type A behavior pattern, and its impact on coronary artery disease. Maladaptive personality traits or coping styles are particularly likely to interfere with the physician–patient relationship as well as the patient's relationships with other caregivers.

Maladaptive Health Behaviors Affecting a General Medical Condition

Many maladaptive health behaviors have significant effects on the course and treatment of many medical conditions. Examples include sedentary lifestyle, smoking, abuse of alcohol or other substances, and unsafe sexual practices. If the maladaptive behaviors can be better accounted for by an Axis I or Axis II disorder, the first subcategory (mental disorder affecting a medical condition) should be used instead.

Stress-related Physiological Response Affecting a General Medical Condition

Examples of stress-related physiological responses affecting a medical condition include the precipitation by psychological stress of angina, cardiac arrhythmia, migraine, or attack of colitis in medically vulnerable individuals. In such cases, stress is not the cause of the illness or symptoms; the patient has a medical condition that etiologically accounts for the symptoms (e.g., coronary artery disease, migraine, or ulcerative colitis), and the stressor instead represents a precipitating or aggravating factor.

Other or Unspecified Psychological Factors Affecting a General Medical Condition

There are other psychological phenomena that may not fit within one of these subcategories. An interpersonal example is marital dysfunction. A cultural example is the extreme discomfort women from some cultures may experience being alone with a male physician, even while they are fully dressed. A religious example is a Jehovah's Witness who ambivalently refuses blood transfusion. These fall under the residual category of other or unspecified psychological factors affecting a medical condition.

Differential Diagnosis

As noted before, the close temporal association between psychiatric symptoms and a medical condition does not always reflect PFAMC. If the two are considered merely coincidental, then separate psychiatric and medical diagnoses should be made. In some cases of coincident psychiatric and medical illness, the mental symptoms are actually the result of the medical condition (i.e., the causality is in a direction opposite from that of PFAMC). When a medical condition is judged to be pathophysiologically causing the mental disorder (e.g., hypothyroidism causing depression), the correct diagnosis is the appropriate mental disorder due to a general medical condition (e.g., mood disorder due to hypothyroidism, with depressive features). In PFAMC, the psychological or behavioral factors are judged to precipitate or aggravate the medical condition.

Substance use disorders may adversely affect many medical conditions, and this can be described through PFAMC. However, in some patients, all of the psychiatric and medical symptoms are direct consequences of substance abuse, and it is usually parsimonious to use just the substance use disorder diagnosis. For example, a patient with delirium tremens after alcohol withdrawal would receive a diagnosis of alcohol withdrawal delirium, not PFAMC, but a patient with alcohol dependence who repeatedly missed hemodialysis treatments because of intoxication would receive diagnoses of alcohol dependence and PFAMC (mental disorder affecting end stage renal disease).

Patients with somatoform disorders (e.g., somatization disorder, hypochondriasis) present with physical complaints which may mimic a medical illness, but the somatic symptoms are actually accounted for by the psychiatric disorder. In principle, it might seem that somatoform disorders are easily distinguished from PFAMC, because PFAMC requires the presence of a diagnosable medical condition. The distinction in practice is sometimes difficult because the patient may have both a somatoform disorder and one or more medical disorders. For example, a patient with seizures regularly precipitated by emotional stress might have true epilepsy aggravated by stress (PFAMC), pseudoseizures (conversion disorder), or both.

Epidemiology and Comorbidity

Because this diagnosis describes a variety of possible interactions between the full range of psychiatric disorders (as well as symptoms and behaviors) on the one hand and the complete range of medical diseases on the other, it is impossible to estimate overall rates of prevalence or incidence. We can start, however, by noting how frequently medical and psychiatric disorders coexist. Psychiatric problems are common in medical patients, although the measured frequency varies, depending on the criteria and method of measurement used. A reasonable estimate is that 25 to 30% of medical outpatients and 40 to 50% of general medical inpatients have diagnosable psychiatric disorders (Table 63.1). Most common in medical outpatients are depression, anxiety and substance abuse; medical inpatients most often have cogni-

Table 63.1	Prevalence of Selected Psychiatric Disorders		
Disorder	Community	Primary Care Patients	Medical Inpatients
All psychiatric disorders	15–20%	25–30%	40–50%
Depression			
Depressive symptoms	10–15%	10–30%	20–35%
Major depressive disorder	2–4%	5–10%	5–25%
Anxiety			
Anxiety symptoms	10–20%	12–20%	20–30%
Panic disorder	1–2%	2–15%	—
Cognitive disorders			
	1%	—	15–20%
	5–10% (>65 yr)	—	30–50% (>65 yr)

Source: Levenson JL (1994) Common psychological reactions to medical illness and treatment, in *Clinical Psychiatry for Medical Students*, 2nd edn. (ed Stoudemire A). JB Lippincott, Philadelphia, pp. 580–609.

tive impairment (delirium, dementia), depression and substance abuse. Depression, both as a diagnosis and as a symptom, has been better studied in the medically ill than any other psychiatric syndrome. Major depressive disorder occurs in 18 to 25% of patients with serious coronary disease, in 25% of those with cancer, and at three times the normal rate in diabetic patients. Individuals presenting with symptoms of chronic fatigue have a 50 to 75% lifetime prevalence of major depression.

Nonpsychiatric physicians under diagnose and under treat psychiatric disorders in the medically ill. Medical disorders are also common in patients seen for mental health treatment, and mental health specialists often under recognize the presence and significance of coexisting medical disorders. Regardless of whether the patient has come seeking medical care or mental health care, medical and psychiatric problems are often both present. Such coincidence by itself is not sufficient for the diagnosis of PFAMC. In some cases, the illnesses may coexist with little effect on each other; in other cases, the effects of the medical illness on the psychiatric condition may be more important. The diagnosis of PFAMC in DSM-IV is reserved for patients in whom psychological factors adversely affect a medical condition in a specifiable way.

Course

Given the wide range of psychiatric disorders and psychological factors that may affect medical illness and the large number of different medical disorders that may be influenced, there are no general rules about the course of the PFAMC interaction. Psychological factors may have minor or major effects at a particular point or throughout the course of a medical illness. We do know in general that patients with medical disorders who also have significant psychological symptoms have poorer outcomes and higher medical care costs than those patients with the same medical disorders but without psychological distress. A number of studies now document that psychological or psychiatric problems (particularly cognitive disorder, depression and anxiety) in general medical inpatients are associated with significant increases in length of hospital stay. Psychosocial interventions have been able to improve outcomes in medical illness, sometimes with an attendant savings in health care costs.

The impact of psychological factors on the course and natural history of medical disorders is discussed further in this chapter in the context of specific diseases.

Treatment

Management of psychological factors affecting the patient's medical condition should be tailored both to the particular psychological factor of relevance and to the medical outcome of concern. Some general guidelines, however, can be helpful. The physician, whether in primary care or a specialty, should not ignore apparent psychiatric illness. Unfortunately, this occurs all too often because of discomfort, stigma, lack of training, or disinterest. Referring the patient to a mental health specialist for evaluation is certainly better than ignoring the psychological problem but should not be regarded as "disposing" of it, because the physician must still attend to its potential impact on the patient's medical illness. Similarly, psychiatrists and other mental health practitioners should not ignore coincident medical disease and should not assume that referral to a nonpsychiatric physician absolves them of all responsibility for the patient's medical problem.

Mental Disorder Affecting a Medical Condition

If the patient has a treatable Axis I disorder, treatment for it should be provided. Whereas this is obviously justified on the basis of providing relief from the Axis I disorder, psychiatric treatment is further supported by the myriad ways in which the psychiatric disorder may currently or in future adversely affect the medical illness. The same psychopharmacological and psychotherapeutic treatments used for Axis I mental disorders are normally appropriate when an affected medical condition is also present. However, even well-established psychiatric treatments supported by randomized controlled trials have seldom been validated in the medically ill, who are typically excluded from the controlled trials. Thus, psychiatric treatments may not always be directly generalizable to, and often must be modified for, the medically ill.

When prescribing psychiatric medications for patients with significant medical comorbidity, the psychiatrist should keep in mind potential adverse effects on impaired organ systems (e.g., anticholinergic exacerbation of postoperative ileus; tricyclic antidepressant causing completion of heart block), changes in pharmacokinetics (absorption, protein binding, metabolism and excretion) and drug–drug interactions. Psychotherapy may also require modification in patients with comorbid medical illness, including greater flexibility regarding the length and frequency of appointments, and deviations from standard therapeutic abstinence and neutrality. Psychotherapists treating patients with PFAMC should usually be much more active in communicating with other health care professionals caring for the patient (with the patient's consent) than is usually the case in psychotherapy.

If the patient has an Axis II personality disorder or other prominent personality or coping style, the psychiatrist should modify the patient's treatment accordingly, which is usually more easily accomplished than trying to change the patient's personality. For example, patients who tend to be paranoid or mistrustful should receive more careful explanations, particularly before invasive or anxiety-provoking procedures. With narcissistic patients, the psychiatrist should avoid relating in ways that may seem excessively paternalistic or authoritarian to the patient. With some dependent patients, it may be advisable to be more directive, without overdoing it and fostering excessive dependency.

Psychological Symptoms Affecting a General Medical Condition

In some instances, psychiatric symptoms not meeting the threshold for an Axis I diagnosis will respond positively to the same treatments used for the analogous Axis I psychiatric disorder, with appropriate modifications as noted before. There is not a great amount of treatment research on subsyndromal psychiatric symptoms, and even less in patients with comorbid medical illness, so this area of practice remains less evidence-based. Some psychiatric symptoms affecting a medical condition may be amenable to stress management and other behavioral techniques as well as appropriate reassurance.

Any intervention directed by the psychiatrist at a particular patient's psychological symptoms or behavior should be grounded in exploratory discussion with the patient. Interventions without such grounding tend to seem at best superficial and artificial and at worst are entirely off the mark. For example, if the psychiatrist wrongly presumes to know why a particular patient seems anxious without asking, the patient is likely to feel misunderstood. Facile, nonspecific reassurance can undermine the physician–patient relationship because the patient is likely to feel that the psychiatrist is out of touch with and not really interested in the patient's experience. It is especially important with depressed patients that psychiatrists avoid premature or unrealistic reassurance or an overly cheerful attitude; this tends to alienate depressed patients, who feel that their psychiatrist is insensitive and either does not understand or does not want to hear about their sadness. Physicians **should** provide specific and realistic reassurance, emphasize on a constructive treatment plan and mobilize the patient's support system.

Personality Traits or Coping Style Affecting a General Medical Condition

As with Axis II disorders affecting a medical condition, psychiatrists should be aware of the personality style's effects on the physician–patient relationship and modify management better to fit the patient. For example, with type A "time urgent" patients, psychiatrists may need to be more sensitive to issues of appointment scheduling and waiting times. Group therapy interventions can enhance active coping with serious medical illnesses like cancer, heart disease and renal failure but to date have usually been designed to be broadly generalizable rather than targeted to one particular trait or style (with the exception of type A behavior).

Another general guideline is not to attack or interfere with a patient's defensive style unless the defense is having an adverse impact on the medical illness or its management. Psychiatrists are particularly tempted to intervene when the defense is dramatic, breaks with reality, or makes the psychiatrist uncomfortable.

For example, denial is a defense mechanism that reduces anxiety and conflict by blocking conscious awareness of thoughts, feelings, or facts that an individual cannot face. Denial is common in the medically ill but varies in its timing, strength and adaptive value. Some patients are aware of what is wrong with them but consciously suppress this knowledge by avoiding thinking about or discussing it. Others cope with the threat of being overwhelmed by their illness by unconsciously repressing it and thereby remain unaware of their illness. Marked denial, in which the patient emphatically refuses to accept the existence or significance of obvious symptoms and signs of the disease, may be seen by the psychiatrist as an indication that the patient is "crazy" because the patient seems impervious to rational persuasion. In the absence of signs of another major psychiatric disorder (e.g., paranoid delusions), such denial is not often a sign of psychosis but rather represents a defense against overwhelming fear.

The adaptive value of denial may vary, depending on the nature or stage of illness. When a patient's denial does not preclude cooperation with treatment, the psychiatrist should leave it alone. The psychiatrist does have an ethical and professional obligation to ensure that the patient has been informed about the illness and treatment. After that, if the patient accepts treatment but persists with an irrationally optimistic outlook, the psychiatrist should respect the patient's need to use denial to cope. For some, the denial is fragile, and the psychiatrist must decide whether the defense should be supported and strengthened, or if the patient had better give up the denial to discuss fears directly and receive reassurance from the psychiatrist. The psychiatrist should not support denial by giving the patient false information, but rather encourage hope and optimism. When denial is extreme, patients may refuse vital treatment or threaten to leave against medical advice. Here, the psychiatrist must try to help reduce denial but not by directly assaulting the patient's defenses. Because such desperate denial of reality usually reflects intense underlying anxiety, trying to scare the patient into cooperation will intensify denial and the impulse to flight. A better strategy for the psychiatrist is to avoid directly challenging the patient's claims while simultaneously reinforcing concern for the patient and maximizing the patient's sense of control.

Clinical Vignette 1

Mr B is a 60-year-old married judge with coronary artery disease. He was referred for psychiatric evaluation by his cardiologist because he declined coronary artery bypass surgery despite strong and repeated recommendations for surgery by the cardiologist. The cardiologist perceived that the patient's resistance to surgery was not due to lack of information or understanding.

Mr B had no acute psychiatric symptoms, although he had several lifelong phobias including fear of cats, fear of being buried alive and claustrophobia (recent episodes in the hospital elevator and during magnetic resonance imaging). His only previous psychiatric contact was some marital therapy 20 years earlier. His coronary artery disease was severe, with two myocardial infarctions and recurrent malignant arrhythmias. He continued to have recurrent angina despite maximal medical management; his pain occurred mainly at night as "a predictable consequence of pushing too hard at work" (he typically worked 12-hour days). He had also had a stroke 3 months ago, from which he had made a complete recovery with no sequelae. Twenty years earlier, he had surgery for a renal stone that was complicated postoperatively with five pulmonary emboli. He said that he has had "eight near-death experiences" amidst his various illnesses.

Mr B was eager to discuss his reluctance to have coronary bypass surgery. He had not decided against the surgery but had been unable to reach a decision. He brought to the appointment with the psychiatrist a two-page list of arguments for and against surgery and other variables that could influence the decision and outcome. He was aware that he was approaching the question of surgery with the same style of carefully balanced consideration of all sides of an issue that he prided himself on in his occupation as a judge. He worked longer days than his colleagues because he believed it took more time to make fair, proper and legally correct decisions. His analysis of the pros and cons of surgery, as well as intervening factors affecting and affected by the decision, appeared to the psychiatrist to be well informed, accurate, flexible and appropriate. There was no evidence of rigidity in his thinking, premature closure, or distorted perceptions. Whereas the thought processes were logical, they had not enabled him to reach a decision, despite extensive discussions with the cardiologist over a period of months. He was aware that this was another decision in his life that was taking much longer than average, but he thought it could not be resolved any other way.

This case represents an example of personality trait or coping style affecting a general medical condition. His obsessional style was largely adaptive in his chosen occupation, although it reduced his efficiency. Now confronted with a major health care decision, and mindful of major complications he had suffered after surgery in the past, the need to weigh all sides of an issue had paralyzed his decision-making. The presence of phobias in his history raised the possibility of these too affecting his decision-making, but he denied feeling fearful of the surgery, anesthesia, intubation and the like. The anxiety he was experiencing was entirely focused around making the right decision.

Maladaptive Health Behavior Affecting a General Medical Condition

This is an area of research with many promising approaches. To achieve smoking cessation, bupropion, nicotine replacement, behavioral therapies and other pharmacological strategies all warrant consideration. Behavioral strategies are also useful in promoting better dietary practices, sleep hygiene, safe sex and exercise. For some patients, change can be achieved efficiently through support groups, whereas others change more effectively through a one-to-one relationship with a health care professional.

Stress-related Physiological Response Affecting a Medical Condition

Biofeedback, relaxation techniques, hypnosis and other stress management interventions have been helpful in reducing stress-induced exacerbations of medical illness including cardiac, gastrointestinal, headache and other symptoms. Pharmacological interventions have also been useful (e.g., the widespread practice of prescribing benzodiazepines during acute myocardial infarction to prevent stress-induced increase in myocardial work).

Psychological Factors in Specific Medical Disorders

In the remainder of this chapter, the effects of psychological factors on selected medical disorders are reviewed. The primary focus is on those effects for which there is reasonable evidence from controlled studies. Space considerations preclude inclusion of all valuable studies and all medical disorders.

Most of the early research suffers from serious methodological flaws, including use of small biased samples, limited or no statistical analysis, poor (if any) controls and retrospective designs subject to recall and other biases. This early work generated excitement and interest in psychosomatic medicine but also produced ideas that in retrospect were intellectually appealing but erroneous and simplistic regarding the special designation of certain diseases as psychosomatic.

Later research has shown improvements in methodology, but problems in design and interpretation continue. Several studies that seem to show significant effects of psychological factors on medical disease are inconclusive because of nonequivalence in groups at baseline either in medical disease severity or in treatments received (many studies do not even monitor this possibility). Some studies fail to attend to important potential confounding factors such as smoking or diet. A number of studies measure too many psychological variables and then overly emphasize the few "discovered" positive associations in the published results. Failure to standardize measures of initial psychological factors and measures of medical outcome has also been frequent. Despite these and other critiques, a large and growing body of disease-specific research is illuminating the full range of PFAMC.

Psychological Factors in Oncology

Many health professionals and lay people believe that psychological factors play a major role in cancer onset and progression. The media have promoted popular ideas of overcoming cancer through "mind over body". Enthusiasm for these optimistic theories and practices should be tempered by the recognition that scientific evidence clarifying the relationship between psychological factors and cancer lags far behind. Nevertheless, there is an exciting frontier of exploration of immune and endocrine mechanisms that may provide a pathophysiological basis for some PFAMC in cancer. In this section, aspects of PFAMC in oncology that have received support in the research literature are reviewed.

Mental Disorders and Psychological Symptoms Affecting Cancer

The most active area of study has been the linking of affective states, particularly depression (as a symptom or as a disorder), with the onset and course of cancer. A meta-analysis of studies relating depression to later cancer development found a small statistically significant but clinically insignificant association (McGee et al., 1994). The interpretation of epidemiologic studies is complex with many methodological problems.

Besides epidemiologic studies, other research has focused on the impact of affective states on outcome in cancer patients. Emotional distress may predict lower survival with lung cancer as may anger in metastatic melanoma patients. Other studies have found positive, negative, or mixed associations between depression and mortality in cancer patients. Besides survival, depression in cancer patients may result in poorer pain control, poorer compliance and less desire for life-sustaining therapy. Neither cancer onset nor progression have been clearly shown to be influenced by bereavement.

Personality Traits or Coping Style Affecting Cancer

A large body of literature has described cancer patients' degree of emotional expressiveness and its purported effect on prognosis. Epidemiological studies, however, have not supported a relationship between emotional suppression and cancer occurrence or mortality.

Other Psychological Factors in Cancer

An enormous literature documents the adverse effects of maladaptive health behaviors as risk factors for the development of various cancers, especially smoking but also excessive alcohol use, unsafe sex and dietary practices. Relatively less research has examined the effects of interpersonal variables on cancer, but there is some evidence that the quality of relationships may affect cancer onset and its course. Social relations and social support and their effects on cancer patients (as with other diseases) are complex phenomena and may vary with cancer site and extent of disease.

A number of human studies have shown an increased frequency of stressful life events preceding the onset of cervical, pancreatic, gastric, lung, colorectal and breast cancer. Many other studies have failed to find any association between preceding stressful life events and cancer onset, relapse, or progression.

Psychosocial Intervention and Cancer Outcome

A number of studies have shown improvement in the quality of life in cancer patients receiving group therapy including improved mood and vigor, decreased pain and better. The possibility that cancer patients receiving psychotherapy might have increased survival time as well as improved quality of life has generated intense study with more evidence showing improvement in pain control and mood than for increased survival.

Psychological Factors in Cardiology

Coronary Disease

One of the most studied examples of PFAMC is the type A behavior pattern and its relationship to coronary artery disease. Type A is a complex set of traits including impatience, hostility, intense achievement drive and time urgency, among others. However, the relationship between type A behavior pattern and coronary disease has come under serious question. Later epidemiological studies have not strongly supported type A behavior pattern as a coronary risk factor, and most angiographic studies have failed to find an association between type A behavior and the extent of coronary artery disease. The possibility that type A behavior pattern is nevertheless an important risk factor should be kept in mind, considering that the evidence for other risk factors (e.g., exercise or cholesterol) has often been ambiguous. Whereas global type A behavior ratings are probably not reliable predictors of coronary artery disease outcome, the component behavior of hostility may be although here too there are conflicted studies. Only one large randomized study has been reported, in which men were assigned after myocardial infarction to receive cardiac group counseling with or without type A counseling. The coronary artery disease recurrence rate was 7.2% in the group that received type A behavior counseling and 13% in the control subjects, with no difference in mortality (Friedman et al., 1986).

Although it has received less media attention than type A, the evidence that depression is a risk factor affecting both the onset and course of coronary artery disease is stronger than that for type A. The weighting of depression as an independent risk factor in coronary artery disease has had to adjust for its interrelationships with other risk factors, especially smoking. Depression in coronary artery disease is associated with increased morbidity and mortality, which cannot be accounted for by other variables including severity of cardiac disease. Frasure-Smith and coworkers (1993) reported a fourfold increase in mortality 6 months after myocardial infarction in patients with major depression compared with those without depression. In a large epidemiologic study, major depression tripled the relative risk of cardiac mortality in those without heart disease, and quadrupled it in those who did have heart disease (Penninx et al., 2001). Depression is also associated with an increased risk for serious arrhythmia. The severity of depressive symptoms has more impact on disability than does the number of stenosed coronary arteries. Depression also reduces the return to work in patients with coronary artery disease. A recent randomized trial of 1834 post-MI subjects who were categorized as depressed and/or socially isolated were treated with antidepressant medication (Taylor et al., 2005). Subjects taking SSRIs were at lower risk of death and recurrent MI compared with untreated subjects.

Although the mechanisms by which depression increases morbidity and mortality in coronary artery disease has not been firmly established, evidence is mounting regarding depression's adverse effects on heart rate variability, autonomic imbalance and arrhythmia, and platelet activation. In coronary artery disease, depression also reduces functional capacity, amplifies somatic symptoms (especially pain), and reduces motivation and compliance with medication, lifestyle change and cardiac rehabilitation

One specific mechanism by which psychological factors can affect coronary artery disease (CAD) has been demonstrated experimentally. Silent myocardial ischemia (ischemic changes on the electrocardiogram without symptoms of angina) can be precipitated by acute mental stress. Those who experience it are twice as likely to have major cardiac events compared with those who do not. Silent ischemia may be partly a consequence of cognitive or defensive traits such as denial, hyposensitivity to somatic sensation, or systematic misperception of angina. Psychological stress also changes the balance between procoagulation and fibrinolysis. Psychological factors may also affect outcome in CAD via differences in health care received. After myocardial infarction, patients with mental disorders are less likely to undergo cardiac catheterization and coronary revascularization than those without mental disorder.

Although the diagnosis and treatment of anxiety in patients with cardiac symptoms have received much attention, there has been less examination of anxiety as a risk factor affecting CAD. Increases in myocardial infarction and/or sudden death have been documented in epidemiologic studies of populations undergoing missile attacks, earthquakes and other disasters. A cohort study of 34 000 initially healthy men showed that phobic anxiety predicted deaths from CAD, although not nonfatal myocardial infarctions (MI) (Kawachi et al., 1994). Anxiety following MI may lead to more frequent readmission for unstable angina and more MI recurrences as well as higher mortality. Anxiety's adverse effects on CAD outcome may occur via effects on heart rate variability, QT prolongation, or other autonomically-mediated phenomena, like the stress-induced silent ischemia described above.

Denial is another common and significant psychological factor in patients with coronary disease. Denial may prevent individuals from acknowledging acute cardiac symptoms and promptly seeking medical care. The length of delay between the onset of symptoms of a myocardial infarction and hospitalization is a powerful predictor of morbidity and mortality, so denial at the onset of symptoms has an adverse impact on acute coronary disease. In contrast, denial **during** hospitalization may have adaptive value, perhaps even reducing morbidity and mortality.

There are other psychological factors deserving of study. Women with severe marital stress have triple the risk of recurrent coronary events than those without marital stress. Many studies have also examined maladaptive health behaviors as risk factors in coronary disease, with the effects of smoking better established than those of sedentary lifestyle, obesity, or specific diet. The effects of psychopathology and of smoking on heart disease are easily confounded, as persons with psychiatric disorders are overall twice as likely to smoke as others, with the increased risk found with all the major anxiety, mood and psychotic disorders.

Arrhythmias

There is evidence that psychological stressors can also play an important role in precipitating serious ventricular arrhythmias. Sudden cardiac death after psychological distress has been reported anecdotally for a long time but is difficult to study scientifically. A systematic review of published cases of ventricular fibrillation in patients without known cardiac disease could identify preceding psychological distress in 22% (Viskin and Belhassen, 1990). A recent review of 96 published studies investigating psychosocial risk factors for arrhythmia found that 92% were positive (Hemingway et al., 2001). Whether type A personality traits predict sudden cardiac death after myocardial infarction remains controversial.

Congestive Heart Failure

Depression is especially common in patients with congestive heart failure. In patients hospitalized for congestive heart failure, major depression is independently associated with increased mortality and readmission 3 and 12 months later.

Hypertension

The stress-related physiological response subcategory of PFAMC is particularly relevant to hypertension. There are some data suggesting that blood pressure reactivity to stress is a risk factor for the development of hypertension and may influence progression of disease as well. Many studies have examined relationships between personality, coping style, blood pressure reactivity and hypertension, but conflicting results and methodological limitations have precluded any consensus conclusions. Findings regarding the effects of stress, anger, hostility, or anxiety on blood pressure in normotensive individuals are not necessarily relevant to clinical hypertension. A high level of anxiety at baseline evaluation independently predicted twice the risk for development of hypertension in middle-aged men but not in women in one study, but in another study by the same investigators, anxiety did predict hypertension in women (Markovitz et al., 1991). Some epidemiologic studies have found depression and/or anxiety symptoms predictive of later development of hypertension even after controlling for confounding factors. Several measures of occupational stress appear to be independent risk factors for hypertension in the general population. Some of the apparent association between psychological distress and hypertension is chiefly attributable to health risk behaviors (obesity, smoking, alcohol and sedentary lifestyle).

Studies of psychological treatments for hypertension (mainly biofeedback and relaxation techniques) have demonstrated the possibility of modest but clinically significant sustained reduction in blood pressure but less effectively than with drug therapy. The major limiting factor in using behavioral treatments for hypertension is compliance, because the treatments must be self-administered indefinitely. Behavioral therapies may be helpful as an adjunctive treatment in patients receiving antihypertensive drugs; psychological treatment should seldom be given as the sole treatment for hypertension.

Psychological Factors in Endocrinology

Diabetes Mellitus

Despite some of the early psychosomatic literature, there is no unique diabetic personality, but physicians who take care of diabetic patients attest to a close interrelationship between psychological factors and glucose control. There is conflicting evidence whether psychological factors directly affect the onset of diabetes. That psychological stress can adversely affect glucose control in diabetics seems expectable because the hormones of the stress response are part of the counterregulatory response to insulin. A number of studies have shown that glycemic control is poorer in those diabetic patients who have more perceived stress. As assessed by hemoglobin A1c, metabolic control was poorer in depressed children and in adult depressed type 1 but not type 2 diabetics. A recent meta-analysis of 24 studies concluded that depression consistently is associated with a small-to-moderate increase in hyperglycemia in both type 1 and type 2 diabetes (Lustman et al., 2000). Depression is associated with more diabetic complications. Most such research has been retrospective or cross-sectional, leaving it unclear which came first – poor metabolic control and complications or the psychological factor – and what is the relationship between them.

When psychiatric illness antedates and adversely affects the course of diabetes, it may be mediated by noncompliance (diet, medication, activity, visits to the physician, self-care) (Ciechanowski et al., 2000) or by neurohumoral mechanisms. The adverse effects in diabetic control cannot all be attributed to noncompliance. Psychological stress administered under laboratory conditions can impair glucose control in both insulin-dependent and noninsulin-dependent diabetes. In insulin-dependent diabetes, this effect appears to be mediated by mental stress-induced insulin resistance.

Randomized controlled trials have demonstrated improvements in glucose control in diabetics receiving psychological interventions. Antidepressants are effective in the treatment of depression in diabetics, but can cause increases or decreases in blood glucose by themselves. Deterioration in glucose control in schizophrenic diabetics may be due to some of the newer antipsychotic drugs, but diabetes was a major problem for schizophrenics before their advent, presumably because of obesity (a side effect of almost every antipsychotic), unhealthy diet and poorer health care. Optimal management of diabetes requires a degree of organization very difficult for most patients with schizophrenia.

Thyroid Disease

It is well established that too little or too much thyroid hormone can result in disturbances in mood and activity. In the other direction, the effects of emotion and stress on thyroid function, although long a focus of interest, are less well established. Recent studies have supported stressful life events as a risk factor for Graves' disease. Psychological stress may also be a result of less optimal control of hyperthyroidism.

Whereas there has been little well-substantiated evidence of the impact of psychological factors on thyroid disease, alterations in thyroid function or its hypothalamic–pituitary control have been demonstrated in relation to affective disorders, schizophrenia and post traumatic stress disorder. Depression has been most studied, revealing a variety of thyroid abnormalities, most frequently a relative increase in thyroxine without changes in the activated (triiodothyronine) and inactive (reverse triiodothyronine) forms and a blunting of the thyroid-stimulating hormone response to thyrotropin-releasing hormone. There is no agreement regarding the relationship between these endocrine changes and depressive pathophysiological processes, and it remains unknown whether depression modifies endocrine measures in clinical thyroid disease.

Psychological Factors in Pulmonary Disease

Although asthma was once regarded as a classic psychosomatic disorder, it is currently viewed as a primary respiratory disease with varying immunological and autonomic pathophysiological changes. Many physicians still believe that psychological factors play an important role in the precipitation and aggravation of asthma, particularly anxiety. One must remember, however, that respiratory distress itself causes a wide array of anxiety symptoms (panic attacks, generalized and anticipatory anxiety, phobic avoidance), and most of the drugs used to treat asthma have anxiety as a potential side effect. Brittle asthmatic patients, like brittle diabetic patients, are more likely to have current or past psychiatric disorder (particularly anxiety disorders) than are other asthmatic individuals, but which came first is not established. There is no typical personality type susceptible to development of asthma. Studies have shown that anxiety and depression are associated in asthmatic patients with more respiratory symptom complaints but no differences in objective measures of respiratory function. However, psychological factors and psychosocial problems in hospitalized asthmatics were a more powerful predictor of which ones required intubation than any other examined variable (e.g., smoking, infection, prior hospitalization, etc.) (Le Son and Gershwin, 1996). Psychological morbidity is associated with high levels of denial and delays in seeking medical care, which may be life-threatening in severe asthma as well as less medication adherence and consequently poorer control of the condition. Not surprisingly then psychopathology in severe asthmatics is associated with increased health care utilization including hospitalizations, and outpatient and emergency room visits, independent of asthma severity.

Similar problems exist in interpreting relationships between anxiety or depression and other chronic obstructive pulmonary diseases (COPD) (chronic bronchitis, emphysema). Depression and anxiety are common in COPD though this partly reflects their increased prevalence in past or current smokers. As in asthma, psychological distress in COPD amplifies dyspnea without usually causing changes in objective pulmonary functions. Depression and anxiety do lead to lower exercise tolerance, noncompliance with treatment, and increased disability in COPD. Anxious COPD patients can improve their exercise tolerance through cognitive–behavioral therapy and pulmonary rehabilitation. Smoking is a well-established maladaptive health behavior causing and exacerbating chronic obstructive pulmonary disease, and its elimination is the most beneficial intervention available.

Psychological Factors in Rheumatoid Arthritis

There is no particular personality type susceptible to development of RA and earlier research suggesting that stressful events play a role in the development or onset of RA has not been supported by more recent studies. Psychological factors and disease manifestations account for comparable proportions of disability. Psychological morbidity in RA results in more pain, poorer quality of life, more joint surgery, lower compliance and increased use of health care resources.

Depression has been the most frequently studied psychological disturbance in RA; depression is very common, as in other chronic medical conditions. Depression appears to adversely affect outcome in rheumatoid arthritis, aggravating chronic pain, increasing health care use and increasing social isolation.

Randomized controlled trials of antidepressants in depressed RA patients demonstrate improvements in pain, morning stiffness and disability in addition to depression.

There is a consensus among investigators that passive, avoidant, emotion-laden coping strategies (e.g., wish-fulfilling fantasy, self-blame) are associated with poorer adjustment to illness in RA compared with active, problem-focused coping (e.g., information seeking, cognitive restructuring). Rheumatoid arthritis patients with high helplessness are more likely to receive psychotropic, analgesic and anti-inflammatory drugs and to be less adherent with treatment than those with low helplessness. Patients with RA may be more vulnerable to stress-induced increases in immune and endocrine function. A randomized controlled trial of cognitive–behavioral therapy as an adjunct to standard treatment in recently diagnosed patients with rheumatoid arthritis showed it efficacious in reducing both psychological and physical morbidity (Sharpe *et al.*, 2001).

Psychological Factors in Neurology

Depression is frequent after stroke, particularly in the acute phase during hospitalization and the first few weeks after stroke. The presence of depression is associated with poorer outcome, including higher later mortality and functional status is improved with treatment of depression after stroke. A negative attitude after stroke (i.e., feeling there is nothing one can do to help oneself) is associated with decreased survival. Research has focused on depression as a complication of stroke but there is also evidence that depression and other psychological factors constitute risks for stroke, consistent with widespread lay and folk beliefs regarding stress and stroke. There is preliminary evidence that anger and hostility may pose a risk for carotid atherosclerosis just as it may for coronary disease. Recent studies have found depressive symptoms increase the risk of stroke in older adults. As with many other major medical illnesses, stroke patients with extensive social support have better functional outcomes than those who do not.

Depression is common in Parkinson's disease, may antedate the development of motor symptoms and is associated with cognitive dysfunction. Physicians observe that depression and other psychological factors interact to affect the course and outcome of Parkinson's disease, but there has been little formal study of such relationships. Depression is also common and erodes quality of life in multiple sclerosis (MS) and in epilepsy. The study of depression as an independent risk factor affecting the onset or course of neurological diseases is challenging because depression may also be consequence of the disease, a psychological reaction to the illness, or a complication of pharmacotherapy. In MS depression may increase and its treatment decrease production of proinflammatory cytokines. Depression is especially difficult to study in MS because of its uncertain relationship to the MS-fatigue syndrome.

Patients with chronic migraine headaches have often been described as having a "typical" personality characterized as conscientious, perfectionistic, ambitious, rigid, tense and resentful, but controlled studies have not supported any consistent conclusion. Specific personality traits in migraine appear more likely to be a consequence rather than a cause of suffering from recurrent headaches. Migraine and depression are highly comorbid. But there is no relationship between headache frequency and the severity of psychological distress or personality abnormality. Thus, the relationship between psychological factors and migraine remains to be worked out.

Psychological Factors in End-stage Renal Disease

Studies of the influence of psychological factors upon the course of end-stage renal disease (ESRD) have nearly all focused on depression or noncompliance. There has been essentially no investigation of psychological factors in chronic renal failure before end stage. Depression is associated with smoking, alcoholism and other forms of substance abuse that are highly prevalent in ESRD patients. It is clear that depression predicts higher mortality.

Compliance is a complex, multidimensional array of behaviors, and its relationship with health outcomes in dialysis patients is difficult to study. Thus, whereas effects of noncompliance on dialysis patients' outcomes are well recognized by physicians, they have not been adequately characterized empirically. Nevertheless, the widespread belief among physicians and nurses that noncompliance results in worse outcomes including higher mortality in ESRD is supported by a large multicenter study (Leggat *et al.*, 1998). The chronic overuse of nonsteroidal anti-inflammatory agents and analgesics is a maladaptive health behavior recognized as a fairly common contributing cause of chronic renal insufficiency.

Psychological Factors in Gastroenterology

Inflammatory Bowel Disease

Ulcerative colitis is another disorder that was described in the early literature as a psychosomatic disease, but no specific psychogenic factor contributing to the development of ulcerative colitis or Crohn's disease has ever been substantiated. As with other chronic medical diseases, patients with more psychological distress tend to be those with more severe physical disease and poorer functional capacity, but the causal relationships are not clear. Psychological stress does appear to aggravate both symptom complaints and mucosal disease activity in ulcerative colitis. Disability and distress in patients with inflammatory bowel disease are increased by the presence of a concurrent psychiatric disorder. In fact, depression is a better predictor of subjective impairment in inflammatory bowel disease than is inflammatory activity. Psychotherapy has the potential to improve outcomes in inflammatory bowel disease, as suggested by controlled trials.

Peptic Ulcer Disease

The central role of the bacterium *Helicobacter pylori* in the etiology of peptic ulcer disease (PUD) has been clearly established. Many physicians have consequently discarded the longstanding belief that stress causes PUD, and concluded that PUD is an infectious disease, except when attributable to nonsteroidal anti-inflammatory drugs (NSAIDS). Nevertheless, psychological factors appear to be a significant part of the explanation for why only a fraction of those colonized by *H. pylori* or taking NSAIDS develop ulcers. Psychological stress is an independent risk factor for the development and recurrence of duodenal ulcer. The frequency of peptic ulcer increases following catastrophic stressful events, including bombardment, earthquake, economic crisis, or being a prisoner of war or "boat people" refugee. Overall, psychosocial factors contribute between 30 and 65% of peptic ulcers (Levenstein, 2000), and are most likely to be present in patients with duodenal ulcers who do not have conventional medical risk factors (*H. pylori*, NSAIDS). Occupational stress, family conflicts, depression, maladjustment and hostility also are prospectively associated with PUD.

Psychological factors appear to influence PUD through both health risk behaviors (smoking, alcohol abuse, overuse of NSAIDS, poor diet, poor sleep) and psychophysiologic mechanisms (pepsinogen and acid secretion, altered blood flow, impairment of mucosal defenses, and slowing of healing related to the action of cortisol) (Levenstein, 2000).

Irritable Bowel Syndrome

Irritable bowel syndrome (IBS) is a heterogeneous condition with a high frequency of comorbid anxiety especially panic attacks, depression and somatization. Whereas patients with IBS are psychologically more distressed than normal subjects, they do not have a common profile of psychological symptoms or personality traits. Patients with IBS are more likely to have a history of childhood sexual abuse than are those with other gastrointestinal disorders in studies of patients seeking care at tertiary referral centers. In fact, almost all psychological characteristics and psychopathology thought to be more common in IBS are differentially increased only in those who seek medical care for their symptoms.

Both IBS patients and their physicians observe that their gastrointestinal symptoms seem aggravated by stress, but there is no clear evidence that stress causes a different gastrointestinal smooth muscle response than in control subjects. Instead, psychological factors' effects on IBS appear predominantly on perception of pain and other somatic symptoms, and on health care seeking behaviors. After an acute episode of infectious gastroenteritis, individuals with more life stress, and who were more hypochondriacal, were the ones most likely to go on to develop IBS, without any differences in intestinal physiology (Gwee *et al.*, 1999).

Psychological Factors in Dermatology

Dermatologists routinely observe the effect of psychological factors, especially anxiety, in the aggravation of a wide variety of dermatological conditions. There are few systematic studies, and perhaps the most important relationships are not uniquely related to particular dermatological disorders. Both anxiety and depression appear to worsen pruritus (itching). So-called neurotic excoriation complicates many dermatological disorders and is aggravated by anxiety, depression and other behavioral factors. That so many skin diseases appear to be precipitated or exacerbated by psychological stress also suggests a nonspecific impairment of cutaneous function. There is now evidence in both animals and humans that stress negatively affects skin's function as a permeability barrier.

Dermatologists clinically observe important relationships between psychological factors and urticaria, angioedema, atopic dermatitis, hyperhidrosis, acne and psoriasis, but controlled studies are lacking. Excessive sun exposure is a maladaptive health behavior contributing to skin cancer and various other dermatological conditions.

Psychological Factors Affecting Infectious Diseases

HIV infection is the most destructive example of unsafe sexual practices, as a maladaptive health behavior, contributing to development and transmission of an infectious medical condition. Once contracted, HIV infection appeared to be a likely candidate for important effects of psychological factors, because of the work demonstrating changes in normal immune function after stress, bereavement and depression. The effects of stress and depression on disease progression, immune function and mortality in HIV infection have been an active field of investigation, with varying conclusions. There is less doubt that anxiety worsens symptoms and functioning in HIV patients. No research has demonstrated that depression predicts the onset of somatic symptoms in HIV infection, acquired immunodeficiency syndrome, or death.

Psychological factors influence other infectious diseases as well, including the common cold, pneumonia, genital herpes and recurrent urinary tract infections. A number of studies have convincingly shown that psychological stress suppresses the secondary (but not primary) antibody response to immunization.

Psychological Factors in Obstetrics

While much more attention has been paid to postpartum depression, antepartum depression also adversely affects pregnancy outcome. Both antepartum anxiety and depression have been associated with growth retardation and premature birth, resulting in lower birth weights, but potential confounding factors have often not been adequately controlled for. Whether depression and other psychological dysfunction cause poorer obstetric outcomes through poor nutrition, substance abuse (including tobacco), poor adherence or no prenatal care, and/or physiological (hormonal, vascular) effects require further investigation.

Psychological Factors in Infertility

Psychological factors are likely to affect fertility because frequency and timing of sexual intercourse are important determinants of fertility. Nonconsummation, avoidance of intercourse, vaginismus and psychogenic amenorrhea are attributable to psychological origins. Psychogenic causes do not account for most male impotence but may play a secondary role in many cases.

Whereas some prospective data support psychological factors influencing fertility in the general population, psychological factors appear less potent in predicting pregnancy outcome in couples receiving treatment for infertility. In general, measures of stress, but not of psychopathology, have been associated with infertility. This is a particularly complex subject for study because it involves potential psychological factors in both members of the couple and interactions between them as well as their effects on sexual behavior and fertility. Most psychological distress seen in infertile couples is a result of, rather than a cause of, infertility.

Comparison of DSM-IV/ICD-10 Diagnostic Criteria

Although the corresponding ICD-10 category ("Psychological and behavioural factors associated with disorders or diseases classified elsewhere") does not have specified diagnostic criteria, it is defined in essentially the same way as DSM-IV-TR.

References

Ciechanowski PS, Katon WJ and Russo JE (2000) Depression and diabetes: Impact of depressive symptoms on adherence, function, and costs. *Arch Intern Med* 160, 3278–3285.

DiMatteo MR, Lepper HS and Croghan TW (2000) Depression is a risk factor for noncompliance with medical treatment: Meta-analysis of the effects of anxiety and depression on patient adherence. *Arch Intern Med* 160, 2101–2107.

Druss BG, Bradford WD, Rosenheck RA *et al.* (2001a) Quality of medical care and excess mortality in older patients with mental disorders. *Arch Gen Psychiatr* 58, 565–572.

Druss BG, Rohrbaugh RM, Levinson CM *et al.* (2001b) Integrated medical care for patients with serious psychiatric illness. *Arch Gen Psychiatr* 58, 861–868.

Frasure-Smith N, Lesperance F and Talajic M (1993) Depression following myocardial infarction: Impact on 6-month survival. *JAMA* 270, 1819–1825.

Friedman M, Thoresen CE, Gill JJ *et al.* (1986) Alteration of type A behavior and its effect on cardiac recurrences in postmyocardial infarction patients: Summary results of the Recurrent Coronary Prevention Project. *Am Heart J* 112, 653–665.

Gwee KA, Leong YL, Graham C *et al.* (1999) The role of psychological and biological factors in postinfective gut dysfunction. *Gut* 44, 400–406.

Hemingway H, Malik M and Marmot M (2001) Social and psychosocial influences on sudden cardiac death, ventricular arrhythmia and cardiac autonomic function. *Eur Heart J* 22, 1082–1101.

Herran A, Amado JA, Garcia-Unzueta MT *et al.* (2000) Increased bone remodeling in first-episode major depressive disorder. *Psychosom Med* 62, 779–782.

Kawachi I, Colditz GA, Acherio A *et al.* (1994) Prospective study of phobic anxiety and risk of coronary heart disease in men. *Circulation* 89, 1992–1997.

Leggat JE Jr, Orzol SM, Hulbert-Shearin TE *et al.* (1998) Noncompliance in hemodialysis: Predictors and survival analysis. *Am J Kidney Dis* 32, 139–145.

Le Son S and Gershwin ME (1996) Risk factors for asthmatic patients requiring intubation. III. Observations in young adults. *J Asthma* 33, 27–35.

Levenson JL (1994) Common psychological reactions to medical illness and treatment, in *Clinical Psychiatry for Medical Students*, 2nd edn. (ed Stoudemire A). JB Lippincott, Philadelphia, pp. 580–609.

Levenstein S (2000) The very model of a modern etiology: A biopsychosocial view of peptic ulcer. *Psychosom Med* 62, 176–185.

Lustman PJ, Anderson RJ, Freedland KE *et al.* (2000) Depression and poor glycemic control: A meta-analytic review of the literature. *Diabet Care* 23, 934–942.

Markovitz JH, Matthews KA, Wing RR, *et al.* (1991) Psychological biological, and health behavior predictors of blood pressure changes in middle-aged women. *J Hypertens* 7, 399–406.

McGee R, Williams S and Elwood M (1994) Depression and the development of cancer: A meta-analysis. *Soc Sci Med* 38, 187–192.

Penninx BW, Beekman AT, Honig A *et al.* (2001) Depression and cardiac mortality: Results from community-based longitudinal study. *Arch Gen Psychiatr* 58, 221–227.

Sharpe K, Sensky T, Timberlake N *et al.* (2001) A blind, randomized, controlled trial of cognitive–behavioral intervention for patients with recent onset rheumatoid arthritis: Preventing psychological and physical morbidity. *Pain* 89, 275–283.

Taylor CB, Youngbood ME, Catellier D *et al.* (2005) Effects of antidepressant medication on morbidity and mortality in depressed patients after myocardial infarction. *Arch Gen Psychiatry* 62, 792–798.

Viskin S and Belhassen B (1990) Idiopathic ventricular fibrillation. *Am Heart J* 120, 661–671.

64 Medication-induced Movement Disorders

Introduction

Perhaps the most uncomfortable side effects from psychotropic medications (especially antipsychotics or neuroleptics) are the acute and chronic movement disorders. Any psychiatrist in clinical practice has witnessed the intense distress that medication-induced movement disorders may bring to patients. Perhaps most disturbing is that unlike other medications, antipsychotics can produce "tardive" or late-occurring movement disorders that may be persistent or even irreversible. Patients in whom movement disorders develop may have more than subjective distress; they may suffer psychosocial embarrassment that makes them avoid being seen in public, and they may even suffer occupational impairment in severe cases. The responsibility this places on the prescribing psychiatrist is significant. Careful and reasoned thought must go into the analysis of whether the benefit of treatment with a medication exceeds the risk to the patient. This includes adequately explaining and obtaining informed consent from patients.

When a psychiatrist prescribes a medication that has the potential to induce a movement disorder, the physician–patient relationship is of paramount importance. Patients who require these medications are sometimes not amenable to trusting relationships (i.e., the paranoid patient). Working with a patient who has a psychotic illness requires that the psychiatrist establish a strong therapeutic bond with the patient.

Historical Background

Approximately 5 years after chlorpromazine was observed to be effective for psychotic disorders, orobuccal dyskinesias after prolonged exposure to chlorpromazine were noted. This condition lasted nearly 3 months after the medication was stopped. This was in marked contrast to the parkinsonism-like EPS that had been previously described to reverse on discontinuation of antipsychotics. The term **tardive dyskinesia** (TD) was first used in the 1960s to describe this condition. The number of reports grew rapidly in a period of years, and many of the cases were reported to be irreversible.

Classification

There are different types of movement disorders that may result from treatment with psychotropic (especially neuroleptic) medications. They can generally be divided into those that occur acutely or subacutely and those that occur late in treatment (tardive). For the purpose of this discussion, we group the movement disorders into the relatively acute neuroleptic-induced disorders (acute dystonia,

parkinsonism, and akathisia) neuroleptic-induced TD and neuroleptic malignant syndrome (NMS). We also devote a section to the discussion of medication-induced postural tremor that predominantly focuses on lithium-induced tremor. This covers the major diagnostic groupings contained within the *Diagnostic and Statistical Manual of Mental Disorders*, Fourth Edition, Text Revision (DSM-IV-TR) under the general title medication-induced movement disorders.

A time line for the emergence of the neuroleptic-induced movement disorders is provided in Table 64.1.

Informed Consent and Medicolegal Issues

In general, the more a patient is able to understand the nature of his or her illness and the reason that a particular medication is being prescribed, the more likely he or she is to be adherent. When the psychiatrist does not devote adequate time to informing and instructing the patient, the result may be poor trust, poor communication and possible legal difficulties for everyone involved. Unless declared incompetent by a court of law, a patient is considered to be legally competent to consent to or refuse psychotropic medications. The only exception to this rule is when an emergency situation exists and a patient must be medicated to prevent harm to self or others. The psychiatrist must provide information to the patient or the patient's decision-maker about the nature and purpose of the medication, its risks and benefits, alternatives to the proposed treatment, and prognosis without treatment. Obtaining a written informed consent is one way of documenting the consent process. Another way is noting in the chart a summary of the discussion with a patient (or caregiver) about the consent to neuroleptic treatment.

Although the antipsychotics can produce unpleasant side effects, a patient who has been prepared openly and honestly for their possibility is more likely to view the side effects as evidence of the psychiatrist's excellent fund of knowledge rather than as a terrible surprise thrust on him or her by a dishonest or ignorant physician. On a final note, it may not be assumed that a patient already receiving antipsychotics prescribed by another physician has received an adequate informed consent. The process must begin anew with the new treating physician. A new twist in the legal issues surrounding antipsychotic agents is the lower incidence of EPS and TD with atypical agents. The question of what is standard of care and how this relates to patients' prescribed conventional antipsychotics who are at a higher risk of developing a movement disorder such as TD presents interesting legal issues.

Essentials of Psychiatry   Jerald Kay and Allan Tasman
© 2006 John Wiley & Sons, Ltd.

Table 64.1	Time of Emergence of Neuroleptic-induced Movement Disorders
Condition	**Highest Risk of Emergence**
Acute dystonia	Days 0–7
Neuroleptic malignant syndrome	Days 0–7 (continues at lesser degree until end of first mo)
Akathisia	Days 7–14 (continues at lesser degree until 2.5 mo)
Parkinsonism	Days 14–30 (continues at lesser degree until 2.5 mo)
Tardive dyskinesia	Month 3* → onward (risk increases with increasing time on neuroleptic)

*In patients older than 60 yr, month 1 → onward.

In general, the literature continues to expand with trials demonstrating reduced incidence of new onset neuroleptic-induced movement disorders with atypical antipsychotics and at least partial improvement of existing movement disorders caused by conventional antipsychotics. While atypical antipsychotics are not without a risk of movement disorders, the improved motor side-effect profile of the atypical agents provides a compelling argument for the use of atypical antipsychotics when initiating therapy, especially in susceptible populations such as the elderly. Switching to an atypical agent should be considered for those patients maintained on a conventional agent who develop or have a high risk of movement disorders.

Acute Neuroleptic-induced Movement Disorders

A summary of the treatment of these disorders is provided in Table 64.2.

Neuroleptic-induced Acute Dystonia

Etiology and Pathophysiology

This long-lasting contraction or spasm of musculature develops in conjunction with the use of antipsychotic medication. The pathophysiological mechanism of neuroleptic-induced acute dystonia is presently unknown. The finding that anticholinergic medication reverses the dystonia consistently may suggest that a hypercholinergic state is a correlate of dystonia. There is some suggestion of a correlation with changing blood–brain levels of antipsychotic medication. It is also possible that dystonia is related to the changing ratio of dopamine D_2 to D_1 receptors that accompany the normal aging process.

Abnormalities in dopamine–acetylcholine balance have been suggested as a possible mechanism because cholinergic antagonists and dopaminergic agonists seem to improve the dystonia in many patients, in contrast to dopaminergic antagonists, which seem to exacerbate or even cause dystonia. In contrast, some investigators have proposed that dopaminergic excess may be the responsible factor.

Epidemiology and Comorbidity

Acute dystonia is generally less common than most other extrapyramidal side effects of antipsychotics. Its frequency has been reported to range from 2 to 12% of patients taking conventional antipsychotic medication. For patients who receive high doses of high-potency conventional agents, however, the frequency may be as high as 50%. Incidence of acute dystonia can probably be reduced

Table 64.2	Treatment of Acute Neuroleptic-induced Movement Disorders		
Condition	**First Choice**	**Second Choice**	**Third Choice**
Acute dystonia	Anticholinergic medication, e.g., 2 mg benztropine PO, IM, IV 50 mg diphenhydramine PO, IM, IV	Benzodiazepine, e.g., lorazepam 1 mg IM, IV	—
Parkinsonism	Decrease neuroleptic to lowest effective dose	Anticholinergic, e.g., benztropine at 2 mg/d	Consider high-dose anticholinergic
	Consider change to lower potency neuroleptic		Consider discontinuation of neuroleptic
			Consider experimental treatment
Akathisia			
with high-potency neuroleptic	β-blocker, e.g., propranolol 10–30 mg t.i.d.	Anticholinergic, e.g., 2 mg/d benztropine	Benzodiazepine, e.g., lorazepam, e.g., 1 mg t.i.d.
with low-potency neuroleptic	β-blocker	Benzodiazepine	Anticholinergic
with other extrapyramidal signs	Anticholinergic	Anticholinergic plus β-blocker	Anticholinergic plus benzodiazepine

Reprinted with permission from Arana GW and Rosenbaum JF (2000) *Handbook of Psychiatric Drug Therapy*, 4th edn. Lippincott, Williams & Wilkins, Philadelphia, pp. 6–52.

to approximately 2% if low-dose treatment strategies are employed. Furthermore, acute dystonia is considerably less likely to occur with atypical antipsychotic medications (i.e., less than 5% of individuals) (American Psychiatric Association, 2000). For example, dystonic reactions occurred in less than 5% of patients in a study of ziprasidone and 1% in a dose comparison study with quetiapine.

Large doses of high-potency conventional antipsychotics appear to be the most consistent risk factor reported for acute dystonia. Other factors that also seem to predispose to dystonia are young age and male sex. A prior dystonic reaction is a good predictor of a repeated episode when the same antipsychotic at the same dose is reapplied.

DSM-IV-TR Criteria 333.7

Neuroleptic-induced Acute Dystonia

A. One (or more) of the following signs or symptoms has developed in association with the use of neuroleptic medication:

  (1) abnormal positioning of the head and neck in relation to the body (e.g., retrocollis, torticollis)

  (2) spasms of the jaw muscles (trismus, gaping, grimacing)

  (3) impaired swallowing (dysphagia), speaking, or breathing (laryngeal–pharyngeal spasm, dysphonia)

  (4) thickened or slurred speech due to hypertonic or enlarged tongue (dysarthria, macroglossia) tongue protrusion or tongue dysfunction

  (5) eyes deviated up, down, or sideward (oculogyric crisis)

  (6) abnormal positioning of the distal limbs or trunk

The signs or symptoms in B. criterion A developed within 7 days of starting or rapidly raising the dose of neuroleptic medication, or of reducing a medication used to treat (or prevent) acute extrapyramidal symptoms (e.g., anticholinergic agents).

C. The symptoms in criterion A are not better accounted for by a mental disorder (e.g., catatonic symptoms in schizophrenia). Evidence that the symptoms are better accounted for by a mental disorder might include the following: the symptoms precede the exposure to neuroleptic medication or are not compatible with the pattern of pharmacological intervention (e.g., no improvement after neuroleptic lowering or anticholinergic administration).

D. The symptoms in criterion A are not due to a nonneuroleptic substance or to a neurological or other general medical condition. Evidence that the symptoms are due to a general medical condition might include the following: the symptoms precede the exposure to the neuroleptic medication, unexplained focal neurological signs are present, or the symptoms progress in the absence of change in medication.

Assessment and Differential Diagnosis

Neuroleptic-induced dystonia (sometimes referred to as a dystonic reaction) usually begins 12 to 36 hours after a new antipsychotic is started or the dosage of a preexisting one is increased. It is unusual to see a dystonia after 2 weeks of antipsychotic treatment, and probably 90% of all neuroleptic-induced dystonias occur within the first 5 days of antipsychotic treatment. Patients may report a sense of tongue "thickness" or difficulty in swallowing in the 3 to 6 hours preceding the acute dystonia.

Acute dystonia presents as a sustained, painful muscle spasm that produces twisting, squeezing and pulling movements of the muscle groups involved. The most common muscle groups affected are the eyes, jaw, tongue and neck, but any muscle group in the body can be involved. On occasion, the larynx or pharynx may be involved, and this can result in rapid respiratory compromise (American Psychiatric Association, 2000).

Neuroleptic-induced acute dystonias are dramatic and usually easy to diagnose. There are, however, a number of other conditions that can present similarly and need to be ruled out. Spontaneously occurring focal or segmental dystonias may persist for days to weeks independent of medication. Neurological conditions such as temporal lobe seizures, infections, trauma, or tumors can produce symptoms similar to the neuroleptic-induced acute dystonia. A number of medications, while generally less common than antipsychotics, can cause dystonias (e.g., anticonvulsant medications and selective serotonin reuptake inhibitors) (American Psychiatric Association, 2000).

Neuroleptic malignant syndrome (NMS) can produce muscle contractions that look similar to acute dystonia but can be distinguished by generalized "lead pipe" type of rigidity, fever, fluctuating consciousness and unstable vital signs. Catatonia associated with an affective or psychotic disorder can be difficult to distinguish from dystonia clinically but does not respond to the administration of anticholinergic or antihistaminic medication. Furthermore, patients with catatonia are typically not concerned about their stiffness, whereas the patient with dystonia are likely to be extremely distressed (American Psychiatric Association, 2000).

On occasion, an acute dystonic reaction may resemble tardive dyskinesia (TD). This is easily clarified by administering anticholinergic medications, which rapidly clear dystonia and do not affect (or may worsen) TD. Making a differential diagnosis between an acute dystonia and tardive dystonia can be difficult. Tardive dystonia (similar to TD) is a diagnosis made late in the course of antipsychotic treatment and is generally a chronic condition compared with acute dystonia, which occurs early in the course of medication treatment and typically responds rapidly to pharmacological intervention.

Course

A neuroleptic-induced acute dystonia typically subsides spontaneously within hours after onset. However, treatment should be started as soon as the dystonia is diagnosed because the experience is "intensely" distressing to the patient.

Treatment

The standard approach to treatment is the immediate administration of an anticholinergic or antihistaminic agent. In most cases, this medication may be administered orally, intramuscularly, or intravenously. The first dose of medication should be the equivalent of 2 mg of benztropine or 50 mg of diphenhydramine. This should be repeated if the first dose does not produce a robust response within 30 minutes. This standard approach is usually successful in resolving the dystonia.

In the unusual refractory case, intramuscular or intravenous anticholinergic or antihistaminic drugs should be used at more frequent dosing intervals, and consideration should be given to adding an intramuscular injection of lorazepam for additional sedation. Since even the milder dystonias respond much more quickly to intramuscular or intravenous medication, it may therefore be worth avoiding the use of oral medication in treating dystonia. Oral medication takes much longer to work and is likely to result in unnecessarily prolonged distress of the patient.

In cases of laryngeal or pharyngeal dystonias with airway compromise, repeated dosing of medication should occur at shorter intervals until resolution is achieved. Arana and Rosenbaum (2000) recommended that the patient receive 4 mg of intravenous benztropine within 10 minutes followed by 1 to 2 mg of intravenous lorazepam. If airway compromise continues for any appreciable amount of time, emergent support from an anesthesiologist should be obtained and the patient should receive general anesthesia with airway protection. Fortunately, the need for such measures is rare.

After a dystonia, a patient should be maintained with oral anticholinergic or antihistaminic medication for at least 48 hours. If there is a history of previous dystonias, the medication should be continued for 2 weeks. Consideration should be given to decreasing the previous dose of the antipsychotic or possibly switching to a low-potency neuroleptic or atypical agent if the patient has been prescribed a conventional antipsychotic. The use of prophylactic anticholinergic medication will be discussed later.

Neuroleptic-induced Parkinsonism

Etiology and Pathophysiology

Neuroleptic-induced parkinsonism (NIP) is defined as parkinsonian signs or symptoms (tremor, muscle rigidity, or akinesia) that develop in association with the use of an antipsychotic medication. NIP is presumed to result from blockade of postsynaptic dopamine (D_2) receptors in the corpus striatum causing a pathological state functionally resembling the loss of dopaminergic cells in the striatum in idiopathic Parkinson's disease (PD). However, it is not clear whether nigrostriatal dopamine loss is adequate to explain the clinical symptoms seen in NIP or PD. It is possible that other neurochemical abnormalities may coexist with dopaminergic depletion to produce the syndrome. Abnormalities in norepinephrine and serotonin have also been reported to be involved in the mechanism.

Positron emission tomography (PET) and other technologies have been utilized to examine the relationship between D_2 receptor blockade in the basal ganglia with antipsychotic efficacy and NIP. Clinically effective doses of conventional antipsychotics have been shown to block 70 to 90% of D_2 receptors in the basal ganglia. Of note are findings that with conventional agents at least 60% occupancy is needed for satisfactory antipsychotic response but that NIP tends to occur with 80% or greater occupancy of the D_2 receptors. With regard to atypical agents, the lower D_2 receptor blockade at recommended dosages with some agents and the serotonergic blockade seen with these medications are believed to lead to the reduced risk of NIP. Similar to conventional antipsychotics, higher doses of some atypical agents also appear to be related to an increase in NIP, as greater D_2 receptor blockade has been reported.

Neuroleptic-induced Parkinsonism

A. One (or more) of the following signs or symptoms has developed in association with the use of neuroleptic medication:

   (1) parkinsonian tremor (i.e., a coarse, rhythmic, resting tremor with a frequency between 3 and 6 cycles per second, affecting the limbs, head, mouth, or tongue)

   (2) parkinsonian muscular rigidity (i.e., cogwheel rigidity or continuous "lead-pipe" rigidity)

   (3) akinesia (i.e., a decrease in spontaneous facial expressions, gestures, speech, or body movements)

B. The symptoms in criterion A developed within a few weeks of starting or raising the dose of a neuroleptic medication, or of reducing a medication used to treat (or prevent) acute extrapyramidal symptoms (e.g., anticholinergic agents).

C. The symptoms in criterion A are not better accounted for by a mental disorder (e.g., catatonic or negative symptoms in schizophrenia, psychomotor retardation in a major depressive episode). Evidence that the symptoms are better accounted for by a mental disorder might include the following: the symptoms precede the exposure to neuroleptic medication or are not compatible with the pattern of pharmacological intervention (e.g., no improvement after lowering the neuroleptic dose or administering anticholinergic medication).

D. The symptoms in criterion A are not due to a nonneuroleptic substance or to a neurological or other general medical condition (e.g., Parkinson's disease, Wilson's disease). Evidence that the symptoms are due to a general medical condition might include the following: the symptoms precede the exposure to neuroleptic medication, unexplained focal neurological signs are present, or the symptoms progress despite a stable medication regimen.

Epidemiology and Comorbidity

The reported frequency of NIP varies from 5 to 90%, depending on the study reviewed. This wide variation is due to different definitions of parkinsonism in different studies as well as the inclusion of mild bradykinesia as a sign of NIP in some investigations. The usual incidence of "clinically significant" NIP with conventional antipsychotics is 10 to 15. When, however, high-potency conventional agents are used without anticholinergic drugs and signs of rigidity are carefully assessed, one is likely to find that the majority of patients have some NIP. Rates of parkinsonism induced by atypical antipsychotics are considerably lower (American Psychiatric Association, 2000). The incidence of NIP in older psychiatric patients is considerably greater. A study of newly medicated older patients on low doses of conventional antipsychotics found 32% of patients met criteria for NIP (Caligiuri *et al.*, 1999). In an investigation of extrapyramidal side effects in patients with Alzheimer disease treated with very low dose conventional antipsychotics, 67% of patients met criteria for NIP at some time during the 9-month follow-up period (Caligiuri *et al.*, 1998).

A number of patient-related and medication-related risk factors have been proposed. A history of prior episodes of NIP, older age, and concomitant dementia or delirium are thought to predispose to NIP (American Psychiatric Association, 2000). Neuroleptic potency and preexisting extrapyramidal symptoms may also increase the risk of NIP.

Rapid increases in antipsychotic dosage, administration of higher absolute doses of antipsychotics and absence of concurrent anticholinergic medication represent other risk factors for NIP initiation (American Psychiatric Association, 2000). Highly anticholinergic antipsychotics (i.e., chlorpromazine and thioridazine) are less likely to cause NIP than less anticholinergic agents (i.e., haloperidol and fluphenazine).

Assessment and Differential Diagnosis

NIP symptoms may develop quickly after the initiation of an antipsychotic or insidiously during the course of treatment. It most typically develops 2 to 4 weeks after antipsychotic initiation. The three cardinal symptoms of NIP are tremor, muscle rigidity and akinesia.

Parkinsonian tremor is a steady, rhythmical, oscillatory motion generally at an alternating rhythm of 3 to 6 Hz. The most affected body area tends to be the upper extremities, but the tremor may spread to the head, neck, jaw, face, tongue, legs and trunk. The tremor is typically suppressed during action and increases during times of anxiety, stress, or fatigue (American Psychiatric Association, 2000).

Parkinsonian muscle rigidity appears clinically as a firmness and spasm of muscles at rest that may affect all skeletal muscles or be confined to just a few specific muscle groups. It can appear as a continuous lead pipe-type rigidity that resists movement or a cogwheel-type rigidity that presents a "ratchet-like" resistance when a muscle is moved around a joint. Cogwheeling may represent an extremely high frequency (8–12 Hz) "action" tremor that is physiologically imposed on the rigidity. The psychiatrist may diagnose cogwheel rigidity by placing his or her hand over the joint that is being passively moved. Generalized muscle pain, body aches and discoordination are features associated with NIP rigidity (American Psychiatric Association, 2000).

Parkinsonian akinesia is seen clinically as decreased spontaneous motor activity and a global slowness in the initiation and execution of movements. It can be associated with drooling, bent over neck, stooped shoulders and masked facial expression (the so-called masked facies) (American Psychiatric Association, 2000). Parkinsonism occurs in numerous medical and neurological conditions and can be caused by many medications or substances. Idiopathic PD can be difficult to distinguish from NIP.

The tremor of NIP must be distinguished from tremor caused by other conditions. In general, nonparkinsonian tremors are finer, faster and worse on intention. Tremor associated with substance withdrawal typically presents with associated hyperreflexia and increased autonomic signs. Cerebellar disease-induced tremor may present with associated nystagmus, ataxia, or scanning speech. Strokes and other central nervous system lesions usually have associated focal neurological symptoms. NMS can often present with akinesia and lead pipe-type rigidity but also has other associated findings, such as fever, elevated creatine kinase and fluctuating consciousness (American Psychiatric Association, 2000). It appears that TD and NIP frequently coexist in the same patient.

A number of primary psychiatric illnesses may mimic symptoms of NIP and may be difficult to separate. These include major depressive disorder, catatonic-type schizophrenia, mood disorder with catatonic features, schizophrenia with a predominance of negative features, delirium, dementia, anxiety disorders and certain conversion disorders (American Psychiatric Association, 2000). It may be particularly easy to confuse negative symptoms of schizophrenia and depression with the akinesia and rigidity of NIP. Catatonia and NIP may also be difficult to differentiate, and there is evidence that the two conditions are related to each other. Often, the diagnosis of NIP should be made provisionally and clarified by a dosage reduction of antipsychotic or trial of anticholinergic medication (American Psychiatric Association, 2000).

Course

NIP symptoms usually continue unchanged or diminish slowly in 2 to 3 months after onset. The signs and symptoms typically improve with a dose reduction, discontinuation of antipsychotic medication, or switch to an atypical antipsychotic in patients previously receiving a conventional antipsychotic. Improvement is also seen with the addition of antiparkinsonian agents.

Treatment

Many milder cases of NIP do not require treatment because they are not bothersome to the patient. A switch to an atypical agent should be strongly considered if troublesome NIP develops while on a conventional antipsychotic. Large randomized controlled trials have demonstrated reductions in parkinsonian symptoms in patients treated with atypical antipsychotics. If symptoms become troublesome, the initial step should be to decrease the dose of antipsychotic to the lowest effective dose for the patient. The next step is to add a low dosage of an anticholinergic medication. The equivalent of 2 mg/day of benztropine generally represents a reasonable starting point. Periodic attempts should be made to wean the patient from the anticholinergic agent. As many as 90% of patients do not require anticholinergic medication at the end of 3 months. Anticholinergic medication should always be tapered slowly to avoid the rapid redevelopment of parkinsonian symptoms as well as the possibility of uncomfortable cholinergic rebound symptoms.

Refractory cases of NIP do occur and may require more aggressive management. Increasing the dose of the anticholinergic medication is a good starting point because some patients may require up to the equivalent of 20 mg/day of benztropine to achieve relief from NIP. If such high doses are to be employed, they should be used for the shortest possible time, and rigorous attention should be paid to the possibility of untoward anticholinergic effects (i.e., delirium, urinary retention, fecal impaction). Consideration may be given to starting a dopamine-releasing agent, such as amantadine or perhaps even levodopa. A major concern with this treatment approach is the possibility of exacerbating the psychosis for which the antipsychotic medication was prescribed in the first place. Trials of dopaminergic agents are therefore best attempted in an inpatient setting or with careful outpatient observation and assessment. A number of experimental treatment strategies have been proposed for the treatment of the refractory cases including vitamin E, calcium supplementation, electroconvulsive therapy and L-deprenyl.

Another treatment approach for the refractory case is to lower the dose of the antipsychotic medication or even discontinue it until the NIP resolves, then resume the antipsychotic (preferably a different one) at a lower dose. This treatment strategy may also need to be carried out in an inpatient setting to monitor early emergence of psychotic symptoms.

Neuroleptic-induced Acute Akathisia

Etiology and Pathophysiology

Neuroleptic-induced acute akathisia is defined as a subjective feeling of restlessness and an intensely unpleasant need to move occurring secondary to antipsychotic treatment. The pathophysiological mechanism of akathisia remains unknown. Marsden and Jenner (1980) suggested that dopamine blockade in the mesocortical system may account for the hyperactive symptoms of akathisia. Mesocortical dopaminergic neurons that innervate the prefrontal cortex seem to be resistant to depolarization induced by long-term antipsychotic treatment, suggesting a possible explanation for why akathisia often does not improve with time.

The possibility that excessive noradrenergic activity plays a role in the pathogenesis of akathisia is supported by the efficacy of beta-adrenergic blockers in improving some cases of akathisia. Additionally, opioid mechanisms have been proposed to contribute to akathisia on the basis of reported therapeutic effects of opioid drugs. The lower likelihood of akathisia with atypical antipsychotics and reports of selective serotonin reuptake inhibitors causing akathisia have implicated serotonin as having a possible role in akathisia, however this is still under investigation.

Epidemiology and Comorbidity

Akathisia is a common side effect of antipsychotic treatment. It is estimated to occur in 20 to 75% of all patients treated with conventional agents. The wide discrepancy in reported prevalence may result from a lack of consistency in the definition of akathisia, different prescribing practices, different study designs and differences in population demographics (American Psychiatric Association, 2000). While atypical antipsychotics are less likely to cause akathisia compared with typical agents, prevalence rates have varied. Clozapine-induced akathisia has ranged from 0 to 39% and a point prevalence of 13% has been reported for risperidone. Akathisia is thought by many psychiatrists to be a leading cause of nonadherence.

Higher doses of high-potency conventional antipsychotics appear to be most frequently associated with the appearance of akathisia (American Psychiatric Association, 2000). Previous episodes of neuroleptic-induced akathisia increase the risk for future episodes if antipsychotics are restarted.

Assessment and Differential Diagnosis

Akathisia tends to occur within the first 4 weeks of initiating or increasing the dose of antipsychotic medication. It can develop rapidly after the initiation or the dose increase of an antipsychotic. Patients with akathisia tend to have subjective complaints of "inner restlessness", most often in the legs. It may be difficult for the patients to describe their feelings. They feel that they must move, and this manifests as fidgeting, frequent changes in posture, crossing and uncrossing of the legs, rocking while sitting and shuffling when walking (American Psychiatric Association, 2000).

Akathisia is often associated with severe dysphoria, anxiety and irritability. When the akathisia is particularly severe,

aggression or suicide attempts may be a possible result, although this is controversial. Akathisia in a psychotic patient can easily be mistaken for worsening of psychotic features, resulting in an increase in antipsychotic dose and an exacerbation of the akathisia.

The strange subjective discomfort associated with akathisia is the feature that seems to be most useful in making a differential diagnosis between neuroleptic-induced akathisia and other neuroleptic-induced movement disorders. TD is often associated with a lack of sensory perception of having a movement disorder. This contrasts with akathisia in which patients tend to be acutely aware of their distress. When patients with TD are uncomfortable, it is usually a result of social factors such as embarrassment and functional factors such as frustration over not being able to perform certain tasks. Another differentiating factor is that TD usually involves the face, mouth and upper extremities, whereas akathisia more commonly involves the lower extremities.

The rhythmical appearance of akathisia may sometimes suggest a tremorous condition. Thus, the tremor of NIP and idiopathic PD may be mistaken for akathisia, especially if the feet and legs are involved. Iron deficiency anemia can also present with symptoms phenomenologically similar to neuroleptic-induced akathisia. A number of other medications but particularly selective serotonin reuptake inhibitor antidepressant medications may produce akathisia clinically identical to that produced by antipsychotics (American Psychiatric Association, 2000).

It is critical to differentiate akathisia from other psychiatric disorders presenting with agitation, such as depressive episodes, manic episodes, anxiety disorders, schizophrenia, dementia, delirium, substance intoxication or withdrawal and attention-deficit/hyperactivity disorder. The reason for the importance of this differentiation is that mistaking akathisia for a primary psychiatric disorder can result in an intervention that would be the exact opposite of what is appropriate (i.e., increasing the dose of an antipsychotic instead of decreasing it because akathisia is mistaken for worsening psychosis) (American Psychiatric Association, 2000).

Course

Neuroleptic-induced akathisia typically lasts as long as antipsychotic treatment is continued but may have variable intensity in time (American Psychiatric Association, 2000). Treatment of akathisia may or may not alter the course of the akathisia.

Treatment

Akathisia may be difficult to treat effectively. The best initial approach is to try and reduce the chance of developing akathisia by minimizing the dosage of antipsychotic medication. The use of atypical antipsychotics should be considered as a result of their lower risk of akathisia. If using conventional antipsychotics, a switch to a low-potency agent such as thioridazine or chlorpromazine may prove helpful because these antipsychotics seem to have somewhat lower propensity to cause akathisia than high-potency conventional antipsychotics. After these initial steps, consideration should be given to initiation of an antiakathisic drug regimen. A number of agents have been reported to be effective, including beta-adrenergic blockers, anticholinergic drugs, benzodiazepines and clonidine (American Psychiatric Association, 2000).

When choosing an agent to treat akathisia, a beta-blocker such as propranolol should generally be considered first-line as its efficacy has been proven and it has been shown to be superior to other possible treatments such as benztropine and lorazepam. In terms of antiakathisic effects, the beta-blocker chosen should be lipophilic so as to cross the blood–brain barrier and should also have activity at the beta-2 receptor. Benzodiazepines such as clonazepam and lorazepam have been shown to be efficacious in the treatment of akathisia and are also a reasonable therapeutic option, especially when considering the interplay between anxiety and akathisia, however, their side effects and abuse potential should be considered. Anticholinergic agents such as benztropine may also be tried, but less evidence exists to supports their use. A limited number of studies have also shown possible roles for clonidine and amantadine in the treatment of akathisia. Agents with serotonin receptor blocking activity (i.e., ritanserine, mianserin) have also been reported to be of benefit in akathisia.

Clinical Vignette 1

Confusion Between Neuroleptic-Induced Akathisia and Psychotic Agitation

Ms B, a 77-year-old widow, lived in a nursing home. As a result of severe degenerative arthritis and neuropathic pain due to type 2 diabetes, she was confined mainly to her bed and a wheelchair. She had a past psychiatric history significant for Alzheimer-type dementia diagnosed at age 74. Ms B was started on haloperidol 1 mg b.i.d. 6 weeks ago due to frequent, bothersome delusions regarding her roommate and health care personnel.

Two weeks ago, Ms B's roommate complained that Ms B was increasingly agitated, restless and boisterous throughout the day while in bed. Believing that her behavioral disturbance was inadequately controlled, Ms B's physician increased her haloperidol to 2 mg b.i.d. A few days later, Ms B was noted to be increasingly agitated and restless. Subjective discomfort was noted upon further interviews with the patient. Since the haloperidol-induced akathisia worsened by increased dosages of haloperidol, Ms B was started on low-dose risperidone and haloperidol was stopped over the course of 1 week. Ms B is currently receiving risperidone 0.5 mg b.i.d. without any symptoms of akathisia and noted reductions in her delusions.

Prophylactic Anticholinergic Medication?

One issue that remains controversial among researchers and psychiatrists is whether preventive anticholinergic medication should be given to patients who are starting antipsychotics. Arguments against this practice include the risk of anticholinergic side effects such as dry mouth, blurry vision, constipation and urinary retention. Further, anticholinergic medication is associated with cognitive side effects, such as memory impairment, confusion and delirium. The relationship between anticholinergic medications and TD is not definitive.

Arguments in favor of initiating prophylactic anticholinergic therapy point to the decrease in the frequency of EPS (including dystonias, akathisia and akinesia) when anticholinergic drugs are prescribed prophylactically. Furthermore, medication nonadherence and decompensation may relate to inadequately treated NIP, especially akathisia and akinesia. With the introduction and increased use of atypical antipsychotics, the risk of EPS and TD has decreased, thus reducing the need for prophylactic anticholinergic medication for many patients prescribed atypical agents.

Although this complicated issue remains unresolved, some basic guidelines can be proposed. When psychosis is severe and unmanageable and adherence with medications needs to be rigorously enforced, antipsychotic and anticholinergic medication may be administered concurrently, with the anticholinergic medication tapered slowly within the next few weeks. When the psychosis is milder and antipsychotic medication may be gradually increased, it may be best to avoid anticholinergic medications until such time as they become clinically necessary. In patients with any degree of cognitive impairment (especially the elderly or demented patient with agitation or psychosis), it is best to aim for the administration of less anticholinergic medication. In younger patients, especially young men (who have a high frequency of dystonia), it may be preferable to use anticholinergic medication prophylactically because it may prevent an uncomfortable dystonic reaction and can generally be used with relative impunity of serious side effects. In general, long-term prophylactic use of anticholinergic medication is not recommended nor its use in the elderly.

Neuroleptic-induced tardive dyskinesia

Etiology and Pathophysiology

Neuroleptic-induced tardive dyskinesia (TD) is a syndrome consisting of abnormal, involuntary movements caused by long-term treatment with antipsychotic medication. The movements are typically choreoathetoid in nature and principally involve the mouth, face, limbs and trunk. TD, by definition, occurs late in the course of drug treatment. It is likely that a number of separate neurotransmitter systems are involved in the pathogenesis of TD. There may be different subtypes of TD, each perhaps involving a unique profile of neurochemical imbalance. Neuroleptic-induced striatal pathological change represents another possibility for explaining mechanisms of TD and some have suggested that long-term antipsychotic use may produce "toxic free radicals" that damage neurons and result in persistent TD.

Epidemiology and Comorbidity

The reported prevalence of TD has been somewhat variable as a result of differences in populations of patients and in the methods used. Yassa and Jeste (1992) reviewed 76 studies of the prevalence of TD published from 1960 to 1990. In a total population of approximately 40 000 patients, the overall prevalence of TD was 24.2%, although it was much higher (about 50%) in studies of elderly patients treated with antipsychotics.

There have been relatively few studies of the incidence of TD. Kane and coworkers (1988) prospectively studied more than 850 patients (mean age 29 years) and found the incidence of TD after cumulative exposure to conventional antipsychotics to be 5% after 1 year, 18.5% after 4 years and 40% after 8 years. Incidence in older populations has been found to be much higher. Saltz and colleagues (1991) reported an incidence of 31% after 43 weeks of conventional antipsychotic treatment in a population of elderly patients. Jeste and colleagues (1999) evaluated 439 psychiatric patients with a mean age of 65 years and found that 28.8% of the sample met criteria for TD during the first 12 months of study treatment; 50.1% had TD by the end of 24 months; and 63.1% by the end of 36 months. The risk of severe TD has also been reported to be higher in older patients.

Evidence supporting a reduced risk of TD with atypical antipsychotics is beginning to emerge. The lower risk of EPS with atypical agents has led to the widespread conclusion that these agents will also have reduced TD risk. The low risk of tardive dyskinesia in clozapine-treated individuals has been well established. In addition, a lower incidence of TD has been reported in patients treated with risperidone and olanzapine. More long-term prospective studies are needed with the atypical agents.

Aging consistently appears to be the most important risk factor for the development of TD. Prevalence and severity of TD seem to increase with age. The reasons for this increased risk of TD with aging are not known but may be related to the propensity of the nigrostriatal system to degenerate with age as well as pharmacokinetic and pharmacodynamic factors.

Gender (female) was thought to be a risk factor for TD. A meta-analysis of the published reports demonstrated a greater

---

DSM-IV-TR Criteria 333.82

Neuroleptic-induced Tardive Dyskinesia

A. Involuntary movements of the tongue, jaw, trunk, or extremities have developed in association with the use of neuroleptic medication.

B. The involuntary movements are present over a period of at least 4 weeks and occur in any of the following patterns:

  (1) choreiform movements (i.e., rapid, jerky, nonrepetitive)

  (2) athetoid movements (i.e., slow, sinuous, continual)

  (3) rhythmic movements (i.e., stereotypies)

C. The signs or symptoms in criteria A and B develop during exposure to a neuroleptic medication or within 4 weeks of withdrawal from an oral (or within 8 weeks of withdrawal from a depot) neuroleptic medication.

D. There has been exposure to neuroleptic medication for at least 3 months (1 month if age 60 years or older).

E. The symptoms are not due to a neurological or general medical condition (e.g., Huntington's disease, Sydenham's chorea, spontaneous dyskinesia, hyperthyroidism, Wilson's disease), ill-fitting dentures, or exposure to other medications that cause acute reversible dyskinesia (e.g., L-dopa, bromocriptine). Evidence that the symptoms are due to one of these etiologies might include the following: the symptoms precede the exposure to the neuroleptic medication or unexplained focal neurological signs are present.

F. The symptoms are not better accounted for by a neuroleptic-induced acute movement disorder (e.g., neuroleptic-induced acute dystonia, neuroleptic-induced acute akathisia).

Reprinted with permission from the *Diagnostic and Statistical Manual of Mental Disorders*, Fourth Edition, Text Revision. Copyright 2000 American Psychiatric Association.

---

prevalence of TD in women (26.6%) compared with that in men (21.6%) (Yassa and Jeste, 1992). Interestingly, studies of incidence of TD in older patients failed to confirm the reported propensity of women to have TD at a higher rate than men. A possible relationship between gender and age of onset of schizophrenia to severity of dyskinesia has been reported as women with late-onset schizophrenia (LOS) and men with early-onset schizophrenia (EOS) had more severe dyskinesia than men with LOS and women with EOS.

There are conflicting reports regarding ethnicity as a risk factor for TD and people with diabetes mellitus may be at a higher risk for development of TD. Some have proposed that diabetes mellitus might be a risk factor for TD in patients treated with metoclopramide.

Patients who experience an acute neuroleptic-induced movement disorder (especially parkinsonism or akathisia) are likely to be at a greater risk for development of TD if antipsychotic treatment is continued. Total exposure to typical antipsychotic agents has been correlated with TD risk and within elderly populations, cumulative amount of typical antipsychotics has also been associated with TD risk, especially with high-potency conventional agents. The observation that anticholinergic drugs exacerbate some symptoms of TD does not appear to indicate that the drugs promote the onset of the disorder.

Assessment and Differential Diagnosis

TD may develop at any age and typically has an insidious onset. It may develop during exposure to antipsychotic medication or within 4 weeks of withdrawal from an oral antipsychotic (or within 8 weeks of withdrawal from a depot neuroleptic). There must be a history of at least 3 months of antipsychotic use (or 1 month in the elderly) before TD may be diagnosed (American Psychiatric Association, 2000).

The most common features of TD are involuntary movements of the tongue, face and neck muscles. Less common are movements in the upper and lower extremities as well as in the trunk. Most rare of all are involuntary movements of the muscle groups involved with breathing and swallowing. The earliest symptoms typically involve buccolingual–masticatory movements. The movements of TD are choreiform (rapid, jerky), athetoid (slow, sinuous), or rhythmical (stereotypical) (American Psychiatric Association, 2000).

Severe choreoathetoid dyskinesia differs from the milder forms, mainly in the frequency and amplitude of the abnormal movements. Some cases of severe dyskinesia consist of generalized choreoathetosis of the face, trunk and all four limbs. TD may be accompanied by dystonias, parkinsonism and akathisia. TD is worsened by stimulants, short-term withdrawal of antipsychotic medication, anticholinergic medication, emotional arousal, stress and voluntary movements of other parts of the body. It is improved by relaxation, voluntary movements of the involved parts of the body, sleep and increased dose of antipsychotics.

The differential diagnosis of TD is extensive. The major task for the psychiatrist is to rule out other causes of dyskinesia. It may be useful for the psychiatrist to keep in mind three questions for the facilitation of the differential diagnosis: 1) Does the patient have dyskinesia? 2) Does another disorder fully explain the cause of the dyskinesia? 3) If the dyskinesia is related to antipsychotic use, is it TD?

A number of nondyskinetic movement disorders are part of the differential diagnosis of TD. Tremor can be confused with TD, including the tremor of neuroleptic-induced parkinsonism, rabbit syndrome, Wilson's disease and cerebellar disease. Further, fine tremors of the fingers and hands are produced by anxiety states, alcoholism, hyperthyroidism and drugs. Acute dystonias, myoclonus, tics, mannerisms, compulsions and akathisia must be differentiated from TD. The differentiation is made on the basis of the clinical assessment.

Once it has been established that the patient suffers from a dyskinesia, the main cause must be determined. In children and young adults, a number of conditions may cause dyskinesia besides antipsychotic treatment. The use of drugs, especially amphetamines and antihistamines, are associated with dyskinesia. Sydenham's chorea can produce choreiform movements. Conversion disorder and malingering are conditions that can present with apparently involuntary movements. Hyperthyroidism and hypoparathyroidism are two endocrinological conditions that can produce dyskinesias similar to TD. Huntington's disease is a condition that can be difficult to distinguish clinically from TD, but certain characteristics may aid in the diagnosis, including 1) a family history of Huntington's disease, 2) the presence of dementia, 3) a slowly progressive downhill course, and 4) atrophy of the caudate nucleus on computed tomography scan.

In the middle-aged or elderly patient, denture or dental problems may commonly mimic TD. Lesions of the basal ganglia may result in dyskinesias. The use of antiparkinsonian medications such as levodopa, amantadine and bromocriptine can cause dyskinetic movements. The presence of spontaneous dyskinesias must also be ruled out.

When it has been established that antipsychotics are responsible for the dyskinesia, it does not follow that the dyskinesia is necessarily TD. Acute dyskinesia occurring early in antipsychotic treatment is common and responds well to antihistaminic or anticholinergic medications. Withdrawal–emergent dyskinesia also occurs in a variable proportion of patients. This phenomenon refers to the appearance or worsening of dyskinetic movements on reduction or discontinuation of antipsychotic medication. Withdrawal–emergent dyskinesia is phenomenologically similar to TD and often has the full range of involuntary choreiform and athetoid movements. A typical case may begin within a few days after a sudden decrease in dosage and worsen as the antipsychotic is withdrawn. This phase is followed by rapid improvement in a period of weeks to months. A history of antipsychotic exposure and remission of dyskinetic symptoms within 3 months of antipsychotic withdrawal are suggestive of the diagnosis of withdrawal–emergent dyskinesia.

Finally, tardive Tourette's disorder must be differentiated from TD. A number of cases of tardive Tourette's disorder have been reported as a result of treatment with antipsychotics, emerging during treatment or after cessation of treatment. Tardive Tourette's disorder presents with symptoms similar to those of idiopathic Tourette's disorder. Motor tics are usually compulsive organized stereotypies that may, in certain cases, be difficult to distinguish from the choreoathetoid movements of TD. Typically, vocal tics (including barks, grunts, coughs and yelps) represent part of tardive Tourette's disorder but not TD. Tardive Tourette's disorder seems to show a pharmacological response similar to that of TD, leading to the assumption that the syndrome may be a type of the more commonly seen TD. Thus, tardive Tourette's disorder may be masked by an increase in antipsychotics and exacerbated by withdrawal.

Course

One-third of the TD patients experience remission within 3 months of discontinuation of antipsychotic medication, and approximately half have remission within 12 to 18 months of antipsychotic discontinuation (American Psychiatric Association, 2000). Elderly patients are reported to have lower rates of remission, especially if antipsychotics are continued. When TD patients must be maintained with antipsychotics, TD seems to be stable in 50%, worsen in 25% and improve in the rest. Time may be the most important factor in outcome of TD. In studies that have followed up patients for longer than 5 years, TD seems to improve in half of patients with or without antipsychotic treatment. Furthermore, TD may improve as slowly as it develops and may exist on a spectrum between resolution and persistence.

Severe TD may lead to numerous physical complications and psychosocial problems. Dental and denture problems are common sequelae of severe oral dyskinesia as are ulcerations of the tongue, cheeks and lips. Hyperkinetic dysarthria has been described. Swallowing disorders represent another complication. Respiratory disturbances, although fairly rare, have been reported by a number of investigators. These disturbances are usually manifested by shortness of breath at rest, irregularities in respiration, and various grunts, snorts and gasps. Respiratory alkalosis may be seen on laboratory tests. Gastrointestinal complications of severe TD may involve vomiting and dysphagia secondary to disruption of the normal activity of the esophagus; weight loss may result from such a disturbance.

Subjective distress is a common accompaniment of severe dyskinesia. Suicidal ideation may result from distress over the dyskinesia, and there have been reports of some successful suicides. General impairment of functioning may be related to the severity of the dyskinetic disorder. Social embarrassment as a result of TD may represent a reason that some patients with TD tend to be reluctant to leave their homes. Even mild dyskinesia may lead to anxiety, guilt, shame and anger. These symptoms can lead to severe depressive episodes.

Treatment

Despite intense effort, there is as yet no consistently reliable therapy for TD. As a result, the psychiatrist must focus primary efforts toward prevention of the disorder. The use of atypical antipsychotics are recommended due to their probable lower risk of TD. Antipsychotic use should be minimized in all patients. Patients with nonpsychotic mood or other disorders who need antipsychotics should receive the minimal necessary amounts of antipsychotic treatment and should have the medication tapered and then stopped once the clinical need is no longer present. In general, there must be enough clinical evidence to show that the benefits outweigh the potential risks of TD development. Antipsychotics should be used with particular caution in elderly patients because of their high risk for development of TD (Figure 64.1).

Gradual taper of the antipsychotic medication may be attempted as long as the risk/benefit ratio of antipsychotic maintenance versus withdrawal does not preclude such a strategy. A slow taper of medication to the lowest effective dose is probably the preferred strategy for the treatment of chronic schizophrenia in a large number of stable patients.

Paradoxically, antipsychotics themselves represent the most effective short-term treatment for TD. An increase in dosage of a conventional agent usually (approximately 66% of patients) results in a clinically significant but temporary reduction in TD symptoms. The most exciting development in the treatment of TD has been the use of the atypical antipsychotics. Clozapine has been shown to be effective in reducing TD in patients with existing TD, however, side effects such as agranulocytosis and clozapine's affinity for anticholinergic side effects limits its use. Additional studies have noted a beneficial effect of other atypical agents (i.e., risperidone and olanzapine) on preexisting TD. The reduced risk of TD with all atypical agents (when used at appropriate doses) supports their use as preventive measures and as therapeutic options for those who develop TD on a conventional antipsychotic.

A number of experimental studies have attempted to treat TD with alternative strategies. One treatment that has demonstrated some efficacy has been the use of vitamin E alpha-tocopherol. If antipsychotic treatment results in the production of free radicals that damage the neuronal components, an antioxidant such as vitamin E would therefore, theoretically, result in improvement in the symptoms of TD. Vitamin E is a possible agent for the treatment and prophylaxis of TD. A number of studies of varying design have shown benefit of vitamin E in TD

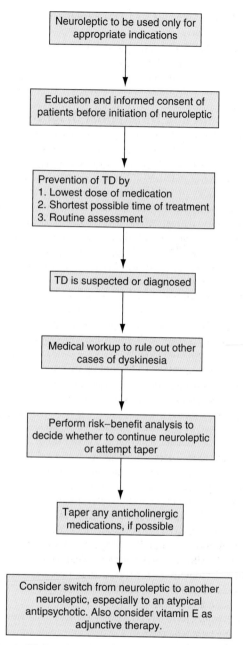

Figure 64.1 *Management of tardive dyskinesia (TD).*

however, a recent double-blind, placebo-controlled multicenter trial failed to show a difference between vitamin E and placebo after 1 year of treatment (Adler *et al.*, 1999). Although the results are far from conclusive, vitamin E remains a reasonably safe treatment modality for a patient with recently diagnosed TD. Doses are usually in the range of 1200 to 1600 mg/day. Other agents have been investigated, such as calcium channel blockers (i.e., diltiazem, verapamil, nifedipine) and clonazepam, but more studies are warranted.

Psychiatrists must regularly assess for the presence and progression of TD and present the patient (or the patient's guardian, when appropriate) with information about the risks of treatment; they may also give written information sheets, assess understanding by the patient or guardian, and accurately record evidence of the informed consent in the patient's record.

Neuroleptic Malignant Syndrome

Etiology and Pathophysiology

Neuroleptic Malignant Syndrome (NMS) is a potentially fatal reaction to antipsychotic medications that is characterized clinically by muscle rigidity, fever, autonomic instability and changes in level of consciousness. The pathophysiological mechanism of NMS remains unclear. The hypothesis of most interest is that of reduced dopaminergic activity secondary to neuroleptic-induced dopamine blockade. This reduced dopamine activity in different parts of the brain (hypothalamus, nigrostriatal system and corticolimbic tracts) may serve to explain the various clinical features of NMS. Dopamine reduction in the hypothalamus may cause fever and autonomic instability; in the nigrostriatal system, dopamine reduction may lead to the rigidity; and the reduction in corticolimbic dopamine activity may explain the altered consciousness. This hypothesis is based on the fact that antipsychotics are dopamine-blocking agents, whereas certain dopamine agonists are reported to help resolve NMS.

The dopaminergic blocking theory does not, however, explain why NMS may develop at a given time and in a given patient. There are probably other genetic (possibly a predisposition similar to that seen in malignant hyperthermia), constitutional, environmental, and pharmacological factors that interact to produce the syndrome. A number of investigators have proposed that other neurotransmitter abnormalities may be responsible for the syndrome, including serotonergic hyperfunction in the hypothalamus, excessive catecholamine secretion, and gamma-aminobutyric acid deficiency.

Epidemiology and Comorbidity

The exact frequency of NMS is unknown. A number of retrospective and prospective studies have found 0.02 to 3.2% of patients treated with antipsychotics to be affected with NMS. Several factors probably account for this large variability in frequency, including differences in study methods and diagnostic criteria for NMS. A prior episode of NMS appears to predispose to future episodes of NMS. Any preexisting medical problems, especially those associated with agitation or dehydration, may increase the likelihood of NMS development when antipsychotics are used. Patients with a neurological condition as well as patients with presumed psychosis due to human immunodeficiency virus infection may be at higher risk for development of NMS. A number of potential risk factors related to antipsychotic treatment have been identified. Higher doses of antipsychotic, rapid increases in dosage (especially "rapid neuroleptization") and intramuscular injections of high-potency conventional agents (e.g., haloperidol and fluphenazine) have been reported to be risk factors for NMS. NMS can occur (but rarely) in patients prescribed atypical antipsychotics and a review of atypical-induced NMS concluded that symptoms appear similar to NMS induced by conventional antipsychotics.

NMS is more frequently reported in men than in women and is more frequently seen in a younger population. A previous diagnosis of a mood disorder may place patients at a higher risk for NMS. Warm, humid climates may also predispose to the disorder (American Psychiatric Association, 2000).

Assessment and Differential Diagnosis

NMS usually presents in the first month of antipsychotic treatment but may develop at any time. Two-thirds of the cases manifest within the first week of treatment (American Psychiatric

---

DSM-IV-TR Criteria 333.92

Neuroleptic Malignant Syndrome

A. The development of severe muscle rigidity and elevated temperature associated with the use of neuroleptic medication.

B. Two (or more) of the following:

   (1) diaphoresis

   (2) dysphagia

   (3) tremor

   (4) incontinence

   (5) changes in level of consciousness ranging from confusion to coma

   (6) mutism

   (7) tachycardia

   (8) elevated or labile blood pressure

   (9) leukocytosis

   (10) laboratory evidence of muscle injury (e.g., elevated CPK [creatine kinase])

C. The symptoms in criteria A and B are not due to another substance (e.g., phencyclidine) or a neurological or other general medical condition (e.g., viral encephalitis).

D. The symptoms in criteria A and B are not better accounted for by a mental disorder (e.g., mood disorder with catatonic features).

Reprinted with permission from the *Diagnostic and Statistical Manual of Mental Disorders*, Fourth Edition, Text Revision.Copyright 2000 American Psychiatric Association.

Association, 2000). The two key diagnostic features for the disorder are severe muscle rigidity (classically referred to as lead pipe rigidity) and elevated temperature. A number of other features are also seen (see DSM-IV-TR criteria). For the psychiatrist, the most suggestive features are fluctuating consciousness (from confusion to coma), labile vital signs (tachycardia, unstable or elevated blood pressure), laboratory evidence of muscle injury (elevation of creatine kinase) and leukocytosis. Other features include diaphoresis, dysphagia, tremor, incontinence and mutism (American Psychiatric Association, 2000).

The differential diagnosis of NMS can be difficult (Table 64.3). The most important point is that the psychiatrist must start by suspecting NMS and then carefully rule out other possible organic problems. Because medical illness is a likely predisposing factor, it is important to consider that NMS may be present even if a definitive organic disease is found to explain the NMS-like symptoms.

Numerous general medical and neurological conditions can present with symptoms that may resemble NMS. Examples include central nervous system infection, status epilepticus, subcortical brain lesions, porphyria and tetanus (American Psychiatric Association, 2000). The presence of significantly elevated temperature and severe muscle rigidity makes the diagnosis of NMS more likely.

Table 64.3   **Differential Diagnosis of Neuroleptic Malignant Syndrome**

	Diagnosis				
Feature	Lethal Catatonia	Heat Stroke	Malignant Hyperthermia	Serotonin Syndrome	Neuroleptic Malignant Syndrome
Previous psychiatric illness	Yes	No	No	Yes	Yes
Onset of symptoms	+ Prodromal psychotic symptoms	− Prodromal symptoms; development in several hours	− Prodromal symptoms; development after anesthesia	− Prodromal symptoms; development days to months after serotoninergic medication	− Prodromal symptoms; development hours to months after neuroleptic
Preceding anesthesia with muscle cell-depolarizing agents	No	No	Yes	No	No
Preceding neuroleptics	Maybe	Maybe	Maybe	Maybe	Yes
Preceding serotoninergic agents	Maybe	Maybe	Maybe	Yes	Maybe
Autonomic dysfunction	Maybe	No	No	No	Yes
Episodes: stupor mixed with episodes of excitement	Yes	No	No	No	Maybe
Diaphoresis	Maybe	No	Maybe	Maybe	Yes
Rigidity	Fluctuating	No	Yes	Yes	Yes

Reprinted with permission form *J Neuropsychiatr Clin Neurosci* 4, 265–269, Sewell DD and Jeste DV. Distinguishing neuroleptic malignant syndrome (NMS) from NMS-like acute medical illnesses: A study of 34 cases. Copyright 1991.

The syndrome of lethal catatonia (seen in patients with uncontrolled manic excitement or catatonic schizophrenia) can mimic NMS (with increased temperature, autonomic irregularities and elevated creatine kinase), and the differential diagnosis can be difficult. It is obviously important to determine whether the patient is indeed being treated with an antipsychotic. Although NMS may clinically look like catatonia, NMS does not typically have alternating periods of catatonic excitement and catatonic mutism. A past history of catatonic episodes is also important in making the differential diagnosis. Lorazepam may be useful in alleviating the symptoms of catatonia but it has not been shown to be useful in treatment of NMS. Therefore, it is possible that a brief lorazepam trial could provide a useful and relatively easy method of distinguishing between these two conditions. The problem, of course, is that not all cases of catatonia respond to lorazepam.

Heat stroke may also look like NMS but typically differs in that it presents with hypotension, dry skin and limb flaccidity (American Psychiatric Association, 2000). Malignant hyperthermia can also have a similar presentation but generally occurs within the context of a patient's receiving halogenated anesthetic agents or succinylcholine. This condition typically begins immediately after administration of the anesthetic agent and only in genetically susceptible individuals (American Psychiatric Association, 2000).

Medications can cause a number of conditions that may present as syndromes similar to NMS. Allergic drug reactions may produce fever and autonomic instability but not rigidity. Serotonin syndrome, with common clinical characteristics including fever, resting tremor, rigidity, myoclonus and generalized seizures should also be considered. A medication history can usually help distinguish between the two syndromes, but patients receiving antipsychotics may also be treated with selective serotonin reuptake inhibitors, thus making the clinical picture more confusing. Lithium intoxication and anticholinergic delirium can both resemble NMS, as can intoxication with amphetamines, cocaine and phencyclidine as well as rapid termination of antiparkinsonian medication.

Course

The course of NMS is variable. Some cases may progress to fatality, whereas others may follow a mild self-limited course. Once the syndrome is recognized and the antipsychotic medication is discontinued, the syndrome usually resolves between 2 weeks and 1 month (American Psychiatric Association, 2000).

Mortality rate is reported to be 4 to 25%. The most common medical complications leading to morbidity and mortality are respiratory failure and renal failure. Shalev and coworkers (1989) reported that myoglobinemia and renal failure are the best predictors of mortality in NMS; the presence of either condition imparted a 50% mortality risk. In general, complications are a result of physiologic consequences of severe rigidity and immobilization such as deep vein thrombosis, pulmonary embolism, dehydration and an increased risk for rhabdomyolysis.

Treatment

The most critical step in treatment (Table 64.4) is to recognize the clinical features of the syndrome and rapidly discontinue the antipsychotic. The importance of this initial step mandates that psychiatrists who use antipsychotics in their practice be cognizant of the early clinical features and recognize that the syndrome can occur at any time during the course of treatment. Once the antipsychotic has been stopped, supportive care remains the core of treatment and often must be carried out in the context of a medical intensive care unit. Each supportive intervention should be targeted to a specific symptom. Examples of interventions include cooling blankets for fever, cardiac monitoring for arrhythmias, parenteral hydration for dehydration and monitoring for urine output and renal function. Dialysis may also be considered for acute renal failure.

It should be noted that despite their widespread use, the efficacy of the muscle relaxant dantrolene and the dopamine agonist bromocriptine has not been thoroughly established. Electroconvulsive therapy is another treatment option in NMS presumably because it increases dopamine turnover in the brain. Electroconvulsive therapy is particularly indicated when there is difficulty in distinguishing between NMS and lethal catatonia and when there seems to be a significant risk of recurrence of NMS on restarting neuroleptics. Some psychiatrists report rapid

Table 64.4	Treatment of Neuroleptic Malignant Syndrome
Step 1	Assess medication regimen • Stop dopamine antagonists • Restart any recently stopped dopamine agonists
Step 2	Supportive care • Monitor vital signs • Administer intravenous fluids • Provide cooling blankets • Administer antipyretics • Consider dialysis for acute renal failure
Step 3	No improvement within 24–28 h • Administer oral bromocriptine 5 mg PO t.i.d. to be increased daily by 5 mg increments until positive response • Continue bromocriptine for 10 d, then withdraw in period of 1 wk • Monitor for relapse
Step 4	If patient cannot tolerate bromocriptine or cannot take oral medications • Administer intravenous dantrolene 1–3 mg/kg/body weight q.i.d. • Gradually increase dose until positive response
Step 5	Consider adding bromocriptine to dantrolene
Step 6	Consider discontinuing all medications and giving supportive care only
Step 7	Consider electroconvulsive therapy after 3–4 d, if no improvement

Reprinted with permission form *J Neuropsychiatr Clin Neurosci* 4, 265–269, Sewell DD and Jeste DV. Distinguishing neuroleptic malignant syndrome (NMS) from NMS-like acute medical illnesses: A study of 34 cases. Copyright 1991.

and dramatic success in the use of electroconvulsive therapy for NMS.

At present, the appropriate course is to begin with antipsychotic discontinuation and supportive care and to consider antidote therapy only if improvement in symptoms is not seen within the first few days. The treatment of NMS should be individualized for each patient based on clinical signs and symptoms. For example, supportive care may be sufficient in mild and early cases of NMS. Trials of bromocriptine, dantrolene, or amantadine are suggested for patients with moderate symptoms. Anticholinergics can be used in managing afebrile patients with neuroleptic-induced parkinsonian symptoms and benzodiazepines may be useful for agitation in NMS. ECT is recommended in situations where lethal catatonia is suspected, when NMS symptoms are treatment refractory, and in patients who remain psychotic in the immediate post-NMS period.

A particular difficulty for the psychotic patient who has NMS is that rechallenge with antipsychotics may cause NMS to recur. Successful rechallenge seems to be positively related to the length of time elapsed after resolution of NMS. There is some evidence to suggest that clozapine may have relatively little propensity to induce NMS. Clozapine, therefore, may represent one option for the patient who has experienced NMS with a conventional agent. It is likely but not yet known definitively that atypical antipsychotics will prove to have a lower frequency of NMS. In general, it is recommended to switch to an agent in a different chemical class and with a lower D_2 affinity compared with the causal agent.

Medication-induced Postural Tremor

Etiology and Pathophysiology

This category refers to fine postural action tremor that develops as a result of a medication. Medications that have been reported to cause such an effect are lithium, beta-adrenergic agonist medications, stimulants, dopaminergic medications, anticonvulsant medications, antipsychotics, antidepressant medications and methylxanthines (e.g., caffeine) (American Psychiatric Association, 2000). The psychotropic medication most typically associated with such tremor is lithium, and most of the available information on medication-induced tremor relates to that caused by lithium.

Normal muscle contractions are accompanied by tremor as a result of contractions of muscle fiber recruitment. This tremor is typically low in amplitude and is referred to as a physiological tremor. When these contractions are maintained, the amplitude of the tremor increases and it becomes visible. This is referred to as an enhanced physiological tremor. A number of medications, including lithium and bronchodilators, produce an enhanced physiological tremor. The pathophysiological mechanism of these tremors is not well understood but seems to relate to adrenergic changes (probably mediated in the locus coeruleus) in the mechanical properties of the skeletal muscle. The response of these tremors to beta-adrenergic blocking agents and their exacerbation as a result of beta-adrenergic agonists seem to lend support to the notion of adrenergic mediation.

Epidemiology and Comorbidity

Estimates of the frequency of lithium-induced tremor vary widely across the literature and range between 4 and 65%. Lifetime

DSM-IV-TR Criteria 333.1

Medication-induced Postural Tremor

A. A fine postural tremor that has developed in association with the use of a medication (e.g., lithium, antidepressant medication, valproic acid).

B. The tremor (i.e., a regular, rhythmic oscillation of the limbs, head, mouth, or tongue) has a frequency between 8 and 12 cycles per second.

C. The symptoms are not due to a preexisting nonpharmacologically induced tremor. Evidence that the symptoms are due to a preexisting tremor might include the following: the tremor was present prior to the introduction of the medication, the tremor does not correlate with serum levels of the medication, and the tremor persists after discontinuation of the medication.

D. The symptoms are not better accounted for by neuroleptic-induced parkinsonism.

Reprinted with permission from the *Diagnostic and Statistical Manual of Mental Disorders*, Fourth Edition, Text Revision. Copyright 2000 American Psychiatric Association.

incidence of tremor is estimated to be 25 to 50% of patients starting lithium therapy. A number of possible risk factors have been proposed to predispose a person to development of a lithium-induced tremor. These include older age, greater serum lithium levels, concomitant use of antidepressant or antipsychotic medication, greater caffeine intake, history of tremor, alcohol dependence and anxiety (American Psychiatric Association, 2000).

Assessment and Differential Diagnosis

Lithium-induced tremor may appear as soon as treatment is initiated. As the lithium level increases, the tremor becomes more severe and coarse and may have associated muscle twitching or fasciculations (American Psychiatric Association, 2000). Complaints about the tremor are typically greatest at the beginning of therapy. There is disagreement as to whether the tremor typically remains stable or improves with time on lithium.

The lithium-induced tremor is reasonably easy to diagnose. It is a rhythmical action tremor. It is most commonly seen in the hands or fingers but can occasionally be seen in the head, mouth, or tongue (American Psychiatric Association, 2000). The frequency of the tremor is typically 8 to 12 Hz and is similar in appearance to an essential tremor. It may usually be seen by asking the patient to hold the affected body part in a stable position. The tremor is made worse by anxiety, stress, fatigue, hypoglycemia, thyrotoxicosis, pheochromocytoma, hypothermia, alcohol withdrawal, performance of voluntary movements and concomitant administration of cyclic antidepressant medications.

The most difficult differential diagnosis involves distinguishing a lithium-induced tremor from a tremor that was preexisting. To be classified as a medication-induced tremor, it must have a temporal relationship to the medication, it must relate to the serum level of the medication, and it must not persist after the medication is discontinued. A similar postural tremor is essential tremor, and differentiation between the two is nearly

impossible clinically without the medication history. Any of the factors listed that may exacerbate a medication-induced tremor can also cause a similar tremor in the absence of the medication. Medication-induced tremor may resemble NIP. NIP, however, is generally worse at rest, is lower in frequency, and has other associated features of parkinsonism (American Psychiatric Association, 2000).

Course

The literature suggests that there is some risk that tremor may be embarrassing for certain patients and could impair activities that require delicate movements. The actual percentage of patients who are bothered by their tremor is unknown. There do not appear to be any long-term sequelae as a result of having a medication-induced postural tremor. A sudden worsening of tremor may be indicative of the beginning of lithium intoxication.

Treatment

Most treatment options have been described for treatment of lithium-induced tremor. Typically the tremor is benign, is not bothersome to the patient, and requires no specific intervention. Some cases, however, require treatment because of the patient's concern about the side effect. Preliminary measures include possibly reducing the lithium dose (if clinically feasible), changing the lithium dose to one-time evening administration, or changing the lithium preparation. Caffeine intake should be reduced or eliminated, and anxiety should be pharmacologically or behaviorally treated.

Beta-blockers represent the best-studied method for gaining pharmacological control of the tremor if the preliminary measures are ineffective. Arana and Rosenbaum (2000) recommended starting propranolol on an as-needed basis. They suggested 10 to 20 mg a half-hour before the activity in which the tremor must not be present. If a patient requires chronic relief from the tremor, propranolol should be initiated at 10 to 20 mg b.i.d and increased until adequate dose for suppression of the tremor is attained. Propranolol may decrease glomerular filtration rate and may result in a reduction in renal lithium clearance. This suggests that patients who require long-term beta-blocker suppression for tremor need to have lithium levels checked more regularly even when they are taking a stable dose of lithium.

There is little information in the literature as to the possible treatment of tremor induced by medications other than lithium and further investigations are needed to elucidate this syndrome.

Comparison of DSM-IV/ICD-10 Diagnostic Criteria

Some of these categories are included in Chapter VI of ICD-10 (Diseases of the Nervous System) but no diagnostic criteria or definitions are provided.

References

Adler LA, Rotrosen J, Edson R *et al.* (1999) Vitamin E treatment for tardive dyskinesia. *Arch Gen Psychiatr* 56, 836–841.

American Psychiatric Association (2000) *Diagnostic and Statistical Manual of Mental Disorders*, 4th edn. Text Rev. APA, Washington DC.

Arana GW and Rosenbaum JF (2000) *Handbook of Psychiatric Drug Therapy*, 4th edn. Lippincott, Williams & Wilkins, Philadelphia.

Caligiuri MP, Rockwell E and Jeste DV (1998) Extrapyramidal side effects in patients with Alzheimer's disease treated with low-dose neuroleptic medication. *Am J Geriatr Psychiatr* 6, 75–82.

Caligiuri MP, Lacro JP and Jeste DV (1999) Incidence and predictors of drug-induced parkinsonism in older psychiatric patients treated with very low doses of neuroleptics. *J Clin Psychopharmacol* 19, 322–328.

Jeste DV, Rockwell E, Harris MJ *et al.* (1999) Conventional versus newer antipsychotics in elderly patients. *Am J Geriatr Psychiatr* 7, 70–76.

Kane JM, Woerner M and Lieberman J (1988b) Tardive dyskinesia: Prevalence, incidence, and risk factors. *J Clin Psychopharmacol* 8(4), 52S–56S.

Marsden CD and Jenner P (1980) The pathophysiology of extra-pyramidal side-effects of neuroleptic drugs. *Psychol Med* 10, 55–72.

Saltz BL, Woerner MG, Kane JM *et al.* (1991) Prospective study of tardive dyskinesia incidence in the elderly. *J Am Med Assoc* 266, 2402–2406.

Sewell DD and Jeste DV (1991) Distinguishing neuroleptic malignant syndrome (NMS) from NMS-like acute medical illnesses: A study of 34 cases. *J Neuropsychiatr Clin Neurosci* 4, 265–269.

Shalev A, Hermesh H and Munitz H (1989) Mortality from neuroleptic malignant syndrome. *J Clin Psychiatr* 50, 18–25.

Yassa R and Jeste DV (1992) Gender differences in tardive dyskinesia: A critical review of the literature. *Schizophr Bull* 18(4), 701–715.

65 Relational Problems

Introduction

A relational problem is a situation in which two or more emotionally attached individuals (i.e., family members, romantic partners) engage in communication or behavior patterns that are destructive or unsatisfying, or both, to one or more of the individuals. Relational problems deserve clinical attention because, once initiated, they tend to be perpetuating and chronic, and are frequently contemporaneous with or are followed by other serious problems, such as individual symptoms in the most vulnerable members of the family (e.g., depression) or social unit dissolution (e.g., divorce). They may be diagnosed either in the presence or absence of individual disorders given in the *Diagnostic and Statistical Manual of Mental Disorders* (DSM).

The strength and direction of causality between the individual and the relational problem are empirically undetermined. Few empirical investigations of the relational problems that are "precursors" to individual pathology have been conducted. Most of the existing research selects disturbed family units in which one member has an existing disorder (e.g., schizophrenia, depression) and examines the communication difficulties that accompany the disorder. Thus, cause-and-effect relations between individual disorders and relational difficulties have not been experimentally specified.

There is also the issue of generalization: Do those who manifest relational problems with a spouse or other family member manifest these same problems with others and in other contexts? Only a beginning literature exists on this issue. However, preliminary data suggest that some individuals manifest severe communication difficulties with their spouses or other family members but not with persons outside the family.

Definition

Relational problems are placed in the fourth edition of the DSM (DSM-IV-TR) section on "other conditions that may be a focus of clinical attention". Five specific relational problems are described chiefly in terms of patterns of impaired family interaction related to:

- a mental or general medical condition
- parent–child problem
- partner
- sibling
- not otherwise specified (e.g. difficulties with others outside of the family).

Constructs and Manifestations of Relational Problems

The empirical data substantiate the existence of relational difficulties that can be reliably assessed and have clinical significance. The data are sparse in reference to each DSM disorder and coexisting family relational difficulties, with the exceptions of depression and schizophrenia.

In our examination of the construct of relational problems, we emphasize those constructs that have shown reliable assessment in research and that have been found to 1) distinguish distressed from nondistressed couples or families, or 2) to identify couples or families in which one or more members manifest significant individual pathologic conditions.

Four major constructs (Table 65.1) have been investigated that describe nodal areas of relational difficulty in the family and marital environment: structure, communication, expression of affect and problem solving. Relational difficulties in other environments (e.g., work) have not been described in the clinical literature.

It is interesting to compare the constructs investigated in the couples and family contexts. The areas of affective communication and conflict resolution are almost identical in conceptualization, behavioral criteria and importance in the spouse–spouse and parent–child communication domains. However, three other rather sharply defined constructs in the parent–child literature are not fully represented in the spouse–spouse literature: communication deviance (CD), emotional overinvolvement and coercive process. In the cognitive realm, the CD construct (unclear, amorphous, or fragmented communication) has been investigated primarily among schizophrenic patients and their parents; comparable work has not been done with couples. The more general construct of communication has been explored with marital couples, with no theoretical link to thought disorder and schizophrenia.

Coercive processes – the shaping of the behavior of parents by negative behavior on the part of the child – is similar to negative escalation in couples. Although not yet investigated in couples, it is quite conceivable that one spouse could effectively utilize a coercive process with the other spouse. Overinvolvement, which has been explored in the parent–child literature, may have a related domain in the marital literature, specifically, structure. Indeed, the over involvement construct has been seen as most relevant with children and parents and has little predictive utility in adult couple samples. However, it seems that the concept of structure, with the issues of leadership, dominance and submission, and distribution of functions, is an area that needs further exploration in reference to both couples and the entire family.

Essentials of Psychiatry   Jerald Kay and Allan Tasman
© 2006 John Wiley & Sons, Ltd.

Table 65.1	Empirically Derived Family Relational Constructs
Structure	Leadership and distribution of functions
Overinvolvement	Unclear boundaries; overdependence
Communication	Amount and clarity of information exchange
deviance	Unclear, amorphous, fragmented, and/ or unintelligible communication
Communication	
Coercion	Behavior control by use of aversive communication
Expression of affect	Implicit or explicit verbalization of affective tone
Problem solving	Definition of problems, consideration of alternative lines of action, agreement to use optimal line of action
Conflict resolution and its	Process of resolving differences of opinion

Structure

For a marriage or family to function as a unit requires leadership and distribution of functions. Leadership, dominance and power distribution can all have a profound effect on the quality of interaction satisfaction and on adequate functioning of both couples and families, both in ordinary and in stressful circumstances.

Couples

Dominance as measured by verbal frequency has not distinguished functional and dysfunctional families. When one spouse is depressed, the power distribution is not always as theoretically hypothesized (i.e., depressed spouse submissive to dominance of the nondepressed partner). Contrary to expectation, depressed patients produce substantial control-oriented communication with their spouses during an acute depressed episode. Introversion and interpersonal dependency may reflect enduring abnormalities in the functioning of individuals with remitted depression.

Families

Some parent–offspring relationships are marked by unclear boundaries and overdependence, often inhibiting the offspring's ability to separate, individuate, or recover from illness. With respect to psychiatric and sometimes medical disorders, it is not unusual to see a pairing of an overprotective, overinvolved parent with a highly disabled, passive, withdrawn offspring. Because ill offspring in these families often elicit such responses, an overinvolved relationship is best thought of as a dyadic attribute rather than a problem generated by a parent. Overinvolvement is often difficult to define or assess in parents of school-age or adolescent children. However, among studies of youth, those focusing

on separation anxiety, and school refusal in particular, describe parental overinvolvement and protectiveness as complicating features.

The term **expressed emotion** (EE) is used to refer to critical comments, hostility, and/or overinvolvement as expressed by a family member toward another family member with a mental disorder. Studies suggest that overinvolvement is a risk factor for later episodes of psychosis among patients diagnosed with schizophrenia, independent of the level of criticism demonstrated by the family.

Communication of Information

Verbal communication between two or more individuals involves the various aspects of information exchange, including the amount and clarity of the information and the reception of the information by another. This broad concept of communication implies the willingness to convey information, the accuracy and clarity of the information, and the accurate decoding of the information by the other.

Couples

The amount and quality of verbal communication have differentiated distressed and nondistressed couples, and treatment leads to an improvement in communication.

Five areas of cognitive phenomena are hypothesized to play important roles in marital communication and maladjustment: selective attention, attributions, expectancies, assumptions and standards. Not all of these areas have been equally investigated.

Distressed spouses focus on negative behavior; positive interactions often are ignored. Distressed spouses tend to attribute their partner's undesired communication behavior as global and the partner is blamed for her or his negative behavior, which is seen as intentional, global, stable and originating from internal factors. In contrast, nondistressed individuals give each other credit for positive behavior and overlook or exonerate their spouses for negative behavior. While the evolution or developmental history of these cognitive sets has not been clearly delineated, current evidence suggests that negative attributions for partner behavior may predict marital satisfaction over time.

Families

Many of the same disordered processes (e.g., expression of hostility or excessive criticism, poor information exchange, lack of conflict resolution) in the spousal communication literature are presumed to disrupt healthy family functioning. Unlike in the marital literature, however, the independent variable in family studies is often the presence or absence of a psychopathologic condition in an offspring or parent rather than high or low levels of marital distress.

Diagnosis of Relational Disorders

Although research on structure, expression of affect, communication and problem solving in couples and families has lead to a greater understanding of the difficulties that can afflict these relational units, specific relational problems have only been recently included as a diagnostic entity in the DSM and clear diagnostic criteria have yet to be developed. Current textual descriptions of these conditions refer to impairment in the "pattern of interaction" in these relational units (American Psychiatric Association,

2000, p. 736), reflecting the broad range of specific difficulties subsumed under these diagnostic entities.

Phenomenology

Five specific relational problems are noted in DSM-IV (see the definition section above). Family relational problems and partner relational problems are delineated below. These difficulties may also afflict relational units in the presence of a mental disorder or medical condition. The phenomenology of sibling relational problems and relational problems with other individuals have not been well explored.

Partner Relational Problems

Clinical experience and the research descriptions suggest that marital (and couples) relational problems manifest in the following ways:

1. Couple does not clarify mutual requests, provide information, or accurately describe problems.
2. Spouse or spouses verbalize underlying attributions, assumptions and expectations that are negative (e.g., spouse is globally negatively intentioned) or exaggerated (e.g., couples should never fight).
3. Affective communication is characterized by negative affect (e.g., anger, hostility, jealousy), critical remarks, disagreement with spouse and nonacceptance of what the mate has communicated.
4. There is a low frequency of self-disclosure of thoughts, feelings and wishes.
5. Couple demonstrates inadequate problem solving characterized by poor problem definition, lack of task focus, mutual criticism and complaint, and negative escalation.
6. Couple displays sequences of negative communication characterized by criticism, disagreement, negative listening and refusal to agree.
7. Couple avoids conflict by withdrawal, lack of discussion and subsequent nonresolution.

Associated features of marital communication difficulties or disorders include poor marital satisfaction, psychiatric disorder in one or both spouses, threatened and contemplated separation and divorce, or concentration and job performance difficulties.

Family Relational Problems

Family relational problems manifest as the following:

1. Family is unable to communicate clearly, cannot communicate closure, or cannot share a focus of attention (CD).
2. Family communication is characterized by unidirectional hostility or frequent criticism or by bidirectional, negatively escalating cycles of pejorative or critical comments.
3. Parent–offspring relationships are characterized by overprotectiveness, overconcern, unnecessarily self-sacrificing behaviors, intrusiveness, or overdependence (emotional overinvolvement).
4. Parent–offspring interchanges are marked by negatively reinforcing coercive cycles that tend to perpetuate antisocial or aggressive behavior in one or more family members.

5. A broad array of family problems cannot be solved because of the family's inability to agree to try to solve, define, generate, or evaluate solutions to, or implement solutions to, existing problems.

The associated features of parent–child communication difficulties or disorders include adolescent acting out and disruptive behavior, major psychiatric disorders in one or more family members (i.e., schizophrenia, affective disorder), poor parental morale and parenting dissatisfaction.

Assessment of Relational Disorders

Overall Relationship Functioning

The Global Assessment of Relational Functioning Scale (GARF) (Group for Advancement of Psychiatry, 1996) included in DSM-IV-TR is a 1 to 100 scale of overall relationship functioning, akin to the Global Assessment Scale for individuals. Recent studies have indicated that the GARF is reliable in clinical settings and that changes in GARF scores are positively associated with both patient and therapist-reported change in treatment and with treatment satisfaction.

Epidemiology of Relational Disorders

The raw frequency of relational disorders (broadly defined) in the general population is unknown. No epidemiological studies have been done, in part because of the absence of accepted diagnostic criteria for these disorders. There are rather vague "proxies" of relational disorders that are useful in making estimations of their prevalence, such as the approximate frequencies of divorce in the general populus (40–50% of all couples) or of marital violence (12–33% of couples). Factors such as divorce or violence, however, are best thought of as relational events rather than relational disorders. A single incident of marital violence does not necessarily signal the presence of a family relational disorder (in the absence of confirmatory information), nor is a diagnosable relational disorder in a spousal couple necessarily associated with divorce. Thus, the prevalence of specific types of relational disorders, as described in this chapter, is difficult to estimate.

A further difficulty in making these estimations in the normal population is that certain of the constructs conveyed, such as expressed emotion (EE) assume the presence of a psychiatric disorder in an index family member. Also, the goal of EE and other family psychopathological studies has been to examine family attribute–outcome relationships on a within-group basis in psychiatric disorders rather than to making comparisons between families of psychiatric patients and nonpsychiatric control subjects. Thus, data are lacking on the frequencies of high-EE attitudes or other family attributes in normal control groups.

The paucity of studies on the frequency of family relational disorders points to the need to develop strict operational criteria for these disorders and to conduct epidemiological studies using random sampling techniques, much as is done for individual disorders. The availability of epidemiological data would allow us to determine not only the need for treatment of specific relational disorders, but also their comorbidity with individual or other relational disorders, their associated features, and the social conditions under which they are most likely to arise.

Treatment

Specific Goals of Treatment

The primary goal of treatment is to bring the relational unit to a more satisfying, organized and less conflictual level of functioning. The mediating goals of treatment are focused on improvement in the specific areas of functioning of the relational unit (i.e., structure, communication, affect expression, problem solving). In relational units where one member is suffering from a mental disorder or medical condition (e.g., schizophrenia, depression, childhood disruptive behavior disorder), additional goals include the reduction of individual symptoms and improvements in psychosocial functioning.

Treatment Format

Relational problems are best observed and treated directly in a family format in which the conflicted family members are present with the therapist. However, there may be certain situations in which relational problems are more conducive to change within an individual treatment format. For example, relational problems related to an individual with a mental disorder (e.g., a 25-year-old son with schizophrenia, in conflict with his mother and father) may in some cases best be approached by individual sessions with the affected person. Further, when one adult in a family unit is depressed, individual interpersonal or cognitive psychotherapies may be used and focused on conflict resolution.

Treatment Strategies and Techniques

The specific techniques available to family therapists can be divided into five categories: psychoeducational, cognitive–behavioral, structural, strategic–systemic and insight-oriented. Psychoeducational approaches are most helpful when there is a family member with a specific medical or psychiatric disorder, and the family can utilize information on how to manage the disorder with the least tension and stress on the patient. Cognitive–behavioral techniques are useful in improving communication and problem-solving skills and the positive interactive behaviors in marital-family units. Structural and strategic–systemic approaches are most useful in rearranging the repetitive interactions in a family that constitute the boundaries and alliances in the social system.

In practice, there are many common elements and much eclectic usage of strategies and techniques across the various schools of family intervention. Family therapy shares many of the common treatment elements with other forms of psychotherapy. All psychosocial treatments require the development and maintenance of a good patient–therapist relationship, or therapeutic alliance. There is an assumption that most patients experience some degree of corrective emotional experience, or reliving of significant life experiences in the presence of an empathic therapist who demonstrates new ways of relating. In this context, the patient (or patients) is able to identify with the therapist and utilize the behaviors discussed and modeled. In all forms of psychotherapy, there is a certain degree of transmission of new information. The learning can be about methods of behavior, ways of thinking, or increased awareness of complex emotions. Most therapies involve some shaping of people's behavior through implicit and explicit rewards for behavior considered appropriate, and discouragement of behaviors considered harmful. This shaping can occur through advice, suggestion, persuasion, role-playing and practice.

Standard Approach to Treatment

There is increasing evidence for the efficacy of family and marital interventions in the treatment of a broad range of relational problems and psychopathology. However, several specific questions about treatment efficacy can be asked here in reference to the previous review of relational difficulties:

1. Do the specific relational difficulties (i.e., structure, communication, affect and problem solving) respond to intervention?
2. Do the individual disorders associated with relational problems (e.g., schizophrenia, affective disorders, adolescent delinquent behavior) show improvements in illness course when the relational problems are at least part of the focus of intervention?

Research suggests that family treatment is effective with schizophrenia, affective disorders, adolescent and child acting-out difficulties and eating disorders. In terms of strategies and techniques used in the family and marital treatment formats, there is substantial evidence for the effectiveness of cognitive–behavioral and psychoeducational techniques, with few data on the other approaches. Future studies should compare the efficacy of (and estimate the relative treatment effect sizes attributable to) family therapy versus competing therapies (i.e., individual or group therapies). Future research should also determine the optimal format in which to administer family treatment (i.e., home-based versus clinic-based; individual families versus multifamily educational groups).

Medical Comorbidity

Relational problems can cooccur with virtually any general medical condition. In most cases, it can be convincingly argued that a medical condition in one member (e.g., cancer) can promulgate relational problems between this member and other members or between two other members of the family (e.g., a husband and wife who develop marital problems stemming from disagreements as to how to treat their daughter's juvenile-onset diabetes). In some cases, the relational problems may have prognostic value for the course of the medical condition and thus may become a focus of ancillary treatment.

Numerous attempts have been made to link the family constructs listed earlier (i.e., structure, communication, expression of affect and problem solving) to the concurrent severity or future outcome of various medical conditions. For example, Koenigsberg and coworkers (1993) examined levels of spousal EE in relation to glucose control in diabetic patients. The number of critical comments made by a spouse significantly predicted glycosylated hemoglobin levels (a measure of glucose control) in the patient, the latter having been measured for the 2- to 3-month period before the interview.

There is evidence that enhanced family problem-solving may be a protective factor in the course of certain medical conditions. Using a pattern-recognition procedure, Reiss and associates (1986) examined the problem-solving interactions of families in which one member had end-stage renal disease requiring long-term hemodialysis. High family scores on "delayed closure" during a problem-solving task indicated that a family was "environmentally sensitive", open to new information in choosing solutions, and willing to introduce new solutions when new information was available. The authors found these high scores predicted fewer medical complications in the affected family member during a 9-month follow-up period.

While family-based interventions for medical conditions have not been sufficiently investigated, there is some evidence of their utility, particularly for the treatment of chronic childhood diseases) where families are faced with numerous challenges in promoting health and adjusting to often-complex medical regimens. Family-based psychoeducational interventions in the treatment of sickle cell disease have resulted in greater disease knowledge among participating families when compared with treatment as usual. In a clinical trial, behavior family systems therapy with adolescents with insulin-dependent diabetes mellitus resulted in lower diabetes-specific family conflict and improvements in the parent–child relationship when compared with treatment as usual and to an educational support group.

It is clear that chronic and progressive medical illness cooccurs with a host of relational difficulties that may in some cases bode poorly for the outcome of the medical condition. In most instances, these relational disturbances seem to arise in reaction to the medical condition and are not apparently causally related to the disorder itself. Family or marital intervention in medical conditions may, however, reduce the tension in the household and the level of burden and psychosocial stress experienced by the caretaking family member(s), which could in turn provide a more protective environment for the ill family member.

References

American Psychiatric Association (2000) *Diagnostic and Statistical Manual of Mental Disorders*, 4th edn., Text Rev. APA, Washington DC.

Group for the Advancement of Psychiatry, Committee on the Family (1996) Global assessment of relational functioning scale (GARF): I. Background and rationale. *Fam Process* 35, 155–172.

Koenigsberg HW, Klausner E, Pelino D *et al.* (1993) Expressed emotion and glucose control in insulin-dependent diabetes mellitus. *Am J Psychiatr* 150, 1114–1115.

Reiss D, Gonzalez S and Kramer N (1986) Family process, chronic illness, and death. *Arch Gen Psychiatr* 43, 795–804.

PART

Six

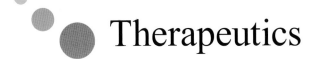

Therapeutics

CHAPTER

66

Individual Psychoanalytic Psychotherapy

Psychoanalytic theory provides the modern clinician with a comprehensive system for the understanding of personality development, the meaningfulness of human conflict and emotional pain, and the mutative factors within the doctor–patient relationship. Psychoanalysis is a general psychology, a developmental theory and a specific treatment. Since its inception, psychoanalytic theory has undergone numerous and substantial revisions. Its history and the movements that contributed to its evolution are described in Chapter 18. With respect to psychoanalysis as a treatment approach, its history has been punctuated by persistent attempts both to simplify psychoanalytic technique and to shorten its duration of treatment. The synonymous terms psychoanalytic psychotherapy, psychoanalytically oriented psychotherapy, psychodynamic psychotherapy and expressive psychotherapy have come to represent the most coherent of these attempts.

What is Psychoanalytic Psychotherapy?

It is customary to define psychotherapy in a broad fashion as being composed of three distinct components: a healing agent, a sufferer and a healing or therapeutic relationship (Frank and Frank, 1991). Strupp (1986) specified that psychotherapy is the systematic use of a human relationship for therapeutic purposes of alleviating emotional distress by effecting enduring changes in a patient's thinking, feelings and behavior. The mutual engagement of the patient and the psychotherapist, both cognitively and emotionally, is the foundation for effective psychotherapeutic work.

Whereas there are many different types of psychotherapy (Figure 66.1), the core task of the psychoanalytic psychotherapist is to make contact with and comprehend, as thoroughly as possible, the patient's subjective inner world to engage in an analytical (i.e., interpretive) conversation about it (Ornstein and Kay, 1990). This core task implies that all psychoanalytic psychotherapies may be further defined in terms of three operations: accepting, understanding and explaining (Ornstein and Ornstein, 1985) (Table 66.1). First, and more specifically, the therapist must engage with the patient by accepting the subjective experience of the patient's emotional pain and conflict. This is achieved through the establishment of a therapeutic dialogue based on an empathic, nonjudgmental rapport. Secondly, within the process of listening to, and feeling with, the patient, the therapist will begin to develop an understanding of the intricacies of the patient's plight. Much of what the therapist observes may at first remain outside of the patient's conscious awareness, manifested in the form of reenactments and reliving of earlier experiences within

the therapy, rather than in deliberate, conscious, descriptive communication. Last, by the sharing of this beginning understanding with the patient through a simultaneously empathic and interpretive mode, both arrive at a deeper appreciation for the genesis of, and the reasons for, the patient's symptoms. The shared relationship in which understanding is gained is no less instrumental in achieving change than are the insights and modified perceptions that may result from the psychotherapeutic experience.

It is appropriate to conceptualize psychoanalytic psychotherapy as being on a continuum of expressive to supportive (Luborsky, 1984; Gabbard, 1994). Traditionally, to the degree that psychoanalytic psychotherapy has focused on the recovery of repressed psychological material, it has been called "expressive" and has been distinguished from the supportive psychotherapies which have concentrated on the shoring up of certain defense mechanisms. This implies that any given treatment might employ more or less expressive and supportive interventions, depending on what is transpiring within the psychotherapeutic process. An important skill of the psychoanalytic psychotherapist is then the ability to employ the appropriate balance of both expressive and supportive interventions as dictated by the needs of the patient. Finally, the conceptualization of an expressive–supportive continuum also facilitates the establishment of therapeutic goals, interventional plans and indications for individual psychoanalytic psychotherapy (Gabbard, 1994) (Table 66.2).

The theoretical concepts that derived from the theory reviewed in Chapter 18 constitute, more or less, the assumptions behind all psychoanalytic psychotherapy. These include, most importantly, the role of the unconscious; the centrality of transference; the characterological defense mechanisms; and the resistance to self-awareness and thereby to progress in the therapeutic setting. Of secondary importance, but nevertheless closely related to the unconscious, is the concept of psychic determinism, namely, that people behave in specific ways for specific reasons. No experience or memory, according to psychoanalysis, is ever lost but resides in the unconscious, which continues to influence current and future ways of experiencing feelings, thoughts and behaviors. Advances in cognitive neuroscience have supported the notion that many significant experiences throughout life remain outside of awareness.

Transference and Resistance, Countertransference and Counterresistance

Transference and resistance constitute the two most distinctive features of psychoanalytic psychotherapies. Transference is

Essentials of Psychiatry   Jerald Kay and Allan Tasman
© 2006 John Wiley & Sons, Ltd.

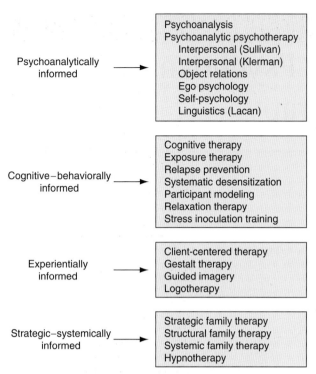

Psychoanalytically informed → Psychoanalysis / Psychoanalytic psychotherapy / Interpersonal (Sullivan) / Interpersonal (Klerman) / Object relations / Ego psychology / Self-psychology / Linguistics (Lacan)

Cognitive–behaviorally informed → Cognitive therapy / Exposure therapy / Relapse prevention / Systematic desensitization / Participant modeling / Relaxation therapy / Stress inoculation training

Experientially informed → Client-centered therapy / Gestalt therapy / Guided imagery / Logotherapy

Strategic–systemically informed → Strategic family therapy / Structural family therapy / Systemic family therapy / Hypnotherapy

Figure 66.1   *Some types of psychotherapy.*

Table 66.2	Comparative Interventions	
Expressive	←Continuum→	Supportive
Confrontation		Suggestion
Clarification		Reassurance
Interpretation		Advice giving
Interpretation of transference		Praise
		Environmental intervention and manipulation

defined as those perceptions of, and responses to, a person in the here and now that more appropriately reflect past feelings about, or responses to, important people earlier in one's life, especially parents and siblings. Psychoanalytic psychotherapy stresses the importance of transference within the treatment relationship, but it differs from psychoanalysis in that it does not, to the same degree, promote the depth and intensity of the transference.

Countertransference is variously defined as 1) the analyst's or psychotherapist's transference reactions to the patient; 2) his or her reactions to the patient's transferences; and 3) any reactions, feelings and attitudes of the analyst or therapist toward the patient, regardless of their source. These responses are manifestations of the requisite engagement by the therapist or analyst in the emotional process of treatment. Moreover, these reactions are a rich source of understanding of the patient's experience as it touches the therapist affectively. Although countertransference feelings are at times uncomfortable for the therapist and a challenge to monitor and process, they are understood as a reflection of the glue of the relationship without which no real connection or significant change can occur.

Resistance is broadly defined as the conscious or, more often, unconscious force within the patient opposing the emergence of unconscious material. Resistance must be understood not as something the patient does to the therapist, but rather as the patient's attempt to protect herself or himself by avoiding the anticipated emotional discomfort that accompanies the emergence of conflictual, dangerous, or painful experiences, feelings, thoughts, memories, needs and desires. Resistance occurs through the use of unconscious mental operations called defense mechanisms, for which there is substantial research support (Vaillant, 1992; Horowitz *et al.*, 1995) (Table 66.3). The recognition, clarification and interpretation of resistance constitute important activities of the psychoanalyst and the psychoanalytic psychotherapist, both of whom must first appreciate how a patient is warding off anxiety before understanding why he or she is so compelled.

Counterresistance refers to those psychological processes within the therapist that impede therapeutic progress. These are reactions to some aspect of the treatment experience that unconsciously create anxiety in the therapist. Such occurrences become accessible first to conscious awareness and then to self-study or self-analytical work often in the form of a mistake or a symptom experienced in a therapy session. As an example, the therapist might forget the patient's appointment time or feel sleepy or bored during a therapy session. Countertransference feelings may also be manifested in dreams or fantasies about the patient. Analysis of such symptoms of countertransference not only can facilitate progress in a stalled treatment but may lead to significant growth in self-understanding by the therapist, as well as improved understanding of the patient.

Table 66.1	Essential Operations of Psychoanalytic Psychotherapy
Accepting	The therapist affirms the patient's past and present subjective experience
Understanding	The therapist appreciates both the conscious and the unconscious contributions to the patient's emotional problems
Explaining	The therapist expresses, through interpretations, his or her understanding to the patient

Adapted with permission from Ornstein PH and Ornstein A (1985) Clinical understanding and explaining: The empathic vantage point, in *Progress in Self Psychology*, Vol. 1 (ed. Goldberg A). Guilford Press, New York, pp. 43–61.

Basic Technique

The analysis of transference by the interpretation of resistance is important for the psychoanalytic psychotherapist. To promote the patient's examination of the phenomena of transference and resistance, both the analyst and the therapist are guided by principles that establish a confidential, safe and predictable environment geared toward maximizing the patient's introspection and focus on the therapeutic relationship. The patient is encouraged to free associate, that is, to notice and report as well as she or he can whatever comes into conscious awareness (Tables 66.4 and 66.5).

Table 66.3	Some Common Defense Mechanisms*
Repression	Relegation of threatening wishes, needs, or impulses into unawareness
Projection	Attribution of conflicted thoughts or feelings to another or to a group of people
Denial	Refusal to appreciate information about oneself or others
Identification	Patterning of oneself after another
Projective identification	Attribution of unacceptable personality characteristics onto another followed by identification with that other
Regression	A partial return to earlier levels of adaptation to avoid conflict
Splitting	Experiencing of others as being all good or all bad, i.e., idealization or devaluation
Reaction formation	Transformation of an unwanted thought or feeling into its opposite
Isolation	Divorcing a feeling from its unpleasant idea
Rationalization	Using seemingly logical explanations to make untenable feelings or thoughts more acceptable
Displacement	Redirection of unpleasant feelings or thoughts onto another object
Dissociation	Splitting off thought or feeling from its original source
Conversion	Transformation of unacceptable wishes or thoughts into body sensations
Sublimation	A mature mechanism whereby unacceptable thoughts and feelings are channeled into socially acceptable ones

*All defense mechanisms are involuntary and unconscious.

Therapeutic neutrality and abstinence are related concepts. Both foster the unfolding and deepening of the transference, as well as the opportunity for its interpretation. The psychoanalytic psychotherapist assumes a neutral position *vis-à-vis* the patient's psychological material by neither advocating for the patient's wishes and needs nor prohibiting against these. The patient is encouraged in the therapeutic relationship to develop the capacity for self-observation. Neutrality does not mean nonresponsiveness; it is nonjudgmental nondirectiveness.

Abstinence refers to the position assumed by the psychoanalytic psychotherapist of recognizing and accepting the patient's wishes and emotional needs, particularly as they emanate from transference distortions, while abstaining from direct gratification of those needs through action. Abstinence is a principle that guards against the therapist's gratification at the patient's expense. For example, as the treatment experience deepens into a more consolidated transference neurosis, there may be a strong tendency by the patient to experience the therapist as **the** important person in the patient's life around whom the characteristic conflictual issues are manifested. By maintaining a neutral and abstinent position with respect to the patient's needs and wishes, the psychotherapist creates a safe atmosphere for the experiencing

Table 66.4	Characteristics of Psychoanalysis
Goals	Personality reorganization Resolution of childhood conflicts
Patient's characteristics	Psychoneuroses and mild to moderate personality disorders Psychological mindedness Introspectiveness Can experience and learn from intense affects or conflicts without acting them out Reasonable object relationships High motivation Can tolerate frustration and therapeutic regression
Techniques	Use of couch Four or five sessions weekly Free association Neutrality Abstinence Analysis of defenses Analysis of transference Dream interpretation Genetic reconstruction Less frequent use of medication
Length of treatment	3–6 yr or longer

Table 66.5	Characteristics of Psychoanalytic Psychotherapy
Goals	Partial personality reorganization Appreciation of conflicts and related defense mechanisms Partial reconstruction of the past Symptom relief Improved interpersonal relationships
Patient's characteristics	Includes all criteria for psychoanalysis Moderate to severe personality disorders (e.g., borderline) Some affective disorders with and without medication (e.g., major depression, dysthymia)
Techniques	Active therapeutic stance Face to face (sitting up) One to three sessions weekly Limited free association Active focus on current life issues Limited transference analysis Some supportive techniques Liberal use of medication Clarification and interpretation
Length of treatment	Months to years (may or may not be shorter than psychoanalysis)

and expression of even highly charged affects, the safety required for the patient's motivation for continued therapeutic work. The position held by the psychiatrist is neither sterile nor overstimulating and promotes the establishment of a meaningful therapeutic relationship.

The rule of free association dictates that the patient should verbalize to the best of her or his ability whatever comes into awareness, including thoughts, feelings, physical sensations, memories, dreams, fears, wishes, fantasies and perceptions of the analyst. Whereas at first glance this requirement appears to be unscientific, in fact, the psychiatrist and patient quickly come to appreciate that no thought or feeling is random or irrelevant but rather that all mental content is relevant to the patient's emotional problems. Indeed, much productive therapeutic work is focused on those instances when the patient is not able to speak about what is on his or her mind.

Many psychoanalytic psychotherapists also use the technique of dream interpretation, although recently there may be less emphasis on this. Freud placed great emphasis on the interpretation of dreams because he discovered that such a technique provided insights into the working of the unconscious. In a similar fashion, slips of the tongue, jokes, puns and some types of forgetfulness are attended to carefully by the therapist because they are nonsleep activities that also provide insight into the patient's unconscious mental processes. Good technique does not necessarily include pointing out to the patient these events each time they occur, for they may often be a source of intense embarrassment. Rather, the slips are noted as helpful data in assessing the patient's inner thoughts.

All of these techniques are embedded in a unique manner of listening to the patient's verbalizations within the context of the treatment situation. In particular, two related but specific components initially attributed to the listening process are worthy of note. First, the concept of the evenly hovering or evenly suspended attention implies that listening to the patient requires of the therapist that he or she be nonjudgmental and give equal attention to every topic and detail that the patient provides. It also embraces the notion that the effective therapist is one who can remain open to her or his own thoughts and feelings as they are evoked while listening to the patient. Such internal responses often supply important insights into the patient's concerns. Secondly, empathic listening is of equal importance to both parties. Empathy permits the patient to feel understood, as well as provides the therapist with a method to achieve vicarious introspection. Indeed, one of the major contributions of self-psychology has been the identification of empathic listening and interpretation (the immersion by the therapist into the subjectivity of the patient's experience) as basic to the methodology of psychoanalysis and psychoanalytic psychotherapy (Kohut, 1978, 1971). Interferences to successful empathic listening are often the product of countertransference reactions, which should be suspected whenever, for example, the therapist experiences irritation, strong erotic feelings, or inattention during a treatment session.

How Does Psychoanalytic Psychotherapy Work?

Psychoanalytic psychotherapy helps by permitting the patient to become increasingly conscious of troublesome feelings, conflicts and wishes that heretofore had remained out of awareness and that produced unhappiness by promoting repetitive self-defeating behaviors, that is to gain "insight".

Whereas insight has always been valued as a goal, insight by itself is insufficient. The process whereby insight is acquired is a lengthy and arduous one that is inextricably linked with the recall of painful affects, memories and traumatic experiences. For treatment to be effective, there must be both cognitive and affective experiences for the patient. Neither a purely intellectual nor a purely cathartic experience is likely to result in relief or behavioral change. The support provided by the treatment relationship, which includes commitment, respect, reliability, honesty and care, is a powerful factor in the curative process. It is this atmosphere that makes bearable the emotional pain that accompanies the healing of the wounds first experienced in isolation, so often inflicted by the first objects of the patient's love, need and trust. All of these considerations are central to psychoanalytic psychotherapy as well.

The concept of "working through" is helpful in appreciating the often lengthy and complex psychotherapeutic processes. Working through is that stage or aspect of treatment characterized by repeated identification of reenactment and reliving of earlier experiences through confrontation, clarification, and interpretation of resistance and transference that ultimately promotes the patient's self-awareness. In effect, the working through process frees the patient from the position of being at the mercy of unconscious conflicts and fears that have compromised interpersonal relationships and achievement. This is accomplished not only through the analysis of the transference but also of current interpersonal relationships outside of the psychotherapy. Ultimately, a thorough understanding of the transference and of current relationships can permit the patient to appreciate their relationship to important early experiences and ultimately to ameliorate the influence of the past on the present.

Therapeutic Alliance

A great deal of research in the outcome of psychoanalytic psychotherapy has focused on the importance of the therapeutic alliance (Docherty, 1985). Increasing appreciation for the role of supportive factors, such as the rapport between the patient and therapist that constitutes the therapeutic relationship, has balanced the earlier and more narrowly defined position that attributed therapeutic success exclusively to insight resulting from specific interpretive activity. The clinical consequences of this appreciation of the helpfulness of nonspecific factors have been the psychoanalytic psychotherapist's paying much greater attention to the initial phases of engaging the patient in psychotherapy and a greater respect for those positive and negative factors that the therapist brings to the working relationship. Currently, approaches to psychoanalytic psychotherapy hold that the psychiatrist's personality and interventional technique have equal influence on the therapeutic process. In essence, the contemporary view is more dyadic, and places greater importance on the contributions of the therapist (both the conscious and the unconscious), as well as of the patient with respect to progress and impasse in the psychotherapeutic process.

Contemporary psychoanalytic psychotherapists still emphasize elucidation of the unconscious, especially within the transference, and still use interpretation as a primary clinical intervention, but recognizes more fully the important role of the mutual emotional engagement of therapist and patient and the curative role of this relationship in addition to other supportive factors. They adhere to a much broader perspective on human development and psychiatric disorders. Psychological problems

Table 66.6	Indications for Psychoanalysis

Psychoanalysis is the treatment of choice for repetitive, longstanding, maladaptive problems involving personality or character and chronic, repetitive behavioral, affective, or mental disturbances or symptoms that do not respond to cheaper or quicker forms of treatment. In general, it is used for all the character disorders or personality disorders, except antisocial and schizotypal disorders, as well as numerous symptom disorders.

The chronic symptoms must reflect both:

1. Intrapsychic conflict
2. Developmental arrest or inhibition

As well, the psychiatrist must expect that:

3. The patient's symptoms are likely to continue unless analysis is undertaken
4. Treatments that are less intensive than analysis would likely result in excessive personal or social cost for the patient or just provide temporary relief of acute symptoms related to a current stress, without dealing with underlying issues, hence predisposing the patient to difficulties in future.

Finally, the patient must be able to use psychoanalysis. In general, this rules out the psychotic disorders and a number, but not all, of the borderline disorders.

Reprinted with permission from the American Psychiatric Association (1985) *Peer Review Manual*, 3rd edn. APA, Washington DC.

can result not only from early intrapsychic conflict but also from developmental deficits or failures as well as from psychological trauma (Table 66.6).

How Does Psychoanalytic Psychotherapy Differ from Psychoanalysis?

The answer to this question has occupied many researchers and psychiatrists throughout the last 50 years. Efforts have been made continually not only to elucidate the differences between the two treatments but, more important, to define the underlying principles of psychoanalytic psychotherapy. Whereas some prefer definitions of psychoanalysis and psychotherapy as distinct separate entities, it is more useful to many psychiatrists to conceptualize psychoanalysis and psychoanalytic psychotherapy as residing on a therapeutic continuum. As discussed, there is much in the conduct of psychoanalytic psychotherapy that has been borrowed from psychoanalysis. Free association, clarification and interpretation in psychoanalytic psychotherapy are such examples. The centrality of transference is another, although early psychiatrists and researchers advocated that transferences were to be recognized and acknowledged in psychoanalytic psychotherapy and "managed" rather than interpreted so that patients were not subject to the intense therapeutic regressions characteristic of psychoanalysis. Today, such a distinction regarding the approach to transference in psychoanalytic psychotherapy is less rigid.

On the other hand, certain supportive and more directive techniques, such as greater activity of the therapist through focusing the patient on specific current problems and relationships, reassuring and affirming the patient, and the giving of advice, are used much more in psychoanalytic psychotherapy than in

Table 66.7	Phases of Psychoanalytic Psychotherapy
Beginning phase	Patient is educated about roles of both parties
	Therapeutic alliance is formed → symptomatic relief from nonspecific relationship factors
Middle phase	Usually the longest phase of therapy
	Reexperiencing of patient's conflicts within dyad
	Interpretation of conscious and previously unconscious material → new insightfulness about current, past and sometimes previously forgotten experiences
Termination phase	Begins with agreed-on end of treatment
	Anxiety evoked by impending loss of therapist
	Initial symptoms may recur
	Integration and consolidation of therapeutic gains
	Therapist is viewed with less distortion

psychoanalysis. Therefore, the adherence to the therapist's neutrality is less strict, and as a result, there is often but not always less frustration for the patient in psychoanalytic psychotherapy. The length of treatment may not distinguish the two approaches, but the frequency of sessions (four or five per week) and the use of the couch, however, are characteristic of psychoanalysis (see Table 66.7).

Overall, it is fair to say that psychoanalytic psychotherapy

- Places greater emphasis on the here and now in terms of the patient's current interpersonal relationships and experiences outside of the therapy; whereas in psychoanalysis, there is greater emphasis on the experiences within the analysis and the relationship between analyst and analysand;
- Incorporates, more than does psychoanalysis, various other techniques from other dynamic and behavioral psychotherapies;
- Emphasizes the usefulness of focusing on current (dynamic) problems and less on genetic issues; and
- Establishes more modest goals of treatment.

The last point is particularly important in that it facilitated the development of brief dynamic psychotherapies which address focal problems generally in up to 20 sessions.

Tasks of the Psychoanalytic Psychotherapist

What are the challenges of the psychotherapist in performing psychoanalytic psychotherapy? First, the therapist must ensure that the patient can feel both emotionally and physically safe within the therapeutic relationship. This is accomplished by acknowledging the goals of the treatment and defining the role of the therapist and through establishing professional boundaries. Boundaries refer to those constant and highly predictable components of the treatment situation that constitute the framework of the working relationship. For example, agreeing to meet with the patient for a specified amount of time, in a professional office, and for an established fee are some of the elements of the professional framework.

Boundaries also have ethical dimensions best summarized as the absolute adherence by the therapist to the rule of never taking advantage of the patient: through sexual behavior; for personal, financial, or emotional gain; or by exploiting the patient's need and love for the therapist in any fashion (e.g., by using the therapy sessions to discuss the therapist's own problems). The concepts of neutrality, abstinence and confidentiality further define the role of the therapist. A critical task of the psychoanalytic psychotherapist is to detect when a breach in either role or boundary has occurred and to restore the patient's security through clarifying and interpreting the meaningfulness of such a breach.

The explication of a boundary violation is but one specific example of the technique of interpretation. Successful interpretation is based on a number of prerequisite skills. These include the capacity to empathize with the patient's plight, the ability to recognize the meaning of one's own fantasies about, and responses to, a patient (countertransference), the ability to maintain the patient's verbal flow through the use of open-ended or focused questions, and the capacity to tolerate a relatively high level of ambiguity within the therapeutic relationship. One important professional characteristic of the skilled psychotherapist is patience. Psychotherapy is often arduous, and the capacity to "stay in the chair" with the patient is critical.

The identification of repeated patterns of behavior both within the therapy and in the patient's outside life is a fundamental technique in making sense of the patient's emotional life. This, of course, involves the appreciation of transference and the art of knowing how and when to share this recognition with the patient. Interpretation relies on both appropriate timing and dosage. That is, the psychoanalytic psychotherapist must appreciate when the patient can best integrate the therapist's observations and must respect the patient's defenses, taking care not to overwhelm the patient by insisting that she or he confront more than is tolerable.

Psychoanalytic psychotherapy requires the successful engagement of the patient and the establishment of a therapeutic or working alliance. The alliance can be threatened by a number of phenomena including, but not limited to, the following:

- The therapist's countertransferences or other limitations in his or her capacity to tolerate the emotions stirred by the patient, resulting in empathic failures and mistakes.
- The emergence of intense feelings and needs within the patient, for example, when an accurate well-timed intervention evokes feelings in relation to the therapist of appreciation and love accompanied by feelings of vulnerability, erotic desire, or inferiority which the patient wants to flee.
- The patient's being reminded of the existence of others in the therapist's life, such as other patients or family (e.g., during interruptions due to the therapist's vacations), triggering painful and embarrassing feelings of jealousy and possessiveness.

The therapist's ability to appreciate and respectfully to acknowledge to the patient the impact of these temporal events is critical to the progress of treatment.

All of the psychotherapist's skills and techniques must be embedded in a consistent and coherent theoretical viewpoint that provides the therapist with a framework to understand the etiology and meaning of a patient's symptoms and dysfunctional behaviors both in the past and in the present in each of the phases of psychotherapy (Table 66.7).

This includes an organized method for understanding the therapist's unconscious and conscious responses to the patient as well. It requires that the therapist listen to the patient's communications in a manner that is markedly different from other forms of social discourse. So-called "process communication" speaks to the therapist on multiple levels and through displacement, through passing remarks and jokes, through shifts in topics, and through metaphors and symbols. To assist in understanding complicated process communication, psychiatrists often ask themselves, Why is the patient telling me this now? What might the patient be trying to say about his or her uncomfortable feelings? Is something being said about the therapeutic relationship?

The objective of this type of treatment is to improve the patient's quality of life largely through enhancing interpersonal relationships by promoting greater insight into perceptual distortion and intrapsychic and interpersonal conflict. Psychoanalytic psychotherapy accomplishes this objective by focusing on the patient's current predicaments as manifested in both life activities and relationship with the therapist. It is at times less concerned with the analysis of transference and the complete discovery of the underlying genetic precursors of the patient's current psychological problems, depending on the specific clinical situation.

Indications for Psychoanalytic Psychotherapy

Although current psychotherapy research attempts to ascertain which specific disorder in which type of patient is most effectively treated by what specific psychotherapeutic approach, studies have not as yet provided the answers to these questions. Conditions and disorders for which psychoanalytic psychotherapy appears to be indicated include personality disorders (except antisocial personality disorder); post traumatic stress disorders; symptom neuroses or neurotic conflicts; adjustment disorders; paraphilias; and **some** mood, anxiety, somatoform, sexual and gender identity, eating, substance abuse and dissociative disorders (Table 66.8). In addition, psychoanalytic psychotherapy is often employed in treating patients who present with relational problems and those

Table 66.8	Putative Indications for Psychoanalytic Psychotherapy
Neuroses	
Personality disorders (except antisocial personality disorder)	
Post traumatic stress disorders	
Adjustment disorders	
Paraphilias*	
Mood disorders*	
Anxiety disorders*	
Somatoform disorders*	
Sexual and gender identity disorders*	
Eating disorders*	
Substance abuse disorders*	
Dissociative disorders*	
Relational problems	
Impulse-control disorders*	
Psychological problems affecting medical illnesses	

*Not indicated for all disorders in these categories.

problems that are the result of abuse or neglect. It may also be useful to patients with certain impulse disorders and to patients whose psychological problems are affecting or are the result of their primary medical illnesses. In short, psychoanalytic psychotherapy, often in combination with medication, is an appropriate intervention in a broad range of disorders, conditions and psychiatric illnesses (Karasu, 1989; Gabbard, 1995).

The characteristics of the patient assumed to be correlated with positive outcome in psychoanalytic psychotherapy include introspectiveness (psychological mindedness); ability to establish and maintain human relationships, even "unhealthy" ones; vocational stability; high degree of motivation; absence of formal thought disorder; and psychological resources sufficient to withstand the possible frustration during the treatment and its characteristic therapeutic regression and accompanying strong affects. Patients with more severe disturbances may be best approached using supportive psychoanalytic psychotherapy discussed below.

Contraindications to Psychoanalytic Psychotherapy

For the most part, contraindications to any psychoanalytic psychotherapy that is heavily weighted toward the expressive end of the therapeutic continuum are as follows (Table 66.9):

- Poor impulse control
- Significant cognitive deficits
- Severely dysfunctional interpersonal relationships
- Little ability to tolerate frustration, anxiety and depression
- Significant lack of introspective capacity

Supportive Psychoanalytic Psychotherapy

Although only recently systematized, this form of psychotherapy provides psychological stabilization to the patient through the vehicle of a consistent and predictable caring therapist–patient relationship (Werman, 1984; Rockland, 1989; Novalis et al., 1993; Hellerstein et al., 1994; Misch, 2000). Supportive psychotherapy attempts to shore up the patient's psychological defenses and enhance his or her ability to cope with the trials of illness or psychological deficits and the challenges they impose on the patient's daily activities (Table 66.10). Not unexpectedly, it also strives to prevent decompensation and regression. As such, psychoanalytic supportive psychotherapy employs a psychodynamic understanding of the patient's difficulties but does not emphasize

Table 66.9   Contraindications to Expressive Psychoanalytic Psychotherapy

Major ego deficits
Poor motivation
Significant cognitive deficits
Inability to obtain symptom relief through understanding
Inability to verbalize affects
Lack of psychological mindedness
Minimal impulse control
No social support network
Low frustration tolerance
Inability to form therapeutic alliance

Table 66.10   Characteristics of Supportive Psychoanalytic Psychotherapy

Goals	Maintain current level of psychological functioning
	Restore premorbid adaptation, if possible
	Enhance coping mechanisms
	Strengthen defense mechanisms unless they are maladaptive
	Support reality testing
	Relieve symptoms
	Decrease mental distress
Patient's characteristics	Severe character disorders
	Chronic ego deficits
	Thought disorders
	Limited psychological mindedness
	Limited motivation
	Poor interpersonal relationships
	Poor impulse control
	Low frustration tolerance
	Regression proneness
	Some potential for therapeutic alliance
	Extreme passivity
	Inability to verbalize affects
	Those in crisis situations (catastrophic loss, acute psychic trauma, medical illness)
	Psychologically healthy
	Effective social network
	High premorbid adaptation
	Flexible defenses
Techniques	Predictability and consistency of therapist
	Conversational style
	Confrontation, clarification, education
	Problem-solving focus
	Provide encouragement, advice, praise, reassurance
	Environmental intervention
	Strengthen reality testing
	Shore up defense mechanisms
	Discourage regression
	Infrequent genetic reconstruction
	Infrequent transference analysis
	Less therapeutic neutrality
	Frequent use of medication
Length of treatment	Usually once weekly or less
	Duration of sessions flexible
	Varies from brief therapy for those reactive disorders in individuals who do not need or are not motivated for further help to lifelong treatment of patients with some chronic disorders

interpretation of the patient's internal world. Rather, supportive psychotherapy focuses on assisting the patient to address interpersonal and environmental challenges in the here and now.

Despite its noninterpretive emphasis, supportive psychotherapy can have a substantial impact in the lives of patients with significant ego deficits and those with major mental illness. These patients may include those with high levels of aggressivity, poor impulse control, overreliance on action rather than verbal expression of emotions, compromised reality testing and limited psychological mindedness. It is also highly effective with higher functioning patients who have experienced recent psychic trauma (e.g., through natural disasters, illness, physical or sexual assault, and unexpected devastating losses).

Supportive psychotherapy techniques consist predominantly of empathically listening to the patient's feelings and experiences; giving advice and reassurance; offering suggestion and helpful coping techniques; and for some patients with severe and chronic maladaptations, gently revealing their misperceptions and how they interfere in daily functioning. Although often unexpressed, the patient's identification with the therapist's values, ideals and approaches to problems is exceptionally therapeutic. Environmental interventions through helping agencies and the patient's significant others are also effective supportive techniques. Although nonspecific to some degree, these interventions are nevertheless based on a comprehensive understanding of the patient's strengths and weaknesses, and are frequently instrumental in curbing self-destructive and self-defeating behaviors. Transference is appreciated but the therapist rarely interprets it in supportive psychoanalytic psychotherapy, choosing rather to foster a positive working relationship through other means (Pinsker et al., 1992).

Although frequently disparaged, effective supportive psychoanalytic psychotherapy is often more challenging to provide than some forms of expressive psychotherapy. Appreciating the psychological forces that are impinging on a marginally functioning patient whose communicative abilities are suboptimal requires a sophisticated clinical approach. Moreover, in supportive psychotherapy, the therapist must assist the patient to modulate intense affective states that are often frightening to the patient and to those in his or her environment. Needless to say, such affects can be directed at the therapist as well. The establishment with the patient of the requisite safe and caring relationship, which may be frequently disrupted by both internal and external forces, is often a significant clinical challenge.

Supportive psychotherapy can produce significant and lasting behavioral change through the reinforcement of health-promoting behaviors; increased capacity for self-reflection; anxiety reduction; and development of new defenses such as intellectualization that enable the patient to acquire a cognitive, anxiety-reducing conceptualization of her or his difficulties.

Gender Issues in Psychotherapy

Does the gender of the psychotherapist have any effect on the psychotherapeutic relationship and treatment outcome? Are certain psychological problems best treated by therapists whose gender is different from that of the patient? Do different phenomena appear in the treatment of those patients whose therapists are of the same gender? Is the duration of treatment affected by the therapist's gender? Does gender have any influence on the choice of therapist by a patient? These are important questions that have been debated in psychotherapy and psychoanalytic literature for more than 50 years.

Although the literature regarding the advantages and disadvantages of gender matching of patients and therapists consists largely of anecdotal and negative reports (Zlotnick et al., 1998), it is nevertheless evocative. A number of common themes have emerged, including that

- The gender of the therapist may be more critical in supportive treatments that rely on identification with the therapist (Cavenar and Werman, 1983).
- The therapist's gender may be less important in psychoanalysis than in face-to-face psychoanalytic psychotherapies because, in the latter, the transference can be less intense (Mogul, 1982).
- Beginning women therapists have less difficulty with empathy but more difficulty with authority issues than do their male counterparts (Kaplan, 1979).

Although there is only one controlled study and it showed no difference regarding the influence of the therapist's gender on the therapeutic process (Zlotnick et al., 1996), there is much to consider about the influence of actual gender and gender-related beliefs of both patient and therapist on the emergence of transference and countertransference. However, the best psychoanalytic psychotherapies will include ample opportunities for the working through of the patient's issues related to important figures of both genders.

Ethnocultural Issues in Psychotherapy

Culture refers to meanings, values and behavioral norms that are learned and transmitted in the dominant society and within its social groups. Culture powerfully influences cognitions, feeling and "self" concept, as well as the diagnostic process and treatment decisions. Ethnicity, a related concept, refers to social groupings which distinguish themselves from other groups based on ideas of shared descent and aspirations, as well as to behavioral norms and forms of personal identity associated with such groups (Mezzich et al., 1993).

Given the increasing multiculturalism of many cities in the USA, how should the psychoanalytic psychotherapist treat patients from cultures other than his or her own? Whereas therapists are obligated to be culturally informed, Foulks and colleagues (1995) have argued against the promotion of culturally specific psychotherapies. Although acknowledging that some cross-cultural psychiatrists believe expressive–supportive psychotherapy to be an ethnotherapy appropriate only to the citizens of the Western world, they emphasized the overwhelming problems in establishing separate therapies and clinics devoted to patients from a multitude of specific cultures. Also, they stated that the principles of psychotherapy elucidated in this chapter – accepting, understanding and explaining – are appropriate for the culturally diverse patient.

Is Psychoanalytic Psychotherapy Effective?

The short answer to this question is yes. Meta-analytical studies of psychotherapy have demonstrated unequivocally that psychotherapy is effective (Luborsky et al., 1975; Smith et al., 1980; Lambert et al., 1986). The study by Smith and coworkers (1980), for example, demonstrated that 80% of those patients treated in psychotherapy fared better on outcome measures than those who received no treatment. Psychological growth achieved through psychotherapy is also enduring (Husby, 1985).

Cost-offset studies have repeatedly demonstrated the helpfulness of psychotherapy in reducing general health care services by as much as one-third (Mumford *et al.*, 1984; Krupnick and Pincus, 1992; Olfson and Pincus, 1994). These include reduction in hospital stays for surgical and cardiac patients (Mumford *et al.*, 1982) and decreased treatment costs for those with respiratory illnesses, diabetes and hypertension (Schlesinger *et al.*, 1983). Brief psychotherapy has also been shown to be effective in general medical clinics, where those patients with significant medical and psychiatric problems improve substantially more than those treated by primary care physicians alone (Meyer *et al.*, 1981).

Luborsky and coworkers (1993) have demonstrated that psychoanalytic psychotherapy is as effective as cognitive, behavioral, experiential, and group therapies and hypnotherapy. For this meta-analysis, rigorous inclusion criteria were established including, but not limited to, adequate sample size with random assignment, suitable length and frequency of sessions, sound outcome measures, adherence by therapists to treatment manuals, and comparable skill levels among therapists. A number of other studies have demonstrated positive benefits in panic disorder depression, personality disorder, drug abuse, eating disorders and others (Willborg and Dahl, 1996; Bateman and Fonagy, 2001.)

The important research questions with respect to brief psychoanalytic psychotherapy have been summarized by Barber (1994) and are relevant to all psychoanalytic psychotherapies (Table 66.11).

Towards a Neurobiology of Psychotherapy

Exciting new research in psychiatry, brain imaging, cognitive neuroscience, genetics, and molecular biology has provided striking insights into how psychotherapy actually changes both brain structure and function (Liggan and Kay, 1999; Gabbard, 2000; Lehrer and Kay, 2002). Learning and memory are associated with alterations in central nervous system (CNS) neuronal plasticity including increased synaptic strength and number of synapses. Neurogenesis, or the creation of new brain cells, occurs daily in the human hippocampus (Eriksson *et al.*, 1998),

the central location for the formation of new explicit memories. Not only does memory consolidation lead to persistent modfications in synaptic plasticity, but psychotherapy, a form of learning, also produces changes in the permanent storage of information acquired throughout an individual's life and provides new resources to address important psychobiological relationships between affect, attachment and memory which is of fundamental importance in psychiatric disorders. Rapidly accruing knowledge about the different types of memory and the role of the amygdala now support the influence of memories that reside outside of the awareness of our patients (LeDoux, 1996). Implicit memories formed in infancy and childhood persistently affect the manner in which patients experience themselves and their worlds as manifested, for example, in transference reactions within and outside of the therapeutic relationship.

The study of psychotherapy from a neurobiological perspective is likely to provide greater understanding of how words in the context of therapeutic relationships can heal. It may be that there are similar mechanisms and anatomical regions that are involved in the successful treatment of psychiatric illness with psychotherapy and pharmacotherapy as monotherapies, as well as in the combined treatment situation (Sacheim, 2001). It is also likely to yield a greater understanding of pathogenesis and delineate helpful interventions to decrease genetic vulnerability to emotional disorders.

Conclusion

At this time, the theory and technique of psychoanalytic psychotherapy provide the most comprehensive orientation to the continuum of expressive–supportive psychotherapy. Psychoanalytic psychotherapy is a potent intervention and, as such, holds great promise when it is used in a sophisticated fashion for appropriate patients with appropriate psychiatric problems. Like medication, psychoanalytic psychotherapy has specific indications, contraindications and, undoubtedly, potentially negative effects. As an effective therapeutic intervention, it requires that the therapist be highly skilled in assessing the inner experience of those who come for help. It also requires extensive training and education in techniques of this treatment modality. As well, the therapist must acquire significant self-knowledge, sophistication and dedication in working so intensively with human pain.

Table 66.11	**Research Challenges for Psychoanalytic Psychotherapy**

Determining efficacy for specific disorders

Developing treatment guidelines for interpersonal problems and personality disorders

Developing reliable and valid self-report measures for core conflicts

Measuring potential cost-offset of different therapies

Determining efficacy of short-term vs. long-term psychotherapies

Matching patients to treatment on basis of personality, functional level, or developmental stage

Examining whether and how experienced therapists can be trained in short-term psychoanalytic treatments

Learning the limits of brief therapy and conditions or symptoms for which longer-term psychotherapy should be recommended

Reprinted with permission from Barber JP (1994) Efficacy of short-term dynamic psychotherapy: Past, present, and future. *J Psychother Pract Res* 3, 108–121. Copyright 1994, American Psychiatric Association.

References

Barber JP (1994) Efficacy of short-term dynamic psychotherapy: Past, present, and future. *J Psychother Pract Res* 3, 108–121.

Bateman A and Fonagy P (2001) Treatment of borderline personality disorder with psychoanalytically oriented partial hospitalization program: An 18-month follow-up. *Am J Psychiatr* 158, 36–42.

Burnand Y, Andreoli A, Kolatte E *et al.* (2002) Psychodynamic psychotherapy and clomipramine in the treatment of major depression. *Psychiatr Serv* 53, 585–590.

Cavenar JO and Werman DS (1983) The sex of the psychotherapist. *Am J Psychiatr* 140, 85–87.

Docherty JP (section ed) (1985) Therapeutic alliance and treatment outcome, in *Psychiatry Update*. American Psychiatric Association Annual Review, Vol. 4 (eds Hales RE and Francis AJ). American Psychiatric Press, Washington DC, pp. 525–633.

Eriksson PS, Perfilieva E, Bjork-Eriksson T *et al.* (1998) Neurogenesis in the adult hippocampus. *Nat Med* 11, 1313–1317.

Foulks EF, Bland IJ and Shervington D (1995) Psychotherapy across cultures, in *American Psychiatric Press Review of Psychiatry*,

Vol. 14 (eds Oldham JM and Riba MB). American Psychiatric Press, Washington DC, pp. 511–528.

Frank JD and Frank JB (1991) *Persuasion and Healing: A Comparative Study of Psychotherapy*, 3rd edn. Johns Hopkins University Press, Baltimore.

Gabbard GO (1994) *Psychodynamic Psychiatry in Clinical Practice*, DSM-IV edn. American Psychiatric Press, Washington DC.

Gabbard GO (ed. in chief) (1995) *Treatments of Psychiatric Disorders*, 2nd edn. American Psychiatric Press, Washington DC.

Gabbard GO (2000) A neurobiologically informed perspective on psychotherapy. *Br J Psychiatr* 177, 117–122.

Hellerstein DJ, Pinsker H, Rosenthal RN *et al.* (1994) Supportive therapy as the treatment model of choice. *J Psychother Pract Res* 3, 300–306.

Horowitz MJ, Milbrath C and Stinson CH (1995) Signs of defensive control locate conflicted topics in discourse. *Arch Gen Psychiatr* 52, 1040–1047.

Husby R (1985) Short-term dynamic psychotherapy IV: Comparison or recorded changes in 33 neurotic patients 2 and 5 years after end of treatment. *Psychother Psychosom* 43, 23–27.

Kaplan A (1979) Toward an analysis of sex-role issues in the therapeutic relationship. *Psychiatry* 42, 112–120.

Karasu TB (ed.) (1989) *Treatment of Psychiatric Disorders*. American Psychiatric Association, Washington DC.

Kohut H (1971) *The Analysis of the Self*. International Universities Press, New York.

Kohut H (1978) Introspection, empathy and psychoanalysis, in *The Search for the Self* (ed Ornstein P). International Universities Press, New York, pp. 205–232.

Krupnick JL and Pincus HA (1992) The cost-effectiveness of psychotherapy: A plan for research. *Am J Psychiatr* 149, 1295–1305.

Lambert MJ, Shapiro DA, and Bergin AE (1986) The effectiveness of psychotherapy. In Handbook of Psychotherapy and Behavior Change, 3rd ed., Garfield SL and Bergin AE (eds). John Wiley, New York, pp. 157–211.

LeDoux J (1996) *The Emotional Brain: The Mysterious Underpinnings of Emotional Life*. Touchstone Books, New York.

Lehrer DS and Kay J (2002) The neurobiology of psychotherapy, in *The Encyclopedia of Psychotherapy* (eds Hersen M and Sledge W). Academic Press, New York, pp. 207–221.

Liggan DY and Kay J (1999) Some neurobiological aspects of psychotherapy. *J Psychother Pract Res* 8, 103–114.

Luborsky L, Singer B, and Luborsky L (1975) Comparative studies of psycotherapies: Is it true that "everyone has won and all must have prizes"? *Arch Gen Psychiatr* 32, 995–1008.

Luborsky L (1984) *Principles of Psychoanalytic Psychotherapy: A Manual for Supportive–Expressive (SE) Treatment*. Basic Books, New York.

Luborsky L, Diguer L, Luborsky E *et al.* (1993) The efficacy of psychodynamic psychotherapy: Is it true that "everyone has won and all must have prizes"? In *Psychodynamic Treatment Research: A Handbook for Clinical Practice* (eds Miller NE, Luborsky L, Barber JP *et al.*). Basic Books, New York, pp. 447–514.

Meyer E, Derogatis LR, Miller MJ *et al.* (1981) Addition of time-limited psychotherapy to medical treatment in a general medical clinic: Results at one-year follow-up. *J Nerv Ment Dis* 169, 780–790.

Mezzich JE, Kleinman A, Fabrega J *et al.* (eds) (1993) *Revised Cultural Proposals for DSM-IV (Technical Report)*. NIMH Cultural and Diagnosis Group, Pittsburgh, PA.

Milrod B, Busch F, Leon AC *et al.* (2001) A pilot open trial of brief psychodynamic pyschotherapy for panic disorder. *J Psychother Pract Res* 10, 239–245.

Misch DA (2000) Basic strategies of dynamic supportive psychotherapy. *J Psychother Pract Res* 9, 173–189.

Mogul KM (1982) Overview: The sex of the therapist. *Am J Psychiatr* 139, 1–11.

Mumford E, Schlesinger HJ and Glass GV (1982) The effects of psychological intervention on recovery from surgery and heart attacks: An analysis of the literature. *Am J Pub Health* 72, 141–152.

Mumford E, Schlesinger HJ, Glass GV *et al.* (1984) A new look at evidence about reduced cost of medical utilization following mental health treatment. *Am J Psychiatr* 141, 1145–1158.

Novalis PN, Rojcewicz SJ and Peele R (1993) *Clinical Manual of Supportive Psychotherapy*. American Psychiatric Press, Washington DC.

Olfson M and Pincus HA (1994) Outpatient psychotherapy in the United States, I: Volume, costs, and user characteristics. *Am J Psychiatr* 151, 1281–1288.

Ornstein PH and Kay J (1990) Development of psychoanalytic self psychology: A historical-conceptual overview, in *American Psychiatric Press Review of Psychiatry*, Vol. 9 (eds Tasman A, Goldfinger SM, and Kaufmann CA). American Psychiatric Press, Washington DC, pp. 303–322.

Ornstein PH and Ornstein A (1985) Clinical understanding and explaining: The empathic vantage point, in Progress in Self Psychology, Vol. 1, (ed Goldberg A). Guilford Press, New York, pp. 43–61.

Pinsker H, Rosenthal R and McCullough L (1992) Dynamic supportive psychotherapy, in *Handbook of Short-term Dynamic Psychotherapy* (eds Crits-Christoph P and Barber JP). Basic Books, New York, pp. 220–247.

Rockland LH (1989) *Supportive Therapy: A Psychodynamic Approach*. Basic Books, New York.

Schlesinger HJ, Mumford E, Glass GV *et al.* (1983) Mental health treatment and medical care utilization in a fee-for-service system: Outpatient mental health treatment following the onset of a chronic disease. *Am J Pub Health* 73, 423–429.

Sacheim HA (2001) Functional brain circuits in major depression and remission. *Arch Gen Psychiatr* 58, 649–650.

Smith ML, Glass GV, and Miller TI (1980) The Benefits of Psychotherapy. The Johns Hopkins University Press, Baltimore.

Strupp HH (1986) The nonspecific hypothesis of therapeutic effectiveness: A current assessment. *Am J Orthopsychiatr* 56, 513–552.

Vaillant GE (1992) *Ego Mechanisms of Defense: A Guide for Clinicians and Researchers*. American Psychiatric Press, Washington DC.

Werman DS (1984) *The Practice of Supportive Psychotherapy*. Brunner/Mazel, New York.

Wilborg IM and Dahl AA (1996) Does brief psychodynamic psychotherapy reduce the relapse rate of panic disorder? *Arch Gen Psychiatr* 53, 689–694.

Woody GE, McLellan AT, Luborsky L *et al.* (1995) Psychotherapy in community methadone programs: A validation study. *Am J Psychiatr* 152, 1302–1308.

Zlotnick C, Shea T, Pilkonis P *et al.* (1996) Gender, type of treatment, dysfunctional attitudes, social support, life events, and depressive symptoms over naturalistic follow-up. *Am J Psychiatr* 153, 10–17.

Zlotnick C, Elkin I and Shea T (1998) Does the gender of a patient or the gender of a therapist affect treatment of patients with major depression? *J Consul Clin Psychol* 66, 655–659.

67 Group Psychotherapy

Human beings live in a social world in which their ability to gain self-esteem and self-definition significantly follows from their success in personal relationships. Psychotherapy in a group setting provides a social arena in which members can learn about their assets and deficits through interactions with peers (fellow members) and authority (the therapist). Members also have opportunities to experiment with newly learned behaviors in the protected atmosphere of the group in preparation for using them in their external world.

A broad spectrum of theoretical approaches informs therapists about which aspects of group behaviors they should attend to. Some focus on individuals as seen through the psychoanalytic lens of transference and resistance; others stress interpersonal transactions in which distortions arising from childhood are played out within the group and are subject to feedback, while others focus on properties of the group as a whole, which emphasize group dynamics and systems theories as the central organizing concepts. Learning principles are contained in almost all of these orientations and are the central emphases in cognitive–behavioral approaches. Successful integration of these approaches has not been accomplished. Therapists may maintain a central theoretical orientation and pragmatically adapt elements from other orientations to address particular problems as they emerge in the treatment process.

The concepts in this chapter primarily address working with adults in an outpatient setting in the psychodynamic tradition. Individuals' internal psychopathologies emerge in the microcosm of the group. They are expressed in interpersonal transactions, which are influenced by the dynamics of the therapeutic system.

Group Development and Group Dynamics

The basic science informing group treatment is group development and dynamics. Understanding of these concepts provides a foundation for the therapist's integration of individual, interpersonal and intrapsychic dynamics with those of group membership (Table 67.1).

Group Development

The seminal work of Bennis and Shepard (1956) produced a spate of studies demonstrating that groups have a natural developmental sequence. Groups must accomplish certain tasks as they move from a collection of individuals to a functioning and working organization. In this discussion, the focus is on developmental sequences in groups conducted along psychodynamic principles.

Table 67.1	Stages of Group Development	
Stage	Theme	Dynamics
Orientation (forming)	Engagement	Dependency Safety Norms
Differentiation (storming)	Power	Testing Competition Autonomy
Maturation (performing)	Work	Affect tolerance Leadership Self–reflection
Termination (departing)	Separation	Loss Hope

Initial (Engagement, Orientation) Phase

Individuals entering a psychotherapy group are faced with two major tasks: they have to decide how they will use the treatment to accomplish their goals and simultaneously they have to determine the limits of emotional safety. Members turn to the therapist in hope of gaining information on how to proceed. They anticipate that the leader, a person they already know and who fulfills a traditional role, will provide guidance and smooth the way in getting to know the strangers in the room. In the main, these "dependency" strivings are frustrated. Members tentatively reveal themselves to others. Gradually, unwritten and primarily unconscious rules (norms) develop, which help contain anxiety and set standards for acceptable behavior. Therapists help shape behavior by providing information on how to proceed and by clarifying (interpreting) underlying anxieties. Common themes and concerns may be highlighted, which serve to diminish members' sense of isolation and enhance cohesion.

Reactive (Power, Differentiation) Phase

Many groups move into this phase by rebelliously rejecting their leader. This may be followed by a relatively short-lived sense of well-being and harmony. However, norms are often experienced as restrictive and members may begin to feel as though they are controlled by the group (group tyranny). In response, they assert individuality and demonstrate their own power. Struggles between members emerge, and angry exchanges are not uncommon. Usual norms against expression of intense intragroup affects are tested and modified in accordance with members' personal capacities. Some members may threaten to quit, or they remain silent during this phase as they grapple with their ability to tolerate

Essentials of Psychiatry   Jerald Kay and Allan Tasman
© 2006 John Wiley & Sons, Ltd.

conflict. The therapist assists in helping members understand and tolerate responses to intense feelings and differences.

Mature (Working) Phase

In this phase, groups have developed considerable cohesion. Members can tolerate differences and they can contain anxiety and allow conflicts to emerge without having to interrupt exchanges. They have learned to provide and receive feedback from others without undue defensiveness. A considerable portion of the group transactions is focused on the here and now, and exchanges are appreciated as containing both reactions to the present and vestiges from prior relationships (transferences). Members attempt to understand one another at both surface and in-depth levels. The therapist no longer is the sole expert, and members are valued for their emotional and cognitive uniqueness. Therapists continue to help patients understand their in-group reactions and assist in broadening their perspectives to include the sources (genetic) of their feelings and their manifestations in their outside world.

Termination Phase

Ending treatment is the final stage. It is filled with mixed feelings: those of success and looking to the future and those surrounding separations (Schermer and Klein, 1996). Often there is a regression as anxieties over departing are addressed. This provides an additional opportunity to explore the problems that emerge. Members respond with pleasure at seeing someone "graduate", but they also experience loss of a valued contributor to the work and envy over a colleague's achievement. A successful termination also offers hope for those who remain. The therapist monitors the dynamic forces and enables members to say their farewells within a context of therapeutic accomplishments and continuing psychological work. In the process, remaining members experience and integrate their responses to the departure.

Summary

Groups do not uniformly traverse these developmental phases, and they undergo shifts to earlier stages under stress, such as vacations or change in membership. A considerable amount of therapeutic work takes place at each developmental level. For instance, a group of individuals experiencing problems with basic trust may spend a good deal of time in an initial stage, where these feelings may be explored. Patients who need to address competitive feelings may alternate between the reactive and the working phases. Understanding group development provides a framework for therapists to appreciate the forces that have an impact on members' feelings and behavior.

Group Dynamics

Group dynamics refer to norms and cultures that are unique to each group. They are influenced by group size, members' race, gender, age and the social environment. Group dynamics are also a product of members' personalities, the leader's functioning and their subsequent interactions. The dynamics emerge as members go about their tasks of determining how they will achieve their goals and maintain personal safety. Norms are rules defining what is acceptable, that is, how people express themselves, what one can do or say. Illustrative of norms are the pressures of using "politically correct" (PC) expressions. There are sanctions, both conscious and unconscious, against violating norms. In part, norms are initially defined in the therapeutic agreement

(discussed later) as presented by the therapist, but they are modified as a result of group development.

The concept of role is intimately linked with group therapy. Roles are essential functions that help the group achieve its goals and support members' emotional tasks. Four general roles can be defined for groups (MacKenzie, 1997): structural, sociable, divergent and cautionary roles. The structural or leadership role helps the group address its work. The therapist is the primary occupant of this role, but members also function in keeping the group on task, organizing the experience and maintaining a perspective of the group process. The social or emotional role helps contain feelings and assists in managing social relationships among the members and with the leader. Some individuals relieve group tensions by changing the topic, making a joke, smoothing ruffled feelings, or by encouraging others to express their less acceptable and/or painful feelings. The divergent role is filled by persons who seem oppositional, who "don't go along with the crowd", or seem to fight authority. They are likely to become a container for unacceptable thoughts or emotions. Such individuals are vulnerable to becoming scapegoated, a process in which inadmissible feelings are seen (or placed) in one person and thereby kept out of awareness in the others. The cautionary or silent role may be played by a member who seldom speaks or keeps his thoughts and feelings hidden. These persons are often a threat to the others because they keep secrets or avoid painful affects. When a group is ready to take action, members often attempt to "recruit" the silent person into their ranks; this process is most frequently seen when there is preparation for fight-or-flight (see discussion of Bion below). Roles may be filled by one or several persons. They are essential for group functioning, and, theoretically, each member has the psychological potential to fill varying roles.

Theories of Group Therapy

The theoretical spectrum informing the practice of group therapy is broad. Within psychodynamics, some emphasize drive theory, object relations, or self-psychology. Other therapists favor interpersonal theory and cognitive–behavioral approaches. Transactional analysis, originating from the work of Berne (1966), and Gestalt therapy (Perls *et al.*, 1951) emphasize interpersonal transactions arising from more traditional psychodynamic theory.

Group theoreticians are generally categorized along a continuum of group as a whole, interpersonal and intrapsychic. Moreover, therapists using object relations, self-psychology or psychodynamic theories integrate their theoretical preferences along this continuum (Kibel, 1992; Harwood and Pines, 1998; Rutan and Stone, 2001). There are few purists and varying degrees of integration is the norm (Table 67.2).

A common thread in many of these theories is that individuals in their interaction and discourse within the group will exhibit their difficulties in relationships, which in turn provides a window into their internal world. In short, the group becomes a microcosm of their external world (Slater, 1966).

Group-as-a-Whole Approaches

These theories emphasize whole-group processes as the primary therapeutic vehicle. They subscribe to notions that members are influenced by the group dynamics and that one or more persons may speak for the entire group, including those who are silent.

Table 67.2 Group Theories

Theory	Authors	Key Phrases
Group-as-a-whole	Bion	Basic assumption, Work group
	Whitaker and Lieberman	Group focal conflict
	Ezriel	Required, Avoided, Calamitous relationship
	Foulkes	Group analysis, Group matrix, Figure/ground
	Horwitz	Integrative, Inductive
Interpersonal	Yalom	Cohesion, Therapeutic factors, Feedback
	Gustafson and Cooper	Unconscious planning
Intrapsychic	Slavson	Limited regression, Transference
	Wolff and Schwartz	Standard analytic, Alternate sessions
	Durkin	Group-as-preoedipal mother, Transference neurosis
	Glatzer	
General system	Durkin	Exchange across boundaries
	Agazarian	Subgrouping
	Ettin	Social and cultural values and attitudes
	Hopper	Social unconscious

Interpersonal Approaches

On the basis of Sullivanian principles, Yalom (1995) emphasized the centrality of transactions in the here and now of the group as the primary, but not exclusive, therapeutic force for change. His formulation of "therapeutic factors" brought into sharp focus the importance of cohesion (which is a dynamic concept that implies that the group is attractive, "safe", and that members have a commitment to the group goals and ideals). Yalom pays particular attention to members' capacity to give and receive feedback. He asserts that maladaptive interpersonal transactions are the consequence of parataxic distortions (having some similarity to transference responses, i.e., arising from childhood experiences) that can be therapeutically altered by authentic human interaction, that is, feedback and consensual validation.

Intrapsychic Approaches

Intrapsychic theories are primarily application of dyadic theory into the group setting. The emphasis is on unconscious processes with the group providing opportunities for patients to regress to a level of internal conflict or developmental arrest. These theories explore individual transferences, resistances and developmental arrests as the primary therapeutic focus. Peers may be experienced as siblings or as displacement objects from parental figures (Slavson, 1950; Wolf and Schwartz, 1962).

Groups may either dilute or intensify transferences to the leader (Horwitz, 1994), which enables "stuck" patients to resolve impasses occurring in dyadic treatment. Regression is limited, and the presence of others creates a balance between the external and the internal worlds (Durkin, 1964). Integration of an intrapsychic framework with that of the group as a whole is contained in descriptions of members' transferences to the group as a preoedipal maternal experience (Glatzer, 1953; Scheidlinger, 1974).

General Systems Approaches

General systems theory is based on open systems theory (von Bertalanffy, 1966). Emphasis is placed on the boundaries separating the group from the external world and members or subgroups from one another (Durkin, 1981). Emphasis on boundaries as worthy of therapeutic concern is evident in the group agreement. Agazarian (1997) elaborated systems concepts into a model of group treatment that focused on subgroups as the primary site of therapeutic attention. She asserted that by focusing on subgroups, which contain individual differences and similarities, members are more prepared to address intrapsychic defenses and resistances.

Beginning a Group

Group Organization

Forming a psychotherapy group is a complex task and attention to organizational details will anticipate some of the potential hazards and smooth the path. Composition, size, fees, place, duration and time of meetings are elements that require decisions in advance of recruiting and preparing potential members.

The size of dynamically-oriented groups ranges from six to 10 members. Groups at the upper size range generally meet for lengthier periods to provide sufficient "airtime" for each person. Smaller groups (four members or less) may be threatened by fears of dissolution (Fulkerson et al., 1981). The duration of meetings is set for 75 to 120 minutes, the norm being 90 minutes. Most groups meet once weekly. Attention must be paid to the group space. An optimal room will comfortably seat eight to 10 persons with unobstructed views of one another. Seats do not have to be identical. Both the position and the type of seat members choose may assume considerable emotional significance. Access to the room needs consideration. Is there time for members to gather in the group room before the meeting, or is a waiting room necessary? In private settings, meetings are occasionally held in a waiting room and therapists must ensure that others do not intrude on that space.

Careful thought must be given to optimal group composition (Table 67.3). Patients chosen for groups that will explore intrapsychic elements should have a capacity for self-reflection and empathy with others. If possible, members with different personality styles should be selected to provide a spectrum of interactive patterns. Other long-term groups may be established with supportive goals and include patients with significant ego deficits. (Groups for the chronically mentally ill are discussed separately later.) Groups designed with a specialized format (e.g., women survivors of sexual abuse, male perpetrators, or individuals with eating disorders) generally are more focused on a symptom or a specific behavior and in such cases balanced membership is of lesser importance.

Table 67.3	Selection of Patients	
Type of Group	Positive Attributes	Negative Attributes
Dynamic	Ego strength	Crisis situation
	Motivation for change	Active substance abuse-related disorder
	Capacity for insight	Sociopathy
	History of satisfying relationship	Cognitive disorder or mental retardation
Supportive	Diminished ego strength	Acute psychosis
	Limited reflective capacity	Disabling cognitive disorders
	Motivation for support	Substance abuse
	Most relationships problematical	
Specialized focus	Common characteristic	Psychosis
	Focus on single problem	Motivation for personality change

Recruiting, Selecting and Preparing Patients

Few applicants requesting psychotherapy consider group treatment. Thus, gathering six to 10 individuals together may not be a simple task. Patients are more likely to agree to enter a group if the rationale is explained to them in some detail. Thus, the therapist needs to be clear about the relationship between group goals and patient goals (to be discussed below). The therapist also needs to be familiar with the patient's history, coping style, symptoms and personality configurations. In obtaining a patient's developmental history, the therapist can specifically search for the person's interaction in group settings, such as school, church, recreation and family. Discussion of the person's typical reactions to group situations helps engage the patient in examining his or her roles in interpersonal situations. The screening and preparatory interviews have five major tasks (Rutan and Stone, 2001):

1. Establish a preliminary alliance between patient and therapist.
2. Define the patients' therapeutic goals.
3. Provide information about the nature of group treatment.
4. Explore the patients' anticipatory anxiety.
5. Discuss the group agreement and gain the patient's acceptance.

Careful screening helps patients anticipate the tasks of entering a group. Such preparation will decrease, but not eliminate premature termination which may range from 20 to 50% of members in newly formed groups.

The Group Agreement

The agreement represents the framework in which treatment will proceed. It promotes a structure that defines boundaries between

Table 67.4	The Group Agreement
Attend all meetings, be on time and remain throughout the session	
Actively work toward treatment goals, remain until they have been achieved and discuss plans to stop treatment	
Observe one's inner reactions to interactions in the group and comment on them	
Use the group for therapeutic and not social purposes	
Put feelings into words and not action	
Be responsible for fees	
Understand the therapist's role	
Protect the confidentiality of the meetings and the anonymity of members	

the group and the environment, among the members and with the therapist. Although members accept the agreement, they also break it. Such disruptions are valuable windows into understanding a person's inner world. The therapist must distinguish between acts that are disruptive to the group and those that carry more benign communications (Nitsun, 1996).

Rutan and Stone (2001) list the elements of the agreement as shown in Table 67.4.

The initial element in the agreement addresses patients' ability to attend all sessions. Those who have responsibilities that interfere with attendance should not be admitted into the group (e.g., executives whose conflicts make them unavailable once every third or fourth week). Similarly, persons who have time conflicts and would consistently come late or leave early should delay entry until their schedule can be adapted to that of the group.

In establishing goals, the patient and therapist enter into a conscious agreement to work toward specified change. However, unconscious elements contributing to a patient's behaviors are likely to emerge in the therapeutic process that may point to additional goals worthy of pursuit. Instructions regarding termination are an additional part of this agreement element. Patients generally have little idea how to stop treatment, and leaders can indicate that sufficient time to take leave of the group is an important part of the therapy. Plans to leave should be discussed and then a date for departure established that allows sufficient time to say goodbye.

The succeeding three elements in the agreement address patient behaviors within the group. Patients slowly learn that one of the major benefits of therapy follows from addressing feelings and reactions to one another and to the therapist. Consistent attainment of this goal suggests that the group is functioning at a mature level. Physical contact and verbal abuse are prohibited. Patients unable to contain these behaviors may be asked to leave the session temporarily. Although physical touching or hugging may seem soothing and reassuring to some individuals, for others it is a threat to their personal boundaries. Those behaviors are open to analysis.

Therapist's Role

The group leader assumes a major, but not the sole, responsibility for the treatment. The therapist's special role is established in part by the agreement. Within that framework, clinicians begin to shape the group to provide participants a way of using their experience to learn about themselves. Assuming that patients'

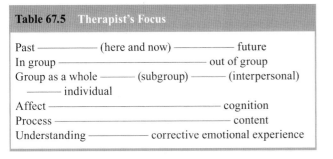

Table 67.5   Therapist's Focus

Past ——————— (here and now) ——————— future
In group ————————————————— out of group
Group as a whole ——— (subgroup) ——— (interpersonal)
————— individual
Affect ————————————————— cognition
Process ————————————————— content
Understanding ————— corrective emotional experience

optimal learning begins with a focus on transactions within the group, psychodynamically-oriented therapists try to find ways of helping members examine resistances and defenses against such engagement. In contrast, clinicians using a more strictly interpersonal (Yalom, 1995) or a system-centered orientation (Agazarian, 1997) may actively instruct members to address one another directly in the here and now of the meeting. The goals of the different approaches are similar: to use the intragroup processes to promote personal change. Therapists always benefit from examining their own contributions to the construction of the group dialogue. The therapist's focus, however, is not exclusively on in-group processes. Rutan and Stone (2001) list six foci for the therapist's attention (Table 67.5):

The major but not exclusive focus promoting change is members learning from the here and now of treatment. Groups develop a rhythm in which members might address outside events as a warm-up to exploring in-group interactions, or they might focus on current feelings and then expand on those experiences in respect to their outside lives, now, in the past, or in the future. Integration of a person's experiences across an extended period enhances feelings of continuity and stability of the self.

The therapist monitors the ebb and flow of affects which reflect the group developmental stage. Members' capacity to tolerate intense feelings is enhanced as trust and cohesion increase. The dialectical tension between affect and cognition is seen in members' roles as they attempt to contain dysphoric states and sustain emotional contacts with one another. Patients may find ways of managing intense feelings through scapegoating or externalizing. These are group-wide processes and should be addressed as such. Some individuals require cognitive understanding before risking immersion into feelings, whereas others search for affective connections before integrating their experience cognitively.

The therapeutic process is fueled by members' searching for new solutions to their developmental arrests and conflicts. In general, members communicate feelings about their in-group experience through associations (not always conscious) to events in their outside world. As such, the associations can be understood as metaphoric communication that informs the treatment process. After a successful interpretation or clarification, associations to external or historical events may represent integration of those experiences into members' psychic structure.

Considerable individual change takes place via the group relationship without overt cognitive integration. The sense of sharing, of being understood, of having needs met, of being responded to in an empathic (corrective) manner may stabilize a shaky psychic structure and, some patients, to their therapist's surprise, may successfully terminate treatment without having achieved understanding (Stone, 1985). These are the powerful forces for change, labeled "corrective emotional" experiences. Patients also strive for cognitive integration of their thoughts and

feelings and, through experiencing and then understanding the here-and-now, external and developmental incidents, they consolidate their learning. Patients are then more prepared to transfer their learning from therapy to situations in their outside world (Ezriel, 1973).

Members' level of self and ego development influence the course of the group as a therapeutic agent. Persons suffering from archaic conflicts of trust or psychic safety, as expressed in a variety of personality disorders (the difficult patient), may require an extended period of therapy exploring these issues. Transferences to the group, leader, or peers emerge that reflect these developmental levels.

Special Treatment Considerations

Scapegoating

Group psychotherapy has been called a hall of mirrors (Foulkes, 1961) where aspects of oneself are seen reflected in others. Scapegoating is the process in which individuals, by "observing" characteristics in another that are unacceptable in themselves, try to deny their feelings and place them in the "offending" person. This process, involving projective identification, is universal and frequently activated during treatment. It is by no means entirely conscious but patients often have an initial awareness that they are attempting to rid themselves of unacceptable feelings or behaviors.

Scapegoating may lead to the "scapegoat's" extrusion from the group. It depletes the group, in the sense that specific emotional responses are not available for examination. Many affects may serve as the stimulus to evoke scapegoating, such as anger, envy, or romantic feelings. Scapegoating becomes virulent because of affect contagion (Freud, 1955), in which feelings become greatly magnified in the communication process and adds a destructiveness to scapegoating.

The therapist's task of protecting the scapegoat is primarily accomplished through assisting members in "taking back" feelings that they are attributing to the scapegoat. A simple illustration is members' anger with an individual who habitually arrives late. That person might be accused of wanting to avoid the group. Analysis of the members' vitriol may reveal that they are also avoiding other intense group feelings. Such an analysis enables the scapegoat to become linked with the others rather than have an isolating experience.

Nonverbal Communication

Patients communicate powerful feelings nonverbally. Discrepancy between verbal and nonverbal messages is confusing, but frequently the latter element is received as the "truth". Patients may tell sad stories and laugh, or they may relate a success in a dreary manner. Members may pull their chairs outside the group circle, sit close to or opposite the therapist, shift position in their chair, or not look at one another during emotionally laden interchanges. White knuckles, crimson blushing, or a black dress are additional colorful communications.

Patients learn to address these meaningful communications as they become comfortable examining in-group behaviors. However, many times the person may be unaware of sending nonverbal messages, and confrontations can be experienced as intrusive and threatening. Stereotyping certain behaviors as carrying predetermined meanings is a common error, and patients learn, sometimes through painful experience, that the sender may have highly personal meanings attached to the behavior.

Exploration of nonverbal behaviors is often a powerful entry into the recipient's and the sender's current and past feelings.

Difficult Patients

A number of individuals appear to be good group candidates, but they prove to benefit little from participation or they seem to obstruct the treatment process. These individuals, generically labeled "difficult patients", can be conceptualized as having significant relational problems that interact with a particular group culture (Roth *et al.*, 1990; Stone and Gustafson, 1982). Although such individuals are often diagnosed as having borderline or narcissistic personality disorder, not all such patients can readily be given those specific diagnoses. Nitsun's (1996) felicitous expression, "the anti-group", characterizes these individuals as having the potential to disrupt the entire therapeutic endeavor.

The difficult patient should be seen in context. Some groups can accept individuals who seldom speak, whereas others see such a person as seriously harming cohesion and, therefore, as "difficult". Difficult patients fill roles and are frequently labeled "monopolizer", "help-rejecting complainer", or "the silent one". The role embodies both the individual personality and a group function. Evidence for this assertion is found when the difficult individual is removed and another rises to fill his or her place, which suggests that, in part, the role was necessary to deal with members' anxieties.

A more careful examination of the processes involved in the emergence of a difficult patient may expose that such individuals are covertly coconstructed by others in the group (Gans and Alonso, 1998). Interactions among members and the therapist tend to evoke and/or exaggerate particular character tendencies of members who often have underlying issues of forming intimate relationships. The therapeutic challenge is to deconstruct the processes so all can see their contributions to the difficult individual. This is similar to scapegoating described previously.

Nevertheless, some patients persist in behaviors that do not change and that become destructive to the treatment process. They evoke responses in others, including the therapist, that interfere with a sense of safety and limit members' willingness to expose their inner thoughts and feelings. Many difficult patients seem unable to process their interactions cognitively but remain enmeshed in emotional exchange. Others may interrupt emotional exchange with intellectual dissertations.

Not infrequently, these individuals prematurely terminate treatment, leaving those remaining with feelings of relief, frustration and anger. Other difficult patients remain in the group and at times the therapist is faced with making a decision that favors the group over an individual. The patient is informed that she or he is not benefiting from the treatment modality and is asked to leave. Such a decision should be reached only after the therapist has completed a thorough self-scrutiny and has sought consultation to explore countertransference contributions to the impasse.

Alternative Treatment Formats

Cotherapy

In some settings, groups are conducted by cotherapists. This format provides opportunities for clinicians to learn from one another, share leadership responsibilities, more readily recruit members and provide continuity in the absence of one leader. Cotherapy uniquely offers therapists chances directly to observe another clinician's work and to learn about countertransferences. The model is utilized for training neophyte group therapists who

can be paired with a more experienced therapist. For patients, this model is thought to offer a recreation of the family, as therapists are cast in parental roles, whether or not the therapists are of the same or different gender.

The conduct of cotherapy is not without special problems (Lang and Halperin, 1989). Cotherapists need to attend to their relationship because they are susceptible to a variety of transference responses to one another, most commonly competitive and narcissistic strivings. They will need to predetermine under what circumstances they might address their inevitable disagreements directly in the session.

Pharmacotherapy and Group Therapy

The inclusion of patients receiving pharmacotherapy in dynamic psychotherapy groups is common practice. Eighty-three percent of surveyed psychiatrists included patients requiring medication in group therapy (Stone *et al.*, 1991).

Combining medications with psychotherapy has become widespread. The evidence for modification, if not cure, of major debilitating symptoms is substantial and yet patients will be left with emotional responses and unexplored meaning of their illness. Moreover, discontinuation of medication is highly correlated with recurrence of symptoms. In my opinion, clinicians' and patients' objections to the combined treatment approach can be sensitively addressed and inclusion of patients receiving medications in groups offers opportunities effectively to treat a wider patient population.

Time-limited Groups

As pressure mounts to conduct therapy in briefer periods, interest in time-limited groups has increased (MacKenzie, 1997). The number of sessions may range from 12 to 30. Many insurance companies limit coverage to 20 sessions and thus a 16-session model allows for preparatory interviews and, if necessary, one or two sessions after termination of the group.

Time-limited goals are established by the therapist. Groups may be organized along specific symptom constellations, such as bereavement, sexual abuse, bulimia, or anorexia nervosa, or they may explore a personality sector with the expectation that the individual will continue to utilize the learning after termination.

Selection of patients for time-limited groups is of central importance. Therapists may opt to organize groups with ability to work with interpretations or one that is primarily supportive. Members should be assessed for their degree of psychological mindedness, that is, are they able to reflect on themselves and their interactions and on their ability to find a focus, not necessarily of recent origin. Difficulties should be formulated in interpersonal terms to facilitate the exploration of the problems in the group setting (e.g., a delayed grief reaction).

In most circumstances, once treatment begins additional members are not accepted. The agreement is similar to that of longer-term groups with the exception that the number of sessions is limited. Using this format, the therapist needs to be more active in defining the focus for the members. In the context of group development, interventions are made that focus on the interpersonal aspects of the particular dynamic stage. These groups can be particularly useful in addressing issues of engagement, trust, unfulfilled hopes, separation and loss. The combination of time pressure, maintaining focus on interpersonal processes and providing encouragement to apply learning in the external world has produced a treatment format that may be as effective as individual treatment (Budman *et al.*, 1988).

Chronically Mentally Ill

This special population of patients requires modification of traditional dynamic approaches (Kanas, 1996; Stone, 1996; Schermer and Pines, 1999). The population is broader than individuals with major psychiatric disorders (schizophrenia or bipolar disorders) and includes some disabling anxiety or personality disorders. Indeed, chronicity is determined primarily by duration and disability rather than by diagnosis. In some instances, groups are organized homogeneously for patients with schizophrenia or bipolar disorder (Cerbone *et al.*, 1992). These groups often emphasize the importance of continuing with medication and include important educational components. They may have greater structure and focus on particular topics, such as managing hallucinations, paranoid thinking, or social relations (Stone, 1996).

More typically, groups are structured to include a spectrum of patients within a relatively small range of disability. Patients are prone to attend erratically and a flexible format that accepts this propensity may serve these individuals well (Stone, 1996). The sessions are usually shorter, 45 to 60 minutes and the group census may range from 12 to 16 persons. In the flexible format, core and peripheral subgroups develop and, over extended periods, groups develop a sense of continuity and cohesion.

Treatment goals should be concordant with patients' strengths and are generally formulated to help in adaptation to everyday problems, improving social relations and managing feelings. The agreement is modified and patients may be encouraged to socialize outside of the meetings. Therapists attempt to help patients manage their isolation and sense of shame over their illness.

Countertransferences require particular attention in part due to the difficulty patients have in linking to their therapists, which may leave the clinician expecting more than the patients can deliver. Moreover, in the current climate, particularly for major mental illness, medications are valorized and therapy is depreciated, a state of affairs that affects the therapist (Della Badia, 1999).

Conclusion

While, historically, group psychotherapy was sometimes misrepresented as a less expensive, watered-down treatment, work by many has helped establish it as an effective, cost efficient and rigorous therapeutic modality applicable to a wide variety of patient problems. It provides a more direct experience for patients working with peers, as well as with those in "authority". The individual's difficulties with people is not limited to the experience of a particular individual therapist but emerges in the relational context of a number of individuals, thereby broadening the entire treatment context. In this era of emphasis on cost containment and efforts to provide rapid, brief therapies, groups can provide for some a positive time-limited treatment and for others an extended opportunity to address and alter significant intrapsychic and interpersonal difficulties.

References

Agazarian YM (1997) *Systems-Centered Therapy for Groups*. Guilford Press, New York.

Bennis WG and Shepard HA (1956) A theory of group development. *Hum Rel* 9, 415–437.

Berne E (1966) *Games People Play*. Grove Press, New York.

Budman SH, Bennett MJ and Wisnecki MJ (1988) Comparative outcome of time-limited individual and group psychotherapy. *Int J Group Psychother* 38, 63–86.

Cerbone MJA, May JA and Cuthbertson BA (1992) Group therapy as an adjunct to medication in the management of bipolar affective disorder. *Group* 16, 174–187.

Della Badia E (1999) Supervision of group psychotherapy with chronic psychotic patients, in *Group Psychotherapy of the Psychoses: Concepts, Interventions and Contexts* (eds Schermer VL and Pines M). Jessica Kingsley, London, pp. 301–323.

Durkin HE (1964) *The Group in Depth*. International Universities Press, New York.

Durkin JE (ed.) (1981) *Living Groups*. Brunner/Mazel, New York.

Ezriel H (1973) Psychoanalytic group therapy, in *Group Therapy: 1973 An Overview* (eds Wolberg LR and Schwartz E). Intercontinental Medical Book, Stratton, New York, pp. 183–210.

Foulkes SH (1961) Group process and the individual in the therapeutic group. *Br J Med* Psychol 34, 23–31.

Freud S (1955) Group psychology and the analysis of the ego, in *The Standard Edition of the Complete Psychological Works of Sigmund Freud*, Vol. 18 (trans-ed Strachey J). Hogarth Press, London, pp. 69–143. (Originally published in 1921.)

Fulkerson CCF, Hawkins DM and Alden AR (1981) Psychotherapy groups of insufficient size. *Int J Group Psychother* 31, 73–81.

Gans JS and Alonso A (1998) Difficult patients: Their construction in group therapy. *Int J Group Psychother* 48, 311–326.

Glatzer HT (1953) Handling transference resistance in group therapy. *Psychoanal Rev* 40, 36–43.

Harwood INH and Pines M (eds) (1998) *Self Experiences in Group: Intersubjective and Self Psychological Pathways to Human Understanding*. Jessica Kingsley, London.

Horwitz L (1994) Depth of transference in groups. *Int J Group Psychother* 44, 271–290.

Kanas N (1996) *Group Therapy for Schizophrenic Patients*. American Psychiatric Press, Washington DC.

Kibel HD (1992) The clinical application of object relations theory, in *Handbook of Contemporary Group Psychotherapy* (eds Klein RH, Bernard HS and Singer DL). International Universities Press, Madison, CT, pp. 141–176.

Lang E and Halperin DA (1989) Coleadership in groups: Marriage a la mode? In *Group Psychodynamics: New Paradigms and New Perspectives* (ed Halperin DA). Year Book Medical Publishers, Chicago, pp. 76–86.

MacKenzie KR (1997) *Time-Managed Group Psychotherapy: Effective Clinical Applications*. American Psychiatric Press, New York.

Nitsun M (1996) *The Anti-Group: Destructive Forces in the Group and Their Creative Potential*. Routledge, London.

Perls F, Hefferline R and Goodman P (1951) *Gestalt Therapy*. Julian, New York.

Roth BE, Stone WN and Kibel HD (eds) (1990) The Difficult Patient in Group: Group Psychotherapy With Borderline and Narcissistic Disorders.

Rutan JS and Stone WN (2001) *Psychodynamic Group Psychotherapy*, 3rd edn. Guilford Press, New York.

Scheidlinger S (1974) On the concept of the mother-group. *Int J Group Psychother* 24, 417–428.

Schermer VL and Klein RH (1996) Termination in group psychotherapy from the perspectives of contemporary object relations theory and self psychology. *Int J Group Psychother* 46, 99–115.

Schermer VL and Pines M (eds) (1999) *Group Psychotherapy of the Psychoses: Concepts, Interventions and Contexts*. Jessica Kingsley, London.

Slater P (1966) *Microcosm: Structural, Psychological and Religious Evolution in Groups*. John Wiley, New York.

Slavson SR (1950) *Analytic Group Psychotherapy*. Columbia University Press, New York.

Stone WN (1985) The curative fantasy in group psychotherapy. *Group* 9, 3–14.

Stone WN (1996) *Group Psychotherapy for People with Chronic Mental Illness*. Guilford Press, New York.

Stone WN and Gustafson JP (1982) Technique in Group Psychotherapy of narcissistic and borderline patients. *Int J Group Psychother* 32, 29–47.

Stone WN, Rodenhauser P and Markert RJ (1991) Combining group psychotherapy and pharmacotherapy: A Survey. *Int J Group Psychother* 34, 401–412.

von Bertalanffy L (1966) General system theory and psychiatry, in *American Handbook of Psychiatry* (ed Arieti S). Basic Books, New York, pp. 705–721.

Wolf A and Schwartz EK (1962) *Psychoanalysis in Groups*. Grune & Stratton, New York.

Yalom ID (1995) *The Theory and Practice of Group Psychotherapy*, 4th edn. Basic Books, New York.

68 Time-limited Psychotherapy (Including Interpersonal Therapy)

In this chapter, we offer an overview of the field of TLP. Given the explosive growth in the field of brief psychotherapy research, it is impossible to review all extant, empirically supported TLPs. Instead, we focus on concepts common to second generation TLPs, practical strategies associated with brief treatments, and problems typical to this modality. To illustrate these principles, we use examples from several evidence-based treatments, with a focus on interpersonal psychotherapy (as it is not covered elsewhere in this text) as a paradigm of TLP.

What is Time-limited Psychotherapy?

Time-limited psychotherapy refers to a psychosocial intervention, usually an individual psychotherapy, of relatively brief duration. Many of the defining features of TLPs follow from the fact that these treatments are intensive or compressed. Over a short period of time, the therapist identifies necessarily circumscribed treatment goals, working actively to maintain the treatment focus and preserve the treatment structure. Thus, TLPs are characterized by 1) specified treatment duration or time limit; 2) narrow treatment focus; 3) rapid and succinct case formulation; 4) structured treatment format; and 5) active therapist role.

Despite these similarities, TLPs comprise a heterogeneous array of treatments used to treat a plethora of conditions over quite variable time periods. "Brief" treatments can last anywhere from a single session to a year, and the therapeutic techniques deployed may range from transference interpretation (in brief psychodynamic psychotherapy) to a fear hierarchy (in behavioral therapy). Brief therapies are not indicated for the management of longstanding character disorders or chronic and persistent mental illness such as schizophrenia or bipolar disorder.

Given that (a) not all TLPs are the same and (b) experience in delivering one treatment does not confer expertise in all TLP modalities, it would be overwhelming to attempt mastery of TLPs in general. Thus, a reasoned approach to acquiring "competence" in brief interventions might include acquainting oneself with the general principles of TLP, learning the techniques and strategies associated with one evidence-based therapy, and then obtaining clinical training (including expert supervision that involves review of audio-recorded or videotaped sessions) in the selected TLP modality. Although standards for "competence" vary across TLP modalities (in some cases, they are not defined

at all), true competence is typically obtained after completion of a course in a specific psychotherapy followed by several carefully supervised cases (Markowitz, 2001). This chapter will facilitate the first step in this process: familiarity with the concepts common to most evidence-based TLPs.

Overview of Interpersonal Psychotherapy

Throughout the chapter, we use examples from interpersonal psychotherapy (IPT) to illustrate many of the general principles of TLP. In order to acquaint the reader with IPT, we offer a brief overview of this modality, introducing IPT-specific concepts such as the interpersonal inventory, the four interpersonal problem areas and the interpersonal formulation. The reader is referred to the treatment manual (Weissman et al., 2000) for a more thorough discussion of IPT.

IPT was developed in the 1970s by Klerman and Weissman as a 16-session psychotherapy for outpatients with nonpsychotic depression (Klerman et al., 1984). IPT grew out of the interpersonal theories of Harry Stack Sullivan and Adolf Meyer as well as several empirical studies demonstrating the bidirectional link between interpersonal stresses and onset of depression. In its original form IPT is an acute treatment for depression. It can be used alone or in combination with medication to treat the patient's depressive symptoms and the interpersonal problems that contribute to or are affected by the depression. IPT makes no inference about causality, simply linking the depressive symptoms to a patient's particular interpersonal issues. Regardless of which came first, IPT assumes, based on empirical evidence, that one can achieve improvement in mood by addressing interpersonal problems.

IPT uses a medical model of psychiatric illness. The therapist explains to the patient that he or she has "major depression" which is a medical illness, like diabetes or heart disease, and instills the hopeful and empirically validated idea that IPT is a good treatment for this specific disorder. Using Parsons's concept of the "sick role" (Parsons, 1951), the patient is assigned the responsibility to work toward better health in exchange for being relieved of unmanageable social obligations. The patient is also educated about the relationship between depression and interpersonal problems and, in collaboration with the therapist, selects an "interpersonal problem area" (see later) as the focus of treatment.

In the process of assessing the patient, the IPT therapist conducts the "interpersonal inventory". The interpersonal inventory consists of a review of all important past and present relationships as they relate to the current depressive episode. The therapist asks about the patient's life circumstances and requests a description of the important people in his or her life. In addition to outlining the "cast of characters" in the patient's life, the therapist probes the quality of those relationships, asking the patient to describe satisfying and unsatisfying aspects, unmet expectations with others, and aspects of relationships that the patient would like to change. The interpersonal inventory helps the therapist establish the "interpersonal problem area".

One of four interpersonal problem areas – grief, role dispute, role transition, or interpersonal deficits – serves as the explicitly agreed upon focus of treatment. It typically consists of issues such as the incompletely mourned loss of a loved one (i.e., complicated bereavement), conflict with a spouse or an employer (i.e., role dispute), an important life event (i.e., role transition) or, in the absence of one of these acute precipitants, longstanding, impoverished interpersonal relationships (i.e., interpersonal deficits). The therapist offers the patient an "interpersonal formulation": having emphasized that depression is a medical disorder with a constellation of psychological and physical symptoms, the therapist links the patient's current interpersonal problem to the depression and offers IPT as a powerful treatment for both the depression and the interpersonal problems. In the ensuing weeks (total of 16 weekly sessions), the therapist uses a variety of techniques outlined in the manual to help the patient work through these "real-life" problems.

General Principles of Time-limited Psychotherapy

The hallmark of TLP is its specified treatment duration. Because of this compression, TLPs share attributes that both link them to one another and distinguish them from long-term treatment modalities. These general principles are summarized in Table 68.1.

Time Limit

Table 68.2 groups psychotherapies commonly administered in a time-limited format by treatment approach and lists representative examples of strategies and typical treatment durations.

TLPs differ from truncated long-term treatments that are interrupted by attrition, noncompliance, or the pressures of managed care organizations. The duration of these latter therapies may coincide with that of a TLP, but they do not constitute fully formed brief treatments. TLPs have distinctly defined beginnings, middles, and ends – regardless of their absolute duration. Knowledge from the outset that therapy has a defined end-point indeed may constitute a key active ingredient of time-limited therapy. It suggests that relief may be near at hand. Marmor speculates that this approach "counters the patient's impulse to see himself as helpless, inadequate, and in need of dependent support" (Marmor 1979, p. 153). Our experience with IPT as a treatment for depression in individuals who are HIV-seropositive suggests that these individuals, despite shortened life spans, use the brevity of treatment as an impetus to effect radical, rapid changes in their lives (Swartz and Markowitz, 1998). The time limit, in a variety of ways, seems to provide an important motivation to speed the patient toward health.

A meta-analysis of many psychotherapy studies (none of them TLPs) found that most (75%) patients achieve symptom relief within 26 sessions of an open-ended treatment (Howard *et al.*, 1986). Most treatments included in this meta-analysis were naturalistic (e.g., not controlled) studies of patients suffering from very heterogeneous symptoms (diagnoses are not specified). This finding suggests that many patients may respond quickly, even if psychotherapy is open-ended. Although no studies have com-

Table 68.1 General Principles of Time-limited Versus Open-ended Psychotherapies		
Principle	Time-limited Psychotherapy	Open-ended Psychotherapy
Duration of treatment	Specified time frame, 1–40 sessions	Duration not specified; may last several years
Scope of treatment	Well-defined treatment focus; circumscribed goals	Flexible treatment goals, varying over time, often not well-defined
Treatment goals	Remission of specific symptoms or intrapsychic conflict	Character change, improved functioning, or ongoing support
Case formulation	Rapid; succinct; drives treatment goals; often explicitly stated to patient	Strives for depth of understanding; subject to ongoing revision and reassessment as treatment unfolds
Characteristics of suitable patients*	Acute illness; good premorbid functioning; limited resources; focused problem area	Chronic illnesses; poor premorbid functioning; extensive resources; multiple targets of change
Treatment structure	Defined stages of treatment; clearly specified termination phase; often specified in a manual	Flexible structure; no specified end point; treatment stages vary widely; not codified as a manual
Therapeutic stance	Active; direct suggestion may be permitted; functions to maintain treatment focus	Less directive; neutral

Adapted from Frances A, Clarkin J and Perry S (1984) *Differential Therapeutics in Psychiatry: The Art and Science of Treatment Selection.* Brunner/Mazel, New York.

Table 68.2   Major Models of Time-limited Psychotherapy

Psychotherapy Type/Major Theorists	Techniques	Typical Time Duration
Interpersonal psychotherapy (IPT) Klerman Weissman	• *Medical model* of illness. • Life events affect mood, and *vice versa.* • Link symptoms to one of four *interpersonal problem areas.* • Work through an affectively meaningful problem area using role-play, communication analysis, and direct suggestion. • Focus on the *here and now*, outside rather than inside the office.	12–16 wk
Cognitive–behavioral therapy (CBT) Beck Rush Barlow	• Identify distorted thoughts that lead to maladaptive feelings and behaviors. • Homework assignments to recognize, test, and challenge underlying *automatic negative thoughts* or maladaptive behaviors. • *Relaxation techniques* to manage anxiety. • Encourage *rational*, scientific, collaboration between patient and therapist.	12–16 wk
Behavior therapy (BT) Foa Mynors-Wallis	• Based on principles of operant conditioning, social learning theory. • Gradual *exposure* to anxiety-producing stimuli. • Self-monitoring, graded task assignment.	8–12 wk
Brief psychodynamic psychotherapy Balint Davanloo Luborsky Malan Mann Sifneos Strupp	• Identify problematic relationship themes that are resolved through *transference interpretations.* • Offer *support* through the formal aspects of treatment such as regular appointments and collaboration. • Select central issue that has current relevance and past antecedent. • *Transference interpretations and clarification* to develop insight and resolve conflict. • *Confront defenses* – despite emergence of anxiety – to uncover underlying impulse. • Explore past *conflicts*, ego *defenses* and *resistances.*	12–20 sessions
Motivational interviewing Miller Rollnick	• Patient-centered, directive method for *enhancing motivation* to change. • Encourage articulation and resolution of *ambivalence.* • Diminish resistance and strengthen patient's *commitment to change.*	2–4 sessions
Psychodynamic–interpersonal Hobson Shapiro	• Less emphasis on interpretation than most psychodynamic treatments. • Greater emphasis on patient–therapist relationship than in IPT. • Help patient learn new ways of relating to therapist and, by extension, others. • Enhance interpersonal skills.	3–8 sessions

pared prospectively response rates of TLPs to open-ended treatments, we predict that treatment response would be more rapid for patients receiving time-limited interventions because of explicit expectations that therapy will conclude within a specified time frame. TLPs are generally dosed with a frequency of once a week, although this varies as well.

The optimal duration and dosage of TLP, although empirical questions, remain largely unanswered to date. In practice, treatment duration is often defined by convention, the exigencies

of a research protocol or managed care organization, or even the inclinations of the therapist.

IPT: Duration of Treatment

IPT was originally designed as a 16-week intervention so that it could be administered over the same period as an acute course of pharmacotherapy, allowing an assessment of the relative efficacy of the two interventions (DiMascio *et al.*, 1979). IPT is also administered as a 14-session intervention (Markowitz unpublished data), a 12-session intervention (Mufson *et al.*, 1999; O'Hara *et al.*, 2000) and an eight-session intervention (Swartz *et al.*, 2002), but there are no data comparing the relative benefits of varying doses of acute IPT.

Treatment Focus

An important characteristic of TLP is careful definition of treatment goals, which are usually agreed upon by the patient and therapist, and often specified at the beginning of treatment. Because therapy is brief, the scope of the treatment is circumscribed and focused. TLPs do not attempt sweeping changes in character. Rather, treatments target a specific diagnosis, set of symptoms, or a narrow aspect of character. Typical and appropriate treatment goals for TLPs include remission of depressive symptoms, reduction in frequency of binge-eating, and resolution of a specific interpersonal conflict.

Most TLPs define treatment goals by diagnostic criteria, in much the manner of pharmacotherapies. IPT focuses on two discrete goals: remission of depressive symptoms and resolution of an interpersonal problem area (Weissman *et al.*, 2000). Cognitive–behavioral therapy for panic disorder focuses on reduction in frequency of panic attacks and relief of general anxiety symptoms (Barlow, 1997). Motivational interviewing, a brief intervention designed to facilitate behavior change, is often administered for the sole purpose of helping patients reduce or eliminate their alcohol consumption (Miller and Rollnick, 1991). Thus, although the treatments vary in their focus, in all cases their treatment goals are narrow and usually specified from the outset.

Case Formulation

Treatment focus is closely allied with the broader concept of case formulation. According to Eells, psychotherapy case formulation is "a hypothesis about the causes, precipitants, and maintaining influences of a person's psychological, interpersonal, and behavioral problems.... It should serve as a blueprint, guiding treatment" (Eells, 1997, pp. 1–2). In TLP, because time is short, the process of generating a case formulation is also compressed. The therapist must identify the most important components of the patient's narrative, balancing the urge to learn more about the patient's life circumstances with the time constraints of the TLP. Thus, the TLP therapist typically conducts an overview of the patient's psychosocial circumstances and then selects a few "hot" topics – relevant both to the current complaint and the nature of the therapy – to consider in greater depth. This approach allows the therapist to develop an informed, timely case formulation. The ability rapidly to develop and deliver such a formulation is for many therapists among the more difficult but also most valuable aspects of learning a TLP.

IPT: Case Formulation

Case formulation in IPT builds on two core IPT concepts: 1) depression is a treatable illness and 2) events in one's psychosocial environment affect one's mood, and vice versa. The IPT therapist defines depression as a medical illness that, like asthma, is both treatable and affected by the patient's circumstances. The therapist notes that, in a biologically vulnerable individual, when painful events occur, mood worsens and depression may result. Conversely, depressed mood compromises one's ability to handle one's social role, generally leading to negative events. IPT therapists use the connections among mood, environment and social

role to help patients understand their depressions within an interpersonal context, and to teach them to handle their social role and environment so as to both solve their interpersonal problems and relieve their depressive syndrome.

The therapist's formulation includes a diagnosis of depression as a medical illness, the provision of reassurance and hope, the assignment of the sick role and, most importantly, the identification of one (or at most two) interpersonal problem areas that become the agenda for the remainder of the treatment. The therapist directly states this case formulation to the patient and elicits his or her agreement with the proposed strategy before moving ahead with the next phase of treatment. Thus, in IPT, case formulation constitutes an important treatment tool that links the patient's mood symptoms to life events and introduces a specific interpersonal problem area as the focus of treatment for the ensuing sessions (Markowitz and Swartz, 1997).

The brevity of treatment leaves little room for error in formulating the IPT case – or any TLP case, for that matter. The therapist must use the initial treatment sessions aggressively to pursue all potential areas and to determine the treatment focus prior to embarking on the middle phase of treatment. If a covert and imposing problem area should arise in the middle phase, however, the therapist would have to renegotiate the treatment contract to address it.

Structured Treatment

In TLP, the structure of the intervention is clearly delineated and referenced throughout the treatment period. The therapist will often call the patient's attention to important landmarks in the treatment: "Today we've reached the halfway point" or "We only have three sessions left". In manualized treatments, each of these time intervals has specified tasks or strategies. For instance, in IPT, the initial phase can last up to three sessions. During that time, the therapist has specific tasks (viz., obtain a psychiatric history and interpersonal inventory, offer a case formulation). Similarly, the middle and end phases of treatment have a specified duration and associated tasks.

In support of the treatment structure, TLP requires the therapists to make formal or informal "treatment contracts" in which the patient and therapist explicitly or implicitly agree to goals, duration and other parameters of treatment. The therapist may discuss with the patient the exact number of sessions planned, rules for missed sessions or rescheduled sessions, fees and so on. Although some aspects of treatment contracts are common to all psychotherapies, TLPs tend to specify more elements in the contract from the outset, including expected treatment responses (e.g., "At the end of 16 weeks, your mood will likely be much better") and specific requirements of the patient (e.g., homework assignments in Prolonged Exposure and CBT). Patients often find the transparent structure of TLPs reassuring, removing some of the unnecessary mystery (and perhaps stigma) historically associated with psychotherapy.

Most TLPs call for serial assessments of symptoms. In clinical practice (and in clinical trials), it is often practical to administer a self-report measure such as the Beck Depression Inventory (Beck and Steer, 1993) or the Beck Anxiety Inventory (Beck and Steer, 1990). Regardless of the instrument chosen, it is important to build into the weekly therapy session time to complete and review a standardized symptom measure and track change over time. Serial symptom assessment provides the patient with additional psychoeducation (i.e., symptom recognition) and a reliable means of tracking improvement (or lack thereof).

Active Therapist

In order to maintain the treatment focus, the therapist must be active in TLP. He or she must move the treatment process forward under the pressure of an inexorably ticking clock. This demands constant attention to the treatment focus and redirection of the patient if the focus falters. The therapist gently keeps the patient on task, shaping the treatment rather than simply following the patient's lead. A challenge in TLP is to balance strict adherence to the treatment focus with an empathic stance that supports the treatment alliance. Although it is important to attend to the agreed upon problem area in IPT, it is also important that the patient feel "heard" and that the therapist allows time in the session for the patient to express his or her feelings unimpeded.

Practical Issues in Time-limited Therapy

Patient Selection

Because of their limited focus, TLPs are ideally suited to patients with acute symptomatology and relatively favorable baseline functioning. Resource availability may also influence decisions to use a time-limited or open-ended approach. Most evidence-based treatments are designed for and have been tested in samples of patients who meet DSM-IV criteria for Axis I disorders (predominantly mood and anxiety disorders, as well as specific behavioral problems such as substance abuse or eating disorders). Thus, it is important to conduct a thorough diagnostic interview, identify target diagnoses and symptoms and select, if possible, a TLP that has been empirically validated for that population. It would be inappropriate to treat a patient with a primary diagnosis of a specific phobia with IPT, as IPT has not been tested in this population; a behavioral approach would be preferable. A patient suffering from major depression, however, might reasonably be treated with CBT, IPT, or brief dynamic therapy.

Engagement

The closely allied concepts of engagement and treatment alliance respectively refer to the patient's commitment to the treatment enterprise and the relationship between therapist and patient. Positive treatment alliance typically correlates with better treatment adherence and engagement. Given the brevity of treatment, one challenge of TLP is to establish rapidly a relationship with the patient in order to facilitate engagement in treatment. Maintaining this alliance throughout treatment is also important because nonattendance, while disruptive to any psychotherapy, is particularly costly in a time-limited treatment.

IPT: Therapeutic Relationship

While many of the so-called "common" factors of psychotherapy function to facilitate this process, in IPT the therapist's stance is specifically intended to create a positive relationship with a depressed patient. The IPT therapist maintains a warm, encouraging stance that counters the depressed patient's pessimism with an equal and opposite optimistic realism. In psychodynamic terms, the IPT therapist cultivates a positive transference. He or she handles negative transference as illness-derived, treatment-interfering behaviors: for instance, tardiness or lack of participation would be defined as sequelae of depression. The therapist might intervene by saying, "It's hard to feel enthusiastic about therapy when your depression makes it hard to enjoy anything". In addition, the therapist might address it on a practical level, saying, "We only have five sessions left. We need all the remaining time

to get to the bottom of your problem with your wife and to treat your depression". These strategies both promote the therapeutic alliance and enhance treatment engagement.

Maintaining the Focus

As previously discussed, it is imperative that the TLP therapist identify clear treatment goals and maintain focus during the brief treatment period. It can be challenging to keep the patient on task and manage material that emerges in sessions unrelated to the primary treatment goal. To address this important issue, the therapist must clarify from the outset the goals and potential limitations of treatment.

IPT: Treatment Focus

In IPT, treatment goals are specifically stated during the initial phase of treatment. The IPT therapist might say, "The goal of this treatment is to help you with this depression and your unresolved feelings about your mother's death last year. At the end of 16 weeks, we can discuss whether you need additional treatment for your bulimia, but let's first see how you feel when the depression has lifted". It is important that the patient explicitly agree to the stated treatment goals. In the case described above, the patient would need to agree to defer treatment for a possible eating disorder, focusing on her depression and grief for the immediate future.

In IPT, a clear treatment contract helps the patient and therapist remain focused. For instance, if the patient brings up feelings of dissatisfaction in the workplace during a therapy designed to address problematic relationships with a spouse (role dispute), the therapist may first briefly explore whether these complaints relate to the treatment focus. Thus, if demands from the spouse lead the patient to accept an unsatisfactory job, or if a dispute at work parallels that at home, the therapist can refocus the comments in light of the ongoing marital dispute. However, if there is no obvious connection to the main treatment focus, the therapist might gently redirect the patient by saying, "Although your work concerns are important too, at the beginning of therapy we agreed that we should spend these few months working through your problems with your spouse. I wonder how that has been going".

Termination

As the end of treatment nears, the therapist reiterates the date and time of the final session, actively eliciting responses to the end of treatment if the patient does not spontaneously offer them. Termination provides an opportunity to review treatment gains (which are often impressive), support the patient's sense of competence and independence, grieve the end of treatment and identify unaddressed problems. The termination phase is more crucial and more complicated in psychodynamic psychotherapies because of their emphasis on the importance of the therapeutic relationship.

IPT: Termination

In IPT, termination is handled as a graduation or role transition. In the termination phase of IPT (typically the last two to three sessions), the therapist helps the patient express expectable sad feelings (which are distinguished from recrudescent depressive affect) about the end of treatment, but underscores patient progress in having treated the depressive episode and problems at work, love relationships, and so on. While concerns about the patient's ability to manage without the therapist's help are inevitable, the therapist counters with examples of the patient's hard therapeutic work outside of the office. The therapist commends the patient's "real world" victories, reminding the patient that IPT has helped him or her to develop new skills that he or she will continue to use after treatment ends. Termination promotes patient independence while grieving the loss of the treatment relationship. The therapist and patient also review the symptoms of depression and identify "warning signs" which might lead the patient to a reevaluation in the future.

In the event of partial response or nonresponse, the therapist suggests alternative treatments and makes appropriate referrals for follow-up. If the therapist judges that additional treatment is warranted for management of persistent symptoms, it is critically important that the therapist blames the therapy rather than the patient for failing to bring about a full remission. The therapist can gently point out that all of our treatments for depression are imperfect and that we cannot yet predict which treatments will work for any individual patient. The therapist confidently reassures the patient that there are other options (i.e., medication, other forms of psychotherapy), helping the patient select follow-up treatment that fits his or her needs. Another reasonable strategy (though not backed by any empirical data) would be to extend the treatment duration of IPT by a fixed number of sessions (e.g., six or eight additional sessions). This option would probably be best for a patient who has had at least a partial response to IPT and may need a few extra sessions to complete therapeutic work that is already underway. In keeping with the spirit of IPT, it would be important to explain this rationale to the patient explicitly and to set a second termination point to help maintain the focus of treatment. See the later section on "nonresponse and partial response" for a fuller discussion of treatment options for patients who are not well at the end of 16 sessions.

When the patient experiences a remission of symptoms by the end of 16 sessions, it may be tempting to refer the patient for additional psychotherapy such as marital treatment or an insight-oriented psychotherapy to address residual interpersonal issues or longstanding personality problems. However, it may be preferable to encourage a treatment-free period of 3 to 6 months to help clarify and consolidate treatment gains, particularly if the patient has presented with a first episode of relatively acute illness. Greater symptom chronicity and number of episodes suggest the need for continuation and maintenance treatment.

Common Problems in Time-limited Psychotherapy

Nonresponse and Partial Response

There are no clear guidelines to determine the optimal next step for patients who fail to respond or do not respond fully to an initial course of psychotherapy. In the case of nonresponse to a given treatment, which may be defined as failure to achieve at least a 25% decrease in baseline symptoms over a 6- to 8-week time period (Nierenberg and DeCecco, 2001), the usual approach would be to stop the unhelpful therapy and consider alternatives. Patients who show no benefit from a TLP should be evaluated for the typical sources of treatment failure such as misdiagnosis, the presence of a comorbid psychiatric disorder, or comorbid general medical conditions (Kornstein and Schneider, 2001), and referred for appropriate treatment. If the TLP psychotherapist is also a physician, it would be reasonable at this point to consider pharmacotherapy. If the clinician decides that it is in the best interest of the patient to abandon a course of TLP, it is important

that the therapist help the patient understand that the "fault" lies with the TLP rather than the patient. The therapist should be certain to offer the patient support during the transition to an alternate treatment, instilling hope that the new treatment will offer relief and making sure that continuity of care is preserved.

In most cases of partial response to a TLP, clinicians choose to add medication as their first strategy. Unless the therapist suspects that psychotherapy may have worsened the patient's condition, continuing psychotherapy usually makes sense. The preexisting therapeutic relationship can provide a supportive holding environment for the patient while medication is initiated that may help the patient tolerate initial medication side effects and the delayed onset of action associated with antidepressant medication. Among depressed patients who fail to respond to an initial course of pharmacotherapy, response rates to a second antidepressant hover around 50% (Marangell, 2001). By contrast, in a sample of depressed women, the addition of an SSRI to IPT among those who failed to respond to IPT alone brought about remission in almost 80% of subjects (Frank *et al.*, 2000). Thus, depressed patients who do not remit with psychotherapy alone may be excellent candidates for combination treatment with psychotherapy and medication.

If a patient refuses medications or prefers a trial of a different psychotherapy, it may be reasonable to change TLP modalities or consider an open-ended treatment. Issues to consider include whether it makes sense to switch therapists, the qualifications of the therapist to administer multiple types of psychotherapy, and the availability of alternate treatments in the patient's geographic area. Whereas psychopharmacologists can easily change prescriptions and proceed with a consistent therapeutic approach, a psychotherapist who suddenly begins acting differently may confuse an already uncomfortable patient.

IPT: Handling Nonresponse to Treatment

In IPT, we make every effort to blame the treatment rather than the patient when symptoms persist beyond termination. Depressed patients are inclined to blame themselves, so it is important for therapists to maintain their objective stance, pointing out treatment successes (there are usually some) and underscoring the fact that not all patients respond to any single treatment. Patients with histories of chronic or recurrent depression who respond to an acute course of IPT are generally considered candidates for continuation and/or maintenance of IPT sessions (usually administered at a reduced frequency) to help achieve a full remission and prevent relapse and/or recurrence (Frank, 1991; Markowitz, 1998).

Mid-treatment Crises

During the course of any psychotherapy, unanticipated crises may occur in the patient's life, temporarily derailing treatment. For instance, if the patient suddenly developed new, life-threatening symptoms such as active suicidal ideation or frank psychosis, the case formulation would be abandoned in order to attend to patient safety. Alternately, if the patient experienced an unexpected life crisis mid-treatment (i.e., the death of an important person, significant changes in socioeconomic status, etc.), it would be reasonable to reevaluate the treatment focus in order to attend to the patient's pressing needs.

Regardless of treatment modality, patient safety supersedes the treatment paradigm. In TLP, it is desirable to address the crisis as quickly as possible in order to return to the treatment focus and complete the treatment within the specified time frame. If the therapist can address the crisis rapidly and resume the prior focus, it may be possible to regain the original treatment trajectory. If multiple sessions are required to address the crisis, the therapist must ask, "Is this TLP salvageable?" and "Can we meet our treatment goals within the remaining allotted time?" If not, the therapist should consider altering the treatment focus or abandoning the current treatment approach entirely. As we have emphasized throughout, changes in treatment approach should be handled carefully, reassuring the patient that they are not to blame and providing support as the patient shifts to a new intervention.

Contraindication to Time-limited Psychotherapy

For all psychoactive treatments it is important to consider instances in which a specific therapy is **not** indicated for a disorder or kind of patient. Unfortunately, thus far there are no well-designed empirical studies of a psychotherapy's potential "toxicities", although there is speculation about the kinds of individuals who would be predicted to respond poorly to time-limited treatments.

In the brief psychodynamic psychotherapy literature, time-limited treatments are generally not recommended for those individuals who might have difficulty in quickly forming a therapeutic alliance or might develop severe difficulties in the face of termination (Marmor 1979). In practice, this usually translates into a reluctance to treat borderline, suicidal, substance abusing, or psychotic patients with brief psychotherapy (Davanloo, 1980; Mann, 1974; Sifneos, 1979). Also excluded are "acting out", cognitively impaired, very dependent, or "unrestrainably" anxious patients (Koss and Shiang, 1994).

Although Sifneos (1979) and Mann (1974) consider severe psychopathology a contraindication to their brief psychodynamic psychotherapies, other time-limited treatments specifically target serious mental disorders. IPT and CBT, for example, were developed for the treatment of major depression; these and other brief psychotherapies have been used to treat a spectrum of significant pathologies including bulimia (Fairburn, 1998), alcohol dependence (Miller *et al.*, 1998), panic disorder (Barlow, 1997; Milrod *et al.*, 2000), and post traumatic stress disorder (Foa *et al.*, 1991).

Table 68.3	**Summary of Empirical Evidence Supporting Efficacy of TLPs for Mood Disorders (Randomized Trials Only)**			
Diagnosis	N	Study Design	Results	Reference
Major depressive disorder	81	16 wk of IPT, amitriptyline (AMI), IPT plus AMI, or nonscheduled control	IPT plus AMI > IPT = AMI > control	DiMascio *et al.* (1979)
Major depressive disorder in the elderly	91	16–20 wk of behavioral (BT), cognitive (CT), or brief psychodynamic (BPT) therapy or wait-list control (WLC)	BT = CT = BPT > WLC	Thompson *et al.* (1987)
Major depressive disorder	250	16 wk of IPT, CBT, imipramine (IMI) or placebo (PLA) plus clinical management (CM)	IMI > IPT > CBT > PLA plus CM (differences were nonsignificant)	Elkin *et al.* (1989)
Recurrent major depressive disorder	128	3 yr of maintenance treatment: monthly maintenance IPT (IPT-M), IMI plus IPT-M, IPT-M plus PLA, CM plus PLA, IMI plus CM	IMI plus IPT-M = IMI plus CM > IPT-M = PT-M plus PLA > CM plus PLA	Frank *et al.* (1990)
Major depressive disorder	107	12 wk of CT, IMI, or CT plus IMI	CT plus IMI > IMI = CT (differences were nonsignificant)	Hollon *et al.* (1992)
Depressive symptoms in HIV-positive individuals	101	16 wk of IPT, CBT, IMI plus supportive therapy (SP), or SP alone	IMI plus SP = IPT > CBT = SP alone (differences were nonsignificant)	Markowitz *et al.* (1998)
Recurrent major depressive disorder in the elderly	180	3 yr of maintenance treatment: nortriptyline (NTP), IPT-M, IPT-M plus NTP, IPT-M plus PLA, or CM plus PLA	NTP plus IPT-M > NTP > IPT-M plus PLA > CM plus PLA	Reynolds *et al.* (1999)
Major depressive disorder in adolescents	48	12 wk of IPT or CM	IPT > CM	Mufson *et al.* (1999)
Severe, refractory, nonpsychotic illness	110	8 wk of psychodynamic interpersonal therapy (PI) or usual care (UC)	PI > UC	Guthrie *et al.* (1999)
Postpartum depression	120	12 wk of IPT or WLC	IPT > WLC	O'Hara *et al.* (2000)
Chronic depression	681	12 wk of nefazodone (NFZ), cognitive–behavioral-analysis system of psychotherapy (CBASP), or NFZ plus CBASP	NFZ plus CBASP > NFZ = CBASP	Keller *et al.* (2000)

Although it is unlikely that a personality disorder will remit following a course of brief psychotherapy, we also know that it is often difficult accurately to diagnose personality disorders in the presence of an Axis I disorder (Hirschfeld *et al.*, 1983). Hence **seeming** Axis II pathology should rarely be an exclusion in the presence of an appropriate Axis I target disorder. Furthermore, the structure and brevity of time-limited treatments may help the therapist to manage or circumvent some of the treatment-interfering behaviors characteristic of cluster B personality disorders. Thus, it may be reasonable to treat patients with moderate character pathology for an Axis I disorder with a TLP and then refer them for a different kind of psychotherapy once the acute symptoms have remitted.

Empirical Data

Because these treatments are relatively short, it is easier (though by no means easy) to conduct psychotherapy outcome studies with TLPs than with longer-term psychotherapies. The past decade has witnessed the publication of relatively large numbers of TLP studies. Because of these studies, we have more confidence that TLPs work, at least for particular indications, than other forms of psychotherapy. In Table 68.3, we summarize findings from empirical studies of TLPs as treatments for mood disorders. In Table 68.4 we summarize population-specific indications for selected TLPs.

Conclusion

In 1975, Luborsky asked the question, "Is it true that 'everyone has won and all must have prizes'?" (Luborsky and Singer, 1975).

In other words, are all psychotherapies equally efficacious for all conditions and all patients all of the time? In the ensuing decades, through more systematic studies of TLPs, we have begun to establish the efficacy of specific psychotherapies for specific disorders. Moving beyond the first generation TLPs that used psychodynamic principles to treat mildly ill patients with heterogeneous diagnoses, the second generation of TLPs are characterized by written manuals that specify treatment interventions for defined disorders and populations.

In the process of focusing the lens, however, we may have lost sight of the big picture. As Guthrie (2000) points out, although patients in real world settings experience chronic symptoms and multiple disorders, psychotherapy researchers have typically excluded these patients from outcome studies. There have been great strides in the field of TLP research over the last two decades, but much work remains. The next challenge will be to develop strategies to disseminate these evidence-based (**efficacy** proven) TLPs into general clinical settings and to conduct new (**effectiveness**) psychotherapy studies of their relevance in general psychiatric populations.

Future empirical work may focus on further defining psychotherapy duration, with the dual goals of establishing the fewest number of sessions that can be used to treat a given problem and identifying those patients for whom longer courses of therapy are indicated.

Acknowledgment

The authors would like to thank Danielle Novick for her assistance in the preparation of the chapter.

Table 68.4	Time-limited Therapies with Demonstrated Efficacy for Specific Disorders	
Disorder	Psychotherapy	Efficacy
Major depression, acute	IPT	1*
	CBT	1
	PI	2
Major depression, recurrent	Maintenance IPT	1
Major depression in the elderly	Cognitive therapy	2
	Behavior therapy	2
	Horowitz's stress-response psychotherapy	2
Depressive symptoms in HIV seropositive men	IPT	2
Chronic depression	Cognitive–behavioral analysis system of psychotherapy	1
Dysthymia	CBT	2
	IPT	2
Opiate addiction	Luborsky's SE plus drug counseling	2
	CBT plus drug counseling	2
Alcohol addiction	CBT	1
	Motivational enhancement therapy	1
	Twelve-step facilitation	1
Bulimia	CBT	1
	IPT	2
PTSD	Prolonged exposure	2
Panic disorder	CBT	1
	Panic-focused psychodynamic therapy	2

*tentative classification; 1, rigorously proven; 2, promising results.

Preparation of this chapter was supported, in part, by a grant from the National Institute of Mental Health, MH-64519 (H.A.S.).

References

Barlow DH (1997) Cognitive–behavioral therapy for panic disorder: Current status. *J Clin Psychiatr* 58(Suppl 2), 32–36; discussion 36–37.

Beck AT and Steer RA (1990) *Manual for the Revised Beck Anxiety Inventory.* Psychological Corporation, San Antonio, TX.

Beck AT and Steer RA (1993) *Manual for the Beck Depression Inventory.* Psychological Corporation, San Antonio, TX.

Davanloo H (ed) (1980) *Short-Term Dynamic Psychotherapy.* Jason Aronson, Northvale, NJ.

DiMascio A, Weissman MM, Prusoff BA *et al.* (1979) Differential symptom reduction by drugs and psychotherapy in acute depression. *Arch Gen Psychiatr* 36(13), 1450–1456.

Eells TD (ed) (1997) *Handbook of Psychotherapy Case Formulation.* Guilford Press, New York.

Elkin I, Shea MT, Watkins JT, *et al.* (1989) National Institute of Mental Health Treatment of Depression Collaborative Research Program: General effectiveness of treatments. *Arch Gen Psychiatr* 46(11), 971–982.

Fairburn CG (1998) Interpersonal psychotherapy for bulimia nervosa in *Interpersonal Psychotherapy.* Review of Psychiatry Series (ed, JC Markowitz). American Psychiatric Press, Washington DC, pp. 99–128.

Foa EB, Rothbaum BO, Riggs DS *et al.* (1991) Treatment of posttraumatic stress disorder in rape victims: A comparison between cognitive–behavioral procedures and counseling. *J Consult Clin Psychol* 59(5), 715–723.

Frank E, Kupfer DJ, Perel JM, *et al.* (1990) Three-year outcomes for maintenance therapies in recurrent depression. *Arch Gen Psychiatr* 47(12), 1093–1099.

Frank E (1991) Interpersonal psychotherapy as a maintenance treatment for patients with recurrent depression. *Psychotherapy* 28(2), 259–266.

Frank E, Grochocinski VJ, Spanier CA *et al.* (2000) Interpersonal psychotherapy and antidepressant medication: Evaluation of a sequential treatment strategy in women with recurrent major depression. *J Clin Psychiatr* 61(1), 51–57.

Guthrie E, Moorey J, Margison F, *et al.* (1999) Cost-effectiveness of brief psychodynamic–interpersonal therapy in high utilizers of psychiatric services. *Arch Gen Psychiatr* 57(6), 519–526.

Guthrie E (2000) Psychotherapy for patients with complex disorders and chronic symptoms. The need for a new research paradigm. *Br J Psychiatr* 177, 131–137.

Hirschfeld RM, Klerman GL, Clayton PJ *et al.* (1983) Assessing personality: Effects of the depressive state on trait measurement. *Am J Psychiatr* 140(6), 695–699.

Hollon SD, DeRubies RJ, Evans MD, *et al.* (1992) Cognitive therapy and pharmacotherapy for depression. Singly and in combination. *Arch Gen Psychiatr* 49(10), 774–781.

Howard KI, Kopta SM, Krause MS *et al.* (1986) The dose–effect relationship in psychotherapy. *Am Psychol* 41(2), 159–164.

Keller MB, McCullough JP, Klein DN, *et al.* (2000) A comparison of nefazodone, the cognitive–behavioral analysis system of psychotherapy, and their combination for the treatment of chronic depression. *New Engl J Med* 342(20), 1462–1470.

Klerman GL, Weissman MM, Rounsaville BJ *et al.* (1984) *Interpersonal Psychotherapy of Depression.* Basic Books, New York.

Kornstein SG and Schneider RK (2001) Clinical features of treatment-resistant depression. *J Clin Psychiatr* 62(Suppl 16), 18–25.

Koss MP and Shiang J (1994) Research on brief psychotherapy in *Handbook of Psychotherapy and Behavior Change* (eds Bergin AE and Garfield SL). John Wiley, New York, pp. 664–700.

Luborsky L and Singer B (1975) Comparative studies of psychotherapies. Is it true that "everyone has won and all must have prizes"? *Arch Gen Psychiatr* 32(8), 995–1008.

Mann J (1974) *Time-Limited Psychotherapy.* Harvard University Press, Cambridge, Mass.

Marangell LB (2001) Switching antidepressants for treatment-resistant major depression. *J Clin Psychiatr* 62(Suppl 18) 12–17.

Markowitz JC (2001) Learning new psychotherapies. In Treatment of Depression: Bridging the 21st Century, (ed MM Weissman). American Psychiatric Press, Washington DC, pp. 281–300.

Markowitz JC (1998) *Interpersonal Psychotherapy for Dysthymic Disorder.* American Psychiatric Press, Washington DC.

Markowitz JC and Swartz HA (1997) Case formulation in interpersonal psychotherapy of depression, in *Handbook of Psychotherapy Case Formulation* (ed Eells TD). Guilford Press, New York, pp. 192–222.

Marmor J (1979) Short-term dynamic psychotherapy. *Am J Psychiatr* 136, 149–155.

Miller WR and Rollnick S (1991) *Motivational Interviewing: Preparing People to Change Addictive Behavior.* Guilford Press, New York.

Miller WR, Andrews NR and Wilbourne P (1998) A wealth of alternatives: Effective treatments for alcohol problems, in *Treating Addictive Behaviors*, 2nd edn. (eds Miller WR and Heather N). Plenum Press, New York, pp. 203–216.

Milrod B, Busch F, Leon AC *et al.* (2000) Open trial of psychodynamic psychotherapy for panic disorder: A pilot study. *Am J Psychiatr* 157(11), 1878–1880.

Mufson L, Weissman MM, Moreau D *et al.* (1999) Efficacy of interpersonal psychotherapy for depressed adolescents. *Arch Gen Psychiatr* 57(6), 573–579.

Nierenberg AA and DeCecco LM (2001) Definitions of antidepressant treatment response, remission, nonresponse, partial response, and other relevant outcomes: A focus on treatment-resistant depression. *J Clin Psychiatr* 62(Suppl 16), 5–9.

O'Hara MW, Stuart S, Gorman LL *et al.* (2000) Efficacy of interpersonal psychotherapy for postpartum depression. *Arch Gen Psychiatr* 57(11), 1039–1045.

Parsons T (1951) Illness and the role of the physician: A sociological perspective. *Am J Orthopsychiatr* 21, 452–460.

Reynolds CF III, Frank E, and Perel JM (1999) Nortriptyline and interpersonal psychotherapy as maintenance therapies for recurrent major depression: A randomized controlled trial in patients older than 59 years. *J Am Med Assoc* 281(1), 39–45.

Sifneos PE (1979) *Short-Term Dynamic Psychotherapy: Evaluation and Technique.* Plenum Press, New York.

Swartz HA and Markowitz JC (1998) Interpersonal psychotherapy for the treatment of depression in HIV-positive men and women, in *Interpersonal Psychotherapy.* Review of Psychiatry Series (ed Markowitz JC). American Psychiatric Press, Washington DC, pp. 129–155.

Swartz HA, Frank E, Shear MK *et al.* (2002) Pilot study of brief interpersonal psychotherapy. Poster presented at the Second Annual Research Day, Western Psychiatric Institute and Clinic, Pittsburgh, PA.

Thompson LW, Gallagher D, and Breckenridge JS (1987) Comparative effectiveness of psychotherapies for depressed elders. *J Consult Clin Psychol* 55(3), 385–390.

Weissman MM, Markowitz JC and Klerman GL (2000) *Comprehensive Guide to Interpersonal Psychotherapy.* Basic Books, New York.

CHAPTER

69

Cognitive and Behavioral Therapies

The family of cognitive and behavioral therapies includes a diverse group of interventions. Nevertheless, the treatments share several pragmatic and theoretical assumptions. First, these therapies emphasize a psychoeducational orientation, by which patients learn about the nature of their difficulties and the rationale for use of particular treatment strategies. Secondly, the cognitive and behavioral therapies typically employ homework and self-help assignments to provide patients the opportunity to practice therapeutic methods to enhance generalization outside of the therapy hour. Thirdly, objective assessment of psychiatric illness is considered an integral part of treatment, and selection of therapeutic strategies derives logically from such assessments. Fourthly, the therapeutic methods used are generally structured, are directive, and require a high level of therapist activity. As such, the cognitive and behavioral therapies tend to be easier than other approaches to describe in treatment manuals. Fifthly, for most disorders, the cognitive and behavioral therapies are time-limited interventions. Sixthly, and perhaps most important, these therapies are built on empirical evidence that validates the theoretical orientation and guides the choice of therapeutic techniques. Specifically, learning theories (i.e., classical, operant and observational models of learning) and the principles of cognitive psychology are relied on heavily in constructing cognitive–behavioral treatment models.

Cognitive Model

The basic theories of the cognitive model are rooted in a long tradition of viewing cognitions as primary determinants of emotion and behavior. For excellent reviews of the historical bases of cognitive therapy, see Dobson and Block (1988) Clark *et al.* (1999). The description of cognitive theories given here is based largely on Beck's concepts. This model of therapy tends to give somewhat more emphasis to cognitive than behavioral factors in treatment interventions, but both are considered to be integral parts of the model (Figure 69.1).

Depending on the case formulation and the phase of therapy, attention may be directed primarily at cognitive or behavioral aspects of the disorder. In most cases, a combination of cognitive and behavioral techniques is used. For this reason, we use the term cognitive–behavioral therapy (CBT) throughout the chapter unless referring to a specific form of behavioral treatment.

Figure 69.2 displays a simplified model for understanding the relationships between environmental events, cognitions, emotion and behavior (Wright and Beck, 1994; Wright, 1988; Thase and Beck, 1993). This model is based on the theoretical assumption

that environmental stimuli trigger cognitive processes and the ensuing cognitions give the event personal meaning and elicit subsequent physiological and affective arousal. These emotions, in turn, have a potent reciprocal effect on cognitive content and information processing, such that cascades of dysfunctional thoughts and emotions can occur. The individual's behavioral responses to stimuli and thoughts are viewed as both a product and a cause of maladaptive cognitions. Thus, treatment interventions may be targeted at any or all components of the model.

Of course, many other factors are involved in psychiatric disorders, including genetic predisposition, state-dependent neurobiological changes and various interpersonal variables. These influences are also included in the case conceptualization in CBT. Wright and Thase (1992) have outlined an expanded cognitive–biological model that can be used for synthesizing cognitive and neurobiological factors in a combined therapy approach. Contemporary psychiatric research is striving to understand how best to combine and/or sequence CBT and pharmacotherapy, and relate CBT technique to new understandings in cognitive neuroscience. Nevertheless, the working model in Figure 69.2 can be used as a practical template to guide the therapist's case formulation and interventions.

Automatic Thoughts and Schemas

Dysfunctional information processing is apparent in many psychiatric disorders at two major levels of cognition–automatic thoughts and schemas (Beck, 1976; Dobson and Shaw, 1986; Teasdale, 1983; Segal, 1988; Alfrod and Correia, 1994). Automatic thoughts are cognitions that stream rapidly through an individual's mind, whether spontaneously or in response to some prompt or stimulus. Automatic thoughts may be triggered by affective arousal (i.e., anger, anxiety, or sadness), or conversely, affective shifts are generally accompanied by automatic negative thoughts (Teasdale, 1983). Their automatic nature refers to their speed of entry into awareness and their implicit believability. In this way, automatic thoughts have emotional validity (Thase and Beck, 1993). For most people, before therapy, automatic thoughts are usually not examined carefully for validity. In fact, many people susceptible to anxiety or depression are likely to use an affectively focused logic referred to as emotional reasoning (i.e., "I *feel* that this is correct, therefore it is correct"). Although we all experience automatic thoughts, in depression, anxiety and other psychiatric disorders the thoughts are distinguished by their greater intensity and frequency (LeFebvre, 1981).

Beck (1967) coined the term **cognitive triad** to describe the content of automatic negative thoughts. Typically, automatic

Essentials of Psychiatry   Jerald Kay and Allan Tasman
© 2006 John Wiley & Sons, Ltd.

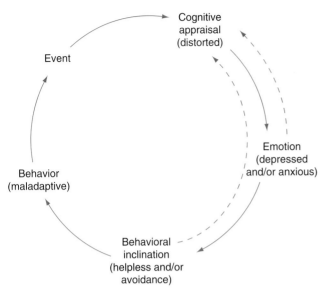

Figure 69.1   *A working model for cognitive–behavioral therapy. Reprinted with permission from the American Psychiatric Press Review of Psychiatry, Vol. 7, pp. 554–590. Cognitive therapy of Depression, Wright JH. Copyright 1988, American Psychiatric Press.*

negative thoughts may be grouped by themes pertaining to self, world (i.e., significant others or people in general) and future. As described subsequently, the themes revealed in one's characteristic automatic negative thoughts may be used to infer deeper levels of cognition: beliefs, rules and schemas. Patients can be taught to examine their beliefs and their operational rules. Although patients are not fully aware of their schemas, these cognitions are usually accessible through the questioning techniques used in CBT (Wright and Beck, 1994).

Beck and coworkers (Beck *et al.*, 1979; Beck and Emery, 1985; Wright and Beck, 1983) have noted that stereotypic errors in logic (termed cognitive errors or cognitive distortions) also shape the content of automatic thoughts (Table 69.1).

Schemas represent the sum of one's beliefs and attitudes. They are the basic assumptions or unspoken rules that act as templates for screening and decoding information from the environment (Segal, 1988; Wright and Beck, 1983; Young and

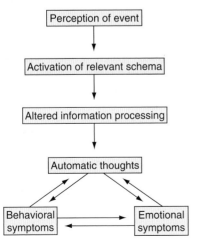

Figure 69.2   *Cognitive model of information processing.*

Table 69.1	Common Patterns of Irrational Thinking in Anxiety and Depression
Cognitive Error	Definition
Overgeneralization	Evidence is drawn from one experience or a small set of experiences that reach an unwarranted conclusion with far-reaching implications.
Catastrophic thinking	An extreme example of overgeneralization, in which the impact of a clearly negative event or experience is amplified to extreme proportions, e.g., "If I have a panic attack, I will lose **all** control and go crazy (or die)."
Maximizing and minimizing	The tendency to exaggerate negative experiences and minimize positive experiences in one's activities and interpersonal relationships.
All-or-none (black or white, absolutistic) thinking	An unnecessary division of complex or continuous outcomes into polarized extremes, e.g., "Either I am a success at this, or I am a total failure."
Jumping to conclusions	Use of pessimism or earlier experiences of failure to prematurely or inappropriately predict failure in a new situation; also known as fortune-telling.
Personalization	Interpretation of an event, situation, or behavior as salient or personally indicative of a negative aspect of self.
Selective negative focus – "ignoring the evidence" or "mental filter"	Undesirable or negative events, memories, or implications are focused on at the expense of recalling or identifying other, more neutral or positive information; in fact, positive information may be ignored *or* disqualified as irrelevant, atypical, or trivial.

Adapted with permission from Beck AT, Rush AJ, Shaw BF *et al.* (1979) *Cognitive Therapy of Depression.* Guilford Press, New York.

Lindermann, 1992). Psychological well-being may be understood in part by development of a set of schemas that yield realistic appraisals of self in relation to world (e.g., "I'm reasonably attractive, but looks aren't everything", "I can be loved under the right circumstances", or "I must work harder to compensate for an average intellect"). Although unspoken, schemas may be inferred from one's beliefs and attitudes. In the cognitive model, dysfunctional attitudes are the structural "bridge" between pathological schemas and automatic negative thoughts. Schemas pertaining to safety, vulnerability to threat, self-evaluation, one's lovability, and one's competence or self-efficacy contain the ground rules for personal behavior that are particularly relevant to the understanding of disorders such as anxiety, depression, or characterological

Table 69.2   Proposed Maladaptive Schemas

Autonomy	
Dependence	The belief that one is unable to function with the constant support of others
Subjugation/lack of individuation	The voluntary or involuntary sacrifice of one's own needs to satisfy others' needs
Vulnerability to harm or illness	The fear that disaster (i.e., natural, criminal, medical, or financial) is about to strike at any time
Fear of losing self-control	The fear that one will involuntarily lose control of one's own impulses, behavior, emotions, mind, and so on

Connectedness	
Emotional deprivation	The expectation that one's needs for nurturance, empathy, or affect will never be adequately met by others
Abandonment/loss	The fear that one will imminently lose significant others or be emotionally isolated forever
Mistrust	The expectation that others will hurt, abuse, cheat, lie, or manipulate you
Social isolation/ alienation	The belief that one is isolated from the rest of the world, is different from other people, or does not belong to any group or community

Worthiness	
Defectiveness/ unlovability	The assumption that one is inwardly defective or that, if the flaw is exposed, one is fundamentally unlovable
Social undesirability	The belief that one is outwardly undesirable to others (e.g., ugly, sexually undesirable, low in status, dull, or boring)
Incompetence/failure	The assumption that one cannot perform competently in areas of achievement, daily responsibilities, or decision-making
Guilt/punishment	The conclusion that one is morally bad or irresponsible and deserving of criticism or punishment
Shame/embarrassment	Recurrent feelings of shame or self-consciousness experienced because one believes that one's inadequacies (as reflected in the preceding maladaption schemas of worthiness) are totally unacceptable to others

Limits and Standards	
Unrelenting standards	The relentless striving to meet extremely high expectation of oneself, at all costs (i.e., at the expense of happiness, pleasure, health, or satisfactory relationships)
Entitlement	Insistence that one should be able to do, say, or have whatever one wants immediately

Reprinted with permission from Thase ME and Beck AT (1992) An overview of cognitive therapy, in *Cognitive Therapy with Inpatients: Developing a Cognitive Milieu* (eds Wright JH, Thase ME, Beck AT *et al.*). Guilford Press, New York, p. 9; adapted from Young (1999) *Cognitive Therapy for Personality Disorders: A Schema-Focused Approach.* Professional Resource Exchange, Sarasota, FL.

disturbances (Segal, 1988; Young and Lindermann, 1992; Blackburn *et al.*, 1986b; Beck *et al.*, 1990). A number of schemas relevant to psychiatric illness are listed in Table 69.2. Bowlby (1985) has noted that most psychopathologically relevant schemas are developed early in life, when the individual is relatively powerless and dependent on caregivers.

The cognitive model of psychiatric illness emphasizes the concept of stress-diathesis (Thase and Beck, 1993; Metalsky *et al.*, 1987). From this perspective, a schema such as "I must be loved to have worth", might remain latent until activated by a relevant life stressor (i.e., a romantic breakup).

Underlying schemas may be buttressed by either maladaptive or adaptive attitudes (e.g., "No matter how hard I try, I'm bound to fail" versus "I'm a survivor; if I just hang in there things will be okay"), but many of these cognitive structures have mixed features (Wright and Beck, 1994). Schemas such as "If I'm not perfect, I'm a failure" may lead to driven obsessional behavior, rigid attitudes and beliefs, and frequent bouts of dysphoric or irritable moods. However, basic perfectionistic beliefs such as these can also result in high levels of performance and success.

The concept of attributional style (Hammen *et al.*, 1989) describes an alternative view of cognitive vulnerability. Derived from human studies of the learned helplessness paradigm (Seligman, 1975), attributional style refers to the characteristic way that people explain the causality, controllability and impact of events. People susceptible to depression are more likely to have an attributional style in which negative events are perceived to be personally controllable (i.e., internality), far-reaching (i.e., globality), and enduring (i.e., stability) (Peterson *et al.*, 1985; Abramson *et al.*, 1989; Sweeney *et al.*, 1986).

The results of many studies suggest that disturbances in information processing are essential features of depression and anxiety (see Chapter 15 on Cognitive Neuroscience).

Behavioral Model

The behavioral model is based on the relatively straightforward chain of events and responses illustrated in Figure 69.3. Through the years, considerable effort and debate have concerned whether stimulus–response and response–reinforcement relationships

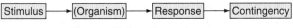

Figure 69.3 *Chain of events.*

could be invoked to account for the complexity of human behavior (Kazdin, 1982; Staats, 1964). In its maturity, behavioral therapy has broadened beyond an exclusive focus on observable behaviors (i.e., radical behaviorism) and now incorporates cognitive processes and other individual variables that affect one's preparedness to learn (Bandura, 1977b; Goldfried and Davison, 1994). For example, in observational learning, the stimulus–response contingency relationship is established vicariously, by watching, reading about, or imagining the event in question. Reinforcement does not have to take place explicitly; it may occur vicariously, or it may simply be imagined. Other factors, such as the individual's past history, inherent talents, or skillfulness of his or her pertinent response repertoire, help account for the wealth of interindividual variability in stimulus–response relationships. Bandura's cognitive–behavioral formulation of self-efficacy is one example of a "mental" construct that has abiding behavioral implications. This modifiable attitude or belief (roughly akin to self-confidence) influences persistence, willingness to try new things, optimism and capacity to endure setbacks (Bandura, 1977a).

Cognitive and Behavioral Treatment Strategies

The cognitive and behavioral therapies are well known for their use of specific treatment techniques. Commonly used CBT procedures are directly linked to the theoretical constructs and empirical research of this school of therapy. Although techniques are given somewhat more emphasis in CBT than in other forms of psychotherapy, there is still considerable room for therapists to be creative and flexible in developing a treatment plan. In fact, novice therapists sometimes focus too much on applying techniques at the expense of nurturing the therapeutic alliance and case formulation. Development of a productive therapeutic relationship and an individualized case conceptualization should always take precedence over the implementation of specific cognitive or behavioral techniques. A number of the more important CBT strategies are described briefly here. More detailed accounts of CBT interventions can be found elsewhere (Beck *et al.*, 1979; Beck 1995; Barlow and Cerny, 1988; Freeman *et al.*, 1989; Persons, 1989).

Collaborative Empiricism

The therapeutic relationship is as important in CBT as in any of the other effective psychotherapies. However, interchanges between therapist and patient often differ from those observed in supportive or dynamically oriented treatment. One difference is that the therapist is responsible for managing the pace of the session and uses an agenda to help make each session as efficient as possible. Cognitive–behavioral therapists strive for a therapeutic relationship that emphasizes: 1) a high degree of collaboration and 2) a scientific attitude toward testing the validity or usefulness of particular cognitions and behavior. This therapeutic stance is referred to as collaborative empiricism. The empirical nature of the relationship reflects that therapist and patient work together as an investigative team to develop hypotheses about cognitive or behavioral patterns, examine data, and explore alternative ways of thinking or behaving. At first, therapists usually spend more time

teaching and explaining in CBT than in other forms of therapy, yet in the course of therapy, patients are actively engaged to become increasingly involved in the work of treatment.

The collaborative empirical stance requires that the therapist and patient work together to make an **honest** appraisal of the validity of cognitions as well as of the adaptive or maladaptive nature of beliefs and behaviors. If a negative assessment proves to be accurate (e.g., the patient actually has made serious mistakes, the individual's spouse is highly likely to leave, or the patient has engaged in a repetitive self-defeating behavior pattern), then the therapist and patient need to work together in a problem-solving mode to develop a plan to cope with the problems at hand or practice more adaptive strategies for use in the future.

Wright and Beck (1994) and others (Clark *et al.* 1999) have recommended several strategies for enhancing collaborative empiricism. These include: 1) adjusting the therapist's level of activity to match the patients' symptom severity or the phase of treatment; 2) encouraging use of self-help procedures; 3) attending to the "nonspecific" variables important in all therapeutic relationships (e.g., empathy, respect, equanimity, kindness and good listening skills); 4) promoting frequent two-way feedback; 5) devising coping strategies to help deal with real losses or implementing a plan of action to address maladaptive behavior; 6) recognizing transference phenomena; 7) customizing therapeutic interventions; and 8) using humor judiciously. It is also important to recognize and account for the wide variety of individual differences in cultural backgrounds, social attitudes and expectations that each patient brings to the therapy encounter (Wright and Davis, 1994).

Psychoeducation

Most forms of CBT integrate explicit psychoeducational procedures as a core element of the treatment process. Psychoeducational procedures are typically blended into treatment sessions in a manner that de-emphasizes formal teaching. There is a concerted effort to teach the patient why it is important to challenge automatic thoughts, identify cognitive errors and practice implementing a more rational thinking style. Behavioral interventions are also preceded by psychoeducation to convey the background for principles such as extinction, reinforcement, self-monitoring, exposure and response prevention.

In the early phases of treatment, special attention is paid to socializing the patient to CBT. The basic cognitive–behavioral model is demonstrated, and expectations for both patient and therapist are conveyed. Some of the frequently used psychoeducational procedures in CBT include brief, impromptu explanations (often written on a chalkboard or a pad of paper to increase the chances of comprehension and retention) and reading assignments, such as *Coping with Depression* (Beck and Greenberg, 1974), *Feeling Good* (Burns, 1980), *Mind Over Mood* (Greenberger and Padesky, 1995) or *Getting Your Life Back* (Wright and Basco, 2001). Psychoeducational initiatives typically become more complex as therapy proceeds. For example, detailed explanations and repeated exercises may be needed before the patient fully grasps abstract concepts such as attributional style or schemas. As therapy progresses, homework assignments continue explicitly to reinforce material covered during therapy sessions.

Modifying Automatic Thoughts

The first step in changing automatic thoughts is to help the patient recognize when she or he is having them. The therapist is often able to illustrate the presence of automatic negative thoughts during the initial session by gently calling attention to a change in the patient's mood. Such "mood shifts" can be excellent learning experiences that give personally relevant illustrations of the linkage between cognitions and feelings.

One common misconception of CBT is that its practitioners disregard the role of affect or feelings in the etiology and treatment of psychiatric disorders. Actually, one of the principal components of CBT is the stimulation and modulation of emotion (see Figure 69.3). In fact, Beck referred to emotion as "the royal road to cognition" (Beck, 1991). In contrast to experiential therapies, variations in emotion are used in CBT to establish links with cognition and identify errors in information processing. Getting in touch with feelings is thus not a goal in CBT but only a means by which therapy helps patients to gain greater control over the processes that influence their moods and behaviors.

Socratic Questioning

The most frequently used technique to uncover and modify automatic negative thoughts is Socratic questioning (or guided discovery) (Beck *et al.*, 1979; Overholser, 1993a, 1993b, 1993c). Socratic questioning teaches the use of rationality and inductive reasoning to challenge whether what is thought or felt is actually true. The therapist models the use of Socratic questioning and encourages the patient to start raising questions about the validity of his or her thinking. There are few formal guidelines for Socratic questioning (Overholser, 1993a). Rather, therapists learn to use their experience and ingenuity to frame good questions that engage the patient in a process aimed at recognizing and modifying a biased or distorted cognitive style. Typical questions include: What ran through your mind at that time? What is the evidence that your impression is accurate? Could there be any alternative explanations? If this were true, what would be the worst thing that would happen? When guided discovery methods are not sufficient to draw out automatic thoughts, the therapist may turn to several alternative ways of eliciting dysfunctional cognitions, as described in the following.

Imagery Techniques and Role-playing

Imagery techniques and role-playing are used when direct questioning does not fully reveal important underlying cognitions. When imagery is used, the therapist sets the scene by asking the patient to visualize the situation that caused distress. Although some patients can readily imagine themselves in a previous scene, many need prompts or imagery induction to encourage their active participation in the exercise. Several types of questions can be used to help frame the scene. These include inquiries about: 1) the physical details of the setting, 2) occurrences immediately before the interaction, and 3) descriptions of the other people in the scene (Wright and Beck, 1994). In role-playing exercises, the therapist and patient act out an interpersonal vignette to uncover automatic thoughts or to try out a revised pattern of thinking. This technique is used less frequently than imagery by most cognitive–behavioral therapists and may be reserved for situations in which transference distortions are unlikely (Wright and Beck, 1994).

Thought Recording

Thought recording is one of the most useful procedures for identifying and changing automatic thoughts. This technique is first presented in relatively simple two- or three-column versions in the early stages of therapy. When the two-column procedure is used, patients are instructed to write down events in one column and thoughts in the other. Alternatively, they can record events, thoughts and emotions in the three columns. The purpose of this exercise is to encourage patients to begin to use self-monitoring to increase awareness of their thought patterns. Next, the strength of the emotion and the believability of the automatic negative thoughts are rated on a scale of 0 to 100. In subsequent sessions, a more complex five-column thought record, the Daily Record of Dysfunctional Thoughts (DRDT) is introduced (Figure 69.4). The fourth column of the DRDT encourages the patient to develop rational alternatives that rebut the automatic negative thoughts; the fifth column is used for a reevaluation of the mood and cognitive ratings. Work on identifying cognitive errors can also be included in this form of thought recording.

Examining the Evidence

The examining the evidence procedure is a collaborative exercise used to test the validity of automatic negative thoughts. Cognitions are set forth as hypotheses rather than established facts. The patient is encouraged to write down evidence that either supports or refutes the automatic thought using a two-column form (i.e., pros and cons). Cognitive errors such as magnification, personalization and all-or-nothing thinking are frequently revealed in these situations.

Next, the therapist helps to guide revision of the automatic negative thought in light of the evidence (e.g., "I **often** feel inferior to others, even when there's no good evidence that they feel that way" or "I have had a number of difficulties with my teachers and employers, but not all relationships have been bad"). The process thus moves from the patient's general and globally negative interpretations to more specific, factually based statements.

When an honest appraisal uncovers evidence in support of negative cognitions, the therapist may choose to focus on the patient's attributions of causality or internality. The patient who posits a negative attribution for poor work evaluation (e.g., "My performance was poor because I don't have what it takes") can usually be aided to consider a more neutral attribution (e.g., "My performance was poor because I was underprepared...my depression also prevented more energetic preparation"). The treatment plan may also be revised to develop better methods of coping in similar situations or to work on ways of remediating skill deficits. Sometimes, particular difficulties cannot be changed (e.g., physical handicaps, markedly unattractive physical looks, or severe financial limitations).

Generating Alternatives

If automatic thoughts prove to be largely dysfunctional, the patient is encouraged to generate alternatives that are more accurate or factual. Many of the techniques discussed earlier can be used to help generate alternatives to automatic thoughts. Socratic questioning is used in therapy sessions to help the patient start to think more creatively. Also, psychoeducational procedures may be employed to teach brainstorming techniques. For example, the patient may be taught to use "expert testimony" or the opinions of someone who knows her or him well (i.e., a sibling, spouse, or best friend) to help develop more rational alternatives. Thought records are often used to record alternatives to automatic thoughts. We often encourage patients to collect their thought records in notebook form for ongoing use. Figure 69.4 illustrates the use of rational alternatives during CBT for a depressed patient.

Date	Event	Automatic thoughts	Emotions	Rational thoughts	Outcome
	a. Describe actual event preceding unpleasant emotion or b. Stream of thoughts, daydream, or memories preceding unpleasant emotion.	a. Write automatic thought(s) that led to emotion(s). b. Rate of belief in automatic thought(s), 0–100%.	a. Specify sad, anxious, angry, tense, and so on. b. Rate degree of emotion, 0–100.	a. Identify cognitive errors. b. Write rational response to automatic thought(s). c. Rate belief in rational response, 0–100%.	a. Specify and rate subsequent emotion(s), 0–100.
1/30/95	My boss asks for a progress report.	I'm in big trouble. (85) I can't handle this job. (90) I've messed everything up. (95)	Anxious (95) Sad (80)	Magnification, ignoring the evidence, overgeneralization. I'm slightly behind schedule, but I can catch up. (95) I've had a good track record with this job. (100) I'm doing O.K. in some other areas of my life. (95)	Anxious (40) Sad (20)
	My son comes home late from a party.	Nobody listens to me. (90) He doesn't care. (75) What's the use of trying? (80)	Angry (75) Sad (85)	All or none thinking, ignoring the evidence, personalizing. My son pays attention a fair amount of the time, but he doesn't always do what I want. (90) There's plenty of evidence that he cares about me. (100) We need to improve how we communicate. (95) I need to tell him that I'm angry. (100)	Angry (30) Sad (25)

Figure 69.4   *Daily record of dysfunctional thoughts.*

Many patients with depression, anxiety and related conditions have relatively rigid cognitive styles that perpetuate dysfunctional thought and behavior patterns. These individuals frequently experience "second-order" automatic negative thoughts, that is, negative thoughts that are triggered by rational alternatives ("that's a cop-out…quit making excuses"). These thoughts about thoughts tend to undermine the credibility of the rational responses and may dampen the patient's enthusiasm for using the procedure. The therapist may notice a particular facial expression or a change in the patient's posture that suggests the existence of second-order thoughts. In such cases, more active therapeutic assistance may be needed. For example, the therapist may need to act as a teacher or coach in the area of adaptive cognitive functioning, rapidly rebutting automatic thoughts as they arise. Coping cards, which are index cards with helpful reminders on the use of CBT methods (in this case, rational responses to repetitive automatic negative thoughts), may be written during sessions and carried by the patient in his or her pocket, wallet, or purse for later use.

Cognitive–Behavioral Rehearsal

Cognitive–behavioral rehearsal is a treatment strategy that is particularly useful for preparing patients to put their experiences in CBT to work in real-life circumstances. After automatic thoughts have been elicited and modified through procedures described before, the therapist guides the patient in a series of rehearsal exercises to try out alternative cognitions in a variety of situations. By using imagery and role-playing scenarios to practice generating more adaptive cognitions, the patient may become aware of problems that could interfere with implementation of the new style of thinking. Further practice and targeted homework assignments may then be needed before alternative cognitions can be fully used. For example, the effects of cognitive–behavioral rehearsal may be extended to real situations by assigning homework to test use of the modified automatic thoughts.

Modifying Schemas

The emphasis in the early phases of therapy is usually on behavioral activation, identifying and changing automatic thoughts, and the reduction of symptoms. However, as the patient gains knowledge of cognitive–behavioral principles and acute symptoms begin to subside, the focus of the treatment sessions usually shifts toward work on the schema level. Because schemas serve as underlying templates for making sense of new information, they play a major role in the modulation of more superficial cognitions (automatic thoughts), regulation of affect, self-esteem and control of the behavioral repertoire. Thus, schema modification is an important component of cognitively oriented therapies.

With Axis I disorders such as major depressive disorder and panic disorder, schema revision efforts are directed at correcting dysfunctional attitudes that may predispose the patient to symptomatic recurrences. After several months of productive therapy, schema modification may be placed in the context of reducing future vulnerability. CBT of personality disorders typically requires that a major portion of therapy be devoted to modifying schemas and related patterns of behavioral dysfunction (Beck *et al.*, 1990). When schematic work cannot be fully addressed in time-limited therapy, the model of ongoing change may be introduced. Thus, the patient may begin to change her or his "life course" by development of a long-term self-help plan. Jarrett and colleagues (2001) have proposed continuation and maintenance phases of CBT treatment of depression, and they argue for focusing on schema change in these phases of treatment if it is not accomplished in the acute phase of treatment.

Many of the techniques used to test and modify automatic thoughts are also used to identify and revise schemas. Psychoeducational interventions are usually required as a first step. Most patients are not aware of their "guiding principles", so the therapist may need to begin by introducing and illustrating this concept. It is often useful to use synonyms for the term schema (such as basic assumptions or core beliefs) and to demonstrate how schemas are linked to automatic negative thoughts using material from the patient's own experience (Wright and Beck, 1994). Socratic questioning is the core procedure used for schema modification (Beck *et al.*, 1979; Overholser, 1993c).

The downward arrow technique (Figure 69.5) is a particularly powerful way to move from surface cognitions to deeper cognitive structures (Thase and Beck, 1993). This technique describes asking the patient a question such as: "If this automatic thought were true, what would it mean about you as a person?" Another useful approach is to examine patterns of automatic thoughts from thought records to sort out common themes. The therapist may suggest a thematic collation based on her or his knowledge of the patient's automatic negative thoughts. In some

situations, it may be helpful to have patients review a description of common pathological schemas to recognize some of their core beliefs (see Table 69.2). On occasion, it may be useful to have the patient write a brief autobiography to help elucidate the historical antecedents of the schema. Computerized learning programs can also be employed to help patients uncover their schemas (Wright *et al.*, 1995, 2002a).

Because schemas are so strongly held (in essence, they have helped define reality and mold behavior for years), they may require intensive work in a number of therapy sessions to undergo significant change. Sometimes long-term continuation and maintenance CBT is required to accomplish schematic restructuring. Therapists can select from a number of CBT techniques, including examining the evidence, listing advantages and disadvantages, generating alternatives, cognitive response prevention and cognitive–behavioral rehearsal, as they attempt to modify schemas (Wright and Beck, 1994). Examining the evidence, generating alternatives and cognitive–behavioral rehearsal were described earlier as methods of changing automatic thoughts.

Cognitive Response Prevention

In cognitive response prevention, the patient agrees to complete a homework assignment in which she or he must behave in a way that is inconsistent with the pathological schema. For example, a person with perfectionistic attitudes may be engaged in an assignment in which she or he must perform in a "so-so" manner. This is intended to activate the schema which is triggering automatic negative thoughts (e.g., "They'll think I'm a sloth" or "I'll never be trusted with an important assignment again"). By not responding to the perfectionistic demands dictated by the schema, the individual thus has the opportunity to cope with the automatic negative thoughts consequent to this "rule violation".

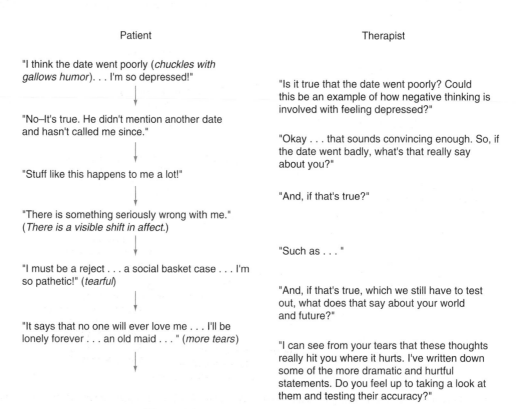

Figure 69.5   *The downward arrow technique.*

Listing Advantages and Disadvantages

The listing advantages and disadvantages procedure is particularly useful when a schema appears to have both adaptive and maladaptive features. Schemas that have damaging effects are often maintained because they also have a positive side. For example, the schema "I must be perfect to be accepted" can have significant benefits (e.g., hard work and attention to detail often lead to success in work or school). Nevertheless, because perfection is seldom possible, the individual may remain vulnerable to setbacks. Other schemas, such as "I'm a complete loser", may not seem to have any advantages at first glance. However, even such a markedly negative basic assumption can have certain behavioral reinforcers associated with it. For example, a person who believes that he or she is a loser may avoid making commitments, withdraw from challenging assignments, or refuse to exert a sustained effort to solve a difficult problem. This strategy may thus protect the person from painful setbacks. The advantages and disadvantages analysis provides the patient and therapist with essential information for planning modifications. Revised schemas are most likely to be used when they take into account both the maladaptive and the adaptive features of the old basic assumption.

In general, it is recommended that patients keep a list of the schemas as they have been identified. The schema list helps to focus the patient's attention on the overarching nature of these maladaptive principles. Because schemas often become manifest only during periods of increased stress or symptom expression, they may appear to fade in significance as the patient begins to improve. For example, behavioral treatment programs that neither endorse nor aim to modify schemas are generally as effective as CBT in the short run. However, there may be a false security engendered by symptom relief. The cognitive model posits that the individual will remain vulnerable to the depressogenic impact of "matching" life events unless schema revision is accomplished (Thase and Beck, 1993).

Behavioral Techniques

In CBT, behavioral methods are usually integrated with cognitive restructuring in a comprehensive treatment plan. Behavioral strategies may be given a greater emphasis earlier in therapy with more severely symptomatic patients such as those with intense depression, bipolar symptoms, or schizophrenia (Beck *et al.*, 1979; Thase and Wright, 1991; Kingdon and Turkingdon, 1995; Basco and Rush, 1996; Scott and Wright, 1997). Some cognitive–behavior therapists may rely primarily on behavioral interventions for conditions such as obsessive–compulsive disorder (OCD) or simple phobias. Commonly used behavioral strategies are described here in alphabetical order.

Activity Scheduling, Graded Tasks and Mastery–Pleasure Exercises

One key to the behavioral approach for treatment of depression is the interruption of the downward spiral linking mood, inactivity and negative cognition (Beck *et al.*, 1979; Lewinsohn *et al.*, 1982) (Figure 69.6). Completing an activity schedule is often the first behavioral homework assignment used in CBT (Beck and Greenberg, 1974). Depressed patients are asked to begin to keep a daily log that is used to chart the relationship between their moods and their activities (Figure 69.7).

The nature of the activities is examined, and deficits in activities that might elicit pleasure or feelings of competence are identified. Next, assignments are made to engage in discrete pleasurable activities (or, in the case of an anhedonic individual, activities that were rewarding before becoming depressed). If needed, a "menu" of reinforcers can be generated by having the patient fill out a Pleasant Events Schedule (Lewinsohn *et al.*, 1982). Following operant principles, activities that have been "high-grade" reinforcers in the past are scheduled during times of low moods or decreased activity. Next, subjective ratings of

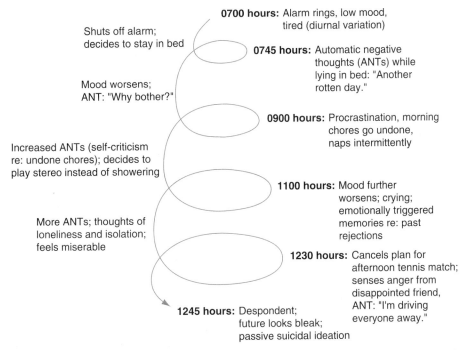

Figure 69.6 *The downward spiral: interaction of affect, behavior, and cognition in severe depression. ANTs, Automatic negative thoughts.*

Note: Grade activities **M** for mastery and **P** for pleasure

		Monday	Tuesday	Wednesday	Thursday	Friday	Saturday	Sunday
AM	6:00 6:30							
	7:00 7:30							
	8:00 8:30							
	9:00 9:30							
	10:00 10:30							
	11:00 11:30							
PM	12:00 12:30							
	1:00 1:30							
	2:00 2:30							
	3:00 3:30							
	4:00 4:30							
	5:00 5:30							

Mastery, accomplished, achieved something
Pleasure, fun, amusement, enjoyment

Scale: 0–5; 0, none, 5, most

Figure 69.7 *Weekly activity schedule.*

mastery or competence and pleasure are added to the activity schedule by use of a simple scale (i.e., 0–5), to avoid the tendency of dichotomous thinking. In this way, achieving a small degree of pleasure or mastery during a scheduled activity may be framed as an accomplishment, particularly early in the course of therapy.

Breathing Control

An important component of CBT for anxiety disorders involves teaching the patient breathing exercises that may be used to counteract hyperventilation and/or reduce tension (Clark *et al.*, 1985). Slow, deep breathing can have a calming effect not unlike progressive muscle relaxation (Bernstein and Borkovec, 1973). These exercises also help to distract the patient from autonomic cues. After initial instruction and practice, the breathing skills are then applied in progressively more anxiety-provoking situations.

A note of caution is in order when teaching patients breathing control exercises. We have seen many patients who have misunderstood instructions and who have developed a pattern of deep overbreathing in response to stress. Instead of helping reduce anxiety, their breathing changes may increase the chances of hyperventilation. Thus, we typically recommend that patients be taught about the pace and form of normal breathing patterns. Next clinicians can model normal, calm breathing as compared with overbreathing during an anxiety attack. The second hand of a watch can be used to time breaths so that they can be slowed to a normal rate. Positive, calming images can also be used to reduce anxiety during the breathing exercises. Finally, we suggest that patients practice breathing exercises regularly to gain mastery of this anxiety management technique.

Contingency Contracting and Behavior Exchange

These strategies use the principles of operant conditioning (Skinner, 1938) to modify the probability of occurrence of either undesired or desired behaviors. An excellent introduction to these methods is presented by Malott and colleagues (1993). One key to applied behavioral analysis is control over the contingencies or reinforcers. Another important factor is that the terms of the contract are negotiated and should be specific and relatively straightforward. The positive contingency or reinforcer should be desirable and available shortly after the terms of the contract have been met. A paycheck is a good example of a contingency contract. Another common strategy is to chain, or pair, a high-frequency behavior (e.g., reading, watching television, or listening to music) to a low-frequency one (e.g., doing paperwork, doing housework, spending time with the children). Contingencies should generally start out relatively "rich" (e.g., 1 hour of video game time after 15 minutes of paperwork) and may be progressively "thinned" in time (Malott *et al.*, 1993). Punishments or "response cost" contingencies are less widely used because of their negative affective responses (Azrin and Holz, 1966).

Behavioral contracts may be particularly useful for assisting patients with medication adherence. For example, the therapist may help the patient identify barriers to taking medication as prescribed and then work out behavioral solutions which are written in contract form. Behavioral methods may include pairing medication taking with routine activities such as brushing teeth or meals, reminder systems and reinforcement from significant others. We recommend explicit discussion of adherence problems and mutual agreement on a plan for taking medications when patients have difficulty in following the pharmacotherapy plan.

Desensitization and Relaxation Training

Systematic desensitization (Wolpe, 1958) was one of the first behavioral strategies to gain wide acceptance. Systematic desensitization relies on exposure through a progressive hierarchy of fear-inducing situations. This procedure may use pairing of progressive deep muscle relaxation and visualization of the target behavior to decondition fearful responses. Systematic desensitization is useful for treatment of simple phobias, social phobia, panic attacks and generalized anxiety (Wolpe, 1982). Some evidence suggests that the active ingredient of systematic desensitization is exposure to the feared situation, first in imagination and later in reality, rather than an actual counterconditioning through the relaxation response (Kazdin and Wilcoxin, 1976). Progressive deep muscle relaxation is also useful as a self-directed coping strategy and for treatment of sleep-onset insomnia (Goldfried and Davison, 1994; Bernstein and Borkovec, 1973).

Exposure and Flooding

The purpose of these strategies is to speed extinction of conditioned fear or anxiety responses. Behavioral theory dictates that fearfulness is reinforced by avoidance and escape behaviors (Rachman *et al.*, 1986). Because the basis of the fear or phobia is irrational, the optimal strategy is to increase exposure to the feared activity without aversive consequences. In obsessive–compulsive disorder, the ritualistic behavior (e.g., handwashing or checking) is presumed to be reinforced by the relief of the anxiety associated with the compulsion (e.g., handwashing temporarily relieves the fear of contamination) (Rachman *et al.*, 1986). In exposure, there are at least three means of fear reduction: autonomic habituation, recognition that the fear is irrational and explicit enhancement of morale or self-efficacy that accompanies mastering the previously dreaded activity.

In graded or progressive exposure, a hierarchy is established, ranging from least to most anxiety-provoking situations. The individual is taught one or more ways to cope with anxiety (e.g., relaxation or self-instruction), and with the help of the therapist, the items on the hierarchy are worked through, one item at a time. Mastery is predicated on maintaining a sufficient duration of exposure for the fear to extinguish or dissipate. In some cases, imagery (exposure *in vitro*) is used before moving to exposure to the actual feared stimulus. Exposure may also be enhanced by guided support (i.e., the therapist's presence during the session) or by use of coping cognitions for the duration of the exposure exercise.

Flooding, which relies on the same principles, dispatches with the hierarchical approach. The individual is exposed to the maximal level of anxiety as quickly as possible. The rationale for this accelerated approach is that it may hasten autonomic habituation. To be effective, flooding needs to be accompanied by response prevention. In response prevention treatment of

OCD, the individual agrees not to perform the compulsion despite strong urges to do so. Because obsessions are more private than compulsions, there can be less certainty that the individual has fully participated in response prevention exercises (Stern, 1978).

Simple phobias may be rapidly treated by an accelerated form of exposure referred to as participant modeling or contact desensitization. The therapist serves as a supportive coach or guide and assists the patient through a progressively more demanding level of exposure to the feared situation. In most cases, lifelong fears of air travel, tunnels, heights, matches, dogs, water, or insects can be fully treated in a few hours of guided exposure.

Social Skills Training

Satisfactory interpersonal relationships require a complex set of skills, including reciprocity, respect for another's opinion, appropriate modulation of self-disclosure, the tempered ability to yield on some occasions and to set limits at other times, the natural use of social reinforcers, and the capacity to express anger and resolve conflicts in a constructive manner (Lewinsohn *et al.*, 1982; Hersen *et al.*, 1984). Many people with psychiatric disorders suffer from either a state-dependent deterioration of these social skills or lifelong deficits of such skills. Once established, social skills deficits can increase the likelihood of experiencing stressful life events as well as "turn off" family members and other sources of social support that may help to buffer people against stressors (Coyne *et al.*, 1987).

Problems as diverse as underassertiveness, temper "attacks", excessive self-disclosure, monopolistic conversational style, underreinforcement of significant others and splitting (i.e., playing one against another) are amenable to social skills training. The methods employed include modeling (i.e., the therapist demonstrates a more effective alternative approach), role-playing and role reversal, behavior rehearsal and specific practice assignments. Often, the interpersonal anxiety and lack of self-confidence that go hand in hand with social skills deficits lessen in response to successful mastery of targeted assignments.

Thought Stopping and Distraction

Automatic negative thoughts and repetitive, intrusive ruminations are sometimes too intense to address with purely cognitive interventions. The technique of thought stopping capitalizes on the individual's ability to use a selectively narrowed attentional focus to suppress the intrusive cognitions. For example, a ruminative individual may be asked to visualize a large red "stop" sign, including its octagonal shape and white lettering. The command "Stop!" is paired with the image. The image and command are then used to interrupt a "run" of ruminations. At first, the technique is practiced in sessions at times when automatic thoughts or ruminations are mild. After initial success, the technique is next applied to more intensely disturbing cognitions. For individuals who find visualization difficult or ineffective, a rubber band may be worn on the wrist as a distractor. In a manner similar to that described before, the command "Stop!" is paired with a brisk snap of the rubber band.

Indications for Treatment

The cognitive and behavioral therapies are indicated as primary treatments for adults suffering from several nonpsychotic, nonorganic disorders including major depressive disorder, dysthymic disorder, panic disorder, social phobia, OCD, post traumatic stress disorder (PTSD), generalized anxiety disorder and bulimia nervosa (Wright *et al.*, 2002b). Cognitive and behavioral therapies are also useful as adjunctive treatments for patients with bipolar disorder (Basco and Rush, 1996; Basco and Thase, 1998; Lam *et al.*, 2000) and schizophrenia (Mueser, 1998; Kingdon and Turkington, 1995; Senky *et al.*, 2000). Although not extensively studied, cognitive and behavioral therapies incorporating coping skills training and relapse prevention strategies may also improve the outcome of individuals with substance abuse disorders (Wright *et al.*, 2002b).

Cognitive and behavioral therapies, like most other types of treatment, have not been studied widely in patients with Axis II disorders. However, the CBT approach to problem specification and explicit training in coping skills may be well suited for treatment of individuals willing to work on changing these habitual, ingrained patterns of thinking and behavior (Beck *et al.*, 1990). Specific cognitive–behavioral formulations have been developed for each of the personality disorders, and modifications of CBT methods have been described for working with patients with Axis II problems (Beck *et al.*, 1990). Linehan's model of CBT (dialectical behavior therapy) has been shown to be efficacious in reducing parasuicidal behavior in patients with borderline personality disorder (Linehan *et al.*, 1991, 1993).

Selection of this Modality

Selection of CBT for an individual patient should be based on the appropriateness of CBT for the treatment situation. Relevant questions include: Is the patient psychotic? If so, are there specific target behaviors and has psychopharmacological treatment been optimized? Does the patient suffer from a disorder known to be responsive to CBT? Within groups of patients with potentially treatable disorders, other indicators of responsivity include chronicity, severity and comorbidity (Whisman, 1993; Thase *et al.*, 1993). A good general rule is that patients with acute, mild to moderately severe, mood and anxiety disorders are the best candidates for treatment with CBT alone (Thase, 1995). Patients with more chronic, severe, or complicated illnesses may be better candidates for combined treatment strategies than for CBT alone (Wright and Thase, 1992; Thase and Howland, 1994; Friedman, 1997). McCullough (2000) has developed a variant of CBT for chronic depression that has shown much promise alone and combined with antidepressant medication.

Preparation of the Patient

The cognitive and behavioral therapies explicitly incorporate strategies to increase involvement and preparedness of the patient for therapy. Patients are typically encouraged to read relevant written materials describing the theory and strategies of the therapy; for common disorders, such as major depressive disorder and panic disorder, self-help manuals for patients are now available (Burns, 1990; Greenberger and Padesky, 1995; Wright and Basco, 2001). Patients beginning CBT need to become acculturated to the following: 1) they will be active participants in trying out new strategies; 2) they will be expected to do homework; 3) the outcome of therapy will be measured and strategies will be altered if they are not helping; 4) therapy will be focused on symptoms and social functioning and generally will be time limited in nature; and 5) the chances of success after treatment termination can be gauged by the patients' incorporation of the therapy into their day-to-day life.

Phases of Treatment

Most cognitive and behavioral therapies may be viewed as using a three-stage process. The initial phase includes the processes of clinical assessment, case formulation, establishment of a therapeutic relationship, socialization of the patient to therapy, psychoeducation and introduction to treatment procedures. The middle stage involves the sequential application and mastery of cognitive and behavioral treatment strategies. The second stage ends when the patient has obtained the desired symptomatic outcome. The final phase of therapy is characterized by preparation for termination. The frequency of sessions is reduced, and there is a steady transfer of the responsibility for the continued use of therapeutic strategies from the therapist to the patient. The third stage of treatment also focuses on relapse prevention. Strategies used at this point include anticipation of reaction to future stressors or high-risk situations, identification of prodromal symptoms, rehearsal of self-help procedures and establishment of guidelines for return to treatment (Otto *et al.*, 1993; Thase, 1993). The failure to achieve a remission of depressive symptoms after 16 to 20 weeks of treatment may indicate a need for continuation phase treatment to achieve these goals and maintenance phase treatment for relapse prevention. Incomplete symptomatic remission after 20 weeks of CBT may also indicate the need for adding pharmacotherapy to the treatment plan as we discuss in greater detail below.

Intensity of Treatment

Outpatient CBT is normally conducted once or twice a week. In selected cases, three-times-weekly or even daily sessions may be useful, but the cost-effectiveness of such a labor-intensive approach is uncertain. Therapists should adjust the frequency and intensity of treatment in concert with the needs of patients as well as the therapy resources that are available.

Duration of Treatment

In most cases, treatment is conducted in a period of 3 to 6 months. For those who begin therapy as inpatients, a similar period of aftercare is strongly recommended (Thase, 1993). Unsuccessful therapy (e.g., failure to effect significant symptomatic improvement) should generally not continue past 12 to 16 weeks for outpatients. Therapy should not be terminated until patients have achieved symptomatic remission. Ideally, at least two or three sessions are planned on an every-other-week basis in preparation for termination.

Outcome Assessment

Cognitive and behavioral therapies are, in part, distinguished by their integrated use of objective assessment methods. For depression and the anxiety disorders, a number of well-established rating scales are available. Therapist-administered scales include the Hamilton Anxiety Rating Scale (Hamilton, 1959) and the Hamilton Depression Rating Scale (Hamilton, 1960) as well as the Yale-Brown Obsessive–Compulsive Scale (Goodman *et al.*, 1989). Self-report assessments of symptoms include the Beck Depression Inventory (Beck *et al.*, 1961), the Beck Anxiety Inventory (Beck *et al.*, 1988), the Fear Survey Schedule (Wolpe and Lang, 1964), the Fear Questionnaire (Marks and Matthews, 1979) and the Hopkins Symptom Checklist (Derogatis *et al.*, 1974). These scales are typically administered before treatment and repeated periodically (e.g., weekly or monthly) to monitor progress. The Dysfunctional Attitudes Scale, the Attributional Style Questionnaire and the Automatic Thoughts Questionnaire may be used to evaluate distorted cognitions (Dobson and Shaw, 1986). As suggested earlier, high residual levels of cognitive symptoms most likely convey an increased risk for relapse after termination of treatment (Thase *et al.*, 1992; Simons *et al.*, 1986). Similarly, high scores on the Hopelessness Scale (Beck *et al.*, 1974) have been associated with a high risk for subsequent suicidal behavior (Beck *et al.*, 1985b).

Augmentation of Therapy

One of the major methods of augmenting a cognitive and behavioral therapy is to add an appropriate form of pharmacotherapy. For example, a depressed or agoraphobic person who has not benefited much from 8 weeks or more of CBT alone should probably be considered for pharmacotherapy. There are no contraindications to combining CBT and pharmacotherapy (Hollon *et al.*, 1991; Wright and Thase, 1992).

Continuation and Maintenance Phase CBT

Because some patients do not completely achieve a remission of symptoms (their return to premorbid well state) and because many patients experience depression as a recurring illness, there is a need for longer-term treatment methods for major depression (Kupfer *et al.*, 1986). Furthermore, incomplete remission of depression leads to recurrence, and this has many adverse economic, interpersonal and medical consequences (Thase, 1992).

Efficacy of CBT

The cognitive and behavioral therapies are, as a class, the best studied type of psychotherapy. Numerous research studies have demonstrated the efficacy for a variety of Axis I DSM IV disorders including mood disorders (Thase, 1995; Dobson, 1989; Depression Guideline Panel, 1993), anxiety disorders (Wolpe, 1982; Clum *et al.*, 1993; Beck and Zebb, 1994; Chambless and Gillis, 1993; Durham and Allan, 1993; Butler *et al.*, 1991; Barlow *et al.*, 2000) and eating disorders (Agras *et al.*, 1992, 1994, 2000; Fairburn *et al.*, 1991, 1992, 1993, 1995; Garner 1992; Goldbloom *et al.*, 1997; Walsh *et al.*, 1997; Wilson, 1999; Ricca *et al.*, 2000). CBT approaches have also been used to treat personality disorders and as part of multimodal treatments for schizophrenia and bipolar disorder.

Conclusion

The cognitive and behavior therapies are based on well-articulated theories that have a strong empirical basis. These therapies emphasize objective assessments and use of directive interventions aimed at reducing symptomatic distress, enhancing interpersonal skills, and improving social and vocational functioning. Cognitive interventions are focused primarily on identifying and modifying distorted thoughts and pathological schemas. Behavioral techniques to increase exposure, increase activity, enhance social skills and improve anxiety management are useful modalities, and can complement or amplify the effects of cognitive strategies. Similarly, the cognitive perspective can add depth to behavioral models for therapy by teaching patients how to recognize and modify their attitudinal vulnerabilities.

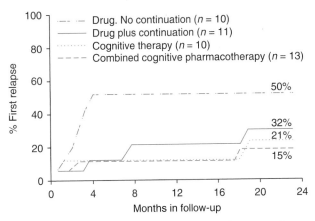

Figure 69.8   *Risk of relapse after cognitive therapy and pharmacotherapy, singly or in combination. Reproduced with permission from Evans MD, Hollon SD, DeRubeis RJ et al. [1992] Differential relapse following cognitive therapy and pharmacotherapy for depression. Arch Gen Psychiatr 49, 802–808. Copyright 1992, American Medical Association.*

The cognitive and behavioral therapies are the best-studied psychological treatments of major depressive, panic, generalized anxiety and obsessive–compulsive disorders. Overall, there is good evidence for the effectiveness of these interventions within these indications. Cognitive and behavioral therapies are being adapted for adjunctive use with pharmacotherapy for treatment of bipolar disorder and schizophrenia. There are no contraindications for use in combination with pharmacotherapy. The cognitive and behavioral therapies have become one of the standard psychosocial treatment approaches for mental disorders.

References

Abramson LY, Metalsky GI and Alloy LB (1989) Hopelessness depression: A theory-based subtype of depression. *Psychol Rev* 96, 358–372.

Agras WS, Rossiter EM, Arnow B *et al.* (1992) Pharmacologic and cognitive–behavioral treatment for bulimia nervosa: A controlled comparison. Am J Psychiatr 149, 82–87.

Agras WS, Telch CF, Arnow B *et al.* (1994) Weight loss, cognitive-behavioral, and desipramine treatments in binge eating disorder: An additive design. *Behav Ther* 25, 225–238.

Agras WS, Walsh BT, Fairburn CG *et al.* (2000) A multicenter comparison of cognitive–behavioral therapy and interpersonal psychotherapy for bulimia nervosa. *Arch Gen Psychiatr* 57(5), 459–466.

Alfrod BA and Correia CJ (1994) Cognitive therapy of schizophrenia: Theory and empirical status. *Behav Ther* 25, 17–33.

Azrin NH and Holz WC (1966) Punishment, in *Operant Behavior: Areas of Research and Application* (ed Honig WK). Appleton-Century-Crofts, New York, pp. 12–32.

Bandura A (1977a) Self-efficacy: Toward a unifying theory of behavioral change. *Psychol Rev* 84, 191–215.

Bandura A (1977b) *Social Learning Theory*. Prentice-Hall, Englewood Cliffs, NJ.

Barlow DH and Cerny JA (1988) *Psychological Treatment of Panic. Treatment Manual for Practitioners*. Guilford Press, New York.

Barlow DH, Gorman JM, Shear MK *et al.* (2000) Cognitive–behavioral therapy, imipramine, or their combination for panic disorder: A randomized controlled trial. *JAMA* 283(19), 2529–2536.

Basco RM and Rush AJ (1996) *Cognitive–Behavior Therapy for Bipolar Disorder*. Guilford Press, New York.

Basco RM and Thase ME (1998) Cognitive–behavioral treatment of bipolar disorder. In International Handbook of Cognitive and

Behavioral Treatments for Psychological Disorders, Caballo VE (ed). Elsevier Science, Oxford, pp. 521–550.

Beck AT (1967) *Depression: Clinical, Experimental, and Theoretical Aspects.* Harper & Row, New York.

Beck AT (1976) *Cognitive Therapy and the Emotional Disorders.* International Universities Press, New York.

Beck AT (1991) Cognitive therapy: A 30-year retrospective. *Am Psychol* 46, 368–375.

Beck AT and Emery G (1985) Anxiety Disorders and Phobias: *A Cognitive Perspective.* Basic Books, New York.

Beck AT and Greenberg RL (1974) *Coping with Depression* [booklet]. Institute for Rational Living, New York.

Beck AT, Epstein N, Brown G *et al.* (1988) An inventory for measuring clinical anxiety: Psychometric properties. *J Consult Clin Psychol* 56, 893–897.

Beck AT, Freeman A and Associates (1990) *Cognitive Therapy of Personality Disorders.* Guilford Press, New York.

Beck AT, Rush AJ, Shaw BF *et al.* (1979) *Cognitive Therapy of Depression.* Guilford Press, New York.

Beck AT, Steer RA, Kovacs M *et al.* (1985b) Hopelessness and eventual suicide: A ten-year prospective study of patients hospitalized with suicidal ideation. *Am J Psychiatr* 142, 559–563.

Beck AT, Ward CH, Mendelson M *et al.* (1961) An inventory for measuring depression. *Arch Gen Psychiatr* 4, 561–571.

Beck AT, Weissman A, Lester D *et al.* (1974) The measurement of pessimism: The hopelessness scale. *J Consult Clin Psychol* 42, 861–865.

Beck JS (1995) *Cognitive Therapy: Basics and Beyond.* Guilford Press, New York.

Beck JS and Zebb BJ (1994) Behavioral assessment and treatment of panic disorder: Current status, future directions. *Behav Ther* 25, 581–611.

Bernstein DA and Borkovec TD (1973) *Progressive Relaxation Training.* Research Press, Champaign, IL.

Blackburn IM, Jones S, and Lewin RJP (1986b) Cognitive style in depression. *Br J Clin Psychol* 25, 241–251.

Bowlby J (1985) The role of childhood experience in cognitive disturbance, in *Cognition and Psychotherapy* (eds Mahoney MJ and Freeman A). Plenum Press, New York, pp. 181–200.

Burns DD (1980) Feeling Good. William Morrow, New York.

Burns DD (1990) *The Feeling Good Handbook.* Penguin Books, New York.

Butler G, Fennell M, Robson P *et al.* (1991) Comparison of behavior therapy and cognitive behavior therapy in the treatment of generalized anxiety disorder. *J Consult Clin Psychol* 59, 167–175.

Chambless DL and Gillis MM (1993) Cognitive therapy of anxiety disorders. *J Consult Clin Psychol* 62, 248–260.

Clark DA, Beck AT and Alford BA (1999) *Scientific Foundations of Cognitive Theory and Therapy of Depression.* John Wiley, New York, pp. 36–76.

Clark DM, Salkovskis PM, and Chalkley AJ (1985) Respiratory control as a treatment for panic attacks. *J Behav Ther Exp Psychiatr* 16, 23–30.

Clum GA, Clum GA and Surls R (1993) A meta-analysis of treatments of panic disorder. *J Consult Clin Psychol* 61, 317–326.

Coyne JC, Kessler RC, Tal M *et al.* (1987) Living with a depressed person. *J Consult Clin Psychol* 55, 347–352.

Depression Guideline Panel (1993) *Depression in Primary Care, Vol. 2, Treatment of Major Depression.* Clinical Practice Guideline, No. 5, US Department of Health and Human Services, Agency for Health Care Policy and Research, publication 93–0551, Rockville, MD.

Derogatis L, Lipman R and Rickels K (1974) The Hopkins Symptom Checklist (HSCL): A self-report symptom inventory. *Behav Sci* 19, 1–16.

Dobson KS (1989) A meta-analysis of the efficacy of cognitive therapy for depression. *J Consult Clin Psychol* 57, 414–419.

Dobson KS and Block L (1988) Historical and philosophical bases of the cognitive–behavioral therapies, in *Handbook of Cognitive Behavioral Therapies* (ed Dobson KS). Guilford Press, New York, pp. 3–38.

Dobson KS and Shaw BF (1986) Cognitive assessment with major depressive disorders. *Cogn Ther Res* 10, 13–29.

Durham RC and Allan T (1993) Psychological treatment of generalized anxiety disorder. A review of the clinical significance of results in outcome studies since 1980. *Br J Psychiatr* 163, 19–26.

Fairburn CG, Jones R, Peveler RC *et al.* (1991) Three psychological treatments for bulimia nervosa. *Arch Gen Psychiatr* 48, 463–469.

Fairburn CG, Agras WS and Wilson GT (1992) The research on treatment of bulimia nervosa: Practical and theoretical implications, in *The Biology of Feast and Famine: Relevance to Eating Disorders* (eds Anderson GH and Kennedy SH). Academic Press, San Diego, pp. 318–340.

Fairburn CG, Jones R, Peveler RC *et al.* (1993) Psychotherapy and bulimia nervosa. *Arch Gen Psychiatr* 50, 419–428.

Fairburn CG, Norman PA, Welch SL *et al.* (1995) A prospective study of outcome in bulimia nervosa and the long-term effects of three psychological treatments. *Arch Gen Psychiatr* 52, 304–312.

Freeman A, Simon KM, Beutler LE *et al.* (eds) (1989) *Comprehensive Handbook of Cognitive Therapy.* Plenum Press, New York.

Friedman ES (1997) Combined therapy for depression. *J Pract Psychiatr Behav Health* 3(4), 211–222.

Garner DM (1992) Psychotherapy for eating disorders. *Curr Opin Psychiatr* 5, 391–395.

Goldbloom DS, Olmsted M, Davis R *et al.* (1997) A randomized controlled trial of fluoxetine and cognitive–behavioral therapy for bulimia nervosa: Short-term outcome. *Behav Res Ther* 35(9), 803–811.

Goldfried MR and Davison GC (1994) *Clinical Behavior Therapy*, Expanded Version. John Wiley, New York.

Goodman WK, Price LH, Rasmussen SA *et al.* (1989) The Yale-Brown Obsessive–Compulsive Scale. II. Validity. *Arch Gen Psychiatr* 46, 1012–1016.

Greenberger D and Padesky CA (1995) *Mind Over Mood: A Cognitive Therapy Treatment Manual for Clients.* Guilford Press, New York.

Hamilton M (1959) The assessment of anxiety states by rating. *Br J Med Psychol* 32, 50–55.

Hamilton M (1960) A rating scale for depression. *J Neurol Neurosur Psychiatr* 23, 56–62.

Hammen C, Ellicott A, Gitlin M *et al.* (1989) Sociotropy/autonomy and vulnerability to specific life events in patients with unipolar depression and bipolar disorders. *J Abnorm Psychol* 98, 154–160.

Hersen M, Bellack AS, Himmelhoch JM *et al.* (1984) Effects of social skill training, amitriptyline, and psychotherapy in unipolar depressed women. *Behav Ther* 15, 21–40.

Hollon SD, Shelton RC and Loosen P (1991) Cognitive therapy and pharmacotherapy for depression. *J Consult Clin Psychol* 59, 88–99.

Jarrett RB, Kraft D, Doyle J *et al.* (2001) Preventing recurrent depression using cognitive therapy with and without a continuation phase: A randomized clinical trial. *Arch Gen Psychiatr* 58, 381–388.

Kazdin AE (1982) History of behavior modification, in *International Handbook of Behavior Modification and Therapy* (eds Bellack AS, Hersen M and Kazdin AE). Plenum Press, New York, pp. 3–32.

Kazdin AE and Wilcoxin LA (1976) Systematic desensitization and nonspecific treatment effects: A methodological consideration. *Psychol Bull* 83, 729–758.

Kingdon DG and Turkington D (1995) *Cognitive–Behavioral Therapy of Schizophrenia.* Guilford Press, New York.

Kupfer DJ, Frank E, Perel JM *et al.* (1986) Five-year outcome for maintenance therapies in recurrent depression. *Arch Gen Psychiatr* 43, 43–50.

Lam DL, Bright J, Jones S, et al. (2000) Cognitive therapy for bipolar illness – A pilot study of relapse prevention. *Cogn Ther Res* 24(5), 503–520.

LeFebvre MF (1981) Cognitive distortion and cognitive errors in depressed psychiatric and low back pain patients. *J Consult Clin Psychol* 49, 517–525.

Lewinsohn PM, Sullivan JM and Grosscup SJ (1982) Behavioral therapy: Clinical applications, in *Short-Term Psychotherapies for Depression* (ed Rush AJ). Guilford Press, New York, pp. 50–87.

Linehan MM, Armstrong HE, Suarez A *et al.* (1991) Cognitive–behavioral treatment of chronically parasuicidal borderline patients. *Arch Gen Psychiatr* 48, 1060–1064.

Linehan MM, Heard HL and Armstrong HE (1993) Naturalistic follow-up of a behavioral treatment for chronically parasuicidal borderline patients. *Arch Gen Psychiatr* 50, 971–974.

Malott RW, Whaley DL and Mallott ME (1993) *Elementary Principles of Behavior*. Prentice-Hall, Englewood Cliffs, NJ.

Marks IM and Matthews AM (1979) Brief standard self-rating for phobic patients. *Behav Res Ther* 17, 263–267.

McCullough JP (2000) *Treatment for Chronic Depression: Cognitive–Behavioral Analysis System of Psychotherapy*. Guilford Press, New York.

Metalsky GI, Halberstadt LJ and Albramson LY (1987) Vulnerability to depressive mood reactions: Toward a more powerful test of the diathesis-stress and causal mediation components of the reformulated theory of depression. *J Pers Soc Psychol* 52, 386–393.

Mueser KT (1998) Cognitive–behavioral treatment of schizophrenia. In International Handbook of Cognitive and Behavioral Treatments for Psychological Disorders, (ed Caballo VE). Elsevier Science, Oxford, pp. 551–570.

Otto MW, Pollack MH, Sachs GS *et al.* (1993) Discontinuation of benzodiazepine treatment: Efficacy of cognitive–behavioral therapy for patients with panic disorder. *Am J Psychiatr* 150(10), 1485–1490.

Overholser JC (1993a) Elements of the Socratic method: I. Systematic questioning. *Psychotherapy* 30, 67–74.

Overholser JC (1993b) Elements of the Socratic method: II. Inductive reasoning. *Psychotherapy* 30, 75–85.

Overholser JC (1993c) Elements of the Socratic method: III. Universal definitions. *Psychotherapy* 31, 286–293.

Persons JB (1989) *Cognitive Therapy in Practice: A Case Formulation Approach*. WW Norton, New York.

Peterson C, Villanova P and Raps CS (1985) Depression and attributions: Factors responsible for inconsistent results in the published literature. *J Abnorm Psychol* 94, 165–168.

Rachman SJ, Craske MG, Tallman K *et al.* (1986) Does escape behavior strengthen agoraphobic avoidance? A replication. *Behav Res Ther* 26, 41–52.

Ricca V, Mannucci E, Zucchi T *et al.* (2000) Cognitive–behavioral therapy for bulimia nervosa and binge eating disorder: A review. *Psychother Psychosom* 69, 287–295.

Scott J and Wright JH (1997) Cognitive therapy for chronic and severe mental disorders, in *American Psychiatric Press Review of Psychiatry*, Vol. 16 (eds Dickstein LJ, Riba MB, and Oldham JM). American Psychiatric Press, Washington DC, pp. 1135–1170.

Segal ZV (1988) Appraisal of the self-schema construct in cognitive models of depression. *Psychol Bull* 103, 147–162.

Seligman MEP (1975) *Helplessness: On Depression, Development, and Death*. WH Freeman, San Francisco.

Senky T, Turkington D, Kingdon D, *et al.* (2000) A randomized controlled trial of cognitive–behavioral therapy for persistent symptoms in schizophrenia resistant to medication. *Arch Gen Psychiatr* 57(2), 176–172.

Simons AD, Murphy GE and Levine JL (1986) Cognitive therapy and pharmacotherapy of depression: Sustained improvement over one year. *Arch Gen Psychiatr* 43, 43–48.

Skinner BF (1938) *The Behavior of Organisms*. Appleton-Century-Crofts, New York.

Staats AW (1964) *Human Learning: Studies Extending Conditioning Principles to Complex Behavior*. Holt, Rinehart & Winston, New York.

Stern RS (1978) Obsessive thoughts: The problem of therapy. *Br J Psychiatr* 133, 200–205.

Sweeney PD, Anderson K and Bailey S (1986) Attributional style in depression: A meta-analysis review. *J Pers Soc Psychol* 50, 974–991.

Teasdale JD (1983) Negative thinking in depression: Cause, effect, or reciprocal relationship? *Adv Behav Res Ther* 5, 3–25.

Thase ME (1992) Long-term treatments of recurrent depressive disorders. *J Clin Psychiatr* 53(Suppl 9), 32–44.

Thase ME (1993) Transition and aftercare, in *Cognitive Therapy with Inpatients* (eds Wright JH, Thase ME, Beck AT *et al.*). Guilford Press, New York, pp. 414–435.

Thase ME (1995) Reeducative psychotherapy, in *Treatments of Psychiatric Disorders: The DSM-IV Edition* (ed Gabbard GO). American Psychiatric Press, Washington DC.

Thase ME and Beck AT (1993) Cognitive therapy: An overview, in *The Cognitive Milieu: Inpatient Applications to Cognitive Therapy* (eds Wright JH, Thase ME, Ludgate J *et al.*). Guilford Press, New York.

Thase ME and Howland R (1994) Refractory depression: Relevance of psychosocial factors and therapies. *Psychiatr Ann* 24, 232–240.

Thase ME and Wright JH (1991) Cognitive–behavior therapy manual for depressed inpatients: A treatment protocol outline. *Behav Ther* 22, 579–595.

Thase ME, Simons AD, McGeary J *et al.* (1992) Relapse after cognitive–behavior therapy of depression: Potential implications for longer courses of treatment? *Am J Psychiatr* 149, 1046–1052.

Thase ME, Simons AD, and Reynolds CF III (1993) Psychobiological correlates of poor response to cognitive–behavior therapy: Potential indications for antidepressant pharmacotherapy. *Psychopharmacol Bull* 29, 293–301.

Walsh BT, Wilson GT, Loeb KL *et al.* (1997) Medication and psychotherapy in the treatment of bulimia nervosa. *Am J Psychiatr* 154(4), 523–531.

Whisman MS (1993) Mediators and moderators of change in cognitive therapy of depression. *Psychol Bull* 114, 248–265.

Wilson GT (1999) Cognitive–behavior therapy for eating disorders: Progress and problems. *Behav Res Ther* 37, S79–S95.

Wolpe J (1958) *Psychotherapy by Reciprocal Inhibition*. Stanford University Press, Stanford, CA.

Wolpe J (1982) *The Practice of Behavior Therapy*. Pergamon Press, New York.

Wolpe J and Lang PJ (1964) A fear survey schedule for use in behavior therapy. *Behav Res Ther* 2, 27–30.

Wright JH (1988) Cognitive therapy of depression, in *The American Psychiatric Press Review of Psychiatry*, Vol. 7 (eds Frances AJ and Hales RE). American Psychiatric Press, Washington DC, pp. 554–590.

Wright JH and Basco MR (2001) *Getting Your Life Back: The Complete Guide to Depression*. The Free Press, New York.

Wright JH and Beck AT (1983) Cognitive therapy of depression: Theory and practice. *Hosp Comm Psychiatr* 34, 1119–1127.

Wright JH and Beck AT (1994) Cognitive therapy, in *American Psychiatric Press Textbook of Psychiatry*, Vol. 13 (eds Hales RE, Yudofsky SC and Talbott JA). American Psychiatric Press, Washington DC, pp. 1083–1114.

Wright JH and Davis D (1994) The therapeutic relationship in cognitive–behavioral therapy: Patient perceptions and therapist responses. *Cogn Behav Pract* 1, 25–45.

Wright JH and Thase ME (1992) Cognitive and biological therapies: A synthesis. *Psychiatr Ann* 22, 451–458.

Wright JH, Salmon P, Wright AS *et al.* (1995) *Cognitive Therapy: A Multimedia Learning Program*. MindStreet Multimedia, Louisville, KY.

Wright JH, Wright AS and Beck AT (2002a) *Good Days Ahead: The Multimedia Program for Cognitive Therapy*. Mindstreet, Louisville, KY.

Wright JH, Wright AS, Salmon P *et al.* (2002b) Development and initial testing of a multimedia program for computer-assisted cognitive therapy. *Am J Psychother* 56(1), 76–86.

Young JE and Lindermann MD (1992) An integrative schema-focused model for personality disorders. *J Cogn Psychother* 6, 11–23.

CHAPTER

70

Family Therapy

Family therapy is psychotherapy that directly involves family members in addition to the identified patient, and/or explicitly attends to the interactions among family members (Pinsof and Wynne, 1995). Family therapy thus engages relational and communicational processes of families and social networks as a primary context for solving clinical problems or treating psychiatric disorders, even though one family member may be the sole bearer of distress or symptoms. By educating family members or altering family patterns of relating or communicating, such clinical problems as depression, anxiety, marital conflict, or disruptive childhood behavior can be resolved or attenuated.

The different family therapy traditions can be usefully contrasted by comparing how each structures perceptual, cognitive, and executive processes when clinicians work with families – from each of these perspectives:

- What does a therapist look for?
- What does a therapist think about?
- What does a therapist do?

Different family therapy traditions are themselves best regarded as different sets of ideas and interventions to be valued as potential tools within comprehensive, multimodality treatment programs. We will illustrate the range of perspectives and interventions available in the different traditions by examining, in turn, how psychodynamic, structural, strategic, cognitive–behavioral and postmodern family therapy traditions each might approach a clinical problem.

Psychodynamic Family Therapy

Psychodynamic psychotherapy helps family members solve relational problems by understanding better how emotional processes influence the perceptions, feelings and actions of those involved. The early psychoanalysts noted that intrapsychic processes of an individual powerfully shape his or her interactions with other people, and most so in emotionally intimate relationships of couples and families. Extending the concepts and language of psychoanalysis to family behavior was a logical next step for those who began meeting with parents and children, couples and whole families. In particular, object relations theory provided a bridge from the individual intrapsychic processes to the interpersonal processes of families (Scharff and Scharff, 1987; Framo, 1991; Slipp, 1991).

What to Think About

In order to understand how one family member acts in relation to other family members, psychodynamic family therapy concen-

trates upon motivations, conflicts, defenses and relationships from the past that currently influence the present. Family interactions are explained in terms of internal processes within individual family members. Therapeutic change is sought through family members gaining conscious insight into previously unconscious processes that have been generating problems in family relationships.

What to Look For

Psychodynamic family therapy grounds its work in historical information. Extensive individual and family histories are elicited in order to understand family members' experiential models of the world. These experiential models govern how meanings are attributed to such family patterns as rules for how people should respond and models for being a man or a woman, husband or wife, or mother or father. These models have developed out of each family member's personal history, the family's history and mythology, and their cultural history. Some of the diagnostic patterns upon which psychodynamic family therapists focus when assessing families include the following:

- **Projective Identification** Projective identification is an ego defense to which psychodynamic family therapists have attributed a crucial role in conflictual family relationships. In projective identification, one family member (a parent or couple partner) relates to another family member (a particular child or the other couple partner) as if he or she embodied a projected part of self. The projecting family member then interacts with, or relates to, the projected part of self as if that part were an internalized part of himself or herself. The projecting family member unconsciously prompts the other to conform to the way in which he or she is being perceived, evoking in the other the associated feelings and behaviors as if they were authentic. When viewed from the outside by the therapist, it appears as if the two are in collusion with one another in order to sustain these mutual, projected perceptions. Projection of disavowed elements of the self, whether positive or negative, has the effect of charging the relationship with emotion that has been transposed from an intrapsychic sphere into an interpersonal one. Acted out interpersonally, it serves to decrease psychic anxiety at the expense of an increase in tension and impasse in the relationship.
- **Unresolved Grief** When a family member, or the family as a whole, has not fully grieved losses, the family can become developmentally frozen. While so preoccupied with the past, it can be difficult to focus enough time and energy on current problems.
- **Clarity of Ego Boundaries and Capacity for Intimacy/ Separateness** Conflicted family relationships can represent an alternative method for stabilizing emotional distance when

Essentials of Psychiatry   Jerald Kay and Allan Tasman
© 2006 John Wiley & Sons, Ltd.

the involved family members lack the emotional maturity to regulate closeness and distance in more differentiated ways. This has been a common model for understanding couples who chronically fight yet never separate.

What to Do

Psychodynamic family therapists employ the fundamental tools of psychodynamic psychotherapy (opening emotional expression, clarifying communications, encouraging family members to speak from the "I" position, and interpretation of unconscious conflicts) to resolve projective processes, cutoff relationships, and difficulties in modulating closeness and distance in family relationships. Psychodramatic techniques, such as doubling and role reversal, can play useful roles in implementing these interventions (Blatner, 1994). Therapeutic rituals are particularly useful in facilitating grief over losses and in facilitating developmental transitions, such as a young adult leaving home or a couple moving into retirement years (Imber-Black and Roberts, 1992).

Structural Family Therapy

Structural family therapy considers problems involving a particular family member to be inextricably linked to the organizational context of the entire family. It solves problems by changing the family's organizational context. Structural family therapy thus emphasizes an understanding of a family in terms of the family rules and roles that shape its members' actions.

Family structure is the internal organization of the family that dictates how, when and to whom family members relate while carrying out the various functions of the family (Aponte and VanDeusen, 1981; Colapinto, 1991). Some important elements of family structure for clinical work are boundaries, hierarchy, alliances and coalitions:

- **Boundaries** Rules defining who participates and how, in particular moments of family life. For example, a boundary around the parental couple means that the children are included in discussions of certain topics but not in others;
- **Hierarchy** Relative influence of each family member upon the outcome of an activity. For example, all family members may have opinions about spending money, but the parents as a couple typically have the final say;
- **Alliances** Family members joining together to support another family member. For example, older children may join the well-parent in organizing to parent younger children if the other parent were to become seriously ill;
- **Coalitions** Family members joining together in opposition to another family member. For example, a grandchild and grandmother might quietly ally together for the child to stay up late at night against the mother's wishes when the child is at grandmother's house.

The family structure should provide cohesive and flexible responses to life stresses so that important family functions – parenting, providing income, marital intimacy, recreation and other activities – can be carried out successfully, and family members can grow and mature in their individual lives.

What to Look For

A structural family therapist observes closely the flow of family structures as family members talk about and interact together around the presenting problem of the therapy. The therapist wishes to witness how sequences of family behaviors are enacted during interactions in the sessions, particularly the occurrence of a symptom as it is embedded within different configurations of organized family interactions. The therapist observes how boundaries, hierarchy, alliances and coalitions are associated with the presenting symptom, as well as any repetitive-behavioral sequences (verbal or nonverbal) that involve symptomatic behavior.

What to Think About

The structural family therapist considers the problem to be sustained by the current family structure and its community ecosystem. Important questions to answer in assessing these relationships include:

- To what elements of family structure – boundaries, hierarchy, alliances, coalitions – do occurrences of the presenting problem appear linked?
- What family functions are blocked by the problem? If not for the problem, what would be happening that is not happening now?
- For whom is the problem a concern? Who is most affected? Who would need to change for the symptom to disappear?

What to Do

Structural family therapists ameliorate symptoms by shifting family structure. Boundaries can be strengthened or weakened by behavioral assignments that exclude a particular family member from certain moments of family life (e.g., an assignment for parents to leave children with a baby sitter to go on a date alone) or include a particular family member where that person had been absent (e.g., involving both parents in collaborative disciplining of a misbehaving child when the father had been only peripherally involved). Alliances are encouraged when they support the individual development of family members and strengthen the family as a whole. Secret coalitions, particularly when they cross generational boundaries, are targeted for therapeutic disruption as when one parent covertly supports a child's oppositional behavior with the other parent.

Strategic Family Therapy

Strategic therapy is built upon the premise that a therapist is responsible for planning a strategy that solves successfully the family's presenting problem. The therapist sets clear goals that intervene by changing relational and communicational processes in the family (Madanes, 1981; Stanton, 1981). Strategic therapy was designed as a counterpoint to psychodynamic psychotherapy by emphasizing "how" people can behave differently in order to solve problems, rather than "why" they behave as they do.

What to Think About

The focus of strategic therapy is upon problem solving. Problems are viewed as persistent efforts by one or more family members to apply a solution that makes sense but is inadequate for the problem at hand, such that "the solution becomes the problem". Common-sense understandings often lead people to pursue unsuccessful strategies even though it ought to be apparent that the problem is not resolving. For example, people intuitively attempt to cheer up a person who is depressed, even though cheering up (a solution) usually makes the depression (the problem) worse.

Strategic therapists commonly view clinical problems as emerging out of difficult life-cycle transitions, both predictable ones (e.g., marriage, birth of a child, separating/individuating of an adolescent) and unpredictable ones (e.g., loss of job, sudden illness, a death in the family) that necessitate shifting to new patterns of perceiving and acting. At such times when innovative problem-solving is needed, people nevertheless persist with once successful strategies that are now outdated.

What to Look For

Strategic therapists are most interested in the here-and-now context of the problem, rather than in its history. They seek to learn what each involved person believes about the problem and how these beliefs are acted upon in efforts to generate a solution. Questions are asked about who, what, when, where and how people are involved, in order to ascertain how moves are sequenced in the family game.

What to Do

The central aim of a strategic therapist is to motivate family members to try novel solutions, rather than repeating what has been tried in the past. Psychoeducation, direct behavioral assignments, and paradoxical or defiance-based directives are the cornerstones of strategic therapy. In-session interventions and out-of-session homework are used. Strategic therapists have become best known for their paradoxical directives. Paradoxical directives include:

- **Reframing or Relabeling the Symptom** By changing the context of actions constituting the symptom, the meaning of the event is reframed. For example, a husband's emotional distancing could be reframed as "his way of getting his wife to notice him".
- **Prescribing the Symptom or Behavioral Sequence** By using a rationale that is plausible in its logic, a therapist can encourage family members to engage in the very behavior that needs to be eliminated. For example, a wife whose husband is emotionally distancing might be told to continue to pursue her husband because "this lets him know that he is the center of her life and that there is nothing else about her life that she finds valuable or interesting". She might be instructed to continue in her behavior for his sake, even though it may give her friends a distorted idea about her. When the reframe "fits", yet the new meaning feels distasteful, the rebound against the directive can paradoxically propel therapeutic change.
- **Restraining the System** The therapist can attempt to discourage or even deny the possibility of change. For example, a therapist may tell couple-partners to "go slow" or may emphasize dangers of improvement. Family members may then react against the therapist's conservative outlook by pressing forward to change.
- **Positioning** The therapist attempts to shift a problematic "position" (usually an assertion that the patient is making about self, the problem, or a partner) by accepting but exaggerating that position. This intervention is used when the partner's position is thought to be maintained by its complementary, reciprocal response from the other partner. For example, when one partner takes an optimistic stance and the other a pessimistic one, a therapist may suggest the pessimistic spouse to worry even more so that the optimistic spouse can feel more secure and even more happily optimistic. Here, too, if a new explanation has a plausible logic, but frames the behavior in a manner that renders it aversive, the behavior will change.

Cognitive–Behavioral Family Therapy

Cognitive–behavioral family therapy applies principles of learning theory to help family members solve problems by modifying cognitive distortions and repetitive problem-inducing interactions, and by learning new knowledge and skills. Cognitive–behavioral family therapy relies heavily upon family psychoeducation and a teaching/coaching stance of the therapist.

Cognitive interventions engage family members as coinvestigators who study the ecology of family problems and symptoms and discern how thoughts, feelings and behaviors interplay. A therapist assists family members in identifying when such cognitive distortions as catastrophic thinking, overgeneralization, or misattributions lead to conflicts in relationships (Epstein *et al.*, 1988; Freeman *et al.*, 1989).

What to Look For

Families presenting problems for therapy often have:

- difficulties in recognizing deviant behavior
- lack of clearly-defined family rules
- problems in emotional communication among family members, usually a paucity of expression of positive feelings coupled with an excess of negative expressions
- relational conflict associated with either a paucity of relational skills or interpretive errors based on faulty assumptions or cognitive distortions.

What to Think About

A cognitive–behavioral family therapist considers each member of the family to be doing his or her best to cope with the behavioral contingencies perceived at that point in time, given the practical and emotional restraints experienced. Family members need to acquire knowledge about cognitive and behavioral principles, to gain skills needed to reinforce desired behaviors, to eliminate reinforcement of undesired behaviors, to modify faulty assumptions and interpretations of others' actions, and to learn skills for communicating clearly and effectively.

What to Do

- **Psychoeducation** Educational modules about the presenting problem are taught when family members appear to lack a significant understanding of issues, ranging from such general topics as developmental milestones of children and principles of learning theory, to specific information about a particular psychiatric disorder (Falloon, 1991).
- **Communication training** Empathic listening, expressing positive feelings, and speaking negative communications more respectfully are taught as skills (Falloon, 1991).
- **Problem-solving training** Family members practice consistent, structured approaches for resolving conflicts (Falloon, 1991).
- **Operant-conditioning strategies** Behavior shaping and time-out procedures are taught to increase desirable behaviors among children (Falloon, 1991).
- **Contingency contracting** Coercive, blaming patterns of family behavior are replaced by contracts that specify what behaviors involved family members each to agree to perform (Falloon, 1991).
- **Thought diaries** Out-of-session, assignments are made to track habitual patterns of thoughts, feelings and behaviors in generating symptoms (Freeman *et al.*, 1989).

Postmodern Family Therapies

Innovations introduced by postmodern therapies including narrative, solution-focused, collaborative language systems and feminist family therapies (Andersen, 1987; Anderson, 1997; de Shazer, 1985; Epston, 1989; Epston and White, 1992; Freedman and Combs, 1995; Griffith and Griffith, 1994; Madsen, 1999; O'Hanlon and Weiner-Davis, 1989; Penn, 2001; Tomm, 1987; Weiner-Davis, 1992; Weingarten, 1995; White, 1989, 1995, 2000) have opened new ways for families to solve problems by valuing and learning from their own experiences, histories, traditions, values and identities, instead of seeking answers from mental health experts. The postmodern therapies have sought to empower families by helping them to develop reflective processes for exercising choice, to build supportive communities with other families, and to clarify undesirable ways in which cultural influences have limited appreciation and utilization of the family's own practical wisdom. In these ways, the postmodern family therapies have rendered family therapy more usable for those whose lives vary from the stereotypic American two-parent, middle-class, nuclear families, traditionally the largest consumers of private-practice family therapy.

The postmodern therapies have made contributions that have broadly influenced the clinical practice of family therapy through:

- the art of crafting interview questions for fostering reflection and creative problem-solving;
- clinical methods that help patients and families to identify and use skills, competencies, and resources from their everyday lived-experiences;
- clinical methods that counter adverse influences of culture in generating and maintaining problems that families face.

What to Think About

Each person makes sense out of his or her life experiences by attributing meaning to them. This meaning is shaped by a canon of personal narratives as they are told and retold to self and to others. Among the most important of these narratives are those of identity about who one is as a person and as a family. There are certain dominant narratives in a person's life that, more than others, organize one's perceptions, cognitions and actions. How a family member views oneself and the other family members is shaped by the limits of the language – the metaphors, stories and beliefs – he or she employs.

Impasses occur in family relationships, and problems emerge when:

- one or more family members lack either the needed emotional vocabulary or the needed narrative skills to make one's personal experience understandable to others;
- the available narratives preclude ways of relating other than conflictual ones;
- specific words hold very different meanings for different family members due to different personal narratives connected to the language (e.g., "loyalty," "trust," "safety");
- family members have become positioned relationally such that they cannot hear, tell and/or expand their stories in conversation, i.e., they have become confused by or habituated to the conflict such that they have stopped listening.

Therapy provides a context where narratives that limit and constrain relationships can be identified. The power of constraining narratives can be attenuated through careful interviewing that renders visible the specific historical, cultural, or political contexts from which they emerged and the hidden interpretive assumptions upon which they rest. Alternatively, more useful narratives often lie unnoticed within forgotten experiences the partners have had with one another, but are now outside their recollection.

What to Look For

- Listen for the exact words and precise manner in which people use language. The focus of therapy is the language itself and the limits of its possibilities, not what this language is interpreted to mean.
- Metaphors, phrases and prominent or repetitive words in the family members' specific uses of language are noted as "doors to be knocked upon" by asking specific questions about stories of lived-experience that have given them meaning.
- "Unique outcomes" or "exceptions" when problems might have been expected to occur, but did not.

What to Do

Narrative approach to therapy consists of two phases:

- First Phases: A first priority is creation of a therapeutic relationship within which important first-person narratives can be safely told, heard and changed. In particular, the therapist carefully watches for nonverbal signs that the dialogue is opening up or closing down, such as family members' breathing, posture, and flow and tone of speech. Creating a relationship and a conversation favorable for the telling of important personal stories is the priority, not gathering data.
- Second Phase: As important first-person narratives relevant to the problem are told, the therapist asks carefully designed questions that facilitate:

  a. retrieval of other forgotten, or unnoticed, narratives that might enhance solving the problem of the therapy, in contrast to the dominant narrative;

  b. cocreation of an alternative narrative to a form that holds more possibilities for resolving the problem of the therapy;

- The therapist utilizes such questions as circular, reflexive, unique outcome, or relative influence questions (Tomm, 1987; White, 1989).
- A solution-focused therapist may assign couple-partners the task of studying segments of time when the problem is "not" occurring, looking for "exceptions…" Examples of solution-focused questions include:

  a. "Between now and the next time we meet, I would like you to observe – so that you can describe to us next time – what happens between both of you that you do value, would NOT want to change, and would like to see continue to happen in the future".

  b. The Miracle Question (de Shazer, 1985): "Suppose that one night, while you were asleep, there was a miracle and this problem was solved. How would you know? What would be different? How would your partner know without your even saying a word about it?" [The therapist then negotiates with the partner(s) what part of this new reality the partner(s) would be willing to implement the next day, as if the miracle had occurred.]

   c. (Weiner-Davis, 1992) "If the problems between you and your partner got resolved all of a sudden, what would you do with the time and energy you have been spending on fixing or worrying about the marriage? Describe what you would do instead".

   d. (Weiner-Davis, 1992) "What might be one or two small things that you can do this week that will take you one step closer to your goal?"

   e. (Weiner-Davis, 1992) "What, if anything, might present a challenge to your taking these steps this week, and how will you meet the challenge?"

Family Psychoeducation Therapies

The earliest approaches to family therapy were built upon individual psychotherapy and simply extended to the family their ideas about diagnosing and treating psychopathology, referring to "family pathology" instead of psychopathology. Early versions of psychodynamic, structural, strategic and cognitive–behavioral family therapies each assessed underlying family pathology and engaged families in corrective treatments. By the 1990s, however, family therapies were shifting to more collaborative therapeutic relationships in which families were regarded as allies, rather than sources of pathology, with education, rather than treatment, as the central focus.

   This shift brought a sea change in how family therapy began to be practiced. Instead of diagnostic scrutiny, clinicians became preoccupied with learning to convey respect to families, to protect them from stigma, and to learn from their real-life experiences coping with illness. A focus on "looking at" families diagnostically in order "to intervene" in the family system, was gradually eclipsed by a commitment to "looking with" families as they coped with illness in order "to collaborate" with them in countering effects of illness on the family.

   By the 1980s, some family therapists working with schizophrenia were proposing that family therapy could be more effectively applied by engaging families as partners in treatment, instead as sources of psychopathology. These efforts were characterized by a fresh set of assumptions (Dixon and Lehman, 1995):

- Severe psychiatric disorders, such as schizophrenia and bipolar disorder, are regarded as illnesses.
- The family environment does not cause the disorder but can influence its course and severity.
- Support is provided to families who are enlisted as partners and collaborators in treatment.
- Family interventions are only one component in a treatment program that includes routine drug treatment and outpatient clinical management.

   These new clinical approaches mixed psychoeducation, behavioral problem-solving training, family support and crisis management in interventions with either individual families or groups of families.

   As a research contribution, the construct of expressed emotion (EE) played a significant role in the evolution of family psychoeducation (Leff and Vaughn, 1985). During a structured interview, families were given an EE rating based on observations of critical comments, hostility and overinvolvement. Over

two decades an enormous body of research suggested that patients living with families characterized by high levels of EE were more vulnerable to relapse (Anderson *et al.*, 1986). Interventions were then designed that relied heavily upon family psychoeducation in order to enable high EE families to change to a low EE status.

   Elements that appeared to be tied to its outcome effectiveness include:

- Creation of social contacts and support;
- Problem-solving with others bearing the burden of the same disorder;
- Countering stigma;
- Cross-parenting of adolescents;
- Normalizing family communications;
- Intervening effectively during crises.

   Family-focused psychoeducational interventions also have been developed for other psychiatric disorders. Family-focused treatment for bipolar disorder, for example, integrates family psychoeducation, communication training and problem-solving into a 20-session therapy extending over most of a year. This intervention in a controlled study has been shown to delay relapse of bipolar disorder (Miklowitz and Goldstein, 1997; Miklowitz *et al.*, 2000).

Family Resilience Therapies

While family psychoeducation approaches have focused on roles that families can play in reducing frequency of illness relapse or buffering its severity, family resilience interventions extend this strategy to identify salutary family processes that not only buffer severity of illness, but prevent its onset for those at risk. Key processes can be identified that enable couples and families facing disruptive crises or persistent stresses to strengthen relationships, regain functioning and further the growth of its individual members (Walsh, 1998; Wolin and Wolin, 1993).

   Family resilience refers to coping and adaptational processes in the family as a functional unit (Walsh, 1998; Wolin and Wolin, 1993). From this perspective, a stressor affects at-risk children only to the extent that they disrupt crucial family processes that otherwise would neutralize or buffer the stressor (Patterson, 1983). Family resilience rests upon several systemic principles (Walsh, 1998, p. 24):

- The hardiness of individuals is best understood and fostered in the context of the family and larger social world, as a mutual interaction of individual, family and environmental processes.
- Crisis events and persistent stresses affect the entire family, posing risks not only for individual dysfunction but for relational conflict and family breakdown.
- Family processes mediate the impact of stress on all members and their relationships, with protective processes fostering resilience by buffering stress and promoting recovery, and maladaptive responses heightening vulnerability and risks for individual and relationship distress.
- All families have the potential for resilience, which can be maximized by encouraging their best efforts and strengthening key processes.

   With programs such as Beardslee's (Beardslee *et al.*, 1999), family resilience programs have moved past treatment of acute illness and relapse prevention, to primary prevention of the

Table 70.1	Resilience Factors That Protect Children At Risk for Depression Due to Living with a Depressed Parent

- Becoming activists and doers
- Becoming heavily involved in school and extracurricular activities
- Developing deep commitments to and involvement in interpersonal relationships
- Seeking self-understanding as a way to deal with a parent's depression
- Expressing articulate understandings of the parent's illness and problems ensuing from it
- Refusing to feel blame or guilt for the parent's illness
- Learning to link life experiences in the family to factual information about depressive disorders
- Acquiring an active voice in family discussions about the illness

Source: Beardslee WR (1998) Prevention and the clinical encounter. *Am J Orthopsychiatr* 69(4), 521–533; Beardslee W, Versage EM, Salt P *et al.* (1999) The development and evaluation of two preventive intervention strategies for children of depressed parents, in *Rochester Symposium on Developmental Psychopathology, Vol. 9, Development Approaches to Prevention and Intervention* (eds Cicchetti D and Toth SL). University of Rochester Press, Rochester, New York.

disorder itself. Such programs identify risk factors and protective factors for onset of illness; relate these factors to family organization, communications, and knowledge of the disorder; and design family interventions that enhance family understanding, attenuate risk factors, and amplify protective factors (see Table 70.1).

Summary

Family therapy has evolved from a treatment modality that searched family relationships for the causes of mental illness to a framework for engaging the strengths and competencies of families in solving clinical problems and treating psychiatric disorders. The various clinical traditions of family that matured during the 1960s and 1970s remain rich sources of ideas and interventions that can be integrated into multimodality programs alongside family psychoeducation, individual psychotherapy and psychopharmacology. Such family-centered approaches as multifamily psychoeducation groups are sufficiently supported by empirical research to be regarded as evidenced-based practices. Family-centered models for primary prevention of major psychiatric disorders and family-centered community mental health programs for immigrant, refugee and international populations represent the developing frontiers of family therapy.

Appendix I

Psychodynamic Family Therapy

What to Look For

- Projective identification
- Unresolved grief
- Clarity of ego boundaries and capacity for intimacy/separateness

What to Think About

- Internal processes within individual family members shape family interactions.
- Family members' motivations, conflicts, defenses and relationships from the past, currently influence present relationships.
- Therapeutic change occurs through family members gaining conscious insight into previously unconscious processes generating problems in family relationships.

What to Do

- Opening emotional expression in family relationships
- Clarifying communications
- Encouraging family members to speak from the "I" position
- Interpretation of unconscious conflicts to resolve projective processes, cutoff relationships, and difficulties in modulating closeness and distance in family relationships
- Psychodramatic techniques, such as doubling and role reversal
- Therapeutic rituals to facilitate developmental transitions and grief over losses
- Family genograms

Structural Family Therapy

What to Look For
Contrasting the particular family structure with that "normal" to the culture and developmental stage in terms of:

- Organization (structure)
- Rules (sequences of action)
- Roles that shape family members' actions
- Boundaries
- Hierarchy of power
- Alliances
- Coalitions
- Verbal and nonverbal behavioral sequences.

What to Think About
Presenting problem results from a family structure out of alignment with the culture and the developmental stage of the family.

What to Do

- Actively shift the family structure
- In-session enactments
- Out-of-session homework assignments

Strategic Family Therapy

What to Look For

- Here-and-now context of the problem
- Who, what, when, where, and how people are involved in trying to solve the problem

What to Think About

- "The solution to the problem is the problem".
- Difficult life-cycle transitions give birth to clinical problems when people persist in old coping strategies but relational and

communication processes need to change to meet new life contexts.

What to Do

- Psychoeducation
- Direct behavioral assignments to adopt new problem-solving strategies
- Defiance-based, paradoxical interventions

Cognitive–Behavioral Family Therapy

What to Look For

- Family member difficulties in recognizing deviant behavior
- Lack of clearly-defined family rules
- Problems in emotional communication among family members, usually a paucity of expression of positive feelings coupled with an excess of negative expressions
- Relational conflict due to a paucity of relational skills
- Relational conflict due to interpretive errors based on faulty assumptions or cognitive distortions

What to Think About

- Each member of the family is assumed to be doing his or her best to cope with the behavioral contingencies perceived at that point in time, given the practical and emotional restraints experienced.
- Family members need to learn cognitive and behavioral principles of learning.
- Family members need to gain skills needed:

  1. To reinforce desired behaviors;
  2. To eliminate reinforcement of undesired behaviors;
  3. To modify faulty assumptions and interpretations about other family member's actions;
  4. To learn skills for communicating clearly and effectively.

What to Do

- Conduct psychoeducation about the presenting problem.
- Conduct skill training in empathic listening expressing positive feelings and speaking negative communications respectfully.
- Conduct training in problem-solving and conflict-resolution skills.
- Teach operant conditioning strategies for behavior shaping with children.
- Teach principles for contingency contracting to replace coercive and blaming behaviors with contracts specifying what each family members agrees to perform.
- Teach family members to utilize behavioral observation and thought diaries in out-of-session assignments to track patterns of thoughts, feelings and behaviors that generate symptoms.

Postmodern Family Therapies

What to Look For

- Listen for exact usage of language expressed as metaphors, stories and beliefs.
- Listen for first-person narratives from family members' lived-experiences that imbue with meaning such abstractions as "love," "trust" and other important language of relationships.
- Note exceptions, or unique outcomes, when problems might have occurred but surprisingly did not.
- Note what is happening at times when problems are absent.

What to Think About

- The limits of a person's language constitutes the limits of his or her experiential world.
- Narratives, or stories, are the basic units of human experience.
- A canon of personal narratives shapes the meaning each family attributes to his or her experience.
- Narratives of identity, about who one is as a family member, and who we are as a family, strongly influence family interactions.
- Family conflicts emerge:

  1. When lack of narrative skills makes their experiences unintelligible to others;
  2. When the available narratives preclude ways of relating other than conflictual ones;
  3. When specific words or expressions hold very different meanings for different family members due to the personal narratives with which they are associated;
  4. When family members become positioned relationally such that they cannot hear, tell, and/or expand their stories in conversation.

What to Do

- Focus on creating a dialogue in which important personal narratives can be safely expressed, heard, and reflected upon by family members.
- Ask questions that elicit forgotten, or unnoticed, narratives of family life that open better possibilities for solving problems than the current narratives that have dominated the family dialogue.
- Engage family members in an inquiry of:

  1. What is happening in family interactions when problems are being solved successfully and symptoms are not occurring.
  2. Skills, practical knowledge, competencies and resources of the family that can be brought to bear upon the problem.

References

Andersen T (1987) The reflecting team: Dialogue and meta-dialogue in clinical work. *Fam Process* 26, 415–428.

Anderson CM, Reiss DJ and Hogarty GE (1986) *Schizophrenia and the Family: A Practitioner's Guide to Psychoeducation and Management*. Guildford Press, New York.

Anderson H (1997) *Conversation, Language, and Possibilities*. Basic Books, New York.

Aponte JH and VanDeusen JM (1981) Structural family therapy, in *The Handbook of Family Therapy* (eds Gurman A and Kniskern D). Brunner/Mazel, New York, pp. 310–360.

Beardslee W, Versage EM, Salt P *et al.* (1999) The development and evaluation of two preventive intervention strategies for children of depressed parents, in *Rochester Symposium on Developmental Psychopathology, Vol. 9, Development Approaches to Prevention and*

Intervention (eds Cicchetti D and Toth SL). University of Rochester Press, Rochester, New York, pp. 111–151.

Blatner A (1994) Psychodramatic methods in family therapy, in *Family Play Therapy* (eds Schaefer CE and Carey LJ). Jason Aronson, Northvale, NJ.

Colapinto J (1991) Structural family therapy, in *The Handbook of Family Therapy*, Vol. 2 (eds Gurman A and Kniskern D). Brunner/Mazel, New York, pp. 417–443.

de Shazer S (1985) *Keys to Solution in Brief Therapy*. WW Norton, New York.

Dixon LB and Lehman AF (1995) Family interventions for schizophrenia. *Schizophr Bull* 21, 631–643.

Epstein N, Schlesinger SE and Dryden W (eds) (1988) *Cognitive–Behavioral Therapy with Families*. Brunner/Mazel, New York.

Epson D (1989) *Collected Papers*. Dulwich Centre Publications, Adelaide, South Australia.

Epston D and White M (eds) (1992) *Experience, Contradiction, Narrative, and Imagination*. Dulwich Centre Publications, Adelaide, South Australia.

Falloon IRH (1991) Behavioral family therapy, in *The Handbook of Family Therapy*, Vol. 2 (eds Gurman A and Kniskern DP). Brunner/Mazel, New York, pp. 65–95.

Framo JL (1991) *Family of Origin Consultations: An Intergenerational Approach*. Brunner/Mazel, New York.

Freeman A, Simon K, Beutler L *et al.* (eds) (1989) *Comprehensive Handbook of Cognitive Therapy*. Plenum Press, New York.

Freedman J and Combs G (1995) *Narrative Therapy: The Social Construction of Preferred Realities*. WW Norton, New York.

Griffith JL and Griffith ME (1994) *The Body Speaks: Therapeutic Dialogues for Mind/Body Problems*. Basic Books, New York.

Imber-Black E and Roberts J (1992) *Rituals for Our Times: Celebrating, Healing, and Changing Our Lives and Our Relationships*. HarperPerennial, New York.

Leff J and Vaughn CE (1985) *Expressed Emotion in Families*. Guilford Press, New York.

Madanes C (1981) *Strategic Family Therapy*. Jossey-Bass, Washington.

Madsen W (1999) *Collaborative Therapy with Multi-Stressed Families: From Old Problems to New Futures*. Guilford Press, New York.

Miklowitz DJ and Goldstein MJ (1997) *Bipolar Disorder: A Family-Focused Treatment Approach*. Guilford Press, New York.

Miklowitz DJ, Simoneau TL, George EL *et al.* (2000) Family-focused treatment of bipolar disorder: One year effects of a psychoeducational program in conjunction with pharmacotherapy. *Biol Psychiatr* 48, 582–592.

O' Hanlon W and Wiener-Davis M (1989) *In Search of Solutions: Creating a Context for Change*. WW Norton, New York.

Patterson G (1983) Stress: A change agent for family processes, in *Stress, Coping, and Development in Children* (eds Garmezy N and Rutter M). McGraw-Hill, New York.

Penn P (2001) Chronic illness: Trauma, language, and writing: Breaking the silence. *Fam Process* 40, 33–52.

Pinsof WM and Wynne LC (1995) The efficacy of marital and family therapy: An empirical overview, conclusions, and recommendations. *J Marital Fam Ther* 21, 585–613.

Scharff DE and Scharff JS (1987) *Object Relations Family Therapy*. Jason Aronson, Northvale, NJ.

Slipp S (1991) *The Technique and Practice of Object Relations Family Therapy*. Jason Aronson, Northvale, NJ.

Stanton MD (1981) Strategic approaches to family therapy, in *The Handbook of Family Therapy* (eds Gurman A and Kniskern D). Brunner/Mazel, New York, pp. 361–402.

Tomm K (1987) Interventive interviewing: Part II. Reflexive questioning as a means to enable self-healing. *Fam Process* 26, 167–183.

Walsh F (1998) *Strengthening Family Resilience*. Guilford Press, New York.

Weiner-Davis M (1992) *Divorce Busting*. Simon & Schuster, New York.

Weingarten K (1995) Radical listening: Challenging cultural beliefs for and about mothers. *J Feminist Fam Ther* 7, 7–22.

White M (1989) *Selected Papers*. Dulwich Centre Publications, Adelaide, South Australia.

White M (1995) *Re-Authoring Lives: Interviews and Essays*. Dulwich Centre Publications, Adelaide, South Australia.

White M (2000) *Reflections on Narrative Practices: Essays and Interviews*. Dulwich Centre Publications, Adelaide, South Australia.

Wolin S and Wolin S (1993) *The Resilient Self: How the Survivors of Troubled Families Rise Above Adversity*. Villard Books, New York.

CHAPTER

71

Couples Therapy

What Is "Couples Therapy?"

Marital or couples therapy can be defined as a format of intervention involving both members of a dyad in which the focus of intervention is the problematic interactional patterns of the couple. In this chapter, we will use marital and couples therapy interchangeably as the majority of the issues are the same. The focus of couples therapy is on the dyad and its intimate emotional and sexual aspects.

Couples therapy is distinguished by the peer relationship of the participants, the ever-present question of commitment, and a need carefully to attend to gender issues. In general, even behaviorally focused couples therapy must attend particularly to the feeling level with the goals being positive feeling between the partners and more reasonable behavior.

It is important to understand that when considering different types of psychotherapy – individual, group and family therapy – "couples therapy" is considered as a subtype of "family therapy". Further, we should make explicit the obvious: a couple is an example of a "family" (broadly defined).

Currently, there are various models and strategies for treating couples. Each may emphasize different assumptions and types of interventions. Some therapists prefer to operate with one strategy in most cases, whereas others intermix these strategies, depending on the presenting problem and the phase of treatment. At times, the type of strategy used is made explicit by the therapist, whereas in other instances it remains covert; irrespective of whether a therapist specializes in one or another approach or is eclectic, some hypotheses will be formed about the nature of the couple's difficulty and the preferable approach to adopt.

Therapists may choose one school or another based on their training or their personality. For example, a very organized and directive person would probably prefer cognitive–behavioral methods, while a person who prefers long-term emotional intensity over problem-solving might gravitate to experiential models. Individuals and families as well may prefer some ways of working over others. This chapter encourages the integration of a variety of techniques depending on the particular problem and personalities of the couple as well as the skill-set of the therapist. It also encourages the therapist to look beyond the problem at hand, that is, the presenting complaint, to issues of power, intimacy and personal growth. Our approach is to emphasize models that have (at least some) empirical data.

With the therapeutic focus on one person, the emphasis is often on the individual's perceptions, reactions and feelings, and also on the equality of status between the individual and the therapist; when two people are the operative system, attention is directed to interactions and relationships. Therapists who think in terms of a unit of three people look at coalitions, structures, and hierarchies

of status and power. The number of people actually involved in the interviews may not be as important as how many people are involved in the therapist's way of thinking about the problem.

Couples Function and Dysfunction

Couples Development

Dym (1993) has described how couples relationships evolve over time. Members of couples are influenced by past and present relationships and tend to form ties that have a distinct character that emerges through regular cycles of conflict and resolution. Dym draws attention to broad, normative changes in couples, characterizing these developmental shifts as periods of expansion, contraction and resolution. For example, in the early expansive years of a committed romantic relationship, the lives of two are in a sense woven into one. Some refer to this period of optimism, promise and fusion as moving from "I" to "We".

In the next years of the relationship, Dym describes a predictable stage of contraction and a feeling of betrayal, in which members of the couple reconnect with a need for an "I". This desire can be marked by experiences of doubts, fears and insecurities, and many couples retreat from their established routines. Partners may find themselves feeling "out of synch" with their own personal ambitions, describe themselves as feeling trapped or lonely, and may believe they are progressing at different tempos from each other. Stormy times may ensue with bitter conflict and blame. During the resolution stage couples may resort to compromise, negotiation, or even a more radical restructuring of their relationship in an effort to make room for both the individual and the relationship. In considering this dialectical movement from expansion to contraction to resolution, this cycle repeats several times over the course of the relationship. Dym notes that many couples have what he calls a "home base" where they tend to reside, in terms of the sense of "We", "I", or "working on it". A home base is the point of the cycle of expansion and contraction where the couples find themselves most often.

Sexual Functioning of Couples

It has been estimated that 50 percent of American marriages have some sexual problems. These can be divided into "difficulties" (such as inability to agree on frequency) which are clearly dyadic issues; and dysfunction which are specific problems with desire, arousal and orgasm, as listed in the DSM-IV (American Psychiatric Association, 1994). Dysfunctions may be organic or psychological at base, and may be lifelong or acquired, generalized or situational. They may be deeply embedded in relational power or

Essentials of Psychiatry   Jerald Kay and Allan Tasman
© 2006 John Wiley & Sons, Ltd.

intimacy struggles, or may be the only problem in an otherwise well-functioning relationship. While most family therapists believe that there is no uninvolved partner when one member of a couple presents with sexual dysfunction, that is different from saying that the relationship itself is the cause of the dysfunction. The job of the therapist is to ascertain as best as possible the etiology of the problem and to choose the most effective therapy, whether medical, individual, or relational. It is also within the therapist's purview to inquire about whether the couple would like to improve a technically functional but not very satisfying sexual relationship, in the same way that the therapist can offer methods or directions to increase intimacy in a couple that wishes personal growth.

Diagnosis/Systems Issues

Sexual dysfunction or dissatisfaction is, in a minority of times, caused by a psychiatric disorder (depression and anxiety may often decrease sexual desire). It is commonly caused by ignorance of sexual anatomy and physiology, negative attitudes and self-defeating behavior, anger, power or intimacy issues with the partners, or medical/physiological problems. Medication side effects are a particularly common cause of sexual dysfunction in patients who are receiving selective serotonin reuptake inhibitors (SSRIs). Male erection problems are proving increasingly amenable to medical forms of treatment. It is also important to remember that people vary enormously in the importance they place on sex or eroticism in their lives. For example, in *The Social Organization of Sexuality: Sexual Practices in the US* (Laumann and Michael, 1994), about a third of the people surveyed have sex at least twice a week, about a third a few times a month, and the rest, sex with a partner a few times a year or not at all. In general, when sex is not part of a marriage over a long period of time, the relationship has less vitality and life. However, even well-functioning marriages may have periods in which sexuality is much less part of their lives (such as after the birth of a first child, or during a family or health crisis). Different people have vastly different tolerance for such periods.

Because sex is a way of each person being vulnerable to the other, it is difficult to have sex when one is angry or not in a mood to be close (although some people can block out other feelings and keep the sexual area more separate). In addition, people who feel abused, mistreated, or ignored in a relationship are less likely to want to please the other. For some who feel that they have no voice in the relationship, lack of desire is sometimes the only way they feel able to manifest displeasure.

Couples who continue in marital or individual treatment for long periods of time can resolve some of their marital problems but can still suffer from specific sexual difficulties in their marriage. It is also true that specific sexual problems may be dramatically reversed after relatively brief periods of sex therapy, even though such problems may have proven intractable following long periods of more customary psychotherapy. However, sexual functioning which is suffering because the partners do not want to be close is not likely to respond to sex therapy unless other issues are also addressed.

Usually, when a marital couple has a generally satisfactory relationship, any minor sexual problems may be only temporary. Resolution of sexual problems, however, will not inevitably produce positive effects in other facets of a relationship as well.

Marital and sexual problems interact in various ways:

1. The sexual dysfunction produces or contributes to secondary marital discord. Specific strategies focused on the sexual dysfunctions would usually be considered the treatment of choice in these situations, especially if the same sexual dysfunction occurred in the person's other relationships.
2. The sexual dysfunction is secondary to marital discord. In such situations, general strategies of marital treatment might be considered the treatment of choice. If the marital relationship is not too severely disrupted, a trial of sex therapy might be attempted because a relatively rapid relief of symptoms could produce beneficial effects on the couple's interest in pursuing other marital issues.
3. Marital discord cooccurs with sexual problems. This situation would probably not be amenable to sex therapy because of the partners' hostility to each other. Marital therapy would usually be attempted first, with later attention given to sexual dysfunction.
4. Sexual dysfunction occurs without marital discord. This case might be found in instances where one partner's medical illness has affected his or her sexual functioning, forcing the couple to learn new ways to manage the change. Another example might be when one partner has a history of sexual abuse or a sexual assault that creates anxiety related to the sexual experience. While individual therapy can be helpful in both of these cases, couples therapy can be especially useful in creating a safe place to address painful feelings and anxious expectations, and to provide education and guidance for couples undergoing these transitions.

Secrets and Confidentiality

Unless a therapist sees both parties together at all times, he/she will eventually face a situation in which family secrets are disclosed in individual sessions. Since secrets are a common source of dysfunction, discovering and dealing with them is a frequent occurrence.

The therapist needs to make a distinction between **secrecy** and **privacy**. Privacy is usually considered to mean information held by one person that they would prefer not to share but that does not directly affect their relationship with others. It usually implies a zone of comfort free from intrusion. Secrets are usually considered to be feelings or information that would directly affect a relationship. They are most often connected to fear, anxiety and shame, and are often shared, that is, some people in the system know, whereas some do not. There is also a gray area in which different people have different ideas about whether the information is important or not. (Does a spouse consider an extramarital affair that ended 10 years ago private or secret?)

In general, the best rule of thumb is that a secret should be disclosed if it is seriously affecting connections between people, posing danger to a family member (sexual abuse), or shaping family coalitions and alliances. In general, keeping secrets is such a serious barrier that it is better to disclose them, even if painful, because otherwise the sense of mystification and isolation in the unaware is very strong.

The therapist must carefully consider the timing and type of disclosure. Premature disclosure, before the therapist has an alliance with the family, can cause the family to leave therapy with no place to deal with potentially explosive material. This is particularly true when there has been a history of violence or abuse.

Although the following guidelines do not sufficiently cover all couples' problems and situations, they do represent a generic set of ideas that therapists may apply to the specifics of many marital issues.

Evaluation of the Couple

The evaluation of a couple involves obtaining data on the current point in the marital and/or family life-cycle, why the couple approaches for assistance at a particular time, and each partner's view of the marital or relationship problem (Table 71.1). Often the couple's therapist will hold one individual session with each partner after the first or second conjoint session. This gives each partner an opportunity to divulge information that might otherwise not be obtainable. Issues of confidentiality need to be carefully addressed.

In formulating the marital difficulties, the evaluator will want to consider the couple's communication, problem-solving, roles, affective expression and involvement, and behavioral expression, especially in sexual and aggressive areas. The clinician will also want to evaluate gender roles, cultural and racial issues, and power inequities resulting from gender, class, age, or financial status. It is critical to ask about alcohol, health and reproductive issues, and violence (Table 71.2).

Even if the partners do not mention their children as a problem, it is wise to spend some time developing a sense of how the children are doing, is there a favored child or problem with any of them, and whether the children are being pulled into marital conflicts. At times children can be the source of a couple's conflict and at other times they may function as the glue that keeps the relationship together. If a large part of the couple's difficulty centers around issues with the children, family therapy may be the preferred treatment modality (see Chapter 70-Family Therapy).

Other areas deserving special attention include each spouse's commitment to the marital union and the couple's sexual life. Assessment is complicated when one spouse is keeping commitment doubts or extramarital sex a secret. Conjoint and individual sessions with each partner may be needed. When infidelity or serious commitment questions arise, the therapist and couple must address whether or not the couple should stay together.

Table 71.1   Outline for Family Evaluation

  I. Current phase of family life-cycle and identifying data
 II. Explicit interview data:
    A. What is the current family problem?
    B. Why does the family come for treatment at the present time?
    C. What is the background of the family problem?
    D. What is the history of past treatment attempts or other attempts at problem solving in the family?
    E. What are the family's goals and expectations of the treatment? What are their motivations and resistances?
III. Formulating the family problem areas:
    A. Rating important dimensions of family functioning:
       1. Communication
       2. Problem-solving
       3. Roles and coalitions
       4. Affective responsiveness and involvement
       5. Behavior control
       6. Operative family beliefs
    B. Family classification and "diagnosis"
IV. Planning the therapeutic approach and establishing the treatment contract

---

Table 71.2   Guidelines for Interviewing Couples: The Process

- Can you tell me about yourself? As individuals? As a couple?
  (Joining, forming an alliance with each member and the couple, creating a safe place)
- What brings you here? How do you understand the problem? What feelings does it elicit for each of you?
  (Developing an interactional problem focus)
- How does the problematic pattern actually work? Can you show me how it works?
  (Observing by staging an "enactment")
- How did this pattern originate? How did you create it?
  (Placing the problem in context of their relationship, family of origin, and their own individual development)
- How have you maintained this pattern? What have you done to keep it going?
  (Placing the pattern or problem under their joint control)
- Tell me about what you believe should be happening.
  (Myths, stories, ideas, expectations about love, sexuality, marriage, and closeness)
- In what other ways is the pattern currently reinforced? What do your family and friends believe is the problem?
  (How do jobs, extended family members, and friends contribute to the pattern's resilience?)
- Is this pattern always occurring or are there exceptions?
  (How pervasive is it, is it chronic, or related to a life transition?)
- What have you done to try to change the pattern?
  (Trying to avoid redundancy by inquiring about solution behavior)
- Have your efforts to change the pattern made things better or worse?
  (Looking at the problem as "attempted solutions")
- What has been the influence of this problem in your lives?
  (Again looking for the "influence" of the problem over their lives)
- How motivated are you to change the pattern now?
  (Assessing individual and couples motivation)
- What would happen if you succeeded in changing the pattern?
  (Anticipating possible consequences of change, both positive and negative)
- What patterns of relating have you created that you want to keep?
  (Identifying and honoring assets and resources)
- Are you ready to make a change? How about trying something different?
  (Preparing the couple for exploring new patterns of interaction)

The therapist is then free to track themes (always keeping an interactional focus), invent tasks and experiments designed to provide new experiences for the couple, and to evaluate the changes that occur or do not occur as a result of the couple's efforts to change their patterns of interaction.

Genograms for Evaluation

A helpful device when evaluating a couple is the use of a genogram. The therapist can collect and organize historical data

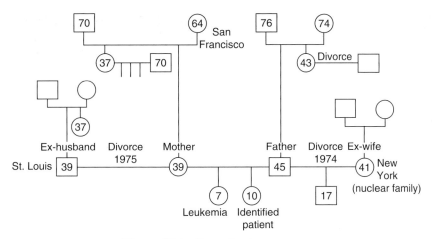

Figure 71.1   *Example of a genogram.*

through the use of a genogram, the three-generational family tree depicting the family's patterns regarding either specific problems or general family functioning. The genogram technique suggests possible connections between present family events and the prior experiences that family members have shared (e.g., regarding the management of serious illnesses, losses and other critical transitions), thereby placing the presenting problem in a historical context (Shorter, 1977; McGoldrick and Gerson, 1985). Constructing a genogram early on in treatment can provide a wealth of data that frequently offers clues about pressures, expectations and hopes regarding the marriage. This pictorial way of gathering a history allows each member of the couple to learn about beliefs or themes that characterize his/her family background. An example of a genogram can be seen in Figure 71.1.

Assessment of Concomitant Psychiatric Illness

Having a spouse with a serious Axis I disorder, such as anxiety disorder, mood disorder, or substance abuse puts realistic strain on the marital relationship. The marital interaction prior to, during and following the onset of the symptoms in the spouse is influenced by numerous factors and is quite variant across dyads. It is incorrect to assume that in all cases the interaction between the spouses brought on, or caused, or even helped trigger the mental disorder and symptoms in the other. Whatever the symptoms in one spouse, the relationship of symptoms to the marital interaction is on a continuum and can take any one of the following forms:

1. The marital interaction neither causes the symptoms nor stresses the psychologically vulnerable spouse.
2. The marital interaction does not stress the vulnerable individual but following onset of symptoms the marital interaction declines and becomes dysfunctional, thus causing more distress.
3. The marital interaction acts as a stressor that contributes to the onset of symptoms in a vulnerable spouse.
4. The symptoms can be explained totally as under the control and function of the interactional patterns between the spouses.

The therapist meeting a new couple therefore can entertain a range of different ideas that may help illuminate and explain their distressing circumstances. The Axis I condition can be a useful focus and often is what brings the couple in for help.

Evaluation of Sexual Disorders

A careful evaluation of the couple's total interactions needs to be done by the therapist as well as a physical assessment when dysfunction is present. When it appears that the basic marriage is a sound one, but that the couple suffers from specific sexual difficulties (which may also lead to various secondary marital consequences), the primary focus might be sex therapy per se. In many cases, however, specific sex therapy cannot be carried out until the relationship between the two partners has been improved in other respects; indeed, the sexual problems may clearly be an outgrowth of the marital difficulties. When marital problems are taken care of, the sexual problems may readily be resolved. It may be difficult to disentangle marital from sexual problems or to decide which came first. The priorities for therapy may not always be clear.

Specific techniques are available which have been devised for eliciting a sexual history and for evaluating sexual functioning. The marital therapist should become familiar with these ideas and obtain experience in their utilization. A systemic assessment of sexual difficulties includes, at the minimum, the following details as listed in Table 71.3.

In addition, in couples where there is any possibility that the problems may have an organic component, it is crucial to insist on a medical work-up. This is particularly key for men, for whom small physiological changes in potency may produce anxiety that exacerbates the problem.

The taking of an intimate sexual history of husband and wife should, of course, be conducted with the couple without children present. The process of taking a sexual history should be handled with care and regard for each person's level of comfort.

What type of language should be used when discussing sexual topics? Obviously, one should not use terms that would be offensive or uncomfortable for either the therapist or the couple. At the same time, care must be taken to avoid using bland generalities which fail to elicit specific sexual information. Frankness is encouraged, and when there is vagueness, the therapist needs to follow-up with more specific questions.

Taking a sexual history of lesbian and gay couples may be particularly difficult for a heterosexual therapist, either because of discomfort with homosexuality or lack of knowledge of homosexual norms and mores. In addition, the couple may have a wider or different set of sexual practices than the therapist is used to (of course, this may be true with heterosexual couples as well). Therapists have the options of educating themselves about homosexual sexuality, either by reading books available in mainstream

Table 71.3	Assessment of Sexual Problems

1. Definition of the problem
   (a) How does the couple describe the problem? What are their theories about its etiology? How do they generally relate to their sexuality, as reflected in their language, attitudes toward sexuality, comfort level, and their permission system?
   (b) How is the problem a problem for them? What is the function of the problem in their relationship system? Is the relationship problem the central problem? Why now?
2. Relationship history
   (a) Current partner
   (b) Previous relationship history
   (c) Psychosexual history, including information about early childhood experiences, nature of sexual encounters prior to the relationship, sexual orientation, and feelings about masculinity and femininity.
   (d) Description of current sexual functioning, focusing on conditions for satisfactory sex, positive behaviors, specific technique, etc. Who initiates sex, who leads, or do both? How does their sexual pattern of intimacy and control reflect on or compensate for other aspects of their relationship?
3. Developmental life-cycle issues (births, deaths, transitions)
4. Medical history, focusing on current physical status, medications and present medical care, especially endocrine, vascular, metabolic.
5. Goals (patients' and therapist's viewpoints): The task is to examine whether goals are realistic and what previous attempted solutions have yielded.

bookstores about gay and lesbian life, and/or asking the couple about their own and other common practices. If the therapist is very anxious in this situation, he/she must decide when the therapy is not proving effective and if he/she should refer to another therapist. Gay and lesbian couples may present with any of the dysfunctions or dissatisfactions of heterosexual couples.

Indications for Couples Therapy

The process of choosing a type of therapy is complex and research is just beginning to develop guidelines for such decisions. The therapist must most often base his or her judgment on clinical intuition, general clinical opinion, and the wishes and judgments of the people involved.

Marital Versus Individual Therapy

One of the most common questions for clinicians who are proficient in both therapies is regarding the decision about type and timing of therapy. The basic theoretical premise of couple/family therapy is that many problems are purely relational, that individual symptoms in one person can be viewed as interpersonal in terms of etiology or problem maintenance, and that they can be changed by altering the system. The basic principle of individual therapy is that problems or symptoms develop because of the biochemistry or dynamics of the individual, and that change occurs in the individual (either behaviorally or because of cognitive understanding of the problems) in the presence of an intense

and exclusive relationship with the therapist. In truth, for many people, both forms of therapy may be useful or necessary. Self-knowledge does not always help the person understand the complex family system and how one's behavior affects and is affected by family members. In addition, family therapy does not allow for intense exploration of psychodynamic issues. Individual therapy also does not allow the clinician to see how the problems of other family members may also be affecting the system.

Since people tend to pick partners at similar stages of differentiation, it is not unusual for people with psychological difficulties to have spouses with similar or complementary but equally severe problems. In addition to the need to evaluate the partner, it must be recognized that such couples create problems maintaining systems that need to be addressed directly. Children in such families often suffer either from genetically based similar illnesses (such as depression) or symptoms as a result of dealing with parental problems. These are often best treated with family therapy, but this does not rule out special time just for the child. For many people, both types of therapy are helpful, allowing for increased pleasure with the partner and also a context for personal and private growth.

The choice of timing of therapy is always of interest. If the person is highly symptomatic and has a problem which is usually amenable to medications, it is often helpful to begin medication and family therapy first, in order to reduce the symptoms and educate the family, as well as to eliminate family sources of stress.

In general, one tries to deal with the most acute problems first. If it is possible in terms of timing and finances, it is easily possible to do individual and couples therapy at the same time. It is often recommended that the therapies be conducted by different therapists, however, in this strategy it is imperative that the therapists remain in contact to avoid splitting or conflicting treatment. Others, including therapists on occasion, have treated both the couple and one member of the couple individually, although this can present some additional challenges to the therapist to remain neutral and unbiased. The therapist's criteria depend more on the characteristics of the couple and how they function than on the particular diagnosis or problem area. The bias of the couple or individual must also be taken into account.

Individual, Couple, or Sex Therapy for Sexual Problems

This distinction was clearer 10 years ago when sex therapy was primarily focused on a specific and highly detailed behavioral protocol. Sex therapy in the last few years has moved in the direction of further understanding of the physiologic causes of sex dysfunction on one hand, and cognitive–behavioral issues on the other. It is clear at this point that, in general, sexual problems do not disappear with couple therapy unless specific attention is paid to the nature and quality of the sexual problems. Usually, it is most effective to deal with severe couple conflict before beginning to deal with sexual issues directly (Table 71.4). Sex therapy includes education, a focus on the intimacy and power aspects of sex, and often homework assignments that in some way deal with sexual anxiety and expansion of sexual options. Individual therapy is indicated if the problems are clearly related to the partner's history (sexual abuse, hatred of women), have occurred in multiple relationships, and are not amenable to being worked on in the couple. Individual therapy is the most inefficient way of dealing with most couple centered sexual problems. It is

Table 71.4	Criteria for Sex and Marital Therapy
Sex Therapy	**Marital Therapy**
The marital problem is clearly focused on sexual dysfunction	Sexuality not an issue, or it is one of many issues in marital dysfunction.
Enabling Factors	
Willingness and ability to carry out the sexual functioning tasks that would be assigned by therapist.	Anger and resistance too intense to carry out extra-session tasks around sexual functioning.
Strong attachment to marital partner; both partners interested in reversing the sexual dysfunction.	Couple not committed to each other; there are covert and/or overt behaviors to dissolve the marriage.

also important to consider the possible role of organic problems in any dysfunction.

Contraindications for Couples Therapy

Couples therapy is not indicated for every couple in distress. In fact, at times, it may even be contraindicated. If one member is keeping an important secret, an attempt to work with them as a pair may fail and the therapist often has to take a strong stand and refuse to treat the couple, as in the case of an HIV positive male who refused to share this information with his wife. At times, one member of a couple may be too ill to benefit from couples therapy. This may be the case when one partner has a bipolar disorder or schizophrenia and is acutely psychotic.

Other couples feel more comfortable when each partner has his or her own therapist. At times it can be more effective to have each member in individual therapy with good coordination between the two therapists. Finally, cases may arise where seeing a couple together may put one member of the couple in physical danger. When one member has a history of violence toward the partner, the therapist must often see each party alone to ensure the safety of a partner. Discussing areas of conflict together may risk increasing the violent behavior of one partner.

Sex therapy may be contraindicated in the same situations as above. In addition, many couples do not feel comfortable in a therapy exclusively focusing on sex. These couples may make more progress if the sex therapy is carefully included in the overall treatment of the couple. When referring to a sex therapist, it is particularly important to be familiar with the skill and credentials of the therapist.

Treatment

We believe that for most people the strongest predictor of overall life satisfaction is the quality of the person's central relationship. In addition, "a good and stable relationship buffers against the genetic vulnerability to both medical and psychiatric disorder". Thus, helping a couple achieve a more satisfying relationship can have widespread and profound influence on their life and lives of those with whom they interact.

The treatment of each couple is unique and may require a combination of couples therapy, individual therapy, group therapy (particularly self-help groups such as Alcoholics Anonymous) family therapy and medication management. By using an integrative approach with each couple, the therapist maximizes the chances for success. Identifying goals of treatment will help determine which modalities will be most effective and in what order they need to be applied. Goals most likely attained by employing couples therapy include the following: specification of the interactional problem, recognition of mutual contributions to the problems, clarification of marital boundaries, clarification and specification of each spouse's needs and desires in the relationship, increased communication skills, decreased coercion and blame, and increased differentiation and resolution of marital transference distortions. Final goals of the marital intervention may involve resolution of presenting problems, reduction of symptoms, increased intimacy, increased role flexibility, balance of power, clear communication, resolution of conflictual interaction, and improved relations with children and families of origin.

The treatment of couples is often conceived of as a relatively brief therapy (though it need not be), usually meeting once weekly, with a focus on the marital interaction. The major indication for marital intervention is the presence of marital conflict but other indications include symptomatic behaviors that impact both parties such as depression, anxiety disorders, substance abuse and illness in a child, marital partner, or other family member.

Strategies and Techniques of Intervention

Couples therapy utilizes strategies for imparting new information, opening up new and expanded individual and marital experiences, psychodynamic strategies for individual and interactional insight, communication and problem-solving strategies, and strategies for restructuring the repetitive interactions between the spouses or partners.

Sometimes, couples present with chronic histories of unresolved and unrelenting conflict. Other couples are in a state of transition, perhaps moving from the initial expansion stage of their marriage to the inevitable crisis related to the reevaluation of the contraction stage. In either case, clarifying the couples' process and their reoccurring patterns of behavior represents the starting place for couples therapy.

The focus should be primarily on the interpersonal distortions between husband and wife, and not on the couple–therapist transference. However, negative transference distortions toward the therapist must be addressed quickly and overtly.

There are three strategies in this focused, active treatment of marital discord:

1. The therapist interrupts collusive processes between the spouses. The interaction may involve either spouse failing to perceive positive or negative aspects of the other that are clear to an outsider (e.g., cruelty or alternately generosity) or when either spouse behaves in a way aimed at protecting the other from experiences that are inconsistent with the spouse's self-perception, (e.g., husband working part time views himself as breadwinner, whereas wife works full time and manages checkbook to shield husband from reality of their income and finances).
2. The therapist links individual experience, including past experience and inner thoughts, to the marital relationships.

3. The therapist creates and allocates tasks that are constructed to (a) encourage the spouses to differentiate between the impact of the other's behavior versus (the other's) intent, (b) to bring into awareness the concrete behavior of the partner that contradicts (anachronistic) past perceptions of that partner, and (c) to encourage each spouse to acknowledge his/her own behavior changes that are incompatible with the maladaptive ways each sees himself/herself and is seen by the marital partner. These tasks also help reconstruct the couple's narrative to make it more positive.

The last (c) is most important. In fact, in the initial stage of marital treatment the authors ask that each partner focus on what they want to change in themselves, not how they want the other spouse to be different.

In an integrative model of couples therapy, the focus is on three related domains: the functional relationships between the antecedents and consequences of discrete interactional sequences; the recurrent patterns of interaction including their implicit rules; and each spouse's individual schemata for intimate relationships. In the initial stage, alliances must be developed between the therapist and each marital partner, with the therapist offering empathy, warmth and understanding. The therapist must also ally with the couple as a whole and learn their shared language as well as their different problem-solving styles and attitudes.

Behavioral techniques, including giving between-session homework, in-session tasks, communication skills and problem-solving training, can facilitate the process of helping marital partners reintegrate denied aspects of themselves and of each other. However, the focus is not on behavioral change alone, as overt behavior is seen as reflecting the interlocking feelings and perceptions of each spouse. Ideally, the process of treatment should be one where each partner can consider what they want to change in themselves as opposed to how they want the other spouse to be different; safely explores new beliefs, feelings and behaviors; and experiments with new patterns of interaction that are unfamiliar and even anxiety-provoking.

Treatment of Sexual Dysfunction

Treatment of psychosexual disorders, in the form developed by Masters and Johnson (1966), consisted of a thorough assessment of the partners and their relationship, education about sexual functioning, and a series of behavioral exercises. There are specific exercises for each of the sexual dysfunctions. Different authors developed different exercises and ways of approaching them. For a complete description of these exercises, we recommend Kaplan (1995), LoPiccolo and Stock (1996) and Zilbergeld (1992). This method works best when there is ignorance, shame, or specific dysfunction such as premature ejaculation. These exercises are difficult to complete if the couple feels angry or unloving toward each other.

Many of the patients who saw Masters and Johnson in the 1970s had issues related to sexual ignorance and inexperience. Two decades later, the increase in premarital sex and the proliferation of easily available articles and books on sexuality and information on the Internet have decreased the number of these couples, and allowed some couples with sexual dysfunction to work on their issues at home. Recent studies of couples requesting sex therapy have shown a higher proportion having concomitant, complicated marital problems. Recent writers in the field,

notably Schnarch (1997), have focused on cognitive/emotional issues in sexuality, and especially on the meanings attached to a particular act, and the level of intimacy involved. Having learned a great deal about the more mechanical and organic issues related to arousal and orgasm, it is important to rethink other aspects of sex, such as eroticism, passion, mystery and dominance/submission which make the act itself meaningful. This is particularly true in areas of sexual boredom or situational lack of desire. These therapists do not use rigidly staged exercises, but focus on the couple's relatedness during sex; they may, however, suggest specific homework to help a couple focus on a particular aspect of their sexuality.

Effectiveness and Efficacy of Couples Therapy

There are two major sources for reviews of efficacy of couples therapy. Shadish and coworkers (1995) summarized 163 randomized studies, 62 marital and 101 family therapy. Pinsof and Wynne (1995) in a commentary have summarized the data. These studies point to the following general conclusions:

1. Family treatment is more effective than no treatment. This conclusion is manifest in studies that contrast family and marital treatment to no-treatment control groups. Roughly 67% of marital cases and 70% of family cases improve. The outcome may be slightly better if the identified patient is a child or an adolescent than if he or she is an adult. These findings were statistically significant. No one therapy method was demonstrated clearly to be better than another.
2. The deterioration rate (i.e., the percentage of patients who become worse or experience negative effects of therapy) is estimated at about 10% – lower than for individual therapy. Pinsof and Wynne (1995) believe the rate is lower than 5 to 10% and describe family therapy as not harmful.
3. In several areas evidence indicates that family treatment is the preferred intervention strategy. In other areas family therapy and individual therapy were tied – often in situations in which the identified patient had a significant Axis I problem (Shadish et al., 1995). These treatments of choice are of great importance for practitioners and students.

Dropouts

The dropout rate in the early stage of couple or family therapy is relatively high. In one study, about 30% of all the families or couples referred for family treatment failed to appear for the first session (defected) and another 30% terminated in the first three sessions, leaving about 40% who continued (Shapiro and Budman, 1973). The main reason families gave for termination was a lack of activity on the part of the therapist, whereas defectors in general had a "change of heart", and denied that a problem existed. The issue usually is that no matter how bad a situation was, it was preferable to what might happen if a couple changed their behaviors. The motivation of the husband appeared to play a crucial role: the more motivated he was, the more likely the family was to continue treatment. The idea that a dropout is "denying a problem" may or may not be true. Because the process of entering therapy is frightening for many people and because the therapist must meet the needs of several people, it is unsurprising that the process of engagement is rocky.

Ethical Issues in Couples Therapy

The fundamental ethical dilemmas inherent in psychotherapy: confidentiality, limits of control, duty to warn/reporting of abuse and therapist–patient boundaries become more complex when the treatment involves more than one person. The couple's therapist has an ethical responsibility to everyone in the family. In some cases, individual needs and system needs may be in conflict. For example, a husband may wish to conceal a brief episode of unprotected sex with another woman, while his wife is better protected, for health reasons as well as psychological reasons, if she knows about it. A wife's wish to be divorced from a psychiatrically ill and demanding husband may conflict with his need for her care. Such clinical situations provide a set of ethical dilemmas for the therapist. The therapist must be clear that his/her job in most cases (such as impending divorce) is to help the partners sort out their values, obligations and options rather than making a decision for them. In some cases, however (such as the reporting of child abuse), the ethical decision must be the therapist's. And in some cases the therapist faces difficult gray areas which must be decided on a case-by-case basis. The therapist also has certain unalterable ethical obligations such as not engaging in "dual relationships" (see later) with patients or exploiting them for their own benefit.

While the operative concept is "first do no harm", the issues of how one defines harm, and who will or will not be harmed by a certain action, are complex and difficult questions, especially when treating a couple or family.

The Conflicting Interests of Family Members

It is not unusual for the interests of each member of the couple to conflict at some point. Boszormenyi-Nagy and Spark (1973) years ago emphasized the contractual obligations and accountability between persons in the multigenerations of a family. Relational ethics are concerned with the balance of equitable fairness between people. To gauge the balance of fairness in the here-and-now, and across time and generations, each member must consider both his/her own interests and the interests of each of their partners. The basic issue is one of equitability, that is, everyone is entitled to have his or her welfare and interests considered in a way that is fair to the related interests of other family members.

There may be times when it is difficult to decide whether a therapeutic action or suggestion may be helpful for one individual, but not helpful or even temporarily harmful to the other individual. In their concern for the healthy functioning of the system as a whole, therapists may inadvertently ignore what is best for one individual. An ethical issue is how the decision is made. Should it be the therapist's concern alone or should it be shared with the couple? How much information should they be given on the pros and cons of modalities? The authors' bias is to negotiate and give the couple all the relevant information so that they can make the most informed decision possible (for further discussion, see also Hare-Mustin et al., 1979; Hare-Mustin, 1980).

Boundaries

The issue of boundaries and dual relationships is a critical one in all forms of psychotherapy. Because couples therapy involves more than one patient in the consulting room, there is less likelihood of inappropriate sexual contact between therapist and patient. However, there have been cases in which a therapist, working with a couple, began an affair with one of the spouses, either during couple's therapy or after the couple separated. The American Association of Marital and Family Therapy (AAMFT) Code of Ethics (1998) has a very sensible code of ethics making clear the inappropriateness of this kind of behavior.

Other confusing issues may arise because the issues that couples face are the same as issues therapists face in their own lives, making it very likely that at some point countertransference issues may become ethical ones. For example, seeing a couple going through a separation at the same time one is going through the early stages of one's own divorce is an extremely difficult thing to do, and the likelihood of remaining neutral to both parties is not great. While it is obviously impossible for a therapist to stop treating patients while going through a divorce, he or she could certainly choose not to accept a new patient whose situation is very similar to their own or who reminds them of their departing spouse. Issues of "confidentiality" and "boundaries" are issues mentioned in the AAMFT Code of Ethics (1998). Three of these have special relevance to couples therapists:

1. Marriage and family therapists are aware of their influential position with respect to clients, and they avoid exploiting the trust and dependency of such persons. Therapists, therefore, make every effort to avoid dual relationships with clients that could impair professional judgment or increase the risk of exploitation. When a dual relationship cannot be avoided, therapists take appropriate professional precautions to ensure judgment is not impaired and no exploitation occurs. Examples of such dual relationships include, but are not limited to business or close personal relationships with clients. Sexual intimacy with clients is prohibited. Sexual intimacy with former clients for 2 years following the termination of therapy is prohibited.
2. Marriage and family therapists respect the right of clients to make decisions and help them understand the consequences of these decisions. Therapists clearly advise a client that a decision on marital status is the responsibility of the client.
3. Marriage and family therapists have unique confidentiality concerns because the client in a therapeutic relationship may be more than one person. Therapists respect and guard confidences of each individual client.

Conclusion

Couples and sex therapy are important forms of psychotherapy. There is little question that developing the skills needed successfully to work with couples presenting with a wide range of difficulties requires an understanding of how normal couples' relationships change over time, how problems emerge and are maintained, and how focused marital treatment can alleviate distress and dysfunction. The rewards, however, are great when therapists can assist couples in recognizing and shifting the patterns that inhibit their abilities to live rich, intimate lives together.

Long-term relationships that are mutually supportive with a high level of intimacy are rare. As societies around the world (including our own) continue to evolve, unexpected events create havoc even for very stable families. What couples ask of their psychiatrists is the basic knowledge and skills, artfully applied to their joint relationships, to improve the quality of their lives.

References

American Association of Marital and Family Therapy (1998) *Code of Ethics*.

American Psychiatric Association (1994) *Diagnostic and Statistical Manual of Mental Disorders*, 4th edn. APA, Washington DC.

Borzormenyi-Nagy I and Spark G (1973) *Invisible Loyalties: Reciprocity in Intergenerational Family Therapy*. Harper & Row, New York.

Dym B (1993) *Couples: Exploring and Understanding the Cycles of Intimate Relationships*. HarperCollins, Boston, MA.

Hare-Mustin R (1980) Family therapy may be dangerous to your health. *Prof Psychol* 11, 935–938.

Hare-Mustin R, Marecek J, Caplan K *et al.* (1979) Rights of clients, responsibilities of therapists. *Am Psychol* 34, 3–16.

Kaplan HS (1995) *The Sexual Desire Disorders: Dysfunctional Regulation of Sexual Motivation*, Ch. 18. Brunner/Mazel, New York.

Laumann E and Michael E (1994) *The Social Organization of Sexuality: Sexual Practices in the US*. University of Chicago Press, Chicago, IL.

LoPiccolo J and Stock W (1996) Treatment of sexual dysfunction. *J Consult Clin Psychol* 54, 158–167.

Masters W and Johnson V (1966) *Human Sexual Response*. Little, Brown, Boston, MA.

McGoldrick M and Gerson R (1985) *Genograms in Family Assessment*. WW Norton, New York.

Pinsof WM and Wynne LC (1995) The efficacy of marital and family therapy: An empirical review, conclusions and recommendations. *J Marital Fam Ther* 21, 585–613.

Schnarch D (1997) *Passionate Marriage*. WW Norton, New York.

Shadish WR, Ragsdale K, Glaser RR *et al.* (1995) The efficacy and effectiveness of marital and family therapy: A perspective from meta-analysis. *J Marital Fam Ther* 21, 345–361.

Shapiro R and Budman S (1973) Defection, termination and continuation in family and individual therapy. *Fam Process* 12, 55–67.

Shorter E (1977) *The Making of the Modern Family*. Basic Books, New York.

Zilbergeld B (1992) *The New Male Sexuality*. Bantam, New York.

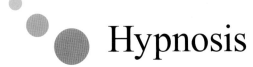

72 Hypnosis

Hypnosis is a natural state of attentive, focused concentration. As such, most individuals are able to experience trance-like states at different times in their daily lives. An example is the alteration of awareness experienced by some persons as they concentrate intently on a movie or a play while disconnecting from awareness of the surrounding environment. Depending on the degree of natural ability to enter a trance state (hypnotic capacity or hypnotizability), a given subject will require more or less help to enter and use his or her hypnotic capacity. That is, highly hypnotizable individuals enter trance states with ease, on many occasions even without being fully aware of it. Individuals with low hypnotizability require more direction or help from the therapist who facilitates the trance experience. High hypnotic capacity may actually become a liability to patients who are unaware of their hypnotic capacity or of their unconscious use of this mechanism, as is the case of individuals suffering from a dissociative disorder. Even when we do not intend to use hypnosis formally, we must remember that the ability to enter a trance state is widely and naturally distributed throughout the normal population. Thus, some of our patients may be experiencing trance states even without our planning.

In 1960, the American Medical Association and the American Psychiatric Association (APA) officially recognized hypnosis as a legitimate therapeutic tool. At present, the uses of hypnosis in clinical and investigational areas continue to grow, as does research on the neuropsychological mechanisms involved in the hypnotic process.

Definition

Hypnosis is a psychophysiological state of attentive, receptive concentration, with a relative suspension of peripheral awareness. Hypnotic phenomena occur spontaneously, and the alteration of consciousness that hypnotized individuals experience has a variety of therapeutic applications. The hypnotic experience may be understood as involving three main factors (Table 72.1).

Hypnosis: What It is and What It is Not

Several principles provide guidance for the use of hypnosis in medicine and psychiatry. We attempt to clarify some of the myths and misconceptions about hypnosis by establishing what hypnosis is and what it is not (Table 72.2).

Hypnotizability is a Stable and Measurable Trait

Not everyone is hypnotizable. Hypnotizability, or hypnotic capacity varies throughout the population. About 75% of the

Table 72.1 Components of the Hypnotic Process

Component	Explanation
Absorption	Refers to the tendency to engage in self-altering and highly focused attention with complete immersion in a central experience at the expense of contextual orientation and more peripheral perceptions, thoughts, memories, or motor activities.
Dissociation	Permits keeping out of conscious awareness many routine experiences that ordinarily would be conscious. Dissociated material may be temporarily and reversibly unavailable to consciousness, but it continues to influence conscious and unconscious experiences and behavior.
Suggestibility	Involves heightened responsiveness to social cues. It allows subjects to suspend the usual conscious curiosity that makes us question the reason for our actions, making subjects more prone to accept suggestions given no matter how irrational.

Table 72.2 What Is Hypnosis?

What It is
Hypnosis is a form of focused concentration.
Hypnotizability is a stable and measurable trait.
Hypnosis is something you do with, rather than to, a subject or patient.
All hypnosis is self-hypnosis.

What It is Not
Hypnosis is not sleep.
There are no apparent sex differences in hypnotizability.
Hypnotizability is not a sign of weak-mindedness.
Hypnosis is not intrinsically dangerous.
Hypnosis is not therapy.
There is nothing you can do with hypnosis that you cannot do without it.

population has some usable hypnotic capacity; of these, about 10% are highly hypnotizable. This means that about one of four adults has no usable hypnotic capacity (Spiegel and Spiegel, 1978). It is advantageous to determine this early and encourage those with the ability to use it; other treatment modalities are offered to those who are not hypnotizable.

Hypnosis is Something You Do *with*, Not Something You Do *to*, a Subject or Patient

A therapist inducing hypnosis is in the position of the Socratic teacher, helping students discover what they already know. A useful metaphor to share with subjects is that of a coach. A correctly performed hypnotic induction allows the patient and physician to assess and explore the patient's hypnotic capacity or lack of it, just as a trainer assesses the athlete's natural capacities and then attempts to maximize them. This approach tends to minimize power struggles between the physician and the patient. For example, there is less chance of misinterpreting a patient's inability to experience a hypnotic trance as resistance.

All Hypnosis is Self-hypnosis

The therapist helps the patient use his or her own hypnotic capacity to undergo a trance state. Helping patients to understand the degree of control they have over their mental processes is a good way to foster mastery and control. By doing this, patients may be able to comprehend the extent to which the unconscious use of their hypnotic abilities may create or contribute to their psychiatric symptoms, as in the case of dissociative disorders (Bliss, 1980, 1984; Spiegel, 1974; Spiegel and Fink, 1979). Similarly, hypnosis may help patients understand how certain physical symptoms may have unconscious etiological factors, as in the case of conversion phenomena (i.e., psychogenic blindness, pseudoseizures) or psychosomatic conditions (i.e., asthma, headache) (Maldonado and Spiegel, 2000).

There are no Apparent Sex Differences in Hypnotizability

Men and women are equally hypnotizable (Hilgard, 1965; Stern *et al.*, 1979).

Hypnosis is Not Sleep

The hypnotized individual is not asleep but rather awake and alert. To an outside observer, hypnotized individuals may appear asleep owing to their apparent lack of responsiveness to the environment. This is due to their intense absorption and concentration on their internal experience, rather than due to their lack of will.

Hypnotizability is Not a Sign of Weak-mindedness

We know that a hypnotic trance requires an intact capacity for focused concentration. If anything, high hypnotizability is associated with the absence of serious psychotic and neurological disorders (Lavoie and Sabourin, 1980; Pettinati, 1982; Spiegel *et al.*, 1982).

Hypnosis is Not Intrinsically Dangerous

For the most part, it is a benign process. The same cognitive flexibility that allows patients to enter the trance facilitates their exit from it with clear structure and support from the therapist. The dangers of hypnosis lay not in the process itself but

in how it is used. There are few contraindications for the use of hypnosis. A schizophrenic patient may incorporate an attempt at inducing hypnosis into a delusional system. A severely depressed individual may interpret a failure to benefit from hypnosis as further evidence of little self-worth. These problems can be avoided in part by use of hypnotizability testing at the beginning of the intervention. The most serious problem involves possible effects of hypnosis on memory. This is discussed under the section "Forensic Applications of Hypnosis" later in the chapter.

Hypnosis is Not Therapy

Entry into a hypnotic state does not have any therapeutic effects of its own, although many find it pleasant and relaxing. Therapeutic change comes not from the state itself but from what happens during it. In this regard, hypnosis is not a treatment itself but rather a facilitator of a variety of treatment strategies. The state of intense concentration elicited in hypnosis can facilitate attention to a variety of strategies that enhance control over somatic function, reduce pain, allow the recovery and restructuring of memories, elicit the reproduction and control of conversion symptoms or fugue episodes, and provide control of dissociated states.

There is Nothing You can Do with Hypnosis that You cannot Do Without it

As an adjuvant to therapy, hypnosis may help speed the process by which information can be accessed and processed because of its ability to heighten concentration and focus attention; however, it is not a treatment in and of itself.

Hypnotizability Scales

Hypnotizability scales have been developed for clinical use (Hypnotic Induction Profile [Spiegel and Spiegel, 1978]; Stanford Hypnotic Clinical Scale [Hilgard and Hilgard, 1975]). These scales are designed for comfortable use even with patients who have severe psychiatric disturbances (Spiegel and Spiegel, 1978; Spiegel *et al.*, 1982, 1988). They are well accepted by patients and help to bypass anxiety by shifting the focus of the interaction from one in which the therapist tries to make the patient have a hypnotic experience to one in which the therapist assesses the patient's response to a set of instructions, like any other medical or psychological test (Spiegel and Spiegel, 1978). The therapist focuses on evaluating the patient's ability to enter the state rather than on getting the person into the state. They all involve a structured hypnotic induction and an assessment of the subject's response to a variety of instructions, such as alterations in the sense of control over body movements, physical sensations, orientation to time and space, and perception. Furthermore, such a standardized testing induction permits an important deduction regarding the hypnotic capacity of the subject. The restricted range of input from the therapist maximizes the information provided by variations in subjects' responses. After the results of the testing are discussed with the subject, both can proceed knowledgeably, choosing to use hypnosis or other techniques in the service of an agreed on treatment goal.

The use of this kind of objective measurement has several clinical advantages and therapeutic implications (Table 72.3).

Hypnosis Induction Profile

The Hypnotic Induction Profile (Figure 72.1) is a useful clinical screening test for hypnotic capacity. It consists of a number

Table 72.3 Benefits of the Use of Hypnotizability Measures

It objectively assesses the patient's natural ability to use his or her hypnotic capacity.
It relieves performance pressure on both therapist and patient.
It provides objective data about the patient's ability to respond to treatment employing hypnosis.
It provides the therapist with scientific data to make rational treatment choices.
It provides helpful information about the subject's interpersonal style and possible psychiatric illness.
It helps predict the patient's likely response to psychotherapeutic treatment.

of the simple instructions that allow the measurement of patients' natural ability to tap into and use their hypnotic capacity. It begins with a simple and quick induction, counting from 1 to 3, accompanied by the eye roll. This involves instructed upward gaze and lowering of the eyelids (Figure 72.2). The dissociation between upward gaze and lowering of the eyelid can be scored (Figure 72.3), providing the therapist with an initial prediction of the subject's hypnotic capacity. The eye roll is then followed by a series of instructions briefly to influence the subject's behavior during and shortly after the test (posthypnotic suggestions). The Hypnotic Induction Profile allows the therapist to rate the subject on five items (Table 72.4) assessing cognitive and behavioral aspects of the single continuous but brief hypnotic experience elicited during the test. These

Hypnotic Induction Profile score sheet

Name ______ Date ______

Sequence ☐ Initial ______ Previous ______ When ______

Position of subject ☐ Standing ______ Supine ______ Chair ______ Chair-stool ______

Item			
A	*Up-gaze*		*0 – 1 – 2 – 3 – 4*
B		Roll:	0 – 1 – 2 – 3 – 4
C		Squint:	0 – 1 – 2 – 3 – 4
D	Eye-roll sign (roll and squint)		0 – 1 – 2 – 3 – 4
E	*Arm (R-L) levitation instruction*		*0 – 1 – 2 – 3 – 4*
F	*Tingle*		*0 – – 1 – 2*
G ______	Dissociation		0 – – 1 – 2
H ______	Levitation (postinduction)	No reinforcement / 1st " / 2nd " / 3rd " / 4th "	3 – 4 / 2 – 3 / 1 – 2 / 1 – / 0 – ; Smile ______ ; Surprise ______
I ______	Control differential		0 – – 1 – 2
J ______	Cut-off		0 – – 1 – 2
K ______	*Amnesia to cut-off or no-test ______*		*0 – – 1 – 2*
L ______	Floating sensation		0 – – 1 – 2

Summary scores

______ Induction score   Profile score 0 – 1 – 2 – 3 – 4 – 5

______ Soft   ______ Zero   ______ Intact

______ Minutes   ______ Decrement   ______ Special zero   ______ Special intact

Figure 72.1 *Hypnotic Induction Profile score sheet. Reprinted with permission from Trance and Treatment: Clinical Use of Hypnosis. Spiegel H and Speigel D (1978) Basic Books, New York, p. 40. Copyright 1987, American Psychiatric Press.*

Eye-roll sign for hypnotizability

Roll	Score

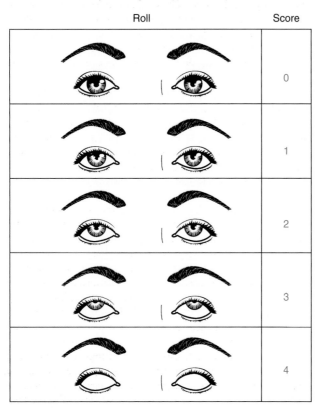

Figure 72.2 *Eye-roll sign for hypnotizability. Reprinted with permission from Trance and Treatment: Clinical Use of Hypnosis. Spiegel H and Speigel D (1978) Basic Books, New York, p. 52. Copyright 1987, American Psychiatric Press.*

are: 1) ability to experience a sense of dissociation of the left hand from the rest of the body; 2) hand levitation, or floating of the hand back up in the air after being pulled down; 3) sense of involuntariness or unconscious compliance while elevating the hand; 4) response to the cutoff signal ending the hypnotic experience; and 5) sensory alteration in the hand or elsewhere in the body.

Scores on the Hypnotic Induction Profile are significantly but moderately correlated with those on the Stanford scales (Orne *et al.*, 1979) and provide useful discrimination among different psychiatric disorders, as described in the following section.

Eye-roll measurement

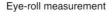
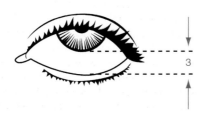

Figure 72.3 *Eye-roll measurement. Reprinted with permission from Trance and Treatment: Clinical Use of Hypnosis. Spiegel H and Speigel D (1978) Basic Books, New York, p. 53. Copyright 1987, American Psychiatric Press.*

Table 72.4	Items Tested by the Hypnotic Induction Profile

Body dissociation
Hand levitation
Level of unconscious compliance
Response to posthypnotic suggestion
Sensory alteration

Hypnotizability in Psychiatric Disorders

Charcot described a relationship between conversion phenomena and hypnotizability. He later incorrectly attributed both phenomena to a pathological process afflicting the central nervous system. Charcot believed that only sick or hysterical people could be hypnotized. Others, including Bernheim, Janet and Breuer, refuted the idea. They attributed the symptoms of conversion to unconscious mechanisms and viewing hypnosis as a tool useful in both the elicitation and removal of such states. Research in hypnosis has lately been directed at understanding the relationship between hypnotizability and psychiatric illness.

Some psychiatric disorders are associated with high hypnotizability scores (Table 72.5).

Several psychiatric syndromes (schizophrenia, generalized anxiety disorder, and to a lesser extent major affective disorder) (DSM-IV-TR) have been associated with generally lower hypnotic responsiveness. It may be that the primary illness process impairs the use of a patient's natural capacity for hypnotic concentration. Because of this, hypnotizability testing can sometimes be used to clarify diagnoses. As always, the presence or absence of hypnotic capacity should be interpreted within the context of the presentation, medical and psychiatric histories, and genetic background. In the case of an acute psychosis in which there is no familial background, the presentation is later in life than normal, there is a past history of physical or sexual abuse, and the patient has a high hypnotizability score, a diagnosis of hysterical psychosis or a dissociative disorder should be strongly considered when the possibility of schizophrenia is evaluated (Spiegel and Fink, 1979; Steingard and Frankel, 1985).

Table 72.5	Psychiatric Disorders Associated with High Hypnotizability

Victims of overwhelming trauma
   Adjustment disorders
   Acute stress disorder
   PTSD
Dissociative disorders
   Fugue states
   Dissociative amnesia
   Dissociative identity disorder
Anxiety disorders
   Phobias
   Performance anxiety
Bulimia nervosa
Borderline personality disorder
Conversion disorder

Table 72.6   Applications of Hypnosis

General Psychiatry

Anxiety disorders
   Phobias
   PTSD
Dissociative disorders
   Dissociative amnesia
   Dissociative identity disorder
Sleep disorders
   Insomnia

General Medicine

Anxiety associated with medical and surgical procedures
Pain control
Psychosomatic disorders
   Bronchial asthma
   Warts and other skin conditions
   Gastrointestinal disturbances (irritable bowel syndrome,
     peptic ulcer disease)
   Cardiovascular diseases
Adjuvant to chemotherapy
Emesis (chemotherapy, hyperemesis gravidarum)

Habit Control

Smoking cessation
Weight control

Forensic Psychiatry

Memory enhancement

Applications of Hypnosis

General Considerations

Because of the intrinsic qualities of the hypnotic state, it can be an effective adjunct to the treatment of a variety of symptoms and problems, both in psychiatry and in medicine in general. The first criterion to consider is the patient's level of hypnotizability. Once it has been determined that the patient has usable hypnotic capacity (defined by high scores in hypnotizability scales), a discussion about the nature of the hypnotic process follows. It is important at this point to dispel any myths and correct misconceptions the patient may have about the process. This includes the cooperative nature of the hypnotic process, rather than the "tell me what to do" most patients expect. Finally, the therapist must decide whether the problem presented by the patient is amenable to hypnotic intervention or whether other steps should be taken instead.

We have divided the discussion of the applications of hypnosis into five areas: general psychiatry, general medicine, psychosomatic disorders, habit control and forensic psychiatry (Table 72.6).

Application in Psychiatric Disorders

The use of hypnosis in the context of conventional psychotherapy can facilitate the therapeutic process in a number of ways. For example, hypnotherapeutic techniques may be used to enhance the patient's sense of self, restructure traumatic and phobic experiences, or access to repressed memories that have not emerged with use of other techniques. This is true not only of painfully repressed memories but also of situations in which both the patient and the therapist have worked on resistance issues and feel that some additional leverage is necessary. In conventional psychotherapy, the transference is observed and analyzed; in hypnosis, the transference is used as part of the therapeutic process.

Conventional psychoanalytic psychotherapy involves observation and analysis of the meaning of the transference reaction that arises during therapeutic interactions. On the other hand, when hypnosis is used, transference is not avoided or bypassed but may be amplified. All the usual therapeutic rules and processes of psychotherapy apply when hypnosis is used in the psychotherapy context, which may intensify or accelerate the therapeutic process.

Because of the intense emotions that are characteristic of the hypnotic retrieval (which facilitates expression of inner fantasies), intense feelings and deep personal experiences may be elicited. Some patients may find that the hypnotic state facilitates a sense of infantile dependency in which the therapist becomes the transferential object. The quality of this transference reaction will be based on the patient's early object relations, just as in any other therapeutic relationship. Indeed, the transference reaction may develop so fast that the inexperienced therapist may not have the opportunity to recognize it or may do so too late. The difference here is the intensity of the feelings developed as a result of the strong emotions that arise during trance. As in the case of victims of abuse, the therapist may use the transference relationship under hypnosis to foster the patient's ability to help herself or himself.

The difficult aspect of doing hypnosis is not the induction of the hypnosis trance, but what happens once the patient is under trance. Remember that all hypnosis is self-hypnosis. Thus, there are two factors which will predict the success of the hypnosis intervention: the patients' hypnotizability and the therapeutic skills of the therapist.

Anxiety Disorders

Anxiety disorders are among the most widely prevalent psychiatric disturbances. They afflict as much as 15% of the population (Myers *et al.*, 1984). Anxiety can be seen as a state of hyperarousal experienced by both emotional and somatic discomfort. Patients describe their experience in physical terms, such as palpitations, gastrointestinal discomfort, chest pain, sweating and motor restlessness. Among anxiety disorders most responsive to hypnotic intervention are generalized anxiety disorder, panic disorder, phobias and post traumatic anxiety disorders (these will be discussed in the section that follows).

Most of the strategies in the treatment of anxiety disorders employing hypnosis combine instructed physical relaxation with a restructuring of cognition, using imagery coupled with physical relaxation. As in the treatment of anxiety disorders by systematic desensitization (Marks *et al.*, 1968) or progressive relaxation, patients are instructed to maintain a physical sense of relaxation (e.g., floating) while picturing the feared situation or stimulus. It is important that the relaxation instruction use an image that connotes reduced somatic tension, such as floating or lightness, rather than being a direct instruction to relax. The more cognitive term "relax" may actually induce more anxiety, whereas affiliation with a somatic metaphor usually produces some reduction in tension. Unlike systematic desensitization, hypnosis produces a physically relaxed state that can be rapidly achieved with a quick induction. Also different from systematic desensitization, the coupling of relaxation to a fearful stimulus does not require the development or working through of a hierarchy.

A typical self-hypnosis induction can be rapid. For example, a patient can be told:

> Now just get as comfortable as you can. There are many ways to enter a state of self-hypnosis. One simple but useful method is to count to yourself from 1 to 3. On 1, do one thing: look up. On 2, do two things: slowly close your eyes and take a deep breath. On 3, do three things: let your eyes relax but keep them closed, let your breath out, and let your body float. Then let one hand or the other float up into the air like a buoyant balloon. This is your signal to yourself and to me that you are ready to concentrate.

Initially, the use of hypnosis in the session can help in demonstrating to patients that they have a greater degree of control over somatic responsiveness than they had imagined. It is often useful to begin by teaching patients to create a place in their mind's eye where they feel safe and secure. On occasion, it helps the subjects to learn how to project their image onto an imaginary screen. Later, they can learn to manipulate the screen by making it either bigger or smaller, having the screen nearer or farther away, as needed:

> Just allow your body to float, as if you were floating in a bath, a lake, or a hot tub. Enjoy this sense of floating lightness. Now, picture in your mind's eye an imaginary screen. It might be a movie screen, a television screen, or a piece of clear blue sky. First picture a pleasant scene, somewhere you enjoy being.

Allow the patient to experience this state for a minute or two, then inquire about the experience:

> With your eyes closed and remaining in this state of concentration, describe how your body is feeling right now. What image are you picturing?

After receiving the answers, add:

> Notice how you can use your store of memories and fantasies to help yourself and your body feel better.

After they have learned to manipulate the screen and their physical sensations, patients may be ready to do therapy work. They may, for example, learn to re-create the physical state of relaxation while projecting the fearful situation onto the screen. This, then, becomes a useful procedure by which to control and obtain mastery over anxiety-producing situations by dissociating the somatic reaction from the psychological response to the feared stimulus. Initially, the patient is asked to re-create the physical feeling of relaxation. Then, the patient projects onto the screen images associated with the feared situation, only this time the somatic reactions associated with anxiety do not develop. On occasion, it helps for patients to foresee likely physical sensations or situations associated with a fearful experience to master them. For example, in the case of plane phobia, the patient can learn to couple the real sensation of floating in the air with the hypnotic experience: "Learn to float with the plane".

Patients may also use the trance state as a means of facing their concerns more directly. As in the preceding cases, they may make use of the screen technique. They can achieve this by placing an image of an upcoming performance or fearful situation on one side of the screen, testing out various strategies for mastering the situation on the other side.

Other approaches using hypnosis have included instructing patients in a trance to imagine that they are literally somewhere else, away from the fearful stimulus, thus separating themselves from the anxiety-producing experience (Erickson and Haley, 1967). Positive reinforcement or "ego-strengthening" techniques have also been used; for example, hypnotic instructions are given to patients suggesting that their capacity to master the situation and their response to it will improve (Crasilneck and Hall, 1985). There is little reason to use uncovering techniques seeking to link anxiety to some early traumatic experience in cases of phobia or generalized anxiety disorders. This is different in cases of PTSD (DSM-IV-TR), however, in which more work may be needed to confront and place into context the traumatic experience.

Certainly, in some cases, understanding the cause of the feared situation may help resolve the conflict. One of the techniques used to facilitate the recovery of traumatic memories associated with fearful situations is the affect bridge technique (Watkins, 1987).

Post Traumatic Stress Disorder

Trauma constitutes a sudden discontinuity in both physical and mental experiences. The effect of the traumatic experience forces the victim to reorganize mental and psychophysiological processes to buffer the immediate impact of the trauma. This process is meant to be an adaptive mechanism to maintain psychological control during a time of enormous stress. Unfortunately, a number of trauma victims go on to suffer acute or chronic symptoms, such as dissociation, intrusive thoughts, anxiety, withdrawal and hyperarousal, leading to a diagnosis of acute stress disorder or PTSD.

There may be a relationship during childhood between stress, such as early trauma, and high hypnotizability. In support of this idea are reports of high hypnotizability in children who were victims of severe punishment during childhood (Nash and Lynn, 1986; Spiegel and Cardeña, 1991). It is possible that the impact of the stress suffered encouraged them to use their self-hypnotic abilities more effectively (Kluft, 1984, 1992; Spiegel et al., 1982).

The major categories of symptoms in PTSD are similar to the components of the hypnotic process (American Psychiatric Association, 1994; Maldonado and Spiegel, 2002a). Hypnotic absorption is similar to the intrusive reliving of traumatic events experienced by these patients. When in a flashback, trauma victims become so absorbed in the memories of the traumatic event, they lose touch with their present surroundings and even forget that the events took place in the past. Likewise, highly hypnotizable individuals may become so intensely absorbed in the trance experience that they can reenact a previous life event (during hypnotic age regression) as if they were reliving it. A hypnotized patient may dissociate a body part to the extent of not recognizing it as part of his or her body. Similarly, PTSD patients may dissociate feelings to the extent of experiencing the so-called psychic numbing. This allows them to disconnect current affects from their everyday experience in an attempt to avoid emotions triggering memories associated with the trauma. Finally, suggestibility is comparable to hyperarousal. The heightened sensitivity to environmental cues observed in those patients suffering from PTSD is similar to that experienced by a hypnotized individual who responds to suggestions of coldness by shivering.

Because many patients suffering from PTSD are highly hypnotizable, and because of the resemblance between the symptoms of PTSD and the hypnotic phenomena, it makes sense to use hypnosis in its treatment. If patients suffering from PTSD are unknowingly using their own hypnotic capacities (Kluft, 1991, 1992; Maldonado and Spiegel, 2002a; Spiegel 1986, 1989; Spiegel *et al.*, 1988), it is therapeutically useful to teach them how to enter, access and control their trance potential. Hypnosis may be invaluable as a tool to access previously dissociated traumatic material.

We do not refer here to uncontrolled abreaction. The purpose is not simply to help the patient remember the trauma, because in a way, every time a patient goes through a flashback, an uncontrolled abreaction is experienced. An abreaction that is not conducted within the context of cognitive restructuring and before new defenses are in place can lead to the further retraumatization of the patient (Kluft, 1992; Spiegel, 1981). At the end of the following section (Dissociative Disorders), we summarize a comprehensive approach to the use of hypnosis in the treatment of psychiatric syndromes associated with severe trauma.

Dissociative Disorders

Hypnosis is one of the most helpful tools in the treatment of patients suffering from dissociative disorders (Maldonado and Spiegel, 2002a; Maldonado *et al.*, 2000). As a rule, these patients experience their symptoms (i.e., fugue states, dissociated identities and blackouts) as occurring unexpectedly and beyond their control. Because these patients are unknowingly using their hypnotic capacities, it makes sense to teach them how to turn their weakness into a strength (Maldonado and Spiegel, 1995). Hypnosis can be used formally both as a diagnostic tool and for therapeutic purposes. The hypnotic state can be seen as a controlled form of dissociation (Nemiah, 1985). Hypnosis is useful in the treatment of these patients, first in determining whether they have a dissociative disorder, and second in providing rapid access to these dissociated states. When used by the therapist in the context of treatment, it can demonstrate to patients the amount of control they have over this state, which they normally experience as "automatic and unpredictable". This not only serves to teach patients how to control dissociation but also allows them to establish a process of communication that will eventually lead to a reduction in spontaneous dissociative symptoms. Therapists must remember that many of these patients have suffered physical, emotional, or sexual abuse. It is imperative that we recognize and take account of the impact of whatever trauma occurred and help patients work through their reactions to it, as in the case of PTSD. Recognizing and teaching patients with dissociative disorders how to master their capacity to dissociate are among the most important psychotherapeutic tasks in the course of their treatment (Maldonado and Spiegel, 2002a; Maldonado *et al.*, 2000).

We can make use of hypnotic techniques as a way to help patients access repressed and dissociated memories. Teaching patients to use self-hypnosis allows them to obtain a sense of control over their symptoms and eventually their lives. The repression or dissociation of traumatic events and

the realities that surround them may serve a defensive purpose of avoiding painful affect associated with the memories. The memories are there, either transformed or interspersed with fantasy. Our approach to the treatment of these victims is directed at helping them acknowledge the extent of the emotional pain caused by the trauma. Then, through therapy, we can assist in the development of mature and adequate coping mechanisms that will allow the patient to place the experience into proper perspective. The goal is to allow the patient to come to terms with the trauma and to redefine herself or himself in view of the past, but with a firm hold on the realities of the present.

Dissociation as a defense serves a dual purpose. It represents an effort to preserve some form of control, safety and identity when faced with overwhelming stress. At the same time, victims use it in an attempt to separate themselves from the full impact of the trauma. Unfortunately, these individuals may ward off memories of the trauma so well that they may act as if it is not happening and later as if it never happened. Some individuals can so effectively repress traumatic memories that they become unable consciously to work through them. As a consequence, they are unable to put the facts surrounding the events associated with the trauma into perspective, but slowly, the dissociated feelings and memories leak into consciousness. This creates some of the classic symptoms associated with PTSD and DID, such as flashbacks or intrusive thoughts.

The advantage of using hypnosis comes from the facilitation of the recovery of affect or memories, the ability to dissociate memories from cognition, and the speed with which the process is achieved. Finally, because of the relationship between a history of childhood abuse and trance, these patients are usually highly hypnotizable (Chu and Dill, 1990; Hilgard, 1984; Nash and Lynn, 1986; Putman, 1993; Spiegel, 1988, 1990; Spiegel *et al.*, 1988).

Many former victims of childhood abuse may unknowingly use their hypnotic capacities to keep out of awareness the content of traumatic memories and in effect create different degrees of psychiatric illness (Sanders and Giola, 1991; Spiegel, 1984, 1986, 1989; Spiegel *et al.*, 1988; Terr, 1991). Teaching these patients self-hypnosis is a way of turning a weakness into a strong tool for self-mastery and control. The controlled use of hypnosis, then, becomes a way systematically to access previously dissociated material.

The Condensed Hypnotic Approach

The use of hypnosis in the treatment of PTSD and dissociative disorders can be conceptualized as having two major goals, which can be achieved by the use of six different techniques (Maldonado and Spiegel, 1994, 1995, 2002b; Spiegel, 1992) (Table 72.7). The goals are to bring into **consciousness** previously repressed memories and to develop a sense of **congruence** between memories associated with the traumatic experience and current self-images. By making conscious previously repressed memories, the patient has the opportunity to understand, accept and restructure them. These goals are achieved by working through six treatment stages: confrontation, condensation, confession, consolation, concentration and control.

First the patient must **confront** the trauma. The therapist helps the patient recognize and understand the factors involved in the development of the symptoms for which help is now being

Table 72.7   Condensed Hypnotic Approach
Goals
To bring into consciousness previously repressed memories
To develop a sense of congruence between the traumatic memories and the self
Treatment Stages
Confrontation
Condensation
Confession
Consolation
Concentration
Control

Table 72.8   Therapeutic Precautions
Traumatic transference
Confabulation
Concreting
Contamination of memories
False memories
Possible compromise of patient's ability to testify in court
Electronic recording of all contacts with patient

sought. Hypnosis is then used to help the patient **condense** the traumatic memories. The hypnotic experience can be used to define a particularly frightening memory during the revision of the patient's history, which summarizes or condenses the main conflicts. The focused concentration achieved during the hypnotic state not only can facilitates recall of traumatic material but also helps place boundaries around it. After memories are recovered, we can help patients restructure them and even "become aware of things you did at the moment of trauma to survive". Once memories are recovered, patients usually need to **confess** feelings and experiences of which they are profoundly ashamed. These are usually things that they may have told no one else before; in fact, they have been running from them all their lives. At this time, the therapist must convey a sense of "being present" for the patient while remaining as neutral as possible. This is followed by the stage of **consolation**. Here, the therapist needs to be emotionally available to the patient. This stage must be carried on with caution and in a most professional manner. Therapists should be aware that the body and emotional boundaries of these patients may have been violated in the past. Then comes the stage of **concentration**. This component of the trance experience allows patients to have access or "turn on" the traumatic memories during the psychotherapeutic session and then "shut them off" once the work has been done. During the final stage, the patient comes to define herself or himself as being in **control** again.

The underlying principle to remember is that the most damaging effect of overwhelming trauma is that it renders its victims defenseless. Because of the lack of physical and emotional control, patients activate dissociative defenses in an attempt to master their experiences. By using self-hypnosis, the therapist can model and teach the patient to regain control over her or his memories. Patients must be encouraged to remember as much as they feel is safe to remember at a given time. The goal is that patients learn how to think about traumatic experiences, rather than negating their existence. The use of self-hypnosis teaches patients that they are in control of their experiences. Patients must dispel the magical beliefs that therapists "can take away the memories". Rather, by modeling this sense of trust in their therapists, patients learn to trust themselves. They relearn trust in their own feelings and perceptions.

The challenge in treating victims of abuse is to achieve a new sense of unity within the patient after the initial fragmentation caused by the traumatic experience. Overwhelming trauma tends to cause sudden and radical discontinuities in consciousness, which leaves the victims with a polarized view of themselves involving, on one hand the old self (before the trauma) and, on the other, the helpless, defenseless and traumatized victim. Our goal is to find ways to integrate these two aspects of the self. Here, the patient's task is to acknowledge and place into perspective painful life events, thereby making them acceptable to conscious awareness.

One of the advantages of the use of hypnosis is that the affect elicited can be so powerful that most patients do not need to remember every single event of abuse or trauma. In fact, through the use of hypnosis, the therapist may help the patient consolidate the memories in a constructive way, thus facilitating recovery. After a condensation of the traumatic experiences, patients become ready to accept the victimized self. Instead of continuing the self-blame and shame because of what happened to them, they can learn to acknowledge and even thank themselves for what they did to survive. This restructuring allows them to shift their perception of self, changing their self-image from that of a victim to that of a survivor.

Therapeutic Precautions Therapeutic precautions are shown in Table 72.8. The strength of transference during the psychotherapy of trauma victims is enormous. The use of hypnosis does not prevent development of a transference reaction; it may actually facilitate its emergence earlier than in regular therapy owing to the intensity with which the material is expressed and memories are recovered (Maldonado and Spiegel, 1994, 1995, 2002b).

Reliving the traumatic experience along with the patient may allow a special feeling of "being there with them" at the moment of trauma. This allows the therapist to provide guidance, support, protection and comfort as the patient goes through the difficult path of reprocessing traumatic memories. On the other hand, this kind of **traumatic transference** between the therapist and the victim of sexual assault is different in the sense that the feelings transferred are related not so much to early object relationships but to the abuser or circumstances that are associated with the trauma (Spiegel, 1992). Instead of seeing this expressed anger at the therapist as a form of negative transference reaction, we should explore the possibility that this may be a healthy attempt for the patient to experience anger toward the perpetrator. As therapists, we should not minimize or shut off these feelings. This will only confirm the patient's former perception that there was something wrong with him or her for having these feelings, which will probably activate further use of primitive defenses, including dissociation or acting out.

A more serious complication of the use of hypnosis with trauma victims is the possible creation of **false memories**. Hypnosis, with its heightened sense of concentration, allows the patient to focus intensely on a given time or place, enhancing memory recall. The principle of state-dependent memory also makes it plausible that the mere entrance into this trance state can facilitate retrieval of memories associated with a similar state of mind that may have occurred during the trauma and subsequent flashbacks. However, not every memory recovered with the use of hypnosis is necessarily true. Hypnosis can facilitate improved recall of true as well as confabulated material (Dywan and Bowers, 1983). Suggestibility is increased in hypnosis, and information can be implanted or imagined and reported as verdict (Laurence and Perry, 1983; McConkey, 1992). Because of this, therapists are warned about "believing" everything a patient is able to recall. Just as we use therapeutic judgment to analyze and interpret our patients' (nontraumatic) childhood memories, fantasies and dreams, so should we treat hypnotically recovered material with caution.

To this date, no evidence proves that the patient's confrontation with alleged perpetrators of childhood abuse or pursuit of legal retribution toward the perpetrator provides any therapeutic benefit. As therapists, we cannot be certain of which memories are real, which are completely confabulated, and which are a combination of both. Because of this, we should not encourage our patients to take legal actions. If, on the other hand, our patients insist in pursuing this avenue, it is our duty to warn them of our concerns but to be supportive of whatever final decision they make. Certainly we will do a service to our patients if we inform them of all the legal ramifications that the use of hypnosis, or any other form of memory enhancement, may have for their defense, including their ability to testify in court or to use the material recovered by such techniques.

Applications in General Medicine

Medical Procedures

Because hypnosis can be used to produce a state of relaxation and to reduce anxiety, it has proved to be valuable as an adjuvant to medical procedures. Once patients have been trained in the use of self-hypnosis, they can use it both in preparation for a hospital visit and while in the clinic or hospital. Once in that state, they can imagine themselves being somewhere they enjoy and feel safe, thereby dissociating their mental experience from the physical (and possibly painful or unpleasant) aspects of the procedure. It can also be used as a way of mastering the anxiety associated with potentially threatening procedures, such as computed tomography, bone marrow aspirations, phlebotomy, needle biopsy, lumbar punctures, or therapeutic interventions, such as chemotherapy, external beam radiation therapy and dental procedures.

Pain Control

Pain is always a psychosomatic phenomenon, combining somatic with subjective distress. It never exists in a vacuum and always represents a combination of tissue injury and the emotional reaction to it.

Despite the organic factors causing pain, it is clear that psychological factors are major variables in the intensity of the pain experience. Beecher (1956) demonstrated that the intensity of pain was directly associated with its meaning. For example, to the extent that pain represented threat and the possibility of future disability, it was more intense than it was among a group of combat soldiers to whom the pain of injury meant that they were likely to get out of combat alive.

Hypnosis can facilitate an alteration in the subjective experience of pain (Brose and Spiegel, 1992). Several techniques can be used to achieve this goal. Most techniques involve the production of physical relaxation coupled with visual or somatic imagery that provides a substitute focus of attention for the painful sensation.

Even though the precise mechanism for hypnotic analgesia is not known, it is suspected to have components of two complementary mechanisms: physical relaxation and attention control. Patients in pain tend to splint the painful area instinctively, which in turn increases muscle tension around the painful area, often resulting in increased pain. Therefore, creating a state of hypnotically induced relaxation may easily decrease their experience or perception of pain.

Studies have also shown the superiority of hypnotic analgesia to the level of analgesia provided by either placebo (McGlashan *et al.*, 1969) or acupuncture (Knox and Shum, 1977). Katz and colleagues (1974) have shown a correlation between hypnotizability and responsiveness to acupuncture, proving that hypnotic mechanisms of pain control may be mobilized by other treatment techniques. Nevertheless, the explicit use of hypnosis with hypnotizable patients has proved to be the most powerful means of controlling pain. Hilgard and Hilgard (1975) estimated a 0.5 correlation between hypnotizability and treatment responsiveness for pain control.

Psychosomatic Disorders

Hypnosis is useful in both the diagnosis and the treatment of psychosomatic illness. By using hypnosis with these patients, the therapist may assist in diagnosing the symptoms as psychosomatic. Under hypnosis, many of the symptoms may improve or be completely reversed. It is important not to "force a cure" in any patient, but rather to allow patients to improve at a pace that feels comfortable, or to give up the symptom when ready. This allows patients not only to feel in control of the treatment and recovery process but also slowly to get back their sense of control over their body. Some patients obtain insight into what is happening to their bodies owing to the ability to explore the meaning and cause of the symptoms hypnotically.

In most instances, it is better if hypnosis is used as an adjuvant to any other medical treatment, including physical rehabilitation or any other treatment modality typically used in the treatment of the "real illness". Most such problems involve a combination of somatic and psychological symptoms. Using a rehabilitation model avoids the trap of humiliating the patient who improves with the inference that the problem was "all in the mind".

Hypnosis can be invaluable in the treatment of a number of psychosomatic conditions. In particular, disorders affecting the gastrointestinal system are among those conditions in which studies demonstrated a dramatic response. In cases of ulcerative colitis and regional enteritis, peptic ulcer disease and side effects of chemotherapy, hypnosis can produce a sense of control over a symptom that causes the patient to feel especially helpless, thereby diminishing the cycle of reactive anxiety.

Applications of Hypnosis in Habit Control

Smoking Cessation

A number of studies demonstrate the efficacy of hypnosis as a tool to facilitate control of smoking, with success rates in cigarette abstinence after treatment with hypnosis ranging from 13 to 64%.

There are several mechanisms by which hypnosis may contribute to success in smoking cessation. The ritualistic process of the hypnotic exercise may provide a kind of substitute physical relaxation for the "breathing exercise" that accompanies the act of smoking; the positive affirmations in self-hypnosis provide positive reinforcement for behavior change and promote positive self-image; its use enhances self-observation and self-monitoring; and finally it can facilitate cognitive restructuring of the smoking habit.

The single-session method developed by Spiegel (1970) emphasizes teaching patients self-hypnosis rather than having multiple sessions with a therapist. It uses a strategy that is intrinsically self-reinforcing and meaningful to the patient. It can be practiced whenever the urge to smoke comes on the patient. This method of cognitive restructuring involves emphasizing that the act of smoking is destructive specifically to the patient's body and thereby limits what the patient can do with his or her life by shortening the life span and deteriorating the quality of life. Hypnosis is used to emphasize the patient's commitment to protect the body from the poison in cigarettes. This approach gives the patient the ability to examine priorities and to balance the urge to smoke against the urge to protect his or her body from damage. Smokers are instructed to focus on what they are **for** – protecting their bodies – rather than what they are **against** – smoking. This reduces the amount of attention they pay to smoking or its absence and provides immediate internal reinforcement for attending to care of the body (Spiegel and Spiegel, 1978).

There is no evidence that treatments employing hypnosis are more effective than other interventions for smoking. Nevertheless, they may be more efficient because they enable patients to employ a self-administered treatment strategy (self-hypnosis) to reinforce a more adaptive cognitive restructuring while providing patients with an exercise in physical relaxation.

Weight Control

Seldom will the use of hypnosis alone be sufficient for the treatment of weight problems. It is usually employed as an adjunct to a comprehensive dietary and exercise control program for weight reduction and management. Similar to the use of self-hypnosis in the control of smoking, the purpose in dietary control is to restructure the patient's experience with overeating. Patients are asked to examine their excess food intake and to pay attention to the damaging effects to their body. This then translates into an exercise about learning to eat with respect for one's body. Once again, the emphasis is on what the patient is **for**, rather than being **against** food.

Unfortunately, long-term outcome studies on the usefulness of hypnosis for weight control are lacking. Clinical experience

suggests that those within 20% of their ideal body weight may obtain some benefit from such restructuring techniques with self-hypnosis, combined with a regimen of a balanced diet and exercise.

Applications in Forensic Psychiatry

The most serious problem involves possible effects of hypnosis on memory. There is evidence that hypnosis can distort memory in two ways: through **confabulation**, the creation of pseudomemories that are reported as real, or through **concreting**, an unwarranted increase in the confidence with which hypnotized individuals report their memories, either true or false (McConkey, 1992; Orne *et al.*, 1985; Spiegel and Spiegel, 1986; Spiegel and Vermutten, 1994). Hypnosis can facilitate the recall of dissociated memories, especially when recall is hampered by the strong affect associated with trauma (Kardiner and Spiegel, 1947; Spiegel, 1984, 1992). However, the research literature indicates that the most clearly reproducible problem is the production of confident errors, exaggerating the true value of memories unearthed in hypnosis.

This is especially a problem when the memories involve witnessing a crime and civil or criminal action in court is a possibility. Most states prohibit the use of hypnotically induced testimony, but some prescribe witnesses who have been hypnotized regarding the content of their potential testimony (Spiegel and Scheflin, 1994). If the possibility exists that a patient may be required to testify, it is wise to discuss the use of hypnosis with the patient and (with the patient's permission) the patient's attorney or the district attorney and obtain written agreement regarding its use. If the patient is likely to be called to testify, the therapist should obtain electronic recording of all contact with the patient (preferably on videotape) so the court can examine for possible suggestive influences. Full guidelines for use of hypnosis in the forensic setting include careful debriefing of the subject before hypnosis is employed, the use of nonleading questions, complete videotaping of all contact with the patient, and careful debriefing afterward (Spiegel and Spiegel, 1986).

The controversies surrounding so-called false memory syndrome have reignited questions regarding the validity of the material recovered by the use of hypnosis. One of the most common applications of hypnosis in the court and legal settings had been refreshing recollection of witnesses and victims of crimes. Even though the current controversy focuses on the dangers of hypnotically induced confabulation or excessive confidence in memories (Diamond, 1980), there have been some positive results. A well-known example is the case involving the driver of a hijacked school bus in Chowchilla, California (*People v. Schoenfeld*, 1980). Under hypnosis, the bus driver was able to recall the license plate number of the car driven by the kidnappers. This information, not consciously available to him before hypnotic intervention, led to the arrest and conviction of the criminals.

Because hypnosis involves a suspension of critical judgment, and therefore a state of heightened suggestibility or responsivity to social cues, it is important that the interview be conducted with a minimum of inserted information. To minimize the risk of contaminating subjects' memories, it is important to use open-ended questions, such as, "What happens next?" rather than, "How did he sexually abuse you?"

Information retrieved with the aide of hypnosis may simply be the result of an additional recall trial (Erdelyi and

Kleinbard, 1978), it may be new and true (Dywan and Bowers, 1983), or it may be a confabulation (Laurence and Perry, 1983). It may indeed be a combination of all three (Orne *et al.*, 1985). As a result, courts have long been unwilling to admit the testimony of a person hypnotized while testifying and have also begun to exclude testimony of witnesses who have previously been hypnotized about the event in question. Even when a subject is acting in good faith, hypnosis can amplify both truth and falsehood. A good guideline is that hypnosis increases the recovery of memories, both true and confabulated.

On the other hand, people do dissociate during trauma, often failing to recall events despite being conscious at the time (Cardeña and Spiegel, 1993; Spiegel and Cardeña, 1991). There is evidence that such memory gaps may persist for years or even decades after such traumatic events as physical or sexual abuse (Williams, 1994).

Therapists treating victims of sexual abuse must be aware that the use of hypnosis may compromise the ability of a witness to testify in court. After much legal battling, some courts now allow witnesses to testify after the use of hypnosis provided that certain guidelines are followed (California Legislature, 1985). These relate primarily to the training and independence of the professional doing the hypnotic interrogation and the electronic recording of the entire process (Spiegel and Spiegel, 1986).

To address this controversial issue, the Council on Scientific Affairs of the American Medical Association convened a panel of experts to examine the research evidence relevant to this problem. The report issued by the panel concluded that the existing evidence indicates that the use of hypnosis tends to increase the productivity of witnesses, resulting in new memories, some of which are true and some of which are incorrect (Orne *et al.*, 1985). The panel recommended that careful guidelines similar to the ones adopted by the state of California be followed when hypnosis is used in the forensic setting (Table 72.9).

As a rule, it is advisable to caution attorneys and witnesses that the use of hypnosis might open the possibility of challenge to the credibility or even the admissibility of a witness. The kind of situation in which hypnosis is most likely to be worth the risk is one in which there is a traumatic amnesia for the events of a crime or in which all other avenues of exploration have been exhausted. Hypnosis is by no means a truth serum, and the courts must weigh the effects of any hypnotic procedure on a witness.

The medico–legal aspects of the use of hypnosis in psychiatric practice have been discussed at length elsewhere (Maldonado and Spiegel, 2002a, 2002b).

Treatment Outcome Studies in Hypnosis

Most outcome studies, of which there have been a number, have resulted in two main conclusions related to the therapeutic uses of hypnosis. First, there is no doubt that hypnosis is effective. Secondly, the degree of hypnotizability is predictive of treatment response (Spiegel *et al.*, 1981b). It also has been observed that hypnosis is particularly useful and yields better results when it is specifically requested by the patient (Glick, 1970; Lazarus, 1973).

Conclusion

Hypnosis is a natural state of mind. As a trait, it can be measured and mastered. Even though it occurs naturally, not everybody has the same hypnotic capacity. It involves the ability to concentrate intensely, the capacity to receive new information, and the flexibility to change behavior. The capacity to experience hypnosis constitutes a therapeutic resource in the patient that can be mobilized by formal hypnosis during the therapy session and self-hypnosis exercises afterward. Strategies such as cognitive restructuring under hypnosis can help patients alter their perspective on their symptoms by experiencing symptom resolution as an occasion to enhance their sense of mastery. Many therapeutic approaches using hypnosis involve changing the patient's perspective on the relationship between the psychological and the physical state, dissociating mental from physical stress and suffering (i.e., pain), adopting a stance of protectiveness toward the body rather than fighting destructive urges (i.e., quality of life versus smoking), or learning to see sudden discontinuities in consciousness (i.e., flashbacks and episodes of dissociation) as understandable and controllable hypnotic phenomena.

Training patients in the use of self-hypnosis can facilitate the therapeutic process. This use of hypnosis can communicate the therapist's desire to enhance the patient's mastery and independence. Thus, patients can learn to use their hypnotic capacity rather than be used by it. This newly developed ability can be understood as an exercise in self-control rather than submission to the will of the therapist. It can be used to enhance control of somatic processes, reactions to anxiety-provoking stimuli and impulsive behavior.

Table 72.9 **Hypnosis and Forensic Psychiatry**
If you consider the use of hypnosis in a trial case, certain guidelines need to be observed:
• Caution attorneys and witnesses that the use of hypnosis might open the possibility of challenge to the credibility or even the admissibility of a witness.
• Carefully document memory before hypnosis of the witness.
• Use an expert psychiatrist or psychologist as a hypnosis consultant.
• Electronically record all interaction preceding, during and after hypnosis sessions. Document and record all contact with the victim.
• Conduct the interview in a neutral tone. Guide the victim through the experience but avoid using leading or suggestive questions. Avoid introducing information during the interrogation.

References

American Psychiatric Association (1994) *Diagnostic and Statistical Manual of Mental Disorders*, 4th edn. APA, Washington DC.

Beecher HK (1956) Relationship of significance of wound to pain experienced. *JAMA* 161, 1609–1616.

Bliss EL (1980) Multiple personalities: A report of 14 cases with implications for schizophrenia and hysteria. *Arch Gen Psychiatr* 37, 1388–1397.

Bliss EL (1984) Hysteria and hypnosis. *J Nerv Ment Dis* 172, 203–206.

Brose WG and Spiegel D (1992) Neuropsychiatric aspects of pain management, in *The American Psychiatric Press Textbook of Neuropsychiatry*, 2nd edn (eds Yudofsky SC and Hales RE). American Psychiatric Press, Washington DC, pp. 245–275.

California Legislature: AB 2669 Chapter 7 (1985) Hypnosis of Witnesses, added to Chapter 7, Division 6 of the Evidence Code, Enacted January 1.

Cardeña E and Spiegel D (1993) Dissociative reactions to the Bay Area earthquake. *Am J Psychiatr* 150, 474–478.

Chu DA and Dill DL (1990) Dissociative symptoms in relation to childhood physical and sexual abuse. *Am J Psychiatr* 147, 887–892.

Crasilneck HD and Hall JA (1985) *Clinical Hypnosis: Principles and Applications*, 2nd edn. Grune & Stratton, New York.

Diamond BL (1980) Inherent problems in the use of pretrial hypnosis on a prospective witness. *Calif Law Rev* 68, 313–349.

Dywan S and Bowers KS (1983) The use of hypnosis to enhance recall. *Science* 222, 184–185.

Erdelyi MH and Kleinbard J (1978) Has Ebbinghaus decayed with time? The growth of recall (hypermnesia) over days. *J Exp Psychol Hum Learn Mem* 4, 275–289.

Erickson MH and Haley J (eds) (1967) *Advanced Techniques of Hypnosis and Therapy. Selected Papers of Milton H. Erickson*, M.D. Grune & Stratton, New York.

Glick BS (1970) Conditioning therapy with phobic patients. Success and failure. *Am J Psychother* 24, 92–101.

Hilgard ER (1965) *Hypnotic Susceptibility*. Harcourt, Brace & World, New York.

Hilgard ER (1984) The hidden observer and multiple personality. *Int J Clin Exp Hypn* 32, 248–253.

Hilgard ER and Hilgard JR (1975) *Hypnosis in the Relief of Pain*. William Kaufmann, Los Altos, CA.

Kardiner A and Spiegel H (1947) *War Stress and Neurotic Illness*. Paul Hoeber, New York.

Katz RL, Kao CY, Spiegel H et al. (1974) Pain, acupuncture, and hypnosis. *Adv Neurol* 4, 819–825.

Kluft RP (1984) Treatment of multiple personality disorder. *Psychiatr Clin N Am* 7, 9–29.

Kluft RP (1991) Clinical presentations of multiple personality disorder. *Psychiatr Clin N Am* 14, 605–629.

Kluft RP (1992) The use of hypnosis with dissociative disorders. *Psychiatr Med* 10, 31–46.

Knox VJ and Shum K (1977) Reduction of cold-processor pain with acupuncture analgesia in high- and low-hypnotic subjects. *J Abnorm Psychol* 86, 639–643.

Laurence JR and Perry C (1983) Hypnotically created memory among highly hypnotizable subjects. *Science* 222, 523–524.

Lavoie G and Sabourin M (1980) Hypnosis and schizophrenia: A review of experimental and clinical studies, in *Handbook of Hypnosis and Psychosomatic Medicine* (eds Burrows GD and Dennerstein L). Elsevier/North-Holland, Amsterdam, pp. 377–420.

Lazarus AA (1973) "Hypnosis" as a facilitator in behavior therapy. *Int J Clin Exp Hypn* 21, 25–31.

Maldonado JR and Spiegel D (1994) Treatment of posttraumatic stress disorder, in *Dissociation: Clinical, Theoretical and Research Perspectives* (eds Lynn SJ and Rhue J). Guilford Press, New York, pp. 215–241.

Maldonado JR and Spiegel D (1995) Using hypnosis, in *Treating Women Molested in Childhood* (ed Classen C). Jossey-Bass, San Francisco, pp. 163–186.

Maldonado JR and Spiegel D (2000) Conversion disorder, in *Review of Psychiatry, Vol. 20, Somatoform and Factitious Disorders* (ed Phillips KA). American Psychiatric Press, Washington DC, pp. 95–128.

Maldonado JR and Spiegel D (2002a) Dissociative disorders, in *Textbook of Psychiatry*, 4th edn (eds Talbot J and Yudofsky S). American Psychiatric Press, Washington DC.

Maldonado JR and Spiegel D (2002b) Hypnosis, in *Textbook of Psychiatry*, 4th edn (eds Talbot J and Yudofsky S). American Psychiatric Press, Washington DC.

Maldonado JR, Butler L and Spiegel D (2000) Treatment of dissociative disorders, in *A Guide to Treatments that Work*, 2nd (eds Nathan PE and Gorman JM). Oxford University Press, New York, pp. 463–496.

Marks IM, Gelder MG and Edwards G (1968) Hypnosis and desensitization for phobias: A controlled prospective trial. *Br J Psychiatr* 114, 1263–1274.

McConkey KM (1992) The effects of hypnotic procedures on remembering, in *Contemporary Hypnosis Research* (eds Fromm E and Nash MR). Guilford Press, New York, pp. 405–426.

McGlashan TD, Evans FJ and Orne MT (1969) The nature of hypnotic analgesia and the placebo response to experimental pain. *Psychosom Med* 31, 227–246.

Myers JK, Weissman MM, Tischler GL et al. (1984) Six-month prevalence of psychiatric disorders in three communities 1980 to 1982. *Arch Gen Psychiatr* 41, 959–967.

Nash MR and Lynn SJ (1986) Child abuse and hypnotic ability. *Imagin Cogn Pers* 5, 211–218.

Nemiah JC (1985) Dissociative disorders, in *Comprehensive Textbook of Psychiatry*, 4th edn. (eds Kaplan H and Sadock B). Williams & Wilkins, Baltimore, pp. 942–957.

Orne MT, Axelrad AD, Diamond BL et al. (1985) Scientific status of refreshing recollection by the use of hypnosis. *JAMA* 253, 1918–1923.

Orne MT, Hilgard ER, Spiegel H et al. (1979) The relation between the Hypnotic Induction Profile and the Stanford Hypnotic Susceptibility Scales, Forms A and C. *Int J Clin Exp Hypn* 27, 85–102.

People v. Schoenfeld (1980) 168 Cal Rptr 762, 111 CA3d 671.

Pettinati HM (1982) Measuring hypnotizability in psychotic patients. *Int J Clin Exp Hypn* 30, 404–416.

Putman FW (1993) Dissociative disorders in children: Behavioral profiles and problems. *Child Abuse Negl* 17, 39–45.

Sanders B and Giolas MH (1991) Dissociation and childhood trauma in psychologically disturbed adolescents. *Am J Psychiatr* 148, 50–54.

Spiegel D (1981) Vietnam grief work using hypnosis. *Am J Clin Hypn* 24, 33–40.

Spiegel D (1984) Multiple personality as a posttraumatic stress disorder. *Psychiatr Clin N Am* 7, 101–110.

Spiegel D (1986) Dissociating damage. *Am J Clin Hypn* 29, 123–131.

Spiegel D (1988) Dissociation and hypnosis in posttraumatic stress disorder. *J Traum Stress* 1, 17–33.

Spiegel D (1989) Hypnosis in the treatment of victims of sexual abuse. *Psychiatr Clin N Am* 12, 295–305.

Spiegel D (1990) Hypnosis, dissociation and trauma: Hidden and overt observers, in *Repression and Dissociation* (ed Singer JL). University of Chicago Press, Chicago, pp. 121–142.

Spiegel D (1992) The use of hypnosis in the treatment of PTSD. *Psychiatr Med* 10, 21–30.

Spiegel D and Cardeña E (1991) Disintegrated experience: The dissociative disorders revisited. *J Abnorm Psychol* 100, 366–378.

Spiegel D and Fink R (1979) Hysterical psychosis and hypnotizability. *Am J Psychiatr* 136, 777–781.

Spiegel D and Scheflin AW (1994) Dissociated or fabricated? Psychiatric aspects of repressed memory in criminal and civil cases. *Int J Clin Exp Hypn* 42, 411–432.

Spiegel D and Spiegel H (1986) Forensic uses of hypnosis, in *Handbook of Forensic Psychology* (eds Weiner IB and Hess AK). John Wiley, New York, pp. 490–507.

Spiegel D and Vermutten E (1994) Physiological correlates of hypnosis and dissociation, in *Dissociation: Culture, Mind and Body* (ed Spiegel D). American Psychiatric Press, Washington DC, pp. 185–209.

Spiegel D, Detrick D and Frischholz EJ (1982) Hypnotizability and psychopathology. *Am J Psychiatr* 139, 431–437.

Spiegel D, Frischholz EJ, Maruffi B *et al.* (1981b) Hypnotic responsivity and the treatment of flying phobia. *Am J Clin Hypn* 23, 239–247.

Spiegel D, Hunt T and Dondershine H (1988) Dissociation and hypnotizability in posttraumatic stress disorder. *Am J Psychiatr* 145, 301–305.

Spiegel H (1970) Termination of smoking by a single treatment. *Arch Environ Health* 20, 736–742.

Spiegel H (1974) The Grade 5 Syndrome. The highly hypnotizable person. *Int J Clin Exp Hypn* 22, 303–319.

Spiegel H and Spiegel D (1978) *Trance and Treatment: Clinical Uses of Hypnosis.* Basic Books, New York. (Reprinted 1987 American Psychiatric Press, Washington DC)

Steingard S and Frankel FH (1985) Dissociation and psychotic symptoms. *Am J Psychiatr* 142, 953–955.

Stern DL, Spiegel H and Nee JCM (1979) The Hypnotic Induction Profile: Normative observations, reliability, and validity. *Am J Clin Hypn* 21, 109–132.

Terr LC (1991) Childhood traumas: An outline and overview. *Am J Psychiatr* 148, 10–20.

Watkins JG (1987) *Hypnotherapeutic Technique: The Practice of Clinical Hypnosis.* Irvington Publishers, New York.

Williams LM (1994) Recall of childhood trauma: A prospective study of women's memories of childhood sexual abuse. *J Consult Clin Psychol* 62, 1167–1176.

Psychosocial Rehabilitation

The developmental consequences of schizophrenia are substantial with typical onset of the first psychotic episode in late adolescence or young adulthood. People with schizophrenia become progressively more removed from their peer group, fail to achieve (or sustain) adult milestones such as marriage, higher education and employment, and often become socially isolated. These functional, psychosocial consequences become more severe and entrenched as illness duration increases, and result in multiple treatment needs that are superimposed on the neurobiological aspects of illness. While innovative new medications could potentially ameliorate (or compensate for) some of the consequences of anomalous neural development, it is unlikely that any pharmacological approach could restore normal brain function. Furthermore, no medication could undo the lifelong consequences of impaired learning, failure to master adult developmental tasks, and social withdrawal. These impairments mandate a multifaceted approach to treatment that includes an array of psychosocial strategies, of which rehabilitation plays a key role (Bellack, 1989).

The term **rehabilitation** is generally used to imply a subcategory of psychosocial treatment in which there is an emphasis on teaching/training, rather than discussion, and the focus is primarily on behaviors and functioning, rather than on intrapsychic processes (thinking and feeling). Reference is made to **psychosocial intervention** when the issues have generality to the broader domain of psychological treatment.

Issues in the Design of Psychosocial Interventions

The potential benefits of psychosocial treatment are often not achieved in the community due to poor understanding of the special needs and liabilities of schizophrenia patients. Five factors need to be taken into account when implementing psychosocial interventions and evaluating the results: 1) timing and duration of treatment; 2) individual differences in treatment needs; 3) the role of the patient in treatment; 4) the limitations imposed by impairments in information processing; and 5) the need to base interventions on a compensatory model.

Timing and Duration of Treatment

The APA *Practice Guidelines for the Treatment of Patients with Schizophrenia* (American Psychiatric Association, 1997, p. 1) makes a number of important points that are germane to rehabilitation programming, not the least of which pertains to the need for multimodal, long-term care: "Schizophrenia is a chronic condition that frequently has devastating effects on many aspects of the patient's life and carries a high risk of suicide

and other life-threatening conditions. The care of most patients involves multiple efforts to reduce the frequency and severity of episodes and to reduce the overall morbidity and mortality of the disorder. Many patients require comprehensive and continuous care over the course of their lives with no limits as to duration of treatment". This guideline is widely reflected in case management and pharmacotherapy but has not been adequately addressed in rehabilitation programs.

The role for psychosocial treatment and rehabilitation increases as the patient becomes more stable and shifts from support and stress reduction to specific rehabilitation strategies such as social skills training and cognitive rehabilitation. This three stage model and associated treatment emphasis has good face validity.

Treatment planning must be individualized. While this might seem like a given, many outpatient treatment systems are designed with a **one-size-fits-all** model, in which most patients are assigned to a standard set of group treatments paired with case management. This is a strategy that maximizes dropouts and minimizes effectiveness. This is a population that is difficult to treat effectively under the best of circumstances. Positive outcomes are likely only if both the content of treatment and the format of treatment are tailored to the individual patient's needs and learning capacities.

The combination of psychosis, thought disorganization and negative symptoms (especially anergia, apathy and anhedonia) often lead to the false assumption that patients are not capable of being active participants in their own treatment. Indeed, many patients seem unmotivated and are noncompliant, but such seeming disinterest and passivity should not be interpreted as accurate reflections of the person's goals and desires or as immutable traits. Negative symptoms are not always stable, and they may be secondary to demoralization, psychotic symptoms, medication side effects and other factors that vary over time (Carpenter *et al.*, 1988; McGlashan and Fenton, 1992). Paul and Lentz (1977) have shown that even extremely withdrawn, chronic schizophrenia patients can be motivated by a systematic incentive program. Similarly, desire to change and inclination to do the work required for treatment also vary over time in the same way that motivation to lose weight or quit smoking varies in nonpatient populations.

As cogently argued by Strauss (1989), schizophrenia patients have an active "will". Much of their behavior is goal directed and reflects an attempt to cope with the illness as best they can. Consequently, it is essential to view the patient as a potentially active partner and involve him or her in goal setting and treatment planning. Too often, treatments are imposed on patients by the treatment team and family members, with little consideration of the patient's own desires or capacities. It should not be surprising in such circumstances if the patient fails to

Essentials of Psychiatry Jerald Kay and Allan Tasman
© 2006 John Wiley & Sons, Ltd.

adhere to treatment recommendations, increasing the risk of relapse and creating tensions in relationships with family members and treatment providers. To be sure, engaging the patient to establish treatment goals can be a long, arduous process, but failure to do so courts the larger risk of undermining the very purpose of the intervention.

Impairments in Information Processing

It is now well established that impaired information processing represents one of the most significant areas of dysfunction in schizophrenia. The illness is marked by neuropsychological deficits in multiple domains, including verbal memory, working memory, attention, speed of processing, abstract reasoning and sensorimotor integration (Braff, 1991; Green and Nuechterlein, 1999). These deficits are highly related to social functioning and role performance in the community, as well as to performance in skills training programs (Green, 1996; Green *et al.*, 2000).

A related issue concerns the impact of neurocognitive deficits on the generalization of treatment effects. A basic assumption of all psychotherapies is that skills acquired in treatment sessions must be transferred or generalized to the patient's natural environment. Yet, such generalization is contingent upon cognitive processes that are often disrupted in schizophrenia, especially "executive functions" mediated by the dorsolateral prefrontal cortex (Weinberger, 1987).

Unfortunately, clinical rehabilitation programs have lagged behind the experimental literature in this arena and neurocognitive deficits generally are not well addressed in a systematic manner.

Adoption of a Compensatory Model

A rehabilitation model is more appropriate for treatment of most patients with schizphrenia than the standard treatment model as: 1) it implies a narrower focus on specific skills and behaviors, and 2) it aims to improve functioning in specific areas, rather than eliminating or curing an entire condition. As indicated above, cognitive impairment is a central feature of the disorder, evident in childhood and progressing sharply with the onset of psychotic illness. It is reasonable to speculate that the impairments observed in ill adult patients are at least of two types: 1) those present from early in development; and 2) those that are related to clinical psychotic illness. The existence of such early, developmentally based impairments suggest that the concept of "premorbid" functioning in schizophrenia may no longer be tenable; rather, there is a prepsychotic period during which there is subtle evidence of the "morbid" process. Thus, the challenge confronting attempts at cognitive enhancement may not be restoration of function, but instead may be the development of critical competencies and strategies for coping with deficits.

Consistent with this hypothesis, a compensatory approach to treatment may be more appropriate than the restorative or reparative approach characteristic of most treatment programs. Cognitive adaptation training (CAT) is a creative compensatory approach developed by Velligan and colleagues (2000). Case managers provide patients with home-based, compensatory environmental strategies to help structure the patient's living environment which maximizes the likelihood that she/he can complete requisite activities of daily living. Examples include posting reminders about appointments on the exit door from the apartment, listing items of clothing to be worn on the closet door, and

---

Clinical Vignette 1

Susan R was a single white woman first diagnosed with schizophrenia when she was 24. She had been working as a clerk in a small store and living with her parents when she first became ill. She had had few friends and dated infrequently. She was 32 when she began to participate in our rehabilitation program. She was living in a group home and had been unable to work since her first psychotic episode. She was described by her case manager as a passive, shy woman who was frequently taken advantage of by other residents in the group home and the day treatment program she attended. She was referred to us because of concerns that: 1) she needed to be more assertive with other patients who were borrowing her money and personal items, and 2) that she had expressed an interest in getting a job but was so quiet that she was unable to get past interviews.

Susan was well-maintained on medication, she did not have significant negative symptoms and she did not manifest behavioral problems that would prevent her from working. Based on the case manager's report and a review of Susan's medical record we focused our attention on social skills. She was appropriately groomed and did not present herself as a "patient" (e.g., no inappropriate mannerisms, no intrusions of psychotic or tangential thoughts, able to track conversation and provide appropriate responses to questions). However, she had a **deer in the headlights** quality. She seemed quite ill at ease; she scarcely made eye contact, looking mostly at the floor; her arms were wrapped round herself and she seemed to be physically tense; her shoulders were hunched and her head tilted toward the floor; she spoke haltingly in a very soft voice, such that the interviewer frequently had to ask her to repeat what she had said and to speak more loudly. When asked about her case manager's concerns about lending things to peers she indicated she didn't always want to give away her money and things, but that she was afraid people would get angry with her if she refused. She expressed the desire to return to work as a clerk, especially if the job did not involve much pressure. She reported that she always felt nervous during job interviews even when she thought she could do the work.

In response to our evaluation and Susan's expressed desire to be more assertive and to be able to get a job, we contracted with her to participate in a social skills training group for 3 months. The group included six other patients and met twice per week for 60 to 90 minutes. Susan's program consisted of three interrelated curriculum units: 1) assertiveness training to teach her how to be more effective in refusing unreasonable requests from peers; 2) job interview skills; and 3) sexual assertion skills. The unit on sex was based on our concern that Susan was vulnerable to unwanted sexual advances, and addressed refusal skills (how to say "no") and safe sex skills (how to get a partner to use a condom). Skills training for all three units consisted primarily of role-play rehearsals. A theme was defined for each sessions (e.g., telling a friend you cannot lend them money) and each patient was prompted to identify a specific situation which had recently occurred or might occur in the near future. Patients then took turns

---

Clinical Vignette 1 (*continued*)

engaging in repeated role plays in which the therapist portrayed someone in the patient's environment. In Susan's case, she identified other patients who frequently asked her for things and she rehearsed saying no to typical requests. Training Susan in job interview skills was coordinated with efforts by her case manager to arrange for interviews, as training is invariably more effective when it has near-term relevance and the new skills can be practiced in the real world. Training in safe sex skills proved to be very relevant as Susan admitted that she was being pressured to have sex by other patients.

Susan responded well to treatment. She was able to secure a part time job as a clerk within a few months of training, and had maintained the job when we followed up some 6 months later. Her case manager reported that she was better able to refuse requests for money, although it was arranged for staff to bank her paychecks and keep a minimal amount of cash on hand just to be safe. The case manager also reported that Susan had a boyfriend, another patient attending the day treatment center. While there is no assurance that Susan was practicing safe sex skills, she had not become pregnant, there was no evidence of an STD, and the boyfriend was known to be taking condoms from the bowl at the reception desk.

placing medications in a location that makes it maximally likely that the patient will see it and be reminded to take it. Prompts and other environmental aides are individually tailored to the patients' level of apathy, disinhibition and executive dysfunction. CAT can be administered in a time limited fashion, but may be a lifelong service for severely impaired patients. Velligan and colleagues found 9-months of CAT to be superior to an attention placebo and standard outpatient care on positive symptoms, negative symptoms, motivation, community functioning, global functioning and incidence of rehospitalization. This is an excellent model for compensatory interventions, and warrants further study (Table 73.1).

Rehabilitation Strategies

The following sections will briefly describe and evaluate the two types of rehabilitation programs that have had the greatest impact on the field in the 1990s, social skills training and cognitive rehabilitation, and promising directions in vocational rehabilitation.

Social Skills Training

The most useful perspective for understanding social functioning and social dysfunction in the illness has been the "social skills model" (Meier and Hope, 1998; Morrison and Bellack, 1984). Social skills are specific response capabilities necessary for effective performance. They include verbal response skills (e.g., the ability to start a conversation or to say "No" when needed), paralinguistic skills (e.g., use of appropriate voice volume and intonation) and nonverbal skills (e.g., appropriate use of gaze, hand gestures and facial expressions). These skills tend to be stable over time and make a unique contribution to the performance of social roles and quality of life (Bellack *et al.*, 1990; Mueser *et al.*, 1991). Increasing social competence and improving social role

functioning has been a major focus of rehabilitation efforts for the past 25 years, and a well-developed technology for teaching social skills has been developed and empirically tested: social skills training (SST) (Bellack *et al.*, 1997; Liberman, 1995).

Social skills training is a highly structured educational procedure that is generally conducted in small groups. Complex social repertoires such as making friends and dating are broken down into steps or component elements such as maintaining eye contact and asking questions. Patients are first taught to perform the elements and then gradually learn smoothly to combine them. Each session has a specific focus such as how to initiate conversations with strangers and how to refuse an unreasonable request. Trainers are more like teachers than traditional therapists. They first give patients simple instructions about how the behavior is to be performed, then they model appropriate behavior in a simulated conversation, and then they engage patients in role playing of simulated social encounters as a vehicle for practicing new skills. The therapists provide social reinforcement after each role played response and shape improved performance.

SST is clearly effective in increasing the use of specific behaviors (e.g., gaze, asking questions, voice volume) and improving functioning in the specific domains that are the primary focus of the treatment (e.g., conversational skill, ability to perform on a job interview). However, it is unclear whether other more diffuse dimensions of social functioning are affected, or the extent to which learning in the clinic translates into improved role functioning in the community. The effects of SST on relapse rate and symptoms appear to be negligible, although this is not surprising given the narrow focus of the intervention. SST is clearly an effective teaching technology that is well-received by both patients and clinicians. Nevertheless, it may well be that no time-limited, compartmentalized, office-based treatment can have broad-based effects. As discussed earlier in this chapter, it may be necessary to employ longer-term treatments that extend into the community and that are integrated with an array of intervention strategies.

Liberman and colleagues (2001) have approached the problem of generalization with an innovative approach referred to as *in vivo* amplified skills training (IVAST). It combines standard skills training with intensive case management, based on the assertive community treatment (ACT) model (Stein and Test, 1985). Office-based SST is supplemented and extended by a case manager who helps guide and reinforce appropriate behaviors in the community such as by helping a patient make a doctor's appointment or learn how to use public transportation. IVAST requires careful assessment of individual skills and needs and the extent to which the living environment is concordant with the patient's capacity to succeed. The case manager/trainer helps develop skills and/or shape the environment as needed, rather than putting the onus for success on the patient. IVAST has not yet been evaluated empirically but it is a creative approach that warrants careful study.

Cognitive Rehabilitation

Recognition of the importance of neurocognitive deficits has stimulated increasing interest in the prospects for cognitive remediation. Results have not been particularly robust but the work has had tremendous heuristic value.

Wykes and colleagues (1999) developed an intervention called **cognitive remediation therapy** that focuses on executive functioning (e.g., cognitive flexibility, working memory and

Table 73.1   Examples of Promising Rehabilitation Strategies

Strategy	Representative Source	Brief Description
Social skills training	Bellack *et al.* (1997)	A small group intervention for teaching patients social skills. Social behaviors are broken down into component units (e.g., making eye contact). Patients receive instruction on how to perform the units, and then rehearse effective social behaviors in simulated social encounters, analogous to learning motor skills.
	In Vivo Amplified Social Skills Training (Liberman *et al.* 2001)	A program designed to foster generalization to the community by combining social skills training with intensive case management.
Cognitive rehabilitation	Integrated Psychological Therapy (Brenner *et al.* 1990)	A small group approach that attempts to reduce cognitive impairment that interferes with social functioning. Program involves a series of stages beginning with basic cognitive processing and ending with social skills training.
	Neuropsychological Educational Approach to Remediation (Medalia and Revheim, 1999)	A training program that employs commercially produced educational software that is selected to be of high **intrinsic** interest to patients. Patients select from a variety of software programs that involve diverse neurocognitive capacities and work at their own pace.
	Cognitive Remediation Therapy (Wykes *et al.*, 1999)	A one-on-one training program that focuses on executive functioning and higher level cognitive capacities using paper and pencil tasks and neurocognitive tests. Emphasis is placed on teaching response strategies (e.g., problem-solving) in a graduated fashion that minimizes errors and frustration.
Vocational rehabilitation	Integrated Placement and Support Model (Drake *et al.*, 1999)	An innovative approach that employs a **train** and **place** model, rather than the traditional **train** and **place** approach. Patients work with a case manager who helps them find a real job in the community, and then provides ongoing support at the workplace to help the person succeed.
Cognitive adaptation training	Velligan *et al.* (2000)	Based on the assumption that many patients cannot monitor and manage their own behavior in the community, a clinician goes to the person's home to help structure the environment in ways that minimize demands on limited cognitive capacity. Techniques include: 1) organizing drawers and closets so person automatically selects appropriate clothing items; 2) placing signs and other prompts in highly visible places in the apartment (e.g., bathroom mirror) to remind patient to perform ADLs (activities of daily life); 3) to take medicine, etc.

planning). The approach employs a sophisticated training model that is based on principles of errorless learning, targeted reinforcement and guided practice on cognitive tasks. Training media consist of a variety of paper and pencil games and neurocognitive tests. A preliminary trial yielded improvement on several neuropsychological measures and modest retention of training effects over a 6-month follow-up interval. A limitation of this program is that it employs a highly tailored individual treatment model and demands high levels of therapist skill slowly to shape patient behavior. However, the focus on executive functioning seems much more likely to lead to transferable effects than narrowly focused programs designed to strengthen working memory or attention.

An alternative approach to cognitive rehabilitation capitalizes on the ease of standardization and flexibility provided by computer software. Wexler and colleagues (1997) and Bell and colleagues (2001) reported positive results for similar programs that provide self-directed practice on basic attention, memory and reasoning tasks (e.g., visual tracking, pyramids). These programs are limited in that patients find the tasks repetitive and boring, and they do not receive training per se. Patients may become more skilled on the specific tasks but they do not necessarily learn effective strategies that normalize dysfunctional neural circuitry or foster generalization to other situations.

Vocational Rehabilitation

The ability to perform productive work, earn money and achieve a degree of independence is generally regarded as a major factor in self-esteem, quality of life and relationships with significant others. Yet it is a domain that is particularly difficult for schizophrenia patients. Rates of competitive employment for persons with schizophrenia are generally less than 25%, and participation in sheltered employment is not much better (Lehman, 1995). There have been numerous hypotheses to explain the poor employment performance of schizophrenia patients, many of which place the onus on symptomatology, especially the sequelae of negative symptoms. Conversely, evidence suggests that employment history, work adjustment and ability to get along or function socially with others are better predictors of employment (Anthony and

Jansen, 1984). Social skill and ability to get along with others appear to be critical factors in both securing work (Charisiou *et al.*, 1989) and maintaining employment (Chadsey-Rusch, 1992; Cook *et al.*, 1994; Lehman, 1995).

There are many forms of vocational programs available in the community, including sheltered workshops, job clubs, transitional employment, the Boston University model and programs of job support. With the exception of programs involving job support, there is little evidence that these types of vocational interventions often result in sustained competitive employment among patients with severe mental illness (Lehman, 1995). Such programs, however, appear to provide many patients with structured opportunities for socialization and meaningful daily activity. Such limited goals may be appropriate for certain patients. However, for patients who are interested in competitive employment, it is clear that traditional approaches to psychiatric rehabilitation have proven to be disappointingly ineffective.

Recent evidence from several well-controlled studies suggests that the integrated placement and support (IPS) model of vocational rehabilitation may provide a distinct advantage in increasing rates of competitive employment among patients with severe mental illness (Drake *et al.*, 1999; Lehman *et al.*, 2002). The IPS model emphasizes the integration of vocational and mental health services by having an employment specialist becoming a member of the multidisciplinary clinical management team. The employment specialist helps patients search for real jobs in the community, rather than for placement in sheltered workshops or training programs. After employment is secured, the specialist provides follow-along support in a time-unlimited manner, including intervening with the employer if necessary. A manual has been developed to ensure fidelity of implementation of the approach. However, job retention is a major problem, that requires different strategies than job finding. Given the high priority placed on employment by patients, family members, and the community, improved employment services should be a major focus of research efforts in the future.

Conclusion

As evidenced by the approaches discussed here, the scientific literature is moving away from long-term, unfocused day treatment approaches to targeted intervention strategies designed to deal with specific problems. This approach, which is much more likely to produce useful outcomes, has not yet had adequate penetration of community services. Further research is required to match interventions with patients to determine when specific interventions should be provided, and to build in sufficient booster or follow-up procedures to maximize the chances for enduring change in the community. It is by now very apparent that neither a **one-size-fits-all** nor a time-limited, up-and-out approach works with the population of major concern, those with schizophrenia.

References

American Psychiatric Association (1997) *Practice Guideline for the Treatment of Patients with Schizophrenia*. APA, Washington DC.

Anthony WA and Jansen MA (1984) Predicting the vocational capacity of the chronically mentally ill. *Am Psychol* 39, 537–544.

Bell M, Bryson G, Tamasine G *et al.* (2001) Neurocognitive enhancement therapy with work: Effects on neuropsychological test performance. *Arch Gen Psychiatr* 58, 763–768.

Bellack AS (1989) A comprehensive model for the treatment of schizophrenia, in *A Clinical Guide for the Treatment of Schizophrenia* (ed Bellack AS). Plenum Press, New York, pp. 1–22.

Bellack AS, Morrison RL, Wixted JT, *et al.* (1990) An analysis of social competence in schizophrenia. *Br J Psychiatr* 156, 809–818.

Bellack AS, Mueser KT, Gingerich S *et al.* (1997) *Social Skills Training for Schizophrenia: A Step-By-Step Guide*. Guilford Press, New York, NY.

Braff DL (1991) Information processing and attentional abnormalities in the schizophrenia disorders, in *Cognitive Bases of Mental Disorders* (ed Magaro PA). Sage Publications, Newbury Park, CA, pp. 262–307.

Brenner HD, Kraemer S, Hermanutz M, *et al.* (1990) Cognitive treatment in schizophrenia. In Schizophrenia: Models and Interventions, Straube E and Hahlweg K (eds). Springer-Verlag, New York, pp. 161–191.

Carpenter WT, Heinrichs DW and Wagman AMI (1988) Deficit and nondeficit forms of schizophrenia: The concept. *Am J Psychiatr* 145, 578–583.

Chadsey-Rusch J (1992) Toward defining and measuring social skills in employment settings. *Am J Ment Retard* 96, 405–418.

Charisiou, J, Jackson HJ, Boyle GJ *et al.* (1989) Which employment interview skills best predict the employability of schizophrenic patients? *Psychol Rep* 64, 683–699.

Cook JA, Razzano LA, Straiton DM *et al.* (1994) Cultivation and maintenance of relationships with employers of people with psychiatric disabilities. *Psychol Rehabil* J 17, 103–116.

Drake RE, McHugo GJ, Bebout RR *et al.* (1999) A randomized clinical trial of supported employment for inner-city patients with severe mental disorders. *Arch Gen Psychiatr* 56, 627–633.

Green MF (1996) What are the functional consequences of neurocognitive deficits in schizophrenia? *Am J Psychiatr* 153, 321–330.

Green MF and Nuechterlein KH (1999) Should schizophrenia be treated as a neurocognitive disorder? *Schizophr Bull* 25, 309–318.

Green MF, Kern RS, Braff DL *et al.* (2000) Neurocognitive deficits and functional outcome in schizophrenia: Are we measuring the "right stuff"? *Schizophr Bull* 26, 119–136.

Lehman A (1995) Vocational rehabilitation in schizophrenia. *Schizophr Bull* 21, 645–656.

Lehman AF, Goldberg R, Dixon LB *et al.* (2002) Improving employment outcomes for persons with severe mental illnesses. *Arch Gen Psychiatr* 59, 165–172.

Liberman RP (1995) *Social and Independent Living Skills: The Community Re-entry Program*. Liberman, Los Angeles.

Liberman RP, Blair KE, Glynn SM *et al.* (2001) Generalization of skills training to the natural environment, in *The Treatment of Schizophrenia: Status and Emerging Trend* (eds Brenner HD, Boker W, and Genner R). Hogrefe & Huber, Seattle, WA, pp. 104–120.

McGlashan TH and Fenton WS (1992) The positive–negative distinction in schizophrenia: Review of natural history validators. *Arch Gen Psychiatr* 49, 63–72.

Medalia A and Revheim N (1999) Computer assisted learning in psychiatric rehabilitation. *Psychiatr Rehabil Skills* 3(1), 77–98.

Meier VJ and Hope DA (1998) Assessment of social skills, in *Behavioral Assessment*, 4th ed. (eds Bellack AS and Hersen M). Allyn & Bacon, Needham Heights, MA, pp. 232–255.

Morrison RL and Bellack AS (1984) Social skills training, in *Schizophrenia: Treatment, Management, and Rehabilitation* (ed Bellack AS). Grune & Stratton, Orlando, FL, pp. 247–279.

Mueser KT, Bellack AS, Douglas MS *et al.* (1991) Prevalence and stability of social skill deficits in schizophrenia. *Schizophr Res* 5, 167–176.

Paul GL and Lentz RJ (1977) *Psychosocial Treatment of Chronic Mental Patients: Milieu Versus Social-Learning Programs*. Harvard University Press, Cambridge, MA.

Stein LI and Test MA (eds) (1985) *The Training in Community Living Model: A Decade of Experience* (New directions for Mental Health Services, No. 26). Jossey-Bass, San Francisco.

Strauss JS (1989) Subjective experiences of schizophrenia: Toward a new dynamic psychiatry II. *Schizophr Bull* 15, 179–187.

Velligan DI, Bow-Thomas CC, Huntzinger C *et al.* (2000) Randomized controlled trial of the use of compensatory strategies to enhance adaptive functioning in outpatients with schizophrenia. *Am J Psychiatr* 157, 1317–1323.

Weinberger DR (1987) Implications of normal brain development for the pathogenesis of schizophrenia. *Arch Gen Psychiatr* 44, 660–669.

Wexler BE, Hawkins KA, Rounsaville B *et al.* (1997) Normal neurocognitive performance after extended practice in patients with schizophrenia. *Schizophr Res* 26, 173–180.

Wykes T, Reeder C, Corner J *et al.* (1999) The effects of neurocognitive remediation on executive processing in patients with schizophrenia. *Schizophr Bull* 25, 291–307.

74 Electroconvulsive Therapy, Transcranial Magnetic Stimulation, and Vagal Nerve Stimulation

Following six decades of uneven use, modern ECT has found a narrow but important niche among contemporary treatments in psychiatry. A large body of controlled data supports the efficacy and safety of ECT in the treatment of major depression and other severe psychiatric disorders (American Psychiatric Association, 2001).

Indications for ECT

General Considerations

In contrast to its origins as a treatment of schizophrenia, ECT today is generally utilized more frequently in patients with depression, especially psychotic depression and in the elderly. Mania and schizophrenia account for most of the remainder of convulsive therapy use. The indications have been most clearly spelled out by the American Psychiatric Association on ECT (American Psychiatric Association, 1990, 2001), which identified "primary " and "secondary" use of convulsive therapy. Primary indications are those for which ECT may appropriately be used as a first-line treatment. These include situations where the patient's medical or psychiatric condition requires rapid clinical response, where the risk of alternative treatments is excessive, or where, based on past history, response to ECT or nonresponse to medications is anticipated. If these conditions are not met, medication or other alternative treatment is recommended first, with ECT reserved for cases of nonresponse to adequate trial(s), unacceptable adverse effects of the alternative treatment, or deterioration of the patient's condition, increasing the urgency of the need for response (American Psychiatric Association, 2001). These general principles in turn require individualized interpretation in the presence of specific psychiatric and medical disorders. Even where ECT is not used as treatment of first choice, its introduction sooner in the decision tree rather than being reserved as a "last resort" may spare the patient multiple unsuccessful medication trials, thereby avoiding months of suffering and possibly reducing the likelihood of treatment resistance (American Psychiatric Association, 2001). Modern diagnostic and clinical considerations in the recommendation of ECT are summarized in Table 74.1.

ECT in Depression

It is well established that major depression is a heterogeneous disorder, encompassing mildly ill, functioning outpatients, as well as profoundly disturbed, dysfunctional, or often psychotic inpatients. Along this spectrum, ECT appears higher in the treatment hierarchy for the more severe presenting depression, usually defined by the presence of neurovegetative signs, psychosis, or suicidality (Abrams, 1982; American Psychiatric Association, 2000, 2001).

While there are no absolute rules, severely melancholic or psychotically depressed patients are often appropriate candidates for ECT as treatment of first choice, whereas more moderately ill individuals might not be considered for ECT until adequate medication trials have failed.

Predictors of Response

The literature describes an overall response rate to ECT of 75 to 85% in depression (Crowe, 1984; O'Connor et al., 2001). Efforts to delineate subtypes of depression particularly responsive to ECT have yielded inconsistent results. ECT is most likely to be helpful in an acute episode of severe depression of relatively brief duration (Rich et al., 1984). Combined data from two simulated-ECT-controlled trials (Brandon et al., 1984; Buchan et al., 1992) identified the presence of delusions and psychomotor retardation as predictive of preferential response.

Psychotic depression, increasingly recognized as a distinct subtype of mood disorder that responds poorly to antidepressants alone, has emerged as a powerful indication for ECT (Potter et al., 1991; Petrides et al., 2001). In this subgroup, ECT is at least as effective as a combination trial of antidepressant and antipsychotic medications. On balance, the evidence supports the early use of ECT in psychotic depression, particularly in lieu of prolonged, complicated medication trials that may be poorly tolerated, especially in the elderly (Khan et al., 1987; Potter et al., 1991; Sackeim, 1993).

While bipolar (discussed below) and unipolar depressions are equally responsive to ECT (American Psychiatric Association, 2002), response may be less likely with secondary than primary depression, in both adults (Kramer, 1982; Zorumski et al., 1986; Zimmerman et al., 1986a), including the elderly

Essentials of Psychiatry   Jerald Kay and Allan Tasman
© 2006 John Wiley & Sons, Ltd.

Table 74.1	Indications for Electroconvulsive Therapy

I. Diagnostic Considerations

A. Major depression: unipolar, especially primary **psychotic** (but other subtypes may respond); bipolar
B. Mania
C. Schizophrenia: acute
D. Schizoaffective disorder
E. Neurologic disorders: Parkinson's disease
   catatonia
   neuroleptic malignant syndrome

II. Clinical Considerations

A. Need for rapid response on medical or psychiatric grounds (e.g. suicidality, inanition)
B. History of treatment-resistance or excessive risk of alternative treatments
C. Severity of illness
D. History of previous positive response to ECT
E. Patient preference
F. Informed consent required

(Zorumski *et al.*, 1988) and adolescents (Schneekloth *et al.*, 1993). This may be especially true when depression is secondary to another psychiatric disorder, rather than to a medical illness.

Bipolar Disorder

ECT is an extremely effective and rapidly acting treatment for both acute mania and bipolar depression (American Psychiatric Association, 2002). However, it is infrequently used for mania, because of the availability of pharmacological strategies. Nonetheless, ECT has been repeatedly endorsed as an accepted second- or third-line treatment for acute manic episodes, particularly in cases of medication resistance, in patients of all ages (NIH/NIMH, 1985; Goodwin and Jamison, 1990; Mukherjee *et al.*, 1994; Van Gerpen *et al.*, 1999; American Psychiatric Association, 2002). In medical emergencies associated with mania, ECT can be regarded as a treatment of first choice (American Psychiatric Association, 2002). The same is true for medical conditions accompanying acute mania (including pregnancy, discussed later) that contraindicate or render intolerable the use of psychotropic medications.

There is little information on which manic patients benefit most from ECT or on optimal ECT treatment in mania. Bipolar depression responds as well as unipolar depression to ECT, in both adult and geriatric patients (American Psychiatric Association, 2002). Hypomania or mania is a risk of using ECT for depression in bipolar patients, but this is not different from the experience with any antidepressant treatment in this disorder (Gormley *et al.*, 1998; American Psychiatric Association, 2001, 2002).

Schizophrenia

Among the changes undergone by convulsive therapy over its 60-year history, few are as striking as those associated with its use in chronic psychotic illness. ECT has evolved from a treatment of

first choice to often a treatment of last resort for DSM-IV schizophrenia. However, the efficacy of ECT for depressive symptoms associated with psychotic illness is reflected in recent nationwide data showing the use of convulsive therapy in almost 12% of patients with recurrent major depression comorbid with schizophrenia (Olfson *et al.*, 1998), a utilization rate higher than that seen in uncomplicated recurrent depressive disorder.

The American Psychiatric Association Task Force on ECT (American Psychiatric Association, 2001) and the Canadian Psychiatric Association (Enns and Reiss, 1992) identified a role for ECT as a second-line treatment for selected patients with schizophrenia, particularly when associated with a brief duration of illness and/or affective symptoms.

It has been consistently found that the schizophrenic patients most likely to respond to ECT are those with good prognosis signs: mood disturbances, short duration of illness, predominance of positive rather than negative symptoms, and overexcitement (Fink and Sackeim, 1996). The potential responsiveness of acute psychotic symptoms in schizophrenia to ECT is more emphatically stated in the 2001 revision of the American Psychiatric Association Task Force Report compared with the previous edition, based on research conducted and compiled in the intervening decade (Fink and Sackeim, 1996).

Other Axis I Disorders

As reiterated in the Surgeon General's report on mental health (US Department of Health and Human Services, 1999), ECT has no demonstrated efficacy in dysthymia, substance abuse, or anxiety disorder. Nonetheless, ECT may play a role when the severity of a secondary major depression is severe and/or treatment refractory (American Psychiatric Association, 2001). In such circumstances, ECT can be expected to improve the comorbid mood component, leaving the underlying primary disorder untreated; in some circumstances, removal of the burden of overlying depression may indirectly benefit the underlying disorder. In the face of a potentially ECT-responsive major depressive episode, the presence of a nonmood Axis I disorder, even substance abuse, should not constitute a contraindication to the use of convulsive therapy (Olfson *et al.*, 1998; American Psychiatric Association, 2001).

Axis II Disorders

There are no evidence-based biological treatments for DSM-IV Axis II personality disorders, including ECT. Given the high incidence of comorbid, often treatment-refractory depression that accompanies Axis II pathology, ECT has been used in personality disordered patients, with inconsistent – but generally negative – reports of success, for many years.

Neurologic Disorders

Only 1% of patients admitted with a primary diagnosis other than a mood disorder or schizophrenia are treated with ECT in this country (Thompson *et al.*, 1994). Nonetheless, individuals with neurologic or other medical problems often suffer from primary or secondary mood or motor disorders that are ECT-responsive.

Catatonia

Over the past decade, benzodiazepines have emerged as the pharmacological treatment of choice for catatonia (Rosebush *et al.*,

1992; Ungavari *et al.*, 1994). However, in medication-unresponsive patients, prolonged drug trials with continuing clinical deterioration can be avoided in favor of a course of ECT (Ungavari *et al.*, 1994). Reflecting current understanding of the syndrome and its treatment, Fricchione (1989) recommended that "given the significant morbidity and mortality associated with catatonia, ECT should be considered if an expeditious 48- to 72-hour benzodiazepine trial is unsuccessful". As a practical point, given the now-common initial use of benzodiazepines in this condition, the catatonic patient may come to ECT with an initially elevated seizure threshold, and treatment parameters should be adjusted accordingly (Fink, 2002).

Other Neurologic Illness

The remaining neurological indications for ECT can be considered to fall into two major categories: 1) those for which, as with any medical illness, ECT is considered for treatment of a secondary depression when benefit–risk analysis favors ECT over antidepressant medications and 2) those for which ECT may play a special role by virtue of its unique actions compared with alternative treatment options.

In the first category are such conditions as poststroke depression (Murray *et al.*, 1986; Currier *et al.*, 1992) and mood disturbance in the context of brain trauma, tumor, or dementia (Hsiao *et al.*, 1987; Liang *et al.*, 1988; Kohler and Burock, 2001). Medication may be difficult to tolerate by these neurologically ill patients, tilting the potential benefit–risk ratio in favor of ECT (Price and McAllister, 1989).

Potential contraindications to ECT are very few and rarely are absolute (American Psychiatric Association, 2001). Although ECT generally should not be performed in the presence of raised intracranial pressure, it has been given safely even in the face of brain tumors and other mass lesions (Hsiao *et al.*, 1987; Fried and Mann, 1988; Abrams, 1991; Kohler and Burock, 2001) with special steps taken to protect against the ECT-associated hemodynamic changes; intracranial pressure may be reduced with the use of oral or parenteral steroids (Beale *et al.*, 1997).

Other Considerations in the Use of ECT

It can be appreciated that while accurate psychiatric diagnosis is essential to prioritize treatment options, it is far from the only consideration for the clinician weighing the advantages and potential problems of prescribing ECT (American Psychiatric Association, 2001). Two often-related variables are the patient's state of physical health and age. A large number of individuals receiving ECT in this country are elderly, many of whom are physically compromised.

Two general points should be made about the use of ECT in the elderly: 1) the physiological changes associated with ECT – cardiovascular (elevated blood pressure, arrhythmias), cognitive (confusion, memory loss), risk of traumatic injury to bones and teeth – that are benign and easily tolerated in young and middle-aged patients are prominent sources of potential ECT-associated morbidity in geriatric patients, and 2) the safety of ECT is appreciably enhanced if the foregoing effects on the older body, whether healthy or diseased, are anticipated and controlled. For example, Casey and Davis (1996) noted that a "rigorous falls prevention protocol" helped protect their elderly ECT patients from a potentially dangerous complication seen in earlier studies.

The very limited use of modern ECT in young people is generally reserved for cases of depression or mania complicated by medication resistance or the need for an urgent clinical response. Nonetheless, where ECT is utilized in younger patients, its efficacy and safety appear comparable to those in adults (Rey and Walter, 1997; Cohen *et al.*, 2000).

A special physical health challenge to the treatment of mental disorders is presented by pregnancy. Guidelines for the administration of ECT in the pregnant patient, incorporating measures such as intravenous hydration, avoidance of hyperventilation and nonessential anticholinergic medication, measures against gastric reflux, proper positioning of the patient during treatment, and uterine and fetal cardiac monitoring, have been developed and incorporated into modern practice (American Psychiatric Association, 2001).

Pretreatment Evaluation

Once the decision has been made to proceed with a course of ECT, specific steps are taken by the treatment team to maximize the benefits and minimize the risks. In some instances these procedures are part of the initial work-up, and the results may influence treatment decisions, as when certain psychiatric or physical disorders are ruled in or out.

The psychiatrist will want to make use of appropriate consultants, especially representing the fields of anesthesiology and, when indicated, internal medicine (often cardiology) or obstetrics. Given the current regulatory climate, the physician needs to be aware of local requirements regarding the need for second opinions or other pretreatment procedures in certain circumstances, or to arrange for guardianship or court proceedings where the patient's capacity to consent to ECT is in question, to assure that the initiation of treatment is not unduly delayed.

Psychiatric Considerations

The pre-ECT evaluation is a good time to confirm psychiatric diagnosis, including Axis II and III. In many settings, a specific ECT consultation may be helpful in evaluating the patient for a potentially ECT-responsive disorder and weighing the various treatment options (Klapheke, 1997). Input from nursing and other professional staff that have been working with the patient should be factored in. Should the indications for ECT remain present, baseline assessments of mental status including evaluation of suicidality, orientation and memory will help monitor changes in both therapeutic and adverse effects over the course of treatment. The history and effects of previous treatment with ECT should be obtained. Also, this time, decisions must be made regarding ongoing psychotropic medications particularly those increasing the risk of toxicity in combination with ECT, for example lithium and those affecting seizure threshold, such as benzodiazepines and anticonvulsants – and steps instituted to adjust, taper, or discontinue these medications, when appropriate.

Other Medical Considerations

History and physical examination should focus on the cardiovascular and neurological systems, the areas of greatest risk. The consulting internist, anesthesiologist, or other physician should advise the treatment team regarding cardiovascular risk of ECT and the need for any modifications in treatment technique, such as medications to moderate hemodynamic changes (Dolinski and

Zvara, 1997). Appropriate pretreatment optimization and monitoring of medical conditions that may be affected by ECT, such as diabetes, should be arranged at this time.

In the uncomplicated situation, the routine laboratory work-up for ECT is that indicated for any procedure involving general anesthesia: complete blood count, serum electrolyte levels and electrocardiogram (ECG) (American Psychiatric Association, 2001; Chaturvedi *et al.*, 2001). Chest X-ray is often obtained as well. The need for further pretreatment work-up, such as serum chemistries, urinalysis, HIV antibody titers and medication blood concentrations, is determined on an individual basis (Lafferty *et al.*, 2001). Given a normal neurologic and fundoscopic examination, computerized tomography (CT) or magnetic resonance imaging (MRI) of the brain is not indicated. Lumbosacral spine films, historically routine prior to institution of muscle relaxation in the ECT premedication protocol, have become optional for many patients. This remains appropriate for older patients with a history of or at risk for osteoporosis, and for any patient with a history of bone trauma. A formal anesthesiology consultation should result in an assignment of the degree of anesthesia risk and recommendations for any necessary modification in the ECT protocol (Folk *et al.*, 2000). A personal or family history of anesthesia complications may call for special assessment. The condition of dentition should be routinely assessed to avoid the treatment-associated risk of aspiration or fracture of loose teeth or bridgework.

Informed Consent

Among the unique features of ECT compared with other standard psychiatric treatments is the requirement for written informed consent by the patient or legal guardian or other substitute. Guidelines regarding the content of a standard informed consent form for ECT have been published (American Psychiatric Association, 2001). Supplemental information regarding ECT for patients and their families in a variety of media is also available and its distribution is encouraged (Fink, 1999; American Psychiatric Association, 2001).

The NIH/NIMH Consensus Development Conference on ECT (1985) emphasized that informed consent is a process that continues throughout the treatment course. Given the transient cognitive impairments common in depression and during an ECT course, it is particularly necessary to maintain a dialogue with the patient as treatment progresses to assure that all of the patient's questions and concerns are addressed, even if repetitive discourse ensues. With appropriate modification of the presentation of information, including use of nonverbal demonstration of the procedure, even patients with mental retardation often can make informed decisions about consent for ECT (Van Waarde *et al.*, 2001).

Initiation of Treatment

Once informed consent has been obtained, the initiation of treatment involves several decisions. These include selection of ECT device, electrode placement, dose of electricity, choice of premedications and frequency of treatment.

In choosing electrode placement there are two important factors to consider: antidepressant efficacy and cognitive side effects. The choices of electrode placement can be divided into unilateral placement over the nondominant (generally right) hemisphere and bilateral electrode placement (Figure 74.1),

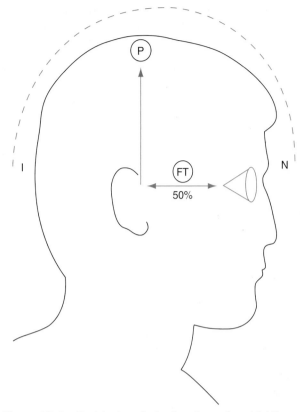

Figure 74.1   *Positioning of stimulus electrodes with bilateral and right unilateral ECT. For the standard bifrontotemporal (bilateral) placement, the electrodes are placed in position FT (frontotemporal). The midpoint of the line connecting the external canthus and the tragus is determined on both sides of the head. The center of the electrode is positioned 1 inch above this point. In the USA, stimulus electrodes are typically 2 inches in diameter, so the bottom of the electrode is adjacent to this point. For the commonly used d'Elia placement with right unilateral ECT, one electrode is in the FT position on the right side. The other electrode (P) is over parietal cortex and is positioned by determining the intersection between the line connecting the left and right tragus and the inion (I) and nasion (N). The center of this electrode is 1 inch below this intersection. (Source: American Psychiatric Association, [2001] The Practice of Electroconvulsive Therapy: Recommendations for Treatment, Training and Privileging – A Task Force Report, 2nd edn. American Psychiatric Press, Washington DC.)*

As potential but still experimental alternatives to traditional bifrontotemporal electrode placement, novel bifrontal and asymmetric placements are undergoing investigation as to whether they confer cognitive advantages by reducing electrical stimulation in left temporal areas while retaining therapeutic efficacy (Bailine et al. 2000). The bifrontal placement of Lawson and coworkers (1990) positions the center of each electrode approximately 5 cm above the lateral angle (external canthus) of each orbit, about 14 to 16 cm apart. The asymmetric (anterior bilateral) placement of Swartz (1994) positions the left-sided electrode above the left eye, with the lateral edge bordering the bony ridge between the forehead and the temple. The right-sided electrode is placed in an identical position to that used for the right-sided electrode in the traditional bifrontotemporal placement.

traditionally bifrontotemporal. The advantage of unilateral placement is that there is less memory loss and confusion than with bilateral electrode placement (Horne *et al.*, 1985; Weiner *et al.*, 1986; Abrams, 1982). The disadvantage of unilateral ECT is that it appears to be less effective when the dose of electricity given is close to seizure threshold (Sackeim *et al.*, 1993), and the seizure threshold can vary more than 40-fold from individual to individual (Sackeim *et al.*, 1987, 1991). With bilateral placement, seizure threshold is less of a concern, and the degree and speed of response appears greater with (high dose) bilateral than unilateral ECT (Nobler *et al.*, 1997; Sackeim *et al.*, 2000). Although bifrontotemporal placement has been more widely used, a limited number of studies suggest that bifrontal electrode placement may offer comparable treatment efficacy with fewer cognitive side effects (Weiner, 1994). Individuals who are unresponsive to several adequately dosed unilateral treatments may benefit from a switch to bilateral electrode placement.

From the start of the treatment procedure (see Table 74.1) EKG, heart rate and blood pressure are monitored and oxygen saturation is measured via pulse oximetry. Oxygen by mask is typically administered after the induction of anesthesia and until the return of spontaneous respiration. Depending upon the preference of the treatment team, patients may or may not be premedicated with an anticholinergic agent. Atropine and glycopyrrolate are the agents most commonly used (Abrams, 1997). The rationale for using these premedications is twofold. First, they reduce the bradycardia observed immediately after the delivery of the stimulus, and secondly, they dry secretions during anesthesia (Sommer *et al.*, 1989). The decrease in heart rate initially observed during seizure induction is the result of increased vagal tone which occurs immediately after the stimulus (Elliot *et al.*, 1982).

The patient is rendered unconscious with a short-acting general anesthetic. Methohexital 0.75 to 1.0 mg/kg given intravenously is the agent most commonly used (Folk *et al.*, 2000). Once the patient is unconscious, a muscle relaxant is administered. Intravenous succinylcholine 0.5 to 1.0 mg/kg is almost always used for this purpose. The goal of the muscle relaxant is to dampen the tonic–clonic movements from the seizure and reduce the risk of musculoskeletal injury (Elliot *et al.*, 1982; Lippmann *et al.*, 1993; Weiner, 1994). The **cuff technique** (Fink and Johnson, 1982) may be applied to an ankle or forearm, preventing localized circulation of the muscle relaxant, thereby facilitating monitoring of the motor seizure duration. The degree of relaxation is somewhat dependent upon the preference of the practitioner; however, when there is a history of skeletal disease the paralysis should be nearly complete. The fasciculations induced by succinylcholine can cause myalgias which can be prevented by administration of a small dose of the nondepolarizing agent, curare, prior to dosing with the succinylcholine. When curare is used in this manner it is necessary to increase the succinylcholine dosage by approximately 25% to achieve the same level of muscle relaxation as previously.

When the patient is unconscious and relaxed, the stimulus is delivered, using the desired electrode placement. Initially, the jaw will clench as a result of direct electrical stimulation. The heart rate will slow and the patient will generally have tonic contraction of the extremities (Elliot *et al.*, 1982). This initial period, which lasts anywhere from 2 to 5 seconds, is usually followed by a marked increase in blood pressure and heart rate (McCall, 1993). This is secondary to a centrally mediated catecholamine surge (Elliot *et al.*, 1982; Swartz, 1993). The extremities change to tonic–clonic contractions, the intensity of which depends on the degree to which they have been modified by the muscle relaxant.

During the treatment, seizure duration should be monitored, if possible, via a one- or two-channel electroencephalogram (EEG), an integral component of most modern ECT devices (Stephens *et al.*, 1991). Combining motor movement timing with EEG monitoring yields the most reliable seizure duration determinations in the clinical setting (Lippmann *et al.*, 1993). Although dose of electricity relative to seizure threshold is the important variable, in general, an adequate seizure is usually between 20 seconds and 2 minutes in duration.

Once the seizure terminates, the patient is continuously supported and monitored until breathing spontaneously and responsive to voice commands, with return of muscle strength. The patient's vital signs are monitored every 15 minutes until stable.

This process is repeated for an average of 6 to 12 sessions in the treatment of depression. In the USA, ECT is usually performed three times per week, while in the UK and Europe twice-a-week schedule is more common. The available data suggest that the twice-a-week schedule produces an equivalent therapeutic response with fewer treatments, but the speed of clinical improvement is slower than the three times per week schedule (Lerer *et al.*, 1995; Shapira *et al.*, 2000). On the other hand, the more rapid therapeutic response to thrice weekly ECT is accompanied by greater cognitive adverse effects than those associated with the slower rate of treatments (Lerer *et al.*, 1995; Shapira *et al.*, 2000).

Regardless of the treatment schedule, the rate of response will vary for each patient. Often, the patient's vegetative symptoms will respond before the patient feels subjectively improved.

Adverse Effects

The potential adverse effects from ECT range from mild complications such as myalgias, to serious events such as fractured bones, to catastrophes such as death. At present, the risk of serious complication is about 1 in 1000 patients. The risk of death is about 1 in 10 000 patients, which approximates the risk of general anesthesia for a minor surgical procedure (NIH/NIMH, 1985) and is actually lower than the spontaneous death rate in the community (Abrams, 1997).

Cardiac complications are the most frequent medical side effects associated with ECT. The arrhythmias range in severity from the common and benign sinus tachycardia to rare life-threatening or fatal ventricular arrhythmias.

Confusion and memory loss are also commonly occurring side effects. These adverse effects are the major factor limiting the use of ECT. Transient confusion occurs universally as a postictal event. Memory disturbance also occurs quite frequently (Calev, 1994). In general, during the acute course of ECT, both retrograde and anterograde memory are impaired to some degree (NIH/NIMH, 1985; Calev, 1994). Retrograde amnesia is generally felt to be more problematic. After the treatments end, the memory difficulties gradually resolve over the ensuing weeks to months (Lisanby *et al.*, 2000). Some patients may have permanent spottiness in memory for events that occurred in the weeks to months before, during and following the ECT course. Rarely, patients have complained of persistent memory difficulties severe enough to interfere with social and/or occupational functioning (NIH/NIMH, 1985). However, the infrequency with which this occurs, and certain technical factors such as the lack of nondepressed pretreatment memory and other neuropsychiatric measures (Coffey, 1994) has made it difficult to study these individuals systematically. Subjective impressions of post-ECT memory deficits appear to correlate more closely with clinical outcome and mood state than with objective cognitive measures (Prudic *et al.*, 2000). Although evidence to date points to only a transient and tolerable degree of cognitive impairment with continuation and maintenance ECT (Datto *et al.*, 2001) as these treatment strategies continue to play an increasing role in the long-term treatment of mood disorders, more definitive research on their effects on memory will help guide clinicians.

Few formal studies of ECT effects on cognitive functioning in children and adolescents have been conducted in the past 50 years.

ECT–Drug Combinations and Interactions

As most patients referred for ECT already are taking psychotropic medications, many ECT–drug interactions result from the inadvertent or intentional continuation of preexisting medication regimens with the initiation of convulsive therapy. Community surveys indicate that fewer than half of patients have discontinued all previous psychotropic medications at the time of ECT (Prudic *et al.*, 2000). While more definitive research is underway, the American Psychiatric Association Task Force recommends that, particularly for patients with a history of treatment resistance, "concurrent treatment with an antidepressant medication and ECT should be considered" (American Psychiatric Association, 2001).

Continuation and Maintenance Treatment

Among the unique features of ECT is the time-limited nature of its use in the treatment of acute episodes of illness. Following completion of an acute treatment course, ECT is generally terminated abruptly, coincident both with clinical response and, in many cases, impending inpatient discharge. It is now clearly established that left untreated after completion of ECT, at least half of patients will relapse, most within 6 months (American Psychiatric Association, 2001; Sackeim *et al.*, 2001a). Antidepressant treatment is now used routinely following a course of ECT to help prevent such relapse. Most contemporary authors adhere to the distinction between **continuation** treatment, over 6 months or so, to prevent relapse into the index episode, and **maintenance** treatment beyond that point, with the goal of avoiding recurrence, that is a new episode of illness. Nearly all published data on continuation and maintenance treatment have dealt with ECT administered for the treatment of depression.

Additional research is necessary to develop even more effective strategies to prevent relapse after completion of ECT.

Although the optimal methodology for an extension of the traditional ECT course – including electrode placement, frequency and duration of treatment – is yet to be determined (Scott *et al.*, 1991) it has become the subject of the ongoing NIMH-supported four-site CORE trial (O'Connor *et al.* 2001). Following an acute course of generally successful bilateral ECT (see earlier), patients in the CORE trial were randomized for the next 6 months to either a weekly to monthly maintenance ECT trial or to an active control pharmacotherapy condition, consisting of the most effective post-ECT medication regimen (combined nortriptyline plus lithium) identified by Sackeim *et al.*, (2001a). Moreover, additional data are required on the

Table 74.2	Typical Electroconvulsive Therapy Schedule of Events
12:00 AM	Patient begins NPO.
7:45 AM	Patient is escorted to the ECT suite.
7:50 AM	Nurse ascertains that patient has voided, has remained NPO, has dentures and jewelry removed, has clean and dry hair, and orders for ECT are completed properly.
7:55 AM	Psychiatrist and anesthesiologist review medical chart and determine any change in medical or mental status or medications.
8:00 AM	An intravenous line is placed; EKG, EEG, blood pressure and oximetry monitoring are instituted; stimulus parameters are selected on the ECT device.
8:02 AM	Sites of the ECT electrodes are prepared to reduce impedance.
8:05 AM	Anticholinergic premedication with glycopyrrolate or atropine is given; other adjunctive medications are administered as needed.
8:07 AM	Short-acting barbiturate anesthetic (e.g., methohexital or thiopental) is administered through IV; positive pressure respiratory support is instituted.
8:08 AM	Loss of consciousness is ascertained (eyelash reflex); blood pressure cuff is inflated over a lower or upper extremity to block distribution of the muscle relaxant (succinylcholine), which is then administered through IV.
8:09 AM	Fasciculations are noted in the cuffed extremity; a nerve stimulator may be used to ensure adequate muscle relaxation.
8:10 AM	Electrodes are positioned and integrity of the electrical circuit is checked; bite block or mouth guard is put in place; electrical stimulus is applied.
8:11 AM	Seizure activity is monitored and duration timed for both motor and EEG manifestations; cardiac status is closely monitored; respiratory support is provided until patient is breathing spontaneously.
8:12 AM	Vital signs are monitored frequently until return to baseline level.
8:20 AM	When the patient is breathing spontaneously, is responsive to commands, and vital signs are stable, the patient is transferred by stretcher to a recovery room.
8:25 AM	Patient is assessed for recovery of orientation; with continued stability of vital signs, the patient is discharged from recovery when reoriented and able to ambulate without assistance, usually 30–60 min following the treatment.

risk of cognitive and other adverse effects of continuation and maintenance ECT, and the best means of minimizing untoward effects of this potentially valuable intervention (Fox, 2001). There is general agreement that new written informed consent, beyond that obtained for the acute series of treatments, must be secured for continuation/maintenance ECT. In the event of prolonged maintenance ECT, the American Psychiatric Association (2001) Task Force recommends that the informed consent process be repeated every 6 months.

Treatment Failure

The total population of patients who are considered ECT treatment failures can be divided into three categories: true nonresponders; relative nonresponders for whom ECT can yet be made to work; and individuals for whom, upon closer inspection and examination, ECT was not the right treatment choice. Thus, the first approach to the ECT-resistant patient is to assure that an appropriately intensive trial of convulsive therapy has been attempted. Then reassessment, removal of any obstacles to treatment responsivity and, in most cases, entry into a treatment-resistant depression algorithm are indicated.

Adequacy of ECT Trial

A course of eight to 12 bilateral ECT treatments should be completed before any patient is declared ECT resistant. Patients who fail to respond to several treatments with unilateral electrode placement should be switched to bilateral ECT and offered an opportunity to respond to a full trial of that modality (Delva et al., 2001). The treatment history of the ECT-refractory patient should be reviewed to ensure that seizures were generalized and of adequate duration, and that in the case of unilateral electrode placement, stimulus intensity was sufficiently above seizure threshold. Some resistant patients may require additional ECT sessions in order to respond (Sackeim et al., 1990).

Re-evaluation

Even in carefully selected patients, lack of response to a course of ECT may occur in 10 to 30% of individuals (NIH/NIMH, 1985). Nonetheless, this degree of refractoriness should trigger a reassessment of the patient, with confirmation of the original diagnosis. The additional information learned during a hospitalization may enable a more accurate assessment of the chronicity of illness, presence of medical disease, degree of mood congruence of symptoms, vegetative functioning, mood reactivity, Axis II pathology, alcohol or other substance abuse, and outstanding psychosocial issues than was available on admission. Such data may both help explain the lack of response to ECT and open avenues to further evaluation or treatment efforts.

New Somatic Treatments

Transcranial Magnetic Stimulation

Coincident with the considerable advances in clinical research aimed at optimizing the use of ECT, the past decade has also witnessed renewed interest in the development of new somatic, nonpharmacologic interventions for mental disorders, particularly depression. Ongoing research supports the antidepressant efficacy of repetitive transcranial magnetic stimulation (rTMS)

(Holtzheimer et al., 2001). These and other related interventions stimulate the brain in manners less direct but more focused than does ECT. In contrast to the application of an electrical stimulus to the scalp, as in ECT, a more precisely localized electrical current can be produced within the brain by pulsing a magnetic wave (generated through a coil on the head), which passes undistorted through the skull. A train of TMS pulses, delivered to the left prefrontal cortex repeatedly but at a subconvulsive rate up to 20 minutes/day to an awake and alert patient, has demonstrated antidepressant efficacy in several small open and sham-controlled trials. To date, antidepressant effects have been relatively modest, and few patients have been medication free or followed systematically beyond a 1- or 2-week rTMS treatment trial.

Vagus Nerve Stimulation

Vagus nerve stimulation (VNS) has been used as an effective treatment of refractory seizure disorders, and now is showing promise as an antidepressant intervention. VNS is now approved by the US Food and Drug Administration for selected cases of depression. The afferent connections of the left vagus nerve with locus coeruleus, dorsal raphe and limbic structures have been implicated in the putative antidepressant effect of this intervention.

An initial surgical procedure is required for implantation of a small pacemaker-like stimulus generator beneath the clavicle, with an attached lead wrapped around the left vagus nerve in the neck. The generator can be programmed automatically to deliver a fixed duration of vagus nerve stimulation, for example 30 seconds of stimulation every 5 minutes. Many patients notice physical concomitants of vagal stimulation, such as coughing or hoarseness (Sackeim et al., 2001b). While this may defeat the masking of no-stimulation programming as a control condition in research studies, the intervention otherwise appears well tolerated. In the event of disturbing adverse effects, a magnet held over the stimulus generator will abort a stimulation. Safety experience thus far with seizure disorder patients has been satisfactory; stimulation of the left vagus nerve has no cardiac effects.

Conclusion

ECT retains a limited but important role in the treatment of selected patients with severe mood and other mental disorders. While efforts to continue to minimize the adverse effects, particularly cognitive, of ECT while retaining its effectiveness, other research is underway at developing additional or alternative nonpharmacologic somatic interventions for depression and other mental illnesses (Rasmussen et al., 2002). Optimal treatment for a given individual continues to require the determination of the benefit–risk ratio for each particular person and situation.

References

Abrams R (1982) Clinical prediction of ECT response in depressed patients. *Psychopharmacol Bull* 18, 48–50.

Abrams R (1991) Electroconvulsive therapy in the medically compromised patient. *Psychiatr Clin N Am* 14, 871–885.

Abrams R (1997) *Electroconvulsive Therapy*, 3rd edn. Oxford University Press, New York.

American Psychiatric Association (1990) *The Practice of ECT: Recommendations for Treatment, Training and Privileging.* American Psychiatric Press, Washington DC.

American Psychiatric Association (2000) *Practice Guideline for the Treatment of Patients With Major Depressive*, 2nd edn. American Psychiatric Publishing, Washington DC.

American Psychiatric Association (2001) *The Practice of Electroconvulsive Therapy: Recommendations for Treatment, Training and Privileging – A Task Force Report*, 2nd edn. American Psychiatric Press, Washington DC.

American Psychiatric Association (2002) Practice guideline for the treatment of patients with bipolar disorder (revision). *Am J Psychiatr* 159(Suppl 4), 1–50.

Bailine SH, Rifkin A, Kayne E, *et al.* (2000) Comparison of bifrontal and bitemporal ECT for major depression. *Am J Psychiatr* 157, 121–123.

Beale MD, Kellner CH and Parsons PJ (1997) ECT for the treatment of mood disorders in cancer patients. *Convuls Ther* 13, 222–226.

Brandon S, Cowley P, McDonald C *et al.* (1984) Electroconvulsive therapy: Results in depressive illness from the Leicestershire trial. *Br Med J* 288, 22–25.

Buchan H, Johnstone E, McPherson K *et al.* (1992) Who benefits from electroconvulsive therapy? Combined results of the Leicester and Northwick Park trials. *Br J Psychiatr* 160, 355–359.

Calev A (1994) Neuropsychology and ECT: Past and future research trends. *Psychopharmacol Bull* 30, 461–469.

Casey DA and Davis MH (1996) Electroconvulsive therapy in the very old. *Gen Hosp Psychiatr* 18, 436–439.

Chaturvedi S, Chadda RK, Rusia U *et al.* (2001) Effect of electroconvulsive therapy on hematological parameters. *Psychiatr Res* 104, 265–268.

Coffey CE (1994) The role of structural brain imaging in ECT. *Psychopharmacol Bull* 30, 477–483.

Cohen D, Taieb O, Flament M, *et al.* (2000) Absence of cognitive impairment as long-term follow-up in adolescents treated with ECT for severe mood disorder. *Am J Psychiatr* 157, 460–462.

Crowe RR (1984) Current concepts. Electroconvulsive therapy – A current perspective. *N Engl J Med* 311, 163–167.

Currier MB, Murray GB and Welch CC (1992) Electroconvulsive therapy for post-stroke depressed geriatric patients. *J Neuropsychiatr Clin Neurosci* 4, 140–144.

Datto CJ, Levy S, Miller DS, *et al.* (2001) Impact of maintenance ECT on concentration and memory. *J ECT* 17, 170–174.

Delva NJ, Brunet DG, Hawken ER *et al.* (2001) Characteristics of responders and nonresponders to brief-pulse right unilateral ECT in a controlled clinical trial. *J ECT* 17, 118–123.

Dolinski SY and Zvara DA (1997) Anesthetic considerations of cardiovascular risk during electroconvulsive therapy. *Convuls Ther* 13, 157–164.

Elliot DL, Linz DH and Kane JA (1982) Electroconvulsive therapy: Pretreatment medical evaluation. *Arch Intern Med* 142, 979–981.

Enns MW and Reiss JP (1992) Electroconvulsive therapy. *Can J Psychiatr* 37, 671–686.

Fink M (1999) *Electroshock: Restoring the Mind.* Oxford University Press, New York.

Fink M (2002) Catatonia and ECT: Meduna's biological antagonism hypothesis reconsidered. *World J Biol Psychiatr* 3, 105–108.

Fink M and Johnson L (1982) Monitoring the duration of electroconvulsive therapy seizures: 'Cuff' and EEG methods compared. *Arch Gen Psychiatr* 39, 1189–1191.

Fink M and Sackeim HA (1996) Convulsive therapy in schizophrenia? *Schizophr Bull* 22, 27–39.

Folk JW, Kellner CH, Beale MD *et al.* (2000) Anesthesia for electroconvulsive therapy: A review. *J ECT* 16, 157–170.

Fox HA (2001) Extended continuation and maintenance ECT for long-lasting episodes of major depression. *J ECT* 17, 60–64.

Fricchione G (1989) Catatonia: A new indication for benzodiazepines? *Biol Psychiatr* 26, 761–765.

Fried D and Mann JJ (1988) Electroconvulsive treatment of a patient with known intracranial tumor. *Biol Psychiatr* 23, 176–180.

Goodwin FK and Jamison KR (1990) *Manic–Depressive Illness.* Oxford University Press, New York.

Gormley N, Cullen C, Walters L *et al.* (1998) The safety and efficacy of electroconvulsive therapy in patients over age 75. *Int J Geriatr Psychiatr* 13, 871–874.

Holtzheimer PE, Russo J and Avery DH (2001) A meta-analysis of repetitive transcranial magnetic stimulation in the treatment of depression. *Psychopharmacol Bull* 35, 149–169.

Horne RL, Pettinati HM, Sugerman AA *et al.* (1985) Comparing bilateral to unilateral electroconvulsive therapy in a randomized study with EEG monitoring. *Arch Gen Psychiatr* 42, 1087–1092.

Hsiao JK, Messenheimer JA and Evans DL (1987) ECT and neurological disorders. *Convuls Ther* 3, 121–136.

Khan A, Cohen S, Stowell M *et al.* (1987) Treatment options in severe psychotic depression. *Convuls Ther* 3, 93–99.

Klapheke MM (1997) Electroconvulsive therapy consultation: An update. *Convuls Ther* 13, 227–241.

Kohler CG and Burock M (2001) ECT for psychotic depression associated with a brain tumor. *Am J Psychiatr* 158, 2089.

Kramer BA (1982) Poor response to electroconvulsive therapy in patients with a combined diagnosis of major depression and borderline personality disorder. *Lancet* II, 1048.

Lafferty JE, North CS, Spitznagel E *et al.* (2001) Laboratory screening prior to ECT. *J ECT* 17, 158–165.

Lawson JS, Inglis J, Delva NJ, *et al.* (1990) Electrode placement in ECT: Cognitive Effects. *Psychol Med* 20, 335–344.

Lerer B, Shapira B, Calev A *et al.* (1995) Antidepressant and cognitive effects of twice-versus three-times-weekly ECT. *Am J Psychiatr* 152, 564–570.

Liang RA, Lam RW and Ancill RJ (1988) ECT in the treatment of mixed depression and dementia. *Br J Psychiatr* 152, 281–284.

Lippmann S, Haas S and Quast G (1993) Procedural complications of electroconvulsive therapy: Assessment and recommendations. *South Med J* 86, 1110–1114.

Lisanby SH, Maddox JH, Prudic J *et al.* (2000) The effects of electroconvulsive therapy on memory of autobiographical and public events. *Arch Gen Psychiatr* 57, 581–590.

McCall WV (1993) Antihypertensive medications and ECT. *Convuls Ther* 9, 317–325.

Mukherjee S, Sackeim HA and Schnur DB (1994) Electroconvulsive therapy of acute manic episodes: A review of 50 years' experience. *Am J Psychiatr* 151, 169–176.

Murray GB, Shea V and Conn DK (1986) Electroconvulsive therapy for poststroke depression. *J Clin Psychiatr* 47, 258–260.

National Institutes of Health/NIMH consensus conference (1985) Electroconvulsive therapy. *JAMA* 254, 2103–2108.

Nobler MS, Sackeim HA, Moeller JR *et al.* (1997) Quantifying the speed of symptomatic improvement with electroconvulsive therapy: Comparison of alternative statistical methods. *Convuls Ther* 13, 208–221.

O'Connor MK, Knapp R, Husain M *et al.* (2001) The influence of age on the response of major depression to electroconvulsive therapy: A C.O.R.E. Report. *Am J Geriatr Psychiatry* 9, 382–390.

Olfson M, Marcus S, Sackeim HA *et al.* (1998) Use of ECT for the inpatient treatment of recurrent major depression. *Am J Psychiatr* 155, 22–29.

Petrides G, Find M, Husain MM *et al.* (2001) ECT remission rates in psychotic versus nonpsychotic depressed patients: A report from CORE. *J ECT* 17, 244–253.

Potter WZ, Rudorfer MV and Manji H (1991) The pharmacologic treatment of depression. *N Engl J Med* 325, 633–642.

Price TR and McAllister TW (1989) Safety and efficacy of ECT in depressed patients with dementia: A review of clinical experience. *Convuls Ther* 5, 61–74.

Prudic J, Peyser S and Sackeim HA (2000) Subjective memory complaints: A review of patient self-assessment of memory after electroconvulsive therapy. *J ECT* 16, 121–132.

Rasmussen KG, Sampson SM and Rummans TA (2002b) Electroconvulsive therapy and newer modalities for the treatment of medication-refractory mental illness. *Mayo Clin Proc* 77, 552–556.

Rey JM and Walter G (1997) Half a century of ECT use in young people. *Am J Psychiatr* 154, 595–602.

Rich CL, Spiker DG, Jewell SW *et al.* (1984) The efficiency of ECT: I. Response rate in depressive episodes. *Psychiatr Res* 11, 167–176.

Rosebush PI, Hildebrand AM and Mazurek MF (1992) The treatment of catatonia: Benzodiazepines or ECT? *Am J Psychiatr* 149, 1279–1280.

Sackeim HA (1993) The use of electroconvulsive therapy in late life depression, in *Diagnosis and Treatment of Depression in Late Life* (eds, Schneider LS, Reynolds III CF, Lebowitz BD *et al.*). American Psychiatric Press, Washington DC, pp. 259–277.

Sackeim HA, Decina P, Prohovnik I *et al.* (1987) Seizure threshold in electroconvulsive therapy: Effects of sex, age, electrode placement and number of treatments. *Arch Gen Psychiatr* 44, 355–360.

Sackeim HA, Prudic J and Devanand DP (1990) Treatment of medication-resistant depression with electroconvulsive therapy, in *Annual Review of Psychiatry*, Vol. 9 (eds Tasman A, Goldfinger SM and Kaufmann CA). American Psychiatric Press, Washington DC, pp. 91–115.

Sackeim HA, Devanand DP and Prudic J (1991) Stimulus intensity, seizure threshold, and seizure duration: Impact on the efficacy and safety of electroconvulsive therapy. *Psychiatr Clin N Am* 14, 803–843.

Sackeim HA, Prudic J, Devanand DP *et al.* (1993) Effects of stimulus intensity and electrode placement on the efficacy and cognitive effects of electroconvulsive therapy. *N Engl J Med* 328, 839–846.

Sackeim HA, Prudic J, Devanand DP *et al.* (2000) A prospective, randomized, double-blind comparison of bilateral and right unilateral electroconvulsive therapy at different stimulus intensities. *Arch Gen Psychiatr* 57, 425–434.

Sackeim HA, Haskett RF, Mulsant BH *et al.* (2001a) Continuation pharmacotherapy in the prevention of relapse following electroconvulsive therapy: A randomized controlled trial. *JAMA* 285, 1299–1307.

Sackeim HA, Rush AJ, George MS *et al.* (2001b) Vagus nerve stimulations (VNS) for treatment-resistant depression: Efficacy, side effects, and predictors of outcome. *Neuropsychopharmacology* 25, 713–728.

Schneekloth TD, Rummans TA and Logan KM (1993) Electroconvulsive therapy in adolescents. *Convuls Ther* 9, 158–166.

Scott AI, Weeks DJ and McDonald CF (1991) Continuation electroconvulsive therapy: Preliminary guidelines and an illustrative case report. *Br J Psychiatr* 159, 867–870.

Shapira B, Tubi N and Lerer B (2000) Balancing speed of response of ECT in major depression and adverse cognitive effects: Role of treatment schedule. *J ECT* 16, 97–109.

Sommer BR, Satlin A, Friedman L *et al.* (1989) Glycopyrrolate versus atropine in post-ECT amnesia in the elderly. *J Geriatr Psychiatr Neurol* 2, 18–21.

Stephens SM, Greenberg RM and Pettinati HM (1991) Choosing an electroconvulsive therapy device. *Psychiatr Clin N Am* 14, 989–1006.

Swartz CM (1993) Anesthesia for ECT. *Convuls Ther* 9, 301–316.

Swartz CM (1994) Asymmetric bilateral right frontotemporal left frontal stimulus electrode placement for electroconvulsive therapy. *Neuropsychobilogy* 29, 174–178.

Thompson JW, Weiner RD and Myers CP (1994) Use of ECT in the United States in 1975, 1980 and 1986. *Am J Psychiatr* 151, 1657–1661.

Ungavari GS, Leung CM, Wong MK *et al.* (1994) Benzodiazepines in the treatment of catatonic syndrome. *Acta Psychiatr Scand* 89, 285–288.

US Department of Health and Human Services (1999) *Mental Health: A Report of the Surgeon General.* US Department of Health and Human Services, Substance Abuse and Mental Health Services Administration/Center for Mental Health Services, National Institutes of Health/National Institute of Mental Health, Rockville, MD.

Van Gerpen MW, Johnson JE and Winstead DK (1999) Mania in the geriatric patient population. *Am J Geriatr Psychiatr* 7, 188–202.

Van Waarde JA, Stolker JJ and van der Mast RC (2001) ECT in mental retardation: A review. *J ECT* 17, 236–243.

Weiner RD (1994) Treatment optimization with ECT. *Psychopharmacol Bull* 30, 313–320.

Weiner RD, Rogers HJ, Davidson JR *et al.* (1986) Effects of stimulus parameters on cognitive side effects. *Ann NY Acad Sci* 462, 315–325.

Zimmerman M, Coryell W, Pfohl B *et al.* (1986a) ECT response in depressed patients with and without a DSM-III personality disorder. *Am J Psychiatr* 143, 1030–1032.

Zorumski CF, Rubin EH and Burke WJ (1988) Electroconvulsive therapy for the elderly: A review. *Hosp Comm Psychiatr* 39, 643–647.

Zorumski CF, Rutherford JL and Burke WJ (1986) ECT in primary and secondary depression. *J Clin Psychiatr* 47, 298–300.

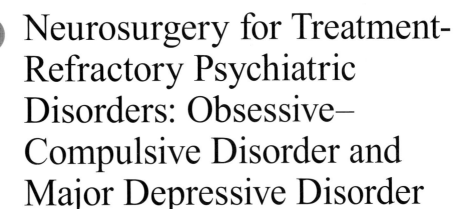

75 Neurosurgery for Treatment-Refractory Psychiatric Disorders: Obsessive–Compulsive Disorder and Major Depressive Disorder

Characteristics of Patients Undergoing Neurosurgery for Treatment-refractory OCD and MDD

Though selection criteria have not been standardized across centers, a review of most reported studies from several countries suggests that only a small number of OCD or MDD patients who have not responded to a variety of exhaustive treatments are considered for palliative neurosurgery. Treatments include multiple adequate medication trials, an adequate trial of behavioral treatment/psychotherapy and electroconvulsive therapy (ECT) for MDD – encompassing patients who remain severely disabled for several years despite these efforts (Table 75.1). In addition to the essential informed consent of the patient, a panel of specialists, usually constituted at the institutional level, carefully reviews all aspects of the patient's condition before making a consensus decision on surgery.

Severe, chronic OCD and MDD referrals commonly present with comorbidities including depression, obsessive–compulsive "psychosis", substance abuse, history of harmful behavior and personality disorders. The decision to offer surgery must be evaluated on a case-by-case basis, carefully considering the benefits and risks of intervention, alongside those of nonintervention. Tables 75.2 and 75.3 contain guidelines for indications and relative contraindications for these procedures evolved in the context of 25 years of experience with the stereotactic cingulotomy procedure for intractable psychiatric disorder at one center. (Massachusetts General Hospital (MGH): OCD Clinic and Cingulotomy Program, Boston, MA, USA).

Interventions

Currently, only a few specialized centers in the world conduct neurosurgical procedures for treatment-refractory OCD and treatment-refractory MDD. These procedures have evolved at particular centers more by convention and experience than by controlled research studies and direct comparison of the various procedures. The modern neurosurgical procedures include 1) cingulotomy, 2) anterior capsulotomy, 3) subcaudate tractotomy

Table 75.1 Suggested Guidelines: Indications for Neurosurgical Intervention for IOCD (Intractable Obsessive–Compulsive Disorder)

1. Patient fulfills the diagnostic criteria for OCD/MDD (SCID derived DSM-IV OR comparable such as ICD-10).
2. The duration of illness exceeds 5 yr.
3. The disorder is severe (while not necessarily reflective of overall disability, OCD patients usually have YBOCS scores of ≥20) and is causing substantial distress.
4. The disorder is causing substantial reduction in the patient's psychosocial functioning (e.g., Global Assessment of Functioning (GAF) of 40 and below).
5. Current treatment options* tried systematically for at least 5 yr either have been without appreciable effect on the symptoms or must be discontinued owing to intolerable side effects.
6. The prognosis, without neurosurgical intervention, is considered poor.
7. The patient gives informed consent.
8. The patient agrees to participate in the preoperative evaluation and postoperative rehabilitation programs respectively.
9. The patients' local referring physician is willing to acknowledge responsibility for the postoperative long-term management of the patient.

*OCD: Adequate trials (at least 12 weeks at the maximally tolerated dose) of all serotoninergic agents (clomipramine, paroxetine, fluoxetine, fluvoxamine, sertraline), and possibly a serotoninergic–noradrenergic agent (venlafaxine) and MAO-I as well; as augmentation of at least one of these drugs for 1 month: lithium, clonazepam, buspirone or other experimental agents; all patients must have had an adequate trial of behavioral therapy (at least 20 hours of "real" exposure and response prevention therapy).

and 4) limbic leukotomy. All four procedures involve magnetic resonance (MR) imaging guided stereotactic lesions placed bilaterally in the various target regions, after which they are named.

Essentials of Psychiatry   Jerald Kay and Allan Tasman
© 2006 John Wiley & Sons, Ltd.

Table 75.2   Suggested Guidelines: Relative Contra-indications to Neurosurgical Intervention

1. Age younger than 18 yr or older than 65 yr.
2. The patient has another current or lifetime Axis I diagnosis (e.g., organic brain syndrome, delusional disorder, somatization or current or recent substance abuse) that substantially complicates diagnosis, treatment, or the patient's ability to comply with treatment or a chronically unstable clinical course (e.g., history of multiple impulsive suicidal attempts).
3. A complicating current DSM-IV Axis II diagnosis from cluster A (e.g., paranoid personality disorder) or B (e.g., borderline, antisocial, or histrionic personality disorder). A current cluster C personality disorder (e.g., avoidant or obsessive–compulsive personality disorder) is generally not a contraindication.
4. The patient has a current Axis III diagnosis with brain pathology, such as moderate or marked cerebral atrophy, stroke, or tumor or has undergone previous neurosurgical procedures that have a high likelihood of producing unacceptable complications.

Results of Comparative Reviews of Outcome

Chiocca and Martuza (1990) reviewed 10 studies ($n = 210$) involving all four current procedures to investigate comparative efficacy. After acknowledging the inherent limitations of such a comparison, the authors concluded that the percentages of patients who improved with each of these four procedures were roughly the same. This latter conclusion may be disputed, however, because the number of outcome categories was not identical (e.g., A, B and C for limbic leukotomy; A and B only for capsulotomy).

Waziri (1990) reviewed 12 studies ($n = 253$) of patients undergoing stereotactic interventions for treatment-refractory OCD and noted that 38% of patients were reported to be symptom free, 29% markedly improved, 10% unchanged and 3% worse or dead on follow-up (including one suicide). An overall figure for satisfactory response to surgery of 67% was found in these 253 OCD patients.

Hodgkiss and colleagues (1995) reported on a 12-month follow-up study of 286 patients who underwent SST between 1979 and 1991 (249 were completely evaluated including 74 who were evaluated by an independent rater); 63/183 (34%) MDD patients and 5/15 (33%) of OCD patients were classified as good outcome. There were six deaths during this period though none was attributed to neurosurgery or suicide. The authors noted that most deaths involved patients over 70 and cautioned the use of this procedure for the elderly.

The methodological issues discussed earlier and the lack of rigorous, controlled and/or head to head comparison studies prevent comment on which of these procedures is superior. This is further complicated by the heterogeneous profile of OCD patients. At present, there is little evidence to suggest the clear superiority of one procedure over another. More research addressing these issues is desirable.

Predictors of Outcome

Most investigators reporting outcome studies concerning various procedures have naturally attempted to identify predictors of outcome, though these have been elusive. Bridges and colleagues (1973) reported that OCD subjects who were considered responders in their study had an older age of onset (mean 28.5 years) versus nonresponders (mean 22 years). In a prospective cingulotomy study, using comprehensive assessment strategies, Baer and colleagues (1995) reported that the presence of symmetry obsessions, ordering and hoarding compulsions were predictive of lower YBOCS score at final follow-up (partial correlations). More recently, Rauch and colleagues (2001) utilizing a retrospective design, reported that higher preoperative metabolic rates in a single right posterior cingulate locus (determined by FDG-PET) was associated with better postcingulotomy outcome in 11 OCD patients. The advantages of predicting response in such invasive palliative procedures are obvious and need further study.

Risks of Neurosurgical Intervention

Surgical Risks

Surgical risks include acute and subacute complications like hemorrhage, postoperative infections and seizures, as well as more serious enduring side effects such as focal neurological deficits, cognitive or personality change and weight gain.

Neuropsychiatric Risks

Cognitive/Intellectual Domain

With regard to cingulotomy, an independent study of a cohort of patients was performed for the US government by the Department of Psychology at the Massachusetts Institute of Technology. The authors reported that they found no evidence of lasting neurological, intellectual, personality, or behavioral deficits after surgery (Corkin et al., 1979; Corkin, 1980). In fact, a comparison of preoperative and postoperative scores revealed modest gains in the Wechsler IQ ratings. The only apparent irreversible decrement identified by these investigators was a decrease in performance on the Taylor Complex Figure Test in patients older than age 40 years. Several authors, using varying assessment strategies and batteries pre and postoperatively, have reported the relative lack of serious adverse cognitive effects following cingulotomy (Corkin et al., 1979; Corkin, 1980), subcaudate tractotomy (Bartlett and Bridges, 1977; Göktepe et al., 1975), limbic leukotomy (Mitchell-Heggs et al., 1976; Kelly, 1980) and capsulotomy (Herner, 1961; Bingley et al., 1977; Vasko and Kullberg, 1979) (Figures 75.1 and 75.2). Nevertheless, the need to include carefully thought out (based on the procedure involved) neurocognitive assessments before and at regular intervals after the surgery/surgeries cannot be overstated. Long-term studies are desirable for the existing procedures better to inform patients and clinicians of the risks as well to help rehabilitative efforts.

Affective/Social and Personality Domains

As these neurosurgical procedures may be expected to influence, directly or indirectly, frontal lobe and other functions comprising one's "personality", it is important that this is an integral part of the pre and postoperative assessment. Important domains that need to be addressed are executive functions, impulsivity/aggressiveness, social propriety and mood changes. Ideally this would involve input from both the patient as well as the family and treating clinician. In general, anecdotal evidence from most reported

Table 75.3 Suggested Guidelines for Neurosurgical Intervention in Neurosurgery for Intractable Psychiatric Illness

1. Center and expertise
Center/s with stereotactic neurosurgical expertise and integrated multidisciplinary expertise in the evaluation, neurosurgical treatment and management of patients with intractable psychiatric disorders.
2. Patient selection
Suggested guidelines for patient selection presented in Tables 75.2 and 75.3. A clinical psychiatrist with OCD expertise evaluates patients and orders a presurgical work-up (below).
3. Profiles
Work-up should be carefully thought out and relevant to the specific procedures as well as to enhance comparability. Information should be collected from multiple sources (patient, family, psychiatrist, etc.).
    Psychiatric:
        Preferably a structured clinical interview (e.g., SCID-CV* for DSM-IV). Reliable and valid scales (inventories and clinician administered) of mood, obsessions and compulsions, and anxiety (e.g., BDI†, HDRS‡; YBOCS§).
    Neuropsychological
        Batteries of both general cognition as well as specific to lesion: (e.g., general intellectual functioning, executive functions, memory, personality assessment)
    Neuromedical
        General surgical risk work-up.
        Specific neurological issues: neurological examination, prelesion MRI (for lesion demarcation), documentation of past neurological problems, especially seizures.
4. Raters and schedule
Assessors and raters should be blinded to the extent possible.
5. Documentation of neurosurgical effects
Documentation of lesion site, size, and extent. Pre and poststructural and functional scans would be highly desirable.
6. Postsurgical follow-up
Should involve administration of selected profiles mentioned above at various intervals (e.g., 1 wk postsurgery, 3, 6, 9, and 12 mo and longer when possible.
Enhancing comparability of data
• Centers should attempt to use universally accepted/equivalent patient selection criteria, psychiatric instruments, neuropsychological batteries and objective quantification and monitoring of lesions.
• Establishment of a database to remove inherent bias of only publishing positive studies.
• Consortium of centers investigating different procedures.

*First MB, Spitzer RL, Gibbon M *et al.* (1996) *Structured Clinical Interview for DSM-IV Axis I Disorders*, Clinical Version (SCID-IV). American Psychiatric Press, Washington DC.
†Beck AT, Steer RA and Brown GK (1996) *Manual for Beck Depression Inventory-II*. Psychological Corporation, San Antonio, TX.
‡Hamilton M (1986) The Hamilton Rating Scale for depression, in *Assessment of Depression* (eds Sartorius N and Ban TA). Springer-Verlag, Berlin.
§Goodman WK, Price LH, Rasmussen SA *et al.* (1989) The Yale-Brown Obsessive–Compulsive Scale. I. Development, use, and reliability. *Arch Gen Psychiatr* 46(11) (Nov), 1006–1011.

studies concerning the different procedures suggest a remarkable freedom from significant adverse personality changes. On the contrary, the few studies that have directly addressed this issue report an improvement in negative personality traits at follow-up.

One of the better researched instruments is the Karolinska Scales of Personality (KSP), developed by Schalling and coworkers (1987). The KSP contains subscales measuring traits related to frontal lobe function as well as those reflecting anxiety proneness. In capsulotomy studies reported from Sweden, the KSP was administered to 24 consecutive patients 1 year and 8 years after radiofrequency capsulotomy. Small changes in mean scores towards normalization were apparent on all 15 KSP subscales at the 1-year follow-up and significant improvement was reported in anxiety proneness at the 8-year follow-up (Mindus *et al.*, 1999).

One would expect that the more precise modern surgical procedures should further reduce this risk. In fact most recent studies report a low incidence of adverse behaviors postsurgery. However, this remains a potential risk and conclusions based on observations made on groups of patients may not preclude negative adverse effects in an individual patient.

Suicide

While suicide is not considered a known complication of neurosurgical procedures in nonpsychiatric patients undergoing these procedures, the possibility of contributing directly or indirectly to this process in psychiatric patients is theoretically present. However, it is important to note that severe major depression is associated with high lifetime suicide rates (approximately 3–8%) (Nierenberg *et al.*, 2001). Thus, of the suicides reported in psychiatric neurosurgical cohorts, it is difficult to ascertain whether these are a result of existing psychopathology or whether the surgery contributed in some way to this process.

For example, Jenike and colleagues (1991) found that four of 33 patients who had undergone cingulotomy for OCD had died by suicide at follow-up that averaged 13 years. Chart reviews revealed that each of these suicide completers had been noted to suffer from extensive comorbid disease (especially

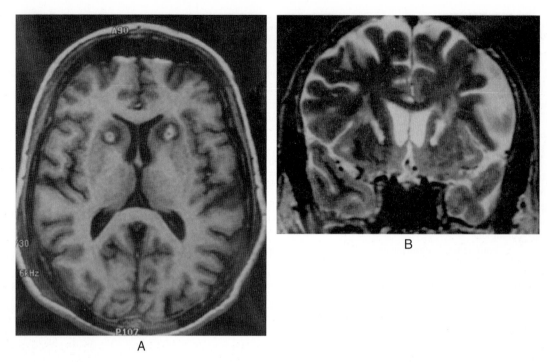

Figure 75.1 *Anterior capsulotomy* (A) *Acute axial view;* (B) *Chronic coronal view.*

severe depression) with prominent suicidal ruminations at initial evaluation for cingulotomy. On the contrary, none of the OCD patients without baseline suicidality became suicidal after the operation. In the large ($n = 44$) prospective long-term follow-up study following one or more cingulotomies, Dougherty and colleagues (2002) reported one suicide (2%) in a patient having severe depression with chronic suicidal ideation and a past history of a suicide attempt. Thus, in most published studies, the suicide rate has been low and these patients have been noted to have had significant presurgical suicidality. This highlights the need

carefully to assess for and monitor suicidality in this severely ill population.

Patients with a poor response to surgery may be at increased risk for suicide (Jenike *et al.*, 1991). Preventative strategies therefore include careful assessment of suicidality at baseline and follow-ups, assessment of family and clinician support networks, clear explanations of the scope of the procedure as well as the long response latency (usually a year for cingulotomy), education that presurgical nonresponders sometimes respond to treatment postsurgery, and the need for secondary or tertiary lesions in case of cingulotomy in some patients to achieve response.

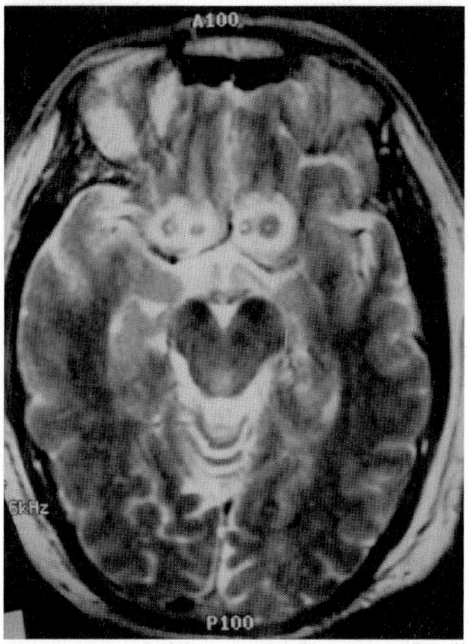

Recent Advances

Neurosurgical Advances and Imaging Strategies

The routine use of MR guided stereotactically placed neurosurgical lesions and the increasing availability of the gamma knife offer more precise procedures with objectively quantifiable lesions. High resolution structural MRI studies are being used to track volumetric changes local and distal to the lesions (Rauch *et al.*, 2000) and PET studies are providing information about blood flow and regional metabolism that may serve as predictors of response (Rauch *et al.*, 2001). Recordings in implicated brain structures such as the cingulum (similar to intracortical recordings and microdialysis in the temporal lobe in surgical epilepsy patients) may provide useful additional information. Strategies such as magnetic resonance spectroscopy (MRS) and newer methods such as diffusion tensor imaging (DT-MRI) can provide information about regional neurochemistry and white matter tract integrity, respectively. They offer the exciting possibility of collecting valuable neurobiological data, which may aid in monitoring changes as well as predicting response.

Figure 75.2 *Subcaudate tractotomy. Acute axial view.*

Newer Strategies

Recently, several new experimental strategies have emerged and are being investigated in refractory OCD and MDD. These are invasive modalities currently being offered only in the context of research studies and thus have not been proven or approved for treatment. They are included in this discussion for the sake of completion.

Deep Brain Stimulation

Deep brain stimulation (DBS) involves stimulation of target regions via stereotactically placed electrodes that can be programmed to deliver low voltage electrical stimulation to modulate transmission of specific brain pathways. While DBS of different regions has been experimentally investigated for treatment-refractory pain syndromes, movement disorders and seizure disorders, only DBS for treatment-refractory Parkinson's disease or essential tremor is currently FDA approved in the USA. Recently following a preliminary report of deep brain stimulation in the anterior limb of the internal capsule in four patients with treatment-refractory OCD (Nuttin et al., 1999), a few specialized centers in the world (including the USA) are conducting ongoing controlled studies of DBS in treatment-refractory OCD patients. Nuttin and colleagues described four patients with treatment-refractory OCD who underwent DBS with bilateral stereotactically implanted quadripolar electrodes in the anterior limb of the internal capsule (instead of anterior capsulotomy) and reported "beneficial effects" in three of the four patients. It is important to note that this remains an experimental procedure at this stage for treatment-refractory OCD. Nevertheless these developments offer the exciting possibility of reversible "lesions" as well as ethically justifiable sham procedures (controls can be implanted but the stimulation not turned on or at lower voltage undetectable by the patient who can subsequently receive the benefit of the treatment) (Greenberg, personal communication).

Vagal Nerve Stimulation

Vagal nerve stimulation, used formerly only as an FDA approved treatment strategy for some patients with drug-resistant, partial-onset epilepsy due to its seizure attenuating effects, has been approved for use in treatment of depression. See the section on new approaches in the chapter on ECT for further discussion of this modality.

Conclusion

A small but significant number of psychiatric patients remain refractory to state-of-the-art treatments and are severely disabled. Based on the existing data, palliative neurosurgery continues to be an option for these patients. The impressive advances in psychiatry as well as stereotactic and radioneurosurgery and neuroimaging have resulted in promising outcomes with a better benefit/risk ratio, suggesting that these options should be further pursued. Improvement of study design as well as improved communication between interested specialized centers is desirable to further advance the field. See Table 75.4 for suggested guidelines. Meanwhile newer, less invasive strategies, such as the gamma knife as well as potentially reversible manipulation of the CNS such as DBS and VNS, have emerged and could potentially change the nature of this field. Until we have data from more sophisticated controlled studies, it is highly recommended that these procedures be carried out only in centers that have the necessary expertise, personnel, and resources to undertake and follow through with such procedures.

Clinical Vignette 1

JS, a 44-year-old, single, Caucasian male, living on a disability income in a semi-independent living facility, was referred for neurosurgical evaluation by his treating psychiatrist. He was first diagnosed to have OCD when he was a 20-year-old sophomore in college and has suffered a progressively deteriorating course despite treatment, leading to his being unable to work as well as care for himself adequately, over the past 10 years. He had failed adequate trials of treatments including fluoxetine, sertraline and clomipramine as well as multiple courses of exposure and response prevention, including long-term intensive residential treatments. His most disabling symptoms have been his fear of contamination and related washing and checking compulsions. He spends most of his day locked in his room engaged in repeatedly washing and showering and often has to be supervised by his family (who live close by) to feed and groom himself. This has taken a significant toll on his family who have constantly to monitor his progress. John has also suffered from several depressive episodes, is chronically dysthymic, and has attempted suicide in the past due to feeling hopeless about his situation.

At the specialized center, a psychiatrist with experience in presurgical evaluations evaluated John. He also underwent neuropsychological and psychosocial evaluations and a medical fitness examination. His case was then discussed by a panel of experts at the institutional level to review his eligibility for anterior cingulotomy. After informed consent from John and his family, he underwent a magnetic resonance guided, stereotactic, bilateral anterior cingulotomy. The immediate postsurgical period was notable for some transient confusion and urinary incontinence. After recovery, John was referred back to his psychiatrist and his medications were continued. At the 3-month follow-up, John did not report any change in his symptoms. At the 6-month and 1-year follow-ups, however, John and his family reported that the frequency of "getting stuck" in his washroom had observably reduced. He still reported contamination obsessions but with less frequency and severity. When they did occur, he was able to "unstick" himself with less difficulty. His mood and self-care was better and he had begun to socialize more. He was considering participating in a day program at the facility. His psychiatrist corroborated these reports.

References

Baer L, Rauch SL, Ballantine HT Jr. et al. (1995) Cingulotomy for treatment refractory obsessive–compulsive disorder: Prospective long-term follow-up of 18 patients. Arch Gen Psychiatr 52, 384–392.

Bartlett JR and Bridges PK (1977) The extended subcaudate tractotomy lesion, in Neurosurgical Treatment in Psychiatry, Pain and Epilepsy (eds Sweet W, Obrador S, and Martin-Rodriguez JG). University Park Press, Baltimore, p. 387.

Bingley T, Leksell L, Meyerson BA et al. (1977) Long term results of stereotactic capsulotomy in chronic obsessive–compulsive neurosis, in Neurosurgical Treatment in Psychiatry, Pain and Epilepsy (eds Sweet W, Obrador S, and Martin-Rodriguez JG). University Park Press, Baltimore, p. 287.

Bridges PK, Goktepe EO and Maratos J (1973) A comparative review of patients with obsessional neurosis and with depression treated by psychosurgery. *Br J Psychiatr* 123(577) (Dec), 663–674.

Chiocca EA and Martuza RL (1990) Neurosurgical therapy of obsessive–compulsive disorder, in *Obsessive–Compulsive Disorders: Theory and Management* (eds Jenike MA, Baer L, and Minichiello WE). Year Book Medical Publishers, Chicago, p. 283.

Corkin S (1980) A prospective study of cingulotomy, in *The Psychosurgery Debate* (ed Valenstein ES). WH Freeman, San Francisco, p. 264.

Corkin S, Twitchell TE and Sullivan EV (1979) Safety and efficacy of cingulotomy for pain and psychiatric disorder, in *Modern Concepts in Psychiatric Surgery* (eds Hitchcock ER, Ballantine HT and Myerson BA). Elsevier/North Holland, New York, pp. 253–272.

Dougherty DD, Baer L, Cosgrove GR *et al.* (2002) Prospective long-term follow-up of 44 patients who received cingulotomy for treatment-refractory obsessive–compulsive disorder. *Am J Psychiatr* 159(2) (Feb), 269–275.

Göktepe EO, Young LB and Bridges PK (1975) A further review of the results of stereotactic subcaudate tractotomy. *Br J Psychiatr* 126, 270.

Herner T (1961) Treatment of mental disorders with frontal stereotactic thermo-lesions. A follow-up of 116 cases. *Acta Psychiatr Scand* 36(Suppl) 158, 1–140.

Hodgkiss AD, Malizia AL, Bartlett JR *et al.* (1995) Outcome after the psychosurgical operation of stereotactic subcaudate tractotomy, 1979–1991. *J Neuropsychiatr Clin Neurosci* 7(2) (Spring), 230–234.

Jenike MA, Baer L, Ballantine HT *et al.* (1991) Cingulotomy for refractory obsessive–compulsive disorder. A long-term follow-up of 33 patients. *Arch Gen Psychiatr* 48, 548–555.

Kelly D (1980) *Anxiety and Emotions. Physiological Basis and Treatment.* Charles C Thomas, Springfield, IL.

Mindus P, Edman G and Andreewitch S (1999) A prospective, long-term study of personality traits in patients with intractable obsessional illness treated by capsulotomy. *Acta Psychiatr Scand* 99(1) (Jan), 40–50.

Mitchell-Heggs N, Kelly D and Richardson A (1976) Stereotactic limbic leucotomy—a follow-up at 16 months. *Br J Psychiatr* 128, 226–240.

Nierenberg AA, Gray SM and Grandin LD (2001) Mood disorders and suicide. *J Clin Psychiatr* 62(Suppl 25), 27–30.

Nuttin B, Cosyns P, Demeulemeester H *et al.* (1999) Electrical stimulation in anterior limbs of internal capsules in patients with obsessive–compulsive disorder. *Lancet* 354(9189) (Oct 30), 1526.

Rauch SL, Kim H, Makris N *et al.* (2000) Volume reduction in the caudate nucleus following stereotactic placement of lesions in the anterior cingulate cortex in humans: A morphometric magnetic resonance imaging study. *J Neurosurg* 93(6) (Dec), 1019–1025.

Rauch SL, Dougherty DD, Cosgrove GR *et al.* (2001) Cerebral metabolic correlates as potential predictors of response to anterior cingulotomy for obsessive–compulsive disorder. *Biol Psychiatr* 50(9) (Nov 1), 659–667.

Schalling D, Åsberg M, Edman G *et al.* (1987) Markers of vulnerability to psychopathy: Temperament traits associated with platelet MAO activity. *Acta Psychiatr Scand* 16, 172.

Vasko T and Kullberg G (1979) Results of psychological testing of cognitive functions in patients undergoing stereotactic psychiatric surgery, in *Modern Concepts in Psychiatric Surgery* (eds Hitchcock ER, Ballantine HT Jr. and Meyerson BA). Elsevier/North Holland Biomedical Press, Amsterdam, p. 303.

Waziri R (1990) Psychosurgery for anxiety and obsessive–compulsive disorders, in *Handbook of Anxiety. Treatment of Anxiety* (eds Noyes R Jr., Roth M and Burrows GD). Elsevier Science, Amsterdam.

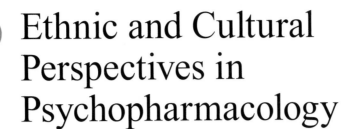

Ethnic and Cultural Perspectives in Psychopharmacology

Dispelling the "Color Blind" Approach

Substantial individual variation in drug responses, at times up to 100-fold in terms of optimal dosing, is the rule rather than the exception. Although the current understanding of such remarkable variability remains incomplete, it is clear that the interplay between genetics and environmental factors plays a pivotal role in pharmacotherapeutic responses, particularly in the context of an individual's ethnic origin, lifestyle and other socio-demographic variables.

As shown in Figure 76.1, virtually all factors affecting pharmacological responses are significantly influenced by culture and ethnicity. Furthermore, patterns of genetic polymorphism, often with substantial ethnic variation, exist in a large number of genes encoding drug metabolizing enzymes as well as receptors and transporters believed to be targets of pharmaceutical agents. The expression of these genes is often significantly modified by a large number of environmental factors, including diet and exposure to various substances (e.g., tobacco). Of even greater importance, the success of any therapy, including pharmacotherapy, depends on the participation of the patient and, as such, depends significantly on the quality of interaction between the clinician and the patient. The importance of culture in this regard is paramount.

Clinicians' Attitudes

A large body of literature indicates that patients' cultural/ethnic backgrounds significantly determine the way clinicians conceptualize and label their problems, which in turn dictate the choices for therapeutic intervention (Mezzich *et al.*, 1995). Using case vignettes that are identical except for ethnic group identification, a number of studies demonstrated that cases identical in every other aspect were nevertheless given significantly more severe diagnoses if the patients were identified as being of ethnic minority origin (Gaw, 1993; Lopez, 1989). Paralleling such a tendency, African-American psychiatric patients are more likely to have been given a diagnosis of schizophrenia as compared with their Caucasian counterparts (Littlewood, 1992; Lopez, 1989). Interestingly, in studies where patients were reassessed with the use of structured interviews, such differences largely disappeared, suggesting that such a differential diagnostic pattern is possibly determined by variables related to clinicians' biases rather than to the patients' clinical conditions (Adebimpe, 1981; Marquez *et al.*, 1985; Mukherjee *et al.*, 1983; Roukema *et al.*, 1984).

Adherence

Most studies exploring correlates of nonadherence have focused on patient and treatment variables, and have shown that a large number of factors significantly predict problems with adherence. These include the sociodemographics of the patient, the financial burden of the treatment, and the side effect profile of the medications (Manne, 1998; Fenton *et al.*, 1997). The health belief model has served as the theoretical framework for a large number of seminal research endeavors, which in aggregate demonstrate that the beliefs held by patients and those significant in their lives to a large extent determine their participation in and response to treatment decisions (Hughes *et al.*, 1997).

Following the logic of the health belief model, one would expect adherence to be an even larger problem in cross-cultural clinical situations. This has been substantiated by a number of clinical observations and reports of the service utilization of particular ethnic minority groups (Sue *et al.*, 1991). Compared with Caucasians, ethnic minority patients are often found to enter treatment at a significantly delayed stage, and they also are more likely to drop out of psychiatric treatment prematurely. Programs aiming at bridging cultural gaps have been shown significantly to improve treatment retention and outcome (Acosta *et al.*, 1982).

Adverse effects of psychotropics are often substantial. Depending on beliefs and expectations, many positive drug effects could be interpreted either as negative or positive. For example, in a study of Hong Kong Chinese bipolar patients treated with lithium, Lee and colleagues (1992) found that, unlike Western patients, the Chinese rarely complained of "missing the highs", and "loss of creativity" and actually regarded polydipsia, polyuria and weight gain as part of the therapeutic effect of the medicine. In contrast, lethargy, drowsiness and poor memory represented serious concerns for many of these patients, and were prominent in their complaints, even though objectively they were not likely to be due to the medications they were taking, since they occurred at similar rates among matched controls. Such findings highlight the importance of culturally based beliefs and expectations in determining how physical and psychological experiences associated with drug treatment and recovery are attributed.

The Explanatory Model (EM) approach, as originally proposed by Kleinman (1988), may be a particularly effective way for the systematic assessment of such beliefs and expectations. By

Essentials of Psychiatry   Jerald Kay and Allan Tasman
© 2006 John Wiley & Sons, Ltd.

937

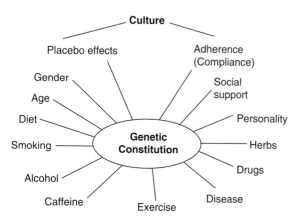

Figure 76.1 *Factors affecting drug response.*

methodically eliciting the patient's perspectives on the symptoms that are most salient and worrisome to them (patterns of distress), their attributions (perceived causes), their help-seeking experiences and preference, as well as their perception on stigma, discrepancy between the patients' and the professionals' EMs could be systematically identified and bridged (Weiss, 1997). Elements of the EM are included in Appendix I of the DSM-IV manual as part of the Outline for Cultural Formulation (American Psychiatric Association, 1994).

Expectation ("Placebo") Effects

The term "expectations effect" reflects the importance and power of expectation and beliefs on treatment effects in determining patients' response to any therapy, whether psychosocial or pharmacological. Expectations regarding the safety and effectiveness of any therapeutic interventions, in turn, are shaped by patients' sociocultural backgrounds as well as individual "idiosyncratic" experiences (e.g., past experiences of side effects). Since patients' beliefs regarding medical treatments are often shaped by their cultural backgrounds, it stands to reason that patients' expectation regarding the therapeutic effect of the offered treatment would be largely affected by their cultural construct of the illness.

Despite rapid modernization, traditional medical theories and practices remain deeply rooted and influential in determining individuals' health beliefs and behaviors in many societies (Wolffers, 1989; Okpaku, 1998; Wig, 1989; Rappaport, 1977). For example, most traditional medical systems emphasize the importance of maintaining a dynamic balance between "coldness" and "hotness" (Castro *et al.*, 1994) or between "Yin" and "Yang" in the case of the Chinese system (Lin, 1981). These principles provide guidance for assessment as well as for formulating treatment approaches. For patients who subscribe to such beliefs, a perceived mismatch between the therapeutic agents and the afflictions may significantly lower the expectation effect. For example, red-colored pills might be regarded as capable of enhancing the "hot" element, and might be regarded as less effective in the treatment of conditions perceived as a result of excessive "hotness" (e.g., fever, anxiety state, or mania). Interestingly, Buckalew and Coffield (1982) reported findings from a well-controlled study showing significant ethnic differences in response to placebo pills with different colors.

The Concomitant Use of Alternative/ Indigenous Treatment and Healing Methods

"Alternative" health care traditions (e.g., Chinese medicine and Ayurvedic medicine) seemed to have responded well to challenges of modern medicines and have continued to evolve and thrive (Landy, 1977; Leslie, 1976). Multiple medical and healing traditions and treatment modalities coexist in all societies, and patients often utilize these services simultaneously or sequentially, frequently without informing their physicians. Problems with drug–drug interactions from such behavior that could potentially arise from such a practice are not limited to particular ethnic groups, and constitute an important consideration for clinicians prescribing medications.

Various herbs utilized by traditional practitioners and healers are biologically active (it has been estimated that approximately 40% of our "modern" pharmacotherapeutic agents originated from natural sources [Balick and Cox, 1996]). Although much remains unclear, herbal preparations do exert significant impact on various biological systems, including those crucial for the functioning of the central nervous system (Cott, 1997; Duke, 1995). Since most patients do not regard herbs as medicines and typically fail to inform their physicians of such uses unless specifically inquired, toxicities or treatment failures due to "herb–drug interactions" are likely widespread and unsuspected. Herbal preparations may modulate the effect of modern therapeutic agents, including psychotropics, both at the pharmacodynamic level (the effect of the drugs on the organism), and at the pharmacokinetic level.

Biological Diversity and Its Consequence in Psychotropic Responses

Emerging data now convincingly demonstrate that for the majority of the genes, polymorphism is the rule rather than the exception. Furthermore, the frequency and distribution of alleles responsible for such polymorphisms often vary substantially across ethnic groups, effectively requiring that ethnicity always be considered in genetic studies (National Institute of Mental Health, 1997). These phenomena have long been known in blood and human lymphocyte antigen (HLA) typing (Polednak, 1989). In recent years, it has become increasingly clear that equally extensive polymorphisms exist in genes governing key aspects of how drugs are metabolized (see Table 76.1) as well as how they affect the target organs. These processes, commonly called pharmacokinetics and pharmacodynamics, are depicted in Figure 76.2 (Greenblatt, 1993). Together, these genetic factors may explain to a large extent the often extensive inter-individual cross-ethnic variations in drug responses (Kalow, 1992; Lin *et al.*, 1993).

Genetic Polymorphism of Genes Encoding "Drug-metabolizing Enzymes": The Cytochrome P-450 System

As shown in Figure 76.2, of the four factors (absorption, distribution, metabolism and excretion) that together determine the fate and disposition of most drugs, variability in the process of metabolism is most substantial and usually is the reason for inter-individual and cross-ethnic variation in drug responses (Lin and Poland, 1995). Most drugs are metabolized via two phases: Phase I, commonly mediated by one or more of the cytochrome

Table 76.1	Genetically Variable Enzymes of Drug Metabolism
*Alcohol dehydrogenase (ADH)	Dopamine β-hydroxylase
*Aldehyde dehydrogenase (ALDH)	Dihydropyrimidine dehydrogenase
Butyryl cholinersterase	*Glucuronyl transferase (UDPGT)
Catalase	*Glutathione-S-transferase (class mu)
*Catechol-O-methyltransferase (COMT)	Monoamine oxidase
CYP1A2	*N-Acetyl transferase (NAT2)
*CYP2A6	*Phenol sulfotransferase
*CYP2C19	*Serum paroxanase/ arylesterase
CYP2D6	Superoxide dismutase
*CYP2E1	*Thiol methyltransferase
*CYP3A4	*Thiopurine methyltransferase

*Indicates polymorphic variation.
Adapted from Kalow W (1992) *Pharmacogenetics of Drug Metabolism*. Pergamon Press, New York; Lin KM and Poland RE (1995) *Ethnicity, Culture, and Psychopharmacology in Psychopharmacology: The Fourth Generation of Progress* (eds Bloom FE and Kupfer DI). Raven Press, New York.

as well as selected substances that are psychoactive and are commonly used by psychiatric patients.

Functionally significant genetic polymorphisms exist in most of the CYPs (Lin and Poland, 1995), leading to extremely large variations in the activity of these enzymes in any given population (Table 76.2). CYP2D6 represents the most dramatic example, with more than 20 mutations that inactivate, impair, or accelerate its function (Daly *et al.*, 1996). Significantly, most of these mutant alleles are to a large extent ethnically specific. For example, CYP2D6*4, which leads to the production of defective proteins, is found in approximately 25% of Caucasians, but is rarely identified in other ethnic groups. This mutation is mainly responsible for the poor metabolizers (PM) in Caucasians (5–9%), who are extremely sensitive to drugs metabolized by CYP2D6. Instead of CYP2D6*4, extremely high frequencies of CYP2D6*17 (Leathart *et al.*, 1998, Masimirembwa and Hasler, 1997) and CYP2D6*10 (Wang *et al.*, 1993; Dahl *et al.*, 1995; Roh *et al.*, 1996) were found among those of African and Asian origins, respectively. Both of these alleles are associated with lower enzyme activities and slower metabolism of CYP2D6 substrates (Figure 76.3), and may be in part responsible for previous findings of slower pharmacokinetic profiles and lower therapeutic dose ranges observed in Asians in regard to both classes of psychotropics, and in African-Americans in regard to tricyclic antidepressants (Lin and Poland, 1995).

Genetic polymorphism also exists in CYP2C19, CYP2C9, CYP2E1, CYP3A4 as well as the majority of other drug metabolizing enzymes. It is interesting to note that, almost without exception, wherever genetic polymorphism is identified, the allele frequency of the mutations typically show substantial ethnic variations (Stephens *et al.*, 1994; Gill *et al.*, 1999; Kidd *et al.*, 1999).

Patients from different ethnic/cultural backgrounds live divergent lifestyles, and are likely to be exposed to unique substances that may have strong effects on the expression and activity of drug metabolizing enzymes. Thus, what we currently know about environmental influences on drug metabolism may represent only the tip of the iceberg. This may be especially true in regard to ethnic minority and other nonWestern populations.

P-450 enzymes (CYPs), leads to the oxidation of the substrate; Phase II involves conjugation and is usually mediated by one of the transferases. There is clear evidence of inter-individual and cross-ethnic variations in the activity of enzymes in both phases, the genetic basis of which has been increasingly elucidated in recent years (Kalow, 1992; Weber, 1997).

Table 76.2 includes a list of major CYPs that are responsible for the Phase I metabolism of commonly used psychotropics

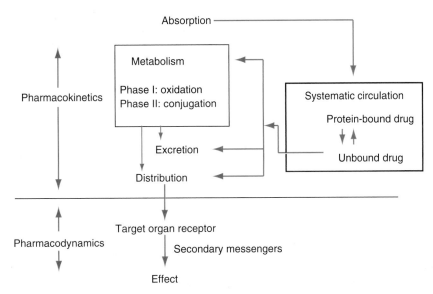

Figure 76.2 *Pharmacokinetics and pharmacodynamics.*

Table 76.2   Major Human Cytochrome P-450 Enzymes and Their Psychotropic Substrates

	Substrates	Genetic Polymorphisms
CYP1A2	Antidepressants: amitriptyline, clomipramine, imipramine, fluvoxamine	No report of polymorphism until 1999; the significance of the following findings remain unclear (Nakajima, 1999)
	Neuroleptics: haloperidol, phenothiazines, thiothixine, clozapine, olanzapine	*1C: reduced activity; 23% in Japanese
	Others: tacrine, caffeine, theophylline, acetominophen, phenacetin	*1F: higher inducibility; 32% in Caucasians
CYP2C19	Benzodiazepines: diazepam	*2: no activity; 23–39% in Asians; 13% in Caucasians; 25% in African-Americans
	Antidepressants: imipramine, amitriptyline, clomipramine, citalopram	*3: no activity; 6–10% in Asians; 0% in others
	Others: propranolol, hexobarbital, mephobarbital, proguanil, omeprazole, S-mephenytoin	*6 *7 and *8 contain mutations that result in the poor metabolizer phenotype in Caucasians (Ibeanu, 1998, 1999)
CYP2D6	Antidepressants: amitriptyline, clomipramine, imipramine, desipramine, nortriptyline, trimipramine, N-desmethyl-clomipramine, fluoxetine, norfluoxetine, paroxetine, venlafaxine, seltraline	*2: accounts for 60% of intermediate metabolizers in Caucasians (Raimundo, 2000).
	Neuroleptics: chlorpromazine, thioridazine, perphenazine, haloperidol, reduced haloperidol, risperidone, clozapine, sertindole	*3: no activity; 1% in Caucasians (Shimada, 2001) *4: no activity; 25% in Caucasians; 0–10% in others
	Others: codeine, opiate, propranolol, dextromethorphan	*5: no activity; 2–10% in all groups
		*10: reduced activity; 47–70% in Asians, ≤5% in others (Mendoza, 2001)
		*17: reduced activity; 25–40% in blacks, 0% in others (Wan, 2001)
		*2XN: increased activity; 19–29% in Arabs and Ethiopians; ≤5% in others
CYP3A4	Antidepressants: mirtazepine, nefazadone, sertraline	Several single nucleotide polymorphisms have been identified with racial variability in their frequency. However, functional significance of these polymorphisms have not been clearly elucidated (Dai et al., 2001)
	Neuroleptics: thioridazine, haloperidol, clozapine, quetiapine, risperidone, sertindole, ziprasidone	
	Mood stabilizers: carbamazepine, gabapentin, lamotrigine	Recent reports of the functional significance of a variant with mutation in the regulatory region (*1B) has been suggested. The prevalence of *1B is 10% in Caucasians, and unknown in other ethnic groups.
	Benzodiazepines: alprazolam, clonazepam, diazepam, midazolam, triazolam, zolpidem	
	Calcium channel blockers: diltiazem, nifedipine, nimodipine, verapamil	
	Steroids: androgens, estrogens, cortisol	
	Others: erthyromycin, terfenadine, cyclosporine, dapsone, ketaconazole, lovastatin, lidocaine, alfentanil, amiodarone, astemiazole, codeine, sildenafil	There are preliminary reports of two other promising alleles (*2 and *3), but details of these mutations are not yet available.
		*4, *5, *6 have been suggested to possibly decrease 3A4 activity in Chinese subjects but the incidences of these mutations are rare and their prevalence in other ethnic groups is unknown (Hsieh, 2001)

Other important human CYPs include CYP2A6, CYP2B6, CYP2C8, CYP2C9, and CYP2E1. CYP2A6 is involved in the metabolism of nicotine and cotinine, CYP2C9 is responsible for the biotransformation of drugs including phenytoin and warfarin, CYP2E1 metabolizes acetaminophen, theophylline as well as alcohol and is associated with the production of free radicals.

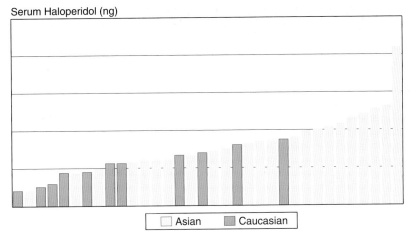

Figure 76.3   *Variability of haloperidol concentrations in normal volunteers after the administration of haloperidol (0.5 mg, IM). The graph shows: 1) substantial interindividual variability within each of the ethnic groups; 2) dramatic differences in the pharmacokinetics of haloperidol between the two ethnic groups; and 3) overlap of the pharmacokinetics between the two groups. (Source: Lin KM, Poland RE, Lan JK et al. [1988] Haloperidol and prolactin concentrations in Asians and Cancasians. J Clin Psychopharmacol 8, 195–201.)*

For example, studies have shown that Asian Indians and Africans were significantly slower in metabolizing substrates of CYP1A2, such as theophylline, antipyrine and clomipramine. However, after they immigrated to Europe and adapted to the new dietary habits, their metabolic profiles for these drugs became indistinguishable from the "native" Westerner's (Allen *et al.*, 1977).

Genetic Polymorphism of Genes Encoding Receptors, Transporters, or Other Therapeutic Targets

Along with the cloning and sequencing of the genes encoding the receptors and transporters that mediate and regulate the function of important neurotransmitters, it has become apparent that, contrary to earlier predictions (Kalow, 1990), these genes are almost without exception highly polymorphic, and the pattern of these polymorphisms vary significantly across ethnicity (Gelenter *et al.*, 1997; Goldman *et al.*, 1996; Hodge, 1994; Dean *et al.*, 1994; Chang *et al.*, 1996). For example, the frequency of the TaqI A RFLP polymorphism of the dopamine D_2 receptor (DRD2), one of the most extensively investigated brain receptors, ranges from 5 to 18% in Caucasians to approximately 36% in African-Americans and 37 to 42% in Asians (Blum *et al.*, 1995). Similarly, dramatic ethnic variations exist in the pattern of genetic polymorphism of many other receptor and transporter genes. These include other DRD2 mutations (Taql B, 311Ser/Cys and exon 8 A/G substitution), other dopamine receptors such as DRD4 and DRD3 (Parsian *et al.*, 1999; Sander *et al.*, 1995; Sullivan *et al.*, 1998), the dopamine transporter gene (DAT1; locus symbol SLC6A3) (Vandenbergh *et al.*, 1992), the serotonin transporter gene (5-HTT), and a number of serotonin receptors (5-HT$_{2A}$-1438 A/G and 5-HT$_{2A}$-102 T/C) (Greenberg *et al.*, 1998; Smeraldi *et al.*, 1998; Michaelovsky *et al.*, 1999).

These polymorphisms may have functional significance and hence might be associated with the risk for psychopathology as well as the response to treatment regimens. We await further research to confirm this possibility.

Summary

This brief discussion serves to highlight the significance as well as the complexity of issues surrounding the influence of cultural and ethnic forces on psychotropic responses. At the same time, it is equally important that any findings regarding ethnic variations in pharmacological responses not be interpreted stereotypically. In this regard, it is useful to keep in mind that almost all ethnic and cultural contrasts are superimposed on usually very substantial inter-individual variations in all human groups. This is true not only in regard to biological traits such as the ones reviewed above, but equally so (or even more so) with regard to "cultural" and psychosocial variables. Stereotypic interpretations of cultural and ethnic differences in either psychological or biological characteristics are not only misleading but also potentially divisive and dangerous.

Further, in interpreting biological diversity, both within and across populations, it is important to keep in mind that biological systems are dynamic rather than static, and the expression of genetic predisposition is constantly modified by environmental exposure. Although it is reasonable to believe that social and psychological events would similarly exert powerful influences on the functioning of relevant genes, such influences are likely to be subtle and complex, and have remained largely unexplored.

Future progress in pharmacogenetics might stimulate research on "nonbiological" issues such as cultural influences on adherence and other factors that determine patients' perception and help-seeking behavior, which in turn contribute toward their sense of satisfaction and their being able maximally to benefit from psychotropic treatment. With such an integrative approach, we would be best able to define elements for optimal pharmacotherapeutic practices that would take both cultural and biological diversity into consideration and tailor treatment to individual characteristics rather than relying on global guidelines.

References

Acosta FX, Yamamoto J and Evans LA (1982) *Effective Psychotherapy for Low-Income and Minority Patients.* Plenum Press, New York.

Adebimpe VR (1981) Overview: White norms and psychiatric diagnosis of Black patients. *Am J Psychiatr* 138, 279–285.

Allen JG, Rack P and Vaddadi K (1977) Differences in the effects of clomipramine on English and Asian volunteers: Preliminary report on a pilot study. *Postgrad Med J* 53, 79–86.

American Psychiatric Association (1994) *Diagnostic and Statistical Manual of Mental Disorders*, 4th edn. APA, Washington, DC.

Balick MJ and Cox PA (1996) *Plants, People, and Culture: The Science of Ethnobotany*. Scientific American Library, New York.

Blum K, Sheridan PJ, Wood RC *et al.* (1995) Dopamine D$_2$ receptor gene variants: Association and linkage studies in impulsive–addictive–compulsive behaviour. *Pharmacogenetics* 5, 121–141.

Buckalew LW and Coffield K (1982) Drug expectations associated with perceptual characteristics: Ethnic factors. *Percept Motor Skills* 55, 915–918.

Castro, FG, Furth P and Karlow H (1994) The health beliefs of Mexican, Mexican-American and Anglo-American women. *Hispanic J Behav Sci* 6, 365–383.

Chang FM, Kidd JR, Livak KJ *et al.* (1996) The world-wide distribution of allele frequencies at the human dopamine D$_4$ receptor locus. *Hum Genet* 98, 91–101.

Cott JM (1997) *In vitro* receptor binding and enzyme inhibition by hypericum perforatum extract. *Pharmacopsychiatry* 30, 108–112.

Dahl ML, Yue QY, Roh HK *et al.* (1995) Genetic analysis of the CYP2D locus in relation to debrisoquine hydroxylation capacity in Korean, Japanese and Chinese subjects. *Pharmacogenetics* 5, 159–164.

Dai D, Tang J, Rose R, *et al.* (2001) Identification of variants of CYP3A4 and characterization of their abilities to metabolize testosterone and chlorpyrifos. *J Pharmacol Exp Ther* 299(3), 825–831.

Daly AK, Brockmoller J, Broly F *et al.* (1996) Nomenclature for human CYP2D6 alleles. *Pharmacogenetics* 6, 193–201.

Dean M, Stephens JC, Winkler C *et al.* (1994) Polymorphic admixture typing in human ethnic populations. *Am J Hum Genet* 55, 788–808.

Duke JA (1995) Commentary – novel psychotherapeutic drugs: A role for ethnobotany. *Psychopharmacol Bull* 31, 177–184.

Fenton WS, Blyler CR and Heinssen RK (1997) Determinants of medication compliance in schizophrenia: Empirical and clinical findings. *Schizophr Bull* 23, 637–651.

Gaw A (1993) *Culture, Ethnicity, and Mental Illness*. American Psychiatric Press, Washington DC.

Gelenter J, Kranzler H, Cubells JF *et al.* (1997) Serotonin transporter protein (SLC6A4) allele and haplotype frequencies and linkage disequilibria in African- and European-American and Japanese populations in alcohol-dependent subjects. *Hum Genet* 101, 243–246.

Gill HJ, Tijia JF, Kitteringham NR *et al.* (1999) The effect of genetic polymorphisms in CYP2C9 on suphamethoxazole N-hydroxylation. *Pharmacogenetics* 9, 43–53.

Goldman D, Lappalainen J and Ozaki N (1996) Direct analysis of candidate genes in impulsive behaviors. *Ceiba Found Sump* 194, 139–152.

Greenberg BD, McMahon FJ and Murphy DL (1998) Serotonin transporter candidate gene studies in affective disorders and personality: Promises and potential pitfalls. Guest Editorial. *Mol Psychiatr* 3, 186–189.

Greenblatt DJ (1993) Basic phamacokinetic principles and their application to psychotropic drugs. *J Clin Psychiatr* 54, 8–13.

Hodge SE (1994) What association analysis can and cannot tell us about the genetics of complex disease. *Am J Med Genet* 54, 318–323.

Hsieh KP, Lin YY, Cheng CL, *et al.* (2001) Novel mutations of CYP3A4 in Chinese. *Drug Metab Dispos* 29(3), 268–273.

Hughes JB, Daily GC and Ehrlich PR (1997) Population diversity: Its extent and extinction. *Science* 278, 689–692.

Ibeanu GC, Blaisdell J, Ferguson RJ, *et al.* (1999) A novel transversion in the intron 5 donor splice junction of CYP2C19 and a sequence polymorphism in exon 3 contribute to the poor metabolizer phenotype for the anticonvulsant drug S-mephenytoin. *J Pharmacol Exp Ther* 290(2), 635–640.

Ibeanu GC, Goldstein JA, Meyer U, *et al.* (1998) Identification of new human CYP2C19 alleles (CYP2C19&6 and CYP2C19*2B) in a Caucasian poor metabolizer of mephenytoin. *J Pharmacol Exp Ther* 286(3), 1490–1495.

Kalow W (1990) Pharmacogenetics: Past and future. *Life Sci* 47, 1385–1397.

Kalow W (1992) *Pharmacogenetics of Drug Metabolism*. Pergamon Press, New York.

Kidd RS, Straughn AB, Meyer MC *et al.* (1999) Pharmacokinetics of chlorpheniramine, phenytoin, glipizide and nifedipine in an individual homozygous for the CYP2C9*3 allele. *Pharmacogenetics* 9, 71–80.

Kleinman A (1988) *Rethinking Psychiatry*. Free Press, New York.

Landy D (1977) *Culture, Disease, and Healing*. Macmillan, New York.

Leathart JB, London SJ, Steward A *et al.* (1998) CYP2D6 phenotype-genotype relationships in African-Americans and Caucasians in Los Angeles. *Pharmacogenetics* 8, 529–541.

Lee S, Wing YK and Wong KC (1992) Knowledge and compliance towards lithium therapy among Chinese psychiatric patients in Hong Kong. *Aust NZ J Psychiatr* 26, 444–449.

Leslie C (1976) *Asian Medical Systems: A Comparative Study*. University of California Press, Berkeley, CA.

Lin KM (1981) Traditional Chinese medical beliefs and their relevance for mental illness and psychiatry, in *Normal and Abnormal Behavior in Chinese Culture* (eds Kleinman S and Lin TY). Dordrecht, Boston, Reidel, Hingham, MA.

Lin KM and Poland RE (1995) *Ethnicity, Culture, and Psychopharmacology in Psychopharmacology: The Fourth Generation of Progress* (eds Bloom FE and Kupfer DI). Raven Press, New York.

Lin KM, Poland RE and Nakasaki G (1993) *Psychopharmacology and Psychobiology of Ethnicity*. American Psychiatric Press, Washington DC.

Littlewood R (1992) Psychiatric diagnosis and racial bias: Empirical and interpretative approaches. *Soc Sci Med* 34, 141–149.

Lopez SR (1989) Patient variable biases in clinical judgment: Conceptual overview and methodological considerations. *Psychol Bull* 106, 184–203.

Manne SL (1998) Treatment adherence and compliance, in *Handbook of Pediatric Psychology and Psychiatric, Vol. 2: Disease, Injury, and Illness*. Allyn & Bacon, Boston, MA.

Marquez C, Taintor Z and Schwartz MA (1985) Diagnosis of manic depressive illness in Blacks. *Compr Psychiatr* 26, 337–341.

Masimirembwa CM and Hasler JA (1997) Genetic polymorphism of drug metabolising enzymes in African populations: Implications for the use of neuroleptics and antidepressants. *Brain Res Bull* 44, 561–571.

Mendoza, R, Wan JJY, Poland RE, *et al.* (2001) CYP2D6 polymorphism in a Mexican American population. *Clin Pharmacol Therap* 70(6), 552–560.

Mezzich JE, Kleinman A, Fabrega H *et al.* (1995) *Culture and Psychiatric Diagnosis*. American Psychiatric Press, Washington DC.

Michaelovsky E, Frisch A, Rockah R *et al.* (1999) A novel allele in the promoter region of the human serotonin transporter gene. *Mol Psychiatr* 4, 97–99.

Mukherjee S, Shukla S, Woodle J *et al.* (1983) Misdiagnosis of schizophrenia in bipolar patients: A multiethnic comparison. *Am J Psychiatr* 140, 1571–1574.

Nakajima M, Yodoi T, Mizutani M, *et al.* (1999) Genetic polymorphism in the 5′-flanking region of human CYP1A2 gene: Effect on the CYP1A2 inducibility in humans. *J Biochem* (Tokyo) 125(4), 803–808.

National Institute of Mental Health (1997) *Genetics and Mental Disorders: Report of the National Institute of Health's Genetics Workgroup.* www.nimh.nih.gov/research/genetics.htm.

Okpaku SO (1998) *Clinical Methods in Transcultural Psychiatry*. American Psychiatric Press, Washington, DC.

Parsian A, Chakraverty S, Fisher L *et al.* (1999) No association between polymorphisms in the human dopamine D$_3$ and D$_4$ receptors genes and alcoholism. *Am J Med Genet* 74, 281–285.

Polednak A (1989) *Racial and Ethnic Differences in Disease*. Oxford University Press, New York.

Raimundo S, Fischer J, Eischelbaum M, *et al.* (2000) Elucidation of the genetic basis of the common 'intermediate metabolizer' phenotype for drug oxidation by CYP2D6. *Pharmacogenetics* 10(7), 577–581.

Rappaport H (1977) The tenacity of folk psychotherapy: A functional interpretation. *Soc Psychiatr* 12(3), 127–132.

Roh HK, Dahl ML, Johansson I *et al.* (1996) Debrisoquine and S-mephenytoin hydroxylation phenotypes and genotypes in a Korean population. *Pharmacogenetics* 6, 441–447.

Roukema R, Fadem BH, James B *et al.* (1984) Bipolar disorder in a low socioeconomic population: Difficulties in diagnosis. *J Nerv Ment Dis* 72, 76–79.

Sander T, Harms H, Podschus J *et al.* (1995) Dopamine D$_1$, D$_2$ and D$_3$ receptor genes in alcohol dependence. *Psychiatr Genet* 5, 171–176.

Shimada T, Tsumura F, Yamazaki H, et al. (2001) Characterization of (+/−)-bufuralol hydroxylation activities in liver microsomes of Japanese and Caucasian subjects genotyped for CYP2D6. *Pharmacogenetics* 1(2), 143–156.

Smeraldi E, Zanardi R, Benedetti F *et al.* (1998) Polymorphism within the promoter of the serotonin transporter gene and antidepressant efficacy of fluvoxamine. *Mol Psychiatr* 3, 508–511.

Stephens EA, Taylor JA, Yang CH *et al.* (1994) Ethnic variation in the CYP2E1 gene: Polymorphism analysis of 695 African-Americans, European-Americans and Taiwanese. *Pharmacogenetics* 4, 185–192.

Sue S, Fujino DC, Hu LT *et al.* (1991) Community mental health services for ethnic minority the cultural responsiveness hypothesis. *J Consult Clin Psychol* 59, 533–540.

Sullivan PF, Fifield WJ, Kennedy MA *et al.* (1998) No association between novelty seeking and the type 4 dopamine receptor gene (DRD4) in two New Zealand samples. *Am J Psychiatr* 155, 98–101.

Vandenbergh DJ, Persico AM, Hawkins AL *et al.* (1992) Human dopamine transporter gene (DAT1) maps to chromosome 5p15.3 and displays a VNTR. *Genomics* 14, 1104–1106.

Wan YJY, Poland RE, Han G, *et al.* (2001) Analysis of the CYP2D6 gene polymorphism and enzyme activity in African-Americans in Southern California. *Pharmacogenetics* 11, 489–499.

Wang SL, Huang JD, Lai MD *et al.* (1993) Molecular basis of genetic variation in debrisoquin hydroxylation in Chinese subjects: Polymorphism in RFLP and DNA sequence of CYP2D6. *Clin Pharmacol Ther* 53, 410–418.

Weber WW (1997) *Pharmacogenetics.* Oxford University Press, New York.

Weiss M (1997) Explanatory Model Interview Catalogue (EMIC): Framework for comparative study of illness. *Transcult Psychiatr* 34, 235–263.

Wig NN (1989) Indian concepts of mental health and their impact on care of the mentally ill. *Int J Ment Health* 18(3), 71–80.

Wolffers I (1989) Traditional practitioners' behavioral adaptations to changing patients' demands in Sri Lanka. *Soc Sci Med* 29(9), 1111–1119.

CHAPTER
77

Antipsychotic Drugs

Introduction

Information about antipsychotic drugs and theoretical developments in the treatment of psychosis is rapidly expanding, and more agents with antipsychotic efficacy are being developed. The advent of newer second-generation antipsychotics in the wake of clozapine represents the first significant advances in the pharmacologic treatment of schizophrenia and related psychotic disorders, and many clinicians in the USA are prescribing these second-generation antipsychotics as the first-choice agent for acute and maintenance therapy for these illnesses (Buckley, 2001; McEvoy *et al.*, 1999).

Pharmacology of Antipsychotic Agents

First-generation Antipsychotic Agents

The first-generation antipsychotic agents are equally effective in the treatment of psychotic symptoms of schizophrenia, while they vary in potency, their pharmacological properties, and their propensity to induce side effects (Davis *et al.*, 1980; American Psychiatric Association, 2000). The effect that is common to all first-generation antipsychotics is a high affinity for dopamine D_2 receptors (Marder and Van Putten, 1995). In addition, all of the first-generation agents produce EPS, including parkinsonism, dystonia, akathisia and TD, to a varying degree and increase serum prolactin concentration in the usual clinical dose range (Meltzer, 1985). These are described in greater detail in the section "Adverse Effects".

The first-generation agents are usually classified into three groups: phenothiazines, butyrophenones (e.g., haloperidol) and others (e.g., thiothixene, molindone and loxapine), based on their structure.

Phenothiazines

The phenothiazine antipsychotics are usually categorized into three classes according to substitutions at position 10 (Marder and Van Putten, 1995). The aliphatic class (e.g., chlorpromazine) consists of agents that have relatively low potency at D_2 receptors compared with other first-generation antipsychotics, more antimuscarinic activity, more sympathetic and parasympathetic activity, and more sedation. The piperidine class (e.g., thioridazine) has a similar clinical profile to the aliphatic class, with somewhat reduced affinity for D_2 sites. The piperazine class (e.g., fluphenazine) has fewer antimuscarinic and autonomic effects, but greater potency at D_2 sites, and thus can produce more EPS.

Butyrophenones

The butyrophenone antipsychotics, represented by haloperidol, tend to be potent D_2 antagonists and have minimal anticholinergic and autonomic effects (Marder and Van Putten, 1995). PET studies demonstrate that low doses of haloperidol (2–5 mg/day) would be expected to induce 60 to 80% dopamine D_2 receptor occupancy (Kapur *et al.*, 1996, 1997). While theoretically this dosage should be enough for optimal clinical efficacy correlated to an optimal D_2 receptor antagonism, dosages five to 20 times as high are prescribed in current clinical practice (Stip, 2000) (see section "Dose of Antipsychotic Agent").

Second-generation and Novel Antipsychotic Agents

The pharmacological properties that confer the unique therapeutic properties of second-generation antipsychotic drugs are poorly understood despite intensive research efforts by the pharmaceutical industry and the psychopharmacology research community. Since clozapine is the prototype "atypical" drug, defining the role of the individual complex actions of this drug, that are responsible for its unique therapeutic profile, is necessary for rational design of new and improved second-generation (clozapine-like) antipsychotics (Miyamoto *et al.*, 2002a). In this chapter, second-generation antipsychotics refer to clozapine, risperidone, olanzapine, quetiapine, ziprasidone, sertindole, amisulpride, zotepine, aripiprazole and iloperidone. The relative receptor affinities for these medications all shown in Table 77.1.

Antipsychotic Medications for Different Indications

Antipsychotic agents are effective for treating nearly every medical and psychiatric condition where psychotic symptom or aggression is the predominant feature. The development of second-generation antipsychotics has been a major clinical advance for the treatment of schizophrenia. At present, these second-generation drugs are being used for schizophrenia as the first-line treatment, and are being used increasingly for various conditions beyond schizophrenia as happened with the first-generation antipsychotics (Marder, 1997; Glick *et al.*, 2001). The low incidence of EPS and TD associated with second-generation agents is highly beneficial in several neuropsychiatric conditions. A summary of various indications for second-generation antipsychotics is shown in Table 77.2. Some uses have gained general acceptance, whereas others depend on moderate or preliminary evidence.

Essentials of Psychiatry   Jerald Kay and Allan Tasman
© 2006 John Wiley & Sons, Ltd.

Table 77.1   Relative Neurotransmitter Receptor Affinities for Some Antipsychotics at Therapeutic Doses

Receptor	Clozapine	Risperidone	Olanzapine	Quetiapine	Ziprasidone	Sertindole	Amisulpride	Zotepine	Aripiprazole	Iloperidone	Haloperidol
D_1	+	+	++	−	+	++	−	+	+	+	+
D_2	++	++++	+++	+	+++	++++	++++	++	++++	+++	++++
D_3	++	++	++	−	++	++	++	+	++	++	+++
D_4	++	−	++	−	++	+	−	++	+	++	+++
$5\text{-}HT_{1A}$	−	−	−	−	+++						−
$5\text{-}HT_{1D}$	−	+	−	−	+++						−
$5\text{-}HT_{2A}$	+++	++++	+++	+	++++	++++	−	+++	+	+++	+
$5\text{-}HT_{2C}$	++	++	++	−	++++	++	−	++		++	−
$5\text{-}HT_6$	++	−	++	−	+			++	++	+	−
$5\text{-}HT_7$	+++	+++	−	−	++			++	++	+++	+++
A_1	+++	+++	++	+++	++	++	−	++		+++	−
A_2	+	++	+	+	−	+	−	++		++	−
H_1	+++	−	+++	++	−	+	−	+		++	−
M_1	++++	−	+++	++	−	−	−				−
DA Transporter	++		++		++			++		−	
NA Transporter	+		++		++					−	
5-HT Transporter										−	

−, minimal to none; +, low; ++, moderate; +++, high; ++++, marked

Adapted and modified with permission from Blin O (1999) A comparative review of new antipsychotics. *Can J Psychiatr* 44, 235–244; Burns MJ (2001) The pharmacology and toxicology of atypical antipsychotic agents. *J Clin Toxicol* 39, 1–14.

Table 77.2   Indications for Second-ieneration Antipsychotic Use Other than Schizophrenia

Strong Evidence	Moderate Evidence	Preliminary Evidence
Risperidone		
Dementia	Bipolar disorder, Stuttering	Pediatric psychoses
Pervasive developmental disorders	Conduct disorder, Tourette's disorder	
Olanzapine		
Bipolar disorder	Dementia	Borderline personality disorder
	Substance-induced psychosis	Depression, Pediatric psychoses
		Childhood schizophrenia
Quetiapine		
Bipolar disorder	Dementia	Borderline personality disorder
L-dopa-induced psychosis		Substance-induced psychosis
Clozapine		
L-dopa-induced psychosis	Pediatric psychoses	
	Prophylaxis of treatment resistant bipolar disorder	
Ziprasidone		Bipolar disorder
		Tourette's disorder
Zotepine		Psychotic depression
Amisulpride		

Schizophrenia and Schizoaffective Disorder

Nearly all acute episodes of schizophrenia and schizoaffective disorder, including first episode psychosis and recurrence in chronic schizophrenia, should be treated with antipsychotic medications (American Psychiatric Association, 2000). The psychiatrist should evaluate the patient's mental status and physical condition before establishing a baseline for the administration of antipsychotic medications. Once the patient is diagnosed, pharmacotherapy should be applied as early in this phase as possible.

Continuous medications may be preferable for most patients with schizophrenia, even if they are symptom free, to reduce the likelihood of relapse.

Major Depression with Psychotic Features

Clear psychotic symptoms, such as delusions or hallucinations, are observed in approximately 25% of patients with major depressive disorder (Rothschild, 1996). These symptoms often respond poorly to antidepressants when they are administered alone, and may require the use of adjunctive antipsychotic agents (Marder, 1997). Conventional antipsychotic drugs are likely to expose patients to the development of TD and EPS, which may occur more frequently in patients with affective disorders than in those with schizophrenia (Casey, 1999). Thus, second-generation antipsychotics may have a more beneficial effect for this patient population.

There is clinical evidence that some of the second-generation antipsychotics may have antidepressant effects in addition to their antipsychotic properties, and thus may improve depressive symptoms in schizophrenia (Tollefson et al., 1999; Buckley, 2001). Although depressive symptoms have traditionally been treated with antidepressants, a number of case reports and open trials have shown risperidone and olanzapine to be efficacious as monotherapy or adjunctive treatment for the treatment of depression without psychotic features (Jacobsen, 1995; Ostroff and Nelson, 1999) (for review, see Buckley, 2001).

Mania

In almost 50% of manic episodes, clear psychotic symptoms, such as delusions or hallucinations, are observed (Goodwin and Jamison, 1990). Antipsychotic medications can effectively treat the symptoms of acute mania, particularly in patients, who present with prominent agitation, in advance of the onset of action of lithium or mood stabilizers (Marder, 1997; Buckley, 2001). Over the past few years, second-generation antipsychotics have gained increasing favor over the conventional neuroleptics for the treatment of bipolar disorder because of their fewer EPS, a presumably lower risk of TD, and antimanic or mood stabilizing effects (Thase and Sachs, 2000). Currently, second-generation antipsychotics are being used as second-choice treatments for bipolar disorder and/or adjunctive therapy with lithium, carbamazepine, or sodium valproate (Ghaemi, 2000).

Tourette's Disorder

Tourettes's disorder is a neurobehavioral disorder characterized clinically by motor and vocal tics (Jimenez-Jimenez and Garcia-Ruiz, 2001). Tics are usually present in childhood and may persist throughout life. The pathophysiology of the illness is not well known. When the tics interfere with the functioning of the patient, an antipsychotic medication can be effective in reducing the severity of both motor and vocal tics (Marder, 1997). Although haloperidol and pimozide have been the most commonly used agents for the disease, second-generation antipsychotics are considered as promising agents for the control of tics, because of their better adverse event profiles.

Substance-related Disorders

A variety of substances, including amphetamines, cocaine, alcohol and phencyclidine, can cause schizophrenia-like symptoms that occur while the patient is intoxicated or during drug withdrawal (Marder, 1997). While clinical trials have not yet established the efficacy of the second-generation antipsychotics for substance use disorders, several case reports and open-labeled studies offer suggestions of the effectiveness of new agents in these off-label uses (Misra and Kofoed, 1997; Smelson *et al.*, 1997).

Behavioral Disturbances in the Elderly

Dementia, whether due to Alzheimer's disease or other causes, is frequently associated with behavioral disturbance, agitation and psychotic phenomena (e.g., persecutory delusions, hallucinations) (Stoppe *et al.*, 1999). The management of behavioral disturbance and psychosis in the elderly is complicated by age-related decline in drug metabolism, vulnerability to drug–drug interactions, high incidence of concomitant physical illnesses and heightened sensitivity to EPS and TD (Marder, 1997; Buckley, 2001). Usually, lower dosages are more necessary for the elderly than for younger patients. Although evidence from a number of double-blind studies supports the efficacy of traditional antipsychotics for treating agitated elderly patients, the use of older agents is limited by EPS, TD, anticholinergic adverse effects, sedation, and orthostatic hypotension, which may result in falls and fractures.

Other Organic Syndromes

Patients with Parkinson's disease (PD) are sometimes accompanied with psychotic symptoms. Second-generation antipsychotics can offer a true benefit to this patient population (Friedman and Factor, 2000). Patients with Huntington's disease (HD) can also benefit from antipsychotic medications (Marder, 1997). As with PD, the use of conventional agents worsens chorea movement disturbance (Buckley, 2001).

Childhood Schizophrenia

Children with schizophrenia may need neuroleptics for a long term. At present, no controlled trials have been published on the use of risperidone, olanzapine, quetiapine, or ziprasidone for the pediatric population with schizophrenia, thus definitive evidence is lacking. A number of open clinical trials and case reports of these new agents, however, indicate a possible effectiveness, though pediatric patients seem to have a greater propensity than adults for side effects, particularly EPS, weight gain and dysphoria, but also prolactin increase and white blood count aberrations (Kumra *et al.*, 1998; Toren *et al.*, 1998; Wudarsky *et al.*, 1999; McConville *et al.*, 2000).

Effects of Antipsychotic Agents on Symptoms of Schizophrenia

Positive Symptoms

Antipsychotic agents have a specific effect on positive symptoms of schizophrenia including hallucinations, delusions and thought disorder (Hirsch and Barnes, 1995). First-generation antipsychotic drugs (e.g., chlorpromazine and haloperidol) are effective for alleviating positive symptoms and in preventing their recurrence in many schizophrenic patients (Miyamoto *et al.*, 2000, 2002a).

Although the proportion of patients who improve and the magnitude of therapeutic effects vary greatly, second-generation antipsychotics appear to be at least as effective for psychotic symptoms as conventional drugs (Markowitz *et al.*, 1999; Remington and Kapur, 2000).

Within a short period of time, clozapine, risperidone, olanzapine, quetiapine and ziprasidone have become the drugs of choice over conventional antipsychotic drugs in the treatment of schizophrenia and schizoaffective disorder (Buckley, 2001). There is, however, still considerable debate with regard to the clinical superiority of second-generation over conventional antipsychotics. The CATIE study (Lieberman, 2005) failed to resolve this debate, with all medications tested demonstrating comparable clinical efficacy.

Negative Symptoms

Negative symptoms can be divided into three components that are usually difficult to distinguish: 1) primary or deficit-enduring negative symptoms, 2) primary nonenduring negative symptoms, and 3) secondary negative symptoms that may be associated with positive symptoms, EPS, depression and environmental deprivation (Buchanan and Gold, 1996; Collaborative Working Group on Clinical Trial Evaluations, 1998a). Studies of the early course of illness have shown that about 70% of schizophrenics develop primary negative symptoms, such as affective blunting, emotional withdrawal, poverty of speech, anhedonia and apathy, before the onset of positive symptoms (Hafner *et al.*, 1992). Negative symptoms may represent core features of the illness, and may be associated with poor outcome and prolonged hospitalization for patients (Buchanan and Gold, 1996).

Conventional antipsychotics are generally less effective against negative than positive symptoms of schizophrenia (Miyamoto *et al.*, 2002a). Thus, the efficacy of second-generation antipsychotics on negative symptoms compared with that of first-generation drugs has received much attention. Although second-generation antipsychotics have been shown to be more effective than conventional agents in treating negative symptoms, there is a continuing debate as to whether these effects are related to a reduction in EPS, or to a direct effect on primary negative symptoms (Marder and Meibach, 1994; Kane *et al.*, 2001; Remington and Kapur, 2000; Carpenter *et al.*, 1995; Conley *et al.*, 1994; Meltzer, 1995).

A summary of the clinical profile of second-generation drugs on a range of symptoms is provided in Table 77.3.

Mood Symptoms and Suicidal Behavior

Depressive symptoms frequently occur in the context of psychotic symptoms or intercurrently between psychotic episodes (Siris, 2001). Antidepressant medication used adjunctively to antipsychotic drugs is generally indicated and effective (Siris, 2001). Atypical antidepressants have been reported to have selective benefits against mood symptoms in schizophrenia, both manic and depressive (Sartorius *et al.*, 2002).

Suicidal behavior presents a particular problem in patients with schizophrenia. Recently the FDA approved clozapine for use in suicidal patients with schizophrenia on the basis of results in the InterSePT study. This study found that clozapine treatment produced a lower rate of suicidal behavior than the comparison treatment olanzapine in patients with active or histories of suicidal behavior (Meltzer *et al.*, 2003).

Treatment of Different Phases of Schizophrenia

Treatment During the Acute Phase

Route of Administration

In clinical situations, antipsychotic medications can be administered in oral forms, including oral tablets, oral liquid concentrates

Table 77.3 Clinical Profile of Second-generation Antipsychotic Drug Efficacy

Drug Clinical effect	Clozapine	Risperidone	Olanzapine	Quetiapine	Ziprasidone	Sertindole	Amisulpride	Aripiprazole	Iloperidone
Psychotic symptoms	+++	+++	+++	++	++	+++	+++	+++	+++
Negative symptoms	+	+	+	+	+	++	++	++	++
Cognitive symptoms	++	++	++	+	?	?	?	++	?
Mood symptoms	+++	++	+++	++	++	++	++	++	?
Refractory symptoms	+++	++	++	++	?	?	++	?	?

+ to +++, weakly to strongly active; ?, questionable to unknown activity.

Source: Adapted with permission and modified from Dawkins K, Lieberman JA, Lebowitz BD *et al.* (1999) Antipsychotics: Past and future. National Institute of Mental Health Division of Services and Intervention Research Workshop (July 14, 1998). *Schizophr Bull* 25, 395–404.

and orally dissolving formulations, as short-acting intramuscular preparations, or as long-acting depot preparations (American Psychiatric Association, 2000). In most cases, patients who are cooperative prefer oral administration to parenteral medications. A summary of dosing recommendations for newer agents is provided in Table 77.4. Oral antipsychotic medications tend to be rapidly and well absorbed from the gastrointestinal tract, and reach a peak plasma concentration in 1 to 10 hours (Burns, 2001). The long average half-life (12–24 hours) and active metabolites of most oral antipsychotic drugs allow for once- to twice-daily dosing (Marder, 1997; Burns, 2001). Among the second-generation agents, quetiapine and ziprasidone have relatively shorter half-lives (Table 77.4), and should be administered in divided doses (Markowitz *et al.*, 1999). A single or twice-daily dose of an oral preparation will result in steady-state blood levels in 2 to 5 days (Dahl, 1990).

Short-acting intramuscular (IM) medications are particularly useful in the management of acute pathologic excitement and agitation (Buckley, 1999). The main indication for the use of a short-acting parenteral form in the acute situation is to treat severely disturbed patients who cannot be verbally redirected, who may be violent, and who may have to be medicated over objection. Short-acting IM preparations can reach a peak concentration 30 to 60 minutes after the medication is administered (Dahl, 1990).

Selection of an Antipsychotic Agent

Selection of an agent in emergency settings for the management of the gross agitation, excitement and violent behavior associated with psychosis might be based on clinical symptoms, differences in efficacy or side effects of candidate drugs, or, more pragmatically, the formulation of a drug as it affects route of administration, onset and duration (Hirsch and Barnes, 1995; Allen, 2000). Most agitated patients will assent to oral medication and, in a survey of 51 psychiatric emergency services, the medical doctors

estimated that only 10% of emergency patients require injectable medications (Currier, 2000). Practice and legal requirements concerning injectable medications differ substantially across the globe. The US Health Care Finance Administration's (HCFA) regulations regarding so-called "chemical restraint" call for it to be a last resort, which would suggest that oral medication should be offered whenever it is possible to speak with the patient (Allen, 2000). Intramuscular treatments, however, remain necessary for some agitated or aggressive patients who refuse oral medications of any kind (Allen *et al.*, 2001). In these situations, many clinicians avoid high doses on antipsychotic medications in favor of a combination of an antipsychotic and a benzodiazepine (Miyamoto *et al.*, 2002b).

Dose of Antipsychotic Agent

Effective Doses of First-generation Antipsychotics The goal of pharmacotherapy is to maximize efficacy and minimize adverse effects with the lowest effective dose. When groups of patients are assigned to higher doses, such as more than 2000 mg chlorpromazine or 40 mg haloperidol equivalent, the rate and amount of improvement are no greater than for those assigned to more moderate doses (Marder, 1996).

Effective Doses of Second-generation Antipsychotics The dosage recommendations for second-generation antipsychotic drugs are summarized in Table 77.4. Although clinical trial data show that second-generation antipsychotics are efficacious and cause fewer EPS than the conventional agents, optimal dosing constitutes a critical issue in their effective use.

Treatment Resistance

Patients with schizophrenia may manifest poor response to treatment because of intolerance to medication, poor compliance, inappropriate dosing, as well as true resistance of their illness to antipsychotic medications. It has been consistently reported

Table 77.4   Recommended Dosages for Second-generation Antipsychotic Agents

	Half-life (hr) (Mean)	Starting Dose (Total mg/day)	Average Dose Range (mg/day)		Average Maintenance Dose (mg/day)	Routes of Administration
			First Episode	**Recurrent Episode**		
Clozapine	10–105 (16)	25–50	150–300	400–600	400	Oral
Risperidone	3–24 (15)	1–2	2–4	3–6	3–6	Oral, depot
Olanzapine	20–70 (30)	5–10	10–20	15–30	10–20	Oral, IM
Quetiapine	4–10 (7)	50–100	300–400	500–800	400–600	Oral
Ziprasidone	4–10	40–80	80–120	120–200	120–160	Oral, IM
Zotepine	12–30 (15)	50–100	75–150	150–450	75–300	Oral
Amisulpride	(12)	50–100	50–300	400–800	400–800	Oral
Aripiprazole	(75–96)	10–15	10–30	15–30	15–30	Oral

Source: Adapted with permission and modified from McEvoy JP, Scheifler PL and Frances A (1999) The expert consensus guideline series: Treatment of schizophrenia 1999. *J Clin Psychiatr* 60, 1–80; Burns MJ (2001) The pharmacology and toxicology of atypical antipsychotic agents. *J Clin Toxicol* 39, 1–14; Worrel JA, Marken PA, Beckman SE *et al.* (2000) Atypical antipsychotic agents: A critical review. *Am J Health Syst Pharm* 57, 238–255.

Table 77.5	**Proposed Guidelines for Determining Treatment Resistance in Schizophrenia**

1. Drug-refractory condition
   At least two prior drug trials of 4- to 6-weeks duration at 400 to 600 mg of chlorpromazine (or equivalent) with no clinical improvement
2. Persistence of illness
   >5 years with no period of good social or occupational functioning
3. Persistent psychotic symptoms
   BPRS total score > 45 (on 18 item scale) and item score >4 (moderate) on at least two of four positive symptom items

BPRS, Brief Psychiatric Rating Scale.
Source: Adapted with permission from Conley RR and Kelly DL (2001) Management of treatment resistance in schizophrenia. *Biol Psychiatr* 50, 898–911.

that approximately 10 to 15% of patients with first-episode schizophrenia are resistant to drug treatment (Lieberman *et al.*, 1993), and between 30 to 60% of patients become only partially responsive or completely unresponsive to treatment during the course of the illness (Davis and Casper, 1977; Essock *et al.*, 1996; Lieberman, 1999). Before a patient is considered treatment-resistant, an optimized medication and treatment trial should be employed (Conley and Kelly, 2001). The most accepted criteria for defining treatment resistance in schizophrenia were initially utilized by Kane and collaborators (1988) in the Multicenter Clozapine Trial (MCT), and the modified criteria have been used to define treatment resistance (Table 77.5). Although most definitions of treatment resistance focus on the persistence of positive symptoms, there is growing awareness of the problems of persistent negative symptoms and cognitive impairments, which may have an important impact on level of functioning, psychosocial integration and quality of life (Conley and Kelly, 2001; Peuskens, 1999).

Only clozapine has consistently demonstrated efficacy for psychotic symptoms in well-defined treatment refractory patients. The mechanism responsible for this therapeutic advantage remains uncertain. Thus, clozapine remains the "gold standard" for treatment of this patient population. The evidence is strongest in support of clozapine monotherapy as an intervention for treatment-resistant patients; serum levels of 350 μg/mL or greater have been associated with maximal likelihood of response (Miller, 1996).

Since the approval of clozapine, attention has shifted to a greater focus on the use of other second-generation antipsychotics for managing treatment resistance in schizophrenia, but the relative efficacy of other second-generation antipsychotics is less clear.

Given the risk of agranulocytosis, the burden of side effects and the requirement of white blood cell monitoring, the second-generation agents (risperidone, olanzapine, quetiapine and ziprasidone) should be tried before proceeding to clozapine in almost all patients (Conley and Kelly, 2001; Miyamoto *et al.*, 2002a). Many clinicians express the impression that certain patients do respond preferentially to a single agent of this class. Sequential controlled trials of the newer agents in treatment-resistant patients will be necessary fully to examine this issue.

Treatment During the Resolving Phase

During the resolving phase, the goals of treatment are to minimize stress on the patient, to facilitate the patient's return to community life, and to establish a long-term maintenance plan (Marder, 1999; American Psychiatric Association, 2000). If a particular antipsychotic medication has improved the acute symptoms, it should be continued at the same dose for the next 6 months, before a lower maintenance dose is considered for continued treatment (American Psychiatric Association, 2000). Rapid dose reduction or discontinuation of the medications during the resolving phase may result in relatively rapid relapse (American Psychiatric Association, 2000). If the psychiatrist has decided to switch the therapy to a long-acting depot antipsychotic agent, this can often be accompanied during this phase. This may also be a reasonable time to educate the patient and family regarding the course and outcome of schizophrenia, as well as factors that influence the outcome such as drug compliance (Marder, 1997; American Psychiatric Association, 2000). Patients should be helped to begin formulating a rehabilitation plan through realistic goal setting (Marder, 1997).

Treatment During the Stable Phase (Maintenance Treatment)

The goals of treatment during the stable or maintenance phase are to maintain symptom remission, to prevent psychotic relapse, to implement a plan for rehabilitation and to improve the patient's quality of life (Marder, 1999; American Psychiatric Associations, 2000). Current guidelines recommend that first-episode patients should be treated for 1 to 2 years; however, 75% of patients will have relapses after their treatment is discontinued (Kissling, 1991; Davis *et al.*, 1994; Lehman and Steinwachs, 1998; American Psychiatric Association, 2000). Patients who have had multiple episodes should receive at least 5 years of maintenance therapy (Kissling, 1991; Davis *et al.*, 1994; American Psychiatric Association, 2000). Patients with severe or dangerous episodes should probably be treated indefinitely (American Psychiatric Association, 2000).

For conventional antipsychotics, the risk of long-term side effects such as the development of TD inspired a search for strategies to reduce patients' exposure to these agents, and strategies for preventing relapse during the maintenance phase has focused on finding dosages that minimize drug adverse effects and provide adequate protection against psychotic relapse (Marder, 1999). Maintenance studies of the dose–response relationship found that lowering the dose prescribed for acute treatment by about 80% may be relatively safe for maintenance, although relapse rates are excessively high when doses are reduced to about 10% of an acute dose (Marder *et al.*, 1987; Hogarty *et al.*, 1988; Kane *et al.*, 1983). The international consensus conference recommended a gradual reduction in antipsychotic dose of approximately 20% every 6 months until a minimal maintenance dose is reached (Kissling, 1991).

Use of Plasma Levels of Antipsychotic Drugs

The use of plasma levels as a guide for dosing or determining lack of response to an antipsychotic medication is relatively common in clinical settings, yet it remains controversial (Marder, 1997). There is a wide interindividual difference in blood levels in patients on the same dose of an antipsychotic drug, and a narrow dose range between therapeutic efficacy and increasing risk of adverse effects (Van Putten *et al.*, 1991; Kane and Marder,

1993; Marder, 1997). Although plasma levels among first-generation antipsychotics have been established for several compounds, there is at best a moderate correlation between these levels and clinical effects (Kane and Marder, 1993).

It may be useful to monitor the plasma level of an antipsychotic medication under certain circumstances (Fleischhacker, 2001). For example, before deciding that the agent is ineffective despite an adequate trial at a sufficient dose, it is important to determine whether it may be due to alterations in the pharmacokinetics of the drug or nonadherence to medications (Van Putten *et al.*, 1991; Conley and Kelly, 2001). A low plasma level (e.g., less than 5 µg/mL of haloperidol) may require raising the dose or addressing compliance issues. A higher plasma level (e.g., greater than 15 µg/mL of haloperidol) may require lowering the dose because medication side effects may be overshadowing therapeutic effects (Marder, 1997). Other instances when plasma level monitoring may be useful is when decreasing the dose of drug during maintenance therapy, since too low plasma levels may indicate an increased risk of relapse (Marder, 1997).

Drug Interactions and Antipsychotic Agents

Most antipsychotics are metabolized by hepatic microsomal oxidases (cytochrome P450 system). The major isoenzyme systems involved are CYP1A2, CYP2C19, CYP2D6 and CYP3A4 (Ereshefsky, 1996). Induction or inhibition of these enzymes by other drugs may occasionally produce clinically important drug interactions (Burns, 2001). Table 77.6 summarizes clinically significant pharmacokinetic drug interactions involving second-generation antipsychotic drugs.

There are other common interactions that will concern clinicians. Antacids can decrease the absorption of the antipsychotic agent from the gut. Antipsychotic medications can antagonize the effects of dopamine agonists or levodopa when these drugs are used to treat parkinsonism. Antipsychotic agents may also enhance the effects of central nervous system depressants such as analgesics, anxiolytics and hypnotics. If patients require preanesthetic medication or general anesthetics, the doses of these drugs may need to be reduced (Marder, 1997).

Antipsychotic Medications and Pregnancy

Most antipsychotic agents readily cross the placenta and are secreted in breast milk to some degree (Trixler and Tenyi, 1997). There is little data to demonstrate whether prenatal exposure to antipsychotic agents is linked to spontaneous abortion, congenital malformations, carcinogenesis, intrauterine growth retardation, or behavioral teratogenicity (Trixler and Tenyi, 1997). It has, however, been suggested that fetal exposure over the course of pregnancy may affect development of the dopamine system (Altshuler *et al.*, 1996). Physicians must consider the benefits of controlling psychotic symptoms during pregnancy versus the possible risks to the mother and the fetus of withdrawing treatment and the risks to the fetus of continuing treatment (Trixler and Tenyi, 1997). Thus far, second-generation antipsychotics have not been shown to be teratogenic in animal studies or in preliminary human reports (Goldstein *et al.*, 2000; Stoner *et al.*, 1997; Trixler and Tenyi, 1997). However, if possible, use of antipsychotic medication should be avoided, at least during the first trimester, especially between weeks 6 and 10, unless the patient's psychosis

---

Table 77.6   Drug Interactions Involving Second-generation Antipsychotic Agents

Drug and Cytochrome P-450 Isoenzyme(s)	Inhibitors	Inducers
Clozapine		
1A2	Fluoroquinolones, fluvoxamine	Smoking, PAHs[a]
3A4	Erythromycin, ketoconazole, ritonavir, sertraline,[b] cimetidine	Carbamazepine, phenytoin
2D6	Ritonavir, quinidine, risperidone,[b] fluoxetine,[b] sertraline[b]	None
Risperidone		
2D6	Paroxetine, fluoxetine	None
Olanzapine		
1A2	Fluvoxamine	Smoking, PAHs, carbamazepine
2D6	None	Phenytoin
Quetiapine		
3A4	Ketoconazole, erythromycin	Rifampin, carbamazepine, phenytoin
Ziprasidone		
3A4	None	None
Aripiprazole	None	None
3A4		
2D6		

[a]PAHs, polycyclic aromatic hydrocarbons.
[b]Case reports of mild to moderate elevations in serum concentration.
Adapted and modified with permission from Worrel JA, Marken PA, Beckman SE *et al.* (2000) Atypical antipsychotic agents: A critical review. *Am J Health Syst Pharm* 57, 238–255.

places the mother and/or her fetus at significant risk (Trixler and Tenyi, 1997; American Psychiatric Association, 2000). Antipsychotic medications may be relatively safe during the second and third trimesters of pregnancy. If a first-generation antipsychotic agent is used, high-potency agents appear to be preferable for first-line management, because they have a lower propensity to cause orthostasis (Trixler and Tenyi, 1997). Low doses should be given, administration of antipsychotic medication should be as brief as possible, and the medication should be discontinued 5 to 10 days before delivery to minimize the chances of the newborn experiencing EPS (Trixler and Tenyi, 1997; American Psychiatric Association, 2000). This notion, however, has been reevaluated (Altshuler *et al.*, 1996), since discontinuation of medication before delivery may put the mother at risk for decompensation (Trixler and Tenyi, 1997). Anticholinergic agents should also be avoided during pregnancy, especially for the first trimester (American Psychiatric Association, 2000). Since antipsychotics are also secreted into breast milk, the infants should not be breast-fed if the mother resumes taking antipsychotic medication postpartum.

Adverse Effects

Acute Extrapyramidal Side Effects (Dystonia, Parkinsonism, Akathisia)

Antipsychotic-induced EPS occur both acutely and after chronic treatment. All antipsychotic medications are capable of producing EPS. In general, first-generation antipsychotics are more likely to cause EPS than second-generation antipsychotics when the drugs are used at usual therapeutic doses. Among second-generation drugs, clozapine and quetiapine have been shown to carry minimal to no risk for EPS within the therapeutic dosage range. The side-effect profiles for second-generation drugs and comparison with selected other agents are summarized in Table 77.7.

Tardive Dyskinesia and Other Tardive Syndromes

TD is a repetitive, involuntary, hyperkinetic movement disorder caused by sustained exposure to antipsychotic medication. TD is characterized by choreiform movements, tics and grimaces of the orofacial muscles, and dyskinesia of distal limbs, often the paraspinal muscles, and occasionally the diaphragm (Glazer, 2000). Younger patients with TD tend to exhibit slower athetoid movements of the trunk, extremities and neck (Marder, 1997). In addition to the more frequently observed orofacial and choreoathetoid signs of TD, tardive dystonias (sustained abnormal postures or positions) and tardive akathisia (persistent subjective and/or objective signs of restlessness) have been described (Casey, 1999). The abnormal movements of TD are usually increased with emotional arousal and are absent when the individual is asleep (Marder, 1997). According to the diagnostic criteria proposed by Schooler and Kane (1982), the movements should be present for at least 4 weeks, and exposure to antipsychotic drugs should have totaled at least 3 months. The onset of the abnormal movements should occur either while the patient is receiving an antipsychotic agent or within a few weeks of discontinuing the offending agent.

Prevalence surveys indicate that mild forms of TD occur in approximately 20% of patients who receive chronic treatment with conventional antipsychotic medication (Kane and Lieberman, 1992; Casey, 1995). Among the most significant predictors

of TD are older age, female gender, presence of EPS, diabetes mellitus, affective disorders and certain parameters of neuroleptic exposure such as dose and duration of therapy (Casey, 1999).

For most patients, TD dose not appear to be progressive or irreversible (Gardos *et al.*, 1994). The onset of TD often tends to be insidious with a fluctuating course (American Psychiatric Association Task Force, 1992). With time, TD will either stabilize or improve even if the antipsychotic medication is continued, although there are reports of TD worsening during continued drug therapy (American Psychiatric Association Task Force on TD, 1992; Gardos *et al.*, 1994). After discontinuation of antipsychotic medication, a significant proportion of patients with TD will have remission of symptoms, especially if the TD is of recent onset or the patient is young (Glazer *et al.*, 1984). Unfortunately, withdrawal of antipsychotic agents is seldom an option for patients with serious psychosis (Marder, 1997).

The American Psychiatric Association Task Force on TD (1992) issued a report in which a number of recommendations were made for preventing and managing TD. These include 1) establishing objective evidence that antipsychotic medications are effective for an individual; 2) using the lowest effective dose of antipsychotic drugs; 3) prescribing cautiously for children, elderly patients, and patients with mood disorders; 4) examining patients on a regular basis for evidence of TD; 5) considering alternatives to antipsychotic drugs, obtaining informed consent and also considering a reduction in dosage when TD is diagnosed; and 6) considering a number of options if the TD worsens, including discontinuing the antipsychotic medication, switching to a different drug, or considering a trial of clozapine.

Although a large number of agents have been studied for their therapeutic effects on TD, there is no definitive drug treatment for it (American Psychiatric Association, 2000). Second-generation antipsychotics, in particular clozapine, have been used in clinical practice to treat TD, but there have been no adequately controlled trials to date support this practice. Casey (1999), however, suggested that second-generation antipsychotics should be used as first-line treatment for patients who have TD or are at risk for TD. Guidelines for treating TD recommend using second-generation agents for mild TD symptoms, and clozapine or a newer agent for more severe symptoms (McEvoy *et al.*, 1999).

Neuroleptic Malignant Syndrome

Neuroleptic malignant syndrome (NMS), another type of acute EPS, is characterized by the triad of rigidity, hyperthermia (101–104°F), and autonomic instability in association with the use of an antipsychotic medication (American Psychiatric Association, 1994). NMS is often associated with elevation of creatine kinase (greater than 300 U/mL), leukocytosis (greater than 15 000 mm^3) and change in level of consciousness (American Psychiatric Association, 2000). NMS can be of sudden and unpredictable onset, usually occurring early in the course of antipsychotic treatment, and can be fatal in 5 to 20% of untreated cases (American Psychiatric Association, 2000).

The incidence of NMS varies from 0.02 to 3.23%, reflecting differences in criteria (Caroff and Mann, 1993). Prevalence rates are unknown, but are estimated to vary from 1 to 2% of patients treated with antipsychotic medication (American Psychiatric Association, 2000). The relative risk of second-generation antipsychotics for NMS is likely to be lower, but conclusive data is not yet available (Burns, 2001). NMS has been reported with clozapine, risperidone, olanzapine and quetiapine (Burns, 2001). Proposed risk factors include prior episode of NMS, younger age,

Table 77.7 Side-Effect Profile of Second-generation Antipsychotic Drugs

Drug Side effect	Conventional Agents	Clozapine	Risperidone	Olanzapine	Quetiapine	Ziprasidone	Sertindole	Amisulpride	Aripiprazole	Iloperidone
Side effect										
EPS[a]	+++	0	++	+	0	+	0	++	+	+
TD	+++	0	++	+	0	+	0 to +	+	+	+
NMS	++	+	+	+	?	+	+	+	?	?
Prolactin elevation	+++	0	+++	0 to +	0	0 to +	0 to +	++	0	0 to +
Weight gain	+ to ++	+++	+	+++	+	0	+	+	0	?
Prolonged QT[a]	+ to +++	0	+	0	+	++	+++	+	0	0
Hypotension[a]	+ to ++	+++	+	++	++	+	+	0	0	+
Sinus tachycardia[a]	+ to +++	+++	+	++	++	+	+	0	0	+
Anticholinergic effects[a]	+ to +++	+++	0	++	+	0	0	0	0	0
Hepatic transaminitis	+ to ++	++	+	++	+	+	+	+	0	+
Agranulocytosis	0 to +	++	0	0	0	0	0	0	0	0
Sedation	+ to +++	+++	+	++	+++	+	+	+	+	+
Seizures[a]	0 to +	+++	0	0 to +	0 to +	0 to +	0 to +	0 to +	0 to +	0 to +

EPS, extrapyramidal side effects; TD, tardive dyskinesia; NMS, neuroleptic malignant syndrome.
+ to +++, active to strongly active; 0, minimal to none; ?, questionable to unknown activity.
[a]Dose dependent.

Adapted and modified with permission from Dawkins K, Lieberman JA, Lebowitz BD et al. (1999) Antipsychotics: Past and future. National Institute of Mental Health Division of Services and Intervention Research Workshop (July 14, 1998). Schizophr Bull 25, 395–404; Burns MJ (2001) The pharmacology and toxicology of atypical antipsychotic agents. J Clin Toxicol 39, 1–14.

953

male gender, physical illness, dehydration, use of high-potency antipsychotics, rapid dose titration, use of parenteral (IM) preparations and preexisting neurological disability (Caroff and Mann, 1993; American Psychiatric Association, 2000).

If NMS is suspected, the offending antipsychotic agent should be discontinued and supportive and symptomatic treatment started (Marder 1997). Both dantrolene and dopamine agonists such as bromocriptine have also been used in the treatment of NMS (American Psychiatric Association, 2000). These agents, however, have not shown greater efficacy compared with supportive treatment (Caroff and Mann, 1993; Levenson, 1985).

The usual course of treatment is between 5 and 10 days. Long-acting depot preparations will prolong recovery time. After several weeks of recovery, treatment may be cautiously resumed with a different antipsychotic medication with gradually increased doses (American Psychiatric Association, 2000).

Metabolic Effects

Various degrees of weight gain have been recognized as a common problem with conventional antipsychotic medications. Weight gain is an important issue in the management of patients, because this adverse effect may be associated with noncompliance and certain medical illnesses, such as diabetes mellitus, cardiovascular disease, certain cancers and osteoarthritis (Lader, 1999; Sussman, 2001; Kurzthaler and Fleischhacker, 2001).

Differences have been discovered among second-generation antipsychotics with respect to their ability to induce weight gain (Table 77.7). There is currently no standard approach to the management of weight gain induced by antipsychotic medication. Patient education prior to initiating treatment should be provided, and regular exercise should be encouraged in all patients receiving antipsychotic medication. Switching to other second-generation antipsychotics with fewer propensities for producing weight gain may be the most efficient way to deal with antipsychotic-induced weight gain.

Hematologic Side Effects

Antipsychotic medications may cause blood dyscrasias, including neutropenia, leukopenia, leukocytosis, thrombopenia and agranulocytosis. Leukopenia, usually transient, commonly occurs early in treatment, and resolves spontaneously. Chlorpromazine has been associated with benign leukopenia, which occurs in up to 10% of patients (American Psychiatric Association, 2000; Kane and Lieberman, 1992). This phenomenon is even more common following clozapine administration (Hummer et al., 1994).

Agranulocytosis (granulocyte count less than 500/mm^3) is a fatal side effect of antipsychotic drugs. Approximately 0.32% of patients receiving chlorpromazine, and 1% treated with clozapine will experience agranulocytosis (American Psychiatric Association, 2000; Lieberman et al., 1989). The risk of agranulocytosis is greatest early in treatment, usually within the first 8 to 12 weeks of treatment (Novartis Pharmaceuticals, 2000). It tends to occur slightly more often in women, the elderly and young patients (less than 21 years old). Agranulocytosis from clozapine is usually reversible if the drug is withdrawn immediately (Lieberman et al., 1988). Olanzapine is not associated with severe agranulocytosis (Beasley et al., 1996a, 1996b; Dossenbach et al., 2000). Despite these encouraging studies, there are a number of case studies reporting agranulocytosis during treatment with olanzapine (and quetiapine) in patients who had suffered this adverse event during previous clozapine exposure (Tolosa-Vilella et al., 2002).

Before initiating treatment with clozapine, patients in the USA must be registered in a program that ensures that they receive weekly monitoring of their white blood cell (WBC) count during the first 6 months of treatment (Marder, 1997). Clozapine is prescribed on a weekly basis unless the WBC count is less than 3500/mm^3 or if there is a substantial drop in the WBC count (Marder, 1997). If the WBC count is 3000 to 3500/mm^3 and the absolute neutrophil count (ANC) is greater than 1500/mm^3, patients should be monitored twice weekly. If the WBC count is 2000 to 3000/mm^3 or the ANC count is 1000 to 1500/mm^3, clozapine treatment should be discontinued and patients should be monitored daily. If the WBC count falls below 2000/mm^3 or the ANC is less than 1000/mm^3, clozapine should be discontinued and bone marrow aspiration should be considered (American Psychiatric Association, 2000). If this occurs, the patient should be given immediate intensive treatment and considered protective isolation. Current guidelines require weekly monitoring for 1 month after the termination of clozapine treatment (American Psychiatric Association, 2000). Guidelines on the use of clozapine vary between different countries.

Other Side Effects

Sedation is the single most common side effect among low-potency conventional antipsychotics, as well as clozapine, zoteapine and quetiapine (American Psychiatric Association, 2000; Young et al., 1998). Although sedation is often beneficial at the beginning of treatment to calm down an anxious or aggressive patient, it usually impairs functioning during long-term treatment (Hummer and Fleischhacker, 2000). Most patients usually develop tolerance over time, or it may be possible to minimize sedation by dose reduction or by shifting most of the medication to night to reduce daytime sleepiness (Hummer and Fleischhacker, 2000).

Antipsychotic medications can lower the seizure threshold to some degree (Kane and Lieberman, 1992). Seizure is more common with low-potency first-generation antipsychotics and clozapine (American Psychiatric Association, 2000). Clozapine is associated with dose-related increase in seizures. For example, Devinsky and colleagues (1991) reported that doses of clozapine below 300 mg/day have a seizure rate of about 1%, doses between 300 and 600 mg/day have a seizure rate of 2.7%, and doses above 600 mg/day have a rate of 4.4%. Strategies to reduce the risk for seizures include slower dose titration, a lower dose and the addition of an anticonvulsant agent (i.e., valproic acid) (Hummer and Fleischhacker, 2000).

References

Allen MH (2000) Managing the agitated psychotic patient: A reappraisal of the evidence. *J Clin Psychiatr* 61(Suppl 14), 11–20.

Allen MH, Currier GW, Hughes DH et al. (2001) The expert consensus guideline series. Treatment of behavioral emergencies. *Postgrad Med* (Spec No) 1–88.

Altshuler LL, Cohen L, Szuba MP et al. (1996) Pharmacologic management of psychiatric illness during pregnancy: Dilemmas and guidelines. *Am J Psychiatr* 153, 592–606.

American Psychiatric Association (1994) Diagnostic and Statistical Manual of Mental Disorders, 4th edn. APA, Washington DC.

American Psychiatric Association (2000) Practice guideline for the treatment of patients with schizophrenia, in *Practice Guidelines for the Treatment of Psychiatric Disorders*. APA, Washington DC, pp. 299–412.

American Psychiatric Association Task Force on TD (1992) *Tardive Dyskinesia: A Task Force Report of the American Psychiatric Association*. APA, Washington DC.

Beasley CMJ, Sanger T, Satterlee W *et al.* (1996a) Olanzapine versus placebo: Results of a double-blind, fixed-dose olanzapine trial. *Psychopharmacology* (Berl) 124, 159–167.

Beasley CMJ, Tollefson G, Tran P *et al.* (1996b) Olanzapine versus placebo and haloperidol: Acute phase results of the North American double-blind olanzapine trial. *Neuropsychopharmacology* 14, 111–123.

Buchanan RW and Gold JM (1996) Negative symptoms: Diagnosis, treatment and prognosis. *Int Clin Psychopharmacol* 11 (Suppl 2), 3–11.

Buckley PF (1999) The role of typical and atypical antipsychotic medications in the management of agitation and aggression. *J Clin Psychiatr* 60(Suppl 10), 52–60.

Buckley PF (2001) Broad therapeutic uses of atypical antipsychotic medications. *Biol Psychiatr* 50, 912–924.

Burns MJ (2001) The pharmacology and toxicology of atypical antipsychotic agents. *J Clin Toxicol* 39, 1–14.

Caroff SN and Mann SC (1993) Neuroleptic malignant syndrome. *Med Clin N Am* 77, 185–202.

Carpenter WT Jr, Conley RR, Buchanan RW *et al.* (1995) Patient response and resource management: Another view of clozapine treatment of schizophrenia. *Am J Psychiatr* 152, 827–832.

Casey DE (1995) Neuroleptic-induced extrapyramidal syndromes and tardive dyskinesia, in *Schizophrenia* (eds Hirsch SR and Weinberger DR). Blackwell, Oxford, UK, pp. 546–565.

Casey DE (1999) Tardive dyskinesia and atypical antipsychotic drugs. *Schizophr Res* 35(Suppl), S61–S66.

Collaborative Working Group on Clinical Trial Evaluations (1998a) Assessing the effects of atypical antipsychotics on negative symptoms. *J Clin Psychiatr* 59(Suppl 12), 28–34.

Conley R, Gounaris C and Tamminga C (1994) Clozapine response varies in deficit versus nondeficit schizophrenic subjects. *Biol Psychiatr* 35, 746–747.

Conley RR and Kelly DL (2001) Management of treatment resistance in schizophrenia. *Biol Psychiatr* 50, 898–911.

Currier GW (2000) Atypical antipsychotic medications in the psychiatric emergency service. *J Clin Psychiatr* 61(Suppl 14), 21–26.

Dahl SG (1990) Pharmacokinetics of antipsychotic drugs in man. *Acta Psychiatr Scand* 358(Suppl), 37–40.

Davis JM and Casper R (1977) Antipsychotic drugs: Clinical pharmacology and therapeutic use. *Drugs* 14, 260–282.

Davis JM, Matalon L, Watanabe MD *et al.* (1994) Depot antipsychotic drugs. Place in therapy. *Drugs* 47, 741–773.

Davis JM, Schaffer CB, Killian GA *et al.* (1980) Important issues in the drug treatment of schizophrenia. *Schizophr Bull* 6, 70–87.

Devinsky O, Honigfeld G and Patin J (1991) Clozapine-related seizures. *Neurology* 41, 369–371.

Dossenbach MRK, Beuzen JN, Avnon M *et al.* (2000) The effectiveness of olanzapine in treatment-refractory schizophrenia when patients are nonresponsive to or unable to tolerate clozapine. *Clin Ther* 22, 1021–1034.

Ereshefsky L (1996) Pharmacokinetics and drug interactions: Update for new antipsychotics. *J Clin Psychiatr* 57(Suppl 11), 12–25.

Essock SM, Hargreaves WA, Dohm FA *et al.* (1996) Clozapine eligibility among state hospital patients. *Schizophr Bull* 22, 15–25.

Fleischhacker WW (2001) Drug treatment of patients with schizophrenia, in *Contemporary Psychiatry*, Vol. 3 (eds Henn F, Sartorius N, Helmchen H *et al.*). Springer-Verlag, Berlin, Heidelberg; New York, pp. 139–158.

Friedman JH and Factor SA (2000) Atypical antipsychotics in the treatment of drug-induced psychosis in Parkinson's disease. *Mov Disord* 15, 201–211.

Gardos G, Casey DE, Cole JO *et al.* (1994) Ten-year outcome of tardive dyskinesia. *Am J Psychiatr* 151, 836–841.

Ghaemi SN (2000) New treatments for bipolar disorder: The role of atypical neuroleptic agents. *J Clin Psychiatr* 61(Suppl 14), 33–42.

Glazer WM (2000) Expected incidence of tardive dyskinesia associated with atypical antipsychotics. *J Clin Psychiatr* 61(Suppl 4), 21–26.

Glazer WM, Moore DC, Schooler NR *et al.* (1984) Tardive dyskinesia: A discontinuation study. *Arch Gen Psychiatr* 41, 623–627.

Glick ID, Murray SR, Vasudevan P *et al.* (2001) Treatment with atypical antipsychotics: New indications and new populations. *J Psychiatr Res* 35, 187–191.

Goldstein DJ, Corbin LA, and Fung MC (2000) Olanzapine-exposed pregnancies and lactation: Early experience. *J Clin Psychopharmacol* 20, 399–403.

Goodwin FK and Jamison KR (1990) *Manic–Depressive Illness*. Oxford University Press, New York.

Hafner H, Riecher-Rossler A, Maurer K *et al.* (1992) First onset and early symptomatology of schizophrenia. A chapter of epidemiological and neurobiological research into age and sex differences. *Eur Arch Psychiatr Clin Neurosci* 242, 109–118.

Hirsch SR and Barnes TRE (1995) The clinical treatment of schizophrenia with antipsychotic medication, in *Schizophrenia* (eds Hirsch SR and Weinberger DR). Blackwell Science, Oxford, pp. 443–468.

Hogarty GE, McEvoy JP, Munetz M *et al.* (1988) Dose of fluphenazine, familial expressed emotion, and outcome in schizophrenia. Results of a two-year controlled study. *Arch Gen Psychiatr* 45, 797–805.

Hummer M and Fleischhacker WW (2000) Non-motor side effects of novel antipsychotics. *Curr Opin CPNS Invest Drugs* 2, 45–51.

Hummer M, Kurz M, Barnas C *et al.* (1994) Clozapine-induced transient white blood count disorders. *J Clin Psychiatr* 55, 429–432.

Jacobsen FM (1995) Risperidone in the treatment of affective illness and obsessive–compulsive disorder. *J Clin Psychiatr* 56, 423–429.

Jimenez-Jimenez FJ and Garcia-Ruiz PJ (2001) Pharmacological options for the treatment of Tourette's disorder. *Drugs* 61, 2207–2220.

Kane J, Honigfeld G, Singer J *et al.* (1988) Clozapine for the treatment-resistant schizophrenic. A double-blind comparison with chlorpromazine. *Arch Gen Psychiatr* 45, 789–796.

Kane JM and Lieberman JA (1992) *Adverse Effects of Psychotropic Drugs*. Guilford Press, New York.

Kane JM and Marder SR (1993) Psychopharmacologic treatment of schizophrenia. *Schizophr Bull* 19, 287–302.

Kane JM, Gunduz H, and Malhortra AK (2001) Second generation antipsychotics in the treatment of schizophrenia: Clozapine, in *Current Issues in the Psychopharmacology of Schizophrenia* (eds Breier A, Tran PV, Herrera JM *et al.*). Lippincott Williams & Wilkins Healthcare, Philadelphia, pp. 209–223.

Kane JM, Rifkin A, Woerner M *et al.* (1983) Low-dose neuroleptic treatment of outpatient schizophrenics. I. Preliminary results for relapse rates. *Arch Gen Psychiatr* 40, 893–896.

Kapur S, Remington G, Jones C *et al.* (1996) High levels of dopamine D_2 receptor occupancy with low-dose haloperidol treatment: A PET study. *Am J Psychiatr* 153, 948–950.

Kapur S, Zipursky R, Roy P *et al.* (1997) The relationship between D_2 receptor occupancy and plasma levels on low dose oral haloperidol: A PET study. *Psychopharmacology (Berl)* 131, 148–152.

Kissling W (1991) *Guidelines for Neuroleptic Relapse Prevention in Schizophrenia*. Springer-Verlag, Berlin.

Kumra S, Jacobsen LK, Lenane M *et al.* (1998) Childhood-onset schizophrenia: An open-label study of olanzapine in adolescents. *J Am Acad Child Adolesc Psychiatr* 37, 377–385.

Kurzthaler I and Fleischhacker WW (2001) The clinical implications of weight gain in schizophrenia. *J Clin Psychiatr* 62(Suppl 7), 32–37.

Lader M (1999) Some adverse effects of antipsychotics: Prevention and treatment. *J Clin Psychiatr* 60, 18–21.

Lehman AF and Steinwachs DM (1998) Translating research into practice: The Schizophrenia Patient Outcomes Research Team (PORT) treatment recommendations. *Schizophr Bull* 24, 1–10.

Levenson JL (1985) Neuroleptic malignant syndrome. *Am J Psychiatr* 142, 1137–1145.

Lieberman J, Jody D, Geisler S *et al.* (1993) Time course and biologic correlates of treatment response in first-episode schizophrenia. *Arch Gen Psychiatr* 50, 369–376.

Lieberman JA (1999) Pathophysiologic mechanisms in the pathogenesis and clinical course of schizophrenia. *J Clin Psychiatr* 60(Suppl 12), 9–12.

Lieberman JA, Johns CA, Kane JM *et al.* (1988) Clozapine-induced agranulocytosis: Non-cross-reactivity with other psychotropic drugs. *J Clin Psychiatr* 49, 271–277.

Lieberman JA, Kane JM and Johns CA (1989) Clozapine: Guidelines for clinical management. *J Clin Psychiatr* 50, 329–338.

Lieberman JA, Stroup T, McEvoy JP, Swartz MS *et al.* (2005) The Clinical Antipsychotic Trials of Intervention Effectiveness (CATIE) Investigators. *N Engl J Med* 2005; 353, 1209–1223.

Marder SR (1996) Pharmacological treatment strategies in acute schizophrenia. *Int Clin Psychopharmacol* 11(Suppl 2), 29–34.

Marder SR (1997) Antipsychotic drugs, in *Psychiatry* (eds Tasman A, Kay J, and Lieberman JA). WB Saunders, Philadelphia, pp. 1569–1585.

Marder SR (1999) Antipsychotic drugs and relapse prevention. *Schizophr Res* 35, S87–S92.

Marder SR and Meibach RC (1994) Risperidone in the treatment of schizophrenia. *Am J Psychiatr* 151, 825–835.

Marder SR and Van Putten T (1995) Antipsychotic medications, in *The American Psychiatric Press Textbook of Psychopharmacology* (eds Schatzberg AF and Nemeroff CB). American Psychiatric Press, Washington DC, pp. 247–261.

Marder SR, Van Putten T, Mintz J *et al.* (1987) Low- and conventional-dose maintenance therapy with fluphenazine decanoate. Two-year outcome. *Arch Gen Psychiatr* 44, 518–521.

Markowitz JS, Brown CS and Moore TR (1999) Atypical antipsychotics Part I: Pharmacology, pharmacokinetics, and efficacy. *Ann Pharmacother* 33, 73–85.

McConville BJ, Arvanitis LA, Thyrum PT *et al.* (2000) Pharmacokinetics, tolerability, and clinical effectiveness of quetiapine fumarate: An open-label trial in adolescents with psychotic disorders. *J Clin Psychiatr* 61, 252–260.

McEvoy JP, Scheifler PL and Frances A (1999) The expert consensus guideline series: Treatment of schizophrenia 1999. *J Clin Psychiatr* 60, 1–80.

Meltzer HY (1985) Long-term effects of neuroleptic drugs on the neuroendocrine system. *Adv Biochem Psychopharmacol* 40, 59–68.

Meltzer HY (1995) Clozapine: Is another view valid? *Am J Psychiatr* 152, 821–825.

Meltzer HY, Alphs L and Green AI (2003) Clozapine Treatment for Suicidality in Schizophrenia: International Suicide Prevention Trial (InterSePT). *Arch Gen Psychiatr* 60(1), 82–91.

Miller DD (1996) The clinical use of clozapine plasma concentrations in the management of treatment-refractory schizophrenia. *Ann Clin Psychiatr* 8, 99–109.

Misra L and Kofoed L (1997) Risperidone treatment of methamphetamine psychosis. *Am J Psychiatr* 154, 1170.

Miyamoto S, Duncan GE, Mailman RB, *et al.* (2000) Developing novel antipsychotic drugs: Strategies and goals. *Curr Opin CPNS Invest Drugs* 2, 25–39.

Miyamoto S, Duncan GE, Goff DC *et al.* (2002a) Therapeutics of schizophrenia, in *Neuropsychopharmacology: The Fifth Generation of Progress* (eds Davis KL, Charney D, Coyle JT *et al.*). Lippincott Williams & Wilkins, Philadelphia, pp. 775–807.

Miyamoto S, Stroup TS, Duncan GE *et al.* (2002b) Acute pharmacologic treatment of schizophrenia, in *Schizophrenia*, 2nd edn. (eds Hirsch SR and Weinberger DR). Blackwell Science, London.

Novartis Pharmaceuticals (2000) Product Information: Clozaril (Clozapine), in *Physicians' Desk Reference*, 54th edn. Anonymous Medical Economics Company, Montvale, NJ, pp. 2008–2012.

Ostroff RB and Nelson JC (1999) Risperidone augmentation of selective serotonin reuptake inhibitors in major depression. *J Clin Psychiatr* 60, 256–259.

Peuskens J (1999) The evolving definition of treatment resistance. *J Clin Psychiatr* 60(Suppl 12), 4–8.

Rothschild AJ (1996) Management of psychotic, treatment-resistant depression. *Psychiatr Clin N Am* 19, 237–252.

Remington G and Kapur S (2000) Atypical antipsychotics: Are some more atypical than others? *Psychopharmacology (Berl)* 148, 3–15.

Sartorius N, Fleischhacker WW, Gjerris A *et al.* (2002) The usefulness and use of Second-Generation Antipsychotic Medications. *Current Opinion in Psychiatry* 15(Suppl 1).

Schooler NR and Kane JM (1982) Research diagnoses for tardive dyskinesia. *Arch of Gen Psychiatr* 39, 486–487.

Siris SG (2001) Depression and Schizophrenia: Perspective in the era of 'Atypical' antipsychotic agents. *Am J Psychiatr* 157(9), 1379–1389.

Smelson DA, Roy A and Roy M (1997) Risperidone and neuropsychological test performance in cocaine-withdrawn patients. *Can J Psychiatr* 42, 431.

Stip E (2000) Novel antipsychotics: Issues and controversies. Typicality of atypical antipsychotics. *J Psychiatr Neurosci* 25, 137–153.

Stoner SC, Sommi RW Jr., Marken PA, *et al.* (1997) Clozapine use in two full-term pregnancies. *J Clin Psychiatr* 58, 364–365.

Stoppe G, Brandt CA and Staedt JH (1999) Behavioural problems associated with dementia: The role of newer antipsychotics. *Drugs Aging* 14, 41–54.

Sussman N (2001) Review of atypical antipsychotics and weight gain. *J Clin Psychiatr* 62(Suppl 23), 5–12.

Thase ME and Sachs GS (2000) Bipolar depression: Pharmacotherapy and related therapeutic strategies. *Biol Psychiatr* 48, 558–572.

Tollefson GD, Andersen SW and Tran PV (1999) The course of depressive symptoms in predicting relapse in schizophrenia: A double-blind, randomized comparison of olanzapine and risperidone. *Biol Psychiatr* 46, 365–373.

Tolosa-Vilella C, Ruiz-Ripoll A, Mari-Alfonso B *et al.* (2002) Olanzapine-induced agranulocytosis: A case report and review of the literature. *Prog Neuropsychopharmacol Biol Psychiatr* 26, 411–414.

Toren P, Laor N and Weizman A (1998) Use of atypical neuroleptics in child and adolescent psychiatry. *J Clin Psychiatr* 59, 644–656.

Trixler M and Tenyi T (1997) Antipsychotic use in pregnancy. What are the best treatment options? *Drug Safety* 16, 403–410.

Van Putten T, Marder SR, Wirshing WC *et al.* (1991) Neuroleptic plasma levels. *Schizophr Bull* 17, 197–216.

Wudarsky M, Nicolson R, Hamburger SD *et al.* (1999) Elevated prolactin in pediatric patients on typical and atypical antipsychotics. *J Child Adolesc Psychopharmacol* 9, 239–245.

Young CR, Bowers MB Jr and Mazure CM (1998) Management of the adverse effects of clozapine. *Schizophr Bull* 24, 381–390.

78   Mood Stabilizers

Acute Mania

General Management Considerations

The goal of treatment should be to suppress completely all symptoms of mania and return the patient to his or her mental status *quo ante*. Mood, thinking and behavior should normalize. The patient should act and feel like herself or himself. For economic or social reasons, it is sometimes necessary to discharge a patient before total remission of symptoms has occurred. In such cases it is imperative that a patient continues to take medication as prescribed and is protected from a recrudescence of manic symptoms or a rapid slide into acute depression.

Pharmacotherapy

The mechanism of action of antimanic drugs is poorly understood. It is not as clear what neural systems are involved in the mechanism of antimanic drugs. That few significant changes in neurotransmitter levels have been measured suggests that the site of action may be at the receptor, intracellular level, or second-messenger systems.

Lithium

For many patients with hypomania, lithium by itself can induce a total remission. For patients with full-blown mania, however, an adjunctive antipsychotic or antianxiety agent may be required to treat intolerable psychosis or excitement.

Lithium is rapidly and completely absorbed after oral administration. It is not protein bound and does not undergo metabolism. Peak plasma levels are achieved within 1.5 to 2 hours for standard preparations or 4 to 4.5 hours for slow-release forms. Lithium's plasma half-life is 17 to 36 hours. Ninety-five percent of the drug is excreted by the kidneys, with excretion proportionate to plasma concentrations. Because lithium is filtered through the proximal tubules, factors that decrease glomerular filtration rates will decrease lithium clearance. Sodium also is filtered through the proximal tubules, so a decrease in plasma sodium can increase lithium reabsorption and lead to increased plasma lithium levels. Conversely, an increase in plasma lithium levels can cause an increase in sodium excretion, depleting plasma sodium. Many other drugs affect lithium levels (Table 78.1).

Tests that should be done before lithium is started include a complete blood count, electrocardiography, electrolyte determinations, and renal and thyroid panels (Table 78.2). Lithium dosage may be based on a plasma concentration sampled 12 hours after the last dose, or the drug may be gradually titrated to a dose that is tolerated and within the range usually considered "therapeutic". As with any drug, approximately five half-lives must elapse for steady state to be achieved. For an average adult, this takes about 5 days for lithium (longer in the elderly or in patients with impaired renal function). To treat acute mania, plasma concentrations should typically be greater than 0.8 mEq/L, but to avoid toxicity, the level should not usually exceed 1.5 mEq/L. It is important to know what other medications a patient may be taking, because many drugs interact with lithium and can lead to increased or decreased lithium levels and possibly adverse effects (Table 78.2).

To reach therapeutic levels rapidly in healthy younger patients with normal renal and cardiac function, the psychiatrist may prescribe 300 mg of lithium carbonate four times daily from the outset, sampling the first plasma level after 5 days (or sooner should toxic signs become apparent). Thereafter, the dose should be adjusted to achieve a 12-hour plasma concentration between 0.8 and 1.3 mEq/L at steady state.

In a patient with mild hypomanic symptoms, by contrast, it may be wiser to begin with a lower lithium dose, such as 300 mg b.i.d., taking longer to achieve therapeutic levels but, at the same time, minimizing side effects that could trouble the patient and hamper cooperation. Once steady state has been achieved at therapeutic concentrations and the patient is clinically stable, lithium can be administered to most patients in a once-daily dose, usually at bedtime. Not only is this schedule easier to remember, but it tends to decrease such common side effects as tremor and polyuria.

The most common acute adverse effects from lithium are nausea, vomiting, diarrhea, postural tremor, polydipsia and polyuria (Table 78.2). If troublesome, these can usually be mitigated by a slower dosage increase or other measures. More severe symptoms and signs, including confusion and ataxia, may herald lithium intoxication and should prompt an immediate blood assay and, if necessary, temporary discontinuation or dosage reduction (see Table 78.3).

Anxiolytic Agents

Among current anxiolytic agents, benzodiazepines are usually selected as adjuncts to treat acute mania because of their safety and efficacy. Benzodiazepines have a wide margin of safety and can be safely administered in even very high doses, suppressing potentially dangerous excitement and allowing patients much needed sleep. When used together with an antipsychotic agent, benzodiazepines counteract the antipsychotic agent's tendency to provoke extrapyramidal reactions and seizures. For lorazepam, 1 to 2 mg can be administered by mouth or intramuscularly as frequently as hourly.

Valproate

Valproate is available in the USA as valproic acid or divalproex sodium, a compound containing equal parts valproic acid and sodium valproate. Divalproex is better tolerated than valproic acid, has been studied more extensively and is more commonly

Essentials of Psychiatry   Jerald Kay and Allan Tasman
© 2006 John Wiley & Sons, Ltd.

Table 78.1   Drug Interactions with Lithium

Increase Levels of Lithium	Decrease Levels of Lithium	Increase Adverse Reactions
Angiotensin-converting enzyme(ACE) inhibitors	Aminophylline (Aminophyllin and others)	Atracurium (Tracurium): prolonged neuromuscular blocking effects
Alprazolam (Xanax)	Caffeine	Carbamazepine (Tegretol and others): antithyriod effects
Amiloride (Midamor)	Carbonic anhydrase inhibitors	Chlorpromazine (Thorazine and others): extrapyramidal symptoms, delirium, cerebellar function impairment
Antipsychotic agents?	Dyphylline (Lufyllin, Dilor)	Clozapine (Clozaril): neurotoxicity
Ethacrynic acid (Edecrin)	Laxatives	Diltiazem (Cardizem): neurotoxicity
Fluoxetine (Prozac)	Osmotic diuretics	Electroconvulsive therapy: confusion
Ibuprofen (Motrin and others)	Oxtriphylline (Choledyl)	Fluoxetine (Prozac): lithium toxicity
Indapamide (Lozol)	Theobromine diuretic (Athenol and others)	Fluvoxamine (Luvox): seizures
Indomethacin (Indocin)	Theophylline (Tedral and others)	Haloperidol (Haldol): neurotoxicity
Mefenamic acid (Ponstel)		Hydroxyzine (Atarax, Vistril, and others): cardiovascular toxicity
Naproxen (Naprosyn)		Iodine: antithyroid effects
Nonsteroidal anti-inflammatory drugs (NSAIDs)		Methyldopa (Aldomet and others): hypertension, toxic symptoms at normal blood levels
Phenylbutazone (Butazolidin and others)		Metronidazole (Flagyl and others): lithium toxicity
Some antibiotics		Neuroleptics: extrapyramidal symptoms, somnambulism, neurotoxicity
Spironolactone (Aldactone, and others)		Pancuronium (Pavulon): prolonged neuromuscular blocking effects
Sulindac (Clinoril)		Succinylcholine (Anectine and others): prolonged neuromuscular blocking effets
Thiazide diuretics		Verapamil (Calan and others): neurotoxicity
Triamterene (Dyrenium and others)		
Zomepirac (no longer available)		

used. All valproate preparations are rapidly absorbed after oral administration, reaching peak plasma levels within 2 to 4 hours of ingestion. Food may delay absorption but does not affect bioavailability. Valproate is rapidly distributed and highly bound (90%) to plasma proteins. Its half-life ranges from 9 to 16 hours, depending on whether it is taken alone or with other medications, and it takes 1 to 4 days to attain steady state.

Experts usually rank lithium as the treatment of choice for a patient with classic mania, but divalproex is an acceptable first-line alternative. It may be used singly in patients who cannot tolerate lithium. For patients who do not respond to lithium, there are no secure data on whether divalproex should be added as an adjunct or substituted, but many psychiatrists would choose the former in a patient who appears to respond at least partially to lithium and the latter in patients for whom lithium seems to afford no benefit. Increasingly, psychiatrists are turning to divalproex first for manic patients with organic brain impairment, rapid cycling, mixed or dysphoric mania, or comorbid substance abuse (Bowden *et al.*, 1994; Calabrese *et al.*, 1993).

Before initiating divalproex, the psychiatrist should obtain a comprehensive medical history and insure that a physical examination has been performed, with particular attention to suggestions of liver disease or bleeding abnormalities (see Table 78.4).

Table 78.2   Adverse Effects of Lithium

Common	Less Common	Rare
Dermatitis	Ataxia	Hyperoarathyroidism
Fatigue	Autonomic slowing of bladder and bowel function	Hyperthyroidism
Gastrointestinal upset		Metallic taste
Headache		Nystagmus
Hypothyroidism	Cardiovascular complications	Organic brain syndrome
Memory and concentration difficulties	Diabetes mellitus	Parathyroid hyperplasia and parathyroid adenomas
	Dysarthria	
Muscle weakness	Edema	Tearing, itching, burning, or blurring of the eyes
	Elevated WBC count	
Polydipsia	Extrapyramidal reactions	Tinnitus
Polyuria		Vertigo
Tremor	Goiter	Visual distortion
Weight gain	Hypercalcemia	

Table 78.3   Lithium Intoxication

Patients Should	When These Symptoms Occur
Call psychiatrist	Gastrointestinal symptoms
Stop lithium and see psychiatrist	Increased tremor, confusion, ataxia

Patients should report any other medications they are considering taking (prescribed or over-the-counter) and be wary of diet changes (especially decreased sodium intake).

Table 78.4 Pretreatment Tests

MEDICATION	TESTING
Any Medication	• Comprehensive medical history • Physical examination including vital signs and weight • Pregnancy test, if applicable
Lithium	• Complete blood count • Electrolytes • Renal panel (blood urea nitrogen, creatinine, and routine urinalysis) • Thyroid panel plus thyroid-stimulating hormone • Electrocardiogram
Valproate	• Complete blood count • Liver function tests
Carbamazepine	• Complete blood count • Liver function tests • Renal panel • Urinalysis
Atypical Antipsychotics	• Blood glucose • Blood lipids

Baseline liver and hematological functions are measured before treatment, every 1 to 4 weeks for the first 6 months, and then every 3 to 6 months. Evidence of hemorrhage, bruising, or a disorder of hemostasis–coagulation suggests a reduction of dosage or withdrawal of therapy. The drug should be discontinued immediately in the presence of significant hepatic dysfunction.

A typical starting dose for healthy adults is 750 mg/day in divided doses. The dose can then be adjusted to achieve a 12-hour serum valproate concentration between 50 and 125 μg/mL. The time of dosing is determined by possible side effects and, if tolerated, once-a-day dosing can be employed. As with lithium, the antimanic response to valproate typically occurs after 1 to 2 weeks.

Adverse effects that appear early in the course of therapy are usually mild and transient, and tend to resolve in time. Gastrointestinal upset is probably the most common complaint in patients taking valproate and tends to be less of a problem with the enteric-coated divalproex sodium preparation. The administration of a histamine H2 antagonist such as famotidine (Pepcid) or cimetidine (Tagamet) may alleviate persistent gastrointestinal problems (Stoll *et al.*, 1991). Other common complaints include tremor, sedation, increased appetite and weight, and alopecia. Weight gain is even more of a problem when other drugs are administered that also promote weight gain, such as lithium, antipsychotic and other antiepileptics. Less common are ataxia, rashes and hematological dysfunction, such as thrombocytopenia and platelet dysfunction. Platelet count usually recovers with a dosage decrease, but the occurrence of thrombocytopenia or leukopenia may necessitate the discontinuation of valproate. Serum hepatic transaminase elevations are common, dose related, and usually

self-limiting and benign. Fatal hepatotoxicity is extremely rare, is usually restricted to young children, and usually develops within the first 6 months of valproate therapy. Other serious problems include pancreatitis and teratogenesis (McElroy *et al.*, 1989). There is also a concern that polycystic ovary syndrome, possibly associated with weight gain, may be a risk for young women who take valproate. If at any point during administration the side effects of valproate become intolerable, the psychiatrist may need to discontinue it and try one of the other treatments described in this section as an alternative. If valproate is tolerated but not totally effective, the psychiatrist might use one of the other treatments as an adjunct.

Carbamazepine

In light of the less well-substantiated evidence for the efficacy of carbamazepine, we place this anticonvulsant fourth in the antimania algorithm – behind lithium, valproate, and olanzapine. The decision to move on to carbamazepine – and whether to use it alone or in addition to lithium, valproate, or olanzapine – hinges on the same treatment considerations listed earlier. If a patient has been treated with one or more of these agents in a previous manic episode, that experience may guide treatment of a current episode.

Carbamazepine's absorption and metabolism are variable. Peak plasma levels occur within 4 to 6 hours after ingestion of the solid dosage form. Bioavailability is estimated at 85% but may be less when the drug is taken with meals. Eighty percent of plasma carbamazepine is protein bound, and its half-life ranges from 5 to 26 hours (after 3–4 weeks of treatment). Carbamazepine's active metabolite, 10,11-epoxide, has a half-life of about 6 hours.

Carbamazepine is metabolized by the hepatic cytochrome P450 2D6 system. It causes an induction of the cytochrome P450 enzymes, often resulting in an increased rate of its own metabolism over several weeks, as well as that of other drugs metabolized by the P450 system (Table 78.5). Because of enzyme induction, the dose of carbamazepine often must be raised after 2 to 4 months of treatment. Steady state may be attained within 4 to 5 days, but when clearance increases as a result of autoinduction, steady state may not be achieved for 3 to 4 weeks. Concomitant administration of drugs that inhibit P450 (see Table 78.6) will increase plasma levels of carbamazepine. Conversely, drugs that induce P450 enzymes – such as phenobarbital, phenytoin, or primidone – can decrease carbamazepine levels. Before carbamazepine is started, baseline blood and platelet counts, urinalysis, and liver and kidney function tests are in order (see Table 78.4). Although earlier guidelines called for routine monitoring of some or all of these indices, and some psychiatrists still obtain blood counts once or twice during the first few months of treatment and when plasma concentrations are sampled, a more general consensus at present is to instruct patients and family members to contact the psychiatrist immediately if petechiae, pallor, weakness, fever, or infection occur, at which time the psychiatrist should order relevant tests.

Used as a monotherapy, the typical starting dose for carbamazepine is 200 to 400 mg/day in three or four divided doses, increased to 800 to 1000 mg/day by the end of the first week. If clinical improvement is insufficient by the end of the second week, and the patient has not had intolerable side effects to the drug, increases to as high as 1600 mg/day may be considered. Although there are no good studies of the correlation between blood level and clinical response, a common target range for mania is 4 to 15 ng/mL. If carbamazepine is combined with lithium

Table 78.5 Drug Interactions with Carbamazepine
Increase Levels of Carbamazepine
Cimetidine (Tagamet)
Diltiazem
Erythromycin
Fluoxetine (Prozac)
Fluvoxamine (Luvox)
Isoniazid (Nydrazid and others)
Propoxyphene (Darvon and others)
Valporic acid
Verapamil
Decrease Levels of Carbamazepine
Phenobarbital
Primidone
Phenytoin (Dilantin and others)
Carbamazepine Decreases Levels of
Antipsychotics
Benzodiazepines (except clonazepam)
Corticosteroids
Hormonal contraceptives
Lamotrigine
Thyroid hormone
Tricyclic antidepressants
Others
Lithium and carbamazepine: may increase neurotoxicity

Table 78.6 Adverse Effects of Carbamazepine
Common Diminish in Time or With Temporary Reduction in Dose
Ataxia
Blurred vision
Diplopia
Dizziness
Drowsiness
Fatigue
Headache
Nausea
Less Common
Cardiovascular complications
Gastrointestinal upset
Hyponatremia
Skin reactions (if severe, may require discontinuation of carbamazepine)
Uncommon
Congnitive impairment
Chills
Genitourinary effects
Fever
Hepatitis
Increased intraocular pressure
Jaundice, cholestatic and hepatocellular
Liver function abnormalities Renal damage leading to oilguria and hypertension
SIADH
Transient leukopenia (carbamzepine may be continued unless infection develops)
Water intoxication
Rare
Agranulocytosis
Aplastic anemia
Lupus erythematosus-like syndrome
Pulmonary hypersensitivity

SIADH, Syndrome of inappropriate secretion of antidiuretic hormone.

or neuroleptics, lower doses and blood levels of carbamazepine are often used. If valproate and carbamazepine are administered simultaneously, blood levels of each should be monitored carefully because of complex interactions between the two agents.

When the dose of carbamazepine is built up rapidly, side effects are more likely. The most common effects in the first couple of weeks are drowsiness, dizziness, ataxia, diplopia, nausea, blurred vision and fatigue (Table 78.6). These tend to diminish in time or to respond to a temporary reduction in dose. Less common reactions include gastrointestinal upset, hyponatremia and a variety of skin reactions, some of which are severe enough to require discontinuation of carbamazepine. About 10% of patients experience transient leukopenia, but unless infection develops, carbamazepine may be continued. More serious hematopoietic reactions, including aplastic anemia and agranulocytosis, are rare.

Other Drug Treatments

Since carbamazepine and valproate are efficacious for acute mania, new antiepileptic medications are often tested for mania. Lamotrigine, which appears useful in maintenance, bipolar depression and rapid-cycling (see below), has not shown efficacy in acute mania, with the exception of one recent double-blind trial (Berk, 1999; Anand *et al.*, 1999; Bowden *et al.*, 2000).

Nonpharmacotherapy: Electroconvulsive Therapy

The specifics about electroconvulsive therapy (ECT), safety data and precautions concerning administration are covered in Chapter 74. When an acutely manic patient is unresponsive to or intolerant of

medication, or if medication presents other risks (e.g., during pregnancy), ECT should be seriously considered and may be lifesaving. Although there are no coherent theories about why ECT is effective in acute mania, it has been used for more than half a century, and there are widespread clinical impressions of its safety and efficacy.

Acute Bipolar Depression

General Management Considerations

Bipolar depression is usually indistinguishable from other forms of major depression, except that the episodes are typically shorter and more frequent. Other clues that the disorder may be bipolar include onset at a young age, a positive family history for bipolar disorder (particularly in first-degree relatives), and the occurrence of a hypomanic phase before the onset of the depressive episode.

For the most part, the treatment of a bipolar patient during an acute episode of depression is similar to that of a nonbipolar

Table 78.7   Treatments for Acute Depression

Treatment	Advantages	Disadvantages
Antidepressants	Efficacious	Possibly trigger switch into mania
Lamotrigine	Efficacious, possibly no switch into mania	Risk of side effects
Mood stabilizers	Enhance effectiveness of antidepressants, possibly protect against switch into mania	Not specifically antidepressant
ECT	Efficacious, safe for patients unable to take medication	More difficult to administer, possible cognitive side effects

Table 78.8   Effects of Combining Lamotrigine with Other Anticonvulsants

Carbamazepine decreases levels 40%
Oxcarbazepine decreases levels 30%
Phenobarbital decreases levels 40%
Phenytoin decreases levels 50%
Valproate increases levels 100%

patient. The same concerns about protecting the patient from suicide and maintaining physical health and safety apply, and for the most part, the same antidepressants or ECT will be useful (Table 78.7). These antidepressants are covered in Chapter 79. Because of fears about speeding up cycling and/or precipitating mania in patients with bipolar disorder, most doctors avoid prescribing tricyclics in bipolar depression. The short section that follows addresses issues unique to treatment of bipolar depression.

Pharmacotherapy

There is a widespread clinical impression that administering some antidepressants to bipolar patients can trigger switches into mania. Some experts also believe that antidepressants speed up mood cycles, although this point is more controversial. Because of both concerns, psychiatrists are often cautious about prescribing an antidepressant at the first sign of depression in a bipolar patient. If symptoms are mild and short-lived, many clinicians choose watchful waiting, while maintaining close contact to detect clinical deterioration.

Current guidelines by the American Psychiatric Association list lithium, as well as the anticonvulsant lamotrigine, as first-line monotherapy for acute bipolar depression (Hirschfeld *et al.*, 2002). This is a result of recent research that suggests that lamotrigine may be an effective treatment for bipolar depression, while carrying a low risk of triggering a switch into mania.

Lamotrigine is completely absorbed after oral administration, with a bioavailability of 98%, which is not affected by food. Peak plasma concentrations occur between 1.4 and 4.8 hours after administration. Lamotrigine is approximately 55% protein bound, making clinical interactions with other protein-bound drugs unlikely. Its half-life is 14 to 49 hours, with steady-state levels reached in 3 to 10 days.

Lamotrigine is metabolized predominantly by glucuronic acid conjugation in the liver, with the conjugate and the remaining 10% of the unmetabolized drug excreted in the urine. Clearance is markedly increased with the administration of other drugs that induce hepatic enzymes, including phenytoin, carbamazepine and phenobarbital (Table 78.8). Adding lamotrigine to carbamazepine can decrease steady-state concentrations of lamotrigine by approximately 40%. Adding lamotrigine to valproate, however, can decrease steady-state levels of valproate by approximately 25%, while the steady-state levels of lamotrigine increases approximately twofold. In this case, the starting dose of lamotrigine should be lowered, and the titration made slowly.

The only contraindication to lamotrigine use is hypersensitivity to the drug, though there is a box warning about dermatologic events, particularly rashes. These rashes, that occurred in approximately 10% of patients, generally occur after 2 to 8 weeks and are usually macular, papular, or erythematous in nature. Of those who develop a rash, one in 1000 adults can precede to a Stephens–Johnson type syndrome. Because it is impossible to distinguish which rashes will develop into this serious condition, it is advised to discontinue the medication at any sign of drug-induced rash. Otherwise the most frequently encountered side effects include dizziness, ataxia, somnolence, headache, blurred vision, nausea, vomiting and diplopia.

To reduce the risk of rash and other side effects lamotrigine should be started at low doses and titrated slowly, especially if combined with valproate therapy. Patients are commonly started on 25 to 50 mg p.o.q.d. doses for 2 weeks, with doses increased by 25 to 50 mg every 1 to 2 weeks until maintenance levels between 100 to 250 mg/day are reached. Maximum doses are lower with valproate at about 100 to 150 mg/day. Initial labs for those undergoing lamotrigine therapy should include liver function tests, renal function tests, a pregnancy test if applicable and a complete medical work-up.

Probably all available antidepressant drugs are effective in alleviating the symptoms of depression in a bipolar patient, and in fact a recent 1-year retrospective chart review by Altshuler and colleagues (2001) suggests that antidepressant discontinuation may increase the risk of depressive relapse in bipolar patients.

When a patient is known to have bipolar disorder, administration of an antidepressant to reverse an acute depression is almost always used together with one of the mood-stabilizing agents, usually lithium, valproate, carbamazepine (or a combination), or possibly one of the newer putative agents. Most bipolar patients will be taking these drugs in maintenance therapy. Moreover, mood stabilizers may enhance the effectiveness of the antidepressant and might protect against the possibility of a switch into mania.

The adverse effects, pharmacology and interactions of antidepressants are covered in Chapter 79.

Nonpharmacotherapy: Electroconvulsive Therapy

ECT is a useful alternative to antidepressants, particularly when a patient appears not to be responding quickly or is intolerant of the medication. Early studies that claimed that ECT works faster than medication in depressed patients are now considered to be methodologically flawed. However, two later studies found a more rapid decrease in depressive symptoms with ECT than is usually observed with medications. In a total of 72 patients with major depression, approximately six ECT treatments administered in a period of about 2 weeks led to a decrease in mean Hamilton Depression Rating Scale scores from between 24 and 30 to below 10 (Abrams *et al.*, 1991; Pettinati, 1994). The authors attributed the efficacy of treatment to the use of high suprathreshold dosages. Sackeim and colleagues (1993) found that higher dosage results in more rapid improvement in both bipolar and unipolar depressed patients. There are indications that bilateral electrode placement is superior to unilateral placement (Abrams *et al.*, 1991; Sackeim *et al.*, 1993), but there may be an increased risk of severe cognitive side effects with bilateral ECT at ultrahigh dosages.

Mixed States

The coexistence of manic and depressive symptoms, the so-called mixed state, is associated with poorer treatment response and prognosis than acute mania or depression (Himmelhoch *et al.*, 1976; Keller *et al.*, 1986; Dilsaver *et al.*, 1993). The optimal treatment of the mixed state has not been rigorously studied, so these recommendations must be considered tentative (Table 78.9).

Maintenance Therapy

General Management Considerations

As in all psychiatric disorders, maintenance therapy of bipolar disorder is a treatment carried out for a long period, with a goal of decreasing the probability, frequency, or severity of future

Table 78.9   Treatments for Mixed Episodes

General	Lithium, valproate, carbamazepine, lamotrigine (alone or in combination)
For severe excitement or psychosis	Antipsychotics
For depressive symptoms	Antidepressants, lamotrigine
Alternative to medication	ECT

episodes. Because bipolar disorder is by its nature a recurrent condition, some would argue that as soon as it is definitively diagnosed (e.g., after a single manic episode not attributable to a medical or neurological cause), maintenance therapy is indicated (Table 78.10). More conservative psychiatrists advocate waiting until the frequency and severity of a patient's disorder become apparent, hoping to avoid long-term exposure to medication that may not be required. The counter to this concern is evidence suggesting that recurrent episodes in themselves may worsen treatment response and long-term outcome (Gelenberg *et al.*, 1989).

Rapid Cycling

Patients with rapid-cycling bipolar disorder – defined as four or more affective episodes in 1 year, with or without an intervening period of euthymia – tend to be less responsive to lithium treatment (Dunner and Fieve, 1974). Whether rapid cycling is a natural progression of the illness or a separate disorder has yet to be determined. The onset of rapid cycling has been associated with

Table 78.10   Advantages and Disadvantages of Specific Maintenance Treatments

Treatment	Advantages	Disadvantages
Lithium	Most robust data set and clearly very effective for prevention of mania Specific anti-suicide effect	Side effects, low therapeutic index Lethality on overdose Risk of renal damage
Valproate	Possibly comparable to lithium May be more effective for patients with rapid cycling, mixed episodes and comorbidity	Weight gain and other side effects Teratogenicity, for female patients in reproductive years
Olanzapine	Possibly comparable to lithium for prevention of mania	Weight gain and metabolic risks Tardive dyskinesia risk
Lamotrigine	Probably more effective than other mood stablizers for depression Generally better tolerated than other mood stablizers	Probably somewhat less effective for prevention of mania
Carbamazepine	Profile comparable to valporoate Less risk of weight gain	More maintenance data needed
Typical antipsychotics	Likely good for prophylaxis of mania	May worsen depression High risk of tardive dyskinesia
Antidepressants	May prevent recurrence of depression	May precipitate mania and provoke rapid cycling
ECT	Accutely effective for both mania and depression	Not adequately studied Maintenance of acute response may be poor
Psychotherapy	As adjunct, increases medication compliance, overall functioning	Not efficacious alone

antidepressant drugs (especially tricyclic antidepressants) and hypothyroidism (Wehr and Goodwin, 1987; Roy-Byrne *et al.*, 1984). Some people also experience ultrarapid cycling, switching between moods in a period of days or even hours. Various therapeutic approaches have been investigated for treating patients with rapid-cycling bipolar disorder.

References

Abrams R, Swartz CM and Vedak C (1991) Antidepressant effects of high-dose right unilateral electroconvulsive therapy. *Arch Gen Psychiatr* 48, 746–748.

Altshuler L, Kiriakos L, Calcagno J *et al.* (2001) The impact of antidepressant discontinuation versus antidepressant continuation on a 1-year risk for relapse of bipolar depression: A retrospective chart review. *J Clin Psychiatr* 62, 612–616.

Anand A, Oren DA, Berman A *et al.* (1999) Lamotrigine treatment of lithium failure outpatient mania: A double-blind placebo-controlled trial. Presented at the Third International Conference on Bipolar Disorder, Pittsburgh, PA.

Berk M (1999) Lamotrigine and the treatment of mania in bipolar disorder. *Eur Neuropsychopharmacol* 9(Suppl 4), S119–S123.

Bowden C, Calabrese JR, Asher J *et al.* (2000) Spectrum of efficacy of lamotrigine in bipolar disorder: Overview of double-blind placebo-controlled studies. Presented at the American College of Neuropsychopharmacolgy, 39th Annual Meeting, San Juan, Puerto Rico.

Bowden CL, Brugger AM, Swann AC *et al.* (1994) Efficacy of divalproex versus lithium and placebo in the treatment of mania. *JAMA* 271, 918–924.

Calabrese JR, Rapport DJ, Kimmel SE *et al.* (1993) Rapid cycling bipolar disorder and its treatment with valproate. *Can J Psychiatr* 38(Suppl 2), S57–S61.

Dilsaver SC, Swann AC, Shoaib AM, *et al.* (1993) Depressive mania associated with nonresponse to antimanic agents. *Am J Psychiatr* 150, 1548–1551.

Dunner DL and Fieve RR (1974) Clinical factors in lithium carbonate prophylaxis failure. *Arch Gen Psychiatr* 30, 229–233.

Gelenberg AJ, Kane JM, Keller MB *et al.* (1989) Comparison of standard and low serum levels of lithium for maintenance treatment of bipolar disorder. *N Engl J Med* 321, 1489–1493.

Himmelhoch JM, Mulla D, Neil JF, *et al.* (1976) Incidence and significance of mixed affective states in a bipolar population. *Arch Gen psychiatr* 33, 1062–1066.

Hirschfeld RMA, Bowden CL, Gitlin MJ *et al.* (2002) Practice guideline for the treatment of patients with bipolar disorder (Revision). American *Journal of Psychiatry* 159(4), 1–50.

Keller MB, Lavori PW, Coryell W, *et al.* (1986) Differential outcome of pure manic, mixed/cycling, and pure depressive episodes in patients with bipolar illness. *JAMA* 255, 3138–3142.

McElroy SL, Keck PE, Pope HG *et al.* (1989) Valproate in psychiatric disorders: Literature review and clinical guidelines. *J Clin Psychiatr* 50(Suppl 3), S23–S29.

Pettinati HM (1994) Speed of ECT? *Convuls Ther* 10, 69–72.

Roy-Byrne PP, Joffe RT, Uhde TW *et al.* (1984) Approaches to the evaluation and treatment of rapid-cycling affective illness. *Br J Psychiatr* 145, 543–550.

Sackeim HA, Prudic J, Devanand DP *et al.* (1993) Effects of stimulus intensity and electrode placement on the efficacy and cognitive effects of electroconvulsive therapy. *N Engl J Med* 328, 839–846.

Stoll AL, Vuckovic A and McElroy SL (1991) Histamine 2-receptor antagonists for the treatment of valproate-induced gastrointestinal distress. *Ann Clin Psychiatr* 3, 301–304.

Wehr TA and Goodwin FK (1987) Can antidepressants cause mania and worsen the course of affective illness? *Am J Psychiatr* 144, 1403–1411.

Antidepressants

The discovery of antidepressants did more than provide a revolutionary therapy for depression; it changed the way we view mood disorders and, by analogy, the mind itself. It permanently transformed the appraisal of our ability to influence areas of existence previously thought unreachable through physical manipulation. Antidepressants are now used to treat a variety of disorders (see Table 79.1).

Mechanisms of Actions

All known antidepressants affect monoamine neurotransmission, and this is believed to be their mechanism of action. As imipramine, iproniazid and related antidepressants shared an ability to augment the monoamine norepinephrine, the early neurochemical theories of depression focused on this neurotransmitter. Later, newer agents were introduced that seemed to exert their primary effect on another monoamine, serotonin. Research into these two neurotransmitters evolved into the monoamine hypothesis of depression. The monoamine theory of depression suggests, in its simplest form, that depression relates to abnormal levels of monoamines: neurotransmitters thought important in the regulation of mood. Antidepressants themselves provide the strongest evidence supporting the role of monoamines in mood, as all known antidepressants affect the levels of monoamines in the brain. Other evidence for the monoamine hypothesis included the observation that reserpine (which depletes norepinephrine and serotonin) frequently causes depression.

The relationship between neurotransmitter activity and the mechanism of antidepressant action is depicted in Figure 79.1.

Antidepressants: Taxonomy and Relation to Mechanism of Action

There are several ways in which antidepressants are grouped. One is historically, in which antidepressants are roughly divided by the period in which they were introduced (e.g., such terms as "first-generation" antidepressants). Another is by chemical structure (e.g., "tricyclic antidepressants"). Alternatively, they are classified by their presumed mechanism of action ("selective serotonin reuptake inhibitors"). In practice, a combination of these is used: thus, some TCAs, which primarily act through serotonin reuptake inhibition (e.g., clomipramine), are usually included with other TCAs rather than as a serotonin reuptake inhibitor, even though they could rightly claim membership in either category.

First-generation Antidepressants

These are, historically, the first antidepressants, and were discovered primarily through serendipity. They include the monoamine antidepressants and the TCAs.

Monoamine Antidepressants (MAOIs)

Historically, these are the first antidepressants discovered. However, owing largely to their side effects, and dietary restrictions, they have rarely enjoyed popular use. They are all characterized by their unique mechanism: they inhibit the action of monoamine oxidase (MAO), the primary catabolic enzyme for the monoamines. The end result is an overall increase in available monoamines.

Tricyclic Antidepressants (TCAs)

These medications all have a structural similarity in common. They are subdivided by the number of amine groups they possess, and are usually referred to as either "tertiary" or "secondary" TCAs. Several are related by metabolism, thus the tertiary amines – amitriptyline and imipramine – are metabolized to the secondary amines – nortriptyline and desipramine – respectively. They all act through reuptake inhibition, and are generally selective for the norepinephrine transporter; several, however, have equal or greater affinity for the serotonin transporter. Normally, excess monoamine is taken up through monoamine transporters into the neuron, where it can be stored, or, more often, catabolized by intracellular MAO. Reuptake inhibitors prevent this through inhibition of the transporter; the excess neurotransmitter remains in the synaptic space where it can bind with receptors. That this is the mechanism of action of these and many other antidepressants is reinforced by the fact that correlations have been demonstrated between transporter inhibition and clinical improvement in depressive symptoms (Hrdina et al., 1997). The TCAs were the drugs of choice for depression through the 1980s. Though very effective, their somewhat nonselective actions, acting on cholinergic, presynaptic adrenergic receptors, for example, resulted in a number of side effects.

Second-generation Antidepressants

These medications were developed using knowledge gained from the first-generation antidepressants. An effort was made to produce medications that were more selective for certain actions. The primary benefit of such selectivity was a decrease in unintended side effects.

Selective Serotonin Receptor Inhibitors (SSRIs)

The SSRIs were first introduced in the late 1980s, and within a few years eclipsed the TCAs as the drugs of choice for depression. As the name suggests, they all act through inhibition of the serotonin transporter. Though very similar, they have some subtle differences, mainly in terms of their half-life, their potency for reuptake inhibition, and their affinity for some other receptors.

Essentials of Psychiatry   Jerald Kay and Allan Tasman
© 2006 John Wiley & Sons, Ltd.

Table 79.1 Various uses of Antidepressants

Major depression
  Acute depression
  Prevention of relapse
  Other depressive syndromes
    Bipolar depression
    Atypical depression
    Dysthymia
Other uses

Tricyclic Antidepressants

Strong evidence
  Panic disorder (most)
  Obsessive-compulsive disorder (clomipramine)
  Bulimia nervosa (imipramine, desipramine)
  Enuresis (imipramine)
Moderate evidence
  Separation anxiety
  Attention-deficit/hyperactivity disorder
  Phobias
  Generalized anxiety disorder
  Anorexia nervosa
  Body dysmorphic disorder
  Migraine (amitriptyline)
  Other headaches
  Diabetic neuropathy, other pain syndromes (amitriptyline, doxepin)
  Sleep apnea (protriptyline)
  Cocaine abuse (desipramine)
  Tinnitus
Evidence for but rarely used for these disorders
  Peptic ulcer disease
  Arrhythmias

Monoamine Oxidase Inhibitors

Strong evidence
  Panic disorder
  Bulimia
Moderate evidence
  Other anxiety disorders
  Anorexia nervosa
  Body dysmorphic disorder

Atypical Agents

Trazodone
  Insomnia
  Dementia with agitation
  Minor sedative-hypnotic withdrawal
Bupropion
  Attention-deficit/hyperactivity disorder

Serotonin Reuptake Inhibitors

Strong evidence
  Obsessive-compulsive disorder (high-dose fluoxetine, sertraline)
  Bulimia (fluoxetine)
  Panic disorder
Moderate evidence
  Generalized anxiety disorder

Table 79.1 Various uses of Antidepressants *Continued*

  Obesity (high-dose fluoxetine)
  Substance abuse
  Impulsivity, anger associated with personality disorders
  Pain syndromes, including diabetic neuropathy
Preliminary evidence
  Obsessive jealousy
  Body dysmorphic disorder
  Hypochondriasis
  Behavioral abnormalities associated with autism and mental retardation
  Anger attack associated with depression
  Depersonalization disorder
  Social phobia
  Attention-deficit/hyperactivity disorder (as an adjunct)
  Chronic enuresis
  Paraphilic sexual disorders
  Nonparaphilic sexual disorders

Selective Serotonin Noradrenaline Reuptake Inhibitors

Duloxetine
  Moderate evidence
    Diabetic peripheral neuropathic pain
Venlafaxine
  Moderate evidence
    Generalized anxiety disorder
    Social phobia
    Panic disorder

These medications are not only the most popular antidepressants, but also some of the most popular drugs of any type. The US sales data demonstrate that the SSRIs remain one of the most lucrative of drugs. In 2001, for example, the producer of sertraline reported global sales of over $2 billion from the product.

Selective Norepinephrine Reuptake Inhibitors (NRIs)

Like the SSRIs, medications in this class share a similar mechanism with the SSRIs, but act on the norepinephrine transporter and have little affinity for the serotonin transporter. Reboxetine (currently available in Europe, and expected to be available soon in the USA) is an example of such a medication.

Other Second-generation Agents

Sometimes referred to as "atypical antidepressants" several were introduced during the same period as the SSRIs. These include bupropion, which seems to exert primarily a dopaminergic effect, and trazodone, which was structurally related to the TCAs but has a primary serotonergic mechanism. Nomifensine, which is not commercially available after international reports of severe hemolytic anemias were reported, would be in a class similar to bupropion.

Third-generation Antidepressant

The next generation of antidepressants involved various attempts to expand the potential of second-generation compounds. One

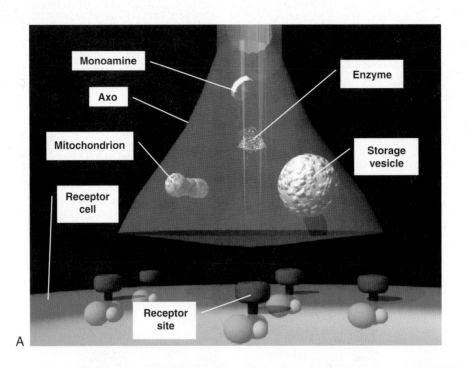

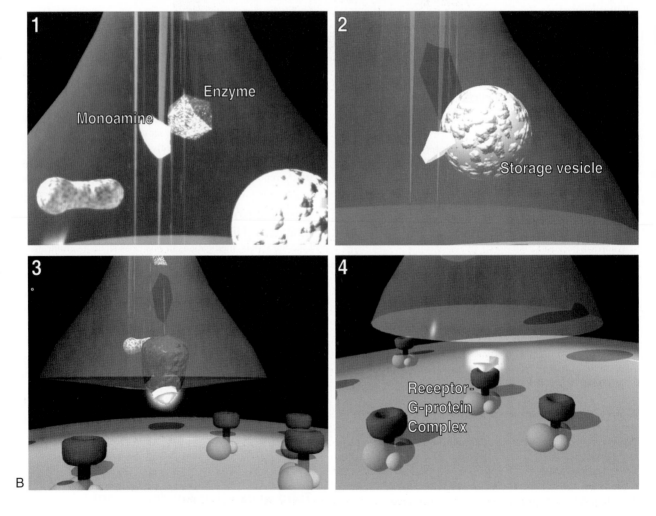

continues

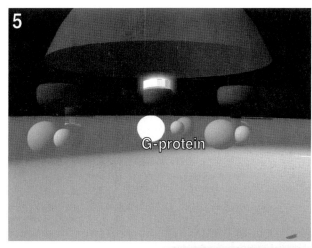
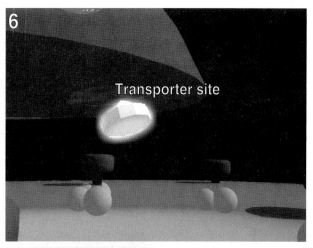
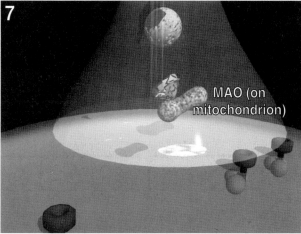

C

Figure 80.1 (A) and (B)   *The "life-cycle" of a monoamine neurotransmitter and potential sites for pharmacological intervention.*

This presents a schematic of monoamine activity. An overview of the neuronal axon–receptor relationship is shown in the overview 1(A), with several key structures pointed out, including the axon and receptor cell, whose membranes are rendered here as transparent to illustrate key intracellular components.

The monoamines – norepinephrine, serotonin, and dopamine – are synthesized within the neuron (1); from dietary amino acids, and then stored within vesicles (2). This vesicle can then bind with the axonal membrane, releasing its contents into the synapse (3).

Upon binding to a receptor complex (4); a resultant cascade of reactions is possible. In general, the binding process causes a destabilization of the subunits comprising the receptor–G-protein complex (5). G-protein, now activated, can then regulate a number of second-messenger systems, such as adenylate cyclase and phospholipase C. The potential results can involve alterations at various levels of neuronal function: from physical structure and membrane permeability to direct regulation of genetic transcription. In this way, it is possible for the many brief and simultaneous inputs to be transduced into coherent and lasting influences on neuronal function. Neurotransmitters can even regulate their own production through binding to presynaptic autoreceptors.

Once the reaction is complete, the receptor–G-protein complex restabilizes, and the monoamine is released from the receptor site. The neurotransmitter can then be metabolized in the extracellular space or, more commonly, taken back in the axon through a transporter site (6). Monoamines undergoing such reuptake can be again stored within vesicles, or be deaminated by intracellular monoamine oxidase (MAO) residing on the wall of mitochondria (7).

Virtually all of these steps can be influenced pharmacologically. For example, enzymatic synthesis can be inhibited by such agents as alpha-methyltyrosine which inhibits tyrosine hydroxylase (1). Reserpine and tetrabenazine can inhibit uptake into the storage vesicles (2), and amphetamines increase the release of norepinephrine from synaptic vesicles (3). A number of drugs can inhibit receptor sites, such as phentolamine and phenoxybenzamine which act at alpha-receptors (4), and most antipsychotics medication, which block dopamine. The lithium ion may act directly on G-protein and second-messenger systems (5).

Most antidepressants appear to act either by inhibiting MAO (e.g., the monoamine oxidase inhibitors [MAOIs] which can inhibit step (7), or by preventing the reuptake on one, or more, monoamines – the TCAs and SSRIs, venlafaxine and bupropion (6). Several of the newer generation antidepressants may have a direct effect on the receptor site (4).

important feature of this group is that many of them have multiple actions. In some cases, this involves actions on multiple neurotransmitters. In other cases, it involves multiple mechanisms of action. Though, in a way this may seem a return to the broader acting first-generation compounds, the attempt with these drugs is to maximize the presumed "clinically relevant" effects of the drugs, while minimizing the less important (and potentially adverse) actions.

Serotonin–Norepinephrine Reuptake Inhibitors (SNRIs)

Medications in this class share a common mechanism with the SSRIs, but differ in that they have equal affinity for the norepinephrine and serotonin transporter. Currently, the only medications of this type available in the USA are venlafaxine and duloxetine. Other medications (available in other countries), such as milnacipran, have similar mechanisms of action. Though, like several of the TCAs, venlafaxine has multiple receptor effects, it is relatively free of the anticholinergic and antihistaminic side effects that are common with the TCAs.

Mixed Serotonin Antagonist/Reuptake Inhibitors

These agents have multiple mechanisms of action, all of which appear to be of clinical importance. Nefazodone is an example of such an agent, with both serotonin (as well as norepinephrine) transporter inhibition as well as antagonism of 5-HT_{2A} and alpha-$_1$-receptors. Trazodone may be similar; however, its effects are somewhat less specific, and as a result, it resembles the TCAs in some respects.

Mixed Serotonin/Noradrenaline Antagonists

Currently, the only agent in this class is mirtazapine. This agent is unique in that it appears to work primarily through receptor blockade, specifically through blockade of the alpha-$_2$-autoreceptors on presynaptic noradrenergic neurons, which enhances noradrenergic output. They may exert a similar effect toward autoreceptors on serotonin neurons. Antagonism of 5-HT_2 and 5-HT_3 receptors may also concentrate the effect of serotonin on 5-HT_{1A} receptors.

Most studies comparing antidepressants have not found significant differences in efficacy between agents. In general, studies comparing TCAs and SSRIs have shown equal efficacy, and meta-analyses of these studies have generally confirmed these findings (Anderson, 2000; Workman and Short, 1993). However, there have been some trends in this data, with TCAs showing, perhaps, greater efficacy in patients with severe depression (Perry, 1996).

Meta-analyses lend some support to the contention that drugs with multiple actions have a greater efficacy than those that are more highly selective. There is some suggestion that the antidepressants that are selective for norepinephrine and serotonin may be more effective than the SSRIs alone. Though these meta-analyses are compelling, the fact that improved efficacy has yet to be demonstrated by the "gold standard" of a placebo-controlled study likely explains why the third generation of antidepressants does not yet enjoy a reputation for improved efficacy. And, even if some of the newer drugs do show improved efficacy, the proposed reason for this – multiplicity of action – may not be correct. In fact, at least one meta-analysis investigating this hypothesis, in which multiple action drugs were compared with selective drugs, did not find a difference between the two (Freemantle et al., 2000). As such, our treatment recommendations, as outlined in the summary, make the assumption that the efficacy of antidepressants is approximately equal for all agents.

The Formulation of Treatment

Indications

All antidepressants are indicated for the treatment of acute major depressive episodes. Beyond the acute period, there is also evidence for the use of antidepressants in the prevention of relapse and recurrence.

There are a number of more minor forms of depression, many of which may also respond to antidepressant medication. Best studied of these is dysthymic disorder. Previously thought to be unresponsive to somatic therapy, a growing literature attests to the responsiveness of this chronic, minor depressive disorder to a variety of medications, including TCAs (Kocsis et al., 1985; Stewart et al., 1993) and serotonin reuptake inhibitors (Hellerstein et al., 1993; Thase et al., 1996; Ravindran et al., 1994; Vanelle, 1997). As with major depression, there is no definitive data to suggest that any one agent is more efficacious than the other. The bulk of data suggests, instead, that any available agent used for major depression is likely to be effective for these other disorders.

Other minor depressive disorders include minor depression and recurrent brief depression. Though rigorous data is largely lacking in the treatment of these disorders, they seem to show an at least modest response to antidepressant medications.

Other Uses for Antidepressants

Although the bulk of this chapter will describe the use of antidepressants in the treatment of major depression, they are also used to treat a number of other conditions (Orsulak and Waller, 1989; Brotman, 1993). Some uses have gained general acceptance while other uses rely on moderate or preliminary evidence. A summary of various indications is presented in Table 79.2.

Selection of an Antidepressant

The decision whether to treat depressive symptoms with pharmacotherapy requires an assessment of both the need for intervention and the likelihood that treatment will be successful. Assessing the need for intervention involves longitudinal and cross-sectional factors. Assessing the likelihood that treatment will be successful is somewhat more difficult, but may rely on clinical, demographical and biological factors.

Assessing the Need for Intervention

This involves assessing the likely result if pharmacological treatment is not given. It is essential in making a useful risk–benefit assessment.

Longitudinal Factors The physician should consider the course and duration of previous episodes of depression. Such episodes can predict the potential severity of the current episode, the likely time to recovery, and the probability of a subsequent recurrence. The physician should also consider the likely complications of depression for the individual patient, which may include substance abuse and suicide.

Cross-sectional Factors The physician should consider the severity of symptoms and the degree of functional impairment. Suicidal ideation is of particular concern and needs rapid and intensive treatment. Such treatment often includes hospitalization. Even with less pressing symptoms, but significant occupational or social impairment, the risk–benefit ratio generally still favors a trial of antidepressants, particularly now that safer and more easily tolerated agents are available.

Table 79.2	SSRI, SNRI and TCA Side Effects

Side Effects of Serotonin Blockade

Jitteriness, activation
Insomnia
Anorexia, weight loss
Nausea, vomiting, diarrhea
Sexual dysfunction
Extrapyramidal-like side effects
Increase in suicidal ideas

Signs And Symptoms of Central Serotonergic Syndrome

Confusion, disorientation
Headache
Autonomic instability
Lethargy
Restlessness
Abdominal cramps, diarrhea
Tremor, myoclonic jerks

Side Effects of Norepinephrine Blockade

Tremors
Jitteriness
Tachycardia
Diaphoresis
Augmentation of pressor effects of sympathomimetics
Sexual dysfunction

Anticholinergic Side Effects

Dry mouth
Constipation (rarely – paralytic ileus)
Urinary hesitancy (rarely – dystonic bladder)
Blurred vision
Sinus tachycardia
Memory impairment
Worsening of narrow-angle glaucoma

Anticholinergic Delirium

"Mad as a hatter": confusion, disorientation, visual
    hallucinations
"Hot as a hare": hyperpyrexia
"Blind as a bat": loss of visual accommodation
"Red as a beet": peripheral vasodilatation
"Dry as a bone": drying of mucous membranes

Selection of a Particular Agent Although, as noted earlier, the various antidepressants seem to have equal efficacy in the treatment of depression, a given patient may respond preferentially to one, or a class of agents. Again, cross-sectional and longitudinal factors should be taken into account.

Pharmacokinetic Concerns

First-generation Antidepressants The pharmacokinetics of TCAs is complex. This complexity is reflected in the diversity of half-lives reported, which vary roughly from 10 to 40 hours. TCAs are primarily absorbed in the small intestine. They are usually well absorbed, and reach peak plasma levels 2 to 6 hours

after oral administration. Absorption can be affected by changes in gut motility. The drugs are extensively metabolized in the liver on first pass through the portal system. They are lipophilic, have a large volume of distribution and are highly protein-bound (85–95%). TCAs are metabolized in the liver by hepatic microsomal enzymes, by demethylation, oxidation, or hydroxylation. They are generally metabolized to active metabolites, and are excreted by the kidneys. There is a large range of elimination half-lives among the antidepressants.

MAOIs are also well absorbed from the gastrointestinal tract. Their metabolism, although quite efficient (they have a half-life of 1 to 2 hours), is not well understood. The short half-life of these compounds is not entirely relevant however, as they bind irreversibly with MAO. Thus, the activity of these drugs depends less on pharmacokinetics, and more on the synthesis of new MAO to restore normal enzyme activity. This synthesis requires approximately 2 weeks.

Second-generation Antidepressants All of the available serotonin reuptake inhibitors are well absorbed, and not generally affected by food administration. Sertraline is an exception to this rule, and its blood level may be increased by food. All serotonin reuptake inhibitors have large volumes of distribution and they are extensively protein-bound. They are metabolized by hepatic microsomal enzymes and are potent inhibitors of these enzymes (a fact which will be discussed later in greater detail).

The only serotonin reuptake inhibitor with an active metabolite is fluoxetine, whose metabolite norfluoxetine has a half-life of 7 to 15 days. Thus, it may take several months to achieve steady state with fluoxetine. This is considerably longer than citalopram, which has a half-life of about 1.5 days, or sertraline and paroxetine, which have half-lives of about a day.

As previously discussed, there is no correlation between half-life and time to onset. Drugs with shorter half-lives have an advantage in cases where rapid elimination is desired (for example, in the case of an allergic reaction). Drugs with a longer half-life may also have advantages: fluoxetine, for example, has been successfully given in a once-weekly dosing during the continuation phase of treatment (Burke *et al.*, 2000), and a once-weekly formulation of this drug is currently available. All serotonin reuptake inhibitors are eliminated in the urine as inactive metabolites. Both fluoxetine and paroxetine are capable of inhibiting their own clearance at clinically relevant doses. As such, they have nonlinear pharmacokinetics: changes in dose can produce proportionately large plasma levels.

As with most of the other antidepressants, bupropion undergoes extensive first pass metabolism in the liver. Although the parent compound has a half-life of 10 to 12 hours, it has three metabolites that appear to be active. One, threohydrobupropion, has a half-life of 35 hours and is relatively free in plasma (it is only 50% protein-bound). There is considerable individual variability in the levels of bupropion and its metabolites. Trazodone has a half-life that is relatively short, having a range of 3 to 9 hours. Given this, and its apparent lack of active metabolites, the plasma levels of trazodone can be quite variable during a day. For this reason, the medication requires divided dosing.

Third-generation Antidepressants Venlafaxine has a short half-life (4 hours); however, it is available in an extended release formulation that allows once-daily dosing. It appears to have a dual effect, in which at lower doses it primarily acts on the serotonin transporter, and clinically significant norepinephrine reuptake inhibition is not seen until higher doses are used (150 mg/day and above).

Table 79.3   Suggested Diet for Patients Taking Monoamine Oxidase Inhibitors (MAOIs)

Proposed Restrictions	Analysis	Can Use
Most cheese and cheese products	M: accounts for most tyramine reactions	Cream, cottage, or ricotta cheese
Sour cream, yogurt	P: except in excess if stored too long	
Fermented meats (sausage, salami, pepperoni)	M: dry fermented sausage (summer sausage) has the most tyramine	Hard sausage has not been associated with hypertensive crises
Aged meats	M: many reports of crises for meats stored for only 2–3 d	Fresh meats
Liver	M: chicken liver has significant tyramine; avoid pate and other prepared dishes	Fresh beef liver
Smoked or pickled herring, caviar	M: high tyramine content	Fresh fish
Broad bean pods (Italian green beans, fava beans)	M: high levodopa content	Other fresh vegetables
Avocado	P: avoid if overripe; no reported reactions	
Sauerkraut	M	
Bananas	P: especially if overripe; peel has highest tyramine (eaten in the only reported case)	Other fresh fruits
Raisins, figs	I: based on one case report	
Chocolate	I: few reported cases	
Yeast extract (brewer's yeast, "Marmite", some packaged soups)	M	Yeast breads
Soy sauce	P: few case reports may be Chinese restaurant syndrome	
Meat tenderizers	I	
Chianti wine	M: most valid of alcohol restrictions	Other wines (moderate amounts)
Vermouth	M: may be similar to Chianti in tyramine	
Beers and ales	P: small amounts allowed; one ration to Irish whiskey	Other alcoholic drinks (moderate amounts)
Other beverages: coffee, tea, caffeinated sodas	I: a nonspecific recommendation (no reports link caffeine to reactions)	

M, must be avoided; P, probably acceptable in moderate amounts; I, insufficient evidence to justify any restriction.

Nefazodone has relatively low bioavailability, and a short half-life (2–8 hours), and thus it is usually given in twice-daily doses. Mirtazapine has a half-life of 13 to 34 hours.

Preparation of the Patient

Side Effects of Antidepressants

General Concerns

Good preparation and reassurance are essential. Side effects – even relatively benign ones – are a major cause of treatment non-adherence. Drop-out rates ranging from 7 to 44% have been reported in various studies of TCAs, and from 7 to 23% in studies of serotonin reuptake inhibitors (Cookson, 1993). Proper education and reassurance about side effects can help reduce this rate. It should help reassure the patient that many of the side effects diminish with time, or with an adjustment of dose. It may also help frame side effects in a positive light, as they represent concrete evidence that the medication is exerting its effect on the body.

The best approach may be to consider both frequency and clinical importance. That is, one should discuss those side effects that are likely to occur, as well as considering the rare but potential dangerous or irreversible side effects that should be discussed (Table 79.3 and Table 79.4).

Specific Side Effects

It is useful to divide side effects into "predictable" and idiosyncratic effects. Predictable side effects result from known pharmacological actions of the drug. Idiosyncratic side effects are not well understood. A number of authors have written important, and very complete reviews of medication-related side effects (e.g., Cookson, 1993; Nierenberg, 1992; Mir and Taylor, 1997; Richelson, 2001); what is intended in the following paragraphs and figures is a brief summary that incorporates data from those works.

Predictable Side Effects

These side effects are the result of the action of the agent at various neurotransmitters and enzyme sites. The major neurotransmitters affected by antidepressants are as follows.

Table 79.4	Antidepressant Drug Interactions	
Inhibitors	Inducers	Substrates
Cytochrome P450 1a2		
Fluvoxamine	Cigarette smoke	Acetaminophen
	Charcoal-broiled beef	Aromatic amines
		Caffeine
		Duloxetine
	Omperazole	Estradiol
		Imipramine
		Theophylline
		Warfarin
Cytochrome P450 2c19		
Fluvoxamine	Rifampin	Citalopram
Tranylcypromine		Diazepam
		Imipramine
		Mephobarbital
		Omperazole
		Propranolol
		Clozapine
Cytochrome P450 2d6		
Moderate	None known	*Antiarrhythmics*
Fluoxetine		Encainide
Paroxetine		Flecainide
Duloxetine		
Mild		Mexiletine
Sertraline		Propafenone
Fluvoxamine		*Antipsychotics*
Yohimbine		Clozapine
Citalopram		Fluphenazine
Escitalopram		Haloperidol
		Perphenazine
		Risperidone
		Thioridazine
		Opiates
		Codeine
		Dextromethorphan
		Other Antidepressants
		Venlafaxine
		Duloxetine
		Trazodone
		Miscellaneous
		Captopril
		Deprenyl
		Mianserin
		Ondansetron
		Beta Blockers
		Alprenolol
		Bufuralol
		Metoprolol
		Propranolol
		Timolol
		TCAs
		Amitriptyline
		Clomipramine
		Desmethylclomipramine

Continues

Table 79.4	Antidepressant Drug Interactions *Continued*	
Inhibitors	Inducers	Substrates
Cytochrome P450 2d6 *Continued*		
		Desipramine
		Imipramine
		Nortriptyline
		SSRIs
		Citalopram
		Fluoxetine
		Paroxetine
Cytochrome P450 3a4		
Ketoconazole	Carbamazepine	*Antiarrhythmics*
Miconazole	Dexamethasone	Lidocaine
Nefazodone	Phenobarbital	Quinidine
Fluvoxamine	Phenytoin	*Antidepressants*
Grapefruit juice	Rifampin	Amitriptyline
		Imipramine
		Nefazodone
		o-Desmethylvenlafaxine
		Antihistamines
		Astemizole
		Terfenadine
		Antipsychotic
		Clozapine
		Benzodiazepines
		Alprazolam
		Diazepam
		Midazolam
		Triazolam
		Calcium Channel Blockers
		Diltiazem
		Nifedipine
		Verapamil
		Miscellaneous
		Acetaminophen
		Carbamazepine
		Dapsone
		Digoxin
		Cortisol
		Tamoxifen
		Theophylline
		Warfarin

Muscarinic Acetylcholine Receptors

Blockade of this receptor produces a variety of peripheral and central effects. Gastrointestinal effects include decreased salivation and decreased peristalsis. Decreased salivation is the most common of these effects and can cause drying of the mucous membranes. Such drying can exacerbate gum disease and dental caries. Decreased peristalsis can cause constipation and, in the extreme, paralytic ileus. Contraction of the bladder wall is inhibited, causing urinary hesitancy and even urinary retention. In the case of TCAs, concomitant sympathomimetic effects that cause constriction of the bladder neck and urethra worsen this effect on urination. Inhibition of the parasympathetically mediated accommodation reflex, in which the ciliary body muscles normally contract to thicken the lens and focus near objects on the retina, results in blurry vision and mydriasis. Such accommodation paresis can occur without other anticholinergic side effects. A more serious ocular effect is the precipitation of acute narrow-angle glaucoma, through pupillary dilatation. The iatrogenic precipitation of narrow-angle glaucoma through antidepressant use is quite rare. Anticholinergic cardiac effects include decreased vagal tone that can cause tachycardia. Central nervous effects include impaired memory and cognition. In severe cases, such cognitive impairment can reach the point of a delirium. Central anticholinergic effects can also worsen existing tardive dyskinesia.

These effects are usually dose-related, and are worse in people with preexisting defects. For example, the cardiac effects are of most concern in those with preexisting cardiac defects, and urinary blockade generally occurs only in the presence of prostatic hypertrophy. These side effects are also more common in patients taking other anticholinergic medications, which is a common feature of many over-the-counter preparations.

MAOIs have little direct effect on receptors, and their side effects relate to enzymatic inhibition, thus they are not included in this section.

Histamine

Blockade of the histamine H_1-receptor is typically associated with sedation. Histamine blockade may also cause orthostatic hypotension and weight gain. It can impair psychomotor coordination and cause falls in the elderly. Cognitive impairment can occur as well. H_2-receptor blockade causes decreased gastric acid production. This is the mechanism of many anti-ulcer medications.

Norepinephrine

Synaptic increases in norepinephrine, through either inhibition of norepinephrine reuptake or decrease in MAO degradation, cause sympathomimetic effects. Increases in norepinephrine can cause anxiety, tremors, diaphoresis and tachycardia. This tachycardia can potentiate anticholinergic cardiac effects. As noted, sympathomimetic effects on the bladder neck and urethra can potentiate the anticholinergic inhibition of normal urinary function.

Receptor Blockade

Blockade of alpha-$_1$-receptors occurs as a chronic effect through both downregulation and desensitization of the beta- and alpha-$_2$-receptors. Blockade of the noradrenergic alpha-$_1$-receptor is responsible for postural hypotension. In the elderly or medically ill, this postural hypotension can be significant, and lead to dizziness or falls. It may also be responsible for ejaculatory delay or impotence. Other potential effects include reflex tachycardia and memory dysfunction.

Serotonin

Potentiation of serotonin can cause anorexia, nausea, vomiting, diarrhea, "jitteriness" and anxiety. Akathisia, a syndrome of motor restlessness usually associated with antipsychotics, may result from either the general effect of serotonin potentiation or the direct effects on the basal ganglia. The latter hypothesis is supported by the fact that the serotonin reuptake inhibitors – fluoxetine (Steur, 1993), sertraline (Shihabuddin and Rapport, 1994) and paroxetine (Choo, 1993) – have all been reported to cause or exacerbate extrapyramidal reactions. Sedation, which has been reported with all serotonin reuptake inhibitors, appears to be a primary serotonin effect (Cookson, 1993). Insomnia, however, is more

common at higher doses, particularly with fluoxetine. A number of sexual side effects have been attributed to serotonin reuptake blockade, including anorgasmia, ejaculatory difficulties and even spontaneous orgasms associated with yawning (Modell, 1989).

Receptor Antagonism

Blockade of the 5-HT_2-receptors may result in hypotension and ejaculatory disturbances. Antagonism of serotonin receptors may also be responsible for weight gain and carbohydrate craving.

Dopamine

Increases in dopamine resulting from reuptake blockade can have an antiparkinsonian effect. It can also cause psychomotor activation and aggravation of psychosis.

Receptor Antagonism

The blockade of dopamine receptors can result in extrapyramidal symptoms. These symptoms include cogwheel-type rigidity, tremor, dyskinesia, masked facies and acute dystonia. Prolonged dopamine blockade appears to be responsible for tardive dyskinesia. Dopamine receptor blockade has also been associated with endocrine changes and sexual dysfunction.

Monoamine Oxidase

MAO is the main enzyme responsible for the metabolism of monoamines. There are two main types of MAOs, identified as types A and B. Type A is selective for serotonin and norepinephrine, and accounts for 80% of the MAO in the brain. Type B selectively deaminates phenylethylamine. Both forms oxidize dopamine and tyramine.

Dietary Restrictions The dietary restrictions required when using MAOIs represent the major limitation to widespread use of these effective antidepressants. Nonselective inhibition of MAO prevents the normal hepatic metabolism of tyramine containing foods or sympathomimetic agents. The increased level of tyramine in the circulation stimulates the release of norepinephrine from sympathetic terminals. This sudden increase in norepinephrine is the basis for the "tyramine–cheese" reaction, so named because cheese is the most common source of the tyramine that causes this reaction. In fact, other pressor amines, such as levodopa, can also cause the reaction, but tyramine – a natural product of food fermentation and bacterial decarboxylation – is the most common in foods. The result of a tyramine–cheese reaction can be a hypertensive crisis. Thus, patients should be well educated as to the foods that must be avoided while using MAOIs. In the past, there has been a tendency towards conservative dietary restrictions, often based on single case reports or indirect analogies. More research and experience have suggested that not all the foods commonly restricted are equally likely to precipitate a reaction (McCabe and Tsuang, 1982). Better compliance is likely if a more reasonable diet is prescribed (as suggested in Table 79.5).

Despite the best of preparation, some patients may err and suffer a hypertensive crisis. This is often experienced as a severe, pulsating, occipital headache that then generalizes. It may be alleviated with 10 mg of nifedipine, either oral or sublingual (Golwyn and Sevlie, 1993).

MAOIs can cause an increase in standing systolic blood pressure, absent of tyramine containing foods or sympathomimetics. Generally, this effect is not clinically significant; however, serious unprovoked hypertensive episodes have been reported

Table 79.5   Typical Antidepressant Therapeutic Doses and Side Effects

Category And Trade Name	Generic Name	Usual Therapeutic Daily Doses (mg)	Sedative Effects	Hypotensive Effects (Decreased Blood Pressure)	Anticholinergic Effects (Dry Mouth, Constipation)	Cardiac Effects (Slowed Heart Rate)
Tricyclic Antidepressants						
Tertiary amines						
Anafranil	Clomipramine	150–300	High	High	High	Yes
Elavil	Amitriptyline	150–300	High	High	High	Yes
Sinequan, Adapin	Doxepin	150–300	High	Moderate	Moderate	Yes
Surmontil	Trimipramine	150–300	High	Moderate	Moderate	Yes
Tofranil	Imipramine	150–300	Moderate	High	Moderate	Yes
Secondary amines						
Norpramin	Desipramine	150–300	Low	Moderate	Low	Yes
Pamelor	Nortriptyline	50–150	Low	Low	Low	Yes
Vivactil	Protriptyline	30–60	Low	Low	High	Yes
Monamine Oxidase Inhibitors						
Marplan	Isocarboxazid	20–60	Low	Moderate	Low	Low
Nardil	Phenelzine	45–90	Low	Moderate	Low	Low
Parnate	Tranylcypromine	30–60	Low	Moderate	Low	Low
Atypical Agents						
Asendin	Amoxapine	200–300	Moderate	Moderate	Low	Yes
Desyrel	Trazodone	300–600	High	Low	Minimal	Low
Ludiomil	Maprotiline	150–200	Moderate	Low	Low	Yes
Wellbutrin	Bupropion	150–450	Minimal	Low	Minimal	Low
Selective Serotonin Reuptake Inhibitors						
Paxil	Paroxetine	20–50	Low	Minimal	Minimal	Low
Prozac	Fluoxetine	20–80	Minimal	Minimal	Minimal	Low
Zoloft	Sertraline	50–200	Minimal	Minimal	Minimal	Low
Luvox	Fluvoxamine	150–300	Low	Low	Low	Low
Celexa	Citalopram	20–50	Low	Minimal	Minimal	Low
Lexapro	Escitalopram	10–20	Low	Minimal	Minimal	Low
Serotonin-norepinephrine Reuptake Inhibitor						
Effexor	Venlafaxine	75–300	Low	None (increased blood pressure)	None	Minimal
Serotonin Transport Blocker And Antagonist						
Serzone	Nefazodone	200–600	Moderate	Low	Minimal	Low

(Lavin *et al.*, 1993), and blood pressure should be monitored for 1 to 2 hours after beginning or increasing an MAOI. Hypotension is also a reported effect of MAO, but the mechanism is not known. MAO inhibition can also cause sedation or overstimulation. Once again, the mechanism of this is not well understood.

Membrane Stabilizing Activity

TCAs have effects on cardiac conduction that are independent of anticholinergic or noradrenergic effects. Destabilization of the cardiac membrane can cause dysrhythmia and asystole, particularly in overdose.

Other Effects

Allergic Reactions

Allergic reactions can occur with any of these agents. Effects include dermatological (rashes, urticaria, photosensitivity, Stevens-Johnson syndrome) and hematological (agranulocytosis) sensitivities. Several case reports have described a photosensitivity reaction apparently caused by desipramine that results in a blue–gray pigmentation (Narurkar *et al.*, 1993; Steele and Ashby, 1993). Fluoxetine has been associated with bleeding, inflammation (Gunzberger and Martinez, 1992), and, most seriously, a fatal systemic vasculitis. It should be stopped if a rash develops.

In most cases of allergic reactions, the primary treatment is to stop the agent. In one report, granulocyte colony stimulating factor was used successfully to treat severe chlomipramine-associated agranulocytosis (Hunt and Resnick, 1993).

Liver Effects

Abnormal liver function tests have been associated with a number of antidepressants, which can be independent of dose. The risk for such effects may be worsened by chronic alcohol or anticonvulsant use.

Seizures

A preexisting seizure disorder increases an antidepressant's likelihood of precipitating a seizure. Other predisposing factors include a family history of a seizure; an abnormal pretreatment electroencephalogram; brain damage; previous electroconvulsive treatment; abuse or withdrawal from sedatives; alcohol, or cocaine; and concurrent use of CNS-activating medications (Rosenstein *et al.*, 1993). Seizures may be more likely to occur early in treatment, or after a large escalation in dose.

The risk of seizure with TCAs is usually reported as 0.1–1.1%. In unselected populations the risk may be as high as 2 to 2.5% (Davidson 1989). Serotonin reuptake inhibitors appear to have a lower incidence of seizures. Bupropion has a high rate of seizures in patients with a preexisting seizure history, and in patients with bulimia. In patients without these predisposing factors, the risk appears to be about 0.4%; thus, it may have a two- to fourfold risk of seizures compared with other antidepressants. Bupropion's effect on the seizure threshold has never been directly compared with other antidepressants.

Precipitation of Mania

Antidepressants have been associated with the precipitation of mania, and rapid cycling bipolar disorder. This appears to be most common in patients with a preexisting history of mania and in unipolar depression the rate of antidepressant-induced mania is very low (<1%). The problem has been most frequently reported in TCAs, but has been seen in SSRIs as well (Cookson, 1993). A similar problem has been found with newer agents, including nefazodone and venlafaxine, though the data for this is more limited. Bupropion may have a lower incidence of mania (Shopsin, 1983).

Sexual Dysfunction

A variety of sexual side effects can be caused by antidepressants, and they can affect all aspects of sexual response. Thus, antidepressants can decrease libido, increase impotence and anorgasmia, and cause delayed or retrograde ejaculation (Segraves, 1992).

SSRIs have a high incidence of delayed orgasm or anorgasmia. Sexual side effects can occur at even low therapeutic doses, and dose reduction may not be possible. A change of agent may be the only alternative. Bupropion appears to have the lowest incidence of sexual side effects among the antidepressants, often not differing from placebo in studies of sexual functioning.

Trazodone has been associated with penile priapism; the risk is around 1 in 6000 to 8000 men. Although rare, it is notable that a third of these cases required surgical intervention, and some resulted in permanent impairment. Clitoral priapism has been reported as well (Pescatori *et al.*, 1993).

Occasionally antidepressants can enhance sexual function. This is usually due to the alleviation of depression; however, there have been case reports of improved libido or potency after initiation of an antidepressant, which occurred independent of any antidepressant effect (Smith and Levitte, 1993).

Miscellaneous

Fine tremors have been noticed with both TCAs and serotonin reuptake inhibitors. The syndrome of inappropriate secretion of antidiuretic hormone has been seen with fluoxetine, as well as with a number of other antidepressants.

Drug Interaction Effects

Drug interactions are summarized in Table 79.4.

First-generation Antidepressants

Tricyclic Antidepressants

As with any combination therapy, the side effects described previously can be additive with other similar drugs. Most problematical are the anticholinergic effects of the TCAs. Such cholinergic – particularly muscarinic – blockade is a property shared by many other medications, including numerous over-the-counter preparations. The general sedative properties of these medications can also augment any soporific. The slowing of cardiac conduction can also potentiate other medications that produce similar effects, such as type IA antiarrhythmics and anticholinergic medications. Adrenergic receptor blockade can worsen the orthostatic hypotension caused by other medications, including vasodilators and low-potency antipsychotic medications.

Absorption of TCAs can be inhibited by cholestyramine, which therefore must be given at different time intervals than the antidepressants. TCA levels can be raised by substances that inhibit enzyme activity, and lowered by substances that induce it. Specific substances reported to increase TCA levels include fluoxetine, antipsychotic medications, methylphenidate and cimetidine. In a controlled trial, methylphenidate was combined with desipramine to treat attention deficits and depression in children. Enzyme "inducers" that can lower tricyclic agent levels include phenobarbital and carbamazepine. The nicotine from cigarettes can also induce enzyme activity.

Guanethidine is contraindicated with TCAs, as it relies on neuronal reuptake for its antihypertensive effect. Clonidine, a presynaptic alpha-$_2$-receptor noradrenergic agonist, is also contraindicated, as it works in an antithetical fashion to tricyclic medications.

Monoamine Oxidase Inhibitors

As with the dietary proscriptions, any medication that increases tyramine can precipitate a hypertensive crisis. Such medications include numerous over-the-counter preparations for coughs, colds and allergies. The same rule applies to sympathomimetic drugs (such as epinephrine and amphetamines) and dopaminergic drugs (such as anti-Parkinsonian medications).

The combination of MAOIs and narcotics – particularly meperidine – may cause a fatal interaction. The reaction can vary from symptoms of agitation and hyperpyrexia to cardiovascular collapse, coma and death. The mechanism of this reaction is poorly understood. A similar reaction has also been reported when propoxyphene, diphenoxylate hydrochloride and atropine are used with MAOIs.

The combination of an MAOI with a potentiator of serotonin (such as a serotonin reuptake inhibitor) can cause the serotonin syndrome (described later in the chapter).

Similar to the dietary restrictions, some of the drug restrictions associated with MAOIs are based on few actual data. Best established are the restrictions against the combination of MAOIs with amines, meperidine, dextromethorphan, hypoglycemic agents, l-dopa, reserpine, tetrabenazine and tryptophan. TCAs are frequently included on this list as causing a "central excitatory syndrome" in combination with MAOIs, although the two have been combined safely. Blackwell (1991) published a comprehensive review of MAOI drug interactions.

Second-generation Antidepressants

Serotonin Reuptake Inhibitors

Serotonin reuptake inhibitors are potent inhibitors of the CYP2D6 pathway, and the drug–drug interactions that can result from this have been the subject of a number of books and articles.

Serotonin reuptake inhibitors can slow the metabolism of any drug that is also metabolized by the same cytochrome P450 pathway. Such drugs include TCAs, carbamazepine, phenothiazines, butyrophenones, opiates, diazepam, alprazolam, verapamil, diltiazem, cimetidine and bupropion. Paroxetine appears to be the most potent inhibitor of this metabolic pathway, with fluoxetine also showing high potency. Sertraline is a somewhat less potent inhibitor.

These pharmacokinetic interactions are best managed with dosage adjustment. Fluoxetine, for example, can be safely used with tricyclic medications if TCA blood levels and, possibly, electrocardiograms are monitored. In the case of bupropion, this relative increase in the blood level can increase the risk for seizures.

Particular caution should be used when a patient using multiple medications starts a serotonin reuptake inhibitor, as the interactions with other drugs can cause dangerous increases in levels. For example, in the cardiac patient, levels of warfarin should be monitored as fluoxetine has been reported to raise these levels (Woolfrey *et al.*, 1993). Several case reports exist of increased antiarrhythmic levels after introduction of fluoxetine, which resulted in potential serious bradyarrhythmias.

Fluoxetine has also been reported to raise lithium levels. The mechanism for this is not clear, as lithium is primarily excreted through the kidneys.

Serotonin Syndrome

Of particular concern is the serotonin syndrome. This syndrome occurs when a serotonin reuptake inhibitor is combined with another drug that can potentiate serotonin, such as MAOIs, pentazocine and l-tryptophan. It has also been reported with the adjunctive use of less obvious serotonergic drugs, such as lithium (Muly *et al.*, 1993) and carbamazepine (Dursun *et al.*, 1993). This creates a toxic effect with symptoms of abdominal pain, diarrhea, diaphoresis, hyperpyrexia, tachycardia, hypertension, myoclonus, irritability, agitation, epileptic seizures and delirium. In its severest form, it can result in coma, cardiovascular shock and death. For this reason, a clearance period is required before switching between a serotonin reuptake inhibitor and an MAOI. Switching from fluoxetine to an MAOI is particularly difficult, given fluoxetine's long clearance time – about 6 weeks. Clearance is considerably more rapid for sertraline or paroxetine, and a 2-week "wash-out" period is advised when changing from one of these agents to an MAOI. Occasionally, case reports have suggested that some patients tolerate a quicker switch; however, a full waiting period remains the most prudent course, as several deaths have occurred after an MAOI was begun too soon after fluoxetine was discontinued (Beasley *et al.*, 1993).

Other Second-generation Antidepressants

Few reports exist of interactions with other drugs and trazodone, although trazodone may increase levels of digoxin, phenytoin and possibly warfarin. Bupropion causes few drug–drug interactions. The main interactions reported have occurred when bupropion is combined with another dopaminergic agent. For example, when bupropion was used with l-dopa, the combination caused excitement, restlessness, nausea, vomiting and tremor (Goetz *et al.*, 1984).

Third-generation Antidepressants

Venlafaxine does not substantially inhibit the CYP enzyme, and is not highly protein-bound, thus it tends to have few clinically significant drug–drug interactions. Nefazodone is highly protein-bound, and has several active metabolites. It is also a strong inhibitor of CYP3A4, and affects other drugs also metabolized by that pathway; however, it has little affinity for the CYP2D6 enzyme. Mirtazapine is highly protein-bound as well, but appears only weakly to affect the cytochrome enzymes.

Initiation of Treatment

Choosing a Drug

On average, all antidepressants are equally effective. Although an individual patient may preferentially respond to a certain antidepressant, it is difficult to predict this in advance. Without a personal or family history of such a response, side effects are the most influential factors in choosing an agent. Side effects may be particularly relevant in the following groups of patients.

Cardiovascular Patients

Tricyclic Antidepressants

There is a high rate of depression in patients who have had a myocardial infarction and the presence of depression adversely affects the prognosis of cardiac disease.

The major cardiovascular side effect of TCAs is orthostatic hypotension. This can be clinically significant in both the hypertensive patient and the elderly patient. Some of the tricyclic medications may have a lower risk of orthostatic hypotension, notably nortriptyline and doxepin. The evidence for nortriptyline causing little or no hypotension is convincing; for doxepin it is weaker (Roose and Dalack, 1992).

TCAs do not show a negative inotropic effect and do not seem to worsen congestive heart failure. Patients with congestive heart failure may, however, be at a higher risk for orthostatic hypotension. Again, nortriptyline is the safest TCA in this case.

TCAs slow conduction at the bundle of His. Their effect is analogous to type 1A antiarrhythmic agents such as quinidine and procainamide. In therapeutic doses they can slow cardiac conduction and in overdose they can cause atrioventricular blockade. These effects are of most concern in patients with preexisting cardiac conduction defects. There is no evidence that any one tricyclic medication is safer than another.

Glassman and coworkers (1993) recommend caution when using TCAs in all patients with ischemic heart disease, particularly patients with ventricular arrhythmias that follow a myocardial infarction.

Serotonin Reuptake Inhibitors

The serotonin reuptake inhibitors differ from the TCAs in that they do not prolong the PR or heart wave (QRS) interval. Thus, they probably lack any of the proarrhythmic and antiarrhythmic activities associated with TCAs. They do not cause orthostatic hypotension. Most studies that exist suggest that SSRIs should be safe in patients with heart disease.

Other Agents

Trazodone has less proarrhythmic effect than the TCAs. However, there have been reports of trazodone-related ventricular ectopy and complete heart block (Martyn *et al.*, 1993). In patients with preexisting heart disease, bupropion does not appear to cause the cardiac side effects attributed to TCAs (Roose *et al.*, 1991).

Elderly Patients

Pharmacokinetic Concerns

Two pharmacokinetic changes are of great importance in aging patients: decreased efficiency of the hepatic microoxidase system and a decreased muscle–fat ratio. Decreased efficiency of hepatic microoxidases results in the slower metabolism of antidepressants and other drugs. Normal increases in body fat and a loss of muscle mass result in an alteration of the volume of distribution for a substance. Thus, lipophilic drugs, including all antidepressants, are more widely distributed in the elderly body.

Both the resulting slower metabolism and the increased volume of distribution increase the half-lives of the various antidepressants. The elderly, therefore, are likely to have a greater incidence of side effects.

The half-lives and steady state concentrations of the serotonin reuptake inhibitors are only minimally affected by age. Paroxetine may be an exception to this, and it may have an increased half-life in the elderly (Leonard, 1993).

Pharmacodynamic Concerns

The assumption that elderly patients require lower blood levels of antidepressant medication is not correct. Although pharmacokinetic concerns may require lowering of the medication dose, plasma levels are comparable to those in young adults.

It appears that antidepressants are as effective in the elderly as in the young, although the elderly may have more difficulty tolerating these medications.

Medically Ill Patients

Few studies are available on the pharmacological treatment of depression in medically ill patients, and even less on medically ill elderly patients. In initiating treatment, the physician should understand the effects of various illnesses on pharmacokinetics and the potential side effects that may result.

Child and Adolescent Patients

Next to stimulants, antidepressants are the most common psychotropic medications prescribed in children (Zito *et al.*, 2000) and adolescents (Jensen *et al.*, 1999) and the trend to use these medications in that group is on an increase. It should be noted that the FDA has placed a "black box" warning related to suicidal ideation in adolescents treated with SSRIs.

In addition to depression, antidepressants are used in a number of nonaffective disorders in children and adolescents, including enuresis, attention-deficit/hyperactivity disorder, OCD and bulimia nervosa. They are used to mitigate behaviors that are not part of a disease, for example, in suicidal adolescents who do not have a concomitant depressive disorder (American Academy of Child and Adolescent Psychiatry, 2001); however, there is little empirical evidence that suggests that they can lower suicide risk (Zametkin *et al.*, 2001). Similarly, they are used to dampen other impulsive behaviors.

Dosage Concerns

Children should generally be treated with levels of medication comparable to those used in adults, with the doses adjusted for body weight. As children have large livers (relative to body weight), they tend to be efficient metabolizers of substances, and may even need higher doses of medications (relative to body weight) than do adults.

Adverse Effects

Well after the introduction of SSRIs, TCAs remained the most popular antidepressants used in children. However, there have been concerns regarding the safety of these medications. Several case studies have documented adverse cardiac affects in children treated with TCAs, especially with desipramine. The Work Group on Research of the American Academy of Child and Adolescent Psychiatry (1990) conducted an extensive review of the available literature and concluded that there is minimal or no increased risk of "sudden death" in children with desipramine. It is probably wise, however, to perform an adequate cardiac work-up before starting an antidepressant in a child.

Given these issues concerning cardiotoxicity, the serotonin reuptake inhibitors have become more popular for the treatment of children and adolescents. Most of the newer agents have evidence for safety and efficacy in children, including fluoxetine (Emslie *et al.*, 1997) and paroxetine (Keller *et al.*, 2001). Others of the SSRIs have data for their usefulness in anxiety disorders, such as fluvoxamine (in OCD) (Riddle *et al.*, 2001) and sertraline (which has open label data for social anxiety disorder and OCD) (Compton *et al.*, 2001). Bupropion has been found safe and effective in children as well, although it may exacerbate tics in Tourette's disorder. Other antidepressants, including most of the first-generation antidepressants, lack any positive efficacy studies in children or adolescents.

Pregnant and Postpartum Patients

Of the commonly used antidepressants, none show compelling evidence of teratogenicity. Nonetheless, as is true for most medications, it is usually best to discontinue antidepressants if a patient becomes pregnant. For all the antidepressants, one must consider a risk–benefit decision, measuring the risk of possible pregnancy-related side effects against the morbidity of a prolonged untreated depressive episode during pregnancy (Wisner *et al.*, 2000). The FDA, in late 2005, classified paroxetine as a class "D" medication, indicating it should be used only with great caution in pregnancy.

Nursing Mothers

All antidepressants are secreted in breast milk. The levels of these agents are difficult to predict, and their effect on the developing infant is not known (Cohen *et al.*, 1991). There are no systematic investigations of this issue. Given the level of uncertainty, nursing should be deferred if antidepressant treatment is required.

Suicidal Patients

Meta-analysis of both world (Mann and Kapur, 1991) and the USA (Kapur *et al.*, 1992) and a more recent study using prospective data (Leon *et al.*, 1999) showed no unique relationship between fluoxetine (or any antidepressant) and suicidal behaviors. However, as with any rare event, one cannot totally discount the possibility that antidepressants may "trigger" suicidal ideation, either through a direct neurochemical effect (e.g., through an acute decrease in serotonergic transmission) or through nonspecific side effects of the drug (e.g., the induction of akathisia). If such a phenomenon exists, it is very uncommon, and probably not specific to any one antidepressant. There is, however, now a "black box" warning regarding the emergence of suicidal ideation in some adolescents taking SSRIs.

These concerns must be balanced over the well-proven and much greater risk of suicidal ideation and attempts when depression is not treated. Given this, and the propensity of suicidal patients to choose medication overdose as the method of suicide, the wide safety margin of the second- and third-generation antidepressants makes them preferable to first-generation agents when suicide is a concern. Bupropion has generally not been fatal in overdose, although about a third of such cases experience a seizure.

Starting Doses

See Table 79.7 for usual therapeutic dosages.

First-generation Antidepressants

Tricyclic Antidepressants

TCAs are usually begun at a relatively low dose. For the majority of TCAs, including imipramine, amitriptyline, desipramine, maprotiline and doxepin, the initial starting dose is in the range of 50 to 75 mg/day. Notable exceptions include nortriptyline and protriptyline, which are more potent agents. In the case of nortriptyline, the usual starting dose is 25 to 50 mg/day, and for protriptyline, 10 to 15 mg/day (Schatzberg and Cole, 1991). The lower doses are preferred in patients who are elderly. In the frail elderly, further dose reductions may be needed (about one-half or less of the usual starting dose).

Once a medication is initiated, it is gradually increased to a therapeutic level. A number of strategies have been suggested for this increase. Most TCAs can be increased to 150 mg/day by the second week, and then to a range of 300 mg/day by the third or fourth week. This can be achieved through small daily increase of 25 mg or weekly increase of 75 mg. Younger patients will tolerate larger and more rapid increases, whereas the elderly benefit from smaller (25 mg/day) and less frequent (every other day) increases with a lower target dose (150 mg/day).

For nortriptyline, increases of 50 mg/week are usually tolerated in the young, with the elderly requiring smaller increases (25 mg/week). Of particular interest is nortriptyline's therapeutic window: doses above and below a certain range appear to be less effective. The effective range is approximately 50 to 150 mg/day. Some authors suggest a lower range (for example, from 30 to 100 mg (Brotman *et al.*, 1987); however, plasma blood monitoring is a more accurate indicator of the proper level.

Monoamine Oxidase Inhibitors

Patients taking MAOIs must adhere to a special diet to reduce the risk of a hypertensive crisis (see Table 79.7) Phenelzine is usually begun at a dose of 30 mg/day. It is increased by 15 mg after 3 days, then weekly to a target range of 45 to 90 mg/day. Tranylcypromine is started at 20 mg/day. It is increased by 10 mg after 3 days, with additional daily increases of 10 mg after 1 week, to a target range of 30 to 60 mg/day. Isocarboxazid is usually begun at 20 mg/day. It is titrated in a manner similar to tranylcypromine to a target of 30 mg/day. Schatzberg and Cole (1991) suggested that most patients require doses in the higher range, and that some may require doses above the normally recommended limits (e.g., phenelzine at 120 mg/day tranylcypromine at 110 to 130 mg/day, and isocarboxazid at 50 mg/day).

Second-generation Antidepressants

Serotonin Reuptake Inhibitors

Although dosing strategies are less well understood with these agents, the wisest choice is to start a patient at the lowest effective dose and increase as indicated by clinical response. Reasonable doses are 20 mg/day for fluoxetine, 50 mg/day for sertraline, 20 mg/day for paroxetine and citalopram. For children, adolescents, the elderly and patients who find medications generally difficult to tolerate, 50% reductions in these doses are reasonable starting doses.

A number of studies have shown increasing response with increasing doses of SSRIs (Leonard, 1993), but the dropout rate due to side effects also increases with increasing dose. Fluoxetine, paroxetine and citalopram should be started at a dose of 10 or 20 mg for 3 weeks (20 mg for a normal healthy adult, 10 mg for patients who are young, elderly, or particularly sensitive to medications), after which they can be increased in 10 or 20 mg increments to a dose of 40 mg/day if there is no response. A maximum dose of 60 mg/day of fluoxetine is recommended for the treatment of depression. A similar strategy can be used for sertraline, which can be begun at 25 to 50 mg, and increased in 25 to 50 mg increments to a target dose of 50 to 150 mg. Other disorders, particularly OCD and bulimia nervosa, may require 80 mg/day or more for maximal effect. The issue of dosage for SSRIs remains complicated, as some studies have suggested that fluoxetine may not have a linear dose–response curve; some patients may respond better to lower doses of the medication, such as 10 mg/day (Leonard, 1993). Other studies have documented responses to fluoxetine at incredible doses and blood levels (320 mg/day and over 2000 ng/mL, respectively) without adverse effects (Stoll *et al.*, 1991).

As with tricyclic medications, there is a significant delay between initiation of medication and response, and there is no reason to believe that increasing the dose hastens response.

Other Second-generation Antidepressants

Trazodone is generally dosed in a manner similar to TCAs, with starting doses of 50 to 75 mg/day, and target ranges of 150 to 300 mg/day, with doses not exceeding 400 mg/day in outpatients and 600 mg/day in inpatients. Unlike many of the TCAs, trazodone's short half-life requires divided doses, usually twice daily.

Bupropion, like trazodone, requires divided doses. It is available in a short acting form that requires three times a day dosing, or a longer acting form that allows twice-daily dosing. It should be begun at 100 mg b.i.d., and increased to a target of 300 mg/day after a few days. The recommended dose of the medication is 300 mg/day; however, patients not responding to that dose can be increased to 450 mg/day. Patients should be instructed to avoid taking more than 150 mg in a single dose. In the elderly, a usual starting dose is 75 mg/day of the shorter acting preparation. This is then increased to 75 mg b.i.d.

Third-generation Antidepressants

Venlafaxine

It is currently available in a slow release preparation that enables once-daily dosing. Venlafaxine is usually begun at a dose of 37.5 mg and is increased within half to 1 week to a dose of 75 mg. If further increases are needed, it can be titrated at a rate of 75 mg every 4 days or more. Though a maximum dose of 225 mg per day is recommended by the manufacturer, doses as much as 300 to 450 mg/day have been employed to good effect in some patients.

Duloxetine

It is available in 20, 30, and 60 mgm capsules. Starting dose is usually 20 mg twice a day. Maximum recommended effective dose is 60 mgm/day.

Mirtazapine

Adults should be started on a dose of 15 mg/day. It is usually given as a before bedtime dose. The dosage generally needs to be increased in 15-mg intervals every half to 1 week to a target dose. The effective dose is usually between 15 and 45 mg/day; however, higher doses, such as 60 mg have been useful in some patients.

Nefazodone

Nefazodone is given in twice-daily doses. Patients can be started at a dose of 100 mg b.i.d. and increased at a rate of 100 to 200 mg a week. The recommended effective dose is 300 to 600 mg/day. Some clinical experience suggests that once-daily doses (given at night) are acceptable for some patients (Marathe *et al.*, 1996).

Therapeutic Drug Monitoring

Although blood levels are available for many antidepressants, those for imipramine, desipramine, and nortriptyline have been best established (see Table 79.6). Imipramine and desipramine appear to have a curvilinear dose–response curve with an optimal range of 150 to 300 ng/mL. Nortriptyline appears to have a therapeutic window in the range of 50 to 150 ng/mL (Preskorn *et al.*, 1993). These blood levels are nominal, as some patients do respond above or below these ranges, and blood level monitoring should not be a substitute for clinical observation.

Drug levels have not been well established for the MAOIs and the serotonin reuptake inhibitors.

Table 79.6	Therapeutic Blood Levels of the TCAs
TCA	**Therapeutic blood level**
Imipramine (IMI)	>225 ng/dl of IMI + DMI
Desipramine (DMI)	>125 ng/dl of DMI
Amitriptyline	Conflicting evidence
Nortriptyline	>50 ng/dl and <150 ng/dl

Antidepressant Augmentation

Typical augmentation strategies (Table 79.7) include the addition of lithium carbonate, thyroid hormone, or a stimulant. These may be considered when response is inadequate to initial treatment using an adequate dose for an adequate time of a single agent.

Changing to a New Agent

For the patient who shows no response or whose condition deteriorates during therapy, the physician should initiate a new trial of an alternative single agent. There remains some debate as to what type of agent should be used next. Some studies have suggested that patients who do not respond to one SSRI may respond to another (Thase *et al.*, 1997). However, the most convincing study continues to support the more commonly held belief that it is best to switch to an agent of a different class, and approximately 50% of patients unresponsive to a first trial respond to an antidepressant of a different class (Phillips and Nierenberg, 1994; Thase *et al.*, 2002).

When the switch involves an MAOI, sufficient time must be given for medication clearance. Although seldom used, MAOIs may

Table 79.7	Augmentation Strategies			
Agent	Dosing Strategy	Length of Trial	Reported Response Rate	Comments
Lithium carbonate	Start at 300 mg b.i.d., increase to therapeutic blood level (0.8–1.2 mEq/L)	3–6 wk	As high as 65%	Best documented strategy; has been combined with most agents
Triiodothyronine	Start at 25 μg/d, may increase to 50 μg/d	At least 3 wk	At 25%	Equal to lithium in one placebo controlled trial
Stimulants (methylphenidate dextroamphetamine)	†	†	†	Few systematic data
Atypical antipsychotics	Begin with low dose (e.g. olanzapine 2.5 mg/day, aripiprazole 5 mg/day, gradually increase to full therapeutic dose if needed)	†	†	Mainly open trials; controlled studies in progress
Combined antidepressant therapy	May need lower doses than usual (due to enzyme inhibition)†	†	†	Mainly open trials; controlled studies in progress
Psychotherapy	N/A	Varies by therapy	Varies by therapy	Good data for both cognitive–behavioral therapy and interpersonal therapy

†Inadequate data.

be very effective in patients not responsive to other classes of antidepressants (McGrath *et al.*, 1993). Generally, 10 to 14 days for either medication is required for clearance of TCAs and MAOIs. Fluoxetine requires a much longer period – 6 weeks – whereas sertraline and paroxetine require about 2 weeks when switching to an MAOI.

Continuation Period

This period usually lasts 5 to 8 months after the end of the acute treatment period. The goal at this phase is the prevention of relapse. There is a high risk of relapse if treatment is discontinued after the acute treatment phase. The National Institutes of Health Consensus Development Conference on the Mood Disorders (1985) reported a cumulative relapse rate of 15% after 6 months and 22% after 12 months. Keller and colleagues (1982) found that the two best predictors of relapse were a high number of previous depressive episodes (greater than three predicted relapses) and underlying dysthymic disorder.

Once a patient has responded to a medication, the medication should be continued for a minimum of 4 to 6 months, beginning from the point of initial response. The World Health Organization (1989) recommended 6 months as a minimum period for continuation of treatment after the acute phase, and the American Psychiatric Association (2000b) recommended a minimum of 16 to 20 weeks of treatment following the full remission of symptoms. This period should be lengthened for the patient with a history of longer depressive episodes.

Surprisingly, few studies exist that directly look at the efficacy of antidepressants for continuation therapy. However, there exists at least one placebo-controlled study for each of the SSRIs (Montgomery *et al.*, 1988, 1993; Montgomery and Dunbar, 1993; Doogan and Caillard, 1992), nefazodone (Feiger *et al.*, 1999) and mirtazapine (Montgomery *et al.*, 1998).

In the past, it was suggested that, on achievement of euthymia, doses could be reduced. However, it is more likely that levels similar to those needed at the acute stage of treatment will be required throughout the continuation period.

Discontinuance of Treatment

After the continuation period, somatic therapy is usually discontinued in the patient with a single episode of major depression. Before discontinuing, however, it is important to remember that depression is often a lifelong disease with a chronic course. One should always weigh the benefits of discontinuance against the risks of recurrent depression.

In the past, a distinction between exogenous and endogenous depression was used to predict the risk of recurrence. Inferences about etiology, however, are not an accurate predictor of recurrence. More useful information are the age of onset during the initial episode and the number of episodes. Patients with a single episode of acute depression, who have an onset before age 50 years, are the best candidates for discontinuance (Greden, 1993).

Tapering and Withdrawal

For the TCAs, the usual strategy is to taper the medications at a rate of 25 to 50 mg/day every 2 to 3 days. Too rapid a discontinuation may produce symptoms of cholinergic "rebound" or supersensitivity. Such a rebound includes severe gastrointestinal symptoms (nausea, vomiting and cramping), other signs of autonomic hyperactivity (diaphoresis, anxiety, agitation, headaches) and insomnia (often with vivid nightmares). In severe cases, a full delirium may result. Cholinergic rebound may occur as early

as 48 hours or as late as 2 weeks after discontinuation. These symptoms may account for some cases of presumed early relapse from antidepressant discontinuation.

MAOIs may also have a withdrawal syndrome, including symptoms of psychosis, on abrupt withdrawal; however, this syndrome is rarer than that seen with TCAs.

Fluoxetine has a long half-life, and abrupt discontinuation should be permissible. Sertraline, citalopram and paroxetine, with shorter half-lives of around a day, may require a 7- to 10-day taper. With the shorter-acting agents, a withdrawal syndrome including symptoms of fatigue, insomnia, abdominal distress and influenza-like symptoms have been reported when they are too abruptly discontinued. The same may be true for venlafaxine.

Some investigators question current tapering schedules, which are based on pharmacokinetic rather than pharmacodynamic (i.e., receptor) effects. Given an antidepressant's long-term effects, they suggest that receptors will "need" more time to readjust to a new medication-free environment. Greden (1993), for instance, recommended a one-fourth reduction in dose every third month for tricyclic medication. For fluoxetine, he recommended slowly increasing the dosing interval: from daily to every other day for 3 months, then every third day for 3 months. After 3 months of dosing every 3 days, he recommended switching to a liquid form to permit 25% dose reductions each quarter year. Obviously, such a strategy would dramatically increase the taper period from several weeks to approximately a year. It will be interesting to see whether studies support the contention that extended tapers are more likely to prevent recurrence.

On discontinuance, the goal is to enable early intervention should symptoms recur. A first episode of depression has a high risk of recurrence, and the risk of recurrence is even higher in patients who show only partial response to medication. The patient should be educated to recognize symptoms of depression. The patient's own history suggests which symptoms were prodromal to the patient's full depressive episode.

Maintenance Period

The goal of the maintenance period is to prevent the recurrence of depression. There are a number of reasons to consider long-term prophylactic therapy for depression rather than medication withdrawal. Depression is a lifelong disease, with recurrence being the norm rather than the exception (Keller *et al.*, 1992). As the number of acute episodes increases, the risk of future episodes increases as well, and the interval between episodes shortens. Each subsequent episode carries a higher morbidity and disability. Although better understood in bipolar disorder, there is a fear that treatment response may decrease with an increasing number of depressive episodes (Greden, 1993).

A number of factors can influence the decision of when it is appropriate to maintain long-term prophylaxis for depression. The seriousness of previous episodes, the severity of impairment caused by such episodes, the degree of response to previous treatments and the ability of the patient to tolerate the drug all play a role. Central in the decision process is the concept of recurrent depression: that some patients are more likely than others to have a recurrence of the disease. Three previous episodes of depression make recurrent depression likely. The best predictors of the likelihood of recurrence appear to be older age of onset and number of episodes. Greden (1993) proposed that long-term maintenance is the treatment of choice for the following groups of patients: 1) those who were 50 years old or more at the time of the first depressive episode, 2) those who were 40 years old or more at first episode and have had at least one subsequent recurrence, and 3) anyone who has had more than three episodes.

The recommended length of maintenance treatment needs further clarification as well. Recommended lengths of time vary from 5 years of treatment to indefinite continuation. There are only a handful of studies on maintenance antidepressant treatment.

Equally important in preventing recurrence of depression is the problem of maintaining adherence to medication long after the acute episode has resolved. Proper education and support will help with compliance. Toleration of side effects is important and evidence suggests that patients are more likely to comply with the agents that have more favorable side-effect profiles. The serotonin reuptake inhibitors are generally the best tolerated antidepressants.

Although lower doses for prophylaxis have been recommended, there are few data to support this contention. Even though lower doses may increase compliance, full doses should be used until new information indicates otherwise.

Treatment Failure

Failure to respond to treatment is most often due to inadequate treatment rather than "true" nonresponse. Inadequate treatment can be due to an inadequate length of treatment or an inadequate dose. These can result from the physician's error (either improper dosing strategies or impatience in waiting an appropriate amount of time) or the patient's error (through misunderstanding or nonadherence).

Patients will often not acknowledge nonadherence as they fear rejection from treatment, and they are certainly unlikely to admit to it if their physician does not ask them. The best remedy for nonadherence is prevention, through proper education of the patient about likely side effects that might otherwise unnerve the patient. A flexible approach is also necessary. Gentle reassurance and encouragement can be helpful; however, dogmatic insistence on adherence to a prescription leaves the patient with no choice except to hide nonadherence, or look elsewhere for treatment.

Thus, "true" nonresponse can be defined as the lack of response to an adequate dose for an adequate time. Many strategies have been suggested for treatment-resistant patients. Electroconvulsive therapy offers a safe, effective alternative somatic therapy for depression. A prior good response to electroconvulsive therapy, a need for rapid response as with life-threatening depressive symptoms (food refusal, suicide attempts) or a medical contraindication to antidepressants warrants early consideration of this treatment. It should be considered for any patient with major depression who has not responded to antidepressant medication.

Summary

There remain a number of important limitations regarding the pharmacotherapy of depression. Some of these limitations can be addressed by continued progress on current research. Other limitations await truly novel research into the mechanism of depression.

Recommendations for the Use of Antidepressants

Allowing for the many limitations, we can generalize from available data to make the following recommendations:

1. All patients with acute major depression should be considered reasonable candidates for pharmacotherapy.
2. There is adequate evidence to make the same recommendation for other forms of depression. This is particularly true for dysthymia, and may be true for other minor forms of depression as well.
3. There is good evidence for the use of antidepressants for non-mood disorders as well, particularly the anxiety disorders.
4. There remains no strong evidence from choosing one medication over another, and treatment recommendations should be made on the basis of tolerability and, if appropriate, cost.
5. Extended treatment should be recommended both for patients with chronic depression and recurrent depression.
6. Maintenance treatment should consist of the same dose of antidepressant as used to achieve acute phase remission.
7. The exact length of maintenance treatment is not known. The decision for indefinite treatment should be a risks–benefit decision, made with the informed consent of the patient, who is entitled to be informed of the limitations in our knowledge.

Finally, cases like this emphasize the art as well as the science of pharmacotherapy. Though some treatment-related decisions have a clear scientific basis, others are more rooted in judgment and experience. Certainly the switch to bupropion to minimize sexual side effects has a clear pharmacodynamic rationale. However, the subsequent adjunctive use of an SSRI likely relied less on science, and more on the psychiatrist's experience in interpreting the irritability as a symptom that might be more amenable to a serotonergic agent. Though the practice of clinical medicine should be informed by research, the greatest clinicians are still those unique individuals who can integrate research into their own observations and wisdom.

References

American Academy of Child and Adolescent Psychiatry (2001) Practice parameter for the assessment and treatment of children and adolescents with suicidal behavior. *J Am Acad Child Adolesc Psychiatr* 40(Suppl), 24S–51S.

American Psychiatric Association (2000b) Practice guideline for the treatment of patients with major depressive disorder (Rev). *Am J Psychiatr* 157(Suppl), 1–45.

Anderson IM (2000) Selective serotonin reuptake inhibitors versus tricyclic antidepressants: A meta-analysis. *Br Med J* 320, 1574–1577.

Beasley CM, Masica DN, Heiligenstein JH *et al.* (1993) Possible monoamine oxidase inhibitor–serotonin uptake inhibitor interaction: Fluoxetine clinical data and preclinical findings. *J Clin Psychopharmacol* 13, 213–320.

Blackwell B (1991) Monoamine oxidase inhibitor interactions with other drugs. *J Clin Psychopharmacol* 11, 55–59.

Brotman AW (1993) What's new with antidepressants? [audiotape], in *Practical Reviews in Psychiatry*. Educational Reviews, Birmingham, AL.

Brotman AW, Falk WE and Gelenberg AJ (1987) Pharmacologic treatment of acute depressive subtypes, in *Psychopharmacology: The Third Generation of Progress* (ed Meltzer HY). Raven Press, New York, pp. 1031–1040.

Burke WJ, Hendricks SE, McArthur-Miller D *et al.* (2000) Weekly dosing of fluoxetine for the continuation phase of treatment of major depression: Results of a placebo-controlled, randomized clinical trial. *J Clin Psychopharmacol* 20, 423–427.

Choo V (1993) Paroxetine and extrapyramidal reactions. *Lancet* 341, 624.

Cohen LS, Heller VL and Rosenbaum JF (1991) Psychotropic drug use in pregnancy: An update, in *Medical Psychiatric Practice*, Vol. 1 (eds Stoudemire A and Fogel BS). American Psychiatric Press, Washington DC, pp. 615–634.

Compton SN, Grant PJ, Chrisman AK *et al.* (2001) Sertraline in children and adolescents with social anxiety disorder: An open trial. *J Am Acad Child Adolesc Psychiatr* 40, 564–571.

Cookson J (1993) Side-effects of antidepressants. *Br J Psychiatr* 163(Suppl), 20–24.

Davidson J (1989) Seizures and bupropion: A review. *J Clin Psychiatr* 50, 256–261.

Doogan DP and Caillard V (1992) Sertraline in the prevention of depression. *Br J Psychiatr* 160, 217–222.

Dursun SM, Mathew VM and Reveley MA (1993) Toxic serotonin syndrome after fluoxetine plus carbamazepine (letter). *Lancet* 342, 442–443.

Emslie GJ, Rush AJ, Weinberg WA *et al.* (1997) A double-blind, randomized, placebo-controlled trial of fluoxetine in children and adolescents with depression. *Arch Gen Psychiatr* 54, 1031–1037.

Feiger AD, Bielski RJ, Bremner J *et al.* (1999) Double-blind placebo-substitution study of nefazodone in the prevention of relapse during continuation treatment of outpatients with major depression. *Clin Psychopharmacol* 114, 19–28.

Freemantle N, Anderson IM and Young P (2000) Predictive value of pharmacological activity for the relative efficacy of antidepressant drugs: Meta-regression analysis. *Br J Psychiatr* 177, 292–302.

Glassman AH, Roose SP and Bigger JT (1993) The safety of tricyclic antidepressants in cardiac patients. *JAMA* 269, 2673–2675.

Goetz CG, Tanner CM and Klawans HL (1984) Bupropion in Parkinson's disease. *Neurology* 34, 1092–1094.

Golwyn D and Sevlie C (1993) Monoamine oxidase inhibitor hypertensive crisis headache and orthostatic hypotension (letter). *J Clin Psychopharmacol* 13, 77–78.

Greden JF (1993) Antidepressant maintenance medication: When to discontinue and how to stop. *J Clin Psychiatr* 54(Suppl), 39–45.

Gunzberger D and Martinez D (1992) Adverse vascular effects associated with fluoxetine (letter). *Am J Psychiatr* 149, 1751.

Hellerstein DJ, Yanowitch P, Rosenthal J *et al.* (1993) A randomized double-blind study of fluoxetine versus placebo in the treatment of dysthymia. *Am J Psychiatr* 150, 1169–1175.

Hrdina PD, Bakish D, Ravindran A *et al.* (1997) Platelet serotonergic indices in major depression: Up-regulation of 5-HT$_{2A}$ receptors unchanged by antidepressant treatment. *Psychiatr Res* 66, 73–85.

Hunt K and Resnick MP (1993) Clomipramine-induced agranulocytosis and its treatment with G-CSF (letter). *Am J Psychiatr* 150, 522–523.

Jensen PS, Bhatara VS, Vitiello B *et al.* (1999) Psychoactive medication prescribing practices for US children: Gaps between research and clinical practice. *J Am Acad Child Adolesc Psychiatr* 38, 557–565.

Kapur S, Mieczkowski T and Mann JJ (1992) Antidepressant medications and the relative risk of suicide attempt and suicide. *JAMA* 268, 3441–3445.

Keller MB, Shapiro RW, Lavori PW *et al.* (1982) Relapse in major depressive disorder: Analysis with the life table. *Arch Gen Psychiatr* 39, 911–915.

Keller MB, Lavori PW, Mueller TI *et al.* (1992) Time to recovery, chronicity, and levels of psychopathology in major depression: A 5-year prospective follow-up of 431 subjects. *Arch Gen Psychiatr* 49, 809–816.

Keller MB, Ryan ND, Strober M *et al.* (2001) Efficacy of paroxetine in the treatment of adolescent major depression: A randomized, controlled trial. *J Am Acad Child Adolesc Psychiatr* 40, 762–772.

Kocsis JH, Frances AJ, Voss C *et al.* (1985) Imipramine treatment for chronic depression. *Arch Gen Psychiatr* 45, 253–257.

Lavin MR, Mendelowitz A and Kronig MH (1993) Spontaneous hypertensive reactions with monoamine oxidase inhibitors. *Biol Psychiatr* 34, 146–151.

Leon AC, Keller MB, Warshaw MG *et al.* (1999) Prospective study of fluoxetine treatment and suicidal behavior in affectively ill subjects. *Am J Psychiatr* 156, 195–201.

Leonard BE (1993) The comparative pharmacology of new antidepressants. *J Clin Psychiatr* 54(Suppl), 3–15.

Mann J and Kapur S (1991) The emergence of suicidal ideation and behavior during antidepressant pharmacotherapy. *Arch Gen Psychiatr* 48, 1027–1033.

Marathe PH, Lee JS, Greene DS *et al.* (1996) Comparison of the steady-state pharmacokinetics of nefazodone after administration of 200 mg twice daily or 400 mg once daily in the morning or evening. *Br J Clin Pharmacol* 41, 21–27.

Martyn R, Somberg JC and Kerin NZ (1993) Proarrhythmia of nonantiarrhythmic drugs. *Am Heart J* 126, 201–205.

McCabe B and Tsuang MT (1982) Dietary consideration in mao inhibitor regimens. *J Clin Psychiatr* 43, 178–181.

McGrath PJ, Stewart JW, Nunes EV *et al.* (1993) A double-blind crossover trial of imipramine and phenelzine for outpatients with treatment-refractory depression. *Am J Psychiatr* 150, 118–123.

Mir S and Taylor D (1997) The adverse effects of antidepressants. *Curr Opin Psychiatr* 10, 88–94.

Modell JG (1989) Repeated observations of yawning, clitoral enlargement, and orgasm associated with fluoxetine administration. *J Clin Psychopharmacol* 9, 63.

Montgomery SA and Dunbar G (1993) Paroxetine is better than placebo in relapse prevention and the prophylaxis of recurrent depression. *Int Clin Psychopharmacol* 8, 189–195.

Montgomery SA, Dunfour H, Brion S *et al.* (1988) The prophylactic efficacy of fluoxetine in unipolar depression. *Br J Psychiatr* 153(Suppl 3), 69–76.

Montgomery SA, Rasmussen JG and Tanghol P (1993) A 24-week study of 20 mg citalopram, 40 mg citalopram and placebo in the prevention of relapse of major depression. *Int Clin Psychopharmacol* 8, 181–188.

Montgomery SA, Reimitz P-E and Zivkov M (1998) Mirtazapine versus amitriptyline in the long-term treatment of depression: A double-blind placebo-controlled study. Int Clin Psychopharmacol 13, 63–73.

Muly EC, McDonald W, Steffens D *et al.* (1993) Serotonin syndrome produced by a combination of fluoxetine and lithium (letter). *Am J Psychiatr* 150, 1565.

Narurkar V, Smoller BR, Hu CH *et al.* (1993) Desipramine-induced blue-gray photosensitive pigmentation. *Arch Dermatol* 129, 474–476.

Nierenberg AA (1992) The medical consequences of the selection of an antidepressant. *J Clin Psychiatr* 53, 19–24.

NIMH/NIH Consensus Development Panel (1985) Mood disorders: Pharmacologic prevention of recurrences (NIMH/NIH Consensus Development Conference Statement). *Am J Psychiatr* 142, 469–476.

Orsulak PJ and Waller D (1989) Antidepressant drugs: Additional clinical uses. *J Fam Pract* 28, 209–216.

Perry PJ (1996) Pharmacotherapy for major depression with melancholic features: Relative efficacy of tricyclic versus selective serotonin reuptake inhibitor antidepressants. *J Affect Disord* 39, 1–6.

Pescatori ES, Engelman JC, Davis C *et al.* (1993) Priapism of the clitoris: A case following trazodone use. *J Urol* 149, 1557–1559.

Phillips KA and Nierenberg AA (1994) The assessment and treatment of refractory depression. *J Clin Psychiatr* 55(Suppl 2), 20–26.

Preskorn SH, Burke MJ and Fast GA (1993) Therapeutic drug monitoring. *Psychiatr Clin N Am* 16, 611–645.

Ravindran AV, Bialik RJ and Lapierre YD (1994) Therapeutic efficacy of specific serotonin reuptake inhibitors (SSRIs) in dysthymia. *Can J Psychiatr* 39, 21–26.

Richelson E (2001) Pharmacology of antidepressants. *Mayo Clin Proc* 76, 511–527.

Riddle MA, Reeve EA, Yaryura-tobias JA *et al.* (2001) Fluvoxamine for children and adolescents with obsessive–compulsive disorder: A randomized, controlled, multicenter trial. *J Am Acad Child Adolesc Psychiatr* 40, 222–229.

Roose SP and Dalack GW (1992) Treating the depressed patient with cardiovascular problems. *J Clin Psychiatr* 53(Suppl 9), 25–31.

Roose SP, Dalack GW, Glassman AH *et al.* (1991) Cardiovascular effects of bupropion in depressed patients with heart disease. *Am J Psychiatr* 148, 512–516.

Rosenstein DL, Nelson JC and Jacobs SC (1993) Seizures associated with antidepressants: A review. *J Clin Psychiatr* 54, 289–299.

Schatzberg AF and Cole JO (1991) *Manual of Clinical Psychopharmacology*, 2nd edn. American Psychiatric Press, Washington DC.

Segraves RT (1992) Overview of sexual dysfunction complicating the treatment of depression. *J Clin Psychiatr* 10, 4–10.

Shihabuddin L and Rapport D (1994) Sertraline and extrapyramidal side effects (letter). *Am J Psychiatr* 151, 288.

Shopsin B (1983) Bupropion's prophylactic efficacy in bipolar illness. *J Clin Psychiatr* 44, 163–169.

Smith D and Levitte S (1993) Association of fluoxetine and return of sexual potency in three elderly men. *J Clin Psychiatr* 54, 317–319.

Steele T and Ashby J (1993) Desipramine-related slate-gray skin pigmentation (letter). *J Clin Psychopharmacol* 13, 76–77.

Steur E (1993) Increase of Parkinson disability after fluoxetine medication. *Neurology* 43, 211–213.

Stewart JW, McGrath PJ, Quitkin FM *et al.* (1993) Chronic depression: Response to placebo, imipramine and phenelzine. *J Clin Psychopharmacol* 13, 391–396.

Stoll AL, Pope HG and McElroy SL (1991) High-dose fluoxetine: Safety and efficacy in 27 cases. *J Clin Psychopharmacol* 11, 225–226.

Thase ME, Fava M, Halbreich U *et al.* (1996) Placebo-controlled, randomized clinical trial comparing sertraline and imipramine for the treatment of dysthymia. *Arch Gen Psychiatr* 53, 777–784.

Thase ME, Blomgren SL, Birkett MA *et al.* (1997) Fluoxetine treatment in patients with major depressive disorder who failed initial treatment with sertraline. *J Clin Psychiatr* 58, 16–21.

Thase ME, Rush AJ, Howland RH *et al.* (2002). Double-blind switch study of imipramine or sertraline treatment of antidepressant-resistant chronic depression. *Arch Gen Psychiatr* 59, 233–239.

Vanelle JM (1997) Controlled efficacy study of fluoxetine in dysthymia. *Br J Psychiatr* 170, 345–350.

WHO Mental Health Collaborating Centers (1989) Pharmacotherapy of depressive disorders: A consensus statement. *J Affect Disord* 17, 197–198.

Woolfrey S, Gammack NS, Dewar MS *et al.* (1993) Fluoxetine–warfarin interaction (letter). *BMJ* 307, 241.

Wisner KL, Zarin DA, Holmboe ES, *et al.* (2000) Risk-benefit decision making for treatment of depression during pregnancy. *Am J Psychiatr* 157, 1933–1940.

Work Group on Research of the American Academy of Child and Adolescent Psychiatry (1990) Desipramine (DMI) and sudden death: A report from the Work Group on Research and the Office of Research. AACAP Member Forum at the Annual Meeting of the American Academy of Child and Adolescent Psychiatry, (Oct 23), Washington DC.

Workman EA and Short DD (1993) Atypical antidepressants versus imipramine in the treatment of major depression: A meta-analysis. *J Clin Psychiatr* 54, 5–12.

Zametkin AJ, Alter MR, and Yemini T (2001) Suicide in teenagers: Assessment, management, and prevention. JAMA 286, 3120–3125.

Zito JM, Safer DJ, dosReis S *et al.* (2000) Trends in the prescribing of psychotropic medications to preschoolers. *JAMA* 283, 1025–1030.

CHAPTER

80   Anxiolytic Drugs

In the last decade, there has been a substantial increase in the number of medications demonstrated to be effective for the treatment of anxiety and anxiety disorders (Table 80.1).

There was a cascade of anxiolytic research in the 1990s. The selective serotonin reuptake inhibitors (SSRIs) as a class were demonstrated to be efficacious treatments for most of the anxiety disorders described in the DSM-IV-TR. Although these agents have a delayed onset when contrasted with the benzodiazepines, they have a broader spectrum of action, no problems with dependence, and much less of a problem with withdrawal syndromes. The 1990s also saw the approval of venlafaxine as a treatment for generalized anxiety disorder.

A General Approach to Using Medication with Anxious Patients

Making an appropriate differential diagnosis which includes a DSMIV-TR anxiety disorder is critical to the success of any psychopharmacological intervention. The diagnosis dictates the class of medication to be used and the length of pharmacotherapy. An important rule in general is "to start low and go slow" when initiating pharmacological treatment for patients with anxiety disorders. Interestingly, although treating patients with anxiety disorders frequently requires a more gradual initial titration schedule, patients frequently attain maintenance dosages of antidepressant medications that are greater than the dosage commonly used to treat major depressive disorder.

Antidepressant Medication

It has been known that medications initially identified because of their antidepressant properties are frequently effective treatments for anxiety disorders as well. The basic action of the majority of the antidepressants is to increase the availability of neurotransmitters in the synaptic cleft. These agents have the broadest spectrum of activity which spans the entire spectrum of DSM-IV-TR anxiety disorders. The relative differences in terms of major pharmacokinetic and pharmacodynamic properties are outlined in Tables 80.2 and 80.4. As illustrated in Table 80.1, a variety of serotonin receptor subtypes have been implicated in the modulation of anxiety disorders, depressive disorders, migraine, pain and neuropsychiatric disorders.

Indications for Selective Serotonin Reuptake Inhibitors

Initial data from randomized, placebo-controlled treatment trials suggest that SSRIs may be useful in the treatment of adults and children with generalized anxiety disorder. SSRIs have emerged

as a first-line treatment for social anxiety disorder. Most of the efficacy data are derived from multicenter, double-blind trials of paroxetine, sertraline and fluvoxamine.

In addition, SSRIs are generally accepted as a first-line treatment for panic disorder. The major advantage of these agents is their tolerability and thus longer-term acceptance by patients. There is evidence that fluoxetine, sertraline, paroxetine, fluvoxamine and citalopram are effective in the acute treatment of panic disorder.

One of the advantages of SSRIs is that they tend to be fairly well tolerated in contrast to some of the other treatments available for panic disorder. Although a few individuals may have some initial problems with restlessness and increased anxiety, data suggest that starting at lower doses such as 25 mg/day of sertraline or 10 mg/day of paroxetine may decrease the risk of antidepressant "jitteriness".

There have been open-label and double-blind, placebo-controlled studies demonstrating that SSRIs are effective for the treatment of post traumatic stress disorder (PTSD). Open-label trials with all of the SSRIs currently available suggest that each may be effective in decreasing the core symptoms of PTSD.

Large, well-designed, double-blind, placebo-controlled trials demonstrate that fluoxetine, paroxetine, fluvoxamine, citalopram and sertraline are effective acute treatments for obsessive–compulsive disorders.

Indications for Serotonin–Norepinephrine Reuptake Inhibitors in Anxiety Disorders

Venlafaxine

There have been a number of placebo-controlled multicentered studies demonstrating that venlafaxine XR is an effective treatment of GAD.

Doses as low as 37.5 mg/day and as high as 225 mg/day are effective in decreasing symptoms of anxiety for patients with GAD. Side effects appear to be mild and tend to decrease in number and intensity over the course of treatment. Nausea, dry mouth and somnolence are the most commonly repeated side effects.

Case reports and open-label studies have been published for use of venlafaxine in social anxiety disorder (Kelsey, 1995).

There is only one double-blind, placebo-controlled study by Pollack and coworkers. (1996) suggesting that venlafaxine may be an effective treatment for patients with panic disorder.

Indications for Tricyclic Antidepressant Medication and Monoamine Oxidase Inhibitors in Anxiety Disorders

A variety of tricyclic antidepressants (TCAs) have been demonstrated to be effective treatments for GAD. However, the side

Essentials of Psychiatry Jerald Kay and Allan Tasman
© 2006 John Wiley & Sons, Ltd.

Table 80.1   The Efficacy of Psychotropic Medications for the Treatment of Anxiety Disorders

	Generalized Anxiety Disorder	Social Anxiety Disorder	Panic Disorder	Post traumatic Stress Disorder	Obsessive–Compulsive Disorder
Strong evidence	SSRIs Venlafaxine Trazodone TCAs Benzodiazepines Buspirone	SSRIs Bupropion-SR MAOIs Benzodiazepines	SSRIs Venlafaxine MAOIs TCAs Benzodiazepines	SSRIs TCAs MAOIs	SSRIs Clomipramine

Some evidence	Nefazodone
	Mirtazapine
		Venlafaxine
		Nefazodone
		
		Gabapentin
			Mirtazepine
			Nefazodone
			Clonazepam +
			  sertraline
			
			Buspirone adjunct to
			  benzodiazepine
			Valproic acid
			Gabapentin
			Tiagabine
			Pagoclone
				Venlafaxine
				Lamotrigine
				Valproate
				
				Nefazodone
				Mirtazapine
				Clonidine
					MAOIs
					Olanzapine
					  augmentation of SSRI
					
					Risperidone
					  augmentation of SSRI
					Venlafaxine
					Mirtazapine

Not effective		TCAs Buspirone Pindolol augmentation of SSRI	Trazodone Bupropion		Trazodone TCAs Buspirone
No data	MAOIs Bupropion	Trazodone Mirtazapine		Duloxetine Bupropion	

effects and difficulty titrating the dosage of these medications have made their use uncommon.

In general, TCAs have not been found to be effective for the treatment of social anxiety disorder, but there is evidence of effectiveness in panic disorder. Although surpassed by the SSRIs as first-line agents, there is no doubt that first-generation MAOIs are effective. Unfortunately, the risk of hypertensive crisis and the need for patients to follow a tyramine-free diet makes this class of drugs unappealing for the majority of patients.

Although TCAs have been widely used for the treatment of panic disorder, their side-effect profile and slow time to onset of action makes them a difficult class of medication for many patients to tolerate.

There have been seven meta-analyses comparing and contrasting clomipramine and SSRIs (Abramowitz, 1997; Cox *et al.*, 1993; Greist, 1998; Kobak *et al.*, 1998; Piccinelli *et al.*, 1995; Stein *et al.*, 1995). In each case, clomipramine has been found to be significantly more effective than the SSRIs. If one takes the entire body of evidence as a whole into account, analyses suggest that clomipramine is at least as effective as the SSRIs and may, in some instances, be more effective (Greist, 1998; Todorov *et al.*, 2000).

Other Antidepressant Medication (Bupropion, Mirtazapine, Nefazodone, Trazodone) in Anxiety Disorders

Most evidence fails to support these medications as a first-line treatment for generalized anxiety disorders, social anxiety disorder, panic disorder, PTSD, or obsessive-compulsive disorder.

Benzodiazepine Medication

The benzodiazepines as a class work by increasing the relative efficiency of the gamma-aminobutyric acid (GABA) receptor when stimulated by GABA. The benzodiazepines bind to a site located adjacent to the GABA receptor and cause an allosteric change to the receptor that facilitates the increased passage of the chloride ions intracellularly when GABA interacts with the receptor complex. This leads to a relative hyperpolarization of the neuronal membrane and inhibition of activity in the brain. The benzodiazepines as a group have different affinities for GABA receptors, in fact some agents bind to only one of the two types of GABA receptors. The relative pharmacodynamic and pharmacokinetic properties of the benzodiazepines are further outlined in comparison to the other medications in Table 80.2. As a class, benzodiazepines are efficacious for the treatment of panic disorder, social anxiety disorder, generalized anxiety disorder, alcohol withdrawal and situational anxiety. The choice of an agent should take into account the age, medical health and comorbid diagnosis of the patient. Although obsessive–compulsive disorder falls within the taxonomy of anxiety disorders, benzodiazepines do not seem to be particularly effective in treating these patients.

The limitations to these drugs are the same as when used in any indication. Due to the potential for abuse and drug withdrawal, their use must be monitored carefully. This is a particularly problematic issue in social anxiety disorder because of the high rate of comorbid substance abuse. Benzodiazepines may be best suited for patients with situational and performance anxiety on an as-needed basis.

Table 80.2   Pharmacokinetic Properties of Psychotropic Medication Used for the Treatment of Anxiety Disorders

				SSRIs			
	Fluoxetine	**Fluvoxamine**	**Paroxetine**	**Paroxetine CR**	**Sertraline**	**Escitalopram**	**Citalopram**
T_{max} h	6–8	3–8	5.2	6–10	4.5–8.4	3–5	2–4
Dose-proportional plasma level	No	No	No	No	Yes	Yes	Yes
$T_{1/2}$ (h)	24–72	15.6	21	15–20	26	30	33
Metabolite activity	Norfluoxetine (equal)	<10%	<2%	<1%	Desmethyl-sertraline 6–15%	None	<10%
Metabolite $T_{1/2}$	4–16 d	–	–	–	62–104 h	50–60	–
Steady state plasma level	4–5 wk	~1 wk	10 d	10–14 d	~1 wk	10d	~1 wk
Usual daily dosage range	10–80 mg	100–300 mg	10–60 mg	12.5–75 mg	50–200 mg	10–20 mg	10–60 mg

			Other Antidepressants		
	Mirtazapine	**Nefazodone**		**Venlafaxine**	**VenlafaxineXR**
T_{max} h	2	1		2	5.5
Dose-proportional plasma level?	Yes	No		Yes	Yes
$T_{1/2}$ (h)	37 (females), 26 (males)	2–4		5±2	
Metabolite activity	Negligible	Hydroxynefazodone		O-desmethyl-venlafaxine	C-desmethyl-venlafaxine
Metabolite $T_{1/2}$ (h)	–	1.5–4		11±2	11±2
Steady state plasma level	5 d	4–5 d		3 d	3 d
Usual oral dosage	15–60 mg	100–800 mg		45–75 mg	75–225 mg

		Antianxiety			
	Buspirone	**Alprazolam**	**AlprazolamXR**	**Clonazepam**	**Lorazepane**
T_{max} h	0.6–1.5	1–2	5–11	1–4	1–15
Dose-proportional plasma level	No	Yes	Yes	Yes	Yes
$T_{1/2}$ (h)	2–3	6.3–26.9	6.3–26.9	30–40	12–15
Metabolite activity	Unimportant	α-hydroxyl-alprazolam 50%	α-hydroxyl-alprazolam and 4- hydroxyl-alprazolam	No	Unimportant
Steady state plasma level	–	3–4 d	3–4 d	1 wk	4 days
Usual oral dosage	15–90 mg	1–10 mg	1–10 mg	1–6 mg	1–6 mg

		Antipsychotics			
	Olanzapine	**Quetiapine**	**Risperidone**	**Ziprasidone**	**Aripiprazole**
T_{max} h	6	1.5	1	6–8	3–5
Dose-proportional plasma level	Yes	Yes	Yes	Yes	Yes
$T_{1/2}$ (h)	21–54	6	21–30	7	75–96
Metabolite activity	No	No	9-hydroxyrisperidone	Yes	Dehydro-aripiprazole
Steady state plasma level	4–6 d	2 d	5–6 d		14 d
Usual oral dosage	5–10 mg	300–400 mg b.i.d.	2–8 mg	20–80 mg b.i.d.	10–30 mg

		Anticonvulsants			
	Gabapentin	**Valproic acid**	**Pregabalin**	**Tiagabine**	**Topiramate**
T_{max} h		4–5	1.5	0.75	4
Dose-proportional plasma level	No	No	No	No	Yes
$T_{1/2}$ (h)	5–7	9–16	6.3	7–9	21
Metabolite activity	No	No	No	No	No
Steady state plasma level	1 d	7 d	24–48 h	2 d	4 d
Usual oral dosage	2,400 mg/d	750–2,500 mg/d	150–600 mg	4–32 mg/d	100–200 mg/d

$T_{1/2}$, terminal half-life.
T_{max}, time of maximum plasma concentration.

Table 80.3	The Proposed Function of Different 5-HT Receptors
1A	Anxiety
	Depression
	Sexual behavior
	Appetite
	Aggression
	Pain
	Emesis
	Obsessions
	Vasoconstriction
1D	Migraine
	Appetite
	Depression
2A	Vasoconstriction
	Migraine
	Anxiety
2B	Depression
	Sleep
	Hallucination
	Suicide
2C	Appetite
	Anxiety
	Depression
	Learning
	Psychosis
3	Emesis
	Anxiety
	Psychosis
	Migraine
	Reward
4	Muscle contraction, gut and heart
	Learning
	Cognition
	Anxiety
	Sleep
	Emesis
5	Unknown
6	OCD
7	Circadian rhythms

Source: Dubovsky SL and Thomas M (1995) Serotonergic mechanisms and current and future psychiatric practice. *J Clin Psychiatr* 56(2), 38–48.

The two high potency benzodiazepines that have been approved by the FDA, alprazolam and clonazepam are widely used in the treatment of panic disorder. They may also be helpful as adjuncts in the treatment of obsessive-compulsive disorder, though not as first-line stand alone treatments.

Buspirone

Buspirone is a member of the group of agents called azaspirodecanediones. It is believed to exert its anxiolytic effect by acting as a partial agonist at the 5-HT$_{1A}$ autoreceptor. Stimulation of the 5-HT$_{1A}$ autoreceptor causes decrease release of serotonin into the synaptic cleft. However, buspirone also exerts another effect through its active metabolite 1-phenyl-piperazine (1-PP) that acts on alpha-2-adrenergic receptors to increase the firing rate of the locus coeruleus. Some not yet **well-characterized** combination of these effects may be re-

sponsible for anxiolytic effect of buspirone. It usually takes approximately 4 weeks for the benefit of buspirone therapy to be noticed in patients with GAD. It may also be a useful adjuvant in some patients with treatment resistant panic disorder. One major advantage of buspirone is that it does not cross react with benzodiazepines. The most common side effects associated with buspirone include dizziness, gastrointestinal distress, headache, numbness and tingling. The most common pharmacokinetic and pharmacodynamic actions of buspirone are described in Table 80.3.

Beta-blocker Medication

Beta-adrenergic blockers competitively antagonize norepinephrine and epinephrine at the beta-adrenergic receptor. It is thought that the majority of positive effects of beta-blockers are due to their peripheral actions. Beta-blockers can decrease many of the peripheral manifestations of anxiety such as tachycardia, diaphoresis, trembling and blushing. The advent of more selective beta-blockers that only block the beta-2-adrenergic receptor has been beneficial since blockade of beta-1 adrenergic receptors can be associated with bronchospasm. Beta-blockers may be useful for individuals who have situational anxiety or performance anxiety. They generally have not been effective in treating anxiety disorders such as generalized social anxiety disorder, panic disorder, or obsessive–compulsive disorder.

Anticonvulsant Medication

One of the areas of increasing research is the study of anticonvulsants in anxiety disorders. Currently, there are few published placebo-controlled studies investigating the efficacy of commonly used anticonvulsants for the treatment of anxiety or anxiety disorders. There is one published report of a large double-blind, placebo-controlled study of gabapentin for the treatment of social anxiety disorder. The precise mechanism of action of gabapentin is not fully appreciated, however, it is thought gabapentin somehow increases brain GABA levels.

Antipsychotic Medication

The conventional or typical antipsychotic medication whose mechanism of action is primarily to block dopamine Type-2 receptors has been used as adjuvant medication for the treatment of anxiety disorders for years. However, because of problems with extrapyramidal side effects and the risk of developing tardive dyskinesia, these agents had fallen out of favor. The newer class of atypical antipsychotic medications have a decreased risk of both extrapyramidal side effects and tardive dyskinesia and so antipsychotic medications are beginning to be used again as adjuvants in patients with treatment resistant anxiety disorders. This simultaneous blockade of both neurotransmitter systems seems to decrease extrapyramidal side effects and the risk of developing tardive dyskinesia. Although the different atypical antipsychotic medications have different affinities for dopamine Type-2 and serotonin Type-2 receptors, this is the common mechanism of action of these agents. The atypical antipsychotic medications also differ dramatically in terms of their pharmacodynamic

Table 80.4	A Summary of Pharmacologic Properties of Medications Commonly Used to Treat Anxiety					
	Onset of Action	Titration	Abuse Liability	Need for Discontinuation Titration	Potential for Withdrawal Syndrome	Probability of Lethality in Overdose
Sertraline	Delayed (In 2 wk)	Yes	Very low	Yes, but not mandatory	Very low	Low
Paroxetine	Delayed (In 2 wk)	Yes	Very low	Yes	Moderate	Low
Fluvoxamine	Delayed (In 2 wk)	Yes	Very low	Yes, but not mandatory	Very low	Low
Fluoxetine	Delayed (In 2 wk)	Yes	Very low	No	Lowest	Low
Citalopram	Delayed (In 2 wk)	Yes	Very low	Yes, but not mandatory	Very low	Low
Escitalopram	Delayed (In 2 wk)	Sometimes	Very low	Yes, probably not mandatory	Very low	Low
Venlafaxine	Delayed (In 2 wk)	Yes	Very low	Yes	Moderate	Low
Duloxetine	Delayed (In 2 wk)	Yes	Very low	Yes	Moderate	Low
Mirtazepine	Delayed	Yes	Very low	Yes	Moderate	Low
Nefazodone	Delayed	Yes	Very low	Yes	Moderate	Low
Bupropion	Delayed	Yes	Very low	Yes	Low	Low
TCAS	Delayed (2 wk)	Yes	Very low	Yes	Moderate	Moderate–high
MAOIs	Delayed (2 wk)	Yes	Very low	Yes	Moderate	Moderate–high
Buspirone	Delayed (2 wk)	Yes	Very low	Yes	Low–moderate	Low
Clonazapam	Rapid	Yes	Moderate	Yes	Moderate–high	Low
Alprazolam	Very rapid	Yes	Moderate	Yes	High	Low
Alprazolam XR	Rapid	Yes	Moderate	Yes	Moderate–high	Low
Lorazepam	Very rapid	Yes	Moderate	Yes	Moderate–high	Low
Diazepam	Rapid	Yes	Moderate	Yes	Moderate	Low
β-blockers	Rapid	Sometimes	Low	No (acute use)	No (acute use)	Low–medium
Gabapentin	Moderate (d)	Yes	Low	Yes	Low–moderate	Low
Risperidone	Rapid	Probably	Low	Yes	Low	Low
Olanzapine	Rapid	Probably	Low	Yes	Low	Low

properties. There are very few published studies investigating atypical antipsychotic medication augmentation for the treatment of anxiety disorders, so it is not possible to recommend their use as a first-line treatment for anxiety disorders.

Conclusion

Clinicians have a wide array of medications available for the treatment of anxiety and anxiety disorders. We have safe and effective treatments for everything from short-term treatment of pathological anxiety to previously intractable anxiety disorders like obsessive–compulsive disorder. Yet, the most important therapeutic agent we possess is still sound clinical skills and judgement. Appropriate diagnosis and rapport are the foundations of any pharmacological intervention we make with our patients.

References

Abramowitz JS (1997) Effectiveness of psychological and pharmacological treatments for obsessive–compulsive disorder: A quantitative review. *J Consult Clin Psychol* 65(1), 44–52.

Cox BJ, Swinson RP, Morrison B *et al.* (1993) Clomipramine, fluoxetine, and behavior therapy in the treatment of obsessive–compulsive disorder: A meta-analysis. *J Behav Ther Exp Psychiatr* 24(2), 149–153.

Greist JH (1998) The comparative effectiveness of treatments for obsessive–compulsive disorder. *Bull Menn Clin* 62(4) (Suppl A), A65–A81.

Kelsey JE (1995) Venlafaxine in social phobia. *Psychopharmacol Bull* 31(4), 767–771.

Kobak KA, Greist JH, Jefferson JW *et al.* (1998) Behavioral versus pharmacological treatments of obsessive–compulsive disorder: A meta-analysis. *Psychopharmacology (Berl)* 136(3), 205–216.

Piccinelli M, Pini S, Bellantuono C *et al.* (1995) Efficacy of drug treatment in obsessive–compulsive disorder. A meta-analytic review. *Br J Psychiatr* 166(4), 424–443.

Pollack MH, Worthington JJ III, Otto MW *et al.* (1996) Venlafaxine for panic disorder: Results from a double-blind, placebo-controlled study. *Psychopharmacol Bull* 32(4), 667–670.

Stein DJ, Spadaccini E and Hollander E (1995) Meta-analysis of pharmacotherapy trials for obsessive–compulsive disorder. *Int Clin Psychopharmacol* 10(1), 11–18.

Todorov C, Freeston MH and Borgeat F (2000) On the pharmacotherapy of obsessive–compulsive disorder: Is a consensus possible? *Can J Psychiatr* 45(3), 257–262.

Sedative–Hypnotic Agents

Insomnia is a significant health care problem. It can create daytime fatigue, impaired social or occupational functioning, and reduced quality of life. Patients with insomnia are less productive workers, more prone to motor vehicle and workplace accidents, and utilize the general medical health care system to a greater degree than patients with normal sleep habits (Simon and VonKorff, 1997).

The elderly and patients with underlying psychiatric disorders are particularly prone to sleep difficulties. Schizophrenia, anxiety disorders and mood disorders frequently cause significant insomnia. Treatment of the underlying psychiatric illness often improves sleep. Sometimes, however, the medications used to treat the psychiatric illness may create insomnia as well. For example, selective serotonin reuptake inhibitors (SSRI) (particularly during the early weeks of treatment) may cause insomnia, even when they effectively treat an underlying depression.

Nonprescription Agents

There are a number of over-the-counter (OTC) sleep aids used by patients suffering from insomnia (see Table 81.1). These agents typically contain the histamine (H_1) receptor antagonist diphenhydramine (e.g., Benadryl, Sominex) or some other sedating antihistamine such as doxylamine (e.g., Nytol, Unisom). While these agents often cause significant drowsiness due to their antihistaminic properties, their effectiveness in treating insomnia has not been clearly established in randomized, placebo-controlled studies. They tend to have a prolonged duration of action leading to sedation and slowed reaction times during the day following their use. In addition, tachyphylaxis often develops within several days to a week or two limiting their use to only those patients with short-term problems with insomnia.

The OTC antihistamines are also highly anticholinergic and therefore may cause dry mouth, constipation, urinary retention and delirium quite easily. Geriatric patients are particularly susceptible to these anticholinergic effects. Patients already on other medications with significant anticholinergic activity should take these compounds quite judiciously as the anticholinergic effects could be magnified.

The common practice of combining an analgesic such as aspirin or acetaminophen and an antihistamine (e.g., Tylenol PM) is no more effective than the use of an antihistamine alone unless pain is present. As such, their use cannot be recommended for patients suffering from insomnia when pain is not a major complaint.

Melatonin is a naturally occurring pineal gland peptide hormone that is available in OTC formulations from a number of manufacturers. The Food and Drug Administration (FDA) classifies melatonin as a nutritive or dietary supplement. The Dietary Supplement Health and Education Act does not require dietary supplements to be reviewed by the FDA and, as a result, the strength and purity of melatonin cannot be guaranteed. When purified or synthesized and taken orally, melatonin alters circadian rhythms, lowers core body temperature, and reduces daytime alerting phenomena originating in the suprachiasmatic nucleus. Some clinicians feel that melatonin may be particularly effective when the normal circadian cycle is disrupted (e.g., jet lag, shift work). A number of studies have yielded conflicting results regarding the efficacy and long-term safety of melatonin. Efficacy data may be somewhat conflicting due to the lack of solid data regarding appropriate dosing strategies. Efficacy has been reported with doses as low as 0.3 mg at bedtime. While there are no known long-term safety issues associated with the use of melatonin, treatment-emergent side effects include pruritus, tachycardia, headache and daytime drowsiness.

Prescription Medications

Prescription medications for patients suffering from insomnia generally should be used only on a short-term basis. Benzodiazepines replaced barbiturates as the mainstay of treatment for much of the past 30 years. Benzodiazepines have a decreased abuse potential, fewer interactions with other drugs, a broader therapeutic index compared with the barbiturates, and pose a much lower risk in overdose. The adverse effect profile of benzodiazepines includes the risk for abuse and physiological dependence that develops with daily use, as well as problems with daytime sedation, motor incoordination and cognitive impairment. More recently the imidazopyridine, zolpidem and the pyrazolopyrimidine, zaleplon, have become increasingly popular as daytime sedation and the risk for abuse and physiological dependence appear to be somewhat less frequent with these two agents.

Benzodiazepines

Benzodiazepines are clearly effective for transient and situational insomnias. A recent meta-analysis demonstrated that benzodiazepine treated patients reported improvement in sleep onset, number of awakenings at night, the total amount of sleep obtained, and the quality of sleep compared with placebo-treated patients (Nowell *et al.*, 1997). Although only five benzodiazepines are marketed as hypnotic agents (Table 81.2), any benzodiazepine could be used to induce sleep provided an appropriate dose is chosen. Benzodiazepines improve sleep by inducing drowsiness, relaxing muscles and decreasing mental agitation. As doses, and consequently brain concentrations, are increased, drowsiness and relaxation shift into decreased wakefulness and then sleep. Benzodiazepines increase total sleep time, increase non-rapid-eye-movement (non-REM) sleep, decrease sleep latency,

Essentials of Psychiatry   Jerald Kay and Allan Tasman
© 2006 John Wiley & Sons, Ltd.

Table 81.1 Some Over-the-Counter Sleep Aids Commonly Available in the USA

Product Name	Active Ingredient*
Benadryl	Diphenhydramine
Compoz Night-time Sleep Aid	Diphenhydramine
Sleepinal	Diphenhydramine
Sominex	Diphenhydramine
Nervine Night-time Sleep Aid	Diphenhydramine
Nytol	Doxylamine
Nytol QuickCaps	Diphenhydramine
Unisom Night-time Sleep Aid	Doxylamine
Unisom SleepGels	Diphenhydramine

*Various strengths and formulations contain between 25 and 50 mg of the active antihistamine.

decrease stage 1 sleep and increase stage 2 sleep. Effects on stage 3 sleep vary based on the individual drug used, but stage 4 sleep is generally reduced.

Benzodiazepines are central nervous system depressants. Their likely mechanism of action relates to their ability to augment the opening of neuronal gamma-aminobutyric acid receptor-related chloride channels. By modulating the effects of gamma-aminobutyric acid, benzodiazepines increase the frequency of chloride channel openings. This effect is in contrast to the effects of barbiturates or alcohol, which seem to increase the duration of chloride channel opening. While this distinction may appear minor, it accounts for the greater safety of benzodiazepines in overdose (i.e., there is less likelihood of respiratory depression or coma). When alcohol is mixed with a benzodiazepine overdose, the synergistic effects of respiratory depression can have potentially fatal consequences.

There is little convincing evidence that the five marketed benzodiazepine hypnotics differ in terms of efficacy or safety when they are administered appropriately (i.e., amounts, dosing intervals and duration of use). The current benzodiazepines marketed as hypnotic agents are similar in their effects on sleep architecture and differ only in onset of action and duration of action. The individual agent chosen should be based on the type of sleep difficulty being experienced, the age of the patient and comorbid diagnoses. Triazolam has a rapid onset and a short duration of action, making it a better choice for patients with sleep initiation difficulties, while flurazepam has a somewhat longer onset of action and a much longer duration of action, making it a better choice for patients with middle or terminal insomnia.

Shorter half-life benzodiazepine hypnotics cause less daytime sedation and residual cognitive affects the day following administration. Rebound insomnia often occurs with these agents, however, especially after use for several consecutive nights. Rebound insomnia can usually be avoided by tapering the dose or using lower dosages during treatment. There is some evidence to suggest that the likelihood of rebound insomnia is greater in patients who experience greater hypnotic efficacy.

Besides rebound insomnia, some patients receiving shorter half-life benzodiazepines have problems with middle or terminal

Table 81.2 Hypnotic Agents

Generic Name	Trade Name	Dose Strengths (mg)	Half-Life (h)	Onset of Action	Comments
Chloral Hydrate	Noctec	500 mg/5ml	8–10	Intermediate	Active metabolite trichloroethanol has CNS depressive effect
Triazolam	Halcion	0.125, 0.25	1.5–5.5	Intermediate	May cause anterograde amnesia
Temazepam	Restoril	7.5, 15, 30	9–12	Slow	No active metabolites
Estazolam	ProSom	1, 2	10–24	Intermediate	Active metabolite has weak sedating properties as well
Flurazepam	Dalmane	15, 30	30–100	Fast	Active metabolite desalkylflurazepam accumulates and causes additive sedation
Quazepam	Doral	7.5, 15	25–40	Intermediate	Same active metabolite as flurazepam
Esczopiclone	Lunesta	1, 2, 3	6	Fast	
Zalepalon	Sonata	5, 10	1	Fast	
Zolpidem	Ambien	5, 10	1.4–4.5	Fast	
Ramelteon	Rozerem	8	1–2.6	Slow	Unique MOA melatonin receptor subtype agonist

insomnia. Plasma levels are quite low several hours after taking these medications and, as a result, if there is a problem with sleep maintenance these agents are not as likely to be as helpful as hypnotics with longer half-lives. In addition, shorter half-life benzodiazepines can sometimes cause an increase in daytime anxiety, particularly in the morning. For at least some patients, this may reflect the development of physiologic dependence and a withdrawal phenomenon.

Shorter half-life hypnotics, particularly triazolam, appear to cause anterograde amnesia more commonly than the longer half-life agents. Numerous reports in the lay press regarding a greatly increased risk of hallucinations, confusion and anterograde amnesia with triazolam use does not appear to be supported by an examination of all available data. All benzodiazepines can cause anterograde amnesia, however, particularly at higher dosages. Anterograde amnesia commonly occurs following a benzodiazepine overdose. The prevalence of anterograde amnesia with appropriate dosing of sedative–hypnotic agents and risk factors for its development in patients are still open questions at this time.

Longer half-life benzodiazepines may be more appropriate for patients who suffer from middle or terminal insomnia since these agents retain significant sedative properties for many hours after initial administration. Some patients may have problems with daytime sedation or decreased reaction time the day following administration. Sedative agents such as flurazepam and quazepam that have active metabolites with long half-lives are particularly prone to causing such problems. The active metabolite often builds up over time causing an increase in daytime drowsiness, decreased reaction time and in coordination with repeated administration, particularly in the elderly. Patients with significant daytime anxiety may benefit from the longer acting benzodiazepines as the residual amount of medication left in the morning may still have anxiolytic benefits.

The elderly use benzodiazepine hypnotic agents to a much greater degree than the general adult population. While this is likely due to the greater prevalence of sleep disorders in the elderly, the use of hypnotic agents in this population poses particular challenges. The elderly as a group have a decrement in hepatically metabolized benzodiazepines (e.g., estazolam, flurazepam, quazepam, triazolam), which is often more pronounced among men. Incoordination, sedation and confusion can occur when such agents build up over time. Ray and colleagues found a much higher rate of falls and hip fractures in the elderly population that received long-acting benzodiazepine hypnotics. The risk of hip fracture increased in direct proportion to the daily dose of the long-acting benzodiazepine. Short-acting benzodiazepines were not found to have a similar problem in their two large case–control studies (Ray *et al.*, 1987, 1989). A generally safe clinical strategy when managing insomnia problems in the elderly is to halve the starting dose and titrate up slowly as tolerated following the longstanding advice "start low, go slow". Avoiding long-acting benzodiazepines appears prudent as well.

Drug interactions with benzodiazepines are quite common. When mixed with other sedating compounds the effects are additive. Narcotic medications, alcohol and antihistamines are examples where the additive sedation can lead to confusion quite easily. In addition, acute alcohol ingestion slows hepatic metabolism and causes transiently higher concentrations of oxidatively metabolized benzodiazepines leading to further sedation. Antacids that slow gastric emptying may decrease the rate of absorption of a hypnotic agent from its primary site of origin, the small intestine. This could alter both onset and peak concentration effects.

Benzodiazepines all undergo some form of hepatic metabolism, although some agents are much more extensively metabolized than others. Medications that inhibit hepatic microsomal oxidative metabolism may cause clinically meaningful drug interactions when combined with benzodiazepines. All currently available triazolobenzodiazepines (e.g., alprazolam, estazolam, midazolam, triazolam) and diazepam are metabolized by hepatic microsomes and are complete or partial substrates of the CYP 3A4 isoform. Medications that are potent inhibitors of this system will cause higher peak concentrations of the triazolobenzodiazepine, particularly triazolam, which is highly hepatically metabolized. Nefazodone, ketaconazole, cimetidine and macrolide antibiotics are examples of clinically relevant CYP 3A4 inhibitors which may cause a reduction in the clearance of these triazolobenzodiazepines and an increase in their blood and brain concentrations. This increase is greatest with higher hepatic clearance drugs such as triazolam or midazolam and somewhat less for drugs such as alprazolam or estazolam.

All benzodiazepine hypnotic agents are FDA Pregnancy Category X, meaning their use should be avoided during pregnancy, especially during the first trimester due to an increased risk of congenital malformations. A variety of congenital malformations, including cleft palate, delayed ossification of a number of bony structures and an increased occurrence of rudimentary ribs have been reported.

Benzodiazepines must be used in patients with obstructive sleep apnea only with extreme caution. Benzodiazepines may cause respiratory depression and can render patients less likely to mount an appropriate respiratory response to hypoxia. Hypnotic agents such as zolpidem, zaleplon, or trazodone are less likely to cause problems for sleep apnea patients and may be preferable alternatives. Aggressive evaluation and treatment of sleep apnea [e.g., (continuous positive airway pressure) CPAP] is extremely important to ensure adequate restorative sleep.

Chloral Hydrate

Chloral hydrate was among the earliest sleeping pills. Its sedating qualities become evident within 30 minutes of administration, as it is rapidly absorbed from the gastrointestinal tract. At dosages between 0.5 and 1.5 g, it is an effective hypnotic agent. The elimination half-life of its active metabolite, trichloroethanol, is 6 to 8 hours, rendering it unlikely to cause significant next-day sedation or functional impairment. Despite the potential benefits of a rapid onset of action and relatively short elimination half-life, chloral hydrate is rarely used as a hypnotic agent today. It has a narrow therapeutic index (toxic dose–therapeutic dose), causes gastric irritation, nausea and vomiting easily, and may cause gastric necrosis at high doses. Overdose can be fatal due to respiratory depression.

Zolpidem

Zolpidem is also a nonbenzodiazepine hypnotic. A member of the imidazopyridine class, it is available in 5 and 10 mg dosages. Its mechanism of action shares much in common with benzodiazepines as it is active at central benzodiazepine (sometimes called ω) receptors. The ω receptor is a subunit of the $GABA_A$

receptor. Benzodiazepines are thought to bind nonselectively and activate all ω receptor subtypes; by contrast, zolpidem appears to bind preferentially to ω_1 receptors. Although this selective binding is not absolute, it may explain the relative absence of myorelaxant, anxiolytic and anticonvulsant effects of zolpidem at hypnotic dose, as well as the preservation of stages 3 and 4 sleep. Polysomnographic experience with zolpidem indicates that zolpidem induces a sleep pattern very similar to that of physiological sleep, and generally produces little effect on sleep architecture following abrupt discontinuation (Darcourt et al., 1999).

Zolpidem is rapidly absorbed through the gastrointestinal tract and has a rapid onset of action. Peak concentration occurs from 30 minutes to 2 hours following administration. It is metabolized in the liver to several inactive metabolites and has an elimination half-life of approximately 2.5 hours. The elimination half-life is prolonged in the elderly and in patients with impaired hepatic or renal function. Zolpidem overdose can cause respiratory depression or coma, especially when combined with other CNS depressants. The benzodiazepine antagonist flumazenil can reverse the effects of an overdose of zolpidem, reflecting its benzodiazepine-like mechanism of action.

Although zolpidem is classified as a schedule IV drug by the FDA, it appears to cause tolerance and withdrawal syndromes somewhat less frequently than benzodiazepine hypnotics do. Withdrawal symptoms occur more frequently at doses higher than listed in the *Physician's Desk Reference* (PDR), which recommends a maximum dose of 10 mg. Cross tolerance with alcohol and benzodiazepines are found at higher doses, and the incidence of adverse effects is much higher. Anecdotal reports of hallucinations and confusion at standard hypnotic dosages have been reported (Toner et al., 1999, Ansseau et al., 1992), but further research is needed to determine the prevalence of such occurrences across a spectrum of dosages and age groups.

Zaleplon

Zaleplon is a nonbenzodiazepine hypnotic of the pyrazolopyrimidine class. Like zolpidem, zaleplon binds preferentially to central benzodiazepine (or ω) receptors. Zaleplon binds to the ω_1, ω_2 and ω_3 subunits, while zolpidem bind only to the ω_1 subunit. Zaleplon is rapidly absorbed from the gastrointestinal tract, reaching peak serum concentrations within 1 hour. Absolute bioavailability is only 30% as it undergoes extensive hepatic first-pass metabolism. Its elimination half-life is approximately 1 hour. Since cimetidine inhibits aldehyde oxidase and CYP 3A4, and may increase zaleplon plasma concentrations by 85%, the initial starting dose of zaleplon should be halved in patients also taking cimetidine. Other potent inhibitors of the CYP 3A4 system such as ketoconazole and erythromycin also may increase zaleplon levels.

Because of the quick onset of action of zaleplon and its short elimination half-life, it can be used for patients who have a difficult time initiating sleep, but are able to remain asleep throughout the remainder of the night. In patients who have difficulty both in initiating and in maintaining sleep, zaleplon may permit the initiation of sleep, but be less effective in maintaining sleep due to its short elimination half-life. On the other hand, this same short half-life can be an advantage, as it can permit middle of the night dosing for those patients who awaken then. The short half-life permits such a dosing schedule without causing significant next-day sedation (Walsh et al., 2000).

Zaleplon, like zolpidem, is classified as a schedule IV drug by the FDA. Higher than standard dosages have been associated with an abuse potential similar to that of triazolam. With dosages of 20 mg or less, abuse and dependence appears to be significantly less than that of benzodiazepine hypnotic agents (Rush et al., 1999). Rebound insomnia has been reported, but it appears to occur less frequently than in the short acting benzodiazepines such as triazolam.

Other Prescription Hypnotics

Barbiturates are commonly prescribed outside the USA for insomnia. Butabarbital, phenobarbital and secobarbital are the most commonly prescribed barbiturates. The barbiturates are potentially lethal in overdose due to the risk of respiratory depression, and they commonly cause induction of hepatic oxidative metabolism. Their use has generally been replaced by other agents with better side-effect profiles such as the benzodiazepines, the imadazopyridines and the pyrazolopyrimidines.

Hydroxyzine hydrochloride and hydroxyzine pamoate are sedating H_1 receptor antagonists that are used occasionally as hypnotic agents. Sedation occurs with these agents due to inhibition of histamine N-methyltransferase and blockage of central histaminergic receptors. Next-day sedation is a common problem with antihistamines as they have a relatively long elimination half-life. These agents are highly anticholinergic and may cause hypotension and are not usually recommended as first-line agents for the treatment of insomnia.

Trazodone, a triazolopyridine compound marketed as an antidepressant, is frequently used as a hypnotic. Hypnotic dosages vary markedly, from 25 to 300 mg, depending on individual susceptibility to its sedating effects. Trazodone increases slow wave sleep and total sleep time and does not appear to affect REM sleep, unlike other antidepressants (Yamadera et al., 1998). Its elimination half-life of between 6 and 9 hours renders trazodone likely to cause daytime drowsiness. Using the lowest effective dosage can minimize this effect, as taking the medication in late evening rather than at bedtime. Trazodone is commonly used to counter the insomnia associated with SSRI use. It is rarely used as a sole antidepressant because of its strong sedating qualities and the need to take the medication more than once per day because of its half-life. Tolerance to its sedating effects develops only rarely with long-term use, making it an excellent option for those with chronic insomnia. Priapism is an exceedingly rare side effect, occurring in less than one in 40 000 cases. Since anticholinergic side effects and postural hypotension are not common, trazodone has some advantages over the tricyclic antidepressants.

Suggested Guidelines for Prescribing Medications

It is often clinically useful to provide patients with information on good sleep hygiene practices. Certain elements are particularly important (e.g., going to another room and waiting until drowsy or looking for clues about waking life events, and issues that may be keeping one awake). Behavioral techniques such as stimulus control and progressive muscle relaxation are quite useful. When a hypnotic agent is prescribed, it is helpful to advise patients to take the medication on an empty stomach and with ample fluids (e.g., a full glass of water) to promote rapid dissolution and absorption, and onset of effect. For patients prone to nocturia the amount of fluids should be lessened substantially. One should always caution patients about potential impairments in memory, coordination, or driving skills and about unsteadiness if they are awakened after having taken a sleep aid. It is also important to remind them that if they use the medication for more than a few nights, some pattern of tapering should be followed when they stop. It is reinforcing to work out a discontinuation schedule at the time of the first prescription. Patients should also be cautioned to avoid the use of alcohol when taking a hypnotic as the effects are additive in nature. Medications such as the benzodiazepines that have a propensity to be abused should be avoided in those patients with drug or alcohol problems.

Universally accepted guidelines for dosing and duration of use for hypnotics are not established. Both dose and duration must be individualized with the goal of finding the lowest dose and the shortest duration. Short-term treatment (i.e., from 1 or 2 nights to 1 or 2 weeks) is reasonable for most patients. However, some patients with chronic insomnia may benefit from longer-term use provided that there is careful monitoring by the prescribing physician. No criteria are presently available to identify this subpopulation. It seems reasonable to consider several short-term trials, with gradual tapering at the end of each period and a drug-free interval between each period, to establish the patient's need for and the appropriateness and value of continued therapy. The drug-free time interval between the initial periods should range from 1 to 3 weeks, depending on the half-life of the agent and its active metabolites and the rapidity of the taper schedule. Reevaluation of such a patient's continued need for hypnotic medication at 3- to 6-month intervals is also reasonable. Because the elderly are particularly susceptible to falls or confusion from hypnotic medication, use of the lowest available dosage strength is advisable. The elderly should also avoid the use of longer half-life agents or those with active metabolites with long half-lives because such medications tend to accumulate over time in older patients due to pharmacodynamic differences in drug metabolism in the elderly.

For those individuals who hope to benefit from behavioral and nonpharmacological approaches to their insomnia, prescribing hypnotics two or three times per week while they are working out such modifications may be beneficial. Because there are few predictable central tendencies that characterize patients with primary insomnia, individual variation is likely.

References

Ansseau M, Pitchot W, Hansenne M et al. (1992) Psychotic reactions to zolpidem. *Lancet* 339, 809.

Darcourt G, Pringuey D, Salliere D, et al. (1999) The safety and tolerability of zolpidem—An update. J Psychopharmacol 13, 81–93.

Nowell PD, Mazumdar S, Buysse DJ, et al. (1997) Benzodiazepines and zolpidem for chronic insomnia. A meta-analysis of treatment effecacy. JAMA 278, 2170–2177.

Ray WA, Griffin MR and Downey W (1989) Benzodiazepines of long and short elimination half-life and the risk of hip fracture. *JAMA* 262, 3303–3307.

Ray WA, Griffin MR, Schaffner W et al. (1987) Psychotropic drug use and the risk of hip fracture. *New Engl J Med* 319, 1701–1707.

Rush CR, Frey JM, and Griffiths and Griffiths RR (1999) Zaleplon and triazolam in humans: Acute behavioral effects and abuse potential. Psychopharmacology 145, 39–51.

Simon GE and VonKorff M (1997) Prevalence, burden, and treatment of insomnia in primary care. *Am J Psychiatr* 154, 1417–1423.

Toner LC, Tsambiras BM, Catalano G et al. (1999) Central nervous system side effects associated with zolpidem treatment. *Clin Neuropharmacol* 23, 54–58.

Walsh JK, Pollak CP, Scharf MB et al. (2000) Lack of residual sedation following middle-of-the-night zaleplon administration in sleep maintenance insomnia. *Clin Neuropharmacol* 23, 17–21.

Yamadera H, Nakumura S, Suzuki H et al. (1998) Effects of trazodone hydrochloride and imipramine on polysomnography in healthy subjects. *Psychiatr Clin Neurosci* 52, 439–443.

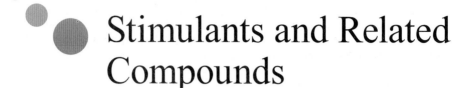

82 Stimulants and Related Compounds

Psychostimulants are highly effective treatment agents that have been used for the treatment of depression, attention-deficit/hyperactivity disorder (ADHD), neurasthenia and acquired immunodeficiency syndrome dementia. However, the greatest clinical application for psychostimulants has been the treatment of childhood disorders, in particular, ADHD. More than 180 placebo-controlled investigations demonstrate that psychostimulants – methylphenidates o-amphetamines are effective in reducing core symptoms of childhood ADHD. Approximately 70% of patients respond to stimulants compared with 13% to placebo. Short-term efficacy is more pronounced for behavioral rather than cognitive and learning abnormalities associated with ADHD. Although psychostimulants are clearly effective in the short term up through 14 months, concern remains that long-term benefits over years have not yet been adequately assessed.

Psychostimulants: Efficacy and Utility

Two groups of stimulants are currently approved by the FDA for treatment of ADHD in children, and are available in both brand and generic. These include: the amphetamines (Adderall, Dextrostat, Dexedrine) and the methylphenidates (Concerta, Metadate-ER, Metadate-CD, methylphenidate, Methylin, Ritalin, Ritalin-SR, Ritalin-LA and Focalin). Characteristics of these stimulants can be found in Table 82.1. Dextroamphetamine (DEX) and methylphenidate (MPH) are structurally related to the catecholamines (DA and NE) (McCracken 1991). Signs of CNS stimulation, including blood pressure and heart rate increases, are more pronounced in adults. The term **psychostimulant** used for these compounds refers to their ability to increase CNS activity in some but not all brain regions. Stimulants ameliorate disruptive ADHD behaviors cross-situationally (classroom, lunchroom, playground and home) when repeatedly administered throughout the day.

Mechanism of Action

The term psychostimulant refers to the ability of these compounds to increase CNS activity in some but not all brain regions. For example, while increasing the activity of striatum and connections between orbitofrontal and limbic regions, stimulants seem to have an inhibitory effect on the neocortex. The CNS psychostimulant effects of DEX and MPH may result in part from their lack of benzene ring substituents. Prominent central effects include activation of the medullary respiratory center and a lessening of central depression from barbiturates.

Psychostimulants have been described as noncatecholamine sympathomimetics. Sympathomimetics show potent agonist

Table 82.1 Side Effects of Stimulants	
Common Side Effects	Uncommon Side Effects
Decreased appetite	Nail biting
Insomnia	Skin rash
Headaches	Psychosis
Stomachaches	Hepatitis and liver failure (pemoline)
Crying spells and irritability	
Tics and other nervous movements	
Dizziness	
Drowsiness	
Raised blood pressure	
Raised heart rate	
Transient weight loss	
Delayed growth	

effects at alpha- and beta-adrenergic receptors. Presynaptically, they cause a stoichiometric displacement of norepinephrine and dopamine from storage sites in the presynaptic terminal. Stimulants also block the reuptake of dopamine by the dopamine transporter (DAT). Postsynaptically, they function as direct agonists at the adrenergic receptor. They also block the action of a degradative enzyme, catechol-o-methyltransferase (COMT).

The putative action of psychostimulants in ADHD has been attributed to the release of DA and their ability to block its reuptake by the DAT at the presynaptic nerve terminal. Radioligand binding studies have demonstrated the direct action of psychostimulants, particularly MPH, on striatal DAT. The dopamine action of psychostimulants also explains the appearance of behavioral stereotypies, seen at high doses. Tritiated MPH binding in rat brain is highest in striatum and is highly dependent on sodium concentration, suggesting that MPH binding is associated with a neurotransmitter transport system.

Yet, no single theory explains the psychostimulant mechanism of action on the CNS which ameliorates ADHD symptoms.

Most hypotheses regarding the neurochemical basis of ADHD have focused on the catecholamines norepinephrine and dopamine. These hypotheses, which posit a dysregulation in

Essentials of Psychiatry   Jerald Kay and Allan Tasman
© 2006 John Wiley & Sons, Ltd.

the norepinephrine or dopamine neurotransmitter systems, or both, are based primarily on the success of these dopaminergic medications in treating ADHD. All stimulant medications used for treating ADHD have their primary effects on these two neurotransmitter systems. Furthermore, the more selective norepinephrine-acting tricyclic medications, such as desipramine and imipramine, as well as the alpha-2-adrenergic agonist clonidine, have all been found to reduce symptoms of ADHD in children. Similarly, although much less commonly used, dopamine-blocking antipsychotic medications also have been found to be effective for treating children with ADHD (Zametkin and Rapoport, 1987).

Pharmacokinetics: Absorption and Metabolism

Psychostimulants are rapidly absorbed from the gut and thus act quickly, often within the first 30 minutes after ingestion. Food enhances absorption. Due, in part, to MPH's low plasma binding rate (15%), it is highly available to cross the blood–brain barrier. Effects on behavior appear during absorption, beginning 30 minutes after ingestion and lasting 3 to 4 hours. Half-lives range between 3 hours for MPH and 6 to 9 hours for *d*-amphetamine. The concentration-enhancing and activity-reducing effects of MPH can disappear well before the medication leaves the plasma, a phenomenon termed **clockwise hysteresis**.

MPH's metabolism is rapid and complete because it is not highly bound to plasma protein and does not disappear into fat stores. MPH peaks in plasma in 2 to 2.5 hours and falls to half the peak (half-life) after 3 hours.

Because MPH's short half-life prevents it from reaching steady state in the plasma, the standard tablet must be given several times a day to maintain behavioral improvement throughout the school day. Although the Physicians' Desk Reference (PDR) suggests giving MPH before meals, standard administration times are after breakfast (8:00 AM), after lunch (noon), and before homework (about 3:30 pm). See Table 82.2 for review of some of the pharmacokinetics of the psychostimulants used to treat children with ADHD.

Effects in Adults

Studies in adults taking *d*-amphetamine have shown a prolongation of performance at repetitive tasks before the onset of fatigue, a decreased sense of fatigue, mood elevation, euphoria, and increased speech rate and initiative (Rapoport *et al.*, 1980). The psychostimulants increase CNS alertness, as shown on tasks requiring vigilance, both in laboratory tasks, such as the CPT, and on the job, such as maintaining the ability to notice new events on a radar screen for periods of hours. These changes have been described as the drug's ability to "increase capacity", although this phrase has been misinterpreted to mean an increase over the person's innate ability.

Substance Abuse of Stimulants

Psychostimulants have been abused by adults, but the risk for addiction by children with ADHD is low. Klein (1980) found that the psychostimulants differ in their ability to induce euphoria, with "dextroamphetamine the most euphorigenic, methylphenidate, less so, and magnesium pemoline, hardly at all." Adolescents and young adults with ADHD do not list the psychostimulants among medications used recreationally, whether or not they had received treatment with psychostimulants. Adolescents previously diagnosed as having ADHD during their school-age years are at greater risk for substance abuse than control subjects, but those who do abuse medications tend not to pick stimulants.

Even though the evidence from the literature suggests that the abuse potential of psychostimulants by children with ADHD is low, DEX and MPH have been classified by the US Food and Drug Administration as potentially drugs of abuse (schedule II) and have warnings concerning abuse in the PDR. MPH was reclassified as a schedule II medication in 1971 because of a concern that the order by the Bureau of Narcotics and Dangerous Drugs to schedule methamphetamine and DEX would direct potential drug abusers to MPH. As a schedule II medication, the annual amount of stimulant medication manufactured must be approved or allocated.

Formulation of Treatment

What Is Being Treated

There are two main indications for the use of MPH: narcolepsy and ADHD. Other stimulants differ somewhat, with the indications for methamphetamine (Desoxyn Gradumets) including ADHD and obesity.

Medication	Stimulant	Effect
Guanethidine	MPH	Decreased hypotensive effect of guanethidine
Coumarin	MPH	Decreased metabolism of coumarin
Antiepileptic medications (phenobarbital, diphenylhydantoin, primidone)	MPH	Decreased metabolism of antiepileptic agents
Phenylbutazone	MPH	Decreased metabolism of phenylbutazone
Tricyclic antidepressants	MPH	Decreased metabolism of antidepressant
Ammonium chloride	DEX	Increased elimination of DEX
Sodium phosphate	DEX	Increased elimination of DEX
Acetazolamide	DEX	Delayed elimination of DEX
Thiazide diuretics	DEX	Delayed elimination of DEX
Sympathomimetics	MPH, DEX	Increased sympathomimetic effects
Sympatholytic antihypertensives (beta-blockers, others)	MPH, DEX	Decreased antihypertensive effect of antihypertensives

Table 82.2 Drug Interactions

Diagnosis of the Stimulant-treatable Disorders

Attention-deficit/Hyperactivity Disorder

ADHD is a heterogeneous behavioral disorder of unknown etiology. As its name suggests, ADHD is characterized by inattention, impulsivity and hyperactivity of varying severity. The disorder, which typically begins in early childhood and lasts into adulthood in a substantial minority, if not a majority, of cases, frequently leads to profound social and academic impairments. For a complete discussion of the ADHD diagnosis, see Chapter 28.

Narcolepsy

Narcolepsy is a chronic neurological disorder that presents with excessive daytime sleepiness and various problems of rapid eye movement physiology, such as cataplexy (unexpected decreases in muscle tone), sleep paralysis and hypnagogic hallucinations, which are intense dream-like imagery before falling asleep (Dahl, 1992). For a more complete discussion of narcolepsy, see Chapter 59. The prevalence is estimated to be 90 in 100000. Treatment can include a regular schedule of naps; counseling of family, school and patient; and use of medications, including stimulants and rapid eye movement-suppressant drugs such as protriptyline. Dahl recommended beginning with standard, short-acting stimulants, such as MPH, 5 mg b.i.d., and increasing the dose up to 30 mg b.i.d. if need be.

Selection of a Stimulant Medication as a Treatment Modality

Deciding to Use Medication

The decision to use stimulant medication in the treatment of ADHD employs different criteria for each developmental stage. The criteria for use of stimulants in school-age children and adolescents are well described in the DSM-IV-TR. More difficulty arises when deciding whether to use these medications in preschool children, adult patients, patients with mental retardation, or children with ADHD and comorbid disorders.

Use of Psychostimulants in Children Younger than 6 Years

Unfortunately, there are only a handful of published treatment studies on preschoolers. No dose-ranging pharmacokinetic studies have been done in this age group to determine if younger children, with their larger liver-to-body size ratio, might show more accelerated metabolism of psychostimulants than seen in older children. Therefore, the optimal doses for this age group are not known. To date there are no studies that would validate or refute clinicians' concerns that preschoolers suffer more pronounced stimulant withdrawal effects.

Adults

The prevalence of ADHD in adults, its severity and indications for treatment are issues that are not known. Although it had been assumed that children with ADHD outgrow their problems, prospective follow-up studies have shown that ADHD signs and symptoms continue into adult life for as many as 60% of children with ADHD (American Psychiatric Association, 1980). However, only a small percent of adults impaired by residual ADHD symptoms actually meet the full DSM-IV childhood criteria for ADHD (Hill and Schoener, 1996). Adults with concentration problems, impulsivity, poor anger control, job instability and marital difficulties sometimes seek help for problems they believe to be the manifestation of ADHD in adult life. Parents may decide that they themselves are impaired by the same attentional and impulse control problems found during an evaluation of their ADHD children.

A variety of medications have been used to treat adults with ADHD. Physicians should be cautious in the use of these agents until proof of efficacy is available. Of particular concern is the danger of using psychostimulants in adults with comorbid substance abuse disorder. It would be wise to use MPH because of its relatively low abuse potential, and because it has been shown in controlled studies to significantly reduce the symptoms of ADHD in adults (see Table 82.3.)

Continuing Stimulant Treatment in Patients with Tic Disorders

Standard package instructions for using MPH warns against its use in patients with tics or in patients with a family history of tics. Patients with Tourette's syndrome often have comorbid ADHD. If the two conditions co-occur, concern arises that stimulant treatment – because of its dopamine agonist actions – might unmask, trigger, accelerate, or precipitate more severe tics.

Tics are unacceptably worsened for a minority of comorbid children, although reversibly, and the majority of such comorbid children can be treated cautiously with low-to-moderate doses of stimulants, particularly MPH (Comings and Comings, 1987).

Patients with Mental Retardation

Many stimulant treatment studies for school-age children with ADHD exclude children with full-scale IQs below 70, who are considered to have mental retardation (MR). This is unfortunate, for the signs of ADHD are far more prevalent in children with IQs in the MR range (Aman et al., 1991). Pharmacotherapy reviews involving patients with MR have reported that institutionalized subjects with severe or profound MR respond poorly to stimulants. However, studies involving community samples of children with MR, have shown that these children do respond to MPH. It appears that children with ADHD who have mild or moderate MR may be more vulnerable to certain stimulant-related adverse side effects.

Does Comorbidity Affect the Indications for the Use of Stimulant Medication?

ADHD children that are referred from other physicians may have other Axis I psychiatric disorders. Extensive literature reviews report that ADHD co-occurs with conduct and oppositional defiant disorder in 30 to 50% of cases, with mood disorders in 15 to 75% of cases, with anxiety disorders in 25% of cases and with learning disabilities in 15 to 30% of cases. Clinicians should be aware that co-morbid ADHD/anxiety disorders may result in lesser response to treatment more side effects.

Treatment with Stimulant Medications

An effective treatment strategy for this chronic disorder of ADHD requires a plan for follow-up and monitoring. Techniques involve regular follow-up visits, the use of rating forms from parent and teacher, and the monitoring of academic progress in the school. Seeing the patient and a family member regularly is essential, often on a once-monthly basis when the medication prescription must be renewed.

Preparation of the Patient

Does the child's attitude about drug treatment influence its success? Concerns that medications may create negative attributions or

Table 82.3   Drugs for ADHD: Doses, and Pharmacodynamics

Medication	Tablets/Dosages	Dose Range	Administration	Peak Effect	Duration of Action
Amphetamines					
Dexedrine®	5 mg	10–40 mg/d	b.i.d. or t.i.d.	1–3 h	5 h
(generic) Adderall	5, 7.5, 10, 12.5, 15, 20, 30 mg	10–40 mg/d	b.i.d. or t.i.d.	1–3 h	5 h
(generic) Dextrostat®	5, 10 mg	10–40 mg/d	b.i.d. or t.i.d.	1–3 h	5 h
Long-duration type					
Dexedrine Spansule®	5, 10, 15 mg spansule	10–45 mg/d	once-daily	1–4 h	6–9 h
Adderall XR®	10, 20, 30 mg capsules	10–40 mg/d	once-daily	1–4 h	9 h
Methylphenidates					
Ritalin®	5, 10, 20 mg	10–60 mg/d	t.i.d.	1–3 h	2–4 h
Methylphenidate	5, 10, 20 mg	10–60 mg/d	t.i.d.	1–3 h	2–4 h
Methylin®	5, 10, 20 mg	10–60 mg/d	t.i.d.	1–3 h	2–4 h
Focalin®	2.5, 5, 10 mg	5–30 mg/d	b.i.d.	1–4 h	2–5 h
Long-duration type					
Ritalin-SR®	20 mg	20–60 mg/d	q.d. in am or b.i.d.	3 h	5 h
Metadate-ER®	10, 20 mg	20–60 mg/d	q.d. in am or b.i.d.	3 h	5 h
Medadate-CD®	20 mg	20–60 mg/d	q.d. in am	5 h	8 h
Concerta®	18, 36, 54 mg	18–54 mg/d	q.d. in am	8 h	12 h
Ritalin-LA®	20, 30, 40 mg	20–60 mg/d	q.d. in am	5 h	8 h
Modafinil	85 mg	1.25–4.5 mg/kg	b.i.d.	2 hours	8 hours

dysphoric effects in children with ADHD have not as a rule been confirmed in direct tests. Excellent studies show that there is considerable variability in children's attributions, as well as their mood response to pills. Pelham and colleagues (1992) found a subgroup of "depressogenic" children who gave external credit for positive events and internal blame for negative events. This group was above the median on attributions of success to their pills. Comorbidity and family history for anxiety and/or depression seemingly are relevant variables in prediction of such attributional effects. During treatment, a small percentage of stimulant-treated children do become dysphoric, weepy and mournful. Children who respond with depressogenic attributions or dysphoria may be children whose depressive diathesis is indistinguishable from ADHD and who are therefore mistakenly diagnosed as ADHD and treated with stimulants. Given the overlap of depression and ADHD, and the findings that depressogenic cognitive styles predict later depression, it could be important to identify those children who may be prone to attribute their success to pills rather than to their own effort, even though most patients do not do so.

Physicians can explain the reasons for taking pills and how the pills can prove helpful in school and at home. Children often have negative attitudes about treatment, thinking of treatment as a punishment. Pill taking can be socially stigmatizing to the child with ADHD if the daily trip to the nurse generates peer ridicule. Discussing the problem of in-school pill administration may be of great interest to the child, and he or she should be included in all discussions about dosing and changing of doses. At best, it may help with compliance.

Consideration of Side Effects

Common side effects and their management are noted in Table 82.4. Stimulant side effects are dose dependent and range from mild to moderate in most children. The management of stimulant-related adverse effects generally involves a temporary

reduction of dose or a change in time of dosing. MPH has an excellent safety record, probably because the duration of action is so brief.

Rebound One adverse effect, commonly known as behavioral rebound, appears when children experience psychostimulant withdrawal at the end of the school day. Children present with afternoon irritability, overtalkativeness, noncompliance, excitability, motor hyperactivity and insomnia about 5 to 15 hours after the last dose. If rebound occurs, many physicians add a small afternoon MPH dose or add a small dose of a tricyclic antidepressant.

Seizure Disorders A commonly held notion is that stimulants lower the seizure threshold. The PDR warns against the use of stimulants in children with preexisting seizure disorders. Both ADHD and seizure disorders are quite prevalent and may occur in the same individual, so the question of the risk of stimulant treatment may frequently arise. Current practice is to give children with ADHD and epilepsy a combination of anticonvulsant and MPH. Plasma levels of the anticonvulsant should be monitored to avoid toxicity resulting from MPH's competitive inhibition of metabolic pathways. At the doses used to treat ADHD in children, the psychostimulants have variable but minimal effects on the seizure threshold.

Long-term Stimulant Effects: Growth Velocity Reductions

Adults taking amphetamines routinely experience weight loss, which can be attributed to reduced appetite and decreased food intake. The drug's action on the lateral hypothalamic feeding center may explain this effect. Appetite suppression differs among different species, with humans showing only mild effects with rapid onset of tolerance. Children with ADHD taking psychostimulants routinely show appetite suppression when starting

Table 82.4	Stimulant Pharmacokinetics and Pharmacodynamics		
Parameter	Dextroamphetamine	Methylphenidate	Adderall
Metabolism	Hepatic to inactive metabolites	Hepatic to inactive metabolites	Hepatic to inactive or weakly active metabolites
Excretion	Renal, of metabolites; rate accelerated by acidification	Renal, of metabolites	Renal; rate accelerated by acidification
T_{max}	2–4 h	1–3 h	2–4 h
Half-life	6–8 h	2–4 h	5–7 h
Effect onset	30–60 min	30–60 min	30 min
Effect peak	1–3 h	1–3 h	1–3 h
Effect duration	3–5 h	2–4 h	3–5 h

treatment. For this reason, dosing should optimally occur after breakfast and lunch. Even though the daytime appetite is reduced, hunger rebounds in the evening. These effects on appetite often decrease within the first 6 weeks of treatment.

The growth effects of MPH appear to be minimal. Height and weight should be measured at 6-month intervals during stimulant treatment and recorded on age-adjusted growth forms to determine the presence of a drug-related reduction in height or weight velocity. If such a decrement is discovered during maintenance therapy with psychostimulants, a reduction in dosage or change to another class of medication can be carried out.

Continuing Stimulant Treatment in Patients with Tic Disorders

The PDR suggests that the presence of tics is a contraindication to stimulant usage. With the comorbidity of ADHD in children with Tourette's disorder estimated to fall between 20 and 54%, there is a concern that a stimulant's dopamine agonist action will unmask, trigger, accelerate, or provoke irreversible Tourette's symptoms. This worry is enhanced by a number of papers, some of them retrospective, that reported onset of tics after stimulant treatment had begun.

Drug Interactions

(See Table 82.5 for a listing of common drug interactions.) Mixing psychostimulants with other psychotropic medications is generally not advisable. Most serious is the addition of a psychostimulant to a monoamine oxidase inhibitor antidepressant regimen, a potentially lethal combination that can elevate blood pressure to dangerous levels. Additive effects between psychostimulants and the systemic agents used to treat asthma can produce feelings of dizziness, tachycardia, palpitation, weakness and agitation. Theophylline, for example, when taken orally (Theo-Dur Sprinkle), can have this undesirable agitating effect. It is best to ask the pediatrician or allergist to switch from the orally ingested preparation to an inhalant to avoid such additive sympathomimetic effects.

Psychostimulants compete with other medications for the same metabolic pathway and have been thought to produce an increase in the plasma concentration of both drugs. The psychostimulants can also interfere with the action of other medications. MPH can block the antihypertensive action of guanethidine. DEX blocks the action of some beta-adrenergic

antagonists (e.g., propranolol) and slows the intestinal absorption of phenytoin and phenobarbital. The renal clearance of DEX is enhanced by urine acidifying agents, so that grapefruit juice will shorten the elimination half-life of the medication. Conversely, urine alkalinizing agents decrease clearance. This is also true for ritalinic acid, although this metabolite is not active in the CNS. MPH may elevate the plasma level of antidepressants, anticonvulsants, coumarin anticoagulants and phenylbutazone. MPH may increase the concentration of the serotonin reuptake blocker fluoxetine, potentially enhancing agitation, although no such side effect was seen in a single case report of the treatment of an 11-year-old boy with both ADHD and obsessive–compulsive disorder. Other medications have been combined successfully with MPH, such as clonazepam to reduce tics. Clonidine has been added to reduce sleep disturbances associated with ADHD and with stimulant medication. Bupropion may exacerbate tics when added to MPH given to children with ADHD.

Initiation of Treatment

Medication treatment begins with a choice of medication. Although the MPH or DEX psychostimulant types have equal efficacy, MPH is often used first.

Titration serves two purposes: acclimatization of the child to the drug and determination of his or her best dose. School-age children should be started with low doses to minimize adverse effects. Psychostimulant medication should be taken at or just after mealtime to lessen the anorectic effects; studies have shown

Table 82.5	Experimental Medication Therapies for Adults with Attention-deficit/Hyperactivity Disorder	
Possible Medication Treatments	Suggested Dose Range	
Methylphenidate (Ritalin)	5 mg b.i.d.–20 mg t.i.d.	
Amphetamine (Dexedrine)	5 mg b.i.d.–20 mg b.i.d.	
Mixed amphetamine salts (Adderall)	5 mg b.i.d.–20 mg. b.i.d.	
Bupropion (Wellbutrin)	100 mg b.i.d.–100 mg t.i.d.	
Selegiline (Eldepryl)	5 mg b.i.d. only	

Table 82.6   Stimulant Side Effects and Management

Side Effect	Management
For all side effects	Unless severe, allow 7–10 d for tolerance to develop. Evaluate dose–response relationships. Evaluate time–action effects and then adjust dosing intervals or switch to sustained-release preparation. Evaluate for concurrent conditions, including comorbidities and environmental stressors. Consider switching stimulant drug.
Anorexia or dyspepsia	Administer before, during, or after meals.
Weight loss	Give drug after breakfast and after lunch. Implement calorie enhancement strategies. Give brief drug holidays.
Slowed growth	Apply weight loss remedies. Give weekend and vacation (longer) drug holidays. Consider another stimulant or nonstimulant drug.
Dizziness	Monitor blood pressure and pulse. Encourage adequate hydration. If associated with only T_{max}, change to sustained-release preparation.
Insomnia or nightmares	Administer earlier in day. Omit or reduce last dose. If giving sustained preparation, switch to tablet drug. Consider adjunctive antihistamine or clonidine.
Dysphoric mood or emotional constriction	Reduce dose or switch to long-acting preparation. Switch stimulants. Consider comorbidity requiring alternative or adjunctive treatment.
Rebound	Switch to stained-release preparation. Combined long- and short-acting preparations.
Tics	Firmly establish correlation between tics and pharmacotherapy by examining dose–response relationship, including no-medication condition. If tics are mild and abate after 7–10 d with medications, reconsider risks and benefits of continued stimulant treatment and renew informed consent. Switch stimulants. Consider nonstimulant treatment (e.g., clonidine or tricyclic antidepressant). If tic disorder and ADHD are severe, consider combining stimulant with a high-potency neuroleptic.
Psychosis	Discontinue stimulant treatment. Assess for comorbid thought disorder. Consider alternative treatments.

that food may enhance drug absorption. MPH treatment can be initiated with a single 5 mg dose at 8:00 am for 3 days; then a 5 mg dose at 8:00 am and at noon for the next 3 days; then 10 mg at 8:00 am and 5 mg at noon for 3 days; and finally 10 mg at 8:00 am and 10 mg at noon are given and maintained for at least 2 weeks. Preschoolers may start as low as 2.5 mg at 8:00 am but build to the same total 20 mg/day dose of MPH. The dosing instructions should be written down for the parent, with dates and times specified in detail. A photocopy of the instructions should be kept in the patient's chart.

Table 82.6 is an inventory of stimulant drugs and doses. DEX is usually started at 2.5 to 5 mg/day and gradually increased in 2.5- to 5-mg increments; MPH is usually started at 5 mg b.i.d. and then titrated in increments of 5 mg/dose every 4 to 7 days. Peak behavioral effects are noted 1 to 3 hours after ingestion and dissipate in 3 to 6 hours for both MPH and DEX.

The Conners Teacher Rating Scale is then repeated. Further dose adjustments up or down depend on the rating scale's scores, teachers' verbal reports, parents' comments, and adverse effects experienced by the child. The minimal effective total daily dose and optimal timing of medication administration should be determined before switching to the sustained-release 20 mg formulation. Eventually, one dose of standard MPH may have to be mixed with one sustained-release 20 mg pill at 8:00 am (to give early- and late-morning coverage), just as one administers short- and long-acting insulin at the same time.

Monitoring

Maintenance plans should include schedules for the regular collection of information that constitutes the child's therapeutic drug monitoring. Each child's response to psychostimulants is different. Likewise, each family's needs are different. Plans for medication vacations and weekend and after-school dosing must be individualized.

Medication **compliance** should be monitored at each visit. The parent is instructed to bring the medication bottle along so that pill counts can be done monthly and compared with the prescription dates. Height and weight should be taken every 6 months, and the child's pediatrician can be requested yearly to perform a complete physical examination and blood work (complete blood count, liver function studies). The frequency of visits depends on the other therapies recommended. These may include once-monthly parental counseling, twice-monthly individual therapy, or weekly meetings for individual psychotherapy or behavioral modification management. A minimal frequency should be once monthly, particularly in the nine states requiring multiple-copy prescription forms, which limit the amount of psychostimulant ordered to a 30-day supply.

The next component of monitoring is the use of **structured rating scales**. These have been the backbone of psychostimulant treatment research but also have utility in clinical practice. Each physician should choose a scale that she or he finds easy to interpret and convenient to use. It should be available in both parent and teacher formats. These scales, however, should not be used as substitutes for an open discussion with the teacher.

These rating forms should be collected every 4 months and whenever the physician needs to make decisions about dosage adjustment, time of dosing, or even continuation of medication. Although the original 39-item Conners Teacher Rating Scale is ubiquitous in the field of child psychopharmacology, Satin and colleagues (1985) have shown the validity of the shorter, 10-item Abbreviated Rating Scale both as a repeated measure and as a screening tool for identifying school-age children with ADHD. This short form is good for tracking children in maintenance treatment. Like most scales, the Abbreviated Rating Scale assigns weights to each scale point. With a 10-item scale, and each point weighted between 0 ("not at all") and 3 ("very much"), 10 checks by a parent in the "very much" column yields a total score of 30.

Unlike the situation with anticonvulsants, it has not proved effective to monitor psychostimulants by maintaining plasma concentrations within a therapeutic range. Alternative medications such as desipramine, however, do lend themselves to regular plasma level monitoring every 3 months.

Phases of Treatment

Medication therapy can be divided into baseline, titration and maintenance phases. Before the first pill is given, baseline data on height, weight, blood pressure and heart rate should be collected as well as a complete blood count. The Conners Teacher Rating Scale and Conners Parent Rating Scale can also be collected. Standardized scoring methods for the teacher rating scale can be used to generate a hyperactivity factor score.

The duration of treatment is an important step in the generation of a treatment plan for a child with ADHD. Although there is no clear-cut recommendation for the length of psychostimulant treatment, many parents have a reasonable expectation that it will not be open-ended. The onset of puberty is one possible stopping point for psychostimulant medication. School-age children were thought to respond "paradoxically", calming down on stimulant medication, an effect that was supposedly lost at puberty. Adolescents with ADHD, who may be at risk for substance abuse, were thought to be particularly vulnerable to psychostimulant euphoria and to abuse of their medications. In addition, more recent prospective follow-up studies suggest that the motor hyperactivity of ADHD disappears between ages 16 and 23 years.

Integration with Other Modalities: Multimodal Treatment

Medication is only one component of a comprehensive therapeutic treatment plan. New standards have been promulgated for the treatment of ADHD recommending multimodal therapy including psychological, educational and social components. This was first reported by Satterfield and colleagues (1980) to be successful in maintaining the short-term stimulant gains for periods of 2 years or more.

Treatment Failure

If a child fails to show improvement as the stimulant dose is being increased, how far should the dose be increased before turning to another medication? The physician is left with the dose range suggested in the PDR and to his or her own standards regarding what constitutes improvement and where to draw the line between a response and failure.

Do true nonresponders exist? Recent studies indicate that many apparent nonresponders to stimulants may simply have been treated with too low a dose. The treating physician is well advised to seek expert consultation with a child and adolescent psychopharmacologist before venturing beyond a total dose of 60 mg/day of MPH and 40 mg/day of DEX.

Use of Long-acting Preparations

There are three reasons for the implementation of longer-acting stimulant preparations. First, children who take medications in school are subject to peer ridicule when they leave activities to go to the nurse. Secondly, some school officials refuse to allow school personnel involvement in the administration of medication. Thirdly, the time–action course of standard stimulant medications allows only a brief 1- to 3-hour window of effect, so some medicated children may experience trough periods of little or no drug action during important parts of the school day.

Sustained-release preparations have been marketed for DEX and MPH. MPH's sustained-release preparation (MPH-SR), which became available in 1984, is manufactured in brand (Ritalin-SR) and generic (MD Pharmaceuticals) versions but only in a single strength of 20 mg (MPH-SR 20). DEX spansules are available in 5-, 10- and 15 mg strengths in the brand version (Dexedrine Spansules). The sustained-release preparations make it possible to give the psychostimulant once in the morning and avoid administration during the school day. Ritalin-SR uses a wax-matrix vehicle for slow release, whereas the DEX "spansule" is a capsule containing small medication particles.

Conclusion

Psychostimulant medications are a mainstay in the US treatment of ADHD. This popularity has resulted from their proven efficacy during short-term controlled studies, as shown by improvements in global ratings by teachers and parents. In fact, the majority of children with ADHD respond to either MPH or DEX, so nonresponders are rare (Elia *et al.*, 1991). Yet, the long-term response of ADHD children to MPH and other psychostimulants is not known; published treatment studies have lasted months, not the years that children take stimulants to adapt to academics in school (Jacobvitz *et al.*, 1990). Optimal treatment involves the planning for a multimodal treatment program that combines educational and psychosocial interventions with medication therapy.

Treatment plans that center on psychostimulant medication have flourished for a number of reasons. The effects of psychostimulants are rapid, dramatic and normalizing. The risk of long-term side effects remains low, and no substantial impairments have emerged to lessen the remarkable therapeutic benefit–risk ratio of these medications. More expensive and demanding treatments, including behavior modification and cognitive–behavioral therapies, have, at best, only equaled the treatment with psychostimulants. In a number of instances, the combination of behavioral and medication therapies is only slightly more effective than the medication alone (Gittelman-Klein, 1987). Current and future studies of multimodal therapies will test whether combined treatment results in better overall functioning in the long run and decreased appearance of comorbid conditions than does monomodal treatment with psychostimulants alone. It is essential to show that the continuation of stimulant medication during long-term maintenance benefits the patient with ADHD.

References

Aman MG, Marks RE, Turbott SH *et al.* (1991) Clinical effects of methylphenidate and thioridazine in intellectually subaverage children. *J Am Acad Child Adolesc Psychiatr* 30(2), 246–256.

American Psychiatric Association (1980) *Diagnostic and Statistical Manual of Mental Disorders*, 3rd edn. APA, Washington DC.

Comings DE and Comings BG (1987) A controlled study of Tourette's syndrome. *Am J Hum Genet* 41, 701–741.

Dahl R (1992) The pharmacologic treatment of sleep disorders. *Child Adolesc Psychiatr Clin* 15(1), 161–178.

Elia J, Borcherding B, Rapoport J *et al.* (1991) Methylphenidate and dextroamphetamine treatments of hyperactivity: Are there true non-responders? *Psychiatr Res* 36, 141–155.

Gittelman-Klein R (1987) Pharmacotherapy of childhood hyperactivity: An update, in *Psychopharmacology: The Third Generation of Progress* (ed Meltzer HY). Raven Press, New York.

Hill J and Schoener E (1996) Age-dependent decline of attention-deficit hyperactivity disorder (abstract). *Am J Psychiatr* 153, 1143–1146.

Jacobvitz D, Srouge LA, Stewart M *et al.* (1990) Treatment of attentional and hyperactivity problems in children with sympathomimetic drugs: A comprehensive review. *J Am Acad Child Adolesc Psychiatr* 29(5), 677–688.

Klein D (1980) Treatment of anxiety, personality, somatoform and factitious disorders, in *Diagnosis and Drug Treatment of Psychiatric Disorders: Adults and Children*, 2nd edn. (eds Klein D, Gittelman R, Quitkin F *et al.*). Williams & Wilkins, Baltimore, pp. 539–573.

McCracken J (1991) A two-part model of stimulant action on attention-deficit hyperactivity disorder in children. *J Neuropsychiatr Clin Neurosci* 3(2), 201–209.

Pelham W, Murphy D, Vanarra K, *et al.* (1992) Methylphenidate and attributions in boys with attention deficit hyperactivity disorder. *J Consult Clin Psychol* 60, 359–369.

Rapoport JL, Buchsbaum MS, Weingartner H *et al.* (1980) Dextroamphetamine: Cognitive and behavioral effects in normal and hyperactive boys and normal men. *Arch Gen Psychiatr* 37, 933–943.

Safer D, Zito M and Gardner JF (2001) Pemoline hepatotoxicity and postmarketing surveillance. *J Am Acad Child Adolesc Psychiatr* 40, 622–629.

Satin M, Winsberg B, Monetti C *et al.* (1985) A general population screen for attention deficit disorder with hyperactivity. *J Am Acad Child Adolesc Psychiatr* 24, 756–764.

Satterfield JH, Satterfield BT and Cantwell DP (1980) Multimodality treatment: A two-year evaluation of 61 hyperactive boys. *Arch Gen Psychiatr* 37(8), 915–919.

Zametkin AJ and Rapoport JL (1987) Neurobiology of attention deficit disorder with hyperactivity: Where have we come in 50 years? *J Am Acad Child Adolesc Psychiatr* 26, 676–686.

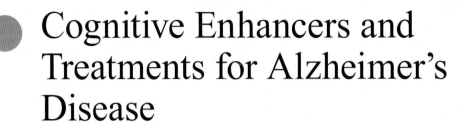

CHAPTER

83

Cognitive Enhancers and Treatments for Alzheimer's Disease

By the late 1980s the advent and general acceptance of research-based diagnostic criteria for the dementia of Alzheimer's disease (AD) (McKhann *et al.*, 1984), an understanding of its underlying pathology along with mechanism-based pharmacological therapeutics provided the framework for clinical trials to exploit a variety of new treatment strategies that might positively impact the illness.

Since AD is defined by the presence of dementia, attempts have been made to identify a predementia state of cognitive impairment, likely to lead to AD. This state of "mild cognitive impairment" (MCI) has now been the target of several clinical trials of medications previously used for AD. However, MCI is not merely a predementia stage of AD, since many people who fulfill criteria do not progress to dementia.

Regulatory Issues

The Food and Drug Administration (FDA) utilizes *de facto* guidelines for establishing that a drug has "antidementia efficacy" (Leber, 2002). These require, in part, that: 1) clinical trials be double-blind and placebo-controlled; 2) patients fulfill the now-accepted criteria for a primary dementia such as AD (e.g., using either DSM-IV-TR or NINCDS-ADRDA (National Institute of Neurological and Communicative Disorders and Stroke-Alzheimer's Disease and Related Disorders Association) Work Group Criteria) (McKhann *et al.*, 1984); and 3) appropriate efficacy instruments be used. Although the *de facto* guidelines avoid specifying that only Alzheimer's dementia can be treated, allowing the possibility that any recognized or accepted conditions can receive approval, at present it is the only dementia for which FDA-approved medications are available. [Note that DSM-IV-TR criteria for Dementia of the Alzheimer's Type very closely reflect the NINCDS-ADRDA Work Group Criteria.]

Limitations to the current guidelines include the failure to recognize improvement in behavior or functional activities **alone** as legitimate therapeutic goals or indications in the prescribing information, despite the fact that behavioral symptoms occur in the majority of dementia patients, and that improvements in functional status may have a major effect on prolonging independence. In addition, these guidelines fail to provide for efficacy measures for severely impaired patients who are unable to perform standard cognitive tests.

Therapeutic Implications of Pathophysiology

Advances in understanding of plaques and tangles over the last few years underscore the biological heterogeneity of the illness, and several clues about definitive therapeutic approaches have appeared. It is likely that there are several stimuli for these abnormal protein processes, genetically, biologically and environmentally determined. These processes need to be understood more fully in order to discover new drugs acting directly on the pathological processes responsible for the neurodegeneration. For example, the finding that amyloid precursor protein processing is in part controlled by a cholinergic mechanism suggests that cholinergically based therapeutic strategies may modify the progress of the disease as well as providing symptomatic relief (Giacobini, 1996).

Other potential interventions in development now include agents that interfere with beta-amyloid formation such as secretase inhibitors, modulators of APP expression, β-secretase and β-secretase inhibitors that prevent cleavage of APP into insoluble β-amyloid protein, inhibitors of β-amyloid protein aggregation or deposition, or the passive or active immunization with antibodies to β-amyloid.

The observed neurotransmitter perturbations in AD, however, provide more immediate and accessible targets for therapeutic interventions. For example, the observation of deficits in noradrenergic or serotoninergic function provide rationales for the use of antidepressants in patients with AD and symptomatic behaviors. Although not the exclusive pathological change, the cholinergic deficits represent the most consistent transmitter depletion and appear to be one of the early events in the disease process (Francis *et al.*, 1985, 1999). Thus, it continues to remain a major focus of applied clinical pharmacological research.

Treatment Paradigms

Approaches to the treatment of AD can be grouped into several conceptual categories (Table 83.1). One approach attempts to treat the behavioral symptoms such as agitation, aggression, psychosis, depression, anxiety, apathy, and sleep or appetite disturbances. A second approach attempts to treat the cognitive or neuropsychological signs symptoms of the illness such as memory, language, praxis, attention, orientation and knowledge. A third

Essentials of Psychiatry   Jerald Kay and Allan Tasman
© 2006 John Wiley & Sons, Ltd.

Table 83.1	Conceptualized Treatment Strategies for Patients with Cognitive Impairment

Symptomatic and/or Restorative

Targets: impaired cognition, depression, psychosis, agitation, aggression, anxiety, insomnia

Examples: cholinesterase inhibitors, various cholinergic agonists, antidepressants, antipsychotics, mood stabilizers, antianxiety agents, hypnotics, NMDA and AMPA receptor modulators, angiotensin converting enzyme inhibitors

Neurotrophic factors: nerve growth factor, brain-derived neurotrophic factors, estrogens

Notes: some substances may have symptomatic or restorative effects but are unproven. These may include Hydergine and neotropics such as piracetam.

Pathophysiologically-directed

Targets: underlying pathophysiology of neurodegeneration, including inflammation, production of oxidizing free radicals, excitatory amino acids.

Examples: anti-inflammatory agents, calcium channel blockers, NMDA and AMPA receptor modulators. Transplantation of hormonally active tissues, or NGF (nerve growth factor) gene therapy using viral vectors have been undertaken experimentally.

Etiologically-directed

Targets: β-amyloid formation or hyperphosphorylated tau protein.

Examples: modulators of APP expression, β- and γ-secretase inhibitors, inhibitors of beta-amyloid protein aggregation or deposition, immunization with antibodies to beta-amyloid.

Note: The interventions listed above include some that are available and marketed, as well as some that have not been demonstrated effective or safe, and some conceptual treatments not yet developed.

approach attempts to slow the rate of progression of the illness, preserving patients' quality of life or autonomy. (Slowing the rate of decline might also be related to treating symptoms.) A fourth conceptual treatment approach is primary prevention, to delay the time to onset of illness. Success at this approach could have considerable impact.

Cholinergic Agents

The primary implication of the cholinergic hypothesis is that potentiation of central cholinergic function should improve the cognitive and behavioral impairment associated with AD. This simple "neurotransmitter replacement" rationale has been made most compelling by the consistent effects of cholinesterase inhibitors as a class of drugs across trials.

While agents with several kinds of procholinergic action have been evaluated for efficacy in AD, the ChIs (cholinesterase inhibitors) are the only agents to have consistently demonstrated efficacy in numerous multicenter, placebo-controlled trials, and thus have been approved by many national regulatory authorities.

Thus ChIs represent the first **class** of efficacious pharmacological approaches for AD, and an approach that is likely to be clinically useful for the indefinite future, especially since research on drugs with other mechanisms has not advanced as rapidly as had been hoped for.

The well-established cholinergic defects in AD include: decline of cholinergic baso-cortical projections; reduced activity of ChAT, the key acetylcholine (ACh) synthesis enzyme, and cholinergic cell body loss in the nucleus basalis. Additionally, there are correlations between cortical ChAT reduction or nucleus basalis cell reduction and cortical plaque density. Such cholinergic deficits correlate with cognitive decline as measured by the Blessed-Roth Dementia Rating Scale (Blessed *et al.*, 1968). The cholinergic hypothesis proposes that cognitive deficits of AD are related to decreases in central acetylcholinergic activity, and that increasing intrasynaptic ACh will enhance cognitive function and clinical well-being. (See Figure 83.1.)

Cholinergic Treatment Approaches

Cholinergic treatment approaches include precursor loading, cholinesterase inhibition, direct cholinergic receptor stimulation and indirect cholinergic stimulation. Unfortunately, most of these cholinergic strategies have thus far proven ineffective, effective but too toxic, or have not been completely developed.

Cholinesterase Inhibitors

ChIs have shown generally consistent symptomatic efficacy in standardized, well-controlled multicenter trials lasting from 6 months to occasionally 12 months. Cholinesterase inhibitors (Table 83.2) have been the most frequently used experimental treatment for AD and the major group of medications to yield consistently positive results in clinical trials. Current marketed ChIs include tacrine, donepezil, rivastigmine and galantamine, although tacrine is now used much less commonly due to the risk of hepatotoxicity.

Mechanisms of Cholinesterase Inhibition

Acetylcholine is inactivated when it is hydrolyzed to choline and acetate by acetylcholinesterase (AChE). By inhibiting the actions of AChE, ChIs effectively increase the amount of ACh available for intrasynaptic cholinergic receptor stimulation. A summary of pharmacokinetics and pharmacodynamics is in Table 83.3.

Individual Cholinesterase Inhibitors – Dosing and Adverse Effects

Tacrine

Tacrine is a noncompetitive reversible inhibitor of ChE. It binds near the catalytically active site of the AChE molecule to inhibit enzyme activity. It has other actions as well including blocking sodium and potassium channels, and direct activity at muscarinic receptors (Adem *et al.*, 1990).

Dosing

Tacrine's FDA-approved dosing regimen is based on the clinical trials. The recommended starting dose is 10 mg q.i.d. to be

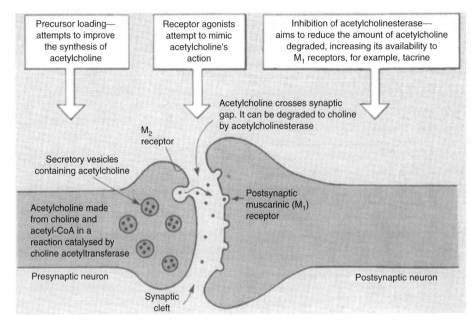

Figure 83.1 *Possible areas of action for therapy in AD. Reprinted with permission from Tariot P, Schneider L, and Coleman PD [1993a] Treatment of Alzheimer's disease: Glimmers of hope? Chem Ind 20, 801–807.*

maintained for 6 weeks, while serum transaminase levels are monitored every other week. If the drug is tolerated and transaminase levels do not increase above three times the upper limit of normal, the dose is then increased to 20 mg q.i.d. After 6 weeks, dosage should be increased to 30 mg q.i.d., again with biweekly monitoring and then, if tolerated, to 40 mg q.i.d. for the next 6

weeks. Due to hepatotoxicity concerns, Tacrine's use greatly decreased.

Donepezil

Donepezil (Aricept™) is a long-acting piperidine-based highly selective and reversible acetylcholinesterase inhibitor.

Dosing

Donepezil is initiated at 5 mg/day and then increased to 10 mg/day after 4 to 6 weeks. Raising the dose earlier increases the risk for cholinergic adverse events. Five or 10 mg/day are effective doses; 10 mg tends to be somewhat more effective than 5 mg when the various trials as a group are evaluated.

Rivastigmine

Rivastigmine (Exelon™) is a pseudo-irreversible, selective AChE subtype inhibitor.

Dosing

The recommended starting dose of rivastigmine is 1.5 mg b.i.d., taken with meals. If this dose is well tolerated after a minimum of 2 weeks of treatment, it may be increased to 3 mg b.i.d. Subsequent increases to 4.5 mg and then 6 mg b.i.d. should be based on good tolerability of the current dose and may be considered after a minimum of 2 weeks of treatment. Higher daily doses, averaging about 9 to 10 mg were associated with better efficacy than lower doses.

Galantamine

Galantamine (Reminyl™), an alkaloid originally extracted from Amaryllidaceae (*Galanthus woronowi*, the Caucasian snowdrop), but now synthesized, is a reversible, competitive inhibitor of AChE with relatively less butyrylcholinesterase activity (Harvey, 1995).

Table 83.2 FDA-Approved Drugs to Improve Cognitive Function in Alzheimer's Disease

Drug	How Supplied	Initial Dosage	Maintenance Dosage
Tacrine	10, 20, 30 and 40 mg capsules	10 mg q.i.d.	30 or 40 mg q.i.d.
Donepezil	5 and 10 mg tablets	5 mg q.i.d.	5–10 mg q.i.d.
Rivastigmine	1.5, 3, 4.5 and 6 mg capsules	1.5 mg b.i.d.	3, 4.5, or 6 mg b.i.d.
Galantamine	4, 8 and 12 mg tablets Solution 4 mg/mL	4 mg b.i.d.	8 or 12 mg b.i.d.
Memantine	5 and 10 mg tablets, oral solution 2 mg/mL	5 mg q.d.	10 mg b.i.d.

Initial dosages should be maintained for at least 2 and preferably 4–6 weeks before increasing. For Memantine, dose may be increased weekly in 5 mgm increments. Adverse events may occur with dosage titration.

Table 83.3   Pharmacodynamic and Pharmacokinetics of Marketed Cholinesterase Inhibitors

Drug	Pharmacodynamics	Absorption	Bioavailability	Peak Plasma (h)	Elimination Half-life (h)	Protein Binding	Metabolism/ Comments
Tacrine (Cognex)	Noncompetitive, reversible ChI, both butryrl and acetyl ChI, also multiple other actions	Delayed by food	17%	1–2	2–4	55%	Via 1A2, nonlinear pharmacokinetics; hepatoxicity requires regular monitoring of serum alamine aminotransferases.
Donepezil (Aricept)	Noncompetitive, reversible acetyl-ChI.	Not affected by food	100%	3–4	70	96%	Via 2D6, 3A4. Nonlinear pharmacokinetics at 10 mg/d
Rivastigmine (Exelon)	Noncompetitive ChI, both butryrl and acetyl ChI, may differentially effect different acetyl ChEs	Delayed by food	40%	1.4–2.6	< 5	40%	Hydrolysis by esterases and excreted in urine (nonhepatic). Duration of cholinesterase inhibition longer than plasma half-life. Nonlinear pharmacokinetics
Galantamine (Reminyl)	Competitive, reversible ChI, modulates nicotine receptors	Delayed by food	90%	1	7	18%	Via 2D6, 3A4

Note: Pharmacodynamic effects of some ChIs are longer than their elimination half-lives. Drugs that inhibit or induce the cytochrome enzymes above might be expected to increase or decrease blood levels. For the most part, clinically however, drug interactions with donepezil, rivastigmine and galantamine have not been clinical problems.

Dosing

Initial dosing is 4 mg b.i.d., and should be raised to 8 mg b.i.d. after 2 to 4 weeks. For patients who are tolerating medication but not responding the dose can be raised to 12 mg b.i.d. after another 4 weeks.

Adverse Effects of Cholinesterase Inhibitors

Most adverse events from ChIs are cholinergically mediated, and are characteristically mild in severity and short-lived, lasting only a few days. Adverse events of the marketed ChIs are summarized in Table 83.4. Significant cholinergic side effects can occur in up to about 25% of patients receiving higher doses. Often they are related to the initial titration of medication. Patients tend rapidly to become tolerant to the adverse events when they occur. Hepatotoxicity with tacrine is a significant concern requiring very close monitoring if the drug is used.

Because of the actions of ChIs, these drugs require caution when used in patients with significant asthma, significant chronic obstructive pulmonary disease, cardiac conduction defects, or clinically significant bradycardia. Appropriate considerations are involved in general anesthesia as well since they may prolong the effects of succinylcholine-type drugs.

Drug interactions with medications which inhibit cytochrome P450 types 3A4 or 2D6 may occur with this class of medications.

Infrequent Adverse Events Worth Noting

A number of infrequent adverse events that may be of particular concern to patients, caregivers and physicians, and are common among the class of ChIs include fatigue, anorexia, weight loss and bradycardia. Myasthenia and respiratory depression occurred in a few patients treated with the higher doses of the organophosphate drug metrifonate leading to its therapeutic demise for AD. Although myasthenia might not be expected to occur with the reversible ChI, physicians should be vigilant for complaints of fatigue and weakness.

An increased but modest incidence of anorexia appears to be a consistent finding across clinical trials and appears to be dose related. The absolute reported incidence varies across trials from approximately 8 to 25% at the highest dose of ChI compared with 3 to 10% in comparable placebo patients. Similarly, there is an increased rate of significant weight loss with higher doses of ChIs compared with placebo patients. The proportion of patients losing greater than 7% of

Table 83.4	Adverse Effects of Cholinesterase Inhibitors

Summary of adverse event data in placebo-controlled, randomized clinical trials. The method of obtaining adverse events and their reporting vary among trials

Drug	Adverse Events
Tacrine	Nausea, vomiting, diarrhea, dyspepsia, myalgia, anorexia, dizziness, confusion, insomnia, rare agranulocytosis
	Many patients will develop direct, reversible hepatotoxicity manifested by elevated transaminases
	Drug interactions may include increased cholinergic effects with bethanacol; increased plasma tacrine levels with cimetidine or fluvoxamine. This may occur by inhibition of P450 1A2. The association of tacrine with haloperidol may increase parkinsonism and tacrine increases theophylline concentration.
Donepezil	Nausea, diarrhea, insomnia, vomiting, muscle cramps, fatigue, anorexia, dizziness, abdominal pain, myasthenia, rhinitis, weight loss, anxiety, syncope (2 vs. 1%)
Rivastigmine	Nausea, vomiting, anorexia, dizziness, abdominal pain, diarrhea, malaise, fatigue, asthenia, headache, sweating, weight loss, somnolence, syncope (3 vs. 2%). Rarely, severe vomiting with esophageal rupture
Galantamine	Nausea, vomiting, diarrhea, anorexia, weight loss, abdominal pain, dizziness, tremor, syncope (2 vs. 1%)

Adverse event estimates vary widely among the cholinesterase inhibitors from study to study and thus relative adverse event rates among drugs are difficult to estimate. Cholinergic side effects generally occur early and are related to initiating or increasing medication. They tend to be mild and self-limited. Medications should be restarted at lowest doses after temporarily stopping. See prescribing information referenced in Table 83.2.

General precautions with cholinesterase inhibitors (as indicated in the prescribing information)

By increasing central and peripheral cholinergic stimulation cholinesterase inhibitors may:

1. increase gastric acid secretion, increasing the risk for GI bleeding especially in patients with ulcer disease or those taking anti-inflammatories
2. produce bradycardia, especially in patients with sick sinus or other supraventricular conduction delay, leading to syncope, falls, and possible injury
3. exacerbate obstructive pulmonary disease
4. cause urinary outflow obstruction
5. increase risk for seizures
6. prolong the effects of succinylcholine-type muscle relaxants

their baseline weight varies from approximately 10 to 24% in the higher doses and from 2 to 10% of the placebo-treated patients in those trials reporting the statistic. Anorexia and weight loss are significant clinical problems for many elderly patients independent of medication effects, and whether or not demented.

Treatment Approach with Cholinesterese Inhibitors

The typical candidates for ChIs are outpatients with AD of mild to moderate cognitive severity. They usually live at home or in an assisted living facility. Dementia is their main clinical problem; concurrent illnesses are not severe or dominating the clinical picture. Nor do behavioral syndromes such as psychosis, agitation, or significant insomnia, apathy, or depression dominate.

As indicated above, dosing should be initiated with 5 mg/day donepezil, 1.5 mg b.i.d. rivastigmine or 4 mg b.i.d. galantamine. Tacrine should be reserved as a second-line medication since it requires q.i.d. dosing and biweekly blood monitoring for elevated transaminase. After a minimum of 2 weeks, but preferably 4 to 6 weeks, the dosages should be doubled although 5 mg of donepezil is an effective dose.

Optimal duration of treatment with continuing efficacy is unknown but overall efficacy extends at least 9 to 12 months based on the clinical trials and open-label extension phases.

Maintenance treatment can be continued as long as a therapeutic benefit for the patient seems apparent. Therefore, the potential clinical benefit of ChIs should be reassessed on a regular basis. Discontinuation should be considered when evidence of a therapeutic effect is no longer present. Because of the great interpatient variability of response, it is not possible to predict individual patient responses to ChIs.

It is difficult to assess individual patient response because of the variability of the deteriorating course of AD, and because most of the effect of medication is due to a stabilization or lack of worsening of symptoms or cognitive function while placebo-treated patients continue to decline. Therefore, the clinical observations of minimal or no clinical worsening may be sufficient reasons to continue medication treatment if patients are tolerating therapy.

Monitoring Side Effects

Cholinergic side effects such as diarrhea, nausea and vomiting, when they occur, tend to occur at initiation of treatment and when titrating to higher doses. They are often transient or self-limited and can often be managed with encouragement and maintenance of the present dose level, by omitting one or more doses, or by temporarily decreasing dosage. Most cholinergic side effects are related to the dose escalation phase of treatment, just after starting or increasing. Patients on maintenance doses should have few and very mild cholinergic side effects if any.

However, anorexia and weight loss may be clinically significant problems over the longer term, especially in older, more medically ill and nursing home patients, so these parameters should be monitored and medication reduced or discontinued if anorexia or weight loss become clinically significant to assess if appetite returns.

Uncommonly, the vagotonic effects of ChIs may cause significant bradycardia, and this can be a particular concern to patients with supraventricular conduction impairments or sick sinus syndrome.

Because gastric acid secretion may be increased with cholinesterase inhibitors, there may be an increased risk for developing ulcers or gastrointestinal bleeding. Patients receiving nonsteroidal anti-inflammatory drugs may be at a particularly additive risk. It is possible that ChIs may cause bladder outflow obstruction, seizures and exacerbate asthma or obstructive pulmonary disease, and interfere with succinylcholinelike anesthetics.

Effect on Behavior

The evidence that ChIs may improve behavior is based on case series and secondary analyses of efficacy trials (Kaufer *et al.*, 1996; Raskind *et al.*, 1997). Nevertheless, clinical experience suggests that they may be effective at least for mildly disturbed behavior, and in delaying the onset of troublesome behaviors, perhaps by maintaining cognitive function or perhaps through enhancing attentional processes and activation.

Neuroprotection

Cholinergic therapies may have effects beyond the short-term symptomatic improvement of cognition and may modify the pathogenetic processes of the illness (Radebaugh *et al.*, 1996; Thal *et al.*, 1997). For example, activation of M_1 muscarinic receptors can stimulate secretion of amyloid precursor proteins via the α-secretase pathway such that there is a decrease in the production of toxic and insoluble β-amyloid, thus theoretically decreasing the formation of amyloid plaques and promoting the normal processing of APP (Inestrosa *et al.*, 1996; Muller *et al.*, 1997; Nitsch *et al.*, 1992). These effects remain to be proven in clinical trials (Buxbaum *et al.*, 1992; Haroutunian *et al.*, 1997; Lahiri *et al.*, 2000).

Memantine

L-glutamate is the main excitatory neurotransmitter in the central nervous system. Enhancement of its activity at the N-methyl-D-aspartate (NMDA) receptor may contribute to the pathogenesis of Alzheimer's disease, a phenomenon known as excitotoxicity. Memantine is a low affinity antagonist that is believed to reduce NMDA receptor overstimulation and restore receptor signalling function to more normal levels. It is also possible that reducing excitotoxicity may be neuroprotective by preventing neuronal calcium overload though there is no evidence that memantine modifies neurodegeneration in patients with Alzheimer's disease.

Unlike the cholinesterase inhibitors, memantine is approved by the FDA for the treatment of moderate to severe Alzheimer's disease (defined as an MMSE score of less than 15).

Dosing

Treatment should be initiated at a dose of 5 mg/day and increased in increments of 5 mg at intervals of one week to a target dose of 20 mg/day; doses of 10 mg/day or more should be divided into two given 12 hours apart. Memantine is well tolerated and is not associated with an increase in treatment discontinuation compared with placebo.

Restorative Approaches: Other Agents

The structural and functional disturbances of central catecholaminergic systems in AD and their important role in brain-related functions provide the rationale for pharmacological enhancement of these systems. The general strategies employed are analogous to those used with cholinergic agents: precursor loading, inhibition of degradative enzymes and use of agonists. Studies of dopamine precursors (e.g., with tyrosine, l-dopa) and agonists (e.g., clonidine, guanefacine, amantadine, bromocriptine) have largely been negative (Schneider and Tariot, 1997).

There have been some positive effects reported with selegiline (l-deprenyl, Eldepryl®, Somerset), a monoamine oxidase (MAO) inhibitor that relatively selectively inhibits MAO type B at a 5 to 10 mg daily dose (Tariot *et al.*, 1993). The overall effect of selegiline at this dose may be to increase CNS levels of dopamine and some trace neurotransmitters such as phenylethylamine without affecting norepinephrine levels. Selegiline is currently marketed for the treatment of Parkinson's disease for which it has demonstrated effects in maintaining motor function (Parkinson Study Group, 1993). However, an adequate efficacy trial has yet to be completed in AD.

Selegiline, 5 mg b.i.d., along with and separately from vitamin E, 1000 IU b.i.d., has been associated with prolonged maintenance of ADLs and survival in the community in moderately to severely impaired AD patients but with no improvement in function (Sano *et al.*, 1997).

Metabolic Enhancement

In view of regional decreases in glucose utilization and abnormal oxidative metabolism, drugs have been employed with the aim of correcting these abnormalities, including ergot alkaloids and nootropics. A discussion of the ergot alkaloids, Hydergine®, can be found in a Cochrane systematic review (Olin *et al.*, 2002). Although once one of the most frequently prescribed medications in the world, it is now uncommonly prescribed. Numerous clinical trials in various elderly patient groups have not clarified its efficacy or clinical role. Another ergoloid derivative available in Europe, nicergoline (Sermion, Pharmacia), was associated with significant improvement on some areas such as orientation and attention and has been undergoing clinical testing (Fioravanti and Flicker, 2002; Winblad *et al.*, 2001).

Nootropics

Piracetam, oxiracetam, pramiracetam, aniracetam, CI 933, and BMY 21502 are pyrrolidone derivatives of γ-aminobutyric acid (GABA), although they do not appear to have GABA-like effects, and are postulated to have a neuroprotective effect on the CNS against hypoxia, electroconvulsive treatment and drug intoxication. These types of drugs may also enhance the CNS microcirculation by reducing platelet activity and by reducing adherence of red blood cells to vessel walls and may stimulate central cholinergic activity. These diverse effects are termed nootropic to indicate the class of drugs that are structurally related to piracetam and may improve learning and memory (Nicholson, 1990). However, a specific mechanism of action relevant for dementia has not been established. Double-blind, multicenter, controlled studies have shown mixed results with piracetam in the treatment of dementia in the elderly (Flicker and Evans, 2002; Vernon and Sorkin, 1991). Pramiracetam and oxiracetam have been evaluated in large scale multicenter studies with no sufficiently significant clinical effects in dementia. Piracetam is undergoing a clinical trial for mild cognitive impairment.

Estrogens

Estrogens may have cholinergic neurotrophic and neuroprotective effects and may enhance cognitive function (Simpkins *et al.*, 1994).

A beneficial role for estrogen in AD, cognitive function, mood and aging is suggested by observations of an inverse relationship of ERT (Estrogen Replacement Therapy) dose and duration with dementia diagnoses on death certificates (Paganini-Hill and Henderson, 1994); by preliminary trials suggesting a cognitive enhancing effect of estradiol, estrone, and conjugated estrogens in AD (Asthana *et al.*, 2001; Fillit *et al.*, 1986; Honjo *et al.*, 1989; Ohkura *et al.*, 1994).

Unfortunately, clinical trials of conjugated equine estrogens (Premarin®) to improve cognition in both hysterectomized and nonhysterectomized women with AD have not led to success, and indeed women treated with Premarin fared somewhat worse both in cognition and safety including 5% developing deep vein thrombosis (Henderson *et al.*, 2000; Mulnard *et al.*, 2000). Thus currently estrogen replacement cannot be recommended as a treatment for women with Alzheimer's dementia.

Etiologically-directed Approaches in AD

Immune and Inflammatory Processes

Inflammatory processess may be seen in various neurodegenerative disorders. Emerging evidence indicates overactivity of aspects of immune function in AD (Aisen and Davis, 1994). Immune/inflammatory reactions may be established by reactive microglia surrounding senile plaques and astrocyte proliferation; and inflammatory cytokines are produced such as tumor necrosis factor alpha, interleukin-1 (IL-1), α-2-macroglobulin and α-1-antichymotrypsin. IL-1 and IL-6 promote the synthesis of β-amyloid precursor protein.

Anti-inflammatory medications

Epidemiological evidence supports the use of nonsteroidal anti-inflammatories as preventative of AD. However, clinical trials data is less encouraging. Thus, overall efficacy of anti-inflammatories agents in AD has yet to be demonstrated.

Antioxidants

There are both theoretical reasons, and empirical findings, to suggest that free radical damage may be one of the mechanisms causing neuronal degeneration in a range of conditions including aging and Alzheimer's disease. Many studies have found evidence of increased level of oxidative damage to neurons in Alzheimer's disease, but neither Vitamin E nor ginkgo biloba can be recommended based on research results to date.

Calcium Channel Blockers

The process of neuronal death in aging and in AD may be mediated by an increase in intracellular free calcium, which activates various destructive enzymes (such as proteases, endonucleases and phospholipases) and disrupts intracellular processes. In principle, blocking the increase in intracellular free calcium may retard these mechanisms of neuronal death and thus slow progression of disease.

Based on this hypothesis, two calcium channel blockers that have been tested in AD patients are nimodipine and a Bristol-Myers Squibb investigational compound. In one trial, the low-dose nimodipine group (30 mg t.i.d.) showed less deterioration on several memory tests over a 10- to 12-week treatment period than the placebo or high-dose nimodipine (60 mg t.i.d.) group (Tollefson, 1990). A larger study showed significant cognitive effects for nimodipine compared with Hydergine® and placebo (Kanowski *et al.*, 1988). It is not clear, however, whether study subjects fulfilled criteria for possible AD. Nimodipine is marketed to reduce the severity of neurological deficits resulting from vasospasm in patients who have had a recent subarachnoid hemorrhage. It is also used off-label as a cognitive enhancer. A continuing interest in calcium blockers is also spurred by results from a French hypertension trial that found that patients taking calcium blockers were less likely to develop dementia.

Combined Therapies

The combination of drugs with different mechanisms of action may be more effective than individual medications alone. The most relevant clinical questions are whether the available ChIs can or should be combined with other drugs. As a past example, choline precursors were combined with ChIs, but with no evident augmenting effect. Most practicing clinicians would take a dim view of combining two ChIs since their actions are additive. Physicians should be skeptical also of combining available anti-inflammatories or hormones with ChIs: first because of the lack of demonstrated efficacy of these drugs, and second because of the additive adverse events, especially gastrointestinal events. Some clinicians are combining memantine with of the ChIs. Clinical experience appears positive but there is no data from controlled trials.

Summary

The prospects for both treatments with greater efficacy for AD, and for cognitive enhancement in elderly patients are encouraging. ChIs are the best proven efficacious symptomatic treatments for AD. They provide consistent effects in many patients with mild to moderate dementia, and have become the current pharmacological standard of treatment. Other therapeutic approaches are not as well tested or as clearly efficacious. Therefore, ChIs are likely to be actively used clinically for at least the next several years.

However, therapeutic results are usually modest, affecting a minority of patients. Patients assessed were usually outpatients with mild to moderately severe dementia and few concomitant medical illnesses. Duration of effect beyond 1 year and long-term safety are not known, except for the uncontrolled observations of patients who continue on these drugs after the controlled trial. It is essential to understand the broad magnitudes of effects and the range of clinical utility. It often takes time, experience and further studies for clinicians to appreciate the overall effectiveness and utility of new drugs. Long-term trials of the cholinesterase inhibitors in patients with mild cognitive impairment will help define the extent and limits of their efficacy, as will trials in vascular dementia. Memantine demonstrates efficacy with very mild adverse events, at least in more severely impaired patients.

Many of the putative cognitive enhancers described in this chapter would not likely be specific for AD and might be expected to be effective in other dementias. The area of cognitive enhancers for people without clinical illness remains to be explored.

References

Adem A, Mohammed AK and Winblad B (1990) Multiple effects of tetrahydroaminoacridine on the cholinergic system: Biochemical and behavioural aspects. *J Neural Transm—Park Dis Dement* Sect 2, 113–128.

Aisen PS and Davis KL (1994) Inflammatory mechanisms in Alzheimer's disease: Implications for therapy. *Am J Psychiatr* 151, 1105–1113.

Asthana S, Baker LD, Craft S et al. (2001) High-dose estradiol improves cognition for women with AD: Results of a randomized study. *Neurology* 57, 605–612.

Blessed G, Tamlinson BE, Roth M (1968) The association between quantitative measures of dementia and of senile change in the cerebral grey matter of elderly subjects. *Br J Psychiatr* 114, 797–811.

Buxbaum JD, Oishi M, Chen HI et al. (1992) Cholinergic agonists and interleukin 1 regulate processing and secretion of the Alzheimer beta/A4 amyloid protein precursor. *Proc Natl Acad Sci USA* 89, 10075–10078.

Fillit H, Weinreb H, Cholst I et al. (1986) Observations in a preliminary open trial of estradiol therapy for senile dementia-Alzheimer's type. *Psychoneuroendocrinology* 11, 337–345.

Fioravanti M and Flicker L (2002) Efficacy of Nicergoline in dementia and other age associated forms of cognitive impairment. *Coch Database Syst Rev* 2.

Flicker L and Evans JG (2002) Piracetam for dementia or cognitive impairment. *Coch Database Syst Rev* 2.

Francis PT, Palmer AM, Sims NR et al. (1985) Neurochemical studies of early-onset Alzheimer's disease. Possible influence on treatment. *New Engl J Med* 313, 7–11.

Francis PT, Palmer AM, Snape M et al. (1999) The cholinergic hypothesis of Alzheimer's disease: A review of progress. *J Neurol Neurosurg Psychiatr* 66, 137–147.

Giacobini E (1996) Cholinesterase inhibitors do more than inhibit cholinesterase, in *Alzheimer's Disease: From Molecular Biology to Therapy* (ed Becker R). Birkhauser, Boston, pp. 187–204.

Haroutunian V, Greig N, Pei XF, Utsuki T, Gluck R, Avecedo LD, Davis KL and Wallace WC (1997) Pharmacological modulation of Alzheimer's β-amyloid precursor protein levels in the CSF of rats with forebrain cholinergic system lesions. *Brain Res Mol Brain Res* 46(1–2), 161–168.

Harvey AL (1995) The pharmacology of galanthamine and its analogues. *Pharmacol Therap* 68, 113–632.

Henderson VW, Paganini-Hill A, Miller BL et al. (2000) Estrogen for Alzheimer's disease in women: Randomized, double-blind, placebo-controlled trial. *Neurology* 54, 295–301.

Honjo H, Ogino Y, Naitoh K et al. (1989) *In vivo* effects by estrone sulfate on the central nervous system-senile dementia (Alzheimer's type). *J Steroid Biochem* 34, 521–525.

Inestrosa NC, Alvarez A, Perez CA, et al. (1196) Acetylcholinesterase accelerates assembly of amyloid-beta-peptides into Alzheimer's fibrils: Possible role of the peripheral site of the enzyme. Neuron 16, 881–891.

Kanowski S, Fischof P and Hiersemenzel R (1988) Wirksamkeitsnachweis von Neotropika am Beispiel von Nimodipin-ein Beitrag zur entwicklung geeigneter klinischer Prufmodelle. *Z Gerontopsychol Psychiatr* 1, 35–44.

Kaufer DI, Cummings JL and Christine D (1996) Effect of tacrine on behavioral symptoms in Alzheimer's disease: An open-label study. *J Geriatr Psychiatr Neurol* 9, 1–6.

Lahiri DK, Farlow MR, Hintz N et al. (2000) Cholinesterase inhibitors, beta-amyloid precursor protein and amyloid beta-peptides in Alzheimer's disease. *Acta Neurol Scand*. 176(Suppl), 60–67.

Leber P (2002) Criteria used by drug regulatory authorities, in *Evidence-Based Dementia Practice* (eds Qizilbash N, Schneider L, Chui H et al.). Blackwell Science, Oxford, pp. 376–387.

McKhann G, Drachman D, Folstein M et al. (1984) Clinical diagnosis of Alzheimer's disease: Report of the NINCDS-ADRDA Work Group under the auspices of Department of Health and Human Services Task Force on Alzheimer's Disease. *Neurology* 34, 939–944.

Muller D, Mendla K, Farber SA et al. (1997) Muscarinic M1 receptor agonists increase the secretion of the amyloid precursor protein ectodomain. *Life Sci* 60, 985–991.

Mulnard RA, Cotman CW, Kawas C et al. (2000) Estrogen replacement therapy for treatment of mild to moderate Alzheimer disease: A randomized controlled trial. Alzheimer's Disease Cooperative Study. *J Am Med Assoc* 283, 1007–1015.

Nicholson CD (1990) Pharmacology of nootropics and metabolically active compounds in relation to their use in dementia. Psychopharmacology 101, 147–159.

Nitsch RM, Slack BE, Wurtman RJ et al. (1992) Release of Alzheimer amyloid precursor derivatives stimulated by activation of muscarinic acetylcholine receptors. *Science* 258, 304–307.

Ohkura T, Isse K, Akazawa K, et al. (1994) Evaluation of estrogen treatment in female patients with dementia of the Alzheimer type Endocr J 41, 361–371.

Olin J and Schneider L (2002) Galantamine for Alzheimer's disease. *Coch Database Syst Rev* 2.

Paganini-Hill A and Henderson VW (1994) Estrogen deficiency and risk of Alzheimer's disease in women. Am J Epidemiol 140, 256–261.

Parkinson Study Group (1993) Effects to tocopherol and deprenyl on the progression of disability in early Parkinson's disease. *New Engl J Med* 328(3), 176–183.

Radebaugh TS, Buckholtz NS and Khachaturian ZS (1996) Fisher symposium: Strategies for the prevention of Alzheimer disease – overview of research planning meeting III. *Alz Dis Assoc Disord* 10, 1–5.

Raskind MA, Sadowsky CH, Sigmund WR et al. (1997) Effect of tacrine on language, praxis, and noncognitive behavioral problems in Alzheimer disease. *Arch Neurol* 54, 836–840.

Sano M, Ernesto C, Thomas RG et al. (1997) A controlled trial of selegiline, alpha-tocopherol, or both as treatment for Alzheimer's disease. The Alzheimer's Disease Cooperative Study. *New Engl J Med* 336, 1216–1222.

Schneider L and Tariot PN (1997) Cognitive enhancers for Alzheimer's Disease, in *Psychiatry* (eds Tasman A, Kay J, Lieberman JA), Vol. 2. WB Saunders, Philadelphia, pp. 1685–1701.

Simpkins JW, Singh M, and Bishop J (1994) The potential role for estrogen replacement therapy in the treatment of the cognitive decline and neurodegeneration associated with Alzheimer's disease. *Neurobiol Aging* 15(Suppl 2), S195–S197.

Thal LJ, Carta A, Doody R, et al. (1997) Prevention protocols for Alzheimer disease. position paper form the International Working Group on Harmonization of Dementia Drug Guidelines. Alz Dis Assoc Disord 11, 46–49.

Tariot P, Schneider L, Patel S et al. (1993) Alzheimer's disease and (−) deprenyl: Rationales and findings, in *Inhibitors of Monoamine Oxidase B: Pharmacology and Clinical Use in Neurodegen-*

erative Disorders (ed Szelenyi I). Birkhauser Verlag, Basel, pp. 301–317.

Tollefson GD (1990) Short-term effects of the calcium channel blocker nimodipine (Bay-e-9736) in the management of primary degenerative dementia (see comments). *Biol Psychiatr* 27, 1133–1142.

Vernon MW and Sorkin EM (1991) Piracetam. An overview of its pharmacological properties and a review of its therapeutic use in senile cognitive disorders. *Drugs Aging* 1, 17–35.

Winblad B, Bonura ML, Rossini BM *et al.* (2001) Nicergoline in the treatment of mild-to-moderate Alzheimer's disease: A European multicentre trial. *Clin Drug Invest* 21, 621–632.

Pharmacotherapies for Substance Abuse

This chapter describes the pharmacologic tools that physicians need to manage syndromes related to intoxication and overdose; syndromes related to withdrawal; relapse prevention once detoxication is complete; and the pharmacotherapy of comorbid psychopathology in substance abusers.

Syndromes Related to Intoxication

An accurate diagnosis is of fundamental importance in the assessment of a patients who may be intoxicated. A full history must be obtained in the awareness that progression to potentially fatal overdose or withdrawal syndromes may occur. The focuse of physical examination should be the acute effects of intoxication (such as vital and neurologic signs) and chronic signs and symptoms associated with drug dependence (size of liver, evidence of venipuncture). Drug use within the previous 4–12 hours can be determined by analysis of blood and breath samples wheareas urinalysis is useful for assessing substance use within the preceding 24–72 hours. With the exception of alcohol testing, urine is generally the body fluid of choice for toxicologic analysis. Urine testing systems for drugs of abuse providing immediate results (e.g. dipsticks) are increasingly available and are handy for rapid office or clinic-based assessment. Saliva testing is also increasingly available.

Alcohol Intoxication

The rate at which blood alcohol levels decline averages 15 mg/dL/hour. Overall, nonpharmacological management is preferred because it avoids the risk of interactions between drugs and alcohol. Lorazepam 1–2 mg orally may be effective in belligerent patients who cannot be managed by supportive limit setting. If, despite these measures, the patient's condition worsens over the next 1–2 hours, an intramuscular injection of haloperidol 5 mg can be safely given.

In patients with significant mental status changes or alterations in sensorium, clinicians should be alert to the possibility of other causes such head trauma or metabolic disturbance (e.g. thiamine deficiency). Further, intoxicated patients with a recent history of regular heavy use and likely physiologic dependence on alcohol, may be at risk for serious alcohol withdrawal (seizures or delirium) as the blood level clears, particularly if there is a past history of such complications. In that case, clinicians should consider starting tapering doses of a long-acting benzodiazepine (e.g. chlordiazepoxide) as acute intoxication begins to clear (see section on alcohol withdrawal below).

Sedative-hypnotic Intoxication

Suspected benzodiazepine overdosage can be reversed with the benzodiazepine antagonist flumazenil, which should be administered intravenously, beginning with 0.2 mg slow push over 30 seconds, followed by increments of 0.3 mg or 0.5 mg if no response, with total dose not to exceed 3 mg to 5 mg. If no response is obtained at those total doses, then another cause stupor or coma should be considered.

As with alcohol, clinicians should be alert to other causes of mental status changes, and for patients with recent regular use and phsysiologic dependence on sedative-hypnotics, particularly short-acting agents (e.g. alprazolam, lorazepam), serious withdrawal can ensure, and prophylactic treatment with taper of a long-acting agent considered (see section on sedative-hypnotic withdrawal below).

Opiate Intoxication

Severe opiate intoxication is a life-threatening condition because of the high likelihood of respiratory depression or arrest. Opiate overdose is a common cause of death, especially among teenagers and young adults, and is particularly likely among individuals with low levels of tolerance, including inexperienced users, or patients who have recently detoxified or been abstinent for a period of time. Death from opiate overdose is an underappreciated risk, and just as one would assess risk of suicide in depressed patients, clinicians evaluating a patient presenting with opiate intoxication should evaluate the risk of overdose, including level of tolerance and past history of overdose episodes.

The presence of miosis and respiratory depression at presentation is an indication for immediate treatment. An intravenous dose of the pure opiate antagonist naloxone HCl 0.4–0.8 mg usually reverses opiate-induced respiratory and CNS depression in 2 minutes. The dose may be repeated every 2–3 min if the previous dose was not effective.

Cocaine and other stimulant use may be associated with serious physical consequences so the cardiac and neurologic status of patients with this type of intoxication must always be evaluated. A management plan for medical emergencies including arrhythmias, hypertension and seizures should be prepared.

The adverse behavioral and psychologic effects of stimulant intoxication should be treated in a quiet environment and in a straightforward and reassuring way. If drug treatment is indicated, lorazepam 2 mg is usually effective. Benzodiazepines are also preferable for treating psychosis because antipsychotic drugs may worsen cardiovascular complications such as tachycardia or neurologic effects such as seizures and hyperthermia. However, a

Essentials of Psychiatry   Jerald Kay and Allan Tasman
© 2006 John Wiley & Sons, Ltd.

high-potency antipsychotic such as haloperidol 5 mg may be used with caution if treatment with a benzodiazepine does not control behavioral escalation. The clearance of amphetamine may be increased by urinary acidification but this is not recommended in cases of cocaine intoxication.

Intoxication by Hallucinogens such as LSD, Mescaline, MDMA ("Ecstasy") and Psilocybin

The usual treatment option is the oral administration of 20 mg of diazepam; this should attenuate the LSD experience and alleviate any associated panic to a halt within 20 minutes and is considered a superior treatment option than the once-common "talking down" method.

Phencyclidine Intoxication

Phencyclidine undergoes entherohepatic recirculation and this is associated with inter-individual variability in the time over which symptoms resolve. As a result, symptoms may re-emerge after a period of apparent quiescence and patients with phencyclidine intoxication should therefore be observed for 12 hours before being discharged.

There is no specific antagonist for the effects of phencyclidine and the aim of drug treatment for phencyclidine intoxication is to produce sedation or relieve psychosis. A benzodiazepine like lorazepam (orally or by intramuscular injection) may be administered for general sedation; if this does not control psychotic agitation, haloperidol is a reasonable choice of antipyschotic agent. Antipsychotics with anticholinergic properties may exacerbate the anticholinergic effects of phencyclidine and others may additively enhance phencyclidine-induced muscle rigidity and dystonias. Although urinary acidification has been suggested as a means to promote the clearance of phencyclidine, there is a risk that it may exacerbate incipient metabolic acidosis and increase the risk of renal failure secondary to rhabdomyolysis.

Drug Treatment of Withdrawal Syndromes

Some general principles apply to drug treatments for specific withdrawal syndromes:

When monitoring treatment:

- Set clear targets.
- Make serial assessments and modify based on these assessments.

Psychosocial factors:

- Prepare the patient.
- Emphasis on detoxification as a beginning to treatment.

From a pharmacologic standpoint, an ideal agent for the treatment of withdrawal should have the following characteristics:

- Efficacy in relieving the complete range of abstinence signs and symptoms for a given type of withdrawal.
- A relatively long duration of action and gradual offset of effects.
- A high degree of safety in the dosage needed to suppress withdrawal (i.e., high therapeutic index).
- It should be available by a variety of routes of administration and have little abuse potential in itself.

Other general but important aspects of detoxification are also frequently overlooked:

- Clear treatment targets should be kept in mind.
- Structured rating scales should be used to measure symptom severity: serial assessment of the clinical response is the best strategy for guiding treatment and detoxification should not be conducted "on autopilot".
- While protocols may offer useful guidance, orders should be rewritten with thought and often daily.

Patients must understand that detoxification is not a treatment for addiction but the beginning of treatment for the chronic problems associated with substance dependence. They should know what they will experience and they should if at all possible be engaged in the effort to relieve their symptoms as safely as possible and with greatest effectiveness. They need to understand, however, that they are likely to experience some distress. Detoxification can be carried out on an outpatient basis for patients who are in relatively good health and have sufficiently stable social support.

Alcohol Withdrawal

Alcohol withdrawal is a medical emergency and can be life-threatening without appropriate supportive medical treatment.

The risk of progressing from uncomplicated withdrawal to seizures or delirium should be greatly reduced by proper management. Patients should be assessed systematically when entering the detoxification protocol and during the process. A widely used but simple tool is the Clinical Institute Withdrawal Assessment – Alcohol Scale (Table 84.1). Starting 6–24 hours after the last drink, this scale should be used to assess the patient initially every 1–2 hours and at regular intervals until two consecutive scores below 8–10 are achieved. It is then safe to end structured assessment. Scores greater than 15 are an indication for monitoring the patient even more closely. Scores in between these limits should be interpreted according to clinical judgment according to the degree of discomfort reported by the patient and their history of withdrawal syndromes.

Undertreatment with doses that are too low or dose intervals that are too long is the commonest error in the drug treatment of withdrawal syndromes. However, striking the balance between withdrawal and intoxication is not complicated provided serial assessments are made.

Benzodiazepines are the drugs of choice for treating alcohol withdrawal because:

- There is cross-tolerance with alcohol (therefore higher than normal doses may be needed).
- They are relatively safe compared with other sedative-hypnotics.
- They have been shown to reduce the frequency of seizures and delirium.

The benzodiazepines can be divided into two major classes according their duration of action. Longer-acting agents, including chlordiazepoxide and diazepam, undergo metabolic oxidation and glucuronidation. Their advantage is that blood levels decline more slowly during the tapering process, increasing patient comfort and reducing the risk of seizures. The disadvantage is that, in older patients and patients with impaired hepatic or pulmonary function, decreased elimination may result in accumulation and toxicity. Chlordiazepoxide may be preferred to diazepam because it may have a lower abuse potential.

Table 84.1   Clinical Institute Withdrawal Assessment – Alcohol Scale

Patient:_____
Time:_____:_____
(24 hour clock, midnight = 00: 00)
Date:_____ /_____ /_____
    y mo d

NAUSEA AND VOMITING: Ask, "Do you feel sick to your stomach? Have you vomited?" Observation.

0—no nausea and no vomiting
1—mild nausea with no vomiting
2
3
4—intermittent nausea with dry heaves
5
6
7—constant nausea, frequent dry heaves and vomiting

TREMOR: Arms extended and fingers spread apart. Observation.

0—no tremor
1—not visible, but can be felt fingertip to fingertip
2
3
4—moderate, with patient's arms extended
5
6
7—severe, even with arms not extended

PAROXYSMAL SWEATS: Observation.

0—no sweat visible
1—barely perceptible sweating, palms moist
2
3
4—beads of sweat obvious on forehead
5
6
7—drenching sweats
Pulse or heart rate, taken for
1 minute:_____
Blood pressure:_____ /_____

TACTILE DISTURBANCES: Ask, "Have you any itching, pins-and-needles sensations, any burning, any numbness, or do you feel bugs crawling on or under your skin?" Observation.

0—none
1—very mild itching, pins and needles, burning, or numbness
2—mild itching, pins and needles, burning, or numbness
3—moderate itching, pins and needles, burning, or numbness
4—moderately severe hallucinations
5—severe hallucinations
6—extremely severe hallucinations
7—continuous hallucinations

AUDITORY DISTURBANCES: Ask, "Are you more aware of sounds around you? Are they harsh? Do they frighten you? Are you hearing anything that is disturbing to you? Are you hearing things that you know aren't there?" Observation.

0—not present
1—very mild harshness or ability to frighten
2—mild harshness or ability to frighten
3—moderate harshness or ability to frighten
4—moderately severe hallucinations
5—severe hallucinations
6—extremely severe hallucinations
7—continuous hallucinations

Table 84.1	Clinical Institute Withdrawal Assessment – Alcohol Scale *continued*

VISUAL DISTURBANCES: Ask, "Does the light appear to be too bright? Is its color different? Does it hurt your eyes? Are you seeing anything that is disturbing you? Are you seeing things that you know aren't there?" Observation.

0—not present
1—very mild sensitivity
2—mild sensitivity
3—moderate sensitivity
4—moderately severe hallucinations
5—severe hallucinations
6—extremely severe hallucinations
7—continuous hallucinations

ANXIETY: Ask, "Do you feel nervous?" Observation.

0—no anxiety, at ease
1—mildly anxious
2
3
4—moderately anxious, or guarded, so anxiety is inferred
5
6
7—equivalent to acute panic states as seen in severe delirium or acute schizophrenic reactions

AGITATION: Observation.

0—normal activity
1—somewhat more than normal activity
2
3
4—moderately fidgety and restless
5
6
7—paces back and forth during most of the interview, or constantly thrashes about

HEADACHE, FULLNESS IN HEAD: Ask, "Does your head feel different? Does it feel like there is a band around your head?" Do not rate dizziness or lightheadedness. Otherwise, rate severity.

0—not present
1—very mild
2—mild
3—moderate
4—moderately severe
5—severe
6—very severe
7—extremely severe

ORIENTATION AND CLOUDING OF SENSORIUM: Ask, "What day is this? Where are you? Who am I?"

0—oriented and can do serial additions
1—cannot do serial additions or is certain about date
2—disoriented for date by no more than 2 calendar days
3—disoriented for date by more than 2 calendar days
4—disoriented for place and/or person

Total CIWA-A score _____
Rater's initials _____
Maximum possible score—67

*This scale is not copyrighted and may be used freely.
See Sullivan JT, Sykora K, Schneiderman J, Narango CA, and Sellers EM (1989) Assessment of alcohol withdrawal: the revised Clinical Institute Withdrawal Instrument for Alcohol Scale (CIWA-AR). *Br J Addiction* 84, 1353–1357.

Shorter-acting agents, such as oxazepam and lorazepam, are metabolized only by glucuronidation. Both drugs are available in oral and intravenous forms though only lorazepam may also be administered by intramuscular injection. These agents are more readily metabolized and eliminated by older patients and they are less likely to accumulate and cause toxicity in patients with liver disease. However, blood levels decline more rapidly and this may cause breakthrough symptoms and seizures between doses.

The treatment response should be assessed serially. Medication should adjusted according to clinical need: if signs of

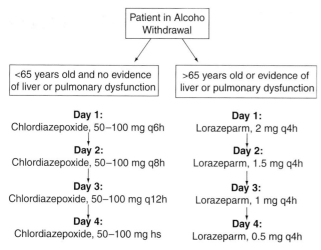

Figure 84.1 *Medication recommendations for treating alcohol withdrawal. Reprinted from Psychiatric Drugs, p. 224. Lieberman JA and Tasman MD (2000). Copyright 2000, Elsevier.*

withdrawal are apparent, the dose should be increased or the dose interval reduced. Some degree of sedation is desirable but medication should be withheld if the patient becomes over-sedated and recommenced when clinically indicated. Recommendations for medication are summarized in Figure 84.1.

Hallucinations that develop as a feature of delirium are relatively refractory to treatment with a benzodiazepine alone. Patients who develop hallucinations despite sedative-hypnotic substitution may be treated with adjunctive haloperidol, 2 to 5 mg.

In the event of persistent tachycardia or hypertension, the possibility of inadequately treated withdrawal should first be excluded. This problem has been managed successfully with beta-blockers and clonidine but while these agents may decrease vital signs and tremor they do not prevent seizures.

An alternative strategy is to "frontload" the patient, achieving sedation by administering diazepam or chlordiazepoxide every 1 to 2 hours. Because these agents have a long elimination half-life, their effects diminish slowly and smoothly over the withdrawal period. However, careful serial assessment remains essential while the patient is vulnerable to the complications of withdrawal.

Thiamine is indicated for every patient with alcoholism to prevent Wernicke's encephalopathy and Korsakoff's amnestic syndrome. It should be administered immediately (typical dose 100 mg daily), before intravenous glucose. Less urgently, nutritional support should include supplementation with folate 1 mg and multivitamins. It has been suggested that magnesium supplementation may prevent withdrawal seizures but there is no consensus on its use in the absence of documented magnesium deficiency.

There are promising reports on the use of carbamazepine and valproate in alcohol withdrawal and they may be helpful in special circumstances. However, the safety and efficacy of benzodiazepines are currently unsurpassed.

Sedative-hypnotic Withdrawal

Similar to the treatment for alcohol withdrawal, benzodiazepine taper (as described above) is a good choice, particularly if the

patients is dependent on benzodiazepines. Another excellent choice for substitution therapy is phenobarbital: it has low potential for abuse, there is a wide margin between therapeutic and lethal blood levels, and it has a long duration of action with relatively little variation in between-dose blood levels. The symptoms of intoxication with phenobarbital (ataxia, slurred speech, nystagmus) are readily observed easy and managed within a detoxication protocol.

For patients dependent on sedative-hypnotics, the first step in management if to take a history. Information about the level of drug consumption can be converted to "phenobarbital equivalents" to provide a guide to the required dose of phenobarbital, as specified in Table 84.2.

The number of phenobarbital equivalents is summed and administered as a thrice-daily dose regimen. The total daily requirement of phenobarbital rarely exceeds 500 mg even in patients with extreme dependency. The first dose of phenobarbital may be administered as an intramuscular injection if signs of withdrawal occur before substitution therapy begins. Symptoms of withdrawal and intoxication should be reassessed after 1 to 2 hours to determine the next dose of phenobarbital.

Table 84.2 Phenobarbital Withdrawal Equivalents of Sedative-Hypnotics

Class/Generic Name	Dose (mg)*
BENZODIAZEPINES	
Alprazolam	1
Chlordiazepoxide	25
Clonazepam	2
Clorazepate	7.5
Diazepam	10
Estazolam	1
Flurazepam	15
Halazepam	40
Lorazepam	2
Oxazepam	10
Prazepam	10
Quazepam	15
Temazepam	15
Triazolam	0.25
BARBITURATES	
Amobarbital	100
Butabarbital	100
Butalbital	100
Pentobarbital	100
Secobarbital	100
OTHER	
Chloral hydrate	500
Ethchlorvynol	500
Glutethimide	250
Meprobamate	1200
Methyprylon	200
Zolpidem	5

*Dose equivalent to 30 mg of phenobarbital for withdrawal
Adapted from Wesson DR, Smith DE, Ling W and Seymour RB: Chapter 17: Sedative-Hypnotics, in *Substance Abuse: A Comprehensive Textbook*, 4th ed. (eds Lowinson JH, Ruiz P, Millman RB, Langrod JG). Philadelphia: Lippincott Williams and Wilkins; 2005.

The degree of dependence can also be assessed by serial challenge with pentobarbital at doses of 200 mg but it is not clear that this method offers any advantage over direct substitution with phenobarbital, which is safe, rapid and simple.

There should be no signs of sedative-hypnotic withdrawal or phenobarbital toxicity after 24 to 48 hours; dose reduction of phenobarbital can then be started. Maintaining the thrice-daily dose regimen, the dose of phenobarbital should be reduced in increments of 30 mg/day. If there is evidence of phenobarbital toxicity (slurred speech, nystagmus, ataxia), the next dose should be withheld and the total daily dose reduced. Conversely, if there are objective signs of withdrawal, the total daily dose of phenobarbital should be increased and dose reduction delayed until the patient is once again stable.

Opiate Withdrawal

Withdrawal from opiates may be intensely uncomfortable but, by contrast with sedative-hypnotic withdrawal, it is not usually life-threatening for adults; important exceptions include adults with little reserve – for example, due to to advanced AIDS – and newborn infants. Nevertheless, reducing withdrawal symptoms may help to engage an addict in a treatment program or facilitate the management of another medical condition.

Methadone is approved by the FDA for treating opiate withdrawal but states may have different regulations governing its use and clinicians need to be aware of local requirements. Methadone use is typically permitted for inpatient detoxification or maintenance treatment but it cannot be prescribed to treat opiate withdrawal in outpatients except as part of a licensed methadone maintenance treatment program.

Methadone is administered orally and has a long duration of action. An initial dose of 15 to 20 mg may be given when signs of opiate withdrawal are seen (not merely when craving is reported). An additional 5 to 10 mg may be given in 1 to 2 hours if symptoms persist or worsen. A dose of 40 mg/day usually controls signs of withdrawal well (note that this is often insufficient for the different indication of long-term maintenance). If oral administration is impossible due to withdrawal symptoms, doses of 5 mg may be administered by intramuscular injection. Having reached a dose at which withdrawal symptoms are alleviated, the dose can be tapered by 5 to 10% per day until full detoxification is achieved.

A newly available option for treatment of opioid withdrawal is the Schedule III opioid partial agonist buprenorphine, which is now available for use in the office based practice by any physician who has taken a brief training and certification. While the use of Schedule II drugs such as methadone for the treatment for opiate dependence is restricted to hospitals or specially licensed clinics (leading to a shortage of facilities where opiate-dependent individuals could receive appropriate treatment), the Drug Addiction Treatment Act of 2000 introduced less stringent regulations, allowing the use of narcotic drugs for the treatment of addiction in the office or any other health care setting by any licensed physician who has taken a brief training course and obtained registration, thereby increasing access to treatment. Two new formulations of the buprenorphine (Subutex and Suboxone sublingual tablets) were the first products to be approved by the FDA under this Act for the treatment of opioid dependence. Subutex contains only buprenorphine in doses of 2 or 8 mg; Suboxone also contains the opioid antagonist naloxone (0.5 and 2 mg respectively); the purpose of the naloxone is to discourage diversion of the medication for abuse intravenously (crushing the pills and injecting them), since naloxone is poorly absorbed after oral or sublingual administration, but if injected would produce precipitated withdrawal.

Buprenorphine is an excellent detoxification agent because of its long duration of action, due to very high affinity for and very slow dissociation from opioid receptors. Starting buprenorphine must be done carefully, because of the partial agonism. If administered too close in time to the last dose of a full agonist such as heroin, buprenorphine will precipitate withdrawal, and the withdrawal produced can be atypical and in rare cases has been observed to include delirium. Precipitated withdrawal is more likely among patients dependent on long-acting agonists (e.g. methadone), or high daily doses of a shorter-acting agonist such as heroin. Thus, when starting buprenorphine, the clinician should wait for symptoms of opioid withdrawal to begin to appear before giving the first dose of buprenorphine, which should be a test dose of 2 mg (Subutex 2 mg, or Suboxone (2 mg buprenorphine/0.5 mg naloxone). If this dose is well tolerated, administer another 2 mg one hour later, and up to 8 mg total on the first day, and up to 16 mg on the second day. After this buprenorphine can be tapered slowly to zero over 10 days to 2 weeks. Considerable flexibility in the taper schedule is possible, including a much faster taper, since the slow dissociation from receptors in itself effectively produces a taper. However, clinicians should also be alert for the emergence of low-grade withdrawal symptoms (fatigue, anxiety, mild flu-like physical symptoms) in the weeks after discontinuing buprenorphine. This subacute or protracted withdrawal can be observed after withdrawal from any opioid drug, but can seem surprisingly with buprenorphine because the taper phase of a buprenorphine detoxification is usually comfortable and uneventful.

If one of the first few doses of buprenorphine administered is followed by a rapid worsening of withdrawal symptoms, this is precipitated withdrawal, and no further buprenorphine should be given; at this point it is probably best to treat with a full agonist (methadone), although one could also wait for precipitated withdrawal to clear and full-blown opiate withdrawal (from whatever the patient was addicted to) to emerge, after which one can try again beginning with a test dose of 2 mg buprenorhine.

A number of nonnarcotic medications are useful in treating the symptoms of opiate withdrawal. These include the α-adrenergic receptor agonist and antihypertensive clonidine, which is particularly helpful with the autonomic symptoms of withdrawal as well as the anxiety, benzodiazepines (clonazepam is typically used), which are particularly helpful for the anxiety and insomnia, antiemetics and NSAIDs for muscle aches (oral agents such as ibuprofen, or Toradol which can be given parenterally). Autonomic symptoms may be well controlled with clonidine alone but patients frequently report greater subjective distress than with methadone or buprenorphine. The role of clonidine is for detoxification from illegal opiates, for example in settings where methadone is not allowed, or to alleviate abstinence symptoms when a patient comes to the end of a methadone maintenance program. Its major side effects are hypotension (which may require dose reduction or discontinuation) and sedation. Hypotension may be worsened by diarrhea, or vomiting, which are common in opiate withdrawal. Patients should be encouraged to take plenty of fluids, and sports drinks such as gatorade are particularly helpful because they also supply electrolytes. Clonidine does not address all aspects of withdrawal and it should therefore be used in combination with the alternatives detailed above. A protocol for clonidine-assisted detoxication is given in Table 84.3.

Table 84.3	Clonidine Detoxification	
Day	Short-acting Opiate*	Long-acting Opiate†
Day 1	0.1 mg q4h	0.1 mg q4h
Days 2–4	0.1–0.2 mg q4h (depending on symptoms)	0.1–0.2 mg q4h (depending on symptoms)
Days 5–10	Reduce daily dose by 0.2–0.4 mg/d	Maintain on 0.4–1.2 mg/d
Day 11		Reduce daily dose by 0.2–0.4 mg/d

Adjunctive medication: oxazepam (in limited supplies) for sleep or agitation; ibuprofen or toradol for muscle or bone pain; bismuth subsalicylate for diarrhea; prochlorperazine or odansetron for nausea.
*For example, heroin.
†For example, methadone.

A combination of clonidine with naltrexone has been used to achieve a more rapid withdrawal, followed by maintenance treatment with naltrexone. However, clinical experience and close monitoring of the patient is necessary to titrate the dose of clonidine against withdrawal symptoms induced by naltrexone. The acceptability of maintenance treatment with naltrexone to opiate addicts is disappointing.

With opiate detoxification, it is particularly important to consider the indications for it, and to establish an adequate treatment plan after detoxification is completed. Chronic opioid use induces tolerance, and detoxification reduces or eliminates tolerance. Because of the loss of tolerance, detoxified opiate addicts are at increased risk for death from opiate overdose; doses that they routine self-administered previously when tolerant, could now be lethal, a problem exacerbated by the variable and sometimes high potency of illicit heroin. In general, the risk of relapse following opioid detoxification is high. Therefore, patients should be assessed for overdose risk, and those with a history of past overdoses, or with multiple past relapses, should be encouraged to take agonist maintenance treatment, with methadone or buprenorphine, rather than undergoing detoxification. For those not entering agonist maintenance, a strong plan for psychosocial treatment is important, for example long-term residential treatment or Therapeutic Community, a good outpatient treatment program, supplemented by self-help group (Alcoholics Anonymous, or Narcotics Anonymous).

Management of Withdrawal in Patients with Drug Dependencies

Medications for Alcohol Dependence

Three medications are now FDA approved for treatment of alcohol dependence, disulfiram, naltrexone and acamprosate.

Disulfiram is an irreversible inhibitor of aldehyde dehydrogenase, the enzyme that catalyzes the conversion of alcohol to acetic acid. Inhibiting aldehyde dehydrogenase alters the body's response to alcohol, leading to an accumulation of acetaldehyde. The resulting reaction is extremely dysphoric but self-limiting and not life-threatening. However, it is associated with hypotension, palpitations, nausea and vomiting, and diaphoresis, which can produce substantial stress to the cardiovascular system, particularly with high doses both of alcohol and of disulfiram. This is generally not dangerous in young, healthy individuals, but could lead to cardiovascular collapse and death in patients with significant cardiovascular or renal disease. Disulfiram has also been associated with liver toxicity, and education of the patient about signs of liver failure, and periodic monitoring of liver functions, are advisable.

Disulfiram was approved by the FDA for treatment of alcoholism in an era that required efficacy studies that would not meet today's standards. The best work to date suggests that disulfiram may reduce the number of drinking days in those alcoholics who drink while taking it. Placebo-controlled studies suggest that compliance with medication taking, rather than the disulfiram itself, is the critical factor in producing a better outcome in persons with alcoholism.

For patients who are well-motivated, disulfiram provides an important disincentive to drink alcohol. It is particularly effective as part of a contract with a spouse, in which the spouse agrees not to comment on the patient's drinking and the patient agrees to allow the spouse to witness disulfiram ingestion. If disulfiram is taken regularly, it will prevent drinking, since even a small amount of intake will make the patient sick.

The usual dose of disulfiram is 250 mg/day. This minimizes side effects such as lethargy while maintaining inhibition of aldehyde dehydrogenase. Some patients will report being able to drink without consequence on 250 mg per day. This may simply mean the patient is not actually taking the medication regularly, and should prompt gentle inquiry into compliance. However, some patients do need higher doses, up to 500 mg per day. Disulfiram inhibits dopamine α-hydroxylase and may rarely cause psychosis. It may affect the blood levels of other drugs (for example, levels of antidepressants and phenytoin are increased). Patients should be made aware that products other than alcholic beverages contain alcohol (e.g. shaving lotions) and that the risk of an acetaldehyde reaction persists for up to 2 weeks after the last dose of disulfiram.

The rationale for prescribing naltrexone to prevent alcohol relapse is based on the hypothesis that the reinforcing effects of alcohol may be mediated via endogenous opiate mechanisms. Naltrexone combined with structured psychosocial treatment has been associated with improvements in complete abstinence, less craving for alcohol when the patient was abstinent, and less drinking once drinking began. Psychosocial treatments that have proven particularly effective in combination with naltrexone are those, such as cognitive-behavioral relapse prevention, that emphasize coping skills for handling various sources of relapse risk. The recommended dose is 50 mg per day. This agent differs from disulfiram in that there is no added ill effect once drinking begins. It may limit the severity of binges, and diminish preoccupation with alcohol in abstinent alcoholics. Nausea has been a common side effect early in naltrexone treatment for alcoholism, but is generally mild and clears with continued use. Naltrexone can produce liver toxicity, which is dose dependent, has mainly been observed at much higher doses (200 or 300 mg per day), and resolves with dose reduction. Elevated liver enzymes which do not resolve with dose reduction or discontinuation likely represent another cause of hepatitis (e.g. viral, alcoholic).

Acamprosate has been approved for a number of years in Europe, and recently received FDA approval. Its mechanism is not well understood, but is thought to involve interference with excitatory amino acid mechanisms that may be involved in relapse. Clinical trials have shown a modest effect in reducing relapse risk, and studies are underway to determine if it may have complementary effects to those of naltrexone and whether the combination of the two may be increase effectiveness. Acamprosate is supplied in 333 mg tablets, and the recommended dosage is two tablets, three times daily. Blister packs, organized according to the daily schedule of dosing, can be helpful to patients in maintaining compliance. Acamprosate is a generally safe and well tolerated. Diarrhea is the most common side effect.

In the same way that any given antidepressant medication will be helpful to some depressed patients, but not others, naltrexone and acamprosate may similarly have little effect in some patients, but work well in others. As of yet, there are no reliable predictors of which alcoho-dependent patient will benefit from these medications, but clinicians should be encouraged to attempt adequate trials (effective dose, for at least a month) of these medications for patients with problem drinking, and not be discouraged by the fact that some patients will not benefit.

Medications for Cocaine Dependence

Given the high relapse rates with psychosocial treatment alone, there has been considerable interest in the development of pharmacotherapies for cocaine dependence. Although case reports and small studies have suggested that a variety of agents may be effective, these findings have not been consistently repeated in double-blind studies and no drug has met the criteria for FDA approval. Nevertheless, survey show that many specialists in the management of addiction prescribe drug treatment for cocaine dependence.

The drugs most frequently prescribed for cocaine dependence are antidepressants. This is based on the observation that depression is relatively frequent among cocaine addicts and the hypothesis that antidepressants may correct underlying abnormalities of neurotransmitter function associated with cocaine use. Although desipramine is the most widely studied, initially encouraging reports of its efficacy in relapse prevention have been followed by studies either challenging its efficacy or suggesting its benefits may not continue beyond 6 to 12 weeks. Typical doses are the same as those used to treat depression. Concurrent use of cocaine and an antidepressant increases the risk of cardiotoxicity; patients who relapse during treatment should be investigated for additive cardiac effects.

It has been suggested that dopamine receptor blockade may attenuate the euphoric response to cocaine and that treatment with an antipsychotic drug may therefore be an appropriate treatment for cocaine dependence. However, experience treating patients with schizophrenia and cocaine dependence do not support this hypothesis. Further cocaine use may increase the risk of extrapyramidal side effects due to dopamine depletion.

Psychomotor stimulants have been suggested as an agonist maintenance treatment strategy. Although early clinical reports suggested stimulants might exacerbate cocaine dependence, more recent placebo controlled trials suggest oral dexedrine may have promise. Patients with attention deficit disorder, which commonly co-occurs with cocaine dependence, may benefit from stimulants. Lithium has only been effective in reducing cocaine use in patients with bipolar disorder and, despite promising early trials, controlled trials have shown that carbamazepine has disappointing efficacy. However, more recently, some of the newer anticonvulsants with GABA-enhancing or excitatory amino acid inhibiting effects (e.g topiramate, gabapentin) have shown promise in small placebo controlled trials.

Interestingly, perhaps the most consistent data so far regarding disulfiram, which has shown promise in a series of small placebo-controlled trials for cocaine dependence, and the effect does not seem to depend on concurrent alcohol use. Since disulfram inhibits dopamine β-hydroxylase, which catalyzes the conversion of dopamine to norepinephrine in the brain, it may promote increased levels of brain dopamine, and combat the dopamine depletion engendered by cocaine.

Another pharmacotherapeutic strategy for cocaine dependence is to treat comorbid psychopathology, most commonly unipolar depression, bipolar disorder, attention deficit hyperactivity disorder and anxiety disorders. Such treatment is most likely to have a direct impact on the psychopathology, followed by indirect effects of improved functioning and reduced drug use; the benefits of pharmacotherapy for patients without comorbid psychopathology remain unclear. The development of an effective pharmacotherapy for cocaine dependence is a research priority of the highest order.

Medications for Opiate Dependence

Agonist maintenance treatment for opiate dependence is a powerful treatment with a large effect size. When properly prescribed, methadone will rapidly induce a dramatic remission in 50% or more of patients. It prevents or reduces illicit opiate use, craving for illicit opiates, criminal behavior associated with acquisition of illicit opiates, and diseases associated with illicit opiate use (such as illness related to infection with human immunodeficiency virus), and improves employment and other aspects of social functioning. Methadone has also been shown to reduce mortality rates among opioid dependent patients, in part by protecting against overdose. Methadone is also sometimes misunderstood as "substituting one drug for another". In fact, methadone works by inducing marked tolerance such that effects of other opiates are blocked, and no euphoric effects of the methadone itself are experienced. When prescribed with careful titration, methadone is neither intoxicating nor sedating, and it does not interfere with performance of functions that are important for responsible adult roles (e.g., studies have shown that methadone does not impair driving ability).

Methadone is a good choice for maintenance treatment:

- it is orally active
- its half-life exceeds 24 hours
- it suppresses opiate withdrawal syndrome for up to 36 hours
- it blocks the euphoriant effects of other opiates
- side effects are minimal during chronic use; the commonest are constipation, excess sweating and decreased sexual interest but they rarely cause discontinuation

Doses of methadone in the early phase of a maintenance program are in the 20 to 40 mg range, primarily to relieve abstinence symptoms. The dose is increased in increments of 5 to 10 mg during the "induction period" over a period of days to weeks until a dose is achieved that prevents opiate craving and blocks the euphoric effects of illicit opiates. Urine toxicology analysis should be carried out regularly and frequently to support subjective reports and interval history. A dose of 40 mg/day is adequate for some patients but there is evidence that most require a dose of 80 mg/day. Under Federal regulations, doses greater than 120 mg/day require permission, though lower ceilings can be specified in individual states. As with many psychopharmacologic treatments, the most common reason for treatment failure in methadone maintenance is inadequate dose, and continued opiate use should prompt consideration of a dosage increase. There is evidence that trough methadone blood levels should be in the range 200 to 400 ng/ml for optimal treatment response, and blood level monitoring may be useful in nonresponders. Some patients are rapid metabolizers, which can be assessed by comparing peak and trough blood levels. Rapid metabolizers may benefit from a divided, twice daily dose schedule.

A pragmatic drawback of methadone maintenance is regulations require that it can only be administered at specially licensed clinics which require frequent attendance (daily at the outset), and are not even available in many geographic regions. This can be a practical constraint or a disincentive for many patients. On the other hand, it has been shown that the effectiveness of methadone maintenance depends upon regular counseling in conjunction with the medication, which is a requirement of methadone clinics, and more severely dysfunctional patients probably benefit from the structure imposed by clinic rules. Further, many of the better methadone clinics offer primary medical and psychiatric care, which is important since chronic opiate dependent patients often have multiple medical (e.g. hepatitis B and C, HIV) and psychiatric (e.g. depression, PTSD) problems.

A recent development is the approval and marketing of the long-acting opiate partial agonist buprenorphine (see also section above on opiate detoxification), which has been shown in clinical trials to have effectiveness equivalent to that of methadone for maintenance treatment. A major difference is that buprenorphine can be prescribed by any physician who has taken a brief training course and received certification, making it more widely available than methadone maintenance. The main regulatory restriction is that individual physicians practicing in an office-based setting are restricted to treating no more than 30 patients with maintenance buprenorphine at any one time.

Buprenorphine has interesting pharmacologic properties. It is a partial agonist, meaning that it binds opiate receptors but only partially activates them. This may translate into lower abuse potential compared with full agonists, although buprenorphine has been abused by intravenous injections in other countries where it was widely available. The sublingual formulations marketed for treatment of opioid dependence do appear to have limited abuse potential by themselves, and the Suboxone formulation, which includes naloxone, discourages attempts to extract and inject the contents, since intravenous naloxone will precipitate withdrawal; the naloxone is poorly absorbed by the sublingual or oral routes. Buprenorphine binds almost irreversibly to opiate receptors, and dissociates very slowly, accounting in part for its long duration of action. When properly dosed, similar to methadone, it induces tolerance, blocks the effects of other opiates, and produces little or no sedating or intoxicating effects.

The buprenorphine/naloxone combination (Suboxone) if preferred for both detoxification and maintenance treatment, although some patients may be more sensitive to the presence of the antagonist (naloxone) and tolerate straight buprenorphine (Subutex) better. Because it is a partial agonist, buprenorphine will precipitate withdrawal in individuals who have recently used any opioid drug; treatment should therefore begin when there are clear signs of withdrawal (or at least 4 hours after last use of a short-acting opioid) (see also section above on buprenorphine for detoxification). There is less experience of induction with buprenorphine in individuals using long-acting agents such as methadone, but the risk of precipitated withdrawal is greater. The daily methadone dose should be below 40 mg per day before buprenorphine induction is attempted, and a delay of around 48 hours or more is advisable to allow withdrawal symptoms from methadone to clearly manifest. Induction is completed over 2 to 4 days, depending on the target dose. The recommended dose on day 1 is 16 mg, increasing to 16 mg on day 2 and thereafter and more gradual induction may be associated with a higher risk of drop-out. The dose should be adjusted in increments of 2 to 4 mg to that which keeps the individual in the treatment program and suppresses withdrawal symptoms; the target maintenance dose is 16 mg/day but may range from 4 to 32 mg/day. Buprenorphine should be administered as part of a psychosocial treatment program. The relative ease of withdrawing from buprenorphine may result in a greater tendency to leave the treatment program compared with methadone.

Due to its long duration of action, buprenorphine can be administered every other day (e.g. 32 mg every other day), or even twice per week; this property can be useful for patients where there are concerns about compliance, since the medication can be held at a clinic or by a significant other and administered under observation on a less than daily basis.

Buprenorphine can produce sedation. However, emergence of sedation should also raise suspicion of use of other drugs or alcohol. Unlike full opiate agonists (heroin, methadone, other narcotic analgesics) where respiratory depression is a serious risk, buprenorphine by itself produce less respiratory depression. The rate of deaths from drug overdose dropped substantially in France after buprenorphine was introduced for treatment of drug dependence. The one exception was overdoses of buprenorphine in combination with benzodiazepines where deaths were observed. This has led to an exaggerated concern that buprenorphine is contraindicated in patients who use benzodiazepines. For patients using benzodiazepines at regular, modest doses, which is the most common pattern even among opiate addicts, buprenorphine is safe. Patients who take large doses or binges of benzodiazepines are at risk for overdose in combination with a variety of other drugs, including buprenorphine, and alcohol. It is likely that the risk of overdose in such patients would be the same on either methadone maintenance or buprenorphine maintenance.

Naltrexone is a long-acting (24 to 48 hour duration) opioid antagonist available in 50 mg tablets. It is effective in blocking the effects of opioids and can be used as a maintenance treatment, but its effectiveness has been limited by poor compliance. Compliance can be improved with behavioral therapy, but rates of retention in treatment still remain well below what can be expected from agonist maintenance with methadone or buprenorpine. Further, naltrexone does not protect against opiate overdose; patients who stop naltrexone are not tolerant and are therefore vulnerable to overdose. Naltrexone is also complicated to manage. It cannot be started until a patient has been fully detoxified, in order not to precipitate withdrawal. Rapid induction methods using buprenorphine, clonidine and clonazepam, have been described, but generally require 5 to 7 days to carry out. Anesthesia assisted rapid detoxification and induction onto naltrexone has been shown to involve the same level of discomfort, with increased risk of serious adverse events, and is not recommended. Once a patient is inducted onto naltrexone, if they stop taking the naltrexone and relapse, naltrexone cannot be resumed without precipitating withdrawal, and repeat detoxification is needed. In summary, while some patients benefit from naltrexone, it is considered a second-line agent, for patients who have failed or refuse agonist treatment. Patients maintained on naltrexone should be warned about the risk of fatal drug overdose if naltrexone is discontinued.

Special Considerations

Methadone-maintained patients on medical-surgical units and pregnant patients merit special comment. After admission to general hospital, the dose of methadone should be verified with the patinet's maintenance program. The dose should be maintained during the stress of an illness and its treatment. Maintenance methadone will suppress opiate withdrawal but it will not provide analgesia. Patients taking methadone who have severe pain should therefore be treated with nonopiate analgesics or short-acting opiates as needed, noting that higher doses and shorter dose intervals may be needed. Drugs with mixed antagonist-agonist activity, such as pentazopcine and buprenorphine, may provoke opiate withdrawal and shoud be avoided.

Women who become pregnant should be encouraged to contiue their methadone maintenance programme. The dose may need to be reduced during the third trimester and neonatal symptoms due to abstinence should be planned for. Longitudinal studies show that infants exposed to methadone in utero develop normally and parents should be reassured.

Medications for Nicotine Dependence

By contrast with methadone, nicotine replacement therapy is not intended as an indefinite maintenance therapy. Instead, the aim is to provide a medically safe source of nicotine while gradually reducing the dose. Nevertheless, it is reasonable to speculate whether, in terms of harm reduction, nicotine replacement is superior to cigarette smoking. Two forms of nicotine are available without prescription: nicotine polacrilex (gum) and a transdermal patch. Both are effective in promoting abstinence.

The FDA has recently approved a sustained-release formulation of bupropion for the treatment of nicotine dependence; efficacy is similar to that of nicotine replacement therapy. The recommended dose is 150 mg twice daily; treatment should begin 2 weeks before the date on which smoking will cease. Combining nicotine replacement and bupropion offers greater efficacy and safety than either agent alone for patients who have not succeeded with monotherapy.

Many patients who succeed in initiating abstinence from cigarettes will relapse within 3 to 6 months. Clinicians and patients should not be discouraged by this. The data suggest that most patients who make repeated quit attempts eventually succeed in achieving sustained abstinence.

Pharmacotherapies for Substance Abusers with Additional Types of Psychiatric Illness

Rates of substance abuse are higher than expecte dmang patients with psychiatric disorders, and psychiatric disorders are higher than expected among people with substance abuse disorders.

Clinical experience shows that:

- treatment should be administered by professionals with considerable experience in both general psychiatry and chemical dependence;
- it is unrealistic to insist on abstinence as a precondition for treatment;
- some symptom stability may be necessary before reductions in substance use are evident;

- abstinence is not a prerequisite for safe and effective treatment with most psychotropic agents;
- unless treated as a disorder in itself, a substance abuse tends to persist after comorbid psychopathology is effectively treated.

This section summarises the management of particular psychiatric illnesses complicated by substance use and some relevant drug interactions.

Drug Treatment for Specific Psychiatric Disorders

There is controversy about the stage at which a mood disorder iunduced by substance abuse becomes a major depressive episode. Most specialists will diagnose a second disorder in a patient who presents with a depressive syndrome only after a 2 week period of sobriety. However, evidence from clinical trials shows that antidepressants may be effective in patients who are not initially abstinent. Clinical judgment is therefore important and, if a nonabstinent patient has persistent depression, a trial of antidepressant therapy may be carried out. Concurrent use of an antidepressant and a substance of abuse may increase the risk of cardiotoxicity (arrhythmias), neurologic effects (seizures) or death from intentional overdose. These risks are greatest with the tricyclic antidepressants whereas the selective serononin reuptake inhibitors have a safer pharmacologic profile. Patients should always be discouraged from substance abuse but significant numbers of those taking antidepressants also use alcohol and other potential drugs of abuse in moderation without harm. Antidepressants seem to have a low risk of abuse, though abuse of amitriptyline (for its sedative effects) and fluoxetine (for stimulant effects) has been reported.

Substance abuse or dependence is a common complication of schizophrenia and psychotic symptoms occurring during drug intoxication or withdrawal also complicate the diagnosis of schizophrenia. An especially high degree of psychiatric sophistication and patience is necessary for this group of patients. Long-term studies (>one year) show that patients with schizophrenia and substance abuse need an energetic treatment strategy to engage them in treatment for psychosis, with an emphasis on compliance with antipsychotic medication and the maladaptive effects of substance abuse. For most patients, the problem of substance abuse diminishes after a year of compliance with medication and treatment for addiction. In this setting, the use of long-acting depot antipsychotic preparations is rational. Medication may also be combined with contingency contracting for patients with schizophrenia, making the unsupervised use of disability benefits contingent on negative urine toxicology analysis.

Substance-induced disorders (particularly stimulant intoxication and alcohol or sedative-hypnotic withdrawal) can resemble generalized anxiety disorder or panic attacks, and thus, as with depression, at least a two week period of abstinence is preferable prior to initiating pharmacotherapy, although again there is room for judgment. Other anxiety disorders, such as social phobia, agoraphobia, PTSD or OCD have distinctive symptoms that do not overlap with symptoms of toxicity or withdrawal. Behavioral approaches are effective for many anxiety disorders, and should be considered, first alone and then as a supplement to pharmacotherapy. Antidepressants are effective in the treatment of panic disorder or generalized anxiety disorder and have less abuse potential than the benzodiazepines. Buspirone may be effective in generalized anxiety disorder, especially at a dose of at least 45 mg/day. If a benzodiazepine is prescribed, clinical opinion supported by experimental evidence suggests that oxazepam and chlordiazepoxide are the safest alternatives because of their gradual onset of action and a lower risk of euphoria. In general, benzodiazepines should be avoided due to their abuse potential.

Substance abuse occurs frequently in patients with bipolar disorder but there is a lack of evidence of the effects of its treatment on substance abuse. Lithium does not appear to have significant interactions with alcohol and cocaine but there is little information about the safety of carbamazepine or valproic acid in pateints with bipolar disorder and substance abuse.

Attention deficithyperactivity disorder (ADHD) occurs more frequently than expected among patients with substance abuse disorders, and high rates of substance abuse occur in children with both ADHD and conduct disorder. It is possible that such patients may preferentially seek stimulants as self-medication of their behavior disorder. The diagnosis of ADHD should be confirmed by evidence of childhood illness and if possible verified by another informant. There is some evidence that methylphenidate may be helpful in such cases and desipramine and bupropion, both of which are used to treat ADHD in children, have also been suggested. Studies are under way to improve our understanding of substance abusers with ADHD.

Drug Interactions in Chemical Dependency

Drug interactions in patients with chemical dependency may be pharmacodynamic or pharmacokinetic, and may occur between drugs of abuse or between drugs of abuse and prescribed medications.

Alcohol

The combination of alcohol and cocaine has been associated with increased hepatotoxicity and fatal cardiotoxicity. Alcohol together with opiates or cannabis causes greater sedation and neurologic impairment than any of these agents alone. Acute alcohol intoxication inhibits hepatic enzymes, increasing blood levels of drugs metabolized by this system. By contrast, chronic alcohol use induces hepatic enzymes and lowers blood levels of antipsychotic drugs, tricyclic antidepressants, valproic acid, carbamazepine and certain benzodiazepines. Griseofulvin, metronidazole, chloramphenical and oral hypoglycemic agents cause a mild disulfiram-like reaction in combination with alcohol. Chloral hydrate and alcohol are both metabolized by a pathway dependent on alcohol dehydrogenase; taken simultaneously, competition for this enzyme results in higher blood levels of both agents (this combination is known as a "Mickey Finn").

Cocaine and Other Stimulants

The combination of cocaine and cannabis is associated with more tachycardia than with either agent alone. Combining heroin and cocaine in a "speedball" more readily produces respiratory depression than either alone. The use of cocaine or amphetamine by someone taking a monoamine oxidase inhibitor may result in hypertensive reactions.

Opiates

Methadone increases blood levels of tricyclic antidepressants and zidovudine. Conversely, methadone levels may be reduced to the point where abstinence occurs by rifampin, phenytoin, barbiturates and carbamazepine. Meperidine taken during treatment with a monoamine oxidase inhibitor may cause extreme reactions ranging from collapse (hypotension and coma) to excitation (hypertension and convulsions).

Nicotine

Smoking cigarettes smoking lowers blood levels of caffeine; caffeine toxicity may be therefore be misinterpreted as nicotine withdrawal in patients who stop smoking. Smoking also lowers blood levels of antipsychotic drugs, tricyclic antidepressants, theophylline and propranolol.

Hallucinogens

Hallucinogens may act partly via serotonergic mechanisms and it is therefore unsurprising that a serotonin reuptake inhibitor reportedly exacerbated hallucinogen-persisting perception disorder (flashbacks) in adolescent LSD users.

For additional readings, the reader is referred to the following:

1) Substance Abuse: A Comprehensive Textbook (4th Edition). Edited by Lowinson JH, Ruiz P, Millman RB, Langrod JG. Philadelphia, Lippincott Williams and Wilkins, 2005.
2) Principles of Addiction Medicine (3rd Edition). Edited by Graham AW, Schultz TK, Mayo-Smith MF, Ries RD, Wilford BB. Chevy Chase, Maryland, American Society of Addiction Medicine, Inc., 2003.
3) Textbook of Substance Abuse Treatment (3rd Edition). Edited by Galanter M, Kleber HD. Washington, D.C., American Psychiatric Publishing, Inc., 2004
4) Clinical Textbook of Addictive Disorders (3rd Edition). Edited by Frances RJ, Miller SI, Mack AH. New York, The Guilford Press, 2005.
5) International Handbook of Alcohol Dependence and Problems. Edited by Heather N, Peters T, Stockwell T. Chichester, England, John Wiley and Sons Ltd., 2001.

85 Therapeutic Management of the Suicidal Patient

According to 1999 data from the Center for Disease Control and Prevention, suicide kills more people than homicide. Suicide was the eleventh leading cause of death (homicide was fourteenth), and the third leading cause of death between ages 15 and 24 years. In the year 1999, 29 199 Americans took their own lives (Hoyert *et al.*, 2001). Suicide and the suicidal patient represent a significant public health problem. The vast majority of people with suicidal intent have a major psychiatric diagnosis. It has been estimated that 90% or more of them can be shown to have a major psychiatric illness (Henriksson *et al.*, 1993; Mann, 2002). Some patients become suicidal, or commit suicide with relatively little warning. Others have communicated their intent to a caregiver or significant other. A significant proportion, estimated as high as 70%, saw a physician within 30 days prior to their death, and nearly 50% had seen a physician in the preceding week (Barraclough *et al.*, 1974). It was noted in the classic studies of Robins and colleagues (1959) that only 18% of suicidal patients communicated their intent to helping professionals, while 69% communicated their intent to an average of three close relatives or associates, 73% within 12 months of their suicide (Robins *et al.*, 1959).

Some patients become acutely suicidal while others are chronically at risk. Suicide leaves in its wake intense suffering among the victim's family and friends, including feelings of grief, anger, shame and frequently guilt. There are relatively limited data on the frequency of suicide attempts. Management of the chronically suicidal is frequently a source of frustration and fear for caregivers. Identifying the risk factors, understanding the suicidal patient and intervening appropriately are key elements in the prevention of suicide. There is a role for parents, families, friends, schools, workplaces and physicians in this task. The suicide rates have fallen since 1993 (Hoyert *et al.*, 2001). However, it remains a given that even with due diligence, not all suicides can be predicted or prevented.

Mann and colleagues (1999) have proposed a stress-diathesis model of suicidal behavior, as "a psychiatric disorder is generally a necessary but insufficient condition for suicide". The model posits that suicidal behavior is a function of an individual's threshold for suicidal acts and the stressors that can lead to vulnerability. The authors believe that the threshold for suicidal acts is trait-dependent (diathesis), and is mediated by factors such as aggression, impulsivity, substance abuse, family history and low brain serotonin function. Stressors include psychiatric illness and interpersonal problems. In this model, intervention should consider the diathesis as well as the stressors (Mann *et al.*, 1999). Low serotonin levels may be the underlying feature of suicidal behavior, aggression and substance abuse (Mann *et al.*, 1999).

Hypotheses

Dynamic

Dynamic theories facilitate the attempt to understand patients and their difficulties. Gabbard (2000) presents an overview to these approaches to understanding the suicidal patient. As he discusses, Freud postulated that suicide could be the result of displaced murderous impulses toward an internalized object, and later in the structural model, the aggression of a sadistic superego against the ego. Menninger believed that suicide was a function of wishes to kill (e.g. an angry act designed to devastate survivors), be killed, and to die. A familiar theme in object relations of the suicidal patient is the conflict between the internalized tormentor and the anguished victim. Patients may either identify with the internalized aggressor and lash out at others or submit to the tormentor through suicide. Fenichel noted the less aggressive reunion fantasy, in which death abates object loss by the imagined joining with a departed loved one, frequently a maternal superego figure. When identity and self-esteem are tied to a lost object, suicide can be viewed as restorative. Pathological grief and anniversaries of losses may be vulnerable times for such patients (Gabbard, 2000).

Cognitive rigidity, especially the inability to revise expectations of the self, can lead to hopelessness and suicidality. Suicidal ideation that is egosyntonic is especially concerning. Four patterns of ego functioning and object relations that differentiate between serious attempters and manipulative gestures are: "(1) an inability to give up infantile wishes for nurturance, associated with a conflict about being overly dependent; (2) a sober but ambivalent view toward death; (3) excessively high self-expectations; and (4) overcontrol of affect, particularly aggression" (Gabbard, 2000).

In contrast to those who are intent on dying, most patients are ambivalent about death, and can come to choose life. Psychotherapy can be an important avenue to understanding why a patient wants to die and what they expect in the aftermath. Gabbard sees this effort as treatment, while providing safety may only be management (Gabbard, 2000).

Neurobiology

There are genetic and biologic correlates of suicidality as well as the underlying psychiatric illnesses that are often associated with suicidal behavior. For example, Ahearn and colleagues (2001) compared MRI studies in 20 pairs of unipolar depressed patients with and without suicide attempts. Subjects were matched on cardiovascular history, ECT treatment and psychosis. There were no statistical differences in age of onset of illness, number of episodes, or depression ratings. It was found that the patients with suicide attempts had more subcortical gray matter intensities. There was a trend toward more periventricular white matter hyperintensities in the patients with suicide attempts. The authors concluded that patients with abnormal MRI, especially gray matter hyperintensities in the basal ganglia, may be at higher risk for mood disorders and suicide attempts secondary to interference in neuroanatomic pathways. These pathways may be crucial to mood regulation (Ahearn et al., 2001). These and other neurobiologic correlates may improve our ability to predict suicide and suicidal behavior. Promising mechanisms include the serotonin system, although adrenergic and dopaminergic systems have also been implicated. Abnormalities in the hypothalamic–pituitary–adrenal (HPA) axis have long been associated with mood disorders.

For example, dysregulation in the serotonin system has been linked to major depression, suicide and violence (see Table 85.1). Disparate findings are a function of the inherent difficulties with association studies. A number of these studies have found an association between reduced serotonin function, including low levels of the serotonin metabolite 5-hydroxyindoleacetic acid (5-HIAA) in cerebrospinal fluid (CSF), with impulsivity, violence and suicide (Mann, 1998; Placidi et al., 2001). Low CSF 5-HIAA levels may also predict future suicide attempts (Roy et al., 1989). Aggressive behavior and, independently, suicidal behavior, may have impulsivity as a common denominator, which may be mediated by serotonergic dysfunction (Placidi et al., 2001).

Small sample sizes, heterogeneous diagnostic groups, retrospective analyses, uncertain impact of psychotropic agents, the continuum of suicidal behaviors (manipulative gestures to self-mutilation without the intent to die to completed suicide), and the "cross talk" between many of the neurobiologic systems targeted for study can all undermine consistency of findings.

Suicide is a multiply determined act, including genetic vulnerabilities, mental illness, environmental and social stressors, impulsivity, and aggressive tendencies.

Psychiatric Diagnoses

A number of psychiatric diagnoses are linked with suicidality. While patients with mood disorders (major depression and bipolar disorder) are commonly assessed for suicidality, anxiety disorders are also associated with significant suicide risk. Psychosis, in both mood disorders and schizophrenia, can heighten risk. Although borderline personality disorder has a high prevalence of suicidal ideation, impulsivity and self-injurious behavior, these patients are at risk for unexpected intentional and accidental death.

Bipolar Disorder

Oquendo and colleagues (2000) evaluated the applicability of their stress-diathesis model to a sample of bipolar patients. As with their other sample of psychiatric patients (Mann et al., 1999), objective illness severity was not a differentiating factor between bipolar attempters and nonattempters, although the symptoms were more severe at the index hospitalization via self-report and research clinician depression ratings. Similarly, bipolar attempters had increased suicidal ideation, hopelessness and decreased reasons for living. In contrast, there were no differences in impulsivity, although bipolar attempters had higher lifetime aggression. Oquendo and Mann (2001) include gender (men more likely to attempt than women, in contrast with other studies); white race; age (no difference in their study); suicidal ideation, hopelessness, fewer reasons for living; life time aggression and impulsivity; smoking, alcoholism and substance abuse, and family history of suicide as possible diathesis-related suicide risk factors for bipolar patients. Stress-related risk factors in

Table 85.1 Summary of Serotonin Mechanisms

Serotonin Mechanisms	Suicide Attempts	Postmortem Studies
5-HIAA	$\downarrow$ CSF (Placidi et al. 2001, Cremniter et al. 1999) $\downarrow$ plasma (Spreaux-Varoquaux et al., 2001) $\downarrow$ urine (Brunner et al., 1993)	
5-HT	$\downarrow$ platelet (Spreaux-Varoquaux et al., 2001)	
SERT		$\downarrow$ binding (Mann et al., 2000)
SERT mRNA		$\downarrow$ dorsal raphe nucleus (Arango et al., 2001)
5-HT_{1A}		$\downarrow$ binding capacity in dorsal raphe nucleus (Arango et al., 2001)
5-HT_{1B}	$\downarrow$ G allele (New et al., 2001)	$\downarrow$ binding sites in frontal cortex (Arranz et al., 1994)
5-HT_{1A}	$\downarrow$ after age 20 (Sheline et al., 2002) + polymorphism (Du et al., 2000) − polymorphism (Bondey et al., 2000; Tsai et al., 1999)	$\uparrow$ receptor, protein, mRNA in prefrontal cortex, hippocampus (Pandey et al., 2002)
5-HT_{2C}		+ differential RNA editing (Niswender et al., 2001)
Tryptophan hydroxylase	+U allele (Mann et al., 1997) − association (Ono et al., 2000; Souery et al., 2001)	

bipolar patients may include depressed or mixed state (Oquendo and Mann, 2001).

Anxiety Disorders

A frequently overlooked risk factor for suicidal behavior is anxiety. The clinical history features that are most predictive of serious suicide attempt in a study of patients with suicide attempts (Hall *et al.*, 1999) are severe anxiety (92%) and panic attacks (80%), partial insomnia (difficulty falling asleep, middle insomnia, early morning awakening) (92%), depressed mood (80%), relationship disruption (78%), substance abuse (68%), pessimism (hopelessness 64%, helplessness 62% and worthlessness 29%), global insomnia (46%) and anhedonia (43%). Severe anxiety and agitation may be an important risk factor for an acute suicide attempt. These "modifiable risk factors" may be responsive to early intervention. Evidence accumulated argues for the assessment of severe anxiety/agitation and aggressive anxiolytic treatment in the management of suicide risk.

Psychosis

Grunebaum and colleagues (2001) reported that about half of the reviewed articles published since 1982 reported a positive association between delusions and suicidal ideation or behavior and about half found a negative association. Approximately half of the subset of studies of delusional depression and suicide risk were negative. Half of the studies of delusions and suicide risk in schizophrenia were negative. A study of delusions and suicidal ideation in bipolar patients was negative.

Although the best predictors of suicidal behavior are past history of suicide attempts, substance abuse, and chronic and/or deteriorating clinical course, clinicians should consider new onset psychosis as a significant risk factor (Verdoux *et al.*, 2001).

Borderline Personality Disorder

Suicidal behavior is frequently associated with affective lability, anger, impulsivity and disruption in interpersonal relationships. Suicidal ideation and suicide attempts are part of the diagnostic criteria for borderline personality disorder. The recurrence and/or chronicity of suicidal ideation, combined with multiple low lethality attempts, have assigned some of these episodes to communicative idioms of distress or suicidal gestures. However, there is evidence (Soloff *et al.*, 2000) that suggests borderline personality disorder may be predictive of the number of attempts, but does not differentiate attempt characteristics, for example intent to die, planning, or lethality. Assumptions about the seriousness of suicidal behavior based on diagnosis alone may be flawed. Comorbid substance abuse and interpersonal disruption/abandonment issues heighten the risk (Soloff *et al.*, 2000).

Risk Factors

Since there are no reliable and specific tests for suicidal behavior, the clinician must rely on clinical, demographic, historical and patient self-report information to guide their judgment and to tailor their intervention. However, the clinician should not be lulled into a false sense of security because of their assessment. The positive predictive value of individual or group of risk factors is low. Stepwise multiple regression was used to develop a statistical model that would predict suicide in 1906 inpatients (admitted between 1970 and 1981). There were 46 suicides at the

Table 85.2	Risk Factors
Gender – male	
Ethnicity – white	
Age – elderly	
Substance abuse	
Past attempts	
Means, especially access to guns	
Family history	
Hopelessness	
Unemployed	
Comorbid medical conditions	
Failed relationship, divorced, widowed	
Irresponsible media coverage of suicides	

end of the follow-up period (1983). Medical illness, substance abuse, personality disorder, marital status were among characteristics that failed to reach significance for the final model. Variables that met significance level criteria (number of prior suicide attempts, suicidal ideation, bipolar disorder, gender, outcome at discharge, unipolar depression with bipolar first-degree relative) were included in the model. The model did not identify any patient who committed suicide. Limitations include the low suicide rate and possible underestimation of suicides (Goldstein *et al.*, 1991). There may be differences in people who attempt suicide versus those who complete it. In 1999, it was estimated that there were 730 000 annual attempts, with an attempt and completion ratio of 25 : 1. It was estimated that 5 million had a history of a suicide attempt (Hoyert *et al.*, 2001). Differential risk factors include gender, ethnicity, age, substance abuse, past suicide attempts, means, family history, hopelessness, comorbid medical conditions, relationship/esteem losses resulting in murder–suicide and media coverage (see Table 85.2).

Assessment of Suicidal Patients

Common presentations include acute, chronic, contingent, and/or potentially manipulative suicidal patient. All are associated with anxiety for the care provider doing the assessment. Careful assessment, use of collateral information and acceptance of predictive limitations can be helpful (see Table 85.3).

As reviewed by Nicholas and Golden (2001), factors to be considered in the assessment of the acutely suicidal patient include the current mental status, with special attention to direct inquiry about suicidal ideation, intent (may be ascertained from family and friends, for example, saying good-byes or putting affairs in order), and plans (well thought out with available means). Sadness, hopelessness, social withdrawal/isolation, anxiety, agitation, impulsivity, insomnia, psychosis (especially command hallucinations or distressing persecutory delusions) are additional concerning symptoms. These factors, coupled with prior high lethality attempts, uncommunicative presentation, recent major loss, active substance abuse, or untreated mood, psychotic, or personality disorder, might indicate that hospitalization is warranted to ensure safety prior to treating the underlying psychiatric disorder (Nicholas and Golden, 2001).

Sachs and colleagues (2001) reviewed suicide prevention strategies for bipolar outpatients, but they can easily be adapted to any potentially suicidal patient. The reader is reminded that "care providers can, however, be fooled by the deceptions of a

Table 85.3	Assessment Factors

Mental status
Suicidal ideation
Intent
Plans
Sadness
Hopelessness
Social withdrawal
Isolation
Anxiety
Agitation
Impulsivity
Insomnia
Psychosis
Prior high lethality attempts
Uncommunicative presentation
Recent major loss
Active substance abuse
Untreated mood, psychotic or personality disorder

clever patient intent on carrying out a lethal act". Individualized treatment plans should be developed after eliciting current symptoms, including suicidal ideation; review of risk factors, stressors, comorbid states like substance use; and past history of suicide attempts. Acute efforts are directed toward safety and treating the underlying disorder, with follow-up monitoring. Adjunctive medications like antipsychotics and anxiolytics can be beneficial. Clinicians must monitor the amounts of medications prescribed and continue to be vigilant during early recovery. Harm reduction strategies can include minimizing access to lethal means, decreasing social isolation, close follow-up and informing of emergency contact procedures. Hospitalization may be warranted if suicide is considered as a solution for problems, for active suicidal ideation, or if there has been a recent attempt. With the caveat that while admission may provide safety, current knowledge of risk factors do not wholly inform when to admit or discharge, overreliance on hospitalization may deter honest reporting, and many acutely depressed patients can be managed as outpatients with sufficient safeguards. Involuntary admission, while not therapy in and of itself, may be lifesaving. ECT remains a safe, typically quick onset, effective option for those at high risk of suicide (Sachs *et al.*, 2001).

There is no evidence that denial of suicidal intent predicts nonsuicide. Review of standard risk factors, additional risk factors (e.g. acute relationship and employment changes), acute versus chronic suicidal ideation, and treatment of readily reversible factors should be undertaken. High risk diagnoses include major depression, bipolar disorder, schizophrenia, alcoholism and substance abuse, and borderline personality disorder. Comorbid alcoholism increases the risk in every diagnostic category. A history of past attempts, hopelessness, previous hospitalizations and recent discharge, while not individually predictive, do heighten concern. Acute risk factors include severe anxiety, panic attacks, global insomnia and agitation. These symptoms should be carefully assessed, with aggressive intervention. Benzodiazepines and antipsychotics can be employed to address anxiety and agitation. Caution must be taken with benzodiazepines to avoid disinhibition and combination with alcohol. Mixed states may require mood stabilizers. Serial assessments should be performed with acute changes as well as chronic suicidal states.

Chronically suicidal patients also require aggressive treatment of anxiety and agitation. DBT and cognitive behavioral therapy (CBT) can be helpful in addressing parasuicidal and suicidal behavior.

A significant number of psychiatrists utilize the no-suicide contract, or the contract for safety. Over half of a sample of psychiatrists acknowledged using them in recent survey, and 41% of them had patients make suicide attempts after entering into one (Kroll, 2000). Sixty-four percent of 14 psychiatric hospital inpatient suicides denied suicidal ideation and half had some form of no-suicide agreement in place in the week before their deaths (Busch *et al.*, 1993). These have not been systematically studied as to whether they have any protective effect (Gray and Otto, 2001). Resnick (2002) cautions that psychiatrists tend to view the patient as a collaborator in treatment. However, the psychiatrist can be less viewed as an "ally" and become an "adversary" when the patient has determined to die by suicide. He notes that failure to recognize this shift in the doctor–patient relationship can have devastating results. Objective evidence, as opposed to patient subjective reports, may be telling. Alliances with family and other caregivers should be maintained, as they can become crucial sources of information. Resnick believes that no-suicide contracts have little credence, especially in an adversarial relationship, cause a false sense of security for the therapist, and have no research literature to suggest efficacy (Resnick, 2002).

Gutheil and Schetky (1998) wrote of a most difficult assessment: the patient who expresses suicidal ideation in terms of a future eventuality. The "if [event or outcome does or does not happen], I will kill myself" contingency poses different challenges from acute suicidality, manipulative suicidal threats and chronic suicidality. Suicidality typically engenders anxiety in the therapist. Contingency suicidality frequently lacks verbalized imminence, may make involuntary commitment difficult, and invites countertransferences which can lead to exaggerated or inappropriately muted responses. For some patients, the contingency is a defense against suicide. For others, it represents the ultimate control. Gutheil and Schetky (1998) make several important points: 1) Some patients almost have an object relationship with death, with death personified as a benevolent bringer of relief. The therapist should approach that tie with caution, as it may be the only one in which the patient has any confidence; 2) Future deadlines should not be accepted literally; 3) Even when the contingency is met positively, the suicidal ideation may not resolve; 4) Some patients view themselves as already dead, cannot conceive of life without depression, and challenge the therapist to resurrect them. This stance undermines any potential relationship; and 5) It is of benefit to negotiate a halt to suicidal acts until depression can be separated from decision-making. Gutheil and Schetky assert "… psychiatrists should never support suicide, but should acknowledge the human impossibility of preventing it". The authors note that in these circumstances, the patient is at least communicating their suicidal ideation. The rationale can be explored and an effort made to maintain the therapeutic relationship. Helplessness should be discussed, as suicidal ideation can be a defense against lack of control or an expression of pain. The countertransference of the therapist should be considered, as it can cloud clinical judgment. Consultation with colleagues can be very helpful. The competency of the patient may be called into question, and has been used as a defense in suicide malpractice cases. The clinician can frequently be justified in involuntary commitment as critical dates or junctures approach. Finally, Gutheil and Schetky state that "accepting the patient's pain and sense of hopelessness is not the same as acceding to his or her wish to commit suicide; the psychiatrist must always hold out hope. At the same time, it may be therapeutic and realistic to let patients know that one can not ultimately prevent their suicides" (Gutheil and Schetky, 1998).

Intervention

Successful suicide prevention strategies include educating the public and primary care providers about mental illness, its common presentations, the availability of treatment and how to access it. Underdiagnosis and undertreatment remain significant problems. Antidepressants, lithium, mood stabilizers and ECT, as well as adjunctive benzodiazepines and antipsychotics, can significantly ameliorate underlying psychiatric diagnoses associated with suicide. Psychosocial interventions have much to add, especially for chronic suicidal ideation, but more intensive outpatient strategies may be limited by resources available.

Education

Educating the public and clinicians about the prevalence, symptoms and available treatment for mood disorders is of crucial importance. It is estimated that half to a quarter of mood disorders go undiagnosed and untreated (Grandin et al., 2001; Nierenberg et al., 2001). Many patients will have spoken to significant others about their distress or have recently seen a health care professional. The US Surgeon General issued a call to action in 1999 to prevent suicide. The linchpins of the strategy include awareness, intervention and methodology. Recommendations include improving public awareness of suicide, including their preventability, enhancing access to prevention resources, and decreasing the stigma of mental illness. Interventions include improved ability of primary care physicians to recognize, treat, or refer the mentally ill; remove barriers; create incentives to treatment; train other professionals, community members and family to recognize or assess risk; develop programs for at risk adolescents; enhance community access to care and support for suicide survivors; and partnering with the media for educated reporting and depictions of mental illness and suicide deaths. Methodology involves researching effective prevention programs, clinical and culture specific interventions; developing evaluation tools to measure efficacy of interventions; and the reduction of access to lethal means of suicide (US Public Health Service, 1999).

Oquendo and colleagues (1999) examined the aggressiveness of antidepressant treatment on patients with major depression, with and without suicide attempts. They included 171 inpatients with major depression, 80 "remote" (defined by the authors as an attempt more than 90 days prior to admission) suicide attempters and 91 nonattempters, in their data analysis. Subjectively and objectively, degrees of major depression were not significantly different. Only 15% of the entire sample was taking antidepressants on admission, and of those who were, 35% were deemed adequately dosed. Almost inexplicably, the patients with a history of suicide attempts, and therefore more likely to have future attempts, were less likely to receive adequate antidepressant therapy. The failure to diagnose and adequately treat major depression warrants ongoing education of all physicians (Oquendo et al., 1999).

Two reports from the NIMH Collaborative Depression Study, 1978–1980 (Keller et al., 1982, 1986), also note undertreatment. Keller and colleagues (1982) described 217 patients

entering the naturalistic study. Only 3% with moderate to severe unipolar depression of a month's duration had been treated with the most intensive dose of tricyclic antidepressants. A quarter of those with psychotic depression received the most intensive therapy and another quarter with psychotic depression received no antipsychotics or antidepressant therapy of any category. The follow-up report (Keller et al., 1986) described treatment of 338 patients in the 2 months after enrollment. Of inpatients, 31% received no or inadequate antidepressant somatotherapy, and only 49% received the equivalent of at 200 mg of imipramine. Of outpatients, 51% received no or inadequate somatotherapy, and 19% received the equivalent of 200 mg of imipramine. As reviewed by Hirshfeld and colleagues (1997), there is "overwhelming evidence" that depression is being undertreated, both before and during the widespread use of SSRIs.

Lithium

Lithium shows consistent antisuicidal effects (Tondo et al., 2001a). Tondo and colleagues (2001b) performed a meta-analysis of the suicide risk with long-term lithium treatment. They included 22 studies, 13 of which provided data on suicide rates with and without lithium ($N = 5647$ patients), and analyzed suicide completions, not attempts. Suicide rates were higher without lithium in all of the studies except one. Four of the studies were exclusive to patients with bipolar disorder. Suicide rates were significantly lower (81.8%) during lithium treatment. Notably, suicide rates in this population were significantly higher than in international general populations. This is probably reflective of differences between clinical and general populations, inclusion of highly suicidal individuals in the study samples, partial or failed treatment, and possible noncompliance (Tondo et al., 2001b).

As reviewed by Goodwin (1999), there has been increasing use of anticonvulsants in the management of bipolar disorder. Anticonvulsants may have an advantage in rapid cycling, mixed states, comorbid substance abuse, or history of poor response to lithium. There is little data about the suicide preventive impact of the anticonvulsants, although a comparison of lithium and carbamazepine was more favorable to lithium (Thies-Flechtner et al., 1996). Both lithium and anticonvulsants can have a positive impact on suicide risk factors of impulsivity and aggression (Goodwin, 1999).

ECT

Electroconvulsive therapy (ECT) has long played a role in the treatment of severe, and treatment refractory depression. Thus, ECT is indicated for illnesses frequently associated with suicidal symptoms, and is noted for relatively quick efficacy. It can have a profound impact on acute suicidal symptoms, in both responders and nonresponders. The authors conclude that although an acute treatment, ECT's long-term impact on mortality may be a function of repeated use in treating or preventing (via continuation and maintenance ECT) relapse and recurrence (Prudic and Sackeim, 1999).

Psychosocial Interventions

Sachs and colleagues (2001) note that psychotherapy is not a cure for suicidal ideation, but may strengthen protective factors and decrease inclination. Gray and Otto (2001) reviewed psychosocial approaches to suicide prevention and their applicability to bipolar patients. An approach tailored toward psychosocial risk factors, for example, hopelessness, poor problem-solving, negative cognitions and dysfunctional coping strategies, may be particularly helpful. Gainful employment and increasing social supports are also appropriate goals. Gray and Otto (2001) reviewed 17 randomized, controlled studies of efforts to decrease suicidal and self-injurious behavior. The studies could be categorized as brief hospitalization, efforts to enhance treatment utilization, problem-solving interventions and intensive treatments. Brief hospitalization was associated with negative to small effect size, while facilitated/rapid hospital reentry was more promising for subjects with initial episodes of self-harm. Studies of some outreach services found no benefits, while those that included home visits had modest to no reductions in suicidal behavior. One in this latter category with noteworthy results (threefold difference compared with treatment as usual) involved 4 months of weekly or biweekly home-based interventions combining psychotherapy, crisis intervention and family therapy (Welu, 1977). This represents a significant commitment of resources. Problem-solving interventions, for example, around interpersonal conflicts or cognitive behavioral therapy, had moderate effect size, and were largely brief, structured and problem-focused. Intensive treatments (1 year) like dialectical behavior therapy (DBT) reflected a large effect size (Gray and Otto, 2001).

Clinicians should consider three effective strategies: lowering barriers to care during times of distress, brief training in problem-solving strategies, and comprehensive strategies that combine problem-solving with intensive rehearsal of cognitive, social, emotional-labeling and tolerance, and coping skills. Patients and families should be educated on procedures for accessing after-hours and emergency care. Cognitive restructuring can address hopelessness, pessimism, cognitive distortions and enhance reasons for living. The development of distress-tolerance skills may be particularly beneficial for patients who feel unable to resist urges to harm themselves or have chronically maladaptive responses to stress (Gray and Otto, 2001).

Aftermath: Clinicians Coping with Patient Suicide

A suicide has repercussions for all parties involved. Primary care providers can be as, or more, vulnerable to patient suicides than psychiatrists. As reviewed by Luoma and colleagues (2002), they are more likely to have been in recent contact with a suicide victim than mental health professionals. In their review of 40 studies, last contacts with mental health services compared with primary care providers within 1 month and 1 year of death were 19% versus 45%, and 32% versus 77%, respectively. The lifetime rate of contact with mental health services averaged 53%.

Kaye and Soreff (1991) had a number of recommendations in the aftermath of a patient suicide, with the caveat that a patient suicide is a very personal event, and the approach has to be individualized in recognition of nuances. They believe that families should be contacted and met with, told realistically of all the efforts on the decedent's behalf, and contact maintained through the funeral and autopsy report. Hospital staff should be contacted and, if possible, informed as a group. Attendance at the funeral can be beneficial. They advocate the psychological autopsy as an opportunity to vent as well as facilitate learning and any policy reform. In some instances, inpatients or surviving group members should meet with staff, with a concern toward patients' devaluing staff and increased suicidal risk to surviving patients.

The treating psychiatrist should seek support, solicit formal or informal consultation with colleagues, consider attending the funeral or sending forms of condolence, and offer expressions of sympathy. The latter is not felt to represent an admission of guilt. A psychological autopsy should be conducted, and attending the autopsy is not verboten in their opinion. Billing for past services, although difficult, is typically appropriate. If affiliated with an institution, cooperation with its risk management is advised, with due caution. Medical records should be accurately completed, with those submitted after the patient's death clearly reflecting so. Although the suicide of a patient reminds the psychiatrist of powerlessness, the psychiatrist should function as team leader in the aftermath (Kaye and Soreff, 1991).

Conclusion

Suicide is a multiple-determined phenomenon, with psychological, dynamic and biologic substrates. Future sophistication in neurobiology and genetics may add greatly to our very limited predictive power as to who is at risk and improve our interventions. Even so, there remains a significant failure appropriately to utilize the knowledge base that we currently have. Too many patients commit suicide because they were undiagnosed, undertreated, or too stigmatized to seek mental health treatment. Those patients who are identified and treated continue to have risk. They require a therapeutic alliance, and frequently our ability to bind anxiety, psychosocial interventions and judicious hospitalization, in addition to our biologic armamentarium.

References

Ahearn EP, Jamison KR, Steffens DC et al. (2001) MRI correlates of suicide attempt history in unipolar depression. *Biol Psychiatr* 50(4), 266–270.

Arango V, Underwood MD, Boldrini M, et al. (2001) Serotonin 1A receptors, serotonin transporter binding and serotonin transporter mRNA expression in the brainstem of depressed suicide victims. *Neuropsychopharmacology* 25(6), 892–903.

Arranz B, Ericksson A, Mellerup E, et al. (1994) Brain 5-HT$_{1A}$, 5-HT$_{1D}$ and 5-HT$_{2A}$ receptors in suicide victims. *Biol Psychiatr* 35, 457–463.

Barraclough B, Bunch J, Nelson B, et al. (1974) A hundred cases of suicide: Clinical aspects. *Br J Psychiatr* 125, 355–373.

Bondy B, Kuznik J, Baghai T, et al. (2000) Lack of association of serotonin-2A receptor gene polymorphism (T102C) with suicidal ideation and suicide. *Am J Med Genet* 96(6), 831–835.

Brunner, HG, Nelen M, Breakefield XO, et al. (1993) Abnormal behavior associated with a point mutation in the structural gene for monoamine oxidase. *Science* 262, 578–580.

Busch K, Clark D, Fawcett J et al. (1993) Clinical features of inpatient suicide. *Psychiatr Ann* 23, 256–262.

Cremniter D, Jamain S, Kollenbach K, et al. (1999) CSF 5-HIAA levels are in lower in impulse violent suicide attempters and control subjects. *Biol Psychiatr* 45, 1572–1579.

Du L, Bakish D, Lapierre YD, et al. (2000) Association of polymorphism of serotonin 2A receptor gene with suicidal ideation in major depressive disorder. *Am J Med Genet* (Neuropsychiatr Genet) 96, 56–60.

Gabbard GO (2000) Affective disorders, in *Psychodynamic Psychiatry in Clinical Practice*. American Psychiatric Press, Washington DC, pp. 203–231.

Goldstein RB, Black DW, Nasrallah A et al. (1991) The prediction of suicide: Sensitivity, specificity, and predictive value of a multivariate model applied to suicide among 1906 patients with affective disorders. *Arch Gen Psychiatr* 48, 418–422.

Goodwin FK (1999) Anticonvulsant therapy and suicide risk in affective disorders. *J Clin Psychiatr* 60(Suppl 2), 89–93.

Grandin LD, Yan LJ, and Gray SM (2001) Suicide prevention: Increasing education and awareness. *J Clin Psychiatr* 62(Suppl 25), 12–16.

Gray SM and Otto MW (2001) Psychosocial approaches to suicide prevention: Applications to patients with bipolar disorder. *J Clin Psychiatr* 62(Suppl 25), 56–64.

Grunebaum MF, Oquendo MA, Harkavy-Friedman JM et al. (2001) Delusions and suicidality. *Am J Psychiatr* 158(5), 742–747.

Gutheil TG and Schetky D (1998) A date with death: Management of the time-based and contingent suicidal intent. *Am J Psychiatr* 155(11), 1502–1507.

Hall RCW, Platt DE and Hall RCW (1999) Suicide risk assessment: A review of risk factors for suicide in 100 patients who made severe suicide attempts. *Psychosomatics* 40(1), 18–27.

Henriksson MM, Aro HM, Marttunen MJ et al. (1993) Mental disorders and comorbidity in suicide. *Am J Psychiatr* 150(6), 935–940.

Hirshfeld RMA, Keller MB, Panico S et al. (1997) The National Depressive and Manic–Depressive Association consensus statement on the undertreatment of depression. *J Am Med Assoc* 277(4), 333–340.

Hoyert DL, Arias E and Smith BL (2001) Deaths: Final Data for 1999. National Vital Statistics Report, 49 (8). National Center for Health Statistics, DHHS Publication No. (PHS) 2001–1120, Hyattsville, MD.

Kaye NS and Soreff SM (1991) The psychiatrist's role, responses, and responsibilities when a patient commits suicide. *Am J Psychiatr* 148, 739–743.

Keller MB, Klerman GL and Lavori PW (1982) Treatment received by depressed patients. *J Am Med Assoc* 248(15), 1848–1855.

Keller MB, Lavori PW, Klerman GL et al. (1986) Low levels and lack of predictors of somatotherapy and psychotherapy received by depressed patients. *Arch Gen Psychiatr* 43, 458–466.

Kroll J (2000) Use of no-suicide contracts by psychiatrists in Minnesota. *Am J Psychiatr* 157, 1684–1686.

Luoma JB, Martin CE and Pearson JL (2002) Contact with mental health and primary care providers before suicide: A review of the evidence. *Am J Psychiatr* 159(6), 909–916.

Mann JJ (1998) The neurobiology of suicide. *Natl Med* 4, 25–30.

Mann JJ (2002) A current perspective of suicide and attempted suicide. *Ann Int Med* 136(4), 302–311.

Mann JJ, Malone KM, Nielson DA, et al. (1997) Possible association of a polymorphism of the tryptophan hydroxylase gene with suicidal behavior in depressed patients. *Am J Psychiatr* 154(10), 1451–1453.

Mann JJ, Huang Y, Underwood MD, et al. (2000) A serotonin transporter gene promoter polymorphism (5-HTTLPR) and prefrontal cortical binding in major depression and suicide. *Arch Gen Psychiatr* 57, 729–738.

Mann JJ, Waternaux C, Haas GL et al. (1999) Toward a clinical model of suicidal behavior in psychiatric patients. *Am J Psychiatr* 156(2), 181–189.

New AS, Gerlernter J, Goodman M, et al. (2001) Suicide, impulsive aggression, and HTR1B genotype. *Biol Psychiatr* 50(1), 62–65.

Nicholas LM and Golden RN (2001) Managing the suicidal patient. *Off Psychiatr* 3(3), 1–8.

Nierenberg AA, Gray SM and Grandin LD (2001) Mood disorders and suicide. *J Clin Psychiatr* 62(Suppl 25), 27–30.

Niswender CM, Herrick-Davis K, Dilley GE, et al. (2001) RNA editing of the human serotonin 5-HT$_{2C}$ receptor. Alterations in suicide and implications for serotonergic pharmacology. *Neuropsychopharmacology* 24(5), 478–491.

Ono H, Shirakawa O, Nishiguch N (2000) Tryptophan hydroxylase gene polymorphisms are not associated with suicide. *Am J Med Genet* 96(6), 861–863.

Oquendo MA and Mann JJ (2001) Identifying and managing suicide risk in bipolar patients. *J Clin Psychiatr* 62(Suppl 25), 31–34.

Oquendo MA, Malone KM, Ellis SP et al. (1999) Inadequacy of antidepressant treatment for patients with major depression who are at risk for suicidal behavior. *Am J Psychiatr* 156(2), 190–194.

Oquendo MA, Waternaux C, Brodsky B et al. (2000) Suicidal behavior in bipolar mood disorder: Clinical characteristics of attempters and nonattempters. *J Affect Disord* 59, 107–117.

Pandey GN, Dwivedi Y, Rizavi HS, et al. (2002) Higher expression of serotonin 5-HT$_{2A}$ receptors in the postmortem brains of teenaged suicide victims. *Am J Psychiatr* 159(3), 419–429.

Placidi GP, Oquendo MA, Malone KM et al. (2001) Aggressivity, suicide attempts, and depression: Relationship to cerebrospinal fluid monoamine metabolite levels. *Biol Psychiatr* 50(10), 783–791.

Prudic J and Sackeim HA (1999) Electroconvulsive therapy and suicide risk. *J Clin Psychiatr* 60(Suppl 2), 104–110.

Resnick PJ (2002) Recognizing that the suicidal patient views you as an "adversary." *Curr Psychiatr* 1, 8.

Robins E, Gassner S, Kayes J et al. (1959) The communication of suicidal intent: A study of 134 consecutive cases of successful (completed) suicide. *Am J Psychiatr* 115, 724–733.

Roy A, De Jong J and Linnoila M (1989) Cerebrospinal fluid monoamine metabolites and suicidal behavior in depressed patients. A 5-year follow-up study. *Arch Gen Psychiatr* 46, 609–612.

Sachs GS, Yan LJ, Swann AC et al. (2001) Integration of suicide prevention into outpatient management of bipolar disorder. *J Clin Psychiatr* 62(Suppl 25), 3–11.

Sheline YI, Mintum MA, and Moerlein SM (2002) Greater loss of 5-HT$_{2A}$ receptors in midlife than in late life. *Am J Psychiatr* 159, 430–435.

Soloff PH, Lynch KG, Kelly TM et al. (2000) Characteristics of suicide attempts of patients with major depressive episode and borderline personality disorder: A comparative study. *Am J Psychiatr* 157(4), 601–608.

Souery D, Van Gestel S, Massat I, et al. (2001) Tryptophan hydroxylase polymorphism and suicidality in unipolar and bipolar affective disorders: A multicenter association study. *Biol Psychiatr* 49(5), 405–409.

Spreux-Varoquaux O, Alvarex JC, Berlin I, et al. (2001) Differential abnormalities in plasma 5-HIAA and platelet serotonin concentrations in violent suicide attempters: Relationships wih impulsivity and depression. *Life Sci* 69(6), 647–657.

Thies-Flechtner K, Müller-Oerlinghausen B, Seibert W et al. (1996) Effect of prophylactic treatment on suicide risk in patients with major affective disorders: Data from a randomized prospective trial. *Pharmacopsychiatry* 29, 103–107.

Tondo L, Ghiani C and Albert M (2001a) Pharmacologic interventions in suicide prevention. *J Clin Psychiatr* 62(Suppl 25), 51–55.

Tondo L, Hennen J and Baldessarini RJ (2001b) Lower suicide risk with long-term lithium treatment in major affective illness: A meta-analysis. *Acta Psychiatr Scand* 104, 163–172.

Tsai SJ, Hong CJ, Hsu CC, et al. (1999) Serotonin-2A receptor polymorphism (102T/C) in mood disorders. *Psychiatr Res* 87, 233–237.

US Public Health Service (1999) The Surgeon General's Call to Action to Prevent Suicide. Washington DC. Available at http://www.surgeongeneral.gov/library/calltoaction/default.htm.

Verdoux H, Liraud F, Gonzales B et al. (2001) Predictors and outcome characteristics associated with suicidal behavior in early psychosis: A two-year follow-up of first-admitted subjects. *Acta Psychiatr Scand* 103, 347–354.

Welu TC (1977) A follow-up program for suicide attempter: Evaluation of effectiveness. *Suicide Life Threat Behav* 7, 17–30.

86 Treatment of Violent Behavior

Introduction

Violent behavior in patients with psychiatric disorders is a frequent reason for presentation to an emergency room and subsequent admission to an inpatient unit, and is often an obstacle to discharge and reintegration back into the community. Aggressive behavior places other patients, mental health workers and family members or other caregivers at risk for harm. Fortunately, within the past 10 years, new treatment approaches have emerged enabling greater opportunities for the successful management of these behaviors.

Some patients are violent only when acutely psychotic, while others may have persistent aggressive behavior unrelated to psychosis. Co-occurring substance use disorders increase the risk of violent behavior. Neuropsychiatric deficits and poor impulse control, underlying character pathology, or a chaotic environment may also be contributing factors.

The management of violent behavior can be divided into short-term and long-term strategies. First, there is a need to manage acute episodes of agitation. Secondly, there is a need to decrease the frequency and intensity of these episodes. The pharmacological treatment of acute agitation requires the use of sedating agents, but long-term use of these same agents would interfere with a patient's level of functioning. Consequently, long-term approaches require the use of medications that target aggressive behavior, without causing undue sedation.

Definitions

Aggression, violence, and hostility are used in the psychiatric literature to denote behaviors that are particularly noxious and a considerable source of concern for those in the field. These terms are used with varying precision and interpretation of research data can be a challenge when different studies use different definitions. Published rating scales may contain their own definitions and these scales may be further modified or adapted to the specific needs of the study in question. In general, "aggression", a term used for both human and animal research, is defined as overt behavior involving intent to deliver noxious stimulation to another organism or to behave destructively toward inanimate objects. Humans demonstrate three main subtypes of aggression: verbal aggression, physical aggression against other people and physical aggression against objects. "Violence" is an exclusively human term, and usually denotes physical aggression against other people and thus can be seen as a subtype of aggression. On the other hand, "hostility" is a loosely defined term in the psychiatric literature. Hostility may include agitation, aggression, irritability, suspicion, uncooperativeness and jealousy, depending on the context in which the word is used.

Agitation can be defined as excessive verbal and/or motor behavior. Mild agitation can escalate to include behaviors such as aggression and violence.

Pathophysiology of Aggressive Behavior

Several principal pathways leading to a predisposition to aggressive behavior are schematically displayed in Figure 86.1. The parents may contribute to the offspring's predisposition via transmitted genes, fetal environment, obstetric complications and rearing environment. Several polymorphisms of genes that control the activity of various neurotransmitters (particularly serotonin and catecholamines) are apparently associated with persistent aggressive behavior. Maternal use of alcohol, smoking and malnutrition during pregnancy were all reported to explain statistically significant (but clinically modest) proportions of the variance of aggressive behavior in adult offspring. Obstetric complications, particularly in interaction with other factors such as early maternal rejection, may lead to elevated rates of violent crime in the offspring. Rearing environment not just limited to overt child abuse is one of the most important factors in the development of predisposition to violence. Detailed explanation of Figure 86.1, as well as the bibliography supporting it, are presented elsewhere (Volavka, 2002).

Mechanisms displayed in Figure 86.2 may operate in persons with or without a diagnosable mental disorder. We will now focus on aggressive behavior in persons with mental disorders.

Substance Use Disorders

Acute effects of alcohol and illicit drugs are involved, perhaps causally, in a large proportion of aggressive incidents. For example, 51.6% of women injured during a physical assault by a male partner reported that the assaulter had been drinking just before the incident (Kyriacou et al., 1999). Positive urine tests for illicit drugs were obtained in a majority of arrested males in the USA (Pastore and Maguire, 2000, p. 380). Epidemiological studies indicate that substance use disorders elevate substantially the prevalence of overt physical aggression (Swanson, 1994).

Psychoses

Most persons diagnosed with a psychosis are not violent. Nevertheless, psychoses are associated with an elevated risk for aggression. It is clear that comorbidity of psychosis and substance use disorder contributes to this risk very substantially. Furthermore, persons with psychoses are more likely to have substance use disorders than other people (Regier et al., 1990). Combination of substance abuse and nonadherence to treatment is the typical prelude to the development of aggressive behavior in persons with severe mental illness living in the community (Swartz et al., 1998).

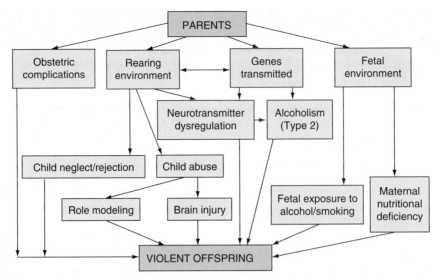

Figure 86.1   *Transmission of violence.*

As every hospital psychiatrist knows, there are many psychotic inpatients who are aggressive without access to alcohol and drugs, and in spite of supervised antipsychotic treatment. Thus, factors other than substance use and nonadherence to treatment must be involved in the pathophysiology of aggression in these patients.

From the standpoint of practical management of aggressive patients with major mental disorders, it seems that it could be fruitful to study in detail individual assaults in order to assess underlying pathophysiology. This is a promising avenue of research since it is generally agreed that aggressive behavior has multiple causes that differ among patients, and perhaps among different incidents in individual patients. Our experience, based on interviews of assailants, victims and witnesses, as well as on observations of videotapes, suggests that most assaults among psychiatric inpatients diagnosed with psychoses are not driven by psychotic symptoms. It appears that many of these assaults are attributable to comorbid personality disorders.

Personality Disorders

Antisocial personality disorder (APD) is partly defined by aggressive behavior and therefore it is not surprising that many violent psychotic patients meet its diagnostic criteria. This circularity of definition makes the use of this diagnosis somewhat unhelpful. The concept of "psychopathy", introduced to modern psychiatry by Cleckley (1976), is less circular since it relies primarily on personality and psychological processes rather than on criminal or aggressive behavior. Psychopathy is assessed by a valid and reliable checklist constructed by Hare and his coworkers (Hart *et al.*, 1992). Table 86.1 shows the screening version of the checklist intended for use in persons with serious mental illness (Hare, 1996; Hart *et al.*, 1995). The first six items in Factor-1 measure the severity of interpersonal and affective symptoms of psychop-

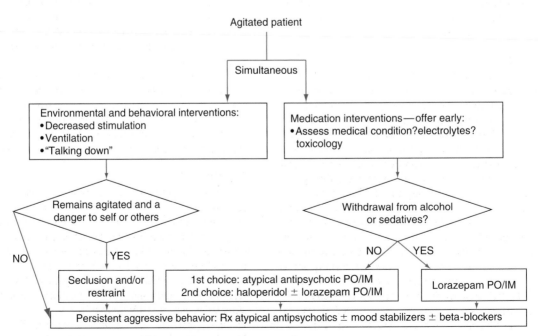

Figure 86.2   *Management of agitation: overview.*

Table 86.1	Hare Psychopathy Checklist (Screening Version)	
Factor 1: Interpersonal/ Affective	Factor 2: Social Deviance	
1. Superficial	7. Impulsive
2. Grandiose	8. Poor behavior controls
3. Manipulative	9. Lacks goals
4. Lacks remorse	10. Irresponsible
5. Lacks empathy	11. Adolescent antisocial behavior
6. Does not accept responsibility	12. Adult antisocial behavior

Table 86.2	Key Issues in Assessment of Acute Agitation/ Aggression/Violence
	1. Somatic conditions
	2. Previous history of violence
	3. Access to weapons
	4. Current ideation, including content of delusions
	5. Active substance abuse, including alcohol
	6. Comorbid antisocial personality disorder/traits or psychopathy
	7. Verbal threats
	8. Premonitory physical signs (clenched fist, pacing)

athy. The next six items in Factor-2 reflect the social deviance symptoms. Psychopathy is a narrower concept than APD. Most psychopaths meet the criteria for APD, but subjects diagnosed as APD do not necessarily meet the criteria for psychopathy. Psychopathy predicts violent behavior in nonpsychotic individuals (Hare and Hart, 1993), as well as in persons with major mental disorders (Hart *et al.*, 1994). The rates of comorbidity of psychopathy and schizophrenia are elevated among violent patients (Nolan *et al.*, 1999).

Differentiating aggressive behavior based on psychopathy from that based on psychotic symptoms has consequences for treatment. It is unlikely that psychopathy will respond to antipsychotics.

Acute Agitation

Agitation can be defined as excessive motor or verbal activity. Common examples include hyperactivity, verbal abuse, and threatening gestures and language. Unmanaged acute agitation can lead to violence. As such, acute agitation is a psychiatric emergency that requires rapid intervention. Oral medication treatment may be impractical or impossible. This section will focus on intramuscular medications within the context of a behavioral management plan.

Assessment

Key points in assessment are outlined in Table 86.2. The time available for patient assessment will be dependent on the acuity of the presentation. For someone who is acutely agitated and an immediate danger to self or others, emergency measures must be taken to avoid harm. Somatic conditions must be ruled out prior to initiating additional treatment, as an underlying metabolic, toxic, infectious, or other nonpsychiatric cause may need to be treated. In these cases the agitation is a symptom to be treated alongside the underlying condition. This is not as great a concern for the physically healthy psychiatric patient whose history is well known to the staff than for the relatively unknown patient presenting to the emergency room. In addition, in the nursing home environment, new-onset agitation may indicate a newly emerging somatic condition. Once the patient is under behavioral control further medical and psychiatric work-ups can be done. Mechanical restraints may be necessary to prevent the agitated patient from injuring himself/herself, or others, while the medical work-up is being conducted.

Care must be taken not to miss comorbid conditions of alcohol or sedative abuse or dependence that may present with acute intoxication or withdrawal. Such conditions will drive the treatment choice towards the use of a benzodiazepine (see later).

Assessment should also include the context of the agitation. Patients may be purposefully using aggressive behavior to intimidate others. Antisocial personality traits may be the most important factor in some instances of patient violence where goal-directed behavior such as extortion of money or cigarettes is present. These antisocial behaviors may not always be evident to staff, as they can occur in unsupervised areas such as hallways, bedrooms and bathrooms. Such predatory behavior may involve victims who are unable to articulate what is happening to them, while the aggressor appears to have an abundance of material goods or undue influence on others.

Where aggressive behavior may appear to be impulsive or random, environmental factors may be a significant factor. Some patients are transiently violent when in a chaotic environment, others are persistently violent no matter the milieu (Krakowski and Czobor, 1997). In contrast to the persistently violent patient, those who were transiently violent were more likely to respond to a new structured environment (Krakowski *et al.*, 1988). Environmental factors leading to increased aggressive behavior on a psychiatric ward include crowding (Palmstierna *et al.*, 1991; Ng *et al.*, 2001). It appears that the transiently violent are more responsive to typical antipsychotic medication and have less neurological impairment than the persistently violent patient (Volavka and Krakowski 1989).

It is generally agreed that it is impossible to predict with absolute certainty if a violent act will occur, but it is possible to assess risks. Past history of violence may be the best predictor of future violent behavior (Blomhoff *et al.*, 1990; Convit *et al.*, 1988; Karson and Bigelow, 1987), and obtaining a history of this, access to weapons, and current ideation are essential elements in risk assessment.

Treatment

Behavioral, psychological, and pharmacological interventions are used simultaneously (Citrome and Green, 1990). Clinicians are urged to survey the environment for potential weapons, not to turn their back on the patient, and to have other staff available. Taking verbal threats seriously and being aware of physical premonitory signs such as a clenched fist and pacing are important. Initially, an agitated patient should be isolated from other patients and from distractions because extraneous stimulation can intensify psychosis in a patient who may be hallucinating, paranoid and agitated. Moreover, other patients may intentionally or inadvertently interfere with treatment. Generally it is easier to clear the area of many calm patients than to move one dangerous individual. Restraint or seclusion may be necessary, and this is the time where the risk for injury for both staff and patients is highest. The technique of the calming blanket, a soft comforter with canvas reinforcements, may be helpful in subduing the patient who is punching, scratching, or kicking.

Psychotherapeutic Approaches

Nonspecific sedation is often used in the management of an acutely agitated patient. In general, intramuscular injection of a sedative has a faster onset of action than oral administration but it has been observed that a patient may calm down readily after an oral dose, knowing that action has been taken and help is being provided. Previously, choice of intramuscular medication for these behavioral emergencies has been limited to typical antipsychotics (such as haloperidol or chlorpromazine) versus benzodiazepines (principally lorazepam) (Table 86.3). The availability of intramuscular formulations of novel atypical antipsychotics provides additional treatment options for the management of acute agitation in patients with psychosis (Citrome, 2002). Lorazepam, the only benzodiazepine that is reliably absorbed when administered intramuscularly, appears to be a good rational choice when treating an acute episode of agitation, especially where the etiology is not clear such as when a patient with a history of schizophrenia may actually be withdrawing from alcohol (Salzman, 1988; Greenblatt *et al.*, 1979, 1982). Caution is required when respiratory depression is a possibility. There may be increased risk of this in patients with sleep apnea (associated with being morbidly obese, history of snoring and daytime drowsiness). Lorazepam is not recommended for long-term daily use because of the problems associated with tolerance, dependence and withdrawal. Paradoxical reactions to benzodiazepines, as exhibited by hostility or violence has been an area of concern (Bond and Lader, 1979), but the evidence is not convincing and, in any event, such reactions are uncommon (Dietch and Jennings, 1988). The possibility of alcohol or sedative withdrawal as a cause of agitation is another point in favor of using lorazepam.

The typical antipsychotics cause sedation, given in a high enough dose. Haloperidol, a high potency butyrophenone, has been frequently used as an intramuscular prn medication for agitation and aggressive behavior in an emergency department setting for a wide variety of patients (Clinton *et al.*, 1987). Depending on the clinical response, subsequent doses may be administered as often as every hour if necessary. However, 4- to 8-hour intervals may be satisfactory. Haloperidol's advantage over the low potency typical antipsychotics (e.g., chlorpromazine) is that it causes less hypotension, fewer anticholinergic side effects, and causes less of a decrease in the seizure threshold. In addition to this nonspecific sedation, a benefit would be its antipsychotic effect (in responsive patients), but this would be evident only after the acute episode of agitation has subsided. High doses of typical antipsychotics may lead to more adverse effects, including akathisia, which may itself provoke violent behavior (Keckich, 1978; Siris, 1985).

The new atypical antipsychotics may emerge as important options in the management of acute agitation in schizophrenia. Although sedation or "calming" remains the primary mode of action when used emergently in the acutely agitated patient, the atypical antipsychotics have several advantages over typical antipsychotics (Citrome, 1997), in particular a lower propensity for extrapyramidal side effects, including akathisia.

Long-term Treatment

The treatment goal is to decrease the frequency and intensity of aggressive behavior. Specialized units such as secure or psychiatric intensive care units (Musisi *et al.*, 1989; Goldney *et al.*, 1985; Warneke, 1986; Citrome *et al.*, 1995) provide a structured environment that optimizes staff and patient safety. In general these specialized units are staffed with persons trained in interacting with volatile and difficult to manage patients (Maier *et al.*, 1987). When available, these units can be a valuable resource for education, training, consultation and referral.

Although pharmacotherapy remains a mainstay of treatment for the persistently aggressive patient, behavioral plans need to be used in tandem. Providing structure, including the use of behavioral contracts, can be useful. Preventive aggression devices (PADS) are a form of ambulatory restraints, which can be used as an alternative to seclusion (Van Rybroek *et al.*, 1987). The technique was first developed for a specialized inpatient unit

Table 86.3   Pharmacological Options for Acute Agitation–Intramuscular Agents

Agent	Dose (mg)	Half-life (h)	Comments
Lorazepam	0.5–2	10–20	There are no active metabolites. Can be administered orally, sublingually, intramuscularly, or intravenously.
Haloperidol	0.5–7.5	12–36	Can combine with lorazepam in the same syringe (combination of haloperidol 5 mg and lorazepam 2 mg is commonly used).
Droperidol	2.5–5	2	QTc prolongation. Withdrawn in UK.
Olanzapine	10 (2.5 for patients with dementia)	34–38	Superiority over haloperidol (schizophrenia) and lorazepam (bipolar disorder) in clinical trials.
Ziprasidone	10–20	2.2–3.4	Superiority over haloperidol (schizophrenia) in clinical trials. QTc prolongation.

with repetitively aggressive patients. Patients in these wrist-to-belt and/or ankle–ankle restraints can remain with their peers on the ward, eat their meals and interact, yet are prevented from striking out and injuring others. In combination with a comprehensive behavior modification program, these patients can be weaned off the use of the ambulatory restraints.

Although pharmacotherapy for the longer-term management of aggressive behavior is somewhat dependent on the patient's underlying diagnosis, clinical management is often complicated and can entail the use of several coprescribed medications. At the core of impulsive aggressive behavior may be a dysregulation of the serotonergic neurotransmitter system and this may explain the possible ameliorative effects of atypical antipsychotics and the selective serotonin reuptake inhibitors (SSRIs). In addition, beta-blockers and moodstabilizers have been used with some success. Table 86.4 outlines the medication strategies useful in patients with aggressive behavior and schizophrenia. Nonadherence to a treatment regimen may require the use of outpatient commitment, now available in many jurisdictions.

Atypical Antipsychotics

The availability of atypical antipsychotics has led to the observation that these agents may act differently from the older antipsychotics in that they may specifically target aggressive behavior. Several retrospective studies have demonstrated a decrease in the number of violent episodes and/or a decrease in the use of seclusion or restraint among inpatients after they began clozapine treatment (Wilson and Claussen, 1995; Ratey *et al.*, 1993; Chiles *et al.*, 1994; Mallya *et al.*, 1992; Spivak *et al.*, 1997; Maier, 1992; Ebrahim *et al.*, 1994). At this time, the weight of the evidence favors clozapine as specific antiaggressive treatment for schizophrenia patients (Glazer and Dickson, 1998), with demonstrated superiority to haloperidol and risperidone (Citrome *et al.*, 2001). More research is needed to compare the other atypical antipsychotics with clozapine for this indication. Ideally, such studies

need to be done double-blind with subjects specially selected because of their aggressive behavior. This is operationally quite difficult because of a number of logistical factors, including the relative rarity of aggressive events and consequent need for a large sample size and lengthy baseline and trial periods, as well as selection/consent bias (Volavka and Citrome, 1999).

Mood Stabilizers

There is an expectation that adjunctive mood stabilizers can reduce aggressive and impulsive behavior (Citrome, 1995). This is understandable when the primary diagnosis is bipolar or schizoaffective disorder where the mood stabilizer is treating the core symptoms of the disorder, but these agents, notably valproate, lithium and carbamazepine, are also used, though less frequently, in patients with schizophrenia.

Beta-blockers

Beta-adrenergic blockers, in particular propranolol, have been used in the treatment of aggressive behavior in brain injured patients (Yudofsky *et al.*, 1981, 1984). Propranolol has also been used as an adjunctive treatment for schizophrenia, and a reduction in symptoms, including aggression, was found (Sheppard, 1979). Nadolol may also be helpful (Ratey *et al.*, 1992; Alpert *et al.*, 1990; Allan *et al.*, 1996). Beta-blockers may exert some of their effects by decreasing akathisia, which in turn may decrease agitation.

Benzodiazepines

Clonazepam, a high potency benzodiazepine, had been reported useful in patients with bipolar disorder. This result is in contrast to a double-blind placebo-controlled trial of adjunctive clonazepam in 13 schizophrenic patients receiving antipsychotics (Karson *et al.*, 1982). In that study no additional therapeutic benefit was observed and, in fact, four patients demonstrated violent behavior during the course of clonazepam treatment.

Table 86.4   Pharmacological Options for Persistent Aggressive Behavior in Schizophrenia

Class of Agent	Basis of Evidence	Comments
Atypical antipsychotics	Case reports, retrospective record reviews, secondary analyses of randomized clinical trials	Best evidence exists for clozapine, some evidence for olanzapine and quetiapine, and conflicting evidence for risperidone. Insufficient information for ziprasidone.
Mood stabilizers	Case reports, retrospective record reviews, few randomized clinical trials	Although mood stabilizers are helpful in bipolar disorder, evidence in schizophrenia is not as strong. Best evidence exists for valproate, some for carbamazepine, and conflicting evidence for lithium. Insufficient information for gabapentin, topiramate, oxcarbazepine.
β-blockers	Case reports, retrospective record reviews, few randomized clinical trials	Best studied in patients with brain injuries. Some evidence demonstrating usefulness in schizophrenia for propranolol and nadolol.
SSRIs	Case reports, one randomized clinical trial	Adjunctive citalopram found helpful in a randomized double-blind study (Vartiainen *et al.*, 1995).
Benzodiazepines	Case reports, one randomized clinical trial	Negative outcomes (patients worsened) in a randomized double-blind study of adjunctive clonazepam (Karson *et al.*, 1982).

Using lorazepam for long-term management (in contrast to acute use as a "prn") can be problematic because of physiological tolerance. Missing scheduled doses of lorazepam may result in withdrawal symptoms that can lead to agitation or excitement, as well as irritability and a greater risk for aggressive behavior.

Antidepressants

The current interest in certain antidepressants' role in aggression is based on the crucial role of serotonergic regulation of impulsive aggression against self and others. A number of reports have emerged that posit a role for fluoxetine (Goldman and Janecek, 1990), citalopram (Vartiainen *et al.*, 1995) and fluvoxamine (Silver and Kushnir, 1998) in the treatment of persistent aggressive behavior.

Adjunctive Electroconvulsive Therapy

Although not often considered as a first-line treatment, adjunctive electroconvulsive therapy (ECT) may be helpful in patients who have inadequately-responsive psychotic symptoms (Fink and Sackeim, 1996). An open trial of ECT in combination with risperidone in male patients with schizophrenia and aggression resulted in a reduction in aggressive behavior for nine of the 10 patients (Hirose *et al.*, 2001). The combination of ECT and clozapine may also be helpful. A review of 36 reported cases treated with this combination, all of whom with a history of treatment-resistance, revealed that approximately two-thirds benefited from this treatment (Kupchik *et al.*, 2000).

Conclusion

The effective management of aggression is a priority for clinicians. Strategies to control acute agitation include the use of mechanical restraints and the administration of parenteral medication. Early intervention is important to avoid further escalation to violence. An overview is presented in Figure 86.2. The new intramuscular formulations of atypical antipsychotics hold promise quickly and efficaciously to control acute agitation, without the side-effect burdens of the older typical antipsychotics. Lorazepam remains a first choice for patients withdrawing from alcohol or sedatives and presenting with agitation. Longer-term management may include the use of a specialized hospital unit, if available. Treatment of the underlying disorder is key, but this may be complicated by a history of poor response to standard treatments. Lorazepam for long-term daily use is not recommended because of problems associated with tolerance, dependence and withdrawal. Clozapine appears to be the most effective antipsychotic in reducing aggressivity in patients with schizophrenia and schizoaffective disorder. Valproate and carbamazepine can be used with antipsychotics to decrease the intensity and frequency of agitation and poor impulse control, but they have not been extensively studied under double-blind placebo-controlled conditions for this indication. Beta-blockers and SSRIs may also be helpful. Adjunctive ECT, together with atypical antipsychotics, may be considered for patients who have failed other approaches.

References

Allan E, Alpert M, Sison C *et al.* (1996) Adjunctive nadolol in the treatment of acutely aggressive schizophrenic patients. *J Clin Psychiatr* 57, 455–459.

Alpert M, Allan ER, Citrome L *et al.* (1990) A double-blind, placebo-controlled study of adjunctive nadolol in the management of violent psychiatric patients. *Psychopharmacol Bull* 26, 367–371.

Arseneault L, Moffitt TE, Caspi A, et al. (2000) Mental disorders and violence in a total birth cohort. *Arch Gen Psychiatr* 57, 979–986.

Blomhoff S, Seim S and Friis S (1990) Can prediction of violence among psychiatric inpatients be improved? *Hosp Comm Psychiatr* 41, 771–775.

Bond A and Lader M (1979) Benzodiazepines and aggression, in *Psychopharmacology of Aggression*, (ed Sandler M). Raven Press, New York, pp. 173–182.

Brennan PA, Sarnoff SA, and Hodgins S (2000) Major mental disorders and criminal violence in a Danish birth cohort. *Arch Gen Psychiatr* 57, 494–500.

Chiles JA, Davidson P and McBride D (1994) Effects of clozapine on use of seclusion and restraint at a state hospital. *Hosp Comm Psychiatr* 45, 269–271.

Citrome L (1995) Use of lithium, carbamazepine, and valproic acid in a state-operated psychiatric hospital. *J Pharm Technol* 11, 55–59.

Citrome L (1997) New antipsychotic medications: What advantages do they offer? *Postgrad Med* 101, 207–214.

Citrome L (2002) Aggression and intramuscular antipsychotics: New options for acute agitation. *Postgrad Med* (in press).

Citrome L and Green L (1990) The dangerous agitated patient: What to do right now. *Postgrad Med* 87, 231–236.

Citrome L, Green L and Fost R (1995) Clinical and administrative consequences of a reduced census on a psychiatric intensive care unit. *Psychiatr Q* 66, 209–217.

Citrome L, Volavka J, Czobor P *et al.* (2001) Effects of clozapine, olanzapine, risperidone, and haloperidol on hostility among patients with schizophrenia. *Psychiatr Serv* 52, 1510–1514.

Cleckley H (1976) *The Mask of Sanity*, 5th edn. The CV Mosby Company, Saint Louis.

Clinton JE, Sterner S, Stelmachers Z *et al.* (1987) Haloperidol for sedation of disruptive emergency patients. *Ann Emerg Med* 16, 319–322.

Convit A, Jaeger J, Lin SP *et al.* (1988) Predicting assaultiveness in psychiatric inpatients: A pilot study. *Hosp Comm Psychiatr* 39, 429–434.

Dietch JT and Jennings RK (1988) Aggressive dyscontrol in patients treated with benzodiazepines. *J Clin Psychiatr* 49, 184–188.

Ebrahim GM, Gibler B, Gacono CB *et al.* (1994) Patient response to clozapine in a forensic psychiatric hospital. *Hosp Comm Psychiatr* 45, 271–273.

Eronen M, Hakola P, and Tiihonen J (1996) Mental disorders and homicidal behavior in Finland. *Arch Gen Psychiatr* 53, 497–501.

Fink M and Sackeim HA (1996) Convulsive therapy in schizophrenia. *Schizophr Bull* 22, 27–39.

Glazer WM and Dickson RA (1998) Clozapine reduces violence and persistent aggression in schizophrenia. *J Clin Psychiatr* 59(Suppl 3), 8–14.

Goldman MB and Janecek HM (1990) Adjunctive fluoxetine improves global function in chronic schizophrenia. *J Neuropsychiatr Clin Neurosci* 2, 429–431.

Goldney R, Bowes J, Spence N *et al.* (1985) The psychiatric intensive care unit. *Br J Psychiatr* 146, 50–54.

Greenblatt DJ, Shader RI, Franke K *et al.* (1979) Pharmacokinetics and bioavailability of intravenous, intramuscular, and oral lorazepam in humans. *J Pharm Sci* 68, 57–63.

Greenblatt DJ, Divoll M, Harmatz JS *et al.* (1982) Pharmacokinetic comparison of sublingual lorazepam with intravenous, intramuscular, and oral lorazepam. *J Pharm Sci* 71, 248–252.

Hare RD (1996) Psychopathy and antisocial personality disorder: A case of diagnostic confusion. *Psychiatr Times* (Feb), 39–40.

Hare RD and Hart SD (1993) Psychopathy, mental disorder, and crime, in *Mental Disorder and Crime* (ed Hodgins S). Sage Publications, Newbury Park, pp. 104–115.

Hart SD, Cox DN and Hare RD (1995) *The Hare PCL: SV: Psychopathy Checklist: Screening Version.* Multi-Health Systems, North Tonowanda, NY.

Hart SD, Hare RD, and Harpur TJ (1992) The psychopathy checklist-revised (PCL-R): An overview for researchers and clinicains. In Advances in Psychological Assessment, Rosen JC and McReynolds P (eds). Plenum Press, New York, pp. 103–130.

Hart SD, Hare RD and Forth AE (1994) Psychopathy as a risk marker for violence: Development and validation of a screening version of the revised psychopathy checklist, in *Violence and Mental Disorder, Developments in Risk Assessment* (eds Monahan J and Steadman HJ). The University of Chicago Press, Chicago, pp. 81–98.

Hirose S, Ashby CR and Mills MJ (2001) Effectiveness of ECT combined with risperidone against aggression in schizophrenia. *J ECT* 17, 22–26.

Hodgins S (1992) Mental disorder, intellectual deficiency, and crime: Evidence from a birth cohort. *Arch Gen Psychiatr* 49, 476–483.

Hodgins S, Mednick SA, Brennan PA, et al. (1996) Mental disorder and crime: Evidence from a Danish birth cohort. *Arch Gen Psychiatr* 53, 489–496.

Karson C and Bigelow LB (1987) Violent behavior in schizophrenic inpatients. *J Nerv Ment Dis* 175, 161–164.

Karson CN, Weinberger DR, Bigelow L *et al.* (1982) Clonazepam treatment of chronic schizophrenia: Negative results in a double-blind, placebo-controlled trial. *Am J Psychiatr* 139, 1627–1628.

Keckich WA (1978) Neuroleptics. Violence as a manifestation of akathisia. *JAMA* 240, 2185.

Krakowski M and Czobor P (1997) Violence in psychiatric patients: The role of psychosis, frontal lobe impairment, and ward turmoil. *Compr Psychiatr* 38, 230–236.

Krakowski M, Convit A and Volavka J (1988) Patterns of inpatient assaultiveness: Effect of neurological impairment and deviant family environment on response to treatment. *Neuropsychiatr Neuropsychol Behav Neurol* 1, 21–29.

Kupchik M, Spivak B, Mester R *et al.* (2000) Combined electroconvulsive-clozapine therapy. *Clin Neuropharmacol* 23, 14–16.

Kyriacou DN, Anglin D, Taliaferro E *et al.* (1999) Risk factors for injury to women from domestic violence against women. *NEJM* 341, 1892–1898.

Link BG, Cullen FT, and Andrews H (1992) The violent and illegal behavior of mental patients reconsidered. *Am Social Rev* 57, 275–292.

Maier GJ (1992) The impact of clozapine on 25 forensic patients. *Bull Am Acad Psychiatr Law* 20, 297–307.

Maier GJ, Stava LJ, Morrow BR *et al.* (1987) A model for understanding and managing cycles of aggression among psychiatric inpatients. *Hosp Comm Psychiatr* 38, 520–524.

Mallya AR, Roos PD and Roebuck-Colgan K (1992) Restraint, seclusion, and clozapine. *J Clin Psychiatr* 53, 395–397.

Musisi SM, Wasylenki DA and Rapp MS (1989) A psychiatric intensive care unit in a psychiatric hospital. *Can J Psychiatr* 34, 200–204.

Ng B, Kumar S, Ranclaud M *et al.* (2001) Ward crowding and incidents of violence on an acute psychiatric inpatient unit. *Psychiatr Serv* 52, 521–525.

Nolan KA, Volavka J, Mohr P *et al.* (1999) Psychopathy and violent behavior among patients with schizophrenia or schizoaffective disorder. *Psychiatr Serv* 50, 787–792.

Palmstierna T, Huitfeldt B and Wistedt B (1991) The relationship of crowding and aggressive behavior on a psychiatric intensive care unit. *Hosp Comm Psychiatr* 42, 1237–1240.

Pastore AL and Maguire K (eds) (2000) *Sourcebook for Criminal Justice Statistics.* US Department of Justice, Bureau of Justice Statistics, Washington DC.

Ratey JJ, Leveroni C, Kilmer D *et al.* (1993) The effects of clozapine on severely aggressive psychiatric inpatients in a state hospital. *J Clin Psychiatr* 54, 219–223.

Ratey JJ, Sorgi P, O'Driscoll GA *et al.* (1992) Nadolol to treat aggression and psychiatric symptomatology in chronic psychiatric inpatients: A double-blind, placebo-controlled study. *J Clin Psychiatr* 53, 41–46.

Regier DA, Farmer ME, Rae DS *et al.* (1990) Comorbidity of mental disorders with alcohol and other drug abuse. Results from the Epidemiologic Catchment Area (ECA) Study. *JAMA* 264, 2511–2518.

Salzman C (1988) Use of benzodiazepines to control disruptive behavior in inpatients. *J Clin Psychiatr* 49(Suppl 12), 13–15.

Sheppard GP (1979) High-dose propranolol in schizophrenia. *Br J Psychiatr* 134, 470–476.

Silver H and Kushnir M (1998) Treatment of aggression in schizophrenia. *Am J Psychiatr* 155, 1298.

Siris SG (1985) Three cases of akathisia and "acting out." *J Clin Psychiatr* 46, 395–397.

Spivak B, Mester R, Wittenberg N *et al.* (1997) Reduction of aggressiveness and impulsiveness during clozapine treatment in chronic neuroleptic-resistant schizophrenic patients. *Clin Neuropharmacol* 20, 442–446.

Steadman HJ, Mulvey EP, Monahan J, et al. (1998) Violence by people discharged from acute psychiatric inpatient facilities and others in the same neighborhoods. *Arch Gen Psychiatr* 55, 393–401.

Swanson JW (1994) Mental disorder, substance abuse, and community violence: An epidemiological approach, in *Violence and Mental Disorder. Developments in Risk Assessment* (eds Monahan J and Steadman HJ). The University of Chicago Press, Chicago, pp. 101–136.

Swartz MS, Swanson JW, Hiday VA *et al.* (1998) Violence and severe mental illness: The effects of substance abuse and nonadherence to medication. *Am J Psychiatr* 155, 226–231.

Tiihonen J, Isohanni M, Rasanen P, et al. (1997) Specific major mental disorders and criminality: A 26-year prospective study of the 1966 Northern Finland birth cohort. *Am J Psychiatr* 154, 840–845.

Van Rybroek GJ, Kuhlman TL, Maier GJ *et al.* (1987) Preventive aggression devices (PADS): Ambulatory restraints as an alternative to seclusion. *J Clin Psychiatr* 48, 401–405.

Vartiainen H, Tiihonen J, Putkonen A *et al.* (1995) Citalopram, a selective serotonin reuptake inhibitor, in the treatment of aggression in schizophrenia. *Acta Psychiatr Scand* 91, 348–351.

Volavka J and Citrome L (1999) Atypical antipsychotics in the treatment of the persistently aggressive psychotic patient: Methodological concerns. *Schizophr Res* 35, S23–S33.

Volavka J (2002) Neurobiology of Violence, 2nd ed. American Psychiatric Publishing, Washington DC.

Volavka J and Krakowski M (1989) Schizophrenia and violence. *Psychol Med* 19, 559–562.

Volavka J, Laska E, Baker S *et al.* (1997) History of violent behavior and schizophrenia in different cultures. *Br J Psychiatr* 171, 9–14.

Warneke L (1986) A psychiatric intensive care unit in a general hospital setting. *Can J Psychiatr* 31(9), 834–837.

Wallace C, Mullen P, Burgess P, et al. (1998) Serious criminal offending and mental disorder. *Br J Psychiatr* 172, 477–484.

Wilson WH and Claussen AM (1995) Eighteen-month outcome of clozapine treatment for 100 patients in a state psychiatric hospital. *Psychiatr Serv* 46, 386–389.

Yudofsky S, Williams D, and Gorman J (1981) Propranolol in the treatment of rage and violent behavior in patients with chronic brain syndrome. *Am J Psychiatr* 138, 218–220.

Yudofsky SC, Stevens L, Silver JM *et al.* (1984) Propranolol in the treatment of rage and violent behavior associated with Korsakoff's psychosis. *Am J Psychiatr* 141, 114–115.

Combined Therapies: Psychotherapy and Pharmacotherapy

The rationale for combining treatment modalities is based on the idea that the strengths of each modality are promoted while the weaknesses are minimized, producing results that are better than with either modality alone (Hollon and Fawcett, 1995). Although intuitively this rings true, psychiatrists have a duty to incorporate evidence-based approaches into their clinical practice. While most evidence-based mental health research in the literature is based on efficacy studies, there has been a recent move towards conducting effectiveness studies that are hoped to be of increased relevance to general outpatient clinical practice (Nathan *et al.*, 2000). Table 87.1 highlights the differences between efficacy and effectiveness research (Barlow, 1996; Nathan *et al.*, 2000). Recent literature examining the efficacies of combined treatment (not necessarily integrated treatment by a psychiatrist) vary by disorder, timing of treatments and whether administered during the acute or maintenance phase. Recent literature has also examined the sequential application of combined treatment (Fava *et al.*, 2001; Frank *et al.*, 2000). Effectiveness studies are far fewer, as mentioned, and do not always demonstrate superiority of combined approaches over either medication or therapy alone.

Hollon and Fawcett (1995) have outlined four ways in which combined treatment may prove advantageous over either treatment alone: increase the magnitude, probability, or breadth of clinical response, and increase the acceptability to the patient of either modality. In general, they feel that there is literature to support the statement that combined treatment enhances the breadth of clinical response. It is within this context that clinical practice guidelines published by the Agency for Health Care Policy and Research support the use of combined treatment in depressive disorders (Depression Guideline Panel, 1993).

Various authors discuss the potential benefits of employing pharmacotherapy within a psychotherapeutic context (Klerman, 1991; Kay, 2001). Pharmacotherapy has been noted to have a quicker onset of action on acute symptoms than most psychotherapies, perhaps with the exclusion of cognitive therapy (Hollon and Fawcett, 2001). It is felt that this rapid dampening of symptoms may enhance the patient's ability to more productively participate in therapy by a variety of mechanisms. These have been described cogently by Klerman (1985, 1991) and include enhancing the patient's self-esteem, creating a safe environment in which emotions are more freely discussed, reducing the stigma of

seeking mental health care through a positive placebo effect, improving cognition (verbalization and abreaction), and functioning as a transitional object during breaks in therapy, among others.

The benefits of employing psychotherapy within a primarily psychopharmacologic relationship have also been described. Empirical evidence exists across the spectrum of mental health disorders to support the following suggested benefits of adding psychotherapy to medications. It decreases the incidence of illness relapse (Hogarty *et al.*, 1986), as well as symptom relapse upon medication discontinuation (Wiborg and Dahl, 1996; Spiegel *et al.*, 1994). It fosters the patient's ability to utilize healthy coping strategies, addresses issues that are not typically targeted by psychopharmacologic treatment such as dysfunctional relationship patterns or negative self-appraisals due to traumatic past events, and enhances psychotropic compliance (Paykel, 1995; Cochran, 1984).

Clinical Applications: Treatment Adherence

Adherence may be enhanced in part through discussion of the patient's metaphor for the medication, either positive or negative (Kay, 2001). Clinical vignettes 1 and 2 illustrate a patient's frequently held conceptions regarding medication use.

The above case highlights one of the beliefs that patients may have regarding medications, that is, they indicate their provider's level of interest in them as a person and the provider truly appreciates the level of their distress. In certain contexts these beliefs may be regarded as a "positive metaphor"; however in others, as demonstrated above, it may hinder the patient's response to treatment, their compliance with the treatment regimen, and their level of trust in their provider.

Clinical Applications: Sequential Treatment

Fava (1999) highlights that sequential treatments may be applied in four ways: 1) using a second type of psychotherapy when the first orientation has not fully achieved treatment goals; 2) introducing a second type of pharmacotherapy when the first medication has not achieved adequate symptom relief; 3) introducing psychotherapy when initial pharmacotherapy has not been fully effective; and 4) introducing pharmacotherapy when initial psychotherapy has not been fully effective. The latter two may include use of combined treatments in a sequential fashion. Clinical Vignette 1 was an example of the third method; Clinical Vignette 2 highlights the fourth method.

Essentials of Psychiatry   Jerald Kay and Allan Tasman
© 2006 John Wiley & Sons, Ltd.

Table 87.1   Efficacy and Effectiveness Research – Comparison

	Efficacy	Effectiveness
Definition	The methodical assessment of an intervention in a controlled clinical trial setting	The assessment of an intervention for pertinence and practicality in a routine clinical practice setting
Type of intervention assessed	Any; may be experimental	Only those with established efficacy
Study population	Homogeneous	Those in need of treatment
Diagnosis	Exclude comorbidity	Comorbidity common
Illness severity, length of illness	Narrow range	Broad range
Inclusion/exclusion criteria	Strict	Few
Need for randomization/control group	Yes	No
Provision of psychotherapy intervention	Strict adherence to intervention, use of treatment manuals common	No requirement for use of/adherence to treatment manuals
Emphasis	Internal validity	External validity
	Replicability	Generalizability

Reprinted with permission from Barlow DH (1996) Health care policy, psychotherapy research, and the future of psychotherapy. *Am Psychol* 51, 1050–1058; Nathan PE, Stuart SP and Dolan SL (2000) Research on psychotherapy efficacy and effectiveness: Between Scylla and charbodis? *Psychol Bull* 126(6) (Nov), 964–981. Copyright, American Psychiatric Press.

Clinical Vignette 1

Ms E, a married 38-year-old with a diagnosis of major depressive disorder, recurrent and severe, and dependent personality disorder presents as a referral to Dr A for continued care due to the retirement of the psychiatrist whom she had been seeing in 15-minute medication management appointments over the past year. Ms E's symptoms included poor energy, anhedonia, lack of libido, intermittent suicidal ideation without a prior history of attempts, trouble concentrating and complaints of "memory loss". Ms E's current stressors include her father's terminal illness and longstanding marital conflicts. Ms E's father, sister and brother all suffer from an affective disorder. A review of the patient's records reveals a complex medication regimen, with frequent medication changes and poor symptom control. Ms E seemed to do well initially on new medications, often responding within a day or two, but then would have her spouse call the psychiatrist on her behalf to report that the effects of the medication had "worn off". Dr A and Ms E agreed to initiate brief psychotherapy, in addition to medication management, due to the persistence of her symptoms despite trials of various psychotropics. During the course of her first session, she revealed a distant relationship with her father, who had been a physician. She found him aloof and unnurturing, except for those times in which she was ill, during which he often directed her medical care. Dr A made no changes to Ms E's medication regimen at the first visit. At her next visit, Ms E commented to Dr A that she greatly missed her former psychiatrist whom she described as "really knew what he was doing with my meds, and understood the depth of my suffering". She asked for a referral to a new psychiatrist as she felt Dr A and herself were "just not a good fit".

Ms E eventually agreed to continue seeing Dr A "for a few more sessions". Dr A explored the psychological meaning that Ms E had been attributing to medication interventions. She was eventually able to recognize that changes in her psychotropic regimen did not have to occur for her to feel that others understood her. Ms E was able to look at connections between her past and her current reactions within the patient–provider relationship (exploration of countertransference issues), as well as within other interpersonal relationships including her marriage. Her medication regimen was simplified, she maintained compliance with her treatment plan, and she achieved remission of her depressive symptoms.

Clinical Vignette 2

Mr B is a 40-year-old executive for a major corporation who has been recently diagnosed with panic disorder with agoraphobia by a psychiatry resident (Dr C). Mr B reports that for the past 6 months he has experienced panic attacks three or four times each day which involve "a sudden intense wave of fear that seems to come out of nowhere", usually during the day, but sometimes waking him up from sleep. During these attacks, he reports symptoms of a racing heart rate, sweating, feelings of nausea, trembling, and a fear of losing control and doing something crazy, like running through his corporate office while yelling at people to get out of his way. Mr B's panic attacks have become so frequent and intense that he can no longer perform his job and relies on other junior executives to manage the company. In fact, he avoids business travel because he fears becoming incapacitated from panic on an airplane. Recently, he has also begun to avoid staff meetings out of concern that a panic attack will occur and that he would have to leave unexpectedly.

Due to the severity of Mr B's panic and avoidance symptoms, the resident suggests a trial of medication for the patient. After discussing medication options with the patient, Mr B decides he would prefer not to take medication because he fears "losing control" or "getting addicted to pills". Although the resident attempted to allay some of the patient's fears about the medication, Mr B persisted in his reluctance to the treatment and even expressed his concern that the resident "must really think I'm crazy if you think I need pills!"

In light of Mr B's resistance to medication, the resident considers the use of cognitive–behavioral therapy (CBT) in order to supply the patient with action-oriented, self-directed behavioral approaches, such as relaxation and exposure exercises. In addition, the resident addresses the patient's cognitive distortions regarding issues of control and beliefs that he is "crazy". Psychotherapy also reveals that Mr B's father was alcoholic and his mother abused benzodiazepines, which explains some of the patient's belief system regarding medications.

After five sessions of CBT, Mr B recognizes only a slight reduction in the frequency of panic attacks and agrees to an "experiment" in which he would start taking medication with a slow increase in dosage. For each subsequent session, the resident follows a structured format by asking the patient for a brief update, check on anxiety, and discussion of the medication's side effects. The resident reviews the previous session and collects Mr B's homework regarding the frequency and severity of self-monitored panic/anxiety; checking for medication treatment results and side effects. The patient practices cognitive reframing regarding any mental or physiological changes he noticed while on the medication. This reframing involves teaching the patient to use self-dialogue to view physiological changes as either expected minor medication side effects that are temporary, or as simply a nonmedication, normal physiological status change that the patient misperceives as a sign of something horribly wrong. The reframing process is accomplished by educating the patient to challenge his distorted belief systems during sessions and then the resident and patient collaboratively set homework assignments. After 15 additional sessions of integrated CT and medication, Mr B is panic-free but continues to receive treatment to address some mild avoidance features.

As demonstrated by the vignettes, the meanings that the patient attributes to medication may have to do with cognitions and feelings in a variety of spheres including the illness, the provider, and themselves (Beck, 2001).

Clinical Applications: Advantages and Challenges

The vignettes also serve to highlight potential benefits and challenges surrounding integrated treatment described by Kay (2001). In Clinical Vignette 2, rapport is well established, precluding the need to reestablish rapport and for the patient to retell his "story"

to yet another provider. Integrated treatment essentially eliminates the communication difficulties encountered in split treatment settings. The practitioner of integrated treatment does face some obstacles. In both cases, the psychiatrist needs to be well trained in a variety of psychotherapy orientations, particularly in the orientation that has evidence to support its use in a particular disorder.

Clinical Vignette 1 highlights the importance of a thorough assessment of the patient using a biopsychosocial approach as described by Engel (1977). To provide a theoretical framework for formulation of the patient and treatment plan, McHugh and Slavney (1983) similarly discuss understanding the psychiatrically ill patient from four "perspectives". These multifactorial models of mental health illnesses serve as conceptual tools with which to understand the whole patient and those forces that together precipitate, perpetuate and modify illness course/progression. It stands to reason that a provider of integrated care should utilize an "integrated" model of illness description, etiology and treatment.

When a single provider directs both forms of treatment, traditional role conflicts may emerge. The role stereotype of a psychotherapist may include one who has a multidimensional understanding of the patient, is interested in intrapsychic/core conflicts and their manifestations in symptoms, behaviors, feelings and thoughts, and whose style is less authoritarian. The pharmacotherapist's traditional role stereotype is of a biological/neurochemical understanding of the patient and a prescriptive, structured, more authoritarian style in approaching diagnosis, medications and other issues. While these roles are, as described, stereotypic, they do have in common the role of the provider in establishing rapport and a therapeutic alliance with the patient. It has been suggested that the psychiatrist who uses an integrated model provides more time for development of the therapeutic alliance thus increasing the patient's comfort in disclosing embarrassing side effects of medication and, perhaps, even aiding in treatment outcome via the strength of the alliance (Gabbard and Kay, 2001). Psychotherapy studies have suggested that therapist variables accounted for 30% of the variance in outcomes, and that therapeutic alliance is perhaps the most important factor in positive treatment outcomes (Lambert, 1992; Svartberg *et al.*, 1998). The therapeutic alliance is crucial; as such, management of transitions between roles, as well as the seamless integration of roles is imperative within the practice of integrated treatment (Gabbard and Kay, 2001). These role transitions may occur rapidly and within a single session.

A familiarity with current literature and clinical practice guidelines concerning when to employ medications alone, therapy alone, or both, and when sequential treatments may lead to a greater probability of remission is a must for any clinician utilizing combined treatment.

Clinical Applications: Managing the Session

This example highlights one way in which to fluidly incorporate both domains (psychotherapy and pharmacotherapy) within each patient visit. The above approach is structured in nature, following cognitive therapy's principle that sessions are structured and remain constant during therapy (Beck, 1995). Providers of psychodynamic therapy, among other types of therapy, often prefer this structured type of approach, advocating that medication use either be discussed at the beginning or at the end of the session. Proponents of the beginning method feel that discussion of medication issues ensures adequate time is spent on concerns and may provide important material for the session. Advocates of the "set aside 5 to 10 minutes at the end of the session" approach feel that it is most important for the patients to set their own agenda, as this allows for time needed for the patient to regain composure/recompensate before the end of the session. Another approach is the nonstructured method. In this case the therapist addresses medication issues only when the need arises. As there are no evidence-based studies to guide clinical practice, it is most important to base the choice on patient and provider preference and to practice consistency with each patient (Kay, 2002).

Clinical Applications: Individualizing Treatment

How can the psychiatrist tailor his/her treatment options to each individual patient? When would sequential approaches be indicated and in which disorders are combined treatments most likely to be helpful? During which phase of treatment (acute versus maintenance) should combined treatments be used versus solo treatments (either medications or therapy)? For what severity of illness are combined treatments preferred? Is there evidence to support sequential approaches and should they be specifically targeted to stages of the illness? How might understanding physiologic changes in the brain, which occur in the context of both medications and psychotherapy, help guide our research and clinical treatment interventions? It should be kept in mind that research regarding these issues is in its infancy, and many recommendations may require further studies definitively to aid with the establishment of critical pathways for each of the disorders In spite of the need for further research, combined treatment appears useful for all major categories of psychotic illness, including

anxiety and mood disorders, psychotic disorders, eating disorders and substance abuse.

Split Treatment

The last few decades have seen an increasing shift from a single relationship between patient and psychiatrist towards a tripartite relationship with the inclusion of medication, or to a four-way or systemic relationship with the addition or deletion of medications (Figure 87.1). Thus, combined treatments are commonly provided by two or more clinicians, hence the term "split".

Positive Aspects

There are several positive aspects of split treatment, including the increased time that patients have with more than one clinician; better utilization of resources; enhanced opportunity for alignment of gender, ethnicity between patient and clinician; more professional support for each clinician; and, perhaps, better adherence of the overall treatment plan by the patient and family.

Increased Time with Clinicians

Within the structure of split treatment, patients actually meet with at least two different clinicians: one for psychotropic medication or other somatic treatment and the other clinician for psychotherapy. Under ideal circumstances, the patient is seen by the nonmedical therapist at appointed intervals between the physician appointments. This could then allow for the patient to get longitudinal care by two clinicians and to therefore be seen on a continuum by both. Under this type of arrangement, there would not be too long an interval in which the patient is not seen by a mental health professional. With good communication, the therapist relays all important information to the physician in a

Dyadic relationship

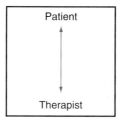

Tripartite relationship

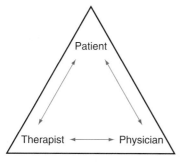

Four-way relationship

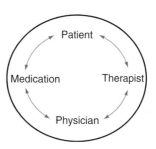

Figure 87.1 *Changes in relationships as therapy and medications are added or deleted. Reprinted with permission from Kay J [2001] Integrated treatment: An overview, in Integrated Treatment for Psychiatric Disorders: Review of Psychiatry, Vol. 20 (ed. Kay J). Copyright, American Psychiatric Press, Washington DC, pp. 1–29.*

timely manner. If there are planned vacations by either clinician, the other clinician is aware and can make different plans accordingly to see the patient. The patient may be able to provide more useful information in this treatment approach, given that she has more time to spend in overall treatment.

Better Utilization of Resources

With the growing realization of the importance of evaluating for emotional problems in the primary care setting, there is better recognition of psychiatric symptoms and disorders. In rural areas where there may not be enough mental health clinicians to serve the needed population, splitting the duties of the various clinicians might be a cost-effective way to ensure allocation of care. Similarly, there are certain types of psychotherapeutic treatments with documented efficacy, such as cognitive–behavioral treatment of depression and behavioral treatment of obsessive–compulsive disorder, panic disorder and phobias, which must be delivered by knowledgeable clinicians (Fawcett, 2001).

Greater Choice of Clinicians

Split treatment allows for more choices in the selection of clinicians based on gender, race or ethnicity, and religion or cultural values. Such matching may help the patient and clinician avoid certain difficulties that arise in psychotherapy when there is not a full appreciation of cultural issues (Foulks and Pena, 1995).

Improved Adherence to the Treatment Plan

Patients attribute certain meanings to the prescription and taking of medication, depending on their illness-belief system (Rolland, 1994; Winer and Andriukatis, 1989). Some patients hear an explanation of the need to take medications as having a "chemical imbalance" and embrace the idea that there is a biochemical reason for the problem. Other patients feel ashamed or guilty over having a defect and develop a strong resistance to taking their medication as prescribed (Paykel, 1995).

It is important for the clinicians involved in split treatment to appreciate how the patient understands the need for medication. Similarly, it is valuable for the physician to be aware of how the nonphysician therapist understands the role of medication in the overall treatment. The physician and therapist must help support medication and psychotherapy so as to help the patient succeed in having a good outcome. In this way, the patient will receive support from both treaters with neither the medication nor the therapy undermined.

Enhanced Support for Clinicians

There are several levels of support that accrue to clinicians involved in split treatment. With particularly difficult patients, such as those with severe personality disorders or hard-to-treat depressions or psychoses, it is very valuable for clinicians to be able to feel a mutual caring for one another and an empathy for the difficult clinical situations that can arise. Split treatment allows for a sharing of information that can help clinicians help patients through crises. As Silk points out, patients with borderline personality disorder, for example, are noted for fueling strong countertransferential feelings of anger, fear, and worry in clinicians (Silk *et al.*, 1995). It is very helpful when clinicians in split treatment can present a unified front to the patient, acknowledging that they are capable of handling the patient's affective storms but also provide support to one another to diminish feelings of burn-out. Balon (1999) has noted

that psychiatry residents, in particular, value the teaching and support they receive from seasoned, mature social workers and psychologists while providing split treatment.

Negative Aspects

Communication

While communication is probably the most important factor in successful split treatment, it is rarely done well (Hansen-Grant and Riba, 1995). Without a systematic way for clinicians and the patient to have regular, documented communication, there often arise misunderstandings and misconceptions. Further, patients are sometimes put in the middle of having to be the messenger between the clinicians. Needing to communicate puts additional burdens and stress on busy clinicians with the telephone or in-person time not usually reimbursable. Poor communication leads to misinterpretation of what should be attributable to psychodynamic issues or medication side effects, or both – a poorly constructed treatment plan, ill-defined plans for discharge from treatment, lack of coordination with family members, neither the clinician nor patient fully understanding vacation or coverage issues, and so on.

Interdisciplinary Issues

The literature demonstrates that when clinicians know one another, they are more comfortable with split treatment (Goldberg *et al.*, 1991; Weiner and Riba, 1997). Unfortunately, often the clinicians do not know one another, which leads to basic mistrust, competition, or inequality in the relationship (Baggs and Schmitt, 1988). Further, this devaluation can be displaced onto the patient during critical treatment decisions, with certain patients exploiting this competition even further (Kelly, 1991). The psychotherapy skills of psychiatrists and nonmedical therapists and the psychopharmacologic education of social workers and psychologists are all highly variable, contributing to mistrust (Neal and Calarco, 1999). In such circumstances, the patient may actually be seen more often by both clinicians and have ill-defined treatment goals.

Transference and Countertransference

When patients are referred by their therapists for medication evaluations, the reactions are variable, but often negative. Such reactions include feeling abandoned or rejected, as if the therapist has lost interest or given up, like a failure because therapy did not work, devaluation of the psychotherapy and the therapist, idealization of the physician, shame, resistance to further psychodynamic exploration of issues and a narcissistic injury (Busch and Gould, 1993). Busch and Gould note the difficulties for the therapist who needs to make the referral: shame that help is needed and anger towards the patient for needing additional help. The psychiatrist could then collude with the patient's negative transference towards the therapist and the psychodynamic process.

Results of such negative transference could lead to premature closure within the therapeutic process (Bradley, 1990). There may be a flight into health by the patient when the medication is first prescribed. The patient and physician may then realize too late that there was an overreliance on biologic interventions. The dyadic relationship between the therapist and patient is changed with the addition of a physician and medication (see Figure 87.1) leading to distortions and transference changes in all the relationships.

Legal Issues

Split treatment means a sharing of authority and control over patient care, meaning a loss of autonomy for each clinician. There is a widespread perception therefore that split treatment is associated with significantly greater risks (Macbeth, 2001).

What are the sources of legal exposure? There is potential liability for all psychiatrists who prescribe psychotropic medications, see patients with depression and anxiety, especially those patients with severe disorders, and treat patients with significant suicide potential. Further, informed consent is an important area of concern.

Since patients are shared in split treatment and it is difficult for clinicians to communicate with one another, there is ample opportunity for there to be a rise in missing information, miscommunication and a decrease in quality of the doctor–patient relationship. Patients are usually seen less frequently by the physician in a split-treatment relationship and the patient is often not clear whom to call in certain emergency situations. Families are usually seen by one of the clinicians, not both. Sometimes there is a supposition that the therapist is being supervised by the physician when the physician believes the relationship to be collaborative rather than supervisory. Macbeth offers the following risk-management strategies:

1. Psychiatrists should familiarize themselves with the operations and routines of all practice settings. The psychiatrist must be knowledgeable about the expertise and authority of those involved in care management.
2. The most problematic practice sites should be weeded out. Issues include looking at staff turnover, peer review procedures and credentials of key staff members. The psychiatrist should find out about opportunities for consultation and staff interaction, system immunities and insurance of nonphysician clinicians.
3. There must be careful coordination with therapists who have greater access to patients. The psychiatrist must inform the therapists what information the psychiatrist needs; when she/he needs to be told about changes in the patient's symptoms and condition, and the strengths and weaknesses of the therapists. The psychiatrist must inform the therapist about the medication regimens (potential side effects). This information must be updated regularly.
4. Psychiatrists must understand the system review and appeals procedures to be able to act quickly when there are problems.
5. Either consultation or supervision schedules should be set up and documented regularly to review specific patients.
6. Personal assessment of individual patients must be set up with reference to her/his condition, status and treatment.
7. Psychiatrists should be extremely careful not to issue an insurance policy to a managed care organization or other system. All proposed contracts must be carefully reviewed and not used to indemnify by accident.

Ethical Issues in Split Treatment

There are many areas of potential ethical conflict when mental health professionals get into split-treatment relationships. These include state licensing laws, competency issues, psychiatrists being used as figureheads, delegation of medical judgment and financial arrangements (Lazarus, 2001).

The potential ethical pitfalls in split treatment arise from economic, manpower and clinical pressures. There is very little research, for example, into whether patients with severe borderline personality disorder should be in split treatment. These patients often do not tell the same story to each clinician (Main, 1957); they externalize their problems (Silk *et al.*, 1995); threaten self-harm (Leibenluft *et al.*, 1987); have emotional lability and substance abuse problems (Springer *et al.*, 1995). If there is no close communication between the clinicians regarding goals, treatment planning, and role of medication and psychotherapy, the clinical and ethical problems in treating such patients are great.

It is important to recognize how complex and difficult split treatment can be for patients and clinicians. Key to this is recognizing the extra time and effort it will take to make obligations and responsibilities of all parties overt rather than covert. Implied duties must be minimized. Some clinicians advocate the use of treatment contracts to cover the various issues and responsibilities that accrue in split-treatment arrangements (Appelbaum, 1991).

Toward Successful Split Treatment

The following suggestions are offered as organizing principles for these three stages (with permission from American Psychiatric Press, Riba and Balon, 2001):

A key aspect of split treatment is how complex and difficult such treatment is for the clinicians, the patient and the patient's family. Unless one works in a clinic or organized setting where relationships between clinicians are well-delineated (e.g., one psychiatrist works with a specific group of nonmedical therapists), much thought must go into managing safe and effective split treatment.

It may be helpful to think of split therapy having a beginning, middle course, and end (Table 87.1). In order to avoid or minimize the pitfalls associated with split treatment, the following clinical suggestions are provided as organizing principles for its three stages (Rand, 1999; Tasman and Riba, 2000):

Beginning of Treatment

- Communication is key to providing excellent care in split treatment. At the beginning, both clinicians should obtain a signed release-of-information form from the patient. Communication must be regular and frequent between the clinicians and the patient should be made aware of these discussions. The forms of regular communication should be decided at the onset – routine telephone calls, faxes, emails, follow-up letters and the like. The patient should not be a messenger between the clinicians.
- Issues of confidentiality should be discussed and reviewed at the beginning of treatment. Confidentiality should not be used as a cover to hide from taking the time to make telephone calls, to send copies of evaluations and follow-up notes, to send emails or faxes, or to have joint sessions with both clinicians and the patient.
- Diagnostic impressions should be independently arrived at, then discussed and agreed upon. If there is a difference of opinion, an understanding must be reached before treatment proceeds.

- The clinicians must work with each other and with the patient to determine the treatment plan. The treatment plan should specify how often each of the clinicians expects to see the patient and what process to pursue if the patient does not follow-up or if there is a missed appointment. If the patient wishes to end either the therapy, the medications, or both, it has to be understood that all parties will discuss this important decision. It is desirable for a written contract to be drawn up between the clinicians and the patient so that all parties understand what the agreement for services will entail. Included in the contract should be a delineation of the clinicians' roles and responsibilities, as well as those of the patient.
- Clinicians vacation schedules and other on-call and coverage issues must be discussed regularly and documented. The patient needs to know whom to call in an emergency. At the beginning of split treatment, both clinicians and the patient should be aware of their respective beliefs regarding medication and psychotherapy.
- There must be a discussion about what type of care would be optimal for the patient and if there are barriers to such care. The patient should be informed of this review; if possible, he or she should participate in it.
- The clinicians should discuss their professional backgrounds and training with each other at the beginning of the patient's treatment. Issues such as licensure, ethics, violations, malpractice claims, hospital privileges, coverage of professional liability insurance, participation on managed care panels and commitment to split treatment should all be made clear.
- The clinicians need to agree who will communicate with third parties regarding the patient's care. Further, each clinician should know the patient's mental health benefits and means of payment. There needs to be an agreement by all parties as to the use of such benefits.
- The clinicians need to understand how best to interface with the patient's family or significant others.
- If the patient has health providers other than the psychiatrist and therapist (e.g., primary care physician, cardiologist a physical therapist), it should be decided which clinician will be the designated communicator or coordinator with those other providers.
- At the beginning of treatment there should be a review of how each clinician will assess and manage the patient's thoughts regarding or attempts at suicide, homicide, violence and domestic abuse.
- It should be made clear to the patient what symptoms or types of issues should be brought to the attention of which clinician.
- It is helpful for the clinicians to decide how problems will be handled as the need arises.
- The clinicians should discuss differences in fee schedules, cancellation policies, length of visits and frequency of visits.

Middle Course

- Special attention must be paid to transference and countertransference in this type of system of care. Disparaging and negative remarks made by the patient concerning either clinician, therapy, or medication must be understood and managed in the context of this complex type of treatment.
- Clinicians should review how many cases of split treatment they have in their practices and whether or not this is a safe

mix. Factors to consider include the clinical complexity of the cases, how busy the practice is, the influence of third-party payers and the hassle factor, the number of different clinicians one is working with, the psychiatric disorders of one's patients, and so on. It may be prudent to determine the risks involved in having a large patient population in split treatment and to weed the number of such patients down to an acceptable level. Further, clinicians should minimize the number of collaborators, since it is virtually impossible to keep track of a large number of clinicians' credentials, vacation schedules, communication patterns, and so on.
- Adherence to medications and to psychotherapy should be addressed equally.
- Treatment plans should be regularly reviewed and updated between the clinicians and the patient.
- Use of the patient's mental health benefits should be regularly reviewed and discussed between the clinicians and the patient when appropriate.
- There must be an agreement that either clinician can terminate the split therapy but that the patient must be provided adequate and appropriate warning and referrals to other clinicians. In other words, the patient cannot be abandoned.

Ending Split Treatment

- After reviewing the treatment plan, both clinicians and the patient will decide together on the goals that have been met or have not been realized and the best time for termination. They should decide how to stagger the discontinuation of therapy and of medication.
- It is important to consider how to manage follow-up and recurrence of symptoms.

The clinicians must have a system for giving each other feedback on the care each is providing to the patient. Ideally, after the treatment is complete, the clinicians should review any aspects of the case that could have been managed or handled differently. Ideally, the patient should be part of this evaluation process as a way of assuring continuous quality improvement. Most importantly, throughout all stages of the split treatment process, clinicians need to respect both the patient and each other's professional understanding.

Although the challenges of split treatment are great, there are many reasons for clinicians and patients to try to surmount the obstacles. Good communication patterns between clinicians and many of the suggestions noted here may be guideposts on the path toward successful split treatment.

References

Appelbaum PS (1991) General guidelines for psychiatrists who prescribe medication for patients treated by nonmedical psychotherapists. *Hosp Comm Psychiatr* 42, 281–282.

Baggs JG and Schmitt MH (1988) Collaboration between nurses and physicians. *Image J Nurs Sch* 20, 145–149.

Balon R (1999) Positive aspects of collaborative treatment, in *Psychopharmacology and Psychotherapy: A Collaborative Approach* (eds Riba MB and Balon R). American Psychiatric Press, Washington DC, pp. 1–31.

Barlow DH (1996) Health care policy, psychotherapy research, and the future of psychotherapy. *Am Psychol* 51, 1050–1058.

Beck JS (1995) *Cognitive Therapy: Basics and Beyond*. Guilford Press, New York, pp. 8–45.

Beck JS (2001) A cognitive therapy approach to medication compliance. In Integrated Treatment for Psychiatric Disorders: Review of Psychiatry, Vol. 20, Kay J (ed American Psychiatric Press). Washington DC, pp. 113–141.

Bradley SS (1990) Nonphysician psychotherapist–physician pharmacotherapist: A new model for concurrent treatment. *Psychiatr Clin N Am* 13, 307–322.

Busch FN and Gould E (1993) Treatment by a psychotherapist and a psychopharmacologist: Transference and countertransference issues. *Hosp Comm Psychiatr* 44, 772–774.

Cochran SD (1984) Preventing medical non-compliance in the outpatient treatment of bipolar affective disorder. *J Consult Clin Psychol* 52, 873–878.

Depression Guideline Panel (1993) Depression in Primary Care, Vol. 2: Treatment of Major Depression (Clinical Practice Guideline No. 5; AHCPR Publ No 93-0551). US Department of Health and Human Services, Public Health Service, Agency for Health Care Policy and Research, Rockville, MD.

Engel GL (1977) The need for a new medical model: A challenge for biomedicine. *Science* 196(4286), 129–136.

Fava GA (1999) Sequential treatment: A new way of integrating pharmacotherapy and psychotherapy. *Psychother Psychosom* 68, 227–229.

Fava GA, Bartolucci G, Rafanelli C et al. (2001) Cognitive-behavioral management of patients with bipolar disorder who relapsed while on lithium prophylaxis. *J Clin Psychiatr* 62 (July), 7.

Fawcett J (2001) An issue that must be addressed, in *Improving the Practice of Split Treatment* (eds Balon R and Riba MB). *Psychiatr Ann* 31(10) (Oct), 582.

Foulks EF and Pena JM (1995) Ethnicity and psychotherapy: A component in the treatment of cocaine addiction in African-Americans. *Psychiatr Clin N Am* 18, 607–620.

Frank E, Shear MK, Rucci P et al. (2000) Influence of panic-agoraphobic spectrum symptoms on treatment response in patients with recurrent major depression. *Am J Psychiatr* 157(7), 1101–1107.

Gabbard GO and Kay J (2001) The fate of integrated treatment: Whatever happened to the biopsychosocial psychiatrist? *Am J Psychiatr* 158(12), 1956–1963.

Goldberg RS, Riba M and Tasman A (1991) Psychiatrists' attitudes toward prescribing medication for patients treated by nonmedical psychotherapists. *Hosp Comm Psychiatr* 42(3) (Mar), 276–280.

Hansen-Grant S and Riba MB (1995) Contact between psychotherapists and psychiatric residents who provide medication back-up. *Psychiatr Serv* 46, 774–777.

Hogarty G, Anderson CM, Reiss DJ et al. (1986) Family education, social skills training, and maintenance chemotherapy in the aftercare of schizophrenia. *Arch Gen Psychiatr* 43, 633–642.

Hollon SD and Fawcett J (1995) Combinde medication and psychotherapy. In Treatments of psychiatric Disorders, Vol. 1, 2nd edn., gabbard Go (ed American Psychiatric Press). Washington DC, pp. 1222–1236.

Hollon SD and Fawcett J (2001) Combined medication and psychotherapy. In Treatments of Psychiatric Disorders, Vol. 1 and 2, 3rd edn. (ed-in-chief Gabbard GO). American Psychiatric Press, Washington DC.

Kay J (2001) Integrated treatment: An overview, in *Integrated Treatment for Psychiatric Disorders: Review of Psychiatry*, Vol. 20 (ed Kay J). American Psychiatric Press, Washington DC, pp. 1–29.

Kay J (2002) Psychopharmacology: Combined treatment, in *Encyclopedia of Psychotherapy* (eds Hersen M and Sledge W). Academic Press, New York.

Kelly KV (1991) Parallel treatment: Therapy with one clinician and medication with another. *Hosp Comm Psychiatr* 43, 778–780.

Klerman GL (1985) Trends in utilization of mental health services. *Med Care* 23, 584.

Klerman GL (1991) Ideologic conflicts, in *Integrating Pharmacotherapy and Psychotherapy* (eds Beitman BB and Klerman G). American Psychiatric Press, Washington DC, pp. 3–20.

Lambert MJ (1992) Psychotherapy outcome research: Implications for integrative and eclectic therapies, in *Handbook of Psychotherapy Integration* (eds Norcross JC and Goldfried MR). Basic Cooks, New York, pp. 94–129.

Lazarus J (2001) Ethics in split treatment, in *Improving the Practice of Split Treatment* (eds Balon R and Riba MB). *Psychiatr Ann* 31(10) (Oct), pp. 611–614.

Leibenluft E, Gardner DI and Cowdrey RW (1987) The inner experience of the borderline self-mutilator. *J Pers Disord* 1, 317–324.

Macbeth JE (2001) Legal aspects of split treatment: How to audit and manage risk, in *Improving the Practice of Split Treatment* (eds Balon R and Riba MB). *Psychiatr Ann* 31(10) (Oct), pp. 605–610.

Main TF (1957) The ailment. *Br J Med Psychol* 30, 129–145.

McHugh PR and Slavney R (1983) *The Perspectives of Psychiatry.* Johns Hopkins University Press, Baltimore, MD.

Nathan PE, Stuart SP and Dolan SL (2000) Research on psychotherapy efficacy and effectiveness: Between scylla and charbodis? *Psychol Bull* 126(6) (Nov), 964–981.

Neal DL and Calarco MM (1999) Mental health providers: Role definitions and collaborative practice issues, in *Psychopharmacology and Psychotherapy: A Collaborative Approach* (eds Riba MB and Balon R). American Psychiatric Press, Washington DC, pp. 85–109.

Paykel ES (1995) Psychotherapy, medication combinations, and compliance. *J Clin Psychiatr* 56(Suppl 1), 24–30.

Rand EH (1999) Guidelines to maximize the process of collaborative treatment, in *Psychopharmacology and Psychotherapy: A Collaborative Approach* (eds Riba MB and Balon R). American Psychiatric Press, Washington DC, pp. 353–380.

Riba MB and Balon R (2001) The challenges of split treatment, in *Integrated Treatment of Psychiatric Disorders: Review of Psychiatry*, Vol. 20 (ed Kay J). APPI, Washington DC, pp. 143–164.

Rolland JS (1994) *Families, Illness, and Disability.* Basic Books, New York.

Silk KR, Lee S, Hill EM et al. (1995) Borderline symptoms and severity of sexual abuse. *Am J Psychiatr* 152, 1059–1064.

Spiegel DA, Bruce TJ, Gregg SF et al. (1994) Does cognitive-behavior therapy assist slow-taper alprazolam discontinuation in panic disorder? *Am J Psychiatr* 151, 876–881.

Springer T, Huth AC, Lohr NE et al. (1995) The quality of depression in personality disorders: An empirical study. Paper presented at the annual meeting of the American Psychological Association (Aug), New York.

Svartberg M, Seltzer MH and Stiles TC (1998) The effects of common and specific factors in short-term anxiety-provoking psychotherapy. *J Nerv Ment Dis* 186, 691–696.

Tasman A and Riba MB (2000) Psychological management in psychopharmacologic treatment, in *Psychiatric Drugs* (eds Lieberman J and Tasman A). WB Saunders, Philadelphia PA, pp. 242–249.

Weiner H and Riba MB (1997) Attitudes and practices in mediation backup. *Psychiatr Serv* 48(4), 536–538.

Wiborg IM and Dahl AA (1996) Does brief dynamic psychotherapy reduce the relapse rate of panic disorder? *Arch Gen Psychiatr* 53, 689–694.

Winer J and Andriukatis S (1989) Interpersonal aspects of initiating pharmacotherapy: How to avoid becoming the patient's feared negative other. *Psychiatr Ann* 19, 318–323

CHAPTER 88 Medication Compliance

Introduction
Compliance, or the degree to which patients' behaviors coincide with the recommendations of health care providers, is an important component in the understanding of patient outcomes, particularly in light of a growing regimen of efficacious and expensive medical treatments. There is an evident gap between the efficacy of regimens tested in tightly controlled clinical trials and their effectiveness when applied to "real world" patient experiences. One explanation for this "efficacy-effectiveness gap", when treatment regimens move from efficacy trials into everyday practice, is the apparent decline in patient compliance. Other terms closely related to compliance include "adherence", "fidelity", and "maintenance".

Compliance is difficult to quantify for several reasons. Completely attributing the difference between an expected and observed treatment effect to problems with medication compliance may be overly simplistic. Several other factors such as differences in population, degree of comorbidity with other psychiatric or medical diagnoses, and severity of illness may all adversely affect the potential benefit to the patient. Poor or partial compliance with treatment may have a variable effect on treatment outcomes depending on the pharmacokinetic profile of the medication in question. For example, occasional missed doses of very long half-life medications will alter serum drug levels to a lesser extent than in short half-life compounds. Therefore, the issue of partial compliance with treatment regimens may become more critical depending on the specific regimen.

A Theoretical Construct for Compliance: The Health Beliefs Model
The health beliefs of individuals play a major role in their decision-making processes regarding participation in recommended treatment. A framework that may be useful in understanding the complex nature of compliance with medical regimens is the health beliefs model (HBM). Derived from social psychological theories of Kurt Lewin, the HBM is grounded in the phenomenological orientation of perception driving action (Rosenstock, 1974). While this model was originally designed to study the utilization of screening tests for detection of asymptomatic diseases, it has been adapted to the areas of medication compliance among psychiatric patients (Kelly *et al.* 1987).

Five components of the HBM apply directly to issues of patient compliance. Figure 88.1 depicts the relationship between these components and ultimate compliance with treatment.

1. Susceptibility: patients must see themselves as vulnerable to a serious illness.

2. Severity: patients must realize that he/she has an illness with health consequences that will continue without medical attention.
3. Perceived benefits: patients must recognize that an effective treatment exists for their condition. Benefits from psychotropic medication treatment may include the understanding that treatment ameliorates mental problems or helps avoid rehospitalization.
4. Barriers: common barriers to pharmacologic interventions involve access to medication, adequate psychiatric follow-up, and adverse effects from the medication.
5. Cues to action: lastly, patients must experience an internal or external motivation or "cue" to engage in the specified action that may benefit them.

Cues that may trigger a patient to participate in their medication regimen typically relate to a return of symptoms attributed to their mental illness such as anxious, depressive, or psychotic states.

Another Conceptual Model of Compliance
Another approach to understanding compliance behavior involves the categorization of problems with compliance along the three domains of psychological problems, planning problems, and medical problems. These three domains have been used to develop a compliance checklist as seen in Table 88.1 (Corrigan *et al.*, 1990, Cramer 1991). **Psychological problems** include issues such as nonacceptance of diagnosis or treatment, negative emotional reactions or negative thoughts, and social criticism from family or friends. **Problems with planning** consist of forgetting to take medications, disruption of usual schedules, and issues with availability of medication. **Medical problems that affect compliance** include adverse reactions, exacerbation of illness that leads to incapacity to administer or tolerate medications, or perceptions that medications may lack efficacy in a given individual. Both HBM and the compliance checklist provide useful starting points to begin the analysis of problems with compliance in specific patients or patient populations.

Interventions to Enhance Compliance
General strategies to enhance compliance take many forms and can be tailored to the specific needs identified in individual patients. Most approaches to enhance compliance involve the introduction of techniques to improve outpatients' self-administration of oral medication therapies. Cramer (1991) identifies several strategies to approach problems with compliance (Table 88.2).

Essentials of Psychiatry Jerald Kay and Allan Tasman
© 2006 John Wiley & Sons, Ltd.

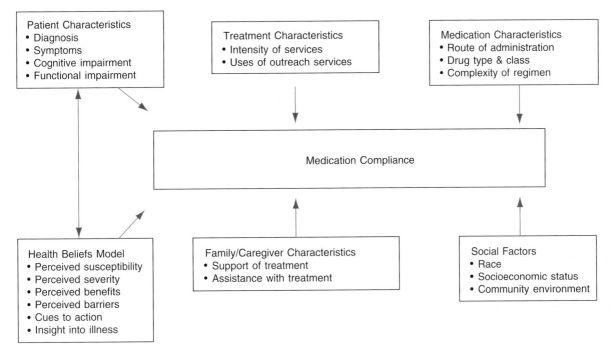

Figure 88.1 *Understanding medication compliance in mental illness.*

Table 88.1	Compliance Checklist

Psychological Problems

- Nonacceptance: Patient does not accept the diagnosis or recommendations for treatment.
- Emotions: Strong emotional reactions (anger, anxiety) prevent the patient from following the treatment plan.
- Other priorities: Patient has placed a higher value on priorities (job, family) other than medication treatment.
- Social criticism: Patient does not take medication due to criticism from others (family, friends, coworkers).

Planning Problems

- Routine forgetfulness: Patient does not follow a standard schedule and often misses doses.
- Disruption of schedule: Extraordinary events prevent patient from following medication regimen.
- No medication: Patient ran out of medication before it could be refilled or medication was no longer available for other reasons, including economic factors.
- Lack of information: Patient received inadequate or incorrect information about medication regimen.

Medical Problems

- Adverse reaction: Patient stopped taking medication due to an adverse reaction.
- Illness: Medical or psychiatric illness interrupted patient's medication regimen.
- Testing efficacy: Patient decided to omit doses in order to determine need for medication.

Table 88.2	Strategies for Improving Compliance

Collect Information

- Understand patient's particular problem with compliance
- Address issues related to compliance in every clinical encounter with the patient

Provide Information

- Education about the illness
- Education about the treatment
- Understanding about problems with compliance

Increase Motivation

- Use motivational interviewing techniques to overcome resistance
- Help the patient overcome psychosocial problems that interfere with compliance

Modify Medication Regimen

- Schedule doses around standard cues (brushing teeth, meals)
- Discuss coping skills regarding potential situations that may interfere with compliance
- Change the dosage schedule or route of administration

Change Contingencies

- Discuss negative consequences of medication compliance (shame, criticism)
- Address adverse reactions
- Specify a formal medication compliance contract
- Associate medication compliance with specific positive reinforcement

The action of monitoring compliance itself may improve adherence to proposed medical regimens, just as frequent weight monitoring may promote weight loss even without a specific diet regimen. Some data indicate that compliance rates improve significantly when outpatients with psychiatric disorders are given continuous feedback on their medication dosing (Cramer and Rosenheck, 1999).

Compliance-enhancement interventions that have been studied include individual, group and family formats and involve diverse theoretical orientations. Unfortunately, many of the studies that investigate compliance therapies do not also assess the distal impact on treatment outcomes leaving the clinician unable to evaluate whether marginal improvements in compliance would in fact lead to cost-effective improvement in treatment outcomes.

One intervention referred to as **compliance therapy** utilizes a specific approach to individual or group psychotherapy with cognitive therapy and motivational interviewing techniques (Goldstein, 1992; Hayward *et al*, 1995). Therapists attempt to help the patients form a cognitive link between discontinuation of medication treatment and relapse of symptoms. Using the patient's frame of reference, therapists seek to instill a sense of cognitive dissonance between discontinuation of medication and achievement of the patient's own goals. Problem-solving techniques are also employed to identify internal and external cues that may compromise future medication compliance.

Other psychosocial interventions to increase compliance in patients with schizophrenia have also been demonstrated to be effective. Kelly and Scott (1990) found that strategies aimed at education of patients' families about compliance and those directed at patients themselves both improved compliance. No significant difference between the two interventions could be demonstrated. It is important to note that, given the multiple factors associated with clinical course, not all improvement in treatment outcomes in schizophrenia is directly attributable to improved medication compliance. Psychosocial interventions that lack a specific focus on treatment compliance may nonetheless have salutatory effects on patient outcomes, regardless of changes in compliance behavior. Zhang and colleagues (1994) found that family therapy without a specific focus on compliance produced improvement in relapse rates in schizophrenic patients independent of changes in medication compliance.

Another approach to increasing compliance involves the change in route of administration of medication from oral preparations that must be taken at least once daily to depot injections, such as haloperidol decanoate and fluphenazine decanoate, that are typically administered every 2 to 4 weeks. The advantages to depot preparations include supervised administration of the medication by health care providers, decreased variability in serum concentrations of the active medication, and no significant difference in adverse effects as compared with similar oral agents. Disadvantages include the limited number of medications available in depot form, the difficulty of scheduling potentially more frequent clinic visits for injections, and the increased cost in clinic staffs' time with administration of the treatments. At the time of this publication, no atypical antipsychotic agents were available in depot form. Therefore, a comparison of compliance with conventional depot agents and atypical oral agents may be limited in utility. Few studies of depot antipsychotic preparations address the issues of long-term compliance and differences in health outcomes when compared with oral agents (Adams and Eisenbruch, 2002; Quraishi and David, 2002). However, some evidence suggests that depot antipsychotic agents do confer a marginal improvement in reducing relapse rates (Glazer and Kane, 1992).

Conclusion

Understanding patient compliance with prescribed medications involves an appreciation of multiple factors pertaining to the specific patient and his/her environment. Likewise, designing interventions to enhance compliance with medications requires an individualized approach in the context of proven therapeutic modalities. In the end, improving patient compliance improves patient outcomes without major modification of existing treatment strategies.

References

Adams CE and Eisenbruch M (2002) Depot fluphenazine for schizophrenia (Cochrane review). The Cochrane Library, Oxford. Update Software.

Corrigan PW, Liberman RP and Engel JD (1990) From noncompliance to collaboration in the treatment of schizophrenia. *Hosp Comm Psychiatr* 41, 1203–1211.

Cramer JA (1991) Identifying and improving compliance patterns: A composite plan for health care providers, in *Patient Compliance in Medical Practice and Clinical Trials* (eds Cramer JA and Spilker B). Raven Press, New York, pp. 387–392.

Cramer JA and Rosenheck R (1999) Enhancing medication compliance for people with serious mental illness. *J Nerv Ment Dis* 187, 53–55.

Glazer WM and Kane JM (1992) Depot neuroleptic therapy: An underutilized treatment option. *J Clin Psychiatr* 53, 426–433.

Goldstein MJ (1992) Psychosocial strategies for maximizing the effects of psychotropic medications for schizophrenia and mood disorder. *Psychopharmacol Bull* 28, 237–240.

Hayward P, Chan N, Kemp R, *et al.* (1995) Medication self-management: A preliminary report on an intervention to improve medication compliance. *J Ment Health* 4, 511–517.

Kelly GR and Scott JE (1990) Medication compliance and health education among outpatients with chronic mental disorders. *Med Care* 28, 1181–1197.

Kelly GR Mamon JA and Scott JE (1987) Utility of the health belief model in examining medication compliance among psychiatric outpatients. *Soc Sci Med* 25, 1205–1211.

Quraishi S and David A (2002) Depot haloperidol decanoate for schizophrenia (Cochrane review). The Cochrane Library, Oxford. Update Software.

Rosenstock IM (1974) Historical origins of the health beliefs model. *Health Educ Monogr* 2, 328–335.

Zhang M, Wang M, Li J *et al.* (1994) Randomised-control trial of family interventions for 78 first-episode male schizophrenic patients. *Br J Psychiatr* 165(Suppl 24), 96–102.

Index